# Contents

**2010**

# the calorie carb and fat bible 2010

Juliette Kellow BSc RD, Lyndel Costain BSc RD & Laurence Beeken

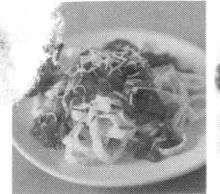 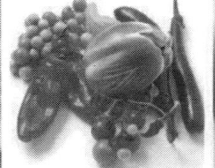 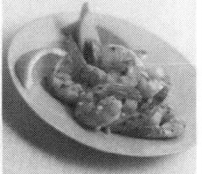 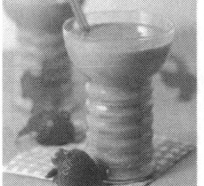 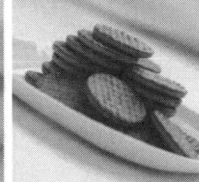 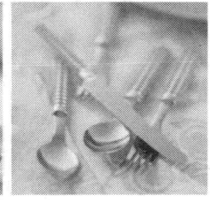

## The UK's Most Comprehensive Calorie Counter

# The Calorie, Carb & Fat Bible 2010

© Weight Loss Resources 2010
Lyndel Costain's contributions © Lyndel Costain 2007

**Published by:**
Weight Loss Resources Ltd
29 Metro Centre
Woodston,
Peterborough
PE2 7UH.

Tel: 01733 345592
www.weightlossresources.co.uk

Companies and other organisations wishing to make bulk purchases of the Calorie, Carb and Fat Bible should contact their local bookstore or Weight Loss Resources direct.

Whilst every effort has been made to ensure accuracy, the publishers cannot be held responsible for any errors or omissions.

**ISBN 978 1 904512 08 0**

Authors:  Lyndel Costain BSc RD
Juliette Kellow BSc RD
Laurence Beeken, Weight Loss Resources

Database Editor: Laurence Beeken

Design & Layout: Jonathan Lansdown

**Printed and bound in Finland by:**
WS Bookwell Oy

# Losing weight – the easy way

Juliette Kellow BSc RD

CHINESE TAKEAWAYS, curries, chocolate, chips and a glass of wine! Imagine being told the best diet to help you lose weight includes all these foods and more. It sounds too good to be true, doesn't it? But the truth is, these are exactly the types of foods you can still enjoy if you opt to lose weight by counting calories.

But you'd be forgiven for not knowing you can still eat all your favourite foods *and* lose weight. In recent years, endless trendy diets that cut carbs, boost protein intake or skip entire groups of foods, have helped to make dieting a complicated business. Added to this, an increasing number of celebrities and so-called nutrition experts have helped mislead us into thinking that dieting is all about restriction and denial. Is it any wonder then that most of us have been left feeling downright confused and miserable about what we should and shouldn't be eating to shift those pounds?

Dieting doesn't have to be complicated or an unhappy experience. In fact, there's really only one word you need to remember if you want to shift those pounds healthily and still eat all your favourite foods. And that's CALORIE!

## It's calories that count

When it comes to losing weight, there's no getting away from the fact that it's calories that count. Ask any qualified nutrition expert or dietitian for advice on how to fight the flab and you'll receive the same reply: quite simply you need to create a calorie deficit or shortfall. In other words, you need to take in fewer calories than you use up so that your body has to draw on its fat stores to provide it with the energy it needs to function properly. The result: you start losing fat and the pounds start to drop off!

Fortunately, it couldn't be easier to create this calorie deficit. Regardless of your age, weight, sex, genetic make up, lifestyle or eating habits, losing weight is as simple as reducing your daily calorie intake slightly by modifying your diet and using up a few more calories by being slightly more active each day.

Better still, it's a complete myth that you need to change your eating and exercise habits dramatically. You'll notice I've said you need to reduce your calorie intake 'slightly' and be 'slightly' more active. It really is just LITTLE differences between the amount of calories we take in and the amount we use up that make BIG differences to our waistline over time. For example, you only need to consume one can of cola more than you need each day to gain a stone in a year. It's no wonder then that people say excess weight tends to 'creep up on them'.

## 10 simple food swaps you can make every day (and won't even notice!)

Make these simple swaps every day and in just 4 weeks you'll lose 7lb!

| SWAP THIS... | FOR THIS... | SAVE... |
|---|---|---|
| 300ml full-fat milk (*195 calories*) | 300ml skimmed milk (*100 calories*) | *95 calories* |
| 1tsp butter (*35 calories*) | 1tsp low-fat spread (*20 calories*) | *15 calories* |
| 1tbsp vegetable oil (*100 calories*) | 10 sprays of a spray oil (*10 calories*) | *90 calories* |
| 1tsp sugar (*16 calories*) | Artificial sweetener (*2 calories*) | *14 calories* |
| 1tbsp mayonnaise (*105 calories*) | 1tbsp fat-free dressing (*10 calories*) | *95 calories* |
| Regular sandwich (*600 calories*) | Low-fat sandwich (*350 calories*) | *250 calories* |
| Can of cola (*135 calories*) | Can of diet cola (*0.5 calories*) | *12.5 calories* |
| Large (50g) packet of crisps (*250 calories*) | Small (25g) packet of crisps (*125 calories*) | *125 calories* |
| 1 chocolate digestive (*85 calories*) | 1 small chocolate chip cookie (*55 calories*) | *30 calories* |
| 1 slice thick-cut wholemeal bread (*95 calories*) | 1 slice medium-cut wholemeal bread (*75 calories*) | *20 calories* |
| | **TOTAL CALORIE SAVING:** | *858.5 calories* |

The good news is the reverse is also true. You only need to swap that daily can of cola for the diet version or a glass of sparking water and you'll lose a stone in a year – it really is as easy as that!

Of course, most people don't want to wait a year to shift a stone. But there's more good news. To lose 1lb of fat each week you need to create a calorie deficit of just 500 calories a day. That might sound like a lot, but you can achieve this by simply swapping a croissant for a wholemeal fruit scone, a regular sandwich for a low-fat variety, a glass of dry white wine for a gin and slimline tonic and using low-fat spread on two slices of toast instead of butter. It is also important to become more active and increase your level of exercise. Losing 1lb a week, amounts to a stone in 14 weeks, or just under 4 stone in a year!

## Taking control of calories

By now you've seen it really is calories that count when it comes to shifting those pounds. So it should be no surprise that a calorie-controlled diet is the only guaranteed way to help you shift those pounds – and that's a scientific fact! But better still, a calorie-controlled diet is one of the few that allows you to include anything, whether it's pizza, wine or chocolate. A healthy diet means including a wide range of foods *(see 'Healthy Eating Made Easy' page 32)*.

And that's where this book can really help. Gone are the days when it was virtually impossible to obtain information about the calorie contents of foods. This book provides calorie information for more than 22,000 different branded and unbranded foods so that counting calories has never been easier.

| **The benefits of counting calories** |
| --- |
| ☐ *It's guaranteed to help you lose weight providing you stick to your daily calorie allowance* |
| ☐ *You can include favourite foods* |
| ☐ *No foods are banned* |
| ☐ *It's a great way to lose weight slowly and steadily* |
| ☐ *Nutrition experts agree that it's a proven way to lose weight* |

# Calorie counting made easy

Forget weird and wacky science, complicated diet rules and endless lists of foods to fill up on or avoid every day! Counting calories to lose weight couldn't be easier. Quite simply, you set yourself a daily calorie allowance to help you lose between ½-2lb (¼-1kg) a week and then add up the calories of everything you eat and drink each day, making sure you don't go over your limit.

To prevent hunger from kicking in, it's best to spread your daily calorie allowance evenly throughout the day, allowing a certain amount of calories for breakfast, lunch, dinner and one or two snacks. For example, if you are allowed 1,500 calories a day, you could have 300 calories for breakfast, 400 calories for lunch, 500 calories for dinner and two snacks or treats of 150 calories each. You'll find more detailed information on p26-31 (Your step-by-step guide to using this book and shifting those pounds).

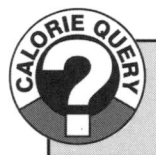

### QUESTION
## What affects the calorie content of a food?

**ANSWER:**
Fat, protein, carbohydrate and alcohol all provide the body with calories, but in varying amounts:

- *1g fat provides 9 calories*

- *1g alcohol provides 7 calories*

- *1g protein provides 4 calories*

- *1g carbohydrate provides 3.75 calories*

The calorie content of a food depends on the amount of fat, protein and carbohydrate it contains. Because fat provides more than twice as many calories as an equal quantity of protein or carbohydrate, in general, foods that are high in fat tend to contain more calories. This explains why 100g of chips (189 calories) contains more than twice as many calories as 100g of boiled potato (72 calories).

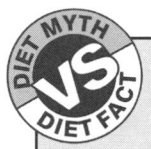

**DIET MYTH:**
# Food eaten late at night stops you losing weight

**DIET FACT:**
It's not eating in the evening that stops you losing weight. It's consuming too many calories throughout the day that will be your dieting downfall! Providing you stick to your daily calorie allowance you'll lose weight, regardless of when you consume those calories. Nevertheless, it's a good idea to spread your calorie allowance throughout the day to prevent hunger from kicking in, which leaves you reaching for high-calorie snack foods.

## Eat for good health

While calories might be the buzz word when it comes to shifting those pounds, it's nevertheless important to make sure your diet is healthy, balanced and contains all the nutrients you need for good health. Yes, you can still lose weight by eating nothing but, for example, chocolate, crisps and biscuits providing you stick to your calorie allowance. But you'll never find a nutrition expert or dietitian recommending this. And there are plenty of good reasons why.

To start with, an unbalanced diet is likely to be lacking in essential nutrients such as protein, vitamins, minerals and fibre, in the long term putting you at risk of nutritional deficiencies. Secondly, research proves that filling up on foods that are high in fat and/or salt and sugar can lead to many different health problems. But most importantly, when it comes to losing weight, it's almost impossible to stick to a daily calorie allowance if you're only eating high-calorie foods.

Filling up on lower-calorie foods also means you'll be able to eat far more with the result that you're not constantly left feeling unsatisfied. For example, six chocolates from a selection box contain around 300 calories, a lot of fat and sugar, few nutrients – and are eaten in just six mouthfuls! For 300 calories, you could have a grilled skinless chicken breast (packed with protein and zinc), a large salad with fat-free dressing (a great source of fibre, vitamins and minerals), a slice of wholemeal bread with low-fat spread (rich in fibre and B vitamins) and a satsuma (an excellent source of vitamin C). That's a lot more food that will take you a lot more time to eat! Not convinced? Then put six chocolates on one plate, and the chicken, salad, bread and fruit on another!

Bottom line: while slightly reducing your calorie intake is the key to losing weight, you'll be healthier and far more likely to keep those pounds off if you do it by eating a healthy diet *(see 'Healthy Eating Made Easy' page 32)*.

---

## Eight steps to a healthy diet

**1** *Base your meals on starchy foods.*

**2** *Eat lots of fruit and vegetables.*

**3** *Eat more fish.*

**4** *Cut down on saturated fat and sugar.*

**5** *Try to eat less salt - no more than 6g a day.*

**6** *Get active and try to be a healthy weight.*

**7** *Drink plenty of water.*

**8** *Don't skip breakfast.*                    SOURCE: FSA www.eatwell.gov.uk

---

## Fat facts

Generally speaking, opting for foods that are low in fat can help slash your calorie intake considerably, for example, swapping full-fat milk for skimmed, switching from butter to a low-fat spread, not frying food in oil and chopping the fat off meat and poultry. But don't be fooled into believing that all foods described as 'low-fat' or 'fat-free' are automatically low in calories or calorie-free. In fact, some low-fat products may actually be higher in calories than standard products, thanks to them containing extra sugars and thickeners to boost the flavour and texture. The solution: always check the calorie content of low-fat foods, especially for things like cakes, biscuits, crisps, ice creams and ready meals. You might be surprised to find there's little difference in the calorie content when compared to the standard product.

# Uncovering fat claims on food labels

Many products may lure you into believing they're a great choice if you're trying to cut fat, but you need to read between the lines on the labels if you want to be sure you're making the best choice. Here's the lowdown on what to look for:

| | |
|---|---|
| **LOW FAT** | by law the food must contain less than 3g of fat per 100g for solids. These foods are generally a good choice if you're trying to lose weight. |
| **REDUCED FAT** | by law the food must contain 25 percent less fat than a similar standard product. This doesn't mean the product is low-fat (or low-calorie) though! For example, reduced-fat cheese may still contain 14g fat per 100g. |
| **FAT FREE** | the food must contain no more than 0.5g of fat per 100g or 100ml. Foods labelled as Virtually Fat Free must contain less than 0.3g fat per 100g. These foods are generally a good choice if you're trying to lose weight. |
| **LESS THAN 8% FAT** | this means the product contains less than 8g fat per 100g. It's only foods labelled 'less than 3% fat' that are a true low-fat choice. |
| **X% FAT FREE** | claims expressed as X% Fat Free shall be prohibited. |
| **LIGHT OR LITE** | claims stating a product is 'light' or 'lite' follows the same conditions as those set for the term 'reduced'. |

## 10 easy ways to slash fat (and calories)

**1** Eat fewer fried foods – grill, boil, bake, poach, steam, roast without added fat or microwave instead.

**2** Don't add butter, lard, margarine or oil to food during preparation or cooking.

**3** Use spreads sparingly. Butter and margarine contain the same amount of calories and fat – only low fat spreads contain less.

**4** Choose boiled or jacket potatoes instead of chips or roast potatoes.

**5** Cut off all visible fat from meat and remove the skin from chicken before cooking.

**6** Don't eat too many fatty meat products such as sausages, burgers, pies and pastry products.

**7** Use semi-skimmed or skimmed milk instead of full-fat milk.

**8** Try low-fat or reduced-fat varieties of cheese such as reduced-fat Cheddar, low-fat soft cheese or cottage cheese.

**9** Eat fewer high-fat foods such as crisps, chocolates, cakes, pastries and biscuits.

**10** Don't add cream to puddings, sauces or coffee.

# Getting Ready for Weight Loss Success

Lyndel Costain BSc RD

THIS BOOK not only provides tools to help you understand more about what you eat and how active you are, but guidance on how to use this information to develop a weight loss plan to suit your needs. Getting in the right frame of mind will also be a key part of your weight control journey, especially if you've lost weight before, only to watch the pounds pile back on.

The fact is that most people who want to lose weight know what to do. But often there is something that keeps stopping them from keeping up healthier habits. The same may be true for you. So what's going on? For many it's a lack of readiness. When the next diet comes along with its tempting promises it's so easy to just jump on board. But if you have struggled with your weight for a while, will that diet actually help you to recognise and change the thoughts and actions that have stopped you shifting the pounds for good?

## Check out your attitude to weight loss programmes

Before starting any new weight loss programme, including the Weight Loss Resources approach, ask yourself:

| | |
|---|---|
| Am I starting out thinking that I like myself as a person right now? | (YES or NO) |
| *OR* I feel I can only like myself once I lose weight? | (YES or NO) |
| Do I want to stop overeating, but at the same time find myself justifying it – in other words I want to be able to eat what I want, but with no consequences? | (YES or NO) |
| Do I believe that I need to take long-term responsibility for my weight? | (YES or NO) |
| *OR* Am I relying on 'it' (the diet) to do it for me? | (YES or NO) |

Keep these questions, and your replies, in mind as you read through this chapter.

## Next Steps

You may have already assessed the healthiness of your weight using the BMI guide on page 37. If not, why not do it now, remembering that the tools are a guide only. The important thing is to consider a weight at which you are healthy and comfortable – and which is realistic for the life you lead *(see opposite - What is a healthy weight?)*.

The next step is to have a long hard think about why you want to lose weight. Consider all the possible benefits, not just those related to how you look. Psychologists have found that if we focus only on appearance we are less likely to succeed in the long-term. This is because it so often reflects low self-esteem or self-worth – which can sabotage success – as it saps confidence and keeps us stuck in destructive thought patterns. Identifying key motivations other than simply how you look - such as health and other aspects of physical and emotional well being - is like saying that you're an OK person right now, and worth making changes for. Making healthy lifestyle choices also has the knock on effect of boosting self-esteem further.

Write down your reasons for wanting to lose weight in your Personal Plan *(see page 42)* – so you can refer back to them. This can be especially helpful when the going gets tough. It may help to think of it in terms of what your weight is stopping you from doing now. Here's some examples: to feel more confident; so I can play more comfortably with my kids; my healthier diet will give me more energy; to improve my fertility.

## What is a Healthy Weight?

With all the 'thin is beautiful' messages in the media it can be easy to get a distorted view about whether your weight is healthy or not. However, as the BMI charts suggest, there is no single 'ideal' weight for anybody. Research also shows that modest amounts of weight loss can be very beneficial to health and are easier to keep off. Therefore, health professionals now encourage us to aim for a weight loss of 5-10%. The ideal rate of weight loss is no more than 1-2 pounds (0.5-1kg) per week – so averaging a pound a week is great, and realistic progress.

**The health benefits of modest weight loss include:**

☐ *Reduced risk of developing heart disease, stroke and certain cancers*

☐ *Reduced risk of developing diabetes and helping to manage diabetes*

☐ *Improvements in blood pressure*

☐ *Improvements in mobility, back pain and joint pain*

☐ *Improvements with fertility problems and polycystic ovarian syndrome*

☐ *Less breathlessness and sleep/snoring problems*

☐ *Increased self esteem and control over eating*

☐ *Feeling fitter and have more energy*

# Are You Really Ready to Lose Weight?

When you think of losing weight, it's easy just to think of what weight you'd like to get to. But weight loss only happens as a result of making changes to your usual eating and activity patterns – which allow you to consume fewer calories than you burn *(see 'It's calories that count' page 5)*.

So here comes the next big question. Are you really ready to do it? Have you thought about the implications of your decision? If you have lost weight in the past, and put it all back on - have you thought about why that was? And how confident do you feel about being successful this time?

To help you answer these questions, try these short exercises.

Where would you place yourself on the following scales?

---

**Importance**

How important is it to you, to make the changes that will allow you to lose weight?

0  1  2  3  4  5  6  7  8  9  10

*Not at all important*　　　　　　　　　*Extremely important*

---

If you ranked yourself over half way along the scale then move on to the next question. If you were half way or less along the scale, you may not be mentally ready to make the required changes to lose weight. To further explore this, go to *'The Pros and Cons of Weight Loss' (page 17)*.

---

**Confidence**

How confident are you in your ability to make the changes that will allow you to lose weight?

0  1  2  3  4  5  6  7  8  9  10

*Not at all confident*　　　　　　　　*Extremely confident*

---

Now ask yourself (regarding your confidence ratings):

1.  Why did I place myself here?

2.  What is stopping me moving further up the scale (if anything)?

3.  What things, information, support would help me move further up the scale? (if not near 10)

If you aren't sure about answers to question 3, then keep reading for some pointers.

# The Pros and Cons of Weight Loss

Making lifestyle changes to lose weight is simpler if there are lots of clear benefits or pros, for example, clothes fit again, more energy, helps back pain - but there will also be associated downsides or cons. For example, some may feel it interferes with their social life, or don't have the time to plan meals or check food labels. Or overeating can help, if only temporarily, as a way of coping with unwanted feelings. Being overweight allows some people to feel strong and assertive, or to control their partner's jealousy. So in these cases there are downsides to losing weight, even if the person says they are desperate to do it.

If you are aware of the possible downsides, as well as the pros, you will be better prepared to deal with potential conflicts. Understanding what could be (or were with past weight loss efforts) barriers to success gives you the chance to address them. This boosts confidence in your ability to succeed this time, which in turn maintains your motivation.

Have a go at weighing up the pros and cons using the charts below and on page 18. Some examples are included. If you decide that the pros outweigh the cons, then great. You can also use the cons as potential barriers to plan strategies for *(see Personal Plan)*. If you find it's the other way around, this may not be the best time to actively lose weight. Try the exercise again in a month or so.

**Making Lifestyle Changes to Lose Weight Now**

| CONS<br>*e.g. Must limit eating out, take aways* | PROS<br>*e.g. Feel more energetic, slimmer* |
|---|---|
|  |  |
|  |  |
|  |  |
|  |  |

**Not Making Changes Now – how would I feel in 6 months time?**

| PROS<br>*e.g. Haven't had to worry about failing;*<br>*Still able to eat take aways a lot* | CONS<br>*e.g. Probably gained more weight;*<br>*Back pain may be worse* |
|---|---|
| | |
| | |
| | |
| | |

# To change your weight, first change your mind

To lose weight you may already have a list of things to change, such as eating more fruit and veg, calculating your daily calorie intake, going for a walk each morning or buying low fat options. Others could also give you tips to try. But knowing what to do isn't the same as feeling motivated or able to do it. To be effective, you have to believe the changes are relevant, do-able and worth it.

What you think, affects how you feel, and in turn the actions you take.

## Self-efficacy

In fact, research is telling us that one of the most important factors that influences weight loss success are your feelings of 'self-efficacy'. Self-efficacy is a term used in psychology to describe a person's belief that any action they take will have an effect on the outcome. It reflects our inner expectation that what we do will lead to the results we want. Not surprisingly, high levels of self-efficacy can enhance motivation, and allow us to deal better with uncertainty and conflict, and recovery from setbacks. But low levels, can reduce our motivation. We fear that whatever we do will not bring about our desired goal. This can lead self-defeating thoughts or 'self-talk', which make it hard to deal with set-backs, meaning we are more likely to give up. Here's some examples.

| Examples: Low self-efficacy |
| --- |
| '*No matter how carefully I diet, I don't lose weight . . .*'<br><br>'*I have eaten that chocolate and as usual blown my diet, so I may as well give up now.*'<br><br>'*I had a rich dessert – I have no willpower to say no. I can't stand not being able to eat what I want.*' |

If you have a strong sense of self-efficacy, your mindset and 'self-talk' will be more like:

| Examples: High self-efficacy |
| --- |
| '*I know from previous weight loss programmes, that if I stay focussed on what I am doing I do lose weight. I have always expected to lose too much too quickly which frustrates me. I know that I will lose weight if I keep making the right changes, and this time it is important to me.*'<br><br>'*The chocolate bar won't ruin my diet, but if I think it has and keep on eating, then my negative self-talk will. So I will get back on track.*'<br><br>'*I don't like having to eat differently from others, but losing weight is very important to me, so I **can** stand it. After all, the world won't stop if I say no to dessert, and I will feel great afterwards. If I think about it, I am not hungry so would just feel bloated and guilty if I ate it.*' |

## Willpower is a Skill

Many people feel that they just need plenty of willpower or a good telling off to lose weight. But willpower isn't something you have or you don't have. Willpower is a skill. Like the dessert example on page 19, it's a sign that you've made a conscious choice to do something, because you believe the benefits outweigh any downsides. In reality everything we do is preceded by a thought. This includes everything we eat. It just may not seem like it because our actions often feel automatic *(see 'Look out for trigger eating' page 21).*

When it comes to weight loss, developing a range of skills – including choosing a lower calorie diet, coping with negative self-talk and managing things that don't go to plan - will boost your sense of self-efficacy to make the changes you want. This is especially important because we live in such a weight-promoting environment.

## Our weight-promoting environment

We are constantly surrounded by tempting food, stresses that can trigger comfort eating and labour-saving devices that make it easy not to be physically active. In other words, the environment we live in makes it easy to gain weight, unless we stop and think about the food choices we make and how much exercise we do. In fact, to stay a healthy weight/maintain our weight, just about all of us need to make conscious lifestyle choices everyday. This isn't 'dieting' but just part of taking care of ourselves in the environment we live in.

It is also true that some people find it more of a challenge than others to manage their weight, thanks to genetic differences in factors such as appetite control, spontaneous activity level and emotional responses to food – rather than metabolic rate, as is often believed. The good news is that with a healthy diet and active lifestyle a healthier weight can still be achieved. But do talk to your doctor if you feel you need additional support.

# Coping with Common Slimming Saboteurs

Lyndel Costain BSc RD

## Look out for 'trigger' eating

Much of the overeating we do or cravings we have are actually down to unconscious, habitual, responses to a variety of triggers. These triggers can be external, such as the sight or smell of food, or internal and emotion-led, such as a response to stress, anger, boredom or emptiness. Your food diary (see page 43) helps you to recognise 'trigger' or 'non-hungry' eating which gives you the chance to think twice before you eat (see below).

## Get some support

A big part of your success will be having someone to support you. It could be a friend, partner, health professional, health club or website. Let them know how they can help you most.

## Make lapses your ally

Don't let a lapse throw you off course. You can't be, nor need to be perfect all the time. Doing well 80-90% of the time is great progress. Lapses are a normal part of change. Rather than feel you have failed and give up, look at what you can learn from a difficult day or week and use it to find helpful solutions for the future.

## Understand why you eat

When I ask people what prompts them to eat, hunger usually comes down near the bottom of their list of reasons. Some people struggle to remember or appreciate what true hunger feels like. We are lucky that we have plenty of food to eat in our society. But its constant presence makes it harder to control what we eat, especially if it brings us comfort or joy.

If you ever find yourself in the fridge even though you've recently eaten, then you know hunger isn't the reason but some other trigger. The urge to eat can be so automatic that you feel you lack willpower or are out of control. But it is in fact a learned or conditioned response. A bit like Pavlov's dogs. He rang a bell every time he fed them, and from then on, whenever they heard the bell ring they were 'conditioned' to salivate in anticipation of food.

Because this 'non-hungry' eating is learned, you can reprogramme your response to the situations or feelings that trigger it. The first step is to identify when these urges strike. When you find yourself eating when you aren't hungry ask yourself 'why do I want to eat, what am I feeling?' If you aren't sure think back to what was happening before you ate. Then ask yourself if there is another way you can feel better without food. Or you could chat to your urge to eat in a friendly way, telling it that you don't want to give into it, you have a planned meal coming soon, and it's merely a learned response. Whatever strategy you choose, the more often you break into your urges to eat, the weaker their hold becomes.

## Practise positive self-talk

Self-talk may be positive and constructive (like your guardian angel) or negative and irrational (like having a destructive devil on your shoulder).

If you've had on-off battles with your weight over the years, it's highly likely that the 'devil' is there more often. 'All or nothing' self-talk for example, 'I ate a "bad food" so have broken my diet', can make you feel like a failure which, can then trigger you into the action of overeating and/or totally giving up *(see 'Diet-binge cycle' page 23)*. One of the most powerful things about it is that the last thoughts we have are what stays in our mind. So if we think 'I still look fat' or 'I will never be slim', these feelings stay with us.

To change your self-talk for the better, the trick is to first recognise it's happening (keeping a diary really helps, *see Keep a Food Diary, page 29*). Then turn it around into a positive version of the same events *(see Self-efficacy, page 18)* where the resulting action was to feel good and stay on track. Reshaping negative self-talk helps you to boost your self-esteem and feelings of self-efficacy, and with it change your self-definition - from someone who can't 'lose weight' or 'do this or that', to someone 'who can'. And when you believe you can…

## The Diet – Binge Cycle

If this cycle looks familiar, use positive self-talk, and a more flexible dietary approach, to help you break free.

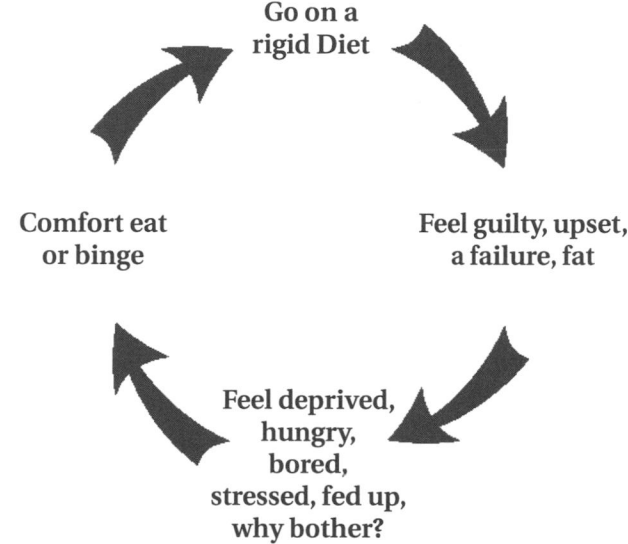

Go on a
rigid Diet

Feel guilty, upset,
a failure, fat

Feel deprived,
hungry,
bored,
stressed, fed up,
why bother?

Comfort eat
or binge

## Really choose what you want to eat

This skill is like your personal brake. It also helps you to manage 'trigger/non-hungry' eating and weaken its hold. It legalises food and stops you feeling deprived. It helps you to regularly remind yourself why you are making changes to your eating habits, which keeps motivation high. But it doesn't just happen. Like all skills it requires practise. Sometimes it will work well for you, other times it won't – but overall it will help. Basically, ask yourself if you really want to eat that food in front of you. This becomes the prompt for you to make a conscious choice, weighing up the pros and cons or consequences of making that choice, and feeling free to have it, reject it or just eat some. Remembering all the while that you can eat this food another time if you want to.

## Action Planning

Successful people don't just wait for things to happen. They believe in themselves, plan ahead, take action and then refine their plan until it gets, and keeps on getting the results they want. Successful slimmers use a very similar approach. They don't rely on quick-fixes or magic formulas, but glean information from reliable sources to develop a plan or approach that suits their needs, tastes and lifestyle. Thinking of weight management as a lifelong project, which has a weight loss phase and a weight maintenance phase, is also a route to success.

## When the Going Gets Tough - Staying on Track

If things start to go off track, don't panic. Learning new habits takes time. And life is never straightforward so there will be times when it all seems too much, or negative 'self- talk' creeps in to try and drag you back into old ways. So if the going gets tough:

- Value what you've achieved so far, rather than only focus on what you plan to do.

- Look back at your reasons to lose weight and refer to the list often .

- Don't expect to change too much, too quickly. Take things a step at a time.

- Accept difficulties as part of the learning and skill building process.

- Enjoy a non-food reward for achieving your goals (including maintaining your weight).

- Use recipes and meal ideas to keep things interesting.

- Talk to your supporters and get plenty of encouragement. This is really vital!

# Strategies of Successful Slimmers

Thanks to research conducted by large studies such as the US National Weight Control Registry and the German Lean Habits Study, we now know more about what works best for people who have lost weight and successfully kept it off. So be inspired!

**The key elements of success are to:**

- Believe that you can control your weight and the changes involved are really worth it.

- Stay realistic and value what you have achieved rather than dwell on a weight you 'dream' of being.

- Be more active – plan ways to fit activity into your daily life – aim for 1 hour of walking daily.

- Plan ahead for regular meals and snacks, starting with breakfast.

- Choose a balanced, low-fat diet with plenty of fruit and vegetables *(see Healthy Eating Made Easy, page 32)*.

- Watch portion size and limit fast food.

- Sit down to eat and take time over meals, paying attention to what you are eating.

- Have a flexible approach – plan in and enjoy some favourite foods without guilt.

- Recognise and address 'all or nothing' thinking and other negative 'self-talk'.

- Keep making conscious choices.

- Learn to confront problems rather than eat, drink, sleep or wish they would go away.

- Enlist ongoing help and support from family, friends, professionals or websites.

- Regularly (at least once a week but not more than once daily) check your weight.

- Take action before your weight increases by more than 4-5lb (2kg).

- Accept that your weight management skills need to be kept up long-term.

- Take heart from successful slimmers, who say that it gets easier over time.

# Your step-by-step guide to using this book and shifting those pounds

Juliette Kellow BSc RD and Rebecca Walton

## 1. Find your healthy weight

Use the weight charts, body mass index table and information on pages 36-43 to determine the right weight for you. Then set yourself a weight to aim for. Research shows it really helps if you make losing 10% of your weight your first overall target. It also brings important health benefits too *(see 'What is a Healthy Weight?' page 15)*. You can break this down into smaller manageable steps, for example, 3kg/6.5lbs at a time. If 10% is too much, then go for a 5% loss – this has important health benefits too. In fact, just keeping your weight stable is a great achievement these days, because of our weight-promoting environment *(see page 20)*.

---

### Waist Management

In addition to BMI, another important way to assess your weight is by measuring your waist just above belly button level. It is especially useful for men as they tend to carry more excess weight around their bellies, but women should test it out too. Having excess weight around your middle (known as being 'apple-shaped') increases your risk of heart disease and type 2 diabetes. A simple way to stay aware of your waist is according to how well, or otherwise, skirts and trousers fit. Talk to your doctor about any weight and health concerns.

#### WAIST MEASUREMENT

|  | Increased Health Risk | High Risk to Health |
|---|---|---|
| Women | 32-35in (81-88cm) | more than 35in (88cm) |
| Men | 37-40in (94-102cm) | more than 40in (102cm) |

---

## 2. Set a realistic time scale

With today's hectic lifestyles, everything tends to happen at breakneck speed, so it's no wonder that when it comes to losing weight, most of us want to shift those pounds in an instant. But it's probably taken years to accumulate that extra weight, with the result that it's unrealistic to expect to lose the excess in just a few weeks! Instead, prepare yourself to lose weight slowly and steadily. It's far healthier to lose weight like this. But better still, research shows you'll be far more likely to maintain your new, lower weight.

If you only have a small amount of weight to lose, aim for a weight loss of around 1lb (½kg) a week. But if you have more than 2 stone (28kg) to lose, you may prefer to aim for 2lb (1kg) each week. Remember though, it's better to keep going at 1lb (½kg) a week than to give up because trying to lose 2lb (1kg) a week is making you miserable! The following words may help you to keep your goal in perspective:

**'Never give up on a goal because of the time it will take to achieve it – the time will pass anyway.'**

---

### Weight Fluctuations

Weight typically fluctuates on a day to day basis. You know that shock/horror feeling when you weigh yourself in the morning then later in the day, or after a meal out, and it looks like youve gained pounds in hours! But this is due to fluid not fat changes. Real changes in body fat can only happen more gradually (remember, to gain 1lb you need to eat 3500 calories more than you usually do). Don't be confused either by seemingly very rapid weight loss in the first week or so.

When calorie intake is initially cut back, the bodys carbohydrate stores in the liver and muscles (known as glycogen) are used up. Glycogen is stored with three times its weight in water, meaning that rapid losses of 4.5- 6.6lb (2 -3 kg) are possible. These stores can be just as rapidly refilled if normal eating is resumed. True weight loss happens more gradually and this book helps you to lose weight at the steady and healthy rate of no more than 1-2 lbs per week.

## 3. Calculate your calorie allowance

Use the calorie tables on pages 39-40 to find out how many calories you need each day to maintain your current weight. Then use the table below to discover the amount of calories you need to subtract from this amount every day to lose weight at your chosen rate. For example, a 35 year-old woman who is moderately active and weighs 12 stone (76kg) needs 2,188 calories a day to keep her weight steady. If she wants to lose ½lb (¼kg) a week, she needs 250 calories less each day, giving her a daily calorie allowance of 1,938 calories. If she wants to lose 1lb (½kg) a week, she needs 500 calories less each day, giving her a daily calorie allowance of 1,688 calories, and so on.

| TO LOSE… | Cut your daily calorie intake by | In three months you could lose… | In six months you could lose… | In one year you could lose… |
|---|---|---|---|---|
| ½lb a week | 250 | 6.5lb | 13lb | 1st 12lb |
| 1lb a week | 500 | 13lb | 1st 12lb | 3st 10lb |
| 1½lb a week | 750 | 1st 5.5lb | 2st 11lb | 5st 8lb |
| 2lb a week | 1,000 | 1st 12lb | 3st 10lb | 7st 6lb |

| TO LOSE… | Cut your daily calorie intake by | In three months you could lose… | In six months you could lose… | In one year you could lose… |
|---|---|---|---|---|
| ¼kg a week | 250 | 3.25kg | 6.5kg | 13kg |
| ½kg a week | 500 | 6.5kg | 13kg | 26kg |
| ¾kg a week | 750 | 9.75kg | 19.5kg | 39kg |
| 1kg a week | 1,000 | 13kg | 26kg | 52kg |

## 4. Keep a food diary

Writing down what you eat and drink and any thoughts linked to that eating helps you become more aware of your eating habits. Recognising what is going on helps you feel in control and is a powerful way to start planning change. Keeping a food diary before you start to change your eating habits will also help you identify opportunities for cutting calories by substituting one food for another, cutting portion sizes of high-calorie foods or eating certain foods less often. Simply write down every single item you eat or drink during the day and use this book to calculate the calories of each item. Then after a few days of eating normally, introduce some changes to your diet to achieve your daily calorie allowance. Remember to spread your daily calorie allowance fairly evenly throughout the day to prevent hunger. You'll find a template for a daily food and exercise diary on page 43. Try to use it as carefully as you can as research shows that people who do, do best.

### Top Tip

If you only fill in your main food diary once a day, keep a pen and notepad with you to write down all those little extras you eat or drink during the day – that chocolate you ate in the office, the sliver of cheese you had while cooking dinner and the few chips you pinched from your husband's plate, for example! It's easy to forget the little things if they're not written down, but they can make the difference between success and failure.

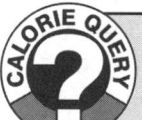

### QUESTION: Why are heavier people allowed more calories than those who have smaller amounts of weight to lose?

**ANSWER:** This confuses a lot of people but is easily explained. Someone who is 3 stone overweight, for example, is carrying the equivalent of 42 small packets of butter with them everywhere they go – up and down the stairs, to the local shops, into the kitchen. Obviously, it takes a lot more energy simply to move around when you're carrying that extra weight. As a consequence, the heavier you are, the more calories you need just to keep your weight steady. In turn, this means you'll lose weight on a higher calorie allowance. However, as you lose weight, you'll need to lower your calorie allowance slightly as you have less weight to carry around.

## 5. Control your portions

As well as making some smart food swaps to cut calories, it's likely you'll also need to reduce your serving sizes for some foods to help shift those pounds. Even 'healthy' foods such as brown rice, wholemeal bread, chicken, fish and low-fat dairy products contain calories so you may need to limit the amount you eat. When you first start out, weigh portions of foods like rice, pasta, cereal, cheese, butter, oil, meat, fish, and chicken rather than completing your food diary with a 'guesstimated' weight! That way you can calculate the calorie content accurately. Don't forget that drinks contain calories too, alcohol, milk, juices and sugary drinks all count.

## 6. Measure your success

Research has found that regular weight checks do help. Weighing yourself helps you assess how your eating and exercise habits affect your body weight. The important thing is to use the information in a positive way – to assess your progress - rather than as a stick to beat yourself up with. Remember that weight can fluctuate by a kilogram in a day, for example, due to fluid changes, premenstrually, after a big meal out, so weigh yourself at the same time of day and look at the trend over a week or two.

People who successfully lose weight and keep it off, also tend to continue weighing themselves at least once a week, and often daily (but not in an obsessive way), because they say it helps them stay 'on track'. Probably because they use it as an early warning system. People who weigh themselves regularly (or regularly try on a tight fitting item of clothing) will notice quickly if they have gained a couple of kilograms and can take action to stop gaining more. Checking your weight less often can mean that you might discover one day that you gained 6kg. That can be pretty discouraging, and it might trigger you to just give up.

### Top Tip

Don't just focus on what the bathroom scales say either – keep a record of your vital statistics, too. Many people find it doubly encouraging to see the inches dropping off, as well as the pounds!

## 7. Stay motivated

Each time you lose half a stone, or reach your own small goal – celebrate! Treat yourself to a little luxury – something new to wear, a little pampering or some other (non-food) treat. It also helps replace the comfort you once got from food and allows you to take care of yourself in other ways. Trying on an item of clothing that used to be tight can also help to keep you feeling motivated. Make sure you keep in touch with your supporters, and if the going gets tough take another look at the 'Coping with Slimming Saboteurs' section. Once you've reviewed how well you've done, use this book to set yourself a new daily calorie allowance based on your new weight to help you lose the next half stone *(see point 3 - page 28 - Calculate your calorie allowance)*.

## 8. Keep it off

What you do to stay slim is just as important as what you did to get slim. Quite simply, if you return to your old ways, you are likely to return to your old weight. The great thing about calorie counting is that you will learn so much about what you eat, and make so many important changes to your eating and drinking habits, that you'll probably find it difficult to go back to your old ways – and won't want to anyway. It's still a good idea to weigh yourself at least once a week to keep a check on your weight. The key is to deal with any extra pounds immediately, rather than waiting until you have a stone to lose (see page 30). Simply go back to counting calories for as long as it takes to shift those pounds and enjoy the new slim you. Page 25 has more information about how successful slimmers keep it off.

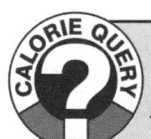

**QUESTION: Do I need to stick to exactly the same number of calories each day or is it OK to have a lower calorie intake during the week and slightly more at the weekend?**

**ANSWER:** The key to losing weight is to take in fewer calories than you need for as long as it takes to reach your target, aiming for a loss of no more than 2lb (1kg) a week. In general, most nutrition experts recommend a daily calorie allowance. However, it's just as valid to use other periods of time such as weeks. If you prefer, simply multiply your daily allowance by seven to work out a weekly calorie allowance and then allocate more calories to some days than others. For example, a daily allowance of 1,500 calories is equivalent to 10,500 calories a week. This means you could have 1,300 calories a day during the week and 2,000 calories a day on Saturday and Sunday.

# Healthy Eating Made Easy

Juliette Kellow BSc RD

GONE ARE THE DAYS when a healthy diet meant surviving on bird seed, rabbit food and carrot juice! The new approach to eating healthily means we're positively encouraged to eat a wide range of foods, including some of our favourites – it's just a question of making sure we don't eat high fat, high sugar or highly processed foods too often.

Eating a healthy diet, together with taking regular exercise and not smoking, has huge benefits to our health, both in the short and long term. As well as helping us to lose or maintain our weight, a healthy diet can boost energy levels, keep our immune system strong and give us healthy skin, nails and hair. Meanwhile, eating well throughout life also means we're far less likely to suffer from health problems such as constipation, anaemia and tooth decay or set ourselves up for serious conditions in later life such as obesity, heart disease, stroke, diabetes, cancer or osteoporosis.

Fortunately, it couldn't be easier to eat a balanced diet. To start with, no single food provides all the calories and nutrients we need to stay healthy, so it's important to eat a variety of foods. Meanwhile, most nutrition experts also agree that mealtimes should be a pleasure rather than a penance. This means it's fine to eat small amounts of our favourite treats from time to time.

To help people eat healthily, the Food Standards Agency recommends eating plenty of different foods from four main groups of foods and limiting the amount we eat from a smaller fifth group. Ultimately, we should eat more fruit, vegetables, starchy, fibre-rich foods and fresh products, and fewer fatty, sugary, salty and processed foods.

The following guidelines are all based on the healthy eating guidelines recommended by the Food Standards Agency.

# Bread, other cereals and potatoes

**Eat these foods at each meal. They also make good snacks.**

Foods in this group include bread, breakfast cereals, potatoes, rice, pasta, noodles, yams, oats and grains. Go for high-fibre varieties where available, such as wholegrain cereals, wholemeal bread and brown rice. These foods should fill roughly a third of your plate at mealtimes.

TYPICAL SERVING SIZES

* *2 slices bread in a sandwich or with a meal*

* *a tennis ball sized serving of pasta, potato, rice, noodles or couscous*

* *a bowl of porridge*

* *around 40g of breakfast cereal*

# Fruit and vegetables

**Eat at least five portions every day.**

Foods in this group include all fruits and vegetables, including fresh, frozen, canned and dried products, and unsweetened fruit juice. Choose canned fruit in juice rather than syrup and go for veg canned in water without added salt or sugar.

TYPICAL PORTION SIZES

* *a piece of fruit eg apple, banana, pear*

* *2 small fruits eg satsumas, plums, apricots*

* *a bowl of fruit salad, canned or stewed fruit*

* *a small glass of unsweetened fruit juice*

* *a cereal bowl of salad*

* *3tbsp vegetables*

# Milk and dairy foods

**Eat two or three servings a day.**

Foods in this group include milk, cheese, yoghurt and fromage frais. Choose low-fat varieties where available such as skimmed milk, reduced-fat cheese and fat-free yoghurt.

TYPICAL SERVING SIZES

- *200ml milk*
- *a small pot of yoghurt or fromage frais*
- *a small matchbox-sized piece of cheese*

# Meat, fish and alternatives

**Eat two servings a day**

Foods in this group include meat, poultry, fish, eggs, beans, nuts and seeds. Choose low-fat varieties where available such as extra-lean minced beef and skinless chicken and don't add extra fat or salt.

TYPICAL SERVING SIZES

- *a piece of meat, chicken or fish the size of a deck of cards*
- *1-2 eggs*
- *3 heaped tablespoons of beans*
- *a small handful of nuts or seeds*

## Healthy Eating on a plate

A simple way to serve up both balance and healthy proportions is to fill one half of your plate with salad or vegetables and divide the other half between protein-rich meat, chicken, fish, eggs or beans, and healthy carbs (potatoes, rice, pasta, pulses, bread or noodles).

# Fatty and sugary foods

## Eat only small amounts of these foods

Foods in this group include oils, spreading fats, cream, mayonnaise, oily salad dressings, cakes, biscuits, puddings, crisps, savoury snacks, sugar, preserves, confectionery and sugary soft drinks.

TYPICAL SERVING SIZES:

• *a small packet of sweets or a small bar of chocolate*

• *a small slice of cake*

• *a couple of small biscuits*

• *1 level tbsp mayo, salad dressing or olive oil*

• *a small packet of crisps*

# Useful Tools

## Body Mass Index

The Body Mass Index (BMI) is the internationally accepted way of assessing how healthy our weight is. It is calculated using an individual's height and weight. Use the Body Mass Index Chart to look up your BMI, and use the table below to see what range you fall into.

| | |
|---|---|
| **BMI** *Under 18.5* | *Underweight* |
| **BMI** *18.5-25* | *Healthy* |
| **BMI** *25-30* | *Overweight* |
| **BMI** *30-40* | *Obese* |
| **BMI** *Over 40* | *Severely Obese* |

This is what different BMI ranges mean.

- **Underweight:** you probably need to gain weight for your health's sake. Talk to your doctor if you have any concerns, or if you feel frightened about gaining weight.

- **Healthy weight:** you are a healthy weight, so aim to stay in this range (note that most people in this range tend to have a BMI between 20-25).

- **Overweight:** aim to lose some weight for your health's sake, or at least prevent further weight gain.

- **Obese:** your health is at risk and losing weight will benefit your health.

- **Severely obese:** your health is definitely at risk. You should visit your doctor for a health check. Losing weight will improve your health.

Please note that BMI is not as accurate for athletes or very muscular people (muscle weighs more than fat), as it can push them into a higher BMI category despite having a healthy level of body fat. It is also not accurate for women who are pregnant or breastfeeding, or people who are frail.

# Body Mass Index Table

## HEIGHT IN FEET / INCHES

| | 4'6 | 4'8 | 4'10 | 5'0 | 5'2 | 5'4 | 5'6 | 5'8 | 5'10 | 6'0 | 6'2 | 6'4 | 6'6 | 6'8 | 6'10 |
|---|---|---|---|---|---|---|---|---|---|---|---|---|---|---|---|
| 6st 7 | 22.0 | 20.5 | 19.1 | 17.8 | 16.7 | 15.7 | 14.7 | 13.9 | 13.1 | 12.4 | 11.7 | 11.1 | 10.6 | 10.0 | 9.5 |
| 7st 0 | 23.7 | 22.1 | 20.6 | 19.2 | 18.0 | 16.9 | 15.9 | 15.0 | 14.1 | 13.3 | 12.6 | 12.0 | 11.4 | 10.8 | 10.3 |
| 7st 7 | 25.4 | 23.6 | 22.0 | 20.6 | 19.3 | 18.1 | 17.0 | 16.0 | 15.1 | 14.3 | 13.5 | 12.8 | 12.2 | 11.6 | 11.0 |
| 8st 0 | 27.1 | 25.2 | 23.5 | 22.0 | 20.6 | 19.3 | 18.1 | 17.1 | 16.1 | 15.2 | 14.4 | 13.7 | 13.0 | 12.3 | 11.8 |
| 8st 7 | 28.8 | 26.8 | 25.0 | 23.3 | 21.8 | 20.5 | 19.3 | 18.2 | 17.1 | 16.2 | 15.3 | 14.5 | 13.8 | 13.1 | 12.5 |
| 9st 0 | 30.5 | 28.4 | 26.4 | 24.7 | 23.1 | 21.7 | 20.4 | 19.2 | 18.1 | 17.2 | 16.2 | 15.4 | 14.6 | 13.9 | 13.2 |
| 9st 7 | 32.2 | 29.9 | 27.9 | 26.1 | 24.4 | 22.9 | 21.5 | 20.3 | 19.2 | 18.1 | 17.1 | 16.2 | 15.4 | 14.7 | 14.0 |
| 10st 0 | 33.9 | 31.5 | 29.4 | 27.4 | 25.7 | 24.1 | 22.7 | 21.4 | 20.2 | 19.1 | 18.0 | 17.1 | 16.2 | 15.4 | 14.7 |
| 10st 7 | 35.6 | 33.1 | 30.8 | 28.8 | 27.0 | 25.3 | 23.8 | 22.4 | 21.2 | 20.0 | 18.9 | 18.0 | 17.0 | 16.2 | 15.4 |
| 11st 0 | 37.3 | 34.7 | 32.3 | 30.2 | 28.3 | 26.5 | 24.9 | 23.5 | 22.2 | 21.0 | 19.8 | 18.8 | 17.9 | 17.0 | 16.2 |
| 11st 7 | 39.0 | 36.2 | 33.8 | 31.6 | 29.6 | 27.7 | 26.1 | 24.6 | 23.2 | 21.9 | 20.7 | 19.7 | 18.7 | 17.8 | 16.9 |
| 12st 0 | 40.7 | 37.8 | 35.2 | 32.9 | 30.8 | 28.9 | 27.2 | 25.6 | 24.2 | 22.9 | 21.6 | 20.5 | 19.5 | 18.5 | 17.6 |
| 12st 7 | 42.3 | 39.4 | 36.7 | 34.3 | 32.1 | 30.1 | 28.3 | 26.7 | 25.2 | 23.8 | 22.5 | 21.4 | 20.3 | 19.3 | 18.4 |
| 13st 0 | 44.0 | 41.0 | 38.2 | 35.7 | 33.4 | 31.4 | 29.5 | 27.8 | 26.2 | 24.8 | 23.5 | 22.2 | 21.1 | 20.1 | 19.1 |
| 13st 7 | 45.7 | 42.5 | 39.6 | 37.0 | 34.7 | 32.6 | 30.6 | 28.8 | 27.2 | 25.7 | 24.4 | 23.1 | 21.9 | 20.8 | 19.8 |
| 14st 0 | 47.4 | 44.1 | 41.1 | 38.4 | 36.0 | 33.8 | 31.7 | 29.9 | 28.2 | 26.7 | 25.3 | 23.9 | 22.7 | 21.6 | 20.6 |
| 14st 7 | 49.1 | 45.7 | 42.6 | 39.8 | 37.3 | 35.0 | 32.9 | 31.0 | 29.2 | 27.6 | 26.2 | 24.8 | 23.5 | 22.4 | 21.3 |
| 15st 0 | 50.8 | 47.3 | 44.0 | 41.2 | 38.5 | 36.2 | 34.0 | 32.0 | 30.2 | 28.6 | 27.1 | 25.7 | 24.4 | 23.2 | 22.0 |
| 15st 7 | 52.5 | 48.8 | 45.5 | 42.5 | 39.8 | 37.4 | 35.2 | 33.1 | 31.2 | 29.5 | 28.0 | 26.5 | 25.2 | 23.9 | 22.8 |
| 16st 0 | 54.2 | 50.4 | 47.0 | 43.9 | 41.1 | 38.6 | 36.3 | 34.2 | 32.3 | 30.5 | 28.9 | 27.4 | 26.0 | 24.7 | 23.5 |
| 16st 7 | 55.9 | 52.0 | 48.5 | 45.3 | 42.4 | 39.8 | 37.4 | 35.2 | 33.3 | 31.4 | 29.8 | 28.2 | 26.8 | 25.5 | 24.2 |
| 17st 0 | 57.6 | 53.6 | 49.9 | 46.6 | 43.7 | 41.0 | 38.6 | 36.3 | 34.3 | 32.4 | 30.7 | 29.1 | 27.6 | 26.2 | 25.0 |
| 17st 7 | 59.3 | 55.1 | 51.4 | 48.0 | 45.0 | 42.2 | 39.7 | 37.4 | 35.3 | 33.3 | 31.6 | 29.9 | 28.4 | 27.0 | 25.7 |
| 18st 0 | 61.0 | 56.7 | 52.9 | 49.4 | 46.3 | 43.4 | 40.8 | 38.5 | 36.3 | 34.3 | 32.5 | 30.8 | 29.2 | 27.8 | 26.4 |
| 18st 7 | 62.7 | 58.3 | 54.3 | 50.8 | 47.5 | 44.6 | 42.0 | 39.5 | 37.3 | 35.3 | 33.4 | 31.6 | 30.0 | 28.6 | 27.2 |
| 19st 0 | 64.4 | 59.9 | 55.8 | 52.1 | 48.8 | 45.8 | 43.1 | 40.6 | 38.3 | 36.2 | 34.3 | 32.5 | 30.8 | 29.3 | 27.9 |
| 19st 7 | 66.1 | 61.4 | 57.3 | 53.5 | 50.1 | 47.0 | 44.2 | 41.7 | 39.3 | 37.2 | 35.2 | 33.3 | 31.7 | 30.1 | 28.6 |
| 20st 0 | 67.8 | 63.0 | 58.7 | 54.9 | 51.4 | 48.2 | 45.4 | 42.7 | 40.3 | 38.1 | 36.1 | 34.2 | 32.5 | 30.9 | 29.4 |
| 20st 7 | 69.4 | 64.6 | 60.2 | 56.3 | 52.7 | 49.4 | 46.5 | 43.8 | 41.3 | 39.1 | 37.0 | 35.1 | 33.3 | 31.6 | 30.1 |
| 21st 0 | 71.1 | 66.2 | 61.7 | 57.6 | 54.0 | 50.6 | 47.6 | 44.9 | 42.3 | 40.0 | 37.9 | 35.9 | 34.1 | 32.4 | 30.9 |
| 21st 7 | 72.8 | 67.7 | 63.1 | 59.0 | 55.3 | 51.9 | 48.8 | 45.9 | 43.3 | 41.0 | 38.8 | 36.8 | 34.9 | 33.2 | 31.6 |
| 22st 0 | 74.5 | 69.3 | 64.6 | 60.4 | 56.5 | 53.1 | 49.9 | 47.0 | 44.4 | 41.9 | 39.7 | 37.6 | 35.7 | 34.0 | 32.3 |
| 22st 7 | 76.2 | 70.9 | 66.1 | 61.7 | 57.8 | 54.3 | 51.0 | 48.1 | 45.4 | 42.9 | 40.6 | 38.5 | 36.5 | 34.7 | 33.1 |
| 23st 0 | 77.9 | 72.5 | 67.5 | 63.1 | 59.1 | 55.5 | 52.2 | 49.1 | 46.4 | 43.8 | 41.5 | 39.3 | 37.3 | 35.5 | 33.8 |
| 23st 7 | 79.6 | 74.0 | 69.0 | 64.5 | 60.4 | 56.7 | 53.3 | 50.2 | 47.4 | 44.8 | 42.4 | 40.2 | 38.2 | 36.3 | 34.5 |
| 24st 0 | 81.3 | 75.6 | 70.5 | 65.9 | 61.7 | 57.9 | 54.4 | 51.3 | 48.4 | 45.7 | 43.3 | 41.0 | 39.0 | 37.0 | 35.3 |
| 24st 7 | 83.0 | 77.2 | 71.9 | 67.2 | 63.0 | 59.1 | 55.6 | 52.3 | 49.4 | 46.7 | 44.2 | 41.9 | 39.8 | 37.8 | 36.0 |
| 25st 0 | 84.7 | 78.8 | 73.4 | 68.6 | 64.2 | 60.3 | 56.7 | 53.4 | 50.4 | 47.6 | 45.1 | 42.8 | 40.6 | 38.6 | 36.7 |
| 25st 7 | 86.4 | 80.3 | 74.9 | 70.0 | 65.5 | 61.5 | 57.8 | 54.5 | 51.4 | 48.6 | 46.0 | 43.6 | 41.4 | 39.4 | 37.5 |
| 26st 0 | 88.1 | 81.9 | 76.3 | 71.3 | 66.8 | 62.7 | 59.0 | 55.5 | 52.4 | 49.5 | 46.9 | 44.5 | 42.2 | 40.1 | 38.2 |
| 26st 7 | 89.8 | 83.5 | 77.8 | 72.7 | 68.1 | 63.9 | 60.1 | 56.6 | 53.4 | 50.5 | 47.8 | 45.3 | 43.0 | 40.9 | 38.9 |
| 27st 0 | 91.5 | 85.1 | 79.3 | 74.1 | 69.4 | 65.1 | 61.2 | 57.7 | 54.4 | 51.5 | 48.7 | 46.2 | 43.8 | 41.7 | 39.7 |
| 27st 7 | 93.2 | 86.6 | 80.8 | 75.5 | 70.7 | 66.3 | 62.4 | 58.7 | 55.4 | 52.4 | 49.6 | 47.0 | 44.7 | 42.4 | 40.4 |
| 28st 0 | 94.9 | 88.2 | 82.2 | 76.8 | 72.0 | 67.5 | 63.5 | 59.8 | 56.4 | 53.4 | 50.5 | 47.9 | 45.5 | 43.2 | 41.1 |
| 28st 7 | 96.5 | 89.8 | 83.7 | 78.2 | 73.2 | 68.7 | 64.6 | 60.9 | 57.5 | 54.3 | 51.4 | 48.7 | 46.3 | 44.0 | 41.9 |
| 29st 0 | 98.2 | 91.4 | 85.2 | 79.6 | 74.5 | 69.9 | 65.8 | 62.0 | 58.5 | 55.3 | 52.3 | 49.6 | 47.1 | 44.8 | 42.6 |
| 29st 7 | 99.9 | 92.9 | 86.6 | 80.9 | 75.8 | 71.1 | 66.9 | 63.0 | 59.5 | 56.2 | 53.2 | 50.5 | 47.9 | 45.5 | 43.3 |

WEIGHT IN STONES / LBS

## Weight Chart

Severely Obese
BMI 40 or more

Obese
BMI 30-40

Overweight
BMI 25-30

HEALTHY WEIGHT
BMI 18.5-25

Underweight
BMI less than 18.5

BMI: 10, 11, 12, 13, 14, 15, 16, 17, 18, 19, 20, 21, 22, 23, 24, 25, 26, 27, 28, 29, 30, 31, 32, 33, 34, 35, 36, 37, 38

Height (left axis):
6ft 6" / 197.5cm
6ft 5" / 195cm
6ft 4" / 192.5cm
6ft 3" / 190cm
6ft 2" / 187.5cm
6ft 1" / 185cm
6ft 0" / 182.5cm
5ft 11" / 180cm
5ft 10" / 177.5cm
5ft 9" / 175cm
5ft 8" / 172.5cm
5ft 7" / 170cm
5ft 6" / 167.5cm
5ft 5" / 165cm
5ft 4" / 162.5cm
5ft 3" / 160cm
5ft 2" / 157.5cm
5ft 1" / 155cm
5ft 0" / 152.5cm
4ft 11" / 150cm
4ft 10" / 147.5cm
4ft 9" / 145cm
4ft 8" / 142.5cm
4ft 7" / 140cm
4ft 6" / 137.5cm

Weight (right axis):
23st 7lb / 149kg
23st 0lb / 146kg
22st 7lb / 143kg
22st 0lb / 140kg
21st 7lb / 137kg
21st 0lb / 133kg
20st 7lb / 130kg
20st 0lb / 127kg
19st 7lb / 124kg
19st 0lb / 121kg
18st 7lb / 118kg
18st 0lb / 114kg
17st 7lb / 111kg
17st 0lb / 108kg
16st 7lb / 105kg
16st 0lb / 102kg
15st 7lb / 98kg
15st 0lb / 95kg
14st 7lb / 92kg
14st 0lb / 89kg
13st 7lb / 86kg
13st 0lb / 83kg
12st 7lb / 79kg
12st 0lb / 76kg
11st 7lb / 73kg
11st 0lb / 70kg
10st 7lb / 67kg
10st 0lb / 64kg
9st 7lb / 60kg
9st 0lb / 57kg
8st 7lb / 54kg
8st 0lb / 51kg
7st 7lb / 48kg
7st 0lb / 45kg
6st 7lb / 41kg
6st 0lb / 38kg
5st 7lb / 35kg
5st 0lb / 32kg
4st 7lb / 29kg

# Calories Required to Maintain Weight
## Adult Females

ACTIVITY LEVEL / AGE

| WEIGHT IN STONES / LBS | VERY SEDENTARY | | | MODERATELY SEDENTARY | | | MODERATELY ACTIVE | | | VERY ACTIVE | | |
|---|---|---|---|---|---|---|---|---|---|---|---|---|
| | <30 | 30-60 | 60+ | <30 | 30-60 | 60+ | <30 | 30-60 | 60+ | <30 | 30-60 | 60+ |
| 7st 7 | 1425 | 1473 | 1304 | 1544 | 1596 | 1412 | 1781 | 1841 | 1630 | 2138 | 2210 | 1956 |
| 8st 0 | 1481 | 1504 | 1338 | 1605 | 1629 | 1450 | 1852 | 1880 | 1673 | 2222 | 2256 | 2008 |
| 8st 7 | 1537 | 1535 | 1373 | 1666 | 1663 | 1487 | 1922 | 1919 | 1716 | 2306 | 2302 | 2059 |
| 9st 0 | 1594 | 1566 | 1407 | 1726 | 1696 | 1524 | 1992 | 1957 | 1759 | 2391 | 2349 | 2111 |
| 9st 7 | 1650 | 1596 | 1442 | 1787 | 1729 | 1562 | 2062 | 1996 | 1802 | 2475 | 2395 | 2163 |
| 10st 0 | 1706 | 1627 | 1476 | 1848 | 1763 | 1599 | 2133 | 2034 | 1845 | 2559 | 2441 | 2214 |
| 10st 7 | 1762 | 1658 | 1511 | 1909 | 1796 | 1637 | 2203 | 2073 | 1888 | 2644 | 2487 | 2266 |
| 11st 0 | 1819 | 1689 | 1545 | 1970 | 1830 | 1674 | 2273 | 2111 | 1931 | 2728 | 2534 | 2318 |
| 11st 7 | 1875 | 1720 | 1580 | 2031 | 1863 | 1711 | 2344 | 2150 | 1975 | 2813 | 2580 | 2370 |
| 12st 0 | 1931 | 1751 | 1614 | 2092 | 1897 | 1749 | 2414 | 2188 | 2018 | 2897 | 2626 | 2421 |
| 12st 7 | 1987 | 1781 | 1648 | 2153 | 1930 | 1786 | 2484 | 2227 | 2061 | 2981 | 2672 | 2473 |
| 13st 0 | 2044 | 1812 | 1683 | 2214 | 1963 | 1823 | 2555 | 2266 | 2104 | 3066 | 2719 | 2525 |
| 13st 7 | 2100 | 1843 | 1717 | 2275 | 1997 | 1861 | 2625 | 2304 | 2147 | 3150 | 2765 | 2576 |
| 14st 0 | 2156 | 1874 | 1752 | 2336 | 2030 | 1898 | 2695 | 2343 | 2190 | 3234 | 2811 | 2628 |
| 14st 7 | 2212 | 1905 | 1786 | 2397 | 2064 | 1935 | 2766 | 2381 | 2233 | 3319 | 2858 | 2680 |
| 15st 0 | 2269 | 1936 | 1821 | 2458 | 2097 | 1973 | 2836 | 2420 | 2276 | 3403 | 2904 | 2732 |
| 15st 7 | 2325 | 1967 | 1855 | 2519 | 2130 | 2010 | 2906 | 2458 | 2319 | 3488 | 2950 | 2783 |
| 16st 0 | 2381 | 1997 | 1890 | 2580 | 2164 | 2047 | 2976 | 2497 | 2362 | 3572 | 2996 | 2835 |
| 16st 7 | 2437 | 2028 | 1924 | 2640 | 2197 | 2085 | 3047 | 2535 | 2405 | 3656 | 3043 | 2887 |
| 17st 0 | 2494 | 2059 | 1959 | 2701 | 2231 | 2122 | 3117 | 2574 | 2449 | 3741 | 3089 | 2938 |
| 17st 7 | 2550 | 2090 | 1993 | 2762 | 2264 | 2159 | 3187 | 2613 | 2492 | 3825 | 3135 | 2990 |
| 18st 0 | 2606 | 2121 | 2028 | 2823 | 2298 | 2197 | 3258 | 2651 | 2535 | 3909 | 3181 | 3042 |
| 18st 7 | 2662 | 2152 | 2062 | 2884 | 2331 | 2234 | 3328 | 2690 | 2578 | 3994 | 3228 | 3093 |
| 19st 0 | 2719 | 2182 | 2097 | 2945 | 2364 | 2271 | 3398 | 2728 | 2621 | 4078 | 3274 | 3145 |
| 19st 7 | 2775 | 2213 | 2131 | 3006 | 2398 | 2309 | 3469 | 2767 | 2664 | 4162 | 3320 | 3197 |
| 20st 0 | 2831 | 2244 | 2166 | 3067 | 2431 | 2346 | 3539 | 2805 | 2707 | 4247 | 3366 | 3249 |
| 20st 7 | 2887 | 2275 | 2200 | 3128 | 2465 | 2383 | 3609 | 2844 | 2750 | 4331 | 3413 | 3300 |
| 21st 0 | 2944 | 2306 | 2235 | 3189 | 2498 | 2421 | 3680 | 2882 | 2793 | 4416 | 3459 | 3352 |
| 21st 7 | 3000 | 2337 | 2269 | 3250 | 2531 | 2458 | 3750 | 2921 | 2836 | 4500 | 3505 | 3404 |
| 22st 0 | 3056 | 2368 | 2303 | 3311 | 2565 | 2495 | 3820 | 2960 | 2879 | 4584 | 3552 | 3455 |
| 22st 7 | 3112 | 2398 | 2338 | 3372 | 2598 | 2533 | 3890 | 2998 | 2923 | 4669 | 3598 | 3507 |
| 23st 0 | 3169 | 2429 | 2372 | 3433 | 2632 | 2570 | 3961 | 3037 | 2966 | 4753 | 3644 | 3559 |
| 23st 7 | 3225 | 2460 | 2407 | 3494 | 2665 | 2608 | 4031 | 3075 | 3009 | 4837 | 3690 | 3611 |
| 24st 0 | 3281 | 2491 | 2441 | 3554 | 2699 | 2645 | 4101 | 3114 | 3052 | 4922 | 3737 | 3662 |
| 24st 7 | 3337 | 2522 | 2476 | 3615 | 2732 | 2682 | 4172 | 3152 | 3095 | 5006 | 3783 | 3714 |
| 25st 0 | 3394 | 2553 | 2510 | 3676 | 2765 | 2720 | 4242 | 3191 | 3138 | 5091 | 3829 | 3766 |
| 25st 7 | 3450 | 2583 | 2545 | 3737 | 2799 | 2757 | 4312 | 3229 | 3181 | 5175 | 3875 | 3817 |
| 26st 0 | 3506 | 2614 | 2579 | 3798 | 2832 | 2794 | 4383 | 3268 | 3224 | 5259 | 3922 | 3869 |
| 26st 7 | 3562 | 2645 | 2614 | 3859 | 2866 | 2832 | 4453 | 3307 | 3267 | 5344 | 3968 | 3921 |
| 27st 0 | 3618 | 2676 | 2648 | 3920 | 2899 | 2869 | 4523 | 3345 | 3310 | 5428 | 4014 | 3973 |
| 27st 7 | 3675 | 2707 | 2683 | 3981 | 2932 | 2906 | 4594 | 3384 | 3353 | 5512 | 4060 | 4024 |
| 28st 0 | 3731 | 2738 | 2717 | 4042 | 2966 | 2944 | 4664 | 3422 | 3397 | 5597 | 4107 | 4076 |
| 28st 7 | 3787 | 2768 | 2752 | 4103 | 2999 | 2981 | 4734 | 3461 | 3440 | 5681 | 4153 | 4128 |

# Calories Required to Maintain Weight
## Adult Males

### ACTIVITY LEVEL / AGE

| WEIGHT IN STONES / LBS | VERY SEDENTARY | | | MODERATELY SEDENTARY | | | MODERATELY ACTIVE | | | VERY ACTIVE | | |
|---|---|---|---|---|---|---|---|---|---|---|---|---|
| | <30 | 30-60 | 60+ | <30 | 30-60 | 60+ | <30 | 30-60 | 60+ | <30 | 30-60 | 60+ |
| 9st 0 | 1856 | 1827 | 1502 | 2010 | 1979 | 1627 | 2320 | 2284 | 1878 | 2784 | 2741 | 2254 |
| 9st 7 | 1913 | 1871 | 1547 | 2072 | 2026 | 1676 | 2391 | 2338 | 1933 | 2870 | 2806 | 2320 |
| 10st 0 | 1970 | 1914 | 1591 | 2134 | 2074 | 1724 | 2463 | 2393 | 1989 | 2955 | 2871 | 2387 |
| 10st 7 | 2027 | 1958 | 1636 | 2196 | 2121 | 1772 | 2534 | 2447 | 2045 | 3041 | 2937 | 2454 |
| 11st 0 | 2084 | 2001 | 1680 | 2258 | 2168 | 1820 | 2605 | 2502 | 2100 | 3127 | 3002 | 2520 |
| 11st 7 | 2141 | 2045 | 1724 | 2320 | 2215 | 1868 | 2677 | 2556 | 2156 | 3212 | 3067 | 2587 |
| 12st 0 | 2199 | 2088 | 1769 | 2382 | 2262 | 1916 | 2748 | 2611 | 2211 | 3298 | 3133 | 2654 |
| 12st 7 | 2256 | 2132 | 1813 | 2444 | 2310 | 1965 | 2820 | 2665 | 2267 | 3384 | 3198 | 2720 |
| 13st 0 | 2313 | 2175 | 1858 | 2506 | 2357 | 2013 | 2891 | 2719 | 2322 | 3470 | 3263 | 2787 |
| 13st 7 | 2370 | 2219 | 1902 | 2568 | 2404 | 2061 | 2963 | 2774 | 2378 | 3555 | 3329 | 2854 |
| 14st 0 | 2427 | 2262 | 1947 | 2630 | 2451 | 2109 | 3034 | 2828 | 2434 | 3641 | 3394 | 2920 |
| 14st 7 | 2484 | 2306 | 1991 | 2691 | 2498 | 2157 | 3106 | 2883 | 2489 | 3727 | 3459 | 2987 |
| 15st 0 | 2542 | 2350 | 2036 | 2753 | 2545 | 2205 | 3177 | 2937 | 2545 | 3813 | 3525 | 3054 |
| 15st 7 | 2599 | 2393 | 2080 | 2815 | 2593 | 2253 | 3248 | 2992 | 2600 | 3898 | 3590 | 3120 |
| 16st 0 | 2656 | 2437 | 2125 | 2877 | 2640 | 2302 | 3320 | 3046 | 2656 | 3984 | 3655 | 3187 |
| 16st 7 | 2713 | 2480 | 2169 | 2939 | 2687 | 2350 | 3391 | 3100 | 2711 | 4070 | 3721 | 3254 |
| 17st 0 | 2770 | 2524 | 2213 | 3001 | 2734 | 2398 | 3463 | 3155 | 2767 | 4155 | 3786 | 3320 |
| 17st 7 | 2827 | 2567 | 2258 | 3063 | 2781 | 2446 | 3534 | 3209 | 2823 | 4241 | 3851 | 3387 |
| 18st 0 | 2884 | 2611 | 2302 | 3125 | 2828 | 2494 | 3606 | 3264 | 2878 | 4327 | 3917 | 3454 |
| 18st 7 | 2942 | 2654 | 2347 | 3187 | 2876 | 2542 | 3677 | 3318 | 2934 | 4413 | 3982 | 3520 |
| 19st 0 | 2999 | 2698 | 2391 | 3249 | 2923 | 2591 | 3749 | 3373 | 2989 | 4498 | 4047 | 3587 |
| 19st 7 | 3056 | 2741 | 2436 | 3311 | 2970 | 2639 | 3820 | 3427 | 3045 | 4584 | 4112 | 3654 |
| 20st 0 | 3113 | 2785 | 2480 | 3373 | 3017 | 2687 | 3891 | 3481 | 3100 | 4670 | 4178 | 3721 |
| 20st 7 | 3170 | 2829 | 2525 | 3434 | 3064 | 2735 | 3963 | 3536 | 3156 | 4756 | 4243 | 3787 |
| 21st 0 | 3227 | 2872 | 2569 | 3496 | 3112 | 2783 | 4034 | 3590 | 3211 | 4841 | 4308 | 3854 |
| 21st 7 | 3285 | 2916 | 2614 | 3558 | 3159 | 2831 | 4106 | 3645 | 3267 | 4927 | 4374 | 3921 |
| 22st 0 | 3342 | 2959 | 2658 | 3620 | 3206 | 2880 | 4177 | 3699 | 3323 | 5013 | 4439 | 3987 |
| 22st 7 | 3399 | 3003 | 2702 | 3682 | 3253 | 2928 | 4249 | 3754 | 3378 | 5098 | 4504 | 4054 |
| 23st 0 | 3456 | 3046 | 2747 | 3744 | 3300 | 2976 | 4320 | 3808 | 3434 | 5184 | 4570 | 4121 |
| 23st 7 | 3513 | 3090 | 2791 | 3806 | 3347 | 3024 | 4392 | 3862 | 3489 | 5270 | 4635 | 4187 |
| 24st 0 | 3570 | 3133 | 2836 | 3868 | 3395 | 3072 | 4463 | 3917 | 3545 | 5356 | 4700 | 4254 |
| 24st 7 | 3627 | 3177 | 2880 | 3930 | 3442 | 3120 | 4534 | 3971 | 3600 | 5441 | 4766 | 4321 |
| 25st 0 | 3685 | 3220 | 2925 | 3992 | 3489 | 3168 | 4606 | 4026 | 3656 | 5527 | 4831 | 4387 |
| 25st 7 | 3742 | 3264 | 2969 | 4054 | 3536 | 3217 | 4677 | 4080 | 3712 | 5613 | 4896 | 4454 |
| 26st 0 | 3799 | 3308 | 3014 | 4116 | 3583 | 3265 | 4749 | 4135 | 3767 | 5699 | 4962 | 4521 |
| 26st 7 | 3856 | 3351 | 3058 | 4177 | 3630 | 3313 | 4820 | 4189 | 3823 | 5784 | 5027 | 4587 |
| 27st 0 | 3913 | 3395 | 3103 | 4239 | 3678 | 3361 | 4892 | 4243 | 3878 | 5870 | 5092 | 4654 |
| 27st 7 | 3970 | 3438 | 3147 | 4301 | 3725 | 3409 | 4963 | 4298 | 3934 | 5956 | 5158 | 4721 |
| 28st 0 | 4028 | 3482 | 3191 | 4363 | 3772 | 3457 | 5035 | 4352 | 3989 | 6042 | 5223 | 4787 |
| 28st 7 | 4085 | 3525 | 3236 | 4425 | 3819 | 3506 | 5106 | 4407 | 4045 | 6127 | 5288 | 4854 |
| 29st 0 | 4142 | 3569 | 3280 | 4487 | 3866 | 3554 | 5177 | 4461 | 4101 | 6213 | 5354 | 4921 |
| 29st 7 | 4199 | 3612 | 3325 | 4549 | 3913 | 3602 | 5249 | 4516 | 4156 | 6299 | 5419 | 4987 |
| 30st 0 | 4256 | 3656 | 3369 | 4611 | 3961 | 3650 | 5320 | 4570 | 4212 | 6384 | 5484 | 5054 |

# Calories Burned in Exercise

This table shows the approximate number of extra* calories that would be burned in a five minute period of exercise activity.

| ACTIVITY | CALORIES BURNED IN 5 MINUTES | ACTIVITY | CALORIES BURNED IN 5 MINUTES |
|---|---|---|---|
| Aerobics, Low Impact | 25 | Situps, Continuous | 17 |
| Badminton, Recreational | 17 | Skiing, Moderate | 30 |
| Cross Trainer | 30 | Skipping, Moderate | 30 |
| Cycling, Recreational, 5mph | 17 | Squash Playing | 39 |
| Dancing, Modern, Moderate | 13 | Tennis Playing, Recreational | 26 |
| Fencing | 24 | Toning Exercises | 17 |
| Gardening, Weeding | 19 | Trampolining | 17 |
| Hill Walking, Up and Down, Recreational | 22 | Volleyball, Recreational | 10 |
| Jogging | 30 | Walking, Uphill, 15% Gradient, Moderate | 43 |
| Kick Boxing | 30 | Walking Up and Down Stairs, Moderate | 34 |
| Netball Playing | 23 | Walking, 4mph | 24 |
| Rebounding | 18 | Weight Training, Moderate | 12 |
| Roller Skating | 30 | Yoga | 13 |
| Rowing Machine, Moderate | 30 | | |
| Running, 7.5mph | 48 | | |

*Extra calories are those in addition to your normal daily calorie needs.

# My Personal Plan

Date: _____

Body Mass Index: _____

Weight: _____

Waist Measurement: _____

Height: _____

Body Fat % (if known) _____

10% Weight Loss Goal:

| Current weight | 16stone (224lb) | 100kg |
| - 10% weight | 1stone 8½lb (22½lb) | 10kg |
| = 10% loss goal | 14stone 5½lb (201½lb) | 90kg |

My smaller weight targets on the way to achieving my 10% goal will be:

_____  _____  _____  _____

Reasons why I want to lose weight:

_____

Changes I will make to help me lose weight:

Diet:

_____

_____

_____

Activity:

_____

_____

_____

Potential saboteurs or barriers will be:

_____

_____

_____

Ways I will overcome these:

_____

_____

_____

My supporters will be:

_____

I will monitor my progress by:

_____    _____

_____    _____

I will reward my progress with:

In the short term:

_____

_____

In the long term:

_____

_____

# Food and Exercise Diary

Date:

[ / / ]

Daily Calorie Allowance: [___] **A**

| Food/Drink Consumed | Serving Size | Calories |
|---|---|---|
| | | |
| | | |
| | | |
| | | |
| | | |
| | | |
| | | |
| | | |
| | | |
| | | |
| | | |
| | | |
| | | |
| | | |
| | | |
| | | |
| | | |

Total calories consumed [___] **B**

| Exercise/Activity | No. mins | Calories |
|---|---|---|
| | | |
| | | |
| | | |
| | | |

Calories used in exercise [___] **C**

Calorie balance [___] **D**

You are aiming for your Calorie Balance (Box D) to be as close to zero as possible - ie. you consume the number of calories you need.

Your Daily Calorie Allowance (Box A) should be set to lose ½-2lb (¼-1kg) a week, or maintain weight, depending on your goals.

Daily Calorie Allowance (A) *plus* Extra Calories used in Exercise (C) *minus* Total Calories Consumed (B) *equals* Calorie Balance (D)

$A + C - B = D$

**You can also write down any comments or thoughts related to your eating if you want to.**

# Food Information

## Nutritional Information

CALORIE AND FAT values are given per serving, plus calorie and nutrition values per 100g of product. This makes it easy to compare the proportions of fat, protein, carbohydrate and fibre in each food.

The values given are for uncooked, unprepared foods unless otherwise stated. Values are also for only the edible portion of the food unless otherwise stated. ie - weighed with bone.

## Finding Foods

The Calorie, Carb & Fat Bible has an Eating Out section which is arranged alphabetically by brand. In the General Foods and Drinks A-Z most foods are grouped together by type, and then put in to alphabetical order. This makes it easy to compare different brands, and will help you to find lower calorie and/or fat alternatives where they are available.

This format also makes it easier to locate foods. Foods are categorised by their main characteristics so, for example, if it is bread, ciabatta or white sliced, you'll find it under "Bread".

This edition is also the first to highlight basic ingredients to make them easier to find at a glance. You'll find all unbranded foods in bold - making the index easier to use, whether it's just an apple or all the components of a home cooked stew.

There are, however, some foods which are not so easy to categorise, especially combination foods like ready meals. The following pointers will help you to find your way around the book until you get to know it a little better.

FILLED ROLLS AND SANDWICHES - Bagels, baguettes, etc which are filled are listed as "Bagels (filled)" etc. Sandwiches are under "Sandwiches".

CURRIES - Popular types of curry, like Balti or Jalfrezi, are listed under their individual types. Unspecified or lesser known types are listed under their main ingredient.

BURGERS - All burgers, including chicken-type sandwiches from fast-food outlets, are listed under "Burgers". CHIPS & FRIES - Are listed separately, depending on the name of the particular brand. All other types of potato are listed under "Potatoes".

SWEETS & CHOCOLATES - Well-known brands, eg. Aero, Mars Bar, are listed under their brand names. Others are listed under "Chocolate" (for bars) and "Chocolates" (for individual sweets).

READY MEALS - Popular types of dishes are listed under their type, eg. "Chow Mein", "Casserole", "Hot Pot", etc. Others are listed by their main ingredient, eg. "Chicken With", "Chicken In", etc.

EATING OUT & FAST FOODS - By popular demand this edition has the major eating out and fast food brands listed separately, at the back of the book. They are alphabetised first by brand, then follow using the same format as the rest of the book.

## Serving Sizes

Many ready-meal type foods are given with calories for the full pack size, so that an individual serving can be worked out by estimating the proportion of the pack that has been consumed. For example, if you have eaten a quarter of a packaged pasta dish, divide the calorie value given for the whole pack by 4 to determine the number of calories you have consumed. Where serving sizes are not appropriate, or unknown, values are given per 1oz/28g. Serving sizes vary greatly from person to person and, if you are trying to lose weight, it's very important to be accurate – especially with foods that are very high in calories such as those that contain a fair amount of fat, sugar, cream, cheese, alcohol etc.

# Food Data

Nutrition information for basic average foods has been compiled by the Weight Loss Resources food data team using many sources of information to calculate the most accurate values possible. Some nutrition information for non-branded food records is from The Composition of Foods 5th Edition (1991). Reproduced under licence from The Controller of Her Majesty's Stationary Office. Where basic data is present for ordinary foodstuffs such as 'raw carrots'; branded records are not included.

Nutrition information for branded goods is from details supplied by retailers and manufacturers, and researched by Weight Loss Resources staff. The Calorie Carb & Fat Bible contains data for over 900 UK brands, including major supermarkets and fast food outlets.

The publishers gratefully acknowledge all the manufacturers and retailers who have provided information on their products. All product names, trademarks or registered trademarks belong to their respective owners and are used only for the purpose of identifying products.

Calorie & nutrition data for all food and drink items are typical values.

| Caution |
| --- |
| The information in The Calorie, Carb and Fat Bible is intended as an aid to weight loss and weight maintenance, and is not medical advice. If you suffer from, or think you may suffer from a medical condition you should consult your doctor before starting a weight loss and/or exercise regime, If you start exercising after a period of relative inactivity, you should start slowly and consult your doctor if you experience pain, distress or other symptons. |

# Weights, Measures and Abbreviations

| ABBREVIATIONS | |
| --- | --- |
| *kcal* | *kilocalories / calories* |
| *prot* | *protein* |
| *carb* | *carbohydrate* |
| *sm* | *small* |
| *med* | *medium* |
| *lge* | *large* |
| *tsp* | *teaspoon* |
| *tbsp* | *tablespoon* |
| *dtsp* | *dessertspoon* |

| BRAND ABBREVIATIONS USED | |
| --- | --- |
| ASDA | |
| *Good for You* | *GFY* |
| MARKS & SPENCER | *M & S* |
| *Count on Us* | *COU* |
| MORRISONS | |
| *Better For You* | *BFY* |
| SAINSBURY'S | |
| *Be Good to Yourself* | *BGTY* |
| *Way to Five* | *WTF* |
| *Taste the Difference* | *TTD* |
| TESCO | |
| *Healthy Eating* | *HE* |
| *Healthy Living* | *HL* |
| WAITROSE | |
| *Perfectly Balanced* | *PB* |

| | Measure INFO/WEIGHT | per Measure KCAL | FAT | Nutrition Values per 100g / 100ml KCAL | PROT | CARB | FAT | FIBRE |
|---|---|---|---|---|---|---|---|---|
| **ABSINTHE** | | | | | | | | |
| *Average* | *1 Shot/35ml* | *127.0* | *0.0* | *363* | *0.0* | *38.8* | *0.0* | *0.0* |
| **ACKEE** | | | | | | | | |
| *Canned, Drained, Average* | *1oz/28g* | *42.0* | *4.0* | *151* | *2.9* | *0.8* | *15.2* | *0.0* |
| **ADVOCAAT** | | | | | | | | |
| *Average* | *1 Shot/35ml* | *91.0* | *2.0* | *260* | *4.7* | *28.4* | *6.3* | *0.0* |
| **AERO** | | | | | | | | |
| Creamy White Centre, Nestle* | 1 Bar/46g | 244.0 | 14.0 | 530 | 7.6 | 57.4 | 30.0 | 0.0 |
| Honeycomb, Nestle* | 1 Serving/40g | 199.0 | 10.0 | 497 | 5.9 | 62.2 | 25.0 | 0.0 |
| Minis, Nestle* | 1 Bar/11g | 57.0 | 3.0 | 518 | 6.8 | 58.1 | 28.7 | 0.8 |
| Mint, Nestle* | 1 Bar/46g | 245.0 | 14.0 | 533 | 4.9 | 61.2 | 29.8 | 0.4 |
| Nestle* | 1 Bar/48g | 255.0 | 15.0 | 536 | 5.0 | 59.8 | 30.8 | 0.8 |
| **ALFALFA SPROUTS** | | | | | | | | |
| *Raw, Average* | *1 Serving/80g* | *19.0* | *1.0* | *24* | *4.0* | *0.4* | *0.7* | *1.7* |
| **ALMONDS** | | | | | | | | |
| *Blanched, Average* | *1oz/28g* | *171.0* | *15.0* | *610* | *24.9* | *7.1* | *53.5* | *8.5* |
| Chocolate Covered, Bonneterre* | 1 Almond/3g | 17.0 | 1.0 | 570 | 11.0 | 43.0 | 40.0 | 0.0 |
| Cocoa Dusted, Organic, Green & Black's* | 1 Pack/110g | 585.0 | 40.0 | 532 | 7.8 | 42.8 | 36.7 | 7.6 |
| *Flaked, Average* | *1oz/28g* | *172.0* | *15.0* | *613* | *24.9* | *6.5* | *54.3* | *7.6* |
| *Flaked, Toasted, Average* | *1oz/28g* | *176.0* | *16.0* | *629* | *24.6* | *5.8* | *56.4* | *7.5* |
| *Ground, Average* | *1 Serving/10g* | *62.0* | *6.0* | *625* | *24.0* | *6.6* | *55.8* | *7.4* |
| *Marcona, Average* | *1 Serving/100g* | *608.0* | *54.0* | *608* | *22.1* | *13.0* | *53.7* | *9.7* |
| Sugared, Co-Op* | 1 Almond/6g | 25.0 | 1.0 | 455 | 7.0 | 74.0 | 14.0 | 2.0 |
| *Toasted, Average* | *1oz/28g* | *178.0* | *16.0* | *634* | *24.9* | *6.6* | *56.4* | *6.6* |
| *Whole, Average* | *1 Serving/20g* | *122.0* | *11.0* | *612* | *23.4* | *8.1* | *54.8* | *8.4* |
| Yoghurt Coated, Holland & Barrett* | 1 Pack/100g | 536.0 | 37.0 | 536 | 10.9 | 45.3 | 37.0 | 2.8 |
| **ALOO TIKKI** | | | | | | | | |
| Budgens* | 1 Serving/25g | 51.0 | 2.0 | 202 | 5.9 | 27.8 | 7.5 | 4.1 |
| Indian Selection, Tesco* | 1 Serving/23g | 49.0 | 3.0 | 211 | 2.3 | 20.1 | 13.5 | 3.5 |
| Mini, from Indian Snack Selection, Sainsbury's* | 1 Piece/25g | 44.0 | 2.0 | 175 | 4.8 | 22.1 | 7.5 | 3.9 |
| Mini, Indian Selection, Somerfield* | 1 Serving/25g | 49.0 | 2.0 | 199 | 4.5 | 30.3 | 6.6 | 0.2 |
| **ANCHOVIES** | | | | | | | | |
| Drained, Finest, Tesco* | 1 Fillet/3g | 7.0 | 0.0 | 220 | 21.3 | 0.8 | 14.6 | 0.5 |
| Fillets, Flat, John West* | 1 Can/50g | 113.0 | 7.0 | 226 | 25.0 | 0.1 | 14.0 | 0.0 |
| Fillets, Tesco* | 1 Serving/15g | 34.0 | 2.0 | 226 | 25.0 | 0.0 | 14.0 | 0.0 |
| *in Oil, Canned, Drained, Average* | *1 Serving/30g* | *58.0* | *3.0* | *194* | *22.9* | *0.0* | *11.3* | *0.0* |
| Marinated, Sainsbury's* | ¼ Pot/44g | 78.0 | 4.0 | 177 | 22.0 | 2.0 | 9.0 | 0.1 |
| Provencale, Finest, Tesco* | 1 Fillet/10g | 20.0 | 1.0 | 201 | 22.0 | 0.0 | 12.6 | 0.0 |
| Salted, Finest, Tesco* | 1 Serving/10g | 9.0 | 0.0 | 93 | 18.2 | 0.0 | 2.2 | 0.0 |
| with Olives, Marinated, H. Forman & Son* | 1 Pack/200g | 320.0 | 17.0 | 160 | 20.2 | 0.2 | 8.7 | 0.0 |
| **ANGEL DELIGHT** | | | | | | | | |
| Banana Flavour, Kraft* | 1 Sachet/59g | 289.0 | 12.0 | 490 | 2.5 | 72.0 | 21.0 | 0.0 |
| Banana Toffee Flavour, No Added Sugar, Kraft* | 1 Sachet/59g | 292.0 | 16.0 | 495 | 4.8 | 58.5 | 26.5 | 0.0 |
| Butterscotch Flavour, Kraft* | 1 Sachet/59g | 280.0 | 11.0 | 475 | 2.4 | 73.5 | 19.0 | 0.0 |
| Butterscotch Flavour, No Added Sugar, Kraft* | 1 Sachet/47g | 226.0 | 11.0 | 480 | 4.5 | 61.0 | 24.0 | 0.0 |
| Chocolate Flavour, Kraft* | 1 Sachet/67g | 305.0 | 12.0 | 455 | 3.7 | 69.5 | 18.0 | 0.4 |
| Chocolate Flavour with Topples, Kraft* | 1 Sachet/59g | 274.0 | 12.0 | 465 | 5.0 | 67.0 | 20.0 | 0.5 |
| Forest Fruit Flavour, Kraft* | 1 Sachet/59g | 289.0 | 13.0 | 490 | 2.5 | 71.5 | 21.5 | 0.0 |
| Raspberry Flavour, Kraft* | 1 Sachet/59g | 289.0 | 12.0 | 490 | 2.5 | 72.0 | 21.0 | 0.0 |
| Raspberry Flavour, No Added Sugar, Kraft* | 1 Sachet/59g | 292.0 | 15.0 | 495 | 4.8 | 59.5 | 26.0 | 0.0 |
| Strawberry Flavour, Kraft* | 1 Sachet/59g | 286.0 | 12.0 | 485 | 2.5 | 71.0 | 21.0 | 0.0 |
| Strawberry Flavour, No Added Sugar, Kraft* | 1 Sachet/47g | 230.0 | 12.0 | 490 | 4.8 | 59.0 | 26.5 | 0.0 |
| Strawberry Flavour with Topples, Kraft* | 1 Sachet/59g | 265.0 | 8.0 | 450 | 2.8 | 74.5 | 14.0 | 0.0 |
| Tangerine Flavour, No Added Sugar, Kraft* | 1 Sachet/59g | 292.0 | 16.0 | 495 | 4.8 | 58.0 | 27.0 | 0.9 |

**A**

| | Measure INFO/WEIGHT | per Measure KCAL | FAT | KCAL | PROT | CARB | FAT | FIBRE |
|---|---|---|---|---|---|---|---|---|
| **ANGEL DELIGHT** | | | | | | | | |
| Toffee Flavour, Kraft* | 1 Sachet/59g | 283.0 | 12.0 | 480 | 2.6 | 70.0 | 21.0 | 0.0 |
| Vanilla Ice Cream Flavour, Kraft* | 1 Sachet/59g | 289.0 | 13.0 | 490 | 2.5 | 71.5 | 21.5 | 0.0 |
| Vanilla Ice Cream Flavour, No Added Sugar, Kraft* | 1 Sachet/59g | 295.0 | 16.0 | 500 | 4.8 | 59.5 | 27.0 | 0.0 |
| **ANGEL HAIR** | | | | | | | | |
| Pasta, Sainsbury's* | 1 Serving/100g | 357.0 | 2.0 | 357 | 12.3 | 73.1 | 1.7 | 2.5 |
| **ANTIPASTO** | | | | | | | | |
| Artichoke, Sainsbury's* | 1 Serving/50g | 67.0 | 6.0 | 135 | 2.0 | 3.6 | 12.5 | 2.3 |
| Mixed, Misto Cotto, Arrosto Erbe, Waitrose* | 1 Slice/9g | 11.0 | 0.0 | 129 | 22.2 | 0.0 | 4.4 | 0.0 |
| Mixed Mushroom, Sainsbury's* | ¼ Jar/72g | 70.0 | 6.0 | 97 | 2.7 | 1.4 | 9.0 | 3.7 |
| Mixed Pepper, Sainsbury's* | ½ Jar/140g | 48.0 | 2.0 | 34 | 1.3 | 4.2 | 1.3 | 3.5 |
| Parma, Salami Milano, Bresaola, Finest, Tesco* | ¼ Pack/30g | 118.0 | 8.0 | 395 | 36.0 | 0.5 | 27.3 | 0.0 |
| Roasted Pepper, Drained, Tesco* | 1 Jar /170g | 127.0 | 9.0 | 75 | 0.9 | 5.5 | 5.5 | 4.1 |
| Seafood, Drained, Sainsbury's* | ½ Jar/84g | 150.0 | 10.0 | 178 | 14.3 | 4.1 | 11.6 | 1.4 |
| Sun Dried Tomato, Sainsbury's* | ¼ Jar/70g | 275.0 | 25.0 | 393 | 4.5 | 13.4 | 35.7 | 6.2 |
| **APPLE & GRAPES** | | | | | | | | |
| Fresh, Morrisons* | 1 Pack/90g | 46.0 | 0.0 | 51 | 0.4 | 12.1 | 0.1 | 2.3 |
| **APPLES** | | | | | | | | |
| Bites, Average | 1 Pack/118g | 58.0 | 0.0 | 49 | 0.3 | 11.6 | 0.1 | 2.2 |
| ***Braeburn, Average*** | *1 Apple/165g* | *79.0* | *0.0* | *48* | *0.4* | *11.3* | *0.1* | *1.8* |
| Cape, Tesco* | 1 Apple/100g | 50.0 | 0.0 | 50 | 0.4 | 11.8 | 0.1 | 1.8 |
| ***Cooking, Baked with Sugar, Flesh Only, Average*** | *1 Serving/140g* | *109.0* | *0.0* | *78* | *0.5* | *20.1* | *0.1* | *1.7* |
| ***Cooking, Raw, Peeled, Average*** | *1oz/28g* | *10.0* | *0.0* | *35* | *0.3* | *8.9* | *0.1* | *1.6* |
| ***Cooking, Stewed with Sugar, Average*** | *1 Serving/140g* | *104.0* | *0.0* | *74* | *0.3* | *19.1* | *0.1* | *1.2* |
| ***Cooking, Stewed without Sugar, Average*** | *1 Serving/140g* | *46.0* | *0.0* | *33* | *0.3* | *8.1* | *0.1* | *1.5* |
| ***Cox, English, Average*** | *1 Apple/108g* | *53.0* | *0.0* | *49* | *0.4* | *11.6* | *0.1* | *2.2* |
| ***Discovery, Average*** | *1 Apple/182g* | *95.0* | *0.0* | *52* | *0.3* | *13.8* | *0.2* | *2.4* |
| ***Dried, Average*** | *1 Pack/250g* | *554.0* | *1.0* | *221* | *1.0* | *57.3* | *0.3* | *6.6* |
| ***Empire, Average*** | *1 Serving/100g* | *48.0* | *0.0* | *48* | *0.4* | *11.8* | *0.1* | *2.0* |
| Fuji, Organic, Sainsbury's* | 1 Apple/130g | 61.0 | 0.0 | 47 | 0.4 | 11.8 | 0.1 | 1.8 |
| ***Gala, Average*** | *1 Apple/152g* | *74.0* | *0.0* | *49* | *0.4* | *11.5* | *0.1* | *1.4* |
| ***Golden Delicious, Average*** | *1 Med/102g* | *49.0* | *0.0* | *48* | *0.4* | *11.5* | *0.1* | *1.7* |
| ***Granny Smith, Average*** | *1 Sm/125g* | *62.0* | *0.0* | *50* | *0.4* | *11.9* | *0.1* | *2.0* |
| ***Green, Average, Raw*** | *1oz/28g* | *13.0* | *0.0* | *47* | *0.3* | *11.3* | *0.1* | *1.7* |
| ***Mackintosh, Red, Average*** | *1 Apple/165g* | *81.0* | *0.0* | *49* | *0.2* | *12.8* | *0.3* | *1.8* |
| ***Pink Lady, Average*** | *1 Apple/125g* | *62.0* | *0.0* | *49* | *0.4* | *11.7* | *0.1* | *1.8* |
| ***Sliced, Average*** | *1oz/28g* | *14.0* | *0.0* | *49* | *0.4* | *11.6* | *0.1* | *1.8* |
| **APPLETISE** | | | | | | | | |
| Schweppes* | 1 Glass/200ml | 98.0 | 0.0 | 49 | 0.0 | 11.8 | 0.0 | 0.0 |
| **APRICOTS** | | | | | | | | |
| & Prunes, in Fruit Juice, Breakfast, Sainsbury's* | 1 Pot/150g | 133.0 | 0.0 | 89 | 1.1 | 21.2 | 0.1 | 0.7 |
| ***Canned, in Syrup, Average*** | *1oz/28g* | *18.0* | *0.0* | *63* | *0.4* | *16.1* | *0.1* | *0.9* |
| ***Dried, Average*** | *1 Apricot/10g* | *17.0* | *0.0* | *171* | *3.6* | *37.4* | *0.5* | *6.3* |
| ***Dried, Soft, Average*** | *1 Serving/100g* | *208.0* | *0.0* | *208* | *3.2* | *47.7* | *0.5* | *6.6* |
| ***Halves, in Fruit Juice, Average*** | *1 Can/221g* | *87.0* | *0.0* | *40* | *0.5* | *9.2* | *0.1* | *1.0* |
| Milk Chocolate Coated, Graze* | 1 Pack/35g | 157.0 | 9.0 | 450 | 6.1 | 55.9 | 24.7 | 0.0 |
| ***Raw, Flesh Only, Average*** | *1 Apricot/37g* | *19.0* | *0.0* | *52* | *1.5* | *12.0* | *0.4* | *2.1* |
| ***Raw, Weighed with Stone, Average*** | *1 Apricot/40g* | *19.0* | *0.0* | *48* | *1.4* | *11.1* | *0.4* | *2.0* |
| Yoghurt Coated, Graze* | 1 Pack/40g | 176.0 | 9.0 | 441 | 3.4 | 58.6 | 22.4 | 0.0 |
| **ARCHERS*** | | | | | | | | |
| Aqua, Peach, Archers* | 1 Bottle/275ml | 206.0 | 0.0 | 75 | 0.3 | 5.1 | 0.0 | 0.0 |
| Peach (Calculated Estimate), Archers* | 1 Shot/35ml | 91.0 | 0.0 | 260 | 0.0 | 0.0 | 0.0 | 0.0 |
| Vea, Tropical, Archers* | 1 Bottle/275ml | 124.0 | 0.0 | 45 | 0.0 | 5.6 | 0.0 | 0.0 |
| Vea, Wildberry, Schnapps, Archers* | 1 Bottle/275ml | 124.0 | 0.0 | 45 | 0.0 | 5.8 | 0.0 | 0.0 |

| | Measure INFO/WEIGHT | per Measure KCAL | FAT | Nutrition Values per 100g / 100ml KCAL | PROT | CARB | FAT | FIBRE |
|---|---|---|---|---|---|---|---|---|
| **ARROWROOT** | | | | | | | | |
| *Fresh, Average* | *1 Root/33g* | *21.0* | *0.0* | *64* | *4.2* | *13.3* | *0.0* | *1.2* |
| **ARTICHOKE** | | | | | | | | |
| *Hearts, Canned, Drained, Average* | *½ Can/117g* | *35.0* | *0.0* | *30* | *1.9* | *5.4* | *0.0* | *2.1* |
| Hearts, Chargrilled in Olive Oil, TTD, Sainsbury's* | ¼ Jar/73g | 150.0 | 15.0 | 205 | 1.0 | 3.4 | 20.8 | 0.0 |
| Hearts, Marinated & Grilled, Tesco* | ½ Pack/100g | 340.0 | 36.0 | 340 | 1.6 | 1.6 | 36.0 | 3.6 |
| Hearts, Marinated & Grilled, Waitrose* | 1 Serving/50g | 57.0 | 5.0 | 114 | 3.0 | 3.0 | 10.0 | 3.0 |
| In Oil, Tesco* | 1 Piece/15g | 18.0 | 2.0 | 120 | 2.0 | 2.2 | 11.0 | 7.5 |
| Marinated, Roasted, M & S* | 1 Pack/200g | 300.0 | 27.0 | 150 | 1.9 | 5.0 | 13.3 | 2.3 |
| *Raw, Fresh, Average* | *1oz/28g* | *13.0* | *0.0* | *47* | *3.3* | *10.5* | *0.1* | *5.4* |
| **ASPARAGUS** | | | | | | | | |
| & Green Vegetables (Steamer Pouch), Waitrose* | ½ Pack/125g | 27.0 | 1.0 | 22 | 2.1 | 2.3 | 0.5 | 2.1 |
| *Boiled, In Salted Water, Average* | *5 Spears/125g* | *32.0* | *1.0* | *26* | *3.4* | *1.4* | *0.8* | *1.4* |
| British, with Butter, Tesco* | 1 Serving/50g | 26.0 | 2.0 | 52 | 2.6 | 1.6 | 4.0 | 2.0 |
| *Canned, Average* | *1 Can/250g* | *47.0* | *0.0* | *19* | *2.3* | *2.0* | *0.2* | *1.6* |
| *Raw, Average* | *1 Serving/80g* | *17.0* | *0.0* | *22* | *2.2* | *3.9* | *0.1* | *2.1* |
| **AUBERGINE** | | | | | | | | |
| Baby, Tesco* | 1 Aubergine/50g | 7.0 | 0.0 | 15 | 0.9 | 2.2 | 0.4 | 2.3 |
| Baked Topped, M & S* | 1 Serving/150g | 165.0 | 12.0 | 110 | 2.4 | 7.4 | 7.7 | 0.9 |
| *Fried, Average* | *1oz/28g* | *85.0* | *9.0* | *302* | *1.2* | *2.8* | *31.9* | *2.3* |
| in Hot Sauce, Yarden* | 1 Serving/35g | 96.0 | 9.0 | 273 | 1.5 | 8.8 | 25.8 | 0.0 |
| Marinated & Grilled, Waitrose* | ½ Pack/100g | 106.0 | 10.0 | 106 | 1.0 | 3.0 | 10.0 | 2.0 |
| Parmigiana, M & S* | 1 Pack/350g | 332.0 | 19.0 | 95 | 4.6 | 7.6 | 5.3 | 1.1 |
| *Raw, Fresh, Average* | *1 Sm/250g* | *37.0* | *1.0* | *15* | *0.9* | *2.2* | *0.4* | *2.0* |
| **AVOCADO** | | | | | | | | |
| *Flesh Only, Average* | *1 Med/145g* | *275.0* | *28.0* | *190* | *1.9* | *1.9* | *19.5* | *3.4* |

A

| | Measure INFO/WEIGHT | per Measure KCAL | FAT | Nutrition Values per 100g / 100ml KCAL | PROT | CARB | FAT | FIBRE |
|---|---|---|---|---|---|---|---|---|
| **BACARDI*** | | | | | | | | |
| & Diet Cola, Bacardi* | 1 Bottle/275ml | 85.0 | 0.0 | 31 | 0.0 | 1.0 | 0.0 | 0.0 |
| *37.5% Volume, Bacardi** | *1 Shot/35ml* | *72.0* | *0.0* | *207* | *0.0* | *0.0* | *0.0* | *0.0* |
| *40% Volume, Bacardi** | *1 Shot/35ml* | *78.0* | *0.0* | *222* | *0.0* | *0.0* | *0.0* | *0.0* |
| Breezer, Apple, Half Sugar, Crisp, Bacardi* | 1 Bottle/275ml | 121.0 | 0.0 | 44 | 0.0 | 3.7 | 0.0 | 0.0 |
| Breezer, Cranberry, Bacardi* | 1 Bottle/275ml | 154.0 | 0.0 | 56 | 0.0 | 7.1 | 0.0 | 0.0 |
| Breezer, Lemon, Diet, Bacardi* | 1 Bottle/275ml | 96.0 | 0.0 | 35 | 0.0 | 1.2 | 0.0 | 0.0 |
| Breezer, Lime, Bacardi* | 1 Bottle/275ml | 181.0 | 0.0 | 66 | 0.0 | 9.1 | 0.0 | 0.0 |
| Breezer, Orange, Bacardi* | 1 Bottle/275ml | 179.0 | 0.0 | 65 | 0.0 | 8.2 | 0.0 | 0.0 |
| Breezer, Orange, Diet, Bacardi* | 1 Bottle/275ml | 80.0 | 0.0 | 29 | 0.0 | 0.0 | 0.0 | 0.0 |
| Breezer, Orange & Vanilla, Diet, Bacardi* | 1 Bottle/275ml | 96.0 | 0.0 | 35 | 0.0 | 1.2 | 0.0 | 0.0 |
| Breezer, Pineapple, Bacardi* | 1 Bottle/275ml | 170.0 | 0.0 | 62 | 0.0 | 8.6 | 0.0 | 0.0 |
| Breezer, Raspberry, Half Sugar, Refreshing, Bacardi* | 1 Bottle/275ml | 99.0 | 0.0 | 36 | 0.0 | 3.3 | 0.0 | 0.0 |
| Breezer, Watermelon, Bacardi* | 1 Bottle/275ml | 151.0 | 0.0 | 55 | 0.0 | 6.8 | 0.0 | 0.0 |
| **BACON** | | | | | | | | |
| *Back, Dry Cured, Average* | *1 Rasher/31g* | *77.0* | *5.0* | *250* | *28.1* | *0.3* | *15.1* | *0.3* |
| *Back, Dry Fried Or Grilled, Average* | *1 Rasher/25g* | *76.0* | *5.0* | *304* | *26.5* | *0.1* | *21.9* | *0.0* |
| *Back, Lean, Average* | *1 Rasher/33g* | *57.0* | *4.0* | *173* | *16.3* | *0.1* | *12.0* | *0.5* |
| *Back, Smoked, Average* | *1 Rasher/25g* | *66.0* | *5.0* | *265* | *20.9* | *0.0* | *19.9* | *0.0* |
| *Back, Smoked, Lean, Average* | *1 Rasher/25g* | *41.0* | *1.0* | *163* | *28.2* | *1.1* | *5.0* | *0.2* |
| *Back, Smoked, Rindless, Average* | *1 Rasher/25g* | *60.0* | *4.0* | *241* | *21.0* | *0.1* | *17.4* | *0.0* |
| *Back, Tendersweet, Average* | *1 Rasher/25g* | *63.0* | *4.0* | *250* | *29.8* | *0.4* | *14.3* | *0.0* |
| *Back, Unsmoked, Average* | *1 Rasher/32g* | *78.0* | *6.0* | *243* | *21.3* | *0.4* | *17.3* | *0.0* |
| *Back, Unsmoked, Rindless, Average* | *1 Rasher/23g* | *56.0* | *4.0* | *241* | *22.5* | *0.0* | *16.9* | *0.0* |
| *Chops, Average* | *1oz/28g* | *62.0* | *4.0* | *222* | *22.3* | *0.0* | *14.8* | *0.0* |
| Chops, Coated in American Style BBQ Glaze, Tesco* | 1 Serving/200g | 480.0 | 36.0 | 240 | 16.1 | 2.1 | 18.1 | 0.0 |
| Chops, in Cheese Sauce, Tesco* | 1 Serving/185g | 405.0 | 26.0 | 219 | 12.6 | 10.0 | 14.3 | 1.1 |
| *Collar Joint, Lean & Fat, Boiled* | *1oz/28g* | *91.0* | *8.0* | *325* | *20.4* | *0.0* | *27.0* | *0.0* |
| *Collar Joint, Lean & Fat, Raw* | *1oz/28g* | *89.0* | *8.0* | *319* | *14.6* | *0.0* | *28.9* | *0.0* |
| *Collar Joint, Lean Only, Boiled* | *1oz/28g* | *53.0* | *3.0* | *191* | *26.0* | *0.0* | *9.7* | *0.0* |
| *Fat Only, Cooked, Average* | *1oz/28g* | *194.0* | *20.0* | *692* | *9.3* | *0.0* | *72.8* | *0.0* |
| *Fat Only, Raw, Average* | *1oz/28g* | *209.0* | *23.0* | *747* | *4.8* | *0.0* | *80.9* | *0.0* |
| *Gammon Rasher, Lean Only, Grilled* | *1oz/28g* | *48.0* | *1.0* | *172* | *31.4* | *0.0* | *5.2* | *0.0* |
| Lardons, Smoked, Sainsbury's* | 1 Serving/200g | 476.0 | 31.0 | 238 | 21.4 | 0.1 | 15.4 | 0.1 |
| *Lean, Average* | *1oz/28g* | *40.0* | *2.0* | *142* | *19.6* | *0.9* | *6.7* | *0.2* |
| *Lean Only, Fried, Average* | *1 Rasher/25g* | *83.0* | *6.0* | *332* | *32.8* | *0.0* | *22.3* | *0.0* |
| *Lean Only, Grilled, Average* | *1 Rasher/25g* | *73.0* | *5.0* | *292* | *30.5* | *0.0* | *18.9* | *0.0* |
| *Loin Steaks, Grilled, Average* | *1 Serving/120g* | *229.0* | *12.0* | *191* | *25.9* | *0.0* | *9.7* | *0.0* |
| *Medallions, Average* | *1 Rasher/18g* | *27.0* | *1.0* | *151* | *29.3* | *0.9* | *3.3* | *0.1* |
| *Middle, Fried* | *1 Rasher/40g* | *140.0* | *11.0* | *350* | *23.4* | *0.0* | *28.5* | *0.0* |
| *Middle, Grilled* | *1 Rasher/40g* | *123.0* | *9.0* | *307* | *24.8* | *0.0* | *23.1* | *0.0* |
| *Middle, Raw* | *1 Rasher/43g* | *104.0* | *9.0* | *241* | *15.2* | *0.0* | *20.0* | *0.0* |
| *Rindless, Average* | *1 Rasher/20g* | *30.0* | *2.0* | *150* | *18.5* | *0.0* | *8.5* | *0.0* |
| *Smoked, Average* | *1 Rasher/28g* | *46.0* | *2.0* | *166* | *24.7* | *0.2* | *7.3* | *0.0* |
| *Smoked, Crispy, Cooked, Average* | *1 Serving/10g* | *46.0* | *3.0* | *460* | *53.0* | *2.1* | *26.9* | *0.0* |
| *Smoked, Rindless, Average* | *1 Rasher/20g* | *21.0* | *1.0* | *106* | *19.8* | *0.0* | *3.0* | *0.0* |
| Steaks, with 3 Cheese Sauce & Mustard Crust, Asda* | ½ Pack/175g | 390.0 | 26.0 | 223 | 20.6 | 2.3 | 14.6 | 2.9 |
| *Streaky, Average* | *1oz/28g* | *76.0* | *6.0* | *270* | *20.0* | *0.0* | *21.0* | *0.0* |
| *Streaky, Cooked, Average* | *1 Rasher/20g* | *68.0* | *6.0* | *342* | *22.4* | *0.3* | *27.8* | *0.0* |
| **BACON BITS** | | | | | | | | |
| *Average* | *1oz/28g* | *66.0* | *5.0* | *235* | *19.6* | *0.0* | *17.4* | *0.0* |
| **BACON VEGETARIAN** | | | | | | | | |
| Rashers, Cheatin, Redwood* | 1 Rasher/16g | 32.0 | 1.0 | 196 | 25.9 | 6.5 | 7.3 | 0.5 |
| Rashers, Tesco* | 1 Rasher/20g | 41.0 | 2.0 | 203 | 22.5 | 3.3 | 11.1 | 3.9 |

| | Measure INFO/WEIGHT | KCAL | FAT | Nutrition Values per 100g / 100ml KCAL | PROT | CARB | FAT | FIBRE |
|---|---|---|---|---|---|---|---|---|
| **BACON VEGETARIAN** | | | | | | | | |
| Realeat* | 1 Rasher/19g | 49.0 | 1.0 | 260 | 27.0 | 25.0 | 5.8 | 1.6 |
| Streaky Style Rashers, Tesco* | 1 Rasher/8g | 17.0 | 1.0 | 215 | 23.7 | 5.0 | 10.6 | 2.2 |
| Strips, Morningstar Farms* | 1 Strip/8g | 30.0 | 2.0 | 375 | 12.5 | 12.5 | 28.1 | 6.2 |
| **BAGEL** | | | | | | | | |
| Bacon, & Soft Cheese, Boots* | 1 Serving/148g | 481.0 | 25.0 | 325 | 12.0 | 31.0 | 17.0 | 2.2 |
| Cream Cheese, & Salmon, Smoked, M & S* | 1 Bagel/23g | 64.0 | 3.0 | 280 | 10.9 | 31.7 | 12.2 | 2.9 |
| Cream Cheese, M & S* | 1 Bagel/23g | 79.0 | 5.0 | 352 | 7.8 | 31.0 | 21.8 | 1.8 |
| Ham, & Pesto, COU, M & S* | 1 Pack/173g | 259.0 | 2.0 | 150 | 11.1 | 23.5 | 1.4 | 1.7 |
| Smoked Salmon, & Cream Cheese, Handmade, Tesco* | 1 Bagel/162g | 380.0 | 13.0 | 235 | 13.1 | 27.7 | 7.8 | 1.5 |
| Smoked Salmon, & Cream Cheese, M & S* | 1 Bagel/19g | 43.0 | 1.0 | 230 | 14.0 | 26.7 | 7.1 | 1.8 |
| Soft Cheese, & Salmon, Smoked, American, Sainsbury's* | 1 Bagel/131g | 356.0 | 16.0 | 272 | 8.3 | 31.8 | 12.4 | 1.7 |
| Soft Cheese, & Salmon, Smoked, Finest, Tesco* | 1 Pack/173g | 396.0 | 10.0 | 229 | 13.1 | 31.2 | 5.8 | 1.7 |
| Tuna, & Salad, BGTY, Sainsbury's* | 1 Bagel/170g | 325.0 | 7.0 | 191 | 10.4 | 26.0 | 4.2 | 1.0 |
| Turkey, Pastrami & American Mustard, Shapers, Boots* | 1 Bagel/146g | 296.0 | 5.0 | 203 | 11.0 | 32.0 | 3.4 | 1.4 |
| **BAGEL CHIPS** | | | | | | | | |
| Sea Salt & Vinegar, Shapers, Boots* | 1 Bag/25g | 94.0 | 1.0 | 378 | 11.0 | 77.0 | 2.9 | 3.1 |
| Smokey Ham Flavour, COU, M & S* | 1 Bag/25g | 91.0 | 1.0 | 365 | 10.5 | 75.6 | 2.5 | 5.2 |
| Sour Cream & Chive, Shapers, Boots* | 1 Bag/25g | 94.0 | 1.0 | 377 | 9.7 | 78.0 | 2.9 | 1.9 |
| **BAGUETTE** | | | | | | | | |
| All Day Breakfast, Darwins Deli* | 1 Serving/184g | 498.0 | 22.0 | 271 | 13.4 | 31.9 | 11.7 | 0.0 |
| Cheese, & Chive, Safeway* | ¼ Baguette/65g | 216.0 | 10.0 | 333 | 7.9 | 37.1 | 14.7 | 1.4 |
| Cheese, & Ham, French, Shell* | 1oz/28g | 82.0 | 3.0 | 292 | 8.9 | 37.2 | 12.0 | 0.0 |
| Cheese, & Ham, Snack 'n' Go, Sainsbury's* | 1 Baguette/178g | 383.0 | 9.0 | 215 | 12.6 | 29.6 | 5.1 | 1.9 |
| Cheese, & Pickle, Fullfillers* | 1 Baguette/280g | 767.0 | 31.0 | 274 | 11.9 | 35.5 | 11.1 | 0.0 |
| Cheese, & Tomato, Tesco* | 1 Baguette/108g | 243.0 | 8.0 | 225 | 9.7 | 29.3 | 7.7 | 1.8 |
| Cheese, Mixed, & Spring Onion, Asda* | 1 Pack/190g | 629.0 | 35.0 | 331 | 9.5 | 32.1 | 18.3 | 1.3 |
| Cheese, Tomato, & Basil, Asda* | ¼ Baguette/42g | 138.0 | 6.0 | 329 | 10.0 | 40.8 | 14.0 | 1.3 |
| Chicken, & Mayonnaise, Asda* | 1 Pack/190g | 407.0 | 17.0 | 214 | 9.7 | 30.5 | 8.7 | 1.3 |
| Chicken, & Salad, Asda* | 1 Serving/158g | 326.0 | 9.0 | 206 | 9.0 | 29.0 | 6.0 | 2.1 |
| Chicken, & Salad, Boots* | 1 Baguette/132g | 202.0 | 2.0 | 153 | 11.0 | 23.0 | 1.8 | 2.0 |
| Chicken, & Salad, Shapers, Boots* | 1 Baguette/132g | 222.0 | 3.0 | 168 | 11.0 | 27.0 | 2.0 | 1.5 |
| Chicken, & Spicy Tomato, Snack, Sainsbury's* | 1 Baguette/160g | 344.0 | 6.0 | 215 | 14.1 | 31.2 | 3.7 | 2.2 |
| Chicken, & Stuffing, Hot, Sainsbury's* | 1 Baguette/227g | 543.0 | 16.0 | 239 | 13.7 | 29.6 | 7.2 | 0.0 |
| Chicken, Honey & Mustard, BGTY, Sainsbury's* | 1 Pack/187g | 340.0 | 4.0 | 182 | 11.0 | 30.0 | 2.0 | 0.0 |
| Chicken, Tikka, Asda* | 1 Pack/190g | 439.0 | 18.0 | 231 | 10.4 | 32.8 | 9.4 | 1.3 |
| Chicken, Tikka, Hot, Sainsbury's* | 1 Pack/190g | 386.0 | 12.0 | 203 | 8.5 | 28.4 | 6.1 | 0.0 |
| Egg, & Tomato, Oldfields* | 1 Pack/198g | 416.0 | 15.0 | 210 | 8.7 | 27.0 | 7.6 | 0.0 |
| Egg Mayonnaise, & Cress, Cafe, Sainsbury's* | 1 Pack/100g | 480.0 | 20.0 | 480 | 13.8 | 60.2 | 20.4 | 0.0 |
| Ham, & Salad, with Mustard Mayonnaise, Sainsbury's* | 1 Baguette/100g | 412.0 | 16.0 | 412 | 17.6 | 49.6 | 15.9 | 0.1 |
| Ham, & Turkey, Asda* | 1 Baguette/360g | 774.0 | 18.0 | 215 | 11.6 | 30.7 | 5.1 | 1.3 |
| Mozzarella, Tomato, & Pesto, Darwins Deli* | 1 Serving/210g | 531.0 | 20.0 | 253 | 11.7 | 29.7 | 9.7 | 0.0 |
| Prawn, French, Shell* | 1 Baguette/63g | 171.0 | 7.0 | 272 | 9.7 | 32.4 | 11.5 | 0.0 |
| Prawn Mayonnaise, Asda* | 1 Pack/190g | 399.0 | 9.0 | 210 | 9.1 | 32.5 | 4.9 | 1.3 |
| Steak, & Onion, Snack 'n' Go, Sainsbury's* | 1 Baguette/177g | 398.0 | 9.0 | 225 | 14.3 | 30.6 | 5.0 | 2.2 |
| Tuna, Crunch, Shapers, Boots* | 1 Pack/138g | 315.0 | 5.0 | 228 | 14.0 | 35.0 | 3.5 | 3.1 |
| Tuna, Melt, Sainsbury's* | 1 Serving/204g | 373.0 | 8.0 | 183 | 11.3 | 25.8 | 3.9 | 0.0 |
| **BAILEYS*** | | | | | | | | |
| Glide, Baileys* | 1 Serving/200ml | 212.0 | 2.0 | 106 | 0.0 | 18.0 | 1.2 | 0.0 |
| *Irish Cream, Original, Baileys** | *1 Glass/37ml* | *121.0* | *5.0* | *327* | *3.0* | *25.0* | *13.0* | *0.0* |
| **BAKE** | | | | | | | | |
| Aubergine & Mozzarella, Finest, Tesco* | 1 Pack/400g | 288.0 | 14.0 | 72 | 3.6 | 6.7 | 3.4 | 2.6 |
| Aubergine & Mozzarella Cheese, BGTY, Sainsbury's* | 1 Pack/360g | 194.0 | 7.0 | 54 | 3.0 | 6.0 | 2.0 | 1.3 |
| Aubergine & Spinach, BGTY, Sainsbury's* | 1 Pack/360g | 148.0 | 6.0 | 41 | 2.2 | 4.0 | 1.8 | 1.3 |

| | Measure INFO/WEIGHT | per Measure KCAL | FAT | Nutrition Values per 100g / 100ml KCAL | PROT | CARB | FAT | FIBRE |
|---|---|---|---|---|---|---|---|---|
| **BAKE** | | | | | | | | |
| Bean & Pasta, Asda* | 1 Pack/450g | 598.0 | 22.0 | 133 | 5.0 | 17.0 | 5.0 | 1.7 |
| Broccoli & Cheese, M & S* | 1 Pack/400g | 380.0 | 23.0 | 95 | 4.8 | 5.6 | 5.7 | 1.1 |
| Cauliflower & Broccoli Bake, Tesco* | ½ Pack/250g | 177.0 | 10.0 | 71 | 2.8 | 5.8 | 4.1 | 1.0 |
| Cheese & Spinach, Tesco* | 1 Bake/140g | 269.0 | 11.0 | 192 | 4.5 | 26.0 | 7.8 | 1.4 |
| Cheesy Brocolli, Asda* | 1 Pack/400g | 400.0 | 18.0 | 100 | 4.5 | 10.6 | 4.4 | 1.4 |
| Chicken, Bacon & Potato, British Classics, Tesco* | ½ Pack/375g | 435.0 | 17.0 | 116 | 7.0 | 12.2 | 4.4 | 1.4 |
| Chicken, Broccoli & Mushroom, Safeway* | 1 Serving/175g | 425.0 | 23.0 | 243 | 8.9 | 22.4 | 13.1 | 3.0 |
| Chicken, Tomato, & Mascarpone, HL, Tesco* | 1 Serving/400g | 468.0 | 11.0 | 117 | 7.6 | 15.5 | 2.7 | 0.8 |
| Chicken, Tomato & Mozzarella, Birds Eye* | 1 Pack/285g | 370.0 | 5.0 | 130 | 7.1 | 14.3 | 1.9 | 0.3 |
| Chicken & Mushroom, COU, M & S* | 1 Serving/360g | 324.0 | 8.0 | 90 | 7.3 | 10.3 | 2.3 | 1.1 |
| Chicken & Pasta, BGTY, Sainsbury's* | 1 Pack/400g | 394.0 | 10.0 | 98 | 9.0 | 10.0 | 2.5 | 2.5 |
| Chicken Arrabbbiata, M & S* | 1 Pack/450g | 540.0 | 13.0 | 120 | 7.6 | 16.0 | 3.0 | 2.0 |
| Chicken Spiralli, M & S* | 1 Serving/400g | 400.0 | 15.0 | 100 | 7.9 | 9.1 | 3.8 | 1.1 |
| Cod & Prawn, COU, M & S* | 1 Pack/400g | 320.0 | 8.0 | 80 | 6.5 | 8.8 | 2.0 | 1.0 |
| Courgette & Tomato, Cauldron Foods* | 1 Pack/285g | 593.0 | 37.0 | 208 | 10.0 | 17.0 | 13.0 | 6.4 |
| Creamy Peppercorn, Vegetarian, Tesco* | 1 Serving/140g | 322.0 | 17.0 | 230 | 3.6 | 27.0 | 12.0 | 1.2 |
| Fish & Vegetable, Youngs* | 1 Serving/375g | 446.0 | 24.0 | 119 | 5.6 | 10.0 | 6.3 | 1.3 |
| Mediterranean Vegetable Bistro, Frozen, Cauldron Foods* | 1 Bake/100g | 190.0 | 10.0 | 190 | 4.0 | 21.0 | 10.0 | 3.0 |
| Minced Beef & Root Vegetable, COU, M & S* | 1 Pack/400g | 320.0 | 12.0 | 80 | 6.6 | 6.0 | 2.9 | 3.0 |
| Mushroom, Cauldron Foods* | 1 Serving/100g | 164.0 | 12.0 | 164 | 6.0 | 15.0 | 12.0 | 6.0 |
| Mushroom, Leek & Cheddar, Asda* | 1 Pack/400g | 348.0 | 18.0 | 87 | 3.7 | 8.1 | 4.4 | 1.9 |
| Mushroom, Leek & Spinach, Cumberland, Sainsbury's* | 1 Pack/450g | 518.0 | 24.0 | 115 | 3.6 | 12.9 | 5.4 | 1.2 |
| Penne Bolognese, BGTY, Sainsbury's* | 1 Pack/450g | 445.0 | 11.0 | 99 | 6.0 | 13.0 | 2.5 | 2.0 |
| Penne Bolognese, Sainsbury's* | 1 Pack/397g | 603.0 | 28.0 | 152 | 7.6 | 14.8 | 7.0 | 2.0 |
| Potato, Cheese, & Bacon, Homepride* | 1 Serving/210g | 277.0 | 26.0 | 132 | 1.6 | 3.2 | 12.5 | 0.0 |
| Potato, Cheese, & Onion, Tesco* | 1 Pack/400g | 376.0 | 20.0 | 94 | 2.4 | 10.0 | 4.9 | 1.0 |
| Potato, Mushroom & Leek, M & S* | 1 Serving/225g | 225.0 | 13.0 | 100 | 3.5 | 10.0 | 5.9 | 2.0 |
| Potato, Tomato & Mozzarella, M & S* | 1 Bake/450g | 585.0 | 34.0 | 130 | 5.2 | 9.8 | 7.6 | 1.8 |
| Potato, with Cheese & Leek, Aunt Bessie's* | ½ Pack/275g | 300.0 | 14.0 | 109 | 3.4 | 12.7 | 5.0 | 2.7 |
| Roast Onion & Potato, COU, M & S* | 1 Pack/450g | 337.0 | 6.0 | 75 | 1.9 | 13.6 | 1.3 | 1.5 |
| Roast Potato, Cheese & Onion, Asda* | ½ Pack/200g | 288.0 | 16.0 | 144 | 4.2 | 14.0 | 8.0 | 1.1 |
| Salmon & Broccoli, Youngs* | 1 Bake/375g | 409.0 | 19.0 | 109 | 6.3 | 9.6 | 5.1 | 1.3 |
| Salmon & Prawn, M & S* | 1 Bake/329g | 460.0 | 31.0 | 140 | 7.4 | 6.6 | 9.5 | 0.7 |
| Smoked Haddock & Prawn, BGTY, Sainsbury's* | 1 Pack/350g | 318.0 | 2.0 | 91 | 7.5 | 13.6 | 0.7 | 1.1 |
| Spicy Bean & Potato, Safeway* | 1 Pack/386g | 405.0 | 12.0 | 105 | 3.9 | 14.2 | 3.2 | 2.1 |
| Spicy Chickpea & Apricot, Safeway* | 1 Pack/400g | 340.0 | 11.0 | 85 | 2.2 | 12.5 | 2.9 | 3.1 |
| Vegetable, M & S* | 1 Pack/300g | 255.0 | 12.0 | 85 | 2.1 | 11.0 | 3.9 | 1.6 |
| Vegetable, Multigrain, Grassington's Food Co* | 1 Bake/106g | 148.0 | 4.0 | 140 | 4.9 | 22.4 | 3.4 | 5.0 |
| Vegetable & Lentil, Somerfield* | 1 Pack/350g | 318.0 | 6.0 | 91 | 4.9 | 13.8 | 1.8 | 2.5 |
| **BAKE MIX** | | | | | | | | |
| Potato, Creamy Cheddar Cheese, Colman's* | 1 Pack/45g | 189.0 | 12.0 | 420 | 11.5 | 34.8 | 26.0 | 9.6 |
| Potato, Ham & Leek, Colman's* | 1 Pack/44g | 181.0 | 11.0 | 412 | 9.9 | 40.4 | 24.0 | 2.1 |
| Tuna & Pasta, Colman's* | 1 Pack/45g | 149.0 | 2.0 | 331 | 10.4 | 60.5 | 5.3 | 4.4 |
| **BAKING POWDER** | | | | | | | | |
| *Average* | *1 Tsp/2g* | *3.0* | *0.0* | *163* | *5.2* | *37.8* | *0.0* | *0.0* |
| **BAKLAVA** | | | | | | | | |
| Assortment, TTD, Sainsbury's* | 1 Pastry/24g | 105.0 | 7.0 | 439 | 10.6 | 33.4 | 29.2 | 4.2 |
| Average | 1 Serving/100g | 393.0 | 21.0 | 393 | 5.0 | 46.0 | 21.0 | 0.0 |
| **BALTI** | | | | | | | | |
| Chick Pea & Spinach, Cauldron Foods* | 1 Pack/400g | 356.0 | 8.0 | 89 | 2.3 | 15.5 | 2.0 | 1.0 |
| Chicken, & Naan Bread, Somerfield* | 1 Pack/335g | 489.0 | 17.0 | 146 | 10.0 | 16.0 | 5.0 | 0.0 |
| Chicken, Asda* | 1 Pack/450g | 324.0 | 10.0 | 72 | 8.0 | 5.0 | 2.2 | 0.0 |
| Chicken, Indian Takeaway, Iceland* | 1 Pack/402g | 362.0 | 19.0 | 90 | 7.8 | 4.0 | 4.8 | 0.7 |

B

| | Measure | per Measure | | Nutrition Values per 100g / 100ml | | | | |
|---|---|---|---|---|---|---|---|---|
| | INFO/WEIGHT | KCAL | FAT | KCAL | PROT | CARB | FAT | FIBRE |
| **BALTI** | | | | | | | | |
| Chicken, M & S* | ½ Pack/175g | 245.0 | 15.0 | 140 | 13.0 | 2.0 | 8.7 | 1.7 |
| Chicken, Ready Meals, M & S* | 1oz/28g | 34.0 | 2.0 | 120 | 10.2 | 4.7 | 6.5 | 1.6 |
| Chicken, Sainsbury's* | ½ Pack/200g | 222.0 | 11.0 | 111 | 11.6 | 3.6 | 5.6 | 1.3 |
| Chicken, Takeaway, Sainsbury's* | 1 Pack/400g | 404.0 | 18.0 | 101 | 10.4 | 4.8 | 4.5 | 1.4 |
| Chicken, Tesco* | 1 Pack/460g | 662.0 | 26.0 | 144 | 6.1 | 17.4 | 5.6 | 1.6 |
| Chicken, Tin, Sainsbury's* | 1 Serving/200g | 168.0 | 7.0 | 84 | 9.4 | 4.0 | 3.4 | 1.0 |
| Chicken, with Garlic & Coriander Naan, Frozen, Patak's* | 1 Pack/375g | 431.0 | 19.0 | 115 | 6.3 | 11.1 | 5.0 | 1.1 |
| Chicken, with Naan Bread, Perfectly Balanced, Waitrose* | 1 Pack/375g | 450.0 | 13.0 | 120 | 12.1 | 9.7 | 3.6 | 2.8 |
| Chicken, with Naan Bread, Sharwood's* | 1 Pack/375g | 529.0 | 23.0 | 141 | 7.3 | 14.1 | 6.2 | 2.2 |
| Chicken, with Pilau Rice, Asda* | 1 Pack/504g | 625.0 | 25.0 | 124 | 5.0 | 15.0 | 4.9 | 1.2 |
| Chicken, with Pilau Rice, Light Choices, Tesco* | 1 Pack/400g | 440.0 | 5.0 | 110 | 6.3 | 17.4 | 1.3 | 1.8 |
| Chicken, with Pilau Rice & Naan Bread, Tesco* | 1 Meal/550g | 660.0 | 20.0 | 120 | 6.1 | 15.5 | 3.6 | 1.4 |
| Chicken, with Potato Wedges, HL, Tesco* | 1 Pack/450g | 387.0 | 9.0 | 86 | 6.0 | 10.8 | 2.1 | 1.1 |
| Chicken, with Rice, Curry Break, Patak's* | 1 Pack/220g | 198.0 | 6.0 | 90 | 4.7 | 11.6 | 2.8 | 0.0 |
| Chicken, with Rice, Patak's* | 1 Pack/370g | 440.0 | 13.0 | 119 | 6.1 | 16.7 | 3.5 | 1.7 |
| Chicken, with Rice, Weight Watchers* | 1 Pack/329g | 253.0 | 6.0 | 77 | 4.8 | 10.7 | 1.7 | 0.5 |
| Chicken & Mushroom, Tesco* | 1 Serving/350g | 325.0 | 10.0 | 93 | 12.3 | 4.2 | 3.0 | 0.7 |
| Chicken Ceylon, Finest, Tesco* | 1 Pack/400g | 588.0 | 38.0 | 147 | 14.4 | 0.9 | 9.5 | 5.0 |
| Chicken Tikka, & Wedges, HL, Tesco* | 1 Pack/450g | 391.0 | 10.0 | 87 | 6.0 | 10.7 | 2.2 | 1.3 |
| Chicken Tikka, Finest, Tesco* | ½ Pack/200g | 280.0 | 17.0 | 140 | 15.8 | 1.1 | 8.6 | 3.2 |
| Chicken,Take Away, Tesco* | ½ Pack/200g | 170.0 | 8.0 | 85 | 8.1 | 4.6 | 3.8 | 1.9 |
| Lamb, Bhuna, Tesco* | 1 Pack/400g | 360.0 | 15.0 | 90 | 9.2 | 4.8 | 3.7 | 1.1 |
| Vegetable, GFY, Asda* | 1 Pack/450g | 324.0 | 4.0 | 72 | 1.9 | 14.0 | 0.9 | 1.5 |
| Vegetable, Indian Meal for 2, Finest, Tesco* | ½ Pack/150g | 144.0 | 11.0 | 96 | 1.6 | 6.1 | 7.2 | 2.9 |
| Vegetable, Naan Bread & Raita, Eat Smart, Safeway* | 1 Pack/371g | 315.0 | 7.0 | 85 | 3.8 | 12.5 | 1.9 | 3.1 |
| Vegetable & Rice, Tesco* | 1 Pack/450g | 378.0 | 7.0 | 84 | 2.0 | 15.6 | 1.6 | 1.3 |
| **BAMBOO SHOOTS** | | | | | | | | |
| *Canned, Average* | *1 Sm Can/120g* | *11.0* | *0.0* | *9* | *1.1* | *0.9* | *0.1* | *0.9* |
| **BANANA** | | | | | | | | |
| *Raw, Flesh Only, Average* | *1 Sm/95g* | *90.0* | *0.0* | *95* | *1.2* | *20.9* | *0.3* | *4.2* |
| *Raw, Weighed with Skin, Average* | *1 Lge/185g* | *176.0* | *1.0* | *95* | *1.2* | *20.9* | *0.3* | *4.2* |
| **BANANA CHIPS** | | | | | | | | |
| *Average* | *1oz/28g* | *143.0* | *9.0* | *511* | *1.0* | *59.9* | *31.4* | *1.7* |
| **BANANA SPLIT** | | | | | | | | |
| Fresh Cream, Tesco* | 1 Serving/240g | 463.0 | 31.0 | 193 | 1.7 | 17.2 | 13.0 | 0.3 |
| **BANGERS & MASH** | | | | | | | | |
| Asda* | 1 Pack/400g | 636.0 | 28.0 | 159 | 9.0 | 15.0 | 7.0 | 1.6 |
| Bitesize, Birds Eye* | 1 Pack/317g | 285.0 | 9.0 | 90 | 2.7 | 13.3 | 2.9 | 1.5 |
| Co-Op* | 1 Pack/300g | 375.0 | 18.0 | 125 | 4.0 | 13.0 | 6.0 | 0.8 |
| Meal for One, M & S* | 1 Pack/431g | 560.0 | 34.0 | 130 | 4.7 | 9.5 | 7.9 | 1.1 |
| Morrisons* | 1 Pack/300g | 306.0 | 15.0 | 102 | 3.0 | 12.3 | 4.9 | 0.8 |
| Sausage, & Cabbage Mash, Eat Smart, Safeway* | 1 Pack/400g | 340.0 | 10.0 | 85 | 6.4 | 9.0 | 2.5 | 1.3 |
| **BARS** | | | | | | | | |
| All Bran, Apple, Kellogg's* | 1 Bar/40g | 158.0 | 8.0 | 395 | 8.0 | 48.0 | 19.0 | 5.0 |
| All Bran, Honey & Oat, Kellogg's* | 1 Bar/27g | 99.0 | 2.0 | 366 | 6.0 | 67.0 | 8.0 | 12.0 |
| All Fruit, Frusli, Passion Fruit, Jordans* | 1 Bar/30g | 92.0 | 0.0 | 307 | 1.3 | 74.0 | 0.7 | 5.0 |
| All Fruit, Frusli, Strawberry, Jordans* | 1 Bar/30g | 94.0 | 0.0 | 313 | 2.3 | 81.3 | 0.3 | 5.0 |
| Almond, Apricot, & Mango, M & S* | 1 Bar/50g | 205.0 | 7.0 | 410 | 9.0 | 60.2 | 14.8 | 5.0 |
| Almond & Apricot, Weight Watchers* | 1 Bar/34g | 151.0 | 7.0 | 443 | 8.6 | 55.9 | 19.4 | 5.2 |
| Am, Breakfast Muffin, Apple & Sultana, McVitie's* | 1 Bar/45g | 168.0 | 8.0 | 373 | 4.4 | 54.9 | 16.7 | 1.6 |
| Am, Cereal, Apple, McVitie's* | 1 Bar/40g | 160.0 | 5.0 | 400 | 4.3 | 65.4 | 13.5 | 3.1 |
| Am, Cereal, Apricot, McVitie's* | 1 Bar/30g | 146.0 | 6.0 | 486 | 6.5 | 68.8 | 20.5 | 0.5 |
| Am, Cereal, Berry, McVitie's* | 1 Bar/30g | 146.0 | 6.0 | 486 | 6.5 | 68.8 | 20.5 | 0.5 |

**B**

## BARS

| | Measure INFO/WEIGHT | per Measure KCAL | per Measure FAT | Nutrition Values per 100g / 100ml KCAL | PROT | CARB | FAT | FIBRE |
|---|---|---|---|---|---|---|---|---|
| Am, Cereal, Fruit & Nut, McVitie's* | 1 Bar/35g | 167.0 | 8.0 | 477 | 6.6 | 64.9 | 21.4 | 3.4 |
| Am, Cereal, Grapefruit, McVitie's* | 1 Bar/35g | 136.0 | 3.0 | 389 | 5.1 | 70.9 | 9.4 | 3.1 |
| Am, Cereal, Orange Marmalade, McVitie's* | 1 Bar/40g | 151.0 | 7.0 | 377 | 4.5 | 53.2 | 18.0 | 1.7 |
| Am, Cereal, Raisin & Nut, McVitie's* | 1 Bar/35g | 148.0 | 6.0 | 422 | 6.4 | 62.1 | 16.4 | 2.4 |
| Am, Cereal, Strawberry, McVitie's* | 1 Bar/35g | 138.0 | 4.0 | 395 | 5.7 | 70.5 | 10.1 | 2.7 |
| Am, Granola, Almond, Raisin & Cranberry, McVitie's* | 1 Bar/35g | 133.0 | 4.0 | 380 | 7.1 | 62.9 | 11.4 | 4.0 |
| Am, Muesli Fingers, McVitie's* | 1 Bar/35g | 154.0 | 7.0 | 440 | 6.0 | 59.8 | 19.6 | 3.1 |
| Apple, Geobar, Traidcraft* | 1 Bar/35g | 132.0 | 3.0 | 376 | 5.3 | 69.0 | 8.8 | 3.5 |
| Apple, Granola, McVitie's* | 1 Bar/35g | 128.0 | 3.0 | 366 | 6.6 | 63.1 | 9.7 | 4.3 |
| Apple, Pear & Berry, Shapers, Boots* | 1 Bar/30g | 78.0 | 0.0 | 261 | 1.2 | 64.0 | 0.1 | 10.0 |
| Apple & Cinnamon, Breakfast Snack, Tesco* | 1 Bar/38g | 137.0 | 5.0 | 365 | 4.3 | 58.8 | 12.5 | 2.0 |
| Apple & Cinnamon, Chewy, GFY, Asda* | 1 Bar/27g | 95.0 | 1.0 | 351 | 6.0 | 76.0 | 2.6 | 3.5 |
| Apple & Custard, Danish, Tesco* | 1 Serving/100g | 268.0 | 15.0 | 268 | 3.6 | 29.5 | 15.1 | 5.6 |
| Apple & Raisin, Snack, Geobar, Traidcraft* | 1 Bar/35g | 127.0 | 2.0 | 362 | 3.3 | 76.4 | 4.8 | 2.3 |
| Apple & Sultana, Goodness, Ryvita* | 1 Bar/23g | 62.0 | 1.0 | 268 | 4.3 | 56.4 | 2.8 | 22.0 |
| Apple Pie, Nakd* | 1 Bar/68g | 221.0 | 6.0 | 325 | 6.8 | 57.2 | 8.7 | 7.3 |
| Apricot, Dried Fruit, Sunsweet* | 1 Bar/33g | 96.0 | 0.0 | 292 | 3.6 | 72.5 | 0.1 | 0.0 |
| Apricot, Fruity Grain, Tesco* | 1 Bar/37g | 135.0 | 3.0 | 366 | 6.5 | 65.0 | 7.0 | 2.5 |
| Apricot & Almond, Chewy & Crisp, Tesco* | 1 Bar/27g | 122.0 | 6.0 | 452 | 6.2 | 60.0 | 20.8 | 2.6 |
| Apricot & Almond, Eat Natural* | 1 Serving/50g | 202.0 | 8.0 | 403 | 11.2 | 53.3 | 16.1 | 0.0 |
| Apricot & Almond, Yoghurt Coated, Eat Natural* | 1 Bar/50g | 228.0 | 12.0 | 456 | 5.7 | 52.8 | 24.7 | 5.7 |
| Apricot & Coconut, Chewy & Crisp, Sainsbury's* | 1 Bar/27g | 123.0 | 6.0 | 457 | 5.2 | 58.8 | 22.3 | 4.0 |
| Apricot & Peach, Multigrain, BGTY, Sainsbury's* | 1 Bar/25g | 70.0 | 1.0 | 282 | 6.6 | 58.2 | 2.5 | 23.1 |
| Banana Break, Breakfast in a Bar, Jordans* | 1 Bar/40g | 152.0 | 4.0 | 381 | 5.7 | 69.1 | 9.1 | 5.0 |
| Banoffee, Weight Watchers* | 1 Bar/18g | 68.0 | 1.0 | 379 | 6.3 | 77.0 | 5.1 | 3.0 |
| Biscuit, Chocolate, Penguin, McVitie's* | 1 Bar/25g | 130.0 | 7.0 | 520 | 5.2 | 62.4 | 27.7 | 2.4 |
| Biscuit, Chocolate Mint, Penguin, McVitie's* | 1 Bar/25g | 133.0 | 7.0 | 531 | 5.4 | 65.0 | 27.7 | 1.5 |
| Biscuit, Chocolate Orange, Penguin, McVitie's* | 1 Bar/25g | 133.0 | 7.0 | 531 | 5.4 | 65.0 | 27.7 | 1.5 |
| Biscuit & Raisin, Reduced Fat, Tesco* | 1 Bar/22g | 90.0 | 3.0 | 410 | 4.9 | 69.5 | 12.5 | 1.8 |
| Black Forest, Weight Watchers* | 1 Bar/23g | 94.0 | 2.0 | 408 | 3.9 | 78.4 | 8.8 | 1.4 |
| Blue Riband, 99 Calories, Nestle* | 1 Bar/19g | 99.0 | 5.0 | 513 | 4.8 | 66.4 | 25.3 | 0.0 |
| Blue Riband, Double Choc, Nestle* | 1 Bar/22g | 113.0 | 6.0 | 513 | 4.8 | 66.4 | 25.3 | 1.1 |
| Blueberry, Fruit & Grain, Asda* | 1 Bar/37g | 124.0 | 3.0 | 335 | 4.1 | 64.0 | 7.0 | 3.9 |
| Blueberry, Weight Watchers* | 1 Bar/25g | 91.0 | 2.0 | 365 | 4.5 | 74.9 | 7.4 | 2.2 |
| Blueberry, Yoghurt & Honey, Altu* | 1 Bar/40g | 129.0 | 5.0 | 323 | 12.9 | 45.5 | 11.7 | 12.0 |
| Blueberry & Yoghurt Nougat, Shapers, Boots* | 1 Bar/23g | 89.0 | 4.0 | 385 | 1.7 | 58.0 | 16.0 | 0.7 |
| Boohbah, Milk & White Chocolate, M & S* | 1 Bar/75g | 405.0 | 24.0 | 540 | 7.9 | 54.7 | 32.3 | 1.2 |
| Breakfast, Blueberry, Free From, Sainsbury's* | 1 Bar/35g | 163.0 | 8.0 | 467 | 3.8 | 62.6 | 22.4 | 0.2 |
| Breakfast, Cherry, Oats & More, Nestle* | 1 Bar/30g | 109.0 | 2.0 | 363 | 6.0 | 70.2 | 6.5 | 3.6 |
| Breakfast, Chocolate Chip Crisp, Morning Start, Atkins* | 1 Bar/37g | 137.0 | 7.0 | 370 | 31.8 | 22.5 | 18.8 | 15.0 |
| Breakfast, Muesli, Country Garden Cakes* | 1 Bar/25g | 94.0 | 2.0 | 376 | 5.6 | 67.6 | 9.2 | 3.6 |
| Breakfast, Vitality, Fruit & Fibre, Asda* | 1 Bar/29g | 113.0 | 3.0 | 390 | 6.0 | 69.0 | 10.0 | 4.1 |
| Breakfast, Vitality, Tropical Fruit, Asda* | 1 Bar/28g | 101.0 | 1.0 | 361 | 6.0 | 75.0 | 4.1 | 4.4 |
| Breakfast, with Cranberries, Asda* | 1 Bar/28g | 105.0 | 1.0 | 376 | 6.0 | 77.0 | 4.9 | 3.0 |
| Breakfast, with Cranberries, Vitality, Asda* | 1 Bar/20g | 103.0 | 1.0 | 509 | 8.4 | 103.7 | 6.4 | 3.9 |
| Brunch, Cranberry & Orange, Cadbury* | 1 Bar/35g | 154.0 | 6.0 | 440 | 5.9 | 67.7 | 15.9 | 0.0 |
| Brunch, Hazelnut, Cadbury* | 1 Bar/35g | 160.0 | 7.0 | 460 | 7.0 | 60.5 | 21.4 | 2.2 |
| Brunch, Snack, Raisin, Cadbury* | 1 Bar/35g | 150.0 | 5.0 | 430 | 5.6 | 66.4 | 15.5 | 1.8 |
| Caramel, Endulge, Atkins* | 1 Bar/24g | 89.0 | 3.0 | 369 | 7.8 | 54.4 | 12.6 | 8.6 |
| Caramel Crisp, Go Ahead, McVitie's* | 1 Bar/33g | 141.0 | 4.0 | 428 | 4.8 | 75.1 | 12.0 | 0.8 |
| Caramel Crunch, Go Ahead, McVitie's* | 1 Bar/24g | 106.0 | 3.0 | 440 | 4.7 | 76.6 | 13.8 | 0.8 |
| Caramel Nougat, Soft, Shapers, Boots* | 1 Bar/25g | 86.0 | 2.0 | 343 | 2.9 | 60.4 | 10.0 | 0.6 |
| Caramel Wafer, Weight Watchers* | 1 Bar/18g | 79.0 | 4.0 | 427 | 5.7 | 64.7 | 20.2 | 1.9 |

| | Measure INFO/WEIGHT | per Measure KCAL | FAT | Nutrition Values per 100g / 100ml KCAL | PROT | CARB | FAT | FIBRE |
|---|---|---|---|---|---|---|---|---|
| **BARS** | | | | | | | | |
| Caramel Whip, Weight Watchers* | 1 Bar/25g | 88.0 | 3.0 | 353 | 2.7 | 72.4 | 10.8 | 1.0 |
| Caramelised Nut & Raisin Crunch, TTD, Sainsbury's* | 1 Bar/50g | 206.0 | 7.0 | 412 | 8.3 | 64.4 | 13.5 | 5.3 |
| Cashew Cookie, Gluten Free, Nakd* | 1 Bar/35g | 143.0 | 8.0 | 410 | 10.0 | 46.0 | 23.0 | 0.0 |
| Cereal, Apple, Chewy, BGTY, Sainsbury's* | 1 Bar/25g | 85.0 | 0.0 | 340 | 4.8 | 76.0 | 2.0 | 2.0 |
| Cereal, Apple & Blackberry, with Yoghurt, Alpen* | 1 Bar/29g | 117.0 | 3.0 | 404 | 5.4 | 71.8 | 10.6 | 5.0 |
| Cereal, Apple & Cinnamon, Fruit 'n' Grain, Asda* | 1 Bar/37g | 131.0 | 3.0 | 353 | 4.5 | 68.0 | 7.0 | 2.9 |
| Cereal, Apple & Cinnamon, Tesco* | 1 Serving/38g | 137.0 | 5.0 | 365 | 4.3 | 58.9 | 12.5 | 2.1 |
| Cereal, Apple & Raisin, Harvest, Quaker* | 1 Bar/22g | 87.0 | 3.0 | 396 | 5.0 | 70.0 | 11.5 | 4.0 |
| Cereal, Apple & Raspberry, Chewy & Crisp, Tesco* | 1 Bar/27g | 123.0 | 5.0 | 456 | 3.3 | 66.7 | 19.6 | 3.0 |
| Cereal, Apple & Raspberry, Waitrose* | 1 Bar/25g | 90.0 | 1.0 | 359 | 5.0 | 77.1 | 3.4 | 4.6 |
| Cereal, Apple & Sultana, Light, Alpen* | 1 Bar/21g | 59.0 | 1.0 | 281 | 5.7 | 56.2 | 3.8 | 22.4 |
| Cereal, Apricot & Yoghurt, Shapers, Boots* | 1 Bar/27g | 99.0 | 2.0 | 366 | 3.7 | 75.0 | 5.7 | 3.3 |
| Cereal, Balance with Fruit, Sainsbury's* | 1 Bar/25g | 100.0 | 2.0 | 401 | 5.8 | 75.2 | 8.6 | 1.9 |
| Cereal, Banana, Value, Tesco* | 1 Bar/21g | 80.0 | 2.0 | 387 | 6.0 | 73.9 | 7.5 | 3.7 |
| Cereal, Banoffee, COU, M & S* | 1 Bar/20g | 75.0 | 0.0 | 375 | 4.5 | 82.5 | 2.0 | 2.5 |
| Cereal, Benefit with Fruit, Aldi* | 1 Bar/27g | 108.0 | 2.0 | 401 | 5.8 | 75.2 | 8.6 | 1.9 |
| Cereal, Berry & Cream, COU, M & S* | 1 Bar/20g | 72.0 | 0.0 | 360 | 5.3 | 79.7 | 2.3 | 3.1 |
| Cereal, Blackcurrant & Apple, GFY, Asda* | 1 Bar/25g | 72.0 | 1.0 | 287 | 7.0 | 59.0 | 2.6 | 22.0 |
| Cereal, Blueberry Flavour, Breakfast, Sweet Mornings* | 1 Bar/38g | 152.0 | 5.0 | 399 | 4.5 | 66.0 | 13.0 | 2.5 |
| Cereal, Cheerios & Milk Bar, Nestle* | 1 Bar/22g | 92.0 | 3.0 | 416 | 7.6 | 66.1 | 13.5 | 2.0 |
| Cereal, Chewy & Crisp with Choc Chips, Tesco* | 1 Bar/27g | 125.0 | 6.0 | 463 | 9.2 | 54.0 | 23.4 | 3.8 |
| Cereal, Chewy & Crisp with Roasted Nuts, Tesco* | 1 Bar/27g | 127.0 | 6.0 | 471 | 9.3 | 57.0 | 22.9 | 2.5 |
| Cereal, Chewy Apple, Fruitus, Lyme Regis Foods* | 1 Bar/35g | 132.0 | 4.0 | 378 | 5.4 | 64.8 | 10.8 | 5.4 |
| Cereal, Choc Chip & Nut, Chewy & Crisp, Sainsbury's* | 1 Bar/27g | 129.0 | 7.0 | 476 | 8.8 | 51.8 | 26.0 | 4.4 |
| Cereal, Chocolate & Orange, Fitnesse, Nestle* | 1 Bar/24g | 87.0 | 1.0 | 370 | 4.7 | 76.2 | 5.1 | 3.8 |
| Cereal, Chocolate & Orange, Light, Alpen* | 1 Bar/21g | 60.0 | 1.0 | 286 | 6.1 | 54.9 | 4.6 | 24.6 |
| Cereal, Chocolate & Orange, Officially Low Fat, Fox's* | 1 Bar/19g | 54.0 | 0.0 | 286 | 5.0 | 61.6 | 2.3 | 17.5 |
| Cereal, Chocolate & Orange, Tesco* | 1 Bar/22g | 78.0 | 1.0 | 355 | 4.5 | 70.2 | 6.0 | 10.3 |
| Cereal, Chocolate & Pear, Fitnesse, Nestle* | 1 Bar/24g | 88.0 | 1.0 | 374 | 4.7 | 76.3 | 5.5 | 3.2 |
| Cereal, Chocolate & Raisin, Geobar, Traidcraft* | 1 Bar/35g | 138.0 | 2.0 | 394 | 4.6 | 81.7 | 5.5 | 1.9 |
| Cereal, Chocolate Chip, Special K, Kellogg's* | 1 Bar/21g | 84.0 | 1.0 | 401 | 9.0 | 76.0 | 7.0 | 1.5 |
| Cereal, Cinnamon Grahams, Nestle* | 1 Bar/25g | 106.0 | 4.0 | 426 | 7.2 | 66.2 | 14.7 | 1.9 |
| Cereal, Citrus Fruits, Light, Alpen* | 1 Bar/21g | 59.0 | 1.0 | 283 | 5.6 | 55.9 | 4.1 | 22.4 |
| Cereal, Coconut, Original Crunchy, Jordans* | 1 Bar/30g | 141.0 | 7.0 | 470 | 6.5 | 60.0 | 22.7 | 6.2 |
| Cereal, Cranberrry & Blackcurrant, HL, Tesco* | 1 Bar/25g | 121.0 | 7.0 | 485 | 7.2 | 50.3 | 27.9 | 3.8 |
| Cereal, Cranberry, Chewy, Safeway* | 1 Bar/25g | 86.0 | 1.0 | 345 | 4.7 | 75.7 | 2.3 | 3.9 |
| Cereal, Cranberry, Eat Smart, Safeway* | 1 Bar/25g | 86.0 | 1.0 | 345 | 4.7 | 75.7 | 2.3 | 3.9 |
| Cereal, Cranberry & Orange, BGTY, Sainsbury's* | 1 Bar/26g | 93.0 | 1.0 | 358 | 2.7 | 75.8 | 4.9 | 2.3 |
| Cereal, Cranberry & Orange, Weight Watchers* | 1 Bar/28g | 102.0 | 1.0 | 365 | 4.5 | 77.6 | 4.1 | 2.3 |
| Cereal, Crunchy Granola, Apple Crunch, Nature Valley* | 1 Bar/21g | 92.0 | 3.0 | 440 | 7.3 | 69.0 | 15.0 | 5.7 |
| Cereal, Fruit & Fibre, Asda* | 1 Bar/29g | 111.0 | 3.0 | 390 | 6.0 | 69.0 | 10.0 | 4.1 |
| Cereal, Fruit & Nut, Alpen* | 1 Bar/28g | 110.0 | 3.0 | 394 | 6.6 | 69.6 | 9.9 | 5.0 |
| Cereal, Fruit & Nut Break, Jordans* | 1 Bar/37g | 138.0 | 4.0 | 374 | 7.0 | 63.2 | 10.4 | 8.1 |
| Cereal, Fruit & Nut with Milk Chocolate, Alpen* | 1 Bar/29g | 124.0 | 4.0 | 427 | 7.1 | 67.8 | 14.1 | 4.0 |
| Cereal, Frusli, Absolutely Apricot, Jordans* | 1 Bar/33g | 120.0 | 3.0 | 365 | 5.0 | 63.8 | 10.0 | 6.3 |
| Cereal, Frusli, Blueberry Burst, Jordans* | 1 Bar/30g | 118.0 | 3.0 | 392 | 5.8 | 70.1 | 9.8 | 5.1 |
| Cereal, Frusli, Cranberry & Apple, Jordans* | 1 Bar/30g | 118.0 | 3.0 | 393 | 5.7 | 70.0 | 10.0 | 5.3 |
| Cereal, Frusli, Raisin & Hazelnut, Jordans* | 1 Bar/30g | 122.0 | 4.0 | 406 | 6.3 | 63.9 | 13.9 | 4.7 |
| Cereal, Frusli, Tangy Citrus, Jordans* | 1 Bar/33g | 124.0 | 3.0 | 376 | 4.4 | 67.7 | 9.8 | 4.8 |
| Cereal, Frusli, Wild Berries, Jordans* | 1 Bar/30g | 118.0 | 3.0 | 392 | 5.7 | 70.0 | 9.8 | 5.0 |
| Cereal, Ginger, Perfectly Balanced, Waitrose* | 1 Bar/26g | 90.0 | 1.0 | 352 | 4.0 | 79.2 | 2.1 | 3.0 |
| Cereal, Ginger & Raisin, BGTY, Sainsbury's* | 1 Bar/40g | 91.0 | 1.0 | 227 | 2.0 | 48.5 | 2.7 | 0.0 |
| Cereal, Golden Grahams, Nestle* | 1 Bar/25g | 106.0 | 3.0 | 425 | 6.5 | 68.8 | 13.7 | 0.0 |

## BARS

| | Measure INFO/WEIGHT | per Measure KCAL | per Measure FAT | Nutrition Values per 100g / 100ml KCAL | PROT | CARB | FAT | FIBRE |
|---|---|---|---|---|---|---|---|---|
| Cereal, Hazelnut & Pistachio, Go Ahead, McVitie's* | 1 Bar/30g | 117.0 | 3.0 | 389 | 4.8 | 66.5 | 11.5 | 2.5 |
| Cereal, Hazelnut & Sultana, Organic, Seeds of Change* | 1 Bar/29g | 116.0 | 4.0 | 399 | 5.9 | 65.5 | 12.6 | 5.1 |
| Cereal, Hazelnuts & Raisins, Organic, Tesco* | 1 Bar/30g | 144.0 | 8.0 | 481 | 7.2 | 50.3 | 27.9 | 3.8 |
| Cereal, Lemon & Sultana, Eat Smart, Safeway* | 1 Bar/25g | 89.0 | 1.0 | 355 | 4.2 | 78.4 | 2.2 | 2.6 |
| Cereal, Maple, Tesco* | 1 Bar/22g | 75.0 | 1.0 | 341 | 4.5 | 70.4 | 2.7 | 12.7 |
| Cereal, Milk Chocolate, Weetos, Weetabix* | 1 Bar/20g | 88.0 | 3.0 | 440 | 5.9 | 70.9 | 14.7 | 1.6 |
| Cereal, Mint Chocolate, Kellogg's* | 1 Bar/22g | 88.0 | 2.0 | 401 | 4.5 | 74.0 | 10.0 | 3.5 |
| Cereal, Mixed Berry, Go Ahead, McVitie's* | 1 Bar/35g | 134.0 | 2.0 | 383 | 4.6 | 77.1 | 6.3 | 3.1 |
| Cereal, Muesli Break, Breakfast in a Bar, Jordans* | 1 Bar/46g | 178.0 | 5.0 | 387 | 5.9 | 66.6 | 10.8 | 4.3 |
| Cereal, Multigrain, Peach & Apricot, BGTY, Sainsbury's* | 1 Bar/28g | 77.0 | 1.0 | 274 | 6.4 | 57.0 | 2.3 | 24.2 |
| Cereal, Multigrain Balance, Maple, BGTY, Sainsbury's* | 1 Bar/27g | 75.0 | 1.0 | 276 | 6.4 | 56.2 | 2.8 | 25.5 |
| Cereal, Nut & Seed, Organic, Green & Black's* | 1 Bar/50g | 258.0 | 16.0 | 516 | 8.4 | 47.2 | 32.6 | 10.0 |
| Cereal, Nutty, Free From, Sainsbury's* | 1 Bar/25g | 114.0 | 5.0 | 454 | 6.8 | 61.8 | 20.0 | 2.3 |
| Cereal, Oat & Raisin, Soft Oaties, Nutri-Grain, Kellogg's* | 1 Bar/40g | 173.0 | 6.0 | 432 | 6.0 | 66.0 | 16.0 | 3.5 |
| Cereal, Oats & More, Chocolate, Nestle* | 1 Bar/30g | 118.0 | 3.0 | 395 | 6.8 | 68.3 | 10.5 | 3.4 |
| Cereal, Oaty, Milk Chocolate, Weetabix* | 1 Bar/23g | 67.0 | 1.0 | 291 | 6.9 | 51.3 | 6.5 | 26.9 |
| Cereal, Oaty, Strawberry, Weetabix* | 1 Bar/23g | 69.0 | 1.0 | 299 | 6.2 | 54.7 | 6.1 | 24.5 |
| Cereal, Oaty, White Chocolate Flavour, Weetabix* | 1 Bar/23g | 67.0 | 1.0 | 290 | 6.5 | 51.9 | 6.3 | 26.9 |
| Cereal, Orange & Grapefruit, HE, Tesco* | 1 Bar/25g | 89.0 | 1.0 | 356 | 4.1 | 79.9 | 2.2 | 2.2 |
| Cereal, Pink Grapefruit, Chewy, BGTY, Sainsbury's* | 1 Bar/25g | 86.0 | 1.0 | 345 | 5.0 | 76.5 | 2.1 | 2.4 |
| Cereal, Pomegranate, with Prebiotic, GFY, Asda* | 1 Bar/22g | 76.0 | 1.0 | 345 | 6.2 | 69.3 | 2.8 | 13.4 |
| Cereal, Raisin & Apricot, Weight Watchers* | 1 Bar/28g | 100.0 | 1.0 | 358 | 6.8 | 72.2 | 4.6 | 3.2 |
| Cereal, Raisin & Nut Snack Bar, Benecol* | 1 Bar/25g | 97.0 | 3.0 | 390 | 3.9 | 68.5 | 11.1 | 2.0 |
| Cereal, Redberry & Chocolate, Sveltesse, Nestle* | 1 Bar/25g | 97.0 | 2.0 | 389 | 5.4 | 69.2 | 9.9 | 6.8 |
| Cereal, Roast Hazelnut, Organic, Jordans* | 1 Bar/33g | 150.0 | 7.0 | 455 | 8.0 | 56.7 | 21.8 | 7.8 |
| Cereal, Special Flake with Chocolate Chips, Tesco* | 1 Bar/21g | 85.0 | 2.0 | 405 | 6.9 | 75.8 | 7.8 | 2.3 |
| Cereal, Special Flake with Cranberries, Tesco* | 1 Bar/23g | 90.0 | 1.0 | 390 | 4.9 | 78.9 | 5.9 | 1.8 |
| Cereal, Strawberry, BGTY, Sainsbury's* | 1 Bar/26g | 100.0 | 1.0 | 385 | 3.8 | 82.0 | 4.6 | 5.2 |
| Cereal, Strawberry, Fitness, Nestle* | 1 Bar/24g | 89.0 | 2.0 | 378 | 4.9 | 73.8 | 7.0 | 4.1 |
| Cereal, Strawberry, Fruit 'n' Grain, Asda* | 1 Bar/37g | 126.0 | 3.0 | 340 | 4.2 | 65.0 | 7.0 | 4.5 |
| Cereal, Strawberry with Yoghurt, Alpen* | 1 Bar/29g | 119.0 | 3.0 | 409 | 5.7 | 72.6 | 10.6 | 0.0 |
| Cereal, Sultana & Apple, Sainsbury's* | 1 Bar/27g | 101.0 | 1.0 | 374 | 6.7 | 75.3 | 5.1 | 4.3 |
| Cereal, Sultana & Honey, Jordans* | 1 Bar/36g | 130.0 | 3.0 | 361 | 6.0 | 65.9 | 8.2 | 9.2 |
| Cereal, Summer Fruits, Light, Alpen* | 1 Bar/21g | 59.0 | 1.0 | 283 | 5.8 | 56.9 | 3.6 | 22.5 |
| Cereal, Toffee Apple, Chewy, Eat Smart, Morrisons* | 1 Bar/25g | 88.0 | 1.0 | 354 | 4.0 | 78.3 | 2.8 | 2.9 |
| Cereal, Toffee Apple, Chewy, Eat Smart, Safeway* | 1 Bar/25g | 89.0 | 1.0 | 355 | 4.0 | 78.3 | 2.8 | 2.9 |
| Cereal, Tropical Fruit & Nut Bar, Delicious, Boots* | 1 Bar/40g | 201.0 | 12.0 | 502 | 7.5 | 52.5 | 30.0 | 2.2 |
| Cereal, White Chocolate & Strawberry, Value, Tesco* | 1 Bar/21g | 85.0 | 2.0 | 405 | 6.2 | 76.2 | 8.1 | 2.4 |
| Cereal, with Fig, Fitness, Nestle* | 1 Bar/24g | 86.0 | 2.0 | 366 | 4.3 | 71.5 | 6.8 | 5.5 |
| Cereal, with Pink Grapefruit, Chewy, Sainsbury's* | 1 Bar/25g | 86.0 | 1.0 | 345 | 5.0 | 76.5 | 2.1 | 2.4 |
| Cherry, Goodness, Ryvita* | 1 Bar/23g | 60.0 | 1.0 | 260 | 6.0 | 52.6 | 2.8 | 23.0 |
| Choc Chip & Nut, Chewy & Crisp, Sainsbury's* | 1 Bar/27g | 129.0 | 7.0 | 476 | 8.8 | 51.8 | 26.0 | 4.4 |
| Chocolate, Caramel, & Biscuit, Asda* | 1 Bar/30g | 150.0 | 8.0 | 508 | 8.0 | 56.0 | 28.0 | 2.5 |
| Chocolate, Caramel, Wacko, Belmont, Aldi* | 1 Bar/21g | 100.0 | 5.0 | 478 | 4.9 | 63.8 | 22.6 | 1.4 |
| Chocolate, Crisp, Weight Watchers* | 1 Bar/25g | 92.0 | 3.0 | 369 | 5.4 | 75.1 | 10.2 | 0.8 |
| Chocolate, Crispy, Free From, Tesco* | 1 Bar/30g | 132.0 | 5.0 | 440 | 4.1 | 71.2 | 15.4 | 0.5 |
| Chocolate, Double Cream, Nestle* | 1 Bar/47g | 250.0 | 15.0 | 531 | 8.5 | 54.8 | 30.9 | 0.0 |
| Chocolate, Fruit & Nut, M & S* | 1 Bar/50g | 235.0 | 12.0 | 470 | 6.5 | 57.1 | 24.1 | 2.5 |
| Chocolate, Geobar, Traidcraft* | 1 Bar/35g | 126.0 | 2.0 | 360 | 5.2 | 72.6 | 5.4 | 4.7 |
| Chocolate, Milk, Crispy, Endulge, Atkins* | 1 Bar/30g | 140.0 | 10.0 | 467 | 14.0 | 30.7 | 32.0 | 2.0 |
| Chocolate, Polar, Sainsbury's* | 1 Bar/25g | 133.0 | 7.0 | 533 | 5.5 | 63.0 | 28.6 | 1.2 |
| Chocolate, Slim Fast* | 1 Bar/39g | 107.0 | 4.0 | 274 | 20.6 | 35.3 | 9.0 | 5.5 |
| Chocolate, Soya, Dairy Free, Free From, Sainsbury's* | 1 Bar/50g | 274.0 | 17.0 | 548 | 10.8 | 47.5 | 35.0 | 4.3 |

|  | Measure INFO/WEIGHT | per Measure | | Nutrition Values per 100g / 100ml | | | | |
|---|---|---|---|---|---|---|---|---|
|  |  | KCAL | FAT | KCAL | PROT | CARB | FAT | FIBRE |
| **BARS** | | | | | | | | |
| Chocolate, Toffee Pecan, M & S* | 1 Bar/36g | 179.0 | 10.0 | 498 | 4.9 | 58.3 | 27.3 | 0.7 |
| Chocolate, Wild & Whippy, Tesco* | 1 Bar/18g | 78.0 | 3.0 | 447 | 3.7 | 72.0 | 16.0 | 0.8 |
| Chocolate & Caramel, Lo Carb, Boots* | 1 Bar/28g | 101.0 | 3.0 | 359 | 2.8 | 82.0 | 11.0 | 1.8 |
| Chocolate & Fudge, Light, Alpen* | 1 Bar/21g | 62.0 | 1.0 | 296 | 5.9 | 54.5 | 6.0 | 25.1 |
| Chocolate & Orange, Crispy, Free From, Sainsbury's* | 1 Bar/30g | 132.0 | 5.0 | 440 | 4.8 | 68.2 | 16.2 | 1.2 |
| Chocolate & Orange, Crispy, Shapers, Boots* | 1 Bar/22g | 93.0 | 3.0 | 425 | 3.6 | 77.0 | 12.0 | 0.8 |
| Chocolate & Orange, Shapers, Boots* | 1 Bar/26g | 98.0 | 3.0 | 378 | 4.2 | 73.0 | 13.0 | 1.5 |
| Chocolate & Raspberry, COU, M & S* | 1 Bar/25g | 90.0 | 1.0 | 360 | 5.4 | 78.2 | 2.7 | 3.2 |
| Chocolate & Toffee, Free From, Sainsbury's* | 1 Bar/30g | 139.0 | 5.0 | 465 | 4.8 | 71.0 | 18.0 | 0.8 |
| Chocolate Caramel, Weight Watchers* | 1 Bar/20g | 80.0 | 2.0 | 400 | 5.0 | 70.0 | 12.5 | 0.0 |
| Chocolate Caramel Whip, Weight Watchers* | 1 Bar/26g | 96.0 | 2.0 | 369 | 2.4 | 75.9 | 9.5 | 1.0 |
| Chocolate Chip, Slim Fast* | 1 Bar/26g | 98.0 | 3.0 | 378 | 4.9 | 70.4 | 11.4 | 1.8 |
| Chocolate Chip, Snack, Slim Fast* | 1 Bar/26g | 99.0 | 3.0 | 382 | 4.9 | 70.4 | 11.4 | 1.8 |
| Chocolate Cookie Dough, Meal, Slim Fast* | 1 Bar/56g | 220.0 | 5.0 | 393 | 14.3 | 64.3 | 8.9 | 3.6 |
| Chocolate Creme, Endulge, Atkins* | 1 Bar/14g | 70.0 | 5.0 | 504 | 12.5 | 38.6 | 34.3 | 2.5 |
| Chocolate Crisp, Weight Watchers* | 1 Bar/25g | 94.0 | 3.0 | 378 | 4.8 | 66.8 | 10.2 | 1.6 |
| Chocolate Decadence, Atkins* | 1 Bar/60g | 227.0 | 12.0 | 378 | 27.1 | 30.7 | 20.4 | 11.6 |
| Chocolate Heaven, Ainsley Harriott* | 1 Bar/26g | 141.0 | 8.0 | 541 | 7.0 | 60.0 | 30.0 | 2.0 |
| Chocolate Muesli, Slim Fast* | 1 Bar/26g | 97.0 | 4.0 | 373 | 4.6 | 53.8 | 14.2 | 6.5 |
| Chocolate Muesli, Snack, Slim Fast* | 1 Bar/26g | 99.0 | 3.0 | 379 | 4.7 | 64.5 | 13.3 | 6.5 |
| Chocolate Peanut, Slim Fast* | 1 Bar/26g | 99.0 | 3.0 | 382 | 5.4 | 67.8 | 12.6 | 1.1 |
| Chocolate Truffle, M & S* | 1 Bar/35g | 168.0 | 11.0 | 480 | 5.9 | 41.7 | 32.5 | 8.3 |
| Club, Fruit, Jacob's* | 1 Biscuit/25g | 124.0 | 6.0 | 496 | 5.6 | 62.2 | 25.0 | 2.3 |
| Club, Milk Chocolate, Jacob's* | 1 Biscuit/24g | 123.0 | 6.0 | 511 | 5.8 | 62.6 | 26.4 | 2.0 |
| Club, Mint, Jacob's* | 1 Biscuit/24g | 124.0 | 7.0 | 517 | 5.6 | 62.5 | 27.2 | 1.7 |
| Club, Orange, Jacob's* | 1 Biscuit/23g | 117.0 | 6.0 | 509 | 5.7 | 61.8 | 26.5 | 2.3 |
| Coco Pops, & Milk, Kellogg's* | 1 Bar/20g | 85.0 | 3.0 | 423 | 7.0 | 70.0 | 13.0 | 1.0 |
| Cocoa Loco, Nakd* | 1 Bar/68g | 226.0 | 7.0 | 332 | 8.0 | 55.0 | 10.0 | 7.0 |
| Cocoa Orange, Gluten Free, Nakd* | 1 Bar/35g | 131.0 | 7.0 | 373 | 9.0 | 48.0 | 20.0 | 0.0 |
| Coconut Chocolate Crisp, Weight Watchers* | 1 Bar/25g | 89.0 | 3.0 | 356 | 3.6 | 71.2 | 10.4 | 3.2 |
| Coconut Whip, Weight Watchers* | 1 Bar/20g | 81.0 | 3.0 | 404 | 2.4 | 70.6 | 14.1 | 1.5 |
| Cookie, Apple Crumble, COU, M & S* | 1 Bar/27g | 90.0 | 1.0 | 335 | 5.8 | 72.6 | 2.6 | 2.3 |
| Corn Flakes, & Chocolate Milk, Kellogg's* | 1 Bar/40g | 176.0 | 6.0 | 440 | 9.0 | 66.0 | 16.0 | 2.0 |
| Cranberry, Perfectly Balanced, Waitrose* | 1 Bar/25g | 91.0 | 1.0 | 363 | 4.5 | 78.3 | 3.5 | 2.9 |
| Cranberry & Honey, Soft & Chewy, Sunny Crunch* | 1 Bar/30g | 115.0 | 2.0 | 382 | 6.0 | 73.1 | 8.3 | 3.1 |
| Cranberry & Raisin, Geobar, Traidcraft* | 1 Bar/35g | 131.0 | 3.0 | 374 | 3.7 | 72.6 | 8.0 | 2.3 |
| Cranberry & Raisin, Goodness, Ryvita* | 1 Bar/23g | 60.0 | 1.0 | 263 | 5.2 | 54.3 | 2.8 | 22.5 |
| Crazy Caramel, Tesco* | 1 Bar/40g | 192.0 | 9.0 | 480 | 3.9 | 64.0 | 23.0 | 1.0 |
| Creme Brulee Chocolate, M & S* | 1 Bar/36g | 178.0 | 11.0 | 495 | 4.4 | 54.0 | 29.2 | 0.4 |
| Crunchy Caramel, Tesco* | 1 Bar/21g | 98.0 | 5.0 | 467 | 4.6 | 56.0 | 25.0 | 1.4 |
| Crunchy Crispy Treat, Kids, Tesco* | 1 Bar/24g | 109.0 | 5.0 | 453 | 3.6 | 62.5 | 20.9 | 1.5 |
| Crunchy Granola, Oats 'n Honey, Nature Valley* | 1 Bar/21g | 97.0 | 3.0 | 460 | 8.3 | 70.4 | 16.1 | 6.2 |
| Crunchy Nut, Chocolate Peanut Crisp, Kellogg's* | 1 Bar/35g | 169.0 | 9.0 | 483 | 12.0 | 53.0 | 25.0 | 3.5 |
| Crunchy Nut, Nuts About Nuts, Kellogg's* | 1 Bar/40g | 212.0 | 14.0 | 530 | 15.0 | 40.0 | 35.0 | 5.0 |
| Dark Chocolate, Cranberries, & Macadamias, Eat Natural* | 1 Bar/45g | 221.0 | 14.0 | 492 | 5.6 | 47.3 | 31.2 | 5.5 |
| Date & Walnut, Eat Natural* | 1 Bar/50g | 220.0 | 10.0 | 441 | 8.0 | 57.1 | 20.1 | 3.3 |
| Digestive, Milk Chocolate, McVitie's* | 1 Bar/23g | 118.0 | 6.0 | 511 | 6.6 | 64.6 | 25.1 | 1.9 |
| Digestive, Milk Chocolate, Tesco* | 1 Bar/19g | 96.0 | 5.0 | 506 | 6.8 | 61.6 | 25.8 | 2.4 |
| Digestive, Milk Chocolate, Value, Tesco* | 1 Bar/19g | 96.0 | 5.0 | 505 | 6.6 | 61.8 | 25.8 | 3.0 |
| Double Chocolate, Breakfast Snack, Tesco* | 1 Bar/37g | 144.0 | 6.0 | 385 | 5.3 | 52.7 | 17.0 | 3.3 |
| Double Chocolate Treat, Shapers, Boots* | 1 Bar/23g | 94.0 | 3.0 | 408 | 3.3 | 75.0 | 11.0 | 0.7 |
| Echo, Fox's* | 1 Bar/25g | 127.0 | 7.0 | 510 | 7.8 | 59.5 | 26.7 | 1.2 |
| Echo, Mint, Fox's* | 1 Bar/25g | 129.0 | 7.0 | 518 | 7.9 | 60.7 | 26.6 | 1.6 |

# BARS

| | Measure INFO/WEIGHT | per Measure KCAL | FAT | Nutrition Values per 100g / 100ml KCAL | PROT | CARB | FAT | FIBRE |
|---|---|---|---|---|---|---|---|---|
| Echo, White Chocolate & Biscuit, Fox's* | 1 Bar/26g | 132.0 | 7.0 | 510 | 7.8 | 59.5 | 26.7 | 1.2 |
| Energy, Cocoa Brownie, Trek* | 1 Bar/68g | 216.0 | 4.0 | 318 | 17.0 | 51.0 | 6.0 | 0.0 |
| Fig & Mango, The Food Doctor* | 1 Bar/35g | 113.0 | 3.0 | 323 | 9.7 | 53.6 | 7.7 | 13.4 |
| Food Bar, Apple & Walnut, The Food Doctor* | 1 Bar/35g | 117.0 | 4.0 | 333 | 10.8 | 46.8 | 11.4 | 15.3 |
| Four Fruits, Organic, Trophy, The Village Bakery* | 1 Bar/43g | 150.0 | 3.0 | 353 | 3.8 | 71.2 | 5.9 | 4.2 |
| Four Seeds, Organic, Trophy, The Village Bakery* | 1 Bar/43g | 164.0 | 4.0 | 385 | 8.1 | 68.7 | 8.7 | 2.5 |
| Frosties, & Milk, Kellogg's* | 1 Bar/25g | 102.0 | 3.0 | 408 | 7.0 | 71.0 | 11.0 | 1.0 |
| Frosties, Chocolate, Kellogg's* | 1 Bar/25g | 103.0 | 3.0 | 412 | 6.0 | 72.0 | 12.0 | 1.6 |
| Fruit, Nut & Seed Bars, The Village Bakery* | 1 Bar/25g | 93.0 | 2.0 | 373 | 5.7 | 73.7 | 6.2 | 0.1 |
| Fruit & Fibre, Whole Grain, Sainsbury's* | 1 Bar/27g | 109.0 | 3.0 | 405 | 6.2 | 70.1 | 11.1 | 3.8 |
| Fruit & Nut, Eat Natural* | 1 Bar/50g | 223.0 | 11.0 | 446 | 11.6 | 49.8 | 22.3 | 5.3 |
| Fruit & Nut, Multigrain, Jordans* | 1 Bar/40g | 164.0 | 6.0 | 410 | 7.0 | 59.1 | 16.2 | 5.7 |
| Fruit & Nut, Organic, Eat Natural* | 1 Bar/50g | 244.0 | 15.0 | 488 | 10.2 | 42.9 | 30.6 | 0.0 |
| Fruit & Nut Crisp, Go Ahead, McVitie's* | 1 Bar/23g | 99.0 | 3.0 | 430 | 5.3 | 71.3 | 13.7 | 1.7 |
| Fruit 'n' Fibre, Kellogg's* | 1 Bar/25g | 95.0 | 2.0 | 380 | 5.0 | 71.0 | 9.0 | 5.0 |
| Fruit 'n' Fibre Bakes, with Sultanas, Kellogg's* | 1 Bar/40g | 146.0 | 5.0 | 365 | 4.5 | 58.0 | 13.0 | 9.0 |
| Fruit to Go, Apple Wildberry, Evernat* | 1 Bar/14g | 49.0 | 0.0 | 350 | 1.4 | 85.7 | 0.0 | 5.7 |
| Fruits of the Forest, Advantage, Atkins* | 1 Bar/60g | 224.0 | 10.0 | 374 | 31.0 | 32.9 | 17.4 | 7.7 |
| Fruitsome, Citrus, Rowntree's* | 1 Bar/35g | 140.0 | 5.0 | 400 | 4.1 | 65.1 | 13.7 | 2.3 |
| Fruity, Oat, Low Fat, Organic, Dove's Farm* | 1 Bar/40g | 142.0 | 1.0 | 354 | 5.0 | 71.5 | 2.7 | 2.4 |
| Fruity Cereal, Go, Soreen* | 1 Bar/40g | 141.0 | 2.0 | 352 | 5.7 | 73.9 | 4.8 | 0.0 |
| Fruity Cereal Bar, Free From, Sainsbury's* | 1 Bar/25g | 100.0 | 3.0 | 399 | 4.4 | 72.3 | 10.2 | 2.6 |
| Fudge Mallow Delight, Whipple Scrumptious, Wonka* | 1 Bar/38g | 205.0 | 12.0 | 537 | 4.6 | 59.2 | 31.3 | 0.6 |
| Ginger, Perfectly Balanced, Waitrose* | 1 Bar/25g | 92.0 | 1.0 | 367 | 4.9 | 79.3 | 3.3 | 3.3 |
| Ginger & Oat, Chocolate Covered, Snack, Waitrose* | 1 Bar/27g | 120.0 | 5.0 | 444 | 4.2 | 65.0 | 18.6 | 2.1 |
| Ginger Truffle, Waitrose* | 1 Bar/38g | 187.0 | 12.0 | 493 | 4.4 | 46.7 | 32.1 | 1.1 |
| Goodies, Cereal & Fruit, Apricot, Organic, Organix* | 1 Bar/30g | 122.0 | 6.0 | 408 | 7.2 | 55.3 | 20.4 | 6.2 |
| Granola, Crunchy, Roasted Almond, Nature Valley* | 1 Bar/42g | 193.0 | 8.0 | 459 | 8.1 | 65.6 | 18.2 | 3.7 |
| Granola, Peanut Butter, Quaker* | 1 Bar/28g | 110.0 | 3.0 | 393 | 7.1 | 64.3 | 12.5 | 3.6 |
| Groove, Lemon, Alpen* | 1 Bar/32g | 124.0 | 2.0 | 389 | 5.6 | 78.4 | 5.9 | 1.9 |
| Groove, Sassy Strawberry, Alpen* | 1 Bar/32g | 124.0 | 2.0 | 386 | 5.6 | 78.8 | 5.4 | 1.9 |
| Harvest Cheweee, Apple & Raisin, Quaker* | 1 Bar/22g | 89.0 | 3.0 | 405 | 5.5 | 68.0 | 12.0 | 3.0 |
| Harvest Cheweee, Choc Chip, Quaker* | 1 Bar/22g | 95.0 | 4.0 | 430 | 5.5 | 68.0 | 16.0 | 3.5 |
| Harvest Cheweee, Toffee, Quaker* | 1 Bar/22g | 94.0 | 3.0 | 427 | 5.0 | 68.0 | 15.0 | 3.0 |
| Harvest Cheweee, White Chocolate Chip, Quaker* | 1 Bar/22g | 93.0 | 3.0 | 425 | 6.0 | 67.0 | 15.5 | 3.5 |
| Honey, Natural, Trail Mix, Kallo* | 1 Bar/40g | 196.0 | 13.0 | 490 | 15.7 | 40.9 | 33.2 | 5.7 |
| Honey Rice Crisp, Lower Fat, Go Ahead, McVitie's* | 1 Bar/22g | 90.0 | 2.0 | 411 | 3.9 | 75.8 | 10.2 | 1.1 |
| K-Time, Honey Nut Crunch, Kellogg's* | 1 Bar/33g | 128.0 | 1.0 | 382 | 5.0 | 82.7 | 2.5 | 1.8 |
| K-Time, Mixed Berry, Kellogg's* | 1 Bar/28g | 104.0 | 1.0 | 372 | 4.9 | 80.1 | 2.2 | 3.8 |
| Luxury, Absolute Nut, Jordans* | 1 Bar/45g | 251.0 | 19.0 | 557 | 12.7 | 33.3 | 41.4 | 7.0 |
| Luxury, Cranberry & Almond, Jordans* | 1 Bar/50g | 217.0 | 10.0 | 434 | 8.6 | 56.6 | 19.2 | 5.8 |
| Luxury, Exotic Fruit & Nut, Jordans* | 1 Bar/50g | 196.0 | 3.0 | 393 | 5.0 | 69.1 | 5.4 | 4.8 |
| Macadamia & Fruit, Eat Natural* | 1 Bar/50g | 242.0 | 15.0 | 485 | 7.3 | 44.6 | 30.8 | 0.0 |
| Mango & Brazil, Tropical Wholefoods* | 1 Bar/40g | 172.0 | 8.0 | 429 | 4.7 | 61.4 | 19.1 | 4.2 |
| Maple & Pecan, Crunchy, Jordans* | 1 Bar/33g | 153.0 | 8.0 | 464 | 7.7 | 56.8 | 22.9 | 6.5 |
| Maple & Pecan, Organic, Jordans* | 1 Bar/25g | 101.0 | 3.0 | 405 | 5.5 | 66.2 | 13.1 | 3.2 |
| Mighty, Asda* | 1 Bar/41g | 189.0 | 10.0 | 462 | 4.8 | 57.1 | 23.8 | 1.4 |
| Milk Chocolate Chip & Hazelnut, Snack, Benecol* | 1 Bar/25g | 99.0 | 3.0 | 395 | 4.7 | 64.5 | 13.1 | 2.5 |
| Milk Chocolate Coated Orange Flavour, Energy, Boots* | 1 Bar/70g | 274.0 | 7.0 | 391 | 5.2 | 70.0 | 10.0 | 2.8 |
| Milk Chocolate Whirls, Asda* | 1 Bar/26g | 116.0 | 4.0 | 447 | 3.7 | 72.0 | 16.0 | 0.8 |
| Mint, Double Take, Sainsbury's* | 1 Bar/20g | 107.0 | 6.0 | 534 | 7.2 | 56.9 | 30.8 | 1.3 |
| Mint Chocolate Whip, Weight Watchers* | 1 Bar/20g | 80.0 | 2.0 | 402 | 3.6 | 74.0 | 9.9 | 0.7 |
| Mixed Berry, Goodness, Ryvita* | 1 Bar/23g | 61.0 | 1.0 | 264 | 4.8 | 54.8 | 2.8 | 23.2 |

| BARS | Measure INFO/WEIGHT | per Measure | | Nutrition Values per 100g / 100ml | | | | |
|---|---|---|---|---|---|---|---|---|
| | | KCAL | FAT | KCAL | PROT | CARB | FAT | FIBRE |
| Mixed Berry, Trek, Natural Balance Foods* | 1 Bar/68g | 204.0 | 1.0 | 300 | 15.6 | 56.5 | 2.2 | 6.0 |
| Muesli, Apricot & Almond, Carmen's* | 1 Bar/45g | 190.0 | 8.0 | 423 | 10.4 | 50.6 | 18.2 | 7.4 |
| Muesli, Cherry & Milk, Sirius* | 1 Bar/25g | 104.0 | 3.0 | 417 | 7.2 | 71.3 | 11.4 | 3.9 |
| Muffin, Cadbury* | 1 Bar/68g | 274.0 | 17.0 | 403 | 5.6 | 38.0 | 25.4 | 0.0 |
| Multigrain, Apple & Sultana, Jordans* | 1 Bar/40g | 141.0 | 2.0 | 353 | 4.4 | 70.0 | 6.2 | 4.8 |
| Multigrain, Cranberry & Raspberry, Jordans* | 1 Bar/37g | 135.0 | 2.0 | 364 | 4.8 | 71.3 | 6.6 | 4.8 |
| Multigrain, Fruit & Nut, Jordans* | 1 Bar/40g | 164.0 | 6.0 | 410 | 7.0 | 59.1 | 16.2 | 5.7 |
| Nougat, Cool Mint, & Dark Chocolate, Shapers, Boots* | 1 Bar/23g | 83.0 | 3.0 | 362 | 2.6 | 70.0 | 14.0 | 1.1 |
| Nougat, Summer Strawberry, Shapers, Boots* | 1 Bar/23g | 83.0 | 3.0 | 361 | 2.7 | 73.0 | 13.0 | 0.6 |
| Nut, Dark Chocolate & Apricot, Natural, Nice & Natural* | 1 Bar/35g | 163.0 | 10.0 | 465 | 15.2 | 35.2 | 29.1 | 5.4 |
| Nutri-Grain, Apple, Kellogg's* | 1 Bar/37g | 131.0 | 3.0 | 355 | 4.0 | 67.0 | 9.0 | 4.0 |
| Nutri-Grain, Blackberry & Apple, Kellogg's* | 1 Bar/37g | 131.0 | 3.0 | 355 | 4.0 | 67.0 | 9.0 | 4.0 |
| Nutri-Grain, Blueberry, Kellogg's* | 1 Bar/37g | 130.0 | 3.0 | 351 | 4.0 | 66.0 | 9.0 | 4.0 |
| Nutri-Grain, Cherry, Kellogg's* | 1 Bar/37g | 129.0 | 3.0 | 348 | 4.0 | 67.0 | 8.0 | 4.0 |
| Nutri-Grain, Chocolate, Kellogg's* | 1 Bar/37g | 136.0 | 4.0 | 367 | 4.5 | 66.0 | 10.0 | 4.0 |
| Nutri-Grain, Chocolate Chip, Chewy, Kellogg's* | 1 Bar/25g | 103.0 | 3.0 | 413 | 4.5 | 73.0 | 12.0 | 2.5 |
| Nutri-Grain, Elevenses, Choc Chip, Kellogg's* | 1 Bar/45g | 179.0 | 6.0 | 397 | 4.0 | 66.0 | 13.0 | 2.0 |
| Nutri-Grain, Elevenses, Ginger, Kellogg's* | 1 Bar/45g | 168.0 | 4.0 | 373 | 5.0 | 68.0 | 9.0 | 3.0 |
| Nutri-Grain, Elevenses, Raisin, Kellogg's* | 1 Bar/45g | 164.0 | 4.0 | 364 | 5.0 | 66.0 | 9.0 | 3.5 |
| Nutri-Grain, Honey Oat & Raisin, Chewy, Kellogg's* | 1 Bar/25g | 98.0 | 2.0 | 393 | 3.5 | 78.0 | 8.0 | 2.5 |
| Nutri-Grain, Oat Bakes, Cherry, Kellogg's* | 1 Bar/50g | 204.0 | 7.0 | 408 | 4.5 | 66.0 | 14.0 | 2.5 |
| Nutri-Grain, Oat Bakes, Totally Oaty, Kellogg's* | 1 Bar/50g | 205.0 | 7.0 | 411 | 5.0 | 64.0 | 15.0 | 3.0 |
| Nutri-Grain, Raspberry, Kellogg's* | 1 Bar/37g | 131.0 | 3.0 | 355 | 4.0 | 67.0 | 9.0 | 4.0 |
| Nutri-Grain, Strawberry, Kellogg's* | 1 Bar/37g | 131.0 | 3.0 | 355 | 4.0 | 67.0 | 9.0 | 3.5 |
| Nuts & Choc Chip, Asda* | 1 Bar/27g | 127.0 | 6.0 | 471 | 8.0 | 58.0 | 23.0 | 2.8 |
| Nutty Crunch Surprise, Wonka* | 1 Bar/37g | 202.0 | 12.0 | 543 | 4.9 | 58.7 | 32.1 | 0.9 |
| Nutty Nougat Caramel, Tesco* | 1 Bar/20g | 99.0 | 5.0 | 493 | 8.5 | 54.0 | 27.0 | 2.4 |
| Oat, Mixed Berry, Quaker* | 1 Bar/38g | 137.0 | 3.0 | 360 | 6.8 | 64.5 | 8.8 | 8.0 |
| Oat, Original with Golden Syrup, Quaker* | 1 Bar/38g | 139.0 | 4.0 | 366 | 7.1 | 64.5 | 9.5 | 7.9 |
| Oats, Raisins, Honey & Apricots, Geobar, Traidcraft* | 1 Bar/35g | 132.0 | 3.0 | 376 | 5.3 | 69.0 | 8.8 | 3.5 |
| Oaty with Cranberry & Blueberry, Tesco* | 1 Bar/38g | 141.0 | 3.0 | 370 | 5.5 | 69.0 | 7.5 | 6.2 |
| Optivita, Berry Oat, Kellogg's* | 1 Bar/28g | 101.0 | 2.0 | 360 | 7.0 | 68.0 | 7.0 | 9.0 |
| Orange Crunch, Go Ahead, McVitie's* | 1 Bar/23g | 99.0 | 3.0 | 430 | 4.1 | 78.0 | 12.8 | 0.8 |
| Orange Truffle, M & S* | 1 Bar/33g | 177.0 | 11.0 | 535 | 6.6 | 55.6 | 31.9 | 1.4 |
| Orchard Fruits & Yoghurt, Fruit & Fibre, Sainsbury's* | 1 Bar/27g | 102.0 | 2.0 | 379 | 5.9 | 75.3 | 6.0 | 4.1 |
| Original, Crunchy, Honey & Almond, Jordans* | 1 Bar/30g | 139.0 | 7.0 | 463 | 8.3 | 56.7 | 22.7 | 6.7 |
| Peanut, Cashew & Thai Sweet Chilli, Altu* | 1 Bar/40g | 172.0 | 8.0 | 430 | 14.7 | 47.0 | 20.3 | 3.1 |
| Peanut, Raisin & Chocolate, Weight Watchers* | 1 Bar/25g | 97.0 | 3.0 | 388 | 7.6 | 60.0 | 11.2 | 12.8 |
| Peanut & Caramel Whip, Weight Watchers* | 1 Bar/20g | 76.0 | 3.0 | 381 | 4.4 | 73.7 | 13.7 | 1.2 |
| Peanut Butter, Chewy, Granola, Slim Fast* | 1 Bar/56g | 123.0 | 3.0 | 220 | 8.0 | 35.0 | 6.0 | 0.0 |
| Pecan Apricot & Peach, M & S* | 1 Bar/50g | 255.0 | 18.0 | 510 | 9.3 | 38.2 | 35.5 | 4.9 |
| Penguin, Chukka, McVitie's* | 1 Bar/28g | 135.0 | 6.0 | 481 | 6.1 | 65.1 | 21.8 | 0.0 |
| Penguin Bigstix, McVitie's* | 1 Biscuit/13g | 63.0 | 3.0 | 508 | 6.4 | 62.8 | 25.7 | 2.6 |
| Raisin, Munch, Tesco* | 1 Bar/30g | 126.0 | 4.0 | 420 | 5.4 | 66.3 | 14.8 | 3.8 |
| Raisin & Apricot, Geobar, Traidcraft* | 1 Bar/35g | 132.0 | 3.0 | 376 | 5.3 | 69.0 | 8.8 | 3.5 |
| Raisin & Hazelnut, Weight Watchers* | 1 Bar/24g | 95.0 | 2.0 | 396 | 5.0 | 71.2 | 10.0 | 2.9 |
| Raisin & Oatmeal, Breakfast Snack, Tesco* | 1 Bar/38g | 133.0 | 4.0 | 355 | 5.6 | 56.8 | 11.7 | 2.8 |
| Rice, Crispy Orange, Milk Chocolate, Reduced Fat, Tesco* | 1 Bar/22g | 95.0 | 3.0 | 432 | 3.6 | 75.4 | 12.7 | 0.4 |
| Rice Crisp, Cranberry & Orange, Go Ahead, McVitie's* | 1 Bar/22g | 92.0 | 2.0 | 417 | 3.9 | 77.0 | 10.4 | 1.0 |
| Rice Krispies & Milk, Kellogg's* | 1 Bar/20g | 83.0 | 2.0 | 416 | 7.0 | 71.0 | 12.0 | 0.3 |
| Rich Toffee, Weight Watchers* | 1 Bar/26g | 83.0 | 3.0 | 319 | 3.6 | 52.3 | 10.6 | 0.8 |
| Roasted Nut, Chewy & Crisp, Sainsbury's* | 1 Bar/27g | 120.0 | 7.0 | 446 | 10.1 | 46.6 | 24.3 | 3.9 |
| Roasted Peanut, Weight Watchers* | 1 Bar/25g | 104.0 | 3.0 | 415 | 9.6 | 65.3 | 12.8 | 3.7 |

**B**

| | Measure INFO/WEIGHT | per Measure KCAL | FAT | Nutrition Values per 100g / 100ml KCAL | PROT | CARB | FAT | FIBRE |
|---|---|---|---|---|---|---|---|---|
| **BARS** | | | | | | | | |
| Sandwich, Milk Chocolate, SmartPrice, Asda* | 1 Bar/25g | 132.0 | 7.0 | 528 | 6.0 | 63.0 | 28.0 | 0.0 |
| Sandwich, Milk Chocolate, Value, Tesco* | 1 Bar/26g | 130.0 | 6.0 | 504 | 5.4 | 64.5 | 24.9 | 2.4 |
| School, Apple, Fruit Bowl* | 1 Bar/20g | 67.0 | 1.0 | 337 | 0.7 | 75.0 | 3.0 | 6.0 |
| School, Apricot, Fruit Bowl* | 1 Bar/20g | 67.0 | 1.0 | 337 | 0.7 | 75.0 | 3.0 | 6.0 |
| School, Blackcurrant, Fruit Bowl* | 1 Bar/20g | 67.0 | 1.0 | 337 | 0.7 | 75.0 | 3.0 | 2.0 |
| School, Cherry, Fruit Bowl* | 1 Bar/20g | 67.0 | 1.0 | 337 | 0.7 | 75.0 | 3.0 | 6.0 |
| Sesame Snaps, Anglo-Dal* | 1 Pack/30g | 163.0 | 9.0 | 542 | 2.8 | 61.8 | 31.5 | 0.0 |
| Sesame Snaps, in Chocolate, Anglo-Dal* | 1 Pack/40g | 211.0 | 12.0 | 527 | 9.3 | 55.6 | 29.7 | 0.0 |
| Sesame Snaps, with Coconut, Anglo-Dal* | 1 Pack/30g | 155.0 | 9.0 | 517 | 9.7 | 52.9 | 29.5 | 0.0 |
| Smarties, Nestle* | 1 Bar/45g | 238.0 | 13.0 | 528 | 6.2 | 58.2 | 30.0 | 0.9 |
| Special Fruit Muesli, Jordans* | 1 Bar/40g | 140.0 | 2.0 | 349 | 5.0 | 68.8 | 6.0 | 5.0 |
| Special K, Apple & Pear, Kellogg's* | 1 Bar/23g | 92.0 | 2.0 | 400 | 8.0 | 73.0 | 8.0 | 2.0 |
| Special K, Bliss Bar, Raspberry & Chocolate, Kellogg's* | 1 Bar/22g | 88.0 | 2.0 | 399 | 4.0 | 74.0 | 10.0 | 4.0 |
| Special K, Chocolate Chip, Kellogg's* | 1 Bar/22g | 90.0 | 2.0 | 401 | 9.0 | 76.0 | 7.0 | 1.5 |
| Special K, Fruits of the Forest, Kellogg's* | 1 Bar/22g | 87.0 | 2.0 | 397 | 8.0 | 74.0 | 8.0 | 2.5 |
| Special K, Peach & Apricot, Kellogg's* | 1 Bar/21g | 84.0 | 2.0 | 400 | 8.0 | 73.0 | 9.0 | 2.5 |
| Special K, Red Fruits, Kellogg's* | 1 Bar/22g | 84.0 | 1.0 | 390 | 8.0 | 78.0 | 5.0 | 1.5 |
| Special Muesli, Jordans* | 1 Bar/40g | 152.0 | 5.0 | 379 | 6.0 | 61.6 | 12.1 | 5.8 |
| Strawberry, Breakfast, Carb Control, Tesco* | 1 Bar/37g | 144.0 | 9.0 | 389 | 7.0 | 40.5 | 23.2 | 4.0 |
| Strawberry, Morning Shine, Atkins* | 1 Bar/37g | 145.0 | 8.0 | 392 | 28.9 | 24.9 | 21.6 | 14.1 |
| Strawberry, Organic, Seeds of Change* | 1 Bar/26g | 102.0 | 2.0 | 390 | 5.4 | 75.7 | 7.3 | 0.0 |
| Strawberry, Shapers, Boots* | 1 Bar/22g | 75.0 | 2.0 | 343 | 2.5 | 77.0 | 11.0 | 0.9 |
| Sultana, Apple & Yoghurt, Balance, Sainsbury's* | 1 Bar/27g | 104.0 | 2.0 | 387 | 6.1 | 77.4 | 5.9 | 2.3 |
| Superfoods, Jordans* | 1 Bar/45g | 171.0 | 5.0 | 379 | 7.0 | 63.3 | 10.9 | 6.7 |
| Three Musketeer, Candy, Mars* | 1 Bar/60g | 260.0 | 8.0 | 430 | 3.3 | 76.2 | 13.2 | 1.7 |
| Toffee, Slim Fast* | 1 Bar/39g | 122.0 | 3.0 | 314 | 19.7 | 47.1 | 8.5 | 5.6 |
| Toffee & Banana, Weight Watchers* | 1 Bar/18g | 67.0 | 1.0 | 372 | 6.1 | 77.2 | 3.9 | 1.7 |
| Tracker, Breakfast, Banana, Mars* | 1 Bar/37g | 176.0 | 8.0 | 476 | 4.7 | 63.3 | 22.6 | 9.4 |
| Tracker, Breakfast, Lemon, Mars* | 1 Bar/26g | 124.0 | 6.0 | 477 | 4.6 | 64.3 | 22.4 | 0.0 |
| Tracker, Chocolate Chip, Mars* | 1 Bar/37g | 178.0 | 9.0 | 480 | 6.8 | 58.0 | 23.6 | 3.8 |
| Tracker, Forest Fruits, Mars* | 1 Bar/26g | 123.0 | 6.0 | 474 | 4.6 | 64.1 | 22.2 | 0.0 |
| Tracker, Yoghurt, Mars* | 1 Bar/27g | 133.0 | 6.0 | 491 | 6.3 | 64.2 | 23.2 | 0.0 |
| Triple Dazzle, Wonka* | 1 Bar/39g | 195.0 | 10.0 | 504 | 5.9 | 61.9 | 25.9 | 0.0 |
| Very Berry, Cookie, Big Softies, Fox's* | 1 Bar/26g | 85.0 | 1.0 | 325 | 5.7 | 69.7 | 2.5 | 2.5 |
| Wafer, Chocolate Flavour Crisp, Carbolite* | 1 Bar/25g | 120.0 | 9.0 | 482 | 8.5 | 52.3 | 34.8 | 2.0 |
| Wafer Biscuit, Milk Chocolate Coated, Value, Tesco* | 1 Bar/24g | 126.0 | 7.0 | 526 | 6.9 | 61.4 | 28.1 | 1.7 |
| Walnuts, Sultanas, Almond & Pumpkin Seeds, Eat Natural* | 1 Bar/50g | 204.0 | 9.0 | 408 | 9.6 | 51.8 | 18.0 | 5.4 |
| With Brazils, Sultanas, Almonds & Hazelnuts, Eat Natural* | 1 Bar/50g | 234.0 | 14.0 | 469 | 12.1 | 40.5 | 28.7 | 5.8 |
| **BASIL** | | | | | | | | |
| *Dried, Ground* | *1 Tsp/1.4g* | *4.0* | *0.0* | *251* | *14.4* | *43.2* | *4.0* | *0.0* |
| *Fresh, Average* | *1 Tbsp/5g* | *2.0* | *0.0* | *40* | *3.1* | *5.1* | *0.8* | *0.0* |
| **BATTER MIX** | | | | | | | | |
| for Pancakes & Yorkshire Puddings, McDougalls* | 1 Pancake/38g | 83.0 | 4.0 | 218 | 6.3 | 24.8 | 10.4 | 1.9 |
| for Yorkshire Puddings & Pancakes, Morrisons* | 1 Pudding/30g | 43.0 | 1.0 | 143 | 6.4 | 23.1 | 2.8 | 4.1 |
| for Yorkshire Puddings & Pancakes, Tesco* | 1 Serving/17g | 34.0 | 0.0 | 200 | 2.3 | 43.3 | 1.5 | 2.5 |
| **BAY LEAVES** | | | | | | | | |
| *Dried, Average* | *1 Tsp/0.6g* | *2.0* | *0.0* | *313* | *7.6* | *48.6* | *8.4* | *0.0* |
| **BEAN SPROUTS** | | | | | | | | |
| *Mung, Canned, Drained, Average* | *1 Serving/90g* | *9.0* | *0.0* | *10* | *1.6* | *0.8* | *0.1* | *0.7* |
| *Mung, Raw, Average* | *1oz/28g* | *9.0* | *0.0* | *31* | *2.9* | *4.0* | *0.5* | *1.5* |
| *Mung, Stir-Fried in Blended Oil, Average* | *1 Serving/90g* | *65.0* | *5.0* | *72* | *1.9* | *2.5* | *6.1* | *0.9* |
| *Raw, Average* | *1 Serving/150g* | *45.0* | *0.0* | *30* | *3.0* | *5.9* | *0.2* | *1.8* |

| | Measure INFO/WEIGHT | per Measure KCAL | per Measure FAT | Nutrition Values per 100g / 100ml KCAL | PROT | CARB | FAT | FIBRE |
|---|---|---|---|---|---|---|---|---|
| **BEANFEAST** | | | | | | | | |
| Bolognese Style, Dry, Batchelors* | 1 Pack/120g | 362.0 | 7.0 | 302 | 23.9 | 39.0 | 5.6 | 13.5 |
| Mexican Chilli, Batchelors* | 1 Serving/65g | 203.0 | 3.0 | 312 | 24.3 | 42.7 | 4.9 | 13.6 |
| **BEANS** | | | | | | | | |
| & Meatballs, in Tomato Sauce, Sainsbury's* | ½ Can/200g | 216.0 | 7.0 | 108 | 5.5 | 13.3 | 3.6 | 2.6 |
| & Peas, M & S* | 1oz/28g | 13.0 | 0.0 | 48 | 4.2 | 6.5 | 0.5 | 6.1 |
| *Aduki, Cooked in Unsalted Water, Average* | *1 Tbsp/30g* | *37.0* | *0.0* | *123* | *9.3* | *22.5* | *0.2* | *5.5* |
| *Aduki, Dried, Raw* | *1 Tbsp/30g* | *82.0* | *0.0* | *272* | *19.9* | *50.1* | *0.5* | *11.1* |
| Baked, & Pork Sausages, Tesco* | ½ Can/210g | 231.0 | 6.0 | 110 | 5.5 | 15.6 | 2.7 | 3.0 |
| Baked, & Sausage, Asda* | ½ Can/205g | 252.0 | 8.0 | 123 | 6.0 | 16.0 | 3.9 | 3.0 |
| Baked, & Sausage in Tomato Sauce, SmartPrice, Asda* | ½ Can/203g | 256.0 | 12.0 | 126 | 5.0 | 13.0 | 6.0 | 0.0 |
| Baked, & Sausages, Meatfree, Sainsbury's* | 1 Can/420g | 500.0 | 17.0 | 119 | 8.0 | 12.6 | 4.0 | 2.7 |
| Baked, & Sausages, Value, Tesco* | ½ Can/276g | 290.0 | 10.0 | 105 | 5.7 | 11.8 | 3.7 | 3.6 |
| Baked, Barbecue, Smokey, Beanz, Heinz* | 1 Can/420g | 332.0 | 1.0 | 79 | 4.9 | 14.3 | 0.2 | 3.8 |
| Baked, Cheezy, Heinz* | 1oz/28g | 53.0 | 1.0 | 189 | 11.6 | 24.5 | 4.9 | 6.2 |
| *Baked, Curried, Average* | *½ Can/210g* | *203.0* | *2.0* | *96* | *4.8* | *17.2* | *0.9* | *3.6* |
| *Baked, in Tomato Sauce, Average* | *1 Can/400g* | *346.0* | *2.0* | *86* | *4.8* | *15.9* | *0.5* | *3.3* |
| *Baked, in Tomato Sauce, Healthy Range, Average* | *½ Can/210g* | *143.0* | *0.0* | *68* | *3.9* | *12.8* | *0.2* | *2.8* |
| *Baked, in Tom Sauce, Reduced Sugar & Salt, Average* | *½ Can/210g* | *159.0* | *1.0* | *75* | *4.5* | *13.6* | *0.3* | *3.8* |
| Baked, Jalfrezi, Mean, Beanz, Heinz* | 1 Serving/195g | 135.0 | 3.0 | 69 | 4.5 | 9.8 | 1.3 | 3.6 |
| Baked, Mexican, Mean, Beanz, Heinz* | ½ Can/208g | 158.0 | 1.0 | 76 | 5.0 | 12.9 | 0.5 | 4.0 |
| Baked, Sweet Chilli, Mean, Beanz, Heinz* | ½ Can/195g | 142.0 | 1.0 | 73 | 4.5 | 13.0 | 0.3 | 3.6 |
| Baked, Tikka, Mean, Beanz, Heinz* | 1 Serving/195g | 172.0 | 6.0 | 88 | 4.8 | 10.6 | 3.0 | 3.5 |
| Baked, with Chicken Nuggets, Beanz, Heinz* | 1 Can/200g | 210.0 | 6.0 | 105 | 6.7 | 12.4 | 3.1 | 3.2 |
| Baked, with Hidden Veg, Beanz, Heinz* | ½ Can/208g | 156.0 | 1.0 | 75 | 4.7 | 13.5 | 0.3 | 4.1 |
| Baked, with HP Sauce, Beanz, Heinz* | ½ Can/208g | 158.0 | 1.0 | 76 | 4.8 | 13.7 | 0.3 | 3.9 |
| Baked, with Lea & Perrins Sauce, Beanz, Heinz* | 1 Can/415g | 303.0 | 1.0 | 73 | 4.8 | 13.1 | 0.2 | 3.8 |
| Baked, with Spicy Meatballs, Beanz, Heinz* | 1 Can/400g | 372.0 | 10.0 | 93 | 5.8 | 12.0 | 2.4 | 2.9 |
| Baked, with Steak Chunks, Beanz, Heinz* | 1 Can/415g | 340.0 | 3.0 | 82 | 6.9 | 12.1 | 0.7 | 3.5 |
| Baked, with Vegetable Sausages, Beanz, Heinz* | 1 Sm Can/200g | 210.0 | 7.0 | 105 | 6.0 | 12.2 | 3.6 | 2.9 |
| *Black, Cooked, Average* | *1 Cup/172g* | *227.0* | *1.0* | *132* | *8.8* | *23.7* | *0.5* | *8.7* |
| *Black, Dried, Average* | *1 Serving/100g* | *341.0* | *1.0* | *341* | *21.6* | *62.4* | *1.4* | *15.2* |
| *Blackeye, Canned, Average* | *1 Can/172g* | *206.0* | *1.0* | *119* | *8.4* | *19.7* | *0.7* | *3.3* |
| *Blackeye, Dried, Raw* | *1oz/28g* | *87.0* | *0.0* | *311* | *23.5* | *54.1* | *1.6* | *8.2* |
| *Borlotti, Canned, Average* | *1oz/28g* | *29.0* | *0.0* | *103* | *7.6* | *16.9* | *0.5* | *4.7* |
| *Borlotti, Dried, Raw, Average* | *1 Serving/100g* | *335.0* | *1.0* | *335* | *23.0* | *60.0* | *1.2* | *24.7* |
| *Broad, Canned, Drained, Average* | *1 Can/195g* | *136.0* | *1.0* | *70* | *6.9* | *9.2* | *0.6* | *6.8* |
| *Broad, Dried, Raw, Average* | *1oz/28g* | *69.0* | *1.0* | *245* | *26.1* | *32.5* | *2.1* | *27.6* |
| Broad, Frozen, Sainsbury's* | 1 Serving/80g | 64.0 | 0.0 | 80 | 7.9 | 10.7 | 0.6 | 6.5 |
| Broad, in Water, Drained, Asda* | 1 Serving/98g | 73.0 | 0.0 | 75 | 7.4 | 10.1 | 0.5 | 7.1 |
| *Broad, Weighed with Pod, Raw, Average* | *1oz/28g* | *17.0* | *0.0* | *59* | *5.7* | *7.2* | *1.0* | *6.1* |
| *Butter, Canned, Average* | *1oz/28g* | *22.0* | *0.0* | *79* | *5.9* | *12.9* | *0.5* | *4.0* |
| *Butter, Dried, Boiled, Average* | *1oz/28g* | *30.0* | *0.0* | *106* | *7.2* | *18.6* | *0.6* | *5.2* |
| *Butter, Dried, Raw, Average* | *1oz/28g* | *81.0* | *0.0* | *290* | *19.1* | *52.9* | *1.7* | *16.0* |
| *Cannellini, Canned, Average* | *1oz/28g* | *26.0* | *0.0* | *94* | *7.2* | *15.0* | *0.5* | *5.7* |
| Cannellini, with Chorizo & Red Peppers, Morrisons* | ½ Pack/100g | 155.0 | 10.0 | 155 | 6.9 | 9.2 | 10.0 | 2.8 |
| *Chilli, Canned, Average* | *1 Can/420g* | *381.0* | *3.0* | *91* | *5.2* | *15.8* | *0.7* | *4.3* |
| Curried, Mixed, Morrisons* | 1 Can/420g | 420.0 | 16.0 | 100 | 4.2 | 12.1 | 3.9 | 5.6 |
| Dwarf, Sainsbury's* | 1oz/28g | 7.0 | 0.0 | 24 | 1.9 | 3.1 | 0.5 | 2.2 |
| Edamame, Sainsbury's* | 1 Serving/150g | 211.0 | 10.0 | 141 | 12.3 | 6.8 | 6.4 | 4.2 |
| *Edamame, Shelled, Frozen, Raw, Average* | *1 Serving/80g* | *88.0* | *4.0* | *110* | *10.2* | *8.6* | *4.7* | *4.8* |
| *Flageolet, Canned, Average* | *1 Can/265g* | *235.0* | *2.0* | *89* | *6.7* | *14.0* | *0.6* | *3.5* |
| *French, Boiled, Average* | *1 Serving/150g* | *37.0* | *0.0* | *25* | *2.3* | *3.8* | *0.0* | *3.7* |
| *French, Canned, Average* | *1oz/28g* | *6.0* | *0.0* | *22* | *1.6* | *3.5* | *0.3* | *2.5* |

|  | Measure | per Measure | | Nutrition Values per 100g / 100ml | | | | |
| --- | --- | --- | --- | --- | --- | --- | --- | --- |
|  | INFO/WEIGHT | KCAL | FAT | KCAL | PROT | CARB | FAT | FIBRE |
| **BEANS** | | | | | | | | |
| *French, Raw* | *1oz/28g* | *7.0* | *0.0* | *24* | *1.9* | *3.2* | *0.5* | *2.2* |
| *Green, Cut, Average* | *1oz/28g* | *6.0* | *0.0* | *22* | *1.7* | *3.7* | *0.2* | *2.1* |
| *Green, Fine, Average* | *1 Serving/75g* | *18.0* | *0.0* | *24* | *1.8* | *3.4* | *0.4* | *2.6* |
| *Green, Sliced, Average* | *1oz/28g* | *6.0* | *0.0* | *23* | *1.9* | *3.5* | *0.2* | *2.1* |
| *Green, Sliced, Frozen, Average* | *1 Serving/50g* | *13.0* | *0.0* | *26* | *1.8* | *4.4* | *0.1* | *4.1* |
| *Green, Whole, Average* | *1oz/28g* | *6.0* | *0.0* | *22* | *1.6* | *3.0* | *0.4* | *1.7* |
| *Haricot, Dried, Boiled in Unsalted Water* | *1oz/28g* | *27.0* | *0.0* | *95* | *6.6* | *17.2* | *0.5* | *6.1* |
| *Haricot, Dried, Raw* | *1oz/28g* | *80.0* | *0.0* | *286* | *21.4* | *49.7* | *1.6* | *17.0* |
| Haricot, in Water, Canned, Tesco* | ½ Can/118g | 76.0 | 1.0 | 65 | 5.7 | 9.0 | 0.5 | 7.8 |
| *Kidney, Red, Canned, Average* | *½ Can/90g* | *92.0* | *1.0* | *102* | *7.8* | *16.7* | *0.6* | *5.6* |
| *Kidney, Red, Dried, Boiled in Unsalted Water* | *1oz/28g* | *29.0* | *0.0* | *103* | *8.4* | *17.4* | *0.5* | *6.7* |
| *Kidney, Red, Dried, Raw* | *1oz/28g* | *74.0* | *0.0* | *266* | *22.1* | *44.1* | *1.4* | *15.7* |
| Kidney, Red, in Chilli Sauce, Sainsbury's* | 1 Can/420g | 365.0 | 2.0 | 87 | 5.3 | 15.6 | 0.4 | 4.5 |
| *Mixed, Canned, Average* | *1 Can/300g* | *300.0* | *3.0* | *100* | *6.7* | *15.6* | *1.2* | *4.1* |
| Mixed, in Mild Chilli Sauce, Sainsbury's* | 1 Can/420g | 328.0 | 1.0 | 78 | 4.9 | 13.8 | 0.3 | 3.7 |
| *Mixed, Spicy, Average* | *1 Serving/140g* | *108.0* | *1.0* | *77* | *4.8* | *13.4* | *0.5* | *3.9* |
| Mixed, with Lentils, Waitrose* | 1 Pack/300g | 399.0 | 22.0 | 133 | 5.1 | 11.6 | 7.3 | 3.1 |
| Mixed, with Passata, Tesco* | 1 Can/300g | 237.0 | 2.0 | 79 | 6.0 | 12.1 | 0.7 | 3.9 |
| *Mung, Whole, Dried, Boiled in Unsalted Water* | *1oz/28g* | *25.0* | *0.0* | *91* | *7.6* | *15.3* | *0.4* | *3.0* |
| *Mung, Whole, Dried, Raw* | *1oz/28g* | *78.0* | *0.0* | *279* | *23.9* | *46.3* | *1.1* | *10.0* |
| *Pinto, Dried, Boiled in Unsalted Water* | *1oz/28g* | *38.0* | *0.0* | *137* | *8.9* | *23.9* | *0.7* | *0.0* |
| *Pinto, Dried, Raw* | *1oz/28g* | *92.0* | *0.0* | *327* | *21.1* | *57.1* | *1.6* | *14.0* |
| *Refried, Average* | *1 Serving/215g* | *162.0* | *2.0* | *75* | *4.6* | *12.7* | *0.7* | *1.7* |
| *Runner, Average* | *1 Serving/80g* | *16.0* | *0.0* | *20* | *1.4* | *2.8* | *0.4* | *2.2* |
| Runner & Carrots, M & S* | 1 Serving/240g | 60.0 | 0.0 | 25 | 1.0 | 4.8 | 0.1 | 2.1 |
| *Soya, Dried, Average* | *1oz/28g* | *104.0* | *5.0* | *370* | *34.2* | *15.4* | *18.3* | *19.6* |
| *Soya, Dried, Boiled in Unsalted Water* | *1oz/28g* | *39.0* | *2.0* | *141* | *14.0* | *5.1* | *7.3* | *6.1* |
| Soya, Frozen, Birds Eye* | 1 Serving/80g | 120.0 | 5.0 | 150 | 12.3 | 11.0 | 6.3 | 4.0 |
| Soya, in Water, Salt Added, Sainsbury's* | 1 Serving/100g | 102.0 | 7.0 | 102 | 4.0 | 5.1 | 7.3 | 6.1 |
| **BEEF** | | | | | | | | |
| *Brisket, Raw, Lean* | *1oz/28g* | *39.0* | *2.0* | *139* | *21.1* | *0.0* | *6.1* | *0.0* |
| *Brisket, Raw, Lean & Fat* | *1oz/28g* | *61.0* | *4.0* | *218* | *18.4* | *0.0* | *16.0* | *0.0* |
| *Cooked, Sliced, From Supermarket, Average* | *1 Slice/35g* | *35.0* | *1.0* | *101* | *17.4* | *2.6* | *2.4* | *0.4* |
| *Flank, Pot-Roasted, Lean* | *1oz/28g* | *71.0* | *4.0* | *253* | *31.8* | *0.0* | *14.0* | *0.0* |
| *Flank, Pot-Roasted, Lean & Fat* | *1oz/28g* | *87.0* | *6.0* | *309* | *27.1* | *0.0* | *22.3* | *0.0* |
| *Flank, Raw, Lean* | *1oz/28g* | *49.0* | *3.0* | *175* | *22.7* | *0.0* | *9.3* | *0.0* |
| *Flank, Raw, Lean & Fat* | *1oz/28g* | *74.0* | *6.0* | *266* | *19.7* | *0.0* | *20.8* | *0.0* |
| *for Casserole, Lean, Diced, Average* | *1oz/28g* | *35.0* | *1.0* | *126* | *23.0* | *0.0* | *3.8* | *0.0* |
| *Fore Rib, Lean & Fat, Average* | *1oz/28g* | *40.0* | *2.0* | *143* | *21.7* | *0.0* | *6.2* | *0.2* |
| *Fore Rib, Raw, Lean* | *1oz/28g* | *41.0* | *2.0* | *145* | *21.5* | *0.0* | *6.5* | *0.0* |
| *Fore Rib, Roasted, Lean* | *1oz/28g* | *66.0* | *3.0* | *236* | *33.3* | *0.0* | *11.4* | *0.0* |
| *Fore Rib, Roasted, Lean & Fat* | *1oz/28g* | *84.0* | *6.0* | *300* | *29.1* | *0.0* | *20.4* | *0.0* |
| *Grill Steak, Average* | *1 Steak/170g* | *501.0* | *39.0* | *295* | *19.3* | *2.1* | *23.2* | *0.1* |
| *Grill Steak, Peppered, Average* | *1 Serving/172g* | *419.0* | *24.0* | *243* | *23.6* | *5.2* | *14.2* | *0.3* |
| *Joint, for Roasting, Average* | *1oz/28g* | *38.0* | *1.0* | *134* | *24.5* | *1.4* | *3.4* | *0.2* |
| *Joint, Sirloin, Roasted, Lean* | *1oz/28g* | *53.0* | *2.0* | *188* | *32.4* | *0.0* | *6.5* | *0.0* |
| *Joint, Sirloin, Roasted, Lean & Fat* | *1oz/28g* | *65.0* | *4.0* | *233* | *29.8* | *0.0* | *12.6* | *0.0* |
| *Mince, Cooked, Average* | *1 Serving/75g* | *214.0* | *15.0* | *286* | *23.9* | *0.0* | *20.3* | *0.0* |
| *Mince, Extra Lean, Raw, Average* | *1 Serving/100g* | *131.0* | *5.0* | *131* | *21.0* | *0.0* | *5.3* | *0.0* |
| *Mince, Extra Lean, Stewed* | *1oz/28g* | *50.0* | *2.0* | *177* | *24.7* | *0.0* | *8.7* | *0.0* |
| *Mince, Lean, Raw, Average* | *1oz/28g* | *49.0* | *3.0* | *175* | *22.0* | *0.0* | *9.7* | *0.0* |
| *Mince, Raw, Average* | *1oz/28g* | *67.0* | *5.0* | *239* | *18.7* | *0.2* | *18.0* | *0.1* |
| *Mince, Steak, Extra Lean, Average* | *1oz/28g* | *37.0* | *2.0* | *131* | *20.5* | *0.4* | *5.6* | *0.0* |

| | Measure INFO/WEIGHT | per Measure KCAL | FAT | Nutrition Values per 100g / 100ml KCAL | PROT | CARB | FAT | FIBRE |
|---|---|---|---|---|---|---|---|---|
| **BEEF** | | | | | | | | |
| *Mince, Steak, Raw, Average* | 1 Serving/125g | 317.0 | 25.0 | 254 | 17.2 | 0.0 | 20.0 | 0.0 |
| Mince, Stewed | 1oz/28g | 59.0 | 4.0 | 209 | 21.8 | 0.0 | 13.5 | 0.0 |
| *Peppered, Sliced, Average* | 1 Slice/20g | 26.0 | 1.0 | 129 | 18.2 | 1.3 | 5.6 | 1.0 |
| Roast, Sliced, Average | 1 Slice/35g | 48.0 | 1.0 | 136 | 26.1 | 0.4 | 3.6 | 0.2 |
| *Salt, Average* | 1 Serving/70g | 80.0 | 2.0 | 114 | 21.7 | 1.0 | 2.5 | 0.1 |
| Salted, Dried, Raw | 1oz/28g | 70.0 | 0.0 | 250 | 55.4 | 0.0 | 1.5 | 0.0 |
| *Silverside, Pot-Roasted, Lean* | 1oz/28g | 54.0 | 2.0 | 193 | 34.0 | 0.0 | 6.3 | 0.0 |
| Silverside, Pot-Roasted, Lean & Fat | 1oz/28g | 69.0 | 4.0 | 247 | 31.0 | 0.0 | 13.7 | 0.0 |
| *Silverside, Raw, Lean* | 1oz/28g | 38.0 | 1.0 | 134 | 23.8 | 0.0 | 4.3 | 0.0 |
| Silverside, Raw, Lean & Fat | 1oz/28g | 60.0 | 4.0 | 215 | 20.4 | 0.0 | 14.8 | 0.0 |
| *Silverside, Salted, Boiled, Lean* | 1oz/28g | 52.0 | 2.0 | 184 | 30.4 | 0.0 | 6.9 | 0.0 |
| Silverside, Salted, Boiled, Lean & Fat | 1oz/28g | 63.0 | 3.0 | 224 | 27.9 | 0.0 | 12.5 | 0.0 |
| *Silverside, Salted, Raw, Lean* | 1oz/28g | 39.0 | 2.0 | 140 | 19.2 | 0.0 | 7.0 | 0.0 |
| Silverside, Salted, Raw, Lean & Fat | 1oz/28g | 64.0 | 5.0 | 227 | 16.3 | 0.0 | 18.0 | 0.0 |
| *Steak, Braising, Braised, Lean* | 1oz/28g | 63.0 | 3.0 | 225 | 34.4 | 0.0 | 9.7 | 0.0 |
| Steak, Braising, Braised, Lean & Fat | 1oz/28g | 69.0 | 4.0 | 246 | 32.9 | 0.0 | 12.7 | 0.0 |
| *Steak, Braising, Lean, Raw, Average* | 1oz/28g | 40.0 | 1.0 | 144 | 24.8 | 0.0 | 5.0 | 0.0 |
| Steak, Braising, Raw, Lean & Fat | 1oz/28g | 45.0 | 2.0 | 160 | 20.7 | 0.0 | 8.6 | 0.0 |
| *Steak, Economy, Average* | 1oz/28g | 53.0 | 2.0 | 190 | 26.9 | 1.2 | 8.7 | 0.4 |
| Steak, Fillet, Cooked, Average | 1oz/28g | 54.0 | 2.0 | 191 | 28.6 | 0.0 | 8.5 | 0.0 |
| *Steak, Fillet, Lean, Average* | 1oz/28g | 42.0 | 2.0 | 150 | 21.0 | 0.0 | 7.3 | 0.0 |
| Steak, Fillet, Lean, Cooked, Average | 1oz/28g | 52.0 | 2.0 | 186 | 28.6 | 0.0 | 7.9 | 0.0 |
| *Steak, Frying, Average* | 1 Steak/110g | 128.0 | 3.0 | 116 | 23.7 | 0.0 | 2.5 | 0.0 |
| Steak, Rump, Cooked, Average | 1oz/28g | 69.0 | 4.0 | 245 | 29.1 | 0.5 | 14.1 | 0.0 |
| *Steak, Rump, Grilled, Rare, Lean* | 1 Steak/227g | 381.0 | 16.0 | 168 | 26.5 | 0.0 | 6.9 | 0.0 |
| Steak, Rump, Lean, Cooked, Average | 1oz/28g | 50.0 | 2.0 | 179 | 31.0 | 0.0 | 6.1 | 0.0 |
| *Steak, Rump, Raw, Lean* | 1oz/28g | 35.0 | 1.0 | 125 | 22.0 | 0.0 | 4.1 | 0.0 |
| Steak, Rump, Raw, Lean & Fat | 1oz/28g | 49.0 | 3.0 | 174 | 20.7 | 0.0 | 10.1 | 0.0 |
| *Steak, Sirloin, Fried, Rare, Lean* | 1oz/28g | 53.0 | 2.0 | 189 | 28.8 | 0.0 | 8.2 | 0.0 |
| Steak, Sirloin, Fried, Rare, Lean & Fat | 1oz/28g | 65.0 | 4.0 | 233 | 26.8 | 0.0 | 14.0 | 0.0 |
| *Steak, Sirloin, Grilled, Medium-Rare, Lean* | 1oz/28g | 49.0 | 2.0 | 176 | 26.6 | 0.0 | 7.7 | 0.0 |
| Steak, Sirloin, Grilled, Medium-Rare, Lean & Fat | 1oz/28g | 60.0 | 4.0 | 213 | 24.8 | 0.0 | 12.6 | 0.0 |
| *Steak, Sirloin, Grilled, Rare, Lean* | 1oz/28g | 46.0 | 2.0 | 166 | 26.4 | 0.0 | 6.7 | 0.0 |
| Steak, Sirloin, Grilled, Rare, Lean & Fat | 1oz/28g | 60.0 | 4.0 | 216 | 25.1 | 0.0 | 12.8 | 0.0 |
| *Steak, Sirloin, Grilled, Well-Done, Lean* | 1oz/28g | 63.0 | 3.0 | 225 | 33.9 | 0.0 | 9.9 | 0.0 |
| Steak, Sirloin, Grilled, Well-Done, Lean & Fat | 1oz/28g | 72.0 | 4.0 | 257 | 31.8 | 0.0 | 14.4 | 0.0 |
| *Steak, Sirloin, Raw, Lean* | 1oz/28g | 38.0 | 1.0 | 135 | 23.5 | 0.0 | 4.5 | 0.0 |
| Steak, Sirloin, Raw, Lean & Fat | 1oz/28g | 56.0 | 4.0 | 201 | 21.6 | 0.0 | 12.7 | 0.0 |
| *Stewed Steak, Average* | 1 Serving/220g | 258.0 | 10.0 | 117 | 15.8 | 3.3 | 4.6 | 0.0 |
| Stewing Steak, Lean & Fat, Raw, Average | 1oz/28g | 41.0 | 2.0 | 146 | 22.1 | 0.0 | 6.4 | 0.0 |
| *Stewing Steak, Raw, Lean* | 1oz/28g | 34.0 | 1.0 | 122 | 22.6 | 0.0 | 3.5 | 0.0 |
| Stewing Steak, Stewed, Lean | 1oz/28g | 52.0 | 2.0 | 185 | 32.0 | 0.0 | 6.3 | 0.0 |
| *Stewing Steak, Stewed, Lean & Fat* | 1oz/28g | 57.0 | 3.0 | 203 | 29.2 | 0.0 | 9.6 | 0.0 |
| Stir Fry Strips, Raw, Average | 1 Serving/125g | 146.0 | 3.0 | 116 | 23.5 | 0.0 | 2.5 | 0.3 |
| *Topside, Lean & Fat, Average* | 1oz/28g | 61.0 | 3.0 | 219 | 27.5 | 0.0 | 12.2 | 0.0 |
| Topside, Raw, Lean | 1oz/28g | 32.0 | 1.0 | 116 | 23.0 | 0.0 | 2.7 | 0.0 |
| *Wafer Thin Sliced, Cooked, Average* | 1 Slice/10g | 13.0 | 0.0 | 129 | 24.5 | 0.5 | 3.2 | 0.1 |
| **BEEF &** | | | | | | | | |
| Beer, Princes* | ½ Can/205g | 215.0 | 6.0 | 105 | 14.0 | 5.5 | 3.0 | 0.0 |
| Black Bean, Sizzling, Oriental Express* | 1 Pack/400g | 420.0 | 8.0 | 105 | 7.2 | 14.0 | 2.1 | 2.1 |
| Black Bean, with Rice, Weight Watchers* | 1 Pack/320g | 288.0 | 4.0 | 90 | 5.0 | 14.6 | 1.3 | 0.1 |
| Chips, Steak, HE, Tesco* | 1 Pack/450g | 472.0 | 12.0 | 105 | 6.3 | 13.8 | 2.7 | 0.5 |
| Mashed Potato, Braised, Sainsbury's* | 1 Pack/434g | 425.0 | 14.0 | 98 | 7.6 | 9.4 | 3.3 | 0.8 |

**B**

| | Measure INFO/WEIGHT | per Measure KCAL | per Measure FAT | Nutrition Values per 100g / 100ml KCAL | PROT | CARB | FAT | FIBRE |
|---|---|---|---|---|---|---|---|---|
| **BEEF &** | | | | | | | | |
| Onions, Minced, Asda* | ½ Can/196g | 314.0 | 20.0 | 160 | 13.0 | 4.6 | 10.0 | 0.1 |
| Onions, with Gravy, Minced, Lean, Sainsbury's* | 1 Sm Can/198g | 285.0 | 14.0 | 144 | 17.0 | 3.1 | 7.0 | 0.2 |
| Potatoes, Minced, Light Choices, Tesco* | 1 Pack/350g | 210.0 | 3.0 | 60 | 4.6 | 7.7 | 0.9 | 2.1 |
| Yorkshire Pudding, Minced, Sainsbury's* | 1 Pack/350g | 374.0 | 12.0 | 107 | 8.4 | 10.7 | 3.4 | 1.1 |
| **BEEF BORDELAISE** | | | | | | | | |
| Sainsbury's* | 1 Pack/401g | 525.0 | 26.0 | 131 | 8.7 | 9.7 | 6.4 | 1.0 |
| **BEEF BOURGUIGNON** | | | | | | | | |
| Extra Special, Asda* | 1 Serving/300g | 279.0 | 11.0 | 93 | 9.3 | 5.7 | 3.7 | 0.7 |
| Finest, Tesco* | ½ Pack/300g | 247.0 | 8.0 | 82 | 9.9 | 4.8 | 2.6 | 0.5 |
| **BEEF BRAISED** | | | | | | | | |
| & New Potatoes, GFY, Asda* | 1 Pack/448g | 242.0 | 6.0 | 54 | 8.1 | 2.2 | 1.4 | 3.1 |
| in Ale, with Mash & Baby Onions, COU, M & S* | 1 Pack/400g | 380.0 | 9.0 | 95 | 7.4 | 11.0 | 2.3 | 1.4 |
| Steak, & Cabbage, COU, M & S* | 1 Pack/380g | 323.0 | 10.0 | 85 | 8.3 | 6.7 | 2.6 | 1.9 |
| Steak, & Carrots, Mini Favourites, M & S* | 1 Serving/200g | 140.0 | 5.0 | 70 | 8.0 | 4.2 | 2.5 | 1.3 |
| Steak, & Mash, GFY, Asda* | 1 Pack/400g | 260.0 | 3.0 | 65 | 3.4 | 11.0 | 0.8 | 0.7 |
| Steak, & Mash, HL, Tesco* | 1 Pack/450g | 418.0 | 12.0 | 93 | 7.0 | 10.2 | 2.7 | 0.7 |
| Steak, & Red Wine, Veg Mash, HL, Tesco* | 1 Pack/500g | 360.0 | 13.0 | 72 | 5.1 | 6.9 | 2.7 | 1.2 |
| Steak, with Colcannon Mash, Tesco* | 1 Pack/450g | 477.0 | 16.0 | 106 | 9.5 | 9.0 | 3.5 | 0.9 |
| Tender, Pub Specials, Birds Eye* | 1 Pack/450g | 243.0 | 4.0 | 54 | 5.5 | 6.1 | 0.8 | 1.8 |
| with Parsnip Mash, Eat Smart, Safeway* | 1 Pack/400g | 300.0 | 5.0 | 75 | 6.8 | 8.2 | 1.2 | 1.1 |
| **BEEF CANTONESE** | | | | | | | | |
| Sainsbury's* | ½ Pack/175g | 199.0 | 2.0 | 114 | 5.5 | 20.1 | 1.3 | 0.5 |
| **BEEF CHASSEUR** | | | | | | | | |
| & Potato Mash, BGTY, Sainsbury's* | 1 Pack/450g | 387.0 | 11.0 | 86 | 7.8 | 8.4 | 2.4 | 1.3 |
| Somerfield* | 1 Serving/275g | 287.0 | 7.0 | 104 | 14.8 | 5.2 | 2.7 | 2.1 |
| **BEEF CHILLI** | | | | | | | | |
| Crispy, Cantonese, Chilled, Sainsbury's* | 1 Pack/250g | 682.0 | 39.0 | 273 | 11.4 | 22.1 | 15.5 | 1.9 |
| Crispy, Tesco* | 1 Pack/250g | 472.0 | 17.0 | 189 | 10.8 | 21.0 | 6.9 | 0.5 |
| Sweet, Asda* | 1 Pack/400g | 356.0 | 4.0 | 89 | 7.8 | 12.3 | 0.9 | 1.9 |
| **BEEF DINNER** | | | | | | | | |
| British Cuisine, Tesco* | 1 Pack/433g | 390.0 | 10.0 | 90 | 6.3 | 10.0 | 2.3 | 2.3 |
| Roast, Iceland* | 1 Serving/340g | 354.0 | 13.0 | 104 | 8.5 | 9.1 | 3.7 | 1.6 |
| Roast, in Gravy, Yorkshire Pudding & Veg, Birds Eye* | 1 Pack/340g | 367.0 | 9.0 | 108 | 8.8 | 12.3 | 2.6 | 1.4 |
| Roast, Sainsbury's* | 1 Pack/400g | 356.0 | 7.0 | 89 | 6.5 | 12.0 | 1.7 | 1.9 |
| **BEEF ESCALOPE** | | | | | | | | |
| BGTY, Sainsbury's* | 1 Serving/300g | 321.0 | 6.0 | 107 | 22.1 | 0.1 | 2.1 | 0.1 |
| **BEEF HOT & SOUR** | | | | | | | | |
| Chef's Selection, M & S* | 1 Pack/329g | 395.0 | 17.0 | 120 | 9.2 | 8.4 | 5.3 | 1.3 |
| with Garlic Rice, BGTY, Sainsbury's* | 1 Pack/400g | 428.0 | 7.0 | 107 | 5.9 | 17.0 | 1.7 | 0.6 |
| with Vegetable Rice, COU, M & S* | 1 Pack/400g | 360.0 | 6.0 | 90 | 5.5 | 14.4 | 1.4 | 0.6 |
| **BEEF IN** | | | | | | | | |
| Ale Gravy, Chunky, Birds Eye* | 1 Pack/340g | 272.0 | 7.0 | 80 | 7.4 | 8.3 | 2.0 | 1.5 |
| Ale with Mushrooms, BGTY, Sainsbury's* | 1 Pack/251g | 193.0 | 4.0 | 77 | 10.2 | 5.6 | 1.5 | 0.4 |
| Black Bean, with Egg Noodles, M & S* | 1 Pack/400g | 460.0 | 6.0 | 115 | 8.6 | 16.7 | 1.5 | 1.8 |
| Black Bean Sauce, Chinese, Tesco* | 1 Pack/400g | 396.0 | 12.0 | 99 | 9.1 | 8.7 | 3.1 | 0.5 |
| Black Bean Sauce, M & S* | 1 Pack/350g | 402.0 | 22.0 | 115 | 8.9 | 5.7 | 6.4 | 1.1 |
| Black Pepper Sauce & Egg Fried Rice, Tesco* | 1 Pack/451g | 622.0 | 25.0 | 138 | 7.0 | 15.2 | 5.5 | 1.2 |
| Burgundy Red Wine, GFY, Asda* | 1 Pack/405g | 348.0 | 8.0 | 86 | 8.0 | 9.0 | 2.0 | 1.1 |
| Creamy Peppercorn Sauce, Steak, Tesco* | 1 Steak/150g | 189.0 | 8.0 | 126 | 16.5 | 2.6 | 5.5 | 0.1 |
| Gravy, Roast, Birds Eye* | 1 Pack/227g | 177.0 | 4.0 | 78 | 13.4 | 2.2 | 1.7 | 0.0 |
| Gravy, Sliced, Sainsbury's* | 1 Serving/125g | 100.0 | 2.0 | 80 | 13.5 | 2.6 | 1.8 | 0.2 |
| Gravy, Sliced, Tesco* | 1 Serving/200g | 152.0 | 4.0 | 76 | 11.3 | 3.1 | 2.1 | 0.2 |
| Madeira & Mushroom Gravy, Sliced, Finest, Tesco* | 1 Pack/400g | 536.0 | 25.0 | 134 | 15.2 | 4.3 | 6.2 | 1.0 |

| | Measure INFO/WEIGHT | per Measure | | Nutrition Values per 100g / 100ml | | | | |
|---|---|---|---|---|---|---|---|---|
| | | KCAL | FAT | KCAL | PROT | CARB | FAT | FIBRE |
| **BEEF IN** | | | | | | | | |
| Oriental Sauce, Lean Cuisine, Findus* | 1 Pack/350g | 420.0 | 9.0 | 120 | 4.5 | 20.0 | 2.5 | 1.5 |
| Oyster Sauce, Asda* | 1 Serving/100g | 82.0 | 4.0 | 82 | 7.0 | 4.4 | 4.0 | 1.7 |
| Peppercorn Sauce, & Mashed Potato, Weight Watchers* | 1 Pack/400g | 312.0 | 8.0 | 78 | 5.0 | 10.0 | 2.0 | 1.0 |
| Red Wine, Spinach Mash, Perfectly Balanced, Waitrose* | 1 Pack/400g | 380.0 | 10.0 | 95 | 7.4 | 10.1 | 2.6 | 0.8 |
| Red Wine Sauce, Milson's Kitchen, Aldi* | 1 Pack/400g | 256.0 | 6.0 | 64 | 5.6 | 9.6 | 1.5 | 2.1 |
| Strips, Chilli Sauce, Tesco* | 1 Pack/166g | 290.0 | 8.0 | 175 | 23.2 | 9.6 | 4.7 | 0.0 |
| **BEEF MEAL** | | | | | | | | |
| Roast, Mini Favourite, M & S* | 1 Pack/200g | 140.0 | 3.0 | 70 | 9.1 | 6.0 | 1.3 | 0.7 |
| **BEEF SZECHUAN** | | | | | | | | |
| Sizzling Hot Spicy, Oriental Express* | 1 Pack/400g | 380.0 | 8.0 | 95 | 6.4 | 13.2 | 1.9 | 2.0 |
| **BEEF TERIYAKI** | | | | | | | | |
| with Noodles, BGTY, Sainsbury's* | 1 Pack/400g | 320.0 | 4.0 | 80 | 7.7 | 10.1 | 1.0 | 1.0 |
| **BEEF WELLINGTON** | | | | | | | | |
| Extra Special, Asda* | 1 Serving/218g | 605.0 | 37.0 | 277 | 11.0 | 20.0 | 17.0 | 0.9 |
| Finest, Tesco* | 1/3 Pack/216g | 525.0 | 34.0 | 243 | 13.0 | 12.3 | 15.7 | 1.5 |
| Sainsbury's* | 1 Serving/175g | 472.0 | 27.0 | 270 | 14.7 | 18.0 | 15.5 | 0.4 |
| **BEEF WITH** | | | | | | | | |
| Black Bean Sauce, Chilli, Sainsbury's* | 1 Pack/300g | 336.0 | 14.0 | 112 | 8.7 | 8.6 | 4.8 | 1.0 |
| Diane Sauce, Rump Steak, Tesco* | 1 Steak/165g | 181.0 | 8.0 | 110 | 15.1 | 1.1 | 4.9 | 0.3 |
| Honey & Black Pepper, Waitrose* | 1 Pack/350g | 325.0 | 7.0 | 93 | 9.1 | 9.4 | 2.1 | 1.8 |
| Horseradish & Mustard Crust, Joint, Easy, Waitrose* | 1/5 Pack/110g | 153.0 | 6.0 | 139 | 20.9 | 2.5 | 5.1 | 0.7 |
| Horseradish Dressing, Slow Cooked, HL, Tesco* | 1 Pack/356g | 285.0 | 10.0 | 80 | 5.4 | 7.5 | 2.9 | 1.4 |
| Onions & Gravy, Minced, Tesco* | 1 Can/198g | 224.0 | 10.0 | 113 | 14.0 | 2.8 | 5.1 | 0.8 |
| Oyster Sauce, Ooodles of Noodles, Oriental Express* | 1 Pack/425g | 378.0 | 6.0 | 89 | 4.9 | 14.2 | 1.3 | 1.5 |
| Peppercorn Sauce, Steak, Just Cook, Sainsbury's* | ½ Pack/128g | 174.0 | 7.0 | 136 | 17.7 | 3.4 | 5.7 | 1.2 |
| Peppercorn Sauce, Steak, Simply Cook, Tesco* | ½ Pack /167g | 242.0 | 13.0 | 145 | 15.3 | 2.1 | 7.9 | 0.2 |
| Red Wine Sauce, Steaks, Just Cook, Sainsbury's* | ½ Pack/70g | 83.0 | 2.0 | 118 | 20.0 | 2.0 | 3.3 | 0.2 |
| Shiraz Wine Sauce, Pot Roast, Finest, Tesco* | 1 Pack/350g | 350.0 | 9.0 | 100 | 14.1 | 5.1 | 2.6 | 0.9 |
| Vegetables, Tesco* | 1 Pot/300g | 102.0 | 3.0 | 34 | 2.9 | 3.3 | 1.0 | 1.1 |
| Vegetables & Gravy, Minced, Birds Eye* | 1 Pack/178g | 155.0 | 6.0 | 87 | 9.1 | 5.1 | 3.4 | 0.6 |
| Vegetables & Mashed Potato, Braised, BGTY, Sainsbury's* | 1 Pack/450g | 330.0 | 6.0 | 73 | 6.5 | 8.9 | 1.3 | 1.2 |
| Whisky, Collops, Sainsbury's* | 1 Pack/450g | 513.0 | 33.0 | 114 | 8.0 | 4.1 | 7.3 | 1.2 |
| **BEER** | | | | | | | | |
| Ale, Bottled, Old Speckled Hen* | 1 Bottle/330ml | 148.0 | 0.0 | 45 | 0.0 | 0.0 | 0.0 | 0.0 |
| *Bitter, Canned, Average* | *1 Can/440ml* | *141.0* | *0.0* | *32* | *0.3* | *2.3* | *0.0* | *0.0* |
| *Bitter, Draught, Average* | *1 Pint/568ml* | *182.0* | *0.0* | *32* | *0.3* | *2.3* | *0.0* | *0.0* |
| *Bitter, Keg, Average* | *1 Pint/568ml* | *176.0* | *0.0* | *31* | *0.3* | *2.3* | *0.0* | *0.0* |
| *Bitter, Low Alcohol, Average* | *1 Pint/568ml* | *74.0* | *0.0* | *13* | *0.2* | *2.1* | *0.0* | *0.0* |
| *Brown Ale, Bottled, Average* | *1 Bottle/330ml* | *99.0* | *0.0* | *30* | *0.3* | *3.0* | *0.0* | *0.0* |
| *Guinness*, Draught* | *1 Pint/568ml* | *210.0* | *0.0* | *37* | *0.3* | *3.2* | *0.0* | *0.0* |
| *Guinness*, Stout* | *1 Pint/568ml* | *170.0* | *0.0* | *30* | *0.4* | *3.0* | *0.0* | *0.0* |
| *Guinness* Extra Stout, Bottled* | *1 Bottle/500ml* | *215.0* | *0.0* | *43* | *4.0* | *0.0* | *0.0* | *0.0* |
| Kilkenny, Diageo* | 1 Pint/568ml | 210.0 | 0.0 | 37 | 0.3 | 3.0 | 0.0 | 0.0 |
| Low Calorie, Low Carb, Cobra* | 1 Bottle/330ml | 96.0 | 0.0 | 29 | 0.1 | 1.3 | 0.0 | 0.0 |
| *Mackeson, Stout* | *1 Pint/568ml* | *205.0* | *0.0* | *36* | *0.4* | *4.6* | *0.0* | *0.0* |
| *Mild, Draught, Average* | *1 Pint/568ml* | *136.0* | *0.0* | *24* | *0.2* | *1.6* | *0.0* | *0.0* |
| Non Alcoholic, Cobra* | 1 Bottle/330ml | 79.0 | 0.0 | 24 | 0.8 | 2.0 | 0.0 | 0.0 |
| Resolution, Low Carb, Marstons* | 1 Glass/250ml | 77.0 | 0.0 | 31 | 0.3 | 0.6 | 0.1 | 0.0 |
| Ultra, Michelob* | 1 Bottle/275ml | 88.0 | 0.0 | 32 | 0.0 | 0.9 | 0.0 | 0.0 |
| Weissbier, Alcohol Free, Erdinger* | 1 Bottle/500ml | 125.0 | 0.0 | 25 | 0.4 | 5.3 | 0.0 | 0.0 |
| Wheat, Tesco* | 1 Bottle/500ml | 155.0 | 0.0 | 31 | 0.5 | 0.4 | 0.0 | 0.0 |
| **BEETROOT** | | | | | | | | |
| & Roasted Red Onion, M & S* | 1 Serving/125g | 94.0 | 3.0 | 75 | 1.5 | 12.6 | 2.1 | 2.5 |

**B**

| | Measure INFO/WEIGHT | per Measure KCAL | FAT | Nutrition Values per 100g / 100ml KCAL | PROT | CARB | FAT | FIBRE |
|---|---|---|---|---|---|---|---|---|
| **BEETROOT** | | | | | | | | |
| *Baby, Pickled, Average* | *1oz/28g* | *10.0* | *0.0* | *37* | *1.7* | *7.2* | *0.1* | *1.2* |
| *Cooked, Boiled, Drained, Average* | *1 Serving/100g* | *44.0* | *0.0* | *44* | *1.7* | *10.0* | *0.2* | *2.0* |
| *Pickled, in Sweet Vinegar, Average* | *1oz/28g* | *16.0* | *0.0* | *57* | *1.2* | *12.8* | *0.1* | *1.5* |
| *Pickled, in Vinegar, Average* | *1 Serving/50g* | *19.0* | *0.0* | *37* | *1.6* | *7.5* | *0.1* | *1.2* |
| *Raw, Average* | *1oz/28g* | *9.0* | *0.0* | *32* | *1.5* | *6.0* | *0.1* | *1.8* |
| **BHAJI** | | | | | | | | |
| Cauliflower, Fried in Vegetable Oil, Average | 1oz/28g | 60.0 | 6.0 | 214 | 4.0 | 4.0 | 20.5 | 2.0 |
| Onion, Asda* | 1 Bhaji/49g | 96.0 | 5.0 | 196 | 6.0 | 20.0 | 10.0 | 2.0 |
| Onion, Mini, Snack Selection, Sainsbury's* | 1 Bhaji/22g | 49.0 | 3.0 | 226 | 4.1 | 17.4 | 15.5 | 3.5 |
| Onion, Sainsbury's* | 1 Bhaji/38g | 93.0 | 5.0 | 245 | 6.5 | 24.7 | 13.4 | 6.4 |
| Onion, Tesco* | 1 Bhaji/47g | 85.0 | 5.0 | 181 | 5.7 | 16.2 | 10.4 | 4.3 |
| Onion, Waitrose* | 1 Bhaji/45g | 124.0 | 9.0 | 276 | 4.7 | 17.5 | 20.8 | 2.5 |
| Potato, Onion & Mushroom, Fried, Average | 1oz/28g | 58.0 | 5.0 | 208 | 2.0 | 12.0 | 17.5 | 1.5 |
| Potato, Spinach & Cauliflower, Fried, Average | 1oz/28g | 47.0 | 4.0 | 169 | 2.2 | 7.1 | 15.1 | 1.4 |
| Potato & Onion, Fried in Vegetable Oil, Average | 1oz/28g | 45.0 | 3.0 | 160 | 2.1 | 16.6 | 10.1 | 1.6 |
| Spinach, Fried in Vegetable Oil, Average | 1oz/28g | 23.0 | 2.0 | 83 | 3.3 | 2.6 | 6.8 | 2.4 |
| Spinach & Potato, Fried in Vegetable Oil, Average | 1oz/28g | 53.0 | 4.0 | 191 | 3.7 | 13.4 | 14.1 | 2.3 |
| Vegetable, Fried in Vegetable Oil, Average | 1oz/28g | 59.0 | 5.0 | 212 | 2.1 | 10.1 | 18.5 | 2.4 |
| **BHUNA** | | | | | | | | |
| Chicken, & Rice, Sainsbury's* | 1 Pack/501g | 696.0 | 32.0 | 139 | 7.3 | 13.3 | 6.3 | 1.5 |
| Chicken, Curry, Tesco* | 1 Serving/300g | 396.0 | 23.0 | 132 | 11.4 | 4.5 | 7.6 | 0.5 |
| Chicken, Hyderabadi, Sainsbury's* | 1 Pack/400g | 472.0 | 21.0 | 118 | 12.6 | 5.2 | 5.2 | 1.3 |
| Chicken, Indian Takeaway, Tesco* | 1 Pack/350g | 437.0 | 28.0 | 125 | 8.3 | 4.6 | 7.9 | 2.2 |
| Chicken, with Naan Bread, Sharwood's* | 1 Pack/375g | 465.0 | 19.0 | 124 | 6.8 | 12.8 | 5.1 | 2.8 |
| Chicken Tikka, Tesco* | 1 Pack/350g | 437.0 | 23.0 | 125 | 11.3 | 5.0 | 6.7 | 0.9 |
| Lamb, & Rice, Sainsbury's* | 1 Pack/500g | 619.0 | 26.0 | 124 | 7.4 | 11.6 | 5.3 | 2.0 |
| Prawn, Co-Op* | 1 Pack/400g | 300.0 | 16.0 | 75 | 3.0 | 6.0 | 4.0 | 1.0 |
| Prawn, Tandoori, Indian, Sainsbury's* | ½ Pack/200g | 152.0 | 8.0 | 76 | 5.5 | 4.5 | 4.0 | 1.7 |
| **BIERWURST** | | | | | | | | |
| *Average* | *1 Slice/10g* | *25.0* | *2.0* | *252* | *14.4* | *0.9* | *21.2* | *0.0* |
| **BILBERRIES** | | | | | | | | |
| *Fresh, Raw* | *1oz/28g* | *8.0* | *0.0* | *30* | *0.6* | *6.9* | *0.2* | *1.8* |
| **BILTONG** | | | | | | | | |
| *Average* | *1 Serving/25g* | *64.0* | *1.0* | *256* | *50.0* | *0.0* | *4.0* | *0.0* |
| **BIRYANI** | | | | | | | | |
| Chicken, COU, M & S* | 1 Pack/400g | 360.0 | 8.0 | 90 | 6.9 | 10.8 | 2.1 | 1.9 |
| Chicken, Easy Steam, HL, Tesco* | 1 Pack/400g | 424.0 | 7.0 | 106 | 7.0 | 15.5 | 1.8 | 0.6 |
| Chicken, Indian, Asda* | 1 Pack/450g | 778.0 | 22.0 | 173 | 9.0 | 23.0 | 5.0 | 0.7 |
| Chicken, Light Choices, Tesco* | 1 Serving/450g | 495.0 | 10.0 | 110 | 7.0 | 15.0 | 2.3 | 3.4 |
| Chicken, Rice Bowl, Eat Smart, Safeway* | 1 Pack/300g | 255.0 | 5.0 | 85 | 5.5 | 11.3 | 1.6 | 2.4 |
| Chicken, Weight Watchers* | 1 Pack/330g | 308.0 | 4.0 | 93 | 6.2 | 14.6 | 1.1 | 0.6 |
| Chicken Tikka, BGTY, Sainsbury's* | 1 Pack/400g | 384.0 | 4.0 | 96 | 7.1 | 14.6 | 1.0 | 1.5 |
| Chicken Tikka, Northern Indian, Sainsbury's* | 1 Pack/450g | 697.0 | 26.0 | 155 | 9.4 | 16.5 | 5.7 | 1.2 |
| Chicken Tikka, with Basmati Rice, Sharwood's* | 1 Pack/373g | 481.0 | 16.0 | 129 | 6.3 | 16.2 | 4.3 | 0.9 |
| Lamb, HL, Tesco* | 1 Pack/400g | 560.0 | 18.0 | 140 | 5.1 | 19.0 | 4.4 | 3.1 |
| Seafood, M & S* | 1 Pack/450g | 619.0 | 26.0 | 138 | 7.1 | 14.4 | 5.7 | 1.7 |
| Vegetable, & Rice, Sainsbury's* | ½ Pack/125g | 229.0 | 5.0 | 183 | 4.4 | 32.4 | 4.0 | 0.7 |
| Vegetable, HL, Tesco* | 1 Pack/450g | 454.0 | 9.0 | 101 | 2.7 | 17.9 | 2.1 | 1.6 |
| Vegetable, Perfectly Balanced, Waitrose* | 1 Serving/350g | 238.0 | 1.0 | 68 | 2.6 | 14.0 | 0.2 | 2.7 |
| Vegetable, Waitrose* | 1 Pack/450g | 486.0 | 18.0 | 108 | 2.8 | 15.2 | 4.0 | 2.2 |
| Vegetable, with Rice, Patak's* | ½ Pack/125g | 194.0 | 2.0 | 155 | 3.6 | 32.9 | 1.5 | 1.2 |
| **BISCOTTI** | | | | | | | | |
| Almond, Pan Ducale* | 1 Serving/30g | 130.0 | 5.0 | 433 | 10.0 | 60.0 | 16.7 | 3.3 |

| | Measure INFO/WEIGHT | per Measure KCAL | FAT | Nutrition Values per 100g / 100ml KCAL | PROT | CARB | FAT | FIBRE |
|---|---|---|---|---|---|---|---|---|
| **BISCOTTI** | | | | | | | | |
| Chocolate, Heinz* | 1 Biscuit/20g | 80.0 | 2.0 | 398 | 8.5 | 72.0 | 8.7 | 5.8 |
| **BISCUITS** | | | | | | | | |
| Abbey Crunch, McVitie's* | 1 Biscuit/9g | 43.0 | 2.0 | 477 | 6.0 | 72.8 | 17.9 | 2.5 |
| Abernethy, Simmers* | 1 Biscuit/12g | 61.0 | 3.0 | 490 | 5.7 | 69.2 | 21.9 | 0.0 |
| Ace Milk Chocolate, McVitie's* | 1 Biscuit/24g | 122.0 | 6.0 | 510 | 6.1 | 66.2 | 24.5 | 1.6 |
| After Eight, Nestle* | 1 Biscuit/5g | 26.0 | 1.0 | 525 | 6.5 | 62.6 | 27.7 | 1.5 |
| All Butter, Tesco* | 1 Biscuit/9g | 44.0 | 2.0 | 486 | 6.3 | 63.5 | 23.0 | 1.9 |
| Almond, Thins, Morrisons* | 1 Biscuit/4g | 16.0 | 1.0 | 450 | 6.7 | 72.8 | 14.7 | 3.1 |
| Almond Butter Thins, Extra Special, Asda* | 1 Biscuit/4g | 15.0 | 0.0 | 375 | 5.0 | 60.0 | 12.5 | 2.5 |
| Almond Fingers, Tesco* | 1 Finger/46g | 180.0 | 7.0 | 391 | 6.2 | 58.4 | 14.7 | 1.0 |
| Almond Thins, All Butter, TTD, Sainsbury's* | 1 Biscuit/4g | 16.0 | 1.0 | 450 | 6.7 | 72.8 | 14.7 | 3.1 |
| Almond Thins, Continental, Tesco* | 1 Biscuit/3g | 15.0 | 0.0 | 450 | 6.7 | 72.8 | 14.7 | 3.1 |
| Almond Thins, Sainsbury's* | 1 Biscuit/3g | 13.0 | 0.0 | 430 | 7.0 | 80.3 | 9.0 | 1.0 |
| Amaretti, M & S* | 1 Biscuit/6g | 30.0 | 1.0 | 480 | 9.6 | 71.3 | 17.2 | 3.8 |
| Amaretti, Sainsbury's* | 1 Biscuit/6g | 27.0 | 1.0 | 450 | 6.5 | 80.5 | 11.3 | 1.1 |
| Animals, Milk Chocolate, Cadbury* | 1 Biscuit/19g | 94.0 | 4.0 | 493 | 6.6 | 69.8 | 20.9 | 0.0 |
| Animals, Mini Packs, Cadbury* | 1 Pack/25g | 123.0 | 5.0 | 491 | 6.7 | 70.7 | 20.2 | 0.0 |
| Apple & Cinnamon Thins, Finest, Tesco* | 1 Biscuit/5g | 22.0 | 1.0 | 470 | 5.9 | 71.7 | 17.5 | 1.5 |
| Apple & Raspberry, Minis, Officially Low Fat, Fox's* | 1 Bag/40g | 140.0 | 1.0 | 350 | 3.9 | 76.9 | 2.7 | 3.8 |
| Apple & Sultana, Go Ahead, McVitie's* | 1 Biscuit/15g | 56.0 | 1.0 | 386 | 6.0 | 72.7 | 7.9 | 3.3 |
| Apple Crumble, Officially Low Fat, Fox's* | 1 Biscuit/23g | 85.0 | 1.0 | 365 | 5.4 | 80.4 | 2.4 | 2.5 |
| Apple Strudel, Big Softies, Fox's* | 1 Biscuit/23g | 80.0 | 0.0 | 348 | 5.3 | 77.0 | 1.6 | 2.8 |
| Apricot, Low Fat, M & S* | 1 Biscuit/23g | 79.0 | 1.0 | 343 | 6.1 | 69.6 | 4.4 | 7.8 |
| Arrowroot, Thin, Crawfords* | 1 Biscuit/7g | 35.0 | 1.0 | 473 | 7.4 | 76.7 | 15.2 | 2.2 |
| Banana Milk Shake, Creams, Safeway* | 1 Biscuit/13g | 60.0 | 2.0 | 460 | 5.6 | 70.9 | 16.8 | 1.8 |
| Belgian Chocolate, Selection, Finest, Tesco* | 1 Biscuit/10g | 51.0 | 3.0 | 515 | 6.0 | 62.0 | 27.0 | 3.0 |
| Belgian Chocolate, Thins, Extra Special, Asda* | 1 Biscuit/9g | 44.0 | 2.0 | 503 | 7.0 | 67.0 | 23.0 | 0.2 |
| Bisc & Bounty, Master Foods* | 1 Bar/25g | 131.0 | 8.0 | 526 | 4.8 | 52.3 | 33.0 | 0.0 |
| Bisc & M&m's, Master Foods* | 1 Biscuit/17g | 90.0 | 5.0 | 527 | 5.8 | 59.2 | 29.6 | 0.0 |
| Bisc & Mars, Master Foods* | 1 Bar/27g | 141.0 | 8.0 | 523 | 5.3 | 61.4 | 28.5 | 0.0 |
| Bisc & Twix, Master Foods* | 1 Bar/27g | 140.0 | 8.0 | 520 | 5.2 | 61.1 | 28.3 | 0.0 |
| Blackcurrant with Wheat Bran, Bisca* | 1 Biscuit/8g | 31.0 | 1.0 | 420 | 6.0 | 72.0 | 12.0 | 5.5 |
| Blueberry & Vanilla, Oaty, Weight Watchers* | 1 Biscuit/22g | 101.0 | 4.0 | 460 | 7.1 | 65.6 | 18.8 | 4.2 |
| Bn, Chocolate Flavour, McVitie's* | 1 Biscuit/18g | 83.0 | 3.0 | 460 | 6.6 | 71.0 | 16.7 | 2.6 |
| Bn, Strawberry Flavour, McVitie's* | 1 Biscuit/18g | 71.0 | 1.0 | 395 | 5.6 | 78.0 | 6.8 | 0.0 |
| Bn, Vanilla Flavour, McVitie's* | 1 Biscuit/18g | 85.0 | 3.0 | 470 | 5.9 | 74.0 | 16.6 | 1.2 |
| Boasters, Hazelnut & Choc Chip, McVitie's* | 1 Biscuit/16g | 88.0 | 5.0 | 549 | 7.0 | 55.5 | 33.3 | 2.4 |
| Bourbon Creams, Asda* | 1 Biscuit/14g | 67.0 | 3.0 | 482 | 5.0 | 66.0 | 22.0 | 3.4 |
| Bourbon Creams, Sainsbury's* | 1 Biscuit/13g | 60.0 | 2.0 | 476 | 5.7 | 70.4 | 19.1 | 1.7 |
| Bourbon Creams, Tesco* | 1 Biscuit/14g | 68.0 | 3.0 | 485 | 5.4 | 66.2 | 21.6 | 3.4 |
| Bourbon Creams, Value, Multipack, Tesco* | 1 Biscuit/13g | 62.0 | 3.0 | 494 | 5.9 | 68.0 | 22.8 | 1.7 |
| Butter, Covered in Dark 70% Chocolate, Green & Black's* | 1 Biscuit/12g | 62.0 | 4.0 | 520 | 7.1 | 5.6 | 29.4 | 0.1 |
| Butter, Crinkle Crunch, Fox's* | 1 Biscuit/11g | 50.0 | 2.0 | 460 | 5.8 | 69.8 | 17.5 | 2.4 |
| Butter, Thins, Belgian Chocolate, The Best, Safeway* | 1 Biscuit/10g | 49.0 | 2.0 | 487 | 6.4 | 64.0 | 22.8 | 0.8 |
| Cafe Noir, McVitie's* | 1 Biscuit/9g | 39.0 | 1.0 | 420 | 4.5 | 87.0 | 5.5 | 1.1 |
| Cantuccini, with Almonds, Average | 1 Biscotti/30g | 130.0 | 5.0 | 433 | 10.0 | 60.0 | 16.7 | 3.3 |
| Caramels, Milk Chocolate, McVitie's* | 1 Serving/17g | 81.0 | 4.0 | 478 | 5.6 | 65.8 | 21.4 | 1.8 |
| Cheddars, Real Cheddar Cheese, Jacob's* | 1 Biscuit/4g | 19.0 | 1.0 | 509 | 11.6 | 53.2 | 27.7 | 2.7 |
| Cheese, Weight Watchers* | 1 Pack/18g | 73.0 | 1.0 | 405 | 13.7 | 71.0 | 7.4 | 2.0 |
| Cheese Melts, Carr's* | 1 Biscuit/5g | 22.0 | 1.0 | 479 | 11.9 | 58.2 | 22.0 | 2.2 |
| Cheese Sandwich, Ritz* | 1 Biscuit/9g | 50.0 | 3.0 | 530 | 9.5 | 55.0 | 30.2 | 2.0 |
| Cheese Savouries, Sainsbury's* | 1 Serving/50g | 268.0 | 15.0 | 536 | 11.6 | 53.3 | 30.6 | 2.5 |
| Choc Chip, Paterson's* | 1 Biscuit/17g | 79.0 | 4.0 | 474 | 5.6 | 64.0 | 21.6 | 3.1 |

# BISCUITS

| | Measure INFO/WEIGHT | per Measure KCAL | per Measure FAT | Nutrition Values per 100g / 100ml KCAL | PROT | CARB | FAT | FIBRE |
|---|---|---|---|---|---|---|---|---|
| Choco Leibniz, Dark Chocolate, Bahlsen* | 1 Biscuit/14g | 69.0 | 4.0 | 493 | 6.8 | 59.0 | 26.0 | 5.1 |
| Choco Leibniz, Milk, Bahlsen* | 1 Biscuit/10g | 51.0 | 3.0 | 515 | 7.9 | 63.4 | 25.5 | 0.0 |
| Choco Leibniz, Orange Flavour, Bahlsen* | 1 Biscuit/14g | 70.0 | 4.0 | 504 | 7.9 | 58.5 | 26.4 | 0.0 |
| Chocolate, Belgian Chocolate, Weight Watchers* | 1 Biscuit/18g | 87.0 | 4.0 | 481 | 7.1 | 61.8 | 22.8 | 4.5 |
| Chocolate, Golden Crunch, Free From Milk, Tesco* | 1 Biscuit/17g | 85.0 | 5.0 | 510 | 4.2 | 57.2 | 29.4 | 4.6 |
| Chocolate & Coconut, Duchy Originals* | 1 Biscuit/13g | 68.0 | 4.0 | 543 | 6.3 | 52.1 | 34.4 | 2.6 |
| Chocolate Break, Plain Chocolate, Tesco* | 1 Biscuit/21g | 112.0 | 6.0 | 535 | 6.7 | 61.2 | 29.2 | 3.8 |
| Chocolate Chip & Peanut, Trufree* | 1 Biscuit/11g | 55.0 | 3.0 | 496 | 4.0 | 66.0 | 24.0 | 2.0 |
| Chocolate Fingers, Caramel, Cadbury* | 1 Finger/8g | 39.0 | 2.0 | 490 | 5.8 | 63.2 | 23.8 | 0.0 |
| Chocolate Fingers, Milk, Cadbury* | 1 Biscuit/6g | 31.0 | 2.0 | 515 | 6.8 | 60.8 | 27.1 | 1.7 |
| Chocolate Fingers, Plain, Cadbury* | 1 Biscuit/6g | 30.0 | 2.0 | 508 | 6.2 | 60.6 | 26.8 | 0.0 |
| Chocolate Florentine, M & S* | 1 Serving/39g | 195.0 | 10.0 | 500 | 7.4 | 64.5 | 24.9 | 1.7 |
| Chocolate Ginger, Organic, Duchy Originals* | 1 Biscuit/12g | 64.0 | 4.0 | 518 | 4.6 | 59.7 | 29.0 | 2.1 |
| Chocolate Ginger, Thorntons* | 1 Biscuit/19g | 96.0 | 5.0 | 512 | 5.9 | 58.2 | 28.4 | 0.0 |
| Chocolate Kimberley, Jacob's* | 1 Biscuit/20g | 86.0 | 3.0 | 428 | 3.9 | 64.4 | 17.2 | 1.1 |
| Chocolate Nibbles, High Lights, Cadbury* | 1 Pack/16g | 75.0 | 3.0 | 465 | 6.2 | 73.4 | 16.1 | 1.7 |
| Chocolate Seville, Thorntons* | 1 Biscuit/19g | 97.0 | 5.0 | 512 | 5.7 | 59.0 | 28.1 | 0.0 |
| Chocolate Toffee, Crunch, Moments, McVitie's* | 1 Biscuit/17g | 89.0 | 5.0 | 520 | 5.6 | 62.3 | 27.6 | 1.7 |
| Chocolate Viennese, Fox's* | 1 Biscuit/16g | 85.0 | 5.0 | 530 | 6.7 | 56.6 | 30.7 | 1.7 |
| Chocolinis, Milk Chocolate, Go Ahead, McVitie's* | 1 Biscuit/12g | 56.0 | 2.0 | 466 | 7.7 | 77.2 | 14.0 | 2.0 |
| Christmas Shapes, Assorted, Sainsbury's* | 1 Biscuit/15g | 77.0 | 4.0 | 525 | 5.2 | 59.0 | 29.8 | 1.7 |
| Classic, Creams, Fox's* | 1 Biscuit/14g | 72.0 | 4.0 | 516 | 4.4 | 65.2 | 25.8 | 1.7 |
| Classic, Milk Chocolate, Fox's* | 1 Biscuit/13g | 67.0 | 3.0 | 517 | 6.1 | 64.9 | 24.0 | 1.6 |
| Coconut Crinkle, Sainsbury's* | 1 Biscuit/11g | 54.0 | 3.0 | 500 | 6.4 | 59.6 | 26.2 | 3.7 |
| Coconut Ring, Asda* | 1 Biscuit/8g | 37.0 | 2.0 | 486 | 6.0 | 66.0 | 22.0 | 2.6 |
| Coconut Rings, Tesco* | 1 Biscuit/9g | 44.0 | 2.0 | 485 | 6.2 | 66.1 | 21.7 | 2.6 |
| Cracked Black Pepper, Savoury, Weight Watchers* | 1 Serving/16g | 71.0 | 3.0 | 446 | 8.3 | 59.2 | 19.5 | 9.4 |
| Cranberry, Crispy Slices, Light Choices, Tesco* | 1 Biscuit/15g | 54.0 | 1.0 | 370 | 6.0 | 76.0 | 3.9 | 5.5 |
| Cranberry & Pumpkin Seed, BGTY, Sainsbury's* | 1 Biscuit/17g | 68.0 | 3.0 | 410 | 7.2 | 56.6 | 17.1 | 13.9 |
| Cranberry & Sunflower Seed, Oaty, Weight Watchers* | 1 Biscuit/22g | 103.0 | 5.0 | 469 | 7.5 | 62.4 | 21.0 | 5.3 |
| Custard Creams, 25% Less Fat, Asda* | 1 Biscuit/10g | 47.0 | 2.0 | 474 | 6.0 | 72.0 | 18.0 | 1.2 |
| Custard Creams, 25% Less Fat, Sainsbury's* | 1 Biscuit/13g | 59.0 | 2.0 | 469 | 5.8 | 72.7 | 17.3 | 1.3 |
| Custard Creams, 25% Less Fat, Tesco* | 1 Biscuit/13g | 59.0 | 2.0 | 473 | 5.8 | 72.2 | 17.9 | 1.2 |
| Custard Creams, Asda* | 1 Biscuit/12g | 59.0 | 3.0 | 495 | 5.0 | 67.0 | 23.0 | 2.0 |
| Custard Creams, BGTY, Sainsbury's* | 1 Biscuit/12g | 56.0 | 2.0 | 473 | 5.8 | 72.2 | 17.9 | 1.2 |
| Custard Creams, Crawfords* | 1 Biscuit/11g | 57.0 | 3.0 | 517 | 5.9 | 69.2 | 24.1 | 1.5 |
| Custard Creams, Sainsbury's* | 1 Biscuit/13g | 67.0 | 3.0 | 514 | 5.5 | 70.4 | 23.4 | 1.6 |
| Custard Creams, Tesco* | 1 Biscuit/13g | 65.0 | 3.0 | 510 | 5.7 | 65.7 | 24.7 | 1.5 |
| Custard Creams, Value, Tesco* | 1 Biscuit/11g | 51.0 | 2.0 | 450 | 7.2 | 72.5 | 14.3 | 3.0 |
| Dark Chocolate & Stem Ginger, TTD, Sainsbury's* | 1 Biscuit/22g | 112.0 | 6.0 | 504 | 4.4 | 62.3 | 26.4 | 1.8 |
| Dark Chocolate All Butter, M & S* | 1 Biscuit/15g | 72.0 | 4.0 | 480 | 6.9 | 52.4 | 27.2 | 11.4 |
| Dark Chocolate Ginger, M & S* | 1 Biscuit/21g | 105.0 | 6.0 | 505 | 5.0 | 58.8 | 27.6 | 4.2 |
| Digestive, 25% Less Fat, Asda* | 1 Biscuit/16g | 73.0 | 3.0 | 455 | 7.3 | 69.8 | 16.3 | 2.6 |
| Digestive, 25% Less Fat, Tesco* | 1 Biscuit/14g | 65.0 | 2.0 | 462 | 7.3 | 71.0 | 16.5 | 3.8 |
| Digestive, Asda* | 1 Biscuit/14g | 66.0 | 3.0 | 464 | 6.0 | 65.0 | 20.0 | 3.1 |
| Digestive, BGTY, Sainsbury's* | 1 Biscuit/15g | 70.0 | 3.0 | 468 | 7.4 | 71.0 | 17.2 | 3.8 |
| Digestive, Creams, McVitie's* | 1 Biscuit/12g | 60.0 | 3.0 | 502 | 5.6 | 68.2 | 23.0 | 2.1 |
| Digestive, Economy, Sainsbury's* | 1 Biscuit/13g | 65.0 | 3.0 | 498 | 6.8 | 66.3 | 22.8 | 3.3 |
| Digestive, Finger, Reduced Fat, Sainsbury's* | 1 Finger/8g | 39.0 | 2.0 | 482 | 6.8 | 63.6 | 22.2 | 3.2 |
| Digestive, Fingers, Morrisons* | 1 Finger/8g | 39.0 | 2.0 | 482 | 6.8 | 63.6 | 22.2 | 3.2 |
| Digestive, GFY, Asda* | 1 Biscuit/14g | 65.0 | 2.0 | 461 | 6.0 | 71.0 | 17.0 | 3.6 |
| Digestive, Happy Shopper* | 1 Biscuit/13g | 64.0 | 3.0 | 498 | 6.8 | 66.3 | 22.8 | 3.3 |
| Digestive, Jacob's* | 1 Biscuit/14g | 67.0 | 3.0 | 479 | 6.6 | 65.7 | 21.1 | 3.4 |

## BISCUITS

| | Measure INFO/WEIGHT | per Measure KCAL | per Measure FAT | Nutrition Values per 100g / 100ml KCAL | PROT | CARB | FAT | FIBRE |
|---|---|---|---|---|---|---|---|---|
| Digestive, Light, McVitie's* | 1 Biscuit/15g | 67.0 | 2.0 | 445 | 7.1 | 67.9 | 16.1 | 3.5 |
| Digestive, McVitie's* | 1 Biscuit/15g | 70.0 | 3.0 | 470 | 7.2 | 62.7 | 21.5 | 3.6 |
| Digestive, Milk Chocolate, 25% Less Fat, Tesco* | 1 Biscuit/17g | 79.0 | 3.0 | 466 | 7.4 | 69.0 | 17.8 | 2.6 |
| Digestive, Milk Chocolate, 25% Reduced Fat, McVitie's* | 1 Biscuit/17g | 78.0 | 3.0 | 459 | 7.2 | 68.6 | 17.3 | 3.2 |
| Digestive, Milk Chocolate, GFY, Asda* | 1 Biscuit/17g | 78.0 | 3.0 | 457 | 7.0 | 69.0 | 17.0 | 3.2 |
| Digestive, Milk Chocolate, M & S* | 1 Biscuit/17g | 85.0 | 4.0 | 505 | 6.1 | 62.2 | 26.0 | 2.6 |
| Digestive, Milk Chocolate, Sainsbury's* | 1 Biscuit/17g | 87.0 | 6.0 | 511 | 6.9 | 65.9 | 36.8 | 2.5 |
| Digestive, Milk Chocolate, Tesco* | 1 Biscuit/17g | 84.0 | 4.0 | 497 | 6.8 | 62.4 | 24.5 | 2.7 |
| Digestive, Munch Bites, McVitie's* | 1 Pack/40g | 205.0 | 10.0 | 512 | 6.5 | 64.5 | 25.5 | 2.0 |
| Digestive, Oat, Weight Watchers* | 1 Biscuit/11g | 50.0 | 2.0 | 457 | 6.0 | 66.3 | 18.6 | 6.9 |
| Digestive, Organic, Sainsbury's* | 1 Biscuit/12g | 60.0 | 3.0 | 483 | 6.6 | 60.9 | 23.7 | 5.8 |
| Digestive, Organic, Tesco* | 1 Biscuit/13g | 60.0 | 3.0 | 464 | 7.7 | 66.3 | 20.8 | 4.6 |
| Digestive, Plain, M & S* | 1 Biscuit/16g | 80.0 | 4.0 | 490 | 6.5 | 62.7 | 23.8 | 3.3 |
| Digestive, Plain Chocolate, Asda* | 1 Biscuit/17g | 84.0 | 4.0 | 500 | 7.0 | 64.0 | 24.0 | 3.2 |
| Digestive, Plain Chocolate, Tesco* | 1 Biscuit/17g | 85.0 | 4.0 | 499 | 6.2 | 63.5 | 24.4 | 2.8 |
| Digestive, Plain Chocolate, Value, Tesco* | 1 Biscuit/14g | 71.0 | 4.0 | 497 | 6.5 | 62.2 | 24.7 | 3.1 |
| Digestive, Reduced Fat, M & S* | 1 Biscuit/16g | 75.0 | 3.0 | 480 | 7.2 | 73.3 | 17.5 | 3.4 |
| Digestive, Reduced Fat, McVitie's* | 1 Biscuit/15g | 70.0 | 2.0 | 467 | 7.1 | 72.8 | 16.3 | 3.4 |
| Digestive, Reduced Fat, Tesco* | 1 Biscuit/16g | 70.0 | 3.0 | 453 | 7.0 | 69.1 | 16.6 | 3.4 |
| Digestive, SmartPrice, Asda* | 1 Biscuit/14g | 67.0 | 3.0 | 465 | 6.0 | 65.3 | 20.0 | 3.1 |
| Digestive, Sweetmeal, Asda* | 1 Biscuit/14g | 68.0 | 3.0 | 499 | 7.0 | 66.0 | 23.0 | 3.5 |
| Digestive, Sweetmeal, Sainsbury's* | 1 Biscuit/14g | 72.0 | 3.0 | 498 | 6.0 | 66.4 | 23.1 | 3.3 |
| Digestive, Sweetmeal, Tesco* | 1 Biscuit/18g | 80.0 | 3.0 | 444 | 8.4 | 70.0 | 14.5 | 3.1 |
| Digestive, Trufree* | 1 Biscuit/10g | 45.0 | 2.0 | 454 | 2.1 | 71.0 | 21.0 | 2.4 |
| Digestive, Value, Tesco* | 1 Biscuit/15g | 73.0 | 3.0 | 490 | 6.9 | 64.0 | 22.4 | 3.3 |
| Double Choc Chip, Trufree* | 1 Biscuit/11g | 58.0 | 3.0 | 523 | 3.0 | 67.0 | 27.0 | 1.8 |
| for Cheese, Bran Cracker, Christmas, Tesco* | 1oz/28g | 127.0 | 5.0 | 454 | 9.7 | 62.8 | 18.2 | 3.2 |
| for Cheese, Chive Cracker, Christmas, Tesco* | 1oz/28g | 125.0 | 4.0 | 448 | 9.3 | 66.6 | 16.0 | 2.4 |
| for Cheese, Cornish Wafer, Christmas, Tesco* | 1oz/28g | 148.0 | 9.0 | 530 | 8.0 | 56.8 | 31.2 | 2.4 |
| for Cheese, Cream Cracker, Christmas, Tesco* | 1oz/28g | 118.0 | 4.0 | 421 | 9.9 | 71.9 | 12.7 | 5.1 |
| for Cheese, Digestive, Hovis, Christmas, Tesco* | 1oz/28g | 127.0 | 5.0 | 453 | 4.2 | 74.6 | 18.2 | 7.0 |
| for Cheese, Poppy Snack, Christmas, Tesco* | 1oz/28g | 129.0 | 5.0 | 461 | 10.0 | 64.4 | 18.2 | 3.1 |
| Fruit, All Butter, Sainsbury's* | 1 Biscuit/9g | 45.0 | 2.0 | 477 | 5.6 | 66.0 | 21.2 | 1.9 |
| Fruit Bake, Organic, Tesco* | 1 Biscuit/12g | 53.0 | 2.0 | 453 | 7.5 | 65.1 | 18.1 | 5.6 |
| Fruit Shewsbury, Mini Pack, Paterson's* | 1 Biscuit/17g | 81.0 | 4.0 | 483 | 4.9 | 64.9 | 22.7 | 1.9 |
| Fruit Shortcake, McVitie's* | 1 Biscuit/8g | 37.0 | 2.0 | 464 | 5.7 | 65.1 | 20.1 | 2.7 |
| Fruit Shortcake, Sainsbury's* | 1 Biscuit/8g | 39.0 | 2.0 | 483 | 5.9 | 69.6 | 20.1 | 2.1 |
| Fruit Shortcake, Tesco* | 1 Biscuit/9g | 43.0 | 2.0 | 473 | 5.8 | 70.1 | 18.8 | 1.9 |
| Garibaldi, Asda* | 1 Biscuit/10g | 39.0 | 1.0 | 375 | 4.7 | 68.5 | 9.1 | 2.2 |
| Garibaldi, Sainsbury's* | 1 Biscuit/9g | 35.0 | 1.0 | 389 | 5.7 | 67.1 | 10.9 | 3.3 |
| Garibaldi, Tesco* | 1 Biscuit/10g | 40.0 | 1.0 | 400 | 4.7 | 74.0 | 9.1 | 2.2 |
| Ginger, Safeway* | 1 Biscuit/12g | 55.0 | 2.0 | 456 | 5.9 | 73.9 | 15.3 | 1.7 |
| Ginger, Traditional, Fox's* | 1 Biscuit/8g | 33.0 | 1.0 | 404 | 4.4 | 70.1 | 11.7 | 1.4 |
| Ginger Crinkle, Sainsbury's* | 1 Biscuit/11g | 53.0 | 3.0 | 486 | 6.2 | 63.8 | 22.9 | 2.9 |
| Ginger Crinkle Crunch, Fox's* | 1 Biscuit/12g | 50.0 | 1.0 | 435 | 4.7 | 75.3 | 12.5 | 1.6 |
| Ginger Crunch Creams, Fox's* | 1 Biscuit/14g | 73.0 | 4.0 | 518 | 4.6 | 64.8 | 26.7 | 0.0 |
| Ginger Nuts, Asda* | 1 Biscuit/10g | 45.0 | 1.0 | 447 | 5.0 | 73.0 | 15.0 | 0.0 |
| Ginger Nuts, McVitie's* | 1 Biscuit/12g | 55.0 | 2.0 | 456 | 5.8 | 70.9 | 16.5 | 2.2 |
| Ginger Nuts, Milk Chocolate, McVitie's* | 1 Biscuit/14g | 68.0 | 3.0 | 489 | 5.8 | 71.8 | 19.9 | 1.5 |
| Ginger Nuts, Tesco* | 1 Biscuit/8g | 36.0 | 1.0 | 450 | 5.8 | 73.1 | 14.7 | 2.0 |
| Ginger Snap, BGTY, Sainsbury's* | 1 Biscuit/12g | 51.0 | 1.0 | 427 | 6.5 | 78.2 | 9.8 | 1.8 |
| Ginger Snap, Fox's* | 1 Biscuit/8g | 35.0 | 1.0 | 443 | 4.6 | 77.1 | 12.8 | 1.5 |
| Ginger Snap, Less Than 10% Fat, Sainsbury's* | 1 Biscuit/12g | 51.0 | 1.0 | 424 | 6.5 | 78.9 | 9.1 | 1.9 |

# B

## BISCUITS

| | Measure INFO/WEIGHT | per Measure KCAL | FAT | Nutrition Values per 100g / 100ml KCAL | PROT | CARB | FAT | FIBRE |
|---|---|---|---|---|---|---|---|---|
| Ginger Snap, Sainsbury's* | 1 Biscuit/11g | 47.0 | 2.0 | 445 | 5.3 | 73.0 | 14.7 | 2.2 |
| Ginger Snaps, Trufree* | 1 Biscuit/11g | 51.0 | 2.0 | 467 | 2.5 | 76.0 | 17.0 | 1.5 |
| Ginger Thins, Asda* | 1 Biscuit/5g | 23.0 | 1.0 | 462 | 6.0 | 73.0 | 16.0 | 1.9 |
| Gingered, Duchy Originals* | 1 Biscuit/16g | 74.0 | 3.0 | 472 | 6.0 | 64.8 | 21.0 | 2.5 |
| Gingernut | 1 Biscuit/11g | 50.0 | 2.0 | 456 | 5.6 | 79.1 | 15.2 | 1.4 |
| Golden Crunch, Go Ahead, McVitie's* | 1 Biscuit/9g | 38.0 | 1.0 | 419 | 7.7 | 75.2 | 9.7 | 2.1 |
| Golden Crunch, Paterson's* | 1 Biscuit/15g | 69.0 | 3.0 | 474 | 5.1 | 62.5 | 22.6 | 4.8 |
| Golden Crunch Creams, Fox's* | 1 Biscuit/15g | 75.0 | 4.0 | 515 | 4.7 | 64.8 | 26.3 | 1.2 |
| Golden Shortie, Jacob's* | 1 Biscuit/11g | 54.0 | 3.0 | 492 | 6.0 | 64.9 | 23.2 | 0.0 |
| Golden Syrup, McVitie's* | 1 Biscuit/12g | 63.0 | 3.0 | 508 | 5.1 | 67.3 | 24.2 | 2.2 |
| Happy Faces, Jacob's* | 1 Biscuit/16g | 78.0 | 4.0 | 485 | 4.8 | 66.1 | 22.3 | 1.6 |
| Hazelnut Crispies, Occasions, Sainsbury's* | 1 Biscuit/7g | 36.0 | 2.0 | 518 | 6.0 | 64.3 | 26.3 | 0.0 |
| Hazelnut Meringue, Sainsbury's* | 1 Biscuit/6g | 24.0 | 1.0 | 404 | 5.0 | 43.0 | 23.5 | 1.1 |
| Hob Nobs, Chocolate Creams, McVitie's* | 1 Biscuit/12g | 60.0 | 3.0 | 503 | 6.7 | 60.3 | 26.1 | 4.0 |
| Hob Nobs, Light, 25% Reduced Fat, McVitie's* | 1 Biscuit/14g | 62.0 | 2.0 | 435 | 8.1 | 64.6 | 16.1 | 6.2 |
| Hob Nobs, McVitie's* | 1 Biscuit/14g | 67.0 | 3.0 | 466 | 7.1 | 60.8 | 21.7 | 5.5 |
| Hob Nobs, Milk Chocolate, McVitie's* | 1 Biscuit/19g | 92.0 | 4.0 | 479 | 6.8 | 60.7 | 23.3 | 4.5 |
| Hob Nobs, Milk Chocolate, Mini, McVitie's* | 1 Pack/25g | 121.0 | 6.0 | 483 | 6.6 | 61.3 | 23.5 | 4.4 |
| Hob Nobs, Munch Bites, McVitie's* | 1 Pack/40g | 203.0 | 10.0 | 508 | 6.8 | 63.4 | 25.2 | 2.8 |
| Hob Nobs, Plain Chocolate, McVitie's* | 1 Biscuit/16g | 81.0 | 4.0 | 498 | 6.7 | 63.3 | 24.3 | 4.2 |
| Hob Nobs, Vanilla Creams, McVitie's* | 1 Biscuit/12g | 60.0 | 3.0 | 501 | 6.1 | 62.3 | 25.2 | 3.6 |
| Honeycomb Nibbles, High Lights, Cadbury* | 1 Bag/16g | 75.0 | 3.0 | 465 | 6.2 | 73.4 | 16.2 | 1.8 |
| Iced Gems, Jacob's* | 1 Portion/30g | 116.0 | 1.0 | 388 | 5.0 | 85.5 | 2.9 | 1.5 |
| Jaffa Cakes, Asda* | 1 Cake/12g | 43.0 | 1.0 | 368 | 4.7 | 67.5 | 8.8 | 1.9 |
| Jaffa Cakes, Blackcurrant, McVitie's* | 1 Cake/12g | 45.0 | 1.0 | 371 | 4.8 | 69.7 | 8.1 | 2.3 |
| Jaffa Cakes, Dark Chocolate, M & S* | 1 Cake/11g | 45.0 | 2.0 | 395 | 3.7 | 64.9 | 13.2 | 2.8 |
| Jaffa Cakes, Dark Chocolate, Mini, M & S* | 1 Cake/5g | 20.0 | 1.0 | 410 | 3.9 | 62.8 | 15.8 | 1.9 |
| Jaffa Cakes, Lemon & Lime, McVitie's* | 1 Cake/12g | 45.0 | 1.0 | 370 | 4.7 | 69.5 | 8.1 | 2.1 |
| Jaffa Cakes, Lunch Box, McVitie's* | 1 Cake/7g | 26.0 | 1.0 | 395 | 4.2 | 74.3 | 9.0 | 1.4 |
| Jaffa Cakes, McVitie's* | 1 Cake/12g | 45.0 | 1.0 | 374 | 4.8 | 70.6 | 8.0 | 2.1 |
| Jaffa Cakes, Mini, Asda* | 1 Cake/5g | 21.0 | 1.0 | 412 | 3.9 | 63.0 | 16.0 | 1.9 |
| Jaffa Cakes, Mini, Bags, McVitie's* | 1 Cake/5g | 20.0 | 1.0 | 396 | 4.2 | 65.0 | 13.1 | 3.5 |
| Jaffa Cakes, Mini, Orange Pods, McVitie's* | 1 Cake/40g | 150.0 | 3.0 | 380 | 4.3 | 71.2 | 8.7 | 3.5 |
| Jaffa Cakes, Mini, Tesco* | 1 Cake/5g | 19.0 | 1.0 | 380 | 4.0 | 64.0 | 12.0 | 2.0 |
| Jaffa Cakes, Mini Roll, McVitie's* | 1 Cake/30g | 115.0 | 3.0 | 382 | 3.5 | 67.2 | 11.0 | 1.3 |
| Jaffa Cakes, Mini Roll Xl, McVitie's* | 1 Cake/44g | 169.0 | 5.0 | 384 | 3.5 | 66.9 | 11.4 | 0.0 |
| Jaffa Cakes, Plain Chocolate, Sainsbury's* | 1 Cake/13g | 50.0 | 1.0 | 384 | 4.4 | 73.3 | 8.1 | 1.3 |
| Jaffa Cakes, Sainsbury's* | 1 Cake/11g | 41.0 | 1.0 | 373 | 4.3 | 69.3 | 8.8 | 2.0 |
| Jaffa Cakes, Value, Tesco* | 1 Cake/11g | 42.0 | 1.0 | 370 | 4.8 | 67.6 | 8.8 | 1.9 |
| Jam Creams, Jacob's* | 1 Biscuit/15g | 75.0 | 3.0 | 486 | 5.0 | 67.4 | 21.8 | 1.6 |
| Jam Rings, Crawfords* | 1 Biscuit/12g | 56.0 | 2.0 | 470 | 5.5 | 73.0 | 17.2 | 1.9 |
| Jam Sandwich Creams, M & S* | 1 Biscuit/17g | 80.0 | 4.0 | 485 | 5.7 | 64.5 | 22.6 | 1.8 |
| Jam Sandwich Creams, Sainsbury's* | 1 Biscuit/16g | 77.0 | 3.0 | 486 | 5.0 | 67.0 | 21.8 | 1.6 |
| Jammie Dodgers, Minis. Lunchbox, Burton's* | 1 Pack/20g | 90.0 | 3.0 | 452 | 5.5 | 72.7 | 14.7 | 2.5 |
| Jammie Dodgers, Original, Burton's* | 1 Biscuit/19g | 83.0 | 3.0 | 437 | 5.1 | 69.5 | 15.9 | 1.9 |
| Jestives, Milk Chocolate, Cadbury* | 1 Biscuit/17g | 86.0 | 4.0 | 506 | 6.4 | 64.4 | 24.8 | 0.0 |
| Lebkuchen, Sainsbury's* | 1 Biscuit/10g | 39.0 | 1.0 | 400 | 5.7 | 76.1 | 8.0 | 1.3 |
| Lemon, All Butter, Half Coated, Finest, Tesco* | 1 Biscuit/17g | 84.0 | 4.0 | 505 | 5.6 | 60.4 | 26.9 | 3.6 |
| Lemon & Ginger, Weight Watchers* | 1 Biscuit/11g | 49.0 | 2.0 | 450 | 6.4 | 65.0 | 18.2 | 5.0 |
| Lemon Butter, Thins, Sainsbury's* | 1 Biscuit/13g | 65.0 | 4.0 | 515 | 5.3 | 60.7 | 27.9 | 2.2 |
| Lemon Curd Sandwich, Fox's* | 1 Biscuit/14g | 69.0 | 3.0 | 494 | 4.7 | 66.2 | 23.4 | 1.3 |
| Lemon Puff, Jacob's* | 1 Biscuit/13g | 69.0 | 4.0 | 533 | 4.3 | 58.8 | 31.2 | 2.8 |
| Lemon Thins, Sainsbury's* | 1 Biscuit/10g | 47.0 | 2.0 | 468 | 5.6 | 72.3 | 17.3 | 1.7 |

# BISCUITS

| | Measure INFO/WEIGHT | per Measure KCAL | FAT | Nutrition Values per 100g / 100ml KCAL | PROT | CARB | FAT | FIBRE |
|---|---|---|---|---|---|---|---|---|
| Lincoln, McVitie's* | 1 Biscuit/8g | 41.0 | 2.0 | 514 | 6.3 | 69.0 | 23.6 | 2.0 |
| Lincoln, Sainsbury's* | 1 Biscuit/8g | 40.0 | 2.0 | 479 | 7.2 | 66.1 | 20.6 | 2.1 |
| Malt, Basics* | 1 Biscuit/8g | 36.0 | 1.0 | 470 | 7.1 | 73.6 | 15.7 | 0.0 |
| Malted Milk, Asda* | 1 Biscuit/8g | 39.0 | 2.0 | 490 | 7.0 | 66.0 | 22.0 | 2.0 |
| Malted Milk, Chocolate, Tesco* | 1 Biscuit/10g | 52.0 | 2.0 | 500 | 6.7 | 64.4 | 24.0 | 1.9 |
| Malted Milk, Milk Chocolate, Asda* | 1 Biscuit/11g | 56.0 | 3.0 | 509 | 7.0 | 64.0 | 25.0 | 1.7 |
| Malted Milk, Sainsbury's* | 1 Biscuit/8g | 40.0 | 2.0 | 488 | 7.1 | 65.5 | 21.9 | 2.0 |
| Malted Milk, Tesco* | 1 Biscuit/9g | 43.0 | 2.0 | 490 | 6.6 | 66.7 | 21.8 | 2.0 |
| Marie, Crawfords* | 1 Biscuit/7g | 33.0 | 1.0 | 475 | 7.5 | 76.3 | 15.5 | 2.3 |
| Melts, Carr's* | 1 Biscuit/4g | 20.0 | 1.0 | 468 | 11.0 | 58.3 | 21.2 | 4.9 |
| Milk Chocolate, All Butter, M & S* | 1 Biscuit/14g | 70.0 | 4.0 | 490 | 7.9 | 57.4 | 25.5 | 1.4 |
| Milk Chocolate, Assortment, Cadbury* | 1 Serving/10g | 51.0 | 3.0 | 510 | 6.8 | 61.0 | 26.4 | 0.0 |
| Milk Chocolate, Tesco* | 1 Biscuit/25g | 135.0 | 7.0 | 535 | 6.4 | 62.1 | 29.0 | 1.8 |
| Mini Assortment, M & S* | 1 Biscuit/3g | 12.0 | 1.0 | 480 | 6.1 | 63.9 | 22.5 | 2.8 |
| Mint, Plain Chocolate, Tesco* | 1 Biscuit/25g | 136.0 | 7.0 | 538 | 5.1 | 63.0 | 29.5 | 1.7 |
| Mint, Viscount* | 1 Biscuit/13g | 73.0 | 4.0 | 552 | 5.1 | 60.6 | 28.8 | 1.3 |
| Mixed Seed & Honey, Oaty, Weight Watchers* | 1 Biscuit/22g | 106.0 | 5.0 | 482 | 9.2 | 59.0 | 23.2 | 4.9 |
| Morning Coffee, Asda* | 1 Biscuit/5g | 22.0 | 1.0 | 455 | 8.0 | 72.0 | 15.0 | 2.4 |
| Nice, Asda* | 1 Biscuit/8g | 38.0 | 2.0 | 480 | 6.0 | 68.0 | 21.0 | 2.4 |
| Nice, Cream, Tesco* | 1 Serving/10g | 50.0 | 2.0 | 503 | 5.3 | 66.2 | 24.1 | 1.9 |
| Nice, Fox's* | 1 Biscuit/9g | 39.0 | 2.0 | 450 | 6.3 | 62.4 | 19.4 | 5.0 |
| Nice, Jacob's* | 1 Biscuit/7g | 33.0 | 1.0 | 471 | 6.1 | 68.5 | 19.2 | 1.8 |
| Nice, Sainsbury's* | 1 Biscuit/8g | 39.0 | 2.0 | 485 | 6.5 | 68.0 | 20.8 | 2.4 |
| Nice, Value, Tesco* | 1 Biscuit/5g | 24.0 | 1.0 | 489 | 6.9 | 64.6 | 22.6 | 2.4 |
| Nobbles, Milk Chocolate, Trufree* | 1 Biscuit/13g | 71.0 | 4.0 | 544 | 6.3 | 58.0 | 32.0 | 3.6 |
| Oat, Fruit & Spice, Nairn's* | 1 Biscuit/10g | 43.0 | 1.0 | 425 | 7.8 | 65.3 | 14.7 | 7.6 |
| Oat, Mixed Berries, Nairn's* | 1 Biscuit/10g | 43.0 | 1.0 | 430 | 7.7 | 67.0 | 14.6 | 5.9 |
| Oat, Stem Ginger, Nairn's* | 1 Biscuit/10g | 43.0 | 1.0 | 434 | 8.3 | 66.6 | 14.9 | 5.5 |
| Oat & Wholemeal, Crawfords* | 1 Biscuit/14g | 67.0 | 3.0 | 482 | 7.7 | 64.2 | 21.6 | 4.8 |
| Oat & Wholemeal, Dbc Foodservice* | 1 Biscuit/14g | 67.0 | 3.0 | 466 | 7.1 | 60.8 | 21.7 | 5.5 |
| Oat Crunch, Weight Watchers* | 1 Biscuit/12g | 52.0 | 2.0 | 448 | 7.4 | 65.2 | 17.8 | 6.1 |
| Oat Digestives, Nairn's* | 1 Biscuit/11g | 50.0 | 2.0 | 437 | 12.0 | 57.8 | 17.5 | 7.8 |
| Oaten, Organic, Duchy Originals* | 1 Biscuit/16g | 71.0 | 3.0 | 441 | 9.8 | 62.3 | 16.9 | 5.3 |
| Oatmeal, Asda* | 1 Biscuit/12g | 54.0 | 3.0 | 470 | 6.0 | 62.0 | 22.0 | 6.0 |
| Oatmeal Crunch, Jacob's* | 1 Biscuit/8g | 37.0 | 1.0 | 458 | 6.8 | 65.9 | 18.6 | 3.6 |
| Orange Chocolate, Organic, Duchy Originals* | 1 Biscuit/13g | 64.0 | 4.0 | 509 | 5.5 | 60.0 | 28.0 | 3.0 |
| Orange Sultana, Go Ahead, McVitie's* | 1 Biscuit/15g | 58.0 | 1.0 | 400 | 5.1 | 75.7 | 8.1 | 3.0 |
| Parmesan Cheese, Sainsbury's* | 1 Biscuit/3g | 18.0 | 1.0 | 553 | 14.7 | 56.4 | 29.9 | 1.8 |
| Party Rings, Iced, Fox's* | 1 Biscuit/6g | 29.0 | 1.0 | 459 | 5.1 | 75.8 | 15.0 | 0.0 |
| Peanut Butter, American Style, Sainsbury's* | 1 Biscuit/13g | 63.0 | 3.0 | 504 | 5.2 | 68.7 | 23.1 | 2.2 |
| Peanut Butter Cups, Mini, Hershey* | 1 Cup/8g | 44.0 | 2.0 | 564 | 10.3 | 56.4 | 30.8 | 2.6 |
| Petit Beurre, Stella Artois* | 1 Biscuit/6g | 26.0 | 1.0 | 440 | 9.0 | 73.0 | 15.0 | 0.0 |
| Pink Wafers, Crawfords* | 1 Biscuit/7g | 36.0 | 2.0 | 521 | 2.5 | 68.6 | 26.5 | 1.1 |
| Pink Wafers, Sainsbury's* | 1 Biscuit/8g | 36.0 | 2.0 | 486 | 4.6 | 64.2 | 23.4 | 1.7 |
| Puffin, Chocolate, Asda* | 1 Biscuit/25g | 133.0 | 7.0 | 533 | 5.0 | 63.0 | 29.0 | 1.2 |
| Puffin, Orange, Asda* | 1 Biscuit/25g | 133.0 | 7.0 | 529 | 5.0 | 62.0 | 29.0 | 2.2 |
| Redcurrant Puffs, Eat Well, M & S* | 1 Biscuit/7g | 32.0 | 1.0 | 470 | 5.6 | 67.7 | 19.8 | 2.0 |
| Rich Shorties, Asda* | 1 Biscuit/10g | 50.0 | 2.0 | 486 | 6.0 | 66.0 | 22.0 | 2.0 |
| Rich Tea, 25% Less Fat, Tesco* | 1 Biscuit/10g | 43.0 | 1.0 | 435 | 7.1 | 77.0 | 11.0 | 1.3 |
| Rich Tea, Basics, Sainsbury's* | 1 Biscuit/8g | 35.0 | 1.0 | 450 | 7.1 | 71.3 | 15.2 | 2.9 |
| Rich Tea, BGTY, Sainsbury's* | 1 Biscuit/10g | 43.0 | 1.0 | 430 | 7.8 | 75.9 | 10.6 | 2.4 |
| Rich Tea, Classic, McVitie's* | 1 Biscuit/8g | 38.0 | 1.0 | 453 | 7.1 | 71.2 | 15.5 | 2.9 |
| Rich Tea, Light, McVitie's* | 1 Biscuit/8g | 36.0 | 1.0 | 431 | 7.5 | 75.0 | 11.3 | 3.1 |

## BISCUITS

| | Measure INFO/WEIGHT | per Measure KCAL | FAT | Nutrition Values per 100g / 100ml KCAL | PROT | CARB | FAT | FIBRE |
|---|---|---|---|---|---|---|---|---|
| Rich Tea, Low Fat, M & S* | 1 Biscuit/9g | 40.0 | 1.0 | 435 | 8.3 | 76.7 | 10.5 | 2.4 |
| Rich Tea, Milk Chocolate, Sainsbury's* | 1 Biscuit/13g | 66.0 | 3.0 | 504 | 6.3 | 68.5 | 22.7 | 2.1 |
| Rich Tea, Milk Chocolate Covered, Cadbury* | 1 Biscuit/12g | 60.0 | 3.0 | 490 | 6.6 | 67.6 | 21.4 | 0.0 |
| Rich Tea, Plain Chocolate, Sainsbury's* | 1 Biscuit/13g | 65.0 | 3.0 | 497 | 6.6 | 66.0 | 23.0 | 2.6 |
| Rich Tea, Sainsbury's* | 1 Biscuit/8g | 34.0 | 1.0 | 440 | 7.2 | 72.7 | 13.4 | 3.0 |
| Rich Tea, Tesco* | 1 Biscuit/8g | 36.0 | 1.0 | 460 | 7.3 | 72.4 | 15.2 | 2.3 |
| Rich Tea, Value, Tesco* | 1 Biscuit/8g | 35.0 | 1.0 | 453 | 7.2 | 72.4 | 15.0 | 2.3 |
| Rich Tea Creams, Fox's* | 1 Biscuit/11g | 52.0 | 2.0 | 456 | 5.3 | 62.7 | 20.4 | 1.4 |
| Rich Tea Finger, Tesco* | 1 Finger/5g | 23.0 | 1.0 | 451 | 7.4 | 72.9 | 14.4 | 2.3 |
| Rich Tea Fingers, Morrisons* | 1 Finger/4g | 18.0 | 1.0 | 448 | 7.2 | 72.5 | 14.3 | 3.0 |
| Riva Milk, McVitie's* | 1 Biscuit/25g | 136.0 | 8.0 | 540 | 6.4 | 57.7 | 31.5 | 1.6 |
| Rocky, Chocolate, Fox's* | 1 Biscuit/25g | 125.0 | 7.0 | 510 | 7.3 | 58.7 | 27.0 | 1.7 |
| Rocky, Chocolate & Caramel, Fox's* | 1 Biscuit/21g | 107.0 | 4.0 | 507 | 6.9 | 60.3 | 19.3 | 15.5 |
| Rocky, Funki Fudge, Fox's* | 1 Biscuit/24g | 125.0 | 7.0 | 520 | 6.9 | 60.3 | 27.7 | 1.1 |
| Rocky Rounds, Caramel, Fox's* | 1 Biscuit/15g | 72.0 | 3.0 | 480 | 6.2 | 62.3 | 22.9 | 1.1 |
| Rolo, Nestle* | 1 Biscuit/22g | 110.0 | 6.0 | 498 | 5.4 | 62.0 | 25.4 | 0.6 |
| Rosemary & Raisin, M & S* | 1 Biscuit/7g | 35.0 | 2.0 | 490 | 5.1 | 62.5 | 24.1 | 1.8 |
| Rosemary & Thyme, Savoury, Weight Watchers* | 1 Biscuit/8g | 33.0 | 1.0 | 419 | 8.1 | 55.0 | 18.7 | 13.1 |
| Savoury, Gluten, Wheat & Dairy Free, Sainsbury's* | 1 Biscuit/17g | 77.0 | 3.0 | 467 | 11.7 | 65.1 | 17.7 | 2.4 |
| Savoury, Organic, M & S* | 1 Biscuit/7g | 28.0 | 1.0 | 395 | 7.0 | 58.4 | 14.6 | 8.7 |
| Savoury Seed, Organic, The Village Bakery* | 1 Biscuit/14g | 63.0 | 4.0 | 438 | 12.6 | 42.5 | 26.5 | 7.0 |
| Shortcake, Asda* | 1 Biscuit/14g | 73.0 | 4.0 | 518 | 5.0 | 66.0 | 26.0 | 2.0 |
| Shortcake, Caramel, Mr Kipling* | 1 Biscuit/36g | 182.0 | 10.0 | 506 | 4.2 | 57.6 | 28.8 | 1.3 |
| Shortcake, Caramel, Squares, M & S* | 1 Square/40g | 190.0 | 10.0 | 475 | 5.5 | 59.7 | 23.9 | 1.0 |
| Shortcake, Caramel, Squares, Tesco* | 1 Square/54g | 274.0 | 16.0 | 507 | 4.6 | 54.1 | 30.4 | 0.4 |
| Shortcake, Caramel, Tesco* | 1 Biscuit/45g | 217.0 | 12.0 | 482 | 4.6 | 57.8 | 25.8 | 0.5 |
| Shortcake, Chocolate Caramel, TTD, Sainsbury's* | 1 Biscuit/41g | 211.0 | 13.0 | 515 | 4.6 | 50.3 | 32.8 | 1.4 |
| Shortcake, Cranberry & Caramel, TTD, Sainsbury's* | 1 Biscuit/40g | 192.0 | 11.0 | 480 | 4.0 | 55.4 | 26.9 | 1.3 |
| Shortcake, Dutch, M & S* | 1 Biscuit/17g | 90.0 | 5.0 | 530 | 5.7 | 58.2 | 30.6 | 0.9 |
| Shortcake, Fruit Biscuits, Crawfords* | 1 Biscuit/8g | 34.0 | 2.0 | 419 | 5.4 | 55.9 | 19.3 | 2.4 |
| Shortcake, Jacob's* | 1 Biscuit/10g | 48.0 | 2.0 | 485 | 6.7 | 65.6 | 21.8 | 2.0 |
| Shortcake, Organic, Waitrose* | 1 Biscuit/13g | 64.0 | 3.0 | 495 | 5.8 | 63.0 | 24.4 | 1.8 |
| Shortcake, Sainsbury's* | 1 Biscuit/11g | 53.0 | 2.0 | 484 | 7.2 | 66.6 | 21.0 | 2.0 |
| Shortcake, Snack, Cadbury* | 1 Biscuit/10g | 52.0 | 3.0 | 520 | 7.0 | 62.6 | 26.8 | 0.0 |
| Shortcake, Value, Tesco* | 1 Biscuit/10g | 49.0 | 2.0 | 486 | 7.1 | 66.5 | 21.2 | 2.1 |
| Shortcake, with Real Milk Chocolate, Cadbury* | 1 Biscuit/15g | 75.0 | 4.0 | 500 | 6.3 | 65.8 | 23.5 | 0.0 |
| Shortcake Ring, Creations, Fox's* | 1 Biscuit/20g | 105.0 | 6.0 | 515 | 7.8 | 59.1 | 27.4 | 1.0 |
| Shorties, Cadbury* | 1 Biscuit/15g | 77.0 | 4.0 | 511 | 6.5 | 67.3 | 24.0 | 0.0 |
| Shorties, Fruit, Value, Tesco* | 1 Serving/10g | 46.0 | 2.0 | 457 | 5.7 | 69.3 | 17.4 | 3.0 |
| Shorties, Sainsbury's* | 1 Biscuit/10g | 50.0 | 2.0 | 500 | 6.4 | 69.8 | 21.8 | 2.0 |
| Signature Collection, Cadbury* | 1 Biscuit/15g | 79.0 | 4.0 | 530 | 6.2 | 60.1 | 29.5 | 0.0 |
| Sports, Fox's* | 1 Biscuit/9g | 41.0 | 2.0 | 483 | 6.7 | 67.0 | 20.0 | 2.0 |
| Stem Ginger, Brakes* | 1 Biscuit/13g | 62.0 | 3.0 | 495 | 5.6 | 62.6 | 24.7 | 0.0 |
| Strawberry, Cream Tease, McVitie's* | 1 Biscuit/19g | 97.0 | 5.0 | 510 | 4.8 | 65.9 | 25.2 | 1.2 |
| Sultana & Cinnamon, Weight Watchers* | 1 Biscuit/12g | 51.0 | 2.0 | 441 | 4.3 | 72.3 | 15.0 | 3.0 |
| Taxi, McVitie's* | 1 Biscuit/27g | 134.0 | 7.0 | 504 | 4.2 | 63.3 | 26.0 | 0.7 |
| Teddy Bear, Mini, M & S* | 1 Biscuit/17g | 80.0 | 4.0 | 475 | 5.4 | 62.6 | 22.7 | 3.2 |
| Thins, Belgian Chocolate, TTD, Sainsbury's* | 1 Biscuit/10g | 49.0 | 2.0 | 487 | 6.4 | 64.0 | 22.8 | 0.8 |
| Toffee Chip Crinkle Crunch, Fox's* | 1 Biscuit/11g | 51.0 | 2.0 | 460 | 4.6 | 69.6 | 18.2 | 0.0 |
| Treacle Crunch Creams, Fox's* | 1 Biscuit/13g | 65.0 | 3.0 | 502 | 4.5 | 65.3 | 24.8 | 1.4 |
| Triple Chocolate, Fox's* | 1 Biscuit/21g | 100.0 | 5.0 | 478 | 5.7 | 57.3 | 25.1 | 2.5 |
| Viennese, Jaffa, M & S* | 1 Biscuit/17g | 80.0 | 4.0 | 465 | 5.9 | 61.1 | 21.7 | 0.9 |
| Viennese, Sandwich, Chocolate, M & S* | 1 Biscuit/15g | 80.0 | 5.0 | 535 | 7.2 | 58.0 | 30.6 | 1.7 |

| | Measure INFO/WEIGHT | per Measure KCAL | FAT | Nutrition Values per 100g / 100ml KCAL | PROT | CARB | FAT | FIBRE |
|---|---|---|---|---|---|---|---|---|
| **BISCUITS** | | | | | | | | |
| Viennese Creams, Raspberry, M & S* | 1 Biscuit/17g | 90.0 | 5.0 | 520 | 4.6 | 60.4 | 28.6 | 1.3 |
| Viennese Creams, Strawberry, M & S* | 1 Biscuit/17g | 80.0 | 4.0 | 485 | 6.4 | 63.0 | 22.2 | 1.7 |
| Viennese Finger, Mr Kipling* | 1 Finger/32g | 167.0 | 10.0 | 523 | 4.3 | 54.9 | 31.8 | 0.0 |
| Viennese Whirl, Chocolate, Border* | 1 Biscuit/19g | 96.0 | 4.0 | 512 | 6.5 | 61.9 | 23.2 | 0.0 |
| Viennese Whirl, Fox's* | 1 Biscuit/25g | 129.0 | 7.0 | 518 | 6.7 | 60.1 | 27.8 | 0.0 |
| Water, Asda* | 1 Biscuit/6g | 25.0 | 0.0 | 412 | 10.0 | 75.0 | 8.0 | 3.3 |
| Water, Carr's* | 1 Biscuit/8g | 35.0 | 1.0 | 434 | 10.3 | 79.1 | 7.6 | 3.2 |
| Water, High Bake, Jacob's* | 1 Biscuit/5g | 22.0 | 0.0 | 414 | 10.5 | 76.4 | 7.4 | 3.0 |
| Water, High Bake, Sainsbury's* | 1 Biscuit/5g | 21.0 | 0.0 | 412 | 9.8 | 76.3 | 7.5 | 3.2 |
| Water, High Baked, Tesco* | 1 Biscuit/5g | 20.0 | 0.0 | 405 | 10.1 | 75.0 | 7.1 | 4.2 |
| Water, Table, Large, Carr's* | 1 Biscuit/8g | 35.0 | 1.0 | 434 | 10.3 | 79.1 | 7.6 | 3.2 |
| Water, Table, Small, Carr's* | 1 Biscuit/3g | 15.0 | 0.0 | 438 | 10.4 | 80.0 | 7.7 | 3.3 |
| Wholemeal Brans, Fox's* | 1 Biscuit/20g | 90.0 | 4.0 | 451 | 8.5 | 58.8 | 20.2 | 7.5 |
| Yorkie, Nestle* | 1 Biscuit/25g | 127.0 | 7.0 | 510 | 6.7 | 60.4 | 26.8 | 1.3 |
| Yumbles, McVitie's* | 1 Biscuit/11g | 53.0 | 3.0 | 498 | 5.5 | 58.4 | 26.9 | 2.8 |
| Yumbles, Oat Nibbles, Organic, McVitie's* | 1 Biscuit/11g | 50.0 | 3.0 | 449 | 7.9 | 53.2 | 22.7 | 6.6 |
| **BISON** | | | | | | | | |
| *Raw* | *1oz/28g* | *31.0* | *1.0* | *109* | *21.6* | *0.0* | *1.8* | *0.0* |
| *Roasted* | *1oz/28g* | *41.0* | *1.0* | *143* | *28.4* | *0.0* | *2.4* | *0.0* |
| **BITTER LEMON** | | | | | | | | |
| Low Calorie, Tesco* | 1 Glass/200ml | 6.0 | 0.0 | 3 | 0.1 | 0.3 | 0.1 | 0.1 |
| Sainsbury's* | 1 Glass/250ml | 45.0 | 0.0 | 18 | 0.1 | 4.4 | 0.1 | 0.1 |
| Schweppes* | 1 Glass/250ml | 85.0 | 0.0 | 34 | 0.0 | 8.2 | 0.0 | 0.0 |
| **BLACK GRAM** | | | | | | | | |
| *Urad Gram, Dried, Raw* | *1oz/28g* | *77.0* | *0.0* | *275* | *24.9* | *40.8* | *1.4* | *0.0* |
| **BLACK PUDDING** | | | | | | | | |
| *Average* | *1 Serving/40g* | *101.0* | *6.0* | *252* | *10.2* | *19.0* | *14.9* | *0.6* |
| VLH Kitchens* | 1 Serving/40g | 105.0 | 6.2 | 262 | 11.0 | 20.3 | 15.6 | 0.4 |
| **BLACKBERRIES** | | | | | | | | |
| *Fresh, Raw, Average* | *1oz/28g* | *8.0* | *0.0* | *29* | *0.8* | *6.0* | *0.3* | *1.5* |
| *in Fruit Juice, Average* | *½ Can/145g* | *52.0* | *0.0* | *36* | *0.6* | *7.9* | *0.2* | *1.3* |
| **BLACKCURRANTS** | | | | | | | | |
| Dried, Graze* | 1 Pack/30g | 95.0 | 0.0 | 317 | 3.3 | 79.0 | 1.0 | 0.0 |
| *Fresh, Raw* | *1oz/28g* | *8.0* | *0.0* | *28* | *0.9* | *6.6* | *0.0* | *3.6* |
| *in Fruit Juice, Average* | *1 Serving/30g* | *11.0* | *0.0* | *37* | *0.6* | *8.6* | *0.1* | *2.4* |
| *Stewed with Sugar* | *1oz/28g* | *16.0* | *0.0* | *58* | *0.7* | *15.0* | *0.0* | *2.8* |
| *Stewed without Sugar* | *1oz/28g* | *7.0* | *0.0* | *24* | *0.8* | *5.6* | *0.0* | *3.1* |
| **BLINIS** | | | | | | | | |
| Cocktail, M & S* | ½ Pack/81g | 154.0 | 2.0 | 190 | 6.3 | 35.9 | 2.3 | 2.0 |
| Sausage, Cocktail, Waitrose* | 1 Blini/16g | 30.0 | 0.0 | 190 | 6.3 | 35.9 | 2.3 | 2.0 |
| Smoked Salmon, M & S* | 1oz/28g | 67.0 | 4.0 | 240 | 11.9 | 18.9 | 13.0 | 1.8 |
| **BLISS*** | | | | | | | | |
| Berries, Bliss* | 1 Bottle/275ml | 170.0 | 0.0 | 62 | 0.0 | 7.8 | 0.0 | 0.0 |
| **BLUEBERRIES** | | | | | | | | |
| Chocolate Covered, Waitrose* | 1 Serving/25g | 120.0 | 6.0 | 481 | 4.0 | 65.6 | 22.4 | 3.0 |
| Dried, Graze* | 1 Packet/27g | 82.0 | 0.0 | 302 | 1.4 | 73.0 | 0.5 | 0.0 |
| Dried, Whitworths* | 1 Pack/75g | 226.0 | 0.0 | 301 | 0.9 | 74.2 | 0.1 | 11.4 |
| *Fresh, Raw, Average* | *1 Serving/80g* | *43.0* | *0.0* | *53* | *0.8* | *12.6* | *0.3* | *2.1* |
| **BOAR** | | | | | | | | |
| *Wild, Raw, Average* | *1 Serving/200g* | *244.0* | *7.0* | *122* | *21.5* | *0.0* | *3.3* | *0.0* |
| **BOILED SWEETS** | | | | | | | | |
| Average | 1oz/28g | 92.0 | 0.0 | 327 | 0.0 | 87.1 | 0.0 | 0.0 |
| Blackcurrant & Liquorice, Co-Op* | 1 Sweet/8g | 32.0 | 0.0 | 405 | 0.9 | 91.0 | 5.0 | 0.0 |

| | Measure INFO/WEIGHT | per Measure KCAL | FAT | Nutrition Values per 100g / 100ml KCAL | PROT | CARB | FAT | FIBRE |
|---|---|---|---|---|---|---|---|---|
| **BOILED SWEETS** | | | | | | | | |
| Cherry Drops, Bassett's* | 1 Sweet/5g | 18.0 | 0.0 | 390 | 0.0 | 98.1 | 0.0 | 0.0 |
| Clear Fruits, Sainsbury's* | 1 Sweet/7g | 26.0 | 0.0 | 372 | 0.1 | 92.9 | 0.0 | 0.0 |
| Fruit Drops, Co-Op* | 1 Sweet/6g | 24.0 | 0.0 | 395 | 0.2 | 98.0 | 0.0 | 0.0 |
| Fruit Sherbets, Assorted, M & S* | 1 Sweet/8g | 34.0 | 1.0 | 425 | 0.0 | 89.7 | 7.3 | 0.0 |
| Lockets, Mars* | 1 Pack/43g | 165.0 | 0.0 | 383 | 0.0 | 95.8 | 0.0 | 0.0 |
| Mentho-Lyptus, Cherry, Sugar Free, Hall's* | 1 Lozenge/4g | 8.0 | 0.0 | 234 | 0.0 | 62.4 | 0.0 | 0.0 |
| Mentho-Lyptus, Extra Strong, Hall's* | 1 Lozenge/4g | 14.0 | 0.0 | 389 | 0.0 | 96.9 | 0.0 | 0.0 |
| Pear Drops, Bassett's* | 1 Sweet/4g | 16.0 | 0.0 | 390 | 0.0 | 96.4 | 0.0 | 0.0 |
| Soothers, Blackcurrant, Hall's* | 1 Lozenge/5g | 16.0 | 0.0 | 365 | 0.0 | 91.4 | 0.0 | 0.0 |
| Soothers, Cherry, Hall's* | 1 Pack/45g | 165.0 | 0.0 | 365 | 0.0 | 91.3 | 0.0 | 0.0 |
| **BOK CHOY** | | | | | | | | |
| Tesco* | 1 Serving/100g | 11.0 | 0.0 | 11 | 1.0 | 1.4 | 0.2 | 1.2 |
| **BOLOGNESE** | | | | | | | | |
| Beef, 2 Minute Meals, Sainsbury's* | 1 Pack/200g | 144.0 | 7.0 | 72 | 4.2 | 5.6 | 3.6 | 1.8 |
| Beef, Asda* | 1 Pack/392g | 412.0 | 20.0 | 105 | 8.0 | 7.0 | 5.0 | 0.0 |
| Meatless, Granose* | 1 Pack/400g | 400.0 | 16.0 | 100 | 8.0 | 8.0 | 4.0 | 0.0 |
| Pasta Shells, Canned, 98% Fat Free, BGTY, Sainsbury's* | ½ Can/200g | 174.0 | 4.0 | 87 | 5.5 | 11.5 | 2.1 | 0.7 |
| Penne, Heinz* | 1 Pack/300g | 213.0 | 3.0 | 71 | 3.8 | 11.8 | 0.9 | 0.6 |
| Shells, Italiana, Weight Watchers* | 1 Can/395g | 280.0 | 5.0 | 71 | 5.2 | 9.6 | 1.3 | 0.7 |
| Tagliatelle, Weight Watchers* | 1 Serving/300g | 300.0 | 5.0 | 100 | 5.5 | 15.4 | 1.8 | 0.1 |
| Vegetarian, M & S* | 1 Pack/360g | 360.0 | 13.0 | 100 | 4.5 | 12.5 | 3.5 | 2.1 |
| **BOMBAY MIX** | | | | | | | | |
| Average | 1oz/28g | 141.0 | 9.0 | 503 | 18.8 | 35.1 | 32.9 | 6.2 |
| **BON BONS** | | | | | | | | |
| Apple, Lemon & Strawberry, Co-Op* | ¼ Bag/50g | 202.0 | 2.0 | 405 | 1.0 | 88.0 | 5.0 | 0.0 |
| Bassett's* | 1 Sweet/7g | 28.0 | 0.0 | 417 | 1.1 | 85.4 | 7.5 | 0.0 |
| Fruit, Bassett's* | 1 Serving/7g | 25.0 | 0.0 | 380 | 0.1 | 94.2 | 0.0 | 0.0 |
| Lemon, Bassett's* | 1 Sweet/7g | 30.0 | 1.0 | 425 | 0.0 | 83.7 | 9.8 | 0.0 |
| **BOOST** | | | | | | | | |
| Treat Size, Cadbury* | 1 Bar/24g | 130.0 | 7.0 | 535 | 5.3 | 59.6 | 30.5 | 0.0 |
| with Glucose, Cadbury* | 1 Bar/61g | 315.0 | 18.0 | 521 | 5.6 | 58.0 | 29.4 | 4.0 |
| with Glucose & Guarana, Cadbury* | 1 Bar/61g | 314.0 | 18.0 | 515 | 5.5 | 56.7 | 29.5 | 0.0 |
| **BOUILLON** | | | | | | | | |
| Beef, Benedicta* | 1 fl oz/30ml | 22.0 | 0.0 | 73 | 7.5 | 9.5 | 0.5 | 0.0 |
| Chicken, Benedicta* | 1 fl oz/30ml | 22.0 | 1.0 | 75 | 4.0 | 8.0 | 3.0 | 5.6 |
| Fish, Benedicta* | 1 fl oz/30ml | 21.0 | 0.0 | 69 | 7.5 | 9.0 | 0.3 | 0.0 |
| Powder, Miso, Marigold* | 1 Tsp/5g | 12.0 | 0.0 | 248 | 7.0 | 34.0 | 9.3 | 1.4 |
| Powder, Swiss Vegetable, Green Tub, Marigold* | 1 Tsp/5g | 12.0 | 0.0 | 243 | 10.5 | 29.4 | 8.1 | 0.7 |
| Vegetable, Benedicta* | 1 fl oz/30ml | 30.0 | 0.0 | 101 | 7.5 | 17.0 | 0.3 | 0.0 |
| Vegetable, Herbamare Concentre* | 1 Serving/5g | 15.0 | 1.0 | 298 | 4.6 | 13.5 | 25.4 | 0.3 |
| **BOUNTY** | | | | | | | | |
| Calapuno, Mars* | 1 Pack/175g | 919.0 | 55.0 | 525 | 6.3 | 54.3 | 31.4 | 0.0 |
| Dark, Mars* | 1 Funsize/29g | 137.0 | 8.0 | 471 | 3.2 | 54.1 | 26.8 | 0.0 |
| Milk, Mars* | 1 Funsize/29g | 137.0 | 7.0 | 471 | 3.7 | 56.4 | 25.6 | 0.0 |
| **BOURNVITA** | | | | | | | | |
| Powder, Made Up with Semi-Skimmed Milk | 1 Mug/227ml | 132.0 | 4.0 | 58 | 3.5 | 7.8 | 1.6 | 0.0 |
| Powder, Made Up with Whole Milk | 1 Mug/227ml | 173.0 | 9.0 | 76 | 3.4 | 7.6 | 3.8 | 0.0 |
| **BOVRIL** | | | | | | | | |
| Beef Extract, Bovril* | 1 Tsp/5g | 10.0 | 0.0 | 197 | 10.8 | 29.3 | 4.1 | 0.0 |
| Chicken Savoury Drink, Bovril* | 1 Serving/13g | 16.0 | 0.0 | 129 | 9.7 | 19.4 | 1.4 | 2.1 |
| **BOYSENBERRIES** | | | | | | | | |
| *Canned, in Syrup* | *1oz/28g* | *25.0* | *0.0* | *88* | *1.0* | *20.4* | *0.1* | *1.6* |

| | Measure INFO/WEIGHT | per Measure KCAL | FAT | Nutrition Values per 100g / 100ml KCAL | PROT | CARB | FAT | FIBRE |
|---|---|---|---|---|---|---|---|---|
| **BRANDY** | | | | | | | | |
| *37.5% Volume, Average* | *1 Shot/35ml* | *72.0* | *0.0* | *207* | *0.0* | *0.0* | *0.0* | *0.0* |
| *40% Volume, Average* | *1 Shot/35ml* | *78.0* | *0.0* | *222* | *0.0* | *0.0* | *0.0* | *0.0* |
| *Cherry, Average* | *1 Shot/35ml* | *89.0* | *0.0* | *255* | *0.0* | *32.6* | *0.0* | *0.0* |
| **BRAZIL NUTS** | | | | | | | | |
| *Average* | *6 Whole/20g* | *137.0* | *14.0* | *687* | *15.5* | *2.9* | *68.3* | *4.9* |
| Milk Chocolate, Tesco* | 1 Nut/8g | 47.0 | 3.0 | 585 | 9.9 | 38.0 | 43.7 | 1.9 |
| **BREAD** | | | | | | | | |
| 50/50, Wholemeal & White, Medium Sliced, Kingsmill* | 1 Slice/40g | 90.0 | 1.0 | 225 | 9.9 | 41.2 | 2.3 | 4.9 |
| Apricot & Sesame Seed, Lifefibre* | 1 Slice/43g | 148.0 | 4.0 | 344 | 8.1 | 55.0 | 10.3 | 6.2 |
| Bagel, Blueberry, Sara Lee* | 1 Bagel/104g | 290.0 | 1.0 | 279 | 9.6 | 58.6 | 1.4 | 1.9 |
| Bagel, Caramelised Onion & Poppyseed, Waitrose* | 1 Bagel/86g | 222.0 | 2.0 | 258 | 9.7 | 49.2 | 2.5 | 2.4 |
| Bagel, Cinnamon & Raisin, New York Bagel Co* | 1 Bagel/85g | 215.0 | 2.0 | 253 | 7.7 | 51.1 | 2.0 | 4.5 |
| Bagel, Cinnamon & Raisin, Tesco* | 1 Bagel/85g | 223.0 | 2.0 | 262 | 10.3 | 51.0 | 1.9 | 2.1 |
| Bagel, Fruit & Spice, Sainsbury's* | 1 Bagel/85g | 234.0 | 2.0 | 275 | 9.7 | 54.3 | 2.1 | 3.8 |
| Bagel, Granary, Bagel Factory* | 1 Bagel/100g | 288.0 | 2.0 | 288 | 11.9 | 57.4 | 2.1 | 4.5 |
| Bagel, High Bran & Seed, Food Doctor* | 1 Bagel/85g | 239.0 | 7.0 | 281 | 10.7 | 41.3 | 7.8 | 6.3 |
| Bagel, High Bran & Seed, with Cranberry, The Food Doctor* | 1 Bagel/85g | 212.0 | 2.0 | 250 | 10.8 | 47.4 | 1.9 | 6.7 |
| Bagel, Mini, Sainsbury's* | 1 Bagel/25g | 67.0 | 0.0 | 268 | 11.2 | 52.4 | 1.6 | 2.8 |
| Bagel, Multigrain, Sainsbury's* | 1 Bagel/113g | 293.0 | 4.0 | 259 | 10.0 | 49.6 | 3.1 | 2.0 |
| Bagel, Onion, New York Bagel Co* | 1 Bagel/85g | 222.0 | 2.0 | 261 | 10.6 | 50.3 | 1.9 | 3.1 |
| Bagel, Onion, Tesco* | 1 Bagel/85g | 233.0 | 2.0 | 274 | 10.5 | 52.4 | 2.4 | 1.9 |
| Bagel, Onion & Poppy Seed, Tesco* | 1 Bagel/85g | 217.0 | 3.0 | 255 | 10.0 | 46.7 | 3.1 | 3.6 |
| Bagel, Original, Organic, New York Bagel Co* | 1 Bagel/85g | 220.0 | 1.0 | 259 | 9.3 | 52.2 | 1.4 | 4.1 |
| Bagel, Plain | 1 Bagel/104g | 290.0 | 2.0 | 279 | 10.6 | 53.8 | 1.9 | 2.9 |
| Bagel, Plain, Asda* | 1 Bagel/85g | 226.0 | 2.0 | 265 | 15.0 | 46.0 | 2.3 | 2.9 |
| *Bagel, Plain, Average* | *1 Bagel/78g* | *215.0* | *1.0* | *276* | *10.7* | *53.6* | *1.5* | *0.0* |
| Bagel, Plain, Tesco* | 1 Bagel/85g | 220.0 | 2.0 | 259 | 9.8 | 50.2 | 2.1 | 1.8 |
| Bagel, Plain, Value, Tesco* | 1 Bagel/71g | 181.0 | 1.0 | 255 | 10.3 | 51.7 | 0.8 | 3.7 |
| Bagel, Poppy Seed, New York Bagel Co* | 1 Bagel/85g | 233.0 | 2.0 | 274 | 11.4 | 50.8 | 2.8 | 3.2 |
| Bagel, Rye, Bagel Factory* | 1 Bagel/85g | 279.0 | 1.0 | 329 | 14.5 | 64.3 | 1.5 | 6.2 |
| Bagel, Sesame, M & S* | 1 Bagel/87g | 240.0 | 3.0 | 275 | 10.2 | 51.2 | 3.2 | 2.1 |
| Bagel, Sesame, New York Bagel Co* | 1 Bagel/85g | 226.0 | 3.0 | 266 | 10.3 | 49.2 | 3.1 | 4.0 |
| Bagel, Sesame Seed, GFY, Asda* | 1 Bagel/84g | 227.0 | 2.0 | 271 | 11.0 | 51.0 | 2.5 | 2.6 |
| Bagel, Wholemeal, Multiseed, M & S* | 1 Bagel/84g | 215.0 | 6.0 | 255 | 13.1 | 35.4 | 6.6 | 8.3 |
| Baguette, Crusty Brown, M & S* | ½ Loaf/71g | 160.0 | 1.0 | 225 | 9.8 | 42.7 | 1.6 | 6.3 |
| Baguette, Mediterranean Herb, Sainsbury's* | 1 Serving/60g | 203.0 | 9.0 | 339 | 8.5 | 40.8 | 15.7 | 2.3 |
| Baguette, Part Baked, Half, Tesco* | ½ Baguette/75g | 180.0 | 1.0 | 240 | 7.8 | 49.5 | 1.2 | 3.4 |
| Baguette, Ready to Bake, Sainsbury's* | ½ Baguette/62g | 150.0 | 1.0 | 242 | 7.8 | 49.7 | 1.3 | 2.8 |
| Baguette, White, Half, Crusty, M & S* | 1 Baguette/162g | 420.0 | 2.0 | 260 | 8.4 | 53.5 | 1.1 | 2.3 |
| Baguette, White, Homebake, Tesco* | 1 Baguette/135g | 331.0 | 2.0 | 245 | 7.8 | 49.7 | 1.3 | 2.5 |
| Baguette, White, Ready to Bake, Asda* | 1 Serving/60g | 168.0 | 1.0 | 280 | 10.0 | 56.0 | 1.8 | 2.6 |
| Baguette, White, Sainsbury's* | 1 Serving/50g | 131.0 | 1.0 | 263 | 9.3 | 53.1 | 1.5 | 2.7 |
| Baguette, Wholemeal, Part Baked, Asda* | ½ Baguette/75g | 176.0 | 1.0 | 235 | 8.2 | 47.7 | 1.3 | 3.0 |
| Baps, Brown, Large, Asda* | 1 Bap/58g | 140.0 | 1.0 | 242 | 10.0 | 47.0 | 1.6 | 0.0 |
| Baps, Brown, Malted Grain, Large, Tesco* | 1 Bap/93g | 228.0 | 3.0 | 245 | 9.9 | 42.7 | 3.3 | 5.3 |
| Baps, Cheese Topped, White, Tesco* | 1oz/28g | 86.0 | 2.0 | 307 | 12.2 | 48.0 | 7.0 | 0.7 |
| Baps, Floured, M & S* | 1 Bap/60g | 168.0 | 4.0 | 280 | 11.5 | 46.8 | 6.2 | 2.0 |
| Baps, Giant Malted, Sainsbury's* | 1 Bap/109g | 282.0 | 5.0 | 260 | 8.6 | 45.7 | 4.8 | 5.7 |
| Baps, Multigrain, Tesco* | 1 Serving/98g | 238.0 | 3.0 | 244 | 8.7 | 45.1 | 3.2 | 1.9 |
| Baps, White, Floured, Waitrose* | 1 Bap/60g | 147.0 | 1.0 | 244 | 8.0 | 48.6 | 2.0 | 1.1 |
| Baps, White, Giant, Sainsbury's* | 1 Bap/86g | 235.0 | 3.0 | 273 | 8.3 | 51.7 | 3.7 | 3.4 |
| Baps, White, Giant, Waitrose* | 1 Bap/104g | 260.0 | 4.0 | 250 | 9.5 | 45.0 | 3.6 | 4.8 |
| Baps, White, Large, Tesco* | 1 Bap/95g | 252.0 | 4.0 | 265 | 8.7 | 46.2 | 4.5 | 2.4 |

# BREAD

| | Measure INFO/WEIGHT | per Measure KCAL | FAT | Nutrition Values per 100g / 100ml KCAL | PROT | CARB | FAT | FIBRE |
|---|---|---|---|---|---|---|---|---|
| Baps, White, Sliced, Large, Asda* | 1 Bap/58g | 148.0 | 1.0 | 255 | 10.0 | 50.0 | 1.7 | 0.0 |
| Baps, White, Soft, Floured, M & S* | 1 Bap/63g | 176.0 | 4.0 | 280 | 11.5 | 46.8 | 6.2 | 2.0 |
| Baps, White, Warburton's* | 1 Bap/57g | 144.0 | 2.0 | 252 | 9.8 | 43.4 | 4.3 | 2.7 |
| Baps, Wholemeal, Giant, Rathbones* | 1 Bap/110g | 230.0 | 2.0 | 209 | 9.4 | 39.0 | 1.9 | 8.0 |
| Baps, Wholemeal, Tesco* | 1 Bap/46g | 104.0 | 2.0 | 227 | 9.6 | 41.4 | 5.3 | 5.6 |
| Baps, Wholemeal, Waitrose* | 1 Bap/67g | 156.0 | 3.0 | 234 | 10.6 | 37.2 | 4.8 | 6.7 |
| Black Olive, Finest, Tesco* | 1 Serving/72g | 184.0 | 5.0 | 255 | 9.7 | 39.7 | 6.4 | 2.9 |
| Bloomer, COU, M & S* | 1 Slice/33g | 78.0 | 0.0 | 235 | 9.5 | 45.5 | 1.5 | 3.6 |
| Bloomer, Multi Seed, Organic, Sainsbury's* | 1 Serving/60g | 160.0 | 4.0 | 266 | 10.9 | 40.3 | 6.8 | 8.8 |
| Bloomer, Multiseed, Finest, Tesco* | 1 Slice/50g | 100.0 | 2.0 | 200 | 12.8 | 28.4 | 3.8 | 11.1 |
| Bloomer, White, Sliced, Waitrose* | 1 Slice/50g | 129.0 | 1.0 | 259 | 8.5 | 52.1 | 1.8 | 2.6 |
| Bloomer, Wholemeal, Organic, M & S* | 1 Slice/50g | 110.0 | 2.0 | 220 | 10.2 | 35.5 | 4.2 | 6.4 |
| Brioche, Loaf, Butter, Sainsbury's* | 1/8 Loaf/50g | 173.0 | 5.0 | 347 | 8.0 | 55.0 | 10.5 | 2.2 |
| Brioche, Rolls, Butter, Tesco* | 1 Serving/35g | 127.0 | 4.0 | 363 | 8.6 | 56.0 | 11.4 | 3.7 |
| Brioche, Rolls, Chocolate Chip, Tesco* | 1 Serving/35g | 131.0 | 6.0 | 374 | 8.6 | 49.1 | 16.0 | 6.0 |
| Brioche, Rolls, Tesco* | 1 Roll/26g | 92.0 | 3.0 | 349 | 8.5 | 54.0 | 11.0 | 0.0 |
| Brown, Danish, Sliced, Weight Watchers* | 1 Slice/20g | 44.0 | 0.0 | 216 | 11.3 | 38.7 | 2.0 | 7.3 |
| Brown, Danish, Warburton's* | 1 Slice/21g | 44.0 | 0.0 | 213 | 11.1 | 38.9 | 1.9 | 7.2 |
| Brown, Gluten & Wheat Free, Sliced | 1 Slice/25g | 56.0 | 1.0 | 224 | 3.4 | 41.0 | 5.2 | 9.4 |
| Brown, Gluten Free, Genius* | 1 Slice/35g | 97.0 | 5.0 | 277 | 6.7 | 42.2 | 13.3 | 9.5 |
| Brown, High Fibre, Ormo* | 1 Slice/24g | 57.0 | 1.0 | 239 | 9.2 | 42.9 | 2.6 | 7.5 |
| Brown, Kingsmill Gold, Seeds & Oats, Kingsmill* | 1 Slice/45g | 126.0 | 4.0 | 280 | 12.2 | 35.6 | 9.8 | 4.9 |
| *Brown, Medium Sliced* | *1 Slice/34g* | *74.0* | *1.0* | *218* | *8.5* | *44.3* | *2.0* | *3.5* |
| Brown, Medium Sliced, Asda* | 1 Slice/36g | 78.0 | 1.0 | 216 | 8.0 | 42.0 | 1.8 | 4.1 |
| Brown, Medium Sliced, Sainsbury's* | 1 Slice/36g | 81.0 | 1.0 | 225 | 8.2 | 43.8 | 1.9 | 3.9 |
| Brown, Medium Sliced, Tesco* | 1 Slice/36g | 78.0 | 1.0 | 218 | 8.0 | 41.6 | 2.2 | 4.5 |
| Brown, Multi Grain, Wheat Free, Gluten Free | 1 Slice/33g | 76.0 | 2.0 | 229 | 5.1 | 40.8 | 5.1 | 5.6 |
| Brown, Premium Gold Malted, TTD, Sainsbury's* | 1 Slice/43g | 93.0 | 1.0 | 217 | 8.5 | 40.3 | 2.4 | 2.4 |
| Brown, Sainsbury's* | 1 Slice/34g | 81.0 | 1.0 | 239 | 8.4 | 46.8 | 2.1 | 4.2 |
| Brown, Seeded Batch, Large Loaf, 800g, Warburton's* | 1 Slice/46g | 132.0 | 4.0 | 288 | 12.3 | 39.7 | 8.9 | 6.0 |
| Brown, Sliced, Free From, Tesco* | 1 Slice/45g | 121.0 | 4.0 | 268 | 5.4 | 43.2 | 8.2 | 3.6 |
| Brown, Soda, M & S* | 1 Slice/40g | 92.0 | 1.0 | 229 | 9.2 | 43.6 | 3.6 | 4.9 |
| Brown, Thick Slice, Tesco* | 1 Serving/50g | 109.0 | 1.0 | 219 | 10.3 | 38.9 | 2.5 | 5.3 |
| Brown, Thin Sliced, Sainsbury's* | 1 Slice/29g | 65.0 | 1.0 | 225 | 8.2 | 43.8 | 1.9 | 3.9 |
| *Brown, Toasted, Average* | *1 Med Slice/24g* | *65.0* | *1.0* | *272* | *10.4* | *56.5* | *2.1* | *4.5* |
| Brown, Toastie, Thick Sliced, Kingsmill* | 1 Slice/44g | 101.0 | 1.0 | 230 | 9.5 | 40.5 | 3.3 | 4.7 |
| Brown, Wholemeal, Healthy Choice, Warburton's* | 1 Slice/24g | 55.0 | 1.0 | 231 | 10.4 | 40.7 | 2.5 | 6.5 |
| Buns, Burger, Sainsbury's* | 1 Bun/56g | 154.0 | 3.0 | 275 | 9.2 | 47.8 | 5.2 | 4.1 |
| Buns, White, Burger, Waitrose* | 1 Serving/64g | 169.0 | 2.0 | 264 | 10.0 | 47.2 | 3.9 | 2.7 |
| *Challah, Average* | *1 Slice/50g* | *143.0* | *4.0* | *286* | *8.9* | *53.6* | *7.1* | *3.6* |
| Cheese, Onion & Garlic, Tear & Share, Waitrose* | ¼ Bread/112g | 326.0 | 15.0 | 290 | 9.4 | 33.9 | 13.0 | 2.1 |
| Cheese, Onion Mustard Seed, Cluster, Sainsbury's* | 1 Cluster/100g | 276.0 | 8.0 | 276 | 10.0 | 40.6 | 8.1 | 3.1 |
| Cheese, Tear & Share, Tesco* | ¼ Loaf/73g | 225.0 | 8.0 | 310 | 8.8 | 44.0 | 10.7 | 0.8 |
| Cheese & Garlic, Pizza Style, Sainsbury's* | ¼ Bread/63g | 199.0 | 8.0 | 318 | 10.7 | 39.7 | 13.0 | 2.2 |
| Cheese & Garlic, Stonebaked, Morrisons* | ¼ Bread/69g | 228.0 | 10.0 | 331 | 10.9 | 39.5 | 14.4 | 1.9 |
| Cheese & Onion, Tear & Share, Sainsbury's* | ¼ Bread/71g | 202.0 | 7.0 | 285 | 9.8 | 40.6 | 9.3 | 1.9 |
| Cheese & Onion, Toastie, Warburton's* | 1 Slice/42g | 120.0 | 6.0 | 286 | 7.5 | 33.1 | 13.7 | 0.0 |
| Cheese & Tomato, Tear & Share, Sainsbury's* | ¼ Bread/72g | 211.0 | 10.0 | 293 | 8.0 | 35.7 | 13.2 | 1.5 |
| *Cholla, Average* | *1/10 Loaf/154g* | *421.0* | *14.0* | *274* | *6.9* | *40.8* | *9.3* | *1.0* |
| Ciabatta, Black Olive, Part Baked, Sainsbury's* | ¼ Ciabatta/67g | 172.0 | 3.0 | 257 | 8.8 | 46.8 | 3.8 | 2.4 |
| Ciabatta, Finest, Tesco* | 1/6 Ciabatta/45g | 124.0 | 3.0 | 275 | 10.4 | 44.8 | 5.9 | 2.7 |
| Ciabatta, Garlic & Herb, GFY, Asda* | ¼ Ciabatta/60g | 137.0 | 1.0 | 230 | 8.8 | 43.2 | 2.4 | 1.0 |
| Ciabatta, Half, M & S* | 1 Ciabatta/135g | 354.0 | 6.0 | 262 | 10.3 | 48.1 | 4.1 | 2.1 |

# BREAD

| INFO/WEIGHT | Measure KCAL | FAT | Nutrition Values per 100g / 100ml KCAL | PROT | CARB | FAT | FIBRE |
|---|---|---|---|---|---|---|---|
| Ciabatta, Half, Organic, Sainsbury's* | ½ Ciabatta/63g 152.0 | 1.0 | 241 | 9.1 | 48.7 | 1.0 | 2.3 |
| Ciabatta, Half, Tesco* | 1 Ciabatta/135g 351.0 | 5.0 | 260 | 8.9 | 47.7 | 3.5 | 2.2 |
| Ciabatta, Italian Style, Waitrose* | 1 Ciabatta/89g 231.0 | 1.0 | 260 | 10.7 | 51.2 | 1.3 | 2.2 |
| Ciabatta, Olive & Rosemary, Mini, Tesco* | 1 Pack/75g 319.0 | 8.0 | 425 | 17.8 | 63.0 | 10.9 | 3.6 |
| Ciabatta, Oregano & Feta, TTD, Sainsbury's* | ½ Ciabatta/200g 574.0 | 22.0 | 287 | 10.4 | 36.5 | 11.0 | 2.4 |
| Ciabatta, Organic, Tesco* | 1/3 Ciabatta/100g 240.0 | 4.0 | 240 | 8.7 | 43.2 | 3.6 | 2.4 |
| Ciabatta, Plain, Tesco* | ¼ Ciabatta/73g 174.0 | 3.0 | 240 | 9.8 | 41.5 | 3.9 | 2.4 |
| Ciabatta, Ready to Bake, M & S* | 1 Serving/150g 393.0 | 6.0 | 262 | 10.3 | 48.1 | 4.1 | 2.1 |
| Ciabatta, Ready to Bake, Sainsbury's* | ½ Ciabatta/66g 172.0 | 2.0 | 260 | 8.9 | 47.7 | 3.7 | 2.2 |
| Ciabatta, Sun Dried Tomato & Basil, Tesco* | ¼ Ciabatta/75g 193.0 | 4.0 | 257 | 8.9 | 42.4 | 5.7 | 2.4 |
| Ciabatta, Sun Dried Tomato & Olive, TTD, Sainsbury's* | 1 Serving/62g 161.0 | 4.0 | 260 | 10.0 | 39.7 | 6.8 | 2.5 |
| Ciabatta, Sweet Pepper, HE, Tesco^ | 1 Serving/50g 135.0 | 1.0 | 270 | 11.8 | 49.5 | 2.7 | 2.8 |
| Ciabatta, Tomato & Basil, GFY, Asda* | 1 Serving/55g 143.0 | 1.0 | 260 | 9.0 | 51.0 | 2.2 | 0.0 |
| Ciabatta Stick, Organic, M & S* | 1 Stick/140g 315.0 | 2.0 | 225 | 8.9 | 48.5 | 1.4 | 4.2 |
| Cinnamon Swirl, Asda* | 1 Serving/25g 87.0 | 3.0 | 349 | 6.0 | 52.0 | 13.0 | 1.6 |
| Cottage Loaf, Stonebaked, Asda* | 1 Serving/67g 155.0 | 1.0 | 232 | 10.0 | 45.0 | 1.3 | 3.2 |
| Farmhouse, Poppy Seed, Crusty, Loaf, M & S* | 1 Slice/40g 104.0 | 1.0 | 260 | 9.4 | 47.6 | 3.3 | 2.3 |
| Farmhouse, with Oatmeal, Batch, Finest, Tesco* | 1 Slice/50g 122.0 | 2.0 | 245 | 10.5 | 40.8 | 4.3 | 4.9 |
| Fiery Green Pepper & Cheese, The Best, Safeway* | ¼ Loaf/75g 180.0 | 3.0 | 240 | 12.3 | 38.4 | 4.1 | 3.4 |
| Flatbread, Garlic, BGTY, Sainsbury's* | ¼ Bread/56g 177.0 | 6.0 | 316 | 9.6 | 46.6 | 10.1 | 2.7 |
| Flatbread, Garlic, Tesco* | 1 Serving/83g 249.0 | 9.0 | 302 | 6.7 | 45.3 | 10.4 | 3.0 |
| Flatbread, Garlic & Herb, Tear & Share, Sainsbury's* | ¼ Bread/68g 201.0 | 6.0 | 297 | 10.9 | 42.5 | 9.3 | 3.7 |
| Focaccia, Onion & Herb, Tesco* | ½ Pack/190g 547.0 | 24.0 | 288 | 8.7 | 35.2 | 12.5 | 3.7 |
| Focaccia, Oregano, The Best, Safeway* | 1 Serving/56g 150.0 | 3.0 | 270 | 9.1 | 45.0 | 5.7 | 1.8 |
| Focaccia, Roast Cherry Tomato & Olive, GFY, Asda* | ½ Pack/148g 350.0 | 6.0 | 237 | 9.0 | 41.0 | 4.1 | 2.8 |
| Focaccia, Roasted Onion & Cheese, M & S* | 1 Serving/89g 240.0 | 4.0 | 270 | 10.4 | 45.7 | 4.6 | 2.8 |
| Focaccia, Rolls, Rosemary & Rock Salt, TTD, Sainsbury's* | 1 Roll/120g 344.0 | 10.0 | 287 | 10.5 | 42.7 | 8.2 | 3.3 |
| Focaccia, Safeway* | 1/6 Bread/47g 131.0 | 3.0 | 279 | 9.5 | 46.9 | 5.9 | 3.4 |
| Foccacia, Mixed Herb, TTD, Sainsbury's* | 1 Serving/67g 179.0 | 6.0 | 269 | 9.7 | 38.0 | 8.7 | 3.8 |
| Foccacia, Tomato & Cheese, TTD, Sainsbury's* | 1 Serving/67g 167.0 | 5.0 | 251 | 10.4 | 35.5 | 7.5 | 3.8 |
| French | 1.5" Slice/45g 110.0 | 0.0 | 244 | 8.9 | 53.3 | 0.0 | 2.2 |
| French, Sliced, Parisian* | 2 Slices/39g 100.0 | 1.0 | 256 | 5.1 | 48.7 | 2.6 | 0.0 |
| **French Stick, Average** | **1 Serving/60g 162.0** | **2.0** | **270** | **9.6** | **55.4** | **2.7** | **1.5** |
| Fruit, Raisin Swirl, Sun-Maid* | 1 Slice/33g 95.0 | 2.0 | 287 | 8.3 | 50.4 | 5.8 | 2.6 |
| Fruit & Cinnamon Loaf, Finest, Tesco* | 1 Slice/37g 134.0 | 5.0 | 363 | 6.4 | 54.6 | 13.2 | 1.5 |
| Fruit Loaf, Apple, M & S* | 1 Slice/39g 100.0 | 1.0 | 255 | 8.5 | 51.9 | 1.5 | 3.3 |
| Fruit Loaf, Banana, Soreen* | 1 Slice/25g 78.0 | 1.0 | 313 | 6.8 | 60.9 | 4.7 | 0.0 |
| Fruit Loaf, Mixed Berry, Weight Watchers* | 1 Slice/34g 79.0 | 1.0 | 231 | 7.6 | 44.3 | 2.6 | 7.7 |
| Fruit Loaf, Mother's Pride* | 1 Slice/36g 92.0 | 1.0 | 256 | 8.2 | 49.3 | 2.9 | 2.6 |
| Fruit Loaf, Sliced, Sainsbury's* | 1 Slice/40g 104.0 | 1.0 | 260 | 8.9 | 47.9 | 3.6 | 2.4 |
| Fruit Loaf, Sliced, Tesco* | 1 Slice/36g 100.0 | 2.0 | 278 | 6.9 | 51.2 | 5.1 | 3.7 |
| Fruit Loaf, Sultana & Cherry, Sainsbury's* | 1 Slice/50g 178.0 | 6.0 | 357 | 2.7 | 59.0 | 12.2 | 1.7 |
| Fruit Loaf, with Orange, Warburton's* | 1 Slice/33g 89.0 | 1.0 | 268 | 7.7 | 51.5 | 3.4 | 3.0 |
| Fruit Loaf, with Strawberry, Summer, Warburton's* | 1 Slice/35g 92.0 | 1.0 | 262 | 7.7 | 50.3 | 3.3 | 3.0 |
| Garlic, & Herb, Giant Feast, Sainsbury's* | 1 Serving/50g 158.0 | 6.0 | 317 | 8.0 | 42.1 | 12.9 | 2.6 |
| Garlic, & Herb, Tear & Share, Tesco* | 1 Serving/73g 217.0 | 9.0 | 300 | 6.3 | 40.0 | 12.7 | 1.7 |
| Garlic, & Parsley, Tesco* | 1 Loaf/230g 699.0 | 27.0 | 304 | 9.0 | 41.0 | 11.6 | 2.7 |
| Garlic, & Tomato, Pizza, Italiano, Tesco* | ½ Bread/140g 405.0 | 15.0 | 289 | 7.5 | 40.5 | 10.8 | 2.5 |
| Garlic, 25% Less Fat, Sainsbury's* | ½ Baguette/85g 268.0 | 12.0 | 315 | 7.8 | 39.4 | 14.0 | 3.1 |
| Garlic, Baguette, 50% Less Fat, Asda* | ¼ Baguette/43g 123.0 | 3.0 | 287 | 10.0 | 46.0 | 7.0 | 2.5 |
| Garlic, Baguette, Extra Strong, Italiano, Tesco* | ¼ Baguette/53g 178.0 | 9.0 | 340 | 7.9 | 39.8 | 16.6 | 2.8 |
| Garlic, Baguette, Extra Strong, Sainsbury's* | ½ Baguette/85g 278.0 | 13.0 | 327 | 8.4 | 40.0 | 14.8 | 3.4 |
| Garlic, Baguette, Frozen, GFY, Asda* | ¼ Baguette/48g 132.0 | 4.0 | 277 | 7.0 | 42.0 | 9.0 | 2.7 |

| | Measure INFO/WEIGHT | per Measure KCAL | FAT | Nutrition Values per 100g / 100ml KCAL | PROT | CARB | FAT | FIBRE |
|---|---|---|---|---|---|---|---|---|
| **BREAD** | | | | | | | | |
| Garlic, Baguette, GFY, Asda* | ¼ Baguette/43g | 106.0 | 3.0 | 249 | 8.1 | 39.9 | 6.3 | 2.1 |
| Garlic, Baguette, Italiano, Tesco* | ¼ Baguette/53g | 186.0 | 10.0 | 355 | 6.9 | 39.2 | 18.8 | 2.4 |
| Garlic, Baguette, Light Choices, Tesco* | ¼ Baguette/52g | 130.0 | 3.0 | 250 | 7.0 | 42.2 | 5.5 | 2.4 |
| Garlic, Baguette, Mediterannean Herb, Tesco* | ¼ Baguette/54g | 181.0 | 9.0 | 335 | 6.9 | 40.3 | 16.3 | 2.3 |
| Garlic, Baguette, Morrisons* | ½ Baguette/95g | 295.0 | 14.0 | 311 | 6.3 | 37.8 | 15.0 | 1.5 |
| Garlic, Baguette, Reduced Fat, Waitrose* | ½ Baguette/85g | 229.0 | 7.0 | 270 | 8.1 | 41.5 | 8.0 | 2.7 |
| Garlic, Baguette, Sainsbury's* | ½ Baguette/85g | 342.0 | 16.0 | 403 | 8.9 | 48.6 | 19.2 | 2.3 |
| Garlic, Baguette, Slices, Tesco* | 1 Serving/60g | 187.0 | 9.0 | 312 | 9.8 | 33.8 | 15.3 | 1.7 |
| Garlic, Baguette, TTD, Sainsbury's* | ½ Baguette/95g | 301.0 | 11.0 | 317 | 8.3 | 44.5 | 11.7 | 2.8 |
| Garlic, Baguette, Value, Tesco* | ½ Baguette/85g | 270.0 | 11.0 | 318 | 8.1 | 42.0 | 13.1 | 2.3 |
| Garlic, Baguette, Waitrose* | ½ Baguette/85g | 290.0 | 15.0 | 341 | 7.1 | 37.8 | 17.9 | 0.0 |
| Garlic, Caramelised, TTD, Sainsbury's* | ¼ Bread/75g | 217.0 | 7.0 | 290 | 9.8 | 41.5 | 9.4 | 3.0 |
| Garlic, Ciabatta, & Herb Butter, Sainsbury's* | ½ Ciabatta/105g | 345.0 | 16.0 | 329 | 8.5 | 38.8 | 15.5 | 0.0 |
| Garlic, Ciabatta, BGTY, Sainsbury's* | ½ Ciabatta/105g | 306.0 | 13.0 | 291 | 8.7 | 36.2 | 12.4 | 2.7 |
| Garlic, Ciabatta, Hand Stretched, Sainsbury's* | ¼ Pack/75g | 244.0 | 11.0 | 325 | 8.4 | 41.0 | 14.1 | 2.9 |
| Garlic, Ciabatta, HL, Tesco* | ¼ Ciabatta/60g | 151.0 | 3.0 | 251 | 8.6 | 44.6 | 4.2 | 2.6 |
| Garlic, Ciabatta, Italiano, Tesco* | 1 Ciabatta/65g | 211.0 | 9.0 | 324 | 7.7 | 40.9 | 14.4 | 2.2 |
| Garlic, Ciabatta, with Herbs, Weight Watchers* | 1 Pack/88g | 216.0 | 4.0 | 245 | 9.2 | 43.0 | 4.0 | 2.9 |
| Garlic, Finest, Tesco* | ¼ Loaf/60g | 187.0 | 8.0 | 311 | 7.7 | 40.3 | 13.2 | 1.8 |
| Garlic, Focaccia, & Onion, GFY, Asda* | ¼ Focaccia/55g | 150.0 | 2.0 | 272 | 12.0 | 47.0 | 4.0 | 0.0 |
| Garlic, Focaccia, & Rosemary, Sainsbury's* | ¼ Focaccia/75g | 219.0 | 7.0 | 292 | 8.0 | 43.0 | 9.8 | 2.8 |
| Garlic, Foccacia, & Herb, Italian Style, Morrisons* | 1/6 Focaccia/76g | 259.0 | 11.0 | 341 | 8.5 | 44.7 | 14.3 | 2.5 |
| Garlic, Foccacia, & Rosemary, Tesco* | ¼ Loaf/73g | 193.0 | 5.0 | 266 | 9.0 | 42.1 | 6.8 | 3.7 |
| Garlic, GFY, Asda* | 1 Slice/31g | 108.0 | 1.0 | 350 | 12.0 | 65.0 | 4.5 | 4.0 |
| Garlic, Herb, with Garlic & Herb Butter, Tesco* | 1 Serving/73g | 217.0 | 9.0 | 300 | 6.3 | 40.0 | 12.7 | 1.7 |
| Garlic, Italian Style Stone Baked, Morrisons* | ½ Pack/115g | 420.0 | 22.0 | 365 | 7.9 | 40.4 | 19.1 | 1.9 |
| Garlic, Micro, McCain* | ½ Bread/54g | 202.0 | 10.0 | 374 | 7.8 | 45.1 | 18.0 | 0.0 |
| Garlic, Reduced Fat, Waitrose* | 1 Pack/170g | 551.0 | 19.0 | 324 | 6.9 | 49.4 | 11.0 | 0.9 |
| Garlic, Slices, Chilled, Sainsbury's* | 1 Pack/368g | 1369.0 | 60.0 | 372 | 9.1 | 47.3 | 16.3 | 3.2 |
| Garlic, Slices, Italian, Chilled, Tesco* | 1 Slice/27g | 110.0 | 6.0 | 415 | 6.2 | 46.8 | 22.4 | 2.7 |
| Garlic, Stonebaked, M & S* | 1 Loaf/85g | 263.0 | 10.0 | 310 | 9.3 | 41.4 | 11.9 | 3.1 |
| Garlic, to Share, M & S* | ¼ Loaf/82g | 230.0 | 11.0 | 280 | 6.5 | 33.2 | 13.0 | 1.3 |
| Garlic & Cheese Slices, Italiano, Tesco* | 1 Slice/31g | 95.0 | 4.0 | 304 | 9.0 | 39.7 | 11.8 | 2.6 |
| Garlic Slices, Asda* | 1 Slice/27g | 88.0 | 3.0 | 328 | 8.0 | 46.2 | 12.4 | 2.8 |
| ***Granary, Average*** | ***1 Slice/35g*** | ***82.0*** | ***1.0*** | ***235*** | ***9.3*** | ***46.3*** | ***2.7*** | ***4.3*** |
| Granary, Baps, Large, Asda* | 1 Bap/64g | 143.0 | 1.0 | 224 | 10.0 | 41.0 | 2.2 | 4.3 |
| Granary, Country, Multiseeded, Hovis* | 1 Slice/44g | 96.0 | 1.0 | 218 | 11.1 | 37.0 | 2.9 | 6.5 |
| Granary, M & S* | 1 Slice/30g | 75.0 | 1.0 | 250 | 9.5 | 46.4 | 3.1 | 3.2 |
| Granary, Malted, Medium Brown, Asda* | 1 Slice/35g | 81.0 | 1.0 | 231 | 9.0 | 43.0 | 2.6 | 3.3 |
| Granary, Oatmeal, Hovis* | 1 Slice/44g | 104.0 | 1.0 | 236 | 9.2 | 45.3 | 2.1 | 3.1 |
| Granary, Seeded, Sunflower, Hovis* | 1 Slice/44g | 119.0 | 3.0 | 271 | 10.1 | 44.9 | 5.7 | 2.9 |
| Granary, Thick Slice, COU, M & S* | 1 Slice/25g | 60.0 | 1.0 | 240 | 10.5 | 44.1 | 2.2 | 6.0 |
| Granary, Waitrose* | 1 Slice/40g | 88.0 | 1.0 | 220 | 9.4 | 39.9 | 2.5 | 4.3 |
| Granary, Wholemeal, Hovis* | 1 Slice/44g | 98.0 | 1.0 | 223 | 10.6 | 39.8 | 2.4 | 6.8 |
| Granary White, Hovis* | 1 Slice/44g | 102.0 | 2.0 | 233 | 9.7 | 40.8 | 3.5 | 5.6 |
| Hi Bran, M & S* | 1 Slice/26g | 55.0 | 1.0 | 210 | 12.6 | 32.5 | 3.0 | 6.3 |
| Hi Fibre, Seed, Lifefibre* | 1 Slice/35g | 109.0 | 4.0 | 313 | 12.5 | 43.6 | 10.1 | 2.7 |
| Irish Barm Brack, Tesco* | 1 Serving/75g | 232.0 | 5.0 | 310 | 16.0 | 47.6 | 6.9 | 3.0 |
| Irish Brown Soda, Tesco* | 1 Serving/50g | 109.0 | 2.0 | 219 | 9.2 | 36.2 | 3.8 | 6.4 |
| Irish Cottage Wheaten, Tesco* | 1 Serving/40g | 79.0 | 1.0 | 198 | 9.1 | 35.4 | 1.9 | 6.1 |
| Italian Style Pesto, TTD, Sainsbury's* | ¼ Bread/99g | 247.0 | 6.0 | 249 | 9.1 | 39.4 | 6.1 | 4.4 |
| Juvela* | 1 Slice/25g | 60.0 | 1.0 | 240 | 3.3 | 50.0 | 3.0 | 1.7 |
| Khobez, Flatbread, White, Dina Foods Ltd* | 1 Bread/56g | 158.0 | 1.0 | 282 | 10.5 | 57.5 | 1.1 | 3.0 |

| BREAD | Measure INFO/WEIGHT | per Measure KCAL | FAT | Nutrition Values per 100g / 100ml KCAL | PROT | CARB | FAT | FIBRE |
|---|---|---|---|---|---|---|---|---|
| Light Grain, Eat Smart, Safeway* | 1 Slice/27g | 65.0 | 1.0 | 245 | 9.7 | 45.5 | 2.5 | 3.5 |
| Loaf, Tasty Grains & Seeds, Warburton's* | 1 Slice/38g | 100.0 | 2.0 | 264 | 10.6 | 45.6 | 4.3 | 5.2 |
| Malt Loaf, Fruity, Sliced, Soreen* | 1 Slice/33g | 103.0 | 1.0 | 312 | 7.7 | 65.9 | 2.0 | 0.0 |
| Malt Loaf, Fruity, Unsliced, Soreen* | 1 Serving/42g | 130.0 | 1.0 | 310 | 7.4 | 65.6 | 2.0 | 2.7 |
| Malt Loaf, Organic, Tesco* | 1 Slice/28g | 82.0 | 1.0 | 292 | 7.2 | 61.2 | 2.0 | 2.3 |
| Malt Loaf, Sticky, M & S* | 1 Slice/16g | 47.0 | 0.0 | 295 | 6.9 | 64.9 | 2.3 | 3.1 |
| Malt Loaf, Tesco* | 1 Slice/50g | 145.0 | 1.0 | 291 | 8.6 | 58.0 | 2.7 | 4.8 |
| Malt Loaf, Value, Tesco* | 1 Slice/25g | 72.0 | 0.0 | 289 | 8.9 | 60.2 | 1.4 | 3.3 |
| Malt Loaf, Weight Watchers* | 1 Slice/23g | 68.0 | 0.0 | 294 | 8.9 | 60.2 | 1.9 | 3.6 |
| Malted, & Seeded, Batch, Organic, Waitrose* | 1 Slice/50g | 118.0 | 2.0 | 236 | 10.9 | 39.5 | 3.9 | 6.2 |
| Malted, Crusty, Sainsbury's* | 1 Slice/42g | 109.0 | 1.0 | 259 | 8.6 | 48.6 | 3.3 | 4.4 |
| Malted, Floury Batch, Sainsbury's* | 1 Roll/68g | 190.0 | 3.0 | 280 | 8.7 | 51.6 | 4.3 | 4.2 |
| Malted, Sunblest* | 1 Serving/45g | 115.0 | 1.0 | 256 | 9.9 | 49.1 | 2.2 | 3.8 |
| Malted, Wheat Loaf, Crusty, Finest, Tesco* | 1 Slice/50g | 115.0 | 1.0 | 230 | 9.8 | 44.2 | 1.5 | 4.4 |
| Malted Brown, Slice, BGTY, Sainsbury's* | 1 Slice/22g | 53.0 | 1.0 | 239 | 12.1 | 41.4 | 2.8 | 5.8 |
| Malted Brown, Thick Sliced, Organic, Tesco* | 1 Slice/44g | 111.0 | 1.0 | 249 | 8.9 | 48.8 | 2.0 | 3.5 |
| Malted Brown, TTD, Sainsbury's* | 1 Slice/44g | 103.0 | 1.0 | 234 | 8.8 | 42.9 | 3.0 | 3.1 |
| Malted Danish, Weight Watchers* | 1 Slice/20g | 49.0 | 0.0 | 241 | 12.3 | 44.5 | 1.7 | 4.3 |
| Malted Grain, Good As Gold, Kingsmill* | 1 Slice/47g | 114.0 | 1.0 | 243 | 9.5 | 45.4 | 2.6 | 4.2 |
| Malted Wheat, The Best, Safeway* | 1 Slice/44g | 103.0 | 1.0 | 235 | 9.1 | 45.6 | 1.8 | 4.7 |
| Malted Wholegrain, Nimble* | 1 Slice/22g | 49.0 | 0.0 | 222 | 10.4 | 41.9 | 1.4 | 6.7 |
| Mediterranean Olive, Waitrose* | 1 Slice/30g | 82.0 | 3.0 | 273 | 7.4 | 40.1 | 9.2 | 4.9 |
| Mediterranean Style, M & S* | 1/6 Loaf/48g | 150.0 | 5.0 | 315 | 10.9 | 42.5 | 11.1 | 1.2 |
| Milk Roll, Warburton's* | 1 Slice/18g | 46.0 | 1.0 | 253 | 11.0 | 45.1 | 2.7 | 2.7 |
| Mixed Seed, Organic, Duchy Originals* | 1 Slice/43g | 114.0 | 3.0 | 269 | 10.9 | 39.1 | 8.1 | 5.3 |
| Multi Seed, Somerfield* | 1 Slice/45g | 105.0 | 2.0 | 235 | 11.0 | 38.2 | 3.7 | 8.1 |
| Multigrain, Batch, Tesco* | 1 Slice/50g | 117.0 | 1.0 | 235 | 10.8 | 40.4 | 2.9 | 5.5 |
| Multigrain, Brown, Farmhouse Baker's, M & S* | 1 Slice/51g | 115.0 | 3.0 | 225 | 13.0 | 31.2 | 5.4 | 5.1 |
| Multigrain, Crusty, Finest, Tesco* | 1 Slice/40g | 98.0 | 1.0 | 245 | 9.0 | 44.7 | 3.4 | 5.0 |
| Multigrain, Gluten Free, Sainsbury's* | 1 Slice/17g | 39.0 | 1.0 | 229 | 5.1 | 40.8 | 5.0 | 5.6 |
| Multigrain, Soft Batch, Sainsbury's* | 1 Slice/44g | 106.0 | 3.0 | 242 | 11.3 | 34.5 | 6.5 | 5.6 |
| Multigrain, Sunblest* | 1 Slice/30g | 76.0 | 1.0 | 254 | 9.0 | 47.0 | 2.5 | 4.5 |
| Multigrain, TTD, Sainsbury's* | 1 Slice/44g | 106.0 | 3.0 | 242 | 10.2 | 35.9 | 6.4 | 5.3 |
| Multiseeded, Loaf, TTD, Sainsbury's* | 1 Slice/35g | 97.0 | 1.0 | 277 | 13.7 | 46.4 | 4.2 | 5.1 |
| *Naan, Average* | *1 Naan/130g* | *337.0* | *8.0* | *259* | *9.0* | *40.3* | *5.8* | *1.8* |
| Naan, Bombay Brasserie, Sainsbury's* | 1 Naan/140g | 372.0 | 4.0 | 266 | 9.8 | 49.6 | 3.1 | 2.9 |
| Naan, Chilli & Mango, Finest, Tesco* | ½ Naan/90g | 229.0 | 5.0 | 255 | 8.4 | 41.9 | 5.7 | 3.2 |
| Naan, Garlic & Coriander, Free From, Tesco* | 1 Naan/90g | 215.0 | 6.0 | 240 | 5.1 | 38.7 | 6.7 | 4.9 |
| Naan, Garlic & Coriander, Mild, Patak's* | 1 Naan/140g | 452.0 | 15.0 | 323 | 9.0 | 47.5 | 10.8 | 0.0 |
| Naan, Garlic & Coriander, Mini, Asda* | 1 Naan/110g | 320.0 | 13.0 | 291 | 6.9 | 40.2 | 11.4 | 2.5 |
| Naan, Garlic & Coriander, Mini, Sainsbury's* | 1 Naan/50g | 140.0 | 2.0 | 280 | 8.2 | 51.2 | 4.1 | 2.6 |
| Naan, Garlic & Coriander, Mini, Sharwood's* | 1 Naan/59g | 144.0 | 2.0 | 244 | 7.1 | 46.2 | 3.4 | 2.0 |
| Naan, Garlic & Coriander, Mini, Tesco* | 1 Naan/65g | 185.0 | 5.0 | 285 | 7.6 | 45.6 | 7.7 | 2.6 |
| Naan, Garlic & Coriander, Mini, Weight Watchers* | 1 Naan/40g | 98.0 | 1.0 | 245 | 9.4 | 48.3 | 1.6 | 2.7 |
| Naan, Garlic & Coriander, Tesco* | ½ Naan/83g | 235.0 | 6.0 | 285 | 7.6 | 45.6 | 7.7 | 2.6 |
| Naan, Garlic & Coriander, TTD, Sainsbury's* | ½ Naan/70g | 203.0 | 6.0 | 290 | 7.9 | 44.3 | 9.1 | 4.5 |
| Naan, Garlic & Coriander, Weight Watchers* | 1 Naan/60g | 155.0 | 3.0 | 259 | 8.9 | 46.0 | 4.3 | 3.4 |
| Naan, Indian Meal for One, BGTY, Sainsbury's* | 1 Serving/45g | 115.0 | 2.0 | 257 | 10.3 | 44.2 | 4.3 | 2.1 |
| Naan, Light Choices, Tesco* | 1 Naan/71g | 181.0 | 2.0 | 255 | 7.5 | 50.7 | 2.2 | 2.3 |
| Naan, Peshwari, Finest, Tesco* | 1 Naan/130g | 338.0 | 7.0 | 260 | 8.6 | 43.7 | 5.6 | 4.9 |
| Naan, Peshwari, M & S* | 1 Serving/127g | 394.0 | 13.0 | 310 | 9.2 | 45.8 | 10.1 | 1.9 |
| Naan, Peshwari, Sainsbury's* | 1 Naan/166g | 511.0 | 18.0 | 308 | 7.1 | 45.1 | 11.0 | 4.7 |
| Naan, Peshwari, Sharwood's* | 1 Naan/130g | 334.0 | 7.0 | 257 | 7.2 | 45.1 | 5.3 | 2.5 |

**B**

## BREAD

| | Measure INFO/WEIGHT | per Measure KCAL | FAT | Nutrition Values per 100g / 100ml KCAL | PROT | CARB | FAT | FIBRE |
|---|---|---|---|---|---|---|---|---|
| Naan, Peshwari, Tesco* | 1 Naan/215g | 684.0 | 27.0 | 318 | 7.5 | 48.9 | 12.4 | 4.8 |
| Naan, Plain, Average | 1 Naan/160g | 538.0 | 20.0 | 336 | 8.9 | 50.1 | 12.5 | 1.9 |
| Naan, Plain, GFY, Asda* | 1 Naan/130g | 307.0 | 3.0 | 236 | 8.4 | 45.9 | 2.1 | 2.4 |
| Naan, Plain, Mini, Asda* | 1 Naan/58g | 156.0 | 3.0 | 269 | 8.0 | 49.0 | 4.6 | 2.3 |
| Naan, Plain, Mini, BGTY, Sainsbury's* | 1 Naan/50g | 113.0 | 1.0 | 226 | 8.2 | 43.2 | 2.2 | 3.3 |
| Naan, Plain, Mini, Weight Watchers* | 1 Naan/44g | 108.0 | 1.0 | 245 | 9.1 | 46.5 | 2.5 | 4.9 |
| Naan, Plain, Sharwood's* | 1 Naan/120g | 326.0 | 9.0 | 272 | 8.5 | 42.9 | 7.4 | 2.4 |
| Naan, Plain, Tesco* | 1 Naan/150g | 391.0 | 7.0 | 261 | 8.4 | 46.4 | 4.6 | 2.3 |
| Naan, Plain, TTD, Sainsbury's* | 1 Naan/140g | 352.0 | 7.0 | 251 | 8.2 | 43.1 | 5.1 | 2.9 |
| Naan, Take Away, Tesco* | 1 Naan/39g | 97.0 | 1.0 | 248 | 8.7 | 45.6 | 3.4 | 1.7 |
| Naan, Tandoori, Sharwood's* | 1 Naan/130g | 330.0 | 6.0 | 254 | 7.3 | 45.0 | 5.0 | 2.0 |
| Oatmeal, Batch, Finest, Tesco* | 1 Slice/50g | 127.0 | 2.0 | 255 | 10.3 | 43.7 | 4.3 | 4.8 |
| Oatmeal, Farmhouse, Extra Special, Asda* | 1 Slice/44g | 102.0 | 1.0 | 231 | 11.0 | 41.0 | 2.6 | 6.0 |
| Oatmeal, Farmhouse, Soft, M & S* | 1 Slice/45g | 110.0 | 2.0 | 245 | 11.1 | 39.5 | 4.4 | 5.2 |
| Oatmeal, Farmhouse, Waitrose* | 1 Slice/40g | 110.0 | 2.0 | 276 | 9.4 | 47.9 | 5.2 | 4.6 |
| Oatmeal, Sliced Loaf, Tesco* | 1 Slice/50g | 111.0 | 2.0 | 222 | 7.4 | 40.5 | 3.4 | 2.8 |
| Olive, Waitrose* | 1 Slice/28g | 86.0 | 3.0 | 306 | 9.0 | 43.6 | 10.6 | 2.0 |
| Pain Au Raisin, M & S* | 1 Pain/74g | 215.0 | 9.0 | 290 | 5.3 | 38.7 | 12.8 | 1.2 |
| Pave, Walnut, Sainsbury's* | 1 Serving/50g | 140.0 | 5.0 | 280 | 9.0 | 40.0 | 9.5 | 3.5 |
| Petit Pain, Homebake, Mini, Tesco* | 1 Roll/50g | 120.0 | 1.0 | 240 | 7.8 | 48.5 | 1.2 | 3.4 |
| Petit Pain, Organic, Tesco* | 1 Roll/100g | 235.0 | 1.0 | 235 | 7.8 | 49.1 | 0.8 | 1.2 |
| Petit Pain, Part Bake, Weight Watchers* | 1 Roll/50g | 102.0 | 1.0 | 204 | 8.2 | 39.9 | 1.2 | 9.8 |
| Pitta, Brown, Organic, Waitrose* | 1 Pitta/60g | 137.0 | 1.0 | 228 | 6.4 | 47.5 | 1.4 | 6.6 |
| Pitta, Free From, Sainsbury's* | 1 Pitta/55g | 134.0 | 1.0 | 243 | 5.9 | 50.8 | 1.8 | 1.7 |
| Pitta, Garlic, Morrisons* | 1 Pitta/60g | 149.0 | 1.0 | 249 | 9.7 | 51.1 | 1.8 | 0.0 |
| Pitta, Garlic, Sainsbury's* | 1 Pitta/60g | 153.0 | 1.0 | 255 | 9.5 | 52.0 | 1.0 | 2.5 |
| Pitta, Garlic & Coriander, Asda* | 1 Pitta/55g | 116.0 | 0.0 | 212 | 7.0 | 44.0 | 0.9 | 1.8 |
| Pitta, Garlic & Herb, Tesco* | 1 Pitta/60g | 134.0 | 1.0 | 223 | 9.6 | 44.6 | 2.0 | 3.0 |
| Pitta, Multi Seed & Cereal, The Food Doctor* | 1 Pitta/70g | 157.0 | 2.0 | 224 | 10.1 | 39.9 | 2.7 | 10.2 |
| Pitta, Organic, Tesco* | 1 Pitta/60g | 124.0 | 1.0 | 206 | 8.3 | 40.2 | 1.4 | 5.7 |
| Pitta, Pockets, Pride Valley* | 1 Pitta/63g | 151.0 | 1.0 | 239 | 9.3 | 48.4 | 0.9 | 3.2 |
| Pitta, Pockets, Sainsbury's* | 1 Serving/75g | 187.0 | 1.0 | 250 | 8.5 | 52.0 | 1.0 | 3.5 |
| Pitta, Seeded, HL, Tesco* | 1 Pitta/60g | 153.0 | 4.0 | 255 | 10.8 | 39.4 | 6.0 | 12.8 |
| Pitta, Sesame, Sainsbury's* | 1 Pitta/59g | 156.0 | 1.0 | 264 | 9.8 | 50.8 | 2.4 | 3.1 |
| *Pitta, White, Average* | *1 Pitta/75g* | *199.0* | *1.0* | *265* | *9.2* | *57.9* | *1.2* | *2.2* |
| Pitta, White, Greek Style, Asda* | 1 Pitta/50g | 126.0 | 1.0 | 253 | 8.0 | 51.0 | 1.9 | 0.0 |
| Pitta, White, Large, Tesco* | 1 Pitta/90g | 252.0 | 2.0 | 280 | 9.8 | 55.1 | 2.1 | 3.4 |
| Pitta, White, Mini, Sainsbury's* | 1 Pitta/30g | 75.0 | 0.0 | 249 | 10.3 | 49.3 | 1.2 | 3.5 |
| Pitta, White, Mini, Tesco* | 1 Pitta/30g | 84.0 | 1.0 | 280 | 9.8 | 55.1 | 2.1 | 3.4 |
| Pitta, White, Weight Watchers* | 1 Pitta/45g | 102.0 | 0.0 | 227 | 9.3 | 45.3 | 1.0 | 9.3 |
| Pitta, Wholemeal, Asda* | 1 Pitta/56g | 133.0 | 1.0 | 238 | 12.0 | 44.0 | 1.6 | 6.0 |
| *Pitta, Wholemeal, Average* | *1 Pitta/64g* | *170.0* | *2.0* | *266* | *9.8* | *55.0* | *2.6* | *7.4* |
| Pitta, Wholemeal, M & S* | 1 Pitta/61g | 137.0 | 2.0 | 225 | 9.8 | 39.7 | 3.0 | 6.7 |
| Pitta, Wholemeal, Mini, M & S* | 1 Pitta/17g | 40.0 | 1.0 | 230 | 11.1 | 39.2 | 3.1 | 7.0 |
| Pitta, Wholemeal, Mini, Tesco* | 1 Pitta/30g | 76.0 | 1.0 | 255 | 11.8 | 48.2 | 1.7 | 4.2 |
| Pitta, Wholemeal, Sainsbury's* | 1 Pitta/60g | 142.0 | 1.0 | 237 | 9.9 | 45.9 | 1.5 | 5.3 |
| Pitta, Wholemeal, Tesco* | 1 Pitta/60g | 147.0 | 1.0 | 245 | 11.2 | 43.6 | 2.5 | 8.7 |
| Pitta, Wholemeal, Waitrose* | 1 Pitta/60g | 145.0 | 1.0 | 242 | 12.4 | 46.0 | 0.9 | 3.1 |
| Potato & Rosemary, M & S* | 1 Serving/40g | 108.0 | 3.0 | 270 | 9.4 | 42.2 | 6.8 | 2.3 |
| Potato Farls, M & S* | 1 Farl/55g | 79.0 | 0.0 | 144 | 4.2 | 33.8 | 0.4 | 4.7 |
| Potato Farls, Sunblest* | 1 Farl/100g | 156.0 | 1.0 | 156 | 3.8 | 33.2 | 0.9 | 1.9 |
| Pumpernickel, Organic, Bavarian Pumpernickel* | 1 Slice/50g | 90.0 | 0.0 | 180 | 6.0 | 38.0 | 1.0 | 10.0 |
| Pumpernickel Rye, Kelderman* | 1 Slice/50g | 92.0 | 0.0 | 185 | 6.0 | 38.0 | 1.0 | 0.0 |

# BREAD

| | Measure INFO/WEIGHT | per Measure KCAL | FAT | Nutrition Values per 100g / 100ml KCAL | PROT | CARB | FAT | FIBRE |
|---|---|---|---|---|---|---|---|---|
| Pumpkin Seed, Raisin & Sunflower Seed, Sainsbury's* | 1 Slice/30g | 76.0 | 1.0 | 255 | 11.6 | 45.9 | 2.8 | 3.4 |
| Raisin & Pumpkin Seed, Organic, Tesco* | 1 Slice/30g | 76.0 | 2.0 | 253 | 9.7 | 40.6 | 5.8 | 3.8 |
| Raisin Loaf with Cinnamon, Warburton's* | 1 Slice/36g | 96.0 | 1.0 | 267 | 7.2 | 51.1 | 3.7 | 3.2 |
| Roasted Onion, M & S* | 1 Slice/50g | 125.0 | 2.0 | 250 | 9.0 | 46.7 | 3.3 | 2.1 |
| Roasted Shallot & Gruyere, Safeway* | ¼ Loaf/53g | 150.0 | 4.0 | 285 | 11.2 | 43.1 | 7.3 | 9.1 |
| Rolls, 3 Seeded, Sandwich, Warburton's* | 1 Roll/77g | 242.0 | 7.0 | 314 | 13.3 | 41.2 | 8.7 | 6.0 |
| Rolls, American Style Deli, Tesco* | 1 Roll/65g | 162.0 | 2.0 | 249 | 7.8 | 46.8 | 3.4 | 1.6 |
| Rolls, Batched Sandwich, Warburton's* | 1 Roll/60g | 148.0 | 2.0 | 246 | 9.6 | 42.7 | 4.1 | 0.0 |
| Rolls, Best of Both, Hovis* | 1 Roll/65g | 154.0 | 3.0 | 237 | 10.2 | 38.4 | 4.8 | 5.2 |
| Rolls, Brioche, Plain Chocolate Chip, Sainsbury's* | 1 Roll/35g | 131.0 | 6.0 | 374 | 8.5 | 49.0 | 16.0 | 5.9 |
| Rolls, Brioche, Sainsbury's* | 1 Roll/32g | 116.0 | 4.0 | 362 | 8.5 | 56.0 | 11.5 | 3.6 |
| Rolls, Brown, Carb Control, Tesco* | 1 Roll/45g | 98.0 | 3.0 | 218 | 20.5 | 20.7 | 5.9 | 10.7 |
| **Rolls, Brown, Crusty** | **1 Roll/50g** | **127.0** | **1.0** | **255** | **10.3** | **50.4** | **2.8** | **3.5** |
| Rolls, Brown, Free From, Tesco* | 1 Roll/65g | 174.0 | 5.0 | 268 | 5.4 | 43.2 | 8.2 | 3.6 |
| Rolls, Brown, M & S* | 1 Roll/105g | 241.0 | 6.0 | 230 | 9.2 | 37.3 | 6.1 | 4.4 |
| Rolls, Brown, Old Fashioned, Waitrose* | 1 Roll/63g | 152.0 | 3.0 | 241 | 9.6 | 41.3 | 4.1 | 4.7 |
| Rolls, Brown, Seeded, Organic, Sainsbury's* | 1 Roll/70g | 166.0 | 3.0 | 237 | 9.9 | 39.1 | 4.6 | 6.5 |
| **Rolls, Brown, Soft, Average** | **1 Roll/50g** | **134.0** | **2.0** | **268** | **10.0** | **51.8** | **3.8** | **3.5** |
| Rolls, Brown, Soft, Tesco* | 1 Roll/50g | 117.0 | 2.0 | 235 | 9.0 | 41.6 | 3.6 | 4.5 |
| Rolls, Brown, Square, M & S* | 1 Roll/105g | 241.0 | 6.0 | 230 | 9.2 | 37.3 | 6.1 | 4.4 |
| Rolls, Cheese Topped, Sandwich Rolls, Warburton's* | 1 Roll/62g | 168.0 | 4.0 | 270 | 12.1 | 40.7 | 6.5 | 2.6 |
| Rolls, COU, M & S* | 1 Serving/51g | 120.0 | 1.0 | 235 | 9.8 | 44.0 | 2.3 | 3.4 |
| Rolls, Crisp, Original, Organic, Kallo* | 1 Roll/9g | 34.0 | 0.0 | 390 | 11.0 | 74.0 | 5.6 | 3.0 |
| Rolls, Crusty, French, M & S* | 1 Roll/65g | 159.0 | 1.0 | 245 | 8.1 | 50.5 | 1.2 | 3.3 |
| Rolls, Finger, Morrisons* | 1 Roll/46g | 119.0 | 1.0 | 259 | 10.7 | 50.0 | 1.8 | 2.3 |
| Rolls, Finger, White, Sainsbury's* | 1 Roll/40g | 96.0 | 1.0 | 240 | 9.0 | 45.2 | 2.6 | 3.2 |
| Rolls, Granary, Bakers Premium, Tesco* | 1 Roll/65g | 158.0 | 1.0 | 243 | 9.9 | 47.8 | 1.3 | 2.3 |
| Rolls, Granary, Mini, Tesco* | 1 Roll/34g | 92.0 | 2.0 | 271 | 10.0 | 43.5 | 6.5 | 3.8 |
| Rolls, Granary, Original, Hovis* | 1 Roll/70g | 180.0 | 3.0 | 257 | 10.7 | 44.3 | 4.1 | 5.3 |
| Rolls, Granary, Waitrose* | 1 Roll/59g | 160.0 | 4.0 | 271 | 10.0 | 47.2 | 6.4 | 3.8 |
| Rolls, Granary Malted Wheatgrain, Soft, M & S* | 1 Roll/80g | 208.0 | 3.0 | 260 | 9.3 | 47.2 | 3.9 | 2.3 |
| Rolls, Green Olive, M & S* | 1 Roll/75g | 210.0 | 4.0 | 280 | 11.2 | 44.0 | 6.0 | 1.8 |
| Rolls, Hot Dog, Sliced, Asda* | 1 Roll/84g | 197.0 | 3.0 | 234 | 7.0 | 44.0 | 3.3 | 0.0 |
| Rolls, Hot Dog, Tesco* | 1 Roll/85g | 200.0 | 3.0 | 235 | 7.3 | 44.0 | 3.3 | 1.9 |
| Rolls, Malted Grain, Sainsbury's* | 1 Roll/68g | 190.0 | 3.0 | 280 | 8.7 | 51.6 | 4.3 | 4.2 |
| Rolls, Malted Grain, Soft, Weight Watchers* | 1 Roll/57g | 142.0 | 1.0 | 251 | 11.7 | 47.1 | 1.8 | 4.2 |
| Rolls, Malted Grain, Submarine, M & S* | 1 Serving/109g | 300.0 | 5.0 | 275 | 8.9 | 53.6 | 4.3 | 3.0 |
| Rolls, Malted Wheat, Sub, Organic, Tesco* | 1 Serving/108g | 279.0 | 4.0 | 258 | 10.1 | 45.2 | 4.1 | 4.8 |
| Rolls, Mediterranean Style, TTD, Sainsbury's* | 1 Roll/75g | 192.0 | 4.0 | 256 | 8.5 | 41.9 | 6.0 | 5.8 |
| Rolls, Mini Submarine, M & S* | 1 Roll/23g | 63.0 | 1.0 | 275 | 11.4 | 47.7 | 4.9 | 1.1 |
| Rolls, Mixed Seed, Deli, Tesco* | 1 Roll/65g | 166.0 | 2.0 | 255 | 9.4 | 46.8 | 3.3 | 5.2 |
| Rolls, Morning, Tesco* | 1 Roll/48g | 117.0 | 1.0 | 243 | 10.4 | 44.8 | 2.5 | 4.7 |
| Rolls, Multigrain, Torpedo, Sainsbury's* | 1 Roll/112g | 328.0 | 7.0 | 293 | 10.5 | 47.7 | 6.7 | 6.3 |
| Rolls, Multigrain, TTD, Sainsbury's* | 1 Roll/110g | 327.0 | 10.0 | 297 | 11.7 | 41.5 | 9.4 | 6.4 |
| Rolls, Panini, Sainsbury's* | 1 Roll/90g | 249.0 | 6.0 | 276 | 11.0 | 44.1 | 6.2 | 3.0 |
| Rolls, Panini, White, Tesco* | 1 Roll/75g | 210.0 | 5.0 | 280 | 10.1 | 45.2 | 6.1 | 2.7 |
| Rolls, Poppy Seeded Knot, Waitrose* | 1 Roll/60g | 169.0 | 3.0 | 282 | 10.3 | 48.3 | 5.3 | 2.2 |
| Rolls, Seed Sensations, Deli, Hovis* | 1 Roll/70g | 184.0 | 6.0 | 263 | 10.3 | 36.5 | 8.5 | 10.6 |
| Rolls, Seeded, Mixed Mini Loaf Pack, M & S* | 1 Roll/76g | 220.0 | 7.0 | 290 | 10.6 | 39.7 | 9.6 | 4.0 |
| Rolls, Seeded, Sandwich, Warburton's* | 1 Roll/77g | 242.0 | 7.0 | 314 | 13.3 | 41.2 | 8.7 | 6.0 |
| Rolls, Snack, Mini, Tesco* | 1 Roll/35g | 95.0 | 2.0 | 271 | 19.0 | 43.0 | 6.0 | 4.0 |
| Rolls, Submarine, Sainsbury's* | 1 Roll/117g | 305.0 | 5.0 | 261 | 9.1 | 47.4 | 3.9 | 2.4 |
| Rolls, Sun Dried Tomato, Homebake, Tesco* | 1 Roll/50g | 123.0 | 1.0 | 246 | 11.3 | 44.0 | 3.0 | 0.0 |

## BREAD

| | Measure INFO/WEIGHT | per Measure KCAL | per Measure FAT | Nutrition Values per 100g / 100ml KCAL | PROT | CARB | FAT | FIBRE |
|---|---|---|---|---|---|---|---|---|
| Rolls, Tomato & Basil, Sub, COU, M & S* | 1 Roll/33g | 86.0 | 1.0 | 265 | 11.0 | 48.7 | 2.7 | 2.4 |
| Rolls, White, BGTY, Sainsbury's* | 1 Roll/50g | 113.0 | 0.0 | 227 | 9.1 | 45.3 | 1.0 | 3.0 |
| Rolls, White, Cheese Topped, Asda* | 1 Roll/46g | 121.0 | 2.0 | 264 | 10.0 | 46.0 | 4.4 | 2.0 |
| Rolls, White, Cheese Topped, Sainsbury's* | 1 Roll/75g | 218.0 | 6.0 | 291 | 12.1 | 41.6 | 8.5 | 2.0 |
| *Rolls, White, Crusty, Average* | *1 Roll/50g* | *140.0* | *1.0* | *280* | *10.9* | *57.6* | *2.3* | *1.5* |
| Rolls, White, Crusty, Morning, M & S* | 1 Roll/65g | 175.0 | 1.0 | 270 | 8.8 | 53.8 | 1.3 | 2.7 |
| Rolls, White, Finger, Tesco* | 1 Roll/68g | 170.0 | 2.0 | 250 | 8.5 | 45.8 | 3.5 | 2.1 |
| Rolls, White, Finger, Value, Tesco* | 1 Roll/50g | 116.0 | 1.0 | 232 | 8.7 | 45.0 | 1.9 | 2.2 |
| Rolls, White, Floured, Batch, Tesco* | 1 Roll/76g | 193.0 | 3.0 | 254 | 8.8 | 47.3 | 3.3 | 2.2 |
| Rolls, White, Floured, Warburton's* | 1 Roll/50g | 123.0 | 2.0 | 247 | 9.8 | 43.3 | 3.8 | 2.7 |
| Rolls, White, Floury Batch, Sainsbury's* | 1 Roll/68g | 168.0 | 2.0 | 247 | 8.3 | 47.2 | 2.8 | 2.2 |
| Rolls, White, Good Health, Warburton's* | 1 Roll/54g | 122.0 | 1.0 | 226 | 9.6 | 42.0 | 2.0 | 4.1 |
| Rolls, White, Hot Dog, Tesco* | 1 Roll/65g | 169.0 | 2.0 | 260 | 9.6 | 46.1 | 3.7 | 3.2 |
| Rolls, White, Kingsmill* | 1 Roll/60g | 151.0 | 2.0 | 252 | 9.3 | 44.5 | 4.1 | 2.4 |
| Rolls, White, Low Price, Sainsbury's* | 1 Roll/44g | 107.0 | 1.0 | 243 | 8.9 | 48.2 | 1.6 | 2.1 |
| Rolls, White, Old Fashioned, Waitrose* | 1 Roll/64g | 176.0 | 3.0 | 275 | 8.8 | 49.8 | 4.5 | 2.8 |
| Rolls, White, Organic, Sainsbury's* | 1 Roll/65g | 170.0 | 2.0 | 262 | 8.7 | 49.9 | 3.0 | 1.0 |
| Rolls, White, Part Baked, Morrisons* | 1 Roll/75g | 227.0 | 1.0 | 303 | 9.6 | 63.0 | 1.4 | 2.6 |
| Rolls, White, Ploughman's, Sainsbury's* | 1 Roll/65g | 185.0 | 2.0 | 285 | 8.6 | 54.1 | 3.8 | 2.3 |
| Rolls, White, Premium, Hovis* | 1 Roll/62g | 154.0 | 3.0 | 249 | 9.5 | 41.9 | 4.8 | 2.3 |
| Rolls, White, Sandwich, Regular, Warburton's* | 1 Roll/58g | 143.0 | 3.0 | 249 | 9.7 | 42.6 | 4.3 | 2.4 |
| Rolls, White, Scottish, Tesco* | 1 Roll/48g | 117.0 | 1.0 | 243 | 10.4 | 44.8 | 2.5 | 4.7 |
| *Rolls, White, Soft, Average* | *1 Roll/45g* | *121.0* | *2.0* | *268* | *9.2* | *51.6* | *4.2* | *1.5* |
| Rolls, White, Soft, Hovis* | 1 Roll/65g | 164.0 | 3.0 | 253 | 8.8 | 44.2 | 4.6 | 3.7 |
| Rolls, White, Soft, Kingsmill* | 1 Roll/58g | 145.0 | 2.0 | 250 | 9.3 | 44.0 | 4.1 | 2.9 |
| Rolls, White, Soft, M & S* | 1 Roll/60g | 150.0 | 2.0 | 250 | 10.3 | 45.2 | 3.1 | 2.7 |
| Rolls, White, Soft, Tesco* | 1 Roll/72g | 175.0 | 2.0 | 243 | 7.6 | 46.7 | 2.5 | 2.8 |
| Rolls, White, Softgrain, GFY, Asda* | 1 Roll/54g | 128.0 | 1.0 | 237 | 9.0 | 46.0 | 1.9 | 2.9 |
| Rolls, White, Split, Asda* | 1 Roll/45g | 113.0 | 2.0 | 251 | 10.0 | 45.0 | 3.4 | 2.8 |
| Rolls, White, Sub, Tesco* | 1 Roll/100g | 258.0 | 4.0 | 258 | 11.1 | 44.4 | 4.0 | 2.8 |
| Rolls, White, Submarine, M & S* | 1 Serving/109g | 300.0 | 5.0 | 275 | 11.0 | 47.0 | 5.0 | 1.0 |
| Rolls, White, Tesco* | 1 Roll/65g | 180.0 | 2.0 | 277 | 8.7 | 52.0 | 3.8 | 2.7 |
| Rolls, White, Warburton's* | 1 Roll/57g | 141.0 | 2.0 | 248 | 9.7 | 42.8 | 4.2 | 0.0 |
| Rolls, White, Weight Watchers* | 1 Roll/54g | 135.0 | 1.0 | 251 | 11.7 | 47.1 | 1.8 | 4.2 |
| *Rolls, Wholemeal* | *1 Roll 45g* | *108.0* | *1.0* | *241* | *9.0* | *48.3* | *2.9* | *5.9* |
| Rolls, Wholemeal, Asda* | 1 Roll/58g | 130.0 | 2.0 | 225 | 11.0 | 39.0 | 2.8 | 6.0 |
| Rolls, Wholemeal, COU, M & S* | 1 Roll/110g | 225.0 | 3.0 | 205 | 11.3 | 33.4 | 2.8 | 7.1 |
| Rolls, Wholemeal, Floury Batch, Sainsbury's* | 1 Roll/68g | 152.0 | 2.0 | 223 | 9.9 | 37.8 | 3.4 | 6.5 |
| Rolls, Wholemeal, Golden, Hovis* | 1 Roll/50g | 111.0 | 2.0 | 223 | 10.5 | 36.5 | 3.9 | 6.8 |
| Rolls, Wholemeal, HL, Tesco* | 1 Roll/68g | 155.0 | 1.0 | 230 | 10.4 | 41.3 | 2.1 | 6.6 |
| Rolls, Wholemeal, Kingsmill* | 1 Roll/68g | 167.0 | 3.0 | 245 | 10.7 | 41.5 | 4.0 | 5.1 |
| Rolls, Wholemeal, Mini, Assorted, Waitrose* | 1 Roll/36g | 84.0 | 2.0 | 236 | 9.0 | 38.1 | 5.3 | 5.2 |
| Rolls, Wholemeal, Mini, Tesco* | 1 Roll/34g | 82.0 | 2.0 | 240 | 10.9 | 36.4 | 5.6 | 5.8 |
| Rolls, Wholemeal, Morrisons* | 1 Roll/67g | 155.0 | 3.0 | 231 | 10.2 | 38.6 | 4.0 | 6.3 |
| Rolls, Wholemeal, Oat Topped, Tesco* | 1 Roll/65g | 166.0 | 3.0 | 255 | 11.3 | 42.2 | 4.5 | 5.1 |
| Rolls, Wholemeal, Oatbran, HL, Tesco* | 1 Roll/56g | 115.0 | 1.0 | 205 | 11.4 | 33.6 | 2.5 | 7.4 |
| Rolls, Wholemeal, Old Fashioned, Waitrose* | 1 Roll/57g | 135.0 | 3.0 | 236 | 11.1 | 37.2 | 4.8 | 6.6 |
| Rolls, Wholemeal, Organic, Sainsbury's* | 1 Roll/66g | 152.0 | 2.0 | 230 | 10.7 | 41.0 | 2.7 | 6.6 |
| Rolls, Wholemeal, Organic, Tesco* | 1 Roll/65g | 177.0 | 4.0 | 273 | 10.3 | 44.1 | 6.2 | 5.5 |
| Rolls, Wholemeal, Ploughman's, Sainsbury's* | 1 Roll/67g | 153.0 | 2.0 | 229 | 10.7 | 39.3 | 3.2 | 8.6 |
| Rolls, Wholemeal, Soft, Sainsbury's* | 1 Roll/60g | 133.0 | 2.0 | 221 | 9.9 | 37.8 | 3.4 | 6.5 |
| Rolls, Wholemeal, Soft, Seeded, Sainsbury's* | 1 Roll/75g | 193.0 | 6.0 | 257 | 11.8 | 35.6 | 7.4 | 6.2 |
| Rolls, Wholemeal, Submarine, Tesco* | 1 Roll/100g | 221.0 | 3.0 | 221 | 9.3 | 39.0 | 3.1 | 5.2 |

B

## BREAD

| | Measure INFO/WEIGHT | per Measure KCAL | FAT | Nutrition Values per 100g / 100ml KCAL | PROT | CARB | FAT | FIBRE |
|---|---|---|---|---|---|---|---|---|
| Rolls, Wholemeal, Sunflower & Honey, Sainsbury's* | 1 Roll/85g | 225.0 | 4.0 | 265 | 9.2 | 45.4 | 5.1 | 4.5 |
| Rolls, Wholemeal, Tasty, Great Everyday, Kingsmill* | 1 Roll/68g | 158.0 | 3.0 | 232 | 10.6 | 38.8 | 3.8 | 6.5 |
| Rolls, Wholemeal, Tesco* | 1 Roll/46g | 115.0 | 2.0 | 250 | 10.9 | 41.8 | 4.0 | 7.5 |
| Rolls, Wholemeal, Warburton's* | 1 Roll/58g | 124.0 | 2.0 | 214 | 10.2 | 35.1 | 3.7 | 6.6 |
| Rolls, Wholemeal & White, Kingsmill* | 1 Roll/60g | 151.0 | 3.0 | 251 | 9.5 | 43.7 | 4.2 | 3.5 |
| Rolls, Wholemeal with Cracked Wheat, Allinson* | 1 Roll/58g | 134.0 | 2.0 | 231 | 11.0 | 38.0 | 3.9 | 7.0 |
| Rolls, Wholewhite, Kingsmill* | 1 Roll/63g | 158.0 | 3.0 | 251 | 9.5 | 43.7 | 4.2 | 3.5 |
| Rolls, Wholmeal, Deli, Tesco* | 1 Roll/65g | 156.0 | 3.0 | 240 | 9.0 | 40.2 | 4.8 | 5.7 |
| *Rye, Average* | *1 Slice/25g* | *55.0* | *0.0* | *219* | *8.3* | *45.8* | *1.7* | *4.4* |
| Rye, Dark, Sliced, Trianon* | 1 Slice/41g | 74.0 | 1.0 | 180 | 6.5 | 35.0 | 1.5 | 0.0 |
| Rye, German Style, Bolletje* | 1 Slice/60g | 114.0 | 1.0 | 190 | 6.0 | 35.0 | 2.0 | 9.5 |
| Rye, German Style, Kelderman* | 1 Slice/57g | 88.0 | 1.0 | 155 | 5.6 | 30.2 | 1.4 | 7.7 |
| Rye, Light, Finest, Tesco* | 1 Slice/20g | 47.0 | 0.0 | 237 | 10.4 | 44.3 | 2.0 | 3.7 |
| Rye, Swedish Style, Kelderman* | 1 Slice/50g | 92.0 | 2.0 | 185 | 7.2 | 31.5 | 3.2 | 4.3 |
| Rye, Wheat Free, New York Deli, The Stamp Collection* | 1 Slice/33g | 61.0 | 0.0 | 184 | 6.6 | 43.6 | 1.4 | 7.3 |
| Rye, Wholemeal, Organic, House Of Westphalia* | 1 Slice/75g | 121.0 | 1.0 | 162 | 5.1 | 32.8 | 1.2 | 7.8 |
| Rye, Wholemeal, with Sunflower Seeds, Organic, Biona* | 1 Slice/72g | 144.0 | 3.0 | 202 | 7.1 | 35.0 | 3.7 | 0.0 |
| Rye, with Sunflower Seeds, Organic, Schneider Brot* | 1 Slice/72g | 138.0 | 3.0 | 191 | 6.2 | 33.4 | 3.6 | 7.9 |
| Rye with Sunflower Seeds, Organic, Sunnyvale* | 1 Slice/25g | 49.0 | 2.0 | 198 | 5.1 | 30.3 | 6.3 | 0.0 |
| Seeded, Batch, Finest, Tesco* | 1 Slice/65g | 168.0 | 4.0 | 259 | 9.3 | 41.8 | 6.1 | 6.1 |
| Seeded Farmhouse Loaf, Extra Special, Asda* | 1 Slice/44g | 92.0 | 1.0 | 207 | 11.0 | 38.0 | 1.2 | 8.0 |
| Seriously Seeded, Gold, Kingsmill* | 1 Slice/50g | 136.0 | 3.0 | 272 | 10.9 | 41.6 | 6.9 | 6.4 |
| Seven Grain, Hearty, Golden Wonder* | 1 Slice/38g | 80.0 | 1.0 | 211 | 10.5 | 47.4 | 2.6 | 7.9 |
| *Soda* | *1oz/28g* | *72.0* | *1.0* | *258* | *7.7* | *54.6* | *2.5* | *2.1* |
| Soda, M & S* | 1 Slice/40g | 82.0 | 1.0 | 205 | 8.7 | 39.2 | 1.6 | 4.2 |
| Softgrain, Farmhouse, M & S* | 1 Slice/25g | 59.0 | 1.0 | 238 | 8.4 | 42.8 | 3.7 | 3.2 |
| Softgrain, Medium Sliced, GFY, Asda* | 1 Slice/35g | 79.0 | 1.0 | 226 | 7.0 | 46.0 | 1.5 | 3.7 |
| Softgrain, Mighty White* | 1 Slice/36g | 81.0 | 1.0 | 224 | 7.2 | 45.5 | 1.5 | 3.7 |
| Soya & Linseed, Burgen* | 1 Slice/36g | 99.0 | 4.0 | 274 | 15.9 | 29.8 | 10.1 | 6.8 |
| Soya & Linseed, Vogel* | 1 Slice/45g | 107.0 | 3.0 | 238 | 12.2 | 34.0 | 5.9 | 5.4 |
| Stoneground, Small Loaf, Organic, Sainsbury's* | 1 Slice/24g | 50.0 | 0.0 | 208 | 10.0 | 37.9 | 2.1 | 7.9 |
| Sunflower, Multi-Grain, Allinson* | 1 Slice/47g | 113.0 | 2.0 | 240 | 9.8 | 39.6 | 4.7 | 3.9 |
| Sunflower & Honey, Organic, Cranks* | 1 Slice/30g | 64.0 | 1.0 | 215 | 11.6 | 37.2 | 3.0 | 8.3 |
| Sunflower & Pumpin Seed, Batched, Organic, Tesco* | 1 Slice/30g | 73.0 | 2.0 | 243 | 11.0 | 33.1 | 7.4 | 5.2 |
| Sunflower & Pumpkin Seed, So Organic, Sainsbury's* | 1 Slice/30g | 76.0 | 2.0 | 254 | 11.4 | 40.0 | 5.4 | 12.9 |
| Sunflower Seed, Bolletje, Delhaize* | 1 Slice/44g | 106.0 | 3.0 | 240 | 7.5 | 35.0 | 7.0 | 6.0 |
| Tiger Loaf, Tesco* | 1 Slice/40g | 96.0 | 1.0 | 239 | 8.7 | 46.6 | 2.0 | 2.6 |
| Tomato, & Herb, Tear & Share, Tesco* | ¼ Pack/73g | 164.0 | 3.0 | 226 | 6.3 | 40.2 | 4.4 | 2.1 |
| Tomato & Chilli, BGTY, Sainsbury's* | ¼ Bread/65g | 155.0 | 3.0 | 238 | 11.9 | 36.9 | 4.7 | 2.8 |
| Tomato & Garlic, Italian Style, Morrisons* | ½ Pack/155g | 355.0 | 12.0 | 229 | 5.8 | 33.4 | 8.0 | 2.5 |
| Veda Malt, St Michael* | 1 Serving/45g | 99.0 | 0.0 | 219 | 7.1 | 45.3 | 1.1 | 2.2 |
| Walnut, Waitrose* | 1/8 Loaf/50g | 169.0 | 8.0 | 339 | 10.0 | 40.6 | 15.2 | 5.9 |
| *Wheat* | *1 Slice/25g* | *65.0* | *1.0* | *260* | *9.1* | *47.2* | *4.1* | *4.3* |
| Wheaten, M & S* | 1 Slice/33g | 74.0 | 1.0 | 225 | 9.3 | 42.9 | 3.5 | 3.9 |
| Wheatgerm, Hovis, Soft, Sliced, M & S* | 1 Slice/23g | 50.0 | 1.0 | 220 | 10.1 | 38.5 | 3.0 | 4.6 |
| Wheatgrain, Robertson* | 1 Slice/30g | 90.0 | 1.0 | 300 | 9.3 | 57.3 | 4.0 | 4.0 |
| *White, Average* | *1 Slice/25g* | *59.0* | *0.0* | *235* | *8.4* | *49.3* | *1.9* | *1.5* |
| White, Batch, Warburton's* | 1 Slice/42g | 98.0 | 1.0 | 233 | 9.8 | 43.6 | 2.1 | 2.7 |
| White, Batch Loaf, Extra Special, Asda* | 1 Slice/47g | 109.0 | 1.0 | 233 | 9.0 | 45.0 | 1.9 | 2.2 |
| White, Classic, Medium Sliced, Hovis* | 1 Slice/38g | 91.0 | 1.0 | 240 | 11.4 | 40.3 | 2.3 | 6.5 |
| White, COU, M & S* | 1 Slice/26g | 60.0 | 1.0 | 231 | 10.6 | 41.9 | 2.3 | 4.6 |
| White, Crusty, Gold, Kingsmill* | 1 Slice/27g | 70.0 | 1.0 | 258 | 9.4 | 48.5 | 2.9 | 2.7 |
| White, Crusty, Hovis* | 1 Slice/44g | 103.0 | 1.0 | 233 | 8.8 | 44.3 | 2.2 | 2.1 |

**B**

## BREAD

| INFO/WEIGHT | Measure | per Measure KCAL | FAT | Nutrition Values per 100g / 100ml KCAL | PROT | CARB | FAT | FIBRE |
|---|---|---|---|---|---|---|---|---|
| White, Crusty, Sliced Loaf, Tesco* | 1 Slice/50g | 116.0 | 1.0 | 233 | 7.4 | 46.0 | 2.1 | 2.0 |
| White, Danish, Sliced, Weight Watchers* | 1 Slice/21g | 49.0 | 0.0 | 238 | 10.5 | 45.8 | 1.4 | 2.3 |
| White, Danish, Soft & Light, Thick Cut, Asda* | 1 Slice/26g | 60.0 | 0.0 | 230 | 9.0 | 45.0 | 1.6 | 2.1 |
| White, Danish, Warburton's* | 1 Slice/26g | 61.0 | 0.0 | 238 | 10.5 | 45.8 | 1.4 | 2.3 |
| White, Eat Smart, Safeway* | 1 Slice/26g | 60.0 | 0.0 | 230 | 8.8 | 45.0 | 1.8 | 2.3 |
| White, Extra Thick Sliced, Kingsmill* | 1 Slice/58g | 135.0 | 1.0 | 232 | 8.8 | 43.8 | 2.4 | 2.8 |
| White, Farmhouse, Hovis* | 1 Slice/44g | 99.0 | 1.0 | 226 | 8.2 | 44.6 | 1.6 | 3.2 |
| White, Farmhouse, Soft, Warburton's* | 1 Slice/43g | 101.0 | 1.0 | 236 | 9.9 | 43.4 | 2.5 | 2.7 |
| White, Farmhouse Crusty, M & S* | 1 Slice/34g | 82.0 | 1.0 | 240 | 8.9 | 46.6 | 2.2 | 3.0 |
| White, Farmhouse Gold Premium, Morrisons* | 1 Slice/38g | 90.0 | 0.0 | 236 | 8.9 | 47.4 | 1.2 | 2.2 |
| White, Fibre, Morrisons* | 1 Slice/40g | 96.0 | 1.0 | 240 | 8.0 | 48.4 | 1.7 | 0.3 |
| **White, Fried in Blended Oil** | **1 Slice/28g** | **141.0** | **9.0** | **503** | **7.9** | **48.5** | **32.2** | **1.6** |
| White, Gluten & Wheat Free, Free From, Sainsbury's* | 1 Slice/33g | 75.0 | 3.0 | 227 | 1.9 | 35.5 | 8.6 | 1.0 |
| White, Gold Seeded, Kingsmill* | 1 Slice/44g | 108.0 | 3.0 | 245 | 9.7 | 38.8 | 5.7 | 3.5 |
| White, Golden, Square Cut, M & S* | 1 Slice/40g | 85.0 | 1.0 | 215 | 8.9 | 40.7 | 2.1 | 6.1 |
| White, Good Health, Warburton's* | 1 Slice/38g | 84.0 | 1.0 | 220 | 9.4 | 41.6 | 1.8 | 4.1 |
| White, High Fibre, Nimble* | 1 Slice/22g | 48.0 | 0.0 | 219 | 10.1 | 40.6 | 1.8 | 7.5 |
| White, Invisible Crust, Hovis* | 1 Slice/40g | 90.0 | 1.0 | 226 | 8.8 | 44.1 | 1.6 | 2.4 |
| White, Loaf, Crusty, Premium, Warburton's* | 1 Slice/31g | 76.0 | 1.0 | 249 | 10.6 | 46.5 | 2.3 | 2.6 |
| White, Low Carb, Sliced, Tesco* | 1 Slice/16g | 35.0 | 0.0 | 211 | 11.3 | 36.4 | 2.2 | 6.9 |
| White, Medium, Round Top, Kingsmill* | 1 Slice/42g | 97.0 | 1.0 | 232 | 8.8 | 43.8 | 2.4 | 2.8 |
| White, Medium, Stayfresh, Tesco* | 1 Slice/45g | 108.0 | 1.0 | 240 | 8.2 | 47.8 | 1.5 | 3.0 |
| White, Medium, VLH Kitchens* | 1 Slice/30g | 72.0 | 0.6 | 241 | 8.4 | 49.3 | 1.9 | 1.5 |
| White, Medium Sliced, Asda* | 1 Slice/37g | 80.0 | 1.0 | 218 | 8.0 | 43.0 | 1.5 | 3.3 |
| White, Medium Sliced, Basics, Sainsbury's* | 1 Slice/36g | 83.0 | 1.0 | 231 | 8.0 | 46.4 | 1.5 | 2.1 |
| White, Medium Sliced, Long Life, Asda* | 1 Slice/36g | 82.0 | 1.0 | 228 | 8.0 | 45.0 | 1.8 | 2.7 |
| White, Medium Sliced, Sainsbury's* | 1 Slice/36g | 78.0 | 1.0 | 216 | 8.7 | 41.1 | 1.9 | 7.1 |
| White, Medium Sliced, Small Loaf, Warburton's* | 1 Slice/23g | 55.0 | 0.0 | 239 | 10.3 | 45.1 | 1.9 | 2.7 |
| White, Medium Sliced, Square, Kingsmill* | 1 Slice/66g | 88.0 | 1.0 | 133 | 5.0 | 25.1 | 1.4 | 1.7 |
| White, Medium Sliced, Stay Fresh, Tesco* | 1 Slice/35g | 85.0 | 1.0 | 246 | 8.9 | 48.1 | 2.0 | 0.8 |
| White, Medium Sliced, Tesco* | 1 Slice/36g | 86.0 | 1.0 | 240 | 8.2 | 47.8 | 1.5 | 3.0 |
| White, Medium Sliced, Value, Tesco* | 1 Slice/36g | 81.0 | 0.0 | 225 | 7.9 | 46.1 | 1.0 | 2.1 |
| White, Medium Sliced, Warburton's* | 1 Slice/40g | 94.0 | 1.0 | 234 | 9.9 | 43.8 | 2.0 | 2.6 |
| White, Medium Sliced, Weight Watchers* | 1 Slice/12g | 30.0 | 0.0 | 247 | 12.5 | 45.2 | 1.9 | 3.2 |
| White, Oatmeal, Allinson* | 1 Slice/47g | 111.0 | 1.0 | 237 | 9.0 | 43.5 | 3.0 | 2.7 |
| White, Organic, Hovis* | 1 Slice/44g | 108.0 | 1.0 | 246 | 8.6 | 45.8 | 3.2 | 2.3 |
| White, Organic, Sainsbury's* | 1 Slice/36g | 84.0 | 1.0 | 234 | 8.9 | 45.5 | 1.8 | 2.3 |
| White, Plain, Scottish, Sunblest* | 1 Slice/57g | 133.0 | 1.0 | 233 | 10.1 | 42.3 | 2.6 | 2.8 |
| White, Premium, M & S* | 1 Slice/40g | 95.0 | 1.0 | 235 | 8.5 | 45.8 | 1.9 | 2.7 |
| White, Premium Gold, TTD, Sainsbury's* | 1 Slice/44g | 103.0 | 1.0 | 233 | 8.4 | 45.6 | 1.9 | 2.2 |
| White, Sandwich, Bakery, Sainsbury's* | 1 Slice/50g | 121.0 | 0.0 | 242 | 10.3 | 49.0 | 0.6 | 2.9 |
| White, Sandwich, Kingsmill* | 1 Slice/42g | 97.0 | 1.0 | 232 | 8.8 | 43.8 | 2.4 | 2.8 |
| White, Sliced, Roberts Bakery* | 1 Slice/35g | 87.0 | 1.0 | 249 | 10.0 | 48.0 | 2.1 | 2.5 |
| White, Softgrain, Sliced, Tesco* | 1 Med Slice/36g | 81.0 | 1.0 | 224 | 7.2 | 45.5 | 1.5 | 3.7 |
| White, Square, Extra Thick Sliced, Hovis* | 1 Slice/67g | 155.0 | 1.0 | 231 | 8.5 | 44.7 | 2.0 | 2.6 |
| White, Square, Medium Sliced, Hovis* | 1 Slice/40g | 92.0 | 1.0 | 231 | 8.5 | 44.7 | 2.0 | 2.6 |
| White, Square, Thick Sliced, Hovis* | 1 Slice/50g | 116.0 | 1.0 | 231 | 8.5 | 44.7 | 2.0 | 2.6 |
| White, Stay Fresh, Tesco* | 1 Slice/40g | 100.0 | 1.0 | 249 | 8.6 | 48.3 | 2.4 | 1.5 |
| White, Thick, So Organic, Sainsbury's* | 1 Slice/44g | 102.0 | 1.0 | 231 | 8.2 | 44.6 | 2.2 | 3.1 |
| White, Thick Sliced, Bakers Gold, Asda* | 1 Slice/44g | 101.0 | 1.0 | 229 | 8.0 | 45.0 | 1.9 | 2.3 |
| White, Thick Sliced, Healthy, Warburton's* | 1 Slice/38g | 84.0 | 1.0 | 222 | 10.3 | 41.2 | 1.8 | 4.1 |
| White, Thick Sliced, M & S* | 1 Slice/42g | 96.0 | 1.0 | 228 | 7.3 | 46.7 | 1.3 | 2.8 |
| White, Thick Sliced, Organic, Tesco* | 1 Slice/44g | 108.0 | 1.0 | 245 | 8.5 | 46.8 | 2.1 | 3.1 |

## BREAD

| | Measure INFO/WEIGHT | per Measure KCAL | FAT | Nutrition Values per 100g / 100ml KCAL | PROT | CARB | FAT | FIBRE |
|---|---|---|---|---|---|---|---|---|
| White, Thick Sliced, Premium, Tesco* | 1 Slice/44g | 99.0 | 0.0 | 222 | 8.7 | 45.2 | 0.7 | 1.5 |
| White, Thick Sliced, Sainsbury's* | 1 Slice/44g | 95.0 | 1.0 | 216 | 8.7 | 41.1 | 1.9 | 7.1 |
| White, Thick Sliced, Square Cut, Asda* | 1 Slice/44g | 101.0 | 1.0 | 230 | 8.0 | 46.0 | 1.5 | 2.1 |
| White, Thick Sliced, Staysoft, Rathbones* | 1 Slice/38g | 87.0 | 0.0 | 228 | 8.5 | 45.5 | 1.3 | 2.7 |
| White, Thick Sliced, Sunblest* | 1 Slice/40g | 91.0 | 1.0 | 228 | 8.0 | 45.7 | 1.5 | 2.8 |
| White, Thick Sliced, Super Toastie, Morrisons* | 1 Slice/50g | 128.0 | 1.0 | 257 | 8.7 | 48.9 | 3.0 | 2.1 |
| White, Thick Sliced, Tesco* | 1 Slice/44g | 106.0 | 1.0 | 240 | 8.2 | 47.8 | 1.5 | 3.0 |
| White, Thick Sliced, Value, Tesco* | 1 Slice/44g | 106.0 | 1.0 | 240 | 8.2 | 47.8 | 1.5 | 3.0 |
| White, Thick Sliced, Warburtons, Weight Watchers* | 1 Slice/29g | 69.0 | 0.0 | 237 | 10.4 | 48.6 | 0.8 | 2.0 |
| White, Thick Sliced, Warburton's* | 1 Slice/28g | 65.0 | 1.0 | 233 | 9.8 | 43.6 | 2.1 | 2.7 |
| White, Thin Sliced, Sainsbury's* | 1 Slice/29g | 66.0 | 0.0 | 228 | 7.1 | 46.4 | 1.5 | 2.8 |
| White, Thin Sliced, Tesco* | 1 Slice/30g | 68.0 | 0.0 | 228 | 9.5 | 44.5 | 1.3 | 3.4 |
| *White, Toasted, Average* | *1 Slice/33g* | *87.0* | *1.0* | *265* | *9.3* | *57.1* | *1.6* | *1.8* |
| White, Toastie, 800g Loaf, Warburton's* | 1 Slice/47g | 111.0 | 1.0 | 234 | 9.9 | 43.9 | 1.9 | 2.5 |
| White, Toastie, Thick, Love to Toast, Kingsmill* | 1 Slice/50g | 116.0 | 1.0 | 232 | 9.0 | 44.6 | 2.0 | 2.7 |
| White, Toastie, Thick Cut, Hovis* | 1 Slice/50g | 115.0 | 1.0 | 230 | 8.5 | 44.7 | 2.0 | 2.5 |
| White, Weight Watchers* | 1 Serving/5g | 12.0 | 0.0 | 246 | 12.3 | 45.1 | 1.6 | 3.3 |
| White, Wholesome, Medium Sliced, Asda* | 1 Slice/35g | 78.0 | 1.0 | 223 | 7.0 | 43.0 | 2.6 | 5.0 |
| White, Wholesome, Medium Sliced, Premium, Tesco* | 1 Slice/37g | 85.0 | 1.0 | 232 | 8.9 | 43.9 | 2.3 | 4.2 |
| Whole Grain, Batch, Finest, Tesco* | 1 Slice/44g | 112.0 | 1.0 | 254 | 9.8 | 47.7 | 2.7 | 4.2 |
| Whole Grain, Brennans* | 1 Slice/39g | 79.0 | 1.0 | 203 | 9.0 | 40.0 | 1.5 | 4.9 |
| Whole Grain, with Sunflower Seeds, Landgut* | 1 Slice/83g | 183.0 | 4.0 | 221 | 7.0 | 37.0 | 5.0 | 29.0 |
| Whole Grain & Rye, Schneider Brot* | 1 Slice/50g | 93.0 | 1.0 | 186 | 5.8 | 37.7 | 1.3 | 8.4 |
| Whole Wheat, Soft, Trader Joe's* | 1 Slice/37g | 70.0 | 1.0 | 189 | 10.8 | 37.8 | 2.7 | 5.4 |
| Wholegrain, Medium Sliced, Irish Pride* | 1 Slice/38g | 90.0 | 1.0 | 237 | 9.2 | 46.6 | 2.1 | 7.6 |
| Wholegrain, Soft, M & S* | 1 Slice/51g | 115.0 | 3.0 | 225 | 13.0 | 31.2 | 5.4 | 8.2 |
| Wholemeal, & Oat Flakes, Gold, Kingsmill* | 1 Slice/47g | 103.0 | 2.0 | 220 | 10.0 | 37.3 | 3.4 | 7.0 |
| Wholemeal, Allinson* | 1 Slice/47g | 102.0 | 1.0 | 216 | 12.5 | 34.8 | 3.0 | 7.4 |
| *Wholemeal, Average* | *1 Slice/25g* | *54.0* | *1.0* | *215* | *9.2* | *41.6* | *2.5* | *5.8* |
| Wholemeal, BGTY, Sainsbury's* | 1 Slice/20g | 41.0 | 0.0 | 207 | 12.6 | 36.8 | 1.0 | 7.3 |
| Wholemeal, COU, M & S* | 1 Slice/21g | 45.0 | 1.0 | 213 | 13.6 | 33.7 | 2.6 | 7.0 |
| Wholemeal, Crusty, Finest, Tesco* | 1 Slice/50g | 103.0 | 1.0 | 206 | 10.8 | 37.0 | 1.7 | 6.9 |
| Wholemeal, Crusty, Kingsmill* | 1 Slice/42g | 104.0 | 2.0 | 247 | 11.2 | 41.1 | 4.2 | 7.0 |
| Wholemeal, Danish, BFY, Morrisons* | 1 Slice/17g | 39.0 | 0.0 | 228 | 11.2 | 47.9 | 1.8 | 6.2 |
| Wholemeal, Danish, Warburton's* | 1 Slice/25g | 57.0 | 1.0 | 229 | 13.3 | 38.5 | 2.4 | 7.2 |
| Wholemeal, Economy, Sainsbury's* | 1 Slice/28g | 61.0 | 1.0 | 217 | 10.3 | 38.4 | 2.5 | 6.5 |
| Wholemeal, Farmhouse, Hovis* | 1 Slice/44g | 91.0 | 1.0 | 207 | 11.0 | 36.0 | 2.2 | 7.1 |
| Wholemeal, Gold, Kingsmill* | 1 Slice/44g | 95.0 | 1.0 | 217 | 10.9 | 36.8 | 2.9 | 7.0 |
| Wholemeal, Golden, M & S* | 1 Slice/30g | 69.0 | 1.0 | 230 | 10.8 | 36.6 | 4.5 | 7.7 |
| Wholemeal, Golden Wheat, Kingsmill* | 1 Slice/44g | 97.0 | 1.0 | 221 | 10.9 | 37.8 | 2.9 | 6.0 |
| Wholemeal, Keep Fresh, Medium Sliced, Safeway* | 1 Slice/37g | 75.0 | 1.0 | 204 | 9.1 | 36.6 | 2.4 | 6.2 |
| Wholemeal, Little Brown Loaf, Unsliced, Hovis* | 1 Slice/40g | 86.0 | 1.0 | 216 | 10.0 | 37.8 | 2.7 | 6.8 |
| Wholemeal, Loaf, Sliced, Medium, 800g, Hovis* | 1 Slice/40g | 86.0 | 1.0 | 216 | 10.0 | 37.8 | 2.7 | 2.7 |
| Wholemeal, Makes Sense, Somerfield* | 1 Slice/36g | 78.0 | 1.0 | 217 | 10.7 | 38.6 | 2.2 | 6.6 |
| Wholemeal, Medium, 400g Loaf, Warburton's* | 1 Slice/24g | 55.0 | 1.0 | 231 | 10.4 | 40.7 | 2.5 | 6.5 |
| Wholemeal, Medium Sliced, Asda* | 1 Slice/36g | 80.0 | 1.0 | 223 | 9.0 | 39.0 | 3.4 | 6.0 |
| Wholemeal, Medium Sliced, Great Everyday, Kingsmill* | 1 Slice/40g | 91.0 | 2.0 | 227 | 10.5 | 37.7 | 3.8 | 6.2 |
| Wholemeal, Medium Sliced, M & S* | 1 Slice/40g | 80.0 | 1.0 | 200 | 10.5 | 32.7 | 3.1 | 6.7 |
| Wholemeal, Medium Sliced, Morrisons* | 1 Slice/32g | 68.0 | 1.0 | 214 | 9.9 | 38.0 | 2.5 | 5.8 |
| Wholemeal, Medium Sliced, Organic, Asda* | 1 Slice/43g | 94.0 | 1.0 | 217 | 9.0 | 40.0 | 2.3 | 6.0 |
| Wholemeal, Medium Sliced, Sainsbury's* | 1 Slice/36g | 77.0 | 1.0 | 214 | 10.3 | 37.8 | 2.4 | 7.4 |
| Wholemeal, Medium Sliced, Waitrose* | 1 Slice/36g | 76.0 | 1.0 | 213 | 10.1 | 37.6 | 2.4 | 7.0 |
| Wholemeal, Nimble* | 1 Slice/22g | 48.0 | 1.0 | 219 | 12.2 | 37.0 | 2.5 | 6.8 |

| | Measure INFO/WEIGHT | per Measure KCAL | FAT | Nutrition Values per 100g / 100ml KCAL | PROT | CARB | FAT | FIBRE |
|---|---|---|---|---|---|---|---|---|
| **BREAD** | | | | | | | | |
| Wholemeal, Organic, 400g Loaf, Warburton's* | 1 Slice/28g | 63.0 | 1.0 | 223 | 10.3 | 37.9 | 3.2 | 6.7 |
| Wholemeal, Organic, Hovis* | 1 Slice/44g | 92.0 | 1.0 | 209 | 10.2 | 35.6 | 2.9 | 7.6 |
| Wholemeal, Premium, Medium Slice, M & S* | 1 Slice/33g | 65.0 | 1.0 | 200 | 10.5 | 32.9 | 3.1 | 6.7 |
| Wholemeal, Rathbones* | 1 Slice/27g | 57.0 | 0.0 | 211 | 9.4 | 39.2 | 1.8 | 7.1 |
| Wholemeal, Rustic, Tin, Tesco* | 1 Slice/37g | 92.0 | 1.0 | 249 | 12.2 | 44.0 | 3.5 | 3.1 |
| Wholemeal, Sliced, Gluten Free, Glutano* | 1 Slice/56g | 107.0 | 2.0 | 191 | 7.0 | 34.0 | 3.0 | 0.0 |
| Wholemeal, Square Cut, Thick Sliced, Asda* | 1 Slice/44g | 91.0 | 1.0 | 208 | 10.0 | 37.0 | 2.2 | 6.0 |
| Wholemeal, Stayfresh, Tesco* | 1 Slice/36g | 81.0 | 1.0 | 225 | 11.0 | 39.1 | 2.2 | 6.0 |
| Wholemeal, Stoneground, 800g Loaf, Warburton's* | 1 Slice/45g | 95.0 | 1.0 | 210 | 10.4 | 35.8 | 2.6 | 6.8 |
| Wholemeal, Stoneground, Organic, Sainsbury's* | 1 Slice/29g | 61.0 | 1.0 | 210 | 10.2 | 37.9 | 1.9 | 7.8 |
| Wholemeal, Thick Sliced, Great Everyday, Kingsmill* | 1 Slice/44g | 100.0 | 2.0 | 227 | 10.5 | 37.7 | 3.8 | 6.2 |
| Wholemeal, Thick Sliced, Organic, Tesco* | 1 Slice/44g | 98.0 | 1.0 | 220 | 8.8 | 38.8 | 2.8 | 5.9 |
| Wholemeal, Thick Sliced, Sainsbury's* | 1 Slice/48g | 102.0 | 1.0 | 213 | 10.1 | 37.4 | 2.6 | 8.5 |
| Wholemeal, Thick Sliced, Waitrose* | 1 Slice/44g | 94.0 | 1.0 | 213 | 10.1 | 37.6 | 2.4 | 7.0 |
| Wholemeal, Thick Sliced, Weight Watchers* | 1 Slice/29g | 67.0 | 1.0 | 231 | 10.9 | 40.3 | 2.5 | 6.5 |
| **Wholemeal, Toasted, Average** | **1 Med Slice/26g** | **58.0** | **1.0** | **224** | **8.6** | **42.3** | **2.2** | **5.8** |
| Wholemeal, Toastie, 800g Loaf, Warburton's* | 1 Slice/45g | 101.0 | 1.0 | 224 | 9.7 | 39.3 | 2.4 | 6.6 |
| Wholemeal, Value, Tesco* | 1 Slice/36g | 78.0 | 1.0 | 217 | 10.3 | 38.4 | 2.5 | 6.5 |
| Wholewheat, No Crusts, Harry's* | 1 Slice/25g | 58.0 | 1.0 | 233 | 8.0 | 40.0 | 4.5 | 5.5 |
| **BREAD & BUTTER PUDDING** | | | | | | | | |
| 5% Fat, M & S* | 1 Pudding/237g | 367.0 | 10.0 | 155 | 4.4 | 24.8 | 4.2 | 0.4 |
| Asda* | 1 Serving/125g | 280.0 | 15.0 | 224 | 4.9 | 24.0 | 12.0 | 0.0 |
| Average | 1 Serving/190g | 304.0 | 15.0 | 160 | 6.2 | 17.5 | 7.8 | 0.3 |
| BGTY, Sainsbury's* | 1 Serving/125g | 126.0 | 3.0 | 101 | 6.3 | 13.4 | 2.3 | 5.4 |
| COU, M & S* | 1 Pot/140g | 161.0 | 3.0 | 115 | 6.1 | 18.4 | 2.0 | 0.8 |
| Finest, Tesco* | 1 Serving/153g | 379.0 | 22.0 | 248 | 4.9 | 24.6 | 14.4 | 0.9 |
| GFY, Asda* | 1 Serving/125g | 152.0 | 2.0 | 122 | 7.0 | 20.0 | 1.6 | 1.3 |
| HE, Tesco* | 1 Serving/125g | 152.0 | 2.0 | 122 | 7.0 | 20.0 | 1.6 | 1.3 |
| Individual, M & S* | 1 Pudding/130g | 279.0 | 16.0 | 215 | 4.4 | 21.4 | 12.6 | 0.5 |
| Low Fat, Individual, BGTY, Sainsbury's* | 1 Pack/125g | 125.0 | 3.0 | 100 | 6.3 | 13.4 | 2.3 | 5.4 |
| Reduced Fat, Waitrose* | 1 Serving/205g | 299.0 | 5.0 | 146 | 7.4 | 23.3 | 2.6 | 2.0 |
| Sainsbury's* | ½ Pudding/115g | 223.0 | 11.0 | 194 | 4.8 | 21.9 | 9.7 | 0.4 |
| Tesco* | ½ Pack | 494.0 | 32.0 | 250 | 5.0 | 20.8 | 16.1 | 0.4 |
| **BREAD MIX** | | | | | | | | |
| Banana, Graze* | 1 Pack/50g | 209.0 | 7.0 | 419 | 7.0 | 47.6 | 14.4 | 0.0 |
| Brown, Sunflower, Sainsbury's* | 1 Serving/60g | 151.0 | 4.0 | 251 | 10.0 | 38.9 | 6.1 | 4.0 |
| Cheese & Onion, Dry Mix, Sainsbury's* | 1 Serving/100g | 311.0 | 3.0 | 311 | 11.9 | 59.5 | 2.8 | 2.6 |
| Ciabatta, Made Up with Water & Olive Oil, Wrights* | 1 Slice/45g | 113.0 | 2.0 | 251 | 10.0 | 43.6 | 4.0 | 1.8 |
| Crusty White, Made Up, Tesco* | 1 Slice/126g | 316.0 | 2.0 | 251 | 9.4 | 49.3 | 1.8 | 2.5 |
| Focaccia, Garlic & Herb, Asda* | 1 Serving/125g | 385.0 | 10.0 | 308 | 11.0 | 48.0 | 8.0 | 3.3 |
| Italian Ciabatta, Sainsbury's* | 1 Slice/45g | 96.0 | 1.0 | 213 | 8.7 | 40.0 | 2.0 | 2.4 |
| Mixed Grain, Sainsbury's* | 1 Serving/45g | 103.0 | 1.0 | 228 | 7.7 | 46.0 | 1.5 | 4.4 |
| White Loaf, Asda* | 1 Slice/60g | 150.0 | 1.0 | 250 | 10.0 | 49.0 | 1.5 | 3.1 |
| Wholemeal, Made Up, M & S* | 1 Loaf/600g | 1410.0 | 14.0 | 235 | 11.0 | 42.0 | 2.4 | 5.3 |
| **BREADCRUMBS** | | | | | | | | |
| **Average** | **1oz/28g** | **98.0** | **1.0** | **350** | **10.7** | **74.8** | **1.9** | **2.5** |
| **BREADFRUIT** | | | | | | | | |
| **Canned, Drained** | **1oz/28g** | **18.0** | **0.0** | **66** | **0.6** | **16.4** | **0.2** | **1.7** |
| **Raw** | **1oz/28g** | **27.0** | **0.0** | **95** | **1.3** | **23.1** | **0.3** | **0.0** |
| **BREADSTICKS** | | | | | | | | |
| Cheese, Italian, Tesco* | 4 Breadsticks/21g | 84.0 | 2.0 | 399 | 14.2 | 67.5 | 8.0 | 3.4 |
| Chive & Onion Twists, Tesco* | 3 Twists/24g | 115.0 | 5.0 | 480 | 11.6 | 57.6 | 22.1 | 2.2 |
| Farleys* | 1 Serving/12g | 50.0 | 1.0 | 414 | 14.0 | 76.5 | 5.8 | 1.1 |

|  | Measure INFO/WEIGHT | per Measure KCAL | FAT | Nutrition Values per 100g / 100ml KCAL | PROT | CARB | FAT | FIBRE |
|---|---|---|---|---|---|---|---|---|
| **BREADSTICKS** | | | | | | | | |
| GFY, Asda* | 1 Breadstick/5g | 19.0 | 0.0 | 378 | 13.7 | 77.3 | 1.6 | 3.8 |
| Grissini, Italian, Sainsbury's* | 1 Breadstick/5g | 20.0 | 0.0 | 408 | 11.6 | 72.9 | 7.8 | 2.9 |
| Grissini, Thin, with Olive Oil, Forno Bianco* | 1 Stick/5g | 21.0 | 0.0 | 420 | 11.0 | 77.0 | 7.5 | 0.0 |
| Grissini, Waitrose* | 1 Breadstick/6g | 25.0 | 0.0 | 397 | 12.0 | 72.5 | 6.2 | 3.1 |
| Mini, Sainsbury's* | 4 Breadsticks/5g | 20.0 | 0.0 | 404 | 15.6 | 68.7 | 7.4 | 4.8 |
| Mini, Wheat & Gluten Free, Free From, Tesco* | 1 Stick/3g | 11.0 | 0.0 | 414 | 4.0 | 72.1 | 12.2 | 2.2 |
| Olive Oil & Rosemary, Finest, Tesco* | 2 Breadsticks/10g | 42.0 | 1.0 | 427 | 13.9 | 64.4 | 12.6 | 4.1 |
| Onion, M & S* | 1 Serving/40g | 166.0 | 6.0 | 415 | 12.6 | 59.6 | 14.1 | 4.8 |
| Original, Italian, Tesco* | 1 Stick/6g | 23.0 | 0.0 | 410 | 11.6 | 72.9 | 7.8 | 2.9 |
| Original, Organic, Kallo* | 1 Breadstick/6g | 24.0 | 0.0 | 393 | 11.8 | 69.5 | 7.6 | 4.7 |
| Oven Baked, Mini, Quaker* | 1 Pack/35g | 145.0 | 3.0 | 415 | 12.9 | 71.0 | 8.8 | 3.7 |
| Perfectly Balanced, Waitrose* | 1 Breadstick/5g | 20.0 | 0.0 | 378 | 13.7 | 77.3 | 1.6 | 3.8 |
| Pesto Flavour, Safeway* | 1 Stick/6g | 24.0 | 0.0 | 394 | 13.4 | 67.5 | 7.8 | 5.2 |
| Rosemary, Asda* | 1 Breadstick/7g | 29.0 | 1.0 | 439 | 12.0 | 64.0 | 15.0 | 3.5 |
| **BREAKFAST** | | | | | | | | |
| All Day, Kershaws* | 1 Pack/280g | 392.0 | 22.0 | 140 | 7.3 | 9.6 | 8.0 | 1.6 |
| All Day, with Baked Beans, Heinz* | 1 Pack/403g | 463.0 | 17.0 | 115 | 5.8 | 13.3 | 4.3 | 2.4 |
| Farmhouse, Ready Meals, Waitrose* | ½ Pack/250g | 385.0 | 25.0 | 154 | 2.9 | 11.0 | 10.0 | 1.2 |
| Pack, Fruit Pudding, Asda* | 1 Serving/44g | 45.0 | 2.0 | 103 | 1.4 | 15.0 | 4.2 | 0.0 |
| **BREAKFAST CEREAL** | | | | | | | | |
| 3 in One, Raisin & Apple, Jordans* | 1 Serving/50g | 170.0 | 2.0 | 340 | 7.6 | 67.4 | 4.4 | 9.8 |
| 3 in One, Strawberry, Jordans* | 1 Serving/50g | 181.0 | 3.0 | 362 | 9.4 | 68.0 | 5.8 | 11.9 |
| Advantage, Weetabix* | 1 Serving/30g | 105.0 | 1.0 | 350 | 10.2 | 72.0 | 2.4 | 9.0 |
| All Bran, Apricot Bites, Kellogg's* | 1 Serving/45g | 126.0 | 1.0 | 279 | 11.0 | 55.0 | 2.5 | 19.0 |
| All Bran, Asda* | 1 Serving/10g | 110.0 | 1.0 | 276 | 15.0 | 46.0 | 3.5 | 27.0 |
| All Bran, Bran Flakes, & Fruit, Kellogg's* | 1 Serving/40g | 143.0 | 2.0 | 358 | 8.0 | 68.0 | 6.0 | 9.0 |
| All Bran, Bran Flakes, Chocolate, Kellogg's* | 1 Serving/30g | 106.0 | 2.0 | 354 | 10.0 | 65.0 | 6.0 | 13.0 |
| All Bran, Bran Flakes, Yoghurty, Kellogg's* | 1 Serving/40g | 141.0 | 2.0 | 353 | 10.0 | 67.0 | 5.0 | 12.0 |
| All Bran, Fibre Plus, Kellogg's* | 1 Serving/40g | 112.0 | 1.0 | 280 | 14.0 | 48.0 | 3.5 | 27.0 |
| All Bran, Fruitful, Kellogg's* | 1 Serving/40g | 136.0 | 3.0 | 340 | 12.5 | 57.5 | 7.5 | 0.0 |
| All Bran, Original, High Fibre, Kellogg's* | 1 Serving/40g | 112.0 | 1.0 | 280 | 14.0 | 48.0 | 3.5 | 27.0 |
| All Bran, Splitz, Kellogg's* | 1 Serving/40g | 130.0 | 1.0 | 325 | 9.0 | 69.0 | 2.0 | 9.0 |
| All-Bran, Bran Flakes, Kellogg's* | 1 Serving/30g | 98.0 | 1.0 | 326 | 10.7 | 67.0 | 2.0 | 15.0 |
| Almond, Low Carb, Atkins* | 1 Serving/30g | 100.0 | 1.0 | 333 | 50.0 | 26.7 | 5.0 | 0.0 |
| Almond, Oats & More, Nestle* | 1 Serving/30g | 119.0 | 3.0 | 398 | 10.7 | 68.7 | 8.9 | 5.5 |
| Almond, Pecan & Cashew Muesli, Kellogg's* | 1 Bowl/45g | 188.0 | 6.0 | 418 | 11.0 | 62.0 | 14.0 | 8.0 |
| Almond, Raisin & Pecan, Nature's Pleasure, Kellogg's* | 1 Serving/45g | 184.0 | 5.0 | 408 | 10.0 | 65.0 | 12.0 | 8.0 |
| Alpen*, Crunchy Bran* | 1 Serving/40g | 120.0 | 2.0 | 299 | 11.8 | 52.3 | 4.7 | 24.8 |
| Apple, Blackberry, & Raspberry Flakes, GFY, Asda* | 1 Serving/30g | 103.0 | 1.0 | 344 | 9.0 | 73.0 | 1.8 | 11.0 |
| Apple & Cinnamon, Crisp, Sainsbury's* | 1 Serving/50g | 216.0 | 7.0 | 433 | 6.2 | 69.1 | 14.7 | 3.4 |
| Apple & Cinnamon Flakes, M & S* | 1 Serving/30g | 111.0 | 1.0 | 370 | 6.0 | 82.7 | 1.9 | 3.4 |
| Apricot Wheats, Whole Grain, Tesco* | 1 Serving/30g | 130.0 | 1.0 | 326 | 7.6 | 70.6 | 1.4 | 8.0 |
| Balance, Sainsbury's* | 1 Serving/30g | 111.0 | 0.0 | 370 | 11.4 | 77.7 | 1.5 | 3.2 |
| Balance with Red Fruits, Sainsbury's* | 1 Serving/40g | 147.0 | 1.0 | 367 | 11.2 | 77.5 | 1.3 | 2.6 |
| Banana, Papaya & Honey Oat, Crunchy, Waitrose* | 1 Serving/40g | 170.0 | 5.0 | 426 | 9.6 | 69.8 | 12.0 | 5.5 |
| Banana & Toffee Crisp, Mornflake* | 1 Serving/30g | 133.0 | 5.0 | 443 | 5.7 | 68.8 | 16.1 | 5.4 |
| Berry Crunchy, Sainsbury's* | 1 Serving/30g | 122.0 | 4.0 | 408 | 7.7 | 67.3 | 12.0 | 4.8 |
| Bitesize, Weetabix* | 1 Serving/40g | 135.0 | 1.0 | 338 | 11.5 | 68.4 | 2.0 | 10.0 |
| Blackberry & Apple, Alpen* | 1 Serving/40g | 140.0 | 2.0 | 349 | 9.2 | 69.4 | 3.8 | 8.3 |
| Bran, Natural, Sainsbury's* | 1 Serving/30g | 64.0 | 1.0 | 212 | 14.7 | 27.0 | 5.0 | 36.0 |
| Bran Flakes, Crunchy Nut, Sainsbury's* | 1 Serving/40g | 203.0 | 4.0 | 507 | 19.7 | 85.7 | 9.5 | 11.0 |
| Bran Flakes, Harvest Home, Nestle* | 1 Serving/30g | 99.0 | 1.0 | 331 | 10.2 | 67.1 | 2.4 | 14.1 |
| Bran Flakes, HL, Tesco* | 1 Serving/30g | 100.0 | 1.0 | 335 | 10.2 | 67.0 | 2.4 | 14.1 |

B

## BREAKFAST CEREAL

| | Measure INFO/WEIGHT | per Measure KCAL | per Measure FAT | KCAL | PROT | CARB | FAT | FIBRE |
|---|---|---|---|---|---|---|---|---|
| Bran Flakes, Honey Nut, Asda* | 1 Serving/50g | 180.0 | 2.0 | 360 | 10.0 | 70.0 | 4.4 | 11.0 |
| Bran Flakes, Honey Nut, Tesco* | 1 Serving/40g | 143.0 | 2.0 | 358 | 9.6 | 70.0 | 4.4 | 11.0 |
| Bran Flakes, Kellogg's* | 1 Serving/50g | 163.0 | 1.0 | 326 | 10.0 | 67.0 | 2.0 | 15.0 |
| Bran Flakes, Organic, Asda* | 1 Serving/30g | 99.0 | 1.0 | 330 | 10.0 | 67.0 | 2.4 | 14.0 |
| Bran Flakes, Organic, Sainsbury's* | 1 Serving/30g | 100.0 | 1.0 | 332 | 10.2 | 67.4 | 2.4 | 14.1 |
| Bran Flakes, Sainsbury's* | 1 Serving/30g | 100.0 | 1.0 | 333 | 10.3 | 67.5 | 2.5 | 14.3 |
| Bran Flakes, Sultana, Dry, Sainsbury's* | 1 Serving/30g | 97.0 | 1.0 | 325 | 8.3 | 68.6 | 1.9 | 12.1 |
| Bran Flakes, Sultana Bran, Kellogg's* | 1 Serving/30g | 95.0 | 1.0 | 318 | 8.0 | 67.0 | 2.0 | 13.0 |
| Bran Flakes, Tesco* | 1 Serving/30g | 99.0 | 1.0 | 331 | 10.2 | 67.1 | 2.4 | 14.1 |
| Bran Flakes, Value, Tesco* | 1 Serving/50g | 167.0 | 1.0 | 335 | 10.3 | 67.2 | 2.4 | 14.2 |
| Bran Flakes, Whole Grain, Sainsbury's* | 1 Serving/30g | 99.0 | 1.0 | 331 | 10.2 | 67.1 | 2.4 | 14.1 |
| Caribbean Crunch, Alpen* | 1 Serving/40g | 155.0 | 4.0 | 388 | 8.8 | 67.9 | 9.0 | 4.6 |
| Cheerios, Honey Nut, Nestle* | 1 Serving/30g | 112.0 | 1.0 | 374 | 7.0 | 78.3 | 3.7 | 5.2 |
| Cheerios, Nestle* | 1 Serving/30g | 111.0 | 1.0 | 369 | 8.1 | 75.2 | 3.9 | 6.6 |
| Choc & Nut Crisp, Tesco* | 1 Serving/40g | 185.0 | 8.0 | 462 | 8.3 | 62.5 | 19.9 | 4.8 |
| Choco Crackles, Morrisons* | 1 Serving/30g | 115.0 | 1.0 | 383 | 5.5 | 84.8 | 2.4 | 1.9 |
| Choco Flakes, Asda* | 1 Serving/50g | 187.0 | 0.0 | 374 | 6.0 | 86.0 | 0.7 | 2.6 |
| Choco Flakes, Kellogg's* | 1 Serving/30g | 114.0 | 1.0 | 380 | 5.0 | 84.0 | 3.0 | 2.5 |
| Choco Flakes, Sainsbury's* | 1 Serving/30g | 111.0 | 0.0 | 370 | 5.5 | 85.4 | 0.7 | 3.0 |
| Choco Flakes, Tesco* | 1 Serving/30g | 112.0 | 0.0 | 374 | 5.6 | 86.3 | 0.7 | 2.6 |
| Choco Hoops, Asda* | 1 Serving/40g | 154.0 | 2.0 | 385 | 7.0 | 79.0 | 4.5 | 4.0 |
| Choco Hoops, Kids, Tesco* | 1 Serving/30g | 116.0 | 1.0 | 387 | 7.6 | 79.1 | 4.5 | 4.5 |
| Choco Snaps, Asda* | 1 Serving/30g | 115.0 | 1.0 | 382 | 5.0 | 85.0 | 2.4 | 1.9 |
| Choco Snaps, Sainsbury's* | 1 Serving/30g | 115.0 | 1.0 | 383 | 5.5 | 84.8 | 2.4 | 1.9 |
| Choco Snaps, Tesco* | 1 Serving/30g | 115.0 | 1.0 | 383 | 5.5 | 84.8 | 2.4 | 1.9 |
| Choco Squares, Asda* | 1 Serving/30g | 130.0 | 4.0 | 434 | 10.0 | 67.0 | 14.0 | 4.0 |
| Chocolate Cereal, Tesco* | 1 Serving/40g | 169.0 | 6.0 | 423 | 8.0 | 66.3 | 14.0 | 6.0 |
| Chocolate Wheats, Kellogg's* | 1 Serving/40g | 148.0 | 4.0 | 369 | 10.0 | 62.0 | 9.0 | 12.0 |
| Cinnamon & Apple, Sensations, Asda* | 1 Serving/30g | 112.0 | 1.0 | 373 | 10.0 | 72.0 | 5.0 | 7.0 |
| Cinnamon Grahams, Nestle* | 1 Serving/40g | 164.0 | 4.0 | 411 | 4.7 | 76.1 | 9.8 | 4.2 |
| Clusters, Nestle* | 1 Serving/40g | 149.0 | 2.0 | 372 | 9.4 | 70.6 | 5.8 | 8.4 |
| Coco Pops, Kellogg's* | 1 Serving/30g | 116.0 | 1.0 | 387 | 5.0 | 85.0 | 3.0 | 2.0 |
| Coco Pops, Mega Munchers, Kellogg's* | 1 Serving/30g | 112.0 | 1.0 | 375 | 8.0 | 80.0 | 2.5 | 4.5 |
| Coco Snaps, Value, Tesco* | 1 Serving/30g | 117.0 | 1.0 | 390 | 7.0 | 84.1 | 2.4 | 2.4 |
| Cookie Crunch, Nestle* | 1 Serving/40g | 154.0 | 1.0 | 385 | 4.6 | 85.3 | 2.8 | 1.8 |
| Corn Flakes, Asda* | 1 Serving/30g | 111.0 | 0.0 | 370 | 7.0 | 84.0 | 0.7 | 3.0 |
| Corn Flakes, Banana Crunch, Kellogg's* | 1 Serving/40g | 163.0 | 3.0 | 408 | 6.0 | 78.0 | 8.0 | 3.0 |
| Corn Flakes, Crispy Nut, Asda* | 1 Serving/30g | 117.0 | 1.0 | 390 | 7.0 | 81.0 | 4.2 | 2.5 |
| Corn Flakes, Hint of Honey, Kellogg's* | 1 Serving/30g | 113.0 | 0.0 | 377 | 6.0 | 87.0 | 0.6 | 2.5 |
| Corn Flakes, Honey Nut, Morrisons* | 1 Serving/30g | 116.0 | 1.0 | 387 | 7.1 | 80.0 | 4.3 | 3.0 |
| Corn Flakes, Honey Nut, Sainsbury's* | 1 Serving/30g | 119.0 | 1.0 | 397 | 7.4 | 81.7 | 4.5 | 2.5 |
| Corn Flakes, Honey Nut, Tesco* | 1 Serving/30g | 118.0 | 1.0 | 392 | 7.4 | 81.2 | 4.2 | 2.5 |
| Corn Flakes, Honey Nut with Cranberries, Tesco* | 1 Serving/50g | 208.0 | 5.0 | 416 | 7.4 | 74.4 | 9.9 | 3.1 |
| Corn Flakes, Kellogg's* | 1 Serving/30g | 112.0 | 0.0 | 372 | 7.0 | 84.0 | 0.9 | 3.0 |
| Corn Flakes, Organic, Whole Earth* | 1 Serving/40g | 154.0 | 0.0 | 386 | 8.6 | 84.2 | 1.0 | 3.0 |
| Corn Flakes, Sainsbury's* | 1 Serving/25g | 93.0 | 0.0 | 371 | 7.3 | 83.8 | 0.7 | 3.0 |
| Corn Flakes, Tesco* | 1 Serving/25g | 93.0 | 0.0 | 371 | 7.3 | 83.8 | 0.7 | 3.0 |
| Corn Flakes, with 125ml Semi Skimmed Milk, Kellogg's* | 1 Serving/30g | 170.0 | 2.0 | 567 | 20.0 | 106.7 | 8.3 | 3.0 |
| Country Crisp, & Flakes, Red Berry, Jordans* | 1 Serving/50g | 203.0 | 6.0 | 407 | 7.1 | 68.5 | 11.6 | 7.3 |
| Country Crisp, Four Nut Combo, Jordans* | 1 Serving/50g | 240.0 | 12.0 | 480 | 8.9 | 55.4 | 24.7 | 6.9 |
| Country Crisp, Wild About Berries, Jordans* | 1 Serving/50g | 221.0 | 8.0 | 443 | 7.5 | 68.0 | 15.7 | 5.7 |
| Country Crisp, with Real Raspberries, Jordans* | 1 Serving/50g | 214.0 | 8.0 | 429 | 7.5 | 64.1 | 15.8 | 7.1 |
| Country Crisp, with Real Strawberries, Jordans* | 1 Serving/50g | 214.0 | 8.0 | 428 | 7.5 | 64.1 | 15.7 | 7.1 |

## BREAKFAST CEREAL

| INFO/WEIGHT | Measure | per Measure | | Nutrition Values per 100g / 100ml | | | | |
|---|---|---|---|---|---|---|---|---|
| | | KCAL | FAT | KCAL | PROT | CARB | FAT | FIBRE |
| Cranberry Wheats, Tesco* | 1 Serving/40g | 130.0 | 1.0 | 325 | 7.3 | 70.9 | 1.4 | 7.7 |
| Cranberry Wheats, Whole Grain, Sainsbury's* | 1 Serving/50g | 162.0 | 1.0 | 325 | 7.3 | 70.9 | 1.4 | 7.7 |
| Crispy Rice & Wheat Flakes, Asda* | 1 Serving/50g | 185.0 | 1.0 | 370 | 11.0 | 78.0 | 1.5 | 3.2 |
| Crunchy, Carb Control, Tesco* | 1 Serving/35g | 174.0 | 12.0 | 497 | 21.5 | 23.3 | 35.0 | 13.4 |
| Crunchy Bran, Weetabix* | 1 Serving/40g | 122.0 | 1.0 | 306 | 11.9 | 56.6 | 3.6 | 20.0 |
| Crunchy Nut, Clusters, Honey & Nut, Kellogg's* | 1 Serving/40g | 174.0 | 6.0 | 435 | 8.0 | 67.0 | 15.7 | 5.0 |
| Crunchy Nut, Corn Flakes, Kellogg's* | 1 Serving/30g | 118.0 | 1.0 | 392 | 6.0 | 83.0 | 4.0 | 2.5 |
| Crunchy Oat, Co-Op* | 1 Serving/50g | 202.0 | 6.0 | 405 | 8.0 | 64.0 | 13.0 | 10.0 |
| Crunchy Oat, with Raisins, Almonds & Fruit, Tesco* | 1 Serving/50g | 201.0 | 6.0 | 403 | 8.5 | 63.8 | 12.6 | 6.6 |
| Crunchy Oat, with Tropical Fruits, Tesco* | 1 Serving/35g | 146.0 | 5.0 | 417 | 7.8 | 65.3 | 13.8 | 6.1 |
| Crunchy Oats, with Tropical Fruits, Jordans* | 1 Serving/75g | 319.0 | 11.0 | 425 | 8.1 | 65.4 | 14.6 | 6.7 |
| Crunchy Rice & Wheat Flakes, Co-Op* | 1 Serving/30g | 111.0 | 1.0 | 370 | 11.0 | 78.0 | 2.0 | 3.0 |
| Eat Natural* | 1 Serving/40g | 180.0 | 10.0 | 450 | 12.0 | 45.0 | 25.0 | 6.0 |
| Fibre 1, Nestle* | 1 Serving/40g | 107.0 | 1.0 | 267 | 10.8 | 50.2 | 2.6 | 30.5 |
| Fitnesse, with Berries, Nestle* | 1 Portion/30g | 171.0 | 2.0 | 570 | 21.0 | 104.0 | 8.0 | 3.3 |
| Fitnesse & Fruits, Nestle* | 1 Serving/40g | 148.0 | 0.0 | 370 | 6.6 | 83.4 | 1.1 | 3.4 |
| Flakes, Multigrain, with Cranberry & Apple, Tesco* | 1 Serving/30g | 107.0 | 1.0 | 357 | 8.1 | 75.7 | 2.4 | 5.4 |
| Flakes & Grains, Exotic Fruit, BGTY, Sainsbury's* | 1 Serving/30g | 113.0 | 1.0 | 377 | 6.8 | 76.4 | 4.9 | 5.9 |
| Flakes & Orchard Fruits, BGTY, Sainsbury's* | 1 Serving/40g | 154.0 | 0.0 | 385 | 13.0 | 80.6 | 1.2 | 4.5 |
| Force, Nestle* | 1 Serving/40g | 138.0 | 1.0 | 344 | 10.6 | 70.3 | 2.3 | 9.2 |
| Four Berry Crisp, Organic, Jordans* | 1 Serving/50g | 221.0 | 8.0 | 442 | 7.7 | 67.1 | 15.8 | 5.4 |
| Frosted Flakes, Sainsbury's* | 1 Serving/30g | 112.0 | 0.0 | 374 | 4.9 | 87.8 | 0.4 | 2.4 |
| Frosted Flakes, Tesco* | 1 Serving/30g | 112.0 | 0.0 | 374 | 4.9 | 87.8 | 0.4 | 2.4 |
| Frosted Wheats, Kellogg's* | 1 Serving/30g | 104.0 | 1.0 | 346 | 10.0 | 72.0 | 2.0 | 9.0 |
| Frosties, Caramel, Kellogg's* | 1 Serving/30g | 113.0 | 0.0 | 377 | 5.0 | 88.0 | 0.6 | 2.0 |
| Frosties, Chocolate, Kellogg's* | 1 Serving/40g | 158.0 | 2.0 | 394 | 5.0 | 80.0 | 6.0 | 3.5 |
| Frosties, Kellogg's* | 1 Serving/30g | 111.0 | 0.0 | 371 | 4.5 | 87.0 | 0.6 | 2.0 |
| Frosties, Reduced Sugar, Kellogg's* | 1 Serving/30g | 111.0 | 0.0 | 369 | 6.0 | 85.0 | 0.6 | 2.5 |
| Fruit & Fibre, Asda* | 1 Serving/40g | 146.0 | 3.0 | 366 | 8.2 | 68.4 | 6.6 | 8.5 |
| Fruit & Fibre, Flakes, Waitrose* | 1 Serving/40g | 143.0 | 2.0 | 357 | 8.2 | 67.2 | 6.2 | 9.9 |
| Fruit & Fibre, Morrisons* | 1 Serving/30g | 110.0 | 2.0 | 366 | 8.8 | 66.5 | 7.2 | 8.5 |
| Fruit & Fibre, Organic, Sainsbury's* | 1 Serving/40g | 147.0 | 2.0 | 367 | 10.0 | 72.4 | 4.1 | 7.8 |
| Fruit & Fibre, Tesco* | 1 Serving/30g | 111.0 | 2.0 | 370 | 8.0 | 69.1 | 6.6 | 7.7 |
| Fruit & Fibre, Value, Tesco* | 1 Serving/40g | 144.0 | 2.0 | 359 | 11.4 | 65.7 | 5.6 | 8.0 |
| Fruit & Fibre, Whole Grain, Sainsbury's* | 1 Serving/30g | 108.0 | 2.0 | 361 | 8.1 | 68.7 | 6.0 | 8.9 |
| Fruit & Nut Crisp, Minis, Weetabix* | 1 Serving/40g | 144.0 | 2.0 | 359 | 9.3 | 70.0 | 4.6 | 8.9 |
| Fruit 'n' Fibre, Kellogg's* | 1 Serving/40g | 143.0 | 2.0 | 358 | 8.0 | 68.0 | 6.0 | 9.0 |
| Fruit Nuts & Flakes, M & S* | 1 Serving/30g | 117.0 | 3.0 | 391 | 9.1 | 69.6 | 8.5 | 3.5 |
| Golden Grahams, Nestle* | 1 Serving/30g | 112.0 | 1.0 | 375 | 6.0 | 81.0 | 3.0 | 3.4 |
| Golden Honey Puffs, Tesco* | 1 Serving/30g | 115.0 | 0.0 | 382 | 6.6 | 86.3 | 1.2 | 3.0 |
| Golden Nuggets, Nestle* | 1 Serving/40g | 152.0 | 0.0 | 381 | 6.2 | 87.4 | 0.7 | 1.5 |
| Golden Puffs, Sainsbury's* | 1 Serving/28g | 107.0 | 0.0 | 383 | 6.6 | 86.3 | 1.2 | 3.0 |
| Granola, Low Fat, Home Farm* | 1 Serving/55g | 180.0 | 3.0 | 328 | 7.3 | 69.0 | 5.4 | 9.0 |
| Granola, Quaker* | 1 Serving/48g | 210.0 | 7.0 | 437 | 10.4 | 72.9 | 14.6 | 6.2 |
| Granola, Superfoods, Jordans* | 1 Serving/50g | 207.0 | 7.0 | 415 | 9.0 | 64.7 | 13.4 | 8.6 |
| Grape Nuts, Kraft* | 1 Serving/45g | 155.0 | 1.0 | 345 | 11.5 | 70.0 | 2.0 | 11.0 |
| Harvest Crunch, Nut, Quaker* | 1 Serving/40g | 184.0 | 8.0 | 459 | 8.0 | 62.5 | 19.5 | 6.0 |
| Harvest Crunch, Real Red Berries, Quaker* | 1 Serving/50g | 223.0 | 8.0 | 447 | 7.0 | 66.0 | 17.0 | 4.5 |
| Harvest Crunch, Soft Juicy Raisins, Quaker* | 1 Serving/50g | 221.0 | 8.0 | 442 | 6.0 | 67.0 | 16.0 | 4.0 |
| Hawaiian Crunch, Asda* | 1 Serving/50g | 220.0 | 8.0 | 441 | 8.0 | 64.0 | 17.0 | 6.0 |
| Healthy Flakes, Safeway* | 1 Serving/30g | 111.0 | 0.0 | 371 | 11.0 | 78.4 | 1.5 | 4.3 |
| High Fibre Bran, Sainsbury's* | 1 Serving/40g | 109.0 | 1.0 | 272 | 14.7 | 45.5 | 3.5 | 27.0 |
| High Fibre Bran, Tesco* | 1 Serving/40g | 110.0 | 1.0 | 275 | 14.7 | 45.5 | 3.5 | 27.0 |

# BREAKFAST CEREAL

| INFO/WEIGHT | Measure | per Measure | | Nutrition Values per 100g / 100ml | | | | |
|---|---|---|---|---|---|---|---|---|
| | | KCAL | FAT | KCAL | PROT | CARB | FAT | FIBRE |
| Honey, Oats & More, Nestle* | 1 Serving/30g | 114.0 | 2.0 | 379 | 9.7 | 73.1 | 5.3 | 5.9 |
| Honey Nut Flakes with Red Berries, Somerfield* | 1 Serving/30g | 126.0 | 3.0 | 419 | 8.6 | 70.4 | 11.4 | 1.9 |
| Honey Raisin & Almond, Crunchy, Waitrose* | 1 Serving/40g | 170.0 | 5.0 | 425 | 10.5 | 68.8 | 12.0 | 5.7 |
| Hooplas, Sainsbury's* | 1 Serving/30g | 112.0 | 1.0 | 375 | 6.5 | 78.6 | 3.8 | 4.6 |
| Hoops, Multigrain, Tesco* | 1 Serving/30g | 112.0 | 1.0 | 375 | 6.5 | 78.6 | 3.8 | 4.6 |
| Hot Cereal, Flax O Meal* | 1 Serving/40g | 130.0 | 6.0 | 325 | 52.5 | 2.5 | 15.0 | 30.0 |
| Hot Oats, Instant, Tesco* | 1 Serving/30g | 108.0 | 3.0 | 360 | 11.8 | 58.4 | 8.7 | 7.9 |
| Hot Oats, Safeway* | 1 Serving/20g | 71.0 | 2.0 | 356 | 11.6 | 58.8 | 8.3 | 8.9 |
| Hunny B's, Kellogg's* | 1 Serving/28g | 106.0 | 1.0 | 379 | 7.0 | 78.0 | 2.5 | 4.5 |
| Just Right, Kellogg's* | 1 Serving/40g | 145.0 | 1.0 | 363 | 7.0 | 78.0 | 2.5 | 4.5 |
| Kashi, Crunch, Seven Whole Grains, Original, Kellogg's* | 1 Serving/40g | 162.0 | 4.0 | 405 | 8.0 | 73.0 | 9.0 | 5.0 |
| Kashi, Honey, Seven Whole Grains, Kellogg's* | 1 Serving/30g | 110.0 | 1.0 | 367 | 9.0 | 77.0 | 2.5 | 7.0 |
| Malt Bites, Safeway* | 1 Serving/40g | 137.0 | 1.0 | 343 | 10.0 | 69.2 | 2.9 | 10.0 |
| Malt Crunchies, Co-Op* | 1 Serving/50g | 167.0 | 1.0 | 335 | 10.0 | 69.0 | 2.0 | 10.0 |
| Malted Wheaties, Asda* | 1 Serving/50g | 171.0 | 1.0 | 342 | 10.0 | 69.0 | 2.9 | 10.0 |
| Malted Wheats, Waitrose* | 1 Serving/32g | 110.0 | 1.0 | 343 | 9.7 | 71.7 | 1.9 | 9.9 |
| Malties, Sainsbury's* | 1 Serving/40g | 137.0 | 1.0 | 343 | 10.0 | 69.2 | 2.9 | 10.0 |
| Malty Flakes, Peach Melba, Tesco* | 1 Serving/30g | 115.0 | 1.0 | 385 | 8.0 | 79.6 | 3.8 | 1.7 |
| Malty Flakes, Tesco* | 1 Serving/40g | 148.0 | 1.0 | 371 | 11.0 | 78.4 | 1.5 | 4.3 |
| Malty Flakes, with Red Berries, Tesco* | 1 Serving/30g | 111.0 | 1.0 | 369 | 9.9 | 78.1 | 1.9 | 3.1 |
| Malty Flakes with Peach & Raspberry, BGTY, Sainsbury's* | 1 Serving/40g | 146.0 | 1.0 | 364 | 10.8 | 76.4 | 1.7 | 3.3 |
| Malty Flakes with Rasberries, M & S* | 1 Serving/40g | 148.0 | 1.0 | 370 | 7.4 | 77.5 | 3.5 | 3.2 |
| Maple & Pecan, Crisp, Asda* | 1 Serving/30g | 135.0 | 6.0 | 451 | 8.0 | 62.0 | 19.0 | 6.0 |
| Maple & Pecan, Sainsbury's* | 1 Serving/60g | 318.0 | 13.0 | 530 | 13.3 | 69.7 | 22.0 | 5.3 |
| Maple & Pecan Crisp, Sainsbury's* | 1 Serving/50g | 226.0 | 10.0 | 452 | 7.9 | 61.3 | 19.5 | 5.4 |
| Maple & Pecan Crisp, Tesco* | 1 Serving/50g | 215.0 | 8.0 | 430 | 10.5 | 62.5 | 15.2 | 10.2 |
| Maple Frosted Flakes, Whole Earth* | 1 Serving/30g | 112.0 | 0.0 | 375 | 6.2 | 85.6 | 1.0 | 1.6 |
| Millet Rice Oatbran Flakes, Nature's Path* | 1 Serving/56g | 204.0 | 3.0 | 365 | 11.3 | 67.0 | 5.8 | 10.0 |
| Mini Wheats, Sainsbury's* | 1 Serving/45g | 157.0 | 1.0 | 348 | 11.8 | 69.9 | 2.3 | 11.8 |
| Minibix, Weetabix* | 1 Serving/40g | 134.0 | 2.0 | 335 | 8.8 | 71.2 | 3.8 | 8.1 |
| Muddles, Kellogg's* | 1 Serving/30g | 110.0 | 1.0 | 368 | 8.0 | 76.0 | 3.5 | 8.0 |
| Muesli, Apricot, Traidcraft* | 1 Serving/30g | 103.0 | 2.0 | 344 | 8.0 | 68.0 | 6.0 | 5.0 |
| Muesli, Base, Nature's Harvest* | 1 Serving/50g | 179.0 | 3.0 | 358 | 11.0 | 71.2 | 5.1 | 7.4 |
| Muesli, Berries & Cherries, Dorset Cereals* | 1 Serving/70g | 225.0 | 2.0 | 321 | 6.5 | 68.8 | 2.2 | 6.3 |
| Muesli, Carb Control, Tesco* | 1 Serving/35g | 154.0 | 9.0 | 439 | 25.0 | 25.0 | 26.6 | 13.8 |
| Muesli, COU, M & S* | 1 Serving/60g | 201.0 | 1.0 | 335 | 7.6 | 70.2 | 2.5 | 8.1 |
| Muesli, Creamy Tropical Fruit, Finest, Tesco* | 1 Serving/80g | 283.0 | 4.0 | 354 | 7.2 | 68.8 | 5.6 | 6.9 |
| Muesli, Crunchy, Organic, Sainsbury's* | 1 Serving/40g | 168.0 | 6.0 | 420 | 10.6 | 62.0 | 14.4 | 9.2 |
| Muesli, De Luxe, No Added Salt Or Sugar, Sainsbury's* | 1 Serving/40g | 161.0 | 6.0 | 403 | 11.9 | 57.6 | 13.9 | 8.4 |
| Muesli, Fruit, 55%, Asda* | 1 Serving/35g | 111.0 | 1.0 | 318 | 6.0 | 67.0 | 2.9 | 7.0 |
| Muesli, Fruit, GFY, Asda* | 1 Serving/50g | 152.0 | 1.0 | 304 | 8.0 | 64.0 | 1.8 | 10.0 |
| Muesli, Fruit, Luxury, Weight Watchers* | 1 Serving/40g | 127.0 | 1.0 | 318 | 7.2 | 67.7 | 2.0 | 8.1 |
| Muesli, Fruit, Sainsbury's* | 1 Serving/40g | 132.0 | 2.0 | 330 | 8.1 | 64.3 | 4.5 | 9.6 |
| Muesli, Fruit, Waitrose* | 1 Serving/30g | 101.0 | 1.0 | 338 | 7.2 | 66.8 | 4.7 | 6.8 |
| Muesli, Fruit & Nut, COU, M & S* | 1 Serving/40g | 128.0 | 1.0 | 320 | 7.4 | 74.5 | 2.8 | 7.4 |
| Muesli, Fruit & Nut, Jordans* | 1 Serving/50g | 180.0 | 5.0 | 361 | 8.0 | 61.2 | 9.4 | 7.5 |
| Muesli, Fruit & Nut, Luxury, Sainsbury's* | 1 Serving/50g | 177.0 | 5.0 | 355 | 10.3 | 57.9 | 9.1 | 11.3 |
| Muesli, Fruit & Nut, Luxury, Waitrose* | 1 Serving/40g | 145.0 | 4.0 | 363 | 9.0 | 60.3 | 9.5 | 6.5 |
| Muesli, Fruit & Nut, M & S* | 1 Serving/40g | 128.0 | 1.0 | 320 | 7.4 | 74.5 | 2.8 | 7.4 |
| Muesli, Fruit & Nut, Organic, M & S* | 1 Serving/50g | 166.0 | 3.0 | 333 | 8.2 | 61.6 | 6.0 | 7.6 |
| Muesli, Fruit & Nut, Sainsbury's* | 1 Serving/30g | 121.0 | 5.0 | 402 | 10.4 | 51.3 | 17.2 | 9.2 |
| Muesli, Fruit & Nut, Tesco* | 1 Serving/50g | 190.0 | 6.0 | 380 | 8.4 | 60.3 | 11.3 | 5.3 |
| Muesli, Fruit & Nut, Whole Wheat, Organic, Asda* | 1 Serving/50g | 171.0 | 3.0 | 343 | 10.0 | 60.0 | 7.0 | 7.0 |

## BREAKFAST CEREAL

| | Measure INFO/WEIGHT | per Measure KCAL | FAT | Nutrition Values per 100g / 100ml KCAL | PROT | CARB | FAT | FIBRE |
|---|---|---|---|---|---|---|---|---|
| Muesli, Fruit & Spice, Sainsbury's* | 1 Serving/50g | 184.0 | 3.0 | 368 | 7.4 | 69.4 | 6.8 | 7.7 |
| Muesli, Fruit Sensation, M & S* | 1 Serving/50g | 157.0 | 1.0 | 315 | 6.0 | 66.0 | 3.0 | 7.4 |
| Muesli, Fruity Fibre, Jordans* | 1 Serving/50g | 172.0 | 3.0 | 344 | 7.7 | 64.2 | 6.3 | 8.5 |
| Muesli, HL, Tesco* | 1 Serving/40g | 126.0 | 1.0 | 315 | 7.6 | 64.3 | 2.3 | 7.5 |
| Muesli, Light & Crispy, Jordans* | 1 Serving/50g | 171.0 | 2.0 | 343 | 7.7 | 66.7 | 5.0 | 9.5 |
| Muesli, Luxury, Finest, Tesco* | 1 Serving/50g | 197.0 | 7.0 | 394 | 8.3 | 60.8 | 13.1 | 5.4 |
| Muesli, Luxury, Jordans* | 1 Serving/40g | 154.0 | 5.0 | 384 | 9.6 | 58.4 | 12.5 | 8.2 |
| Muesli, Luxury, Sainsbury's* | 1 Serving/40g | 144.0 | 4.0 | 359 | 8.5 | 57.1 | 10.7 | 7.7 |
| Muesli, Luxury Fruit, Perfectly Balanced, Waitrose* | 1 Serving/50g | 162.0 | 2.0 | 324 | 7.1 | 66.4 | 3.3 | 7.0 |
| Muesli, Luxury Fruit, Sainsbury's* | 1 Serving/50g | 162.0 | 2.0 | 324 | 7.1 | 66.4 | 3.3 | 7.0 |
| Muesli, Natural, No Added Sugar Or Salt, Jordans* | 1 Serving/50g | 160.0 | 2.0 | 321 | 8.9 | 60.7 | 4.7 | 5.2 |
| Muesli, No Added Sugar, Morrisons* | 1 Serving/50g | 165.0 | 3.0 | 331 | 11.2 | 64.7 | 5.1 | 6.3 |
| Muesli, No Added Sugar, Waitrose* | 1 Serving/40g | 146.0 | 3.0 | 364 | 12.0 | 64.9 | 6.3 | 6.7 |
| Muesli, No Added Sugar Or Salt, Organic, Jordans* | 1 Serbing/50g | 175.0 | 4.0 | 350 | 9.2 | 58.4 | 8.8 | 9.3 |
| Muesli, Organic, Waitrose* | 1 Serving/50g | 187.0 | 1.0 | 375 | 10.3 | 59.6 | 1.6 | 8.3 |
| Muesli, Original, Holland & Barrett* | 1 Serving/30g | 105.0 | 3.0 | 351 | 11.1 | 61.2 | 8.4 | 7.1 |
| Muesli, Original, Sainsbury's* | 1 Serving/60g | 226.0 | 5.0 | 376 | 9.3 | 65.7 | 8.4 | 7.1 |
| Muesli, Peach & Vanilla, Sainsbury's* | 1 Serving/50g | 162.0 | 3.0 | 324 | 7.6 | 61.4 | 5.3 | 7.6 |
| Muesli, Really Nutty, Dorset Cereals* | 1 Serving/70g | 253.0 | 6.0 | 362 | 9.8 | 61.1 | 8.7 | 6.3 |
| Muesli, Rich, Nature's Harvest* | 1 Serving/40g | 143.0 | 4.0 | 358 | 10.0 | 60.5 | 9.2 | 7.6 |
| Muesli, Special, Fruit, Jordans* | 1 Serving/50g | 161.0 | 1.0 | 323 | 6.6 | 68.0 | 2.7 | 8.4 |
| Muesli, Special, Jordans* | 1 Serving/50g | 183.0 | 5.0 | 366 | 7.9 | 59.5 | 10.7 | 8.5 |
| Muesli, Super Berry, Jordans* | 1 Serving/50g | 174.0 | 4.0 | 348 | 9.0 | 60.8 | 7.6 | 8.1 |
| Muesli, Super High Fibre, Dorset Cereals* | 1 Serving/70g | 250.0 | 7.0 | 357 | 8.0 | 60.1 | 9.4 | 8.4 |
| Muesli, Superfoods, Jordans* | 1 Serving/50g | 173.0 | 4.0 | 346 | 9.2 | 60.9 | 7.3 | 10.2 |
| Muesli, Swiss Style, No Added Salt Or Sugar, Sainsbury's* | 1 Serving/50g | 178.0 | 3.0 | 357 | 10.9 | 64.9 | 6.0 | 6.0 |
| Muesli, Swiss Style, No Added Salt Or Sugar, Tesco* | 1 Serving/50g | 177.0 | 3.0 | 355 | 10.9 | 65.1 | 5.4 | 8.2 |
| Muesli, Swiss Style, No Added Sugar Or Salt, Asda* | 1 Serving/50g | 181.0 | 3.0 | 363 | 11.0 | 64.0 | 7.0 | 8.0 |
| Muesli, Swiss Style, Sainsbury's* | 1 Serving/50g | 180.0 | 3.0 | 361 | 9.2 | 68.1 | 5.8 | 7.1 |
| Muesli, Swiss Style, SmartPrice, Asda* | 1 Serving/60g | 222.0 | 4.0 | 370 | 9.0 | 70.0 | 6.0 | 10.0 |
| Muesli, Swiss Style, Waitrose* | 1 Serving/50g | 180.0 | 3.0 | 361 | 9.2 | 68.1 | 5.8 | 7.1 |
| Muesli, Swiss Style, with Fruit, Tesco* | 1 Serving/40g | 144.0 | 2.0 | 360 | 10.4 | 67.4 | 5.3 | 7.4 |
| Muesli, Tropical, Sainsbury's* | 1 Serving/50g | 182.0 | 3.0 | 365 | 6.5 | 69.4 | 6.8 | 6.4 |
| Muesli, Tropical Fruit, Holland & Barrett* | 1 Serving/60g | 197.0 | 2.0 | 328 | 7.5 | 69.8 | 3.2 | 5.1 |
| Muesli, Tropical Fruits, Jordans* | 1 Serving/50g | 164.0 | 1.0 | 329 | 6.9 | 68.7 | 2.9 | 7.1 |
| Muesli, Twelve Fruit & Nut, Sainsbury's* | 1 Serving/50g | 166.0 | 2.0 | 332 | 8.1 | 64.2 | 4.7 | 7.8 |
| Muesli, Unsweetened, M & S* | 1 Serving/40g | 129.0 | 1.0 | 322 | 8.1 | 68.0 | 2.7 | 9.4 |
| Muesli, Unsweetened Whole Wheat, Safeway* | 1 Serving/50g | 180.0 | 3.0 | 360 | 7.7 | 68.0 | 6.3 | 7.2 |
| Muesli, Value, Tesco* | 1 Serving/50g | 162.0 | 3.0 | 325 | 10.7 | 58.3 | 5.1 | 14.9 |
| Muesli, Whole Wheat, No Added Sugar & Salt, Tesco* | 1 Serving/40g | 154.0 | 5.0 | 386 | 9.5 | 59.1 | 12.4 | 7.4 |
| Muesli, Whole Wheat, Organic, Asda* | 1 Serving/50g | 197.0 | 3.0 | 394 | 10.0 | 75.0 | 6.0 | 9.0 |
| Muesli, Whole Wheat, Sainsbury's* | 1 Serving/40g | 144.0 | 3.0 | 359 | 11.5 | 60.5 | 7.9 | 8.5 |
| Muesli Mix, Perfect Start, Organic, The Food Doctor* | 1 Serving/50g | 196.0 | 7.0 | 392 | 12.1 | 55.5 | 14.2 | 7.1 |
| Multi Fruit & Flake, COU, M & S* | 1 Serving/39g | 142.0 | 0.0 | 365 | 6.5 | 81.8 | 1.1 | 4.0 |
| Multi Fruit & Flake, Perfectly Balanced, Waitrose* | 1 Serving/40g | 134.0 | 1.0 | 335 | 8.2 | 68.8 | 3.0 | 14.0 |
| Multigrain, Fitnesse, Nestle* | 1 Serving/30g | 109.0 | 0.0 | 363 | 8.0 | 79.8 | 1.3 | 5.1 |
| Multigrain Boulders, Tesco* | 1 Serving/30g | 112.0 | 0.0 | 375 | 8.2 | 82.3 | 1.3 | 3.6 |
| Multigrain Flakes, with Fruit & Nuts, Aldi* | 1 Serving/30g | 108.0 | 1.0 | 360 | 7.5 | 77.1 | 2.4 | 4.5 |
| Multigrain Flakes with Apple, Eat Smart, Safeway* | 1 Serving/45g | 160.0 | 1.0 | 355 | 8.0 | 74.7 | 2.5 | 7.0 |
| Natures Whole Grains, Jordans* | 1 Serving/25g | 97.0 | 3.0 | 390 | 9.4 | 61.7 | 11.7 | 7.7 |
| Nesquik, Chocolatey Corn & Rice, Nestle* | 1 Serving/30g | 114.0 | 1.0 | 380 | 7.2 | 79.1 | 3.9 | 5.1 |
| No Added Sugar, Alpen* | 1 Serving/40g | 142.0 | 2.0 | 354 | 10.5 | 64.6 | 6.0 | 7.7 |
| Nutty Crunch, Alpen* | 1 Serving/40g | 159.0 | 4.0 | 398 | 10.7 | 63.6 | 11.2 | 6.5 |

B

## BREAKFAST CEREAL

| | Measure INFO/WEIGHT | per Measure KCAL | FAT | Nutrition Values per 100g / 100ml KCAL | PROT | CARB | FAT | FIBRE |
|---|---|---|---|---|---|---|---|---|
| Nutty Crunch, Deliciously, M & S* | 1 Serving/50g | 238.0 | 11.0 | 476 | 8.8 | 59.6 | 22.5 | 4.4 |
| Oat, Crunchy, Sainsbury's* | 1 Serving/50g | 226.0 | 10.0 | 453 | 8.2 | 59.3 | 20.3 | 6.6 |
| Oat, Raisin, Nut & Honey, Crunchy, Dry, Sainsbury's* | 1 Serving/50g | 201.0 | 7.0 | 402 | 8.5 | 60.2 | 14.1 | 7.6 |
| Oat & Bran Flakes, Sainsbury's* | 1 Serving/30g | 97.0 | 2.0 | 324 | 12.2 | 56.0 | 5.7 | 17.7 |
| Oat Bran, Crispies, Quaker* | 1 Serving/40g | 153.0 | 3.0 | 383 | 11.0 | 69.0 | 6.5 | 9.0 |
| Oat Bran, Hodgson Mill* | 1 Serving/40g | 48.0 | 1.0 | 120 | 6.0 | 23.0 | 3.0 | 6.0 |
| Oat Crisp, Quaker* | 1 Serving/30g | 109.0 | 2.0 | 364 | 10.6 | 60.8 | 6.8 | 12.7 |
| Oat Crunchy, Blueberry & Cranberry, Waitrose* | 1 Serving/60g | 259.0 | 9.0 | 432 | 8.0 | 65.9 | 15.2 | 8.5 |
| Oat Granola, Quaker* | 1 Serving/50g | 205.0 | 4.0 | 411 | 8.6 | 73.0 | 8.8 | 5.2 |
| Oat Krunchies, Quaker* | 1 Serving/30g | 118.0 | 2.0 | 393 | 9.5 | 72.0 | 7.0 | 5.5 |
| Oat Meal, Medium, Heart's Content, Mornflake* | 1 Serving/30g | 108.0 | 2.0 | 359 | 11.0 | 60.4 | 8.1 | 8.5 |
| Oatbran Flakes, Nature's Path* | 1 Serving/30g | 124.0 | 1.0 | 414 | 8.7 | 83.0 | 4.7 | 6.7 |
| Oatibix, Bitesize, Original, Weetabix* | 1 Serving/36g | 133.0 | 2.0 | 370 | 10.6 | 66.5 | 6.8 | 10.1 |
| Oatibix, Flakes, Weetabix* | 1 Serving/50g | 190.0 | 3.0 | 381 | 9.5 | 73.2 | 5.6 | 3.5 |
| Oatibix, Weetabix* | 2 Biscuits/48g | 181.0 | 4.0 | 377 | 12.5 | 63.7 | 8.0 | 7.3 |
| Oatiflakes, with Raisin, Cranberry & Apple, Weetabix* | 1 Serving/40g | 135.0 | 0.0 | 338 | 6.7 | 75.0 | 1.2 | 8.6 |
| Oatmeal, Instant, Heart to Heart, Kashi* | 1 Serving/43g | 150.0 | 2.0 | 349 | 7.0 | 76.7 | 4.6 | 9.3 |
| Oatmeal, Quick Oats, Dry, Quaker* | 1 Serving/30g | 114.0 | 2.0 | 380 | 14.0 | 66.7 | 6.7 | 10.0 |
| Oats, Apple Flavour, Instant, Hot, Waitrose* | 1 Serving/36g | 141.0 | 2.0 | 392 | 8.1 | 76.4 | 6.0 | 6.7 |
| Oats, Apple Flavour, Micro, Tesco* | 1 Sachet/36g | 128.0 | 2.0 | 356 | 6.8 | 70.1 | 5.4 | 5.4 |
| Oats, Golden Syrup, Dry, Micro, Tesco* | 1 Sachet/39g | 144.0 | 2.0 | 370 | 7.8 | 71.6 | 5.7 | 6.4 |
| Oats, Golden Syrup Flavour, Instant, Hot, Waitrose* | 1 Serving/39g | 153.0 | 2.0 | 393 | 7.8 | 77.4 | 5.8 | 6.0 |
| Oats, Jumbo, Organic, Waitrose* | 1 Serving/50g | 180.0 | 4.0 | 361 | 11.0 | 61.1 | 8.1 | 7.8 |
| Oats, Orange & Lemon Flavour, Instant, Hot, Waitrose* | 1 Sachet/38g | 137.0 | 2.0 | 361 | 8.9 | 68.4 | 5.8 | 8.7 |
| Oats, Original, Instant, Hot, Waitrose* | 1 Sachet/27g | 97.0 | 2.0 | 359 | 11.0 | 60.4 | 8.1 | 8.5 |
| Oats, Superfast, Mornflake* | 1 Serving/40g | 144.0 | 3.0 | 359 | 11.0 | 60.4 | 8.1 | 8.5 |
| Oatso Simple, Apple & Cinnamon, Quaker* | 1 Sachet/38g | 136.0 | 2.0 | 358 | 8.0 | 68.0 | 5.5 | 2.5 |
| Oatso Simple, Baked Apple Flavour, Quaker* | 1 Serving/38g | 142.0 | 2.0 | 374 | 8.0 | 71.0 | 6.0 | 5.5 |
| Oatso Simple, Berry Burst, Quaker* | 1 Serving/39g | 144.0 | 2.0 | 370 | 8.0 | 70.0 | 6.0 | 6.5 |
| Oatso Simple, Country Honey, Quaker* | 1 Serving/36g | 134.0 | 2.0 | 373 | 8.5 | 69.0 | 6.5 | 6.0 |
| Oatso Simple, Fruit Muesli, Quaker* | 1 Sachet/39g | 136.0 | 2.0 | 348 | 8.0 | 66.1 | 5.8 | 6.8 |
| Oatso Simple, Golden Syrup Flavour, Quaker* | 1 Sachet/36g | 132.0 | 2.0 | 366 | 8.4 | 68.7 | 6.2 | 6.8 |
| Oatso Simple, Original, Quaker* | 1 Serving/27g | 98.0 | 2.0 | 364 | 11.0 | 60.0 | 8.5 | 9.0 |
| Oatso Simple, Raspberry, Quaker* | 1 Sachet/36g | 130.0 | 2.0 | 361 | 8.5 | 68.0 | 6.3 | 7.2 |
| Oatso Simple, Toffee Flavour, Quaker* | 1 Serving/30g | 122.0 | 4.0 | 407 | 6.5 | 66.0 | 13.0 | 5.0 |
| Optivita, Berry Oat Crisp, Kellogg's* | 1 Serving/30g | 107.0 | 1.0 | 357 | 10.0 | 68.0 | 5.0 | 9.0 |
| Organic, Weetabix* | 2 Biscuits/35g | 116.0 | 1.0 | 331 | 10.9 | 66.8 | 2.2 | 11.0 |
| Original, Crunchy, Raisins & Almonds, Jordans* | 1 Serving/50g | 203.0 | 6.0 | 407 | 8.7 | 64.0 | 12.9 | 6.6 |
| Original, Crunchy, Tropical Fruits, Jordans* | 1 Serving/50g | 211.0 | 7.0 | 423 | 8.1 | 65.1 | 14.5 | 6.7 |
| Original, Dry, Micro Oats, Tesco* | 1 Sachet/27g | 97.0 | 2.0 | 360 | 11.0 | 60.4 | 8.1 | 8.5 |
| Original, Ready Brek* | 1 Serving/40g | 144.0 | 3.0 | 359 | 11.8 | 58.5 | 8.7 | 7.9 |
| Original, with Raisins, Hazelnuts & Almonds, Alpen* | 1 Serving/40g | 144.0 | 2.0 | 359 | 10.5 | 66.6 | 5.8 | 7.3 |
| Pomegranate & Raspberry Wheats, Tesco* | 1 Serving/50g | 165.0 | 1.0 | 330 | 7.5 | 71.8 | 1.4 | 8.2 |
| Porage Oats, Old Fashioned, Thick, Scotts* | 1 Serving/45g | 160.0 | 4.0 | 356 | 11.0 | 60.0 | 8.0 | 9.0 |
| Porage Oats, So Easy, Scotts* | 1 Serving/30g | 109.0 | 3.0 | 364 | 11.0 | 60.0 | 8.5 | 9.0 |
| Porridge, Apple, Sultana & Cinnamon, M & S* | 1 Sachet/40g | 144.0 | 3.0 | 360 | 10.3 | 62.3 | 7.5 | 8.6 |
| Porridge, Apple & Raspberry, Seriously Oaty, Weetabix* | 1 Serving/40g | 142.0 | 2.0 | 354 | 8.3 | 63.7 | 6.0 | 7.8 |
| Porridge, Free From, Sainsbury's* | 1 Serving/50g | 174.0 | 1.0 | 348 | 8.6 | 72.0 | 3.0 | 3.4 |
| Porridge, Fruity, Apple & Raisin, Dorset Cereals* | 1 Serving/70g | 233.0 | 3.0 | 333 | 9.7 | 62.7 | 4.8 | 8.9 |
| Porridge, Fruity, Fruit & Nut, Dorset Cereals* | 1 Serving/70g | 242.0 | 6.0 | 346 | 9.4 | 59.0 | 8.0 | 8.2 |
| Porridge, Fruity, Mixed Berries, Dorset Cereals* | 1 Serving/70g | 243.0 | 4.0 | 347 | 10.8 | 62.6 | 6.0 | 7.9 |
| Porridge, Golden Honey, Oatibix, Weetabix* | 1 Serving/40g | 145.0 | 3.0 | 363 | 9.2 | 66.7 | 6.6 | 7.0 |
| Porridge, Instant, Quaker* | 1 Serving/34g | 124.0 | 3.0 | 364 | 11.0 | 60.0 | 8.5 | 9.0 |

## BREAKFAST CEREAL

| | Measure INFO/WEIGHT | per Measure KCAL | per Measure FAT | Nutrition Values per 100g / 100ml KCAL | PROT | CARB | FAT | FIBRE |
|---|---|---|---|---|---|---|---|---|
| Porridge, Made with Semi Skimmed Milk, Waitrose* | 1 Serving/50g | 277.0 | 7.0 | 554 | 24.6 | 80.4 | 15.0 | 8.6 |
| Porridge, Manuka Honey & Apricot, Vogel* | 1 Packet/35g | 122.0 | 1.0 | 349 | 10.1 | 66.3 | 2.9 | 7.1 |
| Porridge, Multigrain, Jordans* | 1 Serving/40g | 134.0 | 2.0 | 335 | 10.4 | 60.9 | 5.5 | 10.0 |
| Porridge, Original, Oatibix, Weetabix* | 1 Sachet/30g | 104.0 | 2.0 | 347 | 12.5 | 55.6 | 8.3 | 10.1 |
| Porridge, Original, Simply Porridge, Asda* | 1 Sachet/27g | 96.0 | 2.0 | 356 | 11.0 | 60.0 | 8.0 | 8.0 |
| Porridge, Real Fruit, Raisin & Apple, Jordans* | 1 Serving/40g | 133.0 | 3.0 | 332 | 9.1 | 58.8 | 6.7 | 7.4 |
| Porridge, Real Fruit, Sultana & Apricot, Jordans* | 1 Sachet/40g | 127.0 | 2.0 | 317 | 8.5 | 57.7 | 5.8 | 7.2 |
| Porridge, Spiced Apple, Sultana, Oatibix, Weetabix* | 1 Sachet/40g | 138.0 | 2.0 | 345 | 9.7 | 65.4 | 5.7 | 8.5 |
| Porridge, Superfoods, Jordans* | 1 Serving/40g | 145.0 | 4.0 | 362 | 10.4 | 59.8 | 9.0 | 8.3 |
| Porridge, Take Heart, Quaker* | 1 Serving/32g | 194.0 | 6.0 | 606 | 30.9 | 80.3 | 17.8 | 7.8 |
| Porridge Flakes, Organic, Barkat* | 1 Serving/30g | 109.0 | 1.0 | 362 | 8.5 | 74.1 | 3.0 | 0.0 |
| Porridge Oats, Dry Weight, Value, Tesco* | 1 Serving/50g | 179.0 | 4.0 | 359 | 11.0 | 60.4 | 8.1 | 8.5 |
| Porridge Oats, Mornflake* | 1 Serving/50g | 179.0 | 4.0 | 359 | 11.0 | 60.4 | 8.1 | 8.5 |
| Porridge Oats, Organic, Jordans* | 1 Serving/40g | 146.0 | 4.0 | 364 | 11.7 | 58.4 | 9.3 | 9.0 |
| Porridge Oats, Organic, Tesco* | 1 Serving/28g | 100.0 | 2.0 | 358 | 11.0 | 60.4 | 8.1 | 8.5 |
| Porridge Oats, Quaker* | 1 Serving/45g | 160.0 | 4.0 | 356 | 11.0 | 60.0 | 8.0 | 4.0 |
| Porridge Oats, Rolled, Tesco* | 1 Serving/50g | 179.0 | 4.0 | 359 | 11.0 | 60.4 | 8.1 | 8.5 |
| Porridge Oats, Scottish, Tesco* | 1 Serving/50g | 179.0 | 4.0 | 359 | 11.0 | 60.4 | 8.1 | 8.5 |
| Porridge Oats, SmartPrice, Asda* | 1 Serving/50g | 178.0 | 4.0 | 356 | 11.0 | 60.0 | 8.0 | 8.0 |
| Porridge Oats, with Bran, Scottish, Sainsbury's* | 1 Serving/50g | 190.0 | 2.0 | 380 | 9.6 | 74.1 | 5.0 | 10.3 |
| Porridge Oats, with Wheat Bran, Tesco* | 1 Serving/50g | 167.0 | 4.0 | 334 | 12.3 | 55.0 | 7.2 | 13.0 |
| Porridge Oats, with Wheat Bran, Waitrose* | 1 Serving/50g | 168.0 | 4.0 | 336 | 11.2 | 55.8 | 7.6 | 13.0 |
| Porridge Oats & Bran, Co-Op* | 1 Serving/40g | 141.0 | 3.0 | 353 | 12.5 | 60.0 | 7.0 | 12.0 |
| Porridge Oats & Bran, Somerfield* | 1 Serving/40g | 154.0 | 3.0 | 385 | 12.0 | 68.0 | 7.0 | 0.0 |
| Precise, Sainsbury's* | 1 Serving/40g | 148.0 | 1.0 | 371 | 6.4 | 79.9 | 2.9 | 3.5 |
| Puffed Rice, Wholegrain, Brown, Original, Organic, Kallo* | 1 Serving/25g | 95.0 | 1.0 | 380 | 8.0 | 80.0 | 3.0 | 9.0 |
| Puffed Wheat, Quaker* | 1 Serving/15g | 49.0 | 0.0 | 328 | 15.3 | 62.4 | 1.3 | 5.6 |
| Puffed Wheat, Tesco* | 1 Serving/28g | 104.0 | 1.0 | 373 | 13.9 | 72.2 | 3.2 | 5.7 |
| Quaker Oats Crunch, Quaker* | 1 Serving/40g | 146.0 | 2.0 | 366 | 9.1 | 71.1 | 5.0 | 7.4 |
| Raisin, Bran Flakes, Asda* | 1 Serving/50g | 165.0 | 1.0 | 331 | 7.0 | 69.0 | 3.0 | 10.0 |
| Raisin, Honey & Almond Crunch, Asda* | 1 Serving/60g | 220.0 | 7.0 | 366 | 9.2 | 56.6 | 11.4 | 15.5 |
| Raisin, Oats and More, Nestle* | 1 Serving/30g | 112.0 | 1.0 | 373 | 8.9 | 73.7 | 4.7 | 5.8 |
| Raisin & Almond, Crunchy, Jordans* | 1 Serving/56g | 230.0 | 7.0 | 411 | 8.4 | 66.0 | 12.5 | 5.0 |
| Raisin & Coconut, Crunchy, Organic, Jordans* | 1 Serving/50g | 206.0 | 7.0 | 412 | 8.4 | 64.2 | 13.5 | 7.1 |
| Raisin Wheats, Kellogg's* | 1 Serving/30g | 99.0 | 1.0 | 330 | 9.0 | 70.0 | 2.0 | 8.0 |
| Raisin Wheats, Sainsbury's* | 1 Serving/50g | 166.0 | 1.0 | 332 | 8.2 | 71.5 | 1.5 | 8.0 |
| Raisins, Almonds, Mixed Seeds & Crispy Rice, Eat Natural* | 1 Serving/50g | 215.0 | 10.0 | 431 | 14.4 | 49.0 | 19.7 | 3.8 |
| Rasberry Crisp, Mornflake* | 1 Serving/50g | 214.0 | 7.0 | 428 | 6.5 | 68.2 | 14.3 | 6.8 |
| Ready Brek, Banana, Weetabix* | 1 Serving/40g | 146.0 | 3.0 | 365 | 8.9 | 68.0 | 6.4 | 6.7 |
| Ready Brek, Original, Weetabix* | 1 Serving/40g | 158.0 | 3.0 | 395 | 11.8 | 58.4 | 8.7 | 7.9 |
| Red Berries Crisp, Somerfield* | 1 Serving/30g | 134.0 | 5.0 | 448 | 7.3 | 67.0 | 16.8 | 4.3 |
| Red Berry & Almond Luxury Crunch, Jordans* | 1 Serving/40g | 176.0 | 7.0 | 441 | 8.2 | 60.5 | 18.5 | 6.6 |
| Rice & Wheat Flake, Special Choice, Waitrose* | 1 Serving/30g | 111.0 | 0.0 | 370 | 11.4 | 77.7 | 1.5 | 3.2 |
| Rice Krispies, Honey, Kellogg's* | 1 Serving/30g | 114.0 | 0.0 | 380 | 4.0 | 89.0 | 0.7 | 1.0 |
| Rice Krispies, Kellogg's* | 1 Serving/30g | 114.0 | 0.0 | 381 | 6.0 | 87.0 | 1.0 | 1.0 |
| Rice Krispies, Multi-Grain Shapes, Kellogg's* | 1 Serving/30g | 111.0 | 1.0 | 370 | 8.0 | 77.0 | 2.5 | 8.0 |
| Rice Pops, Blue Parrot Cafe, Sainsbury's* | 1 Serving/30g | 111.0 | 0.0 | 370 | 7.2 | 82.3 | 1.3 | 2.2 |
| Rice Pops, Organic, Dove's Farm* | 1 Serving/30g | 107.0 | 0.0 | 357 | 6.8 | 86.1 | 0.8 | 2.0 |
| Rice Pops, Sainsbury's* | 1 Serving/30g | 114.0 | 0.0 | 381 | 7.4 | 84.8 | 1.3 | 1.5 |
| Rice Snaps, Asda* | 1 Serving/28g | 105.0 | 0.0 | 376 | 7.0 | 84.0 | 1.3 | 1.5 |
| Rice Snaps, Harvest Home, Nestle* | 1 Serving/25g | 94.0 | 0.0 | 378 | 7.4 | 84.2 | 1.3 | 1.5 |
| Rice Snaps, Tesco* | 1 Serving/35g | 135.0 | 0.0 | 385 | 7.4 | 84.8 | 1.3 | 1.5 |
| Ricicles, Kellogg's* | 1 Serving/30g | 114.0 | 0.0 | 381 | 4.5 | 89.0 | 0.8 | 0.8 |

## BREAKFAST CEREAL

| | Measure INFO/WEIGHT | per Measure KCAL | FAT | Nutrition Values per 100g / 100ml KCAL | PROT | CARB | FAT | FIBRE |
|---|---|---|---|---|---|---|---|---|
| Right Balance, Morrisons* | 1 Serving/50g | 181.0 | 1.0 | 362 | 6.9 | 78.6 | 2.2 | 5.3 |
| Shredded Wheat, 100% Whole Grain, Nestle* | 2 Biscuits/45g | 153.0 | 1.0 | 340 | 11.6 | 67.8 | 2.5 | 11.8 |
| Shredded Wheat, Bitesize, Nestle* | 1 Serving/45g | 157.0 | 1.0 | 350 | 11.8 | 69.9 | 2.6 | 11.9 |
| Shredded Wheat, Fruitful, No Added Salt, Nestle* | 1 Serving/40g | 142.0 | 2.0 | 354 | 8.3 | 68.7 | 5.1 | 8.9 |
| Shreddies, Coco, Nestle* | 1 Serving/45g | 161.0 | 1.0 | 358 | 8.4 | 76.5 | 2.0 | 8.6 |
| Shreddies, Frosted, Variety Pack, Nestle* | 1 Pack/45g | 163.0 | 1.0 | 363 | 6.7 | 81.1 | 1.3 | 6.8 |
| Shreddies, Malt Wheats, Tesco* | 1 Serving/45g | 151.0 | 1.0 | 335 | 8.3 | 70.7 | 2.1 | 9.7 |
| Shreddies, Nestle* | 1 Serving/50g | 175.0 | 1.0 | 351 | 9.9 | 73.7 | 1.9 | 9.8 |
| Special Crunchy Luxury, Jordans* | 1 Serving/50g | 205.0 | 7.0 | 411 | 7.6 | 63.8 | 13.9 | 6.5 |
| Special Flakes, Tesco* | 1 Serving/20g | 74.0 | 0.0 | 371 | 11.0 | 78.4 | 1.5 | 4.3 |
| Special Flakes with Peach Melba, Tesco* | 1 Serving/30g | 115.0 | 1.0 | 385 | 8.0 | 79.6 | 3.8 | 1.7 |
| Special K, Bliss, Creamy Berry Crunch, Kellogg's* | 1 Serving/30g | 114.0 | 1.0 | 379 | 13.0 | 76.0 | 2.5 | 2.5 |
| Special K, Bliss, Strawberry & Chocolate, Kellogg's* | 1 Serving/30g | 115.0 | 1.0 | 383 | 13.0 | 76.0 | 3.0 | 2.5 |
| Special K, Choco, Kellogg's* | 1 Serving/40g | 160.0 | 3.0 | 400 | 14.0 | 70.0 | 7.0 | 3.5 |
| Special K, Kellogg's* | 1 Serving/30g | 112.0 | 0.0 | 373 | 16.0 | 75.0 | 1.0 | 2.5 |
| Special K, Oats & Honey, Kellogg's* | 1 Serving/50g | 191.0 | 1.0 | 383 | 13.0 | 77.0 | 2.5 | 3.0 |
| Special K, Peach & Apricot, Kellogg's* | 1 Serving/30g | 112.0 | 0.0 | 373 | 14.0 | 77.0 | 1.0 | 2.5 |
| Special K, Protein Plus, Kellogg's* | 1 Serving/29g | 100.0 | 3.0 | 345 | 34.5 | 31.0 | 10.3 | 17.2 |
| Special K, Purple Berries, Kellogg's* | 1 Serving/30g | 112.0 | 0.0 | 374 | 13.0 | 77.0 | 1.0 | 3.5 |
| Special K, Red Berries, Kellogg's* | 1 Serving/30g | 112.0 | 0.0 | 373 | 14.0 | 77.0 | 1.0 | 3.0 |
| Special K, Yoghurty, Kellogg's* | 1 Serving/30g | 115.0 | 1.0 | 383 | 14.0 | 75.0 | 3.0 | 2.5 |
| Start, Kellogg's* | 1 Serving/30g | 112.0 | 1.0 | 375 | 8.0 | 80.0 | 2.5 | 5.0 |
| Strawberry & Maltiflakes, COU, M & S* | 1 Serving/40g | 146.0 | 1.0 | 365 | 12.7 | 73.8 | 2.3 | 3.5 |
| Strawberry Crisp, Asda* | 1 Serving/45g | 194.0 | 7.0 | 431 | 8.1 | 64.7 | 15.5 | 5.9 |
| Sugar Puffs, Quaker* | 1 Serving/30g | 114.0 | 0.0 | 379 | 5.3 | 85.8 | 1.6 | 3.7 |
| Sultana Bran, HL, Tesco* | 1 Serving/30g | 97.0 | 1.0 | 325 | 8.2 | 68.0 | 1.9 | 12.0 |
| Sultana Bran, Sainsbury's* | 1 Serving/30g | 97.0 | 1.0 | 324 | 8.2 | 68.6 | 1.9 | 11.6 |
| Sultana Bran, Waitrose* | 1 Serving/30g | 97.0 | 1.0 | 324 | 8.2 | 68.6 | 1.9 | 11.6 |
| Superfoods, Breakfast Flakes, Jordans* | 1 Serving/40g | 136.0 | 2.0 | 341 | 8.7 | 67.2 | 4.1 | 11.3 |
| Toasted Multi-Grain Flakes with Apple, Weight Watchers* | 1 Serving/30g | 97.0 | 0.0 | 323 | 10.4 | 67.8 | 1.1 | 14.4 |
| Triple Chocolate Crisp, Sainsbury's* | 1 Serving/40g | 180.0 | 7.0 | 451 | 7.7 | 63.8 | 18.3 | 6.0 |
| Tropicana, Weight Watchers* | 1 Serving/50g | 120.0 | 0.0 | 240 | 5.1 | 52.0 | 1.0 | 7.0 |
| Ultra Bran, Soya & Linseed, Vogel* | 1 Serving/45g | 117.0 | 1.0 | 260 | 15.3 | 45.3 | 1.8 | 33.3 |
| Vanilla, Carb Check, Heinz* | 1 Serving/35g | 127.0 | 1.0 | 362 | 56.7 | 27.6 | 2.7 | 0.4 |
| Vitality, Asda* | 1 Serving/30g | 111.0 | 0.0 | 370 | 11.0 | 78.0 | 1.5 | 3.2 |
| Vitality, with Red Fruit, Asda* | 1 Serving/30g | 110.0 | 0.0 | 366 | 11.0 | 77.0 | 1.6 | 3.8 |
| Vitality, with Tropical Fruit, Asda* | 1 Serving/30g | 112.0 | 1.0 | 373 | 9.0 | 73.0 | 5.0 | 4.9 |
| Weetaflakes, Weetabix* | 1 Serving/30g | 102.0 | 0.0 | 340 | 8.9 | 72.9 | 1.4 | 11.0 |
| Weetaflakes, with Raisin, Cranberry & Apple, Weetabix* | 1 Serving/40g | 135.0 | 0.0 | 338 | 6.7 | 75.0 | 1.2 | 8.6 |
| Weetos, Chocolate, Weetabix* | 1 Serving/30g | 113.0 | 1.0 | 378 | 8.4 | 75.1 | 4.9 | 5.8 |
| Wheat Biscuits, HE, Tesco* | 2 Biscuits/38g | 127.0 | 1.0 | 338 | 11.5 | 68.4 | 2.0 | 10.0 |
| Wheat Biscuits, Morrisons* | 2 Biscuits/38g | 129.0 | 1.0 | 340 | 11.2 | 67.6 | 2.7 | 10.5 |
| Wheat Biscuits, Somerfield* | 2 Biscuits/38g | 129.0 | 1.0 | 339 | 11.2 | 67.6 | 2.7 | 10.5 |
| Wheat Bisks, Banana, Mini, Asda* | 1 Serving/50g | 190.0 | 3.0 | 380 | 9.7 | 73.1 | 5.4 | 7.4 |
| Wheat Flakes, Alpen* | 1 Serving/40g | 140.0 | 1.0 | 350 | 10.2 | 72.0 | 2.4 | 9.0 |
| Wheat Flakes, Malted, Toasted, Suma* | 1 Serving/75g | 259.0 | 1.0 | 346 | 10.3 | 72.0 | 1.9 | 10.4 |
| Wheats, Mini, Maple & Brown Sugar, Sainsbury's* | 1 Serving/52g | 99.0 | 1.0 | 190 | 4.0 | 44.0 | 1.0 | 5.0 |
| Whole Wheat Biscuits, Dove's Farm* | 1 Serving/30g | 99.0 | 1.0 | 329 | 11.0 | 65.0 | 2.8 | 11.0 |
| Yoghurt & Raspberry, Crisp, Sainsbury's* | 1 Serving/45g | 191.0 | 7.0 | 424 | 7.5 | 65.2 | 14.8 | 6.4 |

## BREAKFAST COMPOTE

| | Measure INFO/WEIGHT | per Measure KCAL | FAT | Nutrition Values per 100g / 100ml KCAL | PROT | CARB | FAT | FIBRE |
|---|---|---|---|---|---|---|---|---|
| in Apple Juice, Tesco* | 1 Can/300g | 219.0 | 1.0 | 73 | 0.4 | 17.0 | 0.4 | 2.1 |
| Sainsbury's* | 1 Can/300g | 327.0 | 1.0 | 109 | 1.7 | 24.4 | 0.5 | 3.1 |

|  | Measure INFO/WEIGHT | per Measure KCAL | FAT | Nutrition Values per 100g / 100ml KCAL | PROT | CARB | FAT | FIBRE |
|---|---|---|---|---|---|---|---|---|
| **BREAKFAST TOPPER** | | | | | | | | |
| Fruit, Sainsbury's* | 1 Dtsp/15g | 42.0 | 0.0 | 283 | 2.7 | 65.6 | 2.1 | 4.5 |
| Nut, Sainsbury's* | 1 Dtsp/15g | 92.0 | 8.0 | 615 | 20.2 | 19.1 | 51.0 | 6.1 |
| **BRESAOLA** | | | | | | | | |
| Della Valtellina, Sainsbury's* | 1 Slice/14g | 23.0 | 0.0 | 163 | 34.7 | 0.1 | 2.6 | 0.1 |
| Finest, Tesco* | 1 Serving/35g | 64.0 | 1.0 | 182 | 36.0 | 0.5 | 4.0 | 0.0 |
| M & S* | 1oz/28g | 56.0 | 2.0 | 200 | 34.6 | 0.0 | 6.8 | 0.0 |
| **BROCCOLI** | | | | | | | | |
| & Cauliflower, Floret Mix, Fresh, Tesco* | 1 Serving/80g | 27.0 | 1.0 | 34 | 3.9 | 2.5 | 0.9 | 2.7 |
| & Cheese, Morrisons* | 1 Pack/350g | 406.0 | 25.0 | 116 | 6.2 | 6.6 | 7.1 | 0.8 |
| Cauliflower & Baby Carrots, Safeway* | 1 Serving/150g | 37.0 | 1.0 | 25 | 2.0 | 3.0 | 0.6 | 2.3 |
| Cauliflower & Carrots, Tesco* | 1 Pack/320g | 112.0 | 2.0 | 35 | 2.5 | 4.9 | 0.6 | 2.3 |
| Chinese, Kai Lan, Cooked | 1 Serving/80g | 18.0 | 1.0 | 22 | 1.4 | 3.8 | 0.7 | 2.5 |
| Courgette & Peppers, COU, M & S* | 1 Pack/283g | 156.0 | 12.0 | 55 | 1.7 | 2.7 | 4.1 | 1.7 |
| *Green, Boiled, Average* | *1 Serving/80g* | *19.0* | *1.0* | *24* | *3.1* | *1.1* | *0.8* | *2.3* |
| *Green, Raw, Average* | *1 Serving/80g* | *25.0* | *1.0* | *31* | *3.7* | *2.1* | *0.8* | *2.4* |
| *Purple Sprouting, Boiled, Average* | *1 Serving/80g* | *15.0* | *0.0* | *19* | *2.1* | *1.3* | *0.6* | *2.3* |
| *Purple Sprouting, Raw* | *1oz/28g* | *10.0* | *0.0* | *35* | *3.9* | *2.6* | *1.1* | *3.5* |
| Tenderstem, Finest, Tesco* | ½ Pack/100g | 31.0 | 0.0 | 31 | 4.2 | 3.2 | 0.2 | 3.1 |
| **BROWNIES** | | | | | | | | |
| Average | 1 Brownie/60g | 243.0 | 10.0 | 405 | 4.6 | 0.0 | 16.8 | 0.0 |
| Chocolate, Bites, Mini, Weight Watchers* | 1 Brownie/9g | 29.0 | 0.0 | 325 | 5.3 | 63.7 | 5.5 | 2.2 |
| Chocolate, Cadbury* | 1 Brownie/36g | 145.0 | 6.0 | 403 | 6.1 | 59.7 | 15.8 | 0.0 |
| Chocolate, Mini Bites, Asda* | 1 Brownie/15g | 62.0 | 3.0 | 420 | 5.0 | 55.0 | 20.0 | 1.4 |
| Chocolate, Sainsbury's* | 1 Brownie/60g | 265.0 | 14.0 | 442 | 4.6 | 55.0 | 22.6 | 1.6 |
| Chocolate, Tesco* | 1 Brownie/46g | 201.0 | 10.0 | 438 | 6.6 | 55.1 | 21.2 | 1.5 |
| Chocolate, Waitrose* | 1 Brownie/45g | 192.0 | 9.0 | 426 | 6.3 | 55.6 | 19.8 | 2.7 |
| Chocolate, Weight Watchers* | 1 Brownie/47g | 143.0 | 2.0 | 304 | 4.8 | 62.5 | 3.8 | 3.2 |
| Chocolate, Wheat & Gluten Free, Mrs Crimble's* | 1 Slice/48g | 180.0 | 10.0 | 379 | 4.2 | 47.9 | 20.3 | 1.5 |
| Double Chocolate, Mini Bites, Sainsbury's* | 1 Brownie/15g | 49.0 | 2.0 | 326 | 5.8 | 38.9 | 16.4 | 1.6 |
| Pecan & Walnut, Sugar Free, Joseph's* | 1 Brownie/26g | 150.0 | 7.0 | 577 | 7.7 | 57.7 | 26.9 | 3.8 |
| Praline, Mini, Finest, Tesco* | 1 Brownie/12g | 59.0 | 3.0 | 492 | 4.2 | 60.0 | 25.8 | 0.8 |
| TTD, Sainsbury's* | 1 Brownie/33g | 139.0 | 7.0 | 420 | 4.8 | 56.5 | 20.4 | 1.5 |
| **BRUSCHETTA** | | | | | | | | |
| Pane Italia* | 1 Serving/75g | 367.0 | 19.0 | 489 | 12.4 | 53.6 | 25.1 | 1.4 |
| Ploughman's Relish, Brunchetta, Golden Vale* | 1 Pack/90g | 261.0 | 15.0 | 290 | 14.2 | 20.2 | 17.2 | 1.6 |
| Red Pepper & Onion, Brunchetta, Golden Vale* | 1 Pack/90g | 266.0 | 17.0 | 296 | 14.6 | 17.0 | 19.0 | 1.3 |
| Safeway* | ¼ Pack/115g | 420.0 | 7.0 | 365 | 11.8 | 65.5 | 5.8 | 2.8 |
| Soft Cheese & Cranberry, Brunchetta, Golden Vale* | 1 Pack/95g | 200.0 | 9.0 | 211 | 8.2 | 24.8 | 9.0 | 1.3 |
| Toasted, Olive Oil & Sea Salt, Tesco* | 1 Serving/30g | 126.0 | 5.0 | 420 | 11.5 | 58.7 | 15.5 | 4.5 |
| **BRUSSELS SPROUTS** | | | | | | | | |
| & Sweet Chestnuts, Asda* | 1 Serving/100g | 73.0 | 2.0 | 73 | 3.1 | 11.0 | 1.7 | 4.2 |
| *Boiled, Average* | *1 Serving/90g* | *31.0* | *1.0* | *35* | *3.1* | *3.2* | *1.3* | *3.5* |
| Button, & Chestnuts, Tesco* | 1 Serving/100g | 80.0 | 2.0 | 80 | 3.1 | 12.8 | 1.8 | 4.1 |
| *Button, Raw, Average* | *1 Serving/80g* | *30.0* | *1.0* | *37* | *3.5* | *2.9* | *1.3* | *3.2* |
| *Canned, Drained* | *1oz/28g* | *8.0* | *0.0* | *28* | *2.6* | *2.4* | *1.0* | *2.6* |
| Frozen, Morrisons* | 1 Serving/200g | 70.0 | 3.0 | 35 | 3.5 | 2.5 | 1.3 | 4.3 |
| *Raw, Average* | *1 Serving/80g* | *29.0* | *1.0* | *37* | *3.5* | *3.3* | *1.1* | *3.0* |
| **BUBBLE & SQUEAK** | | | | | | | | |
| Aunt Bessie's* | 1 Serving/100g | 145.0 | 7.0 | 145 | 2.7 | 17.5 | 7.1 | 1.3 |
| Fried in Vegetable Oil | 1oz/28g | 35.0 | 3.0 | 124 | 1.4 | 9.8 | 9.1 | 1.5 |
| Safeway* | 1 Serving/200g | 160.0 | 7.0 | 80 | 1.8 | 10.7 | 3.3 | 1.4 |
| Tesco* | ½ Pack/325g | 292.0 | 13.0 | 90 | 1.6 | 11.3 | 3.9 | 0.9 |

| | Measure INFO/WEIGHT | per Measure KCAL | FAT | Nutrition Values per 100g / 100ml KCAL | PROT | CARB | FAT | FIBRE |
|---|---|---|---|---|---|---|---|---|
| **BUCKWHEAT** | | | | | | | | |
| *Average* | *1oz/28g* | *102.0* | *0.0* | *364* | *8.1* | *84.9* | *1.5* | *2.1* |
| **BULGAR WHEAT** | | | | | | | | |
| *Dry Weight, Average* | *1oz/28g* | *99.0* | *0.0* | *353* | *9.7* | *76.3* | *1.7* | *8.0* |
| **BUNS** | | | | | | | | |
| Bath, M & S* | 1 Bun/71g | 217.0 | 6.0 | 305 | 8.3 | 49.8 | 8.0 | 1.9 |
| Bath, Tesco* | 1 Bun/80g | 262.0 | 9.0 | 327 | 8.0 | 48.9 | 11.1 | 5.7 |
| Belgian, Asda* | 1 Bun/133g | 464.0 | 20.0 | 350 | 4.8 | 49.0 | 15.0 | 2.2 |
| Belgian, Sainsbury's* | 1 Bun/110g | 398.0 | 11.0 | 362 | 6.1 | 61.3 | 10.3 | 1.9 |
| Belgian, Tesco* | 1 Bun/123g | 438.0 | 16.0 | 356 | 5.2 | 54.9 | 12.8 | 2.2 |
| Chelsea | 1 Bun/78g | 285.0 | 11.0 | 366 | 7.8 | 56.1 | 13.8 | 1.7 |
| Chelsea, Sainsbury's* | 1 Bun/85g | 239.0 | 4.0 | 281 | 6.9 | 51.6 | 5.2 | 2.9 |
| Chelsea, Tesco* | 1 Bun/85g | 269.0 | 6.0 | 316 | 7.9 | 53.9 | 7.6 | 2.3 |
| Choux, Caramel, Asda* | 1 Bun/189g | 745.0 | 51.0 | 394 | 4.3 | 33.5 | 27.0 | 1.3 |
| Choux, Custard, M & S* | 1 Bun/85g | 234.0 | 19.0 | 275 | 4.2 | 15.0 | 22.0 | 0.3 |
| Choux, Fresh Cream, Tesco* | 1 Bun/95g | 340.0 | 24.0 | 358 | 4.9 | 28.5 | 24.9 | 0.9 |
| Choux, M & S* | 1 Bun/78g | 247.0 | 17.0 | 317 | 5.4 | 25.6 | 22.2 | 0.3 |
| Currant | 1 Bun/60g | 178.0 | 4.0 | 296 | 7.6 | 52.7 | 7.5 | 0.0 |
| Currant, HL, Tesco* | 1 Bun/63g | 159.0 | 2.0 | 252 | 7.1 | 50.2 | 2.5 | 2.4 |
| Currant, Safeway* | 1 Bun/65g | 178.0 | 3.0 | 274 | 7.0 | 50.0 | 5.1 | 2.8 |
| Currant, Sainsbury's* | 1 Bun/72g | 197.0 | 4.0 | 274 | 7.0 | 50.0 | 5.1 | 2.8 |
| Dairy Cream, Somerfield* | 1 Bun/98g | 304.0 | 11.0 | 310 | 6.0 | 46.9 | 10.9 | 0.0 |
| Fruit, Waitrose* | 1 Bun/54g | 155.0 | 2.0 | 287 | 8.1 | 54.0 | 4.3 | 1.6 |
| Hevva, Somerfield* | 1 Bun/75g | 298.0 | 12.0 | 397 | 5.4 | 57.8 | 16.0 | 1.5 |
| Hot Cross | 1 Bun/50g | 155.0 | 3.0 | 310 | 7.4 | 58.5 | 6.8 | 1.7 |
| Hot Cross, 25% Reduced Fat, Asda* | 1 Bun/61g | 153.0 | 1.0 | 253 | 9.0 | 49.0 | 2.3 | 3.0 |
| Hot Cross, Apple & Cinnamon, M & S* | 1 Bun/71g | 170.0 | 1.0 | 240 | 7.6 | 48.7 | 1.7 | 3.1 |
| Hot Cross, Asda* | 1 Bun/60g | 190.0 | 4.0 | 317 | 10.0 | 55.0 | 6.3 | 3.3 |
| Hot Cross, BGTY, Sainsbury's* | 1 Bun/70g | 160.0 | 2.0 | 229 | 7.6 | 44.4 | 2.3 | 2.7 |
| Hot Cross, Chocolate, Mini, Sainsbury's* | 1 Bun/39g | 127.0 | 4.0 | 325 | 7.7 | 48.1 | 11.3 | 2.5 |
| Hot Cross, Chocolate & Raisin, Mini, Tesco* | 1 Bun/40g | 127.0 | 4.0 | 318 | 8.1 | 47.0 | 10.9 | 2.8 |
| Hot Cross, Classics, M & S* | 1 Bun/65g | 159.0 | 1.0 | 245 | 8.5 | 49.1 | 1.8 | 2.2 |
| Hot Cross, Co-Op* | 1 Bun/60g | 165.0 | 4.0 | 275 | 8.0 | 47.0 | 6.0 | 3.0 |
| Hot Cross, Finest, Tesco* | 1 Bun/75g | 210.0 | 4.0 | 280 | 7.8 | 49.5 | 5.4 | 2.8 |
| Hot Cross, Fruity, TTD, Sainsbury's* | 1 Bun/72g | 201.0 | 5.0 | 279 | 6.9 | 47.9 | 6.7 | 3.8 |
| Hot Cross, Golden Wholemeal, 3% Fat, M & S* | 1 Bun/67g | 144.0 | 1.0 | 215 | 8.9 | 39.6 | 2.2 | 6.7 |
| Hot Cross, Less Than 3% Fat, M & S* | 1 Bun/70g | 175.0 | 1.0 | 250 | 8.1 | 49.8 | 1.8 | 2.2 |
| Hot Cross, Low Fat, Good Intentions, Somerfield* | 1 Bun/50g | 135.0 | 1.0 | 270 | 10.0 | 51.8 | 2.6 | 2.8 |
| Hot Cross, Luxury, Cafe, M & S* | 1 Bun/78g | 199.0 | 3.0 | 255 | 8.6 | 46.2 | 4.0 | 2.1 |
| Hot Cross, Luxury, M & S* | 1 Bun/79g | 201.0 | 3.0 | 255 | 8.6 | 46.2 | 4.0 | 2.1 |
| Hot Cross, Luxury White, Safeway* | 1 Bun/76g | 185.0 | 4.0 | 245 | 8.0 | 39.4 | 5.9 | 3.7 |
| Hot Cross, Mini, M & S* | 1 Bun/37g | 91.0 | 1.0 | 245 | 8.5 | 49.1 | 1.8 | 2.2 |
| Hot Cross, Mini, Tesco* | 1 Bun/36g | 99.0 | 2.0 | 274 | 7.9 | 48.1 | 5.5 | 2.7 |
| Hot Cross, Reduced Fat, GFY, Asda* | 1 Bun/61g | 136.0 | 1.0 | 223 | 8.0 | 43.0 | 2.1 | 2.4 |
| Hot Cross, Reduced Fat, Waitrose* | 1 Bun/67g | 171.0 | 1.0 | 255 | 8.1 | 54.3 | 2.1 | 3.3 |
| Hot Cross, Safeway* | 1 Bun/65g | 174.0 | 4.0 | 268 | 7.9 | 46.9 | 5.4 | 2.2 |
| Hot Cross, Tesco* | 1 Bun/70g | 185.0 | 2.0 | 265 | 7.4 | 51.8 | 2.7 | 3.6 |
| Hot Cross, White, Kingsmill* | 1 Bun/25g | 71.0 | 1.0 | 286 | 7.0 | 51.1 | 6.0 | 3.0 |
| Hot Cross, White, Light Choices, Tesco* | 1 Bun/70g | 175.0 | 1.0 | 250 | 7.4 | 50.8 | 1.6 | 3.3 |
| Hot Cross, White, Low Fat, Safeway* | 1 Bun/65g | 161.0 | 2.0 | 248 | 8.7 | 47.4 | 2.6 | 3.0 |
| Hot Cross, White, Waitrose* | 1 Bun/68g | 174.0 | 2.0 | 258 | 8.1 | 49.5 | 3.1 | 3.9 |
| Hot Cross, Wholemeal, Asda* | 1 Bun/70g | 182.0 | 4.0 | 262 | 9.0 | 43.0 | 6.0 | 6.0 |
| Hot Cross, Wholemeal, Organic, Tesco* | 1 Bun/55g | 140.0 | 3.0 | 254 | 7.6 | 44.8 | 4.9 | 4.5 |
| Iced, Filled with Raspberry Jam, M & S* | 1 Bun/48g | 155.0 | 3.0 | 320 | 6.4 | 58.9 | 6.6 | 1.9 |

B

| | Measure INFO/WEIGHT | per Measure KCAL FAT | | Nutrition Values per 100g / 100ml KCAL PROT CARB FAT FIBRE | | | | |
|---|---|---|---|---|---|---|---|---|
| **BUNS** | | | | | | | | |
| Iced, Spiced Fruit, M & S* | 1 Bun/90g | 270.0 | 3.0 | 300 | 7.0 | 60.3 | 3.7 | 1.5 |
| Iced, Tesco* | 1 Bun/35g | 117.0 | 3.0 | 334 | 7.0 | 54.8 | 9.6 | 2.5 |
| Iced Lemon, Tesco* | 1 Bun/48g | 156.0 | 4.0 | 325 | 5.2 | 56.5 | 8.7 | 1.9 |
| Spiced, Carb Control, Tesco* | 1 Bun/45g | 96.0 | 2.0 | 214 | 17.6 | 31.4 | 4.2 | 9.2 |
| Spiced, Perfectly Balanced, Waitrose* | 1 Bun/65g | 177.0 | 2.0 | 272 | 8.0 | 52.3 | 3.4 | 2.9 |
| Swiss, Tesco* | 1 Bun/100g | 334.0 | 12.0 | 334 | 4.0 | 52.8 | 11.9 | 1.4 |
| **BURGERS** | | | | | | | | |
| Beef, 100%, Birds Eye* | 1 Burger/41g | 120.0 | 10.0 | 292 | 17.3 | 0.0 | 24.8 | 0.0 |
| Beef, 100%, Half Pounders, Sainsbury's* | 1 Burger/148g | 462.0 | 33.0 | 313 | 26.0 | 1.7 | 22.4 | 0.2 |
| Beef, 100%, Mega, Birds Eye* | 1 Burger/96g | 280.0 | 24.0 | 293 | 17.3 | 0.0 | 24.9 | 0.0 |
| Beef, 100%, Organic, Waitrose* | 1 Burger/57g | 140.0 | 10.0 | 247 | 23.6 | 0.0 | 16.9 | 0.0 |
| Beef, 100%, Quarter Pounders, Ross* | 1 Burger/74g | 222.0 | 19.0 | 301 | 16.8 | 1.1 | 25.5 | 0.0 |
| Beef, 100%, Sainsbury's* | 1 Burger/44g | 133.0 | 10.0 | 302 | 21.4 | 0.9 | 23.6 | 0.9 |
| Beef, 100%, with Seasoning, No Onion, Birds Eye* | 1 Burger/41g | 134.0 | 12.0 | 326 | 16.1 | 0.2 | 29.0 | 0.0 |
| Beef, 100%, without Onion, Sainsbury's* | 1 Burger/43g | 133.0 | 10.0 | 308 | 21.9 | 0.8 | 24.1 | 0.8 |
| Beef, 100% Pure, Ross* | 1 Burger/56g | 128.0 | 10.0 | 229 | 17.1 | 1.4 | 17.1 | 0.0 |
| Beef, Aberdeen Angus, Asda* | 1 Burger/112g | 249.0 | 13.0 | 222 | 22.2 | 6.7 | 11.8 | 0.9 |
| Beef, Aberdeen Angus, Fresh, Waitrose* | 1 Burger/113g | 269.0 | 21.0 | 238 | 16.4 | 1.2 | 18.6 | 0.0 |
| Beef, Aberdeen Angus, Gourmet, Finest, Tesco* | 1 Burger/118g | 225.0 | 13.0 | 190 | 18.9 | 2.0 | 11.3 | 1.0 |
| Beef, Aberdeen Angus, M & S* | 1 Burger/142g | 298.0 | 19.0 | 210 | 18.3 | 4.1 | 13.3 | 0.1 |
| Beef, Aberdeen Angus, Mega, Birds Eye* | 1 Burger/101g | 279.0 | 23.0 | 276 | 16.3 | 2.4 | 22.4 | 0.1 |
| Beef, Asda* | 1 Burger/114g | 304.0 | 19.0 | 267 | 26.8 | 3.2 | 16.3 | 0.7 |
| Beef, Barbecue, Tesco* | 1 Burger/114g | 295.0 | 23.0 | 260 | 15.6 | 3.5 | 20.0 | 0.5 |
| Beef, BGTY, Sainsbury's* | 1 Burger/110g | 177.0 | 6.0 | 161 | 20.8 | 7.1 | 5.5 | 1.1 |
| Beef, British, Finest, Tesco* | 1 Burger/95g | 185.0 | 12.0 | 195 | 17.2 | 3.3 | 12.4 | 0.9 |
| Beef, British, Organic, Waitrose* | 1 Burger/85g | 226.0 | 17.0 | 266 | 19.0 | 3.5 | 19.5 | 1.0 |
| Beef, Chargrill, Tesco* | 1 Burger/114g | 246.0 | 18.0 | 217 | 17.0 | 0.8 | 16.2 | 2.5 |
| Beef, Chargrilled, Quarter Pounder, Morrisons* | 1 Burger/227g | 590.0 | 45.0 | 260 | 15.0 | 5.3 | 19.9 | 0.2 |
| Beef, Flame Grilled, Dalepak* | 1 Burger/44g | 134.0 | 11.0 | 304 | 15.3 | 2.1 | 26.0 | 0.4 |
| Beef, Morrisons* | 1 Burger/57g | 169.0 | 14.0 | 298 | 12.3 | 5.5 | 25.2 | 0.6 |
| Beef, Organic, M & S* | 1 Burger/110g | 239.0 | 18.0 | 217 | 18.2 | 0.0 | 16.0 | 0.2 |
| Beef, Original & Best, Birds Eye* | 1 Burger/46g | 115.0 | 9.0 | 252 | 14.1 | 5.1 | 19.5 | 0.4 |
| Beef, Quarter Pounder, Chilled, Morrisons* | 1 Burger/115g | 228.0 | 14.0 | 198 | 17.2 | 4.4 | 12.1 | 0.2 |
| Beef, Quarter Pounders, Flame Grilled, Rustlers* | 1 Burger/190g | 557.0 | 29.0 | 293 | 14.9 | 24.3 | 15.1 | 0.0 |
| Beef, Quarter Pounders, Flame Grilled, Tesco* | 1 Burger/88g | 246.0 | 20.0 | 280 | 13.1 | 4.8 | 23.2 | 0.8 |
| Beef, Quarter Pounders, Good Intentions, Somerfield* | 1 Burger/96g | 184.0 | 12.0 | 191 | 18.9 | 1.9 | 12.0 | 0.8 |
| Beef, Quarter Pounders, Morrisons* | 1 Burger/114g | 338.0 | 29.0 | 298 | 12.3 | 5.5 | 25.2 | 0.6 |
| Beef, Quarter Pounders, Reduced Fat, Tesco* | 1 Burger/95g | 171.0 | 12.0 | 180 | 14.0 | 1.8 | 13.0 | 0.8 |
| Beef, Quarter Pounders, Somerfield* | 1 Burger/114g | 319.0 | 25.0 | 280 | 14.7 | 5.6 | 22.1 | 1.2 |
| Beef, Quarter Pounders, Tesco* | 1 Burger/113g | 292.0 | 23.0 | 258 | 17.8 | 0.7 | 20.4 | 1.3 |
| Beef, Quarter Pounders, with Onion, BGTY, Sainsbury's* | 1 Burger/83g | 171.0 | 8.0 | 205 | 26.6 | 3.8 | 9.3 | 0.9 |
| Beef, Quarter Pounders, with Onion, Cooked, Birds Eye* | 1 Burger/100g | 230.0 | 16.0 | 230 | 16.0 | 5.9 | 16.0 | 0.4 |
| Beef, Quarter Pounders, with Onion, Sainsbury's* | 1 Burger/113g | 306.0 | 22.0 | 271 | 18.0 | 5.1 | 19.8 | 1.5 |
| Beef, Sainsbury's* | 1 Burger/57g | 152.0 | 9.0 | 267 | 29.6 | 1.3 | 15.9 | 1.5 |
| Beef, Scotch, 5oz, TTD, Sainsbury's* | 1 Burger/142g | 317.0 | 17.0 | 223 | 23.7 | 4.9 | 12.0 | 1.4 |
| Beef, Scotch, Smoked Jalapeno Chilli, TTD, Sainsbury's* | 1 Burger/142g | 338.0 | 21.0 | 238 | 22.7 | 3.5 | 14.8 | 1.7 |
| Beef, Sundried Tomato, Grilled, Finest, Tesco* | 1 Burger/99g | 170.0 | 7.0 | 172 | 20.5 | 5.8 | 7.4 | 0.5 |
| Beef, Ultimate, Scottish, TTD, Sainsbury's* | 1 Burger/142g | 284.0 | 12.0 | 200 | 26.0 | 4.7 | 8.6 | 1.0 |
| Beef, with Jalapeno Chilli, Finest, Tesco* | 1 Burger /205g | 379.0 | 22.0 | 185 | 17.0 | 3.4 | 10.9 | 0.4 |
| Beef, with Onion, Cooked, Ross* | 1 Burger/41g | 117.0 | 10.0 | 284 | 14.7 | 2.8 | 23.8 | 0.4 |
| Beef, with Peppermix, Danish Crown* | 1 Burger/100g | 250.0 | 19.0 | 250 | 19.0 | 0.0 | 19.0 | 0.0 |
| Beef, with Potato Gratin, Weight Watchers* | 1 Pack/400g | 320.0 | 10.0 | 80 | 3.0 | 10.0 | 2.5 | 0.0 |
| Beef, with Red Onion & Mustard, Finest, Tesco* | 1 Burger/130g | 308.0 | 24.0 | 237 | 17.2 | 0.2 | 18.6 | 2.6 |

## BURGERS

| INFO/WEIGHT | Measure | per Measure KCAL | FAT | Nutrition Values per 100g / 100ml KCAL | PROT | CARB | FAT | FIBRE |
|---|---|---|---|---|---|---|---|---|
| Beef, with Shallots, Finest, Tesco* | 1 Burger/84g | 175.0 | 10.0 | 208 | 20.2 | 6.4 | 11.3 | 0.5 |
| Beef & Mature Cheddar, Asda* | 1 Burger/80g | 178.0 | 10.0 | 223 | 21.5 | 6.2 | 12.5 | 0.5 |
| Beef & Onion, Grilled, Asda* | 1 Burger/81g | 201.0 | 12.0 | 248 | 23.1 | 6.9 | 14.2 | 0.5 |
| Beef with Onion, Sainsbury's* | 1 Burger/42g | 102.0 | 6.0 | 243 | 20.7 | 6.9 | 14.8 | 1.0 |
| Cheeseburger, American, Tesco* | 1 Burger/275g | 660.0 | 26.0 | 240 | 13.6 | 24.9 | 9.6 | 1.6 |
| Cheeseburger, Bacon, with Bun, Chargrilled, Tesco* | 1 Burger/265g | 726.0 | 42.0 | 274 | 13.0 | 19.6 | 15.9 | 1.0 |
| Cheeseburger, Micro Snack, Tesco* | 1 Burger/115g | 309.0 | 15.0 | 269 | 12.6 | 26.4 | 12.6 | 0.0 |
| Cheeseburger, SmartPrice, Asda* | 1 Burger/150g | 374.0 | 14.0 | 249 | 13.3 | 28.0 | 9.3 | 1.4 |
| Cheeseburger, with Relish, American Style, Tesco* | 1 Burger/61g | 132.0 | 6.0 | 215 | 14.2 | 17.5 | 9.8 | 4.2 |
| Cheeseburger, with Sesame Seed Bun, Tesco* | 1 Burger/275g | 644.0 | 32.0 | 234 | 12.2 | 20.1 | 11.7 | 2.0 |
| Chicken, Breaded, Value, Tesco* | 1 Burger/145g | 362.0 | 21.0 | 250 | 12.4 | 16.6 | 14.5 | 1.0 |
| Chicken, Crunch Crumb, Tesco* | 1 Burger/57g | 161.0 | 11.0 | 282 | 12.3 | 15.6 | 18.9 | 0.0 |
| Chicken, Fillet, Cajun, Weighed After Cooking, Birds Eye* | 1 Burger/92g | 128.0 | 4.0 | 140 | 20.1 | 4.8 | 4.7 | 0.2 |
| Chicken, Fresh, Non Coated, Waitrose* | 1 Burger/100g | 141.0 | 4.0 | 141 | 16.0 | 10.4 | 4.0 | 0.9 |
| Chicken, Golden Breadcrumbs, Frozen, Birds Eye* | 1 Burger/56g | 130.0 | 7.0 | 232 | 13.8 | 16.4 | 12.4 | 0.3 |
| Chicken, Quarter Pounders, Birds Eye* | 1 Burger/117g | 280.0 | 16.0 | 239 | 13.5 | 15.2 | 13.8 | 0.6 |
| Chicken, Sainsbury's* | 1 Burger/46g | 115.0 | 7.0 | 247 | 15.6 | 12.2 | 15.1 | 1.3 |
| Chicken, Southern Fried, Sainsbury's* | 1 Burger/52g | 154.0 | 10.0 | 297 | 12.6 | 17.2 | 19.8 | 1.3 |
| Chicken, with Sesame Seed Bun, Breaded, Tesco* | 1 Burger/205g | 588.0 | 32.0 | 287 | 10.2 | 26.2 | 15.7 | 2.9 |
| Chicken Cajun, Fillet, Birds Eye* | 1 Pack/180g | 275.0 | 9.0 | 153 | 21.5 | 5.8 | 4.9 | 0.3 |
| Chicken Crunch & Fries, M & S* | 1 Pack/425g | 915.0 | 48.0 | 215 | 8.8 | 20.8 | 11.2 | 2.1 |
| Chicken Fillet, Weight After Cooking, Birds Eye* | 1 Burger/90g | 126.0 | 4.0 | 140 | 20.0 | 5.1 | 4.6 | 0.2 |
| Chilli, Quarter Pounders, Asda* | 1 Burger/88g | 221.0 | 14.0 | 252 | 25.0 | 2.0 | 16.0 | 0.0 |
| Chilli, Quarter Pounders, Farmfoods* | 1 Burger/115g | 285.0 | 23.0 | 248 | 13.5 | 2.9 | 20.3 | 0.9 |
| Classic, Eddie Rockets* | 1 Burger/295g | 620.0 | 35.0 | 210 | 10.8 | 14.9 | 11.9 | 0.0 |
| Gemüse, Alnatura* | 1 Burger/30g | 44.0 | 1.0 | 148 | 5.1 | 25.7 | 2.8 | 0.0 |
| Lamb, Minted, Asda* | 1 Burger/100g | 234.0 | 14.0 | 234 | 22.0 | 4.9 | 14.0 | 0.3 |
| Lamb, Minted, Quarter Pounders, Asda* | 1 Burger/114g | 241.0 | 14.0 | 212 | 19.2 | 6.1 | 12.3 | 0.0 |
| Lamb, Quarter Pounder, Asda* | 1 Burger/85g | 213.0 | 14.0 | 251 | 20.9 | 5.2 | 16.3 | 0.9 |
| Lamb, Quarter Pounders, Birds Eye* | 1 Burger/112g | 232.0 | 17.0 | 207 | 13.9 | 3.8 | 15.1 | 0.3 |
| Lamb, Waitrose* | 1 Burger/67g | 99.0 | 5.0 | 148 | 15.7 | 5.4 | 7.0 | 0.9 |
| Meat Free, Sainsbury's* | 1 Burger/57g | 86.0 | 3.0 | 151 | 22.0 | 4.4 | 5.0 | 3.4 |
| Pork, Quarter Pounders, Birds Eye* | 1 Burger/122g | 292.0 | 23.0 | 239 | 13.9 | 3.2 | 19.0 | 0.2 |
| Quarter Pounder, with Cheese, Flame Grilled, Feasters* | 1 Burger/200g | 550.0 | 20.0 | 275 | 17.2 | 22.1 | 9.9 | 0.9 |
| Quarter Pounder, with Onion, Tesco* | 1 Burger/87g | 213.0 | 16.0 | 245 | 16.0 | 3.0 | 18.6 | 0.5 |
| Quarter Pounder with Cheese & Buns, Sainsbury's* | 1 Burger/198g | 471.0 | 23.0 | 238 | 15.6 | 19.1 | 11.5 | 1.4 |
| Quarter Pounders, 95% Fat Free, Good Choice, Iceland* | 1 Burger/86g | 150.0 | 4.0 | 174 | 27.8 | 5.0 | 4.8 | 1.1 |
| Quarter Pounders, Chargrilled, BGTY, Sainsbury's* | 1 Burger/114g | 184.0 | 6.0 | 161 | 20.8 | 7.1 | 5.5 | 1.1 |
| Quarter Pounders, Scotch Beef, Sainsbury's* | 1 Burger/114g | 255.0 | 15.0 | 225 | 22.2 | 3.5 | 13.6 | 0.5 |
| Salmon, Quarter Pounders, Morrisons* | 1 Burger/110g | 235.0 | 13.0 | 214 | 21.4 | 5.5 | 11.8 | 1.7 |
| Salmon, Quarter Pounders, Tesco* | 1 Burger/114g | 145.0 | 3.0 | 128 | 15.9 | 10.6 | 2.4 | 1.2 |
| Salmon, Tesco* | 1 Burger/100g | 101.0 | 3.0 | 101 | 18.2 | 0.3 | 3.0 | 0.0 |
| Spicy Bean, Ainsley Harriott* | 1 Burger/200g | 302.0 | 7.0 | 151 | 7.2 | 23.5 | 3.7 | 5.2 |
| Spicy Bean, Cooked, Grassington's Food Co* | 1 Burger/108g | 201.0 | 4.0 | 186 | 6.5 | 32.2 | 3.5 | 2.5 |
| Spicy Bean, Sainsbury's* | 1 Burger/110g | 262.0 | 14.0 | 240 | 5.0 | 27.1 | 12.4 | 2.0 |
| Spicy Bean & Nacho, Morrisons* | 1 Burger/113g | 288.0 | 18.0 | 254 | 5.0 | 23.3 | 15.6 | 3.9 |
| Tuna, Quarter Pounders, Sainsbury's* | 1 Serving/100g | 179.0 | 5.0 | 179 | 24.0 | 10.0 | 4.8 | 0.4 |
| Tuna, Quarter Pounders, Tesco* | 1 Burger/114g | 132.0 | 2.0 | 116 | 18.8 | 6.7 | 1.6 | 0.9 |
| Tuna, Sainsbury's* | 1 Serving/105g | 194.0 | 10.0 | 185 | 20.8 | 3.4 | 9.8 | 1.2 |
| Turkey, Cheeseburgers, Tesco* | 1 Burger/105g | 252.0 | 15.0 | 240 | 15.4 | 12.8 | 14.1 | 1.3 |
| Turkey, Crispy Crumb, Bernard Matthews* | 1 Burger/71g | 222.0 | 14.0 | 313 | 11.3 | 19.3 | 19.8 | 0.9 |
| Venison, Finnebrogue Estate* | 1 Burger/142g | 170.0 | 7.0 | 120 | 19.9 | 4.2 | 4.9 | 0.5 |
| Venison, Grilled, Specially Selected, Tesco* | 1 Burger/127g | 210.0 | 10.0 | 165 | 17.3 | 4.9 | 8.1 | 0.6 |

| | Measure INFO/WEIGHT | per Measure KCAL | FAT | Nutrition Values per 100g / 100ml KCAL | PROT | CARB | FAT | FIBRE |
|---|---|---|---|---|---|---|---|---|
| **BURGERS VEGETARIAN** | | | | | | | | |
| Bean, Mexican Style, Quarter Pounder, Meat Free, Tesco* | 1 Burger/114g | 250.0 | 12.0 | 220 | 5.0 | 25.0 | 10.6 | 2.4 |
| Bean, Tesco* | 1 Burger/90g | 192.0 | 11.0 | 213 | 4.4 | 21.6 | 12.1 | 5.0 |
| Black Bean, Organic, Cauldron Foods* | 1 Burger/88g | 169.0 | 10.0 | 193 | 9.2 | 13.1 | 11.5 | 8.5 |
| Chargrilled Style, Safeway* | 1 Burger/57g | 95.0 | 5.0 | 167 | 18.8 | 3.7 | 8.5 | 4.0 |
| Cheese & Spring Onion, Tesco* | 1 Burger/87g | 178.0 | 10.0 | 204 | 4.4 | 20.0 | 11.8 | 3.2 |
| Chilli, Cauldron Foods* | 1 Burger/88g | 148.0 | 8.0 | 169 | 11.5 | 8.5 | 9.3 | 3.3 |
| Flame Grilled, Linda McCartney* | 1 Burger/60g | 104.0 | 3.0 | 174 | 17.9 | 13.8 | 5.2 | 3.3 |
| Meat Free, Asda* | 1 Burger/60g | 138.0 | 6.0 | 230 | 24.0 | 11.0 | 10.0 | 0.3 |
| Meat Free, Sainsbury's* | 1 Burger/57g | 92.0 | 4.0 | 161 | 19.6 | 3.9 | 7.4 | 4.8 |
| Mushroom, Cauldron Foods* | 1 Burger/88g | 125.0 | 6.0 | 143 | 5.5 | 16.1 | 6.3 | 2.6 |
| Mushroom, Meat Free, Tesco* | 1 Burger/87g | 151.0 | 9.0 | 173 | 3.6 | 15.3 | 10.8 | 3.7 |
| Mushroom, Organic, Cauldron Foods* | 1 Burger/88g | 136.0 | 7.0 | 156 | 7.1 | 18.2 | 8.3 | 2.3 |
| Quarter Pounders, Beef Style, Sainsbury's* | 1 Burger/114g | 216.0 | 11.0 | 190 | 20.0 | 6.0 | 9.5 | 2.5 |
| Quarter Pounders, Chargrilled, Tesco* | 1 Burger/114g | 186.0 | 9.0 | 164 | 16.0 | 7.0 | 8.0 | 2.5 |
| Quarter Pounders, HL, Tesco* | 1 Burger/102g | 117.0 | 2.0 | 114 | 4.0 | 20.7 | 1.7 | 2.0 |
| Spicy Bean, BGTY, Sainsbury's* | 1 Burger/85g | 123.0 | 2.0 | 145 | 6.9 | 23.3 | 2.7 | 3.1 |
| Spicy Bean, Linda McCartney* | 1 Burger/85g | 190.0 | 10.0 | 223 | 4.3 | 26.2 | 11.2 | 2.9 |
| Spicy Bean, Quarter Pounder, Dalepak* | 1 Burger/115g | 237.0 | 13.0 | 206 | 4.6 | 22.3 | 10.9 | 2.6 |
| Traditional, Fry's Special Vegetarian* | 1 Burger/75g | 175.0 | 9.0 | 233 | 19.2 | 12.9 | 12.0 | 0.2 |
| Vegeburger, Linda McCartney* | 1 Burger/59g | 79.0 | 2.0 | 134 | 22.6 | 2.9 | 3.6 | 1.6 |
| Vegetable, Captains, Birds Eye* | 1 Burger/48g | 96.0 | 4.0 | 200 | 4.7 | 25.5 | 8.8 | 2.0 |
| Vegetable, Organic, Tesco* | 1 Burger/90g | 108.0 | 4.0 | 120 | 2.6 | 17.6 | 4.3 | 2.1 |
| Vegetable, Quarter Pounders, Crunchy, Birds Eye* | 1 Burger/114g | 240.0 | 12.0 | 211 | 4.8 | 24.9 | 10.2 | 1.8 |
| Vegetable, Quarter Pounders, Dalepak* | 1 Burger/114g | 227.0 | 10.0 | 200 | 4.8 | 26.3 | 8.5 | 1.8 |
| Vegetable, Quarter Pounders, Tesco* | 1 Burger/108g | 227.0 | 13.0 | 211 | 4.4 | 20.8 | 12.2 | 2.7 |
| Vegetable, Spicy, Asda* | 1 Burger/56g | 108.0 | 6.0 | 193 | 3.4 | 20.0 | 11.0 | 0.0 |
| with Tofu, Organic, Evernat* | 1oz/28g | 52.0 | 2.0 | 186 | 7.9 | 16.9 | 8.3 | 0.0 |
| **BUTTER** | | | | | | | | |
| Brandy, Tesco* | 1oz/28g | 152.0 | 11.0 | 543 | 0.3 | 48.3 | 38.7 | 0.5 |
| Brandy, with Cognac, Sainsbury's* | 1/8 Pot/25g | 137.0 | 9.0 | 549 | 0.2 | 44.1 | 37.6 | 0.0 |
| ***Creamery, Average*** | **1 Serving/10g** | **74.0** | **8.0** | **735** | **0.5** | **0.3** | **81.3** | **0.0** |
| ***Fresh, Average*** | **1 Thin Spread/7g** | **51.0** | **6.0** | **735** | **0.5** | **0.4** | **81.3** | **0.0** |
| Garlic, Somerfield* | 1oz/28g | 192.0 | 21.0 | 686 | 1.0 | 2.0 | 75.0 | 0.0 |
| ***Reduced Fat, Fresh, Average*** | **1 Thin Spread/7g** | **26.0** | **3.0** | **368** | **2.3** | **1.2** | **39.4** | **0.2** |
| ***Salted, Average*** | **1 Thin Spread/7g** | **51.0** | **6.0** | **729** | **0.4** | **0.3** | **81.1** | **0.0** |
| ***Spreadable, Fresh, Average*** | **1 Thin Spread/7g** | **51.0** | **6.0** | **730** | **0.4** | **0.3** | **80.8** | **0.0** |
| ***Spreadable, Reduced Fat, Average*** | **1 Thin Spread/7g** | **38.0** | **4.0** | **540** | **0.5** | **0.5** | **60.0** | **0.0** |
| with Crushed Garlic, Lurpak* | 1 Serving/10g | 70.0 | 7.0 | 700 | 1.0 | 4.0 | 75.0 | 0.0 |
| **BUTTERMILK** | | | | | | | | |
| ***Average*** | **1 Mug/400ml** | **177.0** | **1.0** | **44** | **4.2** | **5.9** | **0.3** | **0.0** |
| **BUTTONS** | | | | | | | | |
| Chocolate, Giant, Dairy Milk, Cadbury* | 1 Button/3g | 15.0 | 1.0 | 525 | 7.7 | 56.7 | 29.9 | 0.7 |
| Dairy Milk, Milk Chocolate, Cadbury* | 1 Pack/32g | 170.0 | 10.0 | 525 | 7.7 | 56.7 | 29.9 | 0.7 |
| Milk Chocolate, Somerfield* | 1 Pack/75g | 390.0 | 21.0 | 520 | 8.0 | 58.0 | 28.0 | 0.0 |
| Milk Chocolate, Tesco* | 1 Bag/70g | 359.0 | 19.0 | 513 | 7.1 | 59.1 | 27.6 | 2.1 |
| White Chocolate, Cadbury* | 1 Pack/32g | 180.0 | 11.0 | 555 | 4.5 | 58.4 | 33.8 | 0.0 |
| White Chocolate, Tesco* | 1 Bag/70g | 388.0 | 23.0 | 554 | 5.1 | 58.0 | 33.5 | 0.0 |

**B**

| | Measure INFO/WEIGHT | per Measure | | Nutrition Values per 100g / 100ml | | | | |
|---|---|---|---|---|---|---|---|---|
| | | KCAL | FAT | KCAL | PROT | CARB | FAT | FIBRE |
| **CABBAGE** | | | | | | | | |
| & Leek, Crunchy Mix, Ready to Cook, Sainsbury's* | 1 Serving/125g | 34.0 | 1.0 | 27 | 1.9 | 3.7 | 0.5 | 2.6 |
| & Leek, Tesco* | 1/3 Pack/100g | 28.0 | 1.0 | 28 | 2.2 | 3.2 | 0.7 | 2.4 |
| *Boiled, Average* | *1 Serving/90g* | *14.0* | *0.0* | *15* | *1.0* | *2.2* | *0.3* | *1.7* |
| Creamed, Sainsbury's* | ½ Pack/150g | 88.0 | 6.0 | 59 | 1.5 | 3.9 | 4.2 | 2.3 |
| *Greens, Trimmed, Average* | *1oz/28g* | *8.0* | *0.0* | *28* | *2.9* | *2.9* | *0.5* | *3.4* |
| Mash, Eat Smart, Safeway* | ½ Pack/225g | 146.0 | 4.0 | 65 | 2.0 | 9.2 | 1.8 | 1.7 |
| Medley, Washed, Ready to Cook, Tesco* | 1 Pack/200g | 60.0 | 1.0 | 30 | 2.3 | 3.7 | 0.6 | 2.8 |
| *Raw, Average* | *1 Serving/100g* | *21.0* | *0.0* | *21* | *1.3* | *3.1* | *0.4* | *1.8* |
| *Red, Average* | *1 Serving/90g* | *19.0* | *0.0* | *21* | *1.0* | *3.7* | *0.3* | *2.2* |
| Red, Braised with Red Wine, M & S* | ½ Pack/150g | 180.0 | 7.0 | 120 | 1.4 | 17.1 | 4.8 | 1.0 |
| *Red, Pickled, Average* | *1 Serving/100g* | *26.0* | *0.0* | *26* | *0.9* | *4.6* | *0.1* | *1.5* |
| Red, Spiced, Steamer, Sainsbury's* | ½ Pack/150g | 105.0 | 3.0 | 70 | 1.0 | 10.5 | 2.2 | 2.9 |
| Red, with Apple, Braised, Sainsbury's* | ½ Pack/117g | 91.0 | 4.0 | 78 | 0.8 | 10.8 | 3.5 | 1.7 |
| Red, with Apple, Finest, Tesco* | ½ Pack/150g | 177.0 | 9.0 | 118 | 1.6 | 14.7 | 5.9 | 4.6 |
| Red, with Apple, Frozen, Sainsbury's* | 1 Serving/75g | 37.0 | 0.0 | 50 | 1.8 | 10.8 | 0.0 | 2.2 |
| Red, with Apple & Cranberry, TTD, Sainsbury's* | ½ Pack/200g | 166.0 | 6.0 | 83 | 1.3 | 12.8 | 2.9 | 1.4 |
| *Savoy, Boiled in Salted Water, Average* | *1 Serving/90g* | *15.0* | *0.0* | *17* | *1.1* | *2.2* | *0.5* | *2.0* |
| *Savoy, Raw, Average* | *1 Serving/90g* | *24.0* | *0.0* | *27* | *2.1* | *3.9* | *0.5* | *3.1* |
| Sweetheart, Tesco* | 1 Serving/100g | 20.0 | 1.0 | 20 | 1.9 | 1.6 | 0.7 | 2.6 |
| *White, Raw, Average* | *1oz/28g* | *8.0* | *0.0* | *27* | *1.4* | *5.0* | *0.2* | *2.1* |
| **CAKE** | | | | | | | | |
| Action Man, Birthday, Memory Lane Cakes* | 1/12 Cake/83g | 322.0 | 14.0 | 388 | 3.0 | 57.0 | 16.4 | 0.8 |
| Almond Flavoured Rounds, Country Garden Cakes* | 1 Cake/45g | 183.0 | 7.0 | 403 | 4.3 | 62.4 | 14.7 | 2.3 |
| Almond Slices, GFY, Asda* | 1 Slice/25g | 67.0 | 1.0 | 268 | 4.0 | 56.0 | 3.1 | 0.7 |
| Almond Slices, Lyons* | 1 Slice/27g | 114.0 | 7.0 | 426 | 7.1 | 41.3 | 25.8 | 1.6 |
| Almond Slices, Mr Kipling* | 1 Slice/33g | 131.0 | 5.0 | 403 | 6.3 | 63.4 | 14.0 | 2.0 |
| Almond Slices, Sainsbury's* | 1 Serving/27g | 120.0 | 7.0 | 444 | 5.9 | 45.9 | 26.3 | 1.5 |
| Almond Slices, Weight Watchers* | 1 Slice/26g | 95.0 | 3.0 | 365 | 5.2 | 63.8 | 9.9 | 2.4 |
| Angel, Co-Op* | 1/8 Cake/35g | 131.0 | 6.0 | 375 | 4.0 | 52.0 | 17.0 | 0.7 |
| Angel, Sainsbury's* | 1/8 Cake/41g | 171.0 | 8.0 | 417 | 4.1 | 55.7 | 19.8 | 0.8 |
| Angel Layer, Tesco* | 1 Serving/25g | 101.0 | 4.0 | 403 | 4.5 | 57.4 | 17.3 | 0.9 |
| Angel Slices, Mr Kipling* | 1 Slice/38g | 153.0 | 7.0 | 403 | 2.9 | 58.8 | 18.3 | 0.6 |
| Apple, Bramley, & Blackberry Crumble, M & S* | 1/8 Cake/56g | 221.0 | 10.0 | 395 | 4.4 | 54.1 | 17.9 | 1.5 |
| Apple, Home Style, M & S* | 1 Cake/54g | 189.0 | 8.0 | 350 | 5.3 | 49.4 | 14.7 | 1.5 |
| Apple Bakes, Go Ahead, McVitie's* | 1 Cake/35g | 126.0 | 3.0 | 361 | 2.6 | 70.0 | 7.8 | 2.0 |
| Apple Crumble, Slices, Weight Watchers* | 1 Slice/26g | 90.0 | 2.0 | 346 | 4.5 | 64.8 | 7.7 | 2.3 |
| Apple Slice, Delightful, Mr Kipling* | 1 Slice/29g | 92.0 | 1.0 | 317 | 4.4 | 66.2 | 3.9 | 1.3 |
| Apricot & Apple, Trimlyne* | 1 Cake/50g | 133.0 | 1.0 | 267 | 4.3 | 58.4 | 2.7 | 1.9 |
| Bakewell Slices, Mr Kipling* | 1 Slice/36g | 163.0 | 7.0 | 454 | 4.2 | 63.4 | 20.4 | 1.2 |
| Banana, Organinc, Loaf, Respect Organics* | ¼ Pack/65g | 254.0 | 14.0 | 391 | 3.9 | 48.6 | 21.0 | 1.5 |
| Banana Loaf, Waitrose* | 1 Slice/70g | 236.0 | 7.0 | 337 | 5.0 | 55.2 | 10.7 | 1.7 |
| Battenberg, Mr Kipling* | 1 Serving/38g | 161.0 | 5.0 | 421 | 5.0 | 73.3 | 12.0 | 1.6 |
| Belgian Chocolate, Slices, Weight Watchers* | 1 Slice/30g | 99.0 | 2.0 | 329 | 5.9 | 61.3 | 6.7 | 2.3 |
| Birthday, M & S* | 1 Serving/60g | 240.0 | 7.0 | 400 | 2.3 | 70.9 | 11.9 | 0.8 |
| Birthday Present, Tesco* | 1 Serving/79g | 347.0 | 14.0 | 439 | 3.5 | 66.6 | 17.6 | 0.4 |
| Butterfly, Mr Kipling* | 1 Cake/29g | 114.0 | 6.0 | 392 | 4.4 | 43.4 | 22.2 | 0.6 |
| Buttons, Happy Birthday, Cadbury* | 1 Slice/50g | 235.0 | 14.0 | 470 | 4.1 | 52.8 | 27.1 | 0.0 |
| Caramel, Milk Chocolate, Holly Lane* | 1 Cake/25g | 110.0 | 5.0 | 441 | 6.9 | 57.6 | 20.3 | 1.1 |
| Caramel Slice, M & S* | 1 Slice/64g | 304.0 | 16.0 | 475 | 4.9 | 60.4 | 25.2 | 2.6 |
| Carrot, Entenmann's* | 1 Serving/40g | 156.0 | 8.0 | 391 | 4.1 | 47.4 | 20.5 | 1.5 |
| Carrot, Handmade, Delicious, Boots* | 1 Slice/75g | 292.0 | 13.0 | 389 | 4.1 | 53.0 | 18.0 | 1.4 |
| Carrot, Iced, Tesco* | 1 Serving/61g | 246.0 | 12.0 | 404 | 3.1 | 53.7 | 19.6 | 1.6 |
| Carrot, Mini, Weight Watchers* | 1 Cake/27g | 105.0 | 3.0 | 388 | 3.7 | 68.9 | 10.8 | 2.7 |

# CAKE

| | Measure INFO/WEIGHT | per Measure KCAL | FAT | Nutrition Values per 100g / 100ml KCAL | PROT | CARB | FAT | FIBRE |
|---|---|---|---|---|---|---|---|---|
| Carrot, Organic, Respect Organics* | 1 Slice/45g | 179.0 | 10.0 | 398 | 3.1 | 47.4 | 22.4 | 1.5 |
| Carrot, Slices, Asda* | 1 Slice/80g | 302.0 | 13.0 | 377 | 3.4 | 53.8 | 16.5 | 1.7 |
| Carrot, The Handmade Flapjack Company* | 1 Cake/75g | 295.0 | 13.0 | 393 | 6.4 | 53.0 | 17.3 | 0.0 |
| Carrot & Orange, Extra Special, Asda* | 1/6 Cake/65g | 240.0 | 12.0 | 369 | 4.7 | 47.0 | 18.0 | 0.9 |
| Carrot & Orange, Finest, Tesco* | 1/8 Cake/50g | 205.0 | 10.0 | 410 | 4.6 | 51.2 | 20.5 | 2.1 |
| Carrot & Orange, Light Choices, Tesco* | 1/6 Cake/63g | 227.0 | 6.0 | 360 | 3.9 | 64.2 | 9.8 | 1.3 |
| Carrot & Orange, Waitrose* | 1/6 Cake/47g | 164.0 | 7.0 | 350 | 5.3 | 46.8 | 15.7 | 1.8 |
| Carrot & Orange Slices, GFY, Asda* | 1 Serving/23g | 77.0 | 1.0 | 334 | 3.4 | 74.0 | 2.7 | 1.0 |
| Carrot & Pecan, M & S* | 1 Slice/90g | 330.0 | 15.0 | 365 | 6.4 | 48.7 | 16.2 | 2.3 |
| Carrot & Walnut, Layered, Asda* | 1 Serving/42g | 172.0 | 8.0 | 409 | 4.6 | 55.0 | 19.0 | 1.0 |
| Carrot & Walnut, Mini Classics, Mr Kipling* | 1 Cake/39g | 172.0 | 10.0 | 440 | 4.5 | 48.6 | 25.2 | 1.0 |
| Carrot & Walnut, TTD, Sainsbury's* | 1 Slice/58g | 208.0 | 10.0 | 358 | 3.6 | 47.3 | 17.2 | 0.9 |
| Carrot Slices, GFY, Asda* | 1 Slice/28g | 83.0 | 1.0 | 298 | 2.8 | 66.4 | 2.3 | 2.1 |
| Carrot Slices, Less Than 3% Fat, BGTY, Sainsbury's* | 1 Slice/30g | 94.0 | 1.0 | 313 | 3.4 | 68.7 | 2.7 | 2.4 |
| Carrot Slices, Weight Watchers* | 1 Slice/27g | 71.0 | 1.0 | 263 | 3.0 | 56.7 | 2.7 | 1.9 |
| Carrot Wedge, Tesco* | 1 Pack/175g | 532.0 | 28.0 | 304 | 3.9 | 36.6 | 15.8 | 1.5 |
| Celebration, Sainsbury's* | 1/12 Cake/100g | 265.0 | 9.0 | 265 | 2.1 | 43.6 | 9.2 | 0.3 |
| Cherry, Asda* | 1 Slice/37g | 131.0 | 4.0 | 351 | 4.7 | 56.0 | 12.0 | 0.6 |
| Cherry, M & S* | 1 Serving/75g | 285.0 | 10.0 | 380 | 5.0 | 60.6 | 12.7 | 0.8 |
| Cherry Bakewell, Co-Op* | 1 Cake/47g | 205.0 | 8.0 | 435 | 3.7 | 67.2 | 16.9 | 1.8 |
| Cherry Bakewell, Gluten Free, Bakers Delight* | 1 Cake/50g | 211.0 | 8.0 | 422 | 2.9 | 66.1 | 16.3 | 0.4 |
| Cherry Bakewell, Layer, Asda* | 1/8 Cake/50g | 210.0 | 11.0 | 420 | 4.4 | 51.0 | 22.0 | 0.6 |
| Cherry Bakewell, M & S* | 1 Cake/44g | 185.0 | 8.0 | 420 | 4.5 | 61.7 | 17.7 | 1.0 |
| Cherry Bakewell, Mini, Sainsbury's* | 1 Cake/27g | 101.0 | 3.0 | 370 | 3.4 | 62.2 | 12.0 | 0.4 |
| Cherry Bakewell, Sainsbury's* | 1 Cake/46g | 200.0 | 8.0 | 436 | 3.1 | 66.3 | 17.6 | 1.4 |
| Cherry Bakewell, Sara Lee* | 1/5 Slice/70g | 228.0 | 8.0 | 326 | 4.1 | 51.9 | 11.3 | 1.4 |
| Cherry Bakewell, Slices, GFY, Asda* | 1 Slice/29g | 96.0 | 1.0 | 331 | 3.3 | 74.0 | 2.4 | 0.7 |
| Cherry Bakewell, SmartPrice, Asda* | 1 Cake/38g | 157.0 | 7.0 | 413 | 2.7 | 60.0 | 18.0 | 2.6 |
| Cherry Bakewell, Tesco* | 1 Cake/39g | 171.0 | 7.0 | 439 | 3.2 | 63.3 | 19.2 | 1.1 |
| Cherry Bakewell, Weight Watchers* | 1oz/28g | 102.0 | 3.0 | 365 | 3.6 | 65.4 | 9.9 | 3.6 |
| Cherry Bakewells, Delightful, Mr Kipling* | 1 Cake/45g | 176.0 | 6.0 | 390 | 3.9 | 66.4 | 12.9 | 1.2 |
| Cherry Bakewells, Mr Kipling* | 1 Cake/45g | 193.0 | 8.0 | 428 | 3.9 | 61.3 | 18.5 | 1.4 |
| Chewy Fruity Corn Flake, Dove's Farm* | 1 Bar/40g | 155.0 | 6.0 | 387 | 5.7 | 64.5 | 14.0 | 4.5 |
| Chewy Rice Pop & Chocolate, Dove's Farm* | 1 Bar/35g | 156.0 | 7.0 | 447 | 3.9 | 69.9 | 20.2 | 2.3 |
| Chocolate, Big, Tesco* | 1 Slice/79g | 311.0 | 13.0 | 396 | 7.4 | 54.1 | 16.7 | 1.8 |
| Chocolate, Birthday, Tesco* | 1 Serving/54g | 229.0 | 13.0 | 425 | 5.9 | 45.5 | 24.4 | 2.1 |
| Chocolate, Caterpillar, Tesco* | 1 Serving/53g | 248.0 | 13.0 | 468 | 5.7 | 55.3 | 24.9 | 1.1 |
| Chocolate, Champagne, Sainsbury's* | 1 Serving/75g | 304.0 | 12.0 | 405 | 2.5 | 62.4 | 16.2 | 0.5 |
| Chocolate, Cup, Mini, Weight Watchers* | 1 Cake/17g | 72.0 | 4.0 | 422 | 6.1 | 52.0 | 21.1 | 1.8 |
| Chocolate, Double Dream, Nestle* | 1 Serving/150g | 637.0 | 38.0 | 425 | 5.0 | 44.7 | 25.1 | 0.9 |
| Chocolate, Fondants, Weight Watchers* | 1 Cake/19g | 70.0 | 2.0 | 368 | 6.1 | 59.0 | 12.0 | 3.2 |
| Chocolate, Fudge, The Cake Shop* | 1 Cake/37g | 178.0 | 11.0 | 480 | 3.7 | 50.5 | 29.2 | 1.3 |
| Chocolate, Happy Birthday, Tesco* | 1 Serving/58g | 241.0 | 13.0 | 415 | 4.7 | 46.9 | 22.7 | 2.9 |
| Chocolate, Iced, Tesco* | 1 Serving/40g | 158.0 | 6.0 | 395 | 4.7 | 58.5 | 15.8 | 1.8 |
| Chocolate, Individual, with Mini Eggs, Cadbury* | 1 Cake/26g | 119.0 | 6.0 | 455 | 4.6 | 57.5 | 23.1 | 1.3 |
| Chocolate, Large, Happy Birthday, Tesco* | 1/18 Cake/63g | 249.0 | 12.0 | 396 | 6.2 | 49.3 | 19.3 | 1.8 |
| Chocolate, Loaf, Moist, McVitie's* | 1 Slice/30g | 119.0 | 6.0 | 398 | 4.8 | 49.0 | 20.3 | 1.9 |
| Chocolate, Mini Roll, Safeway* | 1 Cake/40g | 180.0 | 10.0 | 450 | 0.0 | 53.5 | 23.9 | 2.2 |
| Chocolate, Morrisons* | 1 Serving/32g | 159.0 | 10.0 | 505 | 5.3 | 48.0 | 32.4 | 1.2 |
| Chocolate, Party, Tesco* | 1 Slice/62g | 244.0 | 13.0 | 394 | 4.6 | 46.3 | 21.2 | 0.9 |
| Chocolate, Sainsbury's* | 1 Serving/30g | 118.0 | 6.0 | 395 | 4.1 | 52.6 | 18.5 | 1.3 |
| Chocolate, Sara Lee* | ¼ Cake/88g | 339.0 | 15.0 | 385 | 4.1 | 54.3 | 16.8 | 0.0 |
| Chocolate, Smarties, Celebration, Large, Nestle* | 1/16 Cake/71g | 308.0 | 17.0 | 432 | 5.4 | 48.9 | 24.4 | 1.2 |

## CAKE

| INFO/WEIGHT | per Measure KCAL | FAT | Nutrition Values per 100g / 100ml KCAL | PROT | CARB | FAT | FIBRE |
|---|---|---|---|---|---|---|---|

| | Measure INFO/WEIGHT | per Measure KCAL | FAT | Nutrition Values per 100g / 100ml KCAL | PROT | CARB | FAT | FIBRE |
|---|---|---|---|---|---|---|---|---|
| Chocolate, Thorntons* | 1 Serving/87g | 408.0 | 25.0 | 469 | 5.2 | 47.1 | 28.8 | 0.6 |
| Chocolate, TTD, Sainsbury's* | 1 Serving/207g | 749.0 | 32.0 | 362 | 4.4 | 50.9 | 15.5 | 1.3 |
| Chocolate, Ultimate, TTD, Sainsbury's* | 1 Serving/70g | 263.0 | 11.0 | 375 | 5.4 | 51.5 | 16.4 | 1.9 |
| Chocolate, White Button, Asda* | 1 Cake/30g | 117.0 | 6.0 | 390 | 5.0 | 44.0 | 21.0 | 2.0 |
| Chocolate & Orange Rolls, M & S* | 1 Cake/60g | 228.0 | 17.0 | 380 | 3.6 | 27.0 | 28.4 | 1.3 |
| Chocolate & Orange Slices, GFY, Asda* | 1 Serving/30g | 95.0 | 1.0 | 315 | 3.2 | 70.0 | 2.5 | 1.3 |
| Chocolate Flavour Slices, GFY, Asda* | 1 Slice/28g | 71.0 | 1.0 | 257 | 4.3 | 54.0 | 2.6 | 1.4 |
| Chocolate Flower Pot, M & S* | 1 Serving/69g | 295.0 | 13.0 | 430 | 3.8 | 60.8 | 19.3 | 1.5 |
| Chocolate Fudge, & Vanilla Cream, M & S* | 1/6 Cake/69g | 310.0 | 18.0 | 450 | 5.2 | 49.8 | 26.0 | 1.3 |
| Chocolate Fudge, Classics, M & S* | 1 Serving/71g | 195.0 | 8.0 | 275 | 2.8 | 42.8 | 10.6 | 1.1 |
| Chocolate Fudge, Sainsbury's* | 1/8 Cake/98g | 402.0 | 22.0 | 410 | 5.5 | 47.3 | 22.3 | 1.9 |
| Chocolate Fudge, Tea Time Treats, Asda* | 1 Cake/37g | 157.0 | 8.0 | 424 | 3.6 | 53.0 | 22.0 | 1.7 |
| Chocolate Fudge Slice, Waitrose* | 1 Slice/60g | 230.0 | 10.0 | 383 | 4.7 | 54.6 | 16.2 | 1.5 |
| Chocolate Heaven, Extra Special, Asda* | 1/6 Cake/66g | 255.0 | 13.0 | 388 | 4.0 | 48.0 | 20.0 | 1.0 |
| Chocolate Indulgence, Finest, Tesco* | 1 Slice/51g | 207.0 | 9.0 | 405 | 4.8 | 55.9 | 17.9 | 1.2 |
| Chocolate Log, Fresh Cream, Finest, Tesco* | 1 Slice/85g | 301.0 | 15.0 | 354 | 4.5 | 43.2 | 18.1 | 1.4 |
| Chocolate Orange, Slices, Weight Watchers* | 1 Slice/82g | 249.0 | 2.0 | 304 | 4.9 | 64.9 | 2.7 | 2.6 |
| Chocolate Orange, Sponge, Asda* | 1 Serving/70g | 297.0 | 18.0 | 425 | 4.9 | 42.9 | 26.0 | 3.0 |
| Chocolate Party, M & S* | 1 Serving/61g | 240.0 | 13.0 | 395 | 4.6 | 46.9 | 20.8 | 1.1 |
| Chocolate Roll, Sainsbury's* | 1 Slice/50g | 210.0 | 10.0 | 420 | 5.0 | 54.0 | 20.4 | 3.3 |
| Chocolate Sensation, Sainsbury's* | 1 Serving/92g | 320.0 | 18.0 | 348 | 3.7 | 40.0 | 19.2 | 2.3 |
| Chocolate Slice, Go Ahead, McVitie's* | 1 Slice/32g | 94.0 | 3.0 | 293 | 4.5 | 49.4 | 8.2 | 1.9 |
| Chocolate Slices, Mr Kipling* | 1 Slice/33g | 132.0 | 7.0 | 406 | 5.6 | 50.4 | 20.6 | 2.7 |
| Chocolate Sponge, Less Than 5% Fat, Asda* | 1 Sponge/110g | 198.0 | 4.0 | 180 | 4.4 | 32.0 | 3.8 | 1.1 |
| Chocolate Sponge, Morrisons* | 1 Serving/59g | 179.0 | 8.0 | 303 | 4.4 | 42.5 | 12.8 | 0.7 |
| Chocolate Sponge, Tesco* | 1 Serving/35g | 129.0 | 5.0 | 373 | 5.3 | 54.4 | 14.9 | 1.5 |
| Chocolate Truffle, Extra Special, Asda* | 1 Serving/103g | 402.0 | 27.0 | 390 | 5.0 | 34.0 | 26.0 | 1.8 |
| Chocolate Truffle, Mini, Finest, Tesco* | 1 Cake/28g | 125.0 | 7.0 | 448 | 5.9 | 52.9 | 23.7 | 0.3 |
| Chocolate Truffle, So Good, Somerfield* | 1 Slice/80g | 328.0 | 19.0 | 410 | 6.4 | 44.0 | 23.2 | 1.0 |
| Chocolate with Butter Icing, Average | 1oz/28g | 135.0 | 8.0 | 481 | 5.7 | 50.9 | 29.7 | 0.0 |
| Christmas, Conoisseur, M & S* | 1 Slice/60g | 216.0 | 6.0 | 360 | 4.1 | 64.7 | 9.2 | 3.3 |
| Christmas, Iced, Slices, Tesco* | 1 Slice/45g | 168.0 | 4.0 | 369 | 2.9 | 67.6 | 9.6 | 1.2 |
| Christmas, Rich Fruit, All Iced, Sainsbury's* | 1/16 Cake/85g | 307.0 | 8.0 | 361 | 4.0 | 66.4 | 8.9 | 1.5 |
| Christmas, Rich Fruit, Organic, Tesco* | 1 Serving/76g | 282.0 | 8.0 | 374 | 3.9 | 67.1 | 10.0 | 2.0 |
| Christmas, Rich Fruit, Tesco* | 1 Serving/75g | 256.0 | 6.0 | 342 | 3.9 | 60.3 | 7.4 | 3.1 |
| Christmas, TTD, Sainsbury's* | 1/16 Cake/85g | 315.0 | 8.0 | 371 | 3.7 | 67.1 | 8.9 | 1.3 |
| Christmas Pudding Slices, Mr Kipling* | 1 Slice/51g | 173.0 | 4.0 | 339 | 3.6 | 62.1 | 7.1 | 1.3 |
| Christmas Slices, Mr Kipling* | 1 Slice/52g | 190.0 | 5.0 | 366 | 3.0 | 68.0 | 8.9 | 0.9 |
| Christmas Slices, Weight Watchers* | 1 Slice/40g | 136.0 | 3.0 | 339 | 4.4 | 66.0 | 6.4 | 3.0 |
| Classic Lemon Drizzle, M & S* | 1/6 Cake/68g | 253.0 | 10.0 | 375 | 4.7 | 55.0 | 15.3 | 0.6 |
| Coconut | 1 Slice/70g | 304.0 | 17.0 | 434 | 6.7 | 51.2 | 23.8 | 2.5 |
| Coconut & Raspberry, M & S* | 1 Serving/52g | 231.0 | 14.0 | 445 | 5.0 | 45.5 | 26.8 | 2.3 |
| Coconut Delight, Burton's* | 1 Cake/21g | 89.0 | 4.0 | 424 | 4.0 | 63.0 | 16.9 | 2.0 |
| Coconut Snowball, Bobby's* | 1 Cake/18g | 80.0 | 4.0 | 436 | 2.2 | 57.3 | 22.1 | 0.0 |
| Coconut Sponge, Mini Classics, Mr Kipling* | 1 Cake/38g | 155.0 | 9.0 | 409 | 3.7 | 47.0 | 22.9 | 0.9 |
| Coffee, Entenmann's* | 1 Serving/41g | 159.0 | 7.0 | 388 | 4.0 | 54.7 | 17.3 | 0.6 |
| Coffee, Iced, M & S* | 1 Slice/33g | 135.0 | 6.0 | 410 | 4.4 | 54.5 | 19.6 | 1.6 |
| Coffee & Walnut, Classics, M & S* | 1 Serving/71g | 308.0 | 17.0 | 435 | 4.3 | 50.3 | 24.3 | 1.6 |
| Coffee & Walnut, Mrs Beeton's* | 1 Slice/54g | 219.0 | 13.0 | 405 | 3.7 | 41.4 | 25.0 | 0.3 |
| Coffee & Walnut Slices, HE, Tesco* | 1 Slice/23g | 69.0 | 1.0 | 301 | 4.4 | 65.7 | 2.3 | 2.8 |
| Colin the Caterpillar, M & S* | 1 Slice/60g | 234.0 | 13.0 | 390 | 5.3 | 57.2 | 21.3 | 1.3 |
| Cornflake, Bobby's* | 1/6 Cake/45g | 207.0 | 9.0 | 461 | 3.9 | 65.5 | 20.4 | 0.0 |
| Cornflake, Chocolate Clusters, Asda* | 1 Cake/14g | 64.0 | 3.0 | 460 | 8.2 | 65.2 | 18.5 | 2.7 |

C

# CAKE

| | Measure INFO/WEIGHT | per Measure KCAL | per Measure FAT | Nutrition Values per 100g / 100ml KCAL | PROT | CARB | FAT | FIBRE |
|---|---|---|---|---|---|---|---|---|
| Country Farmhouse, Waitrose* | 1 Serving/80g | 308.0 | 12.0 | 385 | 4.7 | 57.5 | 15.1 | 1.4 |
| Country Slices, Asda* | 1 Serving/27g | 111.0 | 5.0 | 411 | 3.9 | 56.0 | 19.0 | 2.4 |
| Country Slices, Mr Kipling* | 1 Slice/32g | 121.0 | 5.0 | 380 | 4.4 | 56.7 | 15.0 | 1.2 |
| Cream Oysters, M & S* | 1 Cake/72g | 227.0 | 15.0 | 315 | 3.6 | 27.5 | 21.2 | 3.0 |
| Cream Slices, M & S* | 1 Slice/80g | 310.0 | 18.0 | 387 | 2.3 | 45.7 | 22.9 | 0.6 |
| Date & Walnut, Slices, Light Choices, Tesco* | 1 Slice/25g | 70.0 | 1.0 | 280 | 4.9 | 60.1 | 2.2 | 3.6 |
| Date & Walnut, Slices, Weight Watchers* | 1 Slice/27g | 73.0 | 0.0 | 271 | 3.5 | 60.6 | 1.6 | 4.2 |
| Date & Walnut, Trimlyne* | 1 Slice/50g | 134.0 | 2.0 | 269 | 5.7 | 53.8 | 4.9 | 1.8 |
| Date & Walnut Loaf, Sainsbury's* | 1/10 Slice/40g | 148.0 | 8.0 | 371 | 6.7 | 40.1 | 20.4 | 1.0 |
| Date & Walnut Slices, GFY, Asda* | 1 Slice/22g | 62.0 | 0.0 | 281 | 5.0 | 61.8 | 1.5 | 1.8 |
| D'oh Nuts, Asda* | 1 Cake/50g | 186.0 | 9.0 | 372 | 4.0 | 47.0 | 19.0 | 0.0 |
| Double Chocolate Ganache, M & S* | 1/12 Cake/61g | 281.0 | 17.0 | 460 | 5.9 | 46.1 | 27.6 | 2.5 |
| Double Chocolate Wedge, Tesco* | 1 Piece/100g | 416.0 | 20.0 | 416 | 5.0 | 53.4 | 20.3 | 0.9 |
| Dundee, Somerfield* | 1/10 Cake/75g | 254.0 | 8.0 | 339 | 5.0 | 57.0 | 11.0 | 0.0 |
| Eccles | 1 Cake/45g | 214.0 | 12.0 | 475 | 3.9 | 59.3 | 26.4 | 1.6 |
| Eccles, Weight Watchers* | 1 Cake/48g | 190.0 | 8.0 | 396 | 4.4 | 57.5 | 16.5 | 2.0 |
| Fairy, Holly Lane* | 1 Cake/26g | 118.0 | 7.0 | 460 | 3.7 | 52.5 | 26.1 | 3.5 |
| Fairy, Lemon Iced, Tesco* | 1 Cake/24g | 94.0 | 3.0 | 393 | 4.4 | 63.2 | 13.6 | 1.1 |
| Fairy, Mini, Tesco* | 1 Cake/13g | 53.0 | 2.0 | 424 | 6.1 | 54.6 | 20.1 | 1.3 |
| Fairy, SmartPrice, Asda* | 1 Cake/15g | 66.0 | 3.0 | 438 | 6.0 | 54.0 | 22.0 | 1.0 |
| Fairy, Snowman, Christmas, Tesco* | 1 Cake/24g | 114.0 | 7.0 | 471 | 4.6 | 49.8 | 28.1 | 2.9 |
| Fairy, Strawberry Iced, Tesco* | 1 Cake/24g | 94.0 | 3.0 | 392 | 4.9 | 62.9 | 13.4 | 1.4 |
| Fairy, Vanilla Iced, Tesco* | 1 Cake/24g | 93.0 | 3.0 | 388 | 4.4 | 65.1 | 12.2 | 1.2 |
| Figfuls, Go Ahead, McVitie's* | 1 Figful/15g | 56.0 | 1.0 | 365 | 4.2 | 76.8 | 4.6 | 2.9 |
| Flake, Cadbury* | 1 Cake/20g | 90.0 | 5.0 | 445 | 6.3 | 54.5 | 22.3 | 0.0 |
| Fondant Fancies, Lemon, Waitrose* | 1 Cake/40g | 176.0 | 7.0 | 441 | 2.5 | 67.9 | 17.7 | 0.6 |
| Fondant Fancies, Sainsbury's* | 1 Cake/27g | 95.0 | 2.0 | 353 | 2.4 | 65.7 | 9.0 | 0.4 |
| French Fancies, Mr Kipling* | 1 Cake/28g | 103.0 | 3.0 | 369 | 2.8 | 68.3 | 9.4 | 0.6 |
| Fresh Cream Bramley Apple Sponge, Tesco* | 1/6 Slice/43g | 130.0 | 7.0 | 303 | 3.6 | 35.4 | 16.3 | 1.0 |
| Fruit, Parisienne, Rich, Finest, Tesco* | 1 Serving/69g | 262.0 | 10.0 | 380 | 4.7 | 55.2 | 14.1 | 1.9 |
| Fruit, Plain, Average | 1 Slice/90g | 319.0 | 12.0 | 354 | 5.1 | 57.9 | 12.9 | 0.0 |
| Fruit, Rich, Average | 1 Slice/70g | 225.0 | 9.0 | 322 | 4.9 | 50.7 | 12.5 | 1.7 |
| Fruit, Rich, Iced | 1 Slice/70g | 249.0 | 8.0 | 356 | 4.1 | 62.7 | 11.4 | 1.7 |
| Fruit, Rich, M & S* | 1 Serving/50g | 157.0 | 3.0 | 315 | 3.1 | 60.9 | 6.5 | 4.3 |
| Fruit, Rich, Truly Irresistible, Co-Op* | 1/6 Cake/70g | 235.0 | 6.0 | 335 | 3.9 | 59.9 | 8.6 | 2.0 |
| Fruit, Slices, Value, Tesco* | 1 Slice/23g | 84.0 | 4.0 | 372 | 4.0 | 48.7 | 17.7 | 1.3 |
| Fruit & Nut Cluster, Finest, Tesco* | 1 Slice/77g | 262.0 | 10.0 | 338 | 4.5 | 50.1 | 13.3 | 2.7 |
| Fruit Cake with Marzipan & Icing, Asda* | 1/12 Slice/76g | 280.0 | 7.0 | 369 | 3.9 | 68.0 | 9.0 | 0.0 |
| Fudge Brownie, The Handmade Flapjack Company* | 1 Cake/75g | 286.0 | 9.0 | 381 | 4.9 | 62.8 | 12.3 | 0.0 |
| Fudgy Chocolate Slices, COU, M & S* | 1 Slice/36g | 95.0 | 1.0 | 265 | 4.6 | 66.4 | 2.2 | 2.1 |
| Genoa, Tesco* | 1 Serving/50g | 162.0 | 4.0 | 325 | 3.6 | 60.9 | 7.4 | 4.0 |
| Ginger Drizzle, Iced, Co-Op* | 1/6 Cake/65g | 226.0 | 8.0 | 350 | 3.0 | 58.0 | 12.0 | 1.0 |
| Ginger Orange, The Handmade Flapjack Company* | 1 Cake/75g | 289.0 | 15.0 | 385 | 4.3 | 46.3 | 20.3 | 0.0 |
| Glitzy Bag, Birthday, Tesco* | 1 Serving/81g | 314.0 | 7.0 | 388 | 2.1 | 75.9 | 8.5 | 0.6 |
| Happy Birthday, Sainsbury's* | 1 Slice/50g | 207.0 | 8.0 | 414 | 2.8 | 64.5 | 16.1 | 0.6 |
| Holly Hedgehog, Tesco* | 1 Serving/55g | 227.0 | 8.0 | 413 | 2.0 | 69.0 | 14.3 | 0.8 |
| Hot Chocolate Fudge, Sainsbury's* | 1/8 Cake/91g | 343.0 | 16.0 | 376 | 5.1 | 50.3 | 17.1 | 3.5 |
| Iced Madeira, Sainsbury's* | 1/8 Cake/47g | 182.0 | 7.0 | 388 | 3.6 | 61.6 | 14.1 | 0.7 |
| Jamaica Ginger, McVitie's* | 1 Cake/291g | 1048.0 | 31.0 | 360 | 3.5 | 62.2 | 10.8 | 1.4 |
| Jamaica Ginger with Lemon Filling, McVitie's* | 1 Cake/33g | 143.0 | 8.0 | 434 | 4.0 | 48.3 | 25.0 | 0.8 |
| Jammy Strawberry Rolls, Mini, Cadbury* | 1 Cake/29g | 119.0 | 5.0 | 411 | 4.9 | 59.8 | 16.5 | 0.5 |
| Lemon, Half Moon, Bobby's* | 1/6 Cake/60g | 244.0 | 11.0 | 406 | 4.1 | 55.7 | 18.4 | 0.0 |
| Lemon, Mini, Weight Watchers* | 1 Cake/27g | 90.0 | 3.0 | 333 | 3.7 | 66.7 | 11.1 | 11.1 |

C

# CAKE

| INFO/WEIGHT | Measure | per Measure | | Nutrition Values per 100g / 100ml | | | | |
|---|---|---|---|---|---|---|---|---|
| | | KCAL | FAT | KCAL | PROT | CARB | FAT | FIBRE |
| Lemon, The Handmade Flapjack Company* | 1 Cake/75g | 312.0 | 16.0 | 416 | 4.5 | 50.5 | 21.8 | 0.0 |
| Lemon & Orange, Finest, Tesco* | 1 Serving/53g | 216.0 | 11.0 | 410 | 4.5 | 52.4 | 20.3 | 1.1 |
| Lemon Bakewell, Mr Kipling* | 1 Cake/48g | 195.0 | 7.0 | 407 | 2.6 | 65.0 | 15.2 | 0.7 |
| Lemon Buttercream & Lemon Curd, The Cake Shop* | 1 Cake/28g | 124.0 | 8.0 | 444 | 3.5 | 43.4 | 27.8 | 0.6 |
| Lemon Drizzle, M & S* | 1/6 Cake/63g | 230.0 | 9.0 | 365 | 4.2 | 55.8 | 13.9 | 1.4 |
| Lemon Drizzle Cake, Asda* | 1 Serving/50g | 149.0 | 6.0 | 299 | 2.8 | 45.0 | 12.0 | 0.4 |
| Lemon Drizzle Slices, Light Choices, Tesco* | 1 Slice/23g | 67.0 | 0.0 | 290 | 4.8 | 62.7 | 2.0 | 2.8 |
| Lemon Slices, BGTY, Sainsbury's* | 1 Slice/26g | 84.0 | 0.0 | 323 | 3.7 | 74.0 | 1.4 | 1.3 |
| Lemon Slices, Eat Smart, Morrisons* | 1 Slice/26g | 81.0 | 1.0 | 312 | 3.8 | 68.1 | 2.7 | 1.9 |
| Lemon Slices, Low Fat, Weight Watchers* | 1 Slice/26g | 79.0 | 1.0 | 303 | 3.1 | 68.1 | 2.0 | 2.2 |
| Lemon Slices, Mr Kipling* | 1 Slice/29g | 120.0 | 5.0 | 413 | 4.2 | 61.9 | 16.6 | 0.7 |
| Lemon Smoothie Bake, Go Ahead, McVitie's* | 1 Bar/35g | 130.0 | 3.0 | 372 | 3.0 | 75.1 | 8.1 | 1.0 |
| Lemon Tartlette, Go Ahead, McVitie's* | 1 Cake/45g | 161.0 | 4.0 | 357 | 3.7 | 67.9 | 9.5 | 1.1 |
| Leo the Lion, Birthday, Asda* | 1 Slice/81g | 325.0 | 13.0 | 402 | 2.6 | 62.0 | 16.0 | 0.5 |
| Madeira | 1 Slice/40g | 157.0 | 7.0 | 393 | 5.4 | 58.4 | 16.9 | 0.9 |
| Madeira, All Butter, Sainsbury's* | 1 Serving/30g | 116.0 | 6.0 | 388 | 5.2 | 47.4 | 19.7 | 0.8 |
| Madeira, Iced, Tesco* | 1/16 Cake/56g | 218.0 | 7.0 | 389 | 2.6 | 67.2 | 12.2 | 0.4 |
| Madeira, Tesco* | 1 Serving/50g | 197.0 | 8.0 | 394 | 5.5 | 57.9 | 15.6 | 1.2 |
| Magic Roundabout, Dougal, Tesco* | 1 Serving/50g | 214.0 | 8.0 | 428 | 2.3 | 68.7 | 16.0 | 0.2 |
| Manor House, Mr Kipling* | 1 Serving/69g | 277.0 | 14.0 | 400 | 5.3 | 49.7 | 20.0 | 1.4 |
| Marble, Tesco* | 1/8 Cake/45g | 184.0 | 8.0 | 410 | 4.4 | 55.9 | 18.7 | 1.5 |
| Mini Rolls, Cadbury* | 1 Roll/27g | 120.0 | 6.0 | 445 | 4.4 | 56.4 | 22.5 | 1.3 |
| Mini Rolls, Chocolate, Tesco* | 1 Roll/29g | 135.0 | 7.0 | 465 | 5.5 | 58.1 | 23.1 | 1.3 |
| Mini Rolls, Juicy Orange, Cadbury* | 1 Cake/28g | 110.0 | 5.0 | 390 | 5.0 | 55.0 | 16.8 | 0.0 |
| Mini Rolls, Milk Chocolate Orange, Shapers, Boots* | 1 Roll/25g | 97.0 | 3.0 | 386 | 4.6 | 64.0 | 12.0 | 2.4 |
| Orange & Cranberry, Mini Classics, Mr Kipling* | 1 Cake/36g | 164.0 | 7.0 | 455 | 4.5 | 42.2 | 20.2 | 0.7 |
| Orange & Ginger, Oat Break, Go Ahead, McVitie's* | 1 Cake/35g | 121.0 | 2.0 | 347 | 5.2 | 67.1 | 6.4 | 2.6 |
| Orange Marmalade, M & S* | 1 Slice/50g | 195.0 | 9.0 | 390 | 3.6 | 53.2 | 18.3 | 1.8 |
| Panettone, Bauli* | 1 Serving/75g | 313.0 | 15.0 | 418 | 5.9 | 53.5 | 20.1 | 0.0 |
| Panettone, M & S* | 1/8 Loaf/51g | 184.0 | 7.0 | 360 | 6.5 | 53.4 | 13.2 | 2.0 |
| Party, Asda* | 1 Serving/57g | 238.0 | 9.0 | 421 | 2.3 | 67.0 | 16.0 | 0.4 |
| Party Bake, M & S* | 1/15 Cake/60g | 230.0 | 12.0 | 385 | 4.0 | 46.6 | 20.2 | 0.9 |
| Piece of Cake, Birthday, M & S* | 1 Serving/85g | 395.0 | 24.0 | 465 | 4.3 | 39.7 | 28.7 | 0.9 |
| Raisin, Sainsbury's* | 1 Cake/40g | 161.0 | 8.0 | 403 | 4.7 | 53.5 | 18.9 | 3.0 |
| Raisin, Tesco* | 1 Cake/38g | 158.0 | 8.0 | 417 | 5.6 | 53.8 | 19.9 | 1.4 |
| Rich Choc' Roll, Cadbury* | 1/6 Portion/39g | 149.0 | 6.0 | 381 | 4.8 | 50.2 | 15.6 | 1.0 |
| Rich Chocolate, Christmas, Tesco* | 1 Slice/82g | 300.0 | 13.0 | 367 | 7.0 | 47.5 | 16.5 | 1.6 |
| Rich Fruit Slices, Free From, Sainsbury's* | 1 Slice/40g | 144.0 | 5.0 | 361 | 4.5 | 57.4 | 12.6 | 3.7 |
| Rock | 1 Sm Cake/40g | 158.0 | 7.0 | 396 | 5.4 | 60.5 | 16.4 | 1.5 |
| Rock, Tesco* | 1 Serving/87g | 311.0 | 8.0 | 357 | 7.4 | 60.1 | 9.7 | 1.6 |
| Seriously Chocolatey, Large, Sainsbury's* | 1/24 Cake/77g | 352.0 | 19.0 | 457 | 5.4 | 51.0 | 25.3 | 3.0 |
| Seriously Chocolatey Celebration, Sainsbury's* | 1/8 Cake/77g | 336.0 | 20.0 | 437 | 6.3 | 45.0 | 25.7 | 0.3 |
| Shrek Birthday, Tesco* | 1/16 Cake/72g | 248.0 | 9.0 | 344 | 3.3 | 64.0 | 12.2 | 0.5 |
| Slices, Belgian Chocolate, Weight Watchers* | 1 Slice/30g | 99.0 | 2.0 | 329 | 5.9 | 61.3 | 6.7 | 2.3 |
| Slices, Carrot & Orange, Light Choices, Tesco* | 1 Slice/30g | 93.0 | 1.0 | 310 | 3.2 | 68.5 | 2.2 | 1.9 |
| Snowballs, Sainsbury's* | 1 Snowball/18g | 80.0 | 4.0 | 445 | 2.5 | 55.6 | 23.0 | 3.6 |
| Snowballs, Tesco* | 1 Snowball/18g | 79.0 | 4.0 | 432 | 2.5 | 55.8 | 22.1 | 5.4 |
| Sponge | 1 Slice/53g | 243.0 | 14.0 | 459 | 6.4 | 52.4 | 26.3 | 0.9 |
| Sponge, Fatless | 1 Slice/53g | 156.0 | 3.0 | 294 | 10.1 | 53.0 | 6.1 | 0.9 |
| Sponge, Fresh Cream & Strawberry, Asda* | 1/12 Cake/60g | 170.0 | 6.0 | 284 | 4.6 | 44.0 | 10.0 | 1.1 |
| Sponge, Jam Filled | 1 Slice/65g | 196.0 | 3.0 | 302 | 4.2 | 64.2 | 4.9 | 1.8 |
| Sponge Roll, Chocolate, M & S* | ¼ Cake/66g | 251.0 | 12.0 | 380 | 3.9 | 50.5 | 18.4 | 1.8 |
| Sponge Roll, Coffee, M & S* | 1 Serving/40g | 150.0 | 7.0 | 375 | 3.5 | 51.1 | 17.3 | 0.6 |

# CAKE

| | Measure INFO/WEIGHT | per Measure KCAL | FAT | Nutrition Values per 100g / 100ml KCAL | PROT | CARB | FAT | FIBRE |
|---|---|---|---|---|---|---|---|---|
| Sponge with Butter Icing | 1 Slice/65g | 318.0 | 20.0 | 490 | 4.5 | 52.4 | 30.6 | 0.6 |
| Spooky, Birthday, Memory Lane Cakes* | 1 Slice/75g | 295.0 | 15.0 | 393 | 3.5 | 50.8 | 19.5 | 0.7 |
| St. Clements, Finest, Tesco* | 1 Serving/49g | 194.0 | 11.0 | 395 | 3.1 | 47.2 | 21.5 | 0.4 |
| Stem Ginger, 96% Fat Free, Trimlyne* | ¼ Cake/63g | 170.0 | 2.0 | 272 | 4.4 | 58.1 | 3.6 | 1.2 |
| Sticky Toffee Slices, Eat Smart, Safeway* | 1 Cake/85g | 259.0 | 2.0 | 305 | 3.6 | 65.8 | 2.7 | 1.3 |
| Strawberry Sponge Roll, M & S* | 1/6 Cake/49g | 160.0 | 5.0 | 330 | 2.8 | 58.0 | 9.5 | 0.8 |
| Sultana, Apple & Cranberry, 99% Fat Free, Trimlyne* | 1/6 Cake/67g | 130.0 | 1.0 | 195 | 4.6 | 45.5 | 0.9 | 3.3 |
| Sultana, Fair Trade, Co-Op* | 1/8 Cake/45g | 155.0 | 4.0 | 345 | 5.0 | 60.0 | 9.0 | 1.0 |
| Sultana & Cherry, Tesco* | 1 Cake/37g | 124.0 | 4.0 | 334 | 4.7 | 54.4 | 10.8 | 2.5 |
| Summer Fruit Cream, GFY, Asda* | 1 Serving/74g | 165.0 | 4.0 | 223 | 3.6 | 41.0 | 4.9 | 2.5 |
| Swiss Roll, Average | 1oz/28g | 77.0 | 1.0 | 276 | 7.2 | 55.5 | 4.4 | 0.8 |
| Swiss Roll, Chocolate, Jumbo, Safeway* | 1/12 Roll/35g | 129.0 | 6.0 | 369 | 4.1 | 47.1 | 18.2 | 0.9 |
| Swiss Roll, Chocolate, Lyons* | 1 Serving/50g | 189.0 | 10.0 | 379 | 4.3 | 47.0 | 19.3 | 0.9 |
| Swiss Roll, Chocolate, M & S* | 1 Serving/46g | 168.0 | 11.0 | 365 | 4.6 | 32.6 | 24.2 | 1.2 |
| Swiss Roll, Chocolate, Mini, Tesco* | 1 Roll/22g | 87.0 | 3.0 | 396 | 4.6 | 61.0 | 14.8 | 0.0 |
| Swiss Roll, Chocolate, Somerfield* | ¼ Roll/44g | 167.0 | 7.0 | 384 | 6.0 | 55.0 | 16.0 | 0.0 |
| Swiss Roll, Chocolate, Value, Tesco* | 1 Serving/20g | 81.0 | 4.0 | 404 | 5.0 | 54.1 | 18.7 | 2.1 |
| Swiss Roll, Raspberry, Lyons* | 1 Roll/175g | 485.0 | 2.0 | 277 | 5.2 | 60.6 | 1.4 | 0.0 |
| Swiss Roll, Raspberry, Sainsbury's* | 1 Serving/35g | 105.0 | 1.0 | 301 | 3.5 | 67.0 | 2.1 | 1.1 |
| Swiss Roll, Raspberry, Somerfield* | 1 Roll/80g | 245.0 | 2.0 | 306 | 5.0 | 66.0 | 3.0 | 0.0 |
| Swiss Roll, Raspberry, Tesco* | 1 Serving/45g | 132.0 | 1.0 | 294 | 3.2 | 65.4 | 2.1 | 1.0 |
| Swiss Roll, Raspberry & Vanilla, Morrisons* | 1 Serving/28g | 98.0 | 3.0 | 350 | 4.2 | 61.8 | 9.5 | 0.0 |
| Swiss Roll, Raspberry Jam, Mr Kipling* | 1/6 Cake/52g | 184.0 | 5.0 | 355 | 2.8 | 63.0 | 10.2 | 1.0 |
| Syrup & Ginger, Tesco* | 1 Serving/32g | 134.0 | 7.0 | 420 | 4.5 | 51.4 | 21.8 | 0.7 |
| Tangy Lemon Trickle, M & S* | 1 Slice/75g | 281.0 | 14.0 | 375 | 4.7 | 47.4 | 18.8 | 1.1 |
| Toffee, Iced, Tesco* | 1 Serving/35g | 132.0 | 5.0 | 376 | 3.3 | 57.2 | 14.9 | 1.6 |
| Toffee, Slices, BGTY, Sainsbury's* | 1 Slice/27g | 88.0 | 1.0 | 327 | 4.3 | 71.7 | 2.5 | 1.8 |
| Toffee, Slices, HL, Tesco* | 1 Cake/24g | 76.0 | 1.0 | 315 | 4.5 | 65.0 | 2.6 | 1.6 |
| Toffee, Slices, Value, Tesco* | 1 Slice/14g | 62.0 | 3.0 | 440 | 4.2 | 54.9 | 22.6 | 0.6 |
| Toffee, Thorntons* | 1/6 Cake/70g | 302.0 | 17.0 | 431 | 4.6 | 49.2 | 24.0 | 0.8 |
| Toffee & Pecan Slices, M & S* | 1 Slice/36g | 160.0 | 9.0 | 445 | 4.7 | 54.0 | 23.7 | 1.3 |
| Toffee Bakewell, Tesco* | 1 Cake/49g | 203.0 | 8.0 | 414 | 3.9 | 63.5 | 16.1 | 1.4 |
| Toffee Flavour Slices, Low Fat, Weight Watchers* | 1 Slice/27g | 80.0 | 1.0 | 297 | 4.2 | 63.9 | 2.6 | 3.2 |
| Toffee Temptation, Finest, Tesco* | 1 Serving/50g | 211.0 | 12.0 | 423 | 4.7 | 49.0 | 23.1 | 0.6 |
| Triple Chocolate, TTD, Sainsbury's* | 1/8 Cake/52g | 214.0 | 13.0 | 412 | 4.7 | 42.6 | 24.7 | 0.5 |
| Vanilla Sponge, Fresh Cream, Sainsbury's* | 1 Slice/50g | 152.0 | 5.0 | 304 | 7.5 | 45.6 | 10.2 | 0.4 |
| Victoria Sandwich, Classic, Large, M & S* | 1/10 Cake/66g | 260.0 | 13.0 | 395 | 5.1 | 49.5 | 19.6 | 2.3 |
| Victoria Slices, Mr Kipling* | 1 Slice/28g | 122.0 | 4.0 | 432 | 3.9 | 68.8 | 15.7 | 0.4 |
| Victoria Sponge, Fresh Cream, Value, Tesco* | 1 Serving/50g | 168.0 | 9.0 | 337 | 4.4 | 40.7 | 17.4 | 0.6 |
| Victoria Sponge, Lemon, Co-Op* | 1 Slice/42g | 151.0 | 8.0 | 360 | 4.0 | 44.0 | 19.0 | 0.7 |
| Victoria Sponge, Mini, Mr Kipling* | 1 Cake/36g | 152.0 | 7.0 | 420 | 3.9 | 58.5 | 19.0 | 0.8 |
| Victoria Sponge, Mini, Weight Watchers* | 1 Cake/26g | 92.0 | 2.0 | 354 | 5.7 | 64.1 | 8.3 | 1.5 |
| Victoria Sponge, TTD, Sainsbury's* | 1 Serving/69g | 255.0 | 11.0 | 370 | 4.3 | 51.4 | 16.4 | 1.0 |
| Viennese, M & S* | 1 Cake/51g | 250.0 | 14.0 | 495 | 4.1 | 58.9 | 28.0 | 2.8 |
| Viennese Whirl, Lemon, Mr Kipling* | 1 Cake/28g | 115.0 | 4.0 | 409 | 4.2 | 62.2 | 15.9 | 0.7 |
| Viennese Whirl, Mr Kipling* | 1 Cake/28g | 142.0 | 9.0 | 507 | 4.1 | 53.9 | 30.5 | 1.3 |
| Viennese Whirl, Tesco* | 1 Cake/39g | 181.0 | 10.0 | 465 | 4.0 | 53.2 | 26.2 | 1.2 |
| Walnut, Sandwich, Sainsbury's* | 1/8 Cake/48g | 182.0 | 8.0 | 379 | 5.4 | 53.7 | 17.3 | 1.3 |
| Walnut & Coffee, Co-Op* | ¼ Cake/65g | 253.0 | 13.0 | 390 | 5.0 | 47.0 | 20.0 | 0.7 |
| Walnut & Coffee, TTD, Sainsbury's* | 1 Slice/68g | 269.0 | 15.0 | 396 | 4.4 | 45.9 | 21.6 | 0.7 |
| Walnut Layer, Somerfield* | ¼ Cake/78g | 295.0 | 15.0 | 381 | 6.0 | 45.0 | 20.0 | 0.0 |
| Welsh, Average | 1oz/28g | 121.0 | 5.0 | 431 | 5.6 | 61.8 | 19.6 | 1.5 |
| Xmas Pudding, Tesco* | 1 Cake/17g | 58.0 | 2.0 | 349 | 3.3 | 60.5 | 9.3 | 1.4 |

C

| | Measure INFO/WEIGHT | per Measure KCAL | FAT | Nutrition Values per 100g / 100ml KCAL | PROT | CARB | FAT | FIBRE |
|---|---|---|---|---|---|---|---|---|
| **CAKE MIX** | | | | | | | | |
| Carrot Cake, Betty Crocker* | ¼ Pack/125g | 504.0 | 8.0 | 403 | 5.8 | 78.9 | 6.7 | 1.4 |
| Cheesecake, Original, Made Up, Asda* | 1/6 Cake/85g | 228.0 | 10.0 | 268 | 4.1 | 36.0 | 12.0 | 1.4 |
| Cheesecake, Strawberry, Real, Green's* | 1 Serving/100g | 254.0 | 13.0 | 253 | 3.9 | 30.6 | 12.8 | 0.6 |
| Cheesecake, Tesco* | 1 Serving/76g | 199.0 | 8.0 | 262 | 4.1 | 38.0 | 10.4 | 1.6 |
| Chocolate Brownie, Chocolate Chips, Weight Watchers* | 1 Pack/190g | 568.0 | 13.0 | 299 | 3.2 | 55.6 | 7.1 | 2.1 |
| Christmas, Mini, Jane Asher* | 1oz/28g | 104.0 | 3.0 | 372 | 5.2 | 65.8 | 12.0 | 1.3 |
| Dennis, Green's* | 1 Cake/17g | 55.0 | 1.0 | 319 | 4.6 | 57.8 | 7.7 | 0.0 |
| Free From, Sainsbury's* | 1 Serving/50g | 173.0 | 0.0 | 346 | 1.3 | 84.4 | 0.3 | 2.2 |
| Yellow, Super Moist, Betty Crocker* | 1 Cake/128g | 517.0 | 9.0 | 404 | 3.3 | 81.6 | 7.4 | 1.1 |
| **CALZONE** | | | | | | | | |
| Bolognese, Weight Watchers* | 1 Calzone/88g | 178.0 | 3.0 | 202 | 11.7 | 31.2 | 3.4 | 4.3 |
| Cheese & Tomato, Weight Watchers* | 1 Calzone/88g | 191.0 | 4.0 | 217 | 11.3 | 33.4 | 4.3 | 3.4 |
| Ham & Gruyere, Asda* | 1 Serving/280g | 661.0 | 22.0 | 236 | 10.0 | 31.0 | 8.0 | 2.7 |
| **CANAPES** | | | | | | | | |
| Aegean Tomato, Finest, Tesco* | 1 Canape/15g | 45.0 | 2.0 | 300 | 7.2 | 34.3 | 14.7 | 2.1 |
| Caponata, Puff Pastry, Occasions, Sainsbury's* | 1 Square/12g | 30.0 | 2.0 | 249 | 4.1 | 22.9 | 15.7 | 2.1 |
| Salmon & Dill, Finest, Tesco* | 1 Canape/15g | 47.0 | 2.0 | 315 | 9.2 | 32.7 | 16.1 | 1.9 |
| Smoked Salmon, Youngs* | 1 Canape/10g | 21.0 | 2.0 | 210 | 15.9 | 2.0 | 15.2 | 0.7 |
| **CANNELLONI** | | | | | | | | |
| Beef, BGTY, Sainsbury's* | 1 Pack/300g | 249.0 | 7.0 | 83 | 5.5 | 10.1 | 2.3 | 1.7 |
| Beef, Finest, Tesco* | ½ Pack/300g | 399.0 | 22.0 | 133 | 7.1 | 9.4 | 7.4 | 1.9 |
| Beef, Great Value, Asda* | 1 Pack/400g | 384.0 | 11.0 | 96 | 6.0 | 12.0 | 2.7 | 1.6 |
| Beef, HL, Tesco* | 1 Pack/340g | 323.0 | 8.0 | 95 | 6.4 | 11.9 | 2.4 | 1.5 |
| Beef, Italian, Sainsbury's* | 1 Pack/400g | 498.0 | 26.0 | 124 | 5.9 | 10.5 | 6.5 | 1.6 |
| Beef, Italian, Tesco* | 1 Pack/400g | 520.0 | 27.0 | 130 | 5.3 | 11.6 | 6.7 | 0.9 |
| Beef, Sainsbury's* | 1 Pack/400g | 372.0 | 18.0 | 93 | 4.4 | 8.8 | 4.4 | 1.6 |
| Beef & Red Wine, Waitrose* | ½ Pack/170g | 355.0 | 16.0 | 209 | 17.5 | 13.8 | 9.4 | 1.0 |
| Chicken & Pesto, Italian, Sainsbury's* | 1 Pack/450g | 675.0 | 34.0 | 150 | 6.1 | 14.4 | 7.5 | 1.1 |
| Mediterranean Vegetable, Waitrose* | 1 Serving/170g | 330.0 | 15.0 | 194 | 9.7 | 18.7 | 9.0 | 1.9 |
| Mushroom, Italian, Sainsbury's* | 1 Pack/450g | 598.0 | 31.0 | 133 | 5.2 | 12.5 | 6.9 | 0.5 |
| Parmesan & Basil, M & S* | 1 Pack/360g | 504.0 | 28.0 | 140 | 5.9 | 11.4 | 7.9 | 0.8 |
| Pork, M & S* | 1 Pack/400g | 460.0 | 25.0 | 115 | 6.2 | 8.7 | 6.2 | 1.1 |
| Ricotta & Spinach, COU, M & S* | 1 Pack/400g | 320.0 | 8.0 | 80 | 5.3 | 9.7 | 2.0 | 2.8 |
| Ricotta & Spinach, Eat Smart, Morrisons* | 1 Pack/400g | 328.0 | 8.0 | 82 | 5.2 | 10.9 | 2.0 | 1.6 |
| Ricotta & Spinach, Fresh, Waitrose* | ½ Pack/225g | 274.0 | 16.0 | 122 | 5.1 | 8.8 | 7.3 | 1.2 |
| Roasted Vegetable, Morrisons* | 1 Serving/350g | 311.0 | 9.0 | 89 | 3.9 | 12.5 | 2.5 | 2.3 |
| Smoked Salmon & Spinach, Sainsbury's* | 1 Pack/450g | 598.0 | 28.0 | 133 | 5.7 | 13.5 | 6.2 | 0.4 |
| Spinach & Ricotta, BGTY, Sainsbury's* | 1 Pack/300g | 246.0 | 7.0 | 82 | 4.7 | 10.7 | 2.3 | 3.8 |
| Spinach & Ricotta, Finest, Tesco* | 1 Serving/120g | 247.0 | 16.0 | 206 | 8.1 | 13.9 | 13.1 | 2.6 |
| Spinach & Ricotta, Frozen, Sainsbury's* | 1 Pack/350g | 513.0 | 26.0 | 147 | 6.1 | 13.9 | 7.4 | 1.1 |
| Spinach & Ricotta, Good Intentions, Somerfield* | 1 Serving/400g | 366.0 | 10.0 | 91 | 5.3 | 12.2 | 2.4 | 2.1 |
| Spinach & Ricotta, HL, Tesco* | 1 Pack/400g | 320.0 | 11.0 | 80 | 4.0 | 10.0 | 2.8 | 1.1 |
| Spinach & Ricotta, Italian, Sainsbury's* | ¼ Pack/400g | 476.0 | 30.0 | 119 | 4.8 | 8.1 | 7.5 | 1.7 |
| Spinach & Ricotta, Italian Style, Co-Op* | 1 Pack/450g | 540.0 | 27.0 | 120 | 5.0 | 12.0 | 6.0 | 2.0 |
| Spinach & Ricotta, Light Choices, Tesco* | 1 Pack/400g | 340.0 | 11.0 | 85 | 4.0 | 10.0 | 2.8 | 1.1 |
| Spinach & Ricotta, Ross* | 1 Pack/300g | 288.0 | 9.0 | 96 | 3.9 | 13.2 | 3.1 | 1.6 |
| Spinach & Ricotta, Weight Watchers* | 1 Pack/400g | 284.0 | 6.0 | 71 | 3.1 | 10.9 | 1.6 | 1.1 |
| Spinach & Wild Mushroom, Linda McCartney* | 1 Pack/340g | 381.0 | 14.0 | 112 | 4.9 | 14.1 | 4.0 | 1.7 |
| *Tubes, Dry, Average* | *1oz/28g* | *101.0* | *1.0* | *361* | *12.5* | *69.1* | *3.6* | *1.2* |
| **CAPERS** | | | | | | | | |
| Caperberries, Spanish, Waitrose* | 1 Serving/55g | 9.0 | 0.0 | 17 | 1.1 | 2.1 | 0.5 | 2.5 |
| Capucines, Sainsbury's* | 1 Tsp/6g | 1.0 | 0.0 | 14 | 1.4 | 1.3 | 0.3 | 2.2 |
| in Brine, Tesco* | 1 Tsp/2g | 1.0 | 0.0 | 29 | 2.4 | 3.5 | 0.6 | 2.7 |

| | Measure INFO/WEIGHT | per Measure KCAL | FAT | Nutrition Values per 100g / 100ml KCAL | PROT | CARB | FAT | FIBRE |
|---|---|---|---|---|---|---|---|---|
| **CAPPELLETTI** | | | | | | | | |
| Goats Cheese & Red Pesto, Waitrose* | ½ Pack/125g | 374.0 | 11.0 | 299 | 11.6 | 43.5 | 8.7 | 2.2 |
| Meat, Italian, Somerfield* | ½ Pack/125g | 331.0 | 8.0 | 265 | 13.6 | 38.5 | 6.3 | 2.4 |
| Parma Ham, Fresh, Waitrose* | ½ Pack/125g | 367.0 | 11.0 | 294 | 14.1 | 38.6 | 9.2 | 2.2 |
| **CAPRI SUN** | | | | | | | | |
| Orange | 1 Pouch/200ml | 90.0 | 0.0 | 45 | 0.0 | 11.0 | 0.0 | 0.0 |
| Orange, 100%, Juice | 1 Pouch/200ml | 75.0 | 0.0 | 38 | 0.5 | 9.2 | 0.0 | 0.1 |
| **CARAMAC** | | | | | | | | |
| Nestle* | 1 Bar/30g | 169.0 | 11.0 | 563 | 5.8 | 54.4 | 35.8 | 0.0 |
| **CARAMBOLA** | | | | | | | | |
| *Average* | *1oz/28g* | *9.0* | *0.0* | *32* | *0.5* | *7.3* | *0.3* | *1.3* |
| **CARAWAY** | | | | | | | | |
| Seeds, Schwartz* | 1 Pack/38g | 170.0 | 8.0 | 448 | 23.3 | 40.9 | 21.2 | 0.0 |
| **CARDAMOM** | | | | | | | | |
| *Black, Ground, Average* | *1 Tsp/2g* | *6.0* | *0.0* | *311* | *10.8* | *68.5* | *6.7* | *28.0* |
| *Ground, Average* | *1 Tsp/2g* | *6.0* | *0.0* | *314* | *10.7* | *53.6* | *7.1* | *28.6* |
| **CAROB POWDER** | | | | | | | | |
| *Average* | *1 Tsp/2g* | *3.0* | *0.0* | *159* | *4.9* | *37.0* | *0.1* | *0.0* |
| **CARROTS** | | | | | | | | |
| & Cauliflower, M & S* | 1 Serving/335g | 74.0 | 1.0 | 22 | 0.6 | 4.4 | 0.4 | 2.3 |
| & Peas, Sainsbury's* | 1 Serving/200g | 100.0 | 1.0 | 50 | 3.3 | 8.3 | 0.5 | 3.8 |
| *Baby, Canned, Average* | *1 Can/195g* | *40.0* | *1.0* | *21* | *0.5* | *4.2* | *0.3* | *2.1* |
| *Baby, Fresh, Average* | *1 Serving/80g* | *28.0* | *1.0* | *35* | *0.6* | *8.2* | *0.1* | *2.9* |
| Baby, with Fine Beans, Tesco* | 1 Pack/200g | 58.0 | 1.0 | 29 | 1.3 | 4.7 | 0.5 | 2.3 |
| Baby Corn, & Mange Tout, Safeway* | 1 Pack/200g | 48.0 | 1.0 | 24 | 2.1 | 3.2 | 0.3 | 0.0 |
| Batons, & Sliced Runner Beans, Sainsbury's* | 1 Serving/200g | 40.0 | 1.0 | 20 | 1.0 | 3.2 | 0.5 | 3.2 |
| Batons, Broccoli & Cauliflower, Freshly Frozen, Asda* | 1 Bag/156g | 39.0 | 1.0 | 25 | 1.9 | 2.9 | 0.6 | 2.4 |
| Batons, Broccoli Florets & Sweetcorn, Frozen, Asda* | 1 Bag/160g | 82.0 | 2.0 | 51 | 2.4 | 7.8 | 1.1 | 2.7 |
| *Batons, Fresh, Average* | *½ Pack/150g* | *41.0* | *0.0* | *27* | *0.6* | *5.7* | *0.3* | *2.6* |
| *Boiled, Average* | *1oz/28g* | *6.0* | *0.0* | *22* | *0.6* | *4.4* | *0.4* | *2.3* |
| *Canned, Average* | *1oz/28g* | *6.0* | *0.0* | *22* | *0.6* | *4.4* | *0.2* | *2.1* |
| Chantenay, Steamer, Sainsbury's* | ½ Pack/125g | 60.0 | 2.0 | 48 | 0.5 | 7.7 | 1.7 | 2.2 |
| Chantenay, Tesco* | 1oz/28g | 7.0 | 0.0 | 24 | 0.6 | 4.4 | 0.4 | 2.3 |
| Crunchies, Shapers, Boots* | 1 Bag/80g | 28.0 | 0.0 | 35 | 0.6 | 7.5 | 0.3 | 3.0 |
| Dippers, Sainsbury's* | 1 Pot/130g | 182.0 | 16.0 | 140 | 0.9 | 5.7 | 12.5 | 2.2 |
| *Sliced, Canned, Average* | *1 Serving/180g* | *36.0* | *0.0* | *20* | *0.7* | *4.1* | *0.1* | *1.5* |
| *Sliced, Fresh, Average* | *1 Serving/60g* | *17.0* | *0.0* | *28* | *0.7* | *5.7* | *0.3* | *2.0* |
| Sweetcorn & Broccoli, Steam & Serve, Morrisons* | 1 Pack/120g | 54.0 | 1.0 | 45 | 2.3 | 8.9 | 1.1 | 2.6 |
| *Whole, Raw, Peeled, Average* | *1 Carrot/75g* | *21.0* | *0.0* | *29* | *0.6* | *6.3* | *0.3* | *2.2* |
| with Parsley & English Butter, M & S* | ½ Pack/100g | 65.0 | 4.0 | 65 | 0.6 | 7.1 | 3.9 | 2.4 |
| **CASHEW NUTS** | | | | | | | | |
| *Plain, Average* | *¼ Pack/25g* | *146.0* | *12.0* | *584* | *15.7* | *18.7* | *48.9* | *3.4* |
| *Roasted & Salted, Average* | *1 Serving/50g* | *306.0* | *26.0* | *612* | *18.8* | *19.5* | *51.1* | *3.1* |
| **CASHEWS & PEANUTS** | | | | | | | | |
| *Honey Roasted, Average* | *1 Serving/50g* | *289.0* | *21.0* | *579* | *21.6* | *26.6* | *42.9* | *4.2* |
| Salted, Sainsbury's* | 1oz/28g | 169.0 | 14.0 | 603 | 24.2 | 12.7 | 50.6 | 6.9 |
| **CASSAVA** | | | | | | | | |
| *Baked, Average* | *1oz/28g* | *43.0* | *0.0* | *155* | *0.7* | *40.1* | *0.2* | *1.7* |
| *Boiled in Unsalted Water, Average* | *1oz/28g* | *36.0* | *0.0* | *130* | *0.5* | *33.5* | *0.2* | *1.4* |
| *Gari, Average* | *1oz/28g* | *100.0* | *0.0* | *358* | *1.3* | *92.9* | *0.5* | *0.0* |
| *Raw, Average* | *1oz/28g* | *40.0* | *0.0* | *142* | *0.6* | *36.8* | *0.2* | *1.6* |
| *Steamed, Average* | *1oz/28g* | *40.0* | *0.0* | *142* | *0.6* | *36.8* | *0.2* | *1.6* |
| **CASSEROLE** | | | | | | | | |
| Bean, & Lentil, Morrisons* | 1 Can/410g | 287.0 | 2.0 | 70 | 4.1 | 12.5 | 0.4 | 0.0 |

**C**

# CASSEROLE

| | Measure INFO/WEIGHT | per Measure KCAL | FAT | Nutrition Values per 100g / 100ml KCAL | PROT | CARB | FAT | FIBRE |
|---|---|---|---|---|---|---|---|---|
| Bean, Spicy, BGTY, Sainsbury's* | 1 Pack/300g | 171.0 | 3.0 | 57 | 3.0 | 9.1 | 0.9 | 4.2 |
| Beef, & Ale, Finest, Tesco* | ½ Pack/300g | 234.0 | 4.0 | 78 | 11.5 | 5.0 | 1.4 | 1.1 |
| Beef, & Ale, with Dumplings, Sainsbury's* | 1 Pack/450g | 711.0 | 33.0 | 158 | 7.7 | 15.4 | 7.3 | 0.6 |
| Beef, & Ale, with Mashed Potato, HL, Tesco* | 1 Pack/450g | 364.0 | 11.0 | 81 | 5.1 | 10.9 | 2.5 | 0.6 |
| Beef, & Onion, Minced, British Classics, Tesco* | 1 Pack/340g | 367.0 | 19.0 | 108 | 5.0 | 9.3 | 5.6 | 0.8 |
| Beef, & Red Wine, BGTY, Sainsbury's* | 1 Pack/300g | 192.0 | 2.0 | 64 | 8.0 | 6.7 | 0.6 | 0.9 |
| Beef, Canned, Waitrose* | 1 Can/400g | 372.0 | 10.0 | 93 | 10.5 | 7.0 | 2.5 | 1.8 |
| Beef, Fellside, Look What We Found* | 1 Pouch/300g | 219.0 | 5.0 | 73 | 9.1 | 5.3 | 1.7 | 2.1 |
| Beef, Meal for One, Tesco* | 1 Pack/450g | 425.0 | 19.0 | 94 | 3.6 | 10.6 | 4.2 | 1.7 |
| Beef, Mini Favourites, M & S* | 1 Pack/200g | 210.0 | 8.0 | 105 | 7.1 | 9.3 | 4.2 | 1.4 |
| Beef, with Dumplings, Eat Smart, Safeway* | 1 Pack/391g | 215.0 | 7.0 | 55 | 1.6 | 7.3 | 1.9 | 1.2 |
| Beef, with Dumplings, GFY, Asda* | 1 Pack/400g | 416.0 | 9.0 | 104 | 11.0 | 10.0 | 2.2 | 0.9 |
| Beef & Melton Red Ale, Roast Potatoes, Weight Watchers* | 1 Pack/450g | 425.0 | 9.0 | 94 | 6.5 | 12.6 | 2.0 | 1.8 |
| Beef & Red Wine, Weight Watchers* | 1 Pack/330g | 254.0 | 9.0 | 77 | 4.3 | 8.6 | 2.8 | 0.3 |
| Chicken, & Asparagus, in White Wine, Finest, Tesco* | 1 Pack/350g | 683.0 | 42.0 | 195 | 10.0 | 11.6 | 12.1 | 0.3 |
| Chicken, & Asparagus in White Wine, Tesco* | ½ Pack/300g | 444.0 | 24.0 | 148 | 11.5 | 7.7 | 7.9 | 0.8 |
| Chicken, & Dumplings, HL, Tesco* | 1 Pack/450g | 441.0 | 12.0 | 98 | 7.4 | 11.1 | 2.7 | 0.6 |
| Chicken, & Dumplings, Morrisons* | 1 Pack/300g | 291.0 | 13.0 | 97 | 3.4 | 11.4 | 4.2 | 1.3 |
| Chicken, & Dumplings, Weight Watchers* | 1 Pack/400g | 332.0 | 8.0 | 83 | 6.8 | 9.5 | 2.0 | 1.3 |
| Chicken, & Red Wine, Duchy Originals* | ½ Pack/175g | 187.0 | 8.0 | 107 | 14.0 | 5.1 | 4.3 | 1.6 |
| Chicken, & Tomato, Asda* | ¼ Pack/273g | 569.0 | 41.0 | 208 | 16.0 | 2.2 | 15.0 | 0.5 |
| Chicken, & Vegetable, Apetito* | 1 Pack/330g | 286.0 | 10.0 | 87 | 6.3 | 9.4 | 3.0 | 1.6 |
| Chicken, & Vegetable, Long Life, Sainsbury's* | 1 Pack/300g | 186.0 | 4.0 | 62 | 4.6 | 7.4 | 1.5 | 0.8 |
| Chicken, Catalan, TTD, Sainsbury's* | ½ Pack/300g | 324.0 | 16.0 | 108 | 10.8 | 4.4 | 5.2 | 0.6 |
| Chicken, Fillets, Safeway* | ½ Pack/172g | 155.0 | 2.0 | 90 | 15.6 | 2.9 | 1.3 | 0.6 |
| Chicken, Green Isle* | 1 Pack/400g | 300.0 | 7.0 | 75 | 5.7 | 9.2 | 1.7 | 1.0 |
| Chicken, Leek & Mushroom, Tesco* | 1 Pack/350g | 381.0 | 22.0 | 109 | 4.5 | 8.6 | 6.3 | 1.0 |
| Chicken, Mediterranean, Tesco* | 1 Pack/400g | 260.0 | 9.0 | 65 | 6.7 | 4.5 | 2.3 | 0.9 |
| Chicken, Perfectly Balanced, Waitrose* | 1 Pack/400g | 392.0 | 14.0 | 98 | 6.6 | 9.8 | 3.6 | 1.2 |
| Chicken, with Dumplings, M & S* | ½ Pack/227g | 261.0 | 10.0 | 115 | 9.7 | 9.0 | 4.4 | 0.9 |
| Cowboy, Iceland* | 1 Pack/400g | 500.0 | 26.0 | 125 | 5.8 | 10.9 | 6.5 | 1.7 |
| Ham Hock & Mash, Tesco* | 1 Pack/250g | 225.0 | 8.0 | 90 | 6.1 | 9.0 | 3.2 | 0.8 |
| Lamb, & Rosemary, Eat Well, M & S* | 1 Pack/380g | 325.0 | 11.0 | 86 | 7.6 | 7.0 | 2.9 | 2.2 |
| Lamb, Braised, British Classics, Tesco* | 1 Pack/350g | 332.0 | 18.0 | 95 | 7.5 | 4.6 | 5.2 | 1.2 |
| Lamb, COU, M & S* | 1 Pack/390g | 253.0 | 7.0 | 65 | 5.9 | 6.7 | 1.7 | 1.6 |
| Lamb, with Mint Dumplings, Minced, Sainsbury's* | 1 Pack/450g | 558.0 | 31.0 | 124 | 5.4 | 10.4 | 6.8 | 1.1 |
| Lamb, With Rosemary Roast Potatoes, Asda* | 1 Pack/450g | 477.0 | 22.0 | 106 | 8.9 | 6.9 | 4.8 | 1.5 |
| Mediterranean Seafood, HL, Tesco* | 1 Pack/344g | 292.0 | 7.0 | 85 | 5.8 | 10.5 | 2.0 | 3.2 |
| Minced Beef & Dumplings, SmartPrice, Asda* | 1 Pack/299g | 320.0 | 13.0 | 107 | 4.5 | 12.7 | 4.2 | 2.3 |
| Mushroom, & Onion, Iceland* | 1 Pack/400g | 272.0 | 12.0 | 68 | 1.3 | 8.8 | 3.1 | 1.9 |
| Pork, & Apple, with Boiled Potatos & Vegetables, Apetito* | 1 Pack/350g | 251.0 | 4.0 | 72 | 5.1 | 8.5 | 1.1 | 1.1 |
| Pork, Normandy Style, Finest, Tesco* | 1 Pack/450g | 405.0 | 22.0 | 90 | 7.6 | 4.1 | 4.8 | 2.3 |
| Pork, with Apple & Cider, Safeway* | 1 Pack/450g | 729.0 | 38.0 | 162 | 8.3 | 13.4 | 8.4 | 1.1 |
| Rabbit, Average | 1oz/28g | 29.0 | 1.0 | 102 | 11.6 | 2.6 | 5.1 | 0.4 |
| Root Vegetable, with Herb Dumplings, Tesco* | 1 Pack/450g | 373.0 | 11.0 | 83 | 2.1 | 12.8 | 2.5 | 3.3 |
| Steak, & Ale, Sainsbury's* | 1 Pack/300g | 288.0 | 10.0 | 96 | 10.6 | 5.6 | 3.5 | 0.4 |
| Steak, & Mushroom, Asda* | ½ Pack/304g | 411.0 | 30.0 | 135 | 7.0 | 4.2 | 10.0 | 0.3 |
| Steak, & Mushroom with Mustard Mash, Finest, Tesco* | 1 Pack/550g | 522.0 | 21.0 | 95 | 5.9 | 9.0 | 3.9 | 1.1 |
| Steak & Kidney, Mini, Favourites, M & S* | 1 Pack/200g | 240.0 | 11.0 | 120 | 7.9 | 9.5 | 5.4 | 1.5 |
| Vegetable, & Lentil, Canned, Granose* | 1 Can/400g | 272.0 | 8.0 | 68 | 3.5 | 9.0 | 2.0 | 3.0 |
| Vegetable, Chunky, M & S* | 1 Bag/450g | 90.0 | 1.0 | 20 | 0.7 | 3.4 | 0.3 | 1.4 |
| Vegetable, Country, Sainsbury's* | 1 Can/400g | 300.0 | 10.0 | 75 | 2.2 | 11.0 | 2.5 | 1.1 |
| Vegetable, with Herb Dumplings, COU, M & S* | 1 Pack/450g | 270.0 | 5.0 | 60 | 1.6 | 10.1 | 1.2 | 1.0 |

| | Measure INFO/WEIGHT | per Measure KCAL | per Measure FAT | Nutrition Values per 100g / 100ml KCAL | PROT | CARB | FAT | FIBRE |
|---|---|---|---|---|---|---|---|---|
| **CASSEROLE** | | | | | | | | |
| Vegetable, with Potato Crush, Safeway* | 1 Pack/450g | 292.0 | 14.0 | 65 | 1.3 | 7.7 | 3.1 | 2.0 |
| Venison, Scottish Wild, & Beaujolais, Tesco* | 1 Pack/425g | 365.0 | 9.0 | 86 | 11.9 | 4.9 | 2.1 | 0.6 |
| **CASSEROLE MIX** | | | | | | | | |
| Beef, Authentic, Schwartz* | 1 Pack/43g | 111.0 | 0.0 | 257 | 7.4 | 54.5 | 1.0 | 0.4 |
| Beef, Colman's* | 1 Pack/40g | 123.0 | 1.0 | 308 | 7.5 | 66.0 | 1.5 | 2.5 |
| Beef & Ale, Colman's* | 1 Pack/45g | 144.0 | 1.0 | 320 | 9.2 | 66.3 | 2.0 | 2.3 |
| Chicken, Authentic, Schwartz* | 1 Pack/36g | 131.0 | 2.0 | 363 | 10.4 | 70.7 | 4.3 | 2.0 |
| Chicken, Traditional, Colman's* | 1 Pack/40g | 124.0 | 1.0 | 311 | 5.7 | 69.4 | 1.3 | 1.5 |
| Chicken Chasseur, Asda* | 1 Pack/80g | 273.0 | 1.0 | 341 | 9.0 | 74.0 | 1.0 | 1.4 |
| Chicken Chasseur, Morrisons* | 1 Pack/40g | 115.0 | 0.0 | 288 | 9.2 | 59.8 | 1.2 | 0.0 |
| Farmhouse Sausage, Schwartz* | 1 Pack/39g | 124.0 | 1.0 | 317 | 8.1 | 64.6 | 2.9 | 0.5 |
| Honey Chicken, Colman's* | 1 Pack/50g | 128.0 | 1.0 | 257 | 3.4 | 58.3 | 1.1 | 1.8 |
| Lamb, Authentic, Schwartz* | 1 Pack/35g | 116.0 | 1.0 | 332 | 7.7 | 68.0 | 3.3 | 1.3 |
| Liver & Bacon, Colman's* | 1 Pack/40g | 121.0 | 1.0 | 303 | 10.3 | 61.6 | 1.7 | 4.7 |
| Moroccan Lamb, Schwartz* | 1 Pack/35g | 124.0 | 2.0 | 354 | 6.2 | 74.1 | 5.7 | 4.5 |
| Peppered Beef, Schwartz* | 1 Pack/40g | 129.0 | 2.0 | 323 | 7.0 | 62.9 | 4.9 | 7.3 |
| Pork, Colman's* | 1 Pack/40g | 131.0 | 1.0 | 328 | 6.7 | 72.0 | 1.4 | 2.8 |
| Pork, Morrisons* | 1 Pack/36g | 118.0 | 1.0 | 327 | 8.1 | 70.6 | 1.4 | 0.0 |
| Sausage, Asda* | ¼ Pack/25g | 80.0 | 1.0 | 321 | 6.0 | 65.0 | 4.1 | 3.0 |
| Sausage, Classic, Schwartz* | 1 Pack/35g | 96.0 | 1.0 | 275 | 12.4 | 50.1 | 2.7 | 14.9 |
| Sausage, Colman's* | 1 Pack/40g | 144.0 | 1.0 | 361 | 8.9 | 77.7 | 1.6 | 1.6 |
| Sausage & Onion, Colman's* | 1 Pack/45g | 143.0 | 1.0 | 318 | 9.6 | 64.2 | 2.6 | 2.6 |
| Somerset Pork, Colman's* | 1 Pack/45g | 144.0 | 1.0 | 321 | 7.1 | 70.2 | 1.3 | 2.2 |
| Somerset Pork, Schwartz* | 1 Pack/36g | 115.0 | 1.0 | 320 | 9.4 | 61.9 | 3.8 | 7.7 |
| Spicy Chicken, Colman's* | 1 Pack/45g | 151.0 | 1.0 | 336 | 6.5 | 73.4 | 1.8 | 1.5 |
| Turkey, Colman's* | 1 Pack/50g | 156.0 | 1.0 | 313 | 5.9 | 68.0 | 1.9 | 3.5 |
| **CATFISH** | | | | | | | | |
| *Cooked, Average* | *1 Fillet/87g* | *199.0* | *12.0* | *229* | *18.0* | *8.0* | *13.3* | *0.7* |
| *Raw, Average* | *1oz/28g* | *27.0* | *1.0* | *96* | *17.6* | *0.0* | *2.8* | *0.0* |
| **CAULIFLOWER** | | | | | | | | |
| *Boiled, Average* | *1 Serving/80g* | *22.0* | *1.0* | *28* | *2.9* | *2.1* | *0.9* | *1.6* |
| Florets, Peas & Carrots, Frozen, Asda* | 1 Serving/100g | 37.0 | 1.0 | 37 | 3.0 | 5.0 | 0.6 | 2.8 |
| *Raw, Average* | *1 Serving/80g* | *25.0* | *1.0* | *31* | *3.2* | *2.7* | *0.8* | *1.6* |
| **CAULIFLOWER CHEESE** | | | | | | | | |
| & Bacon, Gastropub, M & S* | 1 Pack/300g | 318.0 | 21.0 | 106 | 6.3 | 4.5 | 7.0 | 1.0 |
| & Broccoli, Sainsbury's* | 1 Serving/130g | 83.0 | 2.0 | 64 | 4.8 | 7.6 | 1.6 | 2.7 |
| BFY, Morrisons* | 1 Pack/300g | 231.0 | 12.0 | 77 | 4.5 | 5.4 | 4.1 | 1.2 |
| Birds Eye* | 1 Pack/329g | 355.0 | 21.0 | 108 | 4.8 | 7.7 | 6.4 | 0.8 |
| Eat Smart, Morrisons* | 1 Pack/300g | 192.0 | 6.0 | 64 | 4.9 | 6.7 | 2.0 | 1.5 |
| Extra Special, Asda* | ½ Pack/200g | 166.0 | 12.0 | 83 | 4.0 | 3.7 | 5.8 | 2.1 |
| Finest, Tesco* | 1 Serving/250g | 317.0 | 21.0 | 127 | 6.5 | 6.1 | 8.5 | 0.4 |
| Florets, in a Cheese Sauce, Sainsbury's* | 1 Pack/400g | 400.0 | 26.0 | 100 | 4.8 | 5.4 | 6.6 | 0.9 |
| Frozen, Tesco* | 1 Pack/450g | 427.0 | 30.0 | 95 | 4.2 | 4.3 | 6.7 | 1.3 |
| GFY, Asda* | 1 Pack/300g | 204.0 | 8.0 | 68 | 4.8 | 6.0 | 2.7 | 1.0 |
| Grills, Grassington's Food Co* | 1 Grill/92g | 157.0 | 5.0 | 171 | 6.1 | 25.3 | 5.0 | 2.6 |
| Grills, Meat Free, Tesco* | 1 Grill/91g | 160.0 | 7.0 | 175 | 5.3 | 20.0 | 8.1 | 2.9 |
| Grills, Tesco* | 1 Grill/92g | 207.0 | 11.0 | 225 | 6.5 | 22.2 | 11.9 | 4.0 |
| Light Choices, Tesco* | 1 Pack/500g | 245.0 | 10.0 | 49 | 4.5 | 3.3 | 2.0 | 2.4 |
| M & S* | 1 Serving/150g | 150.0 | 9.0 | 100 | 5.5 | 5.9 | 6.1 | 1.1 |
| Made with Semi-Skimmed Milk | 1oz/28g | 28.0 | 2.0 | 100 | 6.0 | 5.2 | 6.4 | 1.3 |
| Made with Skimmed Milk | 1oz/28g | 27.0 | 2.0 | 97 | 6.0 | 5.2 | 6.0 | 1.3 |
| Made with Whole Milk | 1oz/28g | 29.0 | 2.0 | 105 | 6.0 | 5.2 | 6.9 | 1.3 |
| Ross* | 1 Pack/300g | 300.0 | 20.0 | 100 | 4.9 | 5.5 | 6.6 | 0.1 |

**C**

| | Measure INFO/WEIGHT | per Measure KCAL | per Measure FAT | Nutrition Values per 100g / 100ml KCAL | PROT | CARB | FAT | FIBRE |
|---|---|---|---|---|---|---|---|---|
| **CAULIFLOWER CHEESE** | | | | | | | | |
| Sainsbury's* | ½ Pack/200g | 158.0 | 10.0 | 79 | 5.0 | 3.7 | 4.9 | 2.2 |
| TTD, Sainsbury's* | ½ Pack/150g | 252.0 | 18.0 | 168 | 6.9 | 8.0 | 12.0 | 0.9 |
| Vegetarian, Safeway* | 1 Serving/150g | 138.0 | 9.0 | 92 | 4.7 | 5.2 | 5.8 | 1.4 |
| with Crispy Bacon, Finest, Tesco* | 1/3 Pack/166g | 211.0 | 14.0 | 127 | 6.5 | 6.1 | 8.5 | 0.4 |
| **CAVIAR** | | | | | | | | |
| *Average* | *1oz/28g* | *26.0* | *1.0* | *92* | *11.9* | *0.5* | *4.7* | *0.0* |
| **CELERIAC** | | | | | | | | |
| *Boiled in Salted Water, Average* | *1oz/28g* | *4.0* | *0.0* | *15* | *0.9* | *1.9* | *0.5* | *3.2* |
| *Raw, Average* | *1 Serving/100g* | *42.0* | *0.0* | *42* | *1.5* | *9.2* | *0.3* | *1.8* |
| **CELERY** | | | | | | | | |
| *Boiled in Salted Water* | *1 Med Serving/50g* | *4.0* | *0.0* | *8* | *0.5* | *0.8* | *0.3* | *1.2* |
| *Raw* | *1 Stalk/40g* | *6.0* | *0.0* | *16* | *0.7* | *3.6* | *0.1* | *1.7* |
| **CHAMPAGNE** | | | | | | | | |
| *Average* | *1 Glass/120ml* | *91.0* | *0.0* | *76* | *0.3* | *1.4* | *0.0* | *0.0* |
| **CHANNA MASALA** | | | | | | | | |
| M & S* | 1 Pack/225g | 360.0 | 24.0 | 160 | 5.6 | 11.2 | 10.5 | 8.2 |
| Safeway* | 1 Pack/400g | 540.0 | 22.0 | 135 | 5.3 | 16.2 | 5.4 | 2.5 |
| **CHAPATIS** | | | | | | | | |
| Brown Wheat Flour, Waitrose* | 1 Chapati/42g | 128.0 | 3.0 | 305 | 8.6 | 49.4 | 8.0 | 4.6 |
| Indian Style, Asda* | 1 Chapati/43g | 95.0 | 0.0 | 221 | 8.0 | 45.0 | 1.0 | 2.9 |
| Made with Fat | 1 Chapati/60g | 197.0 | 8.0 | 328 | 8.1 | 48.3 | 12.8 | 0.0 |
| Made without Fat | 1 Chapati/55g | 111.0 | 1.0 | 202 | 7.3 | 43.7 | 1.0 | 0.0 |
| Morrisons* | 1 Chapati/40g | 108.0 | 3.0 | 269 | 8.6 | 49.8 | 6.9 | 0.0 |
| Plain, Wraps, Original, Patak's* | 1 Chapati/42g | 115.0 | 3.0 | 273 | 9.4 | 48.8 | 7.5 | 0.0 |
| Wholemeal, Patak's* | 1 Chapati/42g | 130.0 | 4.0 | 310 | 11.2 | 44.9 | 9.5 | 9.0 |
| **CHARD** | | | | | | | | |
| *Swiss, Boiled in Unsalted Water* | *1oz/28g* | *6.0* | *0.0* | *20* | *1.9* | *4.1* | *0.1* | *2.1* |
| *Swiss, Raw* | *1oz/28g* | *5.0* | *0.0* | *19* | *1.8* | *3.7* | *0.2* | *1.6* |
| **CHEDDARS** | | | | | | | | |
| Baked, Mini, Cheese & Ham Flavour, McVitie's* | 1 Bag/30g | 160.0 | 9.0 | 534 | 11.0 | 55.5 | 29.8 | 2.0 |
| Baked, Mini, Original, Cheddar Cheese, McVitie's* | 1 Bag/30g | 155.0 | 9.0 | 517 | 10.8 | 50.9 | 30.0 | 2.5 |
| Baked, Mini, Peperami, McVitie's* | 1 Bag/30g | 160.0 | 9.0 | 532 | 9.7 | 55.2 | 30.2 | 2.0 |
| Baked, Mini, Tangy Salsa, McVitie's* | 1 Bag/50g | 266.0 | 15.0 | 532 | 11.0 | 54.7 | 29.9 | 2.1 |
| Branston Pickle, McVitie's* | 1 Bag/30g | 155.0 | 9.0 | 517 | 9.1 | 53.1 | 29.8 | 2.7 |
| Saucy BBQ, McVitie's* | 1 Bag/50g | 259.0 | 15.0 | 518 | 9.2 | 53.4 | 29.8 | 2.6 |
| **CHEESE** | | | | | | | | |
| Appenzellar, Sainsbury's* | 1 Serving/25g | 96.0 | 8.0 | 386 | 25.4 | 0.0 | 31.6 | 0.0 |
| Babybel, Emmental, Fromageries Bel* | 1 Serving/20g | 63.0 | 5.0 | 316 | 23.0 | 1.0 | 24.5 | 0.0 |
| Babybel, Mini, Light, Fromageries Bel* | 1 Cheese/20g | 42.0 | 2.0 | 210 | 25.5 | 0.2 | 12.0 | 0.0 |
| Babybel, Original, Mini, Fromageries Bel* | 1 Cheese/20g | 61.0 | 5.0 | 304 | 22.0 | 0.0 | 24.0 | 0.0 |
| Babybel, with Cheddar, Mini, Fromageries Bel* | 1 Cheese/20g | 72.0 | 6.0 | 362 | 23.0 | 0.2 | 30.0 | 0.0 |
| Bavarian, Smoked, Slices, Asda* | 1 Slice/18g | 50.0 | 4.0 | 277 | 17.0 | 0.4 | 23.0 | 0.0 |
| Bavarian, Smoked, with Ham, Sainsbury's* | 1 Serving/30g | 89.0 | 7.0 | 298 | 19.4 | 0.8 | 24.1 | 0.0 |
| Bleu D' Auvergne, Sainsbury's* | 1 Serving/25g | 84.0 | 7.0 | 335 | 22.0 | 2.0 | 26.5 | 0.0 |
| Blue, Castello, Soft, Castello* | ¼ Pack/38g | 162.0 | 16.0 | 432 | 14.0 | 0.5 | 41.5 | 0.0 |
| Blue, Saint Agur* | 1 Serving /30g | 109.0 | 10.0 | 363 | 16.0 | 0.2 | 33.0 | 0.0 |
| Bresse Bleu, M & S* | 1oz/28g | 99.0 | 9.0 | 355 | 19.0 | 0.3 | 31.0 | 0.0 |
| *Brie, Average* | *1 Serving/25g* | *74.0* | *6.0* | *296* | *19.7* | *0.3* | *24.0* | *0.0* |
| *Brie, Reduced Fat, Average* | *1 Serving/50g* | *99.0* | *6.0* | *198* | *23.0* | *0.8* | *11.4* | *0.0* |
| *Caerphilly, Average* | *1 Serving/50g* | *187.0* | *16.0* | *374* | *23.0* | *0.1* | *31.3* | *0.0* |
| Cambazola, Tesco* | 1 Serving/30g | 127.0 | 12.0 | 425 | 13.5 | 0.5 | 41.0 | 0.0 |
| *Camembert, Average* | *1 Serving/50g* | *141.0* | *11.0* | *283* | *20.5* | *0.1* | *22.2* | *0.0* |
| Camembert, Breaded, Average | 1 Serving/90g | 307.0 | 21.0 | 341 | 16.6 | 14.2 | 23.2 | 0.4 |

# CHEESE

| INFO/WEIGHT | Measure | per Measure KCAL | FAT | Nutrition Values per 100g / 100ml KCAL | PROT | CARB | FAT | FIBRE |
|---|---|---|---|---|---|---|---|---|
| Cantal, French, Sainsbury's* | 1 Serving/30g | 106.0 | 9.0 | 353 | 23.0 | 0.1 | 29.0 | 0.0 |
| Cantenaar, M & S* | 1 Serving/28g | 84.0 | 5.0 | 300 | 32.2 | 0.1 | 19.2 | 0.0 |
| *Cheddar, Canadian, Average* | *1 Serving/30g* | *123.0* | *10.0* | *409* | *25.0* | *0.1* | *34.3* | *0.0* |
| *Cheddar, Davidstow, Mature, Average* | *1 Serving/28g* | *115.0* | *10.0* | *410* | *25.0* | *0.1* | *34.4* | *0.0* |
| *Cheddar, Extra Mature, Average* | *1 Serving/30g* | *123.0* | *10.0* | *410* | *25.1* | *0.1* | *34.3* | *0.0* |
| *Cheddar, Grated, Average* | *1 Serving/50g* | *206.0* | *17.0* | *413* | *24.4* | *1.5* | *34.3* | *0.0* |
| *Cheddar, Mature, Average* | *1 Serving/30g* | *123.0* | *10.0* | *410* | *25.0* | *0.1* | *34.4* | *0.0* |
| *Cheddar, Mature, Grated, Average* | *1 Serving/28g* | *113.0* | *9.0* | *404* | *24.7* | *1.6* | *33.2* | *0.0* |
| *Cheddar, Mature, Reduced Fat, Average* | *1 Serving/25g* | *68.0* | *4.0* | *271* | *30.0* | *0.1* | *16.7* | *0.0* |
| *Cheddar, Medium, Average* | *1 Serving/30g* | *123.0* | *10.0* | *411* | *24.9* | *0.1* | *34.5* | *0.0* |
| *Cheddar, Mild, Average* | *1 Serving/30g* | *123.0* | *10.0* | *409* | *25.0* | *0.1* | *34.3* | *0.0* |
| *Cheddar, Reduced Fat, Average* | *1 Serving/30g* | *76.0* | *4.0* | *255* | *32.1* | *0.1* | *13.9* | *0.0* |
| *Cheddar, Smoked, Average* | *1 Serving/30g* | *123.0* | *10.0* | *411* | *25.2* | *0.1* | *34.4* | *0.0* |
| *Cheddar, West Country Farmhouse, Average* | *1 Serving/28g* | *115.0* | *10.0* | *410* | *25.0* | *0.1* | *34.4* | *0.0* |
| *Cheddar, Wexford, Average* | *1 Serving/20g* | *82.0* | *7.0* | *410* | *25.0* | *0.1* | *34.4* | *0.0* |
| Cheddar, with Caramelised Onion, Sainsbury's* | 1 Serving/28g | 109.0 | 9.0 | 391 | 22.8 | 5.1 | 31.0 | 0.0 |
| Cheddar, with Caramelised Onion, Tesco* | 1 Serving/50g | 183.0 | 14.0 | 366 | 21.4 | 7.1 | 28.0 | 0.4 |
| Cheddar, with Onion & Chives, Davidson* | 1 Serving/25g | 100.0 | 8.0 | 400 | 24.3 | 0.6 | 33.3 | 0.0 |
| Cheddar, with Pickled Onion Relish, Christmas, Tesco* | ¼ Cheese/50g | 191.0 | 15.0 | 382 | 23.0 | 2.7 | 31.0 | 0.1 |
| Cheddar & Mozzarella, Spicy, Grated, Tesco* | 1 Serving/40g | 140.0 | 10.0 | 350 | 26.0 | 2.5 | 26.2 | 0.0 |
| Cheestrings, Cheddar, Original, Golden Vale* | 1 Stick/21g | 69.0 | 5.0 | 328 | 28.0 | 0.0 | 24.0 | 0.0 |
| Cheestrings, Double Cheese Flavour, Golden Vale* | 1 Stick/21g | 69.0 | 5.0 | 328 | 28.0 | 0.0 | 24.0 | 0.0 |
| *Cheshire* | *1oz/28g* | *106.0* | *9.0* | *379* | *24.0* | *0.1* | *31.4* | *0.0* |
| Chevre Pave D'affinois, Finest, Tesco* | 1 Pack/150g | 403.0 | 33.0 | 269 | 18.5 | 0.0 | 21.7 | 0.0 |
| Cottage, Bettabuy, Morrisons* | 1 Tub/200g | 210.0 | 10.0 | 105 | 11.0 | 5.0 | 5.0 | 0.0 |
| Cottage, BFY, Morrisons* | 1 Pot/125g | 110.0 | 1.0 | 88 | 13.0 | 6.9 | 0.9 | 0.0 |
| Cottage, Crunchy Vegetable, GFY, Asda* | 1 Serving/50g | 37.0 | 1.0 | 74 | 11.0 | 4.5 | 1.3 | 0.6 |
| Cottage, Danone* | 1 Serving/100g | 89.0 | 4.0 | 89 | 11.2 | 2.3 | 3.9 | 0.0 |
| Cottage, Garlic & Herb, Diet, Yoplait* | 1 Pot/225g | 180.0 | 4.0 | 80 | 12.0 | 3.9 | 1.9 | 0.0 |
| Cottage, Healthy Choice, Nisa Heritage* | 1 Pot/227g | 175.0 | 4.0 | 77 | 11.8 | 3.4 | 1.8 | 0.3 |
| Cottage, Jocca, Kraft* | 1 Serving/50g | 54.0 | 3.0 | 109 | 9.3 | 5.0 | 5.5 | 0.0 |
| Cottage, Less Than 5% Fat, Sainsbury's* | ½ Pot/125g | 131.0 | 5.0 | 105 | 12.3 | 4.4 | 4.2 | 0.0 |
| Cottage, Low Fat, 2% Fat, Natural, Average | 1 Serving/75g | 67.0 | 1.0 | 90 | 13.7 | 3.6 | 1.9 | 0.0 |
| Cottage, Natural, Asda* | ¼ Pot/113g | 118.0 | 5.0 | 104 | 12.0 | 4.0 | 4.2 | 0.0 |
| Cottage, Natural, COU, M & S* | ½ Pot/125g | 100.0 | 2.0 | 80 | 11.9 | 3.3 | 1.8 | 0.3 |
| Cottage, Natural, Eat Smart, Morrisons* | 1 Pot/300g | 264.0 | 3.0 | 88 | 11.0 | 6.9 | 0.9 | 0.3 |
| Cottage, Natural, GFY, Asda* | 1 Serving/113g | 95.0 | 2.0 | 84 | 13.0 | 3.9 | 1.8 | 0.3 |
| Cottage, Natural, Healthy Living, Co-Op* | 1 Pot/250g | 187.0 | 5.0 | 75 | 10.0 | 4.0 | 2.0 | 0.0 |
| Cottage, Natural, HL, Tesco* | 1 Sm Pot/125g | 100.0 | 2.0 | 80 | 12.2 | 4.5 | 1.5 | 0.0 |
| Cottage, Natural, Less Than 1% Fat, BGTY, Sainsbury's* | 1 Serving/125g | 105.0 | 1.0 | 84 | 12.0 | 6.9 | 0.9 | 0.0 |
| Cottage, Natural, Light Choices, Tesco* | 1 Serving/60g | 48.0 | 1.0 | 80 | 12.2 | 4.5 | 1.5 | 0.0 |
| Cottage, Natural, Loseley* | ½ Tub/100g | 115.0 | 7.0 | 115 | 9.4 | 2.9 | 7.1 | 0.0 |
| Cottage, Natural, Organic, Sainsbury's* | 1 Pot/201g | 185.0 | 4.0 | 92 | 12.8 | 6.3 | 1.8 | 0.0 |
| *Cottage, Natural, Plain, Average* | *1oz/28g* | *27.0* | *1.0* | *98* | *11.8* | *3.9* | *3.8* | *0.1* |
| Cottage, Natural, SmartPrice, Asda* | ½ Pot/100g | 86.0 | 2.0 | 86 | 12.0 | 4.3 | 2.0 | 0.0 |
| Cottage, Natural, Tesco* | 1 Serving/50g | 49.0 | 2.0 | 98 | 12.4 | 3.2 | 3.5 | 0.4 |
| Cottage, Natural, Waitrose* | ½ Pot/125g | 120.0 | 4.0 | 96 | 12.4 | 3.6 | 3.5 | 0.4 |
| Cottage, Natural, with Creme Fraiche, Tesco* | ½ Pack/125g | 131.0 | 6.0 | 105 | 12.1 | 2.7 | 4.8 | 0.6 |
| Cottage, Onion & Chive, Waitrose* | 1 Serving/20g | 18.0 | 1.0 | 91 | 10.8 | 4.9 | 3.1 | 0.3 |
| Cottage, Onion & Chives, Light Choices, Tesco* | 1 Serving/60g | 51.0 | 1.0 | 85 | 11.4 | 4.8 | 1.5 | 0.1 |
| Cottage, Pineapple, Light Choices, Tesco* | 1 Serving/60g | 54.0 | 1.0 | 90 | 9.8 | 8.5 | 1.3 | 0.4 |
| Cottage, Pineapple, Perfectly Balanced, Waitrose* | ½ Pot/125g | 106.0 | 2.0 | 85 | 8.4 | 9.7 | 1.4 | 0.5 |
| *Cottage, Plain, Average* | *1oz/28g* | *26.0* | *1.0* | *93* | *12.0* | *3.3* | *3.5* | *0.1* |

# CHEESE

| INFO/WEIGHT | Measure | per Measure | | Nutrition Values per 100g / 100ml | | | | |
|---|---|---|---|---|---|---|---|---|
| | | KCAL | FAT | KCAL | PROT | CARB | FAT | FIBRE |
| *Cottage, Plain, Reduced Fat, Average* | *1oz/28g* | *24.0* | *1.0* | *85* | *12.3* | *4.4* | *1.9* | *0.1* |
| Cottage, Red Onion & Garlic, Sainsbury's* | ½ Tub/125g | 91.0 | 1.0 | 73 | 10.4 | 5.8 | 0.9 | 0.6 |
| Cottage, Red Pepper, GFY, Asda* | ¼ Pot/75g | 66.0 | 2.0 | 88 | 11.1 | 4.3 | 2.5 | 0.1 |
| Cottage, Slimline* | 1 Serving/70g | 43.0 | 0.0 | 62 | 12.0 | 3.0 | 0.2 | 0.0 |
| Cottage, Stilton & Celery, BGTY, Sainsbury's* | ½ Pot/125g | 99.0 | 3.0 | 79 | 10.8 | 4.0 | 2.2 | 1.5 |
| Cottage, Tuna & Sweetcorn, GFY, Asda* | ½ Pot/113g | 104.0 | 3.0 | 92 | 12.4 | 5.3 | 2.4 | 0.3 |
| Cottage, Tuna & Sweetcorn, Morrisons* | ¼ Tub/63g | 59.0 | 1.0 | 94 | 12.8 | 8.2 | 1.2 | 0.0 |
| Cottage, Value, Tesco* | ½ Tub/100g | 75.0 | 0.0 | 75 | 11.6 | 4.6 | 0.4 | 0.0 |
| Cottage, Very Low Fat, Nisa Heritage* | 1 Tub/227g | 193.0 | 3.0 | 85 | 13.8 | 4.4 | 1.4 | 0.0 |
| Cottage, Virtually Fat Free, Longley Farm* | ½ Pot/125g | 84.0 | 0.0 | 67 | 13.4 | 3.0 | 0.1 | 0.0 |
| Cottage, Whole Milk, Natural, Average | 1 Serving/75g | 77.0 | 3.0 | 103 | 12.5 | 2.7 | 4.5 | 0.0 |
| Cottage, with Black Pepper, HE, Tesco* | 1 Pot/125g | 101.0 | 2.0 | 81 | 12.1 | 4.0 | 1.8 | 0.0 |
| Cottage, with Chives, Somerfield* | 1oz/28g | 29.0 | 1.0 | 105 | 12.0 | 5.0 | 4.0 | 0.0 |
| Cottage, with Cucumber & Mint, BGTY, Sainsbury's* | ½ Pot/125g | 102.0 | 1.0 | 82 | 12.0 | 6.6 | 0.9 | 0.0 |
| Cottage, with Cucumber & Mint, COU, M & S* | 1 Pot/113g | 85.0 | 2.0 | 75 | 11.6 | 3.1 | 1.5 | 0.2 |
| Cottage, with Cucumber & Mint, GFY, Asda* | 1 Serving/75g | 54.0 | 1.0 | 72 | 11.0 | 4.1 | 1.3 | 0.5 |
| Cottage, with Cucumber & Mint, HE, Tesco* | ½ Pot/125g | 91.0 | 2.0 | 73 | 10.7 | 3.8 | 1.7 | 0.1 |
| Cottage, with Mango, COU, M & S* | 1 Serving/100g | 100.0 | 1.0 | 100 | 10.3 | 11.0 | 1.1 | 0.5 |
| Cottage, with Mango & Pineapple, BGTY, Sainsbury's* | ½ Pot/125g | 112.0 | 1.0 | 90 | 10.7 | 10.4 | 0.7 | 0.2 |
| Cottage, with Mango & Pineapple, Morrisons* | 1 Pot/125g | 112.0 | 1.0 | 90 | 10.7 | 10.4 | 0.7 | 0.0 |
| Cottage, with Onion & Chive, BGTY, Sainsbury's* | 1 Serving/50g | 41.0 | 0.0 | 83 | 12.4 | 6.4 | 0.9 | 0.1 |
| Cottage, with Onion & Chive, GFY, Asda* | 1 Serving/50g | 42.0 | 1.0 | 85 | 12.0 | 4.4 | 1.9 | 0.1 |
| Cottage, with Onion & Chive, HL, Tesco* | 1 Serving/65g | 55.0 | 1.0 | 85 | 13.9 | 3.6 | 1.5 | 0.3 |
| Cottage, with Onion & Chive, M & S* | ¼ Pot/65g | 88.0 | 6.0 | 135 | 10.4 | 4.0 | 8.5 | 0.1 |
| Cottage, with Onion & Chive, Nisa Heritage* | 1 Pot/227g | 168.0 | 4.0 | 74 | 11.1 | 3.8 | 1.6 | 0.3 |
| Cottage, with Peach & Mango, COU, M & S* | 1 Pot/113g | 96.0 | 1.0 | 85 | 9.1 | 9.7 | 1.0 | 0.4 |
| Cottage, with Pineapple, BGTY, Sainsbury's* | 1 Serving/125g | 105.0 | 1.0 | 84 | 10.5 | 8.9 | 0.7 | 0.1 |
| Cottage, with Pineapple, GFY, Asda* | 1 Pot/227g | 193.0 | 2.0 | 85 | 9.0 | 10.0 | 1.0 | 0.5 |
| Cottage, with Pineapple, HL, Tesco* | ½ Pot/125g | 112.0 | 2.0 | 90 | 12.5 | 6.8 | 1.3 | 0.4 |
| Cottage, with Pineapple, Low Fat, Waitrose* | 1 Serving/40g | 34.0 | 1.0 | 84 | 10.4 | 6.7 | 1.7 | 0.2 |
| Cottage, with Pineapple, Shape, Danone* | 1oz/28g | 20.0 | 0.0 | 73 | 9.8 | 8.0 | 0.2 | 0.1 |
| Cottage, with Pineapple, Tesco* | 1 Serving/150g | 157.0 | 5.0 | 105 | 9.1 | 9.8 | 3.3 | 0.1 |
| Cottage, with Poached Salmon & Dill, GFY, Asda* | 1/3 Pot/75g | 64.0 | 2.0 | 86 | 12.0 | 2.3 | 2.7 | 0.6 |
| Cottage, with Prawn & Cucumber, Safeway* | 1 Serving/200g | 184.0 | 5.0 | 92 | 12.0 | 4.7 | 2.5 | 0.1 |
| Cottage, with Prawn Cocktail, BGTY, Sainsbury's* | 1oz/28g | 25.0 | 0.0 | 91 | 12.3 | 8.3 | 0.9 | 0.1 |
| Cottage, with Roasted Vegetables, Low Fat, Safeway* | 1 Pot/125g | 96.0 | 2.0 | 77 | 10.5 | 4.3 | 1.7 | 1.8 |
| Cottage, with Smoked Cheese & Onion, GFY, Asda* | 1 Serving/50g | 39.0 | 1.0 | 78 | 12.0 | 3.9 | 1.6 | 0.4 |
| Cottage, with Smoked Salmon & Dill, BGTY, Sainsbury's* | 1oz/28g | 25.0 | 0.0 | 89 | 13.8 | 6.4 | 0.9 | 0.1 |
| Cottage, with Sweet Chilli Chicken, M & S* | 1 Serving/200g | 190.0 | 4.0 | 95 | 13.8 | 4.7 | 2.1 | 0.5 |
| Cottage, with Tomato & Cracked Black Pepper, Asda* | ½ Pot/113g | 86.0 | 2.0 | 76 | 10.0 | 3.1 | 2.1 | 1.3 |
| Cottage, with Tuna & Cucumber, Safeway* | 1 Serving/40g | 35.0 | 1.0 | 87 | 12.0 | 3.7 | 2.5 | 0.1 |
| Cottage, with Tuna & Pesto, Asda* | 1 Serving/170g | 184.0 | 10.0 | 108 | 10.0 | 3.5 | 6.0 | 0.7 |
| Cottage, with Tuna & Sweetcorn, HL, Tesco* | 1 Serving/150g | 136.0 | 3.0 | 91 | 12.8 | 4.8 | 2.1 | 0.4 |
| *Cream, Average* | *1 Portion/30g* | *132.0* | *14.0* | *439* | *3.1* | *0.0* | *47.4* | *0.0* |
| Cream, Garlic & Herbs, Light, Boursin* | 1 Portion/20g | 28.0 | 2.0 | 140 | 12.0 | 2.5 | 9.0 | 0.0 |
| *Cream, Reduced Fat, Average* | *1 Seving/20g* | *23.0* | *1.0* | *117* | *13.0* | *4.0* | *5.3* | *0.1* |
| Cream, with Onion & Chives, Morrisons* | 1 Serving/20g | 38.0 | 3.0 | 190 | 11.0 | 3.0 | 15.0 | 0.0 |
| Cream, with Pineapple, Asda* | 1 Serving/40g | 77.0 | 5.0 | 193 | 8.0 | 11.0 | 13.0 | 0.0 |
| Cream, with Red Peppers & Onion, GFY, Asda* | 1 Serving/32g | 42.0 | 2.0 | 130 | 13.0 | 6.0 | 6.0 | 0.0 |
| Creme de Saint Agur, Saint Agur* | 1 Serving/10g | 28.0 | 2.0 | 285 | 13.5 | 2.3 | 24.7 | 0.0 |
| Dairylea, Light, Slices, Kraft* | 1 Slice/25g | 51.0 | 3.0 | 205 | 17.0 | 8.6 | 10.5 | 0.0 |
| Dairylea, Rippers, Straight, Kraft* | 1 Ripper/21g | 60.0 | 4.0 | 285 | 28.0 | 1.0 | 18.5 | 0.0 |
| Dairylea, Slices, Kraft* | 1 Slice/25g | 69.0 | 5.0 | 275 | 13.0 | 8.6 | 20.5 | 0.0 |

## CHEESE

| INFO/WEIGHT | Measure | per Measure | | Nutrition Values per 100g / 100ml | | | | |
|---|---|---|---|---|---|---|---|---|
| | | KCAL | FAT | KCAL | PROT | CARB | FAT | FIBRE |
| *Danish Blue, Average* | *1 Serving/30g* | *106.0* | *9.0* | *352* | *20.7* | *0.0* | *29.1* | *0.0* |
| Demi Pont L'eveque, Finest, Tesco* | 1 Serving/46g | 138.0 | 11.0 | 301 | 21.1 | 0.4 | 23.0 | 0.0 |
| *Dolcelatte, Average* | *1 Serving/30g* | *110.0* | *10.0* | *366* | *17.8* | *0.4* | *32.3* | *0.4* |
| *Double Gloucester, Average* | *1 Serving/30g* | *121.0* | *10.0* | *404* | *24.5* | *0.1* | *34.0* | *0.0* |
| Double Gloucester, with Onion & Chives, Sainsbury's* | 1 Serving/30g | 109.0 | 8.0 | 365 | 22.2 | 5.5 | 28.2 | 0.0 |
| *Doux De Montagne, Average* | *1 Serving/25g* | *88.0* | *7.0* | *352* | *22.9* | *1.5* | *28.3* | *0.0* |
| *Edam, Average* | *1 Serving/10g* | *33.0* | *2.0* | *326* | *25.3* | *0.0* | *24.9* | *0.0* |
| Edam, Dutch, Garlic & Herb Wedge, Asda* | 1 Serving/60g | 197.0 | 15.0 | 329 | 26.0 | 0.0 | 25.0 | 0.0 |
| *Edam, Reduced Fat, Average* | *1 Serving/30g* | *69.0* | *3.0* | *230* | *32.4* | *0.1* | *11.1* | *0.0* |
| *Edam, Slices, Average* | *1 Slice/30g* | *96.0* | *7.0* | *320* | *25.0* | *0.4* | *24.1* | *0.0* |
| *Emmental, Average* | *1 Serving/10g* | *37.0* | *3.0* | *368* | *28.3* | *0.0* | *28.3* | *0.0* |
| Emmental, Light, Slices, President* | 1 Slice/20g | 60.0 | 4.0 | 298 | 34.0 | 0.0 | 18.0 | 0.0 |
| *Farmhouse, Reduced Fat, Healthy Range, Average* | *1 Serving/30g* | *78.0* | *5.0* | *260* | *30.4* | *0.0* | *15.4* | *0.0* |
| *Feta, Average* | *1 Serving/30g* | *79.0* | *6.0* | *262* | *16.3* | *1.0* | *21.5* | *0.0* |
| Feta, Lemon, Asda* | 1 Serving/25g | 75.0 | 7.0 | 302 | 13.2 | 1.0 | 27.2 | 0.6 |
| Fondue, Original, Fromalp* | 1 Pack/400g | 888.0 | 68.0 | 222 | 15.0 | 2.5 | 17.0 | 0.0 |
| Fondue, Swiss, Easy Cook, Tesco* | ¼ Pack/100g | 235.0 | 17.0 | 235 | 15.5 | 4.0 | 17.0 | 0.0 |
| *Fontina, Average* | *1 Serving/28g* | *109.0* | *9.0* | *389* | *25.0* | *0.0* | *32.1* | *0.0* |
| *for Pizza, Grated, Average* | *1 Serving/50g* | *163.0* | *12.0* | *325* | *25.0* | *1.5* | *24.4* | *0.0* |
| *Goats, Average* | *1 Tsp/10g* | *26.0* | *2.0* | *262* | *13.8* | *3.8* | *21.2* | *0.0* |
| Goats, Breaded, Bites, Sainsbury's* | 1 Bite/25g | 84.0 | 6.0 | 337 | 13.0 | 15.1 | 25.0 | 0.8 |
| *Goats, French, Mild, Average* | *1 Serving/30g* | *49.0* | *4.0* | *163* | *11.2* | *3.0* | *11.8* | *0.0* |
| *Goats, Premium, Average* | *1 Serving/30g* | *98.0* | *8.0* | *327* | *20.5* | *0.6* | *26.1* | *0.0* |
| Goats, Welsh, with Garlic & Chives, Tesco* | 1 Serving/32g | 93.0 | 8.0 | 290 | 15.1 | 3.3 | 24.1 | 0.1 |
| Goats, Welsh, with Herbs, Sainsbury's* | 1 Serving/30g | 90.0 | 7.0 | 299 | 15.3 | 3.6 | 24.8 | 0.1 |
| *Gorgonzola, Average* | *1 Serving/30g* | *100.0* | *8.0* | *334* | *20.0* | *0.0* | *27.0* | *0.0* |
| *Gouda, Average* | *1 Serving/30g* | *113.0* | *9.0* | *375* | *24.0* | *0.0* | *31.5* | *0.0* |
| Grana Padano, Italian Cheese, Waitrose* | 1 Serving/14g | 54.0 | 4.0 | 388 | 33.0 | 0.0 | 28.4 | 0.0 |
| *Gruyere* | *1oz/28g* | *115.0* | *9.0* | *409* | *27.2* | *0.0* | *33.3* | *0.0* |
| *Halloumi, Average* | *1 Serving/80g* | *253.0* | *20.0* | *316* | *20.8* | *1.6* | *24.7* | *0.0* |
| Halloumi, Light, Pittas* | 1 Pack/225g | 589.0 | 36.0 | 262 | 27.0 | 2.5 | 16.0 | 0.0 |
| *Italian, Grated, Average* | *1 Serving/30g* | *144.0* | *10.0* | *481* | *44.0* | *1.1* | *33.4* | *0.0* |
| *Jarlsberg, Slices, Average* | *1 Slice/15g* | *54.0* | *4.0* | *360* | *27.0* | *0.0* | *27.0* | *0.0* |
| Lactose Free, Lactofree* | 1 Serving/30g | 103.0 | 8.0 | 344 | 25.3 | 1.0 | 27.0 | 0.0 |
| *Lancashire* | *1oz/28g* | *104.0* | *9.0* | *373* | *23.3* | *0.1* | *31.0* | *0.0* |
| *Manchego* | *1 Serving/70g* | *339.0* | *31.0* | *485* | *22.2* | *0.1* | *44.0* | *0.0* |
| Mascarpone, 25% Less Fat, Sainsbury's* | 1 Portion/30g | 95.0 | 9.0 | 316 | 6.7 | 4.8 | 30.0 | 0.0 |
| *Mascarpone, Average* | *1 Serving/30g* | *131.0* | *13.0* | *437* | *5.6* | *4.1* | *43.6* | *0.0* |
| *Mild, Reduced Fat, Grated, Average* | *1 Serving/30g* | *70.0* | *3.0* | *235* | *31.5* | *2.2* | *11.1* | *0.0* |
| Monterey Jack, Iga* | 1 Serving/28g | 110.0 | 9.0 | 393 | 25.0 | 0.0 | 32.1 | 0.0 |
| Morbier, Sainsbury's* | 1 Serving/10g | 33.0 | 2.0 | 330 | 28.0 | 0.1 | 24.2 | 0.0 |
| *Mozzarella, Average* | *1 Serving/50g* | *137.0* | *10.0* | *275* | *21.2* | *1.2* | *20.6* | *0.0* |
| *Mozzarella, Reduced Fat, Average* | *1 Serving/50g* | *92.0* | *5.0* | *184* | *21.1* | *1.0* | *10.2* | *0.0* |
| Norvegia, Sliced Light, Tine* | 1 Slice/10g | 27.0 | 2.0 | 272 | 32.0 | 0.0 | 16.0 | 0.0 |
| *Ossau-Iraty, Average* | *1 Serving/30g* | *120.0* | *10.0* | *400* | *22.3* | *0.2* | *34.0* | *0.0* |
| *Parmesan, Average* | *1 Tbsp/10g* | *40.0* | *3.0* | *401* | *35.2* | *0.0* | *29.4* | *0.0* |
| Pastrami Flavour, Sandwich, Swiss Processed, Gerber* | 1 Slice/13g | 43.0 | 3.0 | 348 | 24.0 | 0.0 | 28.0 | 0.0 |
| Pecorino, Italian, Tesco* | 1 Serving/30g | 119.0 | 10.0 | 397 | 22.0 | 0.0 | 33.0 | 0.0 |
| Philadelphia, for Salad, Kraft* | 1 Pot/50g | 157.0 | 15.0 | 315 | 6.6 | 2.6 | 30.5 | 0.5 |
| Poivre, Boursin* | 1oz/28g | 116.0 | 12.0 | 414 | 7.0 | 2.0 | 42.0 | 0.0 |
| Port Salut, M & S* | 1oz/28g | 90.0 | 7.0 | 322 | 21.0 | 1.0 | 26.0 | 0.0 |
| Provolone Piccante, Sainsbury's* | 1 Serving/30g | 119.0 | 10.0 | 398 | 25.0 | 0.2 | 33.0 | 0.0 |
| P'tit Louis, St Moret* | 1 Serving/20g | 49.0 | 5.0 | 247 | 5.0 | 5.0 | 23.0 | 0.0 |

C

# CHEESE

| INFO/WEIGHT | Measure | per Measure | | Nutrition Values per 100g / 100ml | | | | |
|---|---|---|---|---|---|---|---|---|
| | | KCAL | FAT | KCAL | PROT | CARB | FAT | FIBRE |
| Quark, Average | 1 Serving/20g | 13.0 | 0.0 | 66 | 11.9 | 4.0 | 0.2 | 0.0 |
| Raclette, Richsmonts* | 1 Slice/28g | 100.0 | 8.0 | 357 | 25.0 | 0.0 | 28.6 | 0.0 |
| Reblochon, Average | 1 Serving/30g | 95.0 | 8.0 | 318 | 19.7 | 0.0 | 26.6 | 0.0 |
| Red Leicester, Average | 1 Serving/30g | 120.0 | 10.0 | 400 | 23.8 | 0.1 | 33.7 | 0.0 |
| Red Leicester, Reduced Fat, Average | 1 Serving/30g | 78.0 | 5.0 | 261 | 30.2 | 0.1 | 15.4 | 0.0 |
| Ricotta, Average | 1 Serving/50g | 67.0 | 5.0 | 134 | 9.3 | 2.9 | 9.5 | 0.0 |
| Roquefort, Average | 1oz/28g | 105.0 | 9.0 | 375 | 19.7 | 0.0 | 32.9 | 0.0 |
| Roule, French, Sainsbury's* | 1 Serving/30g | 96.0 | 9.0 | 321 | 8.5 | 3.0 | 30.5 | 0.0 |
| Roule, Garlic & Parsley, Light, BGTY, Sainsbury's* | 1 Serving/30g | 51.0 | 3.0 | 171 | 16.4 | 2.6 | 10.6 | 0.0 |
| Sage Derby | 1oz/28g | 113.0 | 9.0 | 402 | 24.2 | 0.1 | 33.9 | 0.0 |
| Selles Sur Cher, TTD, Sainsbury's* | 1 Serving/30g | 89.0 | 7.0 | 296 | 20.0 | 0.1 | 24.0 | 0.0 |
| Shropshire, Blue, Average | 1 Serving/50g | 195.0 | 17.0 | 391 | 21.0 | 0.0 | 34.2 | 0.0 |
| Slices, Smoked, with Ham, Aldi* | 1 Slice/21g | 66.0 | 5.0 | 313 | 21.0 | 1.0 | 25.0 | 0.1 |
| Soft, & Creamy with Onions & Garlic, GFY, Asda* | 1 Serving/25g | 31.0 | 1.0 | 126 | 13.0 | 5.0 | 6.0 | 0.0 |
| Soft, & Creamy with Pineapple, Asda* | 1 Serving/32g | 62.0 | 4.0 | 193 | 8.0 | 11.0 | 13.0 | 0.0 |
| Soft, Cracked Pepper, Less Than 5% Fat, M & S* | 1 Serving/30g | 30.0 | 1.0 | 100 | 11.0 | 4.2 | 4.5 | 0.3 |
| Soft, Creamy, with Onion & Chives, BGTY, Sainsbury's* | 1 Serving/20g | 23.0 | 1.0 | 115 | 13.5 | 4.0 | 5.0 | 1.0 |
| Soft, Creamy, with Shallots & Chives, BGTY, Sainsbury's* | 1 Serving/20g | 47.0 | 4.0 | 235 | 5.8 | 2.2 | 22.5 | 0.0 |
| Soft, Double Gloucester, & Chives, M & S* | 1oz/28g | 100.0 | 8.0 | 358 | 20.0 | 9.2 | 26.8 | 0.0 |
| Soft, Extra Light, Average | 1 Serving/20g | 25.0 | 1.0 | 125 | 14.3 | 3.5 | 5.9 | 0.1 |
| Soft, Extra Light, Light Choices, HL, Tesco* | 1 Serving/38g | 49.0 | 2.0 | 130 | 13.5 | 4.1 | 6.1 | 0.0 |
| Soft, Fruit & Rum Halo, Discover* | 1 Serving/25g | 103.0 | 9.0 | 414 | 8.6 | 11.7 | 34.1 | 0.0 |
| Soft, Full Fat, Average | 1 Serving/50g | 156.0 | 15.0 | 312 | 8.2 | 1.7 | 30.3 | 0.0 |
| Soft, Garlic & Herb, Extra Light, Light Choices, Tesco* | 1 Serving/38g | 49.0 | 2.0 | 130 | 12.3 | 5.1 | 6.3 | 0.3 |
| Soft, Garlic & Herb, Lite, Somerfield* | ½ Pot/100g | 191.0 | 15.0 | 191 | 9.0 | 4.9 | 15.0 | 0.0 |
| Soft, Garlic & Herb, Medium Fat, Safeway* | 1 Serving/10g | 19.0 | 1.0 | 195 | 9.3 | 4.9 | 15.0 | 0.0 |
| Soft, Garlic & Herb, Soft & Creamy, Extra Light, Asda* | ¼ Pack/50g | 65.0 | 3.0 | 130 | 13.0 | 6.0 | 6.0 | 0.0 |
| Soft, Goats Milk | 1oz/28g | 55.0 | 4.0 | 198 | 13.1 | 1.0 | 15.8 | 0.0 |
| Soft, Herbs & Garlic, Creamery, Light, Sainsbury's* | 1 Serving/30g | 54.0 | 5.0 | 180 | 7.2 | 3.4 | 15.5 | 0.3 |
| Soft, Less Than 5% Fat, BGTY, Sainsbury's* | 1 Serving/30g | 32.0 | 1.0 | 107 | 14.0 | 3.7 | 4.0 | 0.0 |
| Soft, Light, Average | 1 Serving/30g | 54.0 | 4.0 | 179 | 12.1 | 3.2 | 13.1 | 0.0 |
| Soft, Light, Philadelphia, Kraft* | 1 Serving/30g | 47.0 | 4.0 | 157 | 8.7 | 4.0 | 11.7 | 0.3 |
| Soft, Lighter, Asda* | 1 Serving/33g | 36.0 | 1.0 | 109 | 14.0 | 3.7 | 4.0 | 0.0 |
| Soft, Medium Fat, Average | 1 Serving/30g | 62.0 | 5.0 | 207 | 8.4 | 3.0 | 17.9 | 0.0 |
| Soft, Onion & Chives, Extra Light, Light Choices, Tesco* | 1 Serving/30g | 37.0 | 2.0 | 125 | 11.7 | 5.6 | 6.0 | 0.2 |
| Soft, Onion & Chives, Less Than 5% Fat, M & S* | 1 Serving/30g | 30.0 | 1.0 | 100 | 10.7 | 4.4 | 4.7 | 1.2 |
| Soft, Philadelphia, Extra Light, Kraft* | 1 Serving/30g | 33.0 | 1.0 | 111 | 12.0 | 5.0 | 4.7 | 0.4 |
| Soft, Philadelphia, Garlic & Herb, Light, Kraft* | 1 Serving/30g | 47.0 | 3.0 | 156 | 8.2 | 3.9 | 11.5 | 0.4 |
| Soft, Philadelphia, Kraft* | 1 Serving/30g | 76.0 | 7.0 | 255 | 5.9 | 3.2 | 24.0 | 0.2 |
| Soft, Philadelphia, Light, Basil, Philadelphia, Kraft* | 1 Serving/35g | 51.0 | 4.0 | 146 | 8.0 | 4.0 | 10.5 | 0.5 |
| Soft, Philadelphia, Mini Tubs, Cracked Pepper, Kraft* | 1 Tub/35g | 56.0 | 5.0 | 161 | 7.7 | 2.5 | 13.0 | 0.4 |
| Soft, Philadelphia, Mini Tubs, Extra Light, Kraft* | 1 Tub/35g | 39.0 | 2.0 | 111 | 11.0 | 4.8 | 5.2 | 0.4 |
| Soft, Philadelphia, Mini Tubs, Light, Kraft* | 1 Tub/35g | 57.0 | 5.0 | 163 | 7.1 | 2.9 | 14.0 | 0.0 |
| Soft, Philadelphia, Tomato & Basil, Light, Kraft* | 1 Tbsp/20g | 38.0 | 3.0 | 190 | 7.6 | 4.3 | 16.0 | 0.5 |
| Soft, Philadelphia, with Chive & Onion, Kraft* | 1 Serving/25g | 72.0 | 7.0 | 290 | 6.5 | 6.5 | 29.0 | 0.0 |
| Soft, Philadelphia, with Chives, Light, Kraft* | 1 Serving/30g | 48.0 | 4.0 | 160 | 8.4 | 4.2 | 12.0 | 0.5 |
| Soft, Pineapple, Light, Safeway* | 1 Serving/25g | 47.0 | 3.0 | 190 | 7.6 | 10.8 | 12.5 | 0.0 |
| Soft, Pineapple Halo, Discover* | 1 Serving/25g | 101.0 | 8.0 | 404 | 7.2 | 16.6 | 32.6 | 1.2 |
| Soft, White, Lactofree, Arla* | 1 Spread/10g | 20.0 | 2.0 | 197 | 8.6 | 3.0 | 16.5 | 0.0 |
| Soft, with Black Pepper, Light, Sainsbury's* | ½ Pack/100g | 205.0 | 16.0 | 205 | 11.0 | 3.0 | 16.5 | 0.0 |
| Soft, with Garlic & Herbs, Full Fat, Deli, Boursin* | 1 Serving/28g | 84.0 | 8.0 | 299 | 3.5 | 5.0 | 29.5 | 0.0 |
| Soft, with Garlic & Herbs, Medium Fat, Westacre* | 1 Serving/30g | 56.0 | 5.0 | 188 | 8.0 | 3.0 | 16.0 | 0.1 |
| Soft, with Garlic & Herbs, Sainsbury's* | 1 Serving/33g | 89.0 | 9.0 | 269 | 6.1 | 2.7 | 26.0 | 0.0 |

| CHEESE | Measure INFO/WEIGHT | per Measure KCAL | FAT | Nutrition Values per 100g / 100ml KCAL | PROT | CARB | FAT | FIBRE |
|---|---|---|---|---|---|---|---|---|
| Soft, with Garlic and Herbs, Lighter, Asda* | ½ Pack/100g | 106.0 | 4.0 | 106 | 11.8 | 4.3 | 4.4 | 0.1 |
| Soft, with Onion & Chives, Lighter, Asda* | 1 Serving/30g | 31.0 | 1.0 | 105 | 11.6 | 4.5 | 4.3 | 0.2 |
| Soft & Smooth, Extra Light, HL, Tesco* | 1 Serving/30g | 39.0 | 2.0 | 130 | 14.2 | 3.7 | 6.0 | 0.0 |
| *Soya* | *1oz/28g* | *89.0* | *8.0* | *319* | *18.3* | *0.0* | *27.3* | *0.0* |
| *Stilton, Average* | *1 Serving/30g* | *123.0* | *11.0* | *410* | *22.4* | *0.1* | *35.5* | *0.0* |
| *Stilton, Blue, Average* | *1 Serving/30g* | *124.0* | *11.0* | *412* | *22.8* | *0.1* | *35.7* | *0.0* |
| Stilton, White, & Apricot, M & S* | 1oz/28g | 94.0 | 6.0 | 337 | 13.8 | 18.5 | 23.1 | 0.0 |
| Stilton, White, & Cranberry, M & S* | 1oz/28g | 101.0 | 7.0 | 362 | 18.2 | 15.5 | 25.3 | 0.0 |
| *Stilton, White, Average* | *1oz/28g* | *101.0* | *9.0* | *362* | *19.9* | *0.1* | *31.3* | *0.0* |
| Stilton, White, with Apricot, Somerfield* | 1oz/28g | 103.0 | 8.0 | 369 | 16.0 | 8.0 | 30.0 | 0.0 |
| Stilton, White, with Cranberries, Tesco* | 1 Serving/50g | 184.0 | 15.0 | 368 | 15.8 | 9.5 | 29.7 | 0.7 |
| Stilton, White, with Mango & Ginger, Tesco* | 1/3 Pack/65g | 227.0 | 14.0 | 350 | 13.1 | 25.8 | 21.6 | 0.6 |
| Substitute, Mozzarella Style, Grated, Value, Tesco* | 1 Serving/40g | 120.0 | 8.0 | 300 | 25.0 | 2.5 | 21.1 | 0.0 |
| Supreme Des Ducs, Ligne Et Plaisir* | 1 Serving/50g | 100.0 | 6.0 | 200 | 21.0 | 2.0 | 12.0 | 0.0 |
| Wedge, Camembert, Breaded, Morrisons* | 1 Wedge/25g | 88.0 | 6.0 | 352 | 15.1 | 22.9 | 22.2 | 2.0 |
| Wedge, Leerdammer* | 1 Serving/30g | 112.0 | 9.0 | 373 | 28.3 | 0.0 | 28.6 | 0.0 |
| *Wensleydale, Average* | *1 Serving/25g* | *92.0* | *8.0* | *369* | *22.4* | *0.1* | *31.0* | *0.0* |
| Wensleydale with Cranberries, Sainsbury's* | 1 Serving/50g | 179.0 | 14.0 | 359 | 20.7 | 6.4 | 27.8 | 0.0 |
| **CHEESE ALTERNATIVE** | | | | | | | | |
| Cheezly, Cream, Original Flavour, Redwood* | 1 Pack/113g | 357.0 | 34.0 | 316 | 5.6 | 4.8 | 30.5 | 0.0 |
| Cheezly, Feta Style, in Oil, Redwood* | 1 Serving/25g | 119.0 | 12.0 | 475 | 2.5 | 10.6 | 47.0 | 0.0 |
| Cheezly, Mozzarella Style, Redwood* | 1 Portion/25g | 69.0 | 6.0 | 274 | 5.4 | 5.9 | 25.4 | 1.0 |
| Cheezly, Redwood* | 1 Serving/20g | 49.0 | 4.0 | 247 | 3.5 | 18.5 | 17.6 | 1.7 |
| Vegetarian, Average | 1 Serving/30g | 110.0 | 8.0 | 368 | 28.2 | 0.0 | 28.1 | 0.0 |
| **CHEESE HEADS** | | | | | | | | |
| Cheese, Walkers* | 1 Bag/27g | 128.0 | 6.0 | 475 | 10.8 | 58.0 | 22.3 | 2.8 |
| Cheese & Onion, Walkers* | 1 Bag/27g | 128.0 | 6.0 | 475 | 10.8 | 58.0 | 22.3 | 2.8 |
| **CHEESE ON TOAST** | | | | | | | | |
| Average | 1oz/28g | 106.0 | 7.0 | 380 | 13.8 | 23.8 | 26.3 | 0.7 |
| **CHEESE PUFFS** | | | | | | | | |
| Cheeky, Tesco* | 1 Bag/20g | 108.0 | 7.0 | 542 | 6.7 | 50.2 | 34.9 | 0.0 |
| Morrisons* | 1 Bag/25g | 135.0 | 9.0 | 542 | 6.7 | 50.2 | 34.9 | 1.1 |
| Sainsbury's* | 1 Pack/100g | 530.0 | 32.0 | 530 | 9.1 | 51.4 | 32.0 | 1.9 |
| Shapers, Boots* | 1 Bag/16g | 80.0 | 4.0 | 500 | 7.1 | 64.0 | 24.0 | 0.9 |
| Weight Watchers* | 1 Pack/18g | 75.0 | 2.0 | 417 | 7.8 | 72.4 | 10.7 | 2.2 |
| **CHEESE SINGLES** | | | | | | | | |
| 50% Less Fat, Asda* | 1 Slice/20g | 38.0 | 2.0 | 190 | 19.0 | 6.0 | 10.0 | 0.0 |
| American, 2% Milk, Kraft* | 1 Slice/19g | 45.0 | 3.0 | 237 | 21.0 | 5.3 | 15.8 | 0.0 |
| Cheese Food Slices, 50% Less Fat, BGTY, Sainsbury's* | 1 Slice/20g | 39.0 | 2.0 | 195 | 19.2 | 7.1 | 10.0 | 0.0 |
| Half Fat, Co-Op* | 1 Slice/20g | 47.0 | 2.0 | 235 | 25.0 | 7.0 | 12.0 | 0.0 |
| Kraft* | 1 Slice/20g | 52.0 | 4.0 | 260 | 13.5 | 7.6 | 18.5 | 0.0 |
| **CHEESE SLICES** | | | | | | | | |
| Bettabuy, Morrisons* | 1 Slice/17g | 47.0 | 4.0 | 274 | 14.0 | 4.0 | 22.5 | 0.0 |
| Cheddar, Mild, Value, Tesco* | 1 Slice/24g | 100.0 | 8.0 | 410 | 25.0 | 0.1 | 34.4 | 0.0 |
| Gouda, Tesco* | 1 Serving/95g | 356.0 | 29.0 | 375 | 23.0 | 0.0 | 31.0 | 0.0 |
| Havarti, Tesco* | 1 Slice/25g | 85.0 | 6.0 | 340 | 24.0 | 1.4 | 26.0 | 0.0 |
| Jarlsberg, Tesco* | 1 Slice/25g | 91.0 | 7.0 | 365 | 27.5 | 0.0 | 28.0 | 0.0 |
| Leerdammer* | 1 Slice/25g | 89.0 | 7.0 | 358 | 27.0 | 0.1 | 28.0 | 0.0 |
| Light, The Laughing Cow, Fromageries Bel* | 1 Slice/20g | 41.0 | 2.0 | 203 | 21.0 | 6.0 | 10.5 | 0.0 |
| Light Choices, Tesco* | 1 Slice/20g | 37.0 | 2.0 | 185 | 19.8 | 4.0 | 10.6 | 0.0 |
| Reduced Fat, GFY, Asda* | 1 Slice/20g | 38.0 | 2.0 | 191 | 21.0 | 4.2 | 10.0 | 0.0 |
| **CHEESE SPREAD** | | | | | | | | |
| 60% Less Fat, Asda* | 1 Serving/30g | 52.0 | 3.0 | 174 | 16.0 | 7.3 | 9.0 | 0.0 |

C

| | Measure INFO/WEIGHT | per Measure KCAL | FAT | Nutrition Values per 100g / 100ml KCAL | PROT | CARB | FAT | FIBRE |
|---|---|---|---|---|---|---|---|---|
| **CHEESE SPREAD** | | | | | | | | |
| Asda* | 1 Serving/33g | 92.0 | 8.0 | 280 | 9.0 | 7.0 | 24.0 | 0.0 |
| BFY, Morrisons* | 1 Serving/25g | 43.0 | 2.0 | 172 | 13.5 | 6.5 | 8.5 | 0.0 |
| BGTY, Sainsbury's* | 1 Serving/25g | 28.0 | 1.0 | 111 | 11.0 | 4.3 | 5.5 | 0.4 |
| Cheese & Garlic, Primula* | 1 Serving/20g | 49.0 | 4.0 | 247 | 15.7 | 4.3 | 18.6 | 0.0 |
| Cheese & Salmon with Dill, Primula* | 1 Serving/30g | 78.0 | 6.0 | 261 | 17.6 | 3.8 | 19.5 | 0.0 |
| Cream, Light, Sainsbury's* | 1 Serving/50g | 93.0 | 8.0 | 187 | 7.8 | 4.1 | 15.5 | 0.3 |
| Creamery, Light, Sainsbury's* | 1 Serving/25g | 46.0 | 4.0 | 185 | 9.0 | 3.5 | 15.0 | 0.0 |
| Dairylea, Light, Tub, Kraft* | 1 Serving/30g | 44.0 | 2.0 | 147 | 14.5 | 6.1 | 7.0 | 0.0 |
| Dairylea, Tub, Kraft* | 1 Serving/25g | 60.0 | 5.0 | 240 | 11.0 | 5.3 | 19.5 | 0.0 |
| Garlic & Herbs, Light, Benecol* | 1 Serving/20g | 35.0 | 3.0 | 174 | 7.8 | 4.2 | 14.0 | 0.7 |
| Low Fat, Weight Watchers* | 1 Serving/50g | 56.0 | 1.0 | 112 | 18.1 | 3.4 | 2.9 | 1.2 |
| Mediterranean Soft & Creamy, Extra Light, Asda* | 1 Serving/32g | 42.0 | 2.0 | 130 | 13.0 | 6.0 | 6.0 | 0.0 |
| Original, Primula* | 1 Serving/30g | 68.0 | 6.0 | 227 | 12.9 | 2.1 | 18.7 | 0.6 |
| Soft, Low Fat, M & S* | 1 Pack/100g | 111.0 | 4.0 | 111 | 13.0 | 4.2 | 4.5 | 0.3 |
| Squeeze, Light, The Laughing Cow, Fromageries Bel* | 1 Portion/30g | 42.0 | 2.0 | 139 | 12.0 | 7.0 | 7.0 | 5.0 |
| Squeeze, Original, The Laughing Cow, Fromageries Bel* | 1 Portion/30g | 71.0 | 6.0 | 236 | 9.0 | 5.0 | 20.0 | 0.0 |
| Triangles, 50% Less Fat, Morrisons* | 1 Portion/18g | 29.0 | 1.0 | 166 | 15.0 | 8.5 | 8.0 | 0.0 |
| with Chives, Primula* | 1 Serving/30g | 76.0 | 6.0 | 253 | 15.0 | 1.0 | 21.0 | 0.0 |
| with Garlic & Herb, Soft, Free From, Sainsbury's* | 1 Serving/30g | 91.0 | 9.0 | 302 | 2.5 | 5.5 | 30.0 | 0.1 |
| with Ham, Primula* | 1 Serving/30g | 70.0 | 6.0 | 232 | 13.5 | 2.1 | 18.8 | 0.3 |
| with Shrimp, Primula* | 1 Tbsp/15g | 38.0 | 3.0 | 253 | 15.0 | 1.0 | 21.0 | 0.0 |
| **CHEESE STRAWS** | | | | | | | | |
| & Bacon, Party, Tesco* | 1 Straw/13g | 40.0 | 3.0 | 321 | 10.5 | 23.8 | 20.4 | 2.1 |
| Cheddar, M & S* | 1 Straw/11g | 59.0 | 4.0 | 535 | 14.9 | 40.1 | 34.9 | 2.4 |
| Finest, Tesco* | 1 Straw/7g | 39.0 | 3.0 | 558 | 13.3 | 41.5 | 37.6 | 1.5 |
| Fudges* | 1 Serving/10g | 53.0 | 3.0 | 534 | 14.9 | 40.1 | 34.9 | 0.0 |
| Homemade Or Bakery, Average | 1 Straw/41g | 173.0 | 13.0 | 422 | 11.9 | 24.1 | 30.7 | 0.7 |
| Selection, Sainsbury's* | 1 Straw/7g | 41.0 | 3.0 | 558 | 16.6 | 34.5 | 39.3 | 2.8 |
| **CHEESE TRIANGLES** | | | | | | | | |
| Average | 1 Triangle/14g | 35.0 | 3.0 | 247 | 10.6 | 6.6 | 19.9 | 0.0 |
| Dairylea, Light, Kraft* | 1 Triangle/20g | 30.0 | 1.0 | 148 | 14.5 | 5.5 | 7.0 | 0.0 |
| Eat Smart, Morrisons* | 1 Triangle/18g | 30.0 | 1.0 | 166 | 15.0 | 8.5 | 8.0 | 0.0 |
| Extra Light, The Laughing Cow, Fromageries Bel* | 1 Triangle/18g | 20.0 | 1.0 | 116 | 15.0 | 6.5 | 3.0 | 0.0 |
| Light, Swiss, The Laughing Cow, Fromageries Bel* | 1 Triangle/18g | 25.0 | 1.0 | 141 | 13.0 | 6.5 | 7.0 | 0.0 |
| Light Choices, Tesco* | 1 Triangle/18g | 30.0 | 1.0 | 170 | 17.5 | 8.5 | 7.0 | 0.0 |
| Original, The Laughing Cow, Fromageries Bel* | 1 Triangle/18g | 42.0 | 3.0 | 239 | 11.0 | 6.0 | 19.0 | 0.0 |
| Reduced Fat, Average | 1 Triangle/18g | 30.0 | 2.0 | 170 | 14.8 | 7.4 | 9.0 | 0.0 |
| **CHEESE TWISTS** | | | | | | | | |
| All Butter, M & S* | 1 Pack/125g | 625.0 | 33.0 | 500 | 14.2 | 50.2 | 26.7 | 3.2 |
| Asda* | 1 Twist/8g | 42.0 | 2.0 | 500 | 14.0 | 48.0 | 28.0 | 5.0 |
| Gruyere, & Poppy Seed, Truly Irresistible, Co-Op* | 1 Twist/8g | 42.0 | 2.0 | 520 | 13.2 | 48.8 | 30.1 | 2.5 |
| Safeway* | 1 Twist/6g | 29.0 | 2.0 | 496 | 13.6 | 46.2 | 28.5 | 5.6 |
| **CHEESECAKE** | | | | | | | | |
| American Red White & Blueberry, Sainsbury's* | 1/6 Cake/83g | 264.0 | 15.0 | 318 | 3.8 | 35.1 | 18.5 | 0.4 |
| Apple & Cinnamon, Baked, M & S* | 1 Serving/116g | 390.0 | 22.0 | 335 | 3.7 | 39.7 | 18.9 | 2.1 |
| Apricot, HL, Tesco* | 1 Pot/100g | 179.0 | 2.0 | 179 | 4.9 | 34.7 | 2.3 | 1.6 |
| Average | 1 Slice/115g | 490.0 | 41.0 | 426 | 3.7 | 24.6 | 35.5 | 0.4 |
| Belgian Chocolate, M & S* | 1 Slice/100g | 385.0 | 24.0 | 385 | 5.3 | 39.2 | 23.9 | 2.5 |
| Belgian Chocolate Truffle, TTD, Sainsbury's* | 1/6 Cake/92g | 365.0 | 25.0 | 399 | 4.2 | 35.6 | 26.9 | 3.5 |
| Blackcurrant, Perfectly Balanced, Waitrose* | 1/6 Cake/99g | 212.0 | 4.0 | 214 | 4.0 | 39.6 | 3.6 | 2.4 |
| Blackcurrant, Value, Tesco* | 1 Serving/70g | 174.0 | 9.0 | 248 | 2.8 | 31.4 | 12.3 | 1.0 |
| Blackcurrant, VLH Kitchens* | 1 Serving/120g | 341.0 | 10.8 | 285 | 3.4 | 32.0 | 16.4 | 0.9 |
| Blackcurrant, Weight Watchers* | 1 Cake/103g | 191.0 | 3.0 | 185 | 4.6 | 35.4 | 2.8 | 3.5 |

C

| CHEESECAKE | Measure INFO/WEIGHT | per Measure KCAL | per Measure FAT | Nutrition Values per 100g / 100ml KCAL | PROT | CARB | FAT | FIBRE |
|---|---|---|---|---|---|---|---|---|
| Blackcurrant Devonshire, McVitie's* | 1/6 Cake/67g | 193.0 | 11.0 | 288 | 3.8 | 29.7 | 17.1 | 1.7 |
| Blackcurrant Swirl, Heinz* | 1/5 Cake/87g | 241.0 | 13.0 | 277 | 4.1 | 30.3 | 15.4 | 3.6 |
| Blueberry & Lemon Flavour Wedges, Sainsbury's* | 1 Serving/80g | 262.0 | 17.0 | 327 | 5.1 | 29.2 | 21.1 | 1.2 |
| Caramel Swirl, Cadbury* | 1 Slice/91g | 373.0 | 23.0 | 410 | 6.0 | 40.1 | 25.8 | 0.0 |
| Cherry, BGTY, Sainsbury's* | 1 Serving/91g | 181.0 | 4.0 | 199 | 4.6 | 35.5 | 4.3 | 0.5 |
| Cherry, Low Fat, Tesco* | 1 Serving/91g | 185.0 | 4.0 | 203 | 3.4 | 38.0 | 4.1 | 0.9 |
| Cherry, Low Saturated Fat, Waitrose* | 1/6 Cake/108g | 198.0 | 2.0 | 184 | 3.6 | 37.6 | 2.1 | 0.4 |
| Chocolate, & Irish Cream Liqueur, Tesco* | 1 Serving/93g | 385.0 | 28.0 | 414 | 5.0 | 30.7 | 30.1 | 0.8 |
| Chocolate, M & S* | 1oz/28g | 106.0 | 6.0 | 380 | 6.5 | 40.3 | 21.5 | 0.4 |
| Chocolate, Pure Indulgence, Thorntons* | 1 Serving/75g | 307.0 | 18.0 | 410 | 5.6 | 44.3 | 23.4 | 0.6 |
| Chocolate, Tesco* | 1 Serving/91g | 317.0 | 17.0 | 348 | 6.2 | 37.8 | 19.1 | 1.5 |
| Chocolate, Weight Watchers* | 1 Cake/95g | 143.0 | 4.0 | 151 | 7.5 | 20.7 | 4.0 | 0.7 |
| Chocolate & Hazelnut, Sara Lee* | 1 Serving/65g | 224.0 | 14.0 | 345 | 6.5 | 31.2 | 21.4 | 1.2 |
| Chocolate & Hazlenut, Gold, Sara Lee* | 1 Slice/65g | 205.0 | 13.0 | 316 | 5.9 | 28.7 | 19.7 | 1.1 |
| Chocolate & Vanilla, Reduced Fat, M & S* | 1 Serving/114g | 319.0 | 14.0 | 280 | 7.0 | 37.9 | 12.0 | 1.5 |
| Chocolate Chip, M & S* | 1oz/28g | 109.0 | 7.0 | 391 | 5.1 | 39.7 | 23.6 | 0.2 |
| Chocolate Swirl, Deeply Delicious, Heinz* | 1/5 Cake/82g | 221.0 | 9.0 | 271 | 4.6 | 37.4 | 11.5 | 4.7 |
| Chocolate Truffle, HL, Tesco* | 1 Slice/96g | 250.0 | 13.0 | 260 | 10.3 | 23.7 | 13.8 | 6.5 |
| Commercially Prepared | 1/6 Cake/80g | 257.0 | 18.0 | 321 | 5.5 | 25.5 | 22.5 | 0.4 |
| Devonshire Strawberry, McVitie's* | 1/6 Cake/66g | 192.0 | 11.0 | 291 | 4.4 | 31.8 | 16.2 | 3.6 |
| Double Chocolate Wedge, Sainsbury's* | 1 Serving/75g | 327.0 | 25.0 | 436 | 5.7 | 29.0 | 33.0 | 1.7 |
| Fudge, Tesco* | 1 Serving/102g | 384.0 | 24.0 | 376 | 4.6 | 37.5 | 23.1 | 0.5 |
| Irish Cream, McVitie's* | ¼ Slice/190g | 616.0 | 37.0 | 324 | 4.4 | 33.0 | 19.4 | 0.4 |
| Lemon, Asda* | 1 Slice/90g | 319.0 | 21.0 | 354 | 4.3 | 31.2 | 23.5 | 1.1 |
| Lemon, BGTY, Sainsbury's* | 1/6 Cake/71g | 142.0 | 3.0 | 200 | 4.4 | 37.0 | 3.8 | 0.5 |
| Lemon, Carb Control, Tesco^ | 1 Serving/85g | 269.0 | 23.0 | 316 | 8.6 | 9.6 | 27.1 | 11.1 |
| Lemon, Creamy, Weight Watchers* | 1 Cake/98g | 186.0 | 5.0 | 191 | 5.8 | 31.4 | 4.7 | 1.9 |
| Lemon, Sainsbury's* | 1 Serving/180g | 650.0 | 37.0 | 361 | 4.0 | 39.9 | 20.6 | 1.3 |
| Lemon, Swirl, Asda* | 1 Pack/125g | 445.0 | 30.0 | 356 | 3.1 | 32.1 | 23.9 | 1.8 |
| Lemon, Tesco* | 1 Slice/93g | 315.0 | 21.0 | 339 | 5.2 | 28.6 | 22.6 | 0.3 |
| Lemon Creamy & Light, M & S* | 1/6 Cake/68g | 236.0 | 14.0 | 350 | 3.5 | 32.3 | 20.4 | 0.4 |
| Lemon Meringue, Tesco* | 1 Slice/94g | 352.0 | 25.0 | 375 | 3.8 | 30.1 | 26.6 | 0.3 |
| Mandarin, Light Choices, Tesco* | 1/6 Cake/92g | 170.0 | 3.0 | 185 | 4.1 | 33.1 | 3.8 | 1.5 |
| Mandarin, Morrisons* | 1 Serving/135g | 335.0 | 17.0 | 248 | 3.8 | 32.2 | 12.5 | 0.8 |
| Mandarin, Weight Watchers* | 1 Cake/103g | 180.0 | 3.0 | 175 | 4.6 | 32.9 | 2.8 | 1.5 |
| Praline, Asda* | 1/8 Cake/62g | 226.0 | 15.0 | 364 | 7.0 | 30.0 | 24.0 | 3.2 |
| Raspberry, BGTY, Sainsbury's* | 1 Pot/95g | 154.0 | 2.0 | 163 | 6.6 | 28.2 | 2.6 | 2.8 |
| Raspberry, Creamy, Tesco* | 1 Serving/100g | 365.0 | 23.0 | 365 | 5.9 | 32.1 | 23.4 | 0.9 |
| Raspberry, Light Choices, Tesco* | 1 Cake/95g | 185.0 | 4.0 | 195 | 4.3 | 34.7 | 4.3 | 1.3 |
| Raspberry, Low Saturated Fat, Waitrose* | 1/6 Cake/108g | 187.0 | 2.0 | 174 | 3.6 | 35.4 | 2.0 | 0.4 |
| Raspberry, M & S* | 1 Slice/105g | 331.0 | 22.0 | 315 | 5.0 | 32.2 | 20.5 | 1.0 |
| Raspberry, Perfectly Balanced, Waitrose* | 1 Serving/106g | 212.0 | 4.0 | 200 | 4.0 | 36.2 | 3.5 | 1.7 |
| Raspberry & Mascarpone, Best, Morrisons* | 1 Cake/84g | 257.0 | 14.0 | 306 | 3.9 | 34.8 | 16.7 | 1.0 |
| Raspberry Brulee, M & S* | 1 Serving/100g | 255.0 | 13.0 | 255 | 5.7 | 29.7 | 12.9 | 2.1 |
| Raspberry Rapture, Slices, Tesco* | 1 Slice/110g | 341.0 | 20.0 | 310 | 4.2 | 30.8 | 18.5 | 1.8 |
| Raspberry Ripple, M & S* | 1oz/28g | 84.0 | 4.0 | 300 | 5.9 | 32.8 | 15.6 | 0.3 |
| Raspberry Swirl, Heinz* | 1 Serving/100g | 266.0 | 14.0 | 266 | 3.9 | 30.1 | 14.5 | 2.8 |
| Rhubarb Crumble, Sainsbury's* | 1 Serving/114g | 268.0 | 11.0 | 235 | 3.1 | 34.8 | 9.3 | 2.4 |
| Sticky Toffee, Tesco* | 1 Slice/66g | 247.0 | 16.0 | 375 | 4.0 | 35.3 | 24.2 | 0.5 |
| Strawberries & Cream, Finest, Tesco* | 1 Serving/104g | 325.0 | 22.0 | 312 | 4.3 | 25.3 | 21.5 | 0.5 |
| Strawberries & Devonshire Cream, Heinz* | 1/6 Cake/66g | 184.0 | 10.0 | 279 | 3.9 | 31.4 | 15.3 | 3.7 |
| Strawberry, Baked New York, Sara Lee* | 1 Serving/100g | 248.0 | 10.0 | 248 | 4.7 | 34.9 | 9.9 | 0.7 |
| Strawberry, Creamy, Weight Watchers* | 1 Cake/105g | 187.0 | 3.0 | 178 | 4.7 | 34.2 | 2.5 | 2.2 |

C

| | Measure INFO/WEIGHT | per Measure KCAL | FAT | Nutrition Values per 100g / 100ml KCAL | PROT | CARB | FAT | FIBRE |
|---|---|---|---|---|---|---|---|---|
| **CHEESECAKE** | | | | | | | | |
| Strawberry, Finest, Tesco* | 1 Slice/113g | 383.0 | 25.0 | 339 | 4.8 | 30.1 | 22.2 | 0.9 |
| Strawberry, Frozen, Sainsbury's* | 1/6 Cake/84g | 277.0 | 14.0 | 332 | 4.3 | 40.4 | 17.0 | 2.3 |
| Strawberry, Heinz* | 1 Pack/245g | 588.0 | 31.0 | 240 | 3.4 | 28.1 | 12.7 | 2.4 |
| Strawberry, Tesco* | 1 Serving/100g | 254.0 | 12.0 | 254 | 3.9 | 32.5 | 12.0 | 0.0 |
| Strawberry Shortcake, Sara Lee* | 1/6 Cake/68g | 230.0 | 16.0 | 337 | 4.9 | 27.6 | 23.0 | 0.5 |
| Summerfruit, GFY, Asda* | 1/6 Cake/92g | 175.0 | 4.0 | 191 | 3.7 | 34.5 | 4.2 | 1.4 |
| The Ultimate New York Baked, Entenmann's* | 1 Cake/100g | 347.0 | 21.0 | 347 | 4.2 | 35.7 | 21.3 | 0.9 |
| Toffee, American Style, Asda* | 1 Serving/75g | 269.0 | 16.0 | 359 | 4.5 | 38.0 | 21.0 | 3.8 |
| Toffee, Asda* | 1 Cake/87g | 295.0 | 19.0 | 339 | 4.3 | 31.0 | 22.0 | 3.5 |
| Toffee, M & S* | 1 Serving/105g | 357.0 | 23.0 | 340 | 5.2 | 37.2 | 21.5 | 0.9 |
| Toffee, Tesco* | 1 Serving/100g | 265.0 | 13.0 | 265 | 4.3 | 33.1 | 12.9 | 0.8 |
| Toffee & Pecan, Wedge, Sainsbury's* | 1 Serving/75g | 296.0 | 22.0 | 395 | 5.4 | 28.1 | 29.0 | 3.1 |
| Vanilla, Tesco* | 1 Serving/115g | 417.0 | 28.0 | 363 | 5.7 | 29.4 | 24.7 | 0.6 |
| Vanilla Chocolate, Baked, Slice, Sainsbury's* | 1 Slice/90g | 349.0 | 23.0 | 388 | 5.7 | 33.8 | 25.6 | 2.7 |
| Zesty Lemon, M & S* | 1/6 Cake/97g | 325.0 | 19.0 | 335 | 4.0 | 38.7 | 19.5 | 2.6 |
| **CHEETOS** | | | | | | | | |
| Cheese, Walkers* | 1 Bag/24g | 120.0 | 6.0 | 500 | 6.5 | 61.0 | 26.0 | 1.3 |
| **CHERRIES** | | | | | | | | |
| *Black, Fresh, Average* | *1 Serving/80g* | *41.0* | *0.0* | *51* | *0.9* | *11.5* | *0.1* | *1.6* |
| *Black, in Syrup, Average* | *1 Serving/242g* | *160.0* | *0.0* | *66* | *0.6* | *16.0* | *0.0* | *0.7* |
| Dried, Sainsbury's* | 1 Tbsp/14g | 45.0 | 0.0 | 319 | 3.8 | 72.4 | 1.5 | 6.2 |
| *Glace, Average* | *1oz/28g* | *79.0* | *0.0* | *280* | *0.3* | *71.2* | *0.1* | *1.1* |
| Morello, Dried, Graze* | 1 Pack/30g | 100.0 | 0.0 | 335 | 4.5 | 82.0 | 1.5 | 0.0 |
| *Raw, Average* | *1oz/28g* | *14.0* | *0.0* | *49* | *0.9* | *11.2* | *0.1* | *1.4* |
| *Stewed, with Sugar, Average* | *1oz/28g* | *23.0* | *0.0* | *82* | *0.7* | *21.0* | *0.1* | *0.7* |
| *Stewed, without Sugar, Average* | *1oz/28g* | *12.0* | *0.0* | *42* | *0.8* | *10.1* | *0.1* | *0.8* |
| **CHESTNUTS** | | | | | | | | |
| *Average* | *1 Nut/10g* | *17.0* | *0.0* | *170* | *2.0* | *36.6* | *2.7* | *4.1* |
| **CHEWING GUM** | | | | | | | | |
| Airwaves, Sugar Free, Wrigleys* | 1 Pack/15g | 23.0 | 0.0 | 155 | 0.0 | 62.0 | 0.0 | 0.0 |
| Extra, Peppermint, Sugar Free, Wrigleys* | 1 Piece/2g | 3.0 | 0.0 | 155 | 0.0 | 39.0 | 0.0 | 0.0 |
| Spearmint, Wrigleys* | 1 Piece/3g | 9.0 | 0.0 | 295 | 0.0 | 73.0 | 0.0 | 0.0 |
| Splash, Rapberry & Peach, Trident* | 1 Piece/2g | 4.0 | 0.0 | 180 | 1.6 | 68.5 | 0.5 | 0.0 |
| **CHICK PEAS** | | | | | | | | |
| *Dried, Average* | *1 Serving/100g* | *319.0* | *5.0* | *319* | *21.7* | *47.4* | *5.4* | *8.0* |
| *Dried, Boiled, Average* | *1 Serving/75g* | *85.0* | *2.0* | *114* | *7.3* | *16.4* | *2.2* | *2.5* |
| *in Salted Water, Canned, Average* | *1 Can/179g* | *204.0* | *5.0* | *114* | *7.2* | *14.9* | *2.9* | *4.1* |
| *in Water, Canned, Average* | *1 Can/250g* | *282.0* | *7.0* | *113* | *7.2* | *15.3* | *2.6* | *4.8* |
| **CHICKEN** | | | | | | | | |
| Bites, Battered, Tesco* | 1 Pack/200g | 440.0 | 29.0 | 220 | 15.2 | 7.6 | 14.3 | 2.0 |
| Bites, Hot & Spicy, Tesco* | 1 Pack/110g | 143.0 | 2.0 | 130 | 18.9 | 9.6 | 1.6 | 2.5 |
| Bites, Southern Fried, Tesco* | 1 Pack/300g | 720.0 | 33.0 | 240 | 18.1 | 16.9 | 11.1 | 2.1 |
| Bites, Tikka, Average | 1 Serving/50g | 96.0 | 5.0 | 193 | 20.7 | 3.8 | 10.5 | 1.9 |
| Breast, Chargrilled, Premium, Average | 1 Piece/10g | 20.0 | 1.0 | 197 | 21.6 | 1.5 | 11.2 | 0.3 |
| Breast, Chargrilled, Sliced, Average | 1 Slice/19g | 24.0 | 1.0 | 124 | 24.4 | 0.5 | 2.7 | 0.4 |
| *Breast, Diced, Average* | *1 Serving/188g* | *215.0* | *4.0* | *114* | *25.0* | *0.1* | *2.0* | *0.1* |
| Breast, Eastern Spices, Birds Eye* | 1 Portion/175g | 308.0 | 21.0 | 176 | 13.5 | 3.8 | 11.9 | 1.5 |
| Breast, Escalope, Pesto Chargrilled, M & S* | 1 Serving/100g | 135.0 | 6.0 | 135 | 19.6 | 0.7 | 6.2 | 0.6 |
| *Breast, Escalope, Plain, Average* | *1 Serving/100g* | *110.0* | *2.0* | *110* | *22.3* | *0.7* | *2.2* | *0.5* |
| Breast, Fillets, Breaded, Average | 1 Fillet/112g | 246.0 | 12.0 | 220 | 17.5 | 14.0 | 10.4 | 1.3 |
| Breast, Fillets, Breaded, Lemon & Pepper, Average | 1 Fillet/89g | 133.0 | 2.0 | 150 | 22.0 | 10.1 | 2.3 | 1.3 |
| Breast, Fillets, Cajun, Average | 1 Fillet/93g | 124.0 | 3.0 | 134 | 23.6 | 3.5 | 2.8 | 0.3 |
| Breast, Fillets, Chargrilled, Average | 1 Serving/100g | 120.0 | 1.0 | 120 | 27.3 | 0.3 | 1.1 | 0.3 |

# CHICKEN

| | Measure INFO/WEIGHT | per Measure KCAL | per Measure FAT | Nutrition Values per 100g / 100ml KCAL | PROT | CARB | FAT | FIBRE |
|---|---|---|---|---|---|---|---|---|
| Breast, Fillets, Garlic & Herb, Tesco* | 1 Fillet/135g | 290.0 | 12.0 | 215 | 18.9 | 14.4 | 9.0 | 1.3 |
| Breast, Fillets, Korma Style, Average | 1 Serving/100g | 131.0 | 3.0 | 131 | 27.4 | 0.8 | 2.7 | 0.5 |
| Breast, Fillets, Lemon Parsley, M & S* | ½ Pack/145g | 232.0 | 3.0 | 160 | 14.3 | 20.7 | 2.4 | 4.3 |
| Breast, Fillets, Lime & Coriander, Just Add, M & S* | 1 Pack/140g | 182.0 | 2.0 | 130 | 26.1 | 2.7 | 1.7 | 0.1 |
| Breast, Fillets, Mexican Style, Cooked, Ready to Eat, Asda* | ½ Pack/100g | 147.0 | 1.0 | 147 | 27.8 | 5.5 | 1.5 | 0.1 |
| *Breast, Fillets, Mini, Raw, Average* | *1oz/28g* | *34.0* | *0.0* | *121* | *26.9* | *0.2* | *1.5* | *0.1* |
| *Breast, Fillets, Organic, Average* | *1 Serving/150g* | *153.0* | *1.0* | *102* | *23.9* | *0.0* | *0.7* | *0.0* |
| *Breast, Fillets, Skinless & Boneless, Raw, Average* | *1 Serving/100g* | *126.0* | *2.0* | *126* | *25.1* | *1.2* | *2.3* | *0.2* |
| Breast, Fillets, Smokey Maple, Roast, Waitrose* | 1 Fillet/96g | 140.0 | 2.0 | 146 | 27.9 | 4.2 | 2.0 | 0.1 |
| Breast, Fillets, Smoky Chilli, Tesco* | 1 Fillet/92g | 111.0 | 1.0 | 121 | 21.2 | 6.0 | 1.3 | 0.1 |
| Breast, Fillets, Sundried Tomato & Basil, M & S* | ½ Pack/110g | 165.0 | 5.0 | 150 | 22.5 | 4.7 | 4.1 | 1.1 |
| Breast, Fillets, Sweet & Smokey, Mini, Sainsbury's* | 1 Fillet / 48g | 106.0 | 5.0 | 221 | 19.2 | 14.6 | 9.6 | 1.4 |
| Breast, Fillets, Tikka, Mini, Ready to Eat, Tesco* | 1 Pack/200g | 230.0 | 2.0 | 115 | 23.4 | 2.2 | 1.0 | 0.2 |
| Breast, Garlic & Herb, Premium, Bernard Matthews* | 1 Serving/50g | 50.0 | 1.0 | 101 | 17.9 | 1.6 | 2.5 | 1.8 |
| *Breast, Grilled, Average* | *1 Breast/130g* | *192.0* | *3.0* | *148* | *32.0* | *0.0* | *2.2* | *0.0* |
| Breast, Joint, Lemon & Tarragon, Finest, Tesco* | 1 Serving/175g | 247.0 | 11.0 | 141 | 18.8 | 2.3 | 6.3 | 0.2 |
| Breast, Latino Style, Asda* | 1 Breast/65g | 99.0 | 2.0 | 152 | 27.0 | 4.1 | 3.1 | 0.5 |
| *Breast, Meat & Skin, Raw, Average* | *1 Serving/145g* | *249.0* | *13.0* | *172* | *20.8* | *0.0* | *9.2* | *0.0* |
| *Breast, Meat & Skin, Weighed with Bone, Raw, Average* | *1oz/28g* | *48.0* | *3.0* | *172* | *20.8* | *0.0* | *9.2* | *0.0* |
| *Breast, Meat Only, Fried* | *50g* | *93.0* | *2.0* | *187* | *33.4* | *0.5* | *4.7* | *0.0* |
| Breast, Pieces, Tikka, Average | 1 Serving/100g | 154.0 | 3.0 | 154 | 28.2 | 2.7 | 3.3 | 0.4 |
| *Breast, Roast, Sliced, From Supermarket, Average* | *1 Slice/13g* | *17.0* | *0.0* | *139* | *25.0* | *1.8* | *3.5* | *0.2* |
| *Breast, Roast, without Skin, Average* | *1oz/28g* | *42.0* | *1.0* | *149* | *25.4* | *1.0* | *4.7* | *0.2* |
| *Breast, Roll, Average* | *1 Slice/10g* | *17.0* | *1.0* | *167* | *16.1* | *3.2* | *10.0* | *0.2* |
| Breast, Sage & Onion, Slices, BGTY, Sainsbury's* | 1 Pack/100g | 113.0 | 1.0 | 113 | 22.2 | 2.7 | 1.4 | 0.3 |
| Breast, Short Sliced, Mexican, Sainsbury's* | 1 Pack/130g | 177.0 | 3.0 | 136 | 26.4 | 2.5 | 2.2 | 0.1 |
| Breast, Sliced, Mexican Style, Cooked, Asda* | 1 Pack/234g | 307.0 | 5.0 | 131 | 25.5 | 4.3 | 2.2 | 0.1 |
| Breast, Sliced, Tex, Mex, Sainsbury's* | 1 Serving/140g | 185.0 | 2.0 | 132 | 26.7 | 3.8 | 1.1 | 0.0 |
| Breast, Slices, Roast, Hot 'n' Spicy, Sainsbury's* | ½ Pack/65g | 90.0 | 1.0 | 138 | 26.7 | 2.7 | 2.3 | 0.4 |
| *Breast, Smoked, Sliced, Average* | *1 Slice/20g* | *22.0* | *1.0* | *110* | *20.7* | *0.9* | *2.6* | *0.1* |
| Breast, Southern Fried, in Breadcrumbs, Birds Eye* | 1 Breast/100g | 240.0 | 14.0 | 240 | 15.0 | 14.0 | 14.0 | 0.7 |
| Breast, Southern Fried, Premium, Bernard Matthews* | 1 Serving/60g | 70.0 | 2.0 | 117 | 19.6 | 3.1 | 2.9 | 0.6 |
| *Breast, Strips, Raw, Average* | *1 Serving/280g* | *358.0* | *6.0* | *128* | *27.1* | *0.3* | *2.0* | *0.3* |
| Breast, Tandoori Style, Average | 1 Serving/180g | 237.0 | 7.0 | 131 | 22.3 | 2.3 | 3.7 | 1.0 |
| Breast, Tikka, Sliced, Average | 1oz/28g | 34.0 | 0.0 | 120 | 24.9 | 2.0 | 1.7 | 0.6 |
| Breast, Wafer Thin, Sage & Onion, Bernard Matthews* | 1 Serving/25g | 30.0 | 1.0 | 120 | 19.8 | 3.5 | 3.0 | 0.0 |
| Breasts, Chilli & Ginger, COU, M & S* | 1 Breast/120g | 156.0 | 2.0 | 130 | 19.5 | 8.6 | 2.0 | 1.7 |
| Chargrills, Garlic, Weight After Cooking, Birds Eye* | 1 Chargrill/95g | 182.0 | 10.0 | 192 | 19.0 | 4.0 | 11.0 | 0.1 |
| Chargrills, Garlic, Weight Before Cooking, Birds Eye* | 1 Chargrill/95g | 190.0 | 11.0 | 200 | 20.3 | 4.2 | 11.3 | 0.1 |
| Chargrills, Weight After Cooking, Baked, Birds Eye* | 1 Chargrill/90g | 160.0 | 9.0 | 178 | 18.9 | 3.4 | 9.7 | 0.1 |
| Chargrills, Weight Before Cooking, Birds Eye* | 1 Chargrill/95g | 156.0 | 9.0 | 164 | 17.5 | 3.2 | 9.0 | 0.1 |
| Chicksticks, Captain Birds Eye, Birds Eye* | 1 Chickstick/25g | 64.0 | 4.0 | 257 | 13.3 | 15.0 | 16.0 | 0.8 |
| *Cooked, Sliced, Average* | *1 Slice/15g* | *18.0* | *0.0* | *118* | *22.4* | *1.6* | *2.4* | *0.1* |
| Dippers, Crispy, Average | 5 Dippers/93g | 231.0 | 14.0 | 249 | 13.2 | 14.4 | 15.4 | 0.6 |
| Drumsticks, & Thighs, Garlic & Herb, Sainsbury's* | 1 Serving/120g | 184.0 | 11.0 | 153 | 16.6 | 1.5 | 8.9 | 0.1 |
| Drumsticks, BBQ Flavour, Average | 1 Serving/200g | 348.0 | 16.0 | 174 | 22.6 | 3.1 | 8.0 | 0.4 |
| Drumsticks, Breaded, Fried, Average | 1oz/28g | 70.0 | 4.0 | 248 | 19.6 | 9.9 | 14.6 | 0.6 |
| Drumsticks, Chinese Style, Average | 1 Drumstick/100g | 177.0 | 8.0 | 177 | 22.5 | 3.5 | 8.1 | 0.7 |
| *Drumsticks, Roast, without Skin, Average* | *1 Serving/100g* | *163.0* | *8.0* | *163* | *22.6* | *0.5* | *7.8* | *0.2* |
| Drumsticks, Southern Fried, Sainsbury's* | 1 Serving/87g | 190.0 | 9.0 | 218 | 20.8 | 11.2 | 9.9 | 0.7 |
| *Drumsticks, with Skin, Average* | *1 Piece/125g* | *268.0* | *17.0* | *215* | *22.1* | *1.8* | *13.3* | *0.3* |
| Escalope, Breaded, Average | 1 Escalope/128g | 361.0 | 22.0 | 282 | 13.4 | 19.1 | 16.9 | 0.7 |
| Escalope, Cheese Topped, Asda* | 1 Escalope/173g | 411.0 | 23.0 | 237 | 12.0 | 18.0 | 13.0 | 1.9 |

C

## CHICKEN

| INFO/WEIGHT | Measure | per Measure | | Nutrition Values per 100g / 100ml | | | | |
|---|---|---|---|---|---|---|---|---|
| | | KCAL | FAT | KCAL | PROT | CARB | FAT | FIBRE |
| Escalope, Lemon & Pepper, Sainsbury's* | 1 Escalope/143g | 428.0 | 28.0 | 299 | 12.8 | 18.7 | 19.3 | 1.9 |
| Fillet Strips, Barbeque, Birds Eye* | 4 Strips/101g | 180.0 | 9.0 | 179 | 18.9 | 6.5 | 8.6 | 0.2 |
| Fillet Strips, Dijon Mustard, Birds Eye* | 4 Strips/113g | 155.0 | 6.0 | 137 | 18.9 | 3.7 | 5.2 | 0.1 |
| Fillet Strips, Red Pesto, Birds Eye* | 4 Strips/100g | 135.0 | 5.0 | 135 | 19.1 | 3.2 | 5.1 | 0.2 |
| Fillet Strips, Tomato & Basil, Birds Eye* | 4 Strips/101g | 150.0 | 5.0 | 149 | 19.4 | 5.6 | 5.4 | 0.3 |
| Fillets, Battered, Average | 1 Fillet/90g | 199.0 | 10.0 | 221 | 16.1 | 13.3 | 11.5 | 0.5 |
| Fillets, Breaded, Average | 1 Piece/98g | 214.0 | 10.0 | 219 | 14.2 | 15.9 | 10.7 | 1.9 |
| Fillets, Chilli & Mango, Tesco* | 1 Serving/100g | 130.0 | 1.0 | 130 | 27.1 | 3.7 | 0.7 | 1.0 |
| Fillets, Chinese Style, Average | 1oz/28g | 37.0 | 0.0 | 131 | 24.4 | 4.6 | 1.7 | 0.5 |
| Fillets, Coronation, BGTY, Sainsbury's* | 1 Fillet/100g | 136.0 | 3.0 | 136 | 27.1 | 2.4 | 2.6 | 1.0 |
| Fillets, Hickory Barbecue & Chilli, BGTY, Sainsbury's* | 1 Fillet/100g | 133.0 | 1.0 | 133 | 26.9 | 3.6 | 1.2 | 0.9 |
| Fillets, Hickory Style BBQ, Tesco* | 1 Fillet/80g | 112.0 | 2.0 | 140 | 28.4 | 1.5 | 2.2 | 0.5 |
| Fillets, Honey & Mustard, Average | 1 Serving/100g | 138.0 | 4.0 | 138 | 18.4 | 7.5 | 3.7 | 0.8 |
| Fillets, Hot & Spicy, Average | 1oz/28g | 58.0 | 3.0 | 206 | 16.4 | 10.5 | 11.0 | 1.1 |
| Fillets, Lime & Coriander, Mini, Average | 1 Fillet/42g | 49.0 | 1.0 | 118 | 24.3 | 2.6 | 1.3 | 0.6 |
| Fillets, Mango Salsa, Mini, Sainsbury's* | ½ Pack/100g | 132.0 | 1.0 | 132 | 24.7 | 5.6 | 1.2 | 0.0 |
| Fillets, Mini, Skewers, Sticky Sweet Soy Marinade, M & S* | ½ Pack/124g | 155.0 | 1.0 | 125 | 20.7 | 7.6 | 1.1 | 0.3 |
| Fillets, Red Pepper, Mini, BGTY, Sainsbury's* | 1 Serving/100g | 126.0 | 1.0 | 126 | 26.5 | 3.7 | 0.6 | 0.7 |
| Fillets, Southern Fried, Meat Only, Average | 1 Piece/100g | 222.0 | 12.0 | 222 | 16.4 | 12.2 | 12.0 | 1.1 |
| Fillets, Sweet Chilli, Mini, Sainsbury's* | ½ Pack/100g | 119.0 | 1.0 | 119 | 21.8 | 5.4 | 1.1 | 0.9 |
| Fillets, Sweet Chilli & Lime, Mini, M & S* | 1 Serving/50g | 77.0 | 1.0 | 155 | 28.3 | 5.1 | 2.2 | 0.0 |
| Fillets, Tandoori Style, Mini, Average | 1 Serving/100g | 127.0 | 2.0 | 127 | 24.7 | 2.5 | 2.0 | 0.3 |
| Fillets, Thai, COU, M & S* | 1 Fillet/120g | 160.0 | 2.0 | 133 | 19.5 | 10.4 | 1.6 | 1.3 |
| Fillets, Tikka, Average | 1 Serving/100g | 141.0 | 5.0 | 141 | 22.4 | 1.7 | 5.0 | 1.1 |
| Fillets, Tikka, Mini, Average | 1oz/28g | 35.0 | 1.0 | 124 | 25.1 | 1.3 | 2.1 | 1.1 |
| Fillets, Tomato & Basil, Mini, Average | 1oz/28g | 34.0 | 1.0 | 123 | 23.4 | 2.5 | 2.1 | 0.3 |
| Fingers, Average | 1 Serving/75g | 187.0 | 10.0 | 250 | 13.7 | 18.7 | 13.2 | 1.1 |
| Garlic, Frozen, Tesco* | 1 Serving/95g | 182.0 | 8.0 | 192 | 15.6 | 12.9 | 8.7 | 1.0 |
| Garlic Basted, Morrisons* | 1 Serving/100g | 231.0 | 13.0 | 231 | 23.3 | 0.7 | 13.1 | 0.4 |
| Goujons, Breaded, Average | 1 Serving/114g | 293.0 | 17.0 | 258 | 15.8 | 15.2 | 15.0 | 1.0 |
| Griddlers, BBQ, Captain Birds Eye, Birds Eye* | 1 Serving/77g | 161.0 | 10.0 | 209 | 18.3 | 5.7 | 12.5 | 0.5 |
| Honey & Mustard Seasoned Portions, Birds Eye* | 1 Serving/98g | 155.0 | 8.0 | 159 | 17.4 | 5.0 | 7.7 | 0.1 |
| Honey Roast, Sliced, Average | 1 Slice/13g | 15.0 | 0.0 | 117 | 21.5 | 2.1 | 2.4 | 0.1 |
| *Leg, Meat Only, Raw, Average* | *1oz/28g* | *34.0* | *1.0* | *120* | *20.1* | *0.0* | *3.8* | *0.0* |
| *Leg, Meat Only, Raw, with Skin & Bone, Average* | *1oz/28g* | *38.0* | *1.0* | *134* | *22.5* | *0.0* | *4.3* | *0.0* |
| *Leg, Meat Only, Stewed, with Bone & Skin, Average* | *1oz/28g* | *52.0* | *2.0* | *185* | *26.3* | *0.0* | *8.1* | *0.0* |
| *Leg, with Skin, Raw, Average* | *1oz/28g* | *48.0* | *3.0* | *172* | *19.1* | *0.0* | *10.4* | *0.0* |
| *Leg, with Skin, Roasted, Average* | *1oz/28g* | *66.0* | *5.0* | *234* | *21.5* | *0.1* | *16.4* | *0.0* |
| Leg Or Thigh, Hot & Spicy, Average | 1oz/28g | 50.0 | 3.0 | 179 | 19.4 | 1.0 | 10.8 | 0.4 |
| *Leg Portion, Roast, Skin, Without Bone, Average* | *1 Quarter/120g* | *244.0* | *15.0* | *203* | *21.6* | *0.3* | *12.7* | *0.2* |
| *Light Meat, Raw* | *1oz/28g* | *30.0* | *0.0* | *106* | *24.0* | *0.0* | *1.1* | *0.0* |
| *Light Meat, Roasted* | *1oz/28g* | *43.0* | *1.0* | *153* | *30.2* | *0.0* | *3.6* | *0.0* |
| *Meat, Roasted, Average* | *1oz/28g* | *50.0* | *2.0* | *177* | *27.3* | *0.0* | *7.5* | *0.0* |
| *Meat & Skin, Raw, Average* | *1oz/28g* | *64.0* | *5.0* | *230* | *17.6* | *0.0* | *17.7* | *0.0* |
| *Meat & Skin, Roasted, Average* | *1oz/28g* | *60.0* | *4.0* | *216* | *22.6* | *0.0* | *14.0* | *0.0* |
| Meat & Skin Portions, Deep Fried, Average | 1oz/28g | 73.0 | 5.0 | 259 | 26.9 | 0.0 | 16.8 | 0.0 |
| *Mince, Average* | *1oz/28g* | *39.0* | *2.0* | *140* | *20.9* | *0.1* | *6.0* | *0.2* |
| Nuggets, Battered, Average | 1 Nugget/20g | 50.0 | 3.0 | 251 | 13.5 | 16.9 | 14.4 | 0.9 |
| Nuggets, Breaded, Average | 1 Nugget/14g | 37.0 | 2.0 | 263 | 14.8 | 19.8 | 13.8 | 1.9 |
| Nuggets, Free From Gluten & Wheat, Sainsbury's* | 1 Nugget/19g | 47.0 | 2.0 | 251 | 13.4 | 19.7 | 13.2 | 0.8 |
| O'S, Captain Birds Eye, Birds Eye* | 1 Piece/5g | 12.0 | 1.0 | 248 | 13.2 | 16.4 | 14.4 | 0.8 |
| Peri Peri, Chargrill, Birds Eye* | 1 Serving/92g | 157.0 | 8.0 | 171 | 16.9 | 5.2 | 9.2 | 0.3 |
| Pieces, Boneless, Breaded, Fried, From Restaurant | 1 Piece/17g | 51.0 | 3.0 | 301 | 17.0 | 14.4 | 19.4 | 0.0 |

C

| | Measure INFO/WEIGHT | per Measure KCAL | FAT | Nutrition Values per 100g / 100ml KCAL | PROT | CARB | FAT | FIBRE |
|---|---|---|---|---|---|---|---|---|
| **CHICKEN** | | | | | | | | |
| Pieces, Garlic, Crunchy, Birds Eye* | 1 Piece/99g | 259.0 | 15.0 | 262 | 14.4 | 16.9 | 15.2 | 0.9 |
| Pieces, Spicy, Mexican, Birds Eye* | 1 Piece/103g | 254.0 | 14.0 | 247 | 14.6 | 16.5 | 13.6 | 0.6 |
| Pops, Southern Fried, Frozen, Tesco* | 1 Pack/225g | 517.0 | 26.0 | 230 | 13.1 | 18.1 | 11.5 | 1.9 |
| Shashlik, Patak's* | 1 Serving/250g | 203.0 | 4.0 | 81 | 12.4 | 4.4 | 1.4 | 0.0 |
| Skewers, BBQ, George Foreman's Lean Mean Grillers* | 1 Skewer/60g | 68.0 | 1.0 | 114 | 20.0 | 5.5 | 1.4 | 0.4 |
| Skewers, Marinated, Asda* | 1 Skewer/35g | 50.0 | 0.0 | 142 | 24.9 | 8.0 | 1.2 | 0.9 |
| Spatchcock, Poussin, Sainsbury's* | 1 Serving/122g | 168.0 | 7.0 | 138 | 21.1 | 0.1 | 5.4 | 0.2 |
| Spicy, Fried, Sainsbury's* | 1 Serving/150g | 414.0 | 25.0 | 276 | 28.8 | 2.9 | 16.6 | 2.1 |
| ***Steaks, Average*** | *1 Serving/100g* | *205.0* | *9.0* | *205* | *21.1* | *9.0* | *9.4* | *0.7* |
| Steaks, Garlic & Herb, Tesco* | 1 Serving/138g | 354.0 | 23.0 | 257 | 14.1 | 12.2 | 16.9 | 1.7 |
| Strips, Breast, Grilled, KP Snacks* | 1 Serving/84g | 90.0 | 2.0 | 107 | 25.0 | 0.0 | 1.8 | 0.0 |
| Strips, Mexican, Sliced, M & S* | ½ Pack/70g | 77.0 | 0.0 | 110 | 24.3 | 2.3 | 0.6 | 0.5 |
| Strips Or Tenders, Chinese Style, Average | 1oz/28g | 41.0 | 1.0 | 145 | 19.6 | 7.9 | 4.1 | 1.0 |
| Tenders, Tex Mex, Jumbo, M & S* | 1 Serving/200g | 250.0 | 7.0 | 125 | 22.8 | 0.7 | 3.4 | 0.6 |
| Thai Seasoned, Breast, Birds Eye* | 1 Piece/97g | 161.0 | 8.0 | 166 | 17.3 | 4.5 | 8.5 | 0.2 |
| ***Thigh, Meat & Skin, Average*** | *1 Serving/100g* | *218.0* | *15.0* | *218* | *21.4* | *0.0* | *14.7* | *0.0* |
| ***Thigh, Meat & Skin, Casseroled, Average*** | *1oz/28g* | *65.0* | *5.0* | *233* | *21.5* | *0.0* | *16.3* | *0.0* |
| ***Thigh, Meat Only, Diced, Casseroled*** | *1oz/28g* | *50.0* | *2.0* | *180* | *25.6* | *0.0* | *8.6* | *0.0* |
| ***Thigh, Meat Only, Raw, Average*** | *1 Thigh/90g* | *113.0* | *5.0* | *126* | *19.4* | *0.0* | *5.4* | *0.0* |
| ***Thigh, Roast, Average*** | *1 Serving/100g* | *238.0* | *16.0* | *238* | *23.8* | *0.4* | *15.6* | *0.0* |
| Wafer Thin, Average | 1 Slice/10g | 12.0 | 0.0 | 120 | 19.0 | 2.8 | 3.6 | 0.1 |
| ***Whole, Roast, Average*** | *1oz/28g* | *59.0* | *4.0* | *211* | *21.2* | *1.5* | *13.4* | *0.2* |
| Whole, Roasted, Brown Sugar Marinade, Tesco* | 1 Serving/100g | 195.0 | 11.0 | 195 | 22.1 | 0.1 | 11.3 | 0.1 |
| Wing, Breaded, Fried, Average | 1oz/28g | 82.0 | 5.0 | 294 | 18.4 | 14.0 | 18.5 | 0.4 |
| ***Wing, Meat & Skin, Cooked, Average*** | *1oz/28g* | *67.0* | *4.0* | *241* | *23.3* | *1.9* | *15.6* | *0.3* |
| ***Wing Quarter, Meat Only, Casseroled*** | *1oz/28g* | *46.0* | *2.0* | *164* | *26.9* | *0.0* | *6.3* | *0.0* |
| Wings, BBQ Flavour, Average | 1oz/28g | 61.0 | 3.0 | 219 | 20.3 | 6.5 | 12.4 | 0.6 |
| Wings, Chinese Style, Average | 1oz/28g | 72.0 | 4.0 | 256 | 24.2 | 5.1 | 15.5 | 0.6 |
| Wings, Hot & Spicy, Average | 1oz/28g | 65.0 | 4.0 | 231 | 21.8 | 5.1 | 13.6 | 0.8 |
| ***Wings, Meat & Skin, Raw, Average*** | *1oz/28g* | *52.0* | *3.0* | *184* | *19.0* | *0.5* | *11.8* | *0.2* |
| **CHICKEN &** | | | | | | | | |
| Apricot Rice, COU, M & S* | 1 Pack/400g | 360.0 | 4.0 | 90 | 9.4 | 10.6 | 0.9 | 0.7 |
| Asparagus, Baby Potatoes, Creamy, Sainsbury's* | 1 Pack/450g | 472.0 | 20.0 | 105 | 8.0 | 8.3 | 4.4 | 0.9 |
| Asparagus, BGTY, Sainsbury's* | 1 Pack/400g | 428.0 | 6.0 | 107 | 9.1 | 14.5 | 1.4 | 0.9 |
| Asparagus, in a Champagne Sauce, Finest, Tesco* | 1 Pack/500g | 615.0 | 33.0 | 123 | 8.8 | 7.0 | 6.7 | 0.9 |
| Asparagus, Long Grain & Wild Rice, BGTY, Sainsbury's* | 1 Pack/451g | 555.0 | 9.0 | 123 | 9.2 | 17.1 | 2.0 | 0.8 |
| Bacon, Easy Steam, Tesco* | 1 Pack/400g | 728.0 | 36.0 | 182 | 11.7 | 13.6 | 9.1 | 0.8 |
| Bacon Parcels, Finest, Tesco* | 1 Pack/233g | 379.0 | 22.0 | 163 | 16.1 | 3.7 | 9.3 | 0.5 |
| Bacon Parcels, Sainsbury's* | ½ Pack/170g | 406.0 | 29.0 | 239 | 21.9 | 0.1 | 16.8 | 0.0 |
| Balsamic Roasted Pepper Pasta, M & S* | 1 Pack/310g | 418.0 | 11.0 | 135 | 7.8 | 17.2 | 3.7 | 1.7 |
| Black Bean, Chinese, Tesco* | 1 Pack/350g | 381.0 | 17.0 | 109 | 8.9 | 7.4 | 4.9 | 0.7 |
| Black Bean, Chinese Takeaway, Tesco* | 1 Serving/200g | 190.0 | 7.0 | 95 | 8.3 | 8.0 | 3.3 | 0.5 |
| Black Bean, Special Fried Rice, HL, Tesco* | 1 Pack/450g | 360.0 | 6.0 | 80 | 6.8 | 9.5 | 1.4 | 0.9 |
| Black Bean, with Chinese Rice, COU, M & S* | 1 Pack/400g | 320.0 | 10.0 | 80 | 7.4 | 7.6 | 2.4 | 1.1 |
| Black Bean, with Noodles, Tesco* | 1 Pack/475g | 470.0 | 8.0 | 99 | 7.6 | 13.6 | 1.6 | 0.2 |
| Black Bean, with Rice, Chinese, Tesco* | 1 Serving/450g | 459.0 | 9.0 | 102 | 5.3 | 15.4 | 2.1 | 0.5 |
| Black Bean, with Rice, HL, Tesco* | 1 Pack/450g | 463.0 | 7.0 | 103 | 6.9 | 19.6 | 1.6 | 0.6 |
| Black Bean Noodles, Sainsbury's* | 1 Serving/130g | 155.0 | 1.0 | 119 | 4.3 | 23.9 | 0.7 | 0.8 |
| Blackbean, with Vegetable Egg Rice, COU, M & S* | 1 Packet/400g | 360.0 | 6.0 | 90 | 7.2 | 12.0 | 1.6 | 1.4 |
| Broccoli, with Herb Potatoes, Tesco* | 1 Pack/475g | 499.0 | 11.0 | 105 | 7.8 | 12.5 | 2.3 | 1.5 |
| Cashew Nuts, Chinese, Cantonese, Sainsbury's* | ½ Pack/175g | 171.0 | 9.0 | 98 | 8.4 | 4.9 | 5.0 | 1.3 |
| Cashew Nuts, Chinese, Tesco* | 1 Pack/350g | 378.0 | 20.0 | 108 | 9.5 | 4.9 | 5.6 | 0.6 |
| Cashew Nuts, Easy Steam, Tesco* | 1 Serving/400g | 460.0 | 19.0 | 115 | 8.7 | 9.2 | 4.8 | 1.0 |

| | Measure INFO/WEIGHT | per Measure KCAL | FAT | Nutrition Values per 100g / 100ml KCAL | PROT | CARB | FAT | FIBRE |
|---|---|---|---|---|---|---|---|---|
| **CHICKEN &** | | | | | | | | |
| Cashew Nuts, Oriental, HL, Tesco* | 1 Pack/450g | 436.0 | 4.0 | 97 | 7.0 | 15.1 | 1.0 | 0.7 |
| Cashew Nuts, with Egg Fried Rice, HL, Tesco* | 1 Pack/450g | 441.0 | 6.0 | 98 | 8.9 | 12.7 | 1.3 | 1.3 |
| Cashew Nuts, with Egg Rice, GFY, Asda* | 1 Pack/396g | 396.0 | 9.0 | 100 | 7.0 | 13.0 | 2.2 | 1.3 |
| Chargrilled Vegetable Roll, HL, Tesco* | 1 Pack/221g | 336.0 | 6.0 | 152 | 10.1 | 21.8 | 2.7 | 2.3 |
| Chips, BBQ, BGTY, Sainsbury's* | 1 Pack/381g | 423.0 | 7.0 | 111 | 7.9 | 15.9 | 1.8 | 2.5 |
| Chorizo Paella, Go Cook, Asda* | ½ Pack/475g | 591.0 | 10.0 | 124 | 10.2 | 15.9 | 2.2 | 2.6 |
| Cous Cous, HE, Tesco* | 1 Pack/351g | 263.0 | 2.0 | 75 | 10.3 | 7.3 | 0.5 | 1.4 |
| Cranberry, Perfectly Balanced, Waitrose* | 1 Pack/240g | 161.0 | 1.0 | 67 | 11.8 | 4.1 | 0.4 | 1.1 |
| Fries, Southern Fried, Sainsbury's* | ½ Pack/250g | 562.0 | 22.0 | 225 | 10.5 | 26.2 | 8.7 | 0.8 |
| Fries, Southern Fried Style, Tesco* | 1 Pack/500g | 930.0 | 40.0 | 186 | 11.5 | 16.0 | 8.0 | 1.4 |
| Gravy, COU, M & S* | 1 Pack/300g | 216.0 | 4.0 | 72 | 7.2 | 7.8 | 1.3 | 1.6 |
| Herb Pasta with Lemon, HL, Tesco* | 1 Pack/400g | 520.0 | 8.0 | 130 | 8.2 | 18.8 | 2.0 | 1.6 |
| King Prawn Special Fried Rice, Finest, Tesco* | 1 Pack/450g | 733.0 | 32.0 | 163 | 7.7 | 17.0 | 7.1 | 0.7 |
| Mushroom, Chinese, Sainsbury's* | ½ Pack/175g | 115.0 | 3.0 | 66 | 7.6 | 4.4 | 2.0 | 0.9 |
| Mushroom, Chinese, Tesco* | 1 Pack/460g | 474.0 | 13.0 | 103 | 5.7 | 13.8 | 2.8 | 1.0 |
| Mushroom, in White Wine Sauce, GFY, Asda* | 1 Pack/400g | 272.0 | 7.0 | 68 | 6.0 | 7.0 | 1.8 | 1.2 |
| Mushroom, with Vegetable Rice, BGTY, Sainsbury's* | 1 Pack/400g | 376.0 | 7.0 | 94 | 6.4 | 13.0 | 1.8 | 0.9 |
| Peppers, in a Black Bean Sauce, M & S* | 1 Pack/320g | 256.0 | 5.0 | 80 | 9.4 | 7.3 | 1.5 | 1.2 |
| Peppers, M & S* | 1 Serving/240g | 264.0 | 11.0 | 110 | 14.7 | 2.3 | 4.5 | 0.6 |
| Pineapple, Chilled, Tesco* | 1 Pack/350g | 364.0 | 8.0 | 104 | 9.6 | 11.1 | 2.4 | 5.5 |
| Pineapple, with Egg Fried Rice, HL, Tesco* | 1 Pack/450g | 414.0 | 3.0 | 92 | 6.0 | 15.4 | 0.7 | 0.6 |
| Pineapple, with Egg Fried Rice, Tesco* | 1 Pack/450g | 450.0 | 11.0 | 100 | 7.6 | 12.1 | 2.4 | 1.2 |
| Pineapple, with Rice, HL, Tesco* | 1 Pack/450g | 400.0 | 7.0 | 89 | 6.6 | 12.0 | 1.6 | 1.0 |
| Pineapple, with Vegetable Rice, M & S* | 1 Pack/400g | 400.0 | 8.0 | 100 | 7.2 | 13.0 | 1.9 | 1.6 |
| Red Pepper Dressing, Simple Solutions, Tesco* | 1 Serving/140g | 228.0 | 13.0 | 163 | 19.2 | 0.1 | 9.5 | 0.5 |
| Tomato & Basil, COU, M & S* | ½ Pack/200g | 180.0 | 5.0 | 90 | 14.3 | 3.4 | 2.3 | 0.8 |
| Tomato Saag, with Pilau Rice, BGTY, Sainsbury's* | 1 Pack/400g | 404.0 | 4.0 | 101 | 7.3 | 15.6 | 1.0 | 1.0 |
| Vegetable Medley, Chargrilled, HE, Tesco* | 1 Pack/450g | 270.0 | 5.0 | 60 | 6.5 | 5.8 | 1.2 | 0.9 |
| Vegetable Savoury Rice, Safeway* | ½ Pack/185g | 231.0 | 2.0 | 125 | 2.9 | 25.9 | 1.1 | 0.8 |
| White Wine, with Rice, HE, Tesco* | 1 Pack/450g | 450.0 | 6.0 | 100 | 7.1 | 14.8 | 1.4 | 1.0 |
| **CHICKEN ALFREDO** | | | | | | | | |
| BGTY, Sainsbury's* | 1 Serving/200g | 208.0 | 5.0 | 104 | 18.0 | 1.9 | 2.7 | 0.5 |
| HL, Tesco* | 1 Serving/377g | 388.0 | 10.0 | 103 | 9.4 | 10.6 | 2.6 | 0.9 |
| **CHICKEN ARRABBIATA** | | | | | | | | |
| Al Forno, Sainsbury's* | 1 Pack/900g | 1026.0 | 22.0 | 114 | 6.5 | 16.4 | 2.5 | 1.4 |
| Bistro, Waitrose* | ½ Pack/175g | 156.0 | 5.0 | 89 | 12.9 | 2.5 | 3.0 | 0.5 |
| Easy Steam, HL, Tesco* | 1 Pack/400g | 284.0 | 3.0 | 71 | 8.4 | 7.6 | 0.8 | 1.2 |
| GFY, Asda* | 1 Pack/448g | 394.0 | 3.0 | 88 | 5.2 | 15.1 | 0.7 | 1.1 |
| Perfectly Balanced, Waitrose* | 1 Serving/240g | 211.0 | 6.0 | 88 | 12.4 | 4.0 | 2.4 | 0.6 |
| **CHICKEN BANG BANG** | | | | | | | | |
| Oriental Express* | ½ Pack/200g | 170.0 | 3.0 | 85 | 6.4 | 11.0 | 1.7 | 3.2 |
| Waitrose* | 1 Pack/350g | 367.0 | 17.0 | 105 | 9.4 | 5.9 | 4.9 | 1.2 |
| **CHICKEN BUTTER** | | | | | | | | |
| & Rice, Indian, Finest, Tesco* | 1 Serving/475g | 660.0 | 28.0 | 139 | 7.1 | 14.0 | 6.0 | 1.6 |
| Curry, Fresh, Tesco* | 1 Pack/350g | 486.0 | 24.0 | 139 | 11.8 | 7.1 | 7.0 | 1.8 |
| Indian, with Pilau Rice, Asda* | 1 Pack/500g | 770.0 | 23.0 | 154 | 7.0 | 21.0 | 4.7 | 1.3 |
| Rich & Aromatic, Sainsbury's* | 1 Pack/400g | 592.0 | 36.0 | 148 | 12.1 | 4.4 | 9.1 | 1.2 |
| **CHICKEN CAJUN** | | | | | | | | |
| & Pasta, Safeway* | 1 Pack/455g | 500.0 | 15.0 | 110 | 8.6 | 10.5 | 3.4 | 2.1 |
| & Potato Hash, HL, Tesco* | 1 Pack/450g | 427.0 | 6.0 | 95 | 6.5 | 14.1 | 1.4 | 1.5 |
| **CHICKEN CALYPSO** | | | | | | | | |
| with Turmeric Rice, BGTY, Sainsbury's* | 1 Pack/450g | 495.0 | 9.0 | 110 | 6.7 | 16.3 | 2.1 | 1.0 |

| | Measure INFO/WEIGHT | per Measure KCAL | per Measure FAT | Nutrition Values per 100g / 100ml KCAL | PROT | CARB | FAT | FIBRE |
|---|---|---|---|---|---|---|---|---|
| **CHICKEN CANTONESE** | | | | | | | | |
| & Rice, Sizzler, Tesco* | 1 Serving/450g | 639.0 | 26.0 | 142 | 7.7 | 14.9 | 5.7 | 0.9 |
| Breast, Fillets, Sainsbury's* | 1 Serving/154g | 168.0 | 2.0 | 109 | 20.3 | 3.6 | 1.5 | 0.6 |
| Chinese, Tesco* | ½ Pack/175g | 196.0 | 6.0 | 112 | 10.3 | 9.4 | 3.7 | 0.4 |
| Honey, Sesame, Sainsbury's* | 1/3 Pack/135g | 116.0 | 4.0 | 86 | 9.8 | 5.5 | 2.7 | 0.8 |
| Honey Pepper, Sainsbury's* | ½ Pack/175g | 124.0 | 4.0 | 71 | 6.6 | 6.1 | 2.2 | 0.9 |
| **CHICKEN CARIBBEAN** | | | | | | | | |
| Fruity, with Rice & Peas, New, BGTY, Sainsbury's* | 1 Pack/400g | 352.0 | 4.0 | 88 | 6.9 | 13.1 | 0.9 | 2.2 |
| Style, Breasts, COU, M & S* | 1 Serving/205g | 205.0 | 3.0 | 100 | 14.6 | 7.3 | 1.5 | 1.3 |
| with Potato & Toasted Coconut Rosti, TTD, Sainsbury's* | ½ Pack/200g | 320.0 | 15.0 | 160 | 13.8 | 9.7 | 7.3 | 0.6 |
| **CHICKEN CHASSEUR** | | | | | | | | |
| BGTY, Sainsbury's* | 1 Pack/320g | 243.0 | 4.0 | 76 | 6.8 | 9.5 | 1.1 | 1.0 |
| Breast Fillets, Morrisons* | 1 Pack/380g | 384.0 | 11.0 | 101 | 15.7 | 2.9 | 3.0 | 0.8 |
| Finest, Tesco* | ½ Pack/200g | 200.0 | 6.0 | 100 | 14.3 | 2.4 | 3.2 | 1.1 |
| **CHICKEN CHILLI** | | | | | | | | |
| & Lemongrass, with Egg Noodles, BGTY, Sainsbury's* | 1 Pack/450g | 499.0 | 15.0 | 111 | 10.0 | 10.2 | 3.4 | 1.2 |
| Sweet, & Egg Fried Rice, HL, Tesco* | 1 Serving/450g | 446.0 | 8.0 | 99 | 5.7 | 15.0 | 1.8 | 0.4 |
| Sweet, Findus* | 1 Pack/350g | 420.0 | 12.0 | 120 | 6.0 | 15.0 | 3.5 | 1.5 |
| Sweet, Just Cook, Sainsbury's* | ½ Pack/191g | 200.0 | 1.0 | 105 | 15.2 | 9.4 | 0.7 | 0.5 |
| Sweet, with Noodles, Frozen, HL, Tesco* | 1 Pack/450g | 472.0 | 6.0 | 105 | 4.9 | 17.3 | 1.4 | 1.4 |
| with Lime, Breast, Simple Solutions, Tesco* | 1 Pack/400g | 564.0 | 21.0 | 141 | 22.5 | 0.8 | 5.3 | 1.4 |
| **CHICKEN CHINESE** | | | | | | | | |
| & Prawns, Sizzler, House Special, Tesco* | 1 Serving/450g | 684.0 | 23.0 | 152 | 7.5 | 18.8 | 5.2 | 1.2 |
| Balls, M & S* | 1 Ball/16g | 45.0 | 2.0 | 280 | 10.8 | 29.2 | 13.6 | 2.1 |
| Battered, with Plum Sauce, Tesco* | 1 Pack/350g | 647.0 | 20.0 | 185 | 6.7 | 26.5 | 5.8 | 0.8 |
| Crispy Aromatic, Half, Tesco* | 1 Serving/233g | 524.0 | 24.0 | 225 | 16.3 | 16.7 | 10.4 | 1.2 |
| Fillets, with Sweet Chilli Sauce, Tesco* | 1 Serving/350g | 591.0 | 22.0 | 169 | 8.8 | 19.2 | 6.3 | 0.7 |
| Style, & Noodles, HE, Tesco* | 1 Pack/370g | 277.0 | 4.0 | 75 | 6.9 | 9.4 | 1.1 | 0.7 |
| with Ginger & Spring Onion, Tesco* | 1 Serving/350g | 299.0 | 10.0 | 85 | 7.6 | 7.3 | 2.9 | 0.6 |
| **CHICKEN CIDER** | | | | | | | | |
| COU, M & S* | 1 Pack/400g | 300.0 | 9.0 | 75 | 7.2 | 6.7 | 2.3 | 0.8 |
| with Colcannon, Perfectly Balanced, Waitrose* | 1 Pack/401g | 353.0 | 12.0 | 88 | 6.2 | 8.9 | 3.1 | 1.1 |
| **CHICKEN CORDON BLEU** | | | | | | | | |
| Breast, Fillets, Sainsbury's* | 1 Serving/150g | 304.0 | 14.0 | 203 | 17.5 | 11.5 | 9.5 | 1.6 |
| TTD, Sainsbury's* | 1 Fillet/140g | 339.0 | 16.0 | 242 | 21.3 | 14.1 | 11.2 | 1.1 |
| Waitrose* | 1 Serving/160g | 325.0 | 15.0 | 203 | 20.1 | 9.1 | 9.6 | 2.4 |
| **CHICKEN CORONATION** | | | | | | | | |
| COU, M & S* | 1oz/28g | 34.0 | 1.0 | 120 | 16.3 | 8.6 | 2.2 | 0.7 |
| M & S* | 1 Serving/200g | 420.0 | 26.0 | 210 | 12.6 | 10.6 | 13.2 | 1.3 |
| **CHICKEN DINNER** | | | | | | | | |
| Breast, with Pork, Sage & Onion Stuffing, Tesco* | 1 Serving/180g | 277.0 | 15.0 | 154 | 19.4 | 0.7 | 8.2 | 0.5 |
| Tesco* | 1 Serving/400g | 388.0 | 7.0 | 97 | 9.2 | 10.9 | 1.8 | 1.2 |
| **CHICKEN EN CROUTE** | | | | | | | | |
| Asda* | ½ Pack/174g | 393.0 | 17.0 | 226 | 14.0 | 20.0 | 10.0 | 1.5 |
| Breast, Tesco* | 1 Serving/215g | 555.0 | 33.0 | 258 | 9.4 | 20.4 | 15.4 | 0.6 |
| Just Cook, Sainsbury's* | 1 Serving/180g | 481.0 | 27.0 | 267 | 16.8 | 15.9 | 15.1 | 0.4 |
| **CHICKEN FLORENTINE** | | | | | | | | |
| Asda* | 1 Serving/200g | 322.0 | 18.0 | 161 | 18.0 | 2.1 | 9.0 | 0.9 |
| Finest, Tesco* | ½ Pack/225g | 358.0 | 19.0 | 159 | 11.0 | 9.7 | 8.5 | 1.3 |
| HL, Tesco* | 1 Pack/400g | 340.0 | 11.0 | 85 | 12.1 | 3.0 | 2.7 | 0.9 |
| **CHICKEN FORRESTIERE** | | | | | | | | |
| COU, M & S* | 1 Serving/220g | 187.0 | 4.0 | 85 | 14.5 | 2.2 | 1.7 | 0.6 |
| GFY, Asda* | ½ Pack/225g | 205.0 | 5.0 | 91 | 15.0 | 2.5 | 2.3 | 0.3 |

**C**

| | Measure INFO/WEIGHT | per Measure KCAL | FAT | Nutrition Values per 100g / 100ml KCAL | PROT | CARB | FAT | FIBRE |
|---|---|---|---|---|---|---|---|---|
| **CHICKEN FU YUNG** | | | | | | | | |
| Chinese Takeaway, Tesco* | 1 Pack/350g | 315.0 | 3.0 | 90 | 5.6 | 14.5 | 1.0 | 0.8 |
| **CHICKEN GINGER** | | | | | | | | |
| & Lemon, with Apricot Rice, BGTY, Sainsbury's* | 1 Pack/402g | 438.0 | 6.0 | 109 | 9.7 | 14.5 | 1.4 | 0.3 |
| & Lemon, with Basmati Rice, East Smart, Safeway* | 1 Pack/395g | 395.0 | 7.0 | 100 | 7.3 | 13.4 | 1.7 | 1.4 |
| & Plum, with Rice, Perfectly Balanced, Waitrose* | 1 Pack/400g | 492.0 | 2.0 | 123 | 6.3 | 23.5 | 0.5 | 1.0 |
| & Spring Onion, with Rice, Sharwood's* | 1 Pack/375g | 347.0 | 6.0 | 93 | 5.1 | 14.2 | 1.7 | 1.7 |
| **CHICKEN GLAZED** | | | | | | | | |
| Balsamic, HL, Tesco* | 1 Pack/400g | 288.0 | 4.0 | 72 | 5.1 | 10.8 | 0.9 | 0.9 |
| **CHICKEN HARISSA** | | | | | | | | |
| BGTY, Sainsbury's* | 1 Serving/250g | 211.0 | 3.0 | 84 | 10.4 | 8.0 | 1.2 | 1.5 |
| with Cous Cous, Perfectly Balanced, Waitrose* | 1 Pack/400g | 348.0 | 8.0 | 87 | 7.6 | 9.5 | 2.0 | 1.7 |
| **CHICKEN HAWAIIAN** | | | | | | | | |
| with Rice, Birds Eye* | 1 Pack/350g | 406.0 | 5.0 | 116 | 5.5 | 20.2 | 1.5 | 0.6 |
| **CHICKEN HONEY & MUSTARD** | | | | | | | | |
| HL, Tesco* | 1 Serving/375g | 424.0 | 9.0 | 113 | 5.8 | 17.3 | 2.3 | 1.4 |
| Shapers, Boots* | 1 Pack/241g | 304.0 | 6.0 | 126 | 7.0 | 19.0 | 2.4 | 1.7 |
| Weight Watchers* | 1 Serving/320g | 291.0 | 2.0 | 91 | 5.1 | 16.2 | 0.7 | 0.2 |
| with Baby Potatoes, BGTY, Sainsbury's* | 1 Pack/450g | 391.0 | 3.0 | 87 | 8.5 | 11.7 | 0.7 | 0.8 |
| with Spring Vegetable Rice, Slim Fast* | 1 Pack/375g | 375.0 | 5.0 | 100 | 5.8 | 15.5 | 1.4 | 0.8 |
| **CHICKEN IN** | | | | | | | | |
| a Curry Sauce, Fillets, Safeway* | 1 Serving/124g | 180.0 | 8.0 | 145 | 17.2 | 3.9 | 6.4 | 0.6 |
| Bacon, Mushroom & Red Wine Sauce, Asda* | 1 Serving/151g | 145.0 | 4.0 | 96 | 16.0 | 2.2 | 2.6 | 0.5 |
| Barbecue Sauce, COU, M & S* | 1 Pack/352g | 370.0 | 6.0 | 105 | 8.6 | 13.8 | 1.6 | 1.2 |
| Barbeque Sauce, Breasts, COU, M & S* | 1 Pack/350g | 420.0 | 7.0 | 120 | 8.5 | 20.6 | 1.9 | 0.6 |
| Barbeque Sauce, HE, Tesco* | 1 Breast/170g | 177.0 | 2.0 | 104 | 18.3 | 4.5 | 1.4 | 0.9 |
| Basil Sauce, with Pasta, Easy Steam, BGTY, Sainsbury's* | 1 Pack/380g | 429.0 | 7.0 | 113 | 9.7 | 14.4 | 1.8 | 1.3 |
| BBQ Sauce, Breast, Sainsbury's* | 1 Serving/170g | 199.0 | 1.0 | 117 | 14.5 | 13.1 | 0.7 | 1.3 |
| BBQ Sauce, Chargrilled, Breast, GFY, Asda* | 1 Serving/166g | 214.0 | 6.0 | 129 | 19.0 | 5.0 | 3.7 | 1.0 |
| BBQ Sauce, GFY, Asda* | 1 Pack/380g | 494.0 | 3.0 | 130 | 18.0 | 13.0 | 0.7 | 0.2 |
| BBQ Sauce, Weight Watchers* | 1 Pack/339g | 332.0 | 12.0 | 98 | 5.8 | 10.8 | 3.5 | 0.9 |
| Black Bean Sauce, & Rice, Morrisons* | 1 Pack/400g | 408.0 | 9.0 | 102 | 3.9 | 16.4 | 2.3 | 1.2 |
| Black Bean Sauce, Canned, BGTY, Sainsbury's* | 1 Can/400g | 308.0 | 4.0 | 77 | 9.3 | 7.9 | 0.9 | 0.7 |
| Black Bean Sauce, Frozen, BGTY, Sainsbury's* | 1 Pack/400g | 380.0 | 4.0 | 95 | 4.5 | 16.6 | 1.1 | 0.5 |
| Black Bean Sauce, M & S* | 1 Pack/350g | 297.0 | 7.0 | 85 | 8.7 | 8.0 | 2.0 | 1.1 |
| Black Bean Sauce, Sainsbury's* | 1 Pack/465g | 484.0 | 8.0 | 104 | 5.0 | 17.3 | 1.7 | 0.3 |
| Black Bean Sauce, Tinned, Tesco* | 1 Serving/200g | 164.0 | 3.0 | 82 | 10.0 | 7.7 | 1.3 | 1.1 |
| Black Bean Sauce, with Egg Fried Rice, GFY, Asda* | 1 Serving/416g | 320.0 | 4.0 | 77 | 5.0 | 12.0 | 1.0 | 0.9 |
| Black Bean Sauce, with Rice, Asda* | 1 Pack/400g | 500.0 | 8.0 | 125 | 7.0 | 20.0 | 1.9 | 0.6 |
| Broccoli & Mushroom, with Rice, HE, Tesco* | 1 Pack/400g | 440.0 | 5.0 | 110 | 7.5 | 17.1 | 1.2 | 0.7 |
| Cheese & Bacon, Wrapped, Breast, Tesco* | 1 Serving/300g | 474.0 | 23.0 | 158 | 20.7 | 1.2 | 7.8 | 0.5 |
| Cheesy Salsa, Fillets, Safeway* | ½ Pack/175g | 192.0 | 5.0 | 110 | 17.9 | 2.2 | 3.0 | 1.1 |
| Chilli & Lemon Grass with Rice, Sainsbury's* | 1 Pack/450g | 526.0 | 11.0 | 117 | 6.2 | 17.4 | 2.5 | 0.7 |
| Coconut, Sizzler, HL, Tesco* | 1 Pack/350g | 280.0 | 8.0 | 80 | 9.8 | 4.5 | 2.2 | 2.1 |
| Creamy Madeira Sauce, HL, Tesco* | 1 Pack/400g | 320.0 | 7.0 | 80 | 12.8 | 2.3 | 1.7 | 1.0 |
| Creamy Mushroom Sauce, HL, Tesco* | 1 Pack/400g | 296.0 | 6.0 | 74 | 13.2 | 1.8 | 1.5 | 0.5 |
| Creamy Mustard Sauce, GFY, Asda* | 1 Pack/400g | 468.0 | 9.0 | 117 | 6.0 | 18.0 | 2.3 | 0.4 |
| Creamy Thai Sauce, Somerfield* | 1 Pack/440g | 748.0 | 35.0 | 170 | 22.0 | 2.0 | 8.0 | 0.0 |
| Creamy Tikka Style Sauce, Tesco* | 1 Breast/190g | 215.0 | 10.0 | 113 | 15.1 | 0.7 | 5.5 | 0.8 |
| Creamy Tomato & Mascarpone Sauce, Waitrose* | 1 Serving/400g | 492.0 | 23.0 | 123 | 7.9 | 9.9 | 5.8 | 0.8 |
| Creamy White Wine Sauce, Sainsbury's* | 1 Pack/324g | 285.0 | 12.0 | 88 | 8.9 | 4.7 | 3.7 | 1.0 |
| Garlic & Cream Sauce, Breast Fillet, Morrisons* | 1 Serving/180g | 262.0 | 16.0 | 146 | 14.9 | 1.8 | 8.8 | 0.6 |
| Garlic & Herbs, Breast, Sainsbury's* | 1 Serving/200g | 316.0 | 5.0 | 158 | 28.3 | 5.4 | 2.6 | 0.1 |
| Ginger & Chilli with Veg Noodles, COU, M & S* | 1 Pack/400g | 300.0 | 2.0 | 75 | 6.4 | 10.7 | 0.6 | 1.1 |

## CHICKEN IN

| | Measure INFO/WEIGHT | per Measure KCAL | FAT | Nutrition Values per 100g / 100ml KCAL | PROT | CARB | FAT | FIBRE |
|---|---|---|---|---|---|---|---|---|
| Gravy, Chunky, M & S* | 1 Can/489g | 465.0 | 19.0 | 95 | 13.6 | 1.4 | 3.9 | 0.8 |
| Hot Ginger Sauce, with Jasmine Rice, BGTY, Sainsbury's* | 1 Pack/400g | 400.0 | 6.0 | 100 | 6.6 | 15.4 | 1.4 | 0.5 |
| Hot Ginger Sauce, with Thai Sticky Rice, Sainsbury's* | 1 Pack/450g | 603.0 | 21.0 | 134 | 6.8 | 16.3 | 4.6 | 0.5 |
| Hunter's BBQ Sauce, Asda* | ½ Pack /190g | 348.0 | 14.0 | 183 | 19.1 | 10.3 | 7.4 | 0.0 |
| Leek & Bacon Sauce, with Mash, HL, Tesco* | 1 Pack/450g | 337.0 | 8.0 | 75 | 6.7 | 8.0 | 1.8 | 1.6 |
| Lemon & Garlic Marinade, Thighs, Go Cook, Asda* | ½ Pack/265g | 493.0 | 30.0 | 186 | 19.7 | 1.2 | 11.4 | 0.8 |
| Lemon Sauce with Rice, Sainsbury's* | 1 Pack/450g | 513.0 | 7.0 | 114 | 8.1 | 17.0 | 1.5 | 0.7 |
| Lime & Coriander Marinade, Chargrilled, Asda* | ½ Pack/163g | 286.0 | 15.0 | 175 | 23.0 | 0.5 | 9.0 | 0.0 |
| Madeira Sauce, with Mushrooms, Finest, Tesco* | ½ Pack/200g | 210.0 | 8.0 | 105 | 13.8 | 2.9 | 4.1 | 0.9 |
| Mango Ginger Marinade, Breast, Chargrilled, GFY, Asda* | ½ Pack/190g | 234.0 | 2.0 | 123 | 17.0 | 11.0 | 1.2 | 0.5 |
| Masala with Spiced Indian Lentils, M & S* | 1 Pack/330g | 297.0 | 8.0 | 90 | 10.3 | 6.1 | 2.5 | 5.9 |
| Mediterranean Style Sauce, Breasts, BGTY, Sainsbury's* | ½ Pack/170g | 148.0 | 3.0 | 87 | 14.5 | 2.7 | 2.0 | 0.9 |
| Mexican Salsa, Tesco* | 1 Pack/320g | 368.0 | 9.0 | 115 | 19.5 | 3.1 | 2.7 | 0.6 |
| Mexican Style Sauce, Tesco* | 1 Serving/180g | 128.0 | 1.0 | 71 | 13.3 | 2.6 | 0.8 | 0.7 |
| Mushroom & Ham Sauce with Rice, BGTY, Sainsbury's* | 1 Pack/450g | 580.0 | 7.0 | 129 | 9.7 | 18.9 | 1.6 | 0.3 |
| Mushroom & Red Wine Sauce, Breast Fillets, Morrisons* | 1 Serving/177g | 184.0 | 4.0 | 104 | 15.7 | 4.6 | 2.5 | 0.7 |
| Mushroom & White Wine Sauce, Fillets, Morrisons* | 1 Serving/190g | 243.0 | 10.0 | 128 | 18.8 | 0.9 | 5.5 | 0.5 |
| Mushroom Sauce with Mash, HL, Tesco* | 1 Pack/400g | 384.0 | 11.0 | 96 | 9.9 | 8.0 | 2.7 | 0.6 |
| Oyster Sauce, & Mushrooms, Tesco* | 1 Pack/350g | 252.0 | 6.0 | 72 | 8.0 | 6.3 | 1.6 | 0.7 |
| Oyster Sauce, with Mushrooms, Tesco^ | 1 Pack/350g | 189.0 | 3.0 | 54 | 8.0 | 3.5 | 0.9 | 0.8 |
| Peppercorn Sauce, GFY, Asda* | 1 Serving/399g | 431.0 | 7.0 | 108 | 6.0 | 17.0 | 1.8 | 0.5 |
| Peppers, Fillets, Sainsbury's* | 1 Pack/360g | 378.0 | 13.0 | 105 | 13.7 | 4.2 | 3.7 | 1.1 |
| Pesto Style Dressing, Asda* | 1 Serving/150g | 210.0 | 10.0 | 140 | 18.7 | 1.3 | 6.7 | 0.0 |
| Red Pepper Dressing, Tesco* | 1 Serving/140g | 228.0 | 13.0 | 163 | 19.2 | 0.1 | 9.5 | 0.5 |
| Red Thai Marinade, Breasts, Mini, HE, Tesco* | 1 Serving/200g | 276.0 | 5.0 | 138 | 26.8 | 2.0 | 2.5 | 0.5 |
| Red Wine, with Mash, Eat Smart, Morrisons* | 1 Serving/400g | 288.0 | 5.0 | 72 | 9.1 | 6.1 | 1.3 | 1.4 |
| Red Wine Sauce, Fillets, Safeway* | 1 Serving/175g | 210.0 | 7.0 | 120 | 17.7 | 2.9 | 3.9 | 0.7 |
| Satay Sauce, Safeway* | 1 Serving/250g | 362.0 | 20.0 | 145 | 10.5 | 7.1 | 8.0 | 1.4 |
| Shiraz Wine Sauce, Finest, Tesco* | 1 Pack/600g | 420.0 | 10.0 | 70 | 10.9 | 2.9 | 1.6 | 1.3 |
| Smoky Barbecue Sauce, Breast, Fresh Tastes, Asda* | 1 Breast/160g | 258.0 | 6.0 | 161 | 21.9 | 9.6 | 3.9 | 0.9 |
| Smoky Barbeque Sauce, Tesco* | 1 Serving/185g | 229.0 | 4.0 | 124 | 16.3 | 9.9 | 2.1 | 1.0 |
| Spicy Chilli Sauce, Topped with Cheese, Breast, Asda* | ½ Pack/190g | 241.0 | 7.0 | 127 | 20.0 | 3.4 | 3.7 | 0.0 |
| Sun Dried Tomato & Basil Sauce, Breast, Iceland* | 1 Serving/156g | 134.0 | 2.0 | 86 | 14.6 | 3.3 | 1.6 | 1.0 |
| Sweet Chilli Sauce, Breast, Fresh Tastes, Asda* | ½ Pack/180g | 288.0 | 9.0 | 160 | 18.4 | 10.3 | 5.0 | 0.5 |
| Tarragon Sauce, Lean Cuisine* | 1 Pack/338g | 270.0 | 7.0 | 80 | 4.0 | 11.0 | 2.0 | 1.5 |
| Tomato & Basil, with Roasted Potatoes, BGTY, Sainsbury's* | 1 Pack/450g | 418.0 | 4.0 | 93 | 8.1 | 13.1 | 0.9 | 2.3 |
| Tomato & Basil Sauce, Breast, Fresh Tastes, Asda* | ½ Pack/130g | 136.0 | 3.0 | 105 | 19.3 | 2.3 | 2.1 | 0.7 |
| Tomato & Basil Sauce, Breast, GFY, Asda* | 1 Pack/392g | 447.0 | 13.0 | 114 | 12.0 | 9.0 | 3.4 | 1.5 |
| Tomato & Basil Sauce, Breast Fillets, Morrisons* | ½ Pack/171g | 231.0 | 8.0 | 135 | 21.3 | 2.5 | 4.4 | 1.4 |
| Tomato & Basil Sauce, Eat Smart, Safeway* | 1 Serving/236g | 165.0 | 4.0 | 70 | 10.3 | 2.4 | 1.6 | 1.3 |
| Tomato & Basil Sauce, HL, Tesco* | 1 Breast/200g | 154.0 | 2.0 | 77 | 12.4 | 4.2 | 1.2 | 0.6 |
| Tomato & Herb Sauce, Breasts, Tesco* | ½ Pack/173g | 155.0 | 2.0 | 90 | 15.0 | 3.6 | 1.4 | 0.5 |
| Tomato & Wine Sauce, Potatoes, SteamFresh, Birds Eye* | 1 Pack/400g | 280.0 | 6.0 | 70 | 7.7 | 6.7 | 1.4 | 1.6 |
| White Sauce, BGTY, Sainsbury's* | 1 Can/200g | 162.0 | 4.0 | 81 | 1.2 | 2.4 | 2.1 | 1.1 |
| White Sauce, Canned, Asda* | ½ Can/400g | 644.0 | 44.0 | 161 | 12.0 | 3.5 | 11.0 | 0.0 |
| White Sauce, Canned, HL, Tesco* | ½ Can/200g | 180.0 | 6.0 | 90 | 14.3 | 1.3 | 2.9 | 5.4 |
| White Sauce, Low Fat, Breast, Safeway* | 1 Serving/200g | 190.0 | 9.0 | 95 | 11.5 | 2.1 | 4.5 | 0.2 |
| White Wine, with Pasta, Perfectly Balanced, Waitrose* | 1 Pack/400g | 400.0 | 10.0 | 100 | 8.2 | 12.1 | 2.5 | 2.5 |
| White Wine, with Rice, Eat Smart, Safeway* | 1 Serving/400g | 400.0 | 4.0 | 100 | 8.9 | 13.6 | 1.0 | 1.1 |
| White Wine, with Rice, HE, Tesco* | 1 Serving/450g | 513.0 | 12.0 | 114 | 7.1 | 15.3 | 2.7 | 0.7 |
| White Wine & Asparagus Panzerotti, Asda* | ½ Pack/150g | 238.0 | 3.0 | 159 | 8.0 | 28.0 | 1.7 | 0.0 |
| White Wine & Mushroom Sauce, M & S* | 1 Serving/200g | 260.0 | 14.0 | 130 | 15.6 | 1.6 | 6.8 | 1.0 |
| White Wine & Tarragon Sauce, Breasts, Finest, Tesco* | ½ Pack/200g | 326.0 | 20.0 | 163 | 16.8 | 1.3 | 10.1 | 0.0 |

| | Measure INFO/WEIGHT | per Measure KCAL | FAT | Nutrition Values per 100g / 100ml KCAL | PROT | CARB | FAT | FIBRE |
|---|---|---|---|---|---|---|---|---|
| **CHICKEN IN** | | | | | | | | |
| White Wine & Tarragon Sauce, Somerfield* | ½ Pack/136g | 163.0 | 7.0 | 120 | 18.1 | 0.6 | 5.0 | 0.6 |
| White Wine Sauce, Breasts, Tesco* | 1 Serving/370g | 388.0 | 14.0 | 105 | 16.9 | 0.8 | 3.8 | 0.6 |
| White Wine Sauce, Simple Solutions, Tesco* | ½ Pack/200g | 198.0 | 4.0 | 99 | 19.3 | 0.9 | 2.0 | 0.5 |
| White Wine Sauce, Wild Rice, Pub Specials, Birds Eye* | 1 Pack/450g | 335.0 | 6.0 | 74 | 7.1 | 8.4 | 1.3 | 2.1 |
| White Wine Sauce, with Rice, HL, Tesco* | 1 Pack/450g | 500.0 | 7.0 | 111 | 7.1 | 17.0 | 1.6 | 0.8 |
| Wild Mushroom Sauce, Breasts, HL, Tesco* | 1 Serving/212g | 191.0 | 5.0 | 90 | 15.1 | 2.1 | 2.4 | 1.5 |
| Wild Mushroom Sauce, Extra Special, Asda* | 1 Serving/225g | 319.0 | 19.0 | 142 | 14.2 | 2.2 | 8.4 | 0.3 |
| Zesty Orange Sauce, Breast, Asda* | 1 Serving/200g | 326.0 | 14.0 | 163 | 16.0 | 9.0 | 7.0 | 0.0 |
| **CHICKEN ITALIAN** | | | | | | | | |
| Style, BGTY, Sainsbury's* | 1 Pack/400g | 364.0 | 4.0 | 91 | 6.0 | 14.5 | 1.1 | 0.9 |
| Style, Meal, Asda* | 1 Pack/408g | 241.0 | 3.0 | 59 | 6.0 | 7.0 | 0.8 | 0.8 |
| Style, Sainsbury's* | ½ Pack/190g | 222.0 | 8.0 | 117 | 16.3 | 3.9 | 4.0 | 0.1 |
| with a Spicy Tomato, Chilli & Herb Sauce, Slim Fast* | 1 Pack/371g | 390.0 | 4.0 | 105 | 7.1 | 16.6 | 1.1 | 0.4 |
| **CHICKEN JEERA** | | | | | | | | |
| Sainsbury's* | ½ Pack/201g | 247.0 | 14.0 | 123 | 10.5 | 4.6 | 7.0 | 1.8 |
| **CHICKEN KUNG PO** | | | | | | | | |
| Sainsbury's* | ½ Pack/175g | 131.0 | 4.0 | 75 | 9.2 | 4.0 | 2.5 | 1.0 |
| Waitrose* | 1 Pack/350g | 318.0 | 4.0 | 91 | 8.2 | 12.1 | 1.1 | 1.2 |
| with Egg Fried Rice, Asda* | 1 Pack/450g | 688.0 | 22.0 | 153 | 6.0 | 21.0 | 5.0 | 1.0 |
| **CHICKEN LEMON** | | | | | | | | |
| Balls, Asda* | 1 Ball/15g | 42.0 | 3.0 | 279 | 14.0 | 19.0 | 17.0 | 1.6 |
| Battered, Cantonese, Sainsbury's* | 1 Pack/350g | 560.0 | 20.0 | 160 | 10.7 | 16.6 | 5.6 | 0.9 |
| Battered, Chinese Meal for Two, Tesco* | ½ Serving/175g | 294.0 | 13.0 | 168 | 6.6 | 18.8 | 7.4 | 2.0 |
| Battered, HE, Tesco* | 1 Pack/350g | 399.0 | 9.0 | 114 | 8.8 | 13.9 | 2.6 | 0.4 |
| Cantonese, Sainsbury's* | ½ Pack/140g | 218.0 | 9.0 | 156 | 11.0 | 13.9 | 6.3 | 0.6 |
| Chinese, Tesco* | 1 Serving/350g | 563.0 | 11.0 | 161 | 7.0 | 26.0 | 3.2 | 0.3 |
| COU, M & S* | 1 Pack/150g | 150.0 | 1.0 | 100 | 17.9 | 5.6 | 0.9 | 0.8 |
| Steam Cuisine, COU, M & S* | 1 Pack/400g | 420.0 | 9.0 | 105 | 9.8 | 11.8 | 2.2 | 2.0 |
| Tesco* | ½ Pack/175g | 213.0 | 7.0 | 122 | 11.0 | 10.1 | 4.2 | 0.6 |
| with Rice, HL, Tesco* | 1 Pack/450g | 477.0 | 12.0 | 106 | 5.9 | 14.4 | 2.7 | 0.9 |
| with Vegetable Rice, BGTY, Sainsbury's* | 1 Pack/400g | 428.0 | 6.0 | 107 | 6.5 | 16.8 | 1.6 | 0.8 |
| **CHICKEN LUNCH** | | | | | | | | |
| French Style, Light, John West* | 1 Pack/240g | 194.0 | 6.0 | 81 | 7.2 | 6.9 | 2.7 | 2.1 |
| Italian Style, Light, John West* | 1 Pack/240g | 209.0 | 6.0 | 87 | 6.9 | 9.0 | 2.6 | 0.7 |
| **CHICKEN MEAL** | | | | | | | | |
| American, Fillets, Asda* | 1 Pack/345g | 838.0 | 38.0 | 243 | 9.0 | 27.0 | 11.0 | 2.3 |
| Breast Fillets, Meal For One, Eat Well, M & S* | 1 Pack/400g | 340.0 | 10.0 | 85 | 7.0 | 7.9 | 2.6 | 1.5 |
| Roast, M & S* | 1 Pack/250g | 375.0 | 19.0 | 150 | 14.6 | 5.3 | 7.7 | 0.1 |
| **CHICKEN MEDITERRANEAN** | | | | | | | | |
| with Trotolle Pasta, Easy Steam, BGTY, Sainsbury's* | 1 Pack/400g | 284.0 | 4.0 | 71 | 7.8 | 7.5 | 1.1 | 2.9 |
| **CHICKEN MEXICAN** | | | | | | | | |
| Style, BGTY, Sainsbury's* | 1 Serving/260g | 255.0 | 6.0 | 98 | 6.9 | 12.1 | 2.5 | 2.2 |
| Style, Combo, Asda* | 1 Pack/380g | 562.0 | 17.0 | 148 | 21.0 | 6.0 | 4.4 | 2.0 |
| Style, GFY, Asda* | ½ Pack/200g | 256.0 | 10.0 | 128 | 17.0 | 3.7 | 5.0 | 0.3 |
| Style, with Rice, BFY, Morrisons* | 1 Pack/400g | 360.0 | 5.0 | 90 | 5.1 | 14.1 | 1.3 | 0.8 |
| **CHICKEN MOROCCAN** | | | | | | | | |
| Style, Sainsbury's* | ½ Pack/269g | 334.0 | 7.0 | 124 | 14.7 | 10.4 | 2.6 | 3.1 |
| Style, with Spicy Cous Cous, BGTY, Sainsbury's* | 1 Serving/225g | 304.0 | 4.0 | 135 | 9.2 | 20.6 | 1.7 | 0.0 |
| with Cous Cous, GFY, Asda* | 1 Serving/450g | 414.0 | 6.0 | 92 | 8.0 | 12.0 | 1.3 | 0.8 |
| with Cous Cous & Fruity Sauce, BGTY, Sainsbury's* | 1 Pack/400g | 440.0 | 8.0 | 110 | 10.0 | 13.1 | 2.0 | 2.6 |
| **CHICKEN MUSTARD** | | | | | | | | |
| with Creme Fraiche Mash, Perfectly Balanced, Waitrose* | 1 Pack/400g | 408.0 | 16.0 | 102 | 7.2 | 9.4 | 4.0 | 0.8 |
| with Gratin Potatoes, HL, Tesco* | 1 Pack/450g | 463.0 | 12.0 | 103 | 9.0 | 10.7 | 2.7 | 2.5 |

| | Measure INFO/WEIGHT | per Measure KCAL | FAT | Nutrition Values per 100g / 100ml KCAL | PROT | CARB | FAT | FIBRE |
|---|---|---|---|---|---|---|---|---|
| **CHICKEN ORIENTAL** | | | | | | | | |
| & Pineapple, HL, Tesco* | 1 Serving/450g | 414.0 | 3.0 | 92 | 6.0 | 15.4 | 0.7 | 0.6 |
| Slim Fast* | 1 Pack/385g | 385.0 | 2.0 | 100 | 5.7 | 18.6 | 0.6 | 0.6 |
| with Noodles, SteamFresh, Birds Eye* | 1 Pack/400g | 336.0 | 9.0 | 84 | 7.1 | 9.0 | 2.2 | 0.3 |
| **CHICKEN PAPRIKA** | | | | | | | | |
| COU, M & S* | 1 Pack/400g | 380.0 | 6.0 | 95 | 9.0 | 11.7 | 1.6 | 2.0 |
| with Savoury Rice & Vegetables, BGTY, Sainsbury's* | 1 Pack/400g | 383.0 | 2.0 | 96 | 7.1 | 15.5 | 0.6 | 1.1 |
| **CHICKEN PEPPER** | | | | | | | | |
| Fry, Sainsbury's* | 1 Pack/400g | 508.0 | 25.0 | 127 | 15.0 | 2.9 | 6.2 | 1.6 |
| Hot, & Hash, HL, Tesco* | 1 Pack/450g | 396.0 | 9.0 | 88 | 7.0 | 10.7 | 1.9 | 1.0 |
| Hot, with Minted Mash, BGTY, Sainsbury's* | 1 Serving/450g | 333.0 | 5.0 | 74 | 7.3 | 8.4 | 1.2 | 1.3 |
| **CHICKEN PICCATA** | | | | | | | | |
| HE, Tesco* | 1 Pack/405g | 518.0 | 15.0 | 128 | 15.7 | 7.7 | 3.8 | 0.5 |
| **CHICKEN PIRI PIRI** | | | | | | | | |
| & Rice, HE, Tesco* | 1 Pack/395g | 395.0 | 8.0 | 100 | 8.2 | 12.0 | 2.0 | 1.7 |
| GFY, Asda* | 1 Pack/400g | 360.0 | 2.0 | 90 | 4.7 | 17.0 | 0.4 | 0.5 |
| M & S* | 1 Pack/300g | 420.0 | 23.0 | 140 | 10.0 | 7.3 | 7.7 | 1.3 |
| Sainsbury's* | ½ Pack/200g | 248.0 | 11.0 | 124 | 14.0 | 4.8 | 5.4 | 0.5 |
| with Rice, BGTY, Sainsbury's* | 1 Serving/399g | 395.0 | 4.0 | 99 | 10.3 | 11.9 | 1.1 | 1.6 |
| **CHICKEN ROLL** | | | | | | | | |
| Value, Tesco* | 1 Slice/13g | 30.0 | 2.0 | 223 | 15.4 | 3.9 | 16.2 | 0.1 |
| with Pork, Sage & Onion Stuffing, Value, Tesco* | 1 Roll/125g | 166.0 | 9.0 | 133 | 9.4 | 7.8 | 7.1 | 0.5 |
| **CHICKEN SAFFRON** | | | | | | | | |
| & Rice, M & S* | 1 Pack/400g | 360.0 | 5.0 | 90 | 7.6 | 11.6 | 1.2 | 1.1 |
| **CHICKEN SIZZLER** | | | | | | | | |
| GFY, Asda* | 1 Pack/350g | 289.0 | 5.0 | 83 | 12.9 | 4.6 | 1.4 | 1.4 |
| HL, Tesco* | 1 Serving/350g | 273.0 | 7.0 | 78 | 11.1 | 3.8 | 2.0 | 4.3 |
| **CHICKEN SPANISH** | | | | | | | | |
| Style, Asda* | ½ Pack/275g | 322.0 | 13.0 | 117 | 14.0 | 4.1 | 4.9 | 0.7 |
| **CHICKEN STUFFED** | | | | | | | | |
| Asparagus & Ricotta, with Herb Rice, BGTY, Sainsbury's* | 1 Pack/400g | 444.0 | 10.0 | 111 | 8.1 | 13.8 | 2.6 | 0.3 |
| Breast, with Mushrooms, HE, Tesco* | 1 Serving/175g | 152.0 | 3.0 | 87 | 16.3 | 1.5 | 1.8 | 0.2 |
| with Moroccan Style Cous Cous, GFY, Asda* | ½ Pack/180g | 259.0 | 5.0 | 144 | 20.0 | 10.0 | 2.7 | 0.0 |
| with Mushrooms, Finest, Tesco* | 1 Serving/150g | 177.0 | 8.0 | 118 | 15.9 | 2.0 | 5.1 | 0.6 |
| **CHICKEN SUPREME** | | | | | | | | |
| BGTY, Sainsbury's* | 1 Pack/350g | 416.0 | 5.0 | 119 | 9.4 | 17.2 | 1.4 | 0.5 |
| Breast, Sainsbury's* | 1 Serving/187g | 421.0 | 30.0 | 225 | 20.6 | 0.3 | 15.8 | 0.6 |
| with Rice, Birds Eye* | 1 Pack/376g | 470.0 | 10.0 | 125 | 6.6 | 18.8 | 2.6 | 0.5 |
| with Rice, Weight Watchers* | 1 Pack/300g | 255.0 | 5.0 | 85 | 5.6 | 11.9 | 1.6 | 0.5 |
| **CHICKEN SZECHUAN** | | | | | | | | |
| Chilli & Peppercorn, Sainsbury's* | 1 Pack/400g | 352.0 | 16.0 | 88 | 9.9 | 3.2 | 4.0 | 0.5 |
| Tesco* | 1 Pack/350g | 385.0 | 10.0 | 110 | 7.2 | 13.6 | 3.0 | 0.3 |
| with Noodles, Sainsbury's* | 1 Pack/450g | 423.0 | 14.0 | 94 | 6.0 | 10.4 | 3.1 | 0.9 |
| **CHICKEN TANDOORI** | | | | | | | | |
| Finest, Tesco* | 1 Pack/450g | 495.0 | 18.0 | 110 | 7.4 | 10.2 | 4.1 | 1.3 |
| GFY, Asda* | 1 Pack/400g | 324.0 | 10.0 | 81 | 7.5 | 7.3 | 2.4 | 1.7 |
| Masala, & Rice, HL, Tesco* | 1 Serving/450g | 409.0 | 8.0 | 91 | 6.6 | 12.9 | 1.7 | 0.6 |
| Masala, Asda* | 1 Pack/400g | 580.0 | 20.0 | 145 | 7.0 | 18.0 | 5.0 | 1.3 |
| Masala, Indian, Tesco* | 1 Serving/350g | 430.0 | 26.0 | 123 | 10.2 | 4.0 | 7.4 | 1.8 |
| Masala, Sainsbury's* | 1 Pack/400g | 536.0 | 27.0 | 134 | 13.2 | 5.0 | 6.8 | 0.5 |
| Sizzler, HL, Tesco* | 1 Pack/350g | 275.0 | 7.0 | 79 | 11.1 | 3.8 | 2.0 | 4.3 |
| Sizzler, Sainsbury's* | 1 Pack/400g | 536.0 | 29.0 | 134 | 12.8 | 4.3 | 7.3 | 1.7 |
| Sizzler, Tesco* | 1 Serving/175g | 243.0 | 12.0 | 139 | 10.0 | 10.0 | 6.6 | 1.0 |
| with Rice, Easy Steam, Tesco* | 1 Pack/400g | 484.0 | 12.0 | 121 | 8.7 | 14.7 | 3.0 | 0.7 |

C

| | Measure INFO/WEIGHT | per Measure KCAL | FAT | Nutrition Values per 100g / 100ml KCAL | PROT | CARB | FAT | FIBRE |
|---|---|---|---|---|---|---|---|---|
| **CHICKEN TANDOORI** | | | | | | | | |
| with Spicy Potatoes & Dip, HE, Tesco* | 1 Pack/370g | 322.0 | 3.0 | 87 | 9.7 | 10.3 | 0.8 | 1.3 |
| with Spicy Vegatable Rice, Eat Smart, Safeway* | 1 Serving/350g | 367.0 | 8.0 | 105 | 9.7 | 11.1 | 2.2 | 7.0 |
| **CHICKEN TERIYAKI** | | | | | | | | |
| & Noodles, Asda* | ½ Pack/340g | 445.0 | 9.0 | 131 | 9.0 | 18.0 | 2.6 | 0.9 |
| Asda* | 1 Pack/360g | 299.0 | 5.0 | 83 | 9.1 | 8.6 | 1.4 | 0.8 |
| Japanese, with Ramen Noodles, Sainsbury's* | 1 Pack/450g | 481.0 | 9.0 | 107 | 6.5 | 15.5 | 2.1 | 0.8 |
| **CHICKEN THAI** | | | | | | | | |
| & Siu Mai Dumplings, M & S* | 1 Dumpling/21g | 35.0 | 2.0 | 170 | 16.0 | 9.4 | 7.6 | 0.8 |
| & Vegetables, Eat Positive, Birds Eye* | 1 Packet/400g | 412.0 | 12.0 | 103 | 5.9 | 13.0 | 3.0 | 1.0 |
| Chiang Mai, & Noodles, BGTY, Sainsbury's* | 1 Pack/448g | 484.0 | 18.0 | 108 | 6.9 | 11.0 | 4.0 | 1.7 |
| Green, Fillets, Mini, Sainsbury's* | ½ Pack/100g | 130.0 | 2.0 | 130 | 27.9 | 0.9 | 1.6 | 0.8 |
| Marinated in Lemongrass, Lime Leaves & Chilli, Waitrose* | 1 Serving/390g | 323.0 | 9.0 | 83 | 8.0 | 7.2 | 2.4 | 9.5 |
| Style, with Noodles, Tesco* | 1 Pack/400g | 332.0 | 7.0 | 83 | 7.5 | 9.5 | 1.7 | 1.0 |
| Style Marinade, Breast, Chargrilled, GFY, Asda* | ½ Pack/178g | 178.0 | 5.0 | 100 | 17.0 | 1.3 | 3.0 | 0.5 |
| with Rice, SteamFresh, Birds Eye* | 1 Serving/400g | 380.0 | 8.0 | 95 | 6.7 | 12.7 | 1.9 | 0.9 |
| **CHICKEN TIKKA** | | | | | | | | |
| & Coriander Rice, Weight Watchers* | 1 Pack/400g | 348.0 | 2.0 | 87 | 6.2 | 14.3 | 0.6 | 1.6 |
| & Lemon Rice, Deli Meal, M & S* | 1 Pack/360g | 342.0 | 7.0 | 95 | 9.8 | 10.2 | 2.0 | 0.7 |
| BGTY, Sainsbury's* | 1 Serving/188g | 265.0 | 3.0 | 141 | 10.5 | 21.2 | 1.6 | 0.0 |
| Creamy, Breast, Tesco* | 1 Breast/190g | 215.0 | 10.0 | 113 | 15.1 | 0.7 | 5.5 | 0.8 |
| Masala, with Pilau Rice, Hot, Tesco* | 1 Pack/550g | 797.0 | 32.0 | 145 | 7.4 | 15.0 | 5.8 | 1.4 |
| Masala, with Rice & Naan, Big Dish, Tesco* | 1 Pack/600g | 960.0 | 40.0 | 160 | 6.7 | 18.1 | 6.7 | 1.2 |
| Masala, with Yellow Rice, Light Choices, Tesco* | 1 Pack/441g | 485.0 | 9.0 | 110 | 4.9 | 17.4 | 2.0 | 1.0 |
| Masala & Pilau Rice, Asda* | 1 Serving/500g | 720.0 | 20.0 | 144 | 6.2 | 20.7 | 4.0 | 0.9 |
| with Basmati Rice, GFY, Asda* | 1 Pack/400g | 592.0 | 7.0 | 148 | 9.0 | 24.0 | 1.8 | 1.6 |
| with Pilau Rice, GFY, Asda* | 1 Pack/450g | 382.0 | 3.0 | 85 | 7.0 | 13.0 | 0.6 | 1.8 |
| **CHICKEN VINDALOO** | | | | | | | | |
| Asda* | 1 Pack/411g | 649.0 | 25.0 | 158 | 7.0 | 19.0 | 6.0 | 0.0 |
| Sainsbury's* | 1 Pack/400g | 460.0 | 17.0 | 115 | 14.6 | 4.8 | 4.2 | 0.6 |
| Waitrose* | 1 Pack/340g | 398.0 | 18.0 | 117 | 10.6 | 6.4 | 5.4 | 1.6 |
| **CHICKEN WITH** | | | | | | | | |
| a Sticky Honey & Chilli Sauce, Breast, Asda* | 1 Serving/175g | 247.0 | 6.0 | 141 | 20.0 | 8.0 | 3.2 | 0.0 |
| Apricots & Almonds, HE, Tesco* | 1 Pack/500g | 465.0 | 9.0 | 93 | 11.8 | 7.3 | 1.9 | 0.5 |
| Asparagus & Rice, BGTY, Sainsbury's* | 1 Pack/400g | 428.0 | 6.0 | 107 | 9.1 | 14.5 | 1.4 | 0.9 |
| Bacon & Leeks, GFY, Asda* | 1 Pack/400g | 328.0 | 8.0 | 82 | 13.0 | 3.0 | 2.0 | 0.6 |
| Bacon & Leeks, with Mashed Potato, BGTY, Sainsbury's* | 1 Pack/450g | 435.0 | 11.0 | 97 | 8.4 | 10.1 | 2.5 | 0.7 |
| Basil, Puy Lentils & Spelt, Roasted, The Food Doctor* | 1 Pack/350g | 210.0 | 7.0 | 60 | 9.6 | 0.7 | 2.1 | 10.2 |
| Broccoli & Pesto Pasta, BGTY, Sainsbury's* | 1 Pack/301g | 328.0 | 5.0 | 109 | 10.3 | 13.2 | 1.7 | 2.5 |
| Caesar Melt & Prosciutto, Breast, M & S* | 1 Pack/375g | 487.0 | 19.0 | 130 | 19.6 | 1.3 | 5.0 | 1.0 |
| Caramelised Peppers, Chargrilled, M & S* | ½ Pack/237g | 225.0 | 9.0 | 95 | 12.9 | 2.1 | 3.8 | 1.3 |
| Cheddar & Bacon Filling, Breast, Just Cook, Sainsbury's* | 1 Serving/180g | 346.0 | 15.0 | 192 | 23.2 | 6.5 | 8.1 | 0.1 |
| Cheese, Leek & Bacon, Breasts, Stuffed, Safeway* | ½ Pack/159g | 310.0 | 16.0 | 195 | 24.3 | 1.0 | 9.9 | 0.6 |
| Cheese, Leek & Ham, Breast, Asda* | 1 Pack/430g | 632.0 | 30.0 | 147 | 19.5 | 1.5 | 7.0 | 0.6 |
| Cheese & Chive Sauce, Carb Control, Tesco* | 1 Serving/400g | 400.0 | 26.0 | 100 | 8.4 | 2.0 | 6.4 | 1.6 |
| Cheese Croutons & Onion, Asda* | 1 Serving/200g | 200.0 | 6.0 | 100 | 16.0 | 2.0 | 3.2 | 0.9 |
| Cheesy Salsa, Safeway* | 1 Serving/100g | 180.0 | 5.0 | 180 | 29.2 | 3.6 | 4.9 | 1.8 |
| Cherrywood Barbecue Sauce, Simply Cook, Tesco* | 1 Serving/147g | 165.0 | 2.0 | 112 | 16.6 | 7.6 | 1.7 | 0.4 |
| Chorizo, & Patatas Bravas, COU, M & S* | 1 Pack/400g | 380.0 | 9.0 | 95 | 7.8 | 10.8 | 2.3 | 1.7 |
| Coriander & Lime, Asda* | 1 Serving/105g | 122.0 | 1.0 | 116 | 24.0 | 2.9 | 0.9 | 0.2 |
| Cous Cous, Lemon & Herb, Finest, Tesco* | 1 Pack/370g | 492.0 | 18.0 | 133 | 10.5 | 11.5 | 5.0 | 0.9 |
| Creamy Mushroom Sauce, Eat Smart, Safeway* | 1 Serving/250g | 212.0 | 6.0 | 85 | 12.8 | 2.7 | 2.4 | 0.9 |
| Creamy Mushroom Sauce & Mash, HL, Tesco* | 1 Pack/400g | 384.0 | 11.0 | 96 | 9.9 | 8.0 | 2.7 | 0.6 |
| Creamy Spinach & Parmesan, M & S* | 1 Pack/390g | 468.0 | 17.0 | 120 | 10.8 | 12.3 | 4.4 | 2.5 |

## CHICKEN WITH

| | Measure INFO/WEIGHT | per Measure KCAL | FAT | Nutrition Values per 100g / 100ml KCAL | PROT | CARB | FAT | FIBRE |
|---|---|---|---|---|---|---|---|---|
| Fresh Mango, Chilli & Coriander, British, COU, M & S* | 1 Pack/169g | 270.0 | 4.0 | 160 | 12.1 | 22.8 | 2.3 | 1.9 |
| Fusilli & Courgette, Sainsbury's* | 1 Pack/450g | 675.0 | 29.0 | 150 | 8.6 | 14.6 | 6.4 | 0.5 |
| Garlic & Chilli Balti, Tesco* | 1 Pack/400g | 320.0 | 8.0 | 80 | 11.0 | 4.4 | 1.9 | 0.8 |
| Garlic & Mushrooms, Somerfield* | ½ Pack/100g | 145.0 | 5.0 | 145 | 23.9 | 0.0 | 5.5 | 1.6 |
| Garlic Mushrooms, Breast, Fresh Tastes, Asda* | ½ Pack/160g | 226.0 | 8.0 | 141 | 22.6 | 1.0 | 5.2 | 0.5 |
| Garlic Mushrooms, Breast, Simply Cook, Tesco* | ½ Pack/125g | 170.0 | 7.0 | 136 | 22.0 | 0.1 | 5.3 | 0.1 |
| Garlic Mushrooms, Breast, Tesco* | 1 Breast/125g | 149.0 | 6.0 | 119 | 19.0 | 0.2 | 4.7 | 0.1 |
| Grapes & Asparagus, Sainsbury's* | ½ Pack/200g | 240.0 | 13.0 | 120 | 13.3 | 1.8 | 6.6 | 1.0 |
| Gravy & Stuffing, Breasts, Tesco* | ½ Pack/173g | 257.0 | 11.0 | 149 | 14.4 | 8.3 | 6.4 | 2.2 |
| Gruyere & Smoked Garlic, Breast, TTD, Sainsbury's* | ½ Pack/200g | 444.0 | 30.0 | 222 | 17.3 | 4.2 | 15.1 | 0.1 |
| Gruyere Cheese & Parma Ham, Breast, COOK!, M & S* | 1 Breast/194g | 349.0 | 21.0 | 180 | 18.0 | 2.5 | 11.0 | 0.9 |
| Hoi Sin Sauce, Ooodles of Noodles, Oriental Express* | 1 Pack/425g | 399.0 | 9.0 | 94 | 5.3 | 13.2 | 2.2 | 1.7 |
| Honey & Mustard Sauce, Breasts, Simply Cook, Tesco* | ½ Pack/219g | 230.0 | 1.0 | 105 | 16.3 | 8.0 | 0.6 | 0.3 |
| Honey & Sesame, with Rice, Light Choices, Tesco* | 1 Pack/400g | 432.0 | 12.0 | 108 | 5.3 | 14.9 | 3.0 | 2.2 |
| Leek, Cheese & Bacon, Breasts, Simple Solutions, Tesco* | 1 Serving/200g | 296.0 | 17.0 | 148 | 17.6 | 0.5 | 8.4 | 0.3 |
| Lemon Grass, Thai Greens & Baby Corn, Sainsbury's* | 1 Serving/200g | 196.0 | 7.0 | 98 | 10.0 | 6.9 | 3.4 | 1.4 |
| Lime & Coriander, Easy, Waitrose* | ½ Pack/168g | 203.0 | 8.0 | 121 | 18.9 | 0.7 | 4.7 | 0.5 |
| Lime & Tequila, Asda* | 1 Serving/150g | 193.0 | 3.0 | 129 | 24.0 | 4.3 | 1.8 | 0.5 |
| Lyonnaise Potatoes, M & S* | ½ Pack/260g | 286.0 | 8.0 | 110 | 12.6 | 8.0 | 3.1 | 0.9 |
| Mango, Lime & Coriander, Asda* | 1 Pack/400g | 416.0 | 6.0 | 104 | 6.6 | 15.9 | 1.5 | 1.4 |
| Mango Salsa & Potato Wedges, BGTY, Sainsbury's* | 1 Pack/400g | 336.0 | 6.0 | 84 | 7.0 | 10.4 | 1.6 | 1.5 |
| Mascarpone, Bacon & Roasted Onions, Finest, Tesco* | 1 Serving/200g | 312.0 | 18.0 | 156 | 14.5 | 4.7 | 8.8 | 0.5 |
| Mozzarella & Pancetta, Breast, Finest, Tesco* | ½ Pack/225g | 326.0 | 14.0 | 145 | 14.4 | 7.9 | 6.2 | 1.1 |
| Mozzarella & Pesto Melt, Breasts, COOK!, M & S* | ½ Pack/165g | 206.0 | 10.0 | 125 | 16.4 | 1.3 | 6.2 | 0.7 |
| Mushroom & Bacon, Fillets, M & S* | ½ Pack/188g | 225.0 | 11.0 | 120 | 15.5 | 0.5 | 6.0 | 1.7 |
| Mushroom & Garlic, Breast Fillets, Just Cook, Sainsbury's* | ½ Pack/166g | 330.0 | 17.0 | 199 | 20.0 | 4.6 | 10.3 | 0.1 |
| Mushroom & Madeira Ragout, TTD, Sainsbury's* | ½ Pack/225g | 218.0 | 7.0 | 97 | 13.6 | 3.7 | 3.1 | 0.1 |
| Mushroom & Tomato Sauce, GFY, Asda* | 1 Serving/175g | 180.0 | 4.0 | 103 | 19.0 | 2.0 | 2.1 | 2.7 |
| Mushroom Pilaff, BGTY, Sainsbury's* | 1 Serving/400g | 320.0 | 2.0 | 80 | 8.0 | 10.5 | 0.5 | 1.4 |
| Mushroom Risotto, M & S* | 1 Pack/365g | 493.0 | 27.0 | 135 | 6.9 | 10.4 | 7.4 | 1.3 |
| Mushroom Sauce & Herby Rice, Fillets, M & S* | 1 Pack/380g | 475.0 | 19.0 | 125 | 7.7 | 12.0 | 5.1 | 1.3 |
| Mushrooms, in Madeira Sauce, HE, Tesco* | ½ Pack/200g | 182.0 | 2.0 | 91 | 15.0 | 5.4 | 1.0 | 0.4 |
| Pancakes & Plum Sauce, COU, M & S* | 1 Pack/245g | 257.0 | 6.0 | 105 | 7.9 | 12.7 | 2.3 | 0.3 |
| Pasta, Chianti & Balsamic, BGTY, Sainsbury's* | 1 Pack/400g | 372.0 | 8.0 | 93 | 9.4 | 9.5 | 1.9 | 1.9 |
| Peppercorn Sauce & Chunky Chips, Light Choices, Tesco* | 1 Pack/420g | 357.0 | 8.0 | 85 | 7.1 | 9.9 | 1.8 | 0.9 |
| Pesto & Linguine Pasta, Steamfresh Meal, Birds Eye* | 1 Pack/400g | 440.0 | 16.0 | 110 | 8.5 | 10.0 | 4.0 | 1.3 |
| Plum Sauce, Battered, Tesco* | 1 Serving/175g | 324.0 | 10.0 | 185 | 6.7 | 26.5 | 5.8 | 0.8 |
| Plum Tomatoes & Basil, Breast, Birds Eye* | 1 Serving/172g | 200.0 | 8.0 | 116 | 13.3 | 5.0 | 4.7 | 0.6 |
| Pork, Parsnip Herb Stuffing, Sainsbury's* | 1 Serving/100g | 181.0 | 9.0 | 181 | 22.9 | 2.1 | 9.0 | 0.7 |
| Pork, Sage & Onion Stuffing, Mini Roasts, Tesco* | 1 Serving/240g | 353.0 | 21.0 | 147 | 14.7 | 2.6 | 8.6 | 0.2 |
| Pork Stuffing & Chipolatas, Breast Joint, Tesco* | ½ Pack/340g | 524.0 | 28.0 | 154 | 16.7 | 3.4 | 8.2 | 0.5 |
| Potato & Smoked Bacon Topping, M & S* | 1 Serving/175g | 227.0 | 8.0 | 130 | 17.8 | 3.2 | 4.8 | 1.2 |
| Prosciutio, Dolcelatte & 3 Cheese Sauce, Asda* | ½ Pack/195g | 355.0 | 12.0 | 182 | 30.0 | 1.9 | 6.0 | 1.2 |
| Rice, Breast, Chargrilled, Spicy, Asda* | 1 Pack/400g | 372.0 | 2.0 | 93 | 6.0 | 16.0 | 0.6 | 1.0 |
| Rice, Fiesta, Weight Watchers* | 1 Pack/330g | 307.0 | 7.0 | 93 | 6.1 | 12.8 | 2.0 | 0.4 |
| Rice 'n' Peas, Sainsbury's* | 1 Pack/300g | 489.0 | 18.0 | 163 | 12.5 | 14.4 | 6.1 | 2.1 |
| Roast Potatoes, Eat Smart, Safeway* | 1 Serving/363g | 345.0 | 7.0 | 95 | 8.5 | 10.1 | 1.8 | 1.5 |
| Sage & Onion Stuffing & Chipolatas, Breast Joint, Tesco* | ½ Pack/280g | 507.0 | 33.0 | 181 | 16.2 | 2.8 | 11.7 | 1.9 |
| Salsa & Potato Wedges, GFY, Asda* | 1 Serving/400g | 327.0 | 7.0 | 82 | 6.0 | 10.5 | 1.7 | 1.7 |
| Spinach, Honey Mustard, American Style, Asda* | 1 Serving/240g | 394.0 | 24.0 | 164 | 14.0 | 4.4 | 10.0 | 0.3 |
| Spinach & Pasta, M & S* | 1oz/28g | 64.0 | 4.0 | 228 | 9.4 | 14.0 | 15.0 | 1.3 |
| Spirelli, Steam Meal, Tesco* | 1 Serving/400g | 400.0 | 11.0 | 100 | 6.6 | 12.0 | 2.7 | 1.2 |
| Spring Vegetables, Chargrilled, COU, M & S* | 1 Pack/414g | 290.0 | 4.0 | 70 | 8.8 | 7.3 | 0.9 | 1.8 |

| CHICKEN WITH | Measure INFO/WEIGHT | per Measure KCAL | per Measure FAT | Nutrition Values per 100g / 100ml KCAL | PROT | CARB | FAT | FIBRE |
|---|---|---|---|---|---|---|---|---|
| Stilton & Port Sauce, Breasts, Finest, Tesco* | 1 Serving/400g | 668.0 | 34.0 | 167 | 18.5 | 3.9 | 8.6 | 0.7 |
| Sun Dried Tomato & Basil Butter, Sainsbury's* | 1 Breast/185g | 363.0 | 18.0 | 196 | 25.0 | 2.5 | 9.5 | 0.2 |
| Sun Dried Tomato & Basil Sauce, Bistro, Waitrose* | ½ Pack/175g | 254.0 | 14.0 | 145 | 14.2 | 3.7 | 8.1 | 0.3 |
| Sweet Chilli Noodles, Eat Smart, Morrisons* | 1 Pack/380g | 236.0 | 4.0 | 62 | 5.9 | 7.1 | 1.1 | 1.3 |
| Sweet Chilli Sauce & Egg Fried Rice, Tesco* | 1 Pack/380g | 494.0 | 10.0 | 130 | 7.5 | 18.2 | 2.7 | 1.3 |
| Sweet Potato Mash, Jerk, Super Naturals, Sainsbury's* | 1 Pack/400g | 284.0 | 4.0 | 71 | 6.1 | 9.2 | 1.1 | 2.2 |
| Tagine, Cous Cous, Perfectly Balanced, Waitrose* | 1 Pack/400g | 516.0 | 14.0 | 129 | 8.2 | 16.2 | 3.5 | 1.0 |
| Tangy Lemon Sauce, Breasts, Just Cook, Sainsbury's* | 1 Serving/164g | 244.0 | 3.0 | 149 | 16.2 | 16.9 | 1.8 | 0.1 |
| Tomato & Basil, GFY, Sainsbury's* | 1 Pack/400g | 300.0 | 3.0 | 75 | 13.6 | 3.4 | 0.8 | 1.4 |
| Tomato & Basil Sauce, Carb Control, Tesco* | 1 Serving/400g | 316.0 | 19.0 | 79 | 7.4 | 1.7 | 4.7 | 1.6 |
| **CHICORY** | | | | | | | | |
| *Fresh, Raw, Average* | *1 Av Head/150g* | *30.0* | *1.0* | *20* | *0.6* | *2.8* | *0.6* | *0.9* |
| **CHILLI** | | | | | | | | |
| & Lemongrass Prawns with Noodles, BGTY, Sainsbury's* | 1 Pack/400g | 328.0 | 3.0 | 82 | 5.0 | 13.8 | 0.7 | 1.3 |
| & Potato Wedges, Sainsbury's* | 1 Pack/371g | 393.0 | 15.0 | 106 | 7.2 | 10.1 | 4.1 | 2.2 |
| & Rice, Birds Eye* | 1 Serving/285g | 305.0 | 8.0 | 107 | 3.4 | 17.2 | 2.7 | 1.0 |
| & Rice, Frozen, Sainsbury's* | 1 Pack/400g | 436.0 | 8.0 | 109 | 4.8 | 18.4 | 1.9 | 0.6 |
| & Rice, GFY, Asda* | 1 Pack/400g | 352.0 | 2.0 | 88 | 5.0 | 16.0 | 0.4 | 1.8 |
| & Spicy Wedges, Good Intentions, Somerfield* | 1 Serving/400g | 340.0 | 9.0 | 85 | 5.6 | 10.5 | 2.3 | 1.1 |
| & Wedges, BBQ, HL, Tesco* | 1 Pack/420g | 391.0 | 11.0 | 93 | 5.4 | 12.2 | 2.6 | 1.9 |
| & Wedges, GFY, Asda* | 1 Pack/400g | 364.0 | 10.0 | 91 | 7.0 | 10.1 | 2.5 | 2.5 |
| Beef, & Potato Crush, Weight Watchers* | 1 Pack/400g | 232.0 | 6.0 | 58 | 5.0 | 5.9 | 1.5 | 3.4 |
| Beef, Asda* | ½ Pack/200g | 190.0 | 8.0 | 95 | 7.0 | 8.0 | 3.9 | 1.2 |
| Beef, with Potato Wedges, Naturally Good Food, Tesco* | 1 Pack/440g | 352.0 | 12.0 | 80 | 7.2 | 6.2 | 2.8 | 1.8 |
| Beef, with Rice, GFY, Asda* | 1 Serving/402g | 354.0 | 6.0 | 88 | 4.7 | 14.0 | 1.5 | 0.9 |
| Beef, with Rice, Sainsbury's* | 1 Serving/300g | 360.0 | 5.0 | 120 | 5.6 | 20.6 | 1.7 | 1.1 |
| Beef & Mushrooms, GFY, Asda* | 1 Pack/400g | 364.0 | 6.0 | 91 | 9.1 | 10.2 | 1.5 | 1.2 |
| Chicken Grande, Stagg* | 1 Serving/205g | 168.0 | 1.0 | 82 | 9.7 | 9.4 | 0.6 | 1.6 |
| Con Carne, & Rice, Light Choices, Tesco* | 1 Pack/500g | 485.0 | 7.0 | 97 | 6.1 | 14.8 | 1.5 | 2.3 |
| Con Carne, 2 Minute Meals, Sainsbury's* | 1 Pouch/200g | 146.0 | 3.0 | 73 | 6.0 | 8.6 | 1.6 | 2.7 |
| Con Carne, Asda* | 1 Can/392g | 376.0 | 14.0 | 96 | 7.0 | 9.0 | 3.5 | 0.0 |
| Con Carne, Baked Bean, Heinz* | 1 Can/390g | 324.0 | 6.0 | 83 | 7.0 | 10.3 | 1.5 | 2.8 |
| Con Carne, BGTY, Sainsbury's* | 1 Serving/377g | 430.0 | 6.0 | 114 | 6.9 | 17.8 | 1.7 | 0.8 |
| Con Carne, Canned, Morrisons* | 1 Can/392g | 368.0 | 12.0 | 94 | 8.8 | 8.0 | 3.0 | 2.4 |
| Con Carne, Canned, Sainsbury's* | 1 Can/400g | 324.0 | 8.0 | 81 | 6.6 | 8.9 | 2.1 | 2.5 |
| Con Carne, Canned, Tesco* | ½ Can/200g | 220.0 | 11.0 | 110 | 7.8 | 6.4 | 5.7 | 4.7 |
| Con Carne, Dynamite Hot, Stagg* | 1 Serving/250g | 310.0 | 15.0 | 124 | 7.6 | 9.6 | 6.2 | 2.5 |
| Con Carne, Fluffy White Rice, COU, M & S* | 1 Pack/400g | 360.0 | 8.0 | 90 | 5.7 | 12.3 | 1.9 | 1.5 |
| Con Carne, From Restaurant, Average | 1 Serving/253g | 256.0 | 8.0 | 101 | 9.7 | 8.7 | 3.3 | 0.0 |
| Con Carne, Homepride* | 1 Can/390g | 234.0 | 2.0 | 60 | 2.5 | 11.2 | 0.6 | 0.0 |
| Con Carne, M & S* | 1 Pack/285g | 285.0 | 11.0 | 100 | 8.7 | 7.4 | 3.7 | 2.0 |
| Con Carne, Recipe Mix, Colman's* | 1 Pack/50g | 158.0 | 1.0 | 316 | 10.4 | 62.9 | 2.5 | 6.8 |
| Con Carne, Sainsbury's* | 1 Pack/376g | 459.0 | 6.0 | 122 | 7.4 | 19.6 | 1.6 | 1.0 |
| Con Carne, Slim Fast* | 1 Pack/375g | 394.0 | 7.0 | 105 | 5.5 | 16.2 | 1.9 | 1.5 |
| Con Carne, with Rice, BGTY, Sainsbury's* | 1 Pack/400g | 372.0 | 7.0 | 93 | 4.5 | 14.8 | 1.7 | 2.8 |
| Con Carne, with Rice, Birds Eye* | 1 Pack/285g | 291.0 | 7.0 | 102 | 3.3 | 16.6 | 2.5 | 0.8 |
| Con Carne, with Rice, Eat Smart, Morrisons* | 1 Pack/400g | 328.0 | 5.0 | 82 | 5.3 | 12.2 | 1.3 | 1.4 |
| Con Carne, with Rice, Weight Watchers* | 1 Serving/301g | 262.0 | 3.0 | 87 | 4.6 | 14.7 | 1.1 | 0.4 |
| Con Carne with Rice, Eat Smart, Safeway* | 1 Pack/400g | 340.0 | 5.0 | 85 | 5.3 | 12.2 | 1.3 | 1.4 |
| Con Carne with Rice, GFY, Asda* | 1 Serving/400g | 456.0 | 6.0 | 114 | 6.0 | 19.0 | 1.6 | 0.9 |
| Con Carne with Rice, Healthy Choice, Asda* | 1 Pack/400g | 412.0 | 8.0 | 103 | 6.0 | 15.0 | 2.1 | 0.9 |
| Con Carne with Rice, Organic, Sainsbury's* | 1 Pack/400g | 472.0 | 11.0 | 118 | 5.0 | 18.5 | 2.7 | 1.8 |
| Con Carne with Rice, Perfectly Balanced, Waitrose* | 1 Pack/400g | 404.0 | 7.0 | 101 | 5.8 | 15.3 | 1.8 | 1.7 |

| | Measure INFO/WEIGHT | per Measure KCAL | FAT | Nutrition Values per 100g / 100ml KCAL | PROT | CARB | FAT | FIBRE |
|---|---|---|---|---|---|---|---|---|
| **CHILLI** | | | | | | | | |
| Medium, Uncle Ben's* | 1 Jar/500g | 305.0 | 4.0 | 61 | 1.8 | 11.1 | 0.8 | 0.0 |
| Mexican Chilli with Potato Wedges, Weight Watchers* | 1 Pack/300g | 249.0 | 9.0 | 83 | 4.6 | 9.6 | 2.9 | 1.3 |
| Mixed Vegetable, Tesco* | 1 Pack/400g | 352.0 | 12.0 | 88 | 3.9 | 11.0 | 2.9 | 3.2 |
| Non Carne, Linda McCartney* | 1 Pack/340g | 275.0 | 8.0 | 81 | 5.8 | 9.2 | 2.3 | 1.7 |
| Spicy, & Wedges, Healthy Options, Birds Eye* | 1 Pack/350g | 259.0 | 6.0 | 74 | 4.7 | 9.7 | 1.8 | 1.4 |
| Sweet Potato, Mexican, Tasty Veg Pot, Innocent* | 1 Pot/400g | 368.0 | 8.0 | 92 | 3.1 | 15.5 | 2.0 | 3.7 |
| Vegetable, Canned, Sainsbury's* | 1 Can/400g | 368.0 | 2.0 | 92 | 5.1 | 16.7 | 0.5 | 4.9 |
| Vegetable, Tinned, GFY, Asda* | ½ Can/200g | 140.0 | 2.0 | 70 | 3.5 | 12.0 | 0.9 | 3.5 |
| Vegetable & Rice, BGTY, Sainsbury's* | 1 Pack/450g | 409.0 | 5.0 | 91 | 3.5 | 16.7 | 1.1 | 3.5 |
| Vegetable & Rice, HE, Tesco* | 1 Pack/450g | 391.0 | 5.0 | 87 | 2.8 | 16.1 | 1.2 | 1.5 |
| Vegetable Garden, Stagg* | 1 Can/410g | 254.0 | 2.0 | 62 | 3.6 | 10.8 | 0.5 | 2.3 |
| Vegetarian, with Rice, Tesco* | 1 Pack/500g | 575.0 | 13.0 | 115 | 4.0 | 19.0 | 2.6 | 1.8 |
| **CHILLI MEAT FREE** | | | | | | | | |
| Sainsbury's* | 1 Pack/400g | 308.0 | 20.0 | 77 | 4.0 | 4.1 | 5.0 | 5.2 |
| **CHINESE LEAF** | | | | | | | | |
| *Fresh, Raw, Average* | *1oz/28g* | *4.0* | *0.0* | *14* | *1.5* | *1.5* | *0.2* | *1.7* |
| **CHINESE MEAL** | | | | | | | | |
| for One, GFY, Asda* | 1 Pack/570g | 946.0 | 17.0 | 166 | 7.0 | 28.0 | 2.9 | 0.0 |
| for Two, Tesco* | 1 Pack/500g | 480.0 | 8.0 | 96 | 4.4 | 16.0 | 1.6 | 1.1 |
| House Special, I IL, Tesco* | 1 Pack/450g | 369.0 | 7.0 | 82 | 6.5 | 10.5 | 1.6 | 1.1 |
| House Special, with Egg Fried Rice, Tesco* | 1 Pack/450g | 562.0 | 9.0 | 125 | 7.2 | 19.7 | 1.9 | 0.8 |
| My Very Own, Asda* | 1 Pack/297g | 416.0 | 5.0 | 140 | 7.0 | 24.0 | 1.8 | 0.6 |
| **CHIPS** | | | | | | | | |
| 11mm Fresh, Deep Fried, McCain* | 1oz/28g | 66.0 | 3.0 | 235 | 3.2 | 31.8 | 10.6 | 0.0 |
| 14mm Fresh, Deep Fried, McCain* | 1oz/28g | 59.0 | 2.0 | 209 | 2.7 | 34.2 | 6.8 | 0.0 |
| 14mm Friers Choice, Deep Fried, McCain* | 1oz/28g | 56.0 | 2.0 | 199 | 3.5 | 29.3 | 8.0 | 0.0 |
| 3 Way Cook, Somerfield* | 1 Serving/96g | 145.0 | 5.0 | 151 | 2.5 | 24.0 | 5.0 | 1.6 |
| 9/16" Straight Cut Caterpack, Deep Fried, McCain* | 1oz/28g | 63.0 | 3.0 | 225 | 3.1 | 32.1 | 9.4 | 0.0 |
| American Style, Oven, Co-Op* | 1 Serving/150g | 255.0 | 9.0 | 170 | 2.0 | 26.0 | 6.0 | 3.0 |
| American Style, Oven, Safeway* | 1 Serving/125g | 287.0 | 8.0 | 230 | 4.1 | 38.2 | 6.8 | 3.0 |
| American Style, Oven, Sainsbury's* | 1 Serving/165g | 313.0 | 14.0 | 190 | 5.4 | 23.6 | 8.3 | 1.3 |
| American Style, Thin, Oven, Tesco* | 1 Serving/125g | 210.0 | 8.0 | 168 | 2.7 | 24.6 | 6.5 | 2.1 |
| Basics, Sainsbury's* | 1 Serving/165g | 277.0 | 8.0 | 168 | 1.8 | 29.7 | 4.6 | 0.3 |
| Beefeater, Deep Fried, McCain* | 1oz/28g | 71.0 | 3.0 | 253 | 3.3 | 37.7 | 9.9 | 0.0 |
| Beefeater, Oven Baked, McCain* | 1oz/28g | 55.0 | 2.0 | 195 | 4.0 | 32.2 | 5.6 | 0.0 |
| British Classics, HL, Tesco* | ½ Pack/200g | 250.0 | 2.0 | 125 | 2.6 | 26.9 | 0.8 | 1.3 |
| Chippy, Microwave, McCain* | 1oz/28g | 49.0 | 2.0 | 176 | 2.6 | 25.2 | 7.2 | 1.7 |
| Chunky, COU, M & S* | 1 Serving/150g | 157.0 | 2.0 | 105 | 2.1 | 20.5 | 1.6 | 2.3 |
| Chunky, Eat Smart, Safeway* | 1 Serving/158g | 150.0 | 3.0 | 95 | 1.6 | 18.3 | 1.6 | 1.4 |
| Chunky, Fresh, Chilled, Finest, Tesco* | 1 Pack/450g | 607.0 | 18.0 | 135 | 2.1 | 22.3 | 4.0 | 2.7 |
| Chunky, Ready to Bake, M & S* | 1 Serving/200g | 310.0 | 8.0 | 155 | 2.2 | 26.8 | 4.2 | 2.0 |
| Chunky, Waitrose* | 1 Portion/155g | 200.0 | 9.0 | 129 | 1.9 | 17.6 | 5.7 | 2.8 |
| Chunky Oven, Harry Ramsden's* | 1 Serving/150g | 184.0 | 5.0 | 123 | 2.8 | 19.9 | 3.6 | 1.6 |
| Crinkle Cut, Frozen, Fried in Corn Oil | 1oz/28g | 81.0 | 5.0 | 290 | 3.6 | 33.4 | 16.7 | 2.2 |
| Crinkle Cut, M & S* | 1 Serving/150g | 270.0 | 8.0 | 180 | 3.3 | 29.5 | 5.4 | 2.4 |
| Crinkle Cut, Oven, Asda* | 1 Serving/100g | 134.0 | 4.0 | 134 | 2.0 | 23.0 | 3.8 | 8.0 |
| Crinkle Cut, Oven Baked, Aunt Bessie's* | 1 Serving/100g | 206.0 | 9.0 | 206 | 2.9 | 28.0 | 9.2 | 3.2 |
| Family Fries, Oven, Tesco* | 1 Serving/125g | 164.0 | 5.0 | 131 | 2.0 | 22.4 | 3.7 | 1.8 |
| Fat, with Fluffy Centres, M & S* | 1 Serving/200g | 210.0 | 9.0 | 105 | 1.6 | 14.2 | 4.5 | 1.8 |
| Fine Cut, Frozen, Fried in Blended Oil | 1oz/28g | 102.0 | 6.0 | 364 | 4.5 | 41.2 | 21.3 | 2.4 |
| Fine Cut, Frozen, Fried in Corn Oil | 1oz/28g | 102.0 | 6.0 | 364 | 4.5 | 41.2 | 21.3 | 2.7 |
| Fried, Average | 1 Sm Serving/130g | 296.0 | 12.0 | 228 | 4.4 | 33.3 | 9.5 | 1.7 |
| Fried, Chip Shop, Average | 1 Serving/400g | 956.0 | 50.0 | 239 | 3.2 | 30.5 | 12.4 | 2.2 |

C

# CHIPS

| INFO/WEIGHT | Measure | per Measure KCAL | FAT | Nutrition Values per 100g / 100ml KCAL | PROT | CARB | FAT | FIBRE |
|---|---|---|---|---|---|---|---|---|
| Frozen, Crinkle Cut, Aunt Bessie's* | 1 Serving/100g | 163.0 | 7.0 | 163 | 3.1 | 21.3 | 7.3 | 2.2 |
| Frying, Crinkle Cut, Tesco* | 1 Serving/125g | 161.0 | 4.0 | 129 | 2.6 | 22.2 | 3.3 | 1.9 |
| Frying, Value, Tesco* | 1 Serving/125g | 376.0 | 20.0 | 301 | 4.3 | 35.4 | 15.9 | 2.5 |
| Homefries, Chunky, Weighed Frozen, McCain* | 1 Serving/100g | 123.0 | 2.0 | 123 | 2.5 | 22.6 | 2.5 | 1.6 |
| Homefries, Crinkle Cut, Weighed Frozen, McCain* | 1 Serving/100g | 197.0 | 6.0 | 197 | 3.0 | 31.7 | 6.5 | 2.5 |
| Homefries, Jacket Oven, McCain* | 1 Serving/100g | 220.0 | 7.0 | 220 | 3.9 | 37.9 | 7.4 | 0.0 |
| Homefries, Straight Cut, Weighed Frozen, McCain* | 1 Serving/100g | 134.0 | 5.0 | 134 | 2.2 | 21.0 | 4.6 | 1.7 |
| Homefries, Thin & Crispy, Weighed Frozen, McCain* | 1 Serving/100g | 143.0 | 4.0 | 143 | 2.6 | 24.0 | 4.1 | 1.5 |
| Homemade, Fried in Blended Oil, Average | 1oz/28g | 53.0 | 2.0 | 189 | 3.9 | 30.1 | 6.7 | 2.2 |
| Homemade, Fried in Corn Oil, Average | 1oz/28g | 53.0 | 2.0 | 189 | 3.9 | 30.1 | 6.7 | 2.2 |
| Homemade, Fried in Dripping, Average | 1oz/28g | 53.0 | 2.0 | 189 | 3.9 | 30.1 | 6.7 | 2.2 |
| Homestyle, Frozen, Aunt Bessie's* | 1 Serving/200g | 260.0 | 11.0 | 130 | 2.2 | 17.6 | 5.6 | 2.7 |
| Homestyle, Oven Cooked, Aunt Bessie's* | 1 Serving/100g | 191.0 | 8.0 | 191 | 3.1 | 27.0 | 7.8 | 2.9 |
| Homestyle Oven, Sainsbury's* | 1 Serving/125g | 206.0 | 5.0 | 165 | 2.4 | 29.2 | 4.3 | 2.1 |
| Just Bake, Low Fat, M & S* | 1oz/28g | 37.0 | 1.0 | 133 | 2.0 | 24.7 | 3.7 | 1.7 |
| Micro, Asda* | 1 Serving/112g | 221.0 | 8.0 | 197 | 3.5 | 30.0 | 7.0 | 4.0 |
| Micro, Crinkle Cut, Tesco* | 1 Serving/100g | 203.0 | 8.0 | 203 | 3.3 | 29.5 | 8.0 | 1.8 |
| Micro Chips, Crinkle Cut, Cooked, McCain* | 1 Pack/100g | 166.0 | 4.0 | 166 | 2.9 | 28.9 | 4.2 | 2.4 |
| Micro Chips, Straight Cut, Cooked, McCain* | 1 Pack/100g | 163.0 | 5.0 | 163 | 2.3 | 27.7 | 4.8 | 2.0 |
| Microwave, Cooked | 1oz/28g | 62.0 | 3.0 | 221 | 3.6 | 32.1 | 9.6 | 2.9 |
| Oven, 5% Fat, Frozen, McCain* | 1 Serving/200g | 238.0 | 6.0 | 119 | 1.9 | 21.0 | 3.0 | 1.6 |
| Oven, Champion* | 1 Pack/133g | 210.0 | 6.0 | 158 | 2.5 | 27.0 | 4.5 | 0.0 |
| Oven, Chunky, Extra Special, Asda* | 1 Serving/125g | 237.0 | 7.0 | 190 | 3.4 | 31.5 | 5.6 | 3.2 |
| Oven, Chunky, Ross* | 1 Serving/100g | 177.0 | 6.0 | 177 | 3.1 | 26.6 | 6.5 | 3.9 |
| Oven, Cooked, Value, Tesco* | 1 Serving/125g | 307.0 | 10.0 | 246 | 4.5 | 39.5 | 7.8 | 2.9 |
| Oven, Cooked, Weight Watchers* | 1 Serving/100g | 150.0 | 3.0 | 150 | 2.8 | 33.7 | 3.0 | 5.9 |
| Oven, Crinkle Cut, 5% Fat, Weighed Baked, McCain* | 1 Serving/100g | 163.0 | 4.0 | 163 | 3.1 | 27.9 | 4.3 | 3.0 |
| Oven, Crinkle Cut, 5% Fat, Weighed Frozen, McCain* | 1 Serving/100g | 134.0 | 4.0 | 134 | 2.4 | 23.2 | 3.6 | 2.4 |
| Oven, Crinkle Cut, Safeway* | 1 Serving/130g | 234.0 | 7.0 | 180 | 3.3 | 29.5 | 5.4 | 2.4 |
| Oven, Crinkle Cut, Sainsbury's* | 1 Serving/165g | 297.0 | 9.0 | 180 | 3.3 | 29.5 | 5.5 | 2.4 |
| Oven, Frozen, Baked | 1oz/28g | 45.0 | 1.0 | 162 | 3.2 | 29.8 | 4.2 | 2.0 |
| Oven, Frozen, BGTY, Sainsbury's* | 1 Serving/165g | 226.0 | 5.0 | 137 | 2.9 | 25.0 | 2.8 | 2.7 |
| Oven, Frozen, Value, Tesco* | 1 Serving/125g | 189.0 | 6.0 | 151 | 2.8 | 24.7 | 4.6 | 1.9 |
| Oven, Healthy Choice, Safeway* | 1 Serving/150g | 226.0 | 5.0 | 151 | 2.8 | 27.1 | 3.5 | 2.1 |
| Oven, Homefries, McCain* | 1 Serving/100g | 134.0 | 5.0 | 134 | 2.2 | 21.0 | 4.6 | 1.7 |
| Oven, Morrisons* | 1 Serving/100g | 134.0 | 4.0 | 134 | 2.4 | 22.2 | 3.9 | 0.0 |
| Oven, Organic, Little Big Food Company* | 1 Serving/100g | 164.0 | 4.0 | 164 | 3.0 | 28.5 | 4.2 | 1.2 |
| Oven, Organic, Waitrose* | 1 Serving/165g | 233.0 | 6.0 | 141 | 1.5 | 25.1 | 3.8 | 1.6 |
| Oven, Original, McCain* | 1 Serving/100g | 158.0 | 4.0 | 158 | 2.5 | 28.5 | 3.8 | 2.3 |
| Oven, Original, Straight Cut, 5% Fat, Cooked, McCain* | 1 Serving/100g | 172.0 | 5.0 | 172 | 3.4 | 32.4 | 4.9 | 2.3 |
| Oven, Original, Straight Cut, 5% Fat, Frozen, McCain* | 1 Serving/100g | 138.0 | 4.0 | 138 | 2.5 | 26.2 | 4.0 | 1.9 |
| Oven, Steak Cut, Asda* | 1 Serving/100g | 153.0 | 4.0 | 153 | 2.0 | 27.0 | 4.1 | 2.5 |
| Oven, Steak Cut, Sainsbury's* | 1 Serving/165g | 266.0 | 8.0 | 161 | 2.6 | 27.1 | 4.7 | 2.8 |
| Oven, Steak Cut, Waitrose* | 1 Serving/165g | 218.0 | 6.0 | 132 | 2.7 | 22.7 | 3.4 | 1.7 |
| Oven, Steakhouse, Frozen, Tesco* | 1 Serving/125g | 165.0 | 4.0 | 132 | 2.7 | 22.7 | 3.4 | 1.7 |
| Oven, Straight Cut, 5% Fat, Sainsbury's* | 1 Serving/165g | 280.0 | 8.0 | 170 | 3.4 | 28.0 | 4.9 | 2.5 |
| Oven, Straight Cut, Asda* | 1 Serving/100g | 199.0 | 5.0 | 199 | 3.5 | 35.0 | 5.0 | 3.0 |
| Oven, Straight Cut, BFY, Morrisons* | 1 Serving/165g | 249.0 | 6.0 | 151 | 2.8 | 27.1 | 3.5 | 2.1 |
| Oven, Straight Cut, Budgens* | 1 Portion/180g | 205.0 | 3.0 | 114 | 2.3 | 21.9 | 1.9 | 2.7 |
| Oven, Straight Cut, Frozen Weight, HL, Tesco* | 1 Serving/125g | 132.0 | 2.0 | 106 | 2.1 | 20.0 | 1.9 | 2.3 |
| Oven, Straight Cut, Low Fat, HL, Tesco* | 1 Serving/100g | 132.0 | 3.0 | 132 | 2.7 | 23.9 | 2.8 | 2.8 |
| Oven, Straight Cut, Reduced Fat, Tesco* | 1 Serving/100g | 127.0 | 3.0 | 127 | 2.3 | 22.7 | 3.0 | 2.1 |
| Oven, Straight Cut, Safeway* | 1 Serving/125g | 226.0 | 6.0 | 181 | 3.6 | 30.0 | 5.2 | 2.5 |

C

| | Measure INFO/WEIGHT | per Measure KCAL | FAT | Nutrition Values per 100g / 100ml KCAL | PROT | CARB | FAT | FIBRE |
|---|---|---|---|---|---|---|---|---|
| **CHIPS** | | | | | | | | |
| Oven, Straight Cut, Waitrose* | 1 Serving/165g | 219.0 | 6.0 | 133 | 2.0 | 23.0 | 3.7 | 1.7 |
| Oven, Sweet Potato, Tesco* | 1 ¼ Pack/125g | 169.0 | 6.0 | 135 | 2.6 | 18.9 | 5.2 | 5.0 |
| Oven, Thick Cut, Frozen, Baked | 1oz/28g | 44.0 | 1.0 | 157 | 3.2 | 27.9 | 4.4 | 1.8 |
| Oven, Thin & Crispy, Tesco* | 1 Portion/100g | 205.0 | 5.0 | 205 | 2.7 | 37.6 | 4.9 | 5.8 |
| Oven, Thin Cut, American Style, Asda* | 1 Serving/100g | 240.0 | 10.0 | 240 | 3.4 | 34.0 | 10.0 | 3.0 |
| Oven, Thin Fries, Morrisons* | 1 Serving/100g | 161.0 | 6.0 | 161 | 2.9 | 23.6 | 6.1 | 1.2 |
| Steak Cut, Frying, Asda* | 1 Serving/97g | 181.0 | 7.0 | 187 | 2.9 | 28.0 | 7.0 | 2.8 |
| Steak Cut, Oven, Tesco* | 1 Serving/165g | 233.0 | 6.0 | 141 | 2.0 | 24.4 | 3.9 | 2.0 |
| Steakhouse, Fry, Tesco* | 1 Serving/125g | 278.0 | 15.0 | 222 | 3.1 | 25.2 | 12.1 | 2.0 |
| Straight Cut, Frozen, Fried in Blended Oil | 1oz/28g | 76.0 | 4.0 | 273 | 4.1 | 36.0 | 13.5 | 2.4 |
| Straight Cut, Frozen, Fried in Corn Oil | 1oz/28g | 76.0 | 4.0 | 273 | 4.1 | 36.0 | 13.5 | 2.4 |
| Straight Cut, Low Fat, Tesco* | 1 Serving/125g | 159.0 | 4.0 | 127 | 2.3 | 22.7 | 3.0 | 2.1 |
| Straight Cut, Microwave Baked, McCain* | 1oz/28g | 70.0 | 3.0 | 251 | 3.5 | 35.0 | 10.7 | 0.0 |
| The Big Chip, Frozen, Tesco* | 1 Serving/200g | 220.0 | 5.0 | 110 | 1.8 | 20.3 | 2.4 | 2.1 |
| Thick Cut, Caterpack, Deep Fried, McCain* | 1oz/28g | 60.0 | 3.0 | 215 | 3.1 | 28.8 | 9.7 | 0.0 |
| Thick Cut, Frozen, Fried in Corn Oil, Average | 1oz/28g | 66.0 | 3.0 | 234 | 3.6 | 34.0 | 10.2 | 2.4 |
| Three Way Cook, Skinny, Co-Op* | 1 Serving/100g | 175.0 | 7.0 | 175 | 2.0 | 26.0 | 7.0 | 3.0 |
| Vending 3/8" Straight Cut, Deep Fried, McCain* | 1oz/28g | 62.0 | 3.0 | 220 | 3.3 | 29.6 | 9.8 | 0.0 |
| Waffle, Birds Eye* | 1 Serving/75g | 156.0 | 8.0 | 208 | 2.5 | 24.3 | 11.2 | 2.6 |
| **CHIVES** | | | | | | | | |
| *Fresh, Average* | *1 Tsp/2g* | *0.0* | *0.0* | *23* | *2.8* | *1.7* | *0.6* | *1.9* |
| **CHOC ICES** | | | | | | | | |
| Average | 1 Ice/50g | 138.0 | 9.0 | 277 | 3.5 | 28.1 | 17.5 | 0.0 |
| Belgian Milk, Sainsbury's* | 1 Ice/80ml | 170.0 | 11.0 | 212 | 1.9 | 21.1 | 13.4 | 0.5 |
| Chocolate, Dark, Seriously Creamy, Waitrose* | 1 Icc/82g | 195.0 | 13.0 | 238 | 2.6 | 21.6 | 15.7 | 1.7 |
| Chocolate, Real Milk, Sainsbury's* | 1 Ice/48g | 151.0 | 10.0 | 312 | 3.5 | 30.3 | 19.7 | 0.8 |
| Chunky, Wall's Ice Cream* | 1 Ice/81g | 162.0 | 11.0 | 200 | 2.6 | 18.9 | 13.1 | 0.0 |
| Dark, Sainsbury's* | 1 Ice/43g | 136.0 | 10.0 | 315 | 3.8 | 25.5 | 22.0 | 0.4 |
| Dark, Tesco* | 1 Ice/43g | 141.0 | 9.0 | 325 | 2.8 | 30.2 | 21.0 | 0.1 |
| Light, Sainsbury's* | 1 Ice/43g | 135.0 | 9.0 | 313 | 3.2 | 27.0 | 21.4 | 0.3 |
| Light, Waitrose* | 1 Ice/70ml | 141.0 | 10.0 | 201 | 1.7 | 17.0 | 14.3 | 0.3 |
| Mini Mix, Eis Stern* | 1 Ice/39g | 129.0 | 9.0 | 334 | 4.2 | 29.0 | 23.0 | 0.0 |
| Morrisons* | 1 Ice/31g | 86.0 | 6.0 | 279 | 3.0 | 24.7 | 19.3 | 0.4 |
| Neapolitan, Safeway* | 1 Ice/41g | 120.0 | 8.0 | 290 | 2.6 | 25.4 | 19.5 | 0.3 |
| Neapolitan Chocolate, Co-Op* | 1 Ice/62g | 120.0 | 8.0 | 194 | 2.0 | 16.9 | 13.2 | 0.4 |
| Real Plain, Sainsbury's* | 1 Ice/48g | 150.0 | 10.0 | 310 | 2.9 | 29.5 | 20.0 | 2.2 |
| Rum & Rasin, Safeway* | 1 Ice/45g | 136.0 | 9.0 | 303 | 3.3 | 28.9 | 19.3 | 1.1 |
| Safeway* | 1 Ice/70g | 217.0 | 15.0 | 310 | 2.8 | 25.9 | 21.6 | 0.9 |
| SmartPrice, Asda* | 1 Ice/31g | 81.0 | 6.0 | 262 | 2.8 | 20.0 | 19.0 | 0.0 |
| Vanilla, Co-Op* | 1 Ice/70g | 130.0 | 12.0 | 186 | 3.6 | 3.6 | 17.1 | 0.0 |
| White, Real, Tesco* | 1 Ice/52g | 198.0 | 14.0 | 381 | 4.0 | 26.9 | 27.6 | 1.1 |
| White Chocolate, Sainsbury's* | 1 Ice/48g | 140.0 | 9.0 | 292 | 3.8 | 27.3 | 18.6 | 0.1 |
| **CHOCOLATE** | | | | | | | | |
| Advent Calendar, Dairy Milk, Cadbury* | 1 Chocolate/4g | 22.0 | 1.0 | 525 | 7.5 | 56.6 | 30.1 | 0.7 |
| Advent Calendar, Magic of Christmas, Cadbury* | 1 Chocolate/10g | 48.0 | 3.0 | 510 | 7.0 | 57.7 | 28.0 | 0.7 |
| Advent Calendar, Maltesers, Mars* | 1 Chocolate/4g | 21.0 | 1.0 | 537 | 6.8 | 57.9 | 30.9 | 0.0 |
| Advent Calendar, Milky Bar, Nestle* | 1 Chocolate/4g | 22.0 | 1.0 | 547 | 7.3 | 58.4 | 31.7 | 0.0 |
| Advent Calendar, Pirates of the Caribbean, Kinnerton* | 1 Chocolate/4g | 19.0 | 1.0 | 525 | 5.4 | 61.2 | 28.6 | 1.6 |
| Advent Calendar, The Simpsons, Kinnerton* | 1 Chocolate/4g | 20.0 | 1.0 | 526 | 5.3 | 63.2 | 28.9 | 1.6 |
| Advent Calendar, The Snowman, M & S* | 1 Chocolate/4g | 21.0 | 1.0 | 550 | 6.6 | 60.4 | 31.0 | 0.0 |
| Almond & Honey, Dairy Milk, Cadbury* | 1 Sm Bar/54g | 281.0 | 16.0 | 520 | 8.0 | 57.1 | 28.9 | 1.0 |
| Animal Bar, Nestle* | 1 Bar/19g | 97.0 | 5.0 | 513 | 5.8 | 63.6 | 26.1 | 0.0 |
| Baking, Continental, for Home Baking, Luxury, Tesco* | 1 Pack/150g | 822.0 | 68.0 | 548 | 2.7 | 27.7 | 45.1 | 0.9 |

## CHOCOLATE

| | Measure INFO/WEIGHT | per Measure | | Nutrition Values per 100g / 100ml | | | | |
|---|---|---|---|---|---|---|---|---|
| | | KCAL | FAT | KCAL | PROT | CARB | FAT | FIBRE |
| Baking, Milk, for Home Baking, Luxury, Tesco* | 1 Pack/150g | 838.0 | 54.0 | 559 | 7.0 | 51.4 | 36.2 | 1.7 |
| Bar, Apricot & Raisin, Thorntons* | 1 Bar/40g | 185.0 | 11.0 | 462 | 8.0 | 46.0 | 27.3 | 3.5 |
| Bar, Cappuccino, Thorntons* | 1 Bar/38g | 201.0 | 13.0 | 529 | 5.2 | 49.7 | 34.7 | 0.5 |
| Bar, Dark, Thorntons* | 1 Sm Bar/48g | 250.0 | 18.0 | 521 | 7.3 | 39.9 | 36.9 | 10.9 |
| Bar, Dark, with Ginger, Thorntons* | 1 Bar/100g | 509.0 | 35.0 | 509 | 5.8 | 44.3 | 35.1 | 8.8 |
| Bar, Dark Chocolate, Diabetic, Thorntons* | 1 Bar/75g | 345.0 | 27.0 | 460 | 5.4 | 28.5 | 35.8 | 8.1 |
| Bar, Jazz Orange, Thorntons* | 1 Bar/56g | 304.0 | 18.0 | 543 | 6.8 | 55.7 | 32.3 | 1.2 |
| Bar, Milk, Thorntons* | 1 Sm Bar/50g | 269.0 | 16.0 | 538 | 7.5 | 54.8 | 32.0 | 1.0 |
| Bar, Milk Chocolate, Diabetic, Thorntons* | ½ Bar/37g | 174.0 | 12.0 | 470 | 7.3 | 43.0 | 33.1 | 2.2 |
| Bar, Twisted, Creme Egg, Cadbury* | 1 Bar/45g | 210.0 | 9.0 | 467 | 5.1 | 64.7 | 20.9 | 0.0 |
| Bar, Viennese, Continental, Thorntons* | 1 Bar/38g | 206.0 | 13.0 | 542 | 4.2 | 53.9 | 34.2 | 0.8 |
| Bar, White, Thorntons* | 1 Bar/50g | 273.0 | 16.0 | 547 | 6.5 | 59.5 | 31.3 | 0.0 |
| Bars, Alpini, Continental, Thorntons* | 1 Bar/36g | 192.0 | 11.0 | 538 | 6.9 | 55.3 | 32.0 | 2.7 |
| Bars, Chocolate, Cherry, Lindt* | 1 Bar/100g | 470.0 | 23.0 | 470 | 4.5 | 61.7 | 22.8 | 0.0 |
| Bars, Chocolate, Pistacho, Lindt* | 1 Bar/100g | 585.0 | 41.0 | 585 | 7.1 | 48.2 | 40.5 | 0.0 |
| Bars, Chocolate, Strawberry, Lindt* | 1 Bar/100g | 470.0 | 23.0 | 470 | 4.5 | 61.6 | 22.8 | 0.0 |
| Bars, Chocoletti, Stracciatella, Lindt* | 1 Bar/6g | 32.0 | 2.0 | 590 | 7.7 | 49.0 | 41.0 | 0.0 |
| Bars, Milk Chocolate, Galaxy, Mars* | 1 Bar/46g | 250.0 | 15.0 | 544 | 6.6 | 56.3 | 32.5 | 1.5 |
| Bars, Milk Chocolate, Gold, Lindt* | 1 Bar/300g | 1605.0 | 93.0 | 535 | 6.6 | 58.7 | 31.0 | 0.0 |
| Bars, Milk Chocolate, Hazelnut, Gold, Lindt* | 1 Bar/300g | 1665.0 | 108.0 | 555 | 7.9 | 50.7 | 36.1 | 0.0 |
| Bars, Milk Chocolate, Hazelnut, Lindt* | 1 Bar/100g | 570.0 | 39.0 | 570 | 8.5 | 47.0 | 38.8 | 0.0 |
| Bars, Milk Chocolate, Lindt* | 1 Bar/100g | 535.0 | 31.0 | 535 | 6.6 | 57.6 | 31.0 | 0.0 |
| Bars, Milk Chocolate, Raisin & Hazelnut, Gold, Lindt* | 1 Bar/300g | 1590.0 | 95.0 | 530 | 6.8 | 54.7 | 31.6 | 0.0 |
| Bars, Milk Chocolate, Raisin & Hazelnut, Lindt* | 1 Bar/ 100g | 530.0 | 32.0 | 530 | 3.1 | 54.7 | 31.6 | 0.0 |
| Beans, Coffee, Dark, Solid, M & S* | 1 Serving/10g | 53.0 | 4.0 | 532 | 4.7 | 42.4 | 37.6 | 11.6 |
| Beans, Plain, Carl Brandt* | 4 Beans/5g | 25.0 | 1.0 | 501 | 5.7 | 54.6 | 28.9 | 0.0 |
| Bear, Lindt* | 1 Bear/84g | 480.0 | 29.0 | 572 | 7.5 | 57.7 | 34.6 | 0.0 |
| Belgian, Kschocolat* | 4 Pieces/40g | 212.0 | 12.0 | 530 | 6.0 | 57.5 | 30.5 | 2.3 |
| Belgian, Milk, Mini Eggs, M & S* | 1 Egg/8g | 43.0 | 3.0 | 535 | 7.0 | 55.8 | 31.7 | 2.7 |
| Big Purple One, Nestle* | 1 Chocolate/39g | 191.0 | 10.0 | 489 | 5.0 | 60.2 | 25.4 | 0.6 |
| Breakaway, Nestle* | 1 Bar/21g | 106.0 | 5.0 | 504 | 6.3 | 61.6 | 25.5 | 2.4 |
| Bubbly, Dairy Milk, Cadbury* | 1 Bar/35g | 185.0 | 10.0 | 525 | 7.7 | 56.9 | 29.7 | 0.7 |
| Bunny, Easter, Mars* | 1 Bunny/29g | 155.0 | 9.0 | 535 | 6.2 | 56.2 | 31.7 | 0.0 |
| Bunny, Lindt* | 1 Bunny/84g | 480.0 | 29.0 | 572 | 7.5 | 57.5 | 34.6 | 0.0 |
| Cappuccino, Nestle* | 1 Serving/20g | 109.0 | 7.0 | 545 | 6.1 | 56.0 | 32.9 | 0.0 |
| Caramel, Chunk, Dairy Milk, Cadbury* | 1 Chunk/33g | 158.0 | 8.0 | 480 | 5.0 | 63.0 | 23.0 | 0.0 |
| Caramel, Dairy Milk, Cadbury* | 1 Bar/50g | 240.0 | 12.0 | 480 | 4.9 | 62.1 | 23.5 | 0.4 |
| Choco Swing, Milka* | 1 Square/16g | 89.0 | 6.0 | 555 | 5.7 | 54.0 | 34.5 | 0.0 |
| Chocolat Noir, Lindt* | 1/6 Bar/17g | 87.0 | 5.0 | 510 | 6.0 | 50.0 | 32.0 | 0.0 |
| Chocolate Favourites, Tesco* | ½ Box/227g | 1015.0 | 44.0 | 447 | 4.2 | 64.3 | 19.2 | 0.3 |
| Chomp, Cadbury* | 1 Bar/24g | 112.0 | 5.0 | 465 | 3.3 | 67.9 | 20.0 | 0.2 |
| Christmas Tree Decoration, Cadbury* | 1 Piece/12g | 60.0 | 3.0 | 525 | 7.6 | 56.2 | 29.9 | 0.0 |
| Chunk Bar, Dairy Milk, Cadbury* | 1 Chunk/7g | 35.0 | 2.0 | 525 | 7.5 | 57.0 | 29.8 | 0.1 |
| Chunky Hazelnut Bar, M & S* | 1 Bar/52g | 293.0 | 19.0 | 563 | 8.8 | 48.1 | 37.3 | 1.7 |
| Clusters. Rocky Road, Tesco* | 1 Bite/11g | 49.0 | 2.0 | 445 | 4.5 | 80.0 | 15.4 | 3.6 |
| Coconut, White, Excellence, Lindt* | 1 Square/10g | 61.0 | 4.0 | 610 | 6.0 | 48.0 | 44.0 | 0.0 |
| Coins, Milk, Sainsbury's* | 1 Coin/5g | 26.0 | 1.0 | 502 | 5.5 | 58.8 | 27.1 | 2.5 |
| Cool & Delicious, Dairy Milk, Cadbury* | 1 Bar/21g | 110.0 | 6.0 | 525 | 7.6 | 56.1 | 30.1 | 0.0 |
| Crispies, Chunk, Dairy Milk, Cadbury* | 1 Chunk/31g | 158.0 | 8.0 | 510 | 7.6 | 58.6 | 27.4 | 0.0 |
| Crispies, Dairy Milk, Cadbury* | 1 Bar/49g | 250.0 | 13.0 | 510 | 7.6 | 58.6 | 27.4 | 0.0 |
| Crispy, Sainsbury's* | 4 Squares/19g | 99.0 | 5.0 | 521 | 9.1 | 56.9 | 28.5 | 2.1 |
| Dairy Milk, Cadbury* | 1 Bar/49g | 257.0 | 15.0 | 525 | 7.7 | 56.9 | 29.7 | 0.7 |
| Dark, 70% Cocoa Solida, Extra Fine, Lindt* | 1 Square/10g | 54.0 | 4.0 | 537 | 8.0 | 33.0 | 41.0 | 0.0 |

# CHOCOLATE

| | Measure INFO/WEIGHT | per Measure KCAL | FAT | Nutrition Values per 100g / 100ml KCAL | PROT | CARB | FAT | FIBRE |
|---|---|---|---|---|---|---|---|---|
| Dark, 70% Cocoa Solids, Organic, Green & Black's* | 1 Sm Bar/35g | 193.0 | 14.0 | 551 | 9.3 | 36.0 | 41.1 | 11.5 |
| Dark, 85% Cocoa, Excellence, Lindt* | 1 Serving/40g | 208.0 | 18.0 | 521 | 11.0 | 19.0 | 46.0 | 0.0 |
| Dark, 85% Cocoa, TTD, Sainsbury's* | 1 Piece/10g | 56.0 | 5.0 | 562 | 9.5 | 16.4 | 50.9 | 13.0 |
| Dark, Belgian, Luxury Continental, Sainsbury's* | 1 Bar/100g | 490.0 | 39.0 | 490 | 11.1 | 24.2 | 38.7 | 7.4 |
| Dark, Bittersweet, with Cherries, Organic, Green & Black's* | 1 Bar/100g | 477.0 | 28.0 | 477 | 7.9 | 48.0 | 28.2 | 8.7 |
| Dark, Continental, Luxury, Tesco* | 1 Bar/100g | 571.0 | 38.0 | 571 | 11.3 | 46.5 | 37.8 | 0.1 |
| Dark, Co-Op* | 1 Bar/50g | 252.0 | 14.0 | 505 | 4.0 | 57.0 | 29.0 | 6.0 |
| Dark, Espresso, with Coffee, Organic, Green & Black's* | 1 Bar/150g | 823.0 | 62.0 | 549 | 9.8 | 33.8 | 41.6 | 11.7 |
| Dark, Fair Trade, Co-Op* | 1 Bar/45g | 214.0 | 13.0 | 475 | 4.0 | 49.0 | 29.0 | 6.0 |
| Dark, Feuilles, with Orange, Nestle* | 1 Piece/8g | 42.0 | 3.0 | 524 | 4.6 | 54.4 | 32.0 | 0.0 |
| Dark, Luxury Continental, Sainsbury's* | ½ Bar/50g | 252.0 | 20.0 | 504 | 10.7 | 25.5 | 40.0 | 16.1 |
| Dark, Orange with Slivered Almonds, Excellence, Lindt* | 1 Square/10g | 50.0 | 3.0 | 500 | 6.0 | 46.0 | 30.0 | 0.0 |
| *Dark, Plain, Average* | *1oz/28g* | *143.0* | *8.0* | *510* | *5.0* | *63.5* | *28.0* | *2.5* |
| Dark, Plain, Rich, Co-Op* | 1 Bar/200g | 1010.0 | 58.0 | 505 | 4.0 | 57.0 | 29.0 | 6.0 |
| Dark, Plain, Rich, Sainsbury's* | 1oz/28g | 144.0 | 8.0 | 514 | 3.7 | 65.0 | 29.5 | 0.9 |
| Dark, Raspberry, Ruffles, Jameson's* | 1oz/28g | 123.0 | 5.0 | 441 | 1.9 | 65.9 | 18.9 | 4.4 |
| Dark, Rich, Tesco* | 1 Serving/20g | 98.0 | 6.0 | 491 | 5.8 | 60.0 | 30.4 | 11.5 |
| Dark, Special, Hershey* | 1 Pack/41g | 180.0 | 12.0 | 439 | 4.9 | 61.0 | 29.3 | 7.3 |
| Dark, TTD, Sainsbury's* | 1 Square/10g | 57.0 | 5.0 | 569 | 7.2 | 31.2 | 46.3 | 10.9 |
| Dark, Whole Nut, Tesco* | 1 Serving/13g | 67.0 | 4.0 | 539 | 6.1 | 48.3 | 35.7 | 6.5 |
| Dark, with a Soft Mint Centre, Organic, Green & Black's* | 1 Bar/100g | 478.0 | 27.0 | 478 | 7.4 | 50.5 | 27.3 | 8.6 |
| Dark, with Chilli, Thorntons* | 4 Squares/20g | 107.0 | 8.0 | 533 | 7.2 | 36.3 | 39.5 | 10.4 |
| Dark, with Hazelnuts & Currant, Organic, Green & Black's* | 1 Bar/100g | 513.0 | 33.0 | 513 | 7.6 | 45.4 | 33.5 | 9.2 |
| Dark, with Orange & Spices, Maya Gold, Green & Black's* | 1 Sm Bar/35g | 184.0 | 12.0 | 526 | 7.3 | 48.2 | 33.8 | 8.2 |
| Divine, Milk, Co-Op* | 1 Bar/45g | 243.0 | 14.0 | 540 | 7.0 | 57.0 | 32.0 | 2.0 |
| Double Chocolate, Nestle* | 1 Serving/25g | 133.0 | 8.0 | 532 | 9.1 | 49.4 | 33.1 | 0.0 |
| Dream, with Real Strawberries, Cadbury* | 1 Bar/45g | 250.0 | 15.0 | 555 | 4.5 | 59.6 | 33.1 | 0.0 |
| Drops, Plain, Sainsbury's* | 1 Serving/125g | 637.0 | 34.0 | 510 | 5.3 | 60.1 | 27.6 | 4.0 |
| Egg, Double Cream, Nestle* | 1 Egg/28g | 163.0 | 11.0 | 582 | 6.9 | 49.2 | 39.7 | 0.4 |
| Egg, Galaxy* | 1 Egg/38g | 183.0 | 9.0 | 482 | 5.3 | 59.7 | 24.7 | 0.0 |
| Egg, Mars* | 1 Egg/33g | 166.0 | 9.0 | 503 | 4.5 | 57.3 | 28.2 | 0.0 |
| Egg, Truffle Filled, Dark Chocolate, Black Magic, Nestle* | 1 Egg/28g | 144.0 | 9.0 | 522 | 5.8 | 52.0 | 32.3 | 3.4 |
| Eggs, Party, Mini, Safeway* | 1 Egg/20g | 65.0 | 4.0 | 320 | 11.2 | 18.4 | 21.9 | 0.7 |
| Ferrero Rocher, Ferrero* | 1 Chocolate/13g | 74.0 | 5.0 | 593 | 7.0 | 49.0 | 41.0 | 0.0 |
| Football, Milk Chocolate, Thorntons* | 1 Football/200g | 1088.0 | 67.0 | 544 | 7.6 | 52.9 | 33.5 | 1.0 |
| Freddo, Caramel, Dairy Milk, Cadbury* | 1 Bar/20g | 95.0 | 5.0 | 485 | 5.5 | 60.2 | 24.6 | 0.0 |
| Freddo, Dairy Milk, Cadbury* | 1 Freddo/20g | 105.0 | 6.0 | 525 | 7.5 | 57.0 | 29.8 | 0.7 |
| Fruit & Nut, Belgian, Waitrose* | 1 Serving/50g | 254.0 | 15.0 | 508 | 8.6 | 54.6 | 29.2 | 3.4 |
| Fruit & Nut, Dark, Tesco* | 4 Squares/25g | 123.0 | 7.0 | 494 | 5.8 | 54.8 | 27.9 | 6.5 |
| Fudge, Keto Bar* | 1 Serving/65g | 250.0 | 7.0 | 385 | 36.9 | 36.9 | 10.8 | 32.3 |
| Ginger, Traidcraft* | 1 Bar/50g | 212.0 | 7.0 | 424 | 3.9 | 68.2 | 14.8 | 0.0 |
| Golf Balls, Milk Chocolate, Lindt* | 1 Packet/110g | 619.0 | 39.0 | 563 | 6.5 | 53.6 | 35.9 | 0.0 |
| Hazelnut & Walnut, Dark, Organic, Seeds of Change* | 1 Bar/100g | 559.0 | 42.0 | 559 | 8.4 | 37.5 | 41.7 | 9.2 |
| Kinder, Bueno Bar, Ferrero* | 1 Bar/22g | 121.0 | 8.0 | 563 | 9.8 | 46.6 | 37.5 | 0.0 |
| Kinder, Riegel, Ferrero* | 1 Bar/21g | 117.0 | 7.0 | 558 | 10.0 | 53.0 | 34.0 | 0.0 |
| Kinder Maxi, Ferrero* | 1 Bar/21g | 115.0 | 7.0 | 550 | 10.0 | 51.0 | 34.0 | 0.0 |
| Kinder Surprise, Ferrero* | 1 Egg/20g | 110.0 | 7.0 | 550 | 10.0 | 51.0 | 34.0 | 0.4 |
| King Size, Dairy Milk, Cadbury* | 1 Serving/85g | 446.0 | 25.0 | 525 | 7.6 | 56.4 | 29.7 | 0.0 |
| Kitten, Milk Chocolate, Lindt* | 1 Kitten/84g | 480.0 | 29.0 | 572 | 7.5 | 57.7 | 34.6 | 0.0 |
| Light & Whippy, Bite Sized, Sainsbury's* | 1 Bar/15g | 66.0 | 2.0 | 439 | 3.3 | 69.7 | 16.3 | 0.1 |
| Macadamia Nut. Excellence, Lindt* | 1 Bar/100g | 560.0 | 37.0 | 560 | 7.0 | 51.0 | 37.0 | 0.0 |
| Matchmakers, Mint, Nestle* | 1 Stick/4g | 20.0 | 1.0 | 477 | 4.3 | 69.7 | 20.1 | 0.9 |
| Milk, & Hazelnut, Bar, Swiss, M & S* | 1oz/28g | 156.0 | 10.0 | 556 | 6.4 | 51.9 | 36.0 | 3.3 |

C

# CHOCOLATE

| | Measure INFO/WEIGHT | per Measure KCAL | FAT | Nutrition Values per 100g / 100ml KCAL | PROT | CARB | FAT | FIBRE |
|---|---|---|---|---|---|---|---|---|
| Milk, A Darker Shade of Milk Chocolate, Green & Black's* | 1 Sm Bar/35g | 183.0 | 10.0 | 523 | 9.9 | 54.0 | 29.7 | 3.7 |
| *Milk, Average* | *1oz/28g* | *146.0* | *9.0* | *520* | *7.7* | *56.9* | *30.7* | *0.8* |
| Milk, Belgian, TTD, Sainsbury's* | 2 Squares/20g | 110.0 | 7.0 | 549 | 9.6 | 48.8 | 35.0 | 1.8 |
| Milk, Biscuit Sticks, Mikado, Kraft* | 1 Stick/2g | 11.0 | 0.0 | 475 | 7.8 | 67.0 | 19.8 | 3.1 |
| Milk, Bubbly, Swiss, M & S* | 1 Serving/40g | 218.0 | 14.0 | 545 | 8.0 | 52.0 | 34.3 | 2.5 |
| Milk, Exra Fine, Swiss, M & S* | 1 Serving/25g | 141.0 | 9.0 | 565 | 7.2 | 50.9 | 36.7 | 2.3 |
| Milk, Extra Au Lait, Milch Extra, Lindt* | ½ Bar/50g | 267.0 | 15.0 | 535 | 6.5 | 57.0 | 31.0 | 0.0 |
| Milk, Extra Creamy, Excellence, Lindt* | 1 Bar/100g | 560.0 | 37.0 | 560 | 6.0 | 51.1 | 37.1 | 0.0 |
| Milk, Fair Trade, Tesco* | 1 Serving/45g | 236.0 | 13.0 | 524 | 7.6 | 56.7 | 29.6 | 2.0 |
| Milk, Fimbles Bar, Kinnerton* | 1 Bar/12g | 65.0 | 4.0 | 539 | 5.8 | 57.0 | 31.8 | 1.9 |
| Milk, Honey, Traidcraft* | 1 Bar/50g | 272.0 | 16.0 | 545 | 6.0 | 54.0 | 33.0 | 0.0 |
| Milk, Less Than 99 Calories, M & S* | 1 Bar/16g | 85.0 | 5.0 | 531 | 7.5 | 61.2 | 28.7 | 0.6 |
| Milk, Lindor, Lindt* | 1 Square/11g | 68.0 | 5.0 | 615 | 4.7 | 43.0 | 47.0 | 0.0 |
| Milk, Organic, Tesco* | 1 Serving/25g | 139.0 | 9.0 | 558 | 6.3 | 51.4 | 36.3 | 2.3 |
| Milk, Sainsbury's* | 4 Squares/25g | 133.0 | 8.0 | 533 | 9.2 | 54.6 | 30.8 | 2.2 |
| Milk, Santas, Tesco* | 1 Bag/90g | 433.0 | 22.0 | 481 | 4.5 | 61.4 | 24.2 | 1.4 |
| Milk, Shapes, Easter Friends, Tesco* | 1 Chocolate/13g | 67.0 | 4.0 | 540 | 8.0 | 52.3 | 34.2 | 2.3 |
| Milk, SmartPrice, Asda* | 1 Square/6g | 32.0 | 2.0 | 536 | 8.0 | 54.0 | 32.0 | 1.8 |
| Milk, Super Naturals, Sainsbury's* | 4 Pieces/40g | 85.0 | 5.0 | 212 | 2.4 | 23.0 | 12.2 | 0.9 |
| Milk, Swiss Made, Organic, Traidcraft* | 4 Squares/17g | 91.0 | 6.0 | 550 | 7.0 | 50.0 | 34.0 | 0.0 |
| Milk, Tesco* | 1 Serving/25g | 133.0 | 8.0 | 533 | 9.5 | 54.7 | 30.7 | 2.2 |
| Milk, Value, Tesco* | 1/6 Bar/16g | 83.0 | 4.0 | 520 | 6.8 | 60.0 | 28.0 | 2.3 |
| Milk, Whole Nut, Tesco* | 1 Serving/25g | 129.0 | 8.0 | 517 | 8.7 | 53.4 | 33.8 | 9.0 |
| Milk, Winnie the Pooh, Solid Shapes, M & S* | 1 Chocolate/6g | 32.0 | 2.0 | 540 | 8.1 | 54.1 | 32.4 | 1.3 |
| Milk, with a Soft Caramel Centre, Organic, Green & Black's* | 1 Bar/100g | 495.0 | 26.0 | 495 | 8.3 | 56.2 | 26.4 | 2.8 |
| Milk, with Biscuit Pieces, Asda* | 2 Squares/14g | 73.0 | 4.0 | 521 | 8.0 | 57.0 | 29.0 | 1.9 |
| Milk, with Crunchy Butterscotch, Organic, Green & Black's* | 1 Bar/150g | 793.0 | 46.0 | 529 | 9.2 | 53.4 | 31.0 | 3.4 |
| Milk, with Honey & Almond Nougat, Swiss, Toblerone* | 1 Piece/8g | 42.0 | 2.0 | 525 | 5.4 | 59.0 | 29.5 | 2.2 |
| Milk, with Peanut Butter Filling, Ghirardelli* | 1 Serving/45g | 250.0 | 17.0 | 556 | 8.9 | 48.9 | 37.8 | 2.2 |
| Milk, with Raisins & Hazelnuts, Green & Black's* | 1 Bar/100g | 556.0 | 37.0 | 556 | 9.2 | 46.8 | 36.9 | 3.2 |
| Milk, with Whole Almonds, Organic, Green & Black's* | 1 Bar/100g | 578.0 | 42.0 | 578 | 11.8 | 37.7 | 42.2 | 5.2 |
| Mini Bites, Chunky, Moments, Fox's* | 1 Roll/20g | 90.0 | 5.0 | 450 | 5.7 | 52.4 | 24.6 | 2.2 |
| Mini Eggs, Cadbury* | 1 Egg/3g | 16.0 | 1.0 | 485 | 4.6 | 67.8 | 21.9 | 1.3 |
| Mini Eggs, with Soft White Truffle Centre, M & S* | 1 Egg/6g | 33.0 | 2.0 | 550 | 6.5 | 56.3 | 33.9 | 1.4 |
| Mint Chips, Chunk, Dairy Milk, Cadbury* | 1 Chunk/32g | 162.0 | 8.0 | 505 | 6.5 | 61.2 | 26.1 | 0.0 |
| Mint Chips, Dairy Milk, Cadbury* | 1 Bar/49g | 247.0 | 13.0 | 505 | 6.6 | 61.6 | 26.1 | 0.6 |
| Mint Creme, Sainsbury's* | 1 Serving/20g | 93.0 | 5.0 | 467 | 2.8 | 62.7 | 24.5 | 2.1 |
| Mint Crisp, Cadbury* | 1oz/28g | 141.0 | 6.0 | 505 | 6.4 | 70.3 | 22.2 | 0.0 |
| Mint Crisp, Sainsbury's* | 4 Squares/19g | 95.0 | 5.0 | 501 | 5.0 | 63.7 | 25.0 | 3.6 |
| Mint Crisps, M & S* | 1 Mint/8g | 40.0 | 2.0 | 494 | 5.4 | 54.8 | 29.6 | 3.1 |
| Mints, Twilight, Terry's* | 1 Chocolate/8g | 38.0 | 2.0 | 475 | 2.5 | 56.2 | 26.2 | 3.7 |
| Mistletoe Kisses, Galaxy* | 1 Packet /42g | 209.0 | 11.0 | 498 | 5.3 | 57.0 | 27.3 | 0.0 |
| Mountain Bar, Swiss, M & S* | 1 Bar/100g | 555.0 | 35.0 | 555 | 6.5 | 55.2 | 35.3 | 0.2 |
| Mountain Bar, with Orange, Swiss, M & S* | ½ Bar/50g | 267.0 | 16.0 | 535 | 8.0 | 52.2 | 32.8 | 3.2 |
| Mousse au Chocolat, Dark, Lindt* | 1oz/28g | 158.0 | 10.0 | 563 | 6.0 | 50.0 | 37.0 | 5.6 |
| Natural Orange, Excellence, Lindt* | 1 Bar/100g | 560.0 | 37.0 | 560 | 7.0 | 50.0 | 37.0 | 0.0 |
| Natural Vanilla, Excellence, Lindt* | 1 Bar/100g | 590.0 | 40.0 | 590 | 6.0 | 51.0 | 40.0 | 0.0 |
| Neapolitans, Terry's* | 1oz/28g | 146.0 | 8.0 | 522 | 6.0 | 57.3 | 29.7 | 4.1 |
| Noir, Special, Frey* | 1 Bar/35g | 197.0 | 16.0 | 562 | 8.0 | 30.0 | 45.0 | 0.0 |
| Nuts About Caramel, Cadbury* | 1 Bar/55g | 272.0 | 15.0 | 495 | 5.8 | 56.6 | 27.4 | 0.0 |
| Nutty Nougat, Bite Sized, Sainsbury's* | 1 Bar/23g | 111.0 | 5.0 | 481 | 7.6 | 59.0 | 23.8 | 0.6 |
| Old Jamaica, Cadbury* | 1oz/28g | 129.0 | 7.0 | 460 | 5.8 | 56.9 | 23.3 | 0.0 |
| Orange, Fair Trade, Divine* | 4 Squares/17g | 92.0 | 5.0 | 541 | 6.5 | 57.7 | 31.5 | 0.0 |

## CHOCOLATE

| | Measure INFO/WEIGHT | per Measure KCAL | FAT | KCAL | PROT | CARB | FAT | FIBRE |
|---|---|---|---|---|---|---|---|---|
| Orange, Sainsbury's* | 4 Squares/19g | 100.0 | 6.0 | 531 | 9.2 | 54.3 | 30.7 | 2.2 |
| Orange Cream, Cadbury* | 1 Bar/51g | 217.0 | 8.0 | 425 | 2.6 | 68.6 | 15.4 | 0.0 |
| Orange Cream, Fry's* | 1 Bar/50g | 210.0 | 7.0 | 420 | 2.8 | 72.3 | 13.7 | 0.0 |
| Panna Cotta & Raspberry, M & S* | 1 Bar/36g | 190.0 | 12.0 | 528 | 4.7 | 51.4 | 33.6 | 0.3 |
| Peanut Butter Cup, Big Cup, Reese's, Hershey* | 1 Cup/39g | 210.0 | 12.0 | 538 | 10.3 | 53.8 | 30.8 | 2.6 |
| Peanut Butter Cup, Miniature, Reese's, Hershey* | 1 Cup/7g | 36.0 | 2.0 | 514 | 10.0 | 55.7 | 30.0 | 4.3 |
| Peanut Butter Cup, Reese's, Hershey* | 1 Cup/17g | 90.0 | 5.0 | 529 | 11.8 | 58.8 | 29.4 | 5.9 |
| Peanut Butter Cup, White, Mini, Reese's, Hershey* | 5 Cups/39g | 210.0 | 12.0 | 538 | 12.8 | 53.8 | 30.8 | 2.6 |
| Peppermint, Ritter Sport* | 1 Bar/100g | 483.0 | 26.0 | 483 | 3.0 | 60.0 | 26.0 | 0.0 |
| Peppermint Cream, Fry's* | 1 Bar/51g | 217.0 | 8.0 | 425 | 2.6 | 68.8 | 15.4 | 0.0 |
| Plain, 50% Cocoa Solids Minimum, Tesco* | 4 Squares/22g | 115.0 | 6.0 | 523 | 7.4 | 60.0 | 28.1 | 1.8 |
| Plain, 72% Cocoa Solids, Finest, Tesco* | 1 Square/10g | 60.0 | 4.0 | 603 | 7.7 | 44.0 | 44.0 | 3.7 |
| Plain, Belgian, Organic, Waitrose* | 1 Bar/100g | 505.0 | 38.0 | 505 | 9.6 | 32.0 | 37.6 | 5.6 |
| Plain, Continental, Waitrose* | 1 Square/4g | 23.0 | 2.0 | 558 | 7.7 | 32.9 | 44.0 | 5.9 |
| Plain, Dark, Fruit & Nut, Rich, Sainsbury's* | 4 Squares/25g | 122.0 | 7.0 | 489 | 5.2 | 53.9 | 27.9 | 5.7 |
| Plain, Fair Trade, Tesco* | 1 Bar/40g | 200.0 | 12.0 | 501 | 4.8 | 53.8 | 29.6 | 6.6 |
| Plain, Whole Nut, Belgian, Waitrose* | 4 Squares/25g | 135.0 | 9.0 | 540 | 6.3 | 45.4 | 38.0 | 7.8 |
| Plain, Wholenut, Sainsbury's* | 1 Serving/25g | 142.0 | 9.0 | 567 | 5.7 | 54.6 | 36.2 | 2.5 |
| Plain, with Ginger, Belgian, TTD, Sainsbury's* | 2 Squares/20g | 114.0 | 9.0 | 571 | 7.2 | 31.2 | 46.4 | 10.9 |
| Plain, with Ginger, Swiss, Waitrose* | 4 Squares/17g | 88.0 | 5.0 | 519 | 5.3 | 58.3 | 29.4 | 2.0 |
| Plain, with Hazelnuts, Tesco* | 4 Squares/25g | 135.0 | 9.0 | 539 | 6.1 | 48.3 | 35.7 | 6.5 |
| Planets, Mars* | 1 Pack/37g | 178.0 | 8.0 | 481 | 4.9 | 65.4 | 22.4 | 0.0 |
| Praline, M & S* | 1 Bar/34g | 185.0 | 12.0 | 545 | 7.3 | 49.6 | 35.2 | 3.1 |
| Rafaello, Roche, Ferrero* | 1 Sweet/10g | 60.0 | 5.0 | 600 | 9.7 | 35.4 | 46.6 | 0.0 |
| Rico, Organic, Traidcraft^ | 1 Bar/45g | 270.0 | 20.0 | 599 | 7.0 | 44.1 | 43.9 | 0.0 |
| Shots, Cadbury* | 1 Pack/160g | 752.0 | 37.0 | 470 | 5.9 | 59.7 | 23.2 | 0.0 |
| Snack Size, Dairy Milk, Cadbury* | 1 Bar/30g | 159.0 | 9.0 | 530 | 7.8 | 57.1 | 29.9 | 0.0 |
| Snaps, Milk, Cadbury* | 1 Snap/3g | 15.0 | 1.0 | 505 | 6.3 | 60.5 | 27.0 | 1.0 |
| Snaps, Orange, Cadbury* | 1 Snap/3g | 15.0 | 1.0 | 505 | 6.3 | 60.4 | 27.0 | 1.0 |
| Speckled Eggs, M & S* | 1 Egg/6g | 25.0 | 1.0 | 440 | 6.6 | 63.1 | 18.2 | 1.5 |
| Tasters, Dairy Milk, Cadbury* | 1 Bag/45g | 238.0 | 14.0 | 530 | 7.6 | 56.4 | 30.5 | 0.0 |
| Taz Chocolate Bar, Cadbury* | 1 Bar/25g | 121.0 | 6.0 | 485 | 4.8 | 62.0 | 24.0 | 0.0 |
| Teddy Bear, Milk Chocolate, Thorntons* | 1 Teddy/250g | 1357.0 | 84.0 | 543 | 7.6 | 52.6 | 33.5 | 1.0 |
| Toffifee, Storck* | 1 Sweet/6g | 32.0 | 2.0 | 535 | 6.0 | 58.0 | 31.0 | 0.0 |
| Treatsize, Dairy Milk, Cadbury* | 1 Bar/14g | 73.0 | 4.0 | 525 | 7.5 | 57.0 | 29.8 | 0.7 |
| Turkish Delight, Large Bar, Dairy Milk, Cadbury* | 1 Square/8g | 35.0 | 2.0 | 470 | 5.6 | 63.2 | 21.4 | 0.5 |
| Wafer, Dairy Milk, Cadbury* | 1 Bar/46g | 235.0 | 13.0 | 510 | 7.7 | 57.0 | 28.0 | 0.0 |
| ***White, Average*** | ***1oz/28g*** | ***148.0*** | ***9.0*** | ***529*** | ***8.0*** | ***58.3*** | ***30.9*** | ***0.0*** |
| White, Bar, Swiss, M & S* | 1oz/28g | 152.0 | 9.0 | 543 | 8.0 | 58.3 | 30.9 | 0.0 |
| White, Creamy, Dairyfine* | 1 Bar/40g | 220.0 | 13.0 | 551 | 5.5 | 58.0 | 33.0 | 0.0 |
| White, Creamy, Safeway* | 4 Squares/21g | 113.0 | 6.0 | 537 | 6.9 | 59.9 | 29.5 | 0.0 |
| White, Creamy, Tesco* | 1 Serving/25g | 139.0 | 9.0 | 557 | 5.1 | 55.7 | 34.9 | 3.3 |
| White, Creamy Vanilla, Green & Black's* | 1 Sm Bar/35g | 201.0 | 13.0 | 573 | 7.4 | 53.5 | 36.6 | 0.1 |
| White, Crispy, Fair Trade, Co-Op* | ½ Bar/50g | 277.0 | 17.0 | 555 | 9.0 | 51.0 | 35.0 | 0.1 |
| White, Double Berry, Nestle* | ¼ Bar/30g | 167.0 | 10.0 | 556 | 6.6 | 54.9 | 34.5 | 0.0 |
| White, Nestle* | 4 Pieces/40g | 220.0 | 13.0 | 550 | 7.5 | 55.0 | 32.5 | 0.0 |
| White, No Added Sugar, Belgian, Boots* | 1 Serving/30g | 146.0 | 11.0 | 488 | 6.0 | 47.8 | 36.0 | 7.0 |
| White, SmartPrice, Asda* | 1 Serving/25g | 137.0 | 8.0 | 549 | 7.0 | 56.0 | 33.0 | 0.0 |
| White, Value, Tesco* | 1 Serving/10g | 55.0 | 3.0 | 548 | 4.7 | 62.0 | 31.2 | 0.0 |
| White, with Coffee, Belgian, TTD, Sainsbury's* | 2 Squares/20g | 110.0 | 7.0 | 548 | 6.5 | 56.9 | 32.7 | 0.0 |
| White, with Honey & Almond Nougat, Toblerone* | 1 Serving/25g | 132.0 | 7.0 | 530 | 6.2 | 60.5 | 29.0 | 0.2 |
| White, with Lemon, Belgian, TTD, Sainsbury's* | 2 Squares/20g | 109.0 | 6.0 | 546 | 5.7 | 61.2 | 30.9 | 0.1 |
| White, with Strawberry Pieces, Under 99 Cals, M & S* | 1 Bar/16g | 86.0 | 5.0 | 540 | 6.6 | 60.4 | 30.4 | 0.3 |

| | Measure INFO/WEIGHT | per Measure KCAL | FAT | Nutrition Values per 100g / 100ml KCAL | PROT | CARB | FAT | FIBRE |
|---|---|---|---|---|---|---|---|---|
| **CHOCOLATE** | | | | | | | | |
| Whole Nut, Dairy Milk, Cadbury* | 1 Bar/49g | 270.0 | 17.0 | 550 | 8.9 | 49.5 | 35.4 | 1.7 |
| Whole Nut, Sainsbury's* | 4 Chunks/25g | 141.0 | 9.0 | 566 | 8.5 | 48.5 | 37.6 | 2.6 |
| Whole Nut, SmartPrice, Asda* | ½ Bar/16g | 92.0 | 6.0 | 562 | 8.0 | 47.0 | 38.0 | 3.3 |
| Wildlife Bar, Cadbury* | 1 Bar/21g | 109.0 | 6.0 | 520 | 7.8 | 56.8 | 29.3 | 0.0 |
| with Almonds, Nestle* | 1 Square/20g | 109.0 | 7.0 | 547 | 9.2 | 48.7 | 35.1 | 0.1 |
| with Creme Egg, Dairy Milk, Cadbury* | 1 Bar/45g | 210.0 | 9.0 | 470 | 5.2 | 64.8 | 20.9 | 0.5 |
| with Crunchie Bits, Dairy Milk, Cadbury* | 1 Bar/200g | 1000.0 | 49.0 | 500 | 6.2 | 63.3 | 24.4 | 0.0 |
| with Shortcake Biscuit, Dairy Milk, Cadbury* | 1 Square/6g | 31.0 | 2.0 | 520 | 7.5 | 59.0 | 28.0 | 0.0 |
| **CHOCOLATE DROPS** | | | | | | | | |
| Plain, Asda* | 1 Serving/100g | 489.0 | 29.0 | 489 | 7.0 | 50.0 | 29.0 | 10.0 |
| White, for Cooking & Decorating, Sainsbury's* | 1oz/28g | 152.0 | 9.0 | 544 | 6.5 | 60.3 | 30.8 | 0.0 |
| **CHOCOLATE NUTS** | | | | | | | | |
| Almonds, Dark Chohcolate Covered, Bolero* | 2 Almonds/3g | 15.0 | 1.0 | 510 | 2.6 | 48.8 | 33.5 | 0.0 |
| Peanuts, Assorted, Thorntons* | 1 Bag/140g | 785.0 | 57.0 | 561 | 13.8 | 34.8 | 40.8 | 3.6 |
| Peanuts, Belgian Coated, M & S* | 1 Serving/20g | 109.0 | 8.0 | 545 | 14.7 | 35.6 | 38.0 | 5.8 |
| Peanuts, Milk, Tesco* | 1 Bag/227g | 1221.0 | 86.0 | 538 | 17.5 | 31.8 | 37.9 | 4.4 |
| **CHOCOLATE ORANGE** | | | | | | | | |
| Bar, Montana* | 1 Serving/25g | 131.0 | 7.0 | 523 | 7.0 | 62.2 | 27.4 | 0.0 |
| Crunchball, Terry's* | 1 Segment/9g | 45.0 | 2.0 | 520 | 6.9 | 59.8 | 28.1 | 2.0 |
| Dark, Terry's* | 1 Segment/9g | 45.0 | 3.0 | 511 | 4.3 | 57.0 | 29.3 | 6.2 |
| Egg & Spoon, Terry's* | 1 Egg/34g | 195.0 | 13.0 | 575 | 5.5 | 51.6 | 38.0 | 1.7 |
| Goes Minty, Terry's* | 3 Slices/26g | 133.0 | 8.0 | 510 | 4.3 | 57.0 | 29.5 | 6.2 |
| Milk, Mini Segments, Terry's* | 1 Segment/8g | 42.0 | 2.0 | 527 | 7.7 | 57.9 | 29.4 | 2.1 |
| Milk, Terry's* | 1 Orange/175g | 931.0 | 52.0 | 532 | 7.4 | 57.8 | 29.5 | 2.1 |
| Plain, Terry's* | 1 Orange/175g | 889.0 | 51.0 | 508 | 3.8 | 56.8 | 29.4 | 6.2 |
| Segsations, Terry's* | 1 Segsation/8g | 43.0 | 2.0 | 520 | 6.9 | 58.5 | 28.5 | 2.8 |
| White, Terry's* | 1 Segment/11g | 61.0 | 3.0 | 535 | 6.3 | 60.9 | 29.4 | 0.0 |
| **CHOCOLATE RAISINS** | | | | | | | | |
| Assorted, Thorntons* | 1 Bag/140g | 601.0 | 28.0 | 429 | 4.2 | 58.8 | 19.7 | 2.9 |
| Bonds Sweetstars* | 1 Serving/28g | 109.0 | 4.0 | 391 | 4.7 | 57.0 | 16.0 | 0.0 |
| Californian, Belgian White Chocolate, M & S* | 1 Pack/100g | 450.0 | 21.0 | 450 | 4.3 | 60.6 | 20.9 | 0.8 |
| Californian, Tesco* | ¼ Bag/57g | 268.0 | 12.0 | 472 | 5.2 | 66.2 | 20.7 | 1.3 |
| Clusters, Cadbury* | 1 Bag/37g | 175.0 | 8.0 | 473 | 0.0 | 62.7 | 22.2 | 0.0 |
| Coated, Californian, M & S* | 1 Bag/130g | 520.0 | 19.0 | 400 | 4.3 | 63.2 | 14.7 | 1.9 |
| Co-Op* | ¼ Pack/50g | 205.0 | 7.0 | 410 | 4.0 | 64.0 | 15.0 | 1.0 |
| Jameson's* | 1 Serving/23g | 96.0 | 4.0 | 418 | 4.7 | 62.7 | 16.5 | 1.4 |
| M & S* | 1oz/28g | 116.0 | 4.0 | 414 | 4.5 | 66.5 | 14.6 | 1.2 |
| Milk, Asda* | 1 Serving/28g | 127.0 | 6.0 | 452 | 6.0 | 62.0 | 20.0 | 1.2 |
| Milk, Co-Op* | ½ Bag/100g | 420.0 | 17.0 | 420 | 5.0 | 63.0 | 17.0 | 6.0 |
| Milk, Tesco* | 1 Lge Bag/227g | 933.0 | 35.0 | 411 | 4.8 | 63.3 | 15.4 | 0.9 |
| **CHOCOLATE SPREAD** | | | | | | | | |
| *Average* | *1 Tsp/12g* | *68.0* | *5.0* | *569* | *4.1* | *57.1* | *37.6* | *0.0* |
| Snickers, Mars* | 1 Serving/7g | 38.0 | 3.0 | 548 | 8.7 | 43.3 | 37.8 | 0.0 |
| *with Nuts* | *1 Tsp/12g* | *66.0* | *4.0* | *549* | *6.2* | *60.5* | *33.0* | *0.8* |
| **CHOCOLATES** | | | | | | | | |
| All Gold, Dark, Terry's* | 1 Serving/30g | 151.0 | 9.0 | 505 | 4.0 | 57.5 | 29.0 | 4.3 |
| All Gold, Milk, Terry's* | 1 Serving/30g | 157.0 | 9.0 | 525 | 4.8 | 58.0 | 30.5 | 1.5 |
| Almond Marzipan, Milk Chocolate, Thorntons* | 1 Chocolate/13g | 60.0 | 3.0 | 464 | 6.6 | 59.4 | 22.6 | 5.6 |
| Alpini, Thorntons* | 1 Chocolate/13g | 70.0 | 4.0 | 538 | 7.0 | 54.6 | 32.3 | 2.3 |
| Assortment, Belgian, Waitrose* | 1oz/28g | 127.0 | 8.0 | 453 | 6.3 | 45.5 | 27.3 | 3.8 |
| Assortment, Occasions, Tesco* | 1 Chocolate/15g | 70.0 | 3.0 | 470 | 4.6 | 65.8 | 20.9 | 0.5 |
| Bittermint, Bendicks* | 1 Mint/18g | 80.0 | 3.0 | 440 | 4.3 | 68.9 | 16.3 | 2.4 |
| Brandy Liqueurs, Asda* | 1 Chocolate/8g | 34.0 | 1.0 | 409 | 4.0 | 60.0 | 17.0 | 0.8 |

## CHOCOLATES

| | Measure INFO/WEIGHT | per Measure KCAL | FAT | Nutrition Values per 100g / 100ml KCAL | PROT | CARB | FAT | FIBRE |
|---|---|---|---|---|---|---|---|---|
| Brazil Nut Assortment, M & S* | 1oz/28g | 163.0 | 13.0 | 581 | 9.6 | 37.5 | 45.3 | 1.5 |
| Cafe Au Lait, From Continental Selection, Thorntons* | 1 Chocolate/16g | 77.0 | 4.0 | 481 | 5.3 | 58.1 | 25.0 | 0.6 |
| Cappuccino, From Continental Selection, Thorntons* | 1 Chocolate/13g | 70.0 | 5.0 | 538 | 5.9 | 48.5 | 36.2 | 0.8 |
| Caramels, Sainsbury's* | 1 Sweet/12g | 57.0 | 3.0 | 490 | 3.5 | 69.0 | 22.2 | 0.2 |
| Celebrations, Mars* | 1 Av Sweet/8g | 41.0 | 2.0 | 512 | 5.7 | 61.5 | 27.0 | 1.7 |
| Cherry Liqueur, M & S* | 1 Chocolate/10g | 39.0 | 2.0 | 395 | 2.9 | 52.8 | 17.8 | 4.3 |
| Chocolate Mousse, Thorntons* | 1 Chocolate/13g | 67.0 | 5.0 | 515 | 7.5 | 40.0 | 36.2 | 3.1 |
| Classic Collection, Thorntons* | 1 Chocolate/12g | 58.0 | 3.0 | 472 | 4.3 | 62.7 | 22.8 | 2.4 |
| Coffee Creme, Dark, Thorntons* | 1 Chocolate/13g | 52.0 | 1.0 | 400 | 3.0 | 71.5 | 10.8 | 0.8 |
| Coffee Creme, Milk, Thorntons* | 1 Chocolate/13g | 52.0 | 1.0 | 400 | 2.8 | 74.6 | 10.0 | 0.8 |
| Continental, Belgian, Thorntons* | 1 Chocolate/13g | 67.0 | 4.0 | 514 | 5.8 | 53.5 | 30.3 | 2.9 |
| Continental, Thorntons* | 1 Chocolate/15g | 76.0 | 4.0 | 506 | 5.6 | 54.5 | 29.3 | 2.7 |
| Country Caramel, Milk, Thorntons* | 1 Chocolate/9g | 45.0 | 2.0 | 500 | 4.6 | 62.2 | 26.7 | 0.0 |
| Dairy Box, Milk, Nestle* | 1 Piece/11g | 50.0 | 2.0 | 456 | 4.4 | 65.9 | 19.4 | 0.7 |
| Dark, Elegant, Elizabeth Shaw* | 1 Chocolate/8g | 38.0 | 2.0 | 469 | 2.9 | 62.5 | 23.1 | 0.0 |
| Dark, Swiss Thins, Lindt* | 1 Pack/125g | 681.0 | 46.0 | 545 | 4.7 | 49.2 | 37.0 | 0.0 |
| Fondant, Chocolate Coated, Usda Average* | 1 Chocolate/11g | 40.0 | 1.0 | 366 | 2.2 | 80.4 | 9.3 | 2.1 |
| Gorgeous, Bendicks* | 3 Sweets/15g | 82.0 | 5.0 | 550 | 6.6 | 55.3 | 33.3 | 1.1 |
| Italian Collection, Amaretto, M & S* | 1 Chocolate/13g | 60.0 | 3.0 | 480 | 4.4 | 59.7 | 25.1 | 2.3 |
| Italian Collection, Cappuccino, M & S* | 1 Bag/100g | 545.0 | 37.0 | 545 | 6.3 | 46.7 | 37.0 | 1.8 |
| Italian Collection, Favourites, M & S* | 1 Chocolate/14g | 74.0 | 5.0 | 530 | 5.7 | 50.4 | 33.7 | 1.6 |
| Italian Collection, Panna Cotta, M & S* | 1 Chocolate/13g | 70.0 | 5.0 | 545 | 5.3 | 49.4 | 36.4 | 0.1 |
| Liqueur, Barrels, Cointreau | 1 Chocolate/10g | 43.0 | 2.0 | 435 | 3.5 | 57.0 | 18.0 | 0.0 |
| Liqueurs, Cognac Truffle, Thorntons* | 1 Chocolate/14g | 65.0 | 4.0 | 464 | 7.3 | 40.0 | 27.1 | 2.9 |
| Milk, Swiss Thins, Lindt* | 1 Pack/125g | 687.0 | 43.0 | 550 | 5.8 | 53.6 | 34.6 | 0.0 |
| Milk Tray, Cadbury* | 1 Chocolate/9g | 47.0 | 2.0 | 495 | 4.7 | 61.5 | 25.8 | 0.7 |
| Mingles, Bendicks* | 1 Chocolate/5g | 27.0 | 2.0 | 540 | 6.5 | 58.6 | 31.3 | 0.1 |
| Mint Crisp, Bendicks* | 1 Mint/8g | 38.0 | 2.0 | 494 | 5.2 | 55.0 | 29.9 | 0.0 |
| Mint Crisp, Dark, Elizabeth Shaw* | 1 Chocolate/6g | 27.0 | 1.0 | 458 | 1.9 | 68.0 | 20.7 | 0.0 |
| Mint Crisp, Milk, Elizabeth Shaw* | 1 Chocolate/6g | 30.0 | 1.0 | 493 | 4.0 | 70.9 | 21.4 | 0.0 |
| Mint Crisp, Thorntons* | 1 Chocolate/7g | 34.0 | 2.0 | 486 | 7.7 | 40.0 | 31.4 | 4.3 |
| Misshapes, Assorted, Cadbury* | 1 Chocolate/8g | 41.0 | 2.0 | 515 | 5.2 | 57.5 | 29.1 | 0.0 |
| Moments, Thorntons* | 1 Chocolate/7g | 37.0 | 2.0 | 511 | 5.4 | 59.9 | 27.8 | 1.9 |
| Orange Crisp, Elizabeth Shaw* | 1 Chocolate/6g | 29.0 | 1.0 | 478 | 2.9 | 68.2 | 21.5 | 0.0 |
| Praline, Coffee, Thorntons* | 1 Chocolate/7g | 37.0 | 2.0 | 529 | 7.0 | 47.1 | 34.3 | 2.9 |
| Praline, Hazelnut, Thorntons* | 1 Chocolate/5g | 27.0 | 2.0 | 540 | 7.0 | 48.0 | 36.0 | 4.0 |
| Praline, Marzipan, Thorntons* | 1 Chocolate/14g | 63.0 | 3.0 | 450 | 5.9 | 58.6 | 21.4 | 2.1 |
| Quality Street, Nestle* | 1 Av Sweet/8g | 39.0 | 2.0 | 464 | 4.0 | 66.3 | 20.3 | 0.8 |
| Rocher, Continental, Thorntons* | 1 Chocolate/15g | 76.0 | 5.0 | 507 | 6.8 | 45.3 | 33.3 | 2.0 |
| Roses, Cadbury* | 1 Chocolate/9g | 42.0 | 2.0 | 495 | 4.8 | 62.6 | 25.3 | 0.7 |
| Sea Shells, Belgian, Guylian* | 1 Shell/11g | 65.0 | 4.0 | 574 | 8.0 | 49.0 | 39.0 | 0.0 |
| Seashells, Milk & White, Belgian, Waitrose* | 1 Serving/15g | 77.0 | 5.0 | 511 | 5.0 | 53.1 | 31.0 | 2.8 |
| Strawberrys & Cream, Thorntons* | 1 Chocolate/12g | 64.0 | 4.0 | 533 | 5.1 | 54.2 | 32.5 | 0.8 |
| Swiss Tradition, De Luxe, Lindt* | 1 Packet/250g | 1387.0 | 91.0 | 555 | 6.3 | 51.9 | 36.3 | 0.0 |
| Swiss Tradition, Mixed, Lindt* | 1 Packet/392g | 2215.0 | 149.0 | 565 | 6.1 | 49.8 | 38.1 | 0.0 |
| Tartufo, Thorntons* | 1 Chocolate/15g | 77.0 | 5.0 | 513 | 7.4 | 40.0 | 36.0 | 3.3 |
| Truffle, Amaretto, Thorntons* | 1 Chocolate/14g | 66.0 | 4.0 | 471 | 5.5 | 55.0 | 25.7 | 2.9 |
| Truffle, Belgian, TTD, Sainsbury's* | 1 Truffle/13g | 72.0 | 5.0 | 579 | 4.3 | 51.9 | 39.3 | 0.0 |
| Truffle, Belgian Milk, Waitrose* | 1 Truffle/14g | 73.0 | 5.0 | 525 | 5.8 | 52.9 | 34.1 | 1.2 |
| Truffle, Brandy, Thorntons* | 1 Chocolate/14g | 68.0 | 4.0 | 486 | 6.1 | 52.1 | 27.1 | 0.7 |
| Truffle, Caramel, Thorntons* | 1 Chocolate/14g | 67.0 | 4.0 | 479 | 4.2 | 57.9 | 25.7 | 2.1 |
| Truffle, Champagne, Petit, Thorntons* | 1 Chocolate/6g | 31.0 | 2.0 | 517 | 7.5 | 48.3 | 31.7 | 3.3 |
| Truffle, Champagne, Premier, Thorntons* | 1 Chocolate/17g | 88.0 | 6.0 | 518 | 6.9 | 45.3 | 32.9 | 2.4 |

C

| | Measure INFO/WEIGHT | per Measure KCAL | FAT | Nutrition Values per 100g / 100ml KCAL | PROT | CARB | FAT | FIBRE |
|---|---|---|---|---|---|---|---|---|

## CHOCOLATES

| | Measure INFO/WEIGHT | KCAL | FAT | KCAL | PROT | CARB | FAT | FIBRE |
|---|---|---|---|---|---|---|---|---|
| Truffle, Cherry, Thorntons* | 1 Chocolate/14g | 58.0 | 3.0 | 414 | 4.2 | 50.7 | 21.4 | 1.4 |
| Truffle, Continental Champagne, Thorntons* | 1 Chocolate/16g | 78.0 | 4.0 | 488 | 6.1 | 51.3 | 28.0 | 0.6 |
| Truffle, French Cocoa Dusted, Sainsbury's* | 1 Truffle/10g | 57.0 | 4.0 | 570 | 4.0 | 37.0 | 45.0 | 0.0 |
| Truffle, Grand Marnier, Thorntons* | 1 Chocolate/15g | 77.0 | 5.0 | 513 | 7.2 | 40.7 | 34.0 | 4.0 |
| Truffle, Hazelnut, Balls, Lindor, Lindt* | 1 Ball/12g | 76.0 | 6.0 | 632 | 5.0 | 39.1 | 50.6 | 0.0 |
| Truffle, Irish Milk Chocolate Cream, Elizabeth Shaw* | 1 Chocolate/12g | 57.0 | 3.0 | 477 | 3.9 | 63.4 | 22.8 | 0.0 |
| Truffle, Lemon, White, Thorntons* | 1 Chocolate/14g | 63.0 | 3.0 | 450 | 4.6 | 64.3 | 25.0 | 0.7 |
| Truffle, Milk Chocolate, Balls, Lindor, Lindt* | 1 Ball/12g | 74.0 | 6.0 | 617 | 4.9 | 43.1 | 47.2 | 0.0 |
| Truffle, Rum, Average | 1 Truffle/11g | 57.0 | 4.0 | 521 | 6.1 | 49.7 | 33.7 | 1.9 |
| Truffle, Rum, Thorntons* | 1 Chocolate/13g | 63.0 | 3.0 | 485 | 4.8 | 58.5 | 24.6 | 4.8 |
| Truffle, Selection, Tesco* | 1 Chocolate/14g | 75.0 | 4.0 | 539 | 5.1 | 62.0 | 29.8 | 0.5 |
| Truffle, Seville, Thorntons* | 1 Chocolate/14g | 76.0 | 5.0 | 543 | 7.1 | 53.6 | 33.6 | 1.4 |
| Truffle, Thorntons* | 1 Chocolate/7g | 33.0 | 2.0 | 471 | 6.0 | 48.6 | 27.1 | 1.4 |
| Truffle, Vanilla, Thorntons* | 1 Chocolate/13g | 64.0 | 3.0 | 492 | 4.8 | 57.7 | 26.9 | 1.5 |
| Truffle, Viennese, Dark, Thorntons* | 1 Chocolate/10g | 53.0 | 4.0 | 530 | 5.9 | 47.0 | 36.0 | 3.0 |
| Truffle, Viennese, Milk, Thorntons* | 1 Chocolate/10g | 56.0 | 4.0 | 560 | 4.9 | 54.0 | 36.0 | 0.0 |
| Truffle, White Chocolate, Balls, Lindor, Lindt* | 1 Ball/12g | 78.0 | 6.0 | 649 | 5.2 | 40.2 | 51.9 | 0.0 |
| Truffle Hearts, Baileys* | 1 Chocolate/15g | 76.0 | 4.0 | 506 | 5.2 | 52.6 | 28.9 | 1.3 |
| Truffles, Belgian, Flaked, Tesco* | 1 Truffle/14g | 80.0 | 5.0 | 575 | 4.4 | 52.7 | 38.5 | 2.3 |
| Valentine, Thorntons* | 1 Chocolate/11g | 60.0 | 4.0 | 542 | 5.7 | 52.0 | 34.5 | 2.1 |
| Winter Selection, Thorntons* | 1 Chocolate/10g | 51.0 | 3.0 | 506 | 6.2 | 51.3 | 30.6 | 3.8 |

## CHOCOLATINE

| | | | | | | | | |
|---|---|---|---|---|---|---|---|---|
| All Butter, Sainsbury's* | 1 Serving/58g | 241.0 | 14.0 | 415 | 7.9 | 42.5 | 23.7 | 3.3 |
| Mini, Sainsbury's* | 1 Serving/30g | 120.0 | 7.0 | 400 | 7.7 | 41.0 | 23.0 | 3.3 |
| Sainsbury's* | 1 Serving/58g | 263.0 | 16.0 | 454 | 8.5 | 42.3 | 27.9 | 2.1 |

## CHOP SUEY

| | | | | | | | | |
|---|---|---|---|---|---|---|---|---|
| Chicken, with Noodles, Sainsbury's* | 1 Pack/300g | 300.0 | 7.0 | 100 | 5.7 | 13.6 | 2.5 | 1.2 |
| Chinese, Vegetable, Stir Fry, Sharwood's* | 1 Pack/310g | 223.0 | 3.0 | 72 | 1.5 | 13.9 | 1.1 | 0.6 |

## CHOW MEIN

| | | | | | | | | |
|---|---|---|---|---|---|---|---|---|
| Beef, Sainsbury's* | 1 Pack/450g | 499.0 | 11.0 | 111 | 6.6 | 15.5 | 2.5 | 0.8 |
| Cantonese Vegetable Stir Fry, Sainsbury's* | ¼ Pack/100g | 85.0 | 4.0 | 85 | 2.2 | 10.6 | 3.8 | 1.2 |
| Char Sui, Cantonese, Sainsbury's* | ½ Pack/225g | 205.0 | 7.0 | 91 | 5.7 | 10.0 | 3.1 | 1.1 |
| Chicken, Ainsley Harriott* | 1 Serving/250g | 447.0 | 12.0 | 179 | 14.0 | 21.2 | 4.7 | 2.0 |
| Chicken, Chinese Takeaway, Sainsbury's* | 1 Pack/316g | 338.0 | 9.0 | 107 | 9.1 | 11.6 | 2.7 | 0.7 |
| Chicken, Chinese Takeaway, Tesco* | 1 Serving/350g | 294.0 | 8.0 | 84 | 8.1 | 7.5 | 2.4 | 1.1 |
| Chicken, COOK!, M & S* | 1 Pack/375g | 356.0 | 8.0 | 95 | 7.9 | 10.5 | 2.1 | 1.7 |
| Chicken, COU, M & S* | 1 Pack/200g | 180.0 | 5.0 | 90 | 9.3 | 8.1 | 2.3 | 1.1 |
| Chicken, Frozen, Sainsbury's* | 1 Pack/404g | 424.0 | 12.0 | 105 | 6.1 | 13.4 | 3.0 | 0.9 |
| Chicken, Less Than 3% Fat, BGTY, Sainsbury's* | 1 Pack/450g | 355.0 | 10.0 | 79 | 5.8 | 8.7 | 2.3 | 1.4 |
| Chicken, New, BGTY, Sainsbury's* | 1 Pack/450g | 373.0 | 6.0 | 83 | 6.0 | 11.4 | 1.4 | 1.1 |
| Chicken, New Improved Recipe, Sainsbury's* | 1 Pack/449g | 395.0 | 9.0 | 88 | 5.7 | 11.7 | 2.0 | 1.2 |
| Chicken, Sainsbury's* | 1 Serving/400g | 364.0 | 8.0 | 91 | 5.2 | 12.9 | 2.1 | 1.0 |
| Chicken, Waitrose* | 1 Serving/400g | 384.0 | 12.0 | 96 | 6.0 | 11.4 | 2.9 | 1.3 |
| Chicken with Vegetable Spring Roll, Oriental Express* | 1 Pack/300g | 213.0 | 2.0 | 71 | 5.5 | 12.4 | 0.6 | 1.9 |
| Pork, Perfectly Balanced, Waitrose* | ½ Pack/310g | 332.0 | 3.0 | 107 | 7.6 | 17.2 | 0.9 | 1.6 |
| Special, COU, M & S* | 1 Pack/400g | 320.0 | 4.0 | 80 | 7.4 | 9.9 | 1.0 | 1.0 |
| Special, HL, Tesco* | 1 Pack/450g | 351.0 | 5.0 | 78 | 6.3 | 10.6 | 1.2 | 0.6 |
| Stir Fry, Asda* | 1 Pack/350g | 269.0 | 17.0 | 77 | 2.1 | 6.0 | 5.0 | 0.0 |
| Stir Fry, Tesco* | ½ Pack/240g | 180.0 | 3.0 | 75 | 2.8 | 12.0 | 1.4 | 1.6 |
| Stir Fry with Veg & Noodles, Somerfield* | 1 Serving/200g | 234.0 | 12.0 | 117 | 2.8 | 12.9 | 6.0 | 1.3 |
| Vegetable, Asda* | 1 Pack/400g | 520.0 | 15.0 | 130 | 2.4 | 21.5 | 3.8 | 3.0 |
| Vegetable, Take Away, Meal for One, Tesco* | 1 Serving/345g | 262.0 | 8.0 | 76 | 6.7 | 7.3 | 2.2 | 1.3 |
| Vegetable & Cashew Nut, Eat Smart, Safeway* | 1 Pack/380g | 323.0 | 5.0 | 85 | 7.0 | 11.4 | 1.2 | 1.1 |

| | Measure INFO/WEIGHT | per Measure | | Nutrition Values per 100g / 100ml | | | | |
|---|---|---|---|---|---|---|---|---|
| | | KCAL | FAT | KCAL | PROT | CARB | FAT | FIBRE |
| **CHOW MEIN** | | | | | | | | |
| Vegetables & Noodles in Sauce, Safeway* | 1 Serving/200g | 110.0 | 0.0 | 55 | 3.7 | 9.5 | 0.2 | 1.3 |
| **CHRISTMAS PUDDING** | | | | | | | | |
| Average | 1oz/28g | 81.0 | 3.0 | 291 | 4.6 | 49.5 | 9.7 | 1.3 |
| BGTY, Sainsbury's* | 1 Serving/114g | 302.0 | 3.0 | 266 | 2.8 | 58.2 | 2.5 | 4.6 |
| Luxury, Tesco* | ¼ Pudding/114g | 346.0 | 11.0 | 305 | 3.7 | 50.8 | 9.7 | 1.3 |
| Nut Free & Alcohol Free, HE, Tesco* | 1 Serving/100g | 258.0 | 3.0 | 258 | 2.8 | 55.6 | 2.7 | 4.3 |
| Retail | 1oz/28g | 92.0 | 3.0 | 329 | 3.0 | 56.3 | 11.8 | 1.7 |
| Rich Fruit, Laced with Brandy, Tesco* | 1 Serving/100g | 305.0 | 10.0 | 305 | 3.7 | 50.8 | 9.7 | 1.3 |
| Rich Fruit, Tesco* | 1 Serving/114g | 331.0 | 7.0 | 290 | 2.4 | 55.0 | 5.9 | 0.0 |
| Sticky Toffee, Tesco* | ¼ Pudding/114g | 372.0 | 7.0 | 326 | 2.5 | 64.5 | 6.4 | 0.8 |
| Tesco* | 1 Serving/113g | 305.0 | 7.0 | 270 | 2.4 | 55.0 | 5.9 | 1.5 |
| Toffee Sauce Coated, Morrisons* | 1 Pudding/100g | 324.0 | 6.0 | 324 | 2.5 | 64.5 | 6.4 | 0.0 |
| Traditional Style, Asda* | 1 Pudding/100g | 296.0 | 6.0 | 296 | 2.6 | 58.0 | 6.0 | 1.6 |
| Vintage, M & S* | 1/8 Pudding/113g | 335.0 | 6.0 | 295 | 2.6 | 59.8 | 5.6 | 1.4 |
| VLH Kitchens* | 1 Serving 114g | 310.0 | 2.9 | 272 | 3.1 | 59.3 | 2.5 | 4.6 |
| Wheat Free, Gluten Free, Tesco* | 1oz/28g | 84.0 | 2.0 | 295 | 1.9 | 60.4 | 7.1 | 4.5 |
| with Cider, Value, Tesco* | 1 Serving/100g | 312.0 | 7.0 | 312 | 2.7 | 59.6 | 7.0 | 3.3 |
| with Cider & Sherry, Waitrose* | ¼ Pudding/114g | 344.0 | 7.0 | 303 | 2.5 | 59.0 | 6.3 | 3.2 |
| **CHUTNEY** | | | | | | | | |
| Albert's Victorian, Baxters* | 1 Serving/25g | 37.0 | 0.0 | 150 | 35.0 | 6.0 | 0.1 | 0.0 |
| Apple, Spiced, TTD, Sainsbury's* | 1 Serving/10g | 15.0 | 0.0 | 153 | 0.4 | 36.9 | 0.4 | 1.6 |
| Apple, Tomato & Sultana, Tesco* | 1 Serving/50g | 88.0 | 0.0 | 176 | 1.1 | 42.4 | 0.2 | 1.3 |
| Apricot, Sharwood's* | 1 Tsp/16g | 21.0 | 0.0 | 131 | 0.6 | 32.0 | 0.1 | 2.3 |
| Bengal Hot, Sharwood's* | 1oz/28g | 56.0 | 0.0 | 200 | 0.5 | 48.7 | 0.3 | 1.1 |
| Bengal Spice Mango, Sharwood's* | 1 Tsp/5g | 12.0 | 0.0 | 236 | 0.5 | 58.0 | 0.2 | 1.2 |
| Caramalised Onion, Sainsbury's* | 1 Serving/25g | 28.0 | 0.0 | 111 | 1.1 | 23.5 | 1.4 | 1.1 |
| Caramelised Red Onion, Loyd Grossman* | 1 Serving/10g | 11.0 | 0.0 | 111 | 0.5 | 27.2 | 0.0 | 0.5 |
| Cranberry & Caramelised Red Onion, Baxters* | 1 Serving/20g | 31.0 | 0.0 | 154 | 0.3 | 38.0 | 0.1 | 0.3 |
| Flame Roasted Tomato & Pepper, TTD, Sainsbury's* | 1 Serving/5g | 9.0 | 0.0 | 189 | 1.0 | 45.3 | 0.4 | 1.1 |
| Fruit, Spiced, Baxters* | 1 Tsp/16g | 23.0 | 0.0 | 143 | 6.0 | 34.8 | 0.1 | 0.0 |
| Fruit, Traditional, M & S* | 1oz/28g | 43.0 | 0.0 | 155 | 0.9 | 37.2 | 0.3 | 1.7 |
| Lime & Chilli, Geeta's* | 1 Serving/25g | 69.0 | 0.0 | 277 | 2.0 | 64.0 | 1.4 | 1.9 |
| Mango, Green Label, Sharwood's* | 1 Tsp/10g | 23.0 | 0.0 | 234 | 0.3 | 57.8 | 0.2 | 0.9 |
| Mango, Hot, Patak's* | 1 Jar/340g | 877.0 | 1.0 | 258 | 0.4 | 67.1 | 0.2 | 0.7 |
| Mango, Indian Takeaway, Asda* | 1 Pack/70g | 145.0 | 0.0 | 207 | 0.3 | 50.9 | 0.2 | 1.0 |
| Mango, Sensations, Walkers* | ¼ Jar/57g | 122.0 | 0.0 | 214 | 0.3 | 53.0 | 0.1 | 0.6 |
| Mango, Spiced, M & S* | 1 Serving/15g | 26.0 | 0.0 | 175 | 1.2 | 42.3 | 0.4 | 3.2 |
| Mango, Spicy, Sainsbury's* | 1 Tbsp/15g | 24.0 | 0.0 | 160 | 0.7 | 37.0 | 0.7 | 1.3 |
| **Mango, Sweet** | **1 Heaped Tsp/16g** | **30.0** | **0.0** | **189** | **0.7** | **48.3** | **0.1** | **0.0** |
| Mango, Tesco* | 1 Serving/20g | 45.0 | 0.0 | 224 | 0.4 | 55.5 | 0.1 | 1.3 |
| Mango, Waitrose* | 1 Serving/20g | 43.0 | 0.0 | 215 | 1.0 | 49.0 | 1.5 | 2.0 |
| Mango & Apple, Sharwood's* | 1oz/28g | 65.0 | 0.0 | 233 | 0.4 | 57.6 | 0.1 | 1.1 |
| Mango & Ginger, Baxters* | 1 Jar/320g | 598.0 | 1.0 | 187 | 5.0 | 45.7 | 0.2 | 0.9 |
| Mango & Lime, Sharwood's* | 1oz/28g | 58.0 | 0.0 | 206 | 0.4 | 50.5 | 0.3 | 0.8 |
| **Mixed Fruit** | **1 Heaped Tsp/16g** | **25.0** | **0.0** | **155** | **0.6** | **39.7** | **0.0** | **0.0** |
| Onion, TTD, Sainsbury's* | 1 Serving/20g | 55.0 | 0.0 | 277 | 0.9 | 67.2 | 0.5 | 1.4 |
| Peach, Spicy, Waitrose* | 1 Serving/20g | 43.0 | 0.0 | 215 | 1.0 | 49.0 | 1.5 | 1.5 |
| Peach Fruit, Sharwood's* | 1oz/28g | 48.0 | 0.0 | 172 | 0.4 | 42.3 | 0.1 | 0.9 |
| Ploughman's Plum, The English Provender Co.* | 1 Tsp/10g | 16.0 | 0.0 | 160 | 1.3 | 38.1 | 0.2 | 1.6 |
| Red Onion & Sherry Vinegar, Sainsbury's* | 1 Serving/10g | 24.0 | 0.0 | 236 | 0.5 | 57.1 | 0.6 | 1.4 |
| Spicy Fruit, Baxters* | 1 Serving/15g | 22.0 | 0.0 | 146 | 0.6 | 35.4 | 0.2 | 0.0 |
| Sweet Mango, M & S* | 1oz/28g | 67.0 | 0.0 | 240 | 0.3 | 58.8 | 0.2 | 1.5 |
| Sweet Mango, Patak's* | 1 Tbsp/15g | 39.0 | 0.0 | 259 | 0.3 | 67.4 | 0.1 | 0.7 |

**C**

| | Measure INFO/WEIGHT | per Measure KCAL | FAT | Nutrition Values per 100g / 100ml KCAL | PROT | CARB | FAT | FIBRE |
|---|---|---|---|---|---|---|---|---|
| **CHUTNEY** | | | | | | | | |
| *Tomato* | *1 Heaped Tsp/16g* | *20.0* | *0.0* | *128* | *1.2* | *31.0* | *0.2* | *1.3* |
| Tomato, TTD, Sainsbury's* | 1 Tbsp/15g | 29.0 | 0.0 | 193 | 2.0 | 44.7 | 1.3 | 2.7 |
| Tomato, Waitrose* | 1 Pot/100g | 195.0 | 0.0 | 195 | 1.3 | 46.8 | 0.3 | 0.0 |
| Tomato & Red Pepper, Baxters* | 1 Jar/312g | 512.0 | 1.0 | 164 | 2.0 | 38.0 | 0.4 | 1.5 |
| **CIDER** | | | | | | | | |
| Cyder, Premier Cru, Aspall* | 1 Serving/200ml | 120.0 | 0.0 | 60 | 0.0 | 3.1 | 0.0 | 0.0 |
| Diamond White* | 1 fl oz/30ml | 11.0 | 0.0 | 36 | 0.0 | 2.6 | 0.0 | 0.0 |
| *Dry, Average* | *1 Pint/568ml* | *205.0* | *0.0* | *36* | *0.0* | *2.6* | *0.0* | *0.0* |
| Dry, French, So Good, Somerfield* | 1 Bottle/500ml | 150.0 | 0.0 | 30 | 0.0 | 0.3 | 0.0 | 0.0 |
| Dry, Strongbow* | 1 Bottle/375ml | 161.0 | 0.0 | 43 | 0.0 | 3.4 | 0.0 | 0.0 |
| Light, Bulmers* | 1 Can/500ml | 140.0 | 0.0 | 28 | 0.0 | 0.8 | 0.0 | 0.0 |
| *Low Alcohol* | *1 Pint/568ml* | *97.0* | *0.0* | *17* | *0.0* | *3.6* | *0.0* | *0.0* |
| Low Carb, Stowford* | 1 Bottle/500ml | 140.0 | 0.0 | 28 | 0.0 | 0.2 | 0.0 | 0.0 |
| Magner's* | ½ Pint/284ml | 105.0 | 0.0 | 37 | 0.0 | 2.0 | 0.0 | 0.0 |
| Medium Sweet, Somerfield* | 1 Pint/568ml | 233.0 | 0.0 | 41 | 0.0 | 5.0 | 0.0 | 0.0 |
| Original, Bulmers* | 1 Serving/250ml | 105.0 | 0.0 | 42 | 0.0 | 4.0 | 0.0 | 0.0 |
| *Pear, Average* | *1 Serving/200ml* | *86.0* | *0.0* | *43* | *0.0* | *3.6* | *0.0* | *0.0* |
| *Scrumpy, Average* | *1 Serving/200ml* | *93.0* | *0.0* | *46* | *0.0* | *2.3* | *0.0* | *0.0* |
| Scrumpy, Westons* | 1 Serving/200ml | 94.0 | 0.0 | 47 | 0.0 | 1.8 | 0.0 | 0.0 |
| *Sweet, Average* | *1 Pint/568ml* | *239.0* | *0.0* | *42* | *0.0* | *4.3* | *0.0* | *0.0* |
| *Vintage* | *1 Pint/568ml* | *574.0* | *0.0* | *101* | *0.0* | *7.3* | *0.0* | *0.0* |
| **CINNAMON** | | | | | | | | |
| *Ground, Average* | *1 Tsp/3g* | *8.0* | *0.0* | *261* | *3.9* | *55.5* | *3.2* | *0.0* |
| **CLAMS** | | | | | | | | |
| *in Brine, Average* | *1oz/28g* | *22.0* | *0.0* | *79* | *16.0* | *2.4* | *0.6* | *0.0* |
| *Raw, Average* | *20 Sm/180g* | *133.0* | *2.0* | *74* | *12.8* | *2.6* | *1.0* | *0.0* |
| **CLEMENTINES** | | | | | | | | |
| *Raw, Weighed with Peel, Average* | *1 Med/60g* | *27.0* | *0.0* | *44* | *0.8* | *11.3* | *0.1* | *1.6* |
| *Raw, Weighed without Peel, Average* | *1 Med/46g* | *22.0* | *0.0* | *47* | *0.8* | *12.0* | *0.1* | *1.7* |
| **COCKLES** | | | | | | | | |
| *Boiled* | *1 Cockle/4g* | *2.0* | *0.0* | *53* | *12.0* | *0.0* | *0.6* | *0.0* |
| *Bottled in Vinegar, Drained* | *1oz/28g* | *17.0* | *0.0* | *60* | *13.3* | *0.0* | *0.7* | *0.0* |
| **COCKTAIL** | | | | | | | | |
| Alcoholic, Juice Based, Average | 1 Glass/200ml | 464.0 | 29.0 | 232 | 6.4 | 18.7 | 14.6 | 1.4 |
| Bucks Fizz, Premixed, M & S* | 1 Glass/250ml | 152.0 | 0.0 | 61 | 0.0 | 9.0 | 0.0 | 0.0 |
| Grenadine, Oange Juice, Pineapple Juice | 1 Serving/200ml | 158.0 | 0.0 | 79 | 0.5 | 19.2 | 0.1 | 0.2 |
| Mai Tai, Average | 1 Serving/200ml | 209.0 | 0.0 | 105 | 0.2 | 13.9 | 0.1 | 0.1 |
| Pina Colada | 1 Glass/250ml | 592.0 | 20.0 | 237 | 1.0 | 28.0 | 8.0 | 0.0 |
| **COCOA BUTTER** | | | | | | | | |
| *Average* | *1oz/28g* | *251.0* | *28.0* | *896* | *0.0* | *0.0* | *99.5* | *0.0* |
| **COCOA POWDER** | | | | | | | | |
| Cadbury* | 1 Tbsp/16g | 52.0 | 3.0 | 322 | 23.1 | 10.5 | 20.8 | 0.0 |
| Dry, Unsweetened, Average | 1 Tbsp/5g | 12.0 | 1.0 | 229 | 19.6 | 54.3 | 13.7 | 33.2 |
| Organic, Green & Black's* | 1 Tbsp/15g | 52.0 | 3.0 | 350 | 23.6 | 13.6 | 22.3 | 0.0 |
| Valrhona* | 1 Tsp/5g | 22.0 | 1.0 | 450 | 25.0 | 45.0 | 20.0 | 30.0 |
| **COCONUT** | | | | | | | | |
| *Creamed, Average* | *1oz/28g* | *186.0* | *19.0* | *665* | *6.0* | *6.7* | *68.4* | *7.0* |
| *Desiccated, Average* | *1oz/28g* | *169.0* | *17.0* | *604* | *5.6* | *6.4* | *62.0* | *13.7* |
| *Fresh, Flesh Only, Average* | *1oz/28g* | *98.0* | *10.0* | *351* | *3.2* | *3.7* | *36.0* | *7.3* |
| *Ice, Average* | *1oz/28g* | *104.0* | *4.0* | *371* | *1.7* | *66.7* | *12.7* | *2.6* |
| *Milk, Average* | *1 Can/400ml* | *698.0* | *70.0* | *174* | *1.4* | *2.9* | *17.4* | *2.9* |
| *Milk, Reduced Fat, Average* | *1 Av Serving/100g* | *103.0* | *10.0* | *103* | *0.9* | *2.4* | *10.0* | *0.4* |

| | Measure INFO/WEIGHT | per Measure KCAL | per Measure FAT | Nutrition Values per 100g / 100ml KCAL | PROT | CARB | FAT | FIBRE |
|---|---|---|---|---|---|---|---|---|
| **COD** | | | | | | | | |
| *Baked, Average* | *1oz/28g* | *27.0* | *0.0* | *96* | *21.4* | *0.0* | *1.2* | *0.0* |
| Beer Battered, Crispy, Finest, Tesco* | 1 Portion/250g | 575.0 | 35.0 | 230 | 12.0 | 13.4 | 14.0 | 1.3 |
| *Dried, Salted, Average* | *1oz/28g* | *82.0* | *1.0* | *290* | *62.8* | *0.0* | *2.4* | *0.0* |
| *Dried, Salted, Boiled, Average* | *1oz/28g* | *39.0* | *0.0* | *138* | *32.5* | *0.0* | *0.9* | *0.0* |
| Fillets, Battered, Average | 1 Serving/90g | 158.0 | 7.0 | 175 | 12.5 | 12.9 | 8.1 | 1.0 |
| Fillets, Breaded, Average | 1 Serving/97g | 200.0 | 9.0 | 206 | 13.0 | 16.7 | 9.7 | 1.0 |
| Fillets, Breaded, Chunky, Average | 1 Piece/135g | 204.0 | 8.0 | 151 | 13.7 | 10.9 | 5.9 | 1.4 |
| Fillets, Breaded, Light, Healthy Range, Average | 1 Fillet/135g | 209.0 | 7.0 | 154 | 13.6 | 13.3 | 5.1 | 1.2 |
| *Fillets, Chunky, Average* | *1 Fillet/198g* | *267.0* | *7.0* | *135* | *17.1* | *8.2* | *3.7* | *0.8* |
| *Fillets, Skinless & Boneless, Raw, Average* | *1 Portion/92g* | *90.0* | *2.0* | *98* | *17.8* | *2.7* | *1.7* | *0.4* |
| *Fillets, Smoked, Average* | *1 Serving/150g* | *151.0* | *2.0* | *101* | *21.6* | *0.0* | *1.6* | *0.0* |
| *Loins, Average* | *1 Serving/145g* | *116.0* | *1.0* | *80* | *17.9* | *0.1* | *0.8* | *0.2* |
| *Poached, Average* | *1oz/28g* | *26.0* | *0.0* | *94* | *20.9* | *0.0* | *1.1* | *0.0* |
| *Smoked, Raw, Average* | *1oz/28g* | *22.0* | *0.0* | *79* | *18.3* | *0.0* | *0.6* | *0.0* |
| Steaks, Battered, Chip Shop Style, Average | 1 Serving/150g | 321.0 | 18.0 | 214 | 12.5 | 14.3 | 12.0 | 1.1 |
| *Steamed, Average* | *1oz/28g* | *23.0* | *0.0* | *83* | *18.6* | *0.0* | *0.9* | *0.0* |
| **COD &** | | | | | | | | |
| Cauliflower Bake, Asda* | 1 Pack/400g | 492.0 | 28.0 | 123 | 9.5 | 5.5 | 7.0 | 1.0 |
| Chips, Oven Baked, Safeway* | 1 Pack/250g | 522.0 | 21.0 | 209 | 8.4 | 25.0 | 8.4 | 3.5 |
| Parsley Sauce, Frozen, M & S* | 1 Pack/184g | 156.0 | 7.0 | 85 | 11.1 | 1.9 | 3.9 | 1.0 |
| Salmon, Steam Cuisine, COU, M & S* | 1 Pack/400g | 340.0 | 7.0 | 85 | 6.8 | 8.9 | 1.8 | 1.2 |
| **COD IN** | | | | | | | | |
| a Sweet Red Pepper Sauce, Fillets, GFY, Asda* | ½ Pack/170g | 143.0 | 3.0 | 84 | 15.0 | 2.3 | 1.6 | 0.1 |
| Butter Sauce, Ross* | 1 Serving/150g | 126.0 | 6.0 | 84 | 9.1 | 3.2 | 3.9 | 0.1 |
| Butter Sauce, Steaks, Birds Eye* | 1 Pack/170g | 185.0 | 9.0 | 109 | 9.8 | 5.0 | 5.5 | 0.1 |
| Butter Sauce, Steaks, Morrisons* | 1 Steak/170g | 153.0 | 6.0 | 90 | 10.9 | 4.1 | 3.3 | 0.4 |
| Butter Sauce, Steaks, Sainsbury's* | 1 Serving/170g | 184.0 | 10.0 | 108 | 10.5 | 3.1 | 5.9 | 0.3 |
| Butter Sauce, Tesco* | 1 Pack/150g | 123.0 | 5.0 | 82 | 9.4 | 2.9 | 3.6 | 0.5 |
| Cheese Sauce, BGTY, Sainsbury's* | 1 Serving/170g | 144.0 | 4.0 | 85 | 12.8 | 3.1 | 2.4 | 0.0 |
| Cheese Sauce, Steaks, Birds Eye* | 1 Pack/182g | 175.0 | 6.0 | 96 | 10.9 | 5.2 | 3.5 | 0.1 |
| Mushroom Sauce, BGTY, Sainsbury's* | 1 Serving/170g | 112.0 | 3.0 | 66 | 9.9 | 2.8 | 1.7 | 0.1 |
| Parsley Sauce, BGTY, Sainsbury's* | 1 Pack/170g | 143.0 | 5.0 | 84 | 11.4 | 2.4 | 3.2 | 0.3 |
| Parsley Sauce, Fillets, BGTY, Sainsbury's* | 1 Pack/351g | 316.0 | 15.0 | 90 | 11.6 | 1.3 | 4.3 | 0.7 |
| Parsley Sauce, Frozen, Morrisons* | 1 Serving/170g | 131.0 | 5.0 | 77 | 9.6 | 3.2 | 2.7 | 0.5 |
| Parsley Sauce, GFY, Asda* | ½ Pack/149g | 124.0 | 5.0 | 83 | 12.0 | 1.5 | 3.5 | 0.6 |
| Parsley Sauce, Portions, Asda* | 1 Serving/150g | 115.0 | 3.0 | 77 | 11.0 | 3.8 | 2.0 | 0.1 |
| Parsley Sauce, Portions, Ocean Trader* | 1 Serving/120g | 112.0 | 5.0 | 93 | 9.4 | 4.0 | 3.9 | 0.1 |
| Parsley Sauce, Portions, Sainsbury's* | 1 Pack/170g | 143.0 | 5.0 | 84 | 11.4 | 2.4 | 3.2 | 0.3 |
| Parsley Sauce, Steaks, Birds Eye* | 1 Steak/172g | 155.0 | 5.0 | 90 | 10.5 | 5.6 | 2.8 | 0.1 |
| Parsley Sauce, Steaks, Sainsbury's* | 1 Serving/150g | 126.0 | 5.0 | 84 | 11.4 | 2.4 | 3.2 | 0.3 |
| Parsley Sauce, Tesco* | 1 Serving/150g | 121.0 | 5.0 | 81 | 10.0 | 3.3 | 3.1 | 0.3 |
| Red Pepper Sauce, SteamFresh, Birds Eye* | 1 Serving/125g | 115.0 | 2.0 | 92 | 14.4 | 4.7 | 1.9 | 0.3 |
| **COD MEDITERRANEAN** | | | | | | | | |
| Perfectly Balanced, Waitrose* | 1 Serving/370g | 255.0 | 4.0 | 69 | 13.1 | 1.9 | 1.0 | 1.2 |
| Style, Fillets, GFY, Asda* | 1 Pack/397g | 274.0 | 10.0 | 69 | 9.0 | 2.5 | 2.5 | 0.9 |
| **COD WITH** | | | | | | | | |
| a Mediterranean Pepper Sauce, Fillets, Waitrose* | 1 Pack/370g | 240.0 | 5.0 | 65 | 12.2 | 1.1 | 1.3 | 0.9 |
| a Thai Crust, Perfectly Balanced, Waitrose* | 1 Pack/280g | 249.0 | 7.0 | 89 | 15.1 | 1.6 | 2.5 | 0.6 |
| Chunky Chips, M & S* | 1 Serving/340g | 510.0 | 20.0 | 150 | 6.5 | 17.5 | 6.0 | 1.5 |
| Fish Pesto, Fillets, COOK!, M & S* | ½ Pack/165g | 210.0 | 5.0 | 127 | 16.4 | 8.4 | 3.1 | 4.2 |
| Mediterranean Butter, Sainsbury's* | 1 Pack/170g | 196.0 | 9.0 | 115 | 17.0 | 0.1 | 5.2 | 0.1 |
| Parma Ham & Sardinian Chick Peas, M & S* | ½ Pack/255g | 268.0 | 12.0 | 105 | 9.8 | 5.3 | 4.9 | 0.5 |
| Roasted Vegetables, M & S* | 1 Serving/280g | 238.0 | 11.0 | 85 | 8.0 | 4.9 | 3.8 | 1.7 |

| | Measure INFO/WEIGHT | per Measure KCAL | FAT | Nutrition Values per 100g / 100ml KCAL | PROT | CARB | FAT | FIBRE |
|---|---|---|---|---|---|---|---|---|
| **COD WITH** | | | | | | | | |
| Salsa & Rosemary Potatoes, BGTY, Sainsbury's* | 1 Pack/450g | 355.0 | 4.0 | 79 | 4.7 | 13.1 | 0.9 | 1.6 |
| Sunblush Tomato Sauce, GFY, Asda* | ½ Pack/177g | 117.0 | 3.0 | 66 | 13.0 | 0.1 | 1.5 | 1.0 |
| Sweet Chilli, COU, M & S* | 1 Pack/400g | 360.0 | 2.0 | 90 | 7.7 | 13.1 | 0.5 | 1.6 |
| Tomato Sauce, Fillets, Asda* | 1 Serving/181g | 210.0 | 11.0 | 116 | 13.0 | 2.6 | 6.0 | 2.3 |
| Vegetables, Haches, Steaks, Peche Ocean* | 1 Serving/200g | 184.0 | 8.0 | 92 | 12.0 | 2.1 | 3.9 | 0.0 |
| **COD ZESTY** | | | | | | | | |
| COU, M & S* | 1 Serving/400g | 260.0 | 7.0 | 65 | 7.2 | 5.2 | 1.7 | 1.2 |
| **COFFEE** | | | | | | | | |
| Alternative, Wake Up, Whole Earth* | 1 Cup/5g | 19.0 | 0.0 | 377 | 5.5 | 88.4 | 0.2 | 0.0 |
| Black, Average | 1 Mug/270ml | 5.0 | 0.0 | 2 | 0.2 | 0.3 | 0.0 | 0.0 |
| Cafe Caramel, Cafe Range, Nescafe* | 1 Sachet/17g | 72.0 | 2.0 | 423 | 9.2 | 64.6 | 14.1 | 1.3 |
| Cafe Hazelnut, Nescafe* | 1 Sachet/17g | 73.0 | 2.0 | 428 | 9.3 | 66.0 | 14.1 | 0.0 |
| Cafe Irish Cream, Cafe Range, Nescafe* | 1 Sachet/23g | 98.0 | 3.0 | 425 | 8.2 | 65.2 | 14.1 | 1.2 |
| Cafe Latte, Dry, Douwe Egberts* | 1 Serving/12g | 58.0 | 3.0 | 480 | 10.0 | 60.0 | 22.0 | 0.0 |
| Cafe Latte, Instant, Maxwell House* | 1 Serving/16g | 67.0 | 3.0 | 420 | 17.0 | 45.5 | 18.9 | 0.1 |
| Cafe Mocha, Cafe Range, Nescafe* | 1 Sachet/22g | 92.0 | 3.0 | 418 | 8.5 | 66.6 | 13.1 | 0.0 |
| Cafe Vanilla, Cafe Range, Nescafe* | 1 Sachet/19g | 79.0 | 3.0 | 429 | 9.3 | 64.6 | 14.9 | 1.2 |
| Cappuccino, Cafe Mocha, Dry, Maxwell House* | 1 Serving/23g | 100.0 | 2.0 | 434 | 4.3 | 78.2 | 10.8 | 0.0 |
| Cappuccino, Cafe Specials, Dry, M & S* | 1 Serving/14g | 55.0 | 2.0 | 395 | 14.0 | 59.0 | 11.5 | 0.7 |
| Cappuccino, Cappio, Iced, Kenco* | 1 Can/200ml | 138.0 | 6.0 | 69 | 3.0 | 7.0 | 3.0 | 0.0 |
| Cappuccino, Cappio, Kenco* | 1 Sachet/18g | 79.0 | 2.0 | 439 | 11.7 | 73.9 | 10.6 | 0.6 |
| Cappuccino, Chocolate, Safeway* | 1 Serving/120g | 222.0 | 4.0 | 185 | 5.1 | 32.9 | 3.7 | 0.6 |
| Cappuccino, Co-Op* | 1 Serving/13g | 55.0 | 2.0 | 440 | 16.0 | 64.0 | 16.0 | 8.0 |
| Cappuccino, Decaff, Nescafe* | 1 Sachet/16g | 68.0 | 2.0 | 428 | 11.6 | 62.6 | 14.6 | 0.0 |
| Cappuccino, Decaff, Unsweetened, Nescafe* | 1 Sachet/16g | 76.0 | 4.0 | 472 | 15.1 | 47.4 | 24.6 | 0.0 |
| Cappuccino, Dolce Gusto, Nescafe* | 1 Serving/19g | 84.0 | 4.0 | 444 | 19.8 | 50.4 | 19.2 | 3.7 |
| Cappuccino, Dreamy, Cafe, Options* | 1 Serving/30g | 77.0 | 5.0 | 256 | 12.9 | 58.1 | 16.9 | 0.0 |
| Cappuccino, Dry, Maxwell House* | 1 Serving/15g | 52.0 | 1.0 | 350 | 12.0 | 64.0 | 9.6 | 0.4 |
| Cappuccino, Dry, Waitrose* | 1 Sachet/13g | 58.0 | 2.0 | 439 | 15.1 | 56.0 | 17.2 | 4.4 |
| Cappuccino, for Filter Systems, Kenco* | 1 Sachet/6g | 22.0 | 1.0 | 375 | 19.0 | 44.0 | 13.5 | 0.0 |
| Cappuccino, Instant, Alcafe* | 1 Sachet/13g | 49.0 | 2.0 | 393 | 12.5 | 55.1 | 13.6 | 0.0 |
| Cappuccino, Instant, Asda* | 1 Sachet/15g | 60.0 | 2.0 | 399 | 13.0 | 53.0 | 15.2 | 0.9 |
| Cappuccino, Instant, Kenco* | 1 Sachet/20g | 80.0 | 3.0 | 401 | 13.5 | 55.7 | 13.8 | 0.0 |
| Cappuccino, Instant, Unsweetened, Douwe Egberts* | 1 Serving/12g | 48.0 | 2.0 | 400 | 11.0 | 53.0 | 16.0 | 0.0 |
| Cappuccino, Low Sugar, Tesco* | 1 Serving/13g | 55.0 | 3.0 | 425 | 18.4 | 43.3 | 19.8 | 0.4 |
| Cappuccino, M & S* | 1 Serving/164g | 66.0 | 3.0 | 40 | 1.5 | 4.4 | 1.6 | 0.0 |
| Cappuccino, Organic Chocolate, Traidcraft* | 1 Serving/25g | 139.0 | 9.0 | 555 | 7.0 | 43.0 | 38.0 | 0.0 |
| Cappuccino, Original, Sachets, Nescafe* | 1 Sachet/18g | 80.0 | 3.0 | 444 | 11.7 | 60.3 | 17.4 | 0.0 |
| Cappuccino, Original Mugsticks, Maxwell House* | 1 Serving/18g | 73.0 | 3.0 | 406 | 14.4 | 52.8 | 15.6 | 0.0 |
| Cappuccino, Premium Quality, Ernesto* | 1 Sachet/13g | 46.0 | 0.0 | 372 | 12.0 | 71.0 | 3.0 | 1.0 |
| Cappuccino, Reduced Sugar, Sainsbury's* | 1 Serving/12g | 48.0 | 2.0 | 418 | 18.0 | 41.0 | 20.0 | 0.0 |
| Cappuccino, Sainsbury's* | 1 Serving/12g | 49.0 | 2.0 | 411 | 14.9 | 52.9 | 15.5 | 0.4 |
| Cappuccino, Semi Skimmed Milk, Average | 1 Mug/200ml | 48.0 | 2.0 | 24 | 1.6 | 2.6 | 1.1 | 0.0 |
| Cappuccino, Skinny, Nescafe* | 1 Sachet/16g | 51.0 | 1.0 | 318 | 23.6 | 43.9 | 4.4 | 10.6 |
| Cappuccino, Swiss Chocolate, Nescafe* | 1 Sachet/20g | 81.0 | 2.0 | 404 | 10.5 | 65.3 | 11.5 | 2.9 |
| Cappuccino, to Go, Original, Nescafe* | 1 Serving/19g | 84.0 | 3.0 | 444 | 11.7 | 60.3 | 17.4 | 0.0 |
| Cappuccino, to Go, Unsweetened, Nescafe* | 1 Serving/17g | 79.0 | 4.0 | 464 | 15.0 | 47.3 | 23.8 | 0.0 |
| Cappuccino, Unsweetened, Cappio, Kenco* | 1 Serving/18g | 73.0 | 2.0 | 406 | 12.2 | 66.7 | 10.0 | 0.6 |
| Cappuccino, Unsweetened, Nescafe* | 1 Sachet/16g | 74.0 | 4.0 | 464 | 15.0 | 47.3 | 23.8 | 0.0 |
| Cappuccino, Unsweetened Taste, Maxwell House* | 1 Serving/15g | 65.0 | 3.0 | 434 | 17.4 | 47.6 | 19.3 | 0.3 |
| Cappuccino, Whip, M & S* | 1 Serving/28g | 140.0 | 8.0 | 500 | 7.0 | 57.1 | 27.0 | 1.4 |
| Columbian, Nescafe* | 1 Serving/2g | 2.0 | 0.0 | 111 | 16.7 | 11.1 | 0.0 | 5.6 |
| Compliment* | 1 Serving/14ml | 20.0 | 2.0 | 143 | 1.4 | 6.4 | 12.9 | 0.0 |

| | Measure INFO/WEIGHT | per Measure KCAL | per Measure FAT | Nutrition Values per 100g / 100ml KCAL | PROT | CARB | FAT | FIBRE |
|---|---|---|---|---|---|---|---|---|
| **COFFEE** | | | | | | | | |
| Decaffeinated, Gold Blend, Nescafe* | 1 Tsp/5g | 5.0 | 0.0 | 101 | 14.9 | 10.0 | 0.2 | 8.4 |
| Double Choca Mocha, Cafe Range, Nescafe* | 1 Sachet/23g | 94.0 | 3.0 | 408 | 9.2 | 68.0 | 11.0 | 2.8 |
| Frappe Iced, Nestle* | 1 Sachet/24g | 92.0 | 1.0 | 384 | 15.0 | 72.0 | 4.0 | 0.5 |
| Ice Mocha Drink, Nescafe, Nestle* | 1 Bottle/280ml | 160.0 | 3.0 | 57 | 1.1 | 10.5 | 1.2 | 0.0 |
| Infusion, Average with Semi-Skimmed Milk | 1 Cup/220ml | 15.0 | 0.0 | 7 | 0.6 | 0.7 | 0.2 | 0.0 |
| Infusion, Average with Single Cream | 1 Cup/220ml | 31.0 | 3.0 | 14 | 0.4 | 0.3 | 1.2 | 0.0 |
| Infusion, Average with Whole Milk | 1 Cup/220ml | 15.0 | 1.0 | 7 | 0.5 | 0.5 | 0.4 | 0.0 |
| Instant, Alta Rica, Nescafe* | 1 Tsp/1.8g | 2.0 | 0.0 | 98 | 13.8 | 10.0 | 0.3 | 21.0 |
| Instant, Decaffeinated, Nescafe* | 1 Tsp/1.8g | 2.0 | 0.0 | 101 | 14.9 | 10.0 | 0.2 | 8.4 |
| Instant, Made with Skimmed Milk | 1 Serving/270ml | 15.0 | 0.0 | 6 | 0.6 | 0.8 | 0.0 | 0.0 |
| Instant, Made with Water & Semi-Skimmed Milk | 1 Serving/350ml | 24.0 | 1.0 | 7 | 0.4 | 0.5 | 0.4 | 0.0 |
| Instant, Original, Nescafe* | 1 Tsp/1.8g | 2.0 | 0.0 | 103 | 15.4 | 10.0 | 0.2 | 13.4 |
| Instant, with Skimmed Milk, Costa Rican, Kenco* | 1 Mug/300ml | 17.0 | 0.0 | 6 | 0.6 | 0.8 | 0.0 | 0.0 |
| Latte, Cafe, M & S* | 1 Serving/190g | 142.0 | 5.0 | 75 | 4.3 | 8.3 | 2.8 | 0.0 |
| Latte, Instant, Skinny, Douwe Egberts* | 1 Serving/12g | 35.0 | 1.0 | 290 | 11.0 | 38.0 | 11.0 | 29.0 |
| Latte, Macchiato, Tassimo* | 1 Cup/275ml | 63.0 | 3.0 | 23 | 1.9 | 1.1 | 1.2 | 0.0 |
| Latte, Nescafe* | 1 Sachet/22g | 110.0 | 6.0 | 498 | 14.5 | 45.7 | 28.5 | 0.0 |
| Latte, Non Fat, Tall, Ryvita* | 1 Tall Latte/110ml | 37.0 | 0.0 | 34 | 3.4 | 5.0 | 0.1 | 0.0 |
| Latte, Skinny, Nescafe* | 1 Sachet/20g | 72.0 | 1.0 | 359 | 24.1 | 54.3 | 5.3 | 1.1 |
| Latte Macchiato, Dolce Gusto, Nescafe* | 1 Mug/100g | 89.0 | 4.0 | 89 | 4.3 | 9.1 | 4.2 | 0.6 |
| Mocha, Instant, Skinny, Douwe Egberts* | 1 Serving/12g | 37.0 | 1.0 | 308 | 10.8 | 40.8 | 10.8 | 25.0 |
| Mocha, Sainsbury's* | 1 Serving/22g | 84.0 | 3.0 | 383 | 14.0 | 51.0 | 13.7 | 1.3 |
| Regular, Ground Or Instant | 1 Cup/180ml | 6.0 | 0.0 | 4 | 0.2 | 0.7 | 0.0 | 0.0 |
| **COFFEE MATE** | | | | | | | | |
| Original, Nestle^ | 1 Tsp/4g | 19.0 | 1.0 | 547 | 2.4 | 56.7 | 34.4 | 0.0 |
| Virtually Fat Free, Nestle* | 1 Tsp/5g | 10.0 | 0.0 | 200 | 1.0 | 42.0 | 3.0 | 0.0 |
| **COFFEE SUBSTITUTE** | | | | | | | | |
| Bambu, Vogel* | 1 Tsp/3g | 10.0 | 0.0 | 320 | 3.5 | 75.3 | 0.5 | 0.0 |
| **COFFEE WHITENER** | | | | | | | | |
| Half Fat, Co-Op* | 1 Tsp/5g | 21.0 | 1.0 | 430 | 0.9 | 78.0 | 13.0 | 0.0 |
| Light, Asda* | 1 Serving/3g | 13.0 | 0.0 | 433 | 0.9 | 78.0 | 13.0 | 0.0 |
| Light, Tesco* | 1 Tsp/3g | 13.0 | 0.0 | 429 | 0.9 | 77.7 | 12.7 | 0.0 |
| Tesco* | 1 Tsp/3g | 16.0 | 1.0 | 533 | 1.2 | 61.3 | 31.4 | 0.0 |
| **COGNAC** | | | | | | | | |
| *40% Volume* | *1 Shot/35ml* | *78.0* | *0.0* | *222* | *0.0* | *0.0* | *0.0* | *0.0* |
| **COINTREAU** | | | | | | | | |
| *Liqueur Specialite De France* | *1 Serving/37g* | *80.0* | *0.0* | *215* | *0.0* | *0.0* | *0.0* | *0.0* |
| **COLA** | | | | | | | | |
| Average | 1 Can/330ml | 135.0 | 0.0 | 41 | 0.0 | 10.9 | 0.0 | 0.0 |
| Basics, Sainsbury's* | 1 Glass/250ml | 2.0 | 0.0 | 1 | 0.0 | 0.2 | 0.0 | 0.0 |
| Coke, Cherry, Coca-Cola* | 1 Bottle/500ml | 225.0 | 0.0 | 45 | 0.0 | 11.2 | 0.0 | 0.0 |
| Coke, Coca-Cola* | 1 Can/330ml | 142.0 | 0.0 | 43 | 0.0 | 10.7 | 0.0 | 0.0 |
| Coke, Diet, Caffeine Free, Coca-Cola* | 1 Can/330ml | 1.0 | 0.0 | 0 | 0.0 | 0.1 | 0.0 | 0.0 |
| Coke, Diet, Coca-Cola* | 1 Can/330ml | 1.0 | 0.0 | 0 | 0.0 | 0.0 | 0.0 | 0.0 |
| Coke, Diet, with Cherry, Coca-Cola* | 1 Bottle/500ml | 5.0 | 0.0 | 1 | 0.0 | 0.0 | 0.0 | 0.0 |
| Coke, Vanilla, Coca-Cola* | 1 Bottle/500ml | 215.0 | 0.0 | 43 | 0.0 | 10.7 | 0.0 | 0.0 |
| Coke, with Lemon, Diet, Coca-Cola* | 1 Can/330ml | 5.0 | 0.0 | 1 | 0.0 | 0.0 | 0.0 | 0.0 |
| Coke, with Vanilla, Diet, Coca-Cola* | 1 Glass/200ml | 1.0 | 0.0 | 0 | 0.0 | 0.1 | 0.0 | 0.0 |
| Diet, Classic, Sainsbury's* | 1 Can/330ml | 1.0 | 0.0 | 0 | 0.0 | 0.0 | 0.0 | 0.0 |
| Diet, Pepsi* | 1 Can/330ml | 1.0 | 0.0 | 0 | 0.0 | 0.0 | 0.0 | 0.0 |
| Diet, Tesco* | 1 Glass/200ml | 2.0 | 0.0 | 1 | 0.1 | 0.1 | 0.1 | 0.0 |
| Diet, Virgin* | 1 Glass/250ml | 1.0 | 0.0 | 0 | 0.1 | 0.1 | 0.1 | 0.0 |
| Max, Pepsi* | 1 Can/330ml | 2.0 | 0.0 | 1 | 0.1 | 0.1 | 0.0 | 0.0 |

**C**

| | Measure INFO/WEIGHT | per Measure KCAL | FAT | Nutrition Values per 100g / 100ml KCAL | PROT | CARB | FAT | FIBRE |
|---|---|---|---|---|---|---|---|---|
| **COLA** | | | | | | | | |
| Pepsi* | 1 Can/330ml | 145.0 | 0.0 | 44 | 0.0 | 11.1 | 0.0 | 0.0 |
| Tesco* | 1 Can/330ml | 145.0 | 0.0 | 44 | 0.0 | 10.8 | 0.0 | 0.0 |
| Twist, Light, Pepsi* | 1 Bottle/500ml | 4.0 | 0.0 | 1 | 0.0 | 0.1 | 0.0 | 0.0 |
| Twist, Pepsi* | 1 Bottle/500ml | 235.0 | 0.0 | 47 | 0.0 | 11.7 | 0.0 | 0.0 |
| Zero, Coca-Cola* | 1 Can/330ml | 2.0 | 0.0 | 0 | 0.0 | 0.0 | 0.0 | 0.0 |
| **COLESLAW** | | | | | | | | |
| 20% Less Fat, Asda* | 1 Serving/100g | 88.0 | 6.0 | 88 | 1.5 | 7.0 | 6.0 | 1.7 |
| 50% Less Fat, Asda* | 1oz/28g | 17.0 | 1.0 | 61 | 2.1 | 6.8 | 2.8 | 0.9 |
| 99% Fat Free, Kraft* | 1 Serving/40ml | 50.0 | 0.0 | 126 | 1.0 | 28.9 | 1.0 | 0.0 |
| Apple, M & S* | 1oz/28g | 53.0 | 5.0 | 190 | 1.4 | 9.2 | 16.6 | 1.4 |
| Basics, Sainsbury's* | 1 Serving/25g | 24.0 | 2.0 | 98 | 1.0 | 5.2 | 8.1 | 1.6 |
| Cheese, Asda* | 1 Serving/100g | 242.0 | 22.0 | 242 | 4.8 | 6.3 | 22.0 | 1.6 |
| Cheese, M & S* | 1 Serving/57g | 185.0 | 19.0 | 325 | 4.2 | 2.0 | 33.5 | 1.7 |
| Cheese, Sainsbury's* | 1 Serving/75g | 174.0 | 16.0 | 232 | 3.4 | 5.6 | 21.8 | 0.6 |
| Cheese, Supreme, Waitrose* | ¼ Pack/88g | 197.0 | 18.0 | 225 | 4.5 | 5.0 | 20.8 | 1.2 |
| Chunky, Asda* | 1oz/28g | 54.0 | 5.0 | 194 | 1.0 | 7.1 | 18.0 | 1.6 |
| Coronation, Sainsbury's* | ¼ Pot/75g | 135.0 | 11.0 | 180 | 1.2 | 11.9 | 14.2 | 2.4 |
| COU, M & S* | ½ Pack/125g | 75.0 | 3.0 | 60 | 1.3 | 7.4 | 2.7 | 1.7 |
| Creamy, 30% Less Fat, Sainsbury's* | 1 Tub/300g | 378.0 | 33.0 | 126 | 1.0 | 5.5 | 11.0 | 1.4 |
| Creamy, GFY, Asda* | 1 Serving/100g | 163.0 | 15.0 | 163 | 0.7 | 6.5 | 14.9 | 0.8 |
| Creamy, Light Choices, Tesco* | 1/3 Pot/100g | 105.0 | 9.0 | 105 | 1.2 | 4.9 | 8.8 | 1.6 |
| Creamy, Morrisons* | 1 Serving/40g | 111.0 | 11.0 | 277 | 1.1 | 5.5 | 27.7 | 1.3 |
| Creamy, Tesco* | 1 Serving/75g | 142.0 | 13.0 | 190 | 1.0 | 5.5 | 17.8 | 1.5 |
| Deli Style, BGTY, Sainsbury's* | 1 Serving/75g | 64.0 | 5.0 | 85 | 1.5 | 6.0 | 6.1 | 1.7 |
| Deli Style, Creamy, Sainsbury's* | 1 Serving/75g | 133.0 | 13.0 | 178 | 0.8 | 5.4 | 17.0 | 1.5 |
| Deli Style, M & S* | 1 Serving/320g | 336.0 | 31.0 | 105 | 3.5 | 1.5 | 9.7 | 1.4 |
| Deli Style, Sainsbury's* | ½ Pot/150g | 291.0 | 28.0 | 194 | 0.9 | 5.2 | 18.8 | 1.5 |
| Fruity, Asda* | ½ Pot/125g | 101.0 | 6.0 | 81 | 1.3 | 8.0 | 4.9 | 1.7 |
| Fruity, M & S* | 1 Serving/63g | 151.0 | 14.0 | 240 | 1.1 | 8.3 | 22.7 | 3.1 |
| Garlic & Herb, Asda* | 1 Tbsp/15g | 22.0 | 2.0 | 147 | 0.9 | 5.8 | 13.3 | 1.7 |
| GFY, Asda* | 1 Serving/50g | 27.0 | 1.0 | 55 | 1.3 | 6.0 | 2.9 | 2.3 |
| Half Fat, Waitrose* | 1 Serving/100g | 64.0 | 4.0 | 64 | 1.0 | 4.8 | 4.5 | 2.0 |
| Healthy Choice, Safeway* | 1 Pot/250g | 215.0 | 14.0 | 86 | 1.5 | 7.4 | 5.7 | 1.6 |
| Less Than 5% Fat, Side Salad, M & S* | 1 Serving/80g | 44.0 | 3.0 | 55 | 1.0 | 3.4 | 4.2 | 3.9 |
| Light, Reduced Fat, Morrisons* | 1 Serving/30g | 37.0 | 3.0 | 125 | 0.8 | 7.4 | 10.2 | 0.0 |
| Low Fat Mayonnaise, Tesco* | 1oz/28g | 18.0 | 1.0 | 64 | 1.4 | 4.7 | 4.4 | 1.4 |
| Luxury, Asda* | 1 Serving/50g | 108.0 | 10.0 | 217 | 0.9 | 6.0 | 21.0 | 0.0 |
| Luxury, M & S* | 1oz/28g | 43.0 | 4.0 | 152 | 1.0 | 6.0 | 13.8 | 1.0 |
| Luxury, Morrisons* | 1 Serving/50g | 136.0 | 13.0 | 273 | 1.2 | 6.4 | 27.0 | 0.0 |
| Organic, M & S* | 1oz/28g | 41.0 | 3.0 | 145 | 1.1 | 7.3 | 12.4 | 1.0 |
| Prawn, Asda* | 1oz/28g | 54.0 | 5.0 | 192 | 2.4 | 6.6 | 17.3 | 1.4 |
| Prawn, Safeway* | 1 Serving/113g | 156.0 | 11.0 | 139 | 3.1 | 6.3 | 10.0 | 1.0 |
| Reduced Fat, Asda* | 1 Pot/250g | 217.0 | 16.0 | 87 | 1.5 | 6.0 | 6.3 | 1.6 |
| Reduced Fat, Co-Op* | 1 Serving/50g | 45.0 | 3.0 | 90 | 0.9 | 6.0 | 7.0 | 2.0 |
| Reduced Fat, Healthy Living, Co-Op* | 1 Serving/50g | 47.0 | 3.0 | 95 | 0.8 | 8.0 | 7.0 | 2.0 |
| Reduced Fat, M & S* | ½ Tub/112g | 230.0 | 22.0 | 205 | 1.1 | 5.4 | 20.0 | 2.8 |
| Sainsbury's* | 1 Serving/75g | 103.0 | 9.0 | 138 | 1.4 | 6.1 | 12.0 | 1.7 |
| SmartPrice, Asda* | 1oz/28g | 30.0 | 2.0 | 107 | 0.8 | 8.0 | 8.0 | 2.0 |
| So Good, Somerfield* | 1 Serving/50g | 105.0 | 10.0 | 210 | 1.4 | 6.6 | 20.0 | 1.2 |
| Supreme, Waitrose* | 1oz/28g | 53.0 | 5.0 | 190 | 1.8 | 4.9 | 18.1 | 1.7 |
| Three Cheese, Asda* | 1 Serving/78g | 203.0 | 19.0 | 260 | 5.0 | 6.0 | 24.0 | 1.7 |
| Three Cheese, Finest, Tesco* | 1/3 Pack/100g | 255.0 | 23.0 | 255 | 6.4 | 5.8 | 22.7 | 1.1 |
| TTD, Sainsbury's* | ¼ Tub/75g | 181.0 | 18.0 | 241 | 1.1 | 5.0 | 24.1 | 2.8 |

| | Measure INFO/WEIGHT | per Measure KCAL | per Measure FAT | Nutrition Values per 100g / 100ml KCAL | PROT | CARB | FAT | FIBRE |
|---|---|---|---|---|---|---|---|---|
| **COLESLAW** | | | | | | | | |
| with 60% Less Fat, GFY, Asda* | 1 Serving/41g | 36.0 | 2.0 | 88 | 1.5 | 7.0 | 6.0 | 1.7 |
| with Free Range Egg Mayonnaise, Reduced Fat, M & S* | 1oz/28g | 62.0 | 6.0 | 220 | 1.0 | 7.0 | 21.1 | 1.8 |
| with Mayonnaise, Retail | 1oz/28g | 72.0 | 7.0 | 258 | 1.2 | 4.2 | 26.4 | 1.4 |
| with Reduced Calorie Dressing, Retail | 1oz/28g | 19.0 | 1.0 | 67 | 0.9 | 6.1 | 4.5 | 1.4 |
| **COLEY** | | | | | | | | |
| *Portions, Raw, Average* | *1 Serving/92g* | *75.0* | *1.0* | *81* | *18.4* | *0.0* | *0.7* | *0.0* |
| *Steamed, Average* | *1oz/28g* | *29.0* | *0.0* | *105* | *23.3* | *0.0* | *1.3* | *0.0* |
| **CONCHIGLIE** | | | | | | | | |
| *Cooked, Average* | *1 Serving/185g* | *247.0* | *2.0* | *133* | *4.8* | *26.6* | *0.8* | *0.5* |
| *Dry Weight, Average* | *1 Serving/100g* | *352.0* | *2.0* | *352* | *12.5* | *71.6* | *1.7* | *2.6* |
| *Shells, Dry, Average* | *1 Serving/100g* | *345.0* | *1.0* | *345* | *12.3* | *70.4* | *1.5* | *3.0* |
| *Whole Wheat, Dry Weight, Average* | *1 Serving/75g* | *237.0* | *1.0* | *316* | *12.6* | *62.0* | *2.0* | *10.7* |
| **CONCHIGLIONI** | | | | | | | | |
| Dry, Waitrose* | 1 Serving/75g | 256.0 | 1.0 | 341 | 12.5 | 69.8 | 1.3 | 3.7 |
| **CONSERVE** | | | | | | | | |
| *Apricot, Average* | *1 Tbsp/15g* | *37.0* | *0.0* | *244* | *0.5* | *59.3* | *0.2* | *1.5* |
| Apricot, Reduced Sugar, Streamline* | 1 Tbsp/20g | 37.0 | 0.0 | 184 | 0.5 | 45.0 | 0.2 | 0.0 |
| Black Cherry, with Amaretto, Finest, Tesco* | 1 Serving/10g | 26.0 | 0.0 | 261 | 0.5 | 64.4 | 0.1 | 0.8 |
| *Blackcurrant, Average* | *1 Tbsp/15g* | *37.0* | *0.0* | *245* | *0.6* | *60.0* | *0.1* | *1.9* |
| Blueberry, M & S* | 1 Tsp/8g | 15.0 | 0.0 | 206 | 0.3 | 51.1 | 0.1 | 1.3 |
| Morello Cherry, Waitrose* | 1 Tbsp/15g | 39.0 | 0.0 | 258 | 0.4 | 64.2 | 0.0 | 1.4 |
| *Raspberry, Average* | *1 Tbsp/15g* | *37.0* | *0.0* | *249* | *0.6* | *61.0* | *0.3* | *1.3* |
| Red Cherry, Finest, Tesco* | 1 Tbsp/15g | 42.0 | 0.0 | 277 | 0.6 | 67.6 | 0.1 | 0.8 |
| Rhubarb & Ginger, M & S* | 1 Tbsp/15g | 29.0 | 0.0 | 194 | 0.3 | 47.9 | 0.1 | 1.0 |
| Strawberry, 60% Fruit, Reduced Sugar, M & S* | 1 Tsp/7g | 9.0 | 0.0 | 135 | 0.4 | 30.1 | 0.2 | 1.9 |
| *Strawberry, Average* | *1 Tbsp/15g* | *37.0* | *0.0* | *250* | *0.4* | *61.6* | *0.1* | *0.5* |
| Yellow Plum & Greengage, TTD, Sainsbury's* | 1 Tbsp/15g | 36.0 | 0.0 | 243 | 0.4 | 60.0 | 0.1 | 0.7 |
| **CONSOMME** | | | | | | | | |
| *Average* | *1oz/28g* | *3.0* | *0.0* | *12* | *2.9* | *0.1* | *0.0* | *0.0* |
| Beef, Luxury, Baxters* | 1 Can/415g | 54.0 | 0.0 | 13 | 2.6 | 0.7 | 0.0 | 0.0 |
| **COOKIES** | | | | | | | | |
| All Butter, Almond, Italian Style, M & S* | 1 Cookie/23g | 120.0 | 6.0 | 515 | 6.7 | 59.4 | 27.6 | 3.6 |
| All Butter, Ginger Bread, M & S* | 1 Cookie/23g | 102.0 | 5.0 | 445 | 4.3 | 57.5 | 21.8 | 2.4 |
| All Butter, Italian Style Sorrento Lemon, M & S* | 1 Cookie/24g | 120.0 | 6.0 | 500 | 4.9 | 60.4 | 26.7 | 2.1 |
| All Butter, Melting Moment, M & S* | 1 Cookie/23g | 110.0 | 6.0 | 470 | 4.5 | 51.5 | 27.5 | 3.4 |
| Apple & Raisin, Go Ahead, McVitie's* | 1 Cookie/15g | 66.0 | 2.0 | 443 | 5.3 | 76.8 | 12.7 | 3.4 |
| Apple Crumble, M & S* | 1 Cookie/26g | 90.0 | 1.0 | 345 | 4.6 | 76.8 | 2.0 | 2.9 |
| Apple Pie, The Biscuit Collection* | 1 Cookie/19g | 90.0 | 4.0 | 474 | 3.9 | 65.0 | 22.1 | 0.0 |
| Apricot, COU, M & S* | 1 Cookie/26g | 88.0 | 1.0 | 340 | 5.4 | 75.0 | 2.4 | 2.0 |
| Big Milk Chocolate Chunk, Cookie Coach* | 1 Cookie/35g | 174.0 | 9.0 | 497 | 6.2 | 61.4 | 25.1 | 0.0 |
| Bites, Weight Watchers* | 1 Pack/21g | 97.0 | 4.0 | 464 | 5.8 | 67.0 | 19.2 | 4.3 |
| Brazil Nut, Organic, Traidcraft* | 1 Cookie/17g | 91.0 | 5.0 | 547 | 5.8 | 57.7 | 32.6 | 2.1 |
| Brazil Nut, Prewett's* | 1 Cookie/50g | 122.0 | 7.0 | 244 | 2.6 | 25.2 | 14.8 | 1.0 |
| Butter & Sultana, Sainsbury's* | 1 Cookie/13g | 61.0 | 3.0 | 473 | 4.5 | 68.4 | 20.1 | 1.6 |
| Cherry Bakewell, COU, M & S* | 1 Cookie/25g | 90.0 | 1.0 | 355 | 6.0 | 77.2 | 2.5 | 3.4 |
| Choc Chip, Cadbury* | 1 Cookie/11g | 55.0 | 3.0 | 503 | 5.9 | 62.2 | 25.6 | 0.0 |
| Choc Chip, Lyons* | 1 Cookie/11g | 57.0 | 3.0 | 499 | 5.2 | 68.3 | 23.4 | 1.7 |
| Choc Chip, Maryland* | 1 Cookie/11g | 56.0 | 3.0 | 511 | 6.2 | 68.0 | 23.9 | 1.3 |
| Choc Chip, McVitie's* | 1 Cookie/10g | 50.0 | 3.0 | 496 | 5.8 | 60.2 | 25.8 | 3.0 |
| Choc Chip, Reduced Fat, Maryland* | 1 Cookie/11g | 51.0 | 2.0 | 478 | 5.9 | 73.0 | 18.0 | 0.0 |
| Choc Chip, Sainsbury's* | 1 Cookie/11g | 55.0 | 3.0 | 508 | 6.2 | 67.0 | 23.9 | 1.3 |
| Choc Chip & Coconut, Maryland* | 1 Cookie/10g | 55.0 | 3.0 | 512 | 5.1 | 62.9 | 23.7 | 0.0 |
| Choc Chip & Hazelnut, Maryland* | 1 Cookie/11g | 55.0 | 3.0 | 513 | 6.3 | 65.3 | 25.0 | 0.0 |

## COOKIES

| INFO/WEIGHT | Measure | per Measure KCAL | FAT | Nutrition Values per 100g / 100ml KCAL | PROT | CARB | FAT | FIBRE |
|---|---|---|---|---|---|---|---|---|
| Choc Chip 'n' Chunk, McVitie's* | 1 Cookie/11g | 55.0 | 3.0 | 498 | 5.8 | 59.2 | 26.4 | 3.5 |
| Choc Chunk, Fabulous Bakin' Boys* | 1 Cookie/60g | 270.0 | 13.0 | 450 | 5.0 | 59.0 | 21.0 | 3.0 |
| Choc Chunk, Finest, Tesco* | 1 Cookie/80g | 355.0 | 14.0 | 445 | 5.7 | 65.3 | 17.7 | 1.8 |
| Chocolate, Belgian, Extra Special, Asda* | 1 Cookie/26g | 138.0 | 8.0 | 535 | 6.0 | 58.0 | 31.0 | 2.0 |
| Chocolate, Milk, Free From, Tesco* | 1 Cookie/20g | 100.0 | 6.0 | 500 | 5.6 | 50.4 | 30.7 | 4.1 |
| Chocolate, Quadruple, Sainsbury's* | 1 Cookie/20g | 117.0 | 7.0 | 585 | 6.0 | 66.5 | 33.0 | 1.5 |
| Chocolate, Triple, Half Coated, Finest, Tesco* | 1 Cookie/25g | 131.0 | 7.0 | 525 | 5.7 | 58.7 | 29.3 | 2.3 |
| Chocolate & Nut, Organic, Evernat* | 1 Cookie/69g | 337.0 | 16.0 | 489 | 7.2 | 64.1 | 22.6 | 0.0 |
| Chocolate & Orange, COU, M & S* | 1 Cookie/26g | 90.0 | 1.0 | 350 | 5.7 | 77.2 | 2.6 | 3.2 |
| Chocolate Chip, Asda* | 1 Cookie/12g | 57.0 | 3.0 | 497 | 5.0 | 63.0 | 25.0 | 2.6 |
| Chocolate Chip, Average | 1 Cookie/10g | 49.0 | 2.0 | 489 | 5.5 | 64.1 | 24.7 | 2.9 |
| Chocolate Chip, BGTY, Sainsbury's* | 1 Cookie/17g | 72.0 | 2.0 | 428 | 4.5 | 75.6 | 11.9 | 2.5 |
| Chocolate Chip, Carb Check, Heinz* | 1 Cookie/20g | 91.0 | 5.0 | 457 | 7.2 | 43.1 | 24.9 | 7.2 |
| Chocolate Chip, Chips Ahoy* | 1 Cookie/11g | 55.0 | 3.0 | 500 | 6.0 | 65.0 | 25.0 | 3.0 |
| Chocolate Chip, GFY, Asda* | 1 Cookie/10g | 48.0 | 2.0 | 463 | 5.0 | 68.0 | 19.0 | 3.5 |
| Chocolate Chip, Handbaked, Border* | 1 Cookie/15g | 72.0 | 3.0 | 480 | 5.9 | 67.4 | 22.6 | 0.0 |
| Chocolate Chip, Lyons* | 1 Cookie/12g | 56.0 | 3.0 | 483 | 5.6 | 66.5 | 21.6 | 1.7 |
| Chocolate Chip, M & S* | 1 Cookie/12g | 59.0 | 3.0 | 495 | 5.7 | 62.1 | 24.8 | 2.7 |
| Chocolate Chip, McVitie's* | 1 Cookie/11g | 54.0 | 3.0 | 496 | 5.8 | 60.2 | 25.8 | 3.0 |
| Chocolate Chip, Mini, McVitie's* | 1 Bag/40g | 196.0 | 9.0 | 491 | 5.5 | 65.1 | 23.1 | 2.8 |
| Chocolate Chip, Mini, Tesco* | 1 Bag/30g | 148.0 | 7.0 | 493 | 5.4 | 64.6 | 23.7 | 1.7 |
| Chocolate Chip, Organic, Sainsbury's* | 1 Cookie/17g | 89.0 | 5.0 | 530 | 5.0 | 61.8 | 29.2 | 0.3 |
| Chocolate Chip, Organic, Tesco* | 1 Cookie/17g | 88.0 | 5.0 | 520 | 0.0 | 63.3 | 27.4 | 2.8 |
| Chocolate Chip, Tesco* | 1 Cookie/11g | 55.0 | 3.0 | 500 | 4.7 | 66.7 | 23.4 | 0.6 |
| Chocolate Chip, Value, Tesco* | 1 Cookie/11g | 56.0 | 3.0 | 512 | 4.8 | 64.8 | 26.0 | 1.6 |
| Chocolate Chip, Weight Watchers* | 1 Cookie/11g | 49.0 | 2.0 | 443 | 7.6 | 65.4 | 17.2 | 4.6 |
| Chocolate Chip & Hazelnut, Extra Special, Asda* | 1 Cookie/25g | 130.0 | 8.0 | 516 | 6.0 | 51.0 | 32.0 | 2.5 |
| Chocolate Chunk, All Butter, COU, M & S* | 1 Cookie/24g | 110.0 | 4.0 | 460 | 5.7 | 69.1 | 17.9 | 2.3 |
| Chocolate Chunk, All Butter, M & S* | 1 Cookie/24g | 120.0 | 6.0 | 500 | 5.2 | 62.4 | 25.2 | 2.9 |
| Chocolate Chunk, Cadbury* | 1 Cookie/22g | 119.0 | 7.0 | 540 | 6.5 | 58.0 | 31.2 | 0.0 |
| Chocolate Chunk, Quadruple, TTD, Sainsbury's* | 1 Cookie/23g | 117.0 | 7.0 | 509 | 5.2 | 57.4 | 28.7 | 1.7 |
| Chocolate Chunk & Hazelnut, All Butter, TTD, Sainsbury's* | 1 Cookie/18g | 95.0 | 6.0 | 529 | 6.0 | 53.7 | 32.2 | 2.4 |
| Chocolate Chunk & Hazelnut, Tesco* | 1 Cookie/22g | 118.0 | 7.0 | 538 | 6.2 | 60.2 | 30.3 | 1.9 |
| Chocolate Chunk & Hazlenut, So Good, Somerfield* | 1 Cookie/22g | 118.0 | 7.0 | 530 | 6.3 | 55.7 | 31.3 | 2.4 |
| Chocolate Chunk & Orange, So Good, Somerfield* | 1 Cookie/22g | 117.0 | 7.0 | 525 | 5.3 | 60.0 | 29.3 | 1.8 |
| Chocolate Fruit & Nut, Extra Special, Asda* | 1 Cookie/25g | 125.0 | 7.0 | 509 | 6.0 | 56.0 | 29.0 | 2.0 |
| Chocolate Orange, Half Coated, Finest, Tesco* | 1 Cookie/22g | 107.0 | 6.0 | 488 | 4.9 | 59.6 | 25.5 | 1.2 |
| Cocoa, Organic, Bites, No Junk, Organix* | 1 Bag/25g | 105.0 | 3.0 | 421 | 7.0 | 69.0 | 13.0 | 5.5 |
| Coconut, Gluten-Free, Sainsbury's* | 1 Cookie/20g | 103.0 | 6.0 | 516 | 5.6 | 54.4 | 30.7 | 4.1 |
| Coconut, TTD, Sainsbury's* | 1 Cookie/17g | 88.0 | 5.0 | 527 | 5.3 | 60.0 | 29.5 | 4.9 |
| Coconut & Raspberry, Gluten Free, Sainsbury's* | 1 Cookie/20g | 102.0 | 6.0 | 511 | 5.9 | 56.0 | 29.3 | 6.7 |
| Cranberry & Orange, Finest, Tesco* | 1 Cookie/26g | 125.0 | 6.0 | 490 | 4.1 | 67.4 | 22.6 | 3.2 |
| Cranberry & Orange, Go Ahead, McVitie's* | 1 Cookie/17g | 77.0 | 2.0 | 452 | 5.3 | 78.0 | 13.2 | 2.4 |
| Crunchy Muesli, Mini, Shapers, Boots* | 1 Pack/30g | 134.0 | 4.0 | 448 | 6.7 | 71.0 | 15.0 | 1.8 |
| Danish Butter, Tesco* | 1 Cookie/26g | 133.0 | 7.0 | 516 | 4.7 | 66.7 | 25.6 | 1.3 |
| Dark Chocolate Chunk & Ginger, The Best, Morrisons* | 1 Cookie/25g | 126.0 | 6.0 | 503 | 4.6 | 63.7 | 25.5 | 2.8 |
| Dark Treacle, Weight Watchers* | 1 Cookie/11g | 49.0 | 2.0 | 423 | 5.2 | 66.7 | 15.1 | 1.7 |
| Double Choc, Cadbury* | 1 Cookie/11g | 55.0 | 3.0 | 485 | 7.3 | 64.3 | 22.2 | 0.0 |
| Double Choc, Maryland* | 1 Cookie/10g | 51.0 | 3.0 | 510 | 5.2 | 64.4 | 25.7 | 0.0 |
| Double Choc Chip, Mini, M & S* | 1 Cookie/22g | 108.0 | 5.0 | 490 | 5.3 | 63.6 | 23.7 | 1.8 |
| Double Choc Chip, Tesco* | 1 Cookie/11g | 55.0 | 3.0 | 500 | 4.2 | 65.3 | 24.7 | 3.0 |
| Double Choc Chip, Weight Watchers* | 1 Cookie/11g | 49.0 | 2.0 | 443 | 7.6 | 65.4 | 17.2 | 4.6 |
| Double Chocolate, Premium, Co-Op* | 1 Cookie/17g | 86.0 | 5.0 | 505 | 5.0 | 62.0 | 27.0 | 2.0 |

|  | Measure INFO/WEIGHT | per Measure KCAL | per Measure FAT | Nutrition Values per 100g / 100ml KCAL | PROT | CARB | FAT | FIBRE |
|---|---|---|---|---|---|---|---|---|
| **COOKIES** | | | | | | | | |
| Double Chocolate & Walnut, Soft, Tesco* | 1 Cookie/25g | 116.0 | 6.0 | 463 | 5.8 | 52.1 | 25.7 | 4.7 |
| Double Chocolate Chip, Organic, Waitrose* | 1 Cookie/18g | 96.0 | 6.0 | 535 | 5.1 | 58.6 | 31.0 | 1.9 |
| Double Chocolate Chip, Traidcraft* | 1 Cookie/22g | 114.0 | 6.0 | 520 | 5.8 | 64.1 | 26.7 | 2.4 |
| Double Fudge & Chocolate, Sugar Free, Murray* | 1 Cookie/12g | 47.0 | 2.0 | 400 | 5.7 | 65.7 | 20.0 | 5.7 |
| Fortune, Average | 1 Cookie/8g | 30.0 | 0.0 | 378 | 4.2 | 84.0 | 2.7 | 1.6 |
| Fudge, & White Chocolate, TTD, Sainsbury's* | 1 Cookie/17g | 83.0 | 4.0 | 500 | 5.7 | 60.8 | 26.0 | 2.7 |
| Fudge Brownie, Maryland* | 1 Cookie/11g | 56.0 | 3.0 | 510 | 5.8 | 63.0 | 25.0 | 0.0 |
| Fudge Brownie American Cream, Sainsbury's* | 1 Cookie/12g | 60.0 | 3.0 | 499 | 4.8 | 67.9 | 23.2 | 2.2 |
| Ginger, Half Coated, Finest, Tesco* | 1 Cookie/25g | 124.0 | 6.0 | 495 | 4.7 | 64.2 | 24.4 | 3.8 |
| Ginger, Low Fat, M & S* | 1 Cookie/23g | 82.0 | 1.0 | 358 | 5.1 | 74.9 | 4.3 | 2.4 |
| Ginger & Choc Chip, BGTY, Sainsbury's* | 1 Cookie/17g | 69.0 | 3.0 | 415 | 5.8 | 55.3 | 19.0 | 12.1 |
| Glace Cherry, Border* | 1 Cookie/15g | 74.0 | 4.0 | 493 | 5.4 | 64.3 | 25.6 | 0.0 |
| Hazelnut, Gluten Free, Dove's Farm* | 1 Cookie/17g | 80.0 | 4.0 | 484 | 4.5 | 56.8 | 26.8 | 1.8 |
| Hazelnut & Choc Chip 'n' Chunk, McVitie's* | 1 Cookie/11g | 55.0 | 3.0 | 505 | 6.1 | 57.8 | 27.7 | 3.5 |
| Lemon Meringue, COU, M & S* | 1 Cookie/25g | 89.0 | 1.0 | 355 | 5.6 | 77.6 | 2.6 | 3.0 |
| Oat, Giant Jumbo, Paterson's* | 1 Cookie/60g | 299.0 | 16.0 | 499 | 0.4 | 58.4 | 27.0 | 3.2 |
| Oat & Cranberry, BGTY, Sainsbury's* | 1 Cookie/28g | 126.0 | 5.0 | 449 | 6.8 | 65.0 | 18.0 | 5.1 |
| Oat & Raisin, Health Matters* | 1 Cookie/8g | 33.0 | 1.0 | 414 | 7.0 | 76.6 | 8.8 | 3.3 |
| Oatflake & Honey, Organic, Sainsbury's* | 1 Cookie/17g | 82.0 | 4.0 | 480 | 6.3 | 66.0 | 21.2 | 2.6 |
| Oatflake & Raisin, Waitrose* | 1 Cookie/17g | 80.0 | 4.0 | 469 | 5.8 | 61.7 | 22.1 | 4.7 |
| Oatmeal, Chocolate Chip, Chewy, Dad's* | 1 Cookie/15g | 70.0 | 3.0 | 467 | 6.7 | 66.7 | 20.0 | 3.3 |
| Oreo, Nabisco* | 1 Cookie/11g | 52.0 | 2.0 | 471 | 5.9 | 70.6 | 20.6 | 2.9 |
| Raisin & Cinnamon, Low Fat, M & S* | 1 Cookie/22g | 78.0 | 1.0 | 355 | 6.2 | 73.0 | 4.1 | 3.2 |
| Raspberry & White Chocolate, Weight Watchers* | 1 Cookie/11g | 49.0 | 2.0 | 443 | 5.2 | 71.4 | 17.2 | 4.6 |
| Raspberry Spritz, Heaven Scent* | 1 Cookie/19g | 90.0 | 6.0 | 474 | 5.3 | 52.6 | 31.6 | 0.0 |
| Rolo, Nestle* | 1 Cookie/73g | 242.0 | 11.0 | 331 | 3.4 | 46.0 | 15.2 | 0.6 |
| Spiced Apple, COU, M & S* | 1 Cookie/25g | 82.0 | 1.0 | 330 | 5.0 | 72.8 | 2.5 | 2.1 |
| Stem Ginger, & Oatflake, TTD, Sainsbury's* | 1 Cookie/17g | 84.0 | 4.0 | 496 | 4.5 | 63.4 | 24.9 | 1.7 |
| Stem Ginger, BGTY, Sainsbury's* | 1 Cookie/17g | 73.0 | 2.0 | 431 | 4.5 | 76.5 | 11.9 | 1.7 |
| Stem Ginger, Free From, Sainsbury's* | 1 Cookie/17g | 84.0 | 5.0 | 489 | 6.5 | 58.0 | 28.0 | 6.8 |
| Stem Ginger, Half Coated, Finest, Tesco* | 1 Cookie/25g | 127.0 | 7.0 | 508 | 4.4 | 62.4 | 26.8 | 3.6 |
| Stem Ginger, Less Than 5% Fat, M & S* | 1 Cookie/22g | 79.0 | 1.0 | 360 | 6.2 | 73.9 | 4.3 | 3.0 |
| Stem Ginger, Reduced Fat, Waitrose* | 1 Cookie/17g | 75.0 | 3.0 | 448 | 4.5 | 71.0 | 16.2 | 1.6 |
| Stem Ginger, Tesco* | 1 Cookie/20g | 98.0 | 5.0 | 489 | 4.2 | 64.0 | 24.0 | 2.0 |
| Strawberries & Cream, TTD, Sainsbury's* | 1 Cookie/17g | 84.0 | 4.0 | 504 | 4.7 | 62.7 | 26.0 | 1.9 |
| Sultana, All Butter, Reduced Fat, M & S* | 1 Cookie/17g | 70.0 | 2.0 | 420 | 4.9 | 68.6 | 14.2 | 2.6 |
| Sultana, Soft & Chewy, Sainsbury's* | 1 Cookie/25g | 103.0 | 3.0 | 414 | 4.4 | 67.8 | 13.9 | 2.5 |
| Sultana & Cinnamon, Weight Watchers* | 1 Cookie/12g | 46.0 | 1.0 | 398 | 5.0 | 67.1 | 12.1 | 1.8 |
| Toffee, Weight Watchers* | 1 Cookie/12g | 52.0 | 2.0 | 456 | 5.2 | 71.1 | 16.8 | 2.9 |
| White Chocolate, Maryland* | 1 Cookie/10g | 51.0 | 2.0 | 512 | 5.7 | 64.0 | 25.0 | 0.0 |
| White Chocolate & Raspberry, McVitie's* | 1 Cookie/17g | 87.0 | 4.0 | 512 | 4.7 | 64.1 | 25.9 | 1.8 |
| **COQ AU VIN** | | | | | | | | |
| Finest, Tesco* | 1 Serving/273g | 251.0 | 10.0 | 92 | 14.3 | 0.7 | 3.6 | 1.8 |
| M & S* | 1 Serving/295g | 398.0 | 23.0 | 135 | 14.2 | 1.5 | 7.7 | 1.0 |
| Perfectly Balanced, Waitrose* | 1 Pack/500g | 445.0 | 15.0 | 89 | 12.6 | 2.7 | 3.1 | 0.6 |
| Sainsbury's* | 1 Pack/400g | 484.0 | 18.0 | 121 | 16.8 | 3.5 | 4.4 | 0.2 |
| **CORDIAL** | | | | | | | | |
| Blackcurrant & Elderberry, Diluted, TTD, Sainsbury's* | 1 Glass/250ml | 47.0 | 0.0 | 19 | 0.0 | 4.7 | 0.0 | 0.0 |
| Elderflower, Made Up, Bottle Green* | 1 Glass/200ml | 46.0 | 0.0 | 23 | 0.0 | 5.6 | 0.0 | 0.0 |
| Elderflower, Undiluted, Waitrose* | 1 Serving/20ml | 22.0 | 0.0 | 110 | 0.0 | 27.5 | 0.0 | 0.0 |
| Lime, Sainsbury's* | 1 Serving/50ml | 13.0 | 0.0 | 27 | 0.0 | 6.2 | 0.0 | 0.0 |
| Lime, with Aromatic Bitters & Ginger, Sainsbury's* | 1 Serving/40ml | 12.0 | 0.0 | 29 | 0.0 | 6.9 | 0.3 | 0.3 |
| Lime Juice, Concentrated | 1 Serving/20ml | 22.0 | 0.0 | 112 | 0.1 | 29.8 | 0.0 | 0.0 |

**C**

| | Measure INFO/WEIGHT | per Measure KCAL | FAT | Nutrition Values per 100g / 100ml KCAL | PROT | CARB | FAT | FIBRE |
|---|---|---|---|---|---|---|---|---|
| **CORDIAL** | | | | | | | | |
| Lime Juice, Diluted | 1 Glass/250ml | 55.0 | 0.0 | 22 | 0.0 | 6.0 | 0.0 | 0.0 |
| Pomegreat, Original, Pomegreat* | 1 Serving/50ml | 16.0 | 0.0 | 32 | 0.0 | 7.6 | 0.0 | 0.0 |
| **CORIANDER** | | | | | | | | |
| *Leaves, Dried, Average* | *1oz/28g* | *78.0* | *1.0* | *279* | *21.8* | *41.7* | *4.8* | *0.0* |
| *Leaves, Fresh, Average* | *1 Serving/5g* | *1.0* | *0.0* | *23* | *2.1* | *3.7* | *0.5* | *2.8* |
| Seeds, Ground, Schwartz* | 1 Tsp/5g | 22.0 | 1.0 | 446 | 14.2 | 54.9 | 18.8 | 0.0 |
| **CORN** | | | | | | | | |
| Baby, & Asparagus Tips, Tesco* | 1 Pack/150g | 37.0 | 1.0 | 25 | 2.6 | 2.5 | 0.5 | 1.9 |
| Baby, & Mange Tout, Tesco* | 1 Serving/100g | 27.0 | 0.0 | 27 | 2.9 | 3.3 | 0.2 | 2.1 |
| Baby, & Sugar Snap Peas, Safeway* | ½ Pack/100g | 27.0 | 0.0 | 27 | 2.9 | 3.3 | 0.2 | 0.0 |
| *Baby, Average* | *1 Serving/80g* | *21.0* | *0.0* | *26* | *2.5* | *3.1* | *0.4* | *1.7* |
| *Cobs, Boiled, Weighed with Cob, Average* | *1 Ear/200g* | *132.0* | *3.0* | *66* | *2.5* | *11.6* | *1.4* | *1.3* |
| Creamed Style, Green Giant* | 1 Can/418g | 238.0 | 2.0 | 57 | 1.2 | 11.9 | 0.5 | 3.0 |
| in Brine, for Stir Fry, Braxted Hall* | 1 Can/133g | 25.0 | 0.0 | 19 | 1.5 | 3.0 | 0.0 | 1.5 |
| **CORN CAKES** | | | | | | | | |
| Organic, Kallo* | 1 Cake/5g | 16.0 | 0.0 | 340 | 12.7 | 74.3 | 4.1 | 11.2 |
| Ryvita* | 1 Pack/13g | 48.0 | 0.0 | 366 | 10.0 | 74.3 | 3.2 | 7.2 |
| Slightly Salted, Mrs Crimble's* | 1 Pack/28g | 104.0 | 1.0 | 380 | 7.9 | 80.0 | 3.4 | 5.4 |
| Thick Slices, Orgran* | 1 Cake/11g | 42.0 | 0.0 | 385 | 13.2 | 79.0 | 3.7 | 14.2 |
| **CORN MEAL** | | | | | | | | |
| Yellow, Enriched & Degerminated, Quaker* | 1 Tbsp/9g | 30.0 | 0.0 | 333 | 7.4 | 77.8 | 1.8 | 7.4 |
| **CORN NUTS** | | | | | | | | |
| Roasted, Kraft* | 1 Serving/28g | 120.0 | 4.0 | 429 | 10.7 | 71.4 | 16.1 | 7.1 |
| **CORNED BEEF** | | | | | | | | |
| *Average* | *1 Slice/35g* | *75.0* | *4.0* | *214* | *25.9* | *0.7* | *12.1* | *0.0* |
| *Lean, Healthy Range, Average* | *1 Slice/30g* | *57.0* | *3.0* | *191* | *27.0* | *1.0* | *8.7* | *0.0* |
| *Sliced, Premium, Average* | *1 Slice/31g* | *69.0* | *4.0* | *222* | *26.6* | *0.5* | *12.6* | *0.0* |
| **CORNFLOUR** | | | | | | | | |
| *Average* | *1oz/28g* | *99.0* | *0.0* | *355* | *0.6* | *86.9* | *1.2* | *0.1* |
| **COURGETTE** | | | | | | | | |
| & Sweetcorn, Fresh 'n' Ready, Sainsbury's* | 1oz/28g | 12.0 | 0.0 | 42 | 2.3 | 6.7 | 0.9 | 1.3 |
| *Boiled in Unsalted Water, Average* | *1oz/28g* | *5.0* | *0.0* | *19* | *2.0* | *2.0* | *0.4* | *1.2* |
| *Fried, Average* | *1oz/28g* | *18.0* | *1.0* | *63* | *2.6* | *2.6* | *4.8* | *1.2* |
| *Raw, Average* | *1 Serving/80g* | *14.0* | *0.0* | *18* | *1.8* | *1.8* | *0.4* | *0.9* |
| **COUS COUS** | | | | | | | | |
| & Chargrilled Vegetables, M & S* | 1 Serving/200g | 200.0 | 3.0 | 100 | 3.9 | 17.3 | 1.5 | 1.6 |
| Alle Spices Mediterraneo, Antony Worrall Thompson's* | ½ Pack/100g | 352.0 | 3.0 | 352 | 10.7 | 71.0 | 2.8 | 3.8 |
| Balsamic Roasted Vegetable, TTD, Sainsbury's* | 1 Serving/240g | 281.0 | 13.0 | 117 | 2.8 | 14.3 | 5.4 | 1.1 |
| Chargrilled Red & Yellow Pepper, Tesco* | 1 Pack/200g | 212.0 | 4.0 | 106 | 4.6 | 17.8 | 1.8 | 0.5 |
| Chargrilled Vegetable, Morrisons* | 1 Serving/225g | 227.0 | 5.0 | 101 | 3.3 | 16.5 | 2.4 | 1.3 |
| Citrus Kick, Dry, Ainsley Harriott* | ½ Sachet/50g | 184.0 | 1.0 | 368 | 11.6 | 77.0 | 2.4 | 9.2 |
| *Cooked, Average* | *1 Cup/157g* | *249.0* | *3.0* | *158* | *4.3* | *31.4* | *1.9* | *1.3* |
| Coriander & Lemon, Asda* | 1 Pack/110g | 141.0 | 1.0 | 128 | 5.1 | 24.2 | 1.2 | 2.5 |
| Coriander & Lemon, Sainsbury's* | ½ Pack/137g | 205.0 | 6.0 | 150 | 4.3 | 23.4 | 4.3 | 2.7 |
| *Dry, Average* | *1 Serving/50g* | *178.0* | *1.0* | *356* | *13.7* | *72.8* | *1.5* | *2.6* |
| Garlic & Coriander, Dry, Waitrose* | 1 Serving/70g | 235.0 | 3.0 | 336 | 11.7 | 64.2 | 3.6 | 6.2 |
| Harissa Style Savoury, Sainsbury's* | 1 Serving/260g | 434.0 | 12.0 | 167 | 4.7 | 26.8 | 4.6 | 1.3 |
| Indian Style, Sainsbury's* | ½ Pack/143g | 204.0 | 4.0 | 143 | 4.5 | 25.1 | 2.7 | 1.0 |
| Lemon & Coriander, Cooked, Tesco* | 1 Serving/137g | 207.0 | 3.0 | 151 | 4.0 | 28.3 | 2.4 | 2.0 |
| Lemon & Coriander, Dry, Tesco* | 1 Pack/110g | 375.0 | 3.0 | 341 | 11.0 | 68.2 | 2.7 | 6.1 |
| Mediterranean Style, Dry, Tesco* | 1 Pack/110g | 368.0 | 3.0 | 335 | 11.9 | 65.1 | 3.0 | 5.6 |
| Mediterranean Tomato, GFY, Asda* | ½ Pack/141g | 192.0 | 1.0 | 136 | 5.0 | 27.0 | 0.9 | 1.7 |
| Mint & Coriander Flavour, Dry, Amazing Grains* | 1 Sachet/99g | 349.0 | 3.0 | 353 | 12.2 | 70.0 | 2.7 | 3.2 |

| | Measure | | | Nutrition Values per 100g / 100ml | | | | |
|---|---|---|---|---|---|---|---|---|
| | INFO/WEIGHT | KCAL | FAT | KCAL | PROT | CARB | FAT | FIBRE |
| **COUS COUS** | | | | | | | | |
| Moroccan Medley, Cooked, Ainsley Harriott* | ½ Sachet/130g | 186.0 | 2.0 | 143 | 5.4 | 25.4 | 1.5 | 2.2 |
| Moroccan Style, Break, GFY, Asda* | 1 Pack/150g | 215.0 | 3.0 | 143 | 5.6 | 26.1 | 1.8 | 1.8 |
| Moroccan Style, Finest, Tesco* | 1 Tub/225g | 337.0 | 11.0 | 150 | 3.7 | 23.6 | 4.7 | 3.9 |
| Moroccan Style, Fruity, M & S* | 1 Serving/200g | 370.0 | 5.0 | 185 | 3.4 | 36.7 | 2.7 | 3.4 |
| Moroccan Style, Savoury, Sainsbury's* | ½ Pack/151g | 196.0 | 4.0 | 130 | 5.0 | 21.5 | 2.7 | 1.0 |
| Moroccan Sultana & Pine Nuts, Dry, Sammy's* | 1 Serving/50g | 171.0 | 1.0 | 343 | 12.0 | 72.0 | 3.0 | 6.0 |
| Morroccan, Roast Chicken, Delicious, Shapers, Boots* | 1 Pack/250g | 247.0 | 4.0 | 99 | 9.2 | 12.0 | 1.5 | 2.6 |
| Mushrooms, Onion, Garlic & Herbs, Dry, Tesco* | ½ Pack/50g | 166.0 | 1.0 | 333 | 11.3 | 66.2 | 2.6 | 4.9 |
| Red Pepper & Chilli, Waitrose* | 1 Pack/200g | 344.0 | 14.0 | 172 | 4.5 | 23.0 | 6.9 | 1.3 |
| Roasted Vegetable, Dry, Ainsley Harriott* | ½ Sachet/50g | 138.0 | 1.0 | 276 | 11.2 | 51.0 | 3.0 | 5.2 |
| Roasted Vegetables, Waitrose* | 1 Serving/200g | 328.0 | 13.0 | 164 | 3.9 | 22.0 | 6.6 | 0.9 |
| Spice Sensation, Dry, Ainsley Harriott* | ½ Sachet/50g | 166.0 | 1.0 | 332 | 11.6 | 66.2 | 2.4 | 9.2 |
| Spicy Moroccan Chicken & Veg, COU, M & S* | 1 Pack/400g | 380.0 | 7.0 | 95 | 9.1 | 10.3 | 1.7 | 1.9 |
| Spicy Vegetable, GFY, Asda* | ½ Pack/55g | 71.0 | 1.0 | 129 | 4.7 | 25.0 | 1.1 | 2.0 |
| Spicy Vegetable, Morrisons* | 1 Pack/110g | 187.0 | 5.0 | 170 | 5.1 | 26.2 | 5.0 | 2.9 |
| Sun Dried Tomato, Somerfield* | 1 Jar/110g | 176.0 | 5.0 | 160 | 3.0 | 25.0 | 5.0 | 0.0 |
| Tangy Tomato, Dry, Ainsley Harriott* | ½ Sachet/50g | 166.0 | 1.0 | 332 | 12.2 | 67.2 | 1.6 | 8.8 |
| Tomato & Basil, Made Up, Tesco* | 1 Serving/200g | 348.0 | 17.0 | 174 | 3.9 | 21.0 | 8.3 | 3.4 |
| Tomato & Onion, Dry Weight, Waitrose* | 1 Pack/110g | 376.0 | 4.0 | 342 | 12.6 | 64.9 | 3.6 | 5.1 |
| Tomato & Vegetable, Snack Pack, Dry, Sammy's* | 1 Serving/70g | 228.0 | 2.0 | 326 | 12.0 | 67.9 | 3.5 | 6.3 |
| with Chickpea & Feta, Toasted, TTD, Sainsbury's* | 1 Serving/150g | 273.0 | 18.0 | 182 | 5.2 | 12.6 | 12.3 | 0.0 |
| Zesty Lemon & Coriander, Dry, Sammy's* | 1 Serving/50g | 171.0 | 1.0 | 342 | 13.0 | 74.0 | 2.8 | 6.0 |
| **CRAB** | | | | | | | | |
| ***Boiled, Meat Only, Average*** | ***1 Tbsp/40g*** | ***51.0*** | ***2.0*** | ***128*** | ***19.5*** | ***0.0*** | ***5.5*** | ***0.0*** |
| Claws, Asda* | 1oz/28g | 25.0 | 0.0 | 89 | 11.0 | 9.0 | 1.0 | 0.2 |
| Cocktail, Waitrose* | 1 Serving/100g | 217.0 | 18.0 | 217 | 10.8 | 3.8 | 17.6 | 0.4 |
| ***Dressed, Average*** | ***1 Can/43g*** | ***66.0*** | ***3.0*** | ***154*** | ***16.8*** | ***4.1*** | ***7.9*** | ***0.2*** |
| ***Meat, in Brine, Average*** | ***½ Can/60g*** | ***46.0*** | ***0.0*** | ***76*** | ***17.2*** | ***0.9*** | ***0.4*** | ***0.1*** |
| ***Meat, Raw, Average*** | ***1oz/28g*** | ***28.0*** | ***0.0*** | ***100*** | ***20.8*** | ***2.8*** | ***0.6*** | ***0.0*** |
| **CRAB CAKES** | | | | | | | | |
| Goan, M & S* | 1 Pack/190g | 228.0 | 8.0 | 120 | 8.0 | 12.9 | 4.0 | 1.8 |
| Tesco* | 1 Serving/130g | 281.0 | 16.0 | 216 | 11.0 | 15.4 | 12.3 | 1.1 |
| **CRAB STICKS** | | | | | | | | |
| Average | 1 Stick/15g | 14.0 | 0.0 | 94 | 9.1 | 13.9 | 0.3 | 0.0 |
| **CRACKERBREAD** | | | | | | | | |
| High Fibre, Crackerbread, Ryvita* | 1 Slice/5g | 17.0 | 0.0 | 325 | 12.5 | 62.4 | 2.8 | 15.0 |
| Original, Ryvita* | 1 Slice/6g | 21.0 | 0.0 | 380 | 10.3 | 76.9 | 3.5 | 3.5 |
| Rice, Asda* | 1 Slice/5g | 19.0 | 0.0 | 374 | 9.1 | 79.4 | 2.2 | 1.9 |
| Rice, Ryvita* | 1 Slice/5g | 19.0 | 0.0 | 374 | 9.1 | 79.4 | 2.2 | 1.9 |
| Sainsbury's* | 1 Slice/5g | 19.0 | 0.0 | 380 | 10.0 | 80.0 | 4.0 | 2.0 |
| Wheat, Original, Ryvita* | 1 Slice/5g | 19.0 | 0.0 | 380 | 10.3 | 76.9 | 3.5 | 3.5 |
| **CRACKERS** | | | | | | | | |
| Bath Oliver, Jacob's* | 1 Cracker/12g | 52.0 | 2.0 | 432 | 9.6 | 67.6 | 13.7 | 2.6 |
| Biscuits for Cheese, TTD, Sainsbury's* | 1 Cracker/8g | 39.0 | 2.0 | 493 | 8.6 | 61.0 | 23.8 | 3.1 |
| Black Olive, M & S* | 1 Cracker/4g | 20.0 | 1.0 | 485 | 8.3 | 59.4 | 23.5 | 4.3 |
| Blazing BBQ, Jacobites, Jacob's* | 1 Pack/9g | 41.0 | 2.0 | 461 | 5.2 | 55.8 | 24.2 | 1.7 |
| Bombay, Extra Spicy, Patak's* | 1 Serving/30g | 146.0 | 7.0 | 487 | 1.3 | 66.0 | 24.3 | 0.0 |
| Bran, Jacob's* | 1 Cracker/7g | 32.0 | 1.0 | 454 | 9.7 | 62.8 | 18.2 | 3.2 |
| Butter Puff, Sainsbury's* | 1 Cracker/10g | 54.0 | 3.0 | 523 | 10.4 | 60.7 | 26.5 | 2.5 |
| Chapati Chips, Tikka, Medium Spicy, Patak's* | 1 Serving/25g | 127.0 | 7.0 | 508 | 8.0 | 56.0 | 28.0 | 4.0 |
| Cheddars, McVitie's* | 1 Cracker/4g | 22.0 | 1.0 | 543 | 10.0 | 55.1 | 31.3 | 2.6 |
| Cheese, Cheese Heads, Walkers* | 1 Pack/27g | 128.0 | 6.0 | 475 | 10.8 | 58.0 | 22.3 | 2.8 |
| Cheese, Mini, Heinz* | 1 Pack/25g | 108.0 | 4.0 | 433 | 9.4 | 68.6 | 14.6 | 0.6 |

## CRACKERS

| | Measure INFO/WEIGHT | per Measure | | Nutrition Values per 100g / 100ml | | | | |
|---|---|---|---|---|---|---|---|---|
| | | KCAL | FAT | KCAL | PROT | CARB | FAT | FIBRE |
| Cheese, Ritz* | 1 Cracker/4g | 17.0 | 1.0 | 486 | 10.1 | 55.9 | 24.7 | 2.2 |
| Cheese, Trufree* | 1 Cracker/8g | 42.0 | 3.0 | 524 | 9.0 | 50.0 | 32.0 | 0.5 |
| Cheese Thins, Asda* | 1 Cracker/4g | 21.0 | 1.0 | 532 | 12.0 | 49.0 | 32.0 | 0.0 |
| Cheese Thins, Mini, Snack Rite* | 1 Bag/30g | 144.0 | 7.0 | 480 | 12.9 | 55.9 | 22.7 | 2.5 |
| Cheese Thins, Waitrose* | 1 Cracker/4g | 21.0 | 1.0 | 545 | 11.9 | 52.6 | 31.9 | 2.5 |
| Chives, Jacob's* | 1 Cracker/6g | 28.0 | 1.0 | 457 | 9.5 | 67.5 | 16.5 | 2.7 |
| Choice Grain, Jacob's* | 1 Cracker/8g | 32.0 | 1.0 | 427 | 9.0 | 65.5 | 14.3 | 5.4 |
| Corn Thins, 97% Fat Free, Real Foods* | 1 Cracker/6g | 23.0 | 0.0 | 378 | 10.2 | 81.7 | 3.0 | 8.6 |
| Cream, 45% Less Fat, Morrisons* | 1 Cracker/8g | 32.0 | 1.0 | 403 | 10.5 | 74.2 | 7.1 | 3.3 |
| Cream, Average | 1 Cracker/7g | 31.0 | 1.0 | 440 | 9.5 | 68.3 | 16.3 | 2.2 |
| Cream, BFY, Morrisons* | 1 Cracker/8g | 32.0 | 1.0 | 406 | 10.9 | 74.4 | 7.2 | 2.8 |
| Cream, BGTY, Sainsbury's* | 1 Cracker/8g | 32.0 | 1.0 | 400 | 10.9 | 71.7 | 7.7 | 3.1 |
| Cream, Choice Grain, Jacob's* | 1 Cracker/7g | 30.0 | 1.0 | 400 | 9.0 | 64.5 | 11.8 | 7.0 |
| Cream, Jacob's* | 1 Cracker/8g | 34.0 | 1.0 | 431 | 10.0 | 67.5 | 13.5 | 3.8 |
| Cream, Light, Jacob's* | 1 Cracker/8g | 31.0 | 1.0 | 388 | 10.6 | 72.2 | 6.3 | 4.1 |
| Cream, Lower Fat, Tesco* | 1 Cracker/5g | 20.0 | 0.0 | 393 | 11.0 | 72.4 | 6.6 | 3.1 |
| Cream, Morrisons* | 1 Cracker/8g | 36.0 | 1.0 | 446 | 9.6 | 68.5 | 14.8 | 2.7 |
| Cream, Reduced Fat, Tesco* | 1 Cracker/8g | 31.0 | 1.0 | 406 | 10.9 | 74.4 | 7.2 | 2.8 |
| Cream, Roasted Onion, Jacob's* | 1 Cracker/8g | 35.0 | 1.0 | 441 | 10.2 | 66.8 | 14.8 | 2.9 |
| Cream, Sainsbury's* | 1 Cracker/8g | 35.0 | 1.0 | 422 | 9.5 | 66.7 | 15.2 | 2.8 |
| Cream, Sun Dried Tomato Flavour, Jacob's* | 1 Cracker/8g | 35.0 | 1.0 | 434 | 10.2 | 66.7 | 14.0 | 3.0 |
| Cream, Tesco* | 1 Cracker/8g | 34.0 | 1.0 | 447 | 9.0 | 69.0 | 15.0 | 3.0 |
| Cream with Flaked Salt, TTD, Sainsbury's* | 1 Cracker/7g | 37.0 | 2.0 | 500 | 8.5 | 64.8 | 22.9 | 2.7 |
| Crispy Cheese, M & S* | 1 Cracker/4g | 20.0 | 1.0 | 470 | 9.4 | 58.1 | 22.1 | 3.0 |
| Extra Wheatgerm, Hovis* | 1 Serving/6g | 27.0 | 1.0 | 447 | 10.2 | 60.0 | 18.5 | 4.4 |
| Garden Herbs, Jacob's* | 1 Cracker/6g | 28.0 | 1.0 | 457 | 9.5 | 67.5 | 16.5 | 2.7 |
| Glutafin* | 1 Serving/11g | 52.0 | 2.0 | 470 | 2.4 | 70.0 | 20.0 | 0.7 |
| Harvest Grain, Sainsbury's* | 1 Cracker/6g | 27.0 | 1.0 | 458 | 8.5 | 64.5 | 18.4 | 4.1 |
| Herb & Onion, 99% Fat Free, Rakusen's* | 1 Cracker/5g | 18.0 | 0.0 | 360 | 9.1 | 82.6 | 1.0 | 3.9 |
| Herb & Onion, Trufree* | 1 Cracker/6g | 25.0 | 1.0 | 418 | 2.5 | 75.0 | 12.0 | 10.0 |
| Herb & Spice, Jacob's* | 1 Cracker/6g | 27.0 | 1.0 | 457 | 9.5 | 67.5 | 16.5 | 2.7 |
| Herbs & Spice Selection, Jacob's* | 1 Cracker/6g | 27.0 | 1.0 | 451 | 9.5 | 68.0 | 15.7 | 2.7 |
| Japanese Style Rice Mix, Asda* | 1 Serving/25g | 96.0 | 0.0 | 385 | 6.8 | 88.0 | 0.6 | 0.5 |
| Krackawheat, McVitie's* | 1 Cracker/7g | 33.0 | 1.0 | 446 | 9.7 | 60.0 | 18.6 | 5.8 |
| Light & Crispy, Sainsbury's* | 1 Cracker/11g | 42.0 | 1.0 | 384 | 11.3 | 61.0 | 10.5 | 13.0 |
| Lightly Salted, Crispy, Sainsbury's* | 1 Cracker/5g | 25.0 | 1.0 | 533 | 7.8 | 62.6 | 27.9 | 2.1 |
| Lightly Salted, Italian, Jacob's* | 1 Cracker/6g | 26.0 | 1.0 | 429 | 10.3 | 67.6 | 13.0 | 2.9 |
| Mediterranean, Jacob's* | 1 Cracker/6g | 27.0 | 1.0 | 450 | 9.7 | 66.5 | 16.1 | 2.7 |
| Mixed Seed, Multi Grain, Asda* | 1 Cracker/6g | 28.0 | 1.0 | 445 | 11.0 | 62.0 | 17.0 | 4.4 |
| Multigrain, Tesco* | 1 Cracker/6g | 27.0 | 1.0 | 458 | 8.5 | 64.5 | 18.4 | 4.1 |
| Olive Oil & Oregano, Mediterreaneo, Jacob's* | 1 Cracker/6g | 25.0 | 1.0 | 412 | 12.4 | 65.5 | 11.2 | 6.0 |
| Passionately Pizza, Jacobites, Jacob's* | 1 Pack/150g | 708.0 | 38.0 | 472 | 5.7 | 55.3 | 25.4 | 1.7 |
| Pesto, Jacob's* | 1 Cracker/6g | 27.0 | 1.0 | 450 | 9.7 | 66.5 | 16.1 | 2.7 |
| Poppy & Sesame Seed, Sainsbury's* | 1 Cracker/4g | 21.0 | 1.0 | 530 | 9.6 | 58.9 | 28.4 | 3.4 |
| Ritz, Original, Jacob's* | 1 Cracker/3g | 17.0 | 1.0 | 509 | 6.9 | 55.6 | 28.8 | 2.0 |
| Rye, Organic, Dove's Farm* | 1 Cracker/7g | 28.0 | 1.0 | 393 | 7.0 | 58.4 | 14.6 | 8.7 |
| Salt & Black Pepper, Eat Well, M & S* | 1 Pack/25g | 105.0 | 4.0 | 422 | 9.6 | 62.9 | 14.7 | 5.1 |
| Salt & Black Pepper, Jacob's* | 1 Cracker/6g | 27.0 | 1.0 | 457 | 9.5 | 67.5 | 16.5 | 2.7 |
| Salted, Ritz, Nabisco* | 1 Cracker/3g | 17.0 | 1.0 | 493 | 7.0 | 57.5 | 26.1 | 2.9 |
| Selection, Finest, Tesco* | 1 Serving/30g | 136.0 | 4.0 | 452 | 9.6 | 71.0 | 14.4 | 0.0 |
| Sesame & Poppy Thins, Tesco* | 1 Cracker/4g | 20.0 | 1.0 | 485 | 9.9 | 57.6 | 23.5 | 4.4 |
| Spicy, Trufree* | 1 Cracker/6g | 25.0 | 1.0 | 412 | 3.8 | 70.0 | 13.0 | 12.5 |
| Spicy Indonesian Vegetable, Waitrose* | 1 Pack/60g | 295.0 | 16.0 | 492 | 1.2 | 60.6 | 27.2 | 2.2 |

| | Measure INFO/WEIGHT | per Measure KCAL | FAT | Nutrition Values per 100g / 100ml KCAL | PROT | CARB | FAT | FIBRE |
|---|---|---|---|---|---|---|---|---|
| **CRACKERS** | | | | | | | | |
| Spicy Vegetable, Tesco* | 1 Serving/60g | 340.0 | 23.0 | 566 | 2.6 | 52.4 | 38.4 | 1.2 |
| Sweet Chilli, Thins, Savours, Jacob's* | 1 Cracker/4g | 21.0 | 1.0 | 472 | 8.0 | 62.3 | 21.2 | 3.6 |
| Tempting Tandoori, Jacobites, Jacob's* | 1 Pack/150g | 711.0 | 38.0 | 474 | 5.7 | 55.5 | 25.5 | 1.7 |
| Thai Spicy Vegetable, Sainsbury's* | 1 Pack/50g | 231.0 | 10.0 | 462 | 7.2 | 61.5 | 20.8 | 2.6 |
| Tuc, Cheese Sandwich, Jacob's* | 1 Cracker/14g | 72.0 | 4.0 | 531 | 8.4 | 53.8 | 31.4 | 0.0 |
| Tuc, Jacob's* | 1 Cracker/5g | 24.0 | 1.0 | 522 | 7.0 | 60.5 | 28.0 | 2.9 |
| Tuc, Mini, with Sesame Seeds, Jacob's* | 1 Biscuit/2g | 10.0 | 1.0 | 523 | 9.7 | 63.1 | 25.8 | 3.9 |
| Vegetable, Oriental Snack Selection, Sainsbury's* | 1 Cracker/20g | 42.0 | 2.0 | 209 | 4.5 | 26.2 | 9.6 | 3.4 |
| Veggie, Heinz, Heinz* | 1 Pack/25g | 110.0 | 3.0 | 440 | 7.0 | 76.0 | 12.0 | 3.6 |
| Wheaten, M & S* | 1 Cracker/4g | 20.0 | 1.0 | 450 | 10.2 | 57.0 | 20.2 | 5.0 |
| Whole Wheat, 100%, Oven Baked, Master Choice* | 1 Cracker/4g | 17.0 | 0.0 | 429 | 10.0 | 75.0 | 9.6 | 12.1 |
| Wholemeal, Tesco* | 1 Cracker/7g | 29.0 | 1.0 | 414 | 9.4 | 60.6 | 14.9 | 10.4 |
| Wholmeal, Organic, Nairn's* | 1 Cracker/14g | 58.0 | 2.0 | 413 | 9.0 | 61.4 | 14.6 | 8.7 |
| with Onion, Cumin Seed, & Garlic, GFY, Asda* | 1 Cracker/6g | 22.0 | 0.0 | 380 | 11.0 | 78.0 | 2.7 | 1.7 |
| **CRANBERRIES** | | | | | | | | |
| & Blueberries, Delicious, Boots* | 1 Pack/75g | 220.0 | 1.0 | 293 | 0.7 | 70.0 | 1.3 | 9.1 |
| & Raisins, Dried, Sweetened, Ocean Spray* | 1 Serving/50g | 163.0 | 0.0 | 326 | 0.1 | 80.3 | 0.5 | 4.6 |
| *Dried, Sweetened, Average* | *1 Serving/10g* | *34.0* | *0.0* | *335* | *0.3* | *81.1* | *0.8* | *4.4* |
| *Fresh, Raw* | *1oz/28g* | *4.0* | *0.0* | *15* | *0.4* | *3.4* | *0.1* | *3.0* |
| **CRAYFISH** | | | | | | | | |
| *Raw* | *1oz/28g* | *19.0* | *0.0* | *67* | *14.9* | *0.0* | *0.8* | *0.0* |
| Tails, Chilli & Garlic, Asda* | 1 Serving/140g | 133.0 | 4.0 | 95 | 16.0 | 1.1 | 3.1 | 0.8 |
| Tails, in Brine, Luxury, The Big Prawn Co* | ½ Tub/90g | 46.0 | 1.0 | 51 | 10.1 | 1.0 | 0.7 | 0.0 |
| **CREAM** | | | | | | | | |
| *Aerosol, Average* | *1oz/28g* | *87.0* | *9.0* | *309* | *1.7* | *6.2* | *30.9* | *0.0* |
| *Aerosol, Reduced Fat, Average* | *1 Serving/55ml* | *33.0* | *3.0* | *59* | *0.6* | *1.9* | *5.4* | *0.0* |
| Brandy, Pourable, with Remy Martin*, Finest, Tesco* | ½ Pot/125ml | 460.0 | 35.0 | 368 | 2.7 | 19.8 | 28.4 | 0.0 |
| Brandy, Really Thick, Finest, Tesco* | ½ Pot/125ml | 579.0 | 49.0 | 463 | 1.3 | 19.7 | 39.6 | 0.0 |
| Brandy, Really Thick, Tesco* | 1 Sm Pot/250ml | 1162.0 | 98.0 | 465 | 1.4 | 21.3 | 39.3 | 0.0 |
| *Clotted, Fresh, Average* | *1 Serving/28g* | *162.0* | *18.0* | *579* | *1.6* | *2.3* | *62.7* | *0.0* |
| *Double, Average* | *1 Serving/25ml* | *110.0* | *12.0* | *438* | *1.8* | *2.7* | *46.7* | *0.0* |
| *Double, Reduced Fat, Average* | *1 Serving/30g* | *73.0* | *7.0* | *243* | *2.7* | *5.6* | *23.3* | *0.1* |
| Oat Alternative, Dairy Free, Oatly* | 1 Carton/250ml | 375.0 | 32.0 | 150 | 1.0 | 6.0 | 13.0 | 0.8 |
| *Single, Average* | *1 Tbsp/15ml* | *18.0* | *2.0* | *123* | *2.6* | *4.4* | *10.5* | *0.1* |
| *Single, Extra Thick, Average* | *1 Serving/38ml* | *72.0* | *7.0* | *192* | *2.7* | *4.1* | *18.4* | *0.0* |
| *Soured, Fresh, Average* | *1 Tbsp/15ml* | *29.0* | *3.0* | *191* | *2.7* | *3.9* | *18.4* | *0.0* |
| *Soured, Reduced Fat, Average* | *1 fl oz/30ml* | *36.0* | *3.0* | *119* | *5.2* | *6.7* | *8.6* | *0.4* |
| Strawberry, Light, Real Dairy, Uht, Anchor* | 1 Serving/13g | 25.0 | 2.0 | 198 | 2.6 | 8.7 | 17.0 | 0.0 |
| *Thick, Sterilised, Average* | *1 Tbsp/15ml* | *35.0* | *3.0* | *233* | *2.6* | *3.6* | *23.1* | *0.0* |
| *Uht, Double, Average* | *1 Tbsp/15g* | *41.0* | *4.0* | *274* | *2.2* | *7.3* | *26.3* | *0.0* |
| *Uht, Reduced Fat, Average* | *1 Serving/25ml* | *15.0* | *1.0* | *62* | *0.5* | *2.2* | *5.6* | *0.0* |
| *Uht, Single, Average* | *1 Tbsp/15ml* | *29.0* | *3.0* | *194* | *2.6* | *4.0* | *18.8* | *0.0* |
| *Whipping, Average* | *1 Tbsp/15ml* | *52.0* | *5.0* | *348* | *2.1* | *3.2* | *36.4* | *0.0* |
| **CREAM HORN** | | | | | | | | |
| Fresh, Tesco* | 1 Horn/57g | 244.0 | 16.0 | 428 | 4.1 | 40.3 | 27.8 | 0.3 |
| **CREAM SODA** | | | | | | | | |
| American, with Vanilla, Tesco* | 1 Glass/313ml | 75.0 | 0.0 | 24 | 0.0 | 5.9 | 0.0 | 0.0 |
| Diet, Sainsbury's* | 1 Serving/250ml | 2.0 | 0.0 | 1 | 0.0 | 0.0 | 0.0 | 0.0 |
| No Added Sugar, Sainsbury's* | 1 Can/330ml | 2.0 | 0.0 | 0 | 0.1 | 0.1 | 0.1 | 0.1 |
| Traditional Style, Tesco* | 1 Can/330ml | 139.0 | 0.0 | 42 | 0.0 | 10.4 | 0.0 | 0.0 |
| **CREMA CATALANA** | | | | | | | | |
| Cafe Culture, M & S* | 1 Pot/110g | 385.0 | 35.0 | 350 | 3.5 | 12.2 | 31.7 | 0.4 |

**C**

| | Measure INFO/WEIGHT | per Measure KCAL | FAT | Nutrition Values per 100g / 100ml KCAL | PROT | CARB | FAT | FIBRE |
|---|---|---|---|---|---|---|---|---|
| **CREME BRULEE** | | | | | | | | |
| Gastropub, M & S* | 1 Brulee/84g | 285.0 | 25.0 | 340 | 3.1 | 15.7 | 29.3 | 0.7 |
| M & S* | 1 Pot/100g | 360.0 | 33.0 | 360 | 3.3 | 13.0 | 32.6 | 0.0 |
| Nestle* | 1 Serving/100g | 305.0 | 26.0 | 305 | 4.0 | 14.6 | 25.6 | 0.0 |
| Somerfield* | 1 Pot/100g | 316.0 | 27.0 | 316 | 4.0 | 15.0 | 27.0 | 0.0 |
| **CREME CARAMEL** | | | | | | | | |
| Asda* | 1 Pot/100g | 113.0 | 3.0 | 113 | 2.4 | 20.0 | 2.6 | 0.0 |
| Average | 1 Serving/128g | 140.0 | 3.0 | 109 | 3.0 | 20.6 | 2.2 | 0.0 |
| Carmelle, Green's* | 1 Pack/70g | 82.0 | 3.0 | 117 | 3.0 | 17.0 | 4.0 | 0.0 |
| Sainsbury's* | 1 Pot/100g | 102.0 | 1.0 | 102 | 2.5 | 21.1 | 0.9 | 0.0 |
| Somerfield* | 1 Pot/100g | 114.0 | 1.0 | 114 | 3.0 | 24.0 | 1.0 | 0.0 |
| Tesco* | 1 Pot/100g | 120.0 | 2.0 | 120 | 2.6 | 22.8 | 1.6 | 0.0 |
| **CREME EGG** | | | | | | | | |
| Cadbury* | 1 Egg/39g | 174.0 | 6.0 | 445 | 3.0 | 71.0 | 16.0 | 0.0 |
| Minis, Cadbury* | 1 Egg/11g | 50.0 | 2.0 | 445 | 4.1 | 67.5 | 16.4 | 0.4 |
| **CREME FRAICHE** | | | | | | | | |
| ***Average*** | ***1 Pot/295g*** | ***1067.0*** | ***112.0*** | ***362*** | ***2.2*** | ***2.6*** | ***38.0*** | ***0.0*** |
| Cucumber & Mint, Triangles, Sainsbury's* | 1 Serving/25g | 105.0 | 2.0 | 421 | 11.0 | 72.3 | 9.7 | 2.5 |
| Extra Light, President* | 1 Tub/200g | 182.0 | 10.0 | 91 | 2.7 | 8.7 | 5.0 | 0.0 |
| ***Half Fat, Average*** | ***1 Dtsp/30g*** | ***54.0*** | ***5.0*** | ***181*** | ***3.1*** | ***5.5*** | ***16.2*** | ***0.0*** |
| Lemon & Rocket, Sainsbury's* | 1 Serving/150g | 187.0 | 17.0 | 125 | 2.2 | 3.0 | 11.5 | 0.5 |
| **CREPES** | | | | | | | | |
| Chocolate Filled, Tesco* | 1 Crepe/32g | 140.0 | 6.0 | 437 | 5.9 | 62.5 | 18.1 | 1.6 |
| Lobster, Finest, Tesco* | 1 Serving/160g | 250.0 | 10.0 | 156 | 10.7 | 14.0 | 6.4 | 1.2 |
| Mushroom, M & S* | 1 Pack/186g | 195.0 | 4.0 | 105 | 5.7 | 17.1 | 2.4 | 2.5 |
| **CRISPBAKES** | | | | | | | | |
| Dutch, Asda* | 1 Bake/8g | 31.0 | 0.0 | 388 | 14.7 | 74.9 | 3.3 | 4.2 |
| Dutch, HL, Tesco* | 1 Bake/8g | 30.0 | 0.0 | 385 | 14.7 | 74.9 | 2.7 | 4.2 |
| Dutch, Sainsbury's* | 1 Bake/10g | 38.0 | 0.0 | 392 | 14.5 | 72.3 | 5.0 | 5.8 |
| **CRISPBREAD** | | | | | | | | |
| 3 Seed, Classic, Gourmet, Dr Karg* | 1 Bread/25g | 107.0 | 5.0 | 430 | 16.5 | 46.6 | 19.7 | 10.9 |
| 3 Seed, Organic, Gourmet | 1 Bread/25g | 101.0 | 5.0 | 405 | 15.8 | 48.8 | 18.8 | 14.6 |
| Bran, Scandinavian, Gg* | 1 Bread/8g | 18.0 | 0.0 | 223 | 14.9 | 29.0 | 5.3 | 42.1 |
| Breaks, with Currants, Oats & Honey, Ryvita* | 1 Bread/15g | 48.0 | 0.0 | 332 | 8.0 | 69.7 | 2.3 | 12.0 |
| Corn, Orgran* | 1 Bread/5g | 18.0 | 0.0 | 360 | 7.5 | 83.0 | 1.8 | 3.0 |
| Crisp 'n' Light, Wasa* | 1 Bread/7g | 24.0 | 0.0 | 360 | 12.0 | 73.0 | 2.2 | 5.3 |
| Dark Rye, Morrisons* | 1 Bake/13g | 39.0 | 0.0 | 300 | 11.5 | 61.5 | 3.1 | 16.9 |
| Dark Rye, Ryvita* | 1 Bread/10g | 31.0 | 0.0 | 311 | 8.5 | 65.5 | 1.7 | 18.0 |
| Emmental Cheese & Pumpkin Seed, Gourmet, Dr Karg* | 1 Bread/25g | 100.0 | 4.0 | 402 | 17.7 | 45.5 | 16.6 | 12.3 |
| Emmental Cheese & Pumpkin Seed, Organic, Dr Karg* | 1 Bread/25g | 102.0 | 4.0 | 408 | 17.1 | 50.7 | 14.9 | 9.6 |
| Fruit Crunch, Ryvita* | 1 Bread/16g | 57.0 | 1.0 | 366 | 10.9 | 65.8 | 6.6 | 11.1 |
| Garlic & Rosemary, Wholegrain Rye, Ryvita* | 1 Bread/12g | 39.0 | 0.0 | 325 | 8.3 | 70.0 | 1.7 | 16.7 |
| Gluten Free | 1 Bread/8g | 25.0 | 0.0 | 331 | 6.4 | 72.9 | 1.5 | 0.0 |
| Light, Ryvita* | 1 Bread/5g | 19.0 | 0.0 | 383 | 9.8 | 79.3 | 3.0 | 2.6 |
| Mildly Seasoned, Gourmet, Dr Karg* | 1 Bread/25g | 101.0 | 4.0 | 405 | 16.2 | 48.8 | 16.1 | 11.6 |
| Mildly Seasoned, Organic, Dr Karg* | 1 Bread/25g | 100.0 | 4.0 | 401 | 16.0 | 48.5 | 15.9 | 13.8 |
| Minis, Apple, Ryvita* | 1 Pack/30g | 101.0 | 1.0 | 336 | 6.1 | 71.9 | 2.7 | 12.0 |
| Minis, Caramel, Ryvita* | 1 Pack/30g | 100.0 | 1.0 | 335 | 6.1 | 71.7 | 2.7 | 11.9 |
| Minis, Cheese & Chives, Ryvita* | 1 Pack/30g | 103.0 | 1.0 | 342 | 8.0 | 71.0 | 2.9 | 11.5 |
| Minis, Garlic & Herb, Ryvita* | 1 Bag/30g | 103.0 | 1.0 | 343 | 7.9 | 71.5 | 2.8 | 11.5 |
| Minis, Mature Cheddar & Onion, Ryvita* | 1 Bag/30g | 101.0 | 1.0 | 337 | 9.3 | 68.2 | 3.0 | 11.5 |
| Minis, Salt & Vinegar, Ryvita* | 1 Pack/30g | 94.0 | 1.0 | 312 | 6.8 | 64.8 | 2.8 | 12.1 |
| Minis, Sweet Chilli, Ryvita* | 1 Pack/30g | 100.0 | 1.0 | 335 | 7.0 | 71.0 | 2.6 | 11.9 |
| Minis, Worcester Sauce, Ryvita* | 1 Pack/30g | 102.0 | 1.0 | 339 | 6.9 | 71.9 | 2.6 | 12.0 |

| | Measure INFO/WEIGHT | per Measure KCAL | FAT | Nutrition Values per 100g / 100ml KCAL | PROT | CARB | FAT | FIBRE |
|---|---|---|---|---|---|---|---|---|
| **CRISPBREAD** | | | | | | | | |
| Multigrain, Ryvita* | 1 Bread/11g | 36.0 | 1.0 | 331 | 10.0 | 61.1 | 5.2 | 16.7 |
| Multigrain, Wasa* | 1 Bread/13g | 43.0 | 0.0 | 320 | 12.0 | 62.0 | 2.6 | 14.0 |
| Original Rye, Wasa* | 1 Bread/11g | 35.0 | 0.0 | 315 | 9.0 | 67.0 | 1.4 | 14.0 |
| Poppyseed, Wasa* | 1 Bread/13g | 45.0 | 1.0 | 350 | 13.0 | 56.0 | 8.0 | 14.0 |
| Provita* | 1 Bread/6g | 26.0 | 1.0 | 416 | 12.5 | 68.4 | 9.9 | 0.0 |
| Pumpkin Seeds & Oats, Ryvita* | 1 Bread/12g | 43.0 | 1.0 | 362 | 12.5 | 55.6 | 9.9 | 14.5 |
| Rice, & Cracked Pepper, Orgran* | 1 Bread/5g | 18.0 | 0.0 | 388 | 8.4 | 81.9 | 1.8 | 2.0 |
| Rice, Original, Sakata* | 1 Bread/25g | 102.0 | 1.0 | 410 | 6.9 | 88.0 | 2.6 | 1.3 |
| Rice, Sakata* | 1 Bread/25g | 25.0 | 0.0 | 102 | 1.7 | 22.0 | 0.7 | 0.3 |
| Roasted Onion, Gourmet, Dr Karg* | 1 Bread/25g | 100.0 | 4.0 | 399 | 15.9 | 46.6 | 16.5 | 11.1 |
| Roasted Onion, Organic, Dr Karg* | 1 Bread/25g | 97.0 | 4.0 | 390 | 15.8 | 48.5 | 14.8 | 12.9 |
| Rounds, Multigrain, Finn Crisp* | 1 Bread/13g | 41.0 | 1.0 | 330 | 13.0 | 56.0 | 6.0 | 18.0 |
| Rounds, Original, Rye, Finn Crisp* | 1 Bread/14g | 45.0 | 0.0 | 320 | 11.0 | 60.0 | 2.7 | 16.0 |
| Rounds, Wholegrain Wheat, Finn Crisp* | 1 Bread/13g | 45.0 | 1.0 | 360 | 11.0 | 66.0 | 5.9 | 10.0 |
| Rye, Original, Ryvita* | 1 Bread/10g | 32.0 | 0.0 | 317 | 8.5 | 66.6 | 1.7 | 16.5 |
| Seeded, Spelt, Organic, Dr Karg* | 1 Bread/25g | 102.0 | 4.0 | 408 | 17.2 | 44.4 | 18.0 | 10.4 |
| Sesame Rye, Ryvita* | 1 Bread/10g | 34.0 | 1.0 | 338 | 10.5 | 58.3 | 7.0 | 17.5 |
| Snacks, Caribbean Chicken, Seasons, Quaker* | 1 Pack/28g | 118.0 | 3.0 | 421 | 7.9 | 77.1 | 8.9 | 2.1 |
| Snacks, Cheese, Onion & Chive Flavour, Seasons, Quaker* | 1 Pack/28g | 118.0 | 3.0 | 420 | 8.3 | 76.0 | 9.1 | 2.4 |
| Snacks, Lime & Coriander, Seasons, Quaker* | 1 Pack/28g | 115.0 | 3.0 | 410 | 7.5 | 75.0 | 9.0 | 2.3 |
| Snacks, Sun Dried Tomato & Basil, Seasons, Quaker* | 1 Pack/24g | 101.0 | 2.0 | 420 | 8.0 | 77.0 | 9.0 | 2.3 |
| Spelt, Cheese, Sunflower Seeds, Organic, Dr Karg* | 1 Bread/25g | 103.0 | 5.0 | 411 | 19.2 | 42.8 | 18.1 | 10.4 |
| Spelt, Muesli, Organic, Dr Karg* | 1 Bread/25g | 94.0 | 3.0 | 375 | 14.2 | 54.4 | 11.2 | 10.6 |
| Spelt, Sesame, Sunflower, Amisa* | 1 Bread/29g | 85.0 | 4.0 | 297 | 11.7 | 28.5 | 15.1 | 5.0 |
| Sport, Wasa* | 1 Bread/15g | 46.0 | 0.0 | 310 | 9.0 | 64.0 | 1.5 | 16.0 |
| Sunflower Seeds & Oats, Ryvita* | 1 Bread/12g | 42.0 | 1.0 | 348 | 10.1 | 57.2 | 8.8 | 16.7 |
| Thin Crisps, Original Taste, Finn Crisp* | 1 Bread/6g | 20.0 | 0.0 | 320 | 11.0 | 63.0 | 2.4 | 19.0 |
| Trufree* | 1 Bread/6g | 22.0 | 0.0 | 370 | 6.0 | 82.0 | 2.0 | 1.0 |
| Wheat, with Poppy Seeds, Morrisons* | 1 Serving/12g | 45.0 | 1.0 | 390 | 11.0 | 68.0 | 8.0 | 8.0 |
| Whole Grain, Classic, Organic, Dr Karg* | 1 Bread/25g | 89.0 | 4.0 | 355 | 13.4 | 38.2 | 16.5 | 10.2 |
| Whole Grain, Crispy, Thin, Kavli* | 3 Breads/15g | 50.0 | 0.0 | 333 | 10.0 | 70.0 | 1.7 | 12.7 |
| Wholemeal, Light, Allinson* | 1 Bread/5g | 17.0 | 0.0 | 349 | 11.7 | 69.7 | 2.6 | 11.0 |
| Wholemeal, Organic, Allinson* | 1 Bread/5g | 17.0 | 0.0 | 336 | 14.2 | 66.0 | 1.7 | 12.2 |
| Wholemeal, Rye with Milk, Grafschafter* | 1 Bread/9g | 29.0 | 0.0 | 316 | 11.4 | 64.0 | 1.6 | 15.0 |
| Wholemeal Rye, Organic, Kallo* | 1 Bread/10g | 31.0 | 0.0 | 314 | 9.7 | 65.0 | 1.7 | 15.4 |
| **CRISPS** | | | | | | | | |
| Apple, Thyme & Sage, M & S* | 1 Bag/55g | 253.0 | 13.0 | 460 | 5.5 | 55.3 | 24.3 | 6.1 |
| Bacon, Shapers, Boots* | 1 Bag/23g | 99.0 | 3.0 | 431 | 8.0 | 66.0 | 15.0 | 3.0 |
| Bacon & Cheddar, Baked, Walkers* | 1 Pack/38g | 149.0 | 3.0 | 397 | 6.5 | 73.7 | 8.5 | 4.7 |
| Bacon Crispies, Sainsbury's* | 1 Bag/25g | 117.0 | 6.0 | 468 | 19.9 | 45.8 | 22.8 | 4.8 |
| Bacon Flavour Rashers, BGTY, Sainsbury's* | 1 Pack/10g | 34.0 | 0.0 | 340 | 10.8 | 70.3 | 1.6 | 3.5 |
| Bacon Pillows, Light, Shapers, Boots* | 1 Pack/12g | 44.0 | 0.0 | 367 | 3.7 | 83.0 | 2.3 | 4.0 |
| Bacon Rashers, Blazin, Tesco* | 1 Bag/25g | 121.0 | 7.0 | 485 | 16.5 | 45.7 | 26.3 | 3.8 |
| Bacon Rashers, COU, M & S* | 1 Pack/20g | 72.0 | 1.0 | 360 | 9.4 | 77.5 | 2.9 | 3.5 |
| Bacon Rashers, Tesco* | 1 Serving/25g | 125.0 | 6.0 | 500 | 7.1 | 59.8 | 25.5 | 4.0 |
| Bacon Rice Bites, Asda* | 1 Bag/30g | 136.0 | 5.0 | 452 | 7.0 | 70.0 | 16.0 | 0.4 |
| Baked, Bacon & Cheddar, Walkers* | 1 Bag/25g | 99.0 | 2.0 | 396 | 6.4 | 73.6 | 8.4 | 4.8 |
| Baked, Cheese & Onion, Walkers* | 1 Sm Bag/25g | 99.0 | 2.0 | 396 | 6.5 | 73.8 | 8.3 | 4.7 |
| Baked, Ready Salted, Walkers* | 1 Packet/38g | 146.0 | 3.0 | 390 | 6.0 | 74.0 | 8.0 | 5.5 |
| Baked, Salt & Vinegar, Walkers* | 1 Packet/38g | 146.0 | 3.0 | 390 | 6.0 | 73.0 | 8.0 | 5.0 |
| Baked, Sour Cream & Chive, Walkers* | 1 Packet/38g | 148.0 | 3.0 | 395 | 7.0 | 73.0 | 8.5 | 5.0 |
| Baked Bean Flavour, Walkers* | 1 Bag/35g | 184.0 | 12.0 | 525 | 6.5 | 50.0 | 33.0 | 4.0 |
| Banging BBQ, Shots, Walkers* | 1 Pack/18g | 87.0 | 4.0 | 485 | 5.5 | 60.0 | 25.0 | 1.3 |

## CRISPS

| INFO/WEIGHT | Measure | per Measure KCAL | FAT | Nutrition Values per 100g / 100ml KCAL | PROT | CARB | FAT | FIBRE |
|---|---|---|---|---|---|---|---|---|
| Barbecue, Handcooked, Tesco* | 1 Bag/40g | 187.0 | 10.0 | 468 | 6.6 | 53.8 | 25.1 | 5.2 |
| Barbecue, Savoury Snacks, Weight Watchers* | 1 Pack/22g | 81.0 | 2.0 | 366 | 18.6 | 61.0 | 8.7 | 6.1 |
| Barbecue, Sunseed Oil, Walkers* | 1 Pack/25g | 131.0 | 8.0 | 525 | 6.5 | 50.0 | 33.0 | 4.0 |
| Barbecue Beef, Select, Tesco* | 1 Pack/25g | 134.0 | 9.0 | 536 | 6.4 | 49.2 | 34.8 | 4.4 |
| Barbecue Flavour Waffles, American Style, Shapers, Boots* | 1 Pack/20g | 95.0 | 4.0 | 476 | 4.5 | 65.0 | 22.0 | 3.7 |
| BBQ Chilli & Mesquite, Pan-Fried, TTD, Sainsbury's* | 1 Sm Pack/50g | 239.0 | 13.0 | 478 | 8.0 | 51.3 | 26.7 | 5.4 |
| BBQ Rib, Sunseed, Walkers* | 1 Bag/25g | 131.0 | 8.0 | 525 | 6.5 | 50.0 | 33.0 | 4.0 |
| Beef, Squares, Walkers* | 1 Bag/25g | 105.0 | 4.0 | 420 | 6.0 | 59.0 | 18.0 | 4.6 |
| Beef & Onion, Asda* | 1 Bag/25g | 129.0 | 8.0 | 516 | 5.7 | 53.3 | 31.1 | 3.9 |
| Beef & Onion, Potato, M & S* | 1 Bag/25g | 130.0 | 8.0 | 530 | 6.6 | 48.2 | 34.5 | 5.0 |
| Beef & Onion, Walkers* | 1 Bag/35g | 184.0 | 12.0 | 525 | 6.5 | 50.0 | 33.0 | 4.0 |
| Beefy, Smiths, Walkers* | 1 Bag/25g | 133.0 | 9.0 | 531 | 4.3 | 45.2 | 37.0 | 0.0 |
| Buffalo Mozzarella & Herbs, Walkers* | 1 Serving/35g | 171.0 | 9.0 | 490 | 6.1 | 57.0 | 26.0 | 4.2 |
| Buffalo Mozzarella Tomato & Basil, Kettle Chips* | 1 Serving/50g | 238.0 | 13.0 | 476 | 6.7 | 54.4 | 25.7 | 4.9 |
| Builders Breakfast, Walkers* | 1 Sm Bag/25g | 131.0 | 8.0 | 524 | 5.6 | 50.8 | 33.2 | 4.0 |
| Butter & Chive, COU, M & S* | 1 Bag/26g | 95.0 | 0.0 | 365 | 7.7 | 77.3 | 1.9 | 4.6 |
| Cajun Squirrel, Walkers* | 1 Sm Bag/25g | 130.0 | 8.0 | 522 | 5.8 | 51.2 | 32.7 | 4.2 |
| Chargrilled Chicken Crinkles, Shapers, Boots* | 1 Bag/20g | 96.0 | 5.0 | 482 | 6.6 | 60.0 | 24.0 | 4.0 |
| Chargrilled Steak, Max, Walkers* | 1 Bag/55g | 289.0 | 18.0 | 525 | 6.5 | 50.0 | 33.0 | 4.0 |
| Cheddar, Red Wine & Shallot, TTD, Sainsbury's* | 1 Pack/50g | 238.0 | 13.0 | 476 | 6.5 | 55.6 | 25.2 | 4.7 |
| Cheddar & Red Onion Chutney, Sensations, Walkers* | 1 Bag/40g | 198.0 | 11.0 | 495 | 6.5 | 54.0 | 28.0 | 4.5 |
| Cheddar & Spring Onion, 35% Less Fat, Sainsbury's* | 1 Pack/20g | 93.0 | 4.0 | 463 | 6.3 | 62.4 | 20.9 | 0.9 |
| Cheddar & Spring Onion, TTD, Sainsbury's* | 1 Serving/30g | 139.0 | 8.0 | 465 | 6.7 | 48.3 | 27.2 | 7.8 |
| Cheddar Cheese, Sunseed Oil, Walkers* | 1 Bag/35g | 181.0 | 11.0 | 525 | 6.5 | 50.0 | 33.0 | 4.0 |
| Cheese & Branston Pickle, Walkers* | 1 Bag/35g | 181.0 | 11.0 | 525 | 6.5 | 50.0 | 33.0 | 4.0 |
| Cheese & Chive Flavour, GFY, Asda* | 1 Bag/25g | 119.0 | 6.0 | 476 | 6.0 | 59.0 | 24.0 | 6.0 |
| Cheese & Chives, Walkers* | 1 Bag/35g | 185.0 | 12.0 | 530 | 6.5 | 50.0 | 33.0 | 4.1 |
| Cheese & Onion, 30% Less Fat, Sainsbury's* | 1 Pack/25g | 115.0 | 5.0 | 459 | 7.5 | 58.1 | 21.8 | 5.4 |
| Cheese & Onion, Crinkle Cut, Low Fat, Waitrose* | 1 Bag/25g | 122.0 | 6.0 | 490 | 7.7 | 62.6 | 23.2 | 4.7 |
| Cheese & Onion, Flavour Crinkles, Shapers, Boots* | 1 Bag/20g | 96.0 | 5.0 | 482 | 6.6 | 60.0 | 24.0 | 4.0 |
| Cheese & Onion, Golden Wonder* | 1 Bag/25g | 131.0 | 8.0 | 524 | 6.1 | 49.2 | 33.6 | 2.0 |
| Cheese & Onion, KP Snacks* | 1 Bag/25g | 133.0 | 9.0 | 534 | 6.6 | 48.7 | 34.8 | 4.8 |
| Cheese & Onion, Lights, Walkers* | 1 Sm Bag/24g | 113.0 | 5.0 | 470 | 7.5 | 62.0 | 21.0 | 5.0 |
| Cheese & Onion, Max, Walkers* | 1 Pack/50g | 262.0 | 16.0 | 525 | 6.8 | 52.0 | 32.0 | 5.2 |
| Cheese & Onion, Organic, Tesco* | 1 Bag/25g | 128.0 | 8.0 | 514 | 5.2 | 49.9 | 32.6 | 7.0 |
| Cheese & Onion, Oven Baked, Tesco* | 1 Bag/25g | 102.0 | 2.0 | 410 | 5.3 | 74.7 | 6.6 | 7.7 |
| Cheese & Onion, Potato Heads, Walkers* | 1 Pack/23g | 108.0 | 5.0 | 470 | 6.0 | 60.0 | 23.0 | 5.5 |
| Cheese & Onion, Sainsbury's* | 1 Bag/25g | 132.0 | 9.0 | 527 | 4.6 | 48.8 | 34.8 | 3.9 |
| Cheese & Onion, Sprinters* | 1 Bag/25g | 137.0 | 9.0 | 549 | 5.4 | 49.4 | 36.6 | 0.0 |
| Cheese & Onion, Squares, Walkers* | 1 Bag/25g | 107.0 | 4.0 | 430 | 6.5 | 61.0 | 18.0 | 5.5 |
| Cheese & Onion, Sunseed Oil, Walkers* | 1 Bag/35g | 181.0 | 11.0 | 525 | 7.0 | 50.0 | 33.0 | 4.0 |
| Cheese & Onion, Tesco* | 1 Pack/25g | 132.0 | 8.0 | 530 | 5.8 | 51.6 | 33.2 | 4.4 |
| Cheese & Onion, Value, Tesco* | 1 Bag/20g | 108.0 | 7.0 | 541 | 6.0 | 48.3 | 36.0 | 4.8 |
| Cheese & Onion Rings, Crunchy, Shapers, Boots* | 1 Bag/15g | 56.0 | 0.0 | 374 | 5.9 | 81.0 | 2.9 | 2.0 |
| Cheese Bites, Weight Watchers* | 1 Pack/18g | 73.0 | 1.0 | 406 | 13.9 | 71.1 | 5.6 | 2.2 |
| Cheese Curls, Morrisons* | 1 Bag/14g | 71.0 | 4.0 | 510 | 4.5 | 51.0 | 32.0 | 2.6 |
| Cheese Curls, Red Mill* | ½ Bag/50g | 276.0 | 18.0 | 553 | 6.6 | 50.6 | 36.0 | 2.0 |
| Cheese Curls, Shapers, Boots* | 1 Pack/14g | 68.0 | 4.0 | 489 | 4.5 | 57.0 | 27.0 | 2.7 |
| Cheese Curls, Tesco* | 1 Bag/14g | 75.0 | 4.0 | 520 | 4.5 | 54.4 | 31.1 | 1.9 |
| Cheese Curls, Weight Watchers* | 1 Pack/20g | 78.0 | 2.0 | 392 | 5.0 | 73.8 | 8.6 | 3.4 |
| Cheese Moments, Smiths* | 1 Pack/28g | 148.0 | 9.0 | 530 | 8.0 | 50.0 | 33.0 | 2.0 |
| Cheese Tasters, M & S* | 1 Sm Bag/30g | 154.0 | 9.0 | 515 | 8.1 | 55.0 | 29.3 | 1.7 |
| Cheese Twirls, Boulevard, Simply Delicious* | 1 Pack/25g | 137.0 | 9.0 | 550 | 12.1 | 46.7 | 35.0 | 0.0 |

## CRISPS

| INFO/WEIGHT | Measure per Measure | | Nutrition Values per 100g / 100ml | | | | |
|---|---|---|---|---|---|---|---|
| | KCAL | FAT | KCAL | PROT | CARB | FAT | FIBRE |
| Cheese Xl, Golden Wonder* | 1 Bag/30g | 155.0 10.0 | 516 | 6.2 | 50.6 | 32.1 | 4.2 |
| Cheeses with Onion, Soulmates, Kettle Chips* | 1 Pack/40g | 195.0 12.0 | 488 | 7.7 | 50.2 | 29.0 | 5.4 |
| Chicken, Firecracker, McCoys* | 1 Bag/35g | 177.0 10.0 | 506 | 6.2 | 54.0 | 29.5 | 4.0 |
| Chicken, Oven Roasted with Lemon & Thyme, Walkers* | 1 Bag/40g | 200.0 11.0 | 500 | 6.5 | 55.0 | 28.0 | 4.5 |
| Chicken, Potato Heads, Walkers* | 1 Pack/23g | 106.0 5.0 | 460 | 8.5 | 58.0 | 21.0 | 6.0 |
| Chicken Flavour, HE, Tesco* | 1 Bag/12g | 43.0 0.0 | 357 | 5.1 | 81.0 | 1.4 | 3.4 |
| Chilli & Chocolate, Walkers* | 1 Pack/25g | 131.0 8.0 | 523 | 6.1 | 50.1 | 33.1 | 4.2 |
| Chilli & Lemon, Walkers* | 1 Pack/25g | 131.0 8.0 | 525 | 6.3 | 51.0 | 33.0 | 3.8 |
| Chinese Sizzling Beef, McCoys* | 1 Bag/35g | 178.0 11.0 | 506 | 6.9 | 51.8 | 30.2 | 4.0 |
| Chinese Spare Rib, Walkers* | 1 Bag/25g | 131.0 8.0 | 525 | 6.5 | 50.0 | 33.0 | 4.0 |
| Cider Vinegar & Sea Salt, Tyrells* | 1 Pack/40g | 192.0 10.0 | 481 | 7.2 | 60.1 | 24.6 | 2.4 |
| Cool Cheese Curly, Tesco* | 1 Bag/14g | 71.0 4.0 | 510 | 4.5 | 51.0 | 32.0 | 2.6 |
| Corn Chips, Fritos* | 1 Pack/43g | 240.0 15.0 | 565 | 4.7 | 56.5 | 35.3 | 0.0 |
| Coronation Chicken, Walkers* | 1 Bag/25g | 131.0 8.0 | 525 | 6.5 | 50.0 | 33.0 | 4.0 |
| Cracked Black Pepper Seasoned, TTD, Sainsbury's* | 1 Bag/30g | 145.0 8.0 | 484 | 7.0 | 54.6 | 26.4 | 4.0 |
| Cream Cheese & Chive, Waffles, Spar* | 1 Pack/27g | 132.0 7.0 | 488 | 4.2 | 60.7 | 25.3 | 1.3 |
| Crinkle Cut, Lower Fat, No Added Salt, Waitrose* | 1 Bag/40g | 193.0 10.0 | 483 | 6.5 | 58.0 | 25.0 | 3.9 |
| Curls, Cheesy, Asda* | 1 Pack/17g | 87.0 5.0 | 511 | 3.8 | 59.7 | 28.6 | 1.7 |
| Feta Cheese Flavour, Mediterranean, Walkers* | 1 Pack/25g | 127.0 8.0 | 510 | 6.5 | 49.0 | 33.0 | 4.5 |
| Flame Grilled Steak, Ridge Cut, McCoys* | 1 Bag/32g | 165.0 10.0 | 516 | 7.0 | 53.0 | 30.7 | 4.0 |
| Four Cheese & Red Onion, Sensations, Walkers* | 1 Bag/40g | 194.0 11.0 | 485 | 6.5 | 54.0 | 27.0 | 4.5 |
| Garlic & Herbs Creme Fraiche, Kettle Chips* | 1 Bag/50g | 248.0 14.0 | 497 | 6.0 | 54.7 | 28.3 | 4.2 |
| Greek Kebab, Mediterranean, Walkers* | 1 Pack/25g | 127.0 8.0 | 510 | 6.0 | 49.0 | 33.0 | 4.5 |
| Grilled Chicken Flavour, Golden Lights, Golden Wonder* | 1 Bag/21g | 93.0 4.0 | 444 | 4.4 | 66.2 | 18.0 | 4.3 |
| Heinz Tomato Ketchup, Sunseed, Walkers* | 1 Bag/35g | 179.0 11.0 | 520 | 6.5 | 51.0 | 32.0 | 4.0 |
| Honey & BBQ, Wholgrain, Snacks, M & S* | 1 Serving/30g | 145.0 7.0 | 485 | 7.8 | 57.6 | 24.9 | 5.2 |
| Honey Roasted Ham, Sensations, Walkers* | 1 Bag/40g | 196.0 11.0 | 490 | 6.5 | 55.0 | 27.0 | 4.0 |
| Hot & Spicy Salami, Tesco* | 1 Bag/50g | 215.0 18.0 | 431 | 26.2 | 0.7 | 35.9 | 0.0 |
| Jalapeno Peppers, Fire Roasted, Darling Spuds* | 1 Pack/40g | 191.0 11.0 | 478 | 6.3 | 53.4 | 28.5 | 4.5 |
| Lamb & Mint, Slow Roasted, Sensations, Walkers* | 1 Bag/35g | 170.0 9.0 | 485 | 6.5 | 54.0 | 27.0 | 4.5 |
| Lamb & Mint, Sunseed Oil, Walkers* | 1 Pack/35g | 181.0 11.0 | 525 | 6.5 | 50.0 | 33.0 | 4.0 |
| Lighly Salted, Organic, Kettle Chips* | 1 Serving/40g | 198.0 11.0 | 495 | 5.5 | 54.1 | 28.5 | 4.4 |
| Lightly Salted, Baked, COU, M & S* | 1 Bag/25g | 87.0 1.0 | 350 | 8.5 | 76.4 | 2.3 | 5.7 |
| Lightly Salted, Crinkle Cut, Low Fat, Waitrose* | 1 Pack/35g | 163.0 8.0 | 466 | 5.2 | 60.1 | 22.8 | 5.1 |
| Lightly Salted, Crinkles, Shapers, Boots* | 1 Pack/20g | 96.0 5.0 | 482 | 6.6 | 60.0 | 24.0 | 4.0 |
| Lightly Salted, Handcooked, Finest, Tesco* | ½ Pack/150g | 708.0 39.0 | 472 | 6.4 | 52.9 | 26.1 | 5.1 |
| Lightly Salted, Kettle Chips* | 1 Serving/50g | 242.0 13.0 | 485 | 3.2 | 55.1 | 26.6 | 5.2 |
| Lightly Salted, Potato Bakes, Weight Watchers* | 1 Pack/20g | 78.0 2.0 | 392 | 5.0 | 72.0 | 9.0 | 5.0 |
| Lightly Salted, Reduced Fat, Crinkles, Eat Well, M & S* | 1 Pack/30g | 140.0 7.0 | 460 | 6.7 | 59.4 | 21.8 | 4.5 |
| Lightly Salted, Traditional Pan Fried, TTD, Sainsbury's* | 1 Bag/50g | 236.0 13.0 | 472 | 6.2 | 53.6 | 25.8 | 5.1 |
| Lightly Sea Salted, Jonathan Crisp* | 1 Bag/35g | 176.0 10.0 | 503 | 6.5 | 52.0 | 29.0 | 5.4 |
| Lime & Thai Spices, Gently Infused, Sensations, Walkers* | 1 Pack/40g | 200.0 12.0 | 500 | 6.5 | 54.0 | 29.0 | 4.0 |
| Lincolnshire Sausage, Tyrells* | 1 Pack/100g | 530.0 28.0 | 530 | 8.6 | 60.8 | 28.2 | 3.0 |
| Mango & Chilli, Baked, Walkers* | 1 Packet/38g | 147.0 3.0 | 393 | 6.3 | 73.8 | 8.1 | 4.8 |
| Mango Chilli, Kettle Chips* | 1 Serving/40g | 190.0 10.0 | 475 | 6.3 | 53.9 | 24.0 | 6.1 |
| Marmite, Sunseed, Walkers* | 1 Bag/35g | 179.0 11.0 | 520 | 6.5 | 49.0 | 33.0 | 4.0 |
| Mature Cheddar & Chive, Kettle Chips* | 1 Serving/50g | 239.0 13.0 | 478 | 8.1 | 54.4 | 25.4 | 5.0 |
| Mature Cheddar & Chive, Tyrells* | 1 Bag/40g | 194.0 10.0 | 485 | 8.4 | 58.7 | 25.1 | 2.4 |
| Mediterranean Baked Potato, COU, M & S* | 1 Pack/25g | 90.0 1.0 | 360 | 7.6 | 74.0 | 2.4 | 6.8 |
| Mexian Chilli & Chesse, Golden Wonder* | 1 Pack/45g | 230.0 14.0 | 511 | 6.6 | 50.7 | 31.3 | 0.0 |
| Mexican Chilli, Ridge Cut, McCoys* | 1 Bag/50g | 257.0 15.0 | 514 | 6.9 | 53.0 | 30.5 | 4.5 |
| Mexican Lime with a Hint of Chilli, Kettle Chips* | 1 Serving/50g | 242.0 14.0 | 484 | 5.0 | 54.1 | 27.5 | 5.4 |
| Mixed Pepper Flavour Burst, M & S* | 1 Bag/55g | 286.0 18.0 | 520 | 6.0 | 50.1 | 33.5 | 4.0 |

# CRISPS

| INFO/WEIGHT | Measure | per Measure | | Nutrition Values per 100g / 100ml | | | | |
|---|---|---|---|---|---|---|---|---|
| | | KCAL | FAT | KCAL | PROT | CARB | FAT | FIBRE |
| New York Cheddar, Kettle Chips* | 1 Bag/50g | 241.0 | 13.0 | 483 | 6.7 | 53.9 | 26.7 | 4.5 |
| Nicely Spicy, Shots, Walkers* | 1 Bag/18g | 87.0 | 4.0 | 485 | 5.5 | 60.0 | 25.0 | 1.5 |
| Olive Oil, Mozzarella & Oregano, Walkers* | 1 Serving/30g | 151.0 | 9.0 | 505 | 6.5 | 54.0 | 29.0 | 4.0 |
| Onion Rings, Crunchy, Shapers, Boots* | 1 Bag/12g | 61.0 | 3.0 | 507 | 2.5 | 62.0 | 28.0 | 2.6 |
| Onion Rings, Maize Snacks, Sainsbury's* | ¼ Bag/25g | 122.0 | 7.0 | 488 | 5.6 | 56.9 | 26.4 | 1.7 |
| Onion Rings, Tesco* | 1 Serving/30g | 148.0 | 8.0 | 495 | 8.4 | 57.8 | 25.5 | 2.5 |
| Oriental Ribs, Ridge Cut, McCoys* | 1 Pack/50g | 255.0 | 15.0 | 511 | 7.3 | 52.7 | 30.1 | 4.2 |
| Paprika, Handcooked, Shapers, Boots* | 1 Bag/20g | 99.0 | 5.0 | 493 | 7.2 | 62.0 | 24.0 | 5.0 |
| Paprika, Max, Walkers* | 1 Bag/50g | 260.0 | 16.0 | 520 | 6.5 | 52.0 | 31.9 | 5.1 |
| Paprika, Mini Hoops, Shapers, Boots* | 1 Bag/13g | 64.0 | 4.0 | 494 | 8.7 | 54.0 | 27.0 | 2.2 |
| Parsnip, Passions, Snack Rite* | 1 Serving/25g | 123.0 | 9.0 | 494 | 4.5 | 34.5 | 37.6 | 18.8 |
| Parsnip & Black Pepper, Sainsbury's* | 1 Serving/35g | 166.0 | 11.0 | 473 | 3.2 | 43.6 | 31.8 | 15.2 |
| Pastrami & Cheese, Crinkle, M & S* | 1 Bag/25g | 120.0 | 6.0 | 485 | 6.5 | 61.0 | 24.0 | 3.5 |
| Peri Peri Chicken, Nando's* | ½ Bag/75g | 410.0 | 20.0 | 547 | 5.1 | 57.4 | 27.0 | 3.4 |
| Pickled Onion, Golden Wonder* | 1 Bag/25g | 131.0 | 8.0 | 524 | 5.6 | 49.0 | 34.0 | 2.0 |
| Pickled Onion, M & S* | 1 Bag/20g | 70.0 | 0.0 | 345 | 5.0 | 81.7 | 1.5 | 3.7 |
| Pickled Onion, Monster Bites, Sainsbury's* | 1 Bag/20g | 107.0 | 7.0 | 535 | 5.2 | 53.5 | 33.3 | 1.0 |
| Pickled Onion, Stompers, Morrisons* | 1 Pack/25g | 129.0 | 8.0 | 518 | 6.1 | 52.2 | 31.6 | 1.3 |
| Pickled Onion, Sunseed, Walkers* | 1 Bag/35g | 181.0 | 11.0 | 525 | 6.5 | 50.0 | 33.0 | 4.0 |
| Pickled Onion Rings, BGTY, Sainsbury's* | 1 Bag/10g | 34.0 | 0.0 | 345 | 5.0 | 81.7 | 1.5 | 3.7 |
| Pickled Onion Rings, COU, M & S* | 1 Bag/20g | 69.0 | 0.0 | 345 | 5.0 | 81.7 | 1.5 | 3.7 |
| Potato | 1oz/28g | 148.0 | 10.0 | 530 | 5.7 | 53.3 | 34.2 | 5.3 |
| Potato, Baked, COU, M & S* | 1 Bag/25g | 87.0 | 1.0 | 350 | 8.5 | 76.4 | 2.3 | 5.7 |
| Potato, Low Fat | 1oz/28g | 128.0 | 6.0 | 458 | 6.6 | 63.5 | 21.5 | 5.9 |
| Potato, Tyrells* | 1 Pack/261g | 1362.0 | 73.0 | 522 | 6.1 | 56.5 | 27.9 | 0.0 |
| Potato Chips, Anglesey Sea Salt, Red Sky* | 1 Serving/40g | 185.0 | 9.0 | 463 | 6.8 | 59.8 | 21.8 | 5.0 |
| Potato Chips, Roasted Red Pepper & Lime, Red Sky* | 1 Serving/40g | 187.0 | 9.0 | 467 | 6.8 | 59.5 | 22.4 | 4.8 |
| Potato Chips, Sour Cream & Green Herbs, Red Sky* | 1 Pack/40g | 188.0 | 9.0 | 471 | 6.8 | 58.4 | 23.4 | 4.8 |
| Potato Fries, Sea Salt & Malt Vinegar Flavour, GFY, Asda* | 1 Bag/15g | 54.0 | 0.0 | 358 | 6.3 | 79.6 | 1.7 | 2.1 |
| Potato Squares, Ready Salted, Sainsbury's* | 1 Bag/50g | 192.0 | 8.0 | 384 | 6.5 | 53.8 | 15.9 | 7.8 |
| Potato Thins, Light Choices, Tesco* | 1 Pack/20g | 72.0 | 0.0 | 360 | 5.1 | 79.5 | 2.0 | 4.2 |
| Potato Thins, Lightly Salted, Tesco* | 1 Bag/20g | 72.0 | 16.0 | 360 | 5.1 | 79.5 | 79.5 | 4.2 |
| Potato Triangles, Ready Salted, Sainsbury's* | ½ Pack/50g | 243.0 | 12.0 | 486 | 9.4 | 59.7 | 23.4 | 3.4 |
| Prawn Cocktail, Asda* | 1 Bag/25g | 134.0 | 9.0 | 535 | 6.0 | 49.0 | 35.0 | 4.3 |
| Prawn Cocktail, BGTY, Sainsbury's* | 1 Bag/25g | 118.0 | 6.0 | 473 | 6.3 | 58.6 | 23.7 | 5.7 |
| Prawn Cocktail, Golden Wonder* | 1 Bag/25g | 130.0 | 8.0 | 521 | 5.8 | 49.0 | 33.5 | 2.0 |
| Prawn Cocktail, KP Snacks* | 1 Bag/25g | 133.0 | 9.0 | 531 | 5.9 | 48.4 | 34.9 | 4.7 |
| Prawn Cocktail, Lites, Advantage, Tayto* | 1 Pack/21g | 96.0 | 4.0 | 455 | 5.3 | 65.1 | 19.3 | 3.8 |
| Prawn Cocktail, Lites, Shapers, Boots* | 1 Bag/21g | 92.0 | 4.0 | 438 | 5.1 | 64.0 | 18.0 | 4.1 |
| Prawn Cocktail, Sainsbury's* | 1 Bag/25g | 130.0 | 9.0 | 521 | 4.3 | 47.5 | 34.9 | 3.9 |
| Prawn Cocktail, Seabrook* | 1 Bag/32g | 150.0 | 7.0 | 472 | 5.3 | 66.7 | 22.3 | 3.8 |
| Prawn Cocktail, Sunseed Oil, Walkers* | 1 Bag/35g | 181.0 | 11.0 | 525 | 6.5 | 50.0 | 33.0 | 4.0 |
| Prawn Cocktail, Tesco* | 1 Pack/25g | 135.0 | 8.0 | 540 | 5.2 | 52.0 | 32.8 | 4.0 |
| Prawn Cocktail Flavour, Morrisons* | 1 Bag/25g | 131.0 | 8.0 | 525 | 5.1 | 51.9 | 33.0 | 4.1 |
| Ready Salted, BGTY, Sainsbury's* | 1 Bag/25g | 121.0 | 7.0 | 486 | 6.8 | 55.7 | 26.2 | 6.6 |
| Ready Salted, GFY, Asda* | 1 Bag/23g | 109.0 | 5.0 | 475 | 7.0 | 60.0 | 23.0 | 4.3 |
| Ready Salted, Golden Wonder* | 1 Bag/25g | 135.0 | 9.0 | 539 | 5.5 | 49.9 | 35.3 | 2.0 |
| Ready Salted, KP Snacks* | 1 Bag/24g | 131.0 | 9.0 | 545 | 5.6 | 47.9 | 36.8 | 4.9 |
| Ready Salted, M & S* | 1 Bag/25g | 136.0 | 9.0 | 545 | 5.6 | 47.8 | 36.6 | 4.9 |
| Ready Salted, Morrisons* | 1 Bag/25g | 134.0 | 9.0 | 536 | 4.9 | 50.9 | 34.8 | 4.3 |
| Ready Salted, Organic, Tesco* | 1 Bag/25g | 130.0 | 9.0 | 520 | 4.3 | 49.0 | 34.1 | 7.3 |
| Ready Salted, Oven Baked, Asda* | 1 Bag/25g | 95.0 | 2.0 | 379 | 4.4 | 73.1 | 7.7 | 2.6 |
| Ready Salted, Oven Baked, Tesco* | 1 Bag/25g | 95.0 | 2.0 | 380 | 4.4 | 73.1 | 7.7 | 8.4 |

## CRISPS

| | Measure INFO/WEIGHT | per Measure KCAL | FAT | Nutrition Values per 100g / 100ml KCAL | PROT | CARB | FAT | FIBRE |
|---|---|---|---|---|---|---|---|---|
| Ready Salted, Reduced Fat, Tesco* | 1 Pack/25g | 114.0 | 6.0 | 456 | 6.3 | 52.0 | 24.7 | 5.9 |
| Ready Salted, Ridge Cut, McCoys* | 1 Bag/49g | 257.0 | 16.0 | 524 | 6.6 | 52.6 | 31.9 | 4.1 |
| Ready Salted, Sainsbury's* | 1 Bag/25g | 134.0 | 9.0 | 538 | 4.3 | 47.4 | 36.8 | 4.1 |
| Ready Salted, Select, Tesco* | 1 Bag/25g | 136.0 | 9.0 | 544 | 6.2 | 47.9 | 36.6 | 4.5 |
| Ready Salted, SmartPrice, Asda* | 1 Bag/20g | 111.0 | 7.0 | 553 | 5.0 | 50.0 | 37.0 | 3.0 |
| Ready Salted, Snack Rite* | 1 Bag/25g | 136.0 | 9.0 | 545 | 4.9 | 50.3 | 36.0 | 0.0 |
| Ready Salted, Squares, M & S* | 1 Bag/35g | 150.0 | 6.0 | 430 | 6.8 | 63.5 | 18.1 | 3.9 |
| Ready Salted, Squares, Walkers* | 1 Pack/25g | 109.0 | 5.0 | 435 | 6.5 | 60.0 | 19.0 | 6.0 |
| Ready Salted, Sunseed Oil, Walkers* | 1 Bag/35g | 183.0 | 12.0 | 530 | 6.5 | 49.0 | 34.0 | 4.0 |
| Ready Salted, Thick & Chunky Ridge, Tesco* | 1 Pack/25g | 129.0 | 8.0 | 515 | 5.9 | 53.5 | 30.6 | 4.1 |
| Ready Salted, Value, Tesco* | 1 Bag/21g | 115.0 | 8.0 | 548 | 6.0 | 50.0 | 36.0 | 0.0 |
| Red Leicester & Spring Onion, Handcooked, M & S* | 1 Pack/40g | 194.0 | 11.0 | 485 | 6.8 | 55.0 | 26.4 | 5.1 |
| Roast Beef, KP Snacks* | 1 Bag/25g | 133.0 | 9.0 | 534 | 6.6 | 47.5 | 35.3 | 4.7 |
| Roast Beef & Mustard, Thick Cut, Brannigans* | 1 Bag/40g | 203.0 | 12.0 | 507 | 7.6 | 51.7 | 30.0 | 3.7 |
| Roast Chicken, 30% Less Fat, Sainsbury's* | 1 Pack/25g | 115.0 | 5.0 | 460 | 7.4 | 58.3 | 21.9 | 5.2 |
| Roast Chicken, Golden Wonder* | 1 Bag/25g | 130.0 | 8.0 | 522 | 6.2 | 48.6 | 33.6 | 2.0 |
| Roast Chicken, Select, Tesco* | 1 Bag/25g | 134.0 | 9.0 | 536 | 6.6 | 48.6 | 35.0 | 4.4 |
| Roast Chicken, Snack Rite* | 1 Bag/25g | 131.0 | 8.0 | 526 | 5.3 | 51.3 | 33.3 | 0.0 |
| Roast Chicken, Sunseed Oil, Walkers* | 1 Bag/35g | 181.0 | 11.0 | 525 | 6.5 | 50.0 | 33.0 | 4.0 |
| Roast Chicken & Sage Flavour, M & S* | 1 Bag/25g | 135.0 | 9.0 | 540 | 5.9 | 50.6 | 34.6 | 4.6 |
| Roast Chicken Flavour, BGTY, Sainsbury's* | 1 Bag/25g | 118.0 | 6.0 | 473 | 6.2 | 58.9 | 23.6 | 5.7 |
| Roast Ham & Mustard, Ridge Cut, McCoys* | 1 Pack/35g | 181.0 | 11.0 | 518 | 7.1 | 53.5 | 30.6 | 3.9 |
| Roast Pork & Apple Sauce, Select, Tesco* | 1 Bag/25g | 136.0 | 9.0 | 544 | 6.5 | 50.0 | 35.3 | 3.7 |
| Roasted Lamb, Moroccan Spices, Sensations, Walkers* | 1 Bag/40g | 198.0 | 12.0 | 495 | 6.0 | 53.0 | 29.0 | 4.5 |
| Root Vegetable, TTD, Sainsbury's* | ¼ Pack/25g | 115.0 | 8.0 | 460 | 5.7 | 35.9 | 32.6 | 16.4 |
| Salsa with Mesquite, Kettle Chips* | 1 Serving/50g | 231.0 | 12.0 | 462 | 5.8 | 55.2 | 24.2 | 5.7 |
| Salt & Balsamic Vinegar, Perfectly Balanced, Waitrose* | 1 Bag/20g | 69.0 | 1.0 | 347 | 4.2 | 76.4 | 2.7 | 5.2 |
| Salt & Black Pepper, Handcooked, M & S* | 1 Bag/40g | 180.0 | 9.0 | 450 | 5.7 | 55.0 | 22.9 | 5.2 |
| Salt & Cracked Black Pepper, Shapers, Boots* | 1 Bag/20g | 91.0 | 4.0 | 453 | 7.2 | 57.0 | 22.0 | 5.0 |
| Salt & Malt Vinegar, Ridgecut, McCoys* | 1 Sm Bag/32g | 164.0 | 10.0 | 514 | 6.7 | 53.2 | 30.4 | 3.9 |
| Salt & Malt Vinegar Flavour, Sainsbury's* | 1 Bag/25g | 134.0 | 9.0 | 538 | 4.9 | 50.3 | 35.2 | 2.3 |
| Salt & Shake, Walkers* | 1 Bag/30g | 162.0 | 10.0 | 540 | 6.5 | 50.0 | 35.0 | 4.0 |
| Salt & Vinegar, BGTY, Sainsbury's* | 1 Bag/25g | 120.0 | 6.0 | 482 | 6.5 | 57.3 | 25.2 | 5.2 |
| Salt & Vinegar, Crinkle, M & S* | 1 Pack/25g | 120.0 | 6.0 | 485 | 6.5 | 61.0 | 24.0 | 3.5 |
| Salt & Vinegar, Crinkle Cut, Low Fat, Waitrose* | 1 Bag/25g | 121.0 | 6.0 | 484 | 7.1 | 61.3 | 23.4 | 4.5 |
| Salt & Vinegar, Crinkles, Shapers, Boots* | 1 Pack/20g | 96.0 | 5.0 | 482 | 6.6 | 60.0 | 24.0 | 4.0 |
| Salt & Vinegar, Crispy Discs, Boots* | 1 Bag/92g | 404.0 | 17.0 | 439 | 4.8 | 63.0 | 19.0 | 4.9 |
| Salt & Vinegar, Fish Shapes, Food Explorers, Waitrose* | 1 Bag/20g | 86.0 | 3.0 | 430 | 2.4 | 69.1 | 16.0 | 1.3 |
| Salt & Vinegar, GFY, Asda* | 1 Bag/26g | 120.0 | 6.0 | 466 | 6.0 | 61.0 | 22.0 | 4.1 |
| Salt & Vinegar, Golden Lights, Golden Wonder* | 1 Bag/21g | 94.0 | 4.0 | 446 | 4.2 | 65.7 | 18.5 | 3.7 |
| Salt & Vinegar, Golden Wonder* | 1 Bag/25g | 130.0 | 8.0 | 522 | 5.4 | 48.5 | 34.0 | 2.0 |
| Salt & Vinegar, in Sunflower Oil, Sainsbury's* | 1 Serving/25g | 131.0 | 8.0 | 524 | 5.2 | 49.7 | 33.8 | 3.7 |
| Salt & Vinegar, KP Snacks* | 1 Bag/25g | 133.0 | 9.0 | 532 | 5.5 | 48.7 | 35.0 | 4.7 |
| Salt & Vinegar, Lights, Walkers* | 1 Bag/28g | 133.0 | 6.0 | 475 | 7.0 | 62.0 | 22.0 | 4.5 |
| Salt & Vinegar, Limbos, Ryvita* | 1 Pack/18g | 62.0 | 0.0 | 344 | 9.8 | 72.0 | 1.9 | 7.8 |
| Salt & Vinegar, M & S* | 1 Bag/25g | 131.0 | 9.0 | 525 | 5.4 | 48.8 | 34.5 | 4.6 |
| Salt & Vinegar, Max, Walkers* | 1 Bag/55g | 289.0 | 18.0 | 525 | 6.5 | 50.0 | 33.0 | 4.0 |
| Salt & Vinegar, Potato Bakes, Weight Watchers* | 1 Bag/20g | 81.0 | 2.0 | 404 | 5.3 | 76.0 | 8.8 | 2.3 |
| Salt & Vinegar, Red Mill* | 1 Bag/40g | 174.0 | 7.0 | 436 | 3.9 | 65.8 | 17.5 | 2.4 |
| Salt & Vinegar, Sainsbury's* | 1 Bag/25g | 130.0 | 9.0 | 522 | 4.1 | 46.9 | 35.3 | 3.9 |
| Salt & Vinegar, Select, Tesco* | 1 Bag/25g | 132.0 | 9.0 | 529 | 5.9 | 47.8 | 34.9 | 4.3 |
| Salt & Vinegar, Snack Rite* | 1 Bag/25g | 127.0 | 8.0 | 508 | 4.7 | 48.1 | 33.0 | 0.0 |
| Salt & Vinegar, Squares, Walkers* | 1 Bag/25g | 107.0 | 4.0 | 430 | 6.5 | 61.0 | 18.0 | 5.5 |

## CRISPS

| Measure INFO/WEIGHT | | per Measure | | Nutrition Values per 100g / 100ml | | | | |
|---|---|---|---|---|---|---|---|---|
| | | KCAL | FAT | KCAL | PROT | CARB | FAT | FIBRE |
| Salt & Vinegar, Sunseed Oil, Walkers* | 1 Bag/35g | 181.0 | 11.0 | 525 | 6.5 | 50.0 | 33.0 | 4.0 |
| Salt & Vinegar, Value, Tesco* | 1 Bag/20g | 109.0 | 7.0 | 547 | 5.7 | 47.7 | 37.0 | 4.8 |
| Salt & Vinegar Fries, COU, M & S* | 1 Bag/25g | 85.0 | 0.0 | 340 | 5.0 | 80.0 | 1.6 | 4.0 |
| Salt & Vinegar Spirals, Shapers, Boots* | 1 Pack/15g | 71.0 | 3.0 | 475 | 3.1 | 64.0 | 23.0 | 1.7 |
| Salt Your Own, Jacket, 35% Less Fat, Sainsbury's* | 1 Bag/20g | 98.0 | 4.0 | 490 | 7.5 | 64.5 | 22.5 | 9.5 |
| Salt Your Own, Sainsbury's* | 1 Pack/24g | 127.0 | 8.0 | 520 | 5.0 | 52.2 | 32.3 | 3.7 |
| Salted Tubes, Shapers, Boots* | 1 Bag/15g | 67.0 | 3.0 | 448 | 5.1 | 62.0 | 20.0 | 3.6 |
| Sausage & Tomato, Sainsbury's* | 1 Pack/25g | 131.0 | 8.0 | 525 | 6.0 | 49.3 | 33.8 | 3.8 |
| Sausage & Tomato Flavour, Golden Wonder* | 1 Bag/35g | 174.0 | 11.0 | 505 | 6.1 | 51.3 | 30.6 | 4.5 |
| Sea Salt, Golden Lights, Golden Wonder* | 1 Bag/21g | 94.0 | 4.0 | 448 | 3.9 | 66.4 | 18.5 | 4.4 |
| Sea Salt, Handcooked, Extra Special, Asda* | 1 Pack/31g | 149.0 | 8.0 | 477 | 7.0 | 56.0 | 25.0 | 4.1 |
| Sea Salt, Original, Crinkle Cut, Seabrook* | 1 Bag/32g | 181.0 | 12.0 | 569 | 5.4 | 54.4 | 36.7 | 3.9 |
| Sea Salt, TTD, Sainsbury's* | 1 Serving/50g | 236.0 | 13.0 | 472 | 6.2 | 53.6 | 25.8 | 5.2 |
| Sea Salt & Balsamic Vinegar, Kettle Chips* | 1 Bag/40g | 190.0 | 10.0 | 476 | 5.9 | 56.8 | 25.0 | 4.5 |
| Sea Salt & Balsamic Vineger, Low Fat, Peak* | 1 Serving/25g | 87.0 | 0.0 | 348 | 7.4 | 76.6 | 1.4 | 6.7 |
| Sea Salt & Black Pepper, Shapers, Boots* | 1 Bag/20g | 96.0 | 5.0 | 482 | 6.6 | 60.0 | 24.0 | 4.0 |
| Sea Salt & Black Pepper, Tyrells* | ¼ Pack/38g | 182.0 | 9.0 | 480 | 7.3 | 59.9 | 24.5 | 2.4 |
| Sea Salt & Cracked Black Pepper, Lights, Walkers* | 1 Bag/24g | 115.0 | 5.0 | 480 | 7.0 | 63.0 | 22.0 | 5.0 |
| Sea Salt & Cracked Black Pepper, Sensations, Walkers* | 1 Bag/40g | 196.0 | 11.0 | 490 | 6.5 | 55.0 | 27.0 | 4.0 |
| Sea Salt & Malt Vinegar, Sensations, Walkers* | 1 Bag/40g | 194.0 | 11.0 | 485 | 6.5 | 54.0 | 27.0 | 4.5 |
| Simply Salted, Lights, Walkers* | 1 Bag/24g | 113.0 | 5.0 | 470 | 7.0 | 61.0 | 22.0 | 5.0 |
| Sizzling Beef, Spice, McCoys* | 1 Bag/35g | 175.0 | 10.0 | 501 | 6.4 | 51.7 | 29.8 | 4.0 |
| Sizzling King Prawn, Ridge Cut, McCoys* | 1 Packet/50g | 259.0 | 15.0 | 518 | 6.6 | 54.7 | 30.3 | 4.0 |
| Smoked Ham & Pickle, Thick Cut, Brannigans* | 1 Bag/40g | 203.0 | 12.0 | 507 | 7.0 | 52.8 | 29.8 | 3.8 |
| Smokey Bacon, Crinkle, Shapers, Boots* | 1 Pack/20g | 96.0 | 5.0 | 482 | 6.6 | 60.0 | 24.0 | 4.0 |
| Smokey Bacon, Limbos, Ryvita* | 1 Pack/18g | 63.0 | 0.0 | 350 | 0.0 | 7.8 | 1.7 | 7.8 |
| Smokey Bacon, Seabrook* | 1 Bag/32g | 181.0 | 12.0 | 569 | 5.4 | 54.4 | 36.7 | 3.9 |
| Smokey Bacon, Select, Tesco* | 1 Bag/25g | 134.0 | 9.0 | 536 | 6.4 | 49.0 | 34.9 | 4.3 |
| Smoky Bacon, 30% Lower Fat, Sainsbury's* | 1 Bag/25g | 118.0 | 6.0 | 471 | 6.5 | 58.4 | 23.6 | 5.7 |
| Smoky Bacon, BGTY, Sainsbury's* | 1 Bag/25g | 118.0 | 6.0 | 472 | 6.5 | 58.5 | 23.6 | 5.7 |
| Smoky Bacon, Golden Wonder* | 1 Bag/25g | 131.0 | 8.0 | 523 | 5.9 | 49.1 | 33.7 | 2.0 |
| Smoky Bacon, Sainsbury's* | 1 Bag/25g | 132.0 | 9.0 | 529 | 5.7 | 49.5 | 34.2 | 4.4 |
| Smoky Bacon, Sunseed Oil, Walkers* | 1 Bag/35g | 183.0 | 11.0 | 530 | 6.5 | 51.0 | 33.0 | 4.0 |
| Snaps, Spicy Tomato Flavour, Walkers* | 1 Bag/18g | 91.0 | 5.0 | 508 | 1.5 | 65.5 | 26.8 | 0.0 |
| Snax, Tayto* | 1 Pack/17g | 82.0 | 4.0 | 483 | 2.4 | 70.0 | 21.5 | 1.6 |
| Sour Cream & Chive, Crinkle, Reduced Fat, M & S* | 1 Bag/40g | 178.0 | 8.0 | 445 | 5.6 | 58.8 | 20.6 | 5.6 |
| Sour Cream & Chive, HE, Tesco* | 1 Bag/20g | 72.0 | 1.0 | 362 | 6.7 | 81.1 | 3.8 | 3.4 |
| Sour Cream & Chive, Lights, Walkers* | 1 Bag/24g | 114.0 | 5.0 | 475 | 7.5 | 62.0 | 22.0 | 5.0 |
| Sour Cream & Chive, Potato Bakes, Weight Watchers* | 1 Bag/20g | 83.0 | 2.0 | 417 | 3.8 | 80.7 | 8.8 | 3.6 |
| Sour Cream & Chive Crinkles, Shapers, Boots* | 1 Bag/20g | 96.0 | 5.0 | 482 | 6.6 | 60.0 | 24.0 | 4.0 |
| Sour Cream & Chive Crispy Discs, Shapers, Boots* | 1 Bag/21g | 94.0 | 4.0 | 448 | 5.7 | 61.9 | 19.0 | 4.3 |
| Sour Cream & Chives, Jordans* | 1 Bag/30g | 125.0 | 4.0 | 417 | 7.3 | 69.9 | 12.0 | 2.7 |
| Sour Cream & Onion, Golden Lights, Golden Wonder* | 1 Bag/21g | 93.0 | 4.0 | 442 | 4.1 | 66.0 | 17.9 | 4.4 |
| Space Raiders, Cheese, KP Snacks* | 1 Bag/16g | 76.0 | 4.0 | 473 | 7.1 | 61.6 | 22.0 | 3.1 |
| Space Raiders, Pickled Onion, KP Snacks* | 1 Bag/16g | 77.0 | 4.0 | 480 | 6.7 | 61.3 | 23.3 | 4.0 |
| Space Raiders, Salt & Vinegar, KP Snacks* | 1 Bag/17g | 81.0 | 4.0 | 478 | 6.9 | 61.7 | 22.6 | 2.2 |
| Spare Rib Flavour, Chinese, Walkers* | 1 Bag/35g | 181.0 | 11.0 | 525 | 6.5 | 50.0 | 33.0 | 4.0 |
| Spiced Chilli, McCoys* | 1 Bag/35g | 175.0 | 10.0 | 500 | 6.1 | 54.2 | 28.8 | 4.2 |
| Spicy Chilli, Sunseed, Walkers* | 1 Pack/35g | 183.0 | 11.0 | 530 | 6.5 | 51.0 | 33.0 | 4.0 |
| Spring Onion, Seabrook* | 1 Bag/32g | 182.0 | 12.0 | 569 | 5.4 | 54.4 | 36.7 | 3.9 |
| Spring Onion Flavour, M & S* | 1 Bag/40g | 210.0 | 14.0 | 525 | 5.9 | 48.7 | 34.3 | 5.1 |
| Steak & Onion, Walkers* | 1 Pack/35g | 179.0 | 11.0 | 520 | 6.5 | 49.0 | 33.0 | 4.0 |
| Stilton & Cranberry, TTD, Sainsbury's* | 1 Serving/50g | 238.0 | 13.0 | 477 | 6.7 | 54.6 | 25.7 | 4.6 |

| | Measure INFO/WEIGHT | per Measure KCAL | FAT | KCAL | PROT | CARB | FAT | FIBRE |
|---|---|---|---|---|---|---|---|---|
| **CRISPS** | | | | | | | | |
| Strawberry Raisin Snack, Fruitwonders, Golden Wonder* | 1 Bag/30g | 113.0 | 4.0 | 383 | 3.8 | 62.9 | 12.9 | 0.0 |
| Sun Dried Tomato & Basil, Jonathan Crisp* | 1 Pack/35g | 176.0 | 10.0 | 503 | 5.6 | 52.0 | 29.0 | 5.4 |
| Sun Dried Tomato & Chilli, Asda* | 1 Pack/150g | 700.0 | 34.0 | 467 | 7.0 | 58.0 | 23.0 | 4.1 |
| Sunbites, Sweet Chilli, Sun Ripened, Walkers* | 1 Bag/25g | 117.0 | 5.0 | 467 | 7.3 | 61.1 | 21.5 | 6.6 |
| Sweet Chill, Mexican, Phileas Fogg* | 1 Bag/38g | 193.0 | 11.0 | 507 | 6.7 | 54.8 | 29.0 | 4.2 |
| Sweet Chilli, Crinkle Cut, Weight Watchers* | 1 Sm Bag/20g | 80.0 | 2.0 | 400 | 4.5 | 74.5 | 9.5 | 4.0 |
| Sweet Chilli, Hand Cooked, Asda* | 1 Pack/25g | 120.0 | 7.0 | 479 | 5.7 | 54.5 | 28.3 | 4.5 |
| Sweet Chilli & Red Peppers, Fusion, Tayto* | 1 Bag/28g | 140.0 | 8.0 | 500 | 4.9 | 52.2 | 29.8 | 4.6 |
| T Bone Steak, Roysters* | 1 Pack/28g | 148.0 | 9.0 | 530 | 5.2 | 55.3 | 32.0 | 3.0 |
| Tangy Malaysian Chutney, Sensations, Walkers* | 1 Bag/24g | 116.0 | 6.0 | 485 | 0.9 | 62.0 | 26.0 | 0.0 |
| Tangy Tomato & Red Pepper Salsa, Sensations, Walkers* | 1 Bag/35g | 168.0 | 9.0 | 480 | 6.5 | 53.0 | 27.0 | 4.5 |
| Tangy Toms, Red Mill* | 1 Bag/15g | 76.0 | 4.0 | 507 | 6.0 | 60.0 | 27.3 | 0.7 |
| Thai Curry & Coriander, Tyrrell's* | 1 Pack/50g | 261.0 | 14.0 | 522 | 6.1 | 56.5 | 27.9 | 5.4 |
| Thai Green Curry, TTD, Sainsbury's* | 1 Bag/50g | 235.0 | 12.0 | 470 | 6.1 | 55.6 | 24.8 | 5.2 |
| Thai Sweet Chilli, Sensations, Walkers* | 1 Bag/40g | 202.0 | 12.0 | 505 | 6.5 | 54.0 | 29.0 | 4.5 |
| Tomato, Olive Oil & Basil, TTD, Sainsbury's* | 1 Bag/50g | 234.0 | 13.0 | 469 | 7.5 | 51.4 | 26.0 | 5.4 |
| Tomato & Basil, Mediterranean, Walkers* | 1 Pack/25g | 127.0 | 8.0 | 510 | 6.5 | 49.0 | 33.0 | 4.5 |
| Tomato & Herb, Shapers, Boots* | 1 Bag/20g | 94.0 | 4.0 | 468 | 3.7 | 66.0 | 21.0 | 3.9 |
| Tomato Sauce, Golden Wonder* | 1 Bag/25g | 130.0 | 8.0 | 521 | 5.7 | 49.2 | 33.5 | 2.0 |
| Tortillas, Nacho Cheese Flavour, Weight Watchers* | 1 Pack/18g | 78.0 | 3.0 | 433 | 6.1 | 66.7 | 16.1 | 3.9 |
| Traditional, Hand Cooked, Finest, Tesco* | 1 Bag/150g | 708.0 | 39.0 | 472 | 6.4 | 52.9 | 26.1 | 5.1 |
| Tubes, Salt & Vinegar, HL, Tesco* | 1 Bag/17g | 61.0 | 0.0 | 357 | 3.2 | 82.4 | 1.6 | 3.0 |
| Turkey & Paxo, Walkers* | 1 Bag/35g | 181.0 | 11.0 | 525 | 6.4 | 50.1 | 33.0 | 4.1 |
| Unsalted, Potato Heads, Walkers* | 1 Serving/23g | 106.0 | 5.0 | 460 | 5.0 | 61.0 | 22.0 | 5.0 |
| Vegetable, Crunchy, Asda* | ½ Bag/50g | 251.0 | 12.0 | 502 | 1.4 | 70.0 | 24.0 | 6.0 |
| Vegetable, Finest, Tesco* | 1 Serving/50g | 203.0 | 13.0 | 406 | 5.0 | 39.0 | 25.5 | 14.6 |
| Waffles, Bacon Flavour, BGTY, Sainsbury's* | 1 Serving/12g | 41.0 | 0.0 | 345 | 6.4 | 79.7 | 1.4 | 2.9 |
| Wild Chilli, McCoys* | 1 Bag/50g | 255.0 | 15.0 | 510 | 6.0 | 53.2 | 30.3 | 4.8 |
| Wild Paprika Flavour, Croky* | 1 Pack/45g | 234.0 | 13.0 | 521 | 6.0 | 58.0 | 29.0 | 0.0 |
| Worcester Sauce, Sunseed Oil, Walkers* | 1 Bag/35g | 183.0 | 11.0 | 530 | 6.5 | 52.0 | 33.0 | 4.0 |
| Yoghurt & Green Onion, Kettle Chips* | 1 Serving/50g | 236.0 | 13.0 | 473 | 6.6 | 54.1 | 26.1 | 5.4 |
| **CRISPY PANCAKE** | | | | | | | | |
| Beef Bolognese, Findus* | 1 Pancake/65g | 104.0 | 3.0 | 160 | 6.5 | 25.0 | 4.0 | 1.0 |
| Chicken, Bacon & Sweetcorn, Findus* | 1 Pancake/63g | 101.0 | 3.0 | 160 | 5.5 | 26.0 | 4.0 | 1.1 |
| Minced Beef, Findus* | 1 Pancake/63g | 100.0 | 2.0 | 160 | 6.5 | 25.0 | 4.0 | 1.0 |
| Three Cheeses, Findus* | 1 Pancake/62g | 118.0 | 4.0 | 190 | 7.0 | 25.0 | 6.5 | 0.9 |
| **CROISSANT** | | | | | | | | |
| All Butter, BGTY, Sainsbury's* | 1 Croissant/44g | 151.0 | 7.0 | 343 | 9.3 | 42.7 | 14.8 | 1.8 |
| All Butter, Finest, Tesco* | 1 Croissant/77g | 328.0 | 18.0 | 426 | 8.6 | 44.9 | 23.6 | 1.9 |
| All Butter, M & S* | 1 Croissant/54g | 222.0 | 13.0 | 415 | 7.4 | 45.2 | 23.8 | 1.6 |
| All Butter, Mini, Sainsbury's* | 1 Croissant/35g | 150.0 | 9.0 | 428 | 9.2 | 42.6 | 24.5 | 1.2 |
| All Butter, Mini, Tesco* | 1 Croissant/35g | 150.0 | 8.0 | 430 | 9.3 | 45.2 | 23.5 | 2.0 |
| All Butter, Reduced Fat, Tesco* | 1 Croissant/52g | 164.0 | 6.0 | 315 | 7.5 | 47.4 | 10.6 | 1.8 |
| All Butter, Sainsbury's* | 1 Croissant/44g | 188.0 | 11.0 | 428 | 9.2 | 42.6 | 24.5 | 1.2 |
| All Butter, Tesco* | 1 Croissant/48g | 192.0 | 10.0 | 400 | 8.5 | 41.7 | 21.6 | 2.6 |
| All Butter, TTD, Sainsbury's* | 1 Croissant/75g | 362.0 | 24.0 | 483 | 8.3 | 40.2 | 32.1 | 2.9 |
| Average | 1 Croissant/50g | 180.0 | 10.0 | 360 | 8.3 | 38.3 | 20.3 | 1.6 |
| Butter, Asda* | 1 Croissant/46g | 191.0 | 11.0 | 416 | 8.0 | 42.0 | 24.0 | 1.9 |
| Butter, GFY, Asda* | 1 Croissant/44g | 153.0 | 7.0 | 352 | 6.0 | 46.0 | 16.0 | 2.0 |
| Butter, Part Bake, Morrisons* | 1 Croissant/45g | 179.0 | 8.0 | 397 | 7.3 | 49.6 | 18.8 | 1.9 |
| Cheese & Ham, Mini, Waitrose* | 1 Croissant/17g | 64.0 | 4.0 | 383 | 13.2 | 28.1 | 24.5 | 3.0 |
| Flaky Pastry with a Plain Chocolate Filling, Tesco* | 1 Croissant/78g | 318.0 | 19.0 | 408 | 6.5 | 41.0 | 24.3 | 2.0 |
| Heart Shaped, Breakfast in Bed, M & S* | 1 Croissant/54g | 230.0 | 14.0 | 430 | 8.2 | 43.7 | 25.5 | 1.2 |

C

| | Measure<br>INFO/WEIGHT | | per Measure<br>KCAL FAT | | Nutrition Values per 100g / 100ml<br>KCAL PROT CARB FAT FIBRE | | | | |
|---|---|---|---|---|---|---|---|---|---|

## CROISSANT

| | Measure INFO/WEIGHT | per Measure KCAL | FAT | KCAL | PROT | CARB | FAT | FIBRE |
|---|---|---|---|---|---|---|---|---|
| Homebake, Long Life, Stay Fresh Range, Harvestime* | 1 Croissant/44g | 159.0 | 6.0 | 362 | 7.6 | 51.9 | 13.7 | 1.9 |
| Low Fat, M & S* | 1 Croissant/45g | 180.0 | 9.0 | 400 | 8.2 | 46.0 | 20.2 | 1.8 |
| Organic, Tesco* | 1 Croissant/45g | 195.0 | 12.0 | 433 | 8.2 | 42.0 | 25.8 | 2.2 |
| Reduced Fat, Asda* | 1 Croissant/44g | 159.0 | 7.0 | 361 | 9.7 | 47.2 | 14.8 | 2.0 |
| Reduced Fat, Sainsbury's* | 1 Croissant/44g | 173.0 | 8.0 | 393 | 9.8 | 49.2 | 17.5 | 2.2 |
| Wholesome, Sainsbury's* | 1 Croissant/44g | 192.0 | 12.0 | 436 | 8.8 | 38.3 | 27.5 | 4.0 |
| with Egg, Cheese, & Ham, From Restaurant, Average | 1 Croissant/152g | 474.0 | 34.0 | 312 | 12.4 | 15.9 | 22.1 | 0.0 |

## CROQUETTES

| | Measure INFO/WEIGHT | per Measure KCAL | FAT | KCAL | PROT | CARB | FAT | FIBRE |
|---|---|---|---|---|---|---|---|---|
| Potato, Asda* | 3 Croquettes/81g | 144.0 | 6.0 | 177 | 2.0 | 26.5 | 7.0 | 2.2 |
| Potato, Birds Eye* | 1 Croquette/29g | 44.0 | 2.0 | 152 | 2.6 | 22.6 | 5.7 | 1.2 |
| Potato, Chunky, Aunt Bessie's* | 1 Serving/41g | 62.0 | 3.0 | 152 | 2.3 | 23.9 | 6.1 | 1.8 |
| Potato, Fried in Blended Oil, Average | 1 Croquette/80g | 171.0 | 10.0 | 214 | 3.7 | 21.6 | 13.1 | 1.3 |
| Potato, Gruyere & Rosemary, TTD, Sainsbury's* | 1 Croquette/42g | 102.0 | 6.0 | 245 | 5.7 | 21.8 | 15.0 | 1.8 |
| Potato, M & S* | 1 Croquette/41g | 68.0 | 4.0 | 165 | 2.4 | 19.3 | 8.8 | 2.2 |
| Potato, Sainsbury's* | 1 Croquette/28g | 50.0 | 2.0 | 180 | 2.8 | 22.6 | 8.6 | 2.5 |
| Potato & Parsnip, Finest, Tesco* | 2 Croquettes/74g | 155.0 | 7.0 | 210 | 6.0 | 23.2 | 9.9 | 3.9 |
| Vegetable, Sainsbury's* | 1 Serving/175g | 392.0 | 21.0 | 224 | 5.8 | 23.3 | 11.9 | 2.2 |

## CROUTONS

| | Measure INFO/WEIGHT | per Measure KCAL | FAT | KCAL | PROT | CARB | FAT | FIBRE |
|---|---|---|---|---|---|---|---|---|
| Fresh, M & S* | 1 Serving/10g | 53.0 | 3.0 | 530 | 11.4 | 50.0 | 32.8 | 3.2 |
| Garlic, Waitrose* | 1 Serving/40g | 209.0 | 12.0 | 522 | 10.8 | 52.1 | 30.0 | 2.7 |
| Herb, Sainsbury's* | 1 Serving/15g | 64.0 | 2.0 | 429 | 13.4 | 68.2 | 11.4 | 2.8 |
| Herb & Garlic, La Rochelle* | ¼ Pack/18g | 106.0 | 7.0 | 587 | 6.9 | 49.8 | 40.0 | 2.1 |
| Italian Salad, Sainsbury's* | 1 Pack/40g | 204.0 | 10.0 | 510 | 8.5 | 62.7 | 25.0 | 2.5 |
| La Rochelle* | 1 Bag/70g | 400.0 | 28.0 | 572 | 7.0 | 49.0 | 40.0 | 0.0 |
| Lightly Sea Salted, Asda* | 1 Serving/20g | 83.0 | 2.0 | 414 | 12.9 | 69.7 | 9.3 | 4.3 |
| Sun Dried Tomato, Sainsbury's* | ¼ Pack/15g | 75.0 | 4.0 | 497 | 11.7 | 55.2 | 25.5 | 2.5 |

## CRUDITE

| | Measure INFO/WEIGHT | per Measure KCAL | FAT | KCAL | PROT | CARB | FAT | FIBRE |
|---|---|---|---|---|---|---|---|---|
| Platter, Sainsbury's* | 1 Pack/275g | 96.0 | 1.0 | 35 | 1.4 | 6.6 | 0.3 | 1.6 |
| Selection, Prepared, M & S* | 1 Serving/250g | 75.0 | 1.0 | 30 | 1.4 | 5.8 | 0.4 | 2.0 |

## CRUMBLE

| | Measure INFO/WEIGHT | per Measure KCAL | FAT | KCAL | PROT | CARB | FAT | FIBRE |
|---|---|---|---|---|---|---|---|---|
| Apple | 1 Pot/240g | 497.0 | 12.0 | 207 | 0.9 | 40.5 | 5.0 | 1.1 |
| Apple, Basics, Sainsbury's* | ¼ Crumble/125g | 235.0 | 5.0 | 188 | 1.7 | 36.5 | 3.9 | 1.2 |
| Apple, Fresh, Chilled, Tesco* | ¼ Pack/150g | 367.0 | 13.0 | 245 | 2.8 | 38.0 | 8.9 | 1.4 |
| Apple, Frozen, Tesco* | ¼ Pack/150g | 345.0 | 16.0 | 230 | 2.1 | 30.7 | 10.9 | 3.9 |
| Apple, Sainsbury's* | 1 Crumble/565g | 1034.0 | 33.0 | 183 | 2.3 | 30.5 | 5.8 | 2.9 |
| Apple, Sara Lee* | 1 Serving/200g | 606.0 | 18.0 | 303 | 2.3 | 53.3 | 9.0 | 1.2 |
| Apple, Waitrose* | 1 Serving/125g | 310.0 | 3.0 | 248 | 2.2 | 54.5 | 2.3 | 1.2 |
| Apple, with Sultanas, Weight Watchers* | 1 Dessert/110g | 196.0 | 4.0 | 178 | 1.4 | 34.2 | 3.9 | 1.3 |
| Apple & Blackberry, Budgens* | 1 Serving/240g | 821.0 | 31.0 | 342 | 3.7 | 54.0 | 13.0 | 0.6 |
| Apple & Blackberry, Sainsbury's* | 1 Serving/110g | 232.0 | 6.0 | 211 | 3.0 | 37.1 | 5.6 | 2.1 |
| Apple & Blackberry, Somerfield* | 1 Serving/125g | 315.0 | 11.0 | 252 | 3.4 | 39.4 | 9.0 | 2.4 |
| Apple & Blackberry, Tesco* | 1 Crumble/335g | 737.0 | 32.0 | 220 | 2.8 | 30.7 | 9.6 | 2.0 |
| Apple & Blackberry, with Custard, Somerfield* | 1 Serving/120g | 324.0 | 15.0 | 270 | 2.3 | 36.3 | 12.5 | 1.1 |
| Apple & Custard, Asda* | 1 Serving/125g | 250.0 | 9.0 | 200 | 2.3 | 32.0 | 7.0 | 0.0 |
| Apple with Custard, Green's* | 1 Serving/79g | 171.0 | 5.0 | 216 | 1.9 | 37.0 | 6.7 | 1.2 |
| Apple with Custard, Individual, Sainsbury's* | 1 Pudding/120g | 286.0 | 14.0 | 238 | 2.0 | 31.4 | 11.6 | 2.4 |
| Bramley Apple, Favourites, M & S* | 1 Serving/140g | 390.0 | 14.0 | 279 | 4.6 | 43.2 | 9.9 | 1.2 |
| Bramley Apple, M & S* | 1 Serving/149g | 387.0 | 14.0 | 260 | 4.3 | 40.3 | 9.2 | 1.1 |
| Bramley Apple, Tesco* | 1/3 Pack/155g | 378.0 | 15.0 | 244 | 2.8 | 36.7 | 9.6 | 1.8 |
| Cauliflower & Camembert, Sainsbury's* | 1 Pack/400g | 588.0 | 43.0 | 147 | 5.5 | 6.9 | 10.8 | 0.7 |
| Fruit | 1oz/28g | 55.0 | 2.0 | 198 | 2.0 | 34.0 | 6.9 | 1.7 |
| Fruit, Wholemeal | 1oz/28g | 54.0 | 2.0 | 193 | 2.6 | 31.7 | 7.1 | 2.7 |
| Gooseberry, M & S* | 1 Serving/133g | 379.0 | 14.0 | 285 | 3.5 | 43.3 | 10.7 | 1.7 |

C

| | Measure INFO/WEIGHT | per Measure KCAL | FAT | Nutrition Values per 100g / 100ml KCAL | PROT | CARB | FAT | FIBRE |
|---|---|---|---|---|---|---|---|---|
| **CRUMBLE** | | | | | | | | |
| Rhubarb, Co-Op* | ¼ Crumble/110g | 269.0 | 8.0 | 245 | 2.0 | 42.0 | 7.0 | 1.0 |
| Rhubarb, M & S* | 1 Serving/133g | 366.0 | 13.0 | 275 | 3.4 | 42.6 | 9.9 | 1.4 |
| Rhubarb, Sainsbury's* | 1 Serving/50g | 112.0 | 3.0 | 224 | 3.1 | 40.4 | 5.6 | 1.8 |
| Rhubarb, Tesco* | 1/6 Crumble/117g | 228.0 | 10.0 | 195 | 2.8 | 27.3 | 8.3 | 1.7 |
| Rhubarb, with Custard, Sainsbury's* | 1 Serving/120g | 288.0 | 14.0 | 240 | 2.4 | 31.4 | 11.6 | 2.3 |
| **CRUMBLE MIX** | | | | | | | | |
| Luxury, Tesco* | ¼ Pack/55g | 243.0 | 9.0 | 441 | 5.7 | 67.9 | 16.3 | 3.2 |
| **CRUMBLE TOPPING** | | | | | | | | |
| Morrisons* | 1 Serving/40g | 179.0 | 7.0 | 448 | 5.4 | 69.5 | 16.5 | 2.8 |
| Sainsbury's* | 1 Serving/47g | 188.0 | 9.0 | 401 | 5.9 | 50.3 | 19.6 | 5.3 |
| **CRUMPETS** | | | | | | | | |
| Asda* | 1 Crumpet/45g | 85.0 | 0.0 | 188 | 6.0 | 39.0 | 0.9 | 2.1 |
| Finger, Sainsbury's* | 1 Crumpet/30g | 55.0 | 0.0 | 182 | 7.0 | 36.6 | 0.8 | 1.8 |
| Fruit, From Bakery, Tesco* | 1 Crumpet/73g | 161.0 | 2.0 | 220 | 6.2 | 43.2 | 2.3 | 1.1 |
| Golden Sun* | 1 Crumpet/43g | 83.0 | 1.0 | 193 | 7.8 | 37.1 | 1.6 | 1.6 |
| Kingsmill* | 1 Crumpet/55g | 99.0 | 0.0 | 180 | 5.8 | 37.5 | 0.8 | 1.7 |
| Less Than 2% Fat, M & S* | 1 Crumpet/61g | 116.0 | 1.0 | 190 | 8.0 | 36.9 | 1.3 | 2.1 |
| Morrisons* | 1 Crumpet/40g | 70.0 | 0.0 | 174 | 6.6 | 35.3 | 0.7 | 1.8 |
| Mother's Pride* | 1 Crumpet/43g | 80.0 | 0.0 | 185 | 5.6 | 38.3 | 1.0 | 2.3 |
| Perfectly Balanced, Waitrose* | 1 Crumpet/55g | 94.0 | 0.0 | 171 | 6.1 | 36.1 | 0.3 | 4.4 |
| Premium, TTD, Sainsbury's* | 1 Crumpet/56g | 101.0 | 1.0 | 180 | 7.3 | 34.8 | 1.3 | 5.2 |
| Sainsbury's* | 1 Crumpet/46g | 86.0 | 0.0 | 186 | 5.8 | 39.1 | 0.7 | 2.5 |
| SmartPrice, Asda* | 1 Crumpet/36g | 67.0 | 0.0 | 188 | 6.0 | 39.0 | 0.9 | 2.1 |
| Soldier, Mother's Pride* | 1 Crumpet/30g | 58.0 | 0.0 | 193 | 7.8 | 37.1 | 1.6 | 1.6 |
| Somerfield* | 1 Crumpet/41g | 79.0 | 0.0 | 192 | 5.9 | 39.9 | 1.0 | 2.5 |
| Square, Spongebob Squarepants* | 1 Crumpet/50g | 93.0 | 0.0 | 186 | 7.0 | 37.2 | 1.0 | 1.0 |
| Square, Tesco* | 1 Crumpet/60g | 101.0 | 0.0 | 168 | 6.3 | 33.8 | 0.8 | 2.7 |
| Toasted, Average | 1 Crumpet/40g | 80.0 | 0.0 | 199 | 6.7 | 43.4 | 1.0 | 2.0 |
| Toaster, Organic, Waitrose* | 1 Crumpet/55g | 95.0 | 0.0 | 172 | 7.3 | 34.4 | 0.6 | 4.6 |
| Value, Tesco* | 1 Crumpet/35g | 59.0 | 0.0 | 168 | 6.4 | 33.9 | 0.8 | 1.8 |
| Warburton's* | 1 Crumpet/58g | 100.0 | 0.0 | 172 | 5.5 | 36.0 | 0.7 | 2.2 |
| **CRUNCHIE** | | | | | | | | |
| Blast, Cadbury* | 1 Serving/42g | 199.0 | 8.0 | 480 | 4.7 | 69.6 | 20.1 | 0.7 |
| Cadbury* | 1 Bar/40g | 186.0 | 8.0 | 465 | 4.0 | 69.5 | 18.9 | 0.5 |
| Nuggets, Cadbury* | 1 Bag/125g | 569.0 | 20.0 | 455 | 3.8 | 73.1 | 16.4 | 0.0 |
| Treat Size, Cadbury* | 1 Treat Bar/17g | 80.0 | 3.0 | 470 | 4.0 | 71.5 | 18.4 | 0.0 |
| **CRUNCHY STICKS** | | | | | | | | |
| Ready Salted, M & S* | 1 Pack/75g | 397.0 | 25.0 | 530 | 5.6 | 52.2 | 33.0 | 3.8 |
| Ready Salted, Tesco* | 1 Serving/25g | 119.0 | 6.0 | 475 | 5.6 | 60.3 | 23.5 | 3.0 |
| Salt & Vinegar, BGTY, Sainsbury's* | 1 Bag/15g | 51.0 | 0.0 | 340 | 6.0 | 80.1 | 1.5 | 4.1 |
| Salt & Vinegar, Sainsbury's* | 1 Bag/25g | 118.0 | 6.0 | 474 | 5.9 | 58.0 | 24.3 | 2.4 |
| Salt & Vinegar, Shapers, Boots* | 1 Pack/21g | 96.0 | 4.0 | 457 | 5.7 | 66.7 | 18.1 | 2.4 |
| Salt & Vinegar, Tesco* | 1 Serving/25g | 117.0 | 6.0 | 470 | 6.9 | 55.7 | 24.4 | 2.7 |
| Salt & Vinegar, Value, Tesco* | 1 Bag/22g | 113.0 | 6.0 | 512 | 5.7 | 62.1 | 26.8 | 0.7 |
| **CRUSH** | | | | | | | | |
| Morello Cherry, Finest, Tesco* | 1 Bottle/250ml | 115.0 | 0.0 | 46 | 0.0 | 11.2 | 0.0 | 0.0 |
| Orange, Cool, Diet, Sainsbury's* | 1 Can/330ml | 10.0 | 0.0 | 3 | 0.0 | 0.6 | 0.0 | 0.0 |
| Orange & Raspberry, Safeway* | 1 Serving/100ml | 57.0 | 0.0 | 57 | 0.5 | 13.6 | 0.1 | 0.2 |
| Orange & Strawberry, Finest, Tesco* | 1 Bottle/250ml | 115.0 | 0.0 | 46 | 0.4 | 10.5 | 0.1 | 0.4 |
| Pineapple & Grapefruit, No Added Sugar, Morrisons* | 1 Glass/250ml | 10.0 | 0.0 | 4 | 0.2 | 1.2 | 0.0 | 0.0 |
| **CUCUMBER** | | | | | | | | |
| *Average* | *1 Serving/80g* | *8.0* | *0.0* | *10* | *0.7* | *1.5* | *0.1* | *0.6* |
| Crunchies, with a Yoghurt & Mint Dip, Shapers, Boots* | 1 Serving/110g | 35.0 | 1.0 | 32 | 2.1 | 3.7 | 0.9 | 0.8 |

**C**

| | Measure INFO/WEIGHT | per Measure KCAL | per Measure FAT | Nutrition Values per 100g / 100ml KCAL | PROT | CARB | FAT | FIBRE |
|---|---|---|---|---|---|---|---|---|
| **CUMIN** | | | | | | | | |
| *Seeds, Whole, Average* | *1 Tsp/2g* | *7.0* | *0.0* | *375* | *17.8* | *44.2* | *22.7* | *10.5* |
| **CUPCAKES** | | | | | | | | |
| Assorted, Sainsbury's* | 1 Cake/38g | 130.0 | 2.0 | 341 | 2.2 | 69.3 | 6.1 | 0.4 |
| Chocolate, 5% Fat, Sainsbury's* | 1 Cake/38g | 133.0 | 2.0 | 349 | 2.5 | 74.8 | 4.4 | 1.7 |
| Chocolate, BGTY, Sainsbury's* | 1 Cake/38g | 121.0 | 2.0 | 318 | 2.5 | 66.5 | 4.6 | 0.8 |
| Chocolate, COU, M & S* | 1 Cake/45g | 130.0 | 1.0 | 290 | 4.6 | 62.2 | 2.8 | 4.3 |
| Chocolate, Fabulous Bakin' Boys* | 1 Cupcake/34g | 152.0 | 8.0 | 448 | 4.0 | 54.0 | 24.0 | 1.0 |
| Chocolate, Lyons* | 1 Cake/39g | 125.0 | 2.0 | 321 | 2.4 | 67.5 | 4.6 | 0.8 |
| Lemon, COU, M & S* | 1 Cupcake/43g | 130.0 | 1.0 | 305 | 3.3 | 68.1 | 2.1 | 2.0 |
| Pink, M & S* | 1 Cupcake/39g | 160.0 | 3.0 | 410 | 2.5 | 81.3 | 8.5 | 0.6 |
| **CURACAO** | | | | | | | | |
| *Average* | *1 Shot/35ml* | *109.0* | *0.0* | *311* | *0.0* | *28.3* | *0.0* | *0.0* |
| **CURLY WURLY** | | | | | | | | |
| Cadbury* | 1 Bar/26g | 117.0 | 5.0 | 450 | 3.4 | 69.4 | 17.6 | 0.7 |
| Squirlies, Cadbury* | 1 Squirl/3g | 13.0 | 1.0 | 450 | 3.9 | 69.0 | 17.8 | 0.0 |
| **CURRANTS** | | | | | | | | |
| *Average* | *1oz/28g* | *75.0* | *0.0* | *267* | *2.3* | *67.8* | *0.4* | *1.9* |
| **CURRY** | | | | | | | | |
| & Chips, Curry Sauce, Chipped Potatoes, Kershaws* | 1 Serving/330g | 391.0 | 8.0 | 118 | 10.0 | 14.0 | 2.5 | 2.0 |
| Aubergine | 1oz/28g | 33.0 | 3.0 | 118 | 1.4 | 6.2 | 10.1 | 1.5 |
| Beef, Hot, Canned, M & S* | 1 Can/425g | 446.0 | 22.0 | 105 | 12.2 | 2.8 | 5.1 | 1.0 |
| Beef, Sainsbury's* | 1 Serving/400g | 552.0 | 33.0 | 138 | 10.7 | 5.4 | 8.2 | 0.9 |
| Beef, Thai, Finest, Tesco* | 1 Serving/500g | 770.0 | 29.0 | 154 | 9.0 | 16.5 | 5.8 | 1.2 |
| Beef, with Rice, Asda* | 1 Pack/406g | 548.0 | 16.0 | 135 | 6.0 | 19.0 | 3.9 | 1.2 |
| Beef, with Rice, Birds Eye* | 1 Pack/388g | 524.0 | 11.0 | 135 | 6.9 | 20.8 | 2.8 | 0.8 |
| Beef, with Rice, Healthy Choice, Asda* | 1 Pack/400g | 476.0 | 10.0 | 119 | 6.0 | 18.0 | 2.6 | 0.9 |
| Beef, with Rice, Iceland* | 1 Pack/400g | 404.0 | 7.0 | 101 | 6.7 | 14.7 | 1.7 | 1.0 |
| Beef, with Rice, Morrisons* | 1 Serving/400g | 480.0 | 20.0 | 120 | 6.0 | 12.6 | 5.0 | 0.6 |
| Beef, with Rice, Tesco* | 1 Pack/400g | 456.0 | 13.0 | 114 | 4.5 | 16.7 | 3.3 | 0.6 |
| Beef, with Rice, Weight Watchers* | 1 Pack/328g | 249.0 | 3.0 | 76 | 4.2 | 12.5 | 1.0 | 0.3 |
| Blackeye Bean, Gujerati | 1oz/28g | 36.0 | 1.0 | 127 | 7.2 | 16.1 | 4.4 | 2.8 |
| Cabbage | 1oz/28g | 23.0 | 1.0 | 82 | 1.9 | 8.1 | 5.0 | 2.1 |
| Cauliflower & Potato | 1oz/28g | 17.0 | 1.0 | 59 | 3.4 | 6.6 | 2.4 | 1.8 |
| Chick Pea, Whole, Average | 1oz/28g | 50.0 | 2.0 | 179 | 9.6 | 21.3 | 7.5 | 4.5 |
| Chicken, & Rice, International Cuisine* | 1 Serving/400g | 420.0 | 12.0 | 105 | 3.3 | 16.4 | 2.9 | 0.8 |
| Chicken, & Rice, Value, Tesco* | 1 Pack/300g | 399.0 | 14.0 | 133 | 6.5 | 16.2 | 4.7 | 1.0 |
| Chicken, Asda* | 1 Can/200g | 210.0 | 10.0 | 105 | 10.0 | 5.0 | 5.0 | 0.0 |
| Chicken, Canned, Sainsbury's* | 1 Serving/100g | 136.0 | 6.0 | 136 | 11.1 | 9.1 | 6.1 | 1.0 |
| Chicken, Chinese with Egg Fried Rice, Morrisons* | 1 Pack/500g | 600.0 | 15.0 | 120 | 5.7 | 17.4 | 3.1 | 0.9 |
| Chicken, Frozen, Sainsbury's* | 1 Serving/400g | 528.0 | 16.0 | 132 | 5.8 | 18.0 | 4.1 | 0.7 |
| Chicken, Green Thai, BGTY, Sainsbury's* | 1 Pack/400g | 316.0 | 10.0 | 79 | 10.6 | 3.4 | 2.6 | 1.9 |
| Chicken, Green Thai, Birds Eye* | 1 Pack/450g | 535.0 | 20.0 | 119 | 4.7 | 15.2 | 4.4 | 0.3 |
| Chicken, Green Thai, Breasts, Finest, Tesco* | 1 Serving/200g | 292.0 | 16.0 | 146 | 16.5 | 2.0 | 8.0 | 0.7 |
| Chicken, Green Thai, Jasmine Rice, Weight Watchers* | 1 Pack/320g | 291.0 | 3.0 | 91 | 6.1 | 14.3 | 1.0 | 0.5 |
| Chicken, Green Thai, Sainsbury's* | ½ Pack/200g | 264.0 | 14.0 | 132 | 13.0 | 4.8 | 6.8 | 0.9 |
| Chicken, Green Thai Style, & Sticky Rice, Asda* | 1 Pack/450g | 585.0 | 11.0 | 130 | 7.0 | 20.0 | 2.4 | 0.1 |
| Chicken, Hot, Can, Tesco* | 1 Can/418g | 514.0 | 26.0 | 123 | 9.7 | 6.9 | 6.3 | 0.9 |
| Chicken, Hot, Iceland* | 1 Can/392g | 492.0 | 20.0 | 126 | 9.9 | 9.8 | 5.2 | 0.7 |
| Chicken, Kashmiri, Waitrose* | 1 Serving/400g | 640.0 | 36.0 | 160 | 14.5 | 5.0 | 9.1 | 0.6 |
| Chicken, Medium Hot, M & S* | 1 Serving/200g | 310.0 | 14.0 | 155 | 7.8 | 14.3 | 7.1 | 0.8 |
| Chicken, Mild, Asda* | ½ Can/190g | 239.0 | 11.0 | 126 | 11.0 | 7.0 | 6.0 | 0.5 |
| Chicken, Mild, BGTY, Sainsbury's* | 1 Serving/200g | 184.0 | 5.0 | 92 | 10.0 | 7.2 | 2.6 | 0.5 |
| Chicken, Mild, Sainsbury's* | 1 Can/400g | 472.0 | 28.0 | 118 | 10.5 | 3.5 | 6.9 | 1.3 |

C

# CURRY

| INFO/WEIGHT | Measure | per Measure KCAL | FAT | KCAL | PROT | CARB | FAT | FIBRE |
|---|---|---|---|---|---|---|---|---|
| Chicken, Mild, Tinned, Sainsbury's* | 1 Serving/200g | 214.0 | 7.0 | 107 | 12.7 | 6.1 | 3.5 | 1.1 |
| Chicken, Red Thai, 97% Fat Free, Birds Eye* | 1 Pack/366g | 425.0 | 7.0 | 116 | 5.7 | 19.0 | 1.9 | 0.5 |
| Chicken, Red Thai, Asda* | 1 Pack/360g | 461.0 | 28.0 | 128 | 9.1 | 5.5 | 7.7 | 1.0 |
| Chicken, Red Thai, COU, M & S* | 1 Pack/400g | 420.0 | 9.0 | 105 | 7.1 | 13.4 | 2.3 | 1.4 |
| Chicken, Red Thai, Tesco* | 1 Serving/175g | 215.0 | 12.0 | 123 | 10.5 | 5.5 | 6.6 | 1.4 |
| Chicken, Red Thai, with Jasmine Rice, Weight Watchers* | 1 Pack/400g | 344.0 | 3.0 | 86 | 6.5 | 12.9 | 0.8 | 0.8 |
| Chicken, Red Thai, with Rice, Tesco* | 1 Serving/475g | 746.0 | 32.0 | 157 | 7.2 | 16.8 | 6.8 | 1.1 |
| Chicken, Reduced Fat, Asda* | 1 Pack/400g | 476.0 | 10.0 | 119 | 6.0 | 18.0 | 2.6 | 0.9 |
| Chicken, SmartPrice, Asda* | 1 Can/392g | 282.0 | 5.0 | 72 | 4.0 | 11.0 | 1.3 | 1.0 |
| Chicken, Thai, Red, GFY, Asda* | 1 Serving/400g | 364.0 | 8.0 | 91 | 6.0 | 12.0 | 2.1 | 1.6 |
| Chicken, Thai, Red, HE, Tesco* | 1 Pack/380g | 399.0 | 7.0 | 105 | 7.0 | 14.5 | 1.9 | 0.9 |
| Chicken, Thai, Tom Yum, Sainsbury's* | 1 Pot/400g | 416.0 | 20.0 | 104 | 11.1 | 3.5 | 5.1 | 1.9 |
| Chicken, Thai, with Rice, Oriental Express* | 1 Pack/340g | 303.0 | 4.0 | 89 | 4.1 | 15.3 | 1.3 | 1.2 |
| Chicken, Thai Green, Nutritionally Balanced, M & S* | 1 Pack/400g | 400.0 | 5.0 | 100 | 9.2 | 12.4 | 1.3 | 1.4 |
| Chicken, Thai Mango, Sainsbury's* | ½ Pack/200g | 288.0 | 18.0 | 144 | 11.2 | 4.8 | 8.9 | 1.9 |
| Chicken, Thai Peanut, Sainsbury's* | ½ Pack/200g | 314.0 | 19.0 | 157 | 12.8 | 4.9 | 9.6 | 1.2 |
| Chicken, Value, Tesco* | 1 Pack/300g | 399.0 | 16.0 | 133 | 5.5 | 15.9 | 5.2 | 1.7 |
| Chicken, Weight Watchers* | 1 Pack/300g | 303.0 | 6.0 | 101 | 4.8 | 16.0 | 2.0 | 0.1 |
| Chicken, with Potato Wedges, HE, Tesco* | 1 Pack/450g | 427.0 | 12.0 | 95 | 7.6 | 10.3 | 2.7 | 1.1 |
| Chicken, with Rice, Asda* | 1 Pack/400g | 492.0 | 12.0 | 123 | 6.0 | 18.0 | 3.0 | 1.0 |
| Chicken, with Rice, Birds Eye* | 1 Pack/400g | 408.0 | 8.0 | 102 | 6.5 | 14.6 | 2.0 | 7.6 |
| Chicken, with Rice, Frozen, Tesco* | 1 Pack/400g | 488.0 | 16.0 | 122 | 4.6 | 17.2 | 3.9 | 0.7 |
| Chicken, with Rice, Fruity, HL, Tesco* | 1 Pack/450g | 495.0 | 5.0 | 110 | 6.5 | 18.2 | 1.2 | 1.2 |
| Chicken, with Rice, Hot, Asda* | 1 Pack/400g | 476.0 | 12.0 | 119 | 5.0 | 18.0 | 3.0 | 1.0 |
| Chicken, with Rice, Malaysian, Bernard Matthews* | 1 Pack/400g | 512.0 | 16.0 | 128 | 6.1 | 17.0 | 3.9 | 0.0 |
| Chicken, with Rice, Morrisons* | 1 Pack/300g | 345.0 | 6.0 | 115 | 5.5 | 18.7 | 2.0 | 0.4 |
| Chicken, with Rice, Quick Bite, Asda* | 1 Serving/300g | 294.0 | 10.0 | 98 | 5.0 | 12.0 | 3.3 | 0.5 |
| Chicken, with Rice, Ross* | 1 Serving/320g | 272.0 | 4.0 | 85 | 3.4 | 14.7 | 1.3 | 0.5 |
| Chicken, with Rice, Sainsbury's* | 1 Pack/400g | 500.0 | 15.0 | 125 | 5.4 | 17.5 | 3.7 | 0.8 |
| Chicken, with Rice, Tesco* | 1 Pack/300g | 390.0 | 13.0 | 130 | 4.4 | 17.5 | 4.2 | 1.2 |
| Chicken, with Rice, Weight Watchers* | 1 Serving/320g | 294.0 | 4.0 | 92 | 5.2 | 14.5 | 1.4 | 0.1 |
| Chicken, with Vegetables, Canned, Value, Tesco* | 1 Can/392g | 294.0 | 10.0 | 75 | 4.2 | 7.9 | 2.6 | 1.4 |
| Chicken, with Vegetables, Morrisons* | 1 Can/392g | 392.0 | 16.0 | 100 | 9.0 | 7.0 | 4.0 | 1.0 |
| Chicken, Yellow Thai Style, HL, Tesco* | 1 Pack/450g | 504.0 | 12.0 | 112 | 9.3 | 12.6 | 2.7 | 0.5 |
| Chicken & Vegetable, Big Eat, Heinz* | 1 Pot/350g | 392.0 | 18.0 | 112 | 5.4 | 10.9 | 5.2 | 4.3 |
| Chinese Chicken, Morrisons* | 1 Pack/340g | 347.0 | 16.0 | 102 | 10.3 | 5.0 | 4.6 | 0.8 |
| Chinese Chicken, Oriental Express* | 1 Pack/340g | 286.0 | 2.0 | 84 | 4.8 | 16.2 | 0.6 | 0.8 |
| Chinese Chicken, with Rice, GFY, Asda* | 1 Pack/400g | 444.0 | 12.0 | 111 | 10.7 | 10.6 | 2.9 | 0.5 |
| Chinese Chicken, with Vegetable Rice, M & S* | 1 Pack/400g | 320.0 | 8.0 | 80 | 7.1 | 8.4 | 2.0 | 1.3 |
| Cod, Red Thai, with Rice, Perfectly Balanced, Waitrose* | 1 Pack/400g | 360.0 | 7.0 | 90 | 7.5 | 11.0 | 1.8 | 1.0 |
| Courgette & Potato | 1oz/28g | 24.0 | 1.0 | 86 | 1.9 | 8.7 | 5.2 | 1.2 |
| Dudhi, Kofta | 1oz/28g | 32.0 | 2.0 | 113 | 2.6 | 9.4 | 7.4 | 2.8 |
| Fish, & Vegetable, Bangladeshi, Average | 1oz/28g | 33.0 | 2.0 | 117 | 9.1 | 1.4 | 8.4 | 0.5 |
| Fish, Bangladeshi, Average | 1oz/28g | 35.0 | 2.0 | 124 | 12.2 | 1.5 | 7.9 | 0.3 |
| Fish, Red Thai, Waitrose* | 1 Pack/500g | 275.0 | 11.0 | 55 | 5.2 | 3.7 | 2.2 | 1.0 |
| Gobi Aloo Sag, Retail | 1oz/28g | 27.0 | 2.0 | 95 | 2.2 | 7.1 | 6.9 | 1.4 |
| King Prawn, Coconut & Lime, Sainsbury's* | ½ Pack/351g | 207.0 | 9.0 | 59 | 3.7 | 5.4 | 2.5 | 1.0 |
| King Prawn, Goan, Eat Smart, Safeway* | 1 Pack/400g | 340.0 | 7.0 | 85 | 3.7 | 12.7 | 1.7 | 2.1 |
| King Prawn, Malay with Rice, Sainsbury's* | 1 Pack/400g | 608.0 | 20.0 | 152 | 5.0 | 21.5 | 5.1 | 1.4 |
| King Prawn Malay, Waitrose* | 1 Pack/350g | 364.0 | 19.0 | 104 | 6.6 | 7.1 | 5.5 | 0.9 |
| Lamb, Hot, M & S* | ½ Can/213g | 320.0 | 20.0 | 150 | 14.9 | 6.0 | 9.2 | 2.3 |
| Lamb, with Rice, Birds Eye* | 1 Pack/382g | 520.0 | 13.0 | 136 | 5.6 | 20.8 | 3.4 | 0.9 |
| Masala, Vegalicious, Pick Me* | 1 Pot/400g | 156.0 | 6.0 | 39 | 1.6 | 4.8 | 1.5 | 2.8 |

# C

## CURRY

| INFO/WEIGHT | Measure | per Measure | | Nutrition Values per 100g / 100ml | | | | |
|---|---|---|---|---|---|---|---|---|
| | | KCAL | FAT | KCAL | PROT | CARB | FAT | FIBRE |
| Matar Paneer, Peas & Cheese, Ashoka* | ½ Pack/150g | 183.0 | 10.0 | 122 | 5.3 | 10.0 | 6.7 | 2.0 |
| Potato & Pea | 1oz/28g | 26.0 | 1.0 | 92 | 2.9 | 13.0 | 3.8 | 2.4 |
| Prawn, & Mushroom | 1oz/28g | 47.0 | 4.0 | 168 | 7.3 | 2.5 | 14.4 | 1.0 |
| Prawn, Frozen, Sainsbury's* | 1 Pack/400g | 500.0 | 16.0 | 125 | 3.5 | 19.0 | 3.9 | 0.8 |
| Prawn, King, Goan, M & S* | 1 Pack/400g | 680.0 | 44.0 | 170 | 5.1 | 11.6 | 11.1 | 1.5 |
| Prawn, Red Thai, Sainsbury's* | 1 Pack/300g | 546.0 | 40.0 | 182 | 6.3 | 9.4 | 13.2 | 1.7 |
| Prawn, Red Thai Sauce, Youngs* | 1 Pack/255g | 197.0 | 9.0 | 77 | 4.8 | 6.5 | 3.4 | 0.8 |
| Prawn, Thai, with Jasmine Rice, BGTY, Sainsbury's* | 1 Serving/401g | 353.0 | 6.0 | 88 | 4.2 | 14.5 | 1.5 | 2.0 |
| Prawn, with Rice, Asda* | 1 Pack/400g | 420.0 | 10.0 | 105 | 3.5 | 17.0 | 2.6 | 1.1 |
| Prawn, with Rice, Birds Eye* | 1 Pack/375g | 442.0 | 0.0 | 118 | 3.5 | 20.6 | 0.0 | 0.0 |
| Prawn, with Rice, Morrisons* | 1 Serving/400g | 484.0 | 9.0 | 121 | 3.2 | 21.9 | 2.3 | 0.9 |
| Red Kidney Bean, Punjabi | 1oz/28g | 30.0 | 2.0 | 106 | 4.7 | 10.1 | 5.6 | 3.8 |
| Salmon, Green, Waitrose* | 1 Pack/401g | 581.0 | 40.0 | 145 | 9.1 | 4.5 | 10.1 | 2.7 |
| Thai Coconut, Tasty Veg Pot, Innocent* | 1 Pot/400g | 288.0 | 11.0 | 72 | 3.2 | 8.8 | 2.7 | 3.5 |
| Vegetable, & Pilau Rice, BGTY, Sainsbury's* | 1 Pack/400g | 272.0 | 2.0 | 68 | 2.0 | 14.0 | 0.4 | 2.3 |
| Vegetable, & Rice, Microwaveable, M & S* | 1 Pot/325g | 390.0 | 7.0 | 120 | 2.3 | 22.3 | 2.2 | 2.2 |
| Vegetable, Asda* | 1 Pack/350g | 329.0 | 21.0 | 94 | 1.9 | 8.0 | 6.0 | 1.9 |
| Vegetable, Canned, Sainsbury's* | ½ Can/200g | 200.0 | 12.0 | 100 | 1.4 | 9.8 | 6.1 | 1.8 |
| Vegetable, Frozen, Mixed Vegetables, Average | 1oz/28g | 25.0 | 2.0 | 88 | 2.5 | 6.9 | 6.1 | 0.0 |
| Vegetable, in a Mild & Creamy Curry Sauce, Waitrose* | 1 Pack/400g | 388.0 | 26.0 | 97 | 2.6 | 6.9 | 6.6 | 1.5 |
| Vegetable, in Sweet Sauce, Average | 1 Serving/330g | 162.0 | 7.0 | 49 | 1.4 | 6.7 | 2.1 | 1.3 |
| Vegetable, Indian, Canned, Tesco* | 1 Can/400g | 320.0 | 18.0 | 80 | 2.0 | 6.7 | 4.5 | 1.1 |
| Vegetable, Indian, Tesco* | 1 Serving/225g | 257.0 | 18.0 | 114 | 2.1 | 8.6 | 7.9 | 1.6 |
| Vegetable, Indian Meal for One, Tesco* | 1 Serving/200g | 218.0 | 14.0 | 109 | 2.0 | 9.0 | 7.2 | 1.2 |
| Vegetable, Light Choices, Tesco* | 1 Pack/350g | 350.0 | 4.0 | 100 | 2.3 | 19.4 | 1.2 | 1.5 |
| Vegetable, Medium, Tesco* | 1 Pack/350g | 325.0 | 22.0 | 93 | 2.3 | 7.1 | 6.2 | 1.9 |
| Vegetable, Mild, COU, M & S* | 1 Pack/400g | 340.0 | 2.0 | 85 | 2.6 | 17.0 | 0.5 | 2.8 |
| Vegetable, Mild, Tesco* | 1 Can/425g | 314.0 | 11.0 | 74 | 2.1 | 10.7 | 2.5 | 1.7 |
| Vegetable, Pakistani, Average | 1oz/28g | 17.0 | 1.0 | 60 | 2.2 | 8.7 | 2.6 | 2.2 |
| Vegetable, Sabzi Tarkari, Patak's* | 1 Pack/400g | 500.0 | 31.0 | 125 | 2.5 | 11.1 | 7.8 | 2.2 |
| Vegetable, SmartPrice, Asda* | ½ Can/203g | 132.0 | 1.0 | 65 | 2.0 | 13.0 | 0.5 | 1.7 |
| Vegetable, Takeaway, Average | 1oz/28g | 29.0 | 2.0 | 105 | 2.5 | 7.6 | 7.4 | 0.0 |
| Vegetable, Tinned, Asda* | ½ Can/200g | 206.0 | 12.0 | 103 | 2.2 | 10.0 | 6.0 | 2.5 |
| Vegetable, Way to Five, Sainsbury's* | ½ Pack/344g | 227.0 | 4.0 | 66 | 2.5 | 11.6 | 1.1 | 1.4 |
| Vegetable, with Pilau Rice, Linda McCartney* | 1 Pack/339g | 224.0 | 2.0 | 66 | 1.6 | 13.5 | 0.6 | 0.5 |
| Vegetable, with Rice, Asda* | 1 Pack/393g | 432.0 | 12.0 | 110 | 2.6 | 18.0 | 3.1 | 1.4 |
| Vegetable, with Rice, Birds Eye* | 1 Pack/414g | 455.0 | 10.0 | 110 | 2.3 | 19.6 | 2.3 | 1.1 |
| Vegetable, with Rice, Co-Op* | 1 Pack/340g | 289.0 | 3.0 | 85 | 2.0 | 17.0 | 1.0 | 0.7 |
| Vegetable, with Rice, HL, Tesco* | 1 Pack/450g | 486.0 | 12.0 | 108 | 2.7 | 18.2 | 2.7 | 1.1 |
| Vegetable, with Rice, Light Choices, Tesco* | 1 Pack/350g | 340.0 | 4.0 | 97 | 2.3 | 19.3 | 1.1 | 1.5 |
| Vegetable, with Rice, Retail, Average | 1oz/28g | 29.0 | 1.0 | 102 | 3.3 | 16.4 | 3.0 | 0.0 |
| Vegetable, with Rice, Tesco* | 1 Pack/400g | 440.0 | 12.0 | 110 | 2.1 | 18.7 | 3.0 | 1.0 |
| Vegetable, with Yoghurt, Average | 1oz/28g | 17.0 | 1.0 | 62 | 2.6 | 4.6 | 4.1 | 1.4 |
| Vegetable, Yellow Thai, Sainsbury's* | 1 Pack/400g | 624.0 | 49.0 | 156 | 2.2 | 9.4 | 12.2 | 1.1 |
| **CURRY LEAVES** | | | | | | | | |
| *Fresh* | *1oz/28g* | *27.0* | *0.0* | *97* | *7.9* | *13.3* | *1.3* | *0.0* |
| **CURRY PASTE** | | | | | | | | |
| Balti, Sharwood's* | ¼ Pack/73g | 328.0 | 29.0 | 453 | 5.0 | 19.2 | 39.6 | 3.1 |
| Balti, Tomato & Coriander, Original, Patak's* | 1 Tbsp/15g | 58.0 | 5.0 | 388 | 4.0 | 14.6 | 34.0 | 3.7 |
| Bhuna, Tomato & Tamarind, Patak's* | 1 Serving/10g | 40.0 | 6.0 | 397 | 4.3 | 17.5 | 56.2 | 6.3 |
| Garam Masala, Cinnamon & Ginger, Hot, Patak's* | 1 Serving/30g | 121.0 | 11.0 | 403 | 3.2 | 17.9 | 35.4 | 0.6 |
| Green, Thai, Asda* | 1 Tbsp/25g | 28.0 | 2.0 | 114 | 1.6 | 10.0 | 8.0 | 5.0 |
| Green Thai, Mild, Sainsbury's* | 1 Tbsp/15g | 23.0 | 1.0 | 156 | 2.2 | 14.5 | 9.9 | 2.7 |

| | Measure INFO/WEIGHT | per Measure KCAL | per Measure FAT | Nutrition Values per 100g / 100ml KCAL | PROT | CARB | FAT | FIBRE |
|---|---|---|---|---|---|---|---|---|
| **CURRY PASTE** | | | | | | | | |
| Green Thai, Tesco* | 1 Tbsp/15g | 17.0 | 1.0 | 115 | 2.1 | 8.7 | 7.9 | 3.1 |
| Hot, M & S* | 1oz/28g | 69.0 | 5.0 | 245 | 4.2 | 13.4 | 19.2 | 3.3 |
| Hot, Sharwood's* | 1oz/28g | 123.0 | 11.0 | 439 | 5.1 | 18.6 | 38.3 | 2.6 |
| Jalfrezi, Patak's* | 1 Serving/30g | 165.0 | 15.0 | 549 | 4.1 | 16.8 | 51.6 | 3.5 |
| Korma, Asda* | 1 Tube/100g | 338.0 | 23.0 | 338 | 5.1 | 26.6 | 23.5 | 1.2 |
| Korma, Coconut & Coriander, Original, Patak's* | 1 Serving/30g | 124.0 | 12.0 | 415 | 3.5 | 11.6 | 39.0 | 5.2 |
| Madras, Cumin & Chilli, Hot, Patak's* | ¼ Jar/70g | 364.0 | 36.0 | 520 | 4.8 | 9.4 | 51.1 | 7.3 |
| Medium, Asda* | 1 Tsp/5ml/5g | 18.0 | 2.0 | 364 | 5.0 | 14.0 | 32.0 | 5.0 |
| Medium, Barts Spices* | 1 Serving/30g | 88.0 | 6.0 | 295 | 4.5 | 19.2 | 21.5 | 5.5 |
| Medium, M & S* | 1oz/28g | 64.0 | 5.0 | 230 | 2.5 | 10.7 | 19.5 | 4.9 |
| Medium, Sharwood's* | 1oz/28g | 122.0 | 11.0 | 434 | 4.5 | 16.8 | 38.8 | 2.7 |
| Mild, Asda* | ¼ Jar/46g | 206.0 | 19.0 | 448 | 3.8 | 16.0 | 41.0 | 7.0 |
| Mild, Coriander & Cumin, Original, Patak's* | 1 Serving/30g | 169.0 | 16.0 | 562 | 4.8 | 16.8 | 52.5 | 2.8 |
| Mild, Sharwood's* | 1oz/28g | 78.0 | 6.0 | 279 | 3.6 | 17.7 | 21.5 | 3.4 |
| Red, Thai, Asda* | 1 Tbsp/25g | 31.0 | 2.0 | 124 | 1.6 | 7.0 | 10.0 | 5.0 |
| Red Thai, M & S* | ½ Jar/100g | 150.0 | 11.0 | 150 | 1.3 | 11.9 | 10.8 | 2.8 |
| Red Thai, Sainsbury's* | 1 Jar/250g | 385.0 | 31.0 | 154 | 2.2 | 8.5 | 12.4 | 3.5 |
| Red Thai, Tesco* | 1 Tsp/5g | 5.0 | 0.0 | 110 | 1.5 | 8.9 | 7.3 | 3.7 |
| Rogan Josh, Tomato & Paprika, Patak's* | 1 Serving/30g | 119.0 | 11.0 | 397 | 4.1 | 12.7 | 36.7 | 5.9 |
| Tamarind & Ginger, Original, Patak's* | 1 Tbsp/15g | 20.0 | 0.0 | 133 | 3.4 | 23.1 | 2.0 | 2.9 |
| Tandoori, Sharwood's* | 1oz/28g | 64.0 | 4.0 | 228 | 5.9 | 15.5 | 15.8 | 1.9 |
| Tandoori, Tamarind & Ginger, Patak's* | 1 Serving/30g | 33.0 | 1.0 | 110 | 3.1 | 20.4 | 1.8 | 2.6 |
| Tikka, Asda* | ½ Tube/50g | 117.0 | 8.0 | 235 | 4.5 | 16.1 | 17.0 | 1.6 |
| Tikka Masala, Coriander & Lemon, Medium, Patak's* | 1 Serving/30g | 111.0 | 10.0 | 369 | 3.8 | 16.9 | 31.8 | 2.9 |
| Tikka Masala, Sharwood's* | 1oz/28g | 53.0 | 4.0 | 191 | 3.2 | 9.9 | 15.4 | 2.6 |
| **CURRY POWDER** | | | | | | | | |
| *Average* | *1 Tsp/2g* | *6.0* | *0.0* | *325* | *12.7* | *41.8* | *13.8* | *0.0* |
| **CURRY SAUCE** | | | | | | | | |
| Balti, Asda* | ¼ Jar/125g | 155.0 | 12.0 | 124 | 1.6 | 7.0 | 10.0 | 1.7 |
| Balti, Loyd Grossman* | ½ Jar/213g | 346.0 | 28.0 | 163 | 1.7 | 8.8 | 13.4 | 1.4 |
| Dopiaza, Finest, Tesco* | 1 Jar/350g | 234.0 | 10.0 | 67 | 1.3 | 8.5 | 3.0 | 3.7 |
| Green Curry, Thai, Stir Fry, Blue Dragon* | 1 Sachet/120g | 74.0 | 5.0 | 62 | 0.9 | 5.7 | 4.0 | 0.5 |
| Green Thai, Asda* | 1 Jar/340g | 309.0 | 27.0 | 91 | 0.5 | 4.3 | 8.0 | 0.2 |
| Green Thai, Express, Uncle Ben's* | 1 Pack/170g | 131.0 | 10.0 | 77 | 1.1 | 5.4 | 5.8 | 0.0 |
| Jalfrezi, Loyd Grossman* | ½ Jar/213g | 270.0 | 20.0 | 127 | 2.1 | 8.2 | 9.5 | 1.2 |
| Jalfrezi, Piri Piri, Finest, Tesco* | 1 Serving/175g | 145.0 | 11.0 | 83 | 1.2 | 5.7 | 6.2 | 1.5 |
| Jalfrezi, Tesco* | 1 Jar/500g | 450.0 | 32.0 | 90 | 1.3 | 6.6 | 6.5 | 2.4 |
| Korma, Loyd Grossman* | ½ Jar/222g | 542.0 | 38.0 | 244 | 3.6 | 19.1 | 17.0 | 0.6 |
| Korma, Uncle Ben's* | 1 Jar/500g | 630.0 | 42.0 | 126 | 1.4 | 11.1 | 8.4 | 0.0 |
| Madras, Chilli & Cumin, Canned, Patak's* | 1 Can/283g | 640.0 | 53.0 | 226 | 2.7 | 11.9 | 18.6 | 1.6 |
| Madras, Cooking, Asda* | ¼ Jar/142g | 109.0 | 6.0 | 77 | 1.3 | 8.0 | 4.4 | 1.0 |
| Madras, Cooking, Tesco* | 1/3 Jar/161g | 145.0 | 9.0 | 90 | 1.9 | 6.9 | 5.7 | 2.5 |
| Madras, Cumin & Chilli, Original, in Glass Jar, Patak's* | 1 Jar/540g | 648.0 | 38.0 | 120 | 2.1 | 11.9 | 7.1 | 1.8 |
| Madras, Indian, Sharwood's* | 1 Jar/420g | 433.0 | 26.0 | 103 | 1.8 | 9.7 | 6.3 | 1.9 |
| Madras, Sharwood's* | 1 Jar/420g | 521.0 | 38.0 | 124 | 1.7 | 8.9 | 9.1 | 1.4 |
| Madras, Tesco* | ½ Jar/200g | 168.0 | 13.0 | 84 | 1.1 | 5.2 | 6.5 | 1.3 |
| Makhani, Sharwood's* | 1 Jar/420g | 399.0 | 29.0 | 95 | 0.9 | 7.2 | 6.9 | 0.4 |
| Masala, Red Pepper & Mango, Sainsbury's* | ½ Jar/175g | 142.0 | 9.0 | 81 | 1.4 | 7.8 | 4.9 | 1.1 |
| Medium, Uncle Ben's* | 1 Jar/500g | 330.0 | 10.0 | 66 | 0.9 | 10.9 | 2.0 | 0.0 |
| Moglai Pasanda, Asda* | ½ Jar/170g | 277.0 | 21.0 | 163 | 2.9 | 10.0 | 12.3 | 1.1 |
| Red Curry, Thai, Stir Fry, Blue Dragon* | 1 Sachet/120g | 112.0 | 10.0 | 93 | 0.9 | 4.4 | 8.0 | 0.5 |
| Rogan Josh, Loyd Grossman* | 1 Serving/106g | 206.0 | 17.0 | 194 | 2.4 | 10.5 | 15.8 | 1.5 |
| Rogan Josh, Worldwide Sauces* | 1 Jar/500g | 255.0 | 1.0 | 51 | 1.1 | 11.0 | 0.3 | 0.0 |

| | Measure INFO/WEIGHT | per Measure KCAL | per Measure FAT | Nutrition Values per 100g / 100ml KCAL | PROT | CARB | FAT | FIBRE |
|---|---|---|---|---|---|---|---|---|
| **CURRY SAUCE** | | | | | | | | |
| Singapore, Blue Dragon* | 1 Sachet/120g | 89.0 | 4.0 | 74 | 1.8 | 9.0 | 3.4 | 3.7 |
| Sri Lankan Devil Curry, Sharwood's* | 1 Jar/380g | 220.0 | 11.0 | 58 | 0.5 | 7.2 | 3.0 | 2.1 |
| Tikka, Cooking, Tesco* | 1 Std Jar/500g | 617.0 | 42.0 | 123 | 1.7 | 10.1 | 8.4 | 2.0 |
| Tikka Masala, Cooking, HL, Tesco* | ¼ Jar/125g | 94.0 | 4.0 | 75 | 2.6 | 8.2 | 3.0 | 1.2 |
| Tikka Masala, COU, M & S* | ½ Pack/100g | 80.0 | 3.0 | 80 | 4.5 | 9.9 | 2.6 | 1.7 |
| Tikka Masala, Loyd Grossman* | ½ Jar/213g | 438.0 | 34.0 | 206 | 2.6 | 12.5 | 16.2 | 1.0 |
| Vindaloo, Hot, Patak's* | 1 Jar/540g | 643.0 | 46.0 | 119 | 1.7 | 8.5 | 8.6 | 2.1 |
| **CUSTARD** | | | | | | | | |
| Banana Flavour, Ambrosia* | 1 Sm Pot/135g | 139.0 | 4.0 | 103 | 2.9 | 16.1 | 2.9 | 0.0 |
| Chocolate, COU, M & S* | 1 Pot/140g | 147.0 | 3.0 | 105 | 3.1 | 18.6 | 2.2 | 1.0 |
| Chocolate Flavour, Ambrosia* | 1 Pot/150g | 177.0 | 4.0 | 118 | 3.0 | 20.0 | 2.9 | 0.7 |
| Dairy Free, Sainsbury's* | 1 Serving/250g | 210.0 | 4.0 | 84 | 3.0 | 14.2 | 1.7 | 0.2 |
| *Low Fat, Average* | *1/3 Pot/141g* | *116.0* | *2.0* | *82* | *2.9* | *15.0* | *1.2* | *0.0* |
| Pot, Forest Fruits Flavour, Hot 'n' Fruity, Bird's* | 1 Pot/174g | 171.0 | 4.0 | 98 | 0.9 | 18.5 | 2.4 | 0.1 |
| Pot, Strawberry Flavour, Hot 'n' Fruity, Bird's* | 1oz/28g | 28.0 | 1.0 | 99 | 1.0 | 18.5 | 2.4 | 0.1 |
| *Powder* | *1oz/28g* | *99.0* | *0.0* | *354* | *0.6* | *92.0* | *0.7* | *0.1* |
| *Ready to Serve, Average* | *1 Serving/50g* | *59.0* | *2.0* | *118* | *3.3* | *16.1* | *4.6* | *0.2* |
| Strawberry Flavoured, Ambrosia* | 1 Serving/135g | 139.0 | 4.0 | 103 | 2.8 | 16.7 | 2.8 | 0.0 |
| Strawberry Style, Shapers, Boots* | 1 Pot/148g | 83.0 | 1.0 | 56 | 4.0 | 8.2 | 0.8 | 0.1 |
| Summer, Ambrosia* | 1 Pack/500g | 490.0 | 15.0 | 98 | 2.7 | 15.0 | 3.0 | 0.0 |
| Toffee Flavour, Ambrosia* | 1 Pot/150g | 156.0 | 4.0 | 104 | 2.8 | 17.0 | 2.8 | 0.0 |
| Vanilla, COU, M & S* | 1 Pot/140g | 147.0 | 3.0 | 105 | 4.3 | 16.6 | 2.5 | 0.6 |
| Vanilla, Fresh, Waitrose* | 1 Serving/100g | 214.0 | 15.0 | 214 | 3.2 | 15.8 | 15.3 | 1.1 |
| with Strawberry Sauce, Ambrosia* | 1 Pot/160g | 171.0 | 4.0 | 107 | 2.4 | 19.0 | 2.4 | 0.1 |
| **CUTLETS** | | | | | | | | |
| Nut, Goodlife* | 1 Cutlet/88g | 283.0 | 19.0 | 322 | 9.1 | 21.8 | 22.0 | 3.4 |
| Nut, Meat Free, Tesco* | 1 Cutlet/83g | 224.0 | 14.0 | 270 | 8.1 | 20.5 | 16.9 | 4.3 |
| Nut, Retail, Fried in Vegetable Oil, Average | 1 Cutlet/90g | 260.0 | 20.0 | 289 | 4.8 | 18.7 | 22.3 | 1.7 |
| Nut, Retail, Grilled, Average | 1 Cutlet/90g | 191.0 | 12.0 | 212 | 5.1 | 19.9 | 13.0 | 1.8 |
| Vegetable & Nut, Asda* | 1 Cutlet/88g | 296.0 | 20.0 | 335 | 10.0 | 22.0 | 23.0 | 4.6 |
| **CUTTLEFISH** | | | | | | | | |
| *Raw* | *1oz/28g* | *20.0* | *0.0* | *71* | *16.1* | *0.0* | *0.7* | *0.0* |

**C**

| | Measure INFO/WEIGHT | per Measure KCAL | per Measure FAT | Nutrition Values per 100g / 100ml KCAL | PROT | CARB | FAT | FIBRE |
|---|---|---|---|---|---|---|---|---|
| **DAB** | | | | | | | | |
| Fillets, Lightly Dusted, M & S* | 1 Fillet/112g | 190.0 | 10.0 | 170 | 12.8 | 9.7 | 8.7 | 0.5 |
| *Raw* | *1oz/28g* | *21.0* | *0.0* | *74* | *15.7* | *0.0* | *1.2* | *0.0* |
| **DAIRYLEA DUNKERS** | | | | | | | | |
| Baked Crisps, Dairylea, Kraft* | 1 Pack/45g | 101.0 | 4.0 | 225 | 9.2 | 26.0 | 9.0 | 1.1 |
| Jumbo Munch, Dairylea, Kraft* | 1 Serving/50g | 150.0 | 9.0 | 300 | 7.2 | 26.5 | 18.5 | 1.2 |
| Salt & Vinegar, Dairylea, Kraft* | 1 Tub/42g | 115.0 | 8.0 | 275 | 6.7 | 17.5 | 19.5 | 0.3 |
| Smokey Bacon, Dairylea, Kraft* | 1 Pack/45g | 135.0 | 9.0 | 300 | 7.3 | 24.0 | 19.5 | 0.0 |
| with Ritz Crackers, Dairylea, Kraft* | 1 Tub/46g | 122.0 | 6.0 | 265 | 9.6 | 25.0 | 13.9 | 0.6 |
| **DAIRYLEA LUNCHABLES** | | | | | | | | |
| Cheese & Pizza Crackers, Dairylea, Kraft* | 1oz/28g | 105.0 | 8.0 | 375 | 10.5 | 24.5 | 27.0 | 1.4 |
| Double Cheese, Dairylea, Kraft* | 1 Pack/110g | 412.0 | 29.0 | 375 | 18.0 | 17.0 | 26.0 | 0.3 |
| Ham & Cheese Pizza, Dairylea, Kraft* | 1 Pack/97g | 247.0 | 11.0 | 255 | 11.5 | 26.0 | 11.0 | 1.6 |
| Harvest Ham, Dairylea, Kraft* | 1 Pack/110g | 313.0 | 19.0 | 285 | 16.5 | 16.5 | 17.0 | 0.3 |
| Tasty Chicken, Dairylea, Kraft* | 1 Pack/110g | 313.0 | 18.0 | 285 | 17.0 | 17.5 | 16.5 | 0.3 |
| **DAMSONS** | | | | | | | | |
| *Raw, Weighed with Stones, Average* | *1oz/28g* | *10.0* | *0.0* | *34* | *0.5* | *8.6* | *0.0* | *1.6* |
| *Raw, Weighed without Stones, Average* | *1oz/28g* | *11.0* | *0.0* | *38* | *0.5* | *9.6* | *0.0* | *1.8* |
| **DANDELION & BURDOCK** | | | | | | | | |
| Original, Ben Shaws* | 1 Can/440ml | 128.0 | 0.0 | 29 | 0.0 | 7.0 | 0.0 | 0.0 |
| Sparkling, Diet, Morrisons* | 1 Glass/200ml | 2.0 | 0.0 | 1 | 0.0 | 0.3 | 0.0 | 0.0 |
| **DANISH PASTRY** | | | | | | | | |
| Apple, Bar, Sara Lee* | 1/6 Bar/70g | 160.0 | 4.0 | 229 | 4.3 | 42.1 | 5.7 | 1.7 |
| Apple, Fresh Cream, Sainsbury's* | 1 Pastry/67g | 248.0 | 15.0 | 368 | 3.1 | 40.2 | 21.6 | 0.4 |
| Apple & Cinnamon, Danish Twist, Entenmann's* | 1 Serving/52g | 150.0 | 1.0 | 288 | 5.6 | 62.0 | 1.9 | 1.5 |
| Apple & Sultana, Tesco* | 1 Pastry/72g | 293.0 | 16.0 | 407 | 5.4 | 45.0 | 22.8 | 1.4 |
| Average | 1 Pastry/110g | 411.0 | 19.0 | 374 | 5.8 | 51.3 | 17.6 | 1.6 |
| Cherry, Bar, Sainsbury's* | ¼ Bar/88g | 220.0 | 10.0 | 252 | 4.2 | 33.2 | 11.4 | 1.7 |
| Cherry & Custard, Bar, Tesco* | 1 Bar/350g | 910.0 | 49.0 | 260 | 3.5 | 29.9 | 14.0 | 7.7 |
| Custard, Bar, Sara Lee* | ¼ Bar/100g | 228.0 | 6.0 | 228 | 6.6 | 36.1 | 6.4 | 0.8 |
| Fruit Filled, Average | 1 Pastry/94g | 335.0 | 16.0 | 356 | 5.1 | 47.9 | 16.9 | 0.0 |
| Pecan, M & S* | 1 Serving/67g | 287.0 | 17.0 | 428 | 6.2 | 45.0 | 26.0 | 1.3 |
| Toasted Pecan, Danish Twist, Entenmann's* | 1 Slice/48g | 171.0 | 8.0 | 351 | 7.0 | 47.2 | 15.6 | 1.4 |
| **DATES** | | | | | | | | |
| *Dried, Average* | *1 Date/5g* | *14.0* | *0.0* | *272* | *2.8* | *65.4* | *0.4* | *4.2* |
| *Dried, Medjool, Average* | *1 Date/20g* | *56.0* | *0.0* | *279* | *2.2* | *69.3* | *0.3* | *4.3* |
| *Fresh, Raw, Yellow, Average* | *1 Date/20g* | *23.0* | *0.0* | *115* | *1.4* | *29.1* | *0.1* | *1.6* |
| **DELI FILLER** | | | | | | | | |
| Chicken, Caesar Style, Sainsbury's* | 1 Pack/80g | 212.0 | 18.0 | 265 | 14.0 | 1.0 | 22.7 | 2.6 |
| Chicken & Bacon, Co-Op* | 1 Pack/200g | 420.0 | 30.0 | 210 | 17.6 | 1.0 | 14.8 | 2.6 |
| King Prawn & Avocado, M & S* | 1 Pack/170g | 425.0 | 39.0 | 250 | 9.5 | 1.4 | 22.8 | 0.5 |
| Prawn & Mayonnaise, M & S* | 1 Serving/60g | 150.0 | 14.0 | 250 | 11.3 | 1.0 | 23.0 | 0.5 |
| Smoked Salmon & Soft Cheese, M & S* | 1 Serving/85g | 208.0 | 17.0 | 245 | 11.7 | 3.3 | 20.4 | 0.5 |
| **DELIGHT** | | | | | | | | |
| Blackcurrant, Made Up, Asda* | 1 Serving/100g | 115.0 | 4.0 | 115 | 3.2 | 17.0 | 3.8 | 0.0 |
| Butterscotch Flavour, No Added Sugar, Tesco* | 1 Pack/49g | 225.0 | 10.0 | 460 | 4.8 | 63.3 | 20.5 | 0.0 |
| Chocolate Flavour, Dry, Tesco* | 1 Pack/49g | 220.0 | 9.0 | 450 | 6.2 | 64.2 | 18.4 | 2.3 |
| Ravishing Raspberry, Made Up, Asda* | 1/3 Pack/100g | 112.0 | 4.0 | 112 | 3.2 | 16.0 | 3.9 | 0.0 |
| Strawberry, No Added Sugar, Dry, Tesco* | 1 Pack/49g | 51.0 | 2.0 | 105 | 3.4 | 13.7 | 3.7 | 0.1 |
| Strawberry, Shapers, Boots* | 1 Pot/122g | 96.0 | 1.0 | 79 | 4.5 | 13.0 | 1.0 | 0.1 |
| Vanilla, No Added Sugar, Dry, Tesco* | 1 Pack/49g | 51.0 | 2.0 | 105 | 3.4 | 13.7 | 3.7 | 0.1 |
| **DESSERT** | | | | | | | | |
| Apple Crumble, Sainsbury's* | 1 Pot/136g | 291.0 | 10.0 | 214 | 3.2 | 33.0 | 7.7 | 2.7 |
| Banoffee, Shape, Danone* | 1 Pot/120g | 175.0 | 3.0 | 146 | 3.3 | 28.0 | 2.3 | 0.5 |

**D**

## DESSERT

| | Measure INFO/WEIGHT | per Measure KCAL | FAT | Nutrition Values per 100g / 100ml KCAL | PROT | CARB | FAT | FIBRE |
|---|---|---|---|---|---|---|---|---|
| Banoffee, Weight Watchers* | 1 Dessert/81g | 170.0 | 4.0 | 210 | 4.9 | 37.7 | 4.4 | 1.4 |
| Banoffee Layered, Sainsbury's* | 1 Pot/115g | 270.0 | 15.0 | 235 | 2.2 | 27.8 | 12.8 | 1.0 |
| Berrylicious Overload, Iced, COU, M & S* | 1 Tub/119g | 155.0 | 2.0 | 130 | 3.0 | 24.5 | 2.0 | 3.0 |
| Black Cherry, Dragana, Waitrose* | 1 Pot/125g | 236.0 | 11.0 | 189 | 2.1 | 24.7 | 9.1 | 0.5 |
| Black Cherry & Chocolate, COU, M & S* | 1 Pack/115g | 132.0 | 2.0 | 115 | 3.6 | 22.6 | 1.4 | 1.2 |
| Black Forest, Light Choices, Tesco* | 1 Pot/145g | 188.0 | 2.0 | 130 | 3.2 | 25.8 | 1.6 | 0.9 |
| Black Forest, Tesco* | 1 Pot/100g | 287.0 | 14.0 | 287 | 3.5 | 35.8 | 14.4 | 2.4 |
| Blackcurrant, Yoghurt & Sorbet, Mini, Eat Smart, Safeway* | 1 Pot/75g | 90.0 | 1.0 | 120 | 2.2 | 25.8 | 0.7 | 1.8 |
| Blueberry Muffin, Tesco* | 1 Pot/91g | 265.0 | 19.0 | 291 | 2.0 | 24.5 | 20.6 | 3.0 |
| Bounty, Mars* | 1 Pot/110g | 253.0 | 15.0 | 230 | 5.3 | 23.2 | 13.6 | 0.0 |
| Buttons, Milk Chocolate, Cadbury* | 1 Pot/100g | 280.0 | 15.0 | 280 | 6.2 | 30.8 | 14.9 | 0.0 |
| Cafe Latte, COU, M & S* | 1 Pot/120g | 162.0 | 3.0 | 135 | 5.0 | 24.0 | 2.2 | 0.9 |
| Cafe Mocha, COU, M & S* | 1 Dessert/115g | 155.0 | 3.0 | 135 | 5.5 | 21.8 | 2.7 | 1.0 |
| Cappuccino, BGTY, Sainsbury's* | 1 Pot/119g | 224.0 | 10.0 | 188 | 3.3 | 25.2 | 8.1 | 0.8 |
| Caramel Crunch, Weight Watchers* | 1 Serving/89g | 174.0 | 3.0 | 196 | 4.6 | 37.9 | 2.9 | 1.7 |
| Caramel Flavour, Soya, Dairy Free, Organic, Provamel* | 1 Pot/125g | 122.0 | 2.0 | 98 | 3.0 | 17.5 | 1.7 | 0.6 |
| Caramel Shortcake, Luxury, Weight Watchers* | 1 Pot/100ml | 103.0 | 3.0 | 103 | 1.9 | 17.9 | 3.5 | 0.8 |
| Catalan Cream, Sainsbury's* | 1 Pot/95g | 375.0 | 35.0 | 395 | 4.2 | 11.2 | 37.0 | 0.1 |
| Cherry & Vanilla, BGTY, Sainsbury's* | 1 Pot/115g | 225.0 | 8.0 | 196 | 1.6 | 32.6 | 6.6 | 1.0 |
| Chocolate, Campina* | 1 Pot/125g | 186.0 | 9.0 | 149 | 3.2 | 18.5 | 6.9 | 0.0 |
| Chocolate, HL, Tesco* | 1 Pot/95g | 87.0 | 2.0 | 92 | 3.7 | 14.1 | 2.3 | 1.1 |
| Chocolate, Honeycomb Pieces, Iced, Weight Watchers* | 1 Pot/58g | 92.0 | 2.0 | 159 | 3.1 | 26.2 | 4.3 | 0.8 |
| Chocolate, M & S* | 1 Serving/120g | 168.0 | 3.0 | 140 | 5.6 | 26.4 | 2.1 | 1.1 |
| Chocolate, Triple Delight, Weight Watchers* | 1 Dessert/110g | 183.0 | 3.0 | 166 | 4.9 | 30.8 | 2.6 | 2.6 |
| Chocolate, Value, Tesco* | 1 Pot/115g | 112.0 | 3.0 | 97 | 2.8 | 15.7 | 2.6 | 0.0 |
| Chocolate, Weight Watchers* | 1 Serving/82g | 145.0 | 2.0 | 177 | 5.2 | 32.3 | 3.0 | 2.9 |
| Chocolate & Coconut, COU, M & S* | 1 Pot/125g | 169.0 | 3.0 | 135 | 3.6 | 25.6 | 2.2 | 0.7 |
| Chocolate Brownie, M & S* | ¼ Pack/144g | 610.0 | 39.0 | 425 | 4.7 | 39.6 | 27.5 | 1.0 |
| Chocolate Buttons, Cadbury* | 1 Pack/100g | 275.0 | 14.0 | 275 | 5.0 | 30.5 | 14.5 | 0.0 |
| Chocolate Duetto, Weight Watchers* | 1 Pot/85g | 99.0 | 2.0 | 117 | 4.4 | 18.4 | 2.8 | 0.0 |
| Chocolate Flavour, Soya, Dairy Free, Organic, Provamel* | 1 Pot/125g | 116.0 | 2.0 | 93 | 3.0 | 16.4 | 1.6 | 1.5 |
| Chocolate Fudge Brownie, Tesco* | 1 Pot/125g | 374.0 | 17.0 | 299 | 4.6 | 40.2 | 13.3 | 1.3 |
| Chocolate Honeycomb Crisp, COU, M & S* | 1 Serving/71g | 110.0 | 2.0 | 155 | 4.6 | 27.6 | 2.9 | 1.0 |
| Chocolate Mint Torte, Weight Watchers* | 1 Dessert/88g | 174.0 | 4.0 | 198 | 4.7 | 34.3 | 4.7 | 5.2 |
| Chocolate Mocha, BGTY, Sainsbury's* | 1 Pot/100g | 115.0 | 3.0 | 115 | 3.8 | 19.2 | 2.6 | 2.8 |
| Chocolate Mousse Cake, Weight Watchers* | 1 Dessert/75g | 148.0 | 2.0 | 198 | 5.9 | 37.1 | 2.9 | 1.0 |
| Chocolate Muffin, COU, M & S* | 1 Pot/110g | 154.0 | 3.0 | 140 | 6.1 | 26.1 | 2.5 | 1.5 |
| Chocolate Muffin, Light Choices, Tesco* | 1 Pot/108g | 140.0 | 2.0 | 130 | 4.3 | 22.6 | 2.2 | 1.3 |
| Chocolate Muffin, Tesco* | 1 Serving/104g | 354.0 | 21.0 | 340 | 3.5 | 35.5 | 20.4 | 2.1 |
| Chocolate Profiterole, Taste Temptations, Weight Watchers* | 1 Dessert/88g | 186.0 | 5.0 | 211 | 4.8 | 34.1 | 6.1 | 3.7 |
| Chocolate Raspberry, Taste Temptations, Weight Watchers* | 1 Dessert/110g | 208.0 | 3.0 | 189 | 3.6 | 37.9 | 2.5 | 1.3 |
| Chocolate Toffee, Weight Watchers* | 1 Dessert/89g | 177.0 | 4.0 | 197 | 4.3 | 34.9 | 4.5 | 2.2 |
| Chocolate Top, Weight Watchers* | 1 Pot/75g | 162.0 | 7.0 | 216 | 4.2 | 29.3 | 9.9 | 2.8 |
| Crazy Chocolate Overload, M & S* | 1 Pot/120g | 402.0 | 27.0 | 335 | 3.1 | 30.0 | 22.5 | 0.5 |
| Creme Caramel, Sainsbury's* | 1 Pot/100g | 102.0 | 1.0 | 102 | 2.5 | 21.1 | 0.9 | 0.0 |
| Crunchie, Dairy Milk, Cadbury* | 1 Pot/100g | 260.0 | 12.0 | 260 | 4.4 | 33.4 | 12.2 | 0.0 |
| Custard, with Caramel, Layers, Ambrosia* | 1 Pot/161g | 183.0 | 5.0 | 114 | 2.5 | 19.6 | 2.9 | 0.0 |
| Double Chocolate Brownie, Weight Watchers* | 1 Pot/86g | 163.0 | 3.0 | 189 | 5.1 | 33.7 | 3.8 | 2.4 |
| Double Chocolate Fudge, M & S* | 1 Pot/119g | 387.0 | 25.0 | 325 | 3.0 | 30.6 | 21.4 | 1.6 |
| Dreamy Vanilla, BGTY, Sainsbury's* | 1 Serving/58g | 146.0 | 8.0 | 252 | 3.5 | 27.6 | 14.2 | 5.3 |
| Flake, Milk Chocolate, Cadbury* | 1 Pot/100g | 275.0 | 15.0 | 275 | 6.2 | 29.8 | 14.6 | 0.0 |
| Fruit & Nut, Cadbury* | 1 Pot/100g | 285.0 | 12.0 | 285 | 6.4 | 36.3 | 12.5 | 0.0 |
| Fudge, Cadbury* | 1 Pot/90g | 216.0 | 11.0 | 240 | 4.1 | 28.5 | 12.4 | 0.0 |

**D**

## DESSERT

| | INFO/WEIGHT | KCAL | FAT | KCAL | PROT | CARB | FAT | FIBRE |
|---|---|---|---|---|---|---|---|---|
| Galaxy, Mars* | 1 Pot/75g | 166.0 | 9.0 | 221 | 4.9 | 22.7 | 12.3 | 0.0 |
| Gulabjam Indian, Waitrose* | 1 Pot/180g | 479.0 | 15.0 | 266 | 4.8 | 42.9 | 8.6 | 0.6 |
| Irish Cream Cafe Latte, COU, M & S* | 1 Pot/120g | 160.0 | 3.0 | 133 | 5.0 | 24.0 | 2.2 | 0.9 |
| Jaffa Cake, COU, M & S* | 1 Serving/120g | 138.0 | 3.0 | 115 | 2.4 | 20.1 | 2.6 | 1.0 |
| Lemon, Sainsbury's* | 1 Pot/115g | 136.0 | 2.0 | 118 | 2.8 | 23.2 | 1.5 | 0.9 |
| Lemon & Sultana Sponge, COU, M & S* | 1 Pot/130g | 169.0 | 2.0 | 130 | 2.8 | 26.5 | 1.2 | 0.5 |
| Lemon Meringue, Weight Watchers* | 1 Pot/85g | 161.0 | 0.0 | 189 | 2.4 | 43.1 | 0.5 | 0.6 |
| Lemon Mousse Cake, Weight Watchers* | 1 Serving/90g | 130.0 | 2.0 | 144 | 3.2 | 26.7 | 2.7 | 0.5 |
| Lemoncillo, Tesco* | 1 Pot/100g | 273.0 | 10.0 | 273 | 4.2 | 41.8 | 9.9 | 0.8 |
| Mandarin, COU, M & S* | 1 Serving/150g | 195.0 | 6.0 | 130 | 1.0 | 22.0 | 3.8 | 0.1 |
| Maple & Pecan, American Style, Sainsbury's* | 1 Pot/110g | 287.0 | 16.0 | 261 | 2.6 | 30.6 | 14.2 | 1.2 |
| Mars, Mars* | 1 Pot/110g | 214.0 | 7.0 | 195 | 6.0 | 28.2 | 6.7 | 0.7 |
| Mint Chocolate Top, Weight Watchers* | 1 Pot/75g | 160.0 | 7.0 | 214 | 4.0 | 31.4 | 9.2 | 3.5 |
| Paris Brest, Fresh Cream, TTD, Sainsbury's* | 1 Cake/90g | 315.0 | 22.0 | 350 | 5.9 | 26.2 | 24.6 | 1.0 |
| Peach & Raspberry, COU, M & S* | 1 Pot/90g | 135.0 | 1.0 | 150 | 2.6 | 30.5 | 1.6 | 1.0 |
| Pineapple & Passionfruit, M & S* | 1 Pot/100g | 130.0 | 4.0 | 130 | 0.8 | 21.7 | 3.8 | 0.3 |
| Raspberry & Chardonnay, COU, M & S* | 1 Serving/135g | 155.0 | 1.0 | 115 | 1.6 | 25.5 | 0.5 | 2.7 |
| Raspberry Royale, Finest, Tesco* | ½ Pack/170g | 314.0 | 16.0 | 185 | 1.7 | 22.8 | 9.3 | 1.4 |
| Raspberry with Light Lemon Sponge, Weight Watchers* | 1 Dessert/85g | 152.0 | 4.0 | 178 | 4.1 | 30.4 | 4.4 | 2.8 |
| Rich Chocolate, Weight Watchers* | 1 Pot/70g | 62.0 | 2.0 | 89 | 3.5 | 13.4 | 2.4 | 1.4 |
| Rocky Road, Sainsbury's* | 1 Pot/110g | 328.0 | 22.0 | 298 | 3.6 | 26.8 | 19.6 | 2.1 |
| Rolo, Nestle* | 1 Pot/77g | 187.0 | 9.0 | 243 | 3.1 | 30.0 | 12.3 | 0.5 |
| Simply Strawberry, Sainsbury's* | 1 Pot/150g | 126.0 | 0.0 | 84 | 0.6 | 19.3 | 0.1 | 0,9 |
| Soya, Mocha Flavour, Provamel* | 1 Serving/125g | 117.0 | 2.0 | 94 | 3.0 | 16.3 | 1.8 | 0.6 |
| Strawberries & Cream, BFY, Morrisons* | 1 Serving/200g | 244.0 | 2.0 | 122 | 2.2 | 26.0 | 1.1 | 0.1 |
| Strawberry, BGTY, Sainsbury's* | 1 Pot/115g | 133.0 | 2.0 | 116 | 2.7 | 23.1 | 1.4 | 1.3 |
| Strawberry, HL, Tesco* | 1 Pot/122g | 94.0 | 2.0 | 77 | 2.7 | 12.3 | 1.9 | 1.1 |
| Strawberry, Value, Tesco* | 1 Pot/115g | 113.0 | 3.0 | 98 | 2.4 | 16.9 | 2.3 | 0.0 |
| Strawberry & Rhubarb, COU, M & S* | 1 Pot/110g | 104.0 | 1.0 | 95 | 1.5 | 20.1 | 0.7 | 0.9 |
| Strawberry Flavour, SmartPrice, Asda* | 1 Pot/115g | 113.0 | 3.0 | 98 | 2.4 | 17.0 | 2.3 | 0.0 |
| Strawberry Meringue, Iced, Luxury, Weight Watchers* | 1 Pot/100g | 162.0 | 1.0 | 162 | 2.4 | 34.2 | 1.4 | 1.0 |
| Strawberry Mousse Cake, Weight Watchers* | 1 Serving/90g | 124.0 | 2.0 | 138 | 3.0 | 25.5 | 2.7 | 0.5 |
| Strawberry Swirl, Iced, Weight Watchers* | 1 Pot/100ml | 92.0 | 2.0 | 92 | 1.1 | 18.1 | 1.7 | 0.5 |
| Summer Berry, HL, Tesco* | 1 Pot/93g | 120.0 | 2.0 | 130 | 2.8 | 24.5 | 2.3 | 1.5 |
| Summer Fruits, COU, M & S* | 1 Serving/105g | 110.0 | 1.0 | 105 | 2.1 | 21.6 | 1.1 | 1.2 |
| Summer Fruits, Marbled Cream, Waitrose* | 1 Serving/125g | 214.0 | 11.0 | 171 | 2.1 | 20.2 | 9.1 | 1.1 |
| Tantalising Toffee, COU, M & S* | ¼ Pot/85g | 144.0 | 2.0 | 170 | 3.1 | 32.8 | 2.9 | 0.5 |
| Tantalising Toffee Flavour, Weight Watchers* | 1 Serving/57g | 93.0 | 3.0 | 163 | 2.7 | 26.2 | 4.8 | 0.2 |
| Toffee, with Biscuit Pieces, Iced, Weight Watchers* | 1 Pot/57g | 93.0 | 3.0 | 163 | 2.7 | 26.2 | 4.8 | 0.2 |
| Toffee, with Biscuit Pieces, Weight Watchers* | 1 Pot/57g | 93.0 | 3.0 | 163 | 2.7 | 26.2 | 4.8 | 0.2 |
| Toffee & Honeycomb Sundae, Weight Watchers* | 1 Pot/150g | 222.0 | 5.0 | 148 | 2.1 | 32.7 | 3.1 | 1.6 |
| Toffee & Vanilla, Weight Watchers* | 1 Pot/67g | 107.0 | 1.0 | 159 | 3.1 | 34.8 | 0.8 | 3.9 |
| Toffee Apple, Eat Smart, Safeway* | 1 Pot/100g | 145.0 | 2.0 | 145 | 2.4 | 29.1 | 1.7 | 2.6 |
| Toffee Chocolate, Weight Watchers* | 1 Pot/100g | 197.0 | 4.0 | 197 | 4.3 | 34.9 | 4.5 | 2.2 |
| Toffee Flavour & Toffee Sauce, Weight Watchers* | 1 Pot/57g | 93.0 | 3.0 | 163 | 2.7 | 26.2 | 4.8 | 0.2 |
| Toffee Flavour Custard, Ambrosia* | 1 Pack/135g | 139.0 | 4.0 | 103 | 2.7 | 16.4 | 2.9 | 0.1 |
| Triple Chocolate, Delice, Sainsbury's* | 1 Serving/105g | 399.0 | 27.0 | 380 | 3.8 | 32.4 | 26.1 | 0.7 |
| Triple Chocolate Layered, BGTY, Sainsbury's* | 1 Pot/105g | 147.0 | 3.0 | 140 | 4.2 | 24.4 | 2.8 | 0.5 |
| Vanilla & Caramel, Little Desserts, Petits Filous, Yoplait* | 1 Pot/60g | 90.0 | 3.0 | 150 | 4.7 | 21.0 | 5.3 | 0.2 |
| Vanilla & Strawberry Compote, Weight Watchers* | 1 Pot/57g | 81.0 | 2.0 | 142 | 2.5 | 23.4 | 3.9 | 0.2 |
| Vanilla & Toffee, Heavenly Swirls, Tesco* | 1 Pot/73g | 106.0 | 2.0 | 145 | 2.5 | 28.1 | 2.5 | 0.5 |
| Vanilla Creamed Rice, Weight Watchers* | 1 Pot/100g | 108.0 | 1.0 | 108 | 4.2 | 20.8 | 0.9 | 0.4 |
| Vanilla Flavour, Soya, Dairy Free, Organic, Provamel* | 1 Pot/125g | 114.0 | 2.0 | 91 | 3.0 | 15.5 | 1.8 | 0.6 |

| | Measure INFO/WEIGHT | per Measure KCAL | FAT | Nutrition Values per 100g / 100ml KCAL | PROT | CARB | FAT | FIBRE |
|---|---|---|---|---|---|---|---|---|
| **DESSERT** | | | | | | | | |
| Vanilla Supreme, Sainsbury's* | 1 Pot/95g | 116.0 | 4.0 | 122 | 3.0 | 18.0 | 4.0 | 0.0 |
| Vanilla with Strawberries Swirl, Weight Watchers* | 1 Pot/57g | 46.0 | 1.0 | 81 | 1.5 | 13.3 | 2.2 | 0.2 |
| White Chocolate & Raspberry, Tesco* | 1 Dessert/88g | 180.0 | 9.0 | 204 | 3.4 | 25.0 | 10.1 | 3.1 |
| Wild Blueberry & White Peach, Extra Special, Asda* | 1 Pot/120g | 180.0 | 8.0 | 150 | 1.8 | 20.0 | 7.0 | 1.0 |
| **DESSERT SAUCE** | | | | | | | | |
| Chocolate, M & S* | 1 Dtsp/11g | 35.0 | 1.0 | 330 | 2.1 | 59.3 | 9.4 | 1.9 |
| Raspberry, M & S* | 1 Serving/20g | 24.0 | 0.0 | 120 | 0.5 | 28.7 | 0.3 | 2.6 |
| Toffee, Old English, Asda* | 1 Serving/28g | 99.0 | 2.0 | 355 | 2.3 | 73.0 | 6.0 | 0.0 |
| **DHAL** | | | | | | | | |
| Black Gram, Average | 1oz/28g | 21.0 | 1.0 | 74 | 4.2 | 7.0 | 3.4 | 1.7 |
| Blackeye Bean, Patak's* | 1oz/28g | 29.0 | 1.0 | 102 | 3.6 | 12.4 | 4.6 | 1.8 |
| Chick Pea | 1oz/28g | 42.0 | 2.0 | 149 | 7.4 | 17.7 | 6.1 | 3.8 |
| Chick Pea, Canned, Asda* | ½ Can/194g | 198.0 | 6.0 | 102 | 4.3 | 14.0 | 3.2 | 2.9 |
| Lentil, Patak's* | 1 Can/283g | 156.0 | 3.0 | 55 | 2.8 | 9.3 | 1.0 | 1.0 |
| Lentil, Red, Way to Five, Sainsbury's* | ½ Pack/273g | 254.0 | 4.0 | 93 | 5.5 | 14.4 | 1.5 | 1.4 |
| Lentil, Red Masoor, Punjabi, Average | 1oz/28g | 39.0 | 1.0 | 139 | 7.2 | 19.2 | 4.6 | 2.0 |
| Lentil, Red Masoor & Tomato with Butter, Average | 1oz/28g | 26.0 | 1.0 | 94 | 4.0 | 9.7 | 4.9 | 0.9 |
| Lentil, Red Masoor & Vegetable, Average | 1oz/28g | 31.0 | 1.0 | 110 | 5.8 | 14.7 | 3.8 | 1.8 |
| Lentil, Red Masoorl & Mung Bean, Average | 1oz/28g | 32.0 | 2.0 | 114 | 4.8 | 9.9 | 6.7 | 1.6 |
| Lentil, Tesco* | 1 Serving/200g | 248.0 | 13.0 | 124 | 5.1 | 10.6 | 6.6 | 2.5 |
| Mung Bean, Bengali | 1oz/28g | 20.0 | 1.0 | 73 | 4.2 | 7.4 | 3.3 | 1.7 |
| Mung Beans, Dried, Boiled in Unsalted Water | 1oz/28g | 26.0 | 0.0 | 92 | 7.8 | 15.3 | 0.4 | 0.0 |
| Mung Beans, Dried, Raw | 1oz/28g | 81.0 | 0.0 | 291 | 26.8 | 46.3 | 1.1 | 0.0 |
| Split Peas, Yellow, Chana, Asda* | 1 Serving/275g | 300.0 | 19.0 | 109 | 2.6 | 9.0 | 7.0 | 1.8 |
| Tarka, Asda* | ½ Pack/150g | 216.0 | 12.0 | 144 | 6.0 | 12.0 | 8.0 | 6.0 |
| **DHANSAK** | | | | | | | | |
| Chicken, Ready Meals, M & S* | 1oz/28g | 50.0 | 3.0 | 180 | 12.4 | 6.6 | 11.5 | 1.6 |
| Chicken with Bagara Rice, Waitrose* | 1 Pack/450g | 549.0 | 8.0 | 122 | 8.2 | 18.2 | 1.8 | 1.2 |
| Vegetable, Sainsbury's* | 1 Serving/200g | 148.0 | 6.0 | 74 | 3.1 | 8.9 | 2.8 | 2.8 |
| **DILL** | | | | | | | | |
| *Dried* | *1 Tsp/1g* | *3.0* | *0.0* | *253* | *19.9* | *42.2* | *4.4* | *13.6* |
| *Fresh, Average* | *1 Tbsp Chopped/3g* | *1.0* | *0.0* | *25* | *3.7* | *0.9* | *0.8* | *2.5* |
| **DIM SUM** | | | | | | | | |
| From Restaurant, Average | 1 Piece/12g | 50.0 | 2.0 | 433 | 28.9 | 31.3 | 20.4 | 0.0 |
| **DIME** | | | | | | | | |
| Terry's* | 1oz/28g | 154.0 | 9.0 | 550 | 4.6 | 68.5 | 33.8 | 0.6 |
| **DIP** | | | | | | | | |
| Applewood Cheddar & Onion, Fresh, BGTY, Sainsbury's* | ½ Pot/85g | 85.0 | 4.0 | 100 | 7.3 | 7.3 | 4.6 | 0.5 |
| Aubergine, Fresh, Waitrose* | 1 Serving/85g | 159.0 | 13.0 | 187 | 2.5 | 10.5 | 15.0 | 1.7 |
| Bean & Cheese, Asda* | 1 Serving/50g | 78.0 | 4.0 | 157 | 7.0 | 12.0 | 9.0 | 1.7 |
| Blue Cheese, Fresh, Sainsbury's* | 1/5 Pot/34g | 115.0 | 12.0 | 337 | 3.6 | 3.1 | 34.5 | 0.1 |
| Buffalo Mozzarella, Tomato & Basil, Kettle Chips* | 1 Serving/25g | 119.0 | 6.0 | 476 | 6.7 | 54.4 | 25.7 | 4.9 |
| Cheddar & Spring Onion, M & S* | 1 Pack/125g | 581.0 | 60.0 | 465 | 3.6 | 4.7 | 48.3 | 0.5 |
| Cheese & Chive, 50% Less Fat, Morrisons* | 1 Serving/50g | 86.0 | 6.0 | 172 | 8.8 | 5.2 | 12.7 | 0.2 |
| Cheese & Chive, Asda* | 1 Serving/43g | 190.0 | 20.0 | 447 | 4.9 | 3.4 | 46.0 | 0.0 |
| Cheese & Chive, Fresh, Sainsbury's* | 1oz/28g | 109.0 | 11.0 | 390 | 3.9 | 2.7 | 40.4 | 0.0 |
| Cheese & Chive, M & S* | 1oz/28g | 120.0 | 12.0 | 430 | 4.5 | 3.9 | 44.1 | 0.5 |
| Cheese & Chive, Tesco* | ¼ Pack/50g | 267.0 | 28.0 | 535 | 4.3 | 4.3 | 55.1 | 0.1 |
| Chilli, M & S* | 1 Pot/35g | 103.0 | 0.0 | 295 | 0.4 | 73.2 | 0.2 | 0.4 |
| Chilli Cheese, Asda* | 1 Serving/50g | 131.0 | 11.0 | 262 | 8.0 | 8.0 | 22.0 | 1.1 |
| Chilli Cheese, Max, Walkers* | 1 Jar/300g | 390.0 | 27.0 | 130 | 3.3 | 9.4 | 9.1 | 0.3 |
| Cranberry, Asda* | ½ Pot/40g | 53.0 | 1.0 | 132 | 0.4 | 29.0 | 1.6 | 0.8 |
| Cucumber & Mint, Fresh, Sainsbury's* | 1oz/28g | 34.0 | 3.0 | 123 | 4.5 | 3.7 | 10.0 | 0.0 |

**D**

# DIP

| | Measure INFO/WEIGHT | per Measure KCAL | FAT | Nutrition Values per 100g / 100ml KCAL | PROT | CARB | FAT | FIBRE |
|---|---|---|---|---|---|---|---|---|
| Feta Cheese, Fresh, Tesco* | 1oz/28g | 81.0 | 7.0 | 288 | 6.8 | 7.9 | 25.5 | 0.7 |
| Garlic & Herb, Big Dipper, Morrisons* | ¼ Pot/75g | 277.0 | 28.0 | 370 | 1.3 | 6.9 | 37.5 | 0.4 |
| Garlic & Herb, Reduced Fat, M & S* | 1 Serving/10g | 9.0 | 0.0 | 95 | 6.0 | 8.1 | 4.0 | 0.5 |
| Garlic & Herb, Tesco* | ¼ Pack/43g | 257.0 | 28.0 | 604 | 0.9 | 3.2 | 65.4 | 0.3 |
| Garlic Herb & Rocket, M & S* | 1 Serving/25g | 104.0 | 11.0 | 415 | 2.4 | 4.5 | 43.0 | 0.5 |
| Hot Salsa, Doritos, Walkers* | 1 Jar/300g | 87.0 | 1.0 | 29 | 0.9 | 5.8 | 0.2 | 1.6 |
| Mature Cheddar Cheese & Chive, Fresh, Waitrose* | ½ Pot/85g | 393.0 | 41.0 | 462 | 5.8 | 2.4 | 47.7 | 1.7 |
| Mexican Bean, Doritos, Walkers* | 1 Tbsp/20g | 18.0 | 1.0 | 89 | 2.7 | 12.1 | 3.3 | 2.4 |
| Mustard & Honey, Fresh, Sainsbury's* | 1oz/28g | 100.0 | 10.0 | 356 | 2.2 | 5.1 | 36.3 | 0.0 |
| Nacho Cheese, From Tex-Mex Multipack Selection, Tesco* | 1 Tub/125g | 619.0 | 62.0 | 495 | 5.9 | 5.8 | 49.6 | 0.0 |
| Nacho Cheese, M & S* | 1oz/28g | 76.0 | 7.0 | 270 | 9.8 | 3.8 | 23.7 | 0.4 |
| Nacho Cheese, Sainsbury's* | 1 Serving/50g | 243.0 | 25.0 | 487 | 4.8 | 3.9 | 50.2 | 0.0 |
| Onion & Garlic, Classic, Tesco* | 1 Serving/30g | 133.0 | 14.0 | 442 | 1.7 | 4.6 | 46.3 | 0.2 |
| Onion & Garlic, Fresh, BGTY, Sainsbury's* | 1oz/28g | 56.0 | 5.0 | 201 | 4.4 | 4.8 | 18.2 | 0.8 |
| Onion & Garlic, GFY, Asda* | 1/5 Pot/34g | 56.0 | 5.0 | 166 | 2.1 | 8.0 | 14.0 | 0.2 |
| Onion & Garlic, Half Fat, Safeway* | ½ Pot/85g | 170.0 | 15.0 | 200 | 3.2 | 7.4 | 17.2 | 0.1 |
| Onion & Garlic, Healthy Selection, Somerfield* | 1oz/28g | 62.0 | 6.0 | 222 | 3.0 | 5.0 | 21.0 | 0.0 |
| Onion & Garlic, HL, Tesco* | 1 Serving/43g | 80.0 | 7.0 | 188 | 2.5 | 6.3 | 17.0 | 0.1 |
| Onion & Garlic, Safeway* | ¼ Pack/45g | 216.0 | 23.0 | 480 | 1.7 | 4.7 | 50.4 | 0.1 |
| Onion & Garlic, Tesco* | 1oz/28g | 177.0 | 19.0 | 632 | 2.5 | 4.4 | 67.2 | 0.1 |
| Pea, Yogurt & Mint, Sainsbury's* | ¼ Pack/50g | 119.0 | 11.0 | 238 | 3.4 | 7.5 | 21.6 | 2.1 |
| Peanut, Satay Selection, Occasions, Sainsbury's* | 1 Serving/2g | 4.0 | 0.0 | 186 | 7.1 | 13.8 | 11.4 | 1.1 |
| Pecorino, Basil & Pine Nut, Fresh, Waitrose* | ½ Pot/85g | 338.0 | 34.0 | 398 | 5.1 | 5.1 | 39.7 | 0.0 |
| Raita, Indian, Asda* | 1 Pot/70g | 120.0 | 11.0 | 172 | 2.6 | 3.6 | 16.4 | 0.5 |
| Red Pepper, Sainsbury's* | 1 Pot/100g | 103.0 | 4.0 | 103 | 2.3 | 14.6 | 4.0 | 0.0 |
| Roast Onion, Garlic & Rocket, Reduced Fat, Waitrose* | 1 Serving/25g | 50.0 | 5.0 | 202 | 2.7 | 5.4 | 18.8 | 1.5 |
| Salsa, Chunky Tomato, Tesco* | 1 Pot/170g | 68.0 | 2.0 | 40 | 1.1 | 5.9 | 1.3 | 1.1 |
| Salsa, GFY, Asda* | 1 Pot/170g | 68.0 | 1.0 | 40 | 1.2 | 8.0 | 0.4 | 1.5 |
| Salsa, Kettle Chips* | 1 Serving/25g | 10.0 | 0.0 | 39 | 1.7 | 8.0 | 0.0 | 0.0 |
| Salsa, Less Than 5% Fat, Safeway* | ½ Pot/85g | 47.0 | 2.0 | 55 | 1.5 | 6.1 | 2.4 | 0.9 |
| Smoked Salmon & Dill, Fresh, Waitrose* | ½ Pot/85g | 373.0 | 38.0 | 439 | 5.1 | 4.1 | 44.7 | 0.1 |
| Smoked Salmon & Dill, Reduced Fat, Waitrose* | ½ Pot/85g | 184.0 | 17.0 | 217 | 3.9 | 6.1 | 19.7 | 1.1 |
| Sour Cream, Tesco* | 1 Serving/38g | 111.0 | 11.0 | 297 | 3.4 | 3.9 | 29.8 | 0.2 |
| Sour Cream & Chive, BGTY, Sainsbury's* | 1oz/28g | 46.0 | 4.0 | 165 | 4.9 | 3.4 | 14.6 | 0.7 |
| Sour Cream & Chive, Doritos, Walkers* | 1 Tbsp/20g | 52.0 | 5.0 | 258 | 1.9 | 6.9 | 24.7 | 1.9 |
| Sour Cream & Chive, Fresh, Tesco* | ½ Pot/75g | 305.0 | 32.0 | 407 | 2.1 | 4.1 | 42.4 | 0.0 |
| Sour Cream & Chive, Primula* | 1oz/28g | 97.0 | 10.0 | 346 | 5.0 | 1.8 | 35.3 | 0.0 |
| Sour Cream & Chive, Sainsbury's* | 1 Serving/50g | 141.0 | 14.0 | 282 | 3.1 | 5.4 | 27.5 | 0.1 |
| Sour Cream & Chives, Mexican Style, Morrisons* | ¼ Pack/25g | 68.0 | 7.0 | 274 | 2.2 | 3.4 | 27.9 | 0.4 |
| Soured Cream & Chive, 95% Fat Free, M & S* | 1oz/28g | 25.0 | 1.0 | 90 | 6.5 | 9.6 | 2.8 | 0.5 |
| Soured Cream & Chive, BGTY, Sainsbury's* | 1 Serving/170g | 253.0 | 18.0 | 149 | 4.2 | 9.9 | 10.3 | 0.1 |
| Soured Cream & Chive, Classic, Tesco* | 1 Serving/25g | 81.0 | 8.0 | 323 | 1.7 | 3.2 | 33.7 | 0.2 |
| Soured Cream & Chive, for Skins, Tesco* | 1 Serving/12g | 36.0 | 4.0 | 297 | 3.4 | 3.9 | 29.8 | 0.2 |
| Soured Cream & Chive, HL, Tesco* | 1 Serving/31g | 45.0 | 3.0 | 145 | 3.8 | 7.5 | 10.6 | 0.2 |
| Soured Cream & Chive, Light Choices, Tesco* | ¼ Pot/50g | 65.0 | 4.0 | 130 | 4.3 | 7.4 | 9.0 | 0.1 |
| Spiced Mango, Ginger & Chilli Salsa, Weight Watchers* | 1 Serving/56g | 48.0 | 0.0 | 85 | 1.0 | 19.9 | 0.2 | 2.6 |
| Spicy Moroccan, BGTY, Sainsbury's* | ½ Pot/85g | 56.0 | 2.0 | 66 | 2.1 | 10.0 | 2.0 | 1.7 |
| Sweet & Sour, M & S* | 1oz/28g | 36.0 | 0.0 | 130 | 0.7 | 31.4 | 0.1 | 0.5 |
| Sweet & Zesty, Doritos, Walkers* | 1 Jar/375g | 150.0 | 2.0 | 40 | 1.3 | 8.0 | 0.5 | 1.4 |
| Sweet Chilli, Chinese Snack Selection, Morrisons* | ½ Pot/20g | 64.0 | 0.0 | 320 | 0.1 | 79.4 | 0.2 | 0.6 |
| Sweet Pepper & Ricotta, Asda* | 1 Serving/20g | 74.0 | 7.0 | 370 | 1.0 | 12.0 | 35.0 | 0.0 |
| Tangy Barbecue, M & S* | 1oz/28g | 28.0 | 0.0 | 100 | 1.1 | 22.2 | 0.6 | 0.6 |
| Thousand Island, HL, Tesco* | 1 Serving/31g | 57.0 | 5.0 | 183 | 2.5 | 9.6 | 14.9 | 0.3 |

**D**

| | Measure INFO/WEIGHT | per Measure KCAL | FAT | Nutrition Values per 100g / 100ml KCAL | PROT | CARB | FAT | FIBRE |
|---|---|---|---|---|---|---|---|---|
| **DIP** | | | | | | | | |
| Thousand Island, M & S* | 1oz/28g | 69.0 | 6.0 | 245 | 2.1 | 9.4 | 22.2 | 0.7 |
| Yoghurt & Cucumber Mint, Tesco* | 1oz/28g | 34.0 | 2.0 | 121 | 7.0 | 7.2 | 7.1 | 0.6 |
| **DIPPER** | | | | | | | | |
| Broad Beans & Pea, COU, M & S* | 1 Pack/130g | 91.0 | 3.0 | 70 | 3.7 | 8.9 | 2.4 | 2.8 |
| Celery, M & S* | 1 Pot/130g | 162.0 | 14.0 | 125 | 1.8 | 4.4 | 11.0 | 1.2 |
| Cheese & Bacon, with Breadsticks, Weight Watchers* | 1 Pack/50g | 98.0 | 2.0 | 196 | 16.0 | 24.0 | 4.2 | 1.4 |
| Cheese & Onion, Weight Watchers* | 1 Pack/50g | 93.0 | 2.0 | 186 | 15.2 | 24.8 | 3.8 | 2.0 |
| **DISCOS** | | | | | | | | |
| Beef, KP Snacks* | 1 Pack/28g | 145.0 | 8.0 | 518 | 5.1 | 58.7 | 29.3 | 2.4 |
| Cheese & Onion, KP Snacks* | 1 Pack/28g | 146.0 | 8.0 | 520 | 5.1 | 59.1 | 29.3 | 2.5 |
| Salt & Vinegar, KP Snacks* | 1 Bag/28g | 145.0 | 8.0 | 517 | 4.7 | 58.3 | 29.5 | 2.3 |
| **DOLLY MIXTURES** | | | | | | | | |
| M & S* | 1 Pack/115g | 431.0 | 2.0 | 375 | 1.8 | 89.2 | 1.4 | 0.0 |
| Sainsbury's* | 1 Serving/10g | 40.0 | 0.0 | 401 | 1.4 | 94.4 | 1.9 | 0.1 |
| Tesco* | 1 Pack/100g | 376.0 | 1.0 | 376 | 1.6 | 88.9 | 1.5 | 0.0 |
| **DOPIAZA** | | | | | | | | |
| Chicken, M & S* | 1 Pack/350g | 402.0 | 21.0 | 115 | 11.5 | 3.7 | 6.1 | 2.5 |
| Chicken, Safeway* | 1 Pack/326g | 450.0 | 27.0 | 138 | 10.4 | 5.3 | 8.4 | 1.4 |
| Chicken, Sainsbury's* | ½ Pack/200g | 272.0 | 16.0 | 136 | 13.2 | 3.1 | 7.9 | 0.8 |
| Chicken, Tesco* | 1 Pack/350g | 448.0 | 25.0 | 128 | 10.8 | 5.3 | 7.1 | 0.6 |
| Chicken, with Pilau Rice, Sharwood's* | 1 Pack/375g | 472.0 | 17.0 | 126 | 5.3 | 15.8 | 4.6 | 0.8 |
| Chicken, with Pilau Rice, Tesco* | 1 Pack/400g | 424.0 | 15.0 | 106 | 5.7 | 12.3 | 3.8 | 1.5 |
| Mushroom, Retail | 1oz/28g | 19.0 | 2.0 | 69 | 1.3 | 3.7 | 5.7 | 1.1 |
| Mushroom, Tesco* | 1 Pack/225g | 155.0 | 10.0 | 69 | 2.4 | 5.1 | 4.4 | 1.5 |
| Mushroom, Waitrose* | ½ Pack/150g | 81.0 | 5.0 | 54 | 2.2 | 4.3 | 3.1 | 2.3 |
| **DORITOS** | | | | | | | | |
| Chargrilled BBQ, Walkers* | 1 Bag/35g | 170.0 | 9.0 | 485 | 5.5 | 59.0 | 25.0 | 3.5 |
| Cheesy 3d's, Doritos, Walkers* | 1 Pack/20g | 89.0 | 3.0 | 445 | 7.0 | 68.0 | 16.0 | 3.0 |
| Chilli Heatwave, Walkers* | 1 Bag/35g | 175.0 | 9.0 | 500 | 7.0 | 60.0 | 26.0 | 3.0 |
| Cool, Ranch Chips, Walkers* | 1 Pack/50g | 250.0 | 13.0 | 504 | 8.1 | 64.5 | 26.2 | 4.0 |
| Cool Original, Walkers* | 1 Bag/40g | 200.0 | 11.0 | 500 | 7.5 | 58.0 | 27.0 | 3.0 |
| Cool Spice 3ds, Walkers* | 1 Bag/24g | 108.0 | 4.0 | 450 | 8.0 | 64.0 | 18.0 | 4.4 |
| Dippas, Hint of Chilli, Dipping Chips, Walkers* | 1 Bag/35g | 173.0 | 9.0 | 495 | 7.0 | 61.0 | 25.0 | 3.5 |
| Dippas, Hint of Garlic, Dipping Chips, Walkers* | 1 Serving/35g | 175.0 | 9.0 | 500 | 7.0 | 61.0 | 25.0 | 3.5 |
| Dippas, Hint of Lime, Walkers* | 1 Bag/35g | 173.0 | 9.0 | 495 | 7.0 | 60.0 | 25.0 | 3.5 |
| Dippas, Lightly Salted, Dipping Chips, Walkers* | 1 Serving/35g | 178.0 | 9.0 | 510 | 6.5 | 60.0 | 27.0 | 3.0 |
| Latinos, Chargrilled BBQ, Walkers* | 1 Serving/35g | 170.0 | 9.0 | 485 | 5.5 | 59.0 | 25.0 | 3.5 |
| Latinos, Mexican Grill, Walkers* | 1 Serving/35g | 170.0 | 9.0 | 485 | 6.5 | 59.0 | 25.0 | 3.5 |
| Latinos, Sour Cream & Sweet Pepper, Walkers* | 1 Pack/40g | 194.0 | 10.0 | 485 | 5.5 | 60.0 | 25.0 | 3.5 |
| Lightly Salted Dippas, Doritos, Walkers* | 1 Serving/40g | 204.0 | 11.0 | 510 | 6.5 | 60.0 | 27.0 | 3.0 |
| Mexican Hot, Walkers* | 1 Bag/40g | 202.0 | 11.0 | 505 | 8.0 | 57.0 | 27.0 | 3.5 |
| Tangy Cheese, Walkers* | 1 Bag/40g | 200.0 | 11.0 | 500 | 7.0 | 57.0 | 27.0 | 3.0 |
| **DOUBLE DECKER** | | | | | | | | |
| Cadbury* | 1 Bar/60g | 276.0 | 11.0 | 460 | 4.4 | 68.4 | 18.9 | 0.6 |
| Snack Size, Cadbury* | 1 Bar/36g | 165.0 | 7.0 | 465 | 4.8 | 64.5 | 20.9 | 0.0 |
| with Nuts, Cadbury* | 1 Bar/60g | 291.0 | 15.0 | 485 | 7.9 | 58.6 | 24.5 | 0.0 |
| **DOUGH BALLS** | | | | | | | | |
| Cheese & Garlic, Occasions, Sainsbury's* | 1 Ball/12g | 41.0 | 2.0 | 341 | 10.3 | 33.4 | 18.5 | 2.1 |
| Garlic, GFY, Asda* | 1 Ball/8g | 21.0 | 0.0 | 250 | 9.0 | 49.0 | 2.0 | 2.0 |
| Garlic, HL, Tesco* | 1 Serving/40g | 110.0 | 3.0 | 274 | 8.8 | 42.0 | 7.9 | 2.3 |
| Garlic, Tesco* | 1 Serving/10g | 40.0 | 2.0 | 400 | 7.0 | 40.0 | 23.0 | 1.0 |
| Garlic, Waitrose* | 1 Ball/11g | 38.0 | 2.0 | 347 | 8.5 | 41.4 | 16.4 | 3.3 |
| Garlic & Herb, Asda* | 4 Balls/48g | 173.0 | 9.0 | 361 | 9.2 | 40.9 | 17.8 | 3.6 |

D

| | Measure INFO/WEIGHT | per Measure KCAL | FAT | Nutrition Values per 100g / 100ml KCAL | PROT | CARB | FAT | FIBRE |
|---|---|---|---|---|---|---|---|---|
| **DOUGH BALLS** | | | | | | | | |
| Garlic & Herb, Occasions, Sainsbury's* | 1 Ball/12g | 41.0 | 2.0 | 343 | 8.4 | 38.7 | 17.2 | 2.2 |
| Sainsbury's* | 1 Ball/12g | 41.0 | 2.0 | 343 | 8.4 | 38.7 | 17.2 | 2.2 |
| Supermarket, Pizza Express* | 8 Balls/100g | 363.0 | 2.0 | 363 | 14.3 | 72.9 | 1.7 | 3.3 |
| with Garlic & Herb Butter, Aldi* | 1 Ball/12g | 45.0 | 2.0 | 365 | 7.7 | 46.7 | 18.2 | 1.8 |
| **DOUGHNUTS** | | | | | | | | |
| Apple & Fresh Cream, Sainsbury's* | 1 Doughnut/79g | 216.0 | 11.0 | 273 | 5.4 | 30.5 | 14.4 | 1.9 |
| Baked, HL, Tesco* | 1 Doughnut/67g | 166.0 | 4.0 | 248 | 6.4 | 42.2 | 5.9 | 1.4 |
| Chocolate, Somerfield* | 1 Doughnut/57g | 203.0 | 9.0 | 356 | 7.8 | 43.8 | 16.6 | 1.7 |
| Cream & Jam, Assorted Box, Sainsbury's* | 1 Doughnut/71g | 229.0 | 13.0 | 322 | 6.2 | 34.2 | 17.9 | 2.2 |
| Cream & Jam, Tesco* | 1 Doughnut/90g | 288.0 | 14.0 | 320 | 5.4 | 39.4 | 15.7 | 2.0 |
| Custard, Sainsbury's* | 1 Doughnut/70g | 172.0 | 7.0 | 246 | 5.1 | 32.3 | 10.7 | 2.3 |
| Custard, Tesco* | 1 Doughnut/91g | 266.0 | 14.0 | 292 | 4.1 | 33.4 | 15.8 | 1.1 |
| Custard & Bramley Apple, Sainsbury's* | 1 Doughnut/91g | 256.0 | 13.0 | 282 | 4.5 | 34.6 | 13.9 | 1.0 |
| Custard Filled, Average | 1 Doughnut/75g | 268.0 | 14.0 | 358 | 6.2 | 43.3 | 19.0 | 0.0 |
| Dairy Cream & Jam, Somerfield* | 1 Doughnut/80g | 296.0 | 18.0 | 370 | 4.6 | 35.8 | 23.1 | 1.3 |
| Dairy Cream Finger, Safeway* | 1 Doughnut/98g | 342.0 | 20.0 | 349 | 5.5 | 36.4 | 20.1 | 1.8 |
| Finger, Co-Op* | 1 Doughnut/82g | 299.0 | 15.0 | 365 | 4.0 | 45.0 | 18.0 | 2.0 |
| Jam, American Style, Budgens* | 1 Doughnut/46g | 126.0 | 3.0 | 275 | 7.1 | 46.5 | 6.7 | 0.0 |
| Jam, American Style, Sainsbury's* | 1 Doughnut/65g | 220.0 | 21.0 | 339 | 4.9 | 49.6 | 31.8 | 3.5 |
| Jam, Fresh Cream, Sweet Fresh, Tesco* | 1 Doughnut/74g | 248.0 | 12.0 | 335 | 5.5 | 40.7 | 16.4 | 1.9 |
| Jam, M & S* | 1 Doughnut/49g | 141.0 | 2.0 | 287 | 5.0 | 57.6 | 4.0 | 1.3 |
| Jam, Mini, Somerfield* | 1 Doughnut/45g | 138.0 | 4.0 | 307 | 6.4 | 50.1 | 9.0 | 1.4 |
| Jam Filled, Average | 1 Doughnut/75g | 252.0 | 11.0 | 336 | 5.7 | 48.8 | 14.5 | 0.0 |
| Mini, Sainsbury's* | 1 Doughnut/14g | 53.0 | 3.0 | 379 | 5.2 | 47.9 | 18.9 | 2.1 |
| Plain, Ring, Average | 1 Doughnut/60g | 238.0 | 13.0 | 397 | 6.1 | 47.2 | 21.7 | 0.0 |
| Ring, Iced, Average | 1 Doughnut/70g | 268.0 | 12.0 | 383 | 4.8 | 55.1 | 17.5 | 0.0 |
| Ring, Waitrose* | 1 Doughnut/107g | 396.0 | 21.0 | 370 | 4.2 | 43.5 | 19.9 | 0.7 |
| Strawberry Jam & Cream, Sainsbury's* | 1 Doughnut/80g | 299.0 | 19.0 | 374 | 5.3 | 36.2 | 23.2 | 1.3 |
| Toffee, Tesco* | 1 Doughnut/75g | 235.0 | 9.0 | 313 | 8.0 | 44.2 | 11.6 | 1.6 |
| Yum Yums, Glazed, Sweet, Waitrose* | 1 Doughnut/45g | 172.0 | 10.0 | 382 | 4.0 | 41.6 | 22.2 | 2.0 |
| Yum Yums, M & S* | 1 Doughnut/37g | 155.0 | 9.0 | 420 | 4.9 | 45.7 | 23.9 | 1.6 |
| Yum Yums, Tesco* | 1 Doughnut/61g | 232.0 | 10.0 | 380 | 6.1 | 51.6 | 16.6 | 1.7 |
| **DOVER SOLE** | | | | | | | | |
| *Raw, Average* | *1oz/28g* | *25.0* | *1.0* | *89* | *18.1* | *0.0* | *1.8* | *0.0* |
| **DR PEPPER*** | | | | | | | | |
| Coca-Cola* | 1 Bottle/500ml | 210.0 | 0.0 | 42 | 0.0 | 10.9 | 0.0 | 0.0 |
| Z, Coca-Cola* | 1 Serving/250ml | 10.0 | 0.0 | 4 | 0.0 | 0.0 | 0.0 | 0.0 |
| Zero, Coca-Cola* | 1 Can/330ml | 2.0 | 0.0 | 0 | 0.0 | 0.0 | 0.0 | 0.0 |
| **DRAGON FRUIT** | | | | | | | | |
| Raw, Edible Portion, Average | 1 Serving/100g | 41.0 | 1.0 | 41 | 0.7 | 9.6 | 0.5 | 3.6 |
| **DRAMBUIE** | | | | | | | | |
| *39% Volume* | *1 Shot/35ml* | *95.0* | *0.0* | *272* | *0.0* | *0.0* | *0.0* | *0.0* |
| **DREAM** | | | | | | | | |
| Cadbury* | 1 Bar/45g | 250.0 | 15.0 | 555 | 4.5 | 59.7 | 33.3 | 0.0 |
| Double Fudge, Cadbury* | 1oz/28g | 139.0 | 7.0 | 495 | 6.3 | 61.4 | 25.2 | 0.0 |
| Snowbites, Cadbury* | 1 Serving/31g | 170.0 | 10.0 | 545 | 3.1 | 59.7 | 32.7 | 0.0 |
| White Chocolate, Cadbury* | 1 Piece/8g | 44.0 | 3.0 | 555 | 4.5 | 59.7 | 33.3 | 0.0 |
| **DREAM TOPPING** | | | | | | | | |
| Dry, Bird's* | 1oz/28g | 193.0 | 16.0 | 690 | 6.7 | 32.5 | 58.5 | 0.5 |
| Made Up, Skimmed Milk, Bird's* | 1oz/28g | 21.0 | 1.0 | 75 | 2.0 | 4.8 | 5.3 | 0.0 |
| Sugar Free, Dry, Bird's* | 1oz/28g | 195.0 | 17.0 | 695 | 7.3 | 30.5 | 60.5 | 0.5 |
| **DRESSING** | | | | | | | | |
| Balsamic, Extra Virgin Olive Oil, TTD, Sainsbury's* | 1 Tsp/5ml | 19.0 | 2.0 | 376 | 0.5 | 12.8 | 36.0 | 0.4 |

**D**

## DRESSING

| | Measure INFO/WEIGHT | per Measure KCAL | per Measure FAT | KCAL | PROT | CARB | FAT | FIBRE |
|---|---|---|---|---|---|---|---|---|
| Balsamic, M & S* | 1 Tbsp/15g | 73.0 | 7.0 | 490 | 0.3 | 9.7 | 48.0 | 0.5 |
| Balsamic, Sainsbury's* | 1 Tbsp/15ml | 47.0 | 4.0 | 316 | 0.4 | 13.8 | 28.8 | 0.4 |
| Balsamic, Schwartz* | 1 Tbsp/15ml | 12.0 | 0.0 | 77 | 0.5 | 14.2 | 2.0 | 0.0 |
| Balsamic, Sweet, Finest, Tesco* | 1 Serving/10ml | 15.0 | 0.0 | 155 | 0.4 | 36.9 | 0.1 | 0.4 |
| Balsamic, TTD, Sainsbury's* | 1 Serving/15g | 58.0 | 5.0 | 389 | 0.6 | 18.3 | 34.8 | 0.8 |
| Balsamic, Weight Watchers* | 1 Serving/15ml | 12.0 | 0.0 | 81 | 0.1 | 16.0 | 1.8 | 0.5 |
| Balsamic Bliss, Ainsley Harriott* | 1 Tbsp/15g | 41.0 | 3.0 | 272 | 0.8 | 19.3 | 21.1 | 0.6 |
| Balsamic Vinegar, Olives & Herb, COU, M & S* | 1 Serving/30g | 22.0 | 1.0 | 75 | 0.5 | 14.3 | 2.0 | 0.5 |
| Basil & Pesto, COU, M & S* | 1 Serving/50ml | 30.0 | 1.0 | 60 | 0.6 | 8.3 | 2.2 | 0.8 |
| Blue Cheese, 60% Less Fat, BGTY, Sainsbury's* | 1 Tbsp/15ml | 26.0 | 2.0 | 172 | 1.9 | 7.3 | 15.1 | 0.2 |
| Blue Cheese, Fresh, Sainsbury's* | 1 Dtsp/10ml | 42.0 | 5.0 | 423 | 2.3 | 0.5 | 45.7 | 0.1 |
| Blue Cheese, Hellmann's* | 1 Tbsp/15g | 69.0 | 7.0 | 459 | 0.7 | 6.3 | 47.2 | 1.1 |
| Blue Cheese, Low Fat, Weight Watchers* | 1oz/28g | 17.0 | 1.0 | 59 | 1.5 | 5.8 | 3.4 | 0.0 |
| Blue Cheese, Sainsbury's* | 1 Serving/20g | 64.0 | 6.0 | 321 | 2.3 | 10.6 | 29.9 | 0.4 |
| Blue Cheese, Salad, Waitrose* | 1 Serving/50g | 265.0 | 25.0 | 530 | 2.1 | 17.3 | 50.3 | 4.1 |
| Blue Cheese, Tesco* | 1 Serving/15ml | 75.0 | 8.0 | 500 | 2.5 | 6.9 | 51.4 | 0.2 |
| Caesar, Chilled, Reduced Fat, Tesco* | 1 Tsp/5ml | 13.0 | 1.0 | 252 | 6.5 | 3.1 | 23.7 | 0.1 |
| Caesar, Classic, Sainsbury's* | 1 Tsp/5ml | 22.0 | 2.0 | 442 | 2.7 | 4.6 | 45.9 | 0.5 |
| Caesar, Finest, Tesco* | 1 Tbsp/15ml | 72.0 | 8.0 | 477 | 1.9 | 2.8 | 50.9 | 0.2 |
| Caesar, Fresh, Asda* | 1 Dtsp/10ml | 45.0 | 5.0 | 454 | 2.4 | 3.2 | 48.0 | 0.0 |
| Caesar, Fresh, M & S* | 1 Tsp/6g | 31.0 | 3.0 | 525 | 2.0 | 1.8 | 56.4 | 0.2 |
| Caesar, Fresh, Sainsbury's* | 1 Tbsp/15ml | 72.0 | 7.0 | 477 | 3.7 | 3.7 | 49.7 | 1.9 |
| Caesar, Hellmann's* | 1 Tsp/6g | 30.0 | 3.0 | 499 | 2.5 | 4.5 | 51.7 | 0.3 |
| Caesar, Less Than 3% Fat, BGTY, Sainsbury's* | 1 Serving/20g | 10.0 | 0.0 | 48 | 0.8 | 7.0 | 1.9 | 0.3 |
| Caesar, Light, Kraft* | 1 Serving/15g | 14.0 | 1.0 | 95 | 1.7 | 13.0 | 3.6 | 0.2 |
| Caesar, Light Choices, Tesco* | 1 Serving/15g | 9.0 | 0.0 | 60 | 1.5 | 9.5 | 1.5 | 0.5 |
| Caesar, Loyd Grossman* | 1 Dtsp/10g | 34.0 | 3.0 | 342 | 2.1 | 7.0 | 33.9 | 0.0 |
| Caesar, Luxury, Hellmann's* | 1 Tsp/4g | 20.0 | 2.0 | 498 | 2.5 | 4.4 | 51.7 | 0.3 |
| Caesar, Tesco* | 1 Tbsp/15ml | 71.0 | 7.0 | 475 | 4.6 | 2.1 | 49.8 | 0.1 |
| Caesar, Waitrose* | 1 Serving/15ml | 72.0 | 8.0 | 479 | 4.5 | 0.9 | 50.8 | 0.2 |
| Caesar Style, GFY, Asda* | 1 Sachet/44ml | 34.0 | 1.0 | 77 | 5.0 | 9.0 | 2.3 | 0.0 |
| Citrus Salad, BGTY, Sainsbury's* | 1 Tbsp/15ml | 13.0 | 0.0 | 90 | 0.3 | 14.4 | 3.1 | 0.3 |
| Classic French, Fresh, M & S* | 1 Serving/10ml | 51.0 | 5.0 | 515 | 0.6 | 8.2 | 53.1 | 0.2 |
| Classic Italian, Get Dressed, Kraft* | 1 Serving/25ml | 30.0 | 3.0 | 120 | 0.1 | 5.6 | 10.3 | 0.5 |
| Cream Cheese & Chive, Creamy Ranch, Kraft* | 1 Serving/15ml | 31.0 | 3.0 | 205 | 1.2 | 11.0 | 17.0 | 0.0 |
| Creamy Caesar, Get Dressed, Kraft* | 1 Serving/67g | 68.0 | 2.0 | 102 | 2.1 | 15.0 | 3.5 | 0.1 |
| Creamy Caesar, Waistline, Crosse & Blackwell* | 1 Dtsp/11g | 15.0 | 1.0 | 135 | 1.5 | 11.1 | 9.2 | 0.3 |
| Creamy Roasted Garlic, GFY, Asda* | 1 Tbsp/15g | 10.0 | 1.0 | 70 | 0.8 | 8.0 | 3.9 | 0.6 |
| Creme Fraiche, Salad, Kraft* | 1 Tbsp/15ml | 12.0 | 0.0 | 78 | 0.8 | 12.5 | 2.5 | 0.0 |
| Dijon Honey Mustard, Briannas* | 1 Tbsp/15ml | 65.0 | 6.0 | 433 | 0.0 | 20.0 | 40.0 | 0.0 |
| Fire Roasted Garlic & Thyme, Tesco* | 1 Serving/10ml | 45.0 | 5.0 | 447 | 0.9 | 4.7 | 47.2 | 0.0 |
| Fire Roasted Red Pepper, M & S* | 1 Serving/30g | 13.0 | 0.0 | 45 | 0.5 | 10.7 | 0.1 | 0.9 |
| Fire Roasted Tomato Basil, COU, M & S* | 1 Serving/30g | 13.0 | 0.0 | 45 | 0.6 | 8.1 | 0.9 | 1.1 |
| French, BGTY, Organic, Sainsbury's* | 1 Tbsp/15ml | 11.0 | 1.0 | 71 | 0.2 | 8.3 | 4.1 | 0.5 |
| French, BGTY, Sainsbury's* | 1 Tbsp/15ml | 12.0 | 1.0 | 79 | 1.1 | 8.8 | 4.4 | 0.5 |
| French, Cider Vinegar & Mustard, Tesco* | 1 Tbsp/15ml | 45.0 | 4.0 | 300 | 0.7 | 9.9 | 28.1 | 0.3 |
| French, Classic, Fat Free, Kraft* | 1 Tsp/5ml | 2.0 | 0.0 | 39 | 0.1 | 8.7 | 0.0 | 0.5 |
| French, Classic, Sachet, The English Provender Company* | 1 Sachet/25g | 21.0 | 1.0 | 84 | 0.8 | 14.7 | 2.4 | 0.0 |
| French, Classic, Sainsbury's* | 1 Tbsp/15ml | 71.0 | 7.0 | 473 | 1.0 | 5.7 | 49.6 | 0.5 |
| French, Classics, M & S* | 1 Tbsp/15ml | 77.0 | 8.0 | 516 | 0.6 | 8.2 | 53.1 | 0.2 |
| French, Finest, Tesco* | 1 Tbsp/15g | 55.0 | 6.0 | 370 | 0.4 | 5.1 | 38.7 | 1.0 |
| French, Fresh, Morrisons* | 1 Tbsp/15ml | 75.0 | 7.0 | 499 | 1.5 | 13.6 | 48.7 | 0.0 |
| French, Fresh, Sainsbury's* | 1 Tbsp/15ml | 64.0 | 7.0 | 429 | 0.6 | 6.6 | 44.6 | 0.6 |

## DRESSING

| | Measure INFO/WEIGHT | per Measure KCAL | FAT | KCAL | PROT | CARB | FAT | FIBRE |
|---|---|---|---|---|---|---|---|---|
| French, GFY, Asda* | 1 Tbsp/15g | 7.0 | 0.0 | 50 | 0.7 | 7.0 | 2.1 | 0.1 |
| French, Less Than 3% Fat, M & S* | 1 Tbsp/15ml | 10.0 | 0.0 | 68 | 0.7 | 11.5 | 2.6 | 0.7 |
| French, Light, Heinz* | 1 Sachet/12g | 13.0 | 1.0 | 111 | 0.7 | 15.4 | 5.4 | 0.0 |
| French, Light Choices, Tesco* | 1 Serving/20g | 10.0 | 0.0 | 48 | 0.8 | 7.6 | 1.6 | 1.1 |
| French, Luxury, Hellmann's* | 1 Tbsp/15g | 45.0 | 4.0 | 297 | 0.4 | 14.9 | 25.9 | 0.3 |
| French, Oil Free, Perfectly Balanced, Waitrose* | 1 Serving/15ml | 11.0 | 0.0 | 72 | 2.2 | 12.2 | 1.6 | 1.1 |
| French, Organic, M & S* | 1 Tbsp/15g | 98.0 | 10.0 | 655 | 0.2 | 7.5 | 69.4 | 0.3 |
| French, Organic, Tesco* | 1 Tsp/5g | 23.0 | 2.0 | 451 | 0.6 | 11.0 | 44.9 | 0.2 |
| French, Reduced Fat, M & S* | 1 Tbsp/15g | 10.0 | 0.0 | 70 | 0.7 | 11.5 | 2.8 | 0.7 |
| French, Sainsbury's* | 1 Tbsp/15ml | 33.0 | 3.0 | 219 | 0.6 | 9.8 | 19.1 | 0.5 |
| French, Tesco* | 1 Serving/25ml | 110.0 | 11.0 | 441 | 0.7 | 7.2 | 44.9 | 0.2 |
| French Salad, M & S* | 1 Serving/25ml | 156.0 | 17.0 | 625 | 0.5 | 3.8 | 67.3 | 0.1 |
| French Style Calorie-Wise Salad, Kraft* | 1 Tbsp/15ml | 24.0 | 2.0 | 160 | 0.0 | 18.7 | 10.7 | 0.0 |
| Garlic & Herb, Perfectly Balanced, Waitrose* | 1 Serving/50ml | 67.0 | 1.0 | 135 | 0.6 | 29.9 | 1.4 | 0.8 |
| Garlic & Herb, Reduced Calorie, Hellmann's* | 1 Tbsp/15ml | 35.0 | 3.0 | 232 | 0.6 | 12.8 | 19.3 | 0.4 |
| Garlic & Herb, Tesco* | 1 Tbsp/15g | 31.0 | 3.0 | 210 | 0.9 | 5.8 | 20.2 | 0.8 |
| Herb & Garlic, Light, 5% Fat, Get Dressed, Kraft* | 1 Serving/25ml | 29.0 | 1.0 | 116 | 1.3 | 15.5 | 5.1 | 0.2 |
| Honey, Orange & Mustard, BGTY, Sainsbury's* | 1 Tbsp/15ml | 16.0 | 0.0 | 105 | 1.8 | 18.6 | 2.5 | 1.8 |
| Honey & Mustard, BGTY, Sainsbury's* | 1 Tbsp /20g | 14.0 | 0.0 | 71 | 0.4 | 16.1 | 0.5 | 0.2 |
| Honey & Mustard, Finest, Tesco* | 1 Serving/25ml | 72.0 | 6.0 | 288 | 1.7 | 19.6 | 22.5 | 0.7 |
| Honey & Mustard, Fresh, M & S* | 1 Serving/10ml | 43.0 | 4.0 | 430 | 1.7 | 9.7 | 42.4 | 0.5 |
| Honey & Mustard, GFY, Asda* | 1 Tbsp/15g | 13.0 | 1.0 | 89 | 1.5 | 13.0 | 3.4 | 0.8 |
| Honey & Mustard, Light Choices, Tesco* | 1 Tbsp/14g | 9.0 | 0.0 | 65 | 1.3 | 11.6 | 1.1 | 0.6 |
| Honey & Mustard, Sainsbury's* | 1 Serving/10ml | 37.0 | 3.0 | 366 | 1.0 | 15.4 | 33.0 | 0.1 |
| Honey & Mustard, Tesco* | 1 Serving/10ml | 38.0 | 4.0 | 378 | 0.8 | 13.1 | 35.8 | 0.6 |
| Hot Lime & Coconut, BGTY, Sainsbury's* | 1 Tbsp/15ml | 8.0 | 0.0 | 51 | 0.7 | 5.7 | 2.9 | 1.2 |
| Italian, M & S* | 1 Tbsp/15ml | 62.0 | 6.0 | 415 | 0.9 | 8.9 | 41.5 | 1.0 |
| Italian, Reduced Calorie, Hellmann's* | 1 Serving/25ml | 67.0 | 5.0 | 269 | 0.5 | 19.5 | 20.8 | 0.3 |
| Italian, Waistline, 99% Fat Free, Crosse & Blackwell* | 1 Tsp/6g | 2.0 | 0.0 | 39 | 0.7 | 7.0 | 0.9 | 0.3 |
| Italian Balsamic, Loyd Grossman* | 1 Serving/10g | 36.0 | 3.0 | 357 | 0.9 | 13.1 | 33.5 | 0.1 |
| Italian Balsamic, The English Provender Co.* | 1 Serving/30ml | 20.0 | 1.0 | 67 | 0.8 | 9.9 | 2.7 | 0.2 |
| Italian Salad, Hellmann's* | 1 Serving/50ml | 103.0 | 8.0 | 206 | 0.7 | 12.8 | 16.7 | 0.0 |
| Lemon, Feta & Oregano, M & S* | 1 Tbsp/15ml | 24.0 | 2.0 | 160 | 1.3 | 8.2 | 13.4 | 0.6 |
| Lemon & Cracked Black Pepper, GFY, Asda* | 1 Tbsp/15g | 9.0 | 0.0 | 57 | 0.2 | 14.0 | 0.0 | 0.3 |
| Lemon & Watercress, COU, M & S* | 1 Serving/28g | 14.0 | 1.0 | 50 | 0.4 | 8.5 | 1.8 | 0.5 |
| Lime & Coriander, Oil Free, Waitrose* | 1 Tsp/5ml | 3.0 | 0.0 | 65 | 1.5 | 11.9 | 1.3 | 0.4 |
| Lime & Coriander, Sainsbury's* | 1 Tbsp/15ml | 61.0 | 6.0 | 409 | 0.4 | 10.0 | 40.8 | 0.5 |
| Lime & Coriander, The English Provender Co.* | 1 Serving/50g | 28.0 | 0.0 | 57 | 0.3 | 13.3 | 0.3 | 0.0 |
| Mayonnaise Style, 90% Fat Free, Weight Watchers* | 1 Tsp/11g | 14.0 | 1.0 | 125 | 1.7 | 8.9 | 9.2 | 0.0 |
| Mild Mustard, Low Fat, Weight Watchers* | 1 Tbsp/10g | 6.0 | 0.0 | 63 | 2.0 | 5.7 | 3.6 | 0.0 |
| Miracle Whip, Kraft* | 1 Tbsp/15ml | 60.0 | 6.0 | 400 | 0.3 | 11.0 | 39.0 | 0.1 |
| Mustard & Dill, Perfectly Balanced, Waitrose* | 1 Tbsp/15ml | 24.0 | 0.0 | 159 | 1.1 | 31.5 | 3.2 | 1.1 |
| Oil & Lemon | 1 Tbsp/15g | 97.0 | 11.0 | 647 | 0.3 | 2.8 | 70.6 | 0.0 |
| Olive Oil & Balsamic Vinegar, Sainsbury's* | 1 Serving/25ml | 104.0 | 10.0 | 415 | 0.9 | 9.4 | 41.8 | 0.2 |
| Orange & Cracked Pepper, Tesco* | 1 Tbsp/15ml | 17.0 | 0.0 | 114 | 0.5 | 27.8 | 0.1 | 0.3 |
| Orange & Honey, Luxury, Hellmann's* | 1 Serving/15ml | 16.0 | 1.0 | 110 | 0.8 | 17.5 | 3.5 | 0.8 |
| Pesto, Finest, Tesco* | 1 Serving/30ml | 108.0 | 11.0 | 360 | 3.5 | 2.9 | 37.1 | 0.9 |
| Pesto & Balsamic Vinegar, Extra Special, Asda* | 1 Tbsp/15g | 33.0 | 3.0 | 213 | 0.3 | 8.6 | 19.7 | 0.0 |
| Porcini Mushroom, TTD, Sainsbury's* | 1 Tbsp/15g | 46.0 | 5.0 | 308 | 1.3 | 3.3 | 32.1 | 5.4 |
| Ranch Style, Asda* | 1 Serving/44ml | 37.0 | 2.0 | 85 | 3.5 | 9.0 | 3.9 | 0.0 |
| Raspberry Balsamic Vinegar, The English Provender Co.* | 1 Serving/50g | 33.0 | 0.0 | 67 | 0.4 | 15.7 | 0.1 | 0.6 |
| Red Pepper, M & S* | 1 Tbsp/15ml | 58.0 | 6.0 | 385 | 0.6 | 7.6 | 39.2 | 0.5 |
| Roasted Red Pepper, TTD, Sainsbury's* | 1 Tbsp/15ml | 35.0 | 3.0 | 235 | 1.1 | 14.9 | 19.0 | 1.4 |

**D**

| | Measure INFO/WEIGHT | per Measure KCAL | FAT | Nutrition Values per 100g / 100ml KCAL | PROT | CARB | FAT | FIBRE |
|---|---|---|---|---|---|---|---|---|

## DRESSING

| | Measure INFO/WEIGHT | KCAL | FAT | KCAL | PROT | CARB | FAT | FIBRE |
|---|---|---|---|---|---|---|---|---|
| Salad, Catalina, Kraft* | 1 Serving/34g | 100.0 | 6.0 | 294 | 0.0 | 29.4 | 17.6 | 0.0 |
| Salad, Honey & Mustard, Light, Kraft* | 1 Tbsp/15ml | 19.0 | 1.0 | 126 | 1.2 | 19.0 | 4.6 | 1.1 |
| Salad, Italian, Light, Kraft* | 1 Tbsp/15ml | 5.0 | 0.0 | 31 | 0.1 | 6.8 | 0.0 | 0.6 |
| Salad, Kickin' Mango, Oil Free, Ainsley Harriott* | 1 Tbsp/15ml | 14.0 | 0.0 | 92 | 0.1 | 21.1 | 0.1 | 0.0 |
| Salad, Light, Heinz* | 1 Serving/10g | 24.0 | 2.0 | 244 | 1.8 | 13.5 | 19.9 | 0.0 |
| Salad, Luxury Caesar, Hellmann's* | 1 Serving/10ml | 50.0 | 5.0 | 498 | 2.5 | 4.4 | 51.7 | 0.3 |
| Salad, Raspberry Balsamic, GFY, Asda* | 1 Tbsp/15ml | 6.0 | 0.0 | 40 | 0.7 | 9.3 | 0.7 | 1.3 |
| Salad, Thousand Island, 95% Fat Free, Asda* | 1 Tsp/6g | 6.0 | 0.0 | 99 | 1.6 | 12.6 | 4.7 | 0.5 |
| Salad, Vinaigrette Style, 95% Fat Free, Asda* | 1 Tbsp/15ml | 6.0 | 0.0 | 42 | 0.1 | 10.6 | 0.0 | 0.3 |
| Salad Cream Style, Weight Watchers* | 1 Tbsp/10g | 11.0 | 0.0 | 115 | 1.5 | 16.2 | 4.4 | 0.0 |
| Seafood, M & S* | 1 Tsp/7g | 39.0 | 4.0 | 555 | 0.9 | 4.9 | 59.3 | 0.9 |
| Smoked Garlic & Parmesan, Sainsbury's* | 1 Serving/20ml | 83.0 | 8.0 | 415 | 3.0 | 4.0 | 41.1 | 0.3 |
| Sun Dried Tomato, Sainsbury's* | 1 Serving/15ml | 27.0 | 2.0 | 179 | 1.5 | 10.9 | 14.4 | 0.6 |
| Sweet Balsamic & Smoked Garlic, BGTY, Sainsbury's* | 1 Serving/20g | 10.0 | 0.0 | 51 | 0.2 | 11.9 | 0.3 | 0.2 |
| Sweet Chilli, COU, M & S* | 1 Tbsp/15ml | 9.0 | 0.0 | 60 | 0.5 | 14.5 | 0.5 | 0.4 |
| Texas Ranch, Frank Cooper* | 1 Pot/28g | 128.0 | 13.0 | 457 | 1.9 | 9.4 | 45.8 | 0.2 |
| Thai Lime & Coriander, The English Provender Co.* | 1 Serving/25g | 26.0 | 0.0 | 104 | 1.6 | 22.3 | 0.9 | 1.1 |
| Thousand Island | 1 Tsp/6g | 19.0 | 2.0 | 323 | 1.1 | 12.5 | 30.2 | 0.4 |
| Thousand Island, BGTY, Sainsbury's* | 1 Serving/50g | 52.0 | 1.0 | 105 | 1.2 | 21.6 | 1.1 | 2.9 |
| Thousand Island, COU, M & S* | 1 Serving/30g | 25.0 | 1.0 | 85 | 1.4 | 14.2 | 2.6 | 1.1 |
| Thousand Island, Frank Cooper* | 1 Pot/28g | 122.0 | 13.0 | 437 | 1.2 | 7.2 | 44.8 | 0.3 |
| Thousand Island, Light, Kraft* | 1 Tbsp/15ml | 14.0 | 0.0 | 94 | 0.6 | 21.5 | 0.2 | 3.0 |
| Thousand Island, Original, Kraft* | 1oz/28g | 102.0 | 9.0 | 365 | 0.9 | 19.0 | 31.5 | 0.4 |
| Thousand Island, Reduced Calorie | 1 Tsp/6g | 12.0 | 1.0 | 195 | 0.7 | 14.7 | 15.2 | 0.0 |
| Thousand Island, Tesco* | 1 Tbsp/15g | 55.0 | 5.0 | 360 | 1.1 | 19.5 | 30.5 | 0.3 |
| Tomato & Basil, HL, Tesco* | ½ Pot/75ml | 41.0 | 1.0 | 55 | 0.8 | 9.0 | 1.5 | 0.5 |
| Tomato & Chipotle, TTD, Sainsbury's* | 1 Tbsp/15g | 57.0 | 6.0 | 381 | 0.6 | 6.3 | 39.3 | 2.8 |
| Tomato & Herb, Less Than 1% Fat, Asda* | 1 Tbsp/15g | 6.0 | 0.0 | 43 | 0.7 | 8.0 | 0.9 | 0.4 |
| Tomato & Olive, Eat Smart, Safeway* | 1 Tbsp/15ml | 15.0 | 0.0 | 100 | 0.7 | 22.8 | 0.7 | 1.8 |
| Tomato & Red Pepper, BGTY, Sainsbury's* | 1 Serving/50ml | 41.0 | 2.0 | 83 | 1.1 | 10.0 | 4.3 | 0.6 |
| Tomato Basil, Light, Kraft* | 1 Serving/15ml | 10.0 | 0.0 | 68 | 1.0 | 14.5 | 0.4 | 2.5 |
| True Blue Cheese, Briannas* | 2 Tbsp/30ml | 120.0 | 11.0 | 400 | 3.3 | 16.7 | 36.7 | 0.0 |
| Waistline, Reduced Fat, Crosse & Blackwell* | 1oz/28g | 29.0 | 2.0 | 105 | 0.8 | 11.6 | 6.0 | 0.3 |
| Yoghurt & Mint, HL, Tesco* | 1 Serving/50g | 31.0 | 1.0 | 62 | 4.1 | 6.9 | 2.5 | 0.2 |
| Yoghurt & Mint, Perfectly Balanced, Waitrose* | 1 Serving/100ml | 130.0 | 3.0 | 130 | 4.6 | 22.1 | 2.6 | 0.7 |
| Yoghurt & Mint, Safeway* | 1 Serving/15ml | 54.0 | 5.0 | 360 | 3.3 | 6.7 | 35.3 | 0.0 |

## DRIED FRUIT

| | Measure INFO/WEIGHT | KCAL | FAT | KCAL | PROT | CARB | FAT | FIBRE |
|---|---|---|---|---|---|---|---|---|
| Exotic, Ready to Eat, Sainsbury's* | 1/3 Pack/85g | 241.0 | 0.0 | 284 | 0.2 | 70.6 | 0.1 | 2.4 |
| Juicy Sprinkle, Nature's Harvest* | 1 Serving/20g | 79.0 | 2.0 | 397 | 4.9 | 71.9 | 10.0 | 4.2 |

## DRIED FRUIT & NUT MIX

| | Measure INFO/WEIGHT | KCAL | FAT | KCAL | PROT | CARB | FAT | FIBRE |
|---|---|---|---|---|---|---|---|---|
| Peanuts, Cashews & Mango, Fair Trade, Tesco* | 1/6 Pack | 130.0 | 9.0 | 520 | 16.4 | 33.2 | 34.8 | 4.8 |
| The Mix, Whitworths* | 1 Pot/90g | 341.0 | 13.0 | 379 | 4.1 | 63.1 | 14.6 | 7.3 |

## DRIED FRUIT MIX

| | Measure INFO/WEIGHT | KCAL | FAT | KCAL | PROT | CARB | FAT | FIBRE |
|---|---|---|---|---|---|---|---|---|
| 5 Fruits, Ready to Eat, Sundora* | ½ Pack/100g | 233.0 | 0.0 | 233 | 1.6 | 58.4 | 0.4 | 6.8 |
| Albert Heijn* | 1 Serving/50g | 110.0 | 0.0 | 220 | 2.1 | 51.0 | 0.5 | 0.0 |
| Asda* | 1 Serving/50g | 152.0 | 0.0 | 305 | 2.0 | 74.0 | 0.5 | 0.6 |
| Average | 1 Tbsp/25g | 67.0 | 0.0 | 268 | 2.3 | 68.1 | 0.4 | 2.2 |
| Berry, Whole Foods, Tesco* | 1 Serving/25g | 66.0 | 0.0 | 265 | 3.3 | 60.0 | 0.7 | 7.5 |
| Exotic Mix, Sundora* | 1 Sm Pack/50g | 138.0 | 1.0 | 276 | 2.3 | 60.6 | 2.7 | 3.8 |
| Fruit Salad, Whitworths* | 1 Serving/62g | 113.0 | 0.0 | 183 | 2.9 | 41.8 | 0.5 | 6.6 |
| Luxury, Co-Op* | 1 Serving/40g | 114.0 | 0.0 | 285 | 2.0 | 68.0 | 0.6 | 4.0 |
| Medley, Shapers, Boots* | 1 Serving/50g | 131.0 | 0.0 | 262 | 3.2 | 61.0 | 0.6 | 5.5 |
| Natural, Positively Healthy, The Food Doctor* | 1 Serving/50g | 164.0 | 0.0 | 328 | 2.4 | 77.9 | 0.7 | 3.6 |

| | Measure INFO/WEIGHT | per Measure KCAL | FAT | Nutrition Values per 100g / 100ml KCAL | PROT | CARB | FAT | FIBRE |
|---|---|---|---|---|---|---|---|---|
| **DRIED FRUIT MIX** | | | | | | | | |
| Sultanas, Currants, Raisins & Citrus Peel, Asda* | 1 Serving/100g | 283.0 | 0.0 | 283 | 2.6 | 67.0 | 0.5 | 1.7 |
| Taste of Hawaii, Extra Special, Asda* | 1 Serving/100g | 314.0 | 1.0 | 314 | 1.7 | 75.0 | 0.8 | 4.4 |
| Taste of New England, Asda* | 1 Serving/50g | 158.0 | 1.0 | 316 | 2.2 | 74.0 | 1.2 | 5.0 |
| Tesco* | 1 Tbsp/25g | 71.0 | 0.0 | 284 | 2.3 | 67.9 | 0.4 | 2.2 |
| **DRIFTER** | | | | | | | | |
| Nestle* | 1 Finger/20g | 98.0 | 5.0 | 488 | 4.8 | 62.7 | 24.2 | 0.7 |
| **DRINK MIX** | | | | | | | | |
| Chocolate, Finest, Tesco* | 1 Serving/200ml | 242.0 | 13.0 | 121 | 4.9 | 10.7 | 6.4 | 0.7 |
| Chocolate, Flavia* | 1 Serving/18g | 64.0 | 1.0 | 368 | 15.6 | 67.2 | 4.0 | 0.0 |
| Chocolate Orange, Clipper* | 1 Pack/28g | 98.0 | 0.0 | 350 | 14.6 | 69.7 | 1.5 | 0.0 |
| Milk Chocolate, Instant Break, Cadbury* | 4 Tsp/28g | 119.0 | 4.0 | 425 | 10.9 | 64.2 | 14.0 | 0.0 |
| **DRINKING CHOCOLATE** | | | | | | | | |
| Cadbury* | 1 Heap Tbsp/16g | 64.0 | 0.0 | 402 | 4.4 | 89.3 | 2.4 | 0.0 |
| Dry, Asda* | 1 Serving/30g | 111.0 | 2.0 | 370 | 6.0 | 73.0 | 6.0 | 0.0 |
| Dry, Tesco* | 3 Tsp/25g | 92.0 | 1.0 | 368 | 6.4 | 72.6 | 5.8 | 4.2 |
| Dry, Waitrose* | 3 Tsp/12g | 48.0 | 1.0 | 403 | 7.2 | 79.9 | 6.1 | 2.9 |
| Dry Powder, Cocodirect* | 1 Serving/18g | 67.0 | 2.0 | 372 | 8.9 | 65.1 | 8.4 | 0.0 |
| Granules, Dry, Impress* | 1oz/28g | 102.0 | 1.0 | 365 | 5.6 | 77.0 | 3.7 | 6.0 |
| Made Up, BGTY, Sainsbury's* | 1 Serving/178g | 114.0 | 0.0 | 64 | 3.9 | 11.4 | 0.2 | 0.7 |
| Made Up with Semi-Skimmed Milk, Average | 1 Mug/227ml | 129.0 | 4.0 | 57 | 3.5 | 7.0 | 1.9 | 0.2 |
| Made Up with Skimmed Milk, Average | 1 Mug/227ml | 100.0 | 1.0 | 44 | 3.5 | 7.0 | 0.5 | 0.0 |
| Made Up with Whole Milk, Average | 1 Mug/227ml | 173.0 | 10.0 | 76 | 3.4 | 6.8 | 4.2 | 0.2 |
| Maxpax, Light, Suchard* | 1 Serving/11g | 37.0 | 1.0 | 355 | 20.0 | 56.0 | 5.5 | 9.3 |
| Powder, Made Up with Skimmed Milk | 1 Mug/227ml | 134.0 | 1.0 | 59 | 3.5 | 10.8 | 0.6 | 0.0 |
| Powder, Made Up with Whole Milk | 1 Mug/227ml | 204.0 | 9.0 | 90 | 3.4 | 10.6 | 4.1 | 0.0 |
| **DRIPPING** | | | | | | | | |
| *Beef* | *1oz/28g* | *249.0* | *28.0* | *891* | *0.0* | *0.0* | *99.0* | *0.0* |
| **DUCK** | | | | | | | | |
| *Breast, Meat Only, Cooked, Average* | *1oz/28g* | *48.0* | *2.0* | *172* | *25.3* | *1.8* | *7.0* | *0.0* |
| *Breast, Meat Only, Raw, Average* | *1 Serving/160g* | *206.0* | *7.0* | *128* | *22.5* | *0.0* | *4.2* | *0.2* |
| *Leg, Meat & Skin, Average* | *1oz/28g* | *80.0* | *6.0* | *286* | *17.2* | *9.5* | *20.0* | *0.4* |
| *Raw, Meat, Fat & Skin* | *1oz/28g* | *109.0* | *10.0* | *388* | *13.1* | *0.0* | *37.3* | *0.0* |
| *Roasted, Meat, Fat & Skin* | *1oz/28g* | *118.0* | *11.0* | *423* | *20.0* | *0.0* | *38.1* | *0.0* |
| **DUCK &** | | | | | | | | |
| Plum Sauce, Roasted, Sainsbury's* | ½ Pack/150g | 174.0 | 4.0 | 116 | 6.9 | 16.0 | 2.5 | 1.8 |
| **DUCK A L' ORANGE** | | | | | | | | |
| Roast, M & S* | ½ Pack/270g | 553.0 | 42.0 | 205 | 12.5 | 4.1 | 15.6 | 0.6 |
| **DUCK AROMATIC** | | | | | | | | |
| Crispy, Asda* | 1/3 Pack/166g | 469.0 | 25.0 | 283 | 19.0 | 18.0 | 15.0 | 0.8 |
| Crispy, Half, with Hoisin Sauce & 12 Pancakes, Tesco* | 1/6 Pack/70g | 162.0 | 7.0 | 232 | 18.3 | 15.9 | 10.6 | 1.1 |
| Crispy, Half Duck & Pancakes, M & S* | ½ Pack/311g | 590.0 | 27.0 | 190 | 13.9 | 14.0 | 8.6 | 2.1 |
| Crispy, Quarter, with Hoisin Sauce & 6 Pancakes, Tesco* | 1/6 Pack/40g | 100.0 | 4.0 | 250 | 12.3 | 25.3 | 10.6 | 2.0 |
| Crispy, Somerfield* | 1 Serving/265g | 782.0 | 49.0 | 295 | 18.1 | 14.0 | 18.5 | 0.7 |
| Crispy, Whole, with Hoisin Sauce & 18 Pancakes, Tesco* | 1/9 Pack/100g | 280.0 | 17.0 | 280 | 18.9 | 12.0 | 17.2 | 0.4 |
| with a Plum Sauce, Finest, Tesco* | 1 Serving/250g | 400.0 | 14.0 | 160 | 16.1 | 11.3 | 5.6 | 4.6 |
| with Plum Sauce, Tesco* | ½ Pack/250g | 350.0 | 11.0 | 140 | 9.3 | 15.2 | 4.6 | 0.3 |
| **DUCK CANTONESE** | | | | | | | | |
| Style, Roast, Tesco* | 1 Pack/300g | 375.0 | 7.0 | 125 | 8.2 | 17.9 | 2.3 | 0.5 |
| **DUCK IN** | | | | | | | | |
| a Plum Sauce, Crispy, M & S* | 1 Pack/325g | 569.0 | 31.0 | 175 | 10.7 | 11.2 | 9.6 | 0.9 |
| Chinese Barbecue, Wings, Sainsbury's* | 1 Serving/175g | 430.0 | 25.0 | 246 | 19.4 | 9.7 | 14.3 | 0.0 |
| Orange Sauce, Iceland* | 1 Serving/200g | 336.0 | 21.0 | 168 | 11.3 | 7.4 | 10.4 | 1.2 |
| Plum Sauce, Legs, Asda* | 1 Leg/200g | 452.0 | 23.0 | 226 | 24.1 | 6.4 | 11.5 | 0.5 |

| | Measure INFO/WEIGHT | per Measure KCAL | FAT | Nutrition Values per 100g / 100ml KCAL | PROT | CARB | FAT | FIBRE |
|---|---|---|---|---|---|---|---|---|
| **DUCK IN** | | | | | | | | |
| Red Wine Sauce, Free Range Fillets, Waitrose* | ½ Pack/250g | 377.0 | 19.0 | 151 | 16.4 | 4.1 | 7.7 | 2.2 |
| **DUCK PEKING** | | | | | | | | |
| Crispy, Aromatic, Sainsbury's* | ½ Pack/300g | 1236.0 | 111.0 | 412 | 19.5 | 0.6 | 36.9 | 0.1 |
| Crispy, Cherry Valley* | 1 Serving/270g | 702.0 | 36.0 | 260 | 17.5 | 17.8 | 13.3 | 0.7 |
| **DUCK WITH** | | | | | | | | |
| Apple & Calvados Sauce, GFY, Asda* | 1 Serving/162g | 144.0 | 4.0 | 89 | 13.0 | 4.2 | 2.2 | 1.4 |
| Diuelection, M & S* | 1 Serving/67g | 194.0 | 9.0 | 290 | 7.2 | 34.8 | 13.4 | 2.2 |
| Noodles, Shanghai Roast, Sainsbury's* | 1 Pack/450g | 580.0 | 17.0 | 129 | 5.6 | 18.0 | 3.8 | 1.2 |
| **DUMPLINGS** | | | | | | | | |
| Average | 1oz/28g | 58.0 | 3.0 | 208 | 2.8 | 24.5 | 11.7 | 0.9 |
| Dried Mix, Tesco* | 1 Pack/137g | 404.0 | 17.0 | 295 | 5.4 | 39.9 | 12.2 | 2.8 |
| Homestyle, Baked Weight, Frozen, Aunt Bessie's* | 1 Dumpling/49g | 188.0 | 9.0 | 384 | 9.7 | 44.4 | 17.6 | 2.8 |
| Pork & Garlic Chive, Waitrose* | 1 Pack/115g | 215.0 | 8.0 | 187 | 9.4 | 20.4 | 7.0 | 1.1 |
| Prawn, Cantonese, Crispy, Sainsbury's* | 1 Dumpling/11g | 27.0 | 1.0 | 241 | 9.3 | 20.9 | 13.4 | 1.1 |
| Prawn, Siu Mai, Chinese, M & S* | 8 Dumplings/170g | 170.0 | 3.0 | 100 | 7.8 | 13.1 | 1.7 | 1.3 |

**D**

|  | Measure INFO/WEIGHT | per Measure KCAL | per Measure FAT | Nutrition Values per 100g / 100ml KCAL | PROT | CARB | FAT | FIBRE |
|---|---|---|---|---|---|---|---|---|
| **EASTER EGG** | | | | | | | | |
| Aero, Nestle* | ¼ Egg/30g | 164.0 | 10.0 | 544 | 6.5 | 55.4 | 32.9 | 0.6 |
| Bunny, Chocolate, Malteaser, Mars* | 1 Bunny/29g | 155.0 | 9.0 | 535 | 6.2 | 56.2 | 31.7 | 0.0 |
| Bunny, Milk Chocolate, Belgian, TTD, Sainsbury's* | 1 Serving/40g | 218.0 | 13.0 | 546 | 5.7 | 55.0 | 33.7 | 2.0 |
| Buttons, Cadbury* | 1 Pack/200g | 1060.0 | 60.0 | 530 | 7.7 | 56.6 | 30.1 | 0.7 |
| Chick, Dairy Milk, Cadbury* | 1 Chick/185g | 980.0 | 56.0 | 530 | 7.5 | 56.7 | 30.1 | 0.7 |
| Chocolate Orange, Terry's* | 1 Egg/120g | 636.0 | 37.0 | 530 | 7.4 | 57.0 | 30.5 | 2.4 |
| Creme Egg, Cadbury* | ½ Shell/60g | 315.0 | 18.0 | 525 | 7.5 | 56.8 | 30.0 | 0.0 |
| Crunchie, Cadbury* | 1 Egg/120g | 630.0 | 36.0 | 525 | 7.5 | 56.8 | 30.0 | 0.7 |
| Dark Chocolate, 70%, Green & Black's* | 1 Egg/110g | 606.0 | 45.0 | 551 | 9.3 | 36.0 | 41.1 | 0.0 |
| Dark Chocolate, Thorncroft's* | 1 Egg/360g | 1890.0 | 135.0 | 525 | 6.8 | 39.4 | 37.4 | 9.8 |
| Disney, Nestle* | 1 Egg/65g | 342.0 | 19.0 | 526 | 6.3 | 59.7 | 29.1 | 0.6 |
| Kit Kat, Chunky, Nestle* | 1 Egg/70g | 380.0 | 23.0 | 544 | 6.5 | 55.4 | 32.9 | 0.6 |
| Mars* | 1 Serving/63g | 281.0 | 11.0 | 449 | 4.2 | 69.0 | 17.4 | 0.0 |
| Milk Chocolate, Nestle* | ½ Egg/42g | 205.0 | 10.0 | 489 | 5.0 | 65.2 | 23.1 | 0.5 |
| Milk Chocolate, Swiss, Hollow, M & S* | 1 Egg/18g | 100.0 | 6.0 | 555 | 6.7 | 53.2 | 34.8 | 2.5 |
| Milky Bar, Nestle* | 1 Egg/40g | 182.0 | 7.0 | 454 | 4.2 | 70.8 | 17.2 | 0.0 |
| Roses, Cadbury* | 1 Egg/200g | 1050.0 | 60.0 | 525 | 7.5 | 56.8 | 30.0 | 0.7 |
| Smarties, Nestle* | ½ Egg/38g | 179.0 | 7.0 | 478 | 4.8 | 69.6 | 20.0 | 0.7 |
| Twirl, Cadbury* | 1 Egg/200g | 1050.0 | 60.0 | 525 | 7.5 | 56.8 | 30.0 | 0.7 |
| White Chocolate, Thorntons* | 1 Egg/360g | 1958.0 | 109.0 | 544 | 5.5 | 62.2 | 30.3 | 2.1 |
| Wispa, Cadbury* | 1 Egg/200g | 1050.0 | 60.0 | 525 | 7.5 | 56.8 | 30.0 | 0.7 |
| **ECLAIR** | | | | | | | | |
| Belgian Chocolate, Weight Watchers* | 1 Eclair/30g | 81.0 | 4.0 | 271 | 3.9 | 37.6 | 11.7 | 6.6 |
| Chocolate, 25% Less Fat, Sainsbury's* | 1 Eclair/58g | 171.0 | 9.0 | 295 | 6.8 | 31.1 | 16.0 | 1.2 |
| Chocolate, Asda* | 1 Eclair/33g | 144.0 | 11.0 | 436 | 6.7 | 27.3 | 33.3 | 4.8 |
| Chocolate, Cream, Fresh, Tesco* | 1 Eclair/66g | 285.0 | 20.0 | 430 | 6.0 | 31.1 | 30.9 | 1.8 |
| Chocolate, Cream Filled, VLH Kitchens* | 1 Eclair/66g | 286.0 | 19.3 | 434 | 7.0 | 36.4 | 29.2 | 1.8 |
| Chocolate, Dairy Cream, Co-Op* | 1 Eclair/59g | 227.0 | 17.0 | 385 | 5.0 | 26.0 | 29.0 | 0.3 |
| Chocolate, Filled with Pastry Cream, Average | 1 Eclair/100g | 262.0 | 16.0 | 262 | 6.4 | 24.2 | 15.7 | 0.6 |
| Chocolate, Fresh Cream, M & S* | 1 Eclair/44g | 170.0 | 12.0 | 390 | 6.3 | 28.4 | 27.9 | 2.0 |
| Chocolate, Fresh Cream, Sainsbury's* | 1 Eclair/59g | 212.0 | 14.0 | 360 | 4.2 | 32.7 | 23.6 | 0.5 |
| Chocolate, Frozen, Morrisons* | 1 Eclair/31g | 116.0 | 10.0 | 374 | 5.0 | 18.8 | 31.0 | 1.3 |
| Chocolate, HL, Tesco* | 1 Serving/77g | 192.0 | 10.0 | 249 | 6.8 | 27.1 | 12.6 | 0.9 |
| Chocolate & Fresh Cream, Tempting, Tesco* | 1 Eclair/39g | 158.0 | 11.0 | 405 | 6.5 | 29.1 | 28.8 | 1.1 |
| Double Chocolate, with Fresh Cream, Tesco* | 1 Eclair/69g | 275.0 | 19.0 | 400 | 5.9 | 33.4 | 27.0 | 1.6 |
| **EEL** | | | | | | | | |
| *Cooked Or Smoked, Dry Heat, Average* | *1 Serving/100g* | *236.0* | *15.0* | *236* | *23.6* | *0.0* | *14.9* | *0.0* |
| *Jellied, Average* | *1oz/28g* | *27.0* | *2.0* | *98* | *8.4* | *0.0* | *7.1* | *0.0* |
| *Raw, Average* | *1oz/28g* | *47.0* | *3.0* | *168* | *16.6* | *0.0* | *11.3* | *0.0* |
| **EGG SUBSTITUTE** | | | | | | | | |
| 99% Real Eggs, The Crafty Cook* | ¼ Cup/61g | 30.0 | 0.0 | 49 | 10.0 | 2.0 | 0.0 | 0.0 |
| Original, The Crafty Cook* | ¼ Cup 1oz/28g | 30.0 | 0.0 | 107 | 21.4 | 3.6 | 0.0 | 0.0 |
| **EGGS** | | | | | | | | |
| *Dried, White, Average* | *1 Tbsp/14g* | *41.0* | *0.0* | *295* | *73.8* | *0.0* | *0.0* | *0.0* |
| *Dried, Whole, Average* | *1oz/28g* | *159.0* | *12.0* | *568* | *48.4* | *0.0* | *41.6* | *0.0* |
| Duck, Boiled & Salted, Average | 1 Egg/75g | 148.0 | 12.0 | 198 | 14.6 | 0.0 | 15.5 | 0.0 |
| *Duck, Whole, Raw, Average* | *1 Egg/75g* | *122.0* | *9.0* | *163* | *14.3* | *0.0* | *11.8* | *0.0* |
| *Free Range, Large, Average* | *1 Egg/56g* | *80.0* | *6.0* | *143* | *12.6* | *0.8* | *9.9* | *0.0* |
| Free Range, Medium, Average | 1 Egg/50g | 71.0 | 5.0 | 143 | 12.6 | 0.8 | 9.9 | 0.0 |
| Fried, Average | 1 Med/60g | 107.0 | 8.0 | 179 | 13.6 | 0.0 | 13.9 | 0.0 |
| *Goose, Whole, Fresh, Raw, Average* | *1 Egg/144g* | *267.0* | *19.0* | *185* | *13.9* | *1.3* | *13.3* | *0.0* |
| *Large, Average* | *1 Egg/56g* | *82.0* | *6.0* | *147* | *12.5* | *0.0* | *10.8* | *0.0* |
| *Medium, Average* | *1 Egg/50g* | *71.0* | *5.0* | *143* | *12.6* | *0.8* | *9.9* | *0.0* |

E

| | Measure INFO/WEIGHT | per Measure KCAL | FAT | Nutrition Values per 100g / 100ml KCAL | PROT | CARB | FAT | FIBRE |
|---|---|---|---|---|---|---|---|---|
| **EGGS** | | | | | | | | |
| Medium, Boiled, Average | 1 Egg/50g | 73.0 | 5.0 | 147 | 12.5 | 0.0 | 10.8 | 0.0 |
| Poached | 1 Med/50g | 73.0 | 5.0 | 147 | 12.5 | 0.0 | 10.8 | 0.0 |
| *Quail, Whole, Raw* | *1 Egg/13g* | *20.0* | *1.0* | *151* | *12.9* | *0.0* | *11.1* | *0.0* |
| Scrambled, Average | 1 Egg/68g | 100.0 | 7.0 | 147 | 12.5 | 0.0 | 10.8 | 0.0 |
| Scrambled with Milk, Average | 1 Egg/60g | 148.0 | 14.0 | 247 | 10.7 | 0.6 | 22.6 | 0.0 |
| *Turkey, Whole, Raw* | *1oz/28g* | *46.0* | *3.0* | *165* | *13.7* | *0.0* | *12.2* | *0.0* |
| *Whites Only, Raw, Average* | *1 Lg Egg/33g* | *17.0* | *0.0* | *52* | *10.9* | *0.3* | *0.6* | *0.0* |
| *Yolks, Raw* | *1 Av Yolk/14g* | *47.0* | *4.0* | *339* | *16.1* | *0.0* | *30.5* | *0.0* |
| **ELDERBERRIES** | | | | | | | | |
| *Average* | *1oz/28g* | *10.0* | *0.0* | *35* | *0.7* | *7.4* | *0.5* | *0.0* |
| **ELICHE** | | | | | | | | |
| Dry Weight, Buitoni* | 1 Serving/80g | 282.0 | 2.0 | 352 | 11.2 | 72.6 | 1.9 | 0.0 |
| **ENCHILADAS** | | | | | | | | |
| Beef, Light Choices, Tesco* | 1 Pack/400g | 412.0 | 9.0 | 103 | 7.0 | 13.5 | 2.3 | 2.2 |
| Chicken, American, HL, Tesco* | 1 Serving/240g | 353.0 | 4.0 | 147 | 10.4 | 22.5 | 1.8 | 1.2 |
| Chicken, Asda* | 1 Serving/500g | 690.0 | 30.0 | 138 | 10.0 | 17.0 | 6.0 | 1.0 |
| Chicken, Diner Specials, M & S* | ½ Pack/227g | 340.0 | 12.0 | 150 | 9.9 | 15.4 | 5.3 | 2.0 |
| Chicken, in a Spicy Salsa & Bean Sauce, Asda* | ½ Pack/212g | 373.0 | 17.0 | 176 | 10.0 | 16.0 | 8.0 | 0.0 |
| Chicken, Morrisons* | ½ Pack/275g | 393.0 | 13.0 | 143 | 10.0 | 15.4 | 4.6 | 1.8 |
| Chicken, Perfectly Balanced, Waitrose* | 1 Pack/450g | 481.0 | 14.0 | 107 | 6.9 | 12.7 | 3.2 | 1.1 |
| Chicken, Safeway* | 1 Serving/230g | 384.0 | 11.0 | 167 | 7.9 | 22.9 | 4.9 | 1.0 |
| Chicken, Value, Tesco* | 1 Serving/212g | 297.0 | 8.0 | 140 | 7.0 | 19.3 | 3.9 | 1.1 |
| Three Bean, Vegetarian, Tesco* | 1 Pack/440g | 572.0 | 25.0 | 130 | 4.9 | 14.1 | 5.6 | 3.3 |
| Vegetable, GFY, Asda* | 1 Pack/350g | 399.0 | 16.0 | 114 | 4.4 | 14.0 | 4.5 | 1.3 |
| Vegetable, Morrisons* | 1 Pack/400g | 468.0 | 18.0 | 117 | 4.5 | 14.4 | 4.6 | 1.8 |
| Vegetable & Bean, Eat Smart, Morrisons* | 1 Pack/380g | 475.0 | 10.0 | 125 | 4.7 | 20.7 | 2.6 | 3.2 |
| **ENDIVE** | | | | | | | | |
| *Raw* | *1oz/28g* | *4.0* | *0.0* | *13* | *1.8* | *1.0* | *0.2* | *2.0* |
| **ENERGY DRINK** | | | | | | | | |
| Blue Bolt, Sainsbury's* | 1 Can/250ml | 105.0 | 0.0 | 42 | 0.0 | 10.0 | 0.0 | 0.0 |
| Burn, Coca-Cola* | 1 fl oz/30ml | 13.0 | 0.0 | 44 | 0.0 | 10.5 | 0.0 | 0.0 |
| Lemon, Active Sport, Tesco* | 1 Bottle/500ml | 135.0 | 0.0 | 27 | 0.0 | 6.5 | 0.0 | 0.0 |
| Orange, Active Sport, Tesco* | 1 Bottle/500ml | 135.0 | 0.0 | 27 | 0.0 | 6.5 | 0.0 | 0.0 |
| Powerade, Aqua+* | 1 Bottle/500ml | 80.0 | 0.0 | 16 | 0.0 | 3.7 | 0.0 | 0.0 |
| Red Rooster, Hi Energy Mixer, Cott Beverages Ltd* | 1 Can/250ml | 112.0 | 0.0 | 45 | 0.6 | 10.3 | 0.0 | 0.0 |
| Red Thunder, Aldi* | 1 Can/250ml | 112.0 | 0.0 | 45 | 0.6 | 10.3 | 0.0 | 0.0 |
| Redcard, Britvic* | 1 Can/330ml | 96.0 | 0.0 | 29 | 0.1 | 7.0 | 0.0 | 0.0 |
| V, Frucor Beverages* | 1 Can/250ml | 112.0 | 0.0 | 45 | 0.0 | 11.2 | 0.0 | 0.0 |

**E**

## FAGGOTS

| | Measure INFO/WEIGHT | per Measure KCAL | per Measure FAT | KCAL | PROT | CARB | FAT | FIBRE |
|---|---|---|---|---|---|---|---|---|
| in Rich Gravy, Iceland* | 1 Faggot/81g | 116.0 | 5.0 | 143 | 6.5 | 15.9 | 6.4 | 1.1 |
| Mushy Peas & Mash, Sainsbury's* | 1 Pack/450g | 576.0 | 19.0 | 128 | 6.0 | 16.3 | 4.3 | 1.6 |
| Pork, in a Rich, West Country Sauce, Raw, Mr Brains* | 1 Four Pack/378g | 484.0 | 25.0 | 128 | 5.3 | 11.9 | 6.6 | 0.6 |
| **FAGOTTINI** | | | | | | | | |
| Mushroom, Sainsbury's* | ½ Pack/155g | 339.0 | 12.0 | 219 | 10.2 | 27.7 | 7.5 | 2.7 |
| **FAJITA** | | | | | | | | |
| Beef, GFY, Asda* | ½ Pack/208g | 354.0 | 10.0 | 170 | 11.0 | 21.0 | 4.7 | 1.6 |
| Chicken, American Style, Tesco* | 1 Pack/275g | 388.0 | 14.0 | 141 | 9.5 | 14.2 | 5.1 | 1.0 |
| Chicken, Asda* | ½ Pack/225g | 371.0 | 10.0 | 165 | 11.0 | 20.0 | 4.5 | 3.5 |
| Chicken, BGTY, Sainsbury's* | 1 Pack/172g | 256.0 | 4.0 | 149 | 10.8 | 20.9 | 2.5 | 1.7 |
| Chicken, Char Grilled Style, Safeway* | ½ Pack/235g | 586.0 | 5.0 | 250 | 17.2 | 40.5 | 2.3 | 1.9 |
| Chicken, COU, M & S* | 1 Pack/230g | 287.0 | 5.0 | 125 | 10.0 | 16.5 | 2.3 | 1.5 |
| Chicken, Finest, Tesco* | ½ Pack/288g | 457.0 | 20.0 | 159 | 9.9 | 14.4 | 6.8 | 2.1 |
| Chicken, GFY, Asda* | ½ Pack/225g | 233.0 | 4.0 | 104 | 9.3 | 12.9 | 1.8 | 2.0 |
| Chicken, Just Cook, Sainsbury's* | ½ Pack/200g | 200.0 | 3.0 | 100 | 18.5 | 3.1 | 1.5 | 2.0 |
| Chicken, M & S* | 1 Pack/230g | 345.0 | 12.0 | 150 | 8.6 | 17.7 | 5.3 | 1.0 |
| Chicken, Morrisons* | 1 Serving/300g | 370.0 | 15.0 | 123 | 7.4 | 12.2 | 5.1 | 1.9 |
| Chicken, Sainsbury's* | ½ Pack/275g | 396.0 | 15.0 | 144 | 9.5 | 14.5 | 5.3 | 1.9 |
| Chicken, Salt Balanced, COU, M & S* | 1 Pack/230g | 253.0 | 5.0 | 110 | 9.5 | 13.2 | 2.3 | 1.7 |
| Chicken, Tesco* | ½ Pack /275g | 382.0 | 14.0 | 139 | 9.2 | 13.9 | 5.2 | 1.9 |
| Chicken, Value, Tesco* | 1 Serving/250g | 255.0 | 6.0 | 102 | 6.9 | 13.2 | 2.4 | 1.5 |
| Chicken with Salsa & Sour Cream Dips, Safeway* | 1 Pack/242g | 390.0 | 15.0 | 161 | 9.8 | 16.7 | 6.1 | 1.9 |
| Tuna, Sainsbury's* | 1 Pack/450g | 751.0 | 24.0 | 167 | 11.4 | 18.2 | 5.4 | 1.6 |
| Vegetable, Somerfield* | 1 Pack/500g | 640.0 | 25.0 | 128 | 3.0 | 17.0 | 5.0 | 0.0 |
| Vegetable, Tesco* | 1 Fajita/112g | 133.0 | 6.0 | 119 | 4.2 | 14.3 | 5.0 | 1.1 |
| **FALAFEL** | | | | | | | | |
| Asda* | ½ Pack/50g | 140.0 | 10.0 | 281 | 8.3 | 18.9 | 19.1 | 8.2 |
| Cauldron Foods* | 1 Falafel/25g | 51.0 | 2.0 | 203 | 7.6 | 29.8 | 9.0 | 7.2 |
| Fried in Vegetable Oil, Average | 1 Falafel.25g | 45.0 | 3.0 | 179 | 6.4 | 15.6 | 11.2 | 3.4 |
| Mini, Sainsbury's* | 1 Serving/168g | 499.0 | 30.0 | 297 | 8.0 | 26.8 | 17.6 | 3.2 |
| Mix, Asda* | 1 Packet/120g | 313.0 | 15.0 | 261 | 6.4 | 30.8 | 12.5 | 2.6 |
| Mix, Sainsbury's* | ½ Pack/110g | 197.0 | 7.0 | 179 | 7.7 | 23.5 | 6.0 | 5.2 |
| Organic, Cauldron Foods* | 1 Falafel/25g | 51.0 | 2.0 | 203 | 8.4 | 20.3 | 9.8 | 7.2 |
| **FANTA** | | | | | | | | |
| Apple, Z, Coca-Cola* | 1 Can/330ml | 13.0 | 0.0 | 4 | 0.0 | 0.6 | 0.0 | 0.0 |
| Fruit Twist, Coca-Cola* | 1 Serving/250ml | 132.0 | 0.0 | 53 | 0.0 | 13.0 | 0.0 | 0.0 |
| Icy Lemon, Coca-Cola* | 1 Can/330ml | 165.0 | 0.0 | 50 | 0.0 | 12.2 | 0.0 | 0.0 |
| Icy Lemon, Zero, Coca-Cola* | 1 Can/330ml | 7.0 | 0.0 | 2 | 0.0 | 0.2 | 0.0 | 0.0 |
| Lemon, Coca-Cola* | 1 Can/330ml | 165.0 | 0.0 | 50 | 0.0 | 12.0 | 0.0 | 0.0 |
| Light, Coca-Cola* | 1 Glass/250ml | 5.0 | 0.0 | 2 | 0.0 | 0.5 | 0.0 | 0.0 |
| Orange, Coca-Cola* | 1 Serving/251ml | 108.0 | 0.0 | 43 | 0.1 | 10.6 | 0.0 | 0.0 |
| Orange, Z, Coca-Cola* | 1 Can/330ml | 10.0 | 0.0 | 3 | 0.0 | 0.5 | 0.0 | 0.0 |
| Summer Fruits, Z, Coca-Cola* | 1 fl oz/30ml | 1.0 | 0.0 | 3 | 0.0 | 0.6 | 0.0 | 0.0 |
| **FARFALLE** | | | | | | | | |
| ***Bows, Dry, Average*** | ***1 Serving/75g*** | ***265.0*** | ***1.0*** | ***353*** | ***11.4*** | ***72.6*** | ***1.9*** | ***1.9*** |
| Salmon & Broccoli, Eat Smart, Safeway* | 1 Pack/380g | 361.0 | 9.0 | 95 | 6.4 | 11.6 | 2.4 | 1.1 |
| **FENNEL** | | | | | | | | |
| ***Florence, Boiled in Salted Water*** | ***1oz/28g*** | ***3.0*** | ***0.0*** | ***11*** | ***0.9*** | ***1.5*** | ***0.2*** | ***2.3*** |
| ***Florence, Raw, Unprepared*** | ***1 Bulb/250g*** | ***30.0*** | ***0.0*** | ***12*** | ***0.9*** | ***1.8*** | ***0.2*** | ***2.4*** |
| ***Florence, Steamed*** | ***1 Serving/80g*** | ***9.0*** | ***0.0*** | ***11*** | ***9.0*** | ***1.5*** | ***0.2*** | ***2.3*** |
| **FENUGREEK** | | | | | | | | |
| ***Leaves, Raw, Fresh, Average*** | ***1 Serving/80g*** | ***28.0*** | ***0.0*** | ***35*** | ***4.6*** | ***4.8*** | ***0.2*** | ***1.1*** |

F

| | Measure INFO/WEIGHT | per Measure KCAL | FAT | Nutrition Values per 100g / 100ml KCAL | PROT | CARB | FAT | FIBRE |
|---|---|---|---|---|---|---|---|---|
| **FETTUCINI** | | | | | | | | |
| Cajun Chicken, COU, M & S* | 1 Pack/400g | 380.0 | 8.0 | 95 | 8.0 | 10.8 | 2.0 | 2.9 |
| Chicken, Cajun, GFY, Asda* | 1 Pack/398g | 450.0 | 9.0 | 113 | 8.3 | 14.9 | 2.2 | 1.5 |
| Chicken Mushroom, GFY, Asda* | 1 Pack/400g | 359.0 | 7.0 | 90 | 7.2 | 11.2 | 1.7 | 0.7 |
| Dry Weight, Buitoni* | 1 Serving/90g | 326.0 | 2.0 | 362 | 12.2 | 74.4 | 1.7 | 0.0 |
| with Tomato & Mushroom, Easy Cook, Napolina* | 1 Pack/120g | 461.0 | 9.0 | 384 | 11.8 | 67.9 | 7.2 | 0.0 |
| **FIG ROLLS** | | | | | | | | |
| Asda* | 1 Biscuit/19g | 71.0 | 2.0 | 372 | 4.8 | 68.0 | 9.0 | 0.0 |
| Go Ahead, McVitie's* | 1 Biscuit/15g | 55.0 | 1.0 | 365 | 4.2 | 76.8 | 4.6 | 2.9 |
| Jacob's* | 1 Biscuit/18g | 68.0 | 2.0 | 380 | 4.0 | 71.4 | 8.5 | 3.3 |
| Vitalinea, Jacob's* | 1 Biscuit/18g | 61.0 | 1.0 | 339 | 3.7 | 68.2 | 5.8 | 3.8 |
| **FIGS** | | | | | | | | |
| *Dried, Average* | *1 Fig/14g* | *32.0* | *0.0* | *232* | *3.6* | *53.2* | *1.1* | *8.6* |
| In Light Syrup, Asda* | 1 Serving/100g | 75.0 | 0.0 | 75 | 0.4 | 18.0 | 0.1 | 0.7 |
| *Raw, Average* | *1 Fig/35g* | *16.0* | *0.0* | *45* | *1.3* | *9.8* | *0.2* | *1.5* |
| **FISH** | | | | | | | | |
| Balls, Steamed | 1oz/28g | 21.0 | 0.0 | 74 | 11.8 | 5.5 | 0.5 | 0.0 |
| Battered, Portion, Ross* | 1 Serving/110g | 223.0 | 12.0 | 203 | 10.4 | 16.1 | 10.8 | 0.8 |
| Breaded, Asda* | 1 Serving/150g | 351.0 | 21.0 | 234 | 15.0 | 12.0 | 14.0 | 0.5 |
| Dried, Small, Ogura* | 1 Serving/10g | 32.0 | 0.0 | 320 | 69.0 | 0.3 | 3.0 | 0.0 |
| Fillets, White, Breaded, Tesco* | 1 Piece/95g | 198.0 | 10.0 | 208 | 10.6 | 16.9 | 10.9 | 1.0 |
| Fillets, White, Natural, Tesco* | 1 Fillet/100g | 72.0 | 1.0 | 72 | 16.6 | 0.0 | 0.6 | 0.0 |
| Goujons, Asda* | 1 Serving/125g | 240.0 | 8.0 | 192 | 12.8 | 20.8 | 6.4 | 0.2 |
| in Batter, Morrisons* | 1 Fish/140g | 235.0 | 8.0 | 168 | 14.0 | 15.0 | 5.8 | 0.2 |
| Medley, SteamFresh, Birds Eye* | 1 Bag/170g | 170.0 | 6.0 | 100 | 13.0 | 2.3 | 3.7 | 0.1 |
| Seaside Shapes, Birds Eye* | 2 Pieces/80g | 197.0 | 11.0 | 246 | 11.0 | 19.0 | 14.0 | 1.1 |
| Steaks, Skinless & Boneless, Youngs* | 1 Serving/105g | 224.0 | 12.0 | 214 | 10.5 | 16.6 | 11.8 | 0.8 |
| White, Breaded, Fillets, Ocean Pure* | 1 Fillet/113g | 276.0 | 11.0 | 245 | 20.8 | 16.9 | 10.2 | 1.2 |
| White, Tesco* | 1 Med Fillet/100g | 78.0 | 1.0 | 78 | 16.6 | 0.0 | 0.6 | 0.0 |
| **FISH & CHIPS** | | | | | | | | |
| Breaded, Budgens* | 1 Pack/340g | 544.0 | 18.0 | 160 | 8.6 | 19.3 | 5.3 | 1.5 |
| Cod, HL, Tesco* | 1 Pack/400g | 492.0 | 7.0 | 123 | 5.3 | 21.4 | 1.8 | 1.7 |
| Ross* | 1 Serving/250g | 415.0 | 19.0 | 166 | 6.2 | 18.1 | 7.6 | 1.6 |
| Somerfield* | 1 Serving/283g | 495.0 | 17.0 | 175 | 8.0 | 22.0 | 6.0 | 0.0 |
| Tesco* | 1 Serving/300g | 489.0 | 19.0 | 163 | 5.5 | 21.2 | 6.2 | 1.6 |
| with Mushy Peas, Kershaws* | 1 Pack/315g | 450.0 | 18.0 | 143 | 6.4 | 16.4 | 5.8 | 1.6 |
| **FISH CAKES** | | | | | | | | |
| Breaded, Sainsbury's* | 1 Cake/42g | 75.0 | 3.0 | 179 | 10.0 | 16.2 | 8.1 | 0.7 |
| Bubbly Batter, Youngs* | 1 Cake/44g | 109.0 | 7.0 | 247 | 7.1 | 20.5 | 15.1 | 1.4 |
| Captain's Coins, Mini, Captain Birds Eye, Birds Eye* | 1 Cake/20g | 38.0 | 2.0 | 188 | 9.5 | 18.7 | 8.3 | 1.1 |
| Cod, & Pancetta, Cafe Culture, M & S* | 1 Cake/85g | 166.0 | 13.0 | 195 | 9.2 | 7.2 | 15.5 | 2.0 |
| Cod, Big Time, Birds Eye* | 1 Cake/114g | 223.0 | 12.0 | 196 | 8.3 | 17.8 | 10.2 | 1.0 |
| Cod, Birds Eye* | 1 Cake/51g | 95.0 | 4.0 | 186 | 11.3 | 15.9 | 8.6 | 1.0 |
| Cod, Cheese & Chive, Finest, Tesco* | 1 Cake/100g | 212.0 | 11.0 | 212 | 9.7 | 18.3 | 11.5 | 1.7 |
| Cod, Chunky, Breaded, Chilled, Youngs* | 1 Cake/90g | 192.0 | 12.0 | 213 | 9.5 | 14.9 | 12.8 | 1.2 |
| Cod, Fresh, Asda* | 1 Cake/75g | 164.0 | 8.0 | 219 | 7.0 | 23.0 | 11.0 | 1.6 |
| Cod, Homemade, Average | 1 Cake/50g | 120.0 | 8.0 | 241 | 9.3 | 14.4 | 16.6 | 0.7 |
| Cod, in Crunch Crumb, Birds Eye* | 1 Cake/50g | 93.0 | 4.0 | 187 | 11.4 | 16.0 | 8.6 | 1.0 |
| Cod, King Prawn & Pancetta, Extra Special, Asda* | 1 Cake/115g | 202.0 | 8.0 | 176 | 11.0 | 17.8 | 6.7 | 15.0 |
| Cod, Line Caught, Sainsbury's* | 1 Cake/90g | 161.0 | 7.0 | 179 | 10.4 | 17.1 | 7.7 | 1.3 |
| Cod, Tesco* | 1 Cake/90g | 202.0 | 9.0 | 224 | 8.9 | 23.8 | 10.4 | 0.2 |
| Cod & Parsley, Waitrose* | 1 Cake/85g | 147.0 | 6.0 | 173 | 9.2 | 16.9 | 7.6 | 1.1 |
| Crab, & Prawn, Thai, Tesco* | 1 Cake/115g | 269.0 | 17.0 | 234 | 8.8 | 17.4 | 14.4 | 1.2 |
| Fried in Blended Oil | 1 Cake/50g | 109.0 | 7.0 | 218 | 8.6 | 16.8 | 13.4 | 0.0 |

| FISH CAKES | Measure INFO/WEIGHT | per Measure KCAL | FAT | Nutrition Values per 100g / 100ml KCAL | PROT | CARB | FAT | FIBRE |
|---|---|---|---|---|---|---|---|---|
| Frozen, Average | 1 Cake/85g | 112.0 | 3.0 | 132 | 8.6 | 16.7 | 3.9 | 0.0 |
| Grilled, Average | 1 Cake/50g | 77.0 | 2.0 | 154 | 9.9 | 19.7 | 4.5 | 0.0 |
| Haddock, Breaded, Asda* | 1 Cake/90g | 187.0 | 8.0 | 208 | 10.0 | 22.8 | 8.5 | 1.2 |
| Haddock, Fresh Tastes, Asda* | 1 Cake/75g | 141.0 | 5.0 | 188 | 9.6 | 22.2 | 6.7 | 1.8 |
| Haddock, Sainsbury's* | 1 Cake/83g | 166.0 | 7.0 | 199 | 11.4 | 20.1 | 8.1 | 1.8 |
| Haddock, Smoked, Breaded, Asda* | 1 Cake/90g | 202.0 | 12.0 | 225 | 9.0 | 18.0 | 13.0 | 1.6 |
| Haddock, Smoked, Extra Special, Asda* | 1 Cake/115g | 218.0 | 11.0 | 190 | 12.8 | 13.2 | 9.5 | 1.3 |
| Haddock, Smoked, Frozen, Waitrose* | 1 Cake/85g | 186.0 | 10.0 | 219 | 9.6 | 17.8 | 12.1 | 0.8 |
| Haddock, Smoked, M & S* | 1 Cake/85g | 153.0 | 8.0 | 180 | 10.6 | 13.4 | 9.4 | 2.6 |
| Haddock, Smoked, Sainsbury's* | 1 Cake/63g | 127.0 | 6.0 | 201 | 11.0 | 17.8 | 9.5 | 2.1 |
| Haddock, Smoked, Tesco* | 1 Cake/90g | 198.0 | 9.0 | 220 | 10.3 | 21.0 | 10.4 | 0.2 |
| Haddock, Smoked, TTD, Sainsbury's* | 1 Cake/115g | 201.0 | 11.0 | 175 | 9.8 | 13.0 | 9.3 | 1.4 |
| Haddock in Breadcumbs, Sainsbury's* | 1 Cake/88g | 158.0 | 6.0 | 179 | 10.8 | 18.2 | 7.0 | 1.4 |
| Halibut, TTD, Sainsbury's* | 1 Cake/115g | 289.0 | 18.0 | 251 | 10.0 | 17.6 | 15.6 | 1.3 |
| Halibut Cod Loin, Finest, Tesco* | 1 Cake/115g | 213.0 | 8.0 | 185 | 8.8 | 21.3 | 7.2 | 1.4 |
| Prawn, Battered, Asda* | 1 Cake/90g | 182.0 | 10.0 | 202 | 10.0 | 15.6 | 11.1 | 1.0 |
| Prawn, Sainsbury's* | 1 Cake/90g | 184.0 | 8.0 | 204 | 9.6 | 21.7 | 8.7 | 1.2 |
| Prawn, Tesco* | 1 Cake/90g | 209.0 | 8.0 | 232 | 8.2 | 29.2 | 9.1 | 1.8 |
| Prawn, Thai Style, Finest, Tesco* | 1 Cake/94g | 160.0 | 5.0 | 170 | 9.4 | 19.9 | 5.6 | 2.1 |
| Salmon, & Asparagus, Finest, Tesco* | 1 Cake/115g | 300.0 | 18.0 | 261 | 10.7 | 19.6 | 15.5 | 0.4 |
| Salmon, & Broccoli, Morrisons* | 1 Cake/60g | 126.0 | 7.0 | 210 | 9.8 | 17.2 | 11.9 | 1.3 |
| Salmon, & Dill, COOK* | 1 Cake/95g | 144.0 | 5.0 | 152 | 11.3 | 14.2 | 5.6 | 1.5 |
| Salmon, & Dill, Waitrose* | 1 Cake/85g | 206.0 | 12.0 | 242 | 11.5 | 17.5 | 14.0 | 1.8 |
| Salmon, & Tarragon, Waitrose* | 1 Cake/85g | 179.0 | 10.0 | 211 | 11.9 | 14.3 | 11.8 | 2.2 |
| Salmon, Asda* | 1 Cake/86g | 215.0 | 12.0 | 250 | 8.0 | 23.0 | 14.0 | 1.4 |
| Salmon, Birds Eye* | 1 Cake/50g | 84.0 | 4.0 | 168 | 9.5 | 12.2 | 9.0 | 1.4 |
| Salmon, Breaded, Crispy, Frozen, Sainsbury's* | 1 Cake/60g | 140.0 | 9.0 | 234 | 12.2 | 13.7 | 14.5 | 1.9 |
| Salmon, Chunky, Sainsbury's* | 1 Cake/84g | 192.0 | 11.0 | 228 | 13.2 | 15.8 | 12.5 | 2.9 |
| Salmon, Coated in a Light & Crispy Breadcrumb, Tesco* | 1 Cake/90g | 211.0 | 11.0 | 235 | 9.7 | 21.0 | 12.0 | 1.2 |
| Salmon, Homemade, Average | 1 Cake/50g | 136.0 | 10.0 | 273 | 10.4 | 14.4 | 19.7 | 0.7 |
| Salmon, in Crunch Crumb, Birds Eye* | 1 Cake/50g | 107.0 | 6.0 | 216 | 9.7 | 15.0 | 13.0 | 1.4 |
| Salmon, M & S^ | 1 Cake/86g | 180.0 | 11.0 | 210 | 9.1 | 15.1 | 12.7 | 1.7 |
| Salmon, Melting Middle, M & S* | 1 Pack/290g | 551.0 | 30.0 | 190 | 9.1 | 14.3 | 10.5 | 1.5 |
| Salmon, Sainsbury's* | 1 Cake/88g | 171.0 | 8.0 | 194 | 12.6 | 16.5 | 8.6 | 1.6 |
| Salmon, Spinach & Sicilian Lemon, Finest, Tesco* | 1 Cake/114g | 251.0 | 13.0 | 220 | 10.0 | 18.3 | 11.8 | 4.2 |
| Salmon, Tesco* | 1 Cake/90g | 239.0 | 13.0 | 266 | 11.4 | 21.3 | 15.0 | 0.0 |
| Salmon, VLH Kitchens* | 1 Cake/56g | 155.6 | 11.2 | 278 | 10.5 | 14.4 | 20.0 | 0.6 |
| Salmon, with Lemon Butter Sauce, Finest, Tesco* | 1 Cake/220g | 524.0 | 40.0 | 238 | 7.3 | 10.9 | 18.3 | 1.0 |
| Salmon, with Lemon Butter Sauce, Gastropub, M & S* | 1 Cake/108g | 188.0 | 13.0 | 175 | 7.8 | 8.5 | 12.4 | 1.2 |
| Salmon, with Parsley Sauce, Finest, Tesco* | ½ Pack/170g | 350.0 | 24.0 | 206 | 8.6 | 11.7 | 13.9 | 1.0 |
| Salmon & Leek, Northern Catch, Aldi* | 1 Cake/114g | 212.0 | 9.0 | 186 | 9.5 | 19.3 | 7.9 | 0.9 |
| Salmon & Mozzarella, TTD, Sainsbury's* | 1 Cake/115g | 130.0 | 6.0 | 113 | 12.3 | 4.5 | 5.1 | 0.5 |
| Smoked Mackerel & Rocket, BGTY, Sainsbury's* | 1 Cake/91g | 218.0 | 12.0 | 240 | 10.9 | 19.6 | 13.1 | 1.8 |
| Thai, Finest, Tesco* | 1 Cake/65g | 149.0 | 9.0 | 230 | 7.5 | 20.3 | 13.2 | 1.6 |
| Thai, Frozen, Sainsbury's* | 1 Cake/15g | 28.0 | 1.0 | 187 | 21.3 | 9.3 | 7.3 | 0.7 |
| Thai, Oriental Selection, Waitrose* | 1 Cake/11g | 18.0 | 0.0 | 161 | 17.8 | 15.8 | 3.0 | 1.5 |
| Thai, Tesco* | 1 Cake/22g | 37.0 | 1.0 | 166 | 17.4 | 12.8 | 5.0 | 1.1 |
| Thai Prawn, Morrisons* | 1 Cake/90g | 211.0 | 10.0 | 234 | 7.9 | 26.4 | 10.7 | 0.3 |
| Thai Style, Sainsbury's* | 1 Cake/49g | 69.0 | 2.0 | 141 | 12.0 | 13.8 | 4.2 | 1.7 |
| Tuna, & Red Pepper, Waitrose* | 1 Cake/85g | 175.0 | 10.0 | 206 | 9.5 | 15.4 | 11.8 | 1.6 |
| Tuna, Asda* | 1 Cake/75g | 185.0 | 10.0 | 247 | 14.9 | 16.5 | 13.5 | 1.4 |
| Tuna, Lime & Coriander, BGTY, Sainsbury's* | 1 Cake/91g | 200.0 | 11.0 | 220 | 10.7 | 17.7 | 11.8 | 2.6 |
| Tuna, Sainsbury's* | 1 Cake/90g | 183.0 | 7.0 | 203 | 13.7 | 18.4 | 8.3 | 2.1 |

F

| | Measure INFO/WEIGHT | per Measure KCAL | FAT | Nutrition Values per 100g / 100ml KCAL | PROT | CARB | FAT | FIBRE |
|---|---|---|---|---|---|---|---|---|
| **FISH CAKES** | | | | | | | | |
| Tuna, Tesco* | 1 Cake/90g | 222.0 | 9.0 | 247 | 12.8 | 25.4 | 10.5 | 0.2 |
| Value, Tesco* | 1 Cake/40g | 74.0 | 3.0 | 183 | 7.1 | 21.2 | 7.8 | 1.2 |
| **FISH FINGERS** | | | | | | | | |
| Chip Shop, Youngs* | 1 Finger/30g | 75.0 | 5.0 | 251 | 9.3 | 16.6 | 16.4 | 1.2 |
| Cod, 100% Cod Fillet, Tesco* | 1 Finger/30g | 53.0 | 2.0 | 177 | 12.4 | 14.9 | 7.5 | 1.4 |
| Cod, Chunky, Tesco* | 1 Finger/40g | 70.0 | 3.0 | 175 | 12.3 | 14.3 | 7.6 | 1.6 |
| Cod, Fillet, 100%, Birds Eye* | 1 Finger/31g | 56.0 | 2.0 | 184 | 12.5 | 15.6 | 7.9 | 0.7 |
| Cod, Fillet, Asda* | 1 Finger/31g | 66.0 | 3.0 | 214 | 13.0 | 18.0 | 10.0 | 0.0 |
| Cod, Fillet, Chunky, M & S* | 1 Finger/40g | 70.0 | 2.0 | 175 | 12.0 | 17.2 | 6.0 | 1.0 |
| Cod, Fillet, Waitrose* | 1 Finger/30g | 55.0 | 2.0 | 183 | 11.9 | 16.9 | 7.5 | 0.7 |
| Cod, Fried in Blended Oil, Average | 1 Finger/28g | 67.0 | 4.0 | 238 | 13.2 | 15.5 | 14.1 | 0.6 |
| Cod, Frozen, Average | 1 Finger/28g | 48.0 | 2.0 | 170 | 11.6 | 14.2 | 7.8 | 0.6 |
| Cod, Grilled, Average | 1 Finger/28g | 56.0 | 2.0 | 200 | 14.3 | 16.6 | 8.9 | 0.7 |
| Cod, Morrisons* | 1 Finger/30g | 54.0 | 2.0 | 180 | 11.7 | 16.4 | 7.5 | 1.1 |
| Cod, Sainsbury's* | 1 Finger/28g | 53.0 | 2.0 | 190 | 12.5 | 17.7 | 7.7 | 1.0 |
| Free From, Sainsbury's* | 1 Finger/30g | 56.0 | 2.0 | 188 | 11.4 | 18.0 | 7.8 | 0.7 |
| Haddock, Fillet, Asda* | 1 Finger/30g | 61.0 | 3.0 | 205 | 14.0 | 17.0 | 9.0 | 0.0 |
| Haddock, in Crispy Batter, Birds Eye* | 1 Finger/30g | 56.0 | 2.0 | 188 | 14.3 | 15.1 | 7.8 | 0.7 |
| Haddock, in Crunchy Crumb, Morrisons* | 1 Finger/30g | 57.0 | 2.0 | 190 | 13.1 | 16.3 | 8.0 | 1.1 |
| Hoki, Fillet, Birds Eye* | 1 Finger/30g | 58.0 | 3.0 | 193 | 12.6 | 15.6 | 8.9 | 0.7 |
| Omega 3, Tesco* | 1 Finger/30g | 58.0 | 2.0 | 195 | 12.7 | 16.3 | 8.3 | 1.6 |
| Ross* | 1 Finger/26g | 50.0 | 2.0 | 193 | 10.7 | 17.7 | 8.8 | 0.8 |
| Salmon, Birds Eye* | 1 Finger/28g | 63.0 | 3.0 | 225 | 13.2 | 21.7 | 9.5 | 0.9 |
| Value, Tesco* | 1 Finger/25g | 41.0 | 2.0 | 166 | 11.5 | 11.9 | 8.1 | 1.7 |
| **FISH IN** | | | | | | | | |
| Butter Sauce, Steaks, Ross* | 1 Serving/150g | 126.0 | 6.0 | 84 | 9.1 | 3.2 | 3.9 | 0.1 |
| Butter Sauce, Steaks, Youngs* | 1 Steak/150g | 115.0 | 4.0 | 77 | 10.2 | 2.8 | 2.8 | 0.8 |
| Parsley Sauce, Steaks, Ross* | 1 Serving/150g | 123.0 | 6.0 | 82 | 9.1 | 3.1 | 3.7 | 0.1 |
| **FISH WITH** | | | | | | | | |
| Mushrooms, Carrots & Broccoli, Parcel, Birds Eye* | 1 Pack/250g | 235.0 | 14.0 | 94 | 7.9 | 3.1 | 5.6 | 0.8 |
| **FIVE SPICE** | | | | | | | | |
| Powder, Sharwood's* | 1 Tsp/2g | 3.0 | 0.0 | 172 | 12.2 | 11.6 | 8.6 | 23.4 |
| **FLAKE** | | | | | | | | |
| Cadbury* | 1 Bar/32g | 170.0 | 10.0 | 530 | 8.1 | 55.6 | 30.8 | 0.7 |
| Dipped, Cadbury* | 1 Bar/41g | 215.0 | 13.0 | 530 | 7.6 | 56.1 | 30.8 | 0.8 |
| Luxury, Cadbury* | 1 Bar/45g | 240.0 | 14.0 | 533 | 7.3 | 57.8 | 30.2 | 0.0 |
| Praline, Cadbury* | 1 Bar/38g | 201.0 | 13.0 | 535 | 7.7 | 49.5 | 34.3 | 0.0 |
| Snow, Cadbury* | 1 Bar/36g | 198.0 | 11.0 | 550 | 7.2 | 60.1 | 30.9 | 0.0 |
| **FLAN** | | | | | | | | |
| Cauliflower, Cheese & Broccoli, Hot, Sainsbury's* | ¼ Flan/100g | 303.0 | 20.0 | 303 | 6.4 | 24.7 | 19.8 | 1.2 |
| Cheese & Onion, M & S* | 1oz/28g | 81.0 | 5.0 | 290 | 6.1 | 25.1 | 18.7 | 1.4 |
| Cheese & Potato, Hot, Tesco* | ¼ Flan/100g | 282.0 | 20.0 | 282 | 6.0 | 20.0 | 19.7 | 2.3 |
| Chicken & Smoked Bacon, Hot, Sainsbury's* | ¼ Flan/100g | 293.0 | 18.0 | 293 | 10.2 | 21.5 | 18.5 | 1.2 |
| Mediterranean Vegetable, Co-Op* | ¼ Flan/88g | 188.0 | 10.0 | 215 | 4.0 | 22.0 | 12.0 | 3.0 |
| Parsnip, Broccoli & Gruyere, Safeway* | ½ Flan/200g | 534.0 | 33.0 | 267 | 7.0 | 23.0 | 16.4 | 2.8 |
| Pastry, with Fruit | 1oz/28g | 33.0 | 1.0 | 118 | 1.4 | 19.3 | 4.4 | 0.7 |
| Potato, Cheddar & Onion, Safeway* | 1 Serving/150g | 420.0 | 25.0 | 280 | 6.4 | 25.6 | 16.7 | 2.7 |
| Smoked Ham Cheese & Leek, Safeway* | ½ Flan/200g | 520.0 | 33.0 | 260 | 8.0 | 20.0 | 16.4 | 2.0 |
| Sponge with Fruit | 1oz/28g | 31.0 | 0.0 | 112 | 2.8 | 23.3 | 1.5 | 0.6 |
| **FLAN CASE** | | | | | | | | |
| *Sponge, Average* | *1oz/28g* | *90.0* | *2.0* | *320* | *7.0* | *62.5* | *5.4* | *0.7* |
| **FLAPJACK** | | | | | | | | |
| 90% Fat Free, Cookie Coach* | 1 Flapjack/75g | 287.0 | 7.0 | 383 | 7.0 | 66.2 | 9.9 | 0.0 |

F

# FLAPJACK

| | Measure INFO/WEIGHT | per Measure KCAL | FAT | KCAL | PROT | CARB | FAT | FIBRE |
|---|---|---|---|---|---|---|---|---|
| All Butter, Blackcurrant Jam, M & S* | 1 Serving/65g | 279.0 | 12.0 | 430 | 4.8 | 60.5 | 18.6 | 2.2 |
| All Butter, Organic, Sainsbury's* | 1 Serving/35g | 156.0 | 8.0 | 446 | 5.3 | 54.5 | 23.0 | 2.7 |
| All Butter, Sainsbury's* | 1 Flapjack/35g | 156.0 | 8.0 | 446 | 5.7 | 54.5 | 22.8 | 2.7 |
| All Butter, Squares, M & S* | 1 Flapjack/34g | 150.0 | 7.0 | 441 | 6.2 | 56.2 | 21.2 | 4.4 |
| Apple & Raisin, Lite, Crazy Jack* | 1 Flapjack70g | 227.0 | 1.0 | 324 | 9.8 | 72.0 | 2.1 | 0.0 |
| Apple & Raspberry, Fox's* | 1 Flapjack/26g | 105.0 | 5.0 | 403 | 4.8 | 52.5 | 19.4 | 3.7 |
| Apple & Sultana, Mr Kipling* | 1 Flapjack/27g | 123.0 | 6.0 | 456 | 4.6 | 59.0 | 22.4 | 3.6 |
| Apricot, The Handmade Flapjack Company* | 1 Flapjack/90g | 321.0 | 5.0 | 357 | 5.5 | 71.6 | 5.3 | 0.0 |
| Apricot & Raisin, Waitrose* | 1 Flapjack/38g | 143.0 | 4.0 | 376 | 4.7 | 64.3 | 11.1 | 5.8 |
| Average | 1 Sm/50g | 242.0 | 13.0 | 484 | 4.5 | 60.4 | 26.6 | 2.7 |
| Banana, The Handmade Flapjack Company* | 1 Flapjack/90g | 379.0 | 13.0 | 421 | 5.3 | 67.2 | 14.6 | 0.0 |
| Belgian Chocolate Dipped, Asda* | 1 Serving/67g | 321.0 | 17.0 | 477 | 6.0 | 57.0 | 25.0 | 3.2 |
| Black Cherry, Blackfriars* | 1 Serving/110g | 529.0 | 25.0 | 481 | 5.0 | 63.0 | 23.0 | 0.0 |
| Brazil Nut Cluster, The Handmade Flapjack Company* | 1 Flapjack/90g | 353.0 | 9.0 | 392 | 6.6 | 68.7 | 10.1 | 0.0 |
| Cappuccino, Blackfriars* | 1 Flapjack/110g | 481.0 | 27.0 | 437 | 5.0 | 61.0 | 25.0 | 0.0 |
| Caramel Bake, The Handmade Flapjack Company* | 1 Flapjack/90g | 375.0 | 13.0 | 417 | 6.0 | 65.6 | 14.5 | 0.0 |
| Cherry & Coconut, Blackfriars* | 1 Flapjack/110g | 489.0 | 23.0 | 445 | 5.0 | 58.0 | 21.0 | 0.0 |
| Cherry & Sultana, Cookie Coach* | 1 Pack/90g | 373.0 | 16.0 | 414 | 6.2 | 58.2 | 17.3 | 0.0 |
| Cherry & Sultana, M & S* | 1oz/28g | 111.0 | 4.0 | 395 | 5.4 | 63.7 | 13.0 | 5.1 |
| Chocolate, McVitie's* | 1 Flapjack/85g | 422.0 | 23.0 | 496 | 6.6 | 56.6 | 27.1 | 3.2 |
| Chocolate, The Handmade Flapjack Company* | 1 Flapjack/90g | 391.0 | 18.0 | 435 | 6.0 | 58.6 | 19.5 | 0.0 |
| Chocolate & Hazelnut, M & S* | 1 Flapjack/71g | 330.0 | 18.0 | 465 | 7.3 | 55.6 | 25.5 | 3.8 |
| Chocolate Chip, Boots* | 1 Flapjack/75g | 313.0 | 11.0 | 417 | 5.6 | 65.0 | 15.0 | 3.5 |
| Chocolate Dipped, M & S* | 1 Flapjack/96g | 442.0 | 22.0 | 460 | 6.1 | 61.3 | 22.4 | 3.0 |
| Chocolate Special, The Handmade Flapjack Company* | 1 Flapjack/90g | 392.0 | 18.0 | 436 | 5.7 | 58.7 | 19.8 | 0.0 |
| Chunky Chocolate, M & S* | 1 FlapJack/80g | 348.0 | 15.0 | 435 | 5.8 | 59.9 | 18.9 | 2.2 |
| Cranberry, Apple & Raisin, Light Choices, Tesco* | 1 Flapjack/30g | 97.0 | 2.0 | 325 | 5.7 | 63.1 | 5.6 | 5.7 |
| Date & Walnut, The Handmade Flapjack Company* | 1 Flapjack/90g | 360.0 | 13.0 | 400 | 6.1 | 60.2 | 14.9 | 0.0 |
| Fingers, GFY, Asda* | 1 Finger/37g | 129.0 | 4.0 | 350 | 5.0 | 60.0 | 10.0 | 3.5 |
| Fruit, GFY, Asda* | 1 Flapjack/45g | 173.0 | 4.0 | 384 | 6.0 | 72.0 | 8.0 | 3.4 |
| Fruit, Mr Kipling* | 1 Flapjack/75g | 306.0 | 14.0 | 408 | 4.8 | 56.7 | 18.1 | 3.0 |
| Fruit, Tesco* | 1 Flapjack/33g | 136.0 | 5.0 | 412 | 5.7 | 62.0 | 15.7 | 4.0 |
| Fruit, Weight Watchers* | 1 Serving/30g | 106.0 | 2.0 | 353 | 6.0 | 68.3 | 6.3 | 4.7 |
| Fruity, Waitrose* | 1 Serving/50g | 199.0 | 7.0 | 398 | 6.1 | 62.9 | 13.5 | 3.9 |
| Fudge, Blackfriars* | 1 Serving/110g | 528.0 | 26.0 | 480 | 5.0 | 60.0 | 24.0 | 0.0 |
| Golden Oaty, Fingers, Fabulous Bakin' Boys* | 1 Finger/28g | 126.0 | 6.0 | 450 | 5.7 | 59.6 | 21.1 | 3.4 |
| Golden Oaty Fingers, Tesco* | 1 Finger/25g | 112.0 | 5.0 | 450 | 5.7 | 59.6 | 21.1 | 3.4 |
| Hob Nobs, Milk Chocolate, McVitie's* | 1 Flapjack/35g | 159.0 | 8.0 | 454 | 5.7 | 59.4 | 21.4 | 4.0 |
| Ma Baker* | 1 Serving/90g | 381.0 | 18.0 | 423 | 7.4 | 56.9 | 20.0 | 4.8 |
| Mighty Oat, Fabulous Bakin' Boys* | 1 Bar/85g | 365.0 | 17.0 | 430 | 6.0 | 58.0 | 20.0 | 3.0 |
| Milk Chocolate Digestive, McVitie's* | 1 Flapjack/65g | 293.0 | 14.0 | 451 | 5.4 | 59.7 | 21.2 | 3.4 |
| Mixed Fruit, Fabulous Bakin' Boys* | 1 Serving/90g | 350.0 | 9.0 | 389 | 5.5 | 71.0 | 10.5 | 4.0 |
| Oat & Syrup, Oakjacks, McVitie's* | 1 Bar/34g | 153.0 | 7.0 | 450 | 5.3 | 57.6 | 22.0 | 5.0 |
| Oats, Butter & Syrup, McVitie's* | 1 Bar/79g | 356.0 | 18.0 | 454 | 4.9 | 57.9 | 22.5 | 3.7 |
| Organic, Wholebake* | 1 Bar/90g | 388.0 | 19.0 | 431 | 6.0 | 59.4 | 20.8 | 0.0 |
| Plain, The Handmade Flapjack Company* | 1 Flapjack/90g | 398.0 | 19.0 | 442 | 5.4 | 57.1 | 21.3 | 0.0 |
| Raspberry Preserve, The Handmade Flapjack Company* | 1 Flapjack/90g | 310.0 | 2.0 | 345 | 6.4 | 74.4 | 2.3 | 0.0 |
| Really Raspberry, Fabulous Bakin' Boys* | 1 Flapjack/90g | 378.0 | 16.0 | 420 | 6.0 | 60.0 | 18.0 | 0.0 |
| Snickers, McVitie's* | 1 Flapjack/65g | 315.0 | 19.0 | 484 | 7.9 | 49.0 | 28.5 | 6.0 |
| Sultana, Tesco* | 1 Flapjack/50g | 173.0 | 10.0 | 346 | 5.0 | 36.2 | 20.1 | 3.7 |
| Toffee, Finest, Tesco* | 1 Flapjack/35g | 156.0 | 7.0 | 446 | 4.9 | 63.6 | 19.1 | 1.3 |
| Toffeemac, The Handmade Flapjack Company* | 1 Flapjack/90g | 411.0 | 20.0 | 457 | 6.1 | 59.0 | 21.9 | 0.0 |
| Tropical Mix, Reduced Fat, Fabulous Bakin' Boys* | 1 Flapjack/90g | 346.0 | 11.0 | 385 | 6.0 | 63.0 | 12.0 | 3.0 |

F

| | Measure INFO/WEIGHT | per Measure KCAL | FAT | Nutrition Values per 100g / 100ml KCAL | PROT | CARB | FAT | FIBRE |
|---|---|---|---|---|---|---|---|---|
| **FLAPJACK** | | | | | | | | |
| Weight Watchers* | 1 Slice/30g | 109.0 | 2.0 | 363 | 6.7 | 71.0 | 6.0 | 4.0 |
| with Sultanas, Tesco* | 1 Flapjack/49g | 217.0 | 10.0 | 442 | 5.3 | 57.9 | 21.0 | 3.7 |
| Yoghurt Flavour, Blackfriars* | 1 Bar/110g | 521.0 | 26.0 | 474 | 7.0 | 58.0 | 24.0 | 0.0 |
| **FLATBREAD** | | | | | | | | |
| BBQ Chicken, Improved, Shapers, Boots* | 1 Pack/165g | 268.0 | 4.0 | 162 | 10.0 | 25.0 | 2.3 | 1.2 |
| BBQ Style Chicken, Shapers, Boots* | 1 Serving/108g | 187.0 | 5.0 | 173 | 10.0 | 23.0 | 4.6 | 2.8 |
| Chargrilled Chicken, COU, M & S* | 1 Pack/163g | 245.0 | 3.0 | 150 | 10.8 | 23.0 | 1.9 | 5.2 |
| Cheese & Onion Swedish Style, Shapers, Boots* | 1 Flatbread/127g | 265.0 | 10.0 | 209 | 10.0 | 24.0 | 8.1 | 1.3 |
| Cheese & Tomato, Tesco* | ¼ Pack/56g | 134.0 | 4.0 | 240 | 8.7 | 36.1 | 6.6 | 2.7 |
| Chicken & Mango Salsa, Sainsbury's* | 1 Pack/178g | 251.0 | 2.0 | 141 | 9.5 | 22.7 | 1.4 | 1.4 |
| Chicken Caesar, Shapers, Boots* | 1 Serving/160g | 254.0 | 3.0 | 159 | 13.0 | 22.0 | 2.1 | 2.0 |
| Chicken Tikka, BGTY, Sainsbury's* | 1 Flatbread/188g | 241.0 | 3.0 | 128 | 10.3 | 18.5 | 1.4 | 2.0 |
| Chicken Tikka, Shapers, Boots* | 1 Flatbread/164g | 269.0 | 4.0 | 164 | 11.0 | 24.0 | 2.5 | 1.5 |
| Chinese Chicken, COU, M & S* | 1 Flatbread/156g | 281.0 | 4.0 | 180 | 13.9 | 24.3 | 2.8 | 2.2 |
| Chinese Chicken, Shapers, Boots* | 1 Pack/159g | 274.0 | 2.0 | 172 | 11.0 | 29.0 | 1.3 | 1.8 |
| Feta Cheese, Shapers, Boots* | 1 Pack/166g | 255.0 | 6.0 | 154 | 6.7 | 23.0 | 3.9 | 1.4 |
| Greek Feta Salad, Boots* | 1 Pack/158g | 241.0 | 6.0 | 153 | 6.4 | 24.0 | 3.6 | 1.2 |
| Greek Style, GFY, Asda* | 1 Flatbread/165g | 256.0 | 7.0 | 155 | 7.0 | 22.0 | 4.3 | 2.1 |
| Greek Style Salad, Waitrose* | 1 Pack/172g | 280.0 | 8.0 | 163 | 7.4 | 22.3 | 4.9 | 3.3 |
| Italian Chicken, Improved, Shapers, Boots* | 1 Pack/151g | 263.0 | 7.0 | 174 | 11.0 | 22.0 | 4.5 | 1.8 |
| Italian Chicken, Shapers, Boots* | 1 Pack/168g | 266.0 | 6.0 | 158 | 10.0 | 22.0 | 3.3 | 1.3 |
| King Prawn Tikka, Waitrose* | 1 Pack/165g | 257.0 | 3.0 | 156 | 9.4 | 25.1 | 2.0 | 1.5 |
| Mature Cheddar & Garlic, Finest, Tesco* | ¼ Flatbread/66g | 188.0 | 6.0 | 285 | 7.2 | 41.8 | 9.6 | 2.6 |
| Mediterranean Chicken, Ginsters* | 1 Pack/168g | 302.0 | 7.0 | 180 | 10.6 | 25.5 | 4.0 | 0.0 |
| Mediterranean Tuna, Ginsters* | 1 Pack/167g | 297.0 | 6.0 | 178 | 10.3 | 25.6 | 3.8 | 0.0 |
| Mexican Style Chicken, GFY, Asda* | 1 Pack/161g | 241.0 | 3.0 | 150 | 13.0 | 20.0 | 2.0 | 2.5 |
| Peking Duck, Less Than 3% Fat, Shapers, Boots* | 1 Pack/156g | 246.0 | 4.0 | 158 | 7.2 | 27.0 | 2.4 | 1.9 |
| Prawn Korma, Shapers, Boots* | 1 Pack/169g | 267.0 | 7.0 | 158 | 8.8 | 22.0 | 3.9 | 1.3 |
| Rancher's Chicken, COU, M & S* | 1 Pack/174g | 270.0 | 3.0 | 155 | 10.9 | 23.0 | 2.0 | 1.5 |
| Ranchers Chicken, Shapers, Boots* | 1 Pack/194g | 303.0 | 4.0 | 156 | 12.0 | 22.0 | 2.2 | 1.5 |
| Salsa Chicken, Shapers, Boots* | 1 Pack/191g | 328.0 | 8.0 | 172 | 11.0 | 22.0 | 4.4 | 1.6 |
| Spicy Chicken, Shapers, Boots* | 1 Pack/181g | 292.0 | 5.0 | 161 | 11.0 | 23.0 | 2.5 | 0.0 |
| Spicy Chicken & Salsa, HL, Tesco* | 1 Serving/183g | 251.0 | 3.0 | 137 | 10.1 | 21.1 | 1.4 | 1.2 |
| Spicy Mexican, New, Shapers, Boots* | 1 Pack/184g | 281.0 | 5.0 | 153 | 8.0 | 24.0 | 2.7 | 3.7 |
| Spicy Mexican, Shapers, Boots* | 1 Pack/190g | 296.0 | 8.0 | 156 | 7.0 | 23.0 | 4.0 | 3.7 |
| Sticky BBQ Style Chicken, Shapers, Boots* | 1 Pack/158g | 274.0 | 7.0 | 173 | 10.0 | 23.0 | 4.6 | 2.8 |
| Tomato & Chilli, BGTY, Sainsbury's* | ¼ Flatbread/100g | 155.0 | 3.0 | 155 | 7.7 | 24.0 | 3.1 | 1.8 |
| Tomato & Chilli, Sainsbury's* | ¼ Bread/65g | 155.0 | 3.0 | 238 | 11.9 | 36.9 | 4.7 | 2.8 |
| Vegetable & Salsa, HL, Tesco* | 1 Serving/193g | 263.0 | 3.0 | 136 | 7.9 | 22.2 | 1.8 | 1.2 |
| **FLAXSEED** | | | | | | | | |
| Milled, Organic, Linwoods* | 2 Dtsp/30g | 153.0 | 14.0 | 510 | 21.9 | 1.7 | 46.2 | 28.9 |
| **FLOUR** | | | | | | | | |
| *Arrowroot, Average* | *1oz/28g* | *100.0* | *0.0* | *357* | *0.3* | *88.1* | *0.1* | *3.4* |
| *Bread, Brown, Strong, Average* | *1 Serving/100g* | *311.0* | *2.0* | *311* | *14.0* | *61.0* | *1.8* | *6.4* |
| *Bread, White, Strong, Average* | *1oz/28g* | *94.0* | *0.0* | *336* | *11.8* | *68.4* | *1.5* | *3.4* |
| *Brown, Chapati, Average* | *1 Tbsp/20g* | *67.0* | *0.0* | *333* | *11.5* | *73.7* | *1.2* | *0.0* |
| *Brown, Wheat* | *1oz/28g* | *90.0* | *1.0* | *323* | *12.6* | *68.5* | *1.8* | *6.4* |
| *Chick Pea* | *1oz/28g* | *88.0* | *2.0* | *313* | *19.7* | *49.6* | *5.4* | *10.7* |
| Gram, Stoneground, Doves Farm* | 1 Serving/100g | 336.0 | 5.0 | 336 | 12.8 | 60.0 | 5.0 | 9.7 |
| *Millet* | *1oz/28g* | *99.0* | *0.0* | *354* | *5.8* | *75.4* | *1.7* | *0.0* |
| *Plain, Average* | *1oz/28g* | *98.0* | *0.0* | *349* | *10.3* | *73.8* | *1.5* | *2.2* |
| *Potato* | *1oz/28g* | *92.0* | *0.0* | *328* | *9.1* | *75.6* | *0.9* | *5.7* |
| *Rice* | *1oz/28g* | *102.0* | *0.0* | *366* | *6.4* | *80.1* | *0.8* | *2.0* |

**F**

| | Measure INFO/WEIGHT | per Measure KCAL | FAT | Nutrition Values per 100g / 100ml KCAL | PROT | CARB | FAT | FIBRE |
|---|---|---|---|---|---|---|---|---|
| **FLOUR** | | | | | | | | |
| *Rye, Whole* | *1oz/28g* | *94.0* | *1.0* | *335* | *8.2* | *75.9* | *2.0* | *11.7* |
| *Soya, Full Fat, Average* | *1oz/28g* | *118.0* | *6.0* | *421* | *37.9* | *19.7* | *21.7* | *11.6* |
| *Soya, Low Fat, Average* | *1oz/28g* | *99.0* | *2.0* | *352* | *45.3* | *28.2* | *7.2* | *13.5* |
| Speciality Gluten Free, Dove's Farm* | 1 Serving/100g | 353.0 | 2.0 | 353 | 4.7 | 85.2 | 1.8 | 2.7 |
| *Spelt, Average* | *1 Serving/57g* | *216.0* | *2.0* | *381* | *14.3* | *74.5* | *2.9* | *6.3* |
| *Strong, Wholemeal, Average* | *1 Serving/100g* | *315.0* | *2.0* | *315* | *13.2* | *60.5* | *2.2* | *9.0* |
| *White, Average* | *1oz/28g* | *89.0* | *0.0* | *319* | *9.8* | *66.8* | *1.0* | *2.9* |
| *White, Chapati, Average* | *1 Tbsp/20g* | *67.0* | *0.0* | *335* | *9.8* | *77.6* | *0.5* | *0.0* |
| *White, Self Raising, Average* | *1oz/28g* | *94.0* | *0.0* | *336* | *9.9* | *71.8* | *1.3* | *2.9* |
| *White, Wheat, Average* | *1oz/28g* | *95.0* | *0.0* | *341* | *10.4* | *76.5* | *1.3* | *3.1* |
| *Wholemeal, Average* | *1oz/28g* | *87.0* | *1.0* | *312* | *12.6* | *61.9* | *2.2* | *9.0* |
| Wholemeal, Self Raising, Tesco* | 1oz/28g | 89.0 | 1.0 | 317 | 11.5 | 62.9 | 2.2 | 9.0 |
| **FLYING SAUCERS** | | | | | | | | |
| Asda* | 1 Bag/23g | 82.0 | 1.0 | 355 | 0.1 | 83.0 | 2.5 | 0.8 |
| Co-Op* | 1 Sweet/1g | 4.0 | 0.0 | 370 | 0.5 | 90.0 | 1.0 | 0.6 |
| **FLYTE** | | | | | | | | |
| Mars* | Bar/23g | 99.0 | 3.0 | 441 | 3.4 | 74.8 | 14.2 | 0.0 |
| Snacksize, Mars* | 1 Bar/23g | 98.0 | 3.0 | 436 | 3.8 | 72.5 | 14.5 | 0.0 |
| **FOOL** | | | | | | | | |
| Apricot, BGTY, Sainsbury's* | 1 Pot/113g | 95.0 | 3.0 | 84 | 3.6 | 11.4 | 2.6 | 0.5 |
| Apricot, Fruit, Tesco* | 1 Pot/113g | 200.0 | 13.0 | 177 | 2.6 | 16.4 | 11.2 | 0.3 |
| Blackcurrant, Asda* | 1 Pot/114g | 89.0 | 3.0 | 78 | 3.6 | 10.0 | 2.6 | 0.6 |
| Blackcurrant, BGTY, Sainsbury's* | 1 Pot/113g | 89.0 | 3.0 | 79 | 3.5 | 10.4 | 2.6 | 0.6 |
| Fruit | 1oz/28g | 46.0 | 3.0 | 163 | 1.0 | 20.2 | 9.3 | 1.2 |
| Gooseberry, BFY, Morrisons* | 1 Pot/114g | 99.0 | 4.0 | 87 | 3.4 | 10.7 | 3.4 | 0.4 |
| Gooseberry, Fruit, BGTY, Sainsbury's* | 1 Pot/121g | 93.0 | 3.0 | 77 | 2.9 | 10.0 | 2.8 | 0.8 |
| Gooseberry, Perfectly Balanced, Waitrose* | 1 Pot/113g | 125.0 | 3.0 | 111 | 3.6 | 18.3 | 2.6 | 0.7 |
| Gooseberry, Sainsbury's* | 1 Pot/113g | 214.0 | 13.0 | 189 | 2.6 | 19.1 | 11.4 | 1.1 |
| Gooseberry, Tesco* | 1 Pot/113g | 225.0 | 14.0 | 200 | 3.0 | 17.8 | 12.5 | 0.7 |
| Lemon, BFY, Morrisons* | 1 Pot/114g | 96.0 | 4.0 | 84 | 3.4 | 10.1 | 3.4 | 0.3 |
| Lemon, Fruit, BGTY, Sainsbury's* | 1 Pot/113g | 94.0 | 4.0 | 83 | 3.4 | 9.7 | 3.4 | 0.3 |
| Raspberry, Fruit, Tesco* | 1 Pot/113g | 234.0 | 13.0 | 207 | 2.6 | 23.6 | 11.3 | 0.3 |
| Rhubarb, Fruit, BGTY, Sainsbury's* | 1 Pot/120g | 91.0 | 3.0 | 76 | 3.5 | 9.5 | 2.6 | 0.3 |
| Rhubarb, Fruit, Waitrose* | 1 Pot/114g | 182.0 | 13.0 | 160 | 2.7 | 11.9 | 11.3 | 0.3 |
| Rhubarb, Sainsbury's* | 1 Pot/113g | 180.0 | 13.0 | 159 | 2.6 | 11.5 | 11.4 | 0.4 |
| Strawberry, Fruit, BGTY, Sainsbury's* | 1 Pot/120g | 100.0 | 3.0 | 83 | 3.7 | 11.1 | 2.6 | 0.8 |
| Strawberry, GFY, Asda* | 1 Pot/114g | 95.0 | 3.0 | 83 | 3.8 | 11.0 | 2.6 | 0.8 |
| Strawberry, Perfectly Balanced, Waitrose* | 1 Pot/113g | 110.0 | 3.0 | 97 | 3.5 | 14.9 | 2.6 | 0.4 |
| Strawberry, Real Fruit, Safeway* | 1 Pot/114g | 197.0 | 13.0 | 173 | 2.7 | 15.4 | 11.2 | 0.3 |
| **FOR MILK** | | | | | | | | |
| Peachy Banana, Robinson's* | 1 Serving/50ml | 79.0 | 0.0 | 158 | 0.0 | 39.0 | 0.0 | 0.0 |
| Strawberry & Raspberry, Robinson's* | 1 Serving/50ml | 20.0 | 1.0 | 39 | 2.9 | 4.0 | 1.4 | 0.0 |
| **FRANKFURTERS** | | | | | | | | |
| *Average* | *1 Frankfurter/42g* | *123.0* | *11.0* | *292* | *12.0* | *1.3* | *26.6* | *0.0* |
| **FRANKFURTERS VEGETARIAN** | | | | | | | | |
| Asda* | 1 Frankfurter/27g | 54.0 | 3.0 | 199 | 18.0 | 3.5 | 12.5 | 2.5 |
| Tivall* | 1 Sausage/30g | 73.0 | 5.0 | 244 | 18.0 | 7.0 | 16.0 | 3.0 |
| **FRAZZLES** | | | | | | | | |
| Bacon, Smith's, Walkers* | 1 Bag/23g | 112.0 | 5.0 | 485 | 6.5 | 62.0 | 23.0 | 1.3 |
| **FRENCH FRIES** | | | | | | | | |
| Cheese & Onion, Walkers* | 1 Pack/22g | 95.0 | 4.0 | 430 | 5.0 | 66.0 | 16.0 | 5.0 |
| Ready Salted, Walkers* | 1 Bag/22g | 93.0 | 4.0 | 425 | 5.0 | 65.0 | 16.0 | 5.0 |
| Salt & Vinegar, BGTY, Sainsbury's* | 1 Bag/15g | 51.0 | 0.0 | 340 | 6.0 | 80.1 | 1.5 | 4.1 |

**F**

| | Measure INFO/WEIGHT | per Measure KCAL | FAT | Nutrition Values per 100g / 100ml KCAL | PROT | CARB | FAT | FIBRE |
|---|---|---|---|---|---|---|---|---|
| **FRENCH FRIES** | | | | | | | | |
| Salt & Vinegar, Walkers* | 1 Bag/22g | 95.0 | 4.0 | 430 | 5.0 | 66.0 | 16.0 | 5.0 |
| Worcester Sauce, Walkers* | 1 Bag/22g | 93.0 | 4.0 | 425 | 4.5 | 64.0 | 17.0 | 4.1 |
| **FRENCH TOAST** | | | | | | | | |
| Asda* | 1 Toast/8g | 30.0 | 0.0 | 381 | 10.0 | 74.0 | 5.0 | 4.0 |
| Morrisons* | 1 Toast/8g | 31.0 | 1.0 | 393 | 11.0 | 72.5 | 6.6 | 3.0 |
| Sainsbury's* | 1 Toast/8g | 31.0 | 1.0 | 382 | 10.0 | 72.0 | 6.6 | 5.0 |
| Tesco* | 1 Toast/100g | 393.0 | 7.0 | 393 | 11.0 | 72.5 | 6.6 | 3.0 |
| **FRIES** | | | | | | | | |
| 9/16" Straight Cut Home, Deep Fried, McCain* | 1oz/28g | 65.0 | 3.0 | 233 | 3.2 | 32.7 | 9.9 | 0.0 |
| 9/16" Straight Cut Home, Oven Baked, McCain* | 1oz/28g | 53.0 | 2.0 | 188 | 3.2 | 31.5 | 5.5 | 0.0 |
| American Style, Frozen, Thin, Tesco* | 1 Serving/125g | 207.0 | 10.0 | 166 | 2.2 | 21.1 | 8.1 | 1.9 |
| American Style, Slim, Iceland* | 1 Serving/100g | 187.0 | 6.0 | 187 | 2.4 | 30.6 | 6.1 | 2.4 |
| Crispy French, Weighed Deep Fried, McCain* | 1 Serving/100g | 193.0 | 8.0 | 193 | 1.9 | 27.4 | 8.5 | 0.9 |
| Curly, Cajun, Weighed Frozen, McCain* | 1 Portion/100g | 156.0 | 9.0 | 156 | 1.6 | 17.7 | 8.7 | 1.8 |
| Curly, Southern Style, Tesco* | 1 Serving/50g | 124.0 | 4.0 | 248 | 3.8 | 41.7 | 7.3 | 3.8 |
| Curly, Twisters, Frozen, Lamb Weston* | 1 Serving/150g | 273.0 | 14.0 | 182 | 2.5 | 22.0 | 9.3 | 2.2 |
| Extra Chunky, Oven Baked, Homefries, McCain* | 1 Serving/200g | 306.0 | 6.0 | 153 | 3.2 | 28.0 | 3.1 | 2.3 |
| Oven, American Style, Asda* | 1 Serving/180g | 407.0 | 14.0 | 226 | 3.9 | 34.6 | 8.0 | 4.0 |
| Oven, Straight Cut, Morrisons* | 1 Serving/100g | 149.0 | 4.0 | 149 | 2.8 | 24.6 | 4.3 | 2.6 |
| Seasoned, Lamb Weston* | 1 Serving/150g | 247.0 | 12.0 | 165 | 2.4 | 20.8 | 8.0 | 1.9 |
| Southern, Oven Cook, Baked, Potato Winners, McCain* | 1 Serving/100g | 232.0 | 8.0 | 232 | 3.6 | 35.7 | 8.3 | 2.4 |
| Southern, Oven Cook, Frozen, Potato Winners, McCain* | 1 Serving/100g | 176.0 | 7.0 | 176 | 2.4 | 26.5 | 6.7 | 1.6 |
| Southern Spicy Spiral, Deep Fried, McCain* | 1oz/28g | 58.0 | 3.0 | 208 | 2.7 | 26.4 | 10.2 | 0.0 |
| Southern Spicy Spiral, Oven Baked, McCain* | 1oz/28g | 46.0 | 2.0 | 165 | 1.7 | 24.6 | 6.6 | 0.0 |
| **FRISPS** | | | | | | | | |
| Tangy Salt & Vinegar, KP Snacks* | 1 Bag/30g | 160.0 | 10.0 | 532 | 5.0 | 52.6 | 33.5 | 2.9 |
| Tasty Cheese & Onion, KP Snacks* | 1 Bag/28g | 150.0 | 9.0 | 537 | 5.5 | 53.2 | 33.6 | 3.2 |
| **FROG** | | | | | | | | |
| *Legs, Raw, Meat Only* | *1oz/28g* | *20.0* | *0.0* | *73* | *16.4* | *0.0* | *0.3* | *0.0* |
| **FROMAGE FRAIS** | | | | | | | | |
| 0% Fat, Vitalinea, Danone* | 1 Tbsp/28g | 14.0 | 0.0 | 50 | 7.4 | 4.7 | 0.1 | 0.0 |
| Apple Pie, Low Fat, Sainsbury's* | 1 Pot/90g | 108.0 | 2.0 | 120 | 6.7 | 17.3 | 2.6 | 0.3 |
| Apple Strudel, Safeway* | 1 Pot/100g | 116.0 | 3.0 | 116 | 6.6 | 14.8 | 3.4 | 0.7 |
| Apricot, Layered, Weight Watchers* | 1 Pot/100g | 58.0 | 0.0 | 58 | 5.4 | 8.1 | 0.1 | 1.6 |
| Apricot, Tesco* | 1 Pot/100g | 77.0 | 3.0 | 77 | 6.5 | 6.0 | 3.0 | 1.3 |
| Bakewell Tart Flavour, BGTY, Sainsbury's* | 1 Pot/100g | 54.0 | 0.0 | 54 | 7.6 | 5.5 | 0.2 | 1.1 |
| Banana, Organic, Yeo Valley* | 1 Pot/90g | 118.0 | 5.0 | 131 | 6.6 | 12.6 | 6.0 | 0.2 |
| Banoffee Pie Flavour, Low Fat, Safeway* | 1 Pot/100g | 135.0 | 4.0 | 135 | 6.8 | 17.6 | 4.1 | 0.2 |
| Black Cherry, Asda* | 1 Pot/100g | 113.0 | 5.0 | 113 | 4.1 | 13.0 | 5.0 | 0.0 |
| Black Cherry, GFY, Asda* | 1 Pot/100g | 54.0 | 0.0 | 54 | 6.0 | 7.0 | 0.2 | 0.0 |
| Blackberry, Layered, Weight Watchers* | 1 Pot/100g | 64.0 | 0.0 | 64 | 5.3 | 10.4 | 0.2 | 1.0 |
| Blackcurrant, GFY, Asda* | 1 Pot/100g | 43.0 | 0.0 | 43 | 6.0 | 4.2 | 0.2 | 0.0 |
| Blackcurrant, HL, Tesco* | 1 Pot/100g | 56.0 | 0.0 | 56 | 6.2 | 7.4 | 0.2 | 0.4 |
| Cherry, 0% Fat, Vitalinea, Danone* | 1 Serving/150g | 88.0 | 0.0 | 59 | 6.1 | 8.0 | 0.1 | 1.6 |
| Cherry Pie Flavour, BGTY, Sainsbury's* | 1 Pot/100g | 54.0 | 0.0 | 54 | 7.6 | 5.5 | 0.2 | 1.1 |
| Chocolate Fudge, Smooth & Creamy, Tesco* | 1 Pot/100g | 136.0 | 6.0 | 136 | 6.7 | 13.3 | 6.2 | 0.2 |
| COU, M & S* | 1 Pot/100g | 48.0 | 0.0 | 48 | 7.8 | 4.5 | 0.1 | 0.5 |
| Eat Smart, Safeway* | 1 Pot/100g | 55.0 | 0.0 | 55 | 7.7 | 5.1 | 0.2 | 1.6 |
| Exotic Fruits, Eat Smart, Safeway* | 1 Pot/100g | 60.0 | 0.0 | 60 | 7.9 | 6.6 | 0.2 | 0.4 |
| Fabby, Loved By Kids, M & S* | 1 Pot/43g | 45.0 | 2.0 | 105 | 6.2 | 12.3 | 3.7 | 0.0 |
| *Fat Free, Average* | *1oz/28g* | *16.0* | *0.0* | *58* | *7.7* | *6.8* | *0.2* | *0.0* |
| Fruit on the Bottom, BFY, Morrisons* | 1 Pot/100g | 66.0 | 0.0 | 66 | 5.6 | 10.6 | 0.1 | 0.0 |
| Good Intentions, Somerfield* | 1 Pot/100g | 49.0 | 0.0 | 49 | 7.6 | 4.5 | 0.1 | 0.0 |

| | Measure INFO/WEIGHT | per Measure KCAL | FAT | Nutrition Values per 100g / 100ml KCAL | PROT | CARB | FAT | FIBRE |
|---|---|---|---|---|---|---|---|---|
| **FROMAGE FRAIS** | | | | | | | | |
| Kids, Yeo Valley* | 1 Serving/90g | 111.0 | 5.0 | 123 | 6.6 | 12.6 | 5.3 | 0.0 |
| Lemon, COU, M & S* | 1 Serving/100g | 60.0 | 0.0 | 60 | 7.0 | 7.3 | 0.2 | 0.6 |
| Lemon Pie, Low Fat, Sainsbury's* | 1 Pot/90g | 108.0 | 2.0 | 120 | 6.7 | 17.3 | 2.7 | 0.2 |
| Lemon Sponge Flavour, BGTY, Sainsbury's* | 1 Pot/100g | 52.0 | 0.0 | 52 | 7.6 | 5.0 | 0.2 | 1.1 |
| Mandarin & Orange, HL, Tesco* | 1 Pot/100g | 55.0 | 0.0 | 55 | 6.2 | 7.0 | 0.2 | 0.3 |
| Mandarin & Orange, Tesco* | 1 Pot/100g | 75.0 | 3.0 | 75 | 6.5 | 5.6 | 3.0 | 2.3 |
| Mango & Papaya, HL, Tesco* | 1 Pot/100g | 55.0 | 0.0 | 55 | 6.2 | 7.0 | 0.2 | 0.1 |
| Morello Cherries, Perfectly Balanced, Waitrose* | ½ Pot/250ml | 260.0 | 5.0 | 104 | 2.5 | 19.1 | 1.9 | 1.8 |
| Munch Bunch, Nestle* | 1 Pot/42g | 44.0 | 1.0 | 105 | 6.7 | 12.6 | 3.0 | 0.0 |
| Natural, Fat Free, M & S* | 1 Serving/100g | 60.0 | 0.0 | 60 | 9.8 | 4.8 | 0.1 | 0.0 |
| Natural, GFY, Asda* | ½ Pot/100g | 52.0 | 0.0 | 52 | 7.3 | 5.0 | 0.3 | 0.0 |
| Natural, HL, Tesco* | 1 Serving/65g | 30.0 | 0.0 | 46 | 7.8 | 3.3 | 0.2 | 0.0 |
| Natural, Plain, Fat Free, Normandy, BGTY, Sainsbury's* | 1 Serving/30g | 15.0 | 0.0 | 49 | 8.0 | 4.2 | 0.1 | 0.0 |
| Natural, Virtually Fat Free, French, Waitrose* | 1 Tub/500g | 260.0 | 1.0 | 52 | 7.3 | 5.0 | 0.3 | 0.0 |
| Normandy, Light Choices, Tesco* | 1 Serving/100g | 46.0 | 0.0 | 46 | 7.8 | 3.3 | 0.2 | 0.0 |
| Normandy, Sainsbury's* | 1 Serving/25g | 29.0 | 2.0 | 116 | 7.7 | 3.4 | 8.1 | 0.0 |
| Peach, BGTY, Sainsbury's* | 1 Pot/100g | 53.0 | 0.0 | 53 | 7.2 | 5.5 | 0.2 | 0.5 |
| Peach, Layered, Weight Watchers* | 1 Pot/100g | 57.0 | 0.0 | 57 | 5.4 | 7.9 | 0.1 | 1.2 |
| Pineapple, Eat Smart, Safeway* | 1 Pot/100g | 60.0 | 0.0 | 60 | 7.9 | 6.3 | 0.2 | 0.3 |
| Pineapple & Passion Fruit, HL, Tesco* | 1 Pot/100g | 55.0 | 0.0 | 55 | 6.2 | 7.1 | 0.2 | 0.1 |
| *Plain, Average* | *1oz/28g* | *32.0* | *2.0* | *113* | *6.8* | *5.7* | *7.1* | *0.0* |
| Raspberry, COU, M & S* | 1 Pot/100g | 60.0 | 0.0 | 60 | 7.0 | 8.1 | 0.2 | 0.5 |
| Raspberry, GFY, Asda* | 1 Pot/100g | 43.0 | 0.0 | 43 | 6.0 | 4.2 | 0.2 | 0.0 |
| Raspberry, Layered, Weight Watchers* | 1 Pot/100g | 51.0 | 0.0 | 51 | 5.5 | 6.3 | 0.1 | 1.1 |
| Raspberry, Little Stars, Muller* | 1 Pot/60g | 66.0 | 2.0 | 110 | 5.0 | 12.7 | 4.0 | 0.4 |
| Raspberry, Low Fat, Sainsbury's* | 1 Pot/90g | 96.0 | 2.0 | 107 | 5.8 | 15.1 | 2.6 | 0.1 |
| Raspberry, Organic, Yeo Valley* | 1 Pot/100g | 127.0 | 6.0 | 127 | 6.1 | 11.1 | 6.5 | 0.4 |
| Raspberry, Value, Tesco* | 1 Serving/60g | 56.0 | 1.0 | 93 | 7.2 | 13.5 | 1.3 | 0.0 |
| Raspberry & Redcurrant, BGTY, Sainsbury's* | 1 Pot/100g | 51.0 | 0.0 | 51 | 7.4 | 5.4 | 0.1 | 1.6 |
| Real Fruit, Tesco* | 1 Pot/100g | 54.0 | 0.0 | 54 | 5.6 | 7.6 | 0.1 | 0.1 |
| Red Cherry, HE, Tesco* | 1 Pot/100g | 55.0 | 0.0 | 55 | 6.2 | 7.2 | 0.2 | 0.1 |
| Red Cherry, Tesco* | 1 Pot/100g | 75.0 | 3.0 | 75 | 6.5 | 5.5 | 3.0 | 2.3 |
| Rhubarb & Crumble, Low Fat, Sainsbury's* | 1 Pot/90g | 96.0 | 2.0 | 107 | 6.7 | 14.1 | 2.6 | 0.4 |
| Strawberry, 0% Fat, Vitalinea, Danone* | 1 Serving/150g | 82.0 | 0.0 | 55 | 6.0 | 7.4 | 0.1 | 1.6 |
| Strawberry, 99.9% Fat Free, Onken* | 1 Serving/50g | 45.0 | 0.0 | 91 | 6.9 | 15.3 | 0.1 | 0.0 |
| Strawberry, COU, M & S* | 1 Pot/100g | 60.0 | 0.0 | 60 | 6.5 | 8.0 | 0.2 | 0.5 |
| Strawberry, GFY, Asda* | 1 Pot/100g | 58.0 | 0.0 | 58 | 6.0 | 8.0 | 0.2 | 0.0 |
| Strawberry, Healthy Choice, Asda* | 1 Pot/100g | 41.0 | 0.0 | 41 | 6.0 | 3.7 | 0.2 | 0.0 |
| Strawberry, Langley Farm* | 1 Pot/125g | 189.0 | 10.0 | 151 | 7.0 | 13.3 | 7.8 | 0.0 |
| Strawberry, Layered, Weight Watchers* | 1 Pot/100g | 50.0 | 0.0 | 50 | 5.4 | 6.2 | 0.1 | 0.8 |
| Strawberry, Low Fat, St Ivel* | 1 Pot/100g | 69.0 | 1.0 | 69 | 6.9 | 6.8 | 1.2 | 0.0 |
| Strawberry, Organic, Yeo Valley* | 1 Pot/90g | 116.0 | 5.0 | 129 | 6.3 | 12.5 | 6.0 | 0.2 |
| Strawberry, Puree, Somerfield* | 1 Pot/50g | 60.0 | 2.0 | 120 | 7.0 | 14.0 | 4.0 | 0.0 |
| Strawberry, Tesco* | 1 Pot/100g | 75.0 | 3.0 | 75 | 6.5 | 5.5 | 3.0 | 2.5 |
| Strawberry, Thomas the Tank Engine, Yoplait* | 1 Pot/50g | 50.0 | 1.0 | 101 | 6.8 | 15.4 | 1.3 | 0.0 |
| Strawberry, Value, Tesco* | 1 Pot/60g | 55.0 | 1.0 | 92 | 7.2 | 13.0 | 1.3 | 0.0 |
| Strawberry & Rasberry, Organic, Yeo Valley* | 1 Pot/90g | 118.0 | 5.0 | 131 | 6.3 | 12.9 | 6.0 | 0.2 |
| Strawberry Tart, Sainsbury's* | 1 Pot/100g | 54.0 | 0.0 | 54 | 7.6 | 5.5 | 0.2 | 1.1 |
| Toffee, BGTY, Sainsbury's* | 1 Pot/100g | 60.0 | 0.0 | 60 | 7.2 | 7.0 | 0.3 | 0.2 |
| Toffee & Pecan Pie, Smooth & Creamy, Tesco* | 1 Pot/100g | 148.0 | 7.0 | 148 | 6.9 | 14.8 | 6.8 | 0.2 |
| Tropical Fruit, COU, M & S* | 1 Pot/100g | 60.0 | 0.0 | 60 | 6.5 | 8.4 | 0.2 | 0.5 |
| Virtually Fat Free, Tesco* | 1 Pot/100g | 56.0 | 0.0 | 56 | 5.6 | 8.2 | 0.1 | 0.0 |
| Wildlife, Strawberry, Raspberry Or Peach, Yoplait* | 1 Pot/50g | 46.0 | 1.0 | 93 | 7.1 | 13.2 | 1.3 | 0.2 |

**F**

| | Measure INFO/WEIGHT | per Measure KCAL | FAT | Nutrition Values per 100g / 100ml KCAL | PROT | CARB | FAT | FIBRE |
|---|---|---|---|---|---|---|---|---|
| **FROMAGE FRAIS** | | | | | | | | |
| with Cereal, Shape Rise, Danone* | 1 Serving/165g | 205.0 | 2.0 | 124 | 6.5 | 23.9 | 1.3 | 0.5 |
| with Real Fruit Puree, Nestle* | 1 Serving/50g | 65.0 | 1.0 | 130 | 7.1 | 18.9 | 2.7 | 0.2 |
| **FROZEN DESSERT** | | | | | | | | |
| Banoffee, HL, Tesco* | 1 Serving/60g | 92.0 | 2.0 | 153 | 2.5 | 29.9 | 2.6 | 0.6 |
| Neapolitan, GFY, Asda* | 1 Serving/100g | 64.0 | 2.0 | 64 | 1.2 | 10.0 | 2.1 | 0.1 |
| Toffee, BGTY, Sainsbury's* | 1 Pot/74g | 96.0 | 1.0 | 130 | 3.3 | 26.0 | 1.4 | 4.2 |
| Vanilla, BGTY, Sainsbury's* | 1 Serving/75g | 89.0 | 2.0 | 119 | 3.0 | 19.9 | 3.0 | 3.7 |
| Vanilla, GFY, Asda* | 1 Serving/52g | 72.0 | 2.0 | 139 | 2.7 | 22.0 | 4.5 | 0.0 |
| Vanilla Choc Fudge, Non Dairy Soya, Tofutti* | 1 Tub/500ml | 825.0 | 45.0 | 165 | 1.6 | 20.0 | 9.0 | 0.4 |
| **FROZEN YOGHURT** | | | | | | | | |
| Black Cherry, M & S* | 1 Pot/125g | 164.0 | 1.0 | 131 | 3.1 | 27.1 | 1.1 | 0.5 |
| Raspberry, Handmade Farmhouse, Sainsbury's* | 1 Serving/100g | 132.0 | 4.0 | 132 | 2.7 | 21.8 | 3.8 | 2.2 |
| Raspberry, TTD, Sainsbury's* | ¼ Pot/90g | 119.0 | 3.0 | 132 | 2.7 | 21.8 | 3.8 | 2.2 |
| Strawberry, Organic, Yeo Valley* | 1 Serving/100g | 140.0 | 3.0 | 140 | 4.8 | 23.5 | 3.0 | 0.1 |
| Strawberry, Tesco* | 1 Pot/60g | 82.0 | 1.0 | 136 | 2.6 | 26.5 | 2.2 | 0.8 |
| Vanilla, Less Than 5% Fat, Tesco* | 1 Pot/120g | 179.0 | 3.0 | 149 | 8.1 | 23.8 | 2.4 | 0.7 |
| **FRUIT** | | | | | | | | |
| Berry Medley, Freshly Prepared, M & S* | 1 Pack/180g | 90.0 | 0.0 | 50 | 0.7 | 10.9 | 0.2 | 2.9 |
| Bites, Apple & Grape, Food Explorers, Waitrose* | 1 Pack/80g | 44.0 | 0.0 | 55 | 0.4 | 13.2 | 0.1 | 1.4 |
| Black Forest, Frozen, Tesco* | 1 Serving/80g | 37.0 | 0.0 | 46 | 0.7 | 10.5 | 0.0 | 1.7 |
| Citrus Selection, Fresh, Sainsbury's* | 1 Pack/240g | 79.0 | 0.0 | 33 | 0.9 | 7.1 | 0.1 | 1.6 |
| Collection, Freshly Prepared, M & S* | 1 Pack/400g | 180.0 | 1.0 | 45 | 0.6 | 10.3 | 0.2 | 1.3 |
| Deluxe, Fresh, Rindless, Shapers, Boots* | 1 Pack/168g | 64.0 | 0.0 | 38 | 0.7 | 8.3 | 0.2 | 0.7 |
| Exotic, M & S* | 1 Pack/425g | 212.0 | 1.0 | 50 | 0.7 | 11.8 | 0.3 | 0.0 |
| Grapefruit & Orange Segments, Breakfast, Del Monte* | 1 Can/411g | 193.0 | 0.0 | 47 | 1.0 | 10.2 | 0.1 | 1.0 |
| Melon, Kiwi, & Strawberry, Fully Prepared, Sainsbury's* | 1 Pack/245g | 73.0 | 0.0 | 30 | 0.8 | 6.3 | 0.2 | 1.3 |
| Mixed, Fresh, 5 a Day, Tesco* | 1 Pack/400g | 136.0 | 1.0 | 34 | 0.8 | 7.4 | 0.2 | 1.4 |
| Mixed, Pieces, in Orange Jelly, Fruitini, Del Monte* | 1 Can/140g | 94.0 | 0.0 | 67 | 0.3 | 15.8 | 0.1 | 0.0 |
| Mixed, Tropical, Fruit Express, Del Monte* | 1 Pot/185g | 89.0 | 0.0 | 48 | 0.2 | 11.2 | 0.1 | 1.2 |
| Pieces, Mixed in Fruit Juice, Fruiyini, Del Monte* | 1 Serving/120g | 61.0 | 0.0 | 51 | 0.4 | 12.0 | 0.1 | 0.5 |
| Pineapple, Grape & Kiwi, Asda* | 1 Serving/200g | 98.0 | 1.0 | 49 | 0.6 | 11.0 | 0.3 | 1.7 |
| Snack, Apple & Grape, Blue Parrot Cafe, Sainsbury's* | 1 Pack/80g | 42.0 | 0.0 | 53 | 0.4 | 12.5 | 0.1 | 2.1 |
| Snack Pack, Fresh, Sainsbury's* | 1 Serving/120g | 54.0 | 0.0 | 45 | 0.1 | 11.0 | 0.1 | 1.3 |
| to Go, Del Monte* | 1 Can/113g | 80.0 | 0.0 | 71 | 0.0 | 17.7 | 0.0 | 0.0 |
| Tropical, in Juice, Dole* | 1 Pot/113g | 59.0 | 0.0 | 52 | 0.3 | 14.2 | 0.0 | 1.8 |
| Tropical, Tesco* | 1 Pack/180g | 85.0 | 0.0 | 47 | 0.6 | 10.8 | 0.2 | 1.9 |
| **FRUIT & NUT MIX** | | | | | | | | |
| Almond, Raisin & Berry, Sainsbury's* | 1 Bag/50g | 188.0 | 7.0 | 377 | 6.1 | 57.6 | 14.3 | 4.2 |
| Bear Necessities, Graze* | 1 Box/60g | 274.0 | 12.0 | 456 | 14.0 | 55.5 | 19.7 | 0.0 |
| Born In The Usa, Graze* | 1 Pack/50g | 285.0 | 22.0 | 570 | 10.6 | 33.8 | 43.8 | 0.0 |
| Cinnamon & Prailine, Christmas, Finest, Tesco* | ¼ Pot/106g | 470.0 | 27.0 | 442 | 8.2 | 45.9 | 25.1 | 11.5 |
| Exotic, Waitrose* | 1 Serving/50g | 207.0 | 9.0 | 414 | 9.0 | 54.6 | 17.7 | 4.6 |
| Himalayas & Beyond, Graze* | 1 Pack/45g | 196.0 | 12.0 | 435 | 6.9 | 48.4 | 26.4 | 0.0 |
| Johnny Come Lately, Graze* | 1 Pack/65g | 250.0 | 11.0 | 384 | 8.8 | 54.5 | 16.3 | 0.0 |
| Love Mix, Graze* | 1 Pack/55g | 155.0 | 1.0 | 281 | 4.6 | 70.0 | 1.1 | 0.0 |
| Luxury, Asda* | 1 Serving/50g | 225.0 | 15.0 | 451 | 9.0 | 33.5 | 30.5 | 7.4 |
| M & S* | 1 Serving/30g | 135.0 | 8.0 | 450 | 12.4 | 44.3 | 25.3 | 6.0 |
| Milkshake Mix, Graze* | 1 Pack/60g | 254.0 | 9.0 | 424 | 14.2 | 66.3 | 15.3 | 0.0 |
| Mixed, Unsalted, Tesco* | 1 Serving/25g | 112.0 | 5.0 | 449 | 12.6 | 58.1 | 18.5 | 12.2 |
| New World, Graze* | 1 Serving/50g | 206.0 | 12.0 | 413 | 16.8 | 45.2 | 23.4 | 0.0 |
| Organic, Waitrose* | 1 Pack/100g | 489.0 | 33.0 | 489 | 15.0 | 33.8 | 32.6 | 5.4 |
| Papaya & Cranberry, Sainsbury's* | 1 Serving/75g | 300.0 | 11.0 | 400 | 4.1 | 63.1 | 14.6 | 7.3 |
| Port & Winter Spice, Perenium, Christmas, Finest, Tesco* | ¼ Pot/90g | 379.0 | 24.0 | 421 | 7.8 | 37.9 | 26.5 | 13.9 |

| | Measure INFO/WEIGHT | per Measure KCAL | FAT | Nutrition Values per 100g / 100ml KCAL | PROT | CARB | FAT | FIBRE |
|---|---|---|---|---|---|---|---|---|
| **FRUIT & NUT MIX** | | | | | | | | |
| Rock The Casbah, Graze* | 1 Pack/60g | 284.0 | 18.0 | 473 | 10.0 | 39.7 | 30.3 | 0.0 |
| Swallows & Amazons, Graze* | 1 Pack/60g | 252.0 | 12.0 | 420 | 6.3 | 56.3 | 19.7 | 0.0 |
| TTD, Sainsbury's* | 1 Bag/250g | 900.0 | 39.0 | 360 | 5.1 | 49.5 | 15.7 | 5.9 |
| Ying & Yang, Graze* | 1 Pack/60g | 296.0 | 19.0 | 493 | 6.8 | 41.2 | 32.5 | 0.0 |
| **FRUIT COCKTAIL** | | | | | | | | |
| Fresh & Ready, Sainsbury's* | 1 Pack/300g | 117.0 | 0.0 | 39 | 0.6 | 9.0 | 0.1 | 1.2 |
| in Apple Juice, Asda* | 1/3 Can/80g | 40.0 | 0.0 | 50 | 0.3 | 12.0 | 0.1 | 1.6 |
| in Fruit Juice, Heinz* | 1 Pot/125g | 77.0 | 0.0 | 62 | 0.5 | 15.0 | 0.0 | 1.0 |
| in Fruit Juice, Morrisons* | 1 Can/140g | 64.0 | 0.0 | 46 | 0.4 | 11.0 | 0.0 | 0.0 |
| in Fruit Juice, Sainsbury's* | 1 Serving/198g | 97.0 | 0.0 | 49 | 0.3 | 11.9 | 0.1 | 1.3 |
| in Fruit Juice, Waitrose* | 1 Can/142g | 71.0 | 0.0 | 50 | 0.4 | 12.0 | 0.0 | 1.0 |
| in Juice, Del Monte* | 1 Can/415g | 203.0 | 0.0 | 49 | 0.4 | 11.2 | 0.1 | 0.0 |
| in Light Syrup, Princes* | 1 Serving/206g | 64.0 | 0.0 | 31 | 0.4 | 7.3 | 0.0 | 1.0 |
| in Light Syrup, Sainsbury's* | ½ Can/125g | 72.0 | 0.0 | 58 | 0.4 | 14.0 | 0.1 | 1.3 |
| in Light Syrup, Valfrutta* | 1 Serving/206g | 95.0 | 0.0 | 46 | 0.2 | 11.4 | 0.0 | 1.5 |
| in Pear Juice, Kwik Save* | 1 Can/411g | 189.0 | 0.0 | 46 | 0.5 | 11.0 | 0.0 | 1.0 |
| in Syrup, Del Monte* | 1 Can/420g | 315.0 | 0.0 | 75 | 0.4 | 18.0 | 0.1 | 0.0 |
| in Syrup, Morrisons* | ½ Can/205g | 129.0 | 0.0 | 63 | 0.3 | 14.9 | 0.1 | 0.0 |
| in Syrup, Tesco* | 1 Serving/135g | 85.0 | 0.0 | 63 | 0.4 | 15.0 | 0.0 | 1.0 |
| in Very Light Syrup, Value, Tesco* | 1 Can/410g | 123.0 | 0.0 | 30 | 0.4 | 7.3 | 0.0 | 1.0 |
| No Added Sugar, Asda* | 1 Serving/134g | 67.0 | 0.0 | 50 | 0.3 | 12.0 | 0.1 | 1.6 |
| Tropical, Asda* | ½ Can/135g | 81.0 | 0.0 | 60 | 0.0 | 15.0 | 0.0 | 1.6 |
| Tropical, Heinz* | 1 Pot/113g | 61.0 | 0.0 | 54 | 0.5 | 13.0 | 0.0 | 1.0 |
| Tropical, in Syrup, Sainsbury's* | ½ Can/130g | 95.0 | 0.0 | 73 | 0.5 | 17.6 | 0.1 | 1.4 |
| Tropical, Morrisons* | ½ Can/212g | 144.0 | 0.0 | 68 | 0.0 | 17.0 | 0.0 | 0.0 |
| **FRUIT COMPOTE** | | | | | | | | |
| & Vanilla Sponge, Weight Watchers* | 1 Pack/140g | 202.0 | 3.0 | 144 | 2.2 | 29.0 | 2.1 | 1.8 |
| Apple, Strawberry & Blackberry, Organic, Yeo Valley* | ½ Pot/112g | 73.0 | 0.0 | 65 | 0.5 | 15.5 | 0.1 | 1.9 |
| Apricot & Prune, Yeo Valley* | 1 Pot/225g | 207.0 | 0.0 | 92 | 0.6 | 22.3 | 0.1 | 1.6 |
| Hartley's* | 1 Serving/95g | 63.0 | 0.0 | 66 | 0.8 | 15.5 | 0.1 | 2.4 |
| HE, Tesco* | 1 Pot/140g | 113.0 | 0.0 | 81 | 0.9 | 19.1 | 0.2 | 1.6 |
| Orchard Fruits, GFY, Asda* | 1 Pot/180g | 113.0 | 0.0 | 63 | 0.5 | 15.0 | 0.1 | 0.0 |
| Spiced, Tesco* | 1 Serving/112g | 122.0 | 1.0 | 109 | 1.7 | 24.4 | 0.5 | 3.1 |
| Strawberry & Raspberry, M & S* | 1 Serving/80g | 72.0 | 0.0 | 90 | 0.7 | 23.5 | 0.1 | 2.3 |
| Summerfruit, M & S* | ¼ Pot/125g | 119.0 | 1.0 | 95 | 0.9 | 22.7 | 0.6 | 0.8 |
| **FRUIT FILLING** | | | | | | | | |
| Apricot, Sainsbury's* | 1 Can/400g | 316.0 | 0.0 | 79 | 0.5 | 19.1 | 0.1 | 0.9 |
| Black Cherry, Tesco* | 1 Serving/100g | 110.0 | 0.0 | 110 | 0.4 | 26.9 | 0.1 | 0.4 |
| Bramley Apple, Morton* | 1 Serving/198g | 168.0 | 0.0 | 85 | 0.2 | 21.1 | 0.1 | 0.0 |
| Cherry & Amaretto, Asda* | ¼ Pack/100g | 105.0 | 0.0 | 105 | 0.9 | 23.0 | 0.2 | 0.0 |
| Red Cherry, Morton* | 1 Serving/70g | 69.0 | 0.0 | 98 | 0.4 | 23.9 | 0.0 | 0.0 |
| **FRUIT FLAKES** | | | | | | | | |
| Blackcurrant, with Yoghurt Coating, Fruit Bowl* | 1 Bag/25g | 112.0 | 5.0 | 449 | 1.7 | 64.2 | 20.6 | 0.0 |
| Raisins, with Yoghurt Coating, Fruit Bowl* | 1 Pack/30g | 133.0 | 6.0 | 444 | 2.9 | 66.6 | 18.4 | 0.0 |
| Raspberry, with Yoghurt Coating, Fruit Bowl* | 1 Serving/25g | 112.0 | 5.0 | 449 | 1.7 | 64.2 | 20.6 | 0.0 |
| Strawberry, Fruit Bowl* | 1 Pack/20g | 66.0 | 0.0 | 330 | 1.0 | 78.0 | 2.0 | 2.0 |
| Strawberry, with Yoghurt Coating, Fruit Bowl* | 1 Serving/25g | 112.0 | 5.0 | 449 | 1.7 | 64.2 | 20.6 | 0.0 |
| **FRUIT GUMS** | | | | | | | | |
| Fruit Salad, Tesco* | 6 Sweets/30g | 100.0 | 0.0 | 335 | 8.3 | 73.4 | 0.5 | 0.3 |
| No Added Sugar, Boots* | 1 Sweet/2g | 1.0 | 0.0 | 88 | 0.0 | 22.0 | 0.0 | 0.0 |
| Rowntree's* | 1 Tube/49g | 170.0 | 0.0 | 344 | 4.8 | 81.3 | 0.2 | 0.0 |
| Sugar Free, Sainsbury's* | 1 Serving/30g | 63.0 | 0.0 | 209 | 7.7 | 71.3 | 0.2 | 0.1 |

F

| | Measure INFO/WEIGHT | per Measure KCAL | per Measure FAT | Nutrition Values per 100g / 100ml KCAL | PROT | CARB | FAT | FIBRE |
|---|---|---|---|---|---|---|---|---|
| **FRUIT MEDLEY** | | | | | | | | |
| Citrus, Somerfield* | 1 Serving/81g | 25.0 | 0.0 | 31 | 0.6 | 6.9 | 0.1 | 0.4 |
| Fresh, Tesco* | 1 Pack/200g | 86.0 | 0.0 | 43 | 0.4 | 10.0 | 0.1 | 1.1 |
| Mango, Melon, Kiwi & Blueberry, Fresh, M & S* | 1 Pack/260g | 104.0 | 1.0 | 40 | 0.7 | 9.1 | 0.3 | 1.6 |
| Nectarine, Mango & Blueberry, Fresh, M & S* | 1 Pack/245g | 122.0 | 0.0 | 50 | 1.0 | 11.1 | 0.2 | 2.1 |
| Pineapple, Papaya & Mango, Waitrose* | 1 Pack/550g | 297.0 | 1.0 | 54 | 0.6 | 12.8 | 0.1 | 1.1 |
| Shapers, Boots* | 1 Pack/140g | 55.0 | 0.0 | 39 | 0.7 | 8.6 | 0.2 | 1.0 |
| **FRUIT MIX** | | | | | | | | |
| Apple Strudel, Graze* | 1 Pack/55g | 172.0 | 0.0 | 312 | 2.6 | 63.5 | 0.7 | 0.0 |
| Banana, Coconut & Mango, Dried, Graze* | 1 Punnet/45g | 144.0 | 4.0 | 320 | 18.7 | 57.1 | 8.2 | 0.0 |
| Banana Coins, Graze* | 1 Serving/20g | 49.0 | 0.0 | 245 | 2.4 | 54.0 | 0.6 | 0.0 |
| Beach Bum, Graze* | 1 Pack/40g | 168.0 | 3.0 | 419 | 2.2 | 59.8 | 8.4 | 0.0 |
| Berry, Sainsbury's* | 1 Serving/20g | 64.0 | 0.0 | 319 | 1.0 | 78.1 | 1.9 | 5.5 |
| Caribbean, Dried, Graze* | 1 Box/50g | 187.0 | 6.0 | 374 | 1.2 | 67.6 | 12.8 | 0.0 |
| Cherish, Graze* | 1 Pack/50g | 221.0 | 10.0 | 443 | 5.2 | 52.5 | 20.0 | 0.0 |
| Cherry Oranges, Graze* | 1 Pack/119g | 56.0 | 0.0 | 47 | 1.1 | 11.8 | 0.1 | 1.0 |
| Forest, Dried, Graze* | 1 Pack/50g | 159.0 | 0.0 | 319 | 1.8 | 76.0 | 0.8 | 0.0 |
| Forest Fruit, Dried, Graze* | 1 Pack/50g | 159.0 | 0.0 | 319 | 1.8 | 76.0 | 0.8 | 0.0 |
| Fruit Crumble, Graze* | 1 Pack/50g | 199.0 | 10.0 | 399 | 6.0 | 48.6 | 20.2 | 0.0 |
| Loco In Acapulco, Graze* | 1 Pack /50g | 205.0 | 11.0 | 410 | 4.0 | 53.2 | 21.4 | 0.0 |
| Luxury, Sainsbury's* | 1 Serving/30g | 78.0 | 0.0 | 261 | 1.8 | 62.3 | 0.5 | 2.7 |
| Mango & Cranberry, Way to Five, Sainsbury's* | 1 Serving/50g | 165.0 | 0.0 | 331 | 1.8 | 79.4 | 0.7 | 4.8 |
| Melon, Strawberry & Grape, Sainsbury's* | 1 Pack/180g | 58.0 | 0.0 | 32 | 0.5 | 7.0 | 0.2 | 0.4 |
| Muffin, Dried, Graze* | 1 Box/60g | 221.0 | 7.0 | 368 | 1.7 | 65.8 | 11.3 | 1.7 |
| Pineapple, Melon, Mango, Tesco* | 1 Pack/440g | 242.0 | 1.0 | 55 | 1.1 | 11.4 | 0.2 | 1.3 |
| Pumpkin Pie, Graze* | 1 Pack/65g | 274.0 | 11.0 | 422 | 11.4 | 48.2 | 17.2 | 0.0 |
| Razcherries, Graze* | 1 Pack/50g | 163.0 | 0.0 | 327 | 0.5 | 80.0 | 0.5 | 0.0 |
| Rouge Dried, Graze* | 1 Pack/50g | 164.0 | 1.0 | 328 | 1.6 | 77.6 | 1.4 | 0.0 |
| Strawberries & Cream, Graze* | 1 Pack/70g | 303.0 | 11.0 | 433 | 3.7 | 66.9 | 16.3 | 0.0 |
| Summer Fruits, British, Frozen, Waitrose* | 1 Pack/380g | 99.0 | 1.0 | 26 | 1.0 | 5.2 | 0.2 | 5.5 |
| Super Dried, Graze* | 1 Pack/55g | 176.0 | 1.0 | 320 | 5.6 | 76.4 | 1.6 | 0.0 |
| Tropical, Fresh, Waitrose* | 1 Pack/240g | 122.0 | 0.0 | 51 | 0.6 | 11.6 | 0.2 | 1.9 |
| TTD, Sainsbury's* | 1 Serving/50g | 68.0 | 0.0 | 137 | 0.3 | 36.4 | 0.4 | 1.6 |
| **FRUIT PUREE** | | | | | | | | |
| Apple, & Blueberry, Organix* | 1 Pot/100g | 54.0 | 1.0 | 54 | 0.4 | 11.6 | 0.6 | 2.5 |
| Apple, & Peach, Organix* | 1 Pot/100g | 49.0 | 0.0 | 49 | 0.6 | 11.0 | 0.3 | 2.1 |
| Apple & Blueberry, Clearspring* | 1 Tub/100g | 76.0 | 0.0 | 76 | 0.4 | 17.8 | 0.3 | 0.0 |
| Banana, Apple, & Apricot, Organix* | 1 Pot/100g | 68.0 | 0.0 | 68 | 0.8 | 15.4 | 0.4 | 2.0 |
| **FRUIT SALAD** | | | | | | | | |
| Autumn, Fresh, M & S* | ½ Pack/160g | 64.0 | 0.0 | 40 | 0.7 | 9.4 | 0.1 | 2.9 |
| Berry, Seasonal, Asda* | 1 Pack/300g | 93.0 | 0.0 | 31 | 0.6 | 7.0 | 0.1 | 2.1 |
| Citrus, Asda* | 1 Serving/265g | 88.0 | 0.0 | 33 | 0.9 | 7.2 | 0.1 | 1.5 |
| Citrus, Fresh, M & S* | ½ Pack/225g | 79.0 | 0.0 | 35 | 0.9 | 7.7 | 0.1 | 1.5 |
| Classic, Fresh, Sainsbury's* | 1 Pack/400g | 148.0 | 1.0 | 37 | 0.6 | 8.6 | 0.2 | 1.8 |
| Classic, Shapers, Boots* | 1 Pack/200g | 75.0 | 0.0 | 37 | 0.7 | 8.5 | 0.1 | 1.3 |
| Exotic, Fresh, Tesco* | 1 Serving/225g | 85.0 | 0.0 | 38 | 0.7 | 8.4 | 0.2 | 1.5 |
| Exotic, Fully Prepared, Sainsbury's* | 1 Serving/200g | 74.0 | 0.0 | 37 | 0.6 | 8.3 | 0.2 | 1.3 |
| Exotic, Morrisons* | 1 Serving/150g | 78.0 | 0.0 | 52 | 0.6 | 12.2 | 0.2 | 0.0 |
| Exotic, Waitrose* | 1 Pack/300g | 126.0 | 1.0 | 42 | 0.6 | 9.5 | 0.2 | 1.1 |
| Exotic, with Melon, Mango, Kiwi Fruit & Grapes, Asda* | 1 Pot/300g | 141.0 | 1.0 | 47 | 0.6 | 10.5 | 0.3 | 1.4 |
| Fresh, Budgens* | 1 Pack/250g | 105.0 | 0.0 | 42 | 0.7 | 9.6 | 0.1 | 1.3 |
| Fresh, Morrisons* | 1 Tub/350g | 150.0 | 0.0 | 43 | 0.7 | 9.9 | 0.1 | 0.0 |
| Fresh, Sweet, Ripe & Moist, Tesco* | 1 Serving/750g | 345.0 | 1.0 | 46 | 0.7 | 10.6 | 0.1 | 1.6 |
| Fresh, Tesco* | 1 Pack/200g | 84.0 | 0.0 | 42 | 0.7 | 9.3 | 0.2 | 1.5 |

F

| | Measure INFO/WEIGHT | per Measure KCAL | per Measure FAT | Nutrition Values per 100g / 100ml KCAL | PROT | CARB | FAT | FIBRE |
|---|---|---|---|---|---|---|---|---|
| **FRUIT SALAD** | | | | | | | | |
| Fresh, Washed, Ready to Eat, Tesco* | 1 Pack/200g | 92.0 | 0.0 | 46 | 0.7 | 10.6 | 0.1 | 1.6 |
| Fresh for You, Tesco* | 1 Pack/160g | 59.0 | 0.0 | 37 | 0.6 | 8.2 | 0.2 | 1.1 |
| Freshly Prepared, M & S* | 1 Pack/350g | 140.0 | 1.0 | 40 | 0.5 | 9.3 | 0.2 | 1.0 |
| Fruit, Mediterranean Style, Shapers, Boots* | 1 Pack/142g | 61.0 | 0.0 | 43 | 0.6 | 10.0 | 0.1 | 1.5 |
| Golden, Fresh, Asda* | 1 Pot/147g | 69.0 | 0.0 | 47 | 0.6 | 11.0 | 0.1 | 1.6 |
| Grapefruit & Orange, Fresh, M & S* | 1 Serving/250g | 87.0 | 0.0 | 35 | 0.9 | 7.4 | 0.1 | 1.6 |
| Homemade, Unsweetened, Average | 1 Serving/140g | 77.0 | 0.0 | 55 | 0.7 | 13.8 | 0.1 | 1.5 |
| Juicy Melon, Pineapple & Grapes, Asda* | 1 Pot/300g | 111.0 | 0.0 | 37 | 0.5 | 8.4 | 0.1 | 0.9 |
| Kiwi, Pineapple & Grape, Fresh Tastes, Asda* | 1 Pack/200g | 84.0 | 1.0 | 42 | 0.7 | 9.1 | 0.3 | 1.8 |
| Layered, Rainbow, M & S* | 1 Pack/350g | 140.0 | 1.0 | 40 | 0.5 | 9.3 | 0.2 | 1.0 |
| Layered, Tropical Rainbow, Freshly Prepared, M & S* | 1 Pack/375g | 206.0 | 1.0 | 55 | 0.7 | 12.6 | 0.3 | 1.7 |
| Luxury, Fresh, Tesco* | 1 Serving/400g | 164.0 | 1.0 | 41 | 0.7 | 9.2 | 0.2 | 1.6 |
| Luxury, Frozen, Tesco* | ½ Pack/250g | 115.0 | 0.0 | 46 | 0.7 | 10.7 | 0.1 | 1.3 |
| Luxury, Shearway* | 1 Serving/625g | 271.0 | 1.0 | 43 | 0.6 | 10.0 | 0.1 | 0.0 |
| Mango, Kiwi, Blueberry & Pomegranate, Fresh, M & S* | 1 Pack/350g | 210.0 | 1.0 | 60 | 0.9 | 13.4 | 0.3 | 2.4 |
| Mediterranean Style, Budgens* | 1 Serving/250g | 95.0 | 0.0 | 38 | 0.6 | 8.5 | 0.2 | 0.8 |
| Melon, Kiwi, Strawbery, Way to Five, Sainsbury's* | 1 Pack/245g | 73.0 | 0.0 | 30 | 0.8 | 6.3 | 0.2 | 1.3 |
| Melon, Pineapple & Grapes, Fresh, Tesco* | 1 Pack/300g | 120.0 | 0.0 | 40 | 0.5 | 9.2 | 0.1 | 1.0 |
| Melon & Grapes, Shapers, Boots* | 1 Pack/220g | 75.0 | 0.0 | 34 | 0.6 | 7.7 | 0.1 | 0.8 |
| Melon & Red Grape, Freshly Prepared, M & S* | 1 Pack/450g | 157.0 | 0.0 | 35 | 0.5 | 8.4 | 0.1 | 0.7 |
| Mixed, Fresh, Sainsbury's* | 1 Pack/200g | 84.0 | 0.0 | 42 | 0.7 | 9.4 | 0.2 | 1.9 |
| Oranges, Apple, Pineapple & Grapes, Fresh, Asda* | 1 Pack/260g | 120.0 | 0.0 | 46 | 0.6 | 10.5 | 0.1 | 2.1 |
| Peaches & Pears, Fruit Express, Del Monte* | 1 Serving/185g | 87.0 | 0.0 | 47 | 0.4 | 10.8 | 0.1 | 0.9 |
| Pineapple, Apple & Strawberries, Tesco* | 1 Pack/190g | 80.0 | 0.0 | 42 | 0.4 | 9.8 | 0.1 | 1.4 |
| Pineapple, Mandarin & Grapefruit, Asda* | 1 Serving/200g | 86.0 | 0.0 | 43 | 0.6 | 10.0 | 0.1 | 0.0 |
| Pineapple, Mango & Passion Fruit, Prepared, M & S* | 1 Pack/400g | 200.0 | 1.0 | 50 | 0.7 | 10.8 | 0.2 | 1.8 |
| Rainbow, Asda* | 1 Pack/350g | 140.0 | 1.0 | 40 | 0.6 | 8.8 | 0.3 | 1.4 |
| Rainbow, Fresh, Tesco* | 1 Tub/270g | 105.0 | 1.0 | 39 | 0.5 | 8.8 | 0.2 | 0.9 |
| Seasonal, Fresh, Asda* | 1 Pack/125g | 55.0 | 0.0 | 44 | 0.5 | 10.4 | 0.1 | 1.2 |
| Seasonal Melon & Grapes, Asda* | ½ Pack/200g | 66.0 | 1.0 | 33 | 0.5 | 7.5 | 0.5 | 0.4 |
| Shapers, Boots* | 1 Pack/140g | 55.0 | 0.0 | 39 | 0.7 | 8.6 | 0.2 | 1.0 |
| Summer, Red, Fresh, M & S* | 1 Pack/400g | 160.0 | 1.0 | 40 | 0.0 | 10.0 | 0.2 | 1.2 |
| Summer, Sainsbury's* | 1 Pack/240g | 84.0 | 0.0 | 35 | 0.7 | 7.8 | 0.2 | 1.3 |
| Sunshine, Fresh, M & S* | 1 Serving/200g | 70.0 | 0.0 | 35 | 0.0 | 8.3 | 0.1 | 1.3 |
| Tropical, Budgens* | 1 Pack/250g | 127.0 | 0.0 | 51 | 0.6 | 11.7 | 0.2 | 1.8 |
| Tropical, Fresh, Asda* | 1 Pack/400g | 164.0 | 1.0 | 41 | 0.7 | 9.0 | 0.2 | 1.8 |
| Tropical, Fruit Snacks, Frozen, Sainsbury's* | 1 Serving/175g | 79.0 | 0.0 | 45 | 0.7 | 10.4 | 0.1 | 1.6 |
| Tropical, in Light Syrup, Passion Fruit Juice, Tesco* | ½ Can/216g | 130.0 | 0.0 | 60 | 0.3 | 14.1 | 0.1 | 1.1 |
| Weight Watchers* | 1 Serving/135g | 50.0 | 0.0 | 37 | 0.2 | 9.0 | 0.1 | 0.7 |
| **FRUIT SHOOT** | | | | | | | | |
| Apple & Blackcurrant, Robinson's* | 1 Bottle/200ml | 10.0 | 0.0 | 5 | 0.1 | 0.8 | 0.0 | 0.0 |
| Orange, Pure, Robinson's* | 1 Bottle/250ml | 115.0 | 0.0 | 46 | 0.5 | 9.9 | 0.1 | 0.2 |
| **FRUIT SPREAD** | | | | | | | | |
| Apricot, Pure, Organic, Whole Earth* | 1 Serving/20g | 33.0 | 0.0 | 167 | 0.8 | 40.0 | 0.4 | 0.9 |
| Blackcurrant, Carb Check, Heinz* | 1 Tbsp/15g | 8.0 | 0.0 | 54 | 0.5 | 12.8 | 0.1 | 2.7 |
| Blackcurrant, Weight Watchers* | 1 Tsp/6g | 6.0 | 0.0 | 106 | 0.2 | 26.3 | 0.0 | 0.9 |
| Cherries & Berries, Organic, Meridian Foods* | 1 Tbsp/15g | 16.0 | 0.0 | 109 | 0.5 | 26.0 | 0.3 | 1.1 |
| Cherry & Berry, Meridian Foods* | 1 Serving/10g | 14.0 | 0.0 | 138 | 0.7 | 33.7 | 0.6 | 3.2 |
| High, Blueberry, St Dalfour* | 1 Tsp/15g | 34.0 | 0.0 | 228 | 0.5 | 56.0 | 0.2 | 2.2 |
| Raspberry, Weight Watchers* | 1 Tsp/6g | 7.0 | 0.0 | 111 | 0.4 | 27.1 | 0.1 | 0.9 |
| Raspberry & Cranberry, No Added Sugar, Superjam* | 1 Spread/10g | 22.0 | 0.0 | 216 | 2.1 | 47.0 | 0.3 | 0.0 |
| Seville Orange, Weight Watchers* | 1 Tsp/15g | 17.0 | 0.0 | 111 | 0.2 | 27.5 | 0.0 | 0.3 |
| Strawberry, Carb Check, Heinz* | 1 Tbsp/15g | 8.0 | 0.0 | 56 | 0.3 | 13.6 | 0.0 | 0.5 |

F

| | Measure INFO/WEIGHT | per Measure | | Nutrition Values per 100g / 100ml | | | | |
|---|---|---|---|---|---|---|---|---|
| | | KCAL | FAT | KCAL | PROT | CARB | FAT | FIBRE |
| **FRUIT SPREAD** | | | | | | | | |
| Strawberry, Weight Watchers* | 1 Tbsp/15g | 23.0 | 0.0 | 156 | 0.7 | 39.8 | 0.1 | 1.8 |
| **FRUIT WINDERS** | | | | | | | | |
| Real Fruit, Kellogg's* | 1 Serving/18g | 67.0 | 1.0 | 370 | 0.5 | 77.0 | 7.0 | 3.0 |
| **FU YUNG** | | | | | | | | |
| Egg, Average | 1oz/28g | 67.0 | 6.0 | 239 | 9.9 | 2.2 | 20.6 | 1.3 |
| **FUDGE** | | | | | | | | |
| All Butter, Finest, Tesco* | 1 Sweet/10g | 43.0 | 1.0 | 429 | 1.3 | 73.4 | 14.5 | 0.0 |
| Butter, Milk, Thorntons* | 1 Sweet/13g | 60.0 | 2.0 | 462 | 3.7 | 68.5 | 19.2 | 0.0 |
| Cadbury* | 1 Bar/25g | 110.0 | 4.0 | 435 | 2.5 | 72.7 | 14.9 | 0.0 |
| Cherry & Almond, Thorntons* | 1 Bag/100g | 464.0 | 19.0 | 464 | 3.2 | 70.5 | 19.1 | 0.4 |
| Chocolate, Average | 1 Sweet/30g | 132.0 | 4.0 | 441 | 3.3 | 81.1 | 13.7 | 0.0 |
| Chocolate, Thorntons* | 1 Bag/100g | 459.0 | 19.0 | 459 | 3.1 | 69.0 | 19.1 | 0.6 |
| Clotted Cream, M & S* | 1oz/28g | 133.0 | 6.0 | 474 | 1.7 | 67.6 | 22.1 | 0.0 |
| Clotted Cream, Sainsbury's* | 1 Sweet/8g | 35.0 | 1.0 | 430 | 1.9 | 81.5 | 10.7 | 0.7 |
| Dairy, Co-Op* | 1 Sweet/9g | 39.0 | 1.0 | 430 | 2.0 | 76.0 | 13.0 | 0.0 |
| Devon, Somerfield* | 1 Pack/250g | 1060.0 | 28.0 | 424 | 2.0 | 78.9 | 11.1 | 0.0 |
| Double Chocolate Bar, M & S* | 1 Bar/43g | 202.0 | 9.0 | 470 | 4.2 | 66.9 | 21.0 | 0.7 |
| Maple, TTD, Sainsbury's* | 1 Sweet/10g | 43.0 | 1.0 | 426 | 1.3 | 73.0 | 14.3 | 0.0 |
| Pure Indulgence, Thorntons* | 1 Bar/45g | 210.0 | 10.0 | 466 | 1.8 | 65.9 | 21.9 | 0.0 |
| Vanilla, Bar, Diabetic, Thorntons* | 1 Bar/34g | 156.0 | 6.0 | 460 | 3.3 | 69.2 | 18.8 | 0.6 |
| Vanilla, Bar, M & S* | 1 Bar/43g | 205.0 | 10.0 | 476 | 3.7 | 63.0 | 23.3 | 0.4 |
| Vanilla, Thorntons* | 1 Bag/100g | 465.0 | 22.0 | 465 | 1.8 | 65.9 | 21.9 | 0.0 |
| Vanilla, Whipped, M & S* | 1 Serving/43g | 210.0 | 10.0 | 490 | 3.8 | 65.4 | 23.9 | 0.3 |
| **FUSE** | | | | | | | | |
| Cadbury* | 1 Bar/49g | 238.0 | 12.0 | 485 | 7.6 | 58.2 | 24.8 | 0.0 |
| **FUSILLI** | | | | | | | | |
| Carb Check, Heinz* | 1 Serving/75g | 219.0 | 2.0 | 292 | 52.7 | 15.2 | 2.3 | 20.8 |
| Carb Options, Knorr* | 1oz/28g | 98.0 | 0.0 | 350 | 28.5 | 34.0 | 1.5 | 21.0 |
| *Cooked, Average* | *1 Serving/210g* | *248.0* | *1.0* | *118* | *4.1* | *23.8* | *0.6* | *1.1* |
| *Dry, Average* | *1 Serving/90g* | *316.0* | *1.0* | *351* | *12.3* | *72.0* | *1.6* | *2.2* |
| *Fresh, Cooked, Average* | *1 Serving/200g* | *329.0* | *4.0* | *164* | *6.4* | *30.6* | *1.8* | *1.7* |
| *Fresh, Dry, Average* | *1 Serving/75g* | *208.0* | *2.0* | *277* | *10.9* | *53.4* | *2.7* | *2.1* |
| Tomato, Weight Watchers* | 1 Can/388g | 198.0 | 2.0 | 51 | 1.9 | 10.1 | 0.4 | 0.8 |
| *Tricolore, Dry, Average* | *1 Serving/75g* | *264.0* | *1.0* | *351* | *12.2* | *71.8* | *1.7* | *2.7* |
| *Whole Wheat, Dry Weight, Average* | *1 Serving/90g* | *290.0* | *2.0* | *322* | *13.1* | *62.3* | *2.3* | *9.0* |

**F**

| | Measure<br>INFO/WEIGHT | per Measure<br>KCAL | FAT | Nutrition Values per 100g / 100ml<br>KCAL | PROT | CARB | FAT | FIBRE |
|---|---|---|---|---|---|---|---|---|
| **GALAXY** | | | | | | | | |
| Amicelli, Mars* | 1 Serving/13g | 66.0 | 4.0 | 507 | 6.2 | 59.7 | 27.1 | 0.0 |
| Caramel, Mars* | 1 Bar/49g | 254.0 | 13.0 | 518 | 5.8 | 64.2 | 26.4 | 0.0 |
| Caramel Crunch, Promises, Mars* | 1 Bar/100g | 540.0 | 32.0 | 540 | 6.1 | 57.5 | 31.8 | 0.0 |
| Fruit & Hazelnut, Milk, Mars* | 1 Bar/47g | 235.0 | 13.0 | 501 | 7.1 | 55.2 | 28.0 | 0.0 |
| Hazelnut, Mars* | 1 Piece/6g | 37.0 | 2.0 | 582 | 7.8 | 49.4 | 39.2 | 0.0 |
| Hazelnut, Roast, Promises, Mars* | 1 Bar/100g | 544.0 | 33.0 | 544 | 6.4 | 55.6 | 32.9 | 0.0 |
| Liaison, Mars* | 1 Bar/48g | 233.0 | 12.0 | 485 | 5.4 | 60.3 | 24.7 | 0.0 |
| Rich Coffee, Promises, Mars* | 1 Bar/100g | 535.0 | 33.0 | 535 | 5.7 | 54.4 | 32.8 | 0.0 |
| Swirls, Mars* | 1 Bag/150g | 747.0 | 40.0 | 498 | 4.9 | 60.2 | 26.5 | 0.0 |
| **GAMMON** | | | | | | | | |
| Breaded, Average | 1oz/28g | 34.0 | 1.0 | 120 | 22.5 | 1.0 | 3.0 | 0.0 |
| Dry Cured, Ready to Roast, M & S* | ½ Joint/255g | 255.0 | 4.0 | 100 | 20.5 | 0.5 | 1.5 | 0.5 |
| Honey & Mustard, Average | ½ Pack/190g | 294.0 | 14.0 | 155 | 19.1 | 3.6 | 7.1 | 0.1 |
| Joint, Applewood Smoked, Tesco* | 1 Serving/100g | 152.0 | 9.0 | 152 | 17.5 | 0.2 | 9.0 | 0.0 |
| *Joint, Boiled, Average* | *1 Serving/60g* | *100.0* | *4.0* | *167* | *25.1* | *0.4* | *7.1* | *0.0* |
| *Joint, Raw, Average* | *½ Joint/255g* | *404.0* | *21.0* | *158* | *20.9* | *0.2* | *8.1* | *0.1* |
| *Steaks, Average* | *1 Steak/97g* | *157.0* | *7.0* | *161* | *23.3* | *0.4* | *7.4* | *0.0* |
| *Steaks, Healthy Range, Average* | *1 Serving/110g* | *107.0* | *3.0* | *97* | *18.0* | *0.4* | *3.2* | *0.2* |
| *Steaks, Honey Roast, Average* | *1 Steak/100g* | *142.0* | *5.0* | *142* | *21.5* | *2.3* | *5.3* | *0.0* |
| *Steaks, Smoked, Average* | *1 Steak/110g* | *150.0* | *6.0* | *137* | *22.7* | *0.1* | *5.0* | *0.1* |
| **GAMMON &** | | | | | | | | |
| Parsley Sauce, Steak, Tesco* | ½ Pack/140g | 217.0 | 7.0 | 155 | 23.7 | 2.9 | 5.2 | 0.5 |
| Pineapple, Roast, Dinner, Iceland* | 1 Pack/400g | 360.0 | 6.0 | 90 | 6.2 | 12.7 | 1.6 | 1.7 |
| **GAMMON IN** | | | | | | | | |
| Creamy Cheddar Sauce, Steaks, Fresh Tastes, Asda* | ½ Pack/143g | 270.0 | 14.0 | 189 | 19.1 | 5.4 | 10.1 | 1.5 |
| **GAMMON WITH** | | | | | | | | |
| Cheese Sauce & Crumb, Steaks, Simply Cook, Tesco* | ½ Pack/156g | 218.0 | 12.0 | 140 | 14.2 | 3.1 | 7.7 | 1.0 |
| Orange Glaze, Christmas, Joint, Finest, Tesco* | 1/10 Joint/150g | 214.0 | 10.0 | 143 | 17.6 | 2.4 | 7.0 | 0.0 |
| Pineapple, Steaks, Asda* | ½ Pack/195g | 253.0 | 3.0 | 130 | 17.8 | 11.5 | 1.4 | 0.7 |
| Three Cheese & Mustard Crust, Joint, Asda* | 1 Serving/270g | 351.0 | 12.0 | 130 | 21.7 | 1.2 | 4.3 | 0.0 |
| **GARAM MASALA** | | | | | | | | |
| *Dry, Ground, Average* | *1 Tbsp/15g* | *57.0* | *2.0* | *379* | *15.6* | *45.2* | *15.1* | *0.0* |
| **GARGANELLI** | | | | | | | | |
| Egg, Dry, Waitrose* | 1 Serving/125g | 450.0 | 5.0 | 360 | 13.5 | 66.9 | 4.2 | 3.5 |
| **GARLIC** | | | | | | | | |
| Minced, Nishaan* | 1 Tsp/5g | 5.0 | 0.0 | 97 | 6.0 | 16.2 | 0.9 | 0.0 |
| *Powder, Average* | *1 Tsp/3g* | *7.0* | *0.0* | *246* | *18.7* | *42.7* | *1.2* | *9.9* |
| *Raw, Average* | *1 Clove/3g* | *4.0* | *0.0* | *149* | *6.4* | *33.1* | *0.5* | *2.1* |
| Spice Blend, Gourmet Garden* | 1 Squeeze/10ml | 31.0 | 2.0 | 210 | 4.5 | 10.8 | 16.2 | 10.3 |
| Very Lazy, The English Provender Co.* | 1 Tsp/3g | 3.0 | 0.0 | 111 | 6.0 | 20.9 | 0.4 | 3.0 |
| **GARLIC PUREE** | | | | | | | | |
| *Average* | *1 Tbsp/18g* | *68.0* | *6.0* | *380* | *3.5* | *16.9* | *33.6* | *0.0* |
| in Vegetable Oil, GIA* | 1 Tsp/5g | 20.0 | 2.0 | 391 | 3.3 | 1.6 | 41.3 | 0.0 |
| with Tomato, GIA* | 10g | 7.0 | 0.0 | 70 | 5.1 | 0.5 | 1.2 | 0.0 |
| **GATEAU** | | | | | | | | |
| Black Forest, 500g Size, Tesco* | 1 Cake/500g | 1125.0 | 55.0 | 225 | 4.0 | 27.1 | 11.0 | 1.8 |
| Black Forest, Family Size, 860g, Tesco* | 1 Cake/860g | 1978.0 | 114.0 | 230 | 3.4 | 24.8 | 13.2 | 0.9 |
| Black Forest, Mini, Tesco* | 1 Serving/55g | 136.0 | 5.0 | 247 | 5.7 | 35.3 | 9.2 | 1.0 |
| Black Forest, Sara Lee* | 1 Serving/80g | 221.0 | 10.0 | 276 | 3.6 | 37.9 | 12.3 | 1.2 |
| Blackforest, Sainsbury's* | 1/8 Cake/63g | 163.0 | 11.0 | 259 | 3.9 | 27.7 | 17.1 | 3.5 |
| Chocolate, Asda* | 1 Serving/100g | 176.0 | 10.0 | 176 | 2.4 | 19.0 | 10.0 | 0.4 |
| Chocolate, Swirl, Tesco* | 1 Serving/83g | 230.0 | 13.0 | 277 | 3.8 | 29.3 | 16.0 | 0.2 |
| Chocolate Layer, M & S* | 1 Serving/86g | 278.0 | 16.0 | 323 | 4.2 | 35.9 | 18.3 | 0.9 |

**G**

| | Measure INFO/WEIGHT | per Measure KCAL | FAT | Nutrition Values per 100g / 100ml KCAL | PROT | CARB | FAT | FIBRE |
|---|---|---|---|---|---|---|---|---|
| **GATEAU** | | | | | | | | |
| Chocolate Orange, Co-Op* | 1 Serving/97g | 320.0 | 17.0 | 330 | 5.0 | 37.0 | 18.0 | 1.0 |
| Double Chocolate, Light, Sara Lee* | 1/5 Cake/59g | 139.0 | 3.0 | 237 | 5.7 | 43.3 | 4.6 | 2.0 |
| Double Chocolate, Sara Lee* | 1oz/28g | 93.0 | 5.0 | 331 | 5.6 | 41.3 | 16.5 | 0.9 |
| Double Chocolate, Tesco* | 1 Serving/45g | 124.0 | 6.0 | 276 | 4.4 | 32.1 | 14.4 | 2.2 |
| Double Strawberry, Sara Lee* | 1/8 Cake/199g | 533.0 | 24.0 | 268 | 3.2 | 36.2 | 12.2 | 0.6 |
| Ice Cream, Chocolate & Vanilla, Iceland* | 1 Serving/130g | 252.0 | 12.0 | 194 | 3.3 | 24.1 | 9.4 | 0.6 |
| Profiterole, TTD, Sainsbury's* | 1/6 Cake/112g | 410.0 | 31.0 | 365 | 3.9 | 26.2 | 27.2 | 1.1 |
| Strawberry, Co-Op* | 1 Serving/77g | 222.0 | 13.0 | 288 | 5.1 | 29.2 | 16.7 | 1.0 |
| Strawberry, Family Size, Tesco* | 1 Serving/84g | 197.0 | 11.0 | 235 | 2.9 | 25.2 | 13.6 | 0.6 |
| Swiss, Cadbury* | 1/6 Serving/60g | 228.0 | 10.0 | 380 | 5.2 | 52.0 | 16.8 | 0.9 |
| Toffee Ripple, Sara Lee* | 1 Serving/317g | 1005.0 | 49.0 | 317 | 4.0 | 40.2 | 15.6 | 0.5 |
| Triple Chocolate, Heinz* | ¼ Cake/85g | 209.0 | 9.0 | 245 | 5.1 | 31.2 | 11.1 | 2.4 |
| **GELATINE** | | | | | | | | |
| *Average* | *1oz/28g* | *95.0* | *0.0* | *338* | *84.4* | *0.0* | *0.0* | *0.0* |
| **GEMELLI** | | | | | | | | |
| Durum Wheat, Tesco* | 1 Serving/100g | 354.0 | 2.0 | 354 | 13.2 | 68.5 | 2.0 | 2.9 |
| **GHEE** | | | | | | | | |
| *Butter* | *1oz/28g* | *251.0* | *28.0* | *898* | *0.0* | *0.0* | *99.8* | *0.0* |
| *Palm* | *1oz/28g* | *251.0* | *28.0* | *897* | *0.0* | *0.0* | *99.7* | *0.0* |
| *Vegetable* | *1oz/28g* | *251.0* | *28.0* | *895* | *0.0* | *0.0* | *99.4* | *0.0* |
| **GHERKINS** | | | | | | | | |
| *Pickled, Average* | *1 Gherkin/36g* | *5.0* | *0.0* | *14* | *0.9* | *2.5* | *0.1* | *1.2* |
| **GIN** | | | | | | | | |
| & Tonic, Premixed, Canned, Gordons* | 1 Can/250ml | 213.0 | 0.0 | 85 | 0.0 | 6.7 | 0.0 | 0.0 |
| *37.5% Volume* | *1 Shot/35ml* | *72.0* | *0.0* | *207* | *0.0* | *0.0* | *0.0* | *0.0* |
| *40% Volume* | *1 Shot/35ml* | *78.0* | *0.0* | *222* | *0.0* | *0.0* | *0.0* | *0.0* |
| **GINGER** | | | | | | | | |
| Chunks, Crystallized, Julian Graves* | 1 Serving/10g | 34.0 | 0.0 | 340 | 0.0 | 88.0 | 0.0 | 0.0 |
| Crystalised, Graze* | 1 Pack/25g | 61.0 | 0.0 | 243 | 2.9 | 58.0 | 0.3 | 0.0 |
| *Ground, Average* | *1 Tsp/2g* | *5.0* | *0.0* | *258* | *7.4* | *60.0* | *3.3* | *0.0* |
| Lazy, Minced, The English Provender Co.* | 1 Tsp/5g | 1.0 | 0.0 | 15 | 0.2 | 3.2 | 0.2 | 1.5 |
| *Root, Raw, Pared, Average* | *1 Tsp/2g* | *2.0* | *0.0* | *86* | *2.0* | *19.1* | *0.8* | *2.1* |
| *Root, Raw, Unprepared, Average* | *1oz/28g* | *22.0* | *0.0* | *80* | *1.8* | *17.8* | *0.7* | *2.0* |
| Stem, in Sugar Syrup, Sainsbury's* | 1oz/28g | 76.0 | 0.0 | 271 | 0.2 | 67.3 | 0.1 | 1.4 |
| **GINGER ALE** | | | | | | | | |
| 1870, Siver Spring* | 1 Serving/100ml | 18.0 | 0.0 | 18 | 0.0 | 4.2 | 0.0 | 0.0 |
| American, Finest, Tesco* | 1 Serving/150ml | 68.0 | 0.0 | 45 | 0.0 | 11.0 | 0.0 | 0.0 |
| American, Low Calorie, Tesco* | 1 fl oz/30ml | 0.0 | 0.0 | 1 | 0.0 | 0.0 | 0.0 | 0.0 |
| American, Tesco* | 1 Glass/250ml | 57.0 | 0.0 | 23 | 0.0 | 5.5 | 0.0 | 0.0 |
| Dry | 1 Glass/250ml | 37.0 | 0.0 | 15 | 0.0 | 3.9 | 0.0 | 0.0 |
| Dry, Asda* | 1 Serving/150ml | 55.0 | 0.0 | 37 | 0.0 | 9.0 | 0.0 | 0.0 |
| Dry, Sainsbury's* | 1 Glass/250ml | 95.0 | 0.0 | 38 | 0.1 | 9.1 | 0.1 | 0.1 |
| **GINGER BEER** | | | | | | | | |
| Asda* | 1 Can/330ml | 144.0 | 0.0 | 44 | 0.0 | 10.9 | 0.0 | 0.0 |
| Classic, Schweppes* | 1 Can/330ml | 115.0 | 0.0 | 35 | 0.0 | 8.4 | 0.0 | 0.0 |
| Jamaican, Boots* | 1 Bottle/500ml | 5.0 | 0.0 | 1 | 0.0 | 0.0 | 0.0 | 0.0 |
| Light, Waitrose* | 1 Glass/250ml | 2.0 | 0.0 | 1 | 0.0 | 0.0 | 0.1 | 0.1 |
| Sainsbury's* | 1 Can/330ml | 69.0 | 0.0 | 21 | 0.0 | 5.1 | 0.0 | 0.0 |
| Tesco* | 1 Serving/200ml | 70.0 | 0.0 | 35 | 0.1 | 8.2 | 0.1 | 0.0 |
| Traditional Style, Tesco* | 1 Can/330ml | 218.0 | 0.0 | 66 | 0.0 | 16.1 | 0.0 | 0.0 |
| **GINGERBREAD** | | | | | | | | |
| Average | 1oz/28g | 106.0 | 4.0 | 379 | 5.7 | 64.7 | 12.6 | 1.2 |
| Men, Mini, Asda* | 1 Biscuit/11g | 46.0 | 1.0 | 433 | 5.0 | 74.0 | 13.0 | 1.8 |

G

| | Measure INFO/WEIGHT | per Measure KCAL | FAT | Nutrition Values per 100g / 100ml KCAL | PROT | CARB | FAT | FIBRE |
|---|---|---|---|---|---|---|---|---|
| **GINGERBREAD** | | | | | | | | |
| Men, Mini, M & S* | 1 Biscuit/17g | 78.0 | 3.0 | 470 | 6.2 | 63.9 | 18.6 | 1.7 |
| Men, Mini, Sainsbury's* | 1 Biscuit/12g | 56.0 | 1.0 | 463 | 5.7 | 83.4 | 11.8 | 1.5 |
| **GNOCCHI** | | | | | | | | |
| Aldi* | 1 Serving/100g | 160.0 | 0.0 | 160 | 3.8 | 35.6 | 0.3 | 0.0 |
| Di Patate, Italfresco* | ½ Pack/200g | 296.0 | 0.0 | 148 | 3.3 | 33.2 | 0.2 | 0.0 |
| Fresh, Italian, Chilled, Sainsbury's* | ¼ Pack/125g | 190.0 | 0.0 | 152 | 3.8 | 33.6 | 0.3 | 1.4 |
| *Potato, Average* | *1 Serving/150g* | *199.0* | *0.0* | *133* | *0.0* | *33.2* | *0.0* | *0.0* |
| **GOAT** | | | | | | | | |
| *Raw* | *1oz/28g* | *31.0* | *1.0* | *109* | *20.6* | *0.0* | *2.3* | *0.0* |
| **GOJI BERRIES** | | | | | | | | |
| *Average* | *1 Serving/100g* | *287.0* | *1.0* | *287* | *6.6* | *65.1* | *0.7* | *6.8* |
| **GOOSE** | | | | | | | | |
| *Leg, with Skin, Fire Roasted* | *1 Leg/174g* | *482.0* | *30.0* | *277* | *28.8* | *0.0* | *17.1* | *0.0* |
| *Leg, with Skin, Raw* | *1 Leg/265g* | *943.0* | *84.0* | *356* | *16.3* | *0.0* | *31.8* | *0.0* |
| *Meat, Fat & Skin, Raw* | *1oz/28g* | *101.0* | *9.0* | *361* | *16.5* | *0.0* | *32.8* | *0.0* |
| *Meat, Raw* | *1 Portion/185g* | *298.0* | *13.0* | *161* | *23.0* | *0.0* | *7.0* | *0.0* |
| *Meat, Roasted* | *1 Portion/143g* | *340.0* | *19.0* | *238* | *29.0* | *0.0* | *13.0* | *0.0* |
| *Meat & Skin, Roasted* | *½ Goose/774g* | *2361.0* | *170.0* | *305* | *25.2* | *0.0* | *21.9* | *0.0* |
| **GOOSEBERRIES** | | | | | | | | |
| *Dessert, Raw* | *1oz/28g* | *11.0* | *0.0* | *40* | *0.7* | *9.2* | *0.3* | *2.4* |
| *Stewed with Sugar* | *25g* | *13.0* | *0.0* | *54* | *0.7* | *12.9* | *0.3* | *4.2* |
| *Stewed without Sugar* | *25g* | *4.0* | *0.0* | *16* | *0.9* | *2.5* | *0.3* | *4.4* |
| **GOULASH** | | | | | | | | |
| Beef, Bistro Range, Tesco* | 1 Pack/450g | 544.0 | 15.0 | 121 | 7.9 | 14.6 | 3.4 | 0.6 |
| Beef, Finest, Tesco* | ½ Pack/300g | 297.0 | 9.0 | 99 | 11.6 | 6.2 | 3.1 | 0.6 |
| Beef, Weight Watchers* | 1 Pack/330g | 241.0 | 6.0 | 73 | 4.8 | 9.5 | 1.7 | 0.6 |
| Beef, with Tagliatelle, COU, M & S* | 1 Pack/360g | 414.0 | 8.0 | 115 | 8.5 | 14.5 | 2.3 | 1.0 |
| **GRAPEFRUIT** | | | | | | | | |
| *in Juice, Average* | *1oz/28g* | *13.0* | *0.0* | *46* | *0.5* | *10.6* | *0.0* | *0.4* |
| *in Syrup, Average* | *1oz/28g* | *19.0* | *0.0* | *69* | *0.5* | *16.8* | *0.1* | *0.5* |
| *Raw, Flesh Only, Average* | *½ Grapefruit/160g* | *34.0* | *0.0* | *21* | *0.5* | *4.8* | *0.1* | *0.9* |
| *Raw, Weighed with Skin & Seeds, Average* | *1 Lge/340g* | *109.0* | *0.0* | *32* | *0.6* | *8.1* | *0.1* | *1.1* |
| *Ruby Red, in Juice, Average* | *1 Serving/135g* | *54.0* | *0.0* | *40* | *0.5* | *9.3* | *0.0* | *0.5* |
| **GRAPES** | | | | | | | | |
| *Green, Average* | *1oz/28g* | *17.0* | *0.0* | *61* | *0.4* | *15.2* | *0.1* | *0.7* |
| *Red, Average* | *1 Serving/80g* | *53.0* | *0.0* | *67* | *0.4* | *16.5* | *0.1* | *0.7* |
| *Red & Green Selection, Average* | *1 Serving/80g* | *50.0* | *0.0* | *62* | *0.4* | *15.2* | *0.1* | *0.8* |
| **GRATIN** | | | | | | | | |
| Cauliflower, Findus* | 1 Pack/400g | 340.0 | 20.0 | 85 | 3.5 | 7.0 | 5.0 | 0.0 |
| Dauphinoise, Budgens* | ½ Pack/218g | 277.0 | 16.0 | 127 | 3.0 | 12.5 | 7.2 | 2.5 |
| Leek & Carrot, Findus* | 1 Pack/400g | 440.0 | 26.0 | 110 | 3.5 | 9.5 | 6.5 | 0.0 |
| Potato, Creamy, M & S* | ½ Pack/225g | 360.0 | 25.0 | 160 | 2.2 | 11.9 | 11.1 | 0.9 |
| Potato, HL, Tesco* | 1 Serving/225g | 169.0 | 5.0 | 75 | 2.3 | 11.4 | 2.2 | 0.6 |
| Potato, Sainsbury's* | ½ Pack/225g | 448.0 | 34.0 | 199 | 4.4 | 11.4 | 15.1 | 1.0 |
| Potato, Somerfield* | ½ Pack/225g | 355.0 | 27.0 | 158 | 2.0 | 11.0 | 12.0 | 0.0 |
| Spinach & Mushroom, Safeway* | 1 Packet/520g | 728.0 | 44.0 | 140 | 4.8 | 10.3 | 8.4 | 1.5 |
| Vegetable, Somerfield* | 1 Pack/300g | 417.0 | 39.0 | 139 | 1.0 | 5.0 | 13.0 | 0.0 |
| **GRAVY** | | | | | | | | |
| Beef, Aunt Bessie's* | 1 Serving/100g | 73.0 | 5.0 | 73 | 1.0 | 5.3 | 5.3 | 0.5 |
| Beef, Fresh, Sainsbury's* | 1 Serving/83ml | 47.0 | 3.0 | 56 | 2.4 | 4.5 | 3.2 | 0.6 |
| Beef, Heat & Serve, Morrisons* | 1 Serving/150g | 27.0 | 0.0 | 18 | 0.3 | 3.9 | 0.3 | 0.5 |
| Beef, Home Style, Savoury, Heinz* | ¼ Cup/60g | 30.0 | 1.0 | 50 | 1.7 | 6.7 | 1.7 | 0.0 |
| Beef, Rich, Ready to Heat, Schwartz* | ½ Pack/100g | 31.0 | 2.0 | 31 | 0.8 | 3.4 | 1.6 | 0.5 |

**G**

| | Measure INFO/WEIGHT | per Measure | | Nutrition Values per 100g / 100ml | | | | |
|---|---|---|---|---|---|---|---|---|
| | | KCAL | FAT | KCAL | PROT | CARB | FAT | FIBRE |
| **GRAVY** | | | | | | | | |
| Beef, with Winter Berry & Shallot, Made Up, Oxo* | 1 Serving/105ml | 24.0 | 0.0 | 23 | 0.6 | 4.3 | 0.3 | 0.1 |
| Chicken, Granules For, Dry Weight, Bisto* | 1 Serving/20g | 80.0 | 3.0 | 400 | 1.9 | 62.5 | 15.8 | 0.2 |
| Chicken, Rich, Ready to Heat, Schwartz* | ½ Pack/100g | 27.0 | 1.0 | 27 | 0.8 | 3.3 | 1.2 | 0.5 |
| Favourite, Granules, Made Up, Bisto* | 1 Serving/50ml | 14.0 | 1.0 | 28 | 0.2 | 4.2 | 1.2 | 0.0 |
| Granules, Beef, Dry, Tesco* | 1 Serving/6g | 29.0 | 2.0 | 480 | 5.5 | 36.4 | 34.7 | 1.5 |
| Granules, Beef, Made Up, Tesco* | 1 Serving/140ml | 48.0 | 4.0 | 35 | 0.3 | 2.6 | 2.5 | 0.1 |
| Granules, Chicken, Dry, Oxo* | 1oz/28g | 83.0 | 1.0 | 296 | 11.1 | 54.2 | 4.9 | 0.7 |
| Granules, Chicken, Made Up, Oxo* | 1 fl oz/30ml | 5.0 | 0.0 | 18 | 0.7 | 3.3 | 0.3 | 0.0 |
| Granules, Chicken & Hint of Sage & Onion, Oxo* | 1 Serving/30g | 95.0 | 2.0 | 316 | 11.1 | 54.2 | 6.1 | 0.7 |
| Granules, Dry, Bisto* | 1 Serving/10g | 38.0 | 2.0 | 384 | 3.1 | 56.4 | 16.2 | 1.5 |
| Granules, Dry, Value, Tesco* | 1oz/28g | 111.0 | 5.0 | 397 | 3.2 | 54.4 | 18.5 | 1.0 |
| Granules, for Vegetarian Dishes, Made Up, Sainsbury's* | 1 Serving/50ml | 16.0 | 1.0 | 32 | 0.2 | 2.8 | 2.2 | 0.8 |
| *Granules, Instant, Dry* | *1oz/28g* | *129.0* | *9.0* | *462* | *4.4* | *40.6* | *32.5* | *0.0* |
| *Granules, Instant, Made Up* | *1oz/28g* | *10.0* | *1.0* | *34* | *0.3* | *3.0* | *2.4* | *0.0* |
| Granules, Lamb, Hint of Mint, Made Up, Oxo* | 1 Serving/100ml | 25.0 | 0.0 | 25 | 0.7 | 4.3 | 0.5 | 0.0 |
| Granules, Made Up, Bisto* | 1 Serving/50ml | 15.0 | 1.0 | 30 | 0.2 | 4.2 | 1.4 | 0.2 |
| Granules, Made Up, Oxo* | 1 Serving/150ml | 28.0 | 0.0 | 19 | 0.6 | 3.4 | 0.3 | 0.0 |
| Granules, Onion, Dry, Morrisons* | 1 Serving/25g | 124.0 | 9.0 | 495 | 3.4 | 44.0 | 34.7 | 0.0 |
| Granules, Onion, Dry, Oxo* | 1oz/28g | 92.0 | 1.0 | 328 | 8.2 | 62.3 | 4.8 | 0.8 |
| Granules, Onion, Made Up, Oxo* | 1 fl oz/30ml | 6.0 | 0.0 | 20 | 0.5 | 3.7 | 0.3 | 0.0 |
| Granules, Original, Dry, Oxo* | 1oz/28g | 88.0 | 1.0 | 313 | 10.2 | 57.2 | 4.8 | 1.0 |
| Granules, Vegetable, Dry, Oxo* | 1oz/28g | 88.0 | 1.0 | 316 | 8.4 | 59.5 | 4.9 | 0.9 |
| Granules for Chicken, Made Up, SmartPrice, Asda* | 1 Serving/100ml | 34.0 | 2.0 | 34 | 0.2 | 3.0 | 2.3 | 0.1 |
| Granules for Vegetarian Dishes, Dry Weight, Bisto* | 1 Serving/28g | 100.0 | 4.0 | 356 | 2.7 | 56.0 | 13.3 | 4.5 |
| Onion, Fresh, Asda* | 1/6 Pot/77g | 30.0 | 2.0 | 39 | 1.7 | 3.3 | 2.1 | 0.4 |
| Onion, Fresh, Somerfield* | 1 Pack/300g | 195.0 | 12.0 | 65 | 1.0 | 7.0 | 4.0 | 0.0 |
| Onion, Granules, Made Up, Bisto* | 1 Serving/50ml | 14.0 | 0.0 | 28 | 0.2 | 5.6 | 0.6 | 0.0 |
| Onion, Granules For, Dry Weight, Bisto* | 4 Tsp/20g | 78.0 | 3.0 | 391 | 2.4 | 62.3 | 14.7 | 2.3 |
| Onion, Rich, M & S* | ½ Pack/150g | 60.0 | 2.0 | 40 | 2.0 | 5.9 | 1.2 | 0.3 |
| Onion, Rich, Ready to Heat, Schwartz* | ½ Sachet/100g | 24.0 | 1.0 | 24 | 0.4 | 4.3 | 0.6 | 0.5 |
| Onion, TTD, Sainsbury's* | 1 Serving/100g | 78.0 | 5.0 | 78 | 1.3 | 6.6 | 5.2 | 0.8 |
| Paste, Beef, Antony Worrall Thompson's* | 1 Portion/31g | 104.0 | 6.0 | 334 | 11.8 | 30.3 | 18.4 | 0.6 |
| Paste, Onion, Antony Worrall Thompson's* | 1 Tsp/10g | 26.0 | 0.0 | 262 | 7.0 | 48.7 | 4.4 | 1.4 |
| Powder, Gluten Free, Dry, Allergycare* | 1 Tbsp/10g | 26.0 | 0.0 | 260 | 0.3 | 63.8 | 0.4 | 0.0 |
| Powder, Made Up, Sainsbury's* | 1 Serving/100ml | 15.0 | 0.0 | 15 | 0.4 | 3.2 | 0.1 | 0.1 |
| Powder, Vegetarian, Organic, Marigold* | 1 Serving/22g | 79.0 | 2.0 | 361 | 10.6 | 61.5 | 7.7 | 1.3 |
| Roast Beef, Best, in Glass Jar, Made Up, Bisto* | 1 Serving/50ml | 13.0 | 0.0 | 26 | 0.4 | 5.4 | 0.4 | 0.2 |
| Roast Lamb, Bisto, Best* | 1 Serving/20g | 60.0 | 1.0 | 302 | 3.4 | 62.3 | 4.3 | 0.0 |
| Roast Pork, Best, in Glass Jar, Dry Weight, Bisto* | 4 Tsp/20g | 63.0 | 1.0 | 314 | 4.3 | 64.1 | 4.5 | 0.0 |
| Turkey, Granules, Made Up, Bisto* | 1 Serving/50ml | 14.0 | 1.0 | 28 | 0.2 | 4.0 | 1.2 | 0.2 |
| Turkey, Granules For, Dry Weight, Bisto* | 4 Tsp/20g | 75.0 | 3.0 | 377 | 2.4 | 57.2 | 15.5 | 1.0 |
| Turkey, Rich, Ready to Heat, Schwartz* | 1 Pack/200g | 62.0 | 2.0 | 31 | 1.9 | 3.1 | 1.2 | 0.5 |
| Vegetable, Granules For, Dry Weight, Bisto* | 1 Tsp/4g | 15.0 | 1.0 | 380 | 2.1 | 63.0 | 13.3 | 4.5 |
| Vegetable, Granules For, Made Up, Bisto* | 1 Serving/50ml | 14.0 | 0.0 | 28 | 0.2 | 5.6 | 0.4 | 0.2 |
| **GREENGAGES** | | | | | | | | |
| *Raw, Average* | *1 Fruit/66g* | *26.0* | *0.0* | *39* | *0.7* | *9.4* | *0.1* | *2.0* |
| **GREENS** | | | | | | | | |
| *Spring, Boiled, Average* | *1 Serving/80g* | *16.0* | *1.0* | *20* | *1.9* | *1.6* | *0.7* | *2.6* |
| *Spring, Raw, Average* | *1 Serving/80g* | *26.0* | *1.0* | *33* | *3.0* | *3.1* | *1.0* | *3.4* |
| **GRILLS** | | | | | | | | |
| Bacon & Cheese, Tesco* | 1 Grill/78g | 222.0 | 15.0 | 284 | 15.0 | 13.4 | 18.9 | 1.2 |
| Cheese & Bacon, Danepak* | 1 Grill/85g | 241.0 | 16.0 | 284 | 15.0 | 13.4 | 18.9 | 1.2 |
| Vegetable, Dalepak* | 1 Grill/83g | 125.0 | 4.0 | 151 | 4.0 | 22.5 | 5.0 | 1.6 |

**G**

|  | Measure INFO/WEIGHT | per Measure KCAL | FAT | Nutrition Values per 100g / 100ml KCAL | PROT | CARB | FAT | FIBRE |
|---|---|---|---|---|---|---|---|---|
| **GRILLS** | | | | | | | | |
| Vegetable, Mediterranean, Cauldron Foods* | 1 Grill/88g | 145.0 | 10.0 | 166 | 5.3 | 15.8 | 11.9 | 6.5 |
| Vegetable, Ross* | 1 Grill/114g | 252.0 | 13.0 | 221 | 4.3 | 25.5 | 11.3 | 0.9 |
| Vegetable, Tesco* | 1 Grill/72g | 129.0 | 7.0 | 179 | 4.2 | 18.0 | 10.0 | 2.2 |
| Vegetarian, Mushroom & Oregano, Organic, Waitrose* | 1 Grill/100g | 200.0 | 10.0 | 200 | 7.9 | 19.5 | 10.0 | 4.3 |
| **GRITS** | | | | | | | | |
| Enriched White Hominy, Old Fashioned, Quaker* | ¼ Cup/41g | 140.0 | 1.0 | 341 | 7.3 | 78.0 | 1.2 | 4.9 |
| **GROUSE** | | | | | | | | |
| *Meat Only, Roasted* | *1oz/28g* | *36.0* | *1.0* | *128* | *27.6* | *0.0* | *2.0* | *0.0* |
| **GUACAMOLE** | | | | | | | | |
| Asda* | ½ Pot/57g | 113.0 | 11.0 | 200 | 1.8 | 3.3 | 20.0 | 4.0 |
| Average | 1 Tbsp/17g | 22.0 | 2.0 | 128 | 1.4 | 2.2 | 12.7 | 2.5 |
| Chunky, M & S* | 1 Pot/170g | 221.0 | 19.0 | 130 | 1.5 | 5.1 | 11.3 | 1.7 |
| Chunky, Sainsbury's* | ½ Pot/65g | 120.0 | 12.0 | 185 | 1.6 | 3.2 | 18.4 | 3.8 |
| Doritos, Walkers* | 1 Tbsp/20g | 32.0 | 3.0 | 159 | 1.2 | 2.6 | 16.0 | 0.1 |
| Fresh, Sainsbury's* | 1oz/28g | 59.0 | 6.0 | 210 | 1.8 | 5.3 | 20.2 | 2.5 |
| Fresh, VLH Kitchens* | 1 Tbsp/17g | 26.9 | 2.5 | 158 | 1.5 | 3.0 | 14.6 | 2.5 |
| Fresh, Waitrose* | ½ Pack/100g | 190.0 | 18.0 | 190 | 1.9 | 4.1 | 18.4 | 2.5 |
| GFY, Asda* | 1 Pack/113g | 144.0 | 12.0 | 127 | 2.8 | 4.3 | 11.0 | 2.2 |
| Mexican Style, Dip Selection, Morrisons* | ½ Pack/50g | 102.0 | 10.0 | 204 | 1.5 | 3.7 | 20.4 | 0.9 |
| Reduced Fat, Sainsbury's* | ½ Pot/65g | 87.0 | 8.0 | 134 | 1.5 | 3.5 | 12.6 | 4.0 |
| Reduced Fat, Tesco* | 1 Pack/200g | 280.0 | 23.0 | 140 | 2.7 | 5.7 | 11.4 | 3.0 |
| Reduced Fat, Waitrose* | 1 Serving/25g | 31.0 | 3.0 | 126 | 2.9 | 5.7 | 10.1 | 2.3 |
| **GUAVA** | | | | | | | | |
| *Canned, in Syrup* | *1oz/28g* | *17.0* | *0.0* | *60* | *0.4* | *15.7* | *0.0* | *3.0* |
| *Raw, Flesh Only, Average* | *1 Fruit/55g* | *37.0* | *1.0* | *68* | *3.0* | *14.0* | *1.0* | *5.0* |
| **GUINEA FOWL** | | | | | | | | |
| Boned & Stuffed, Fresh, Fayrefield Foods* | 1 Serving/325g | 650.0 | 39.0 | 200 | 19.1 | 3.3 | 12.1 | 0.5 |
| Fresh, Free Range, Waitrose* | 1 Portion/193g | 258.0 | 12.0 | 134 | 19.5 | 0.0 | 6.2 | 0.3 |
| **GUMBO** | | | | | | | | |
| Cajun Vegetable, Sainsbury's* | 1 Serving/450g | 265.0 | 11.0 | 59 | 1.4 | 7.7 | 2.5 | 1.5 |
| Louisiana Chicken, Perfectly Balanced, Waitrose* | 1 Serving/235g | 207.0 | 7.0 | 88 | 12.2 | 3.5 | 2.8 | 1.3 |
| **GUMS** | | | | | | | | |
| American, Hard, Tesco* | 1 Serving/200g | 646.0 | 0.0 | 323 | 0.0 | 80.8 | 0.0 | 0.0 |
| American Hard, Sainsbury's* | 1 Sweet/6g | 22.0 | 0.0 | 360 | 0.1 | 90.0 | 0.1 | 0.0 |
| Milk, Cow, Sainsbury's* | 1 Sweet/3g | 10.0 | 0.0 | 353 | 6.2 | 78.3 | 1.6 | 0.0 |
| Milk Bottles, Bassett's* | 1 Pack/25g | 88.0 | 0.0 | 353 | 6.2 | 78.3 | 1.6 | 0.0 |

**G**

| | Measure INFO/WEIGHT | per Measure KCAL | FAT | Nutrition Values per 100g / 100ml KCAL | PROT | CARB | FAT | FIBRE |
|---|---|---|---|---|---|---|---|---|
| **HADDOCK** | | | | | | | | |
| Fillets, Battered, Average | 1oz/28g | 64.0 | 3.0 | 228 | 13.4 | 16.3 | 12.2 | 1.1 |
| Fillets, in Breadcrumbs, Average | 1oz/28g | 57.0 | 3.0 | 203 | 13.5 | 14.9 | 9.9 | 1.2 |
| *Fillets, Raw, Average* | *1oz/28g* | *22.0* | *0.0* | *80* | *18.0* | *0.2* | *0.8* | *0.0* |
| *Fillets, Smoked, Cooked, Average* | *1 Pack/300g* | *337.0* | *8.0* | *112* | *21.9* | *0.4* | *2.6* | *0.1* |
| *Fillets, Smoked, Raw, Average* | *1 Pack/227g* | *194.0* | *1.0* | *86* | *20.3* | *0.1* | *0.5* | *0.2* |
| Flour, Fried in Blended Oil | 1oz/28g | 39.0 | 1.0 | 138 | 21.1 | 4.5 | 4.1 | 0.2 |
| Goujons, Batter, Crispy, M & S* | 1 Serving/100g | 250.0 | 14.0 | 250 | 11.7 | 18.5 | 14.1 | 0.8 |
| **HADDOCK EN CROUTE** | | | | | | | | |
| Youngs* | 1 Serving/170g | 432.0 | 29.0 | 254 | 8.0 | 17.1 | 16.9 | 4.3 |
| **HADDOCK FLORENTINE** | | | | | | | | |
| Eat Smart, Safeway* | 1 Serving/250g | 200.0 | 4.0 | 80 | 12.0 | 2.5 | 1.8 | 1.3 |
| HE, Tesco* | 1 Pack/370g | 303.0 | 4.0 | 82 | 8.2 | 10.0 | 1.0 | 0.5 |
| **HADDOCK IN** | | | | | | | | |
| Butter Sauce, Steaks, Youngs* | 1 Serving/150g | 133.0 | 6.0 | 89 | 9.9 | 4.0 | 3.7 | 0.5 |
| Cheese & Chive Sauce, Fillets, Go Cook, Asda* | 1 Pack/360g | 400.0 | 19.0 | 111 | 14.8 | 1.5 | 5.3 | 0.2 |
| Cheese & Chive Sauce, Smoked Fillets, Seafresh* | 1 Serving/170g | 201.0 | 10.0 | 118 | 14.7 | 1.2 | 6.1 | 0.1 |
| Fillets, In Cheese Sauce, Fresh Tastes, Asda* | ½ Pack/180g | 212.0 | 10.0 | 118 | 16.2 | 1.3 | 5.3 | 0.6 |
| in Cheese & Leek Sauce, Fillets, SteamFresh, Birds Eye* | 1 Serving/190g | 165.0 | 7.0 | 87 | 11.0 | 2.4 | 3.7 | 0.2 |
| Smoked Leek & Cheese Sauce, Asda* | ½ Pack/200g | 232.0 | 10.0 | 116 | 14.0 | 3.7 | 5.0 | 1.5 |
| Tomato Herb Sauce, Fillets, BGTY, Sainsbury's* | ½ Pack/165g | 150.0 | 5.0 | 91 | 12.9 | 3.6 | 2.8 | 0.1 |
| Watercress Sauce, GFY, Asda* | 1 Pack/400g | 268.0 | 7.0 | 67 | 6.0 | 7.0 | 1.7 | 1.4 |
| **HADDOCK WITH** | | | | | | | | |
| a Rich Cheese Crust, Smoked, Sainsbury's* | 1 Serving/199g | 295.0 | 19.0 | 148 | 13.0 | 2.5 | 9.5 | 0.9 |
| Broccoli & Cheese, Lakeland* | 1 Serving/150g | 280.0 | 10.0 | 187 | 10.4 | 20.6 | 7.0 | 0.0 |
| Cheese & Chive Sauce, Atlantic, Youngs* | ½ Pack/180g | 184.0 | 9.0 | 102 | 13.0 | 1.7 | 4.8 | 0.2 |
| Creme Fraiche & Chive Sauce, Smoked, Tesco* | 1 Serving/150g | 154.0 | 5.0 | 103 | 16.8 | 2.1 | 3.1 | 0.3 |
| **HAGGIS** | | | | | | | | |
| Neeps & Tatties, M & S* | 1 Pack/300g | 330.0 | 14.0 | 110 | 3.8 | 12.3 | 4.8 | 0.8 |
| *Traditional, Average* | *1 Serving/454g* | *1119.0* | *67.0* | *246* | *12.3* | *17.2* | *14.6* | *1.0* |
| Vegetarian, McSween* | 1 Serving/100g | 216.0 | 10.0 | 216 | 6.6 | 26.8 | 10.2 | 2.4 |
| **HAKE** | | | | | | | | |
| Fillets, Herby Mediterranean Glaze, Sensations, Youngs* | ½ Pack/120g | 106.0 | 3.0 | 88 | 16.8 | 0.4 | 2.2 | 0.0 |
| Fillets, in Breadcrumbs, Average | 1oz/28g | 66.0 | 4.0 | 234 | 12.9 | 15.9 | 13.3 | 1.0 |
| Goujons, Average | 1 Serving/150g | 345.0 | 18.0 | 230 | 12.4 | 18.6 | 11.9 | 1.3 |
| *Raw, Average* | *1oz/28g* | *29.0* | *1.0* | *102* | *20.4* | *0.0* | *2.2* | *0.0* |
| with Tomato & Chilli Salsa, Just Cook, Sainsbury's* | ½ Pack/180g | 112.0 | 2.0 | 62 | 11.4 | 2.2 | 0.9 | 0.0 |
| **HALIBUT** | | | | | | | | |
| *Cooked, Average* | *1oz/28g* | *38.0* | *1.0* | *135* | *24.6* | *0.4* | *4.0* | *0.0* |
| *Raw* | *1oz/28g* | *29.0* | *1.0* | *103* | *21.5* | *0.0* | *1.9* | *0.0* |
| Roasted Pepper Sauce, Fillets, M & S* | 1 Serving/145g | 217.0 | 14.0 | 150 | 12.7 | 2.4 | 9.9 | 0.6 |
| **HALVA** | | | | | | | | |
| *Average* | *1oz/28g* | *107.0* | *4.0* | *381* | *1.8* | *68.0* | *13.2* | *0.0* |
| **HAM** | | | | | | | | |
| *Applewood Smoked, Average* | *1 Slice/28g* | *31.0* | *1.0* | *112* | *21.2* | *0.5* | *2.7* | *0.2* |
| *Baked, Average* | *1 Slice/74g* | *106.0* | *4.0* | *143* | *21.1* | *1.8* | *5.8* | *0.3* |
| Belgian, Sainsbury's* | 1 Serving/100g | 141.0 | 6.0 | 141 | 19.4 | 2.0 | 6.1 | 0.0 |
| *Boiled, Average* | *1 Pack/113g* | *154.0* | *6.0* | *136* | *20.6* | *0.6* | *5.7* | *0.0* |
| *Breaded, Average* | *1 Slice/37g* | *57.0* | *2.0* | *155* | *23.1* | *1.8* | *6.3* | *1.6* |
| *Breaded, Dry Cured, Average* | *1 Slice/33g* | *47.0* | *2.0* | *142* | *22.1* | *1.4* | *5.4* | *0.0* |
| *Brunswick, Average* | *1 Slice/20g* | *32.0* | *2.0* | *160* | *19.5* | *0.6* | *8.8* | *0.0* |
| *Cooked, Sliced, Average* | *1 Serving/50g* | *57.0* | *2.0* | *115* | *19.1* | *0.9* | *3.9* | *0.1* |
| *Crumbed, Sliced, Average* | *1 Slice/28g* | *33.0* | *1.0* | *117* | *21.5* | *0.9* | *3.1* | *0.0* |
| *Danish, Average* | *1 Slice/11g* | *14.0* | *1.0* | *125* | *18.4* | *1.0* | *5.3* | *0.0* |

H

|  | Measure INFO/WEIGHT | per Measure KCAL | FAT | Nutrition Values per 100g / 100ml KCAL | PROT | CARB | FAT | FIBRE |
|---|---|---|---|---|---|---|---|---|
| **HAM** | | | | | | | | |
| *Danish, Lean, Average* | *1 Slice/15g* | *14.0* | *0.0* | *92* | *17.8* | *1.0* | *1.8* | *0.0* |
| *Dry Cured, Average* | *1 Slice/18g* | *26.0* | *1.0* | *144* | *22.4* | *1.0* | *5.5* | *0.2* |
| *Extra Lean, Average* | *1 Slice/11g* | *10.0* | *0.0* | *90* | *18.0* | *1.4* | *1.4* | *0.0* |
| Gammon, Applewood Smoked, Dry Cured, Waitrose* | 1 Slice/20g | 29.0 | 1.0 | 145 | 21.4 | 0.0 | 6.6 | 0.0 |
| *Gammon, Breaded, Average* | *1 Serving/25g* | *31.0* | *1.0* | *122* | *22.0* | *1.5* | *3.1* | *0.0* |
| *Gammon, Dry Cured, Sliced, Average* | *1 Slice/33g* | *43.0* | *1.0* | *131* | *22.9* | *0.4* | *4.2* | *0.0* |
| *Gammon, Honey Roast, Average* | *1 Serving/60g* | *81.0* | *3.0* | *134* | *22.4* | *0.4* | *4.7* | *0.0* |
| Gammon, Mustard, Cured, Waitrose* | 1 Slice/45g | 54.0 | 2.0 | 120 | 21.4 | 0.1 | 4.0 | 0.0 |
| Gammon, Peppered, Waitrose* | 1/3 Pack/36g | 51.0 | 2.0 | 142 | 20.7 | 0.3 | 6.4 | 0.0 |
| *Gammon, Smoked, Average* | *1 Slice/43g* | *59.0* | *2.0* | *137* | *22.3* | *0.7* | *4.9* | *0.2* |
| *German Black Forest, Average* | *½ Pack/35g* | *93.0* | *6.0* | *267* | *27.2* | *1.3* | *17.0* | *0.5* |
| *Honey & Mustard, Average* | *1oz/28g* | *39.0* | *1.0* | *140* | *20.8* | *4.6* | *4.3* | *0.0* |
| *Honey Roast, Average* | *1 Slice/20g* | *25.0* | *1.0* | *123* | *20.3* | *1.5* | *3.8* | *0.1* |
| *Honey Roast, Dry Cured, Average* | *1 Slice/33g* | *46.0* | *1.0* | *140* | *22.7* | *2.3* | *4.4* | *0.2* |
| *Honey Roast, Lean, Average* | *1 Serving/25g* | *28.0* | *1.0* | *111* | *18.1* | *2.7* | *3.1* | *0.0* |
| *Honey Roast, Wafer Thin, Average* | *1 Slice/10g* | *11.0* | *0.0* | *113* | *17.4* | *3.7* | *3.2* | *0.3* |
| *Honey Roast, Wafer Thin, Premium, Average* | *1 Slice/10g* | *15.0* | *1.0* | *149* | *22.0* | *1.6* | *6.0* | *0.0* |
| Joint, Easy Carve, Asda* | 1oz/28g | 41.0 | 2.0 | 146 | 22.8 | 1.2 | 5.9 | 0.6 |
| *Lean, Average* | *1 Slice/18g* | *19.0* | *0.0* | *104* | *19.5* | *1.1* | *2.4* | *0.3* |
| Maple Drycure, Asda* | 1 Slice/37g | 49.0 | 1.0 | 132 | 22.0 | 3.0 | 3.5 | 0.0 |
| *Oak Smoked, Average* | *1 Slice/20g* | *26.0* | *1.0* | *130* | *21.0* | *1.0* | *4.7* | *0.3* |
| *Parma, Average* | *1 Serving/10g* | *21.0* | *1.0* | *213* | *29.3* | *0.0* | *10.6* | *0.0* |
| *Parma, Premium, Average* | *1 Serving/80g* | *206.0* | *13.0* | *258* | *27.9* | *0.3* | *16.1* | *0.0* |
| *Peppered, Average* | *1 Slice/12g* | *13.0* | *0.0* | *109* | *18.5* | *2.0* | *2.7* | *0.0* |
| *Prosciutto, Average* | *1 Slice/12g* | *27.0* | *1.0* | *226* | *28.7* | *0.0* | *12.3* | *0.3* |
| San Daniele, Finest, Tesco* | 1 Slice/10g | 24.0 | 1.0 | 242 | 30.5 | 0.5 | 13.1 | 0.0 |
| *Serrano, Average* | *1 Slice/20g* | *46.0* | *2.0* | *230* | *30.5* | *0.4* | *11.8* | *0.0* |
| *Smoked, Average* | *1 Slice/18g* | *21.0* | *1.0* | *117* | *19.7* | *0.9* | *3.7* | *0.0* |
| *Smoked, Dry Cured, Average* | *1 Slice/28g* | *38.0* | *1.0* | *137* | *23.0* | *1.4* | *4.4* | *0.1* |
| *Smoked, Wafer Thin, Average* | *1 Serving/40g* | *41.0* | *1.0* | *102* | *17.7* | *1.2* | *2.9* | *0.2* |
| *Thick Cut, Average* | *1 Slice/74g* | *94.0* | *3.0* | *127* | *22.4* | *0.6* | *3.9* | *0.1* |
| *Tinned, Average* | *½ Can/100g* | *136.0* | *9.0* | *136* | *12.2* | *2.0* | *8.7* | *0.0* |
| *Tinned, Lean, Average* | *½ Can/100g* | *94.0* | *2.0* | *94* | *18.1* | *0.2* | *2.3* | *0.4* |
| *Wafer Thin, Average* | *1 Slice/10g* | *10.0* | *0.0* | *101* | *17.9* | *1.4* | *2.6* | *0.1* |
| Wholemeal Crumbed, Slices, Light Choices, Tesco* | 1 Slice/21g | 23.0 | 0.0 | 110 | 21.5 | 0.2 | 2.1 | 0.0 |
| *Wiltshire, Average* | *1oz/28g* | *41.0* | *1.0* | *147* | *23.1* | *0.0* | *6.0* | *0.0* |
| *Wiltshire, Breaded, Average* | *1oz/28g* | *41.0* | *1.0* | *145* | *23.9* | *1.0* | *5.0* | *0.0* |
| Wiltshire, Orange Marmalade Roasted, Finest, Tesco* | 1 Slice/40g | 67.0 | 2.0 | 167 | 26.0 | 2.0 | 6.1 | 0.3 |
| **HAM VEGETARIAN** | | | | | | | | |
| Cheatin', Co, Redwood* | 1 Slice/10g | 25.0 | 1.0 | 247 | 19.7 | 8.9 | 14.7 | 0.0 |
| **HARE** | | | | | | | | |
| *Raw, Lean Only, Average* | *1oz/28g* | *35.0* | *1.0* | *125* | *23.5* | *0.2* | *3.5* | *0.0* |
| *Stewed, Lean Only, Average* | *1oz/28g* | *48.0* | *2.0* | *170* | *29.5* | *0.2* | *5.5* | *0.0* |
| **HARIBO*** | | | | | | | | |
| American Hard Gums, Haribo* | 1 Pack/175g | 630.0 | 3.0 | 360 | 0.3 | 85.5 | 1.9 | 0.2 |
| Build a Burger, Haribo* | 1oz/28g | 96.0 | 0.0 | 344 | 6.6 | 79.0 | 0.2 | 0.3 |
| Chamallows, Haribo* | 1oz/28g | 92.0 | 0.0 | 330 | 2.0 | 80.0 | 0.0 | 0.0 |
| Cola Bottles, Haribo* | 1 Sm Pack/16g | 56.0 | 0.0 | 348 | 7.7 | 78.9 | 0.2 | 0.3 |
| Dinosaurs, Haribo* | 1oz/28g | 95.0 | 0.0 | 340 | 6.3 | 78.3 | 0.2 | 0.5 |
| Dolly Mixtures, Haribo* | 1 Pack/175g | 719.0 | 8.0 | 411 | 1.8 | 90.2 | 4.8 | 0.2 |
| Fried Eggs/eggstras, Haribo* | 1oz/28g | 96.0 | 0.0 | 344 | 6.6 | 79.0 | 0.2 | 0.0 |
| Gold Bears, Haribo* | 1 Pack/100g | 348.0 | 0.0 | 348 | 7.7 | 78.9 | 0.2 | 0.3 |
| Horror Mix, Haribo* | 1 Sm Pack/100g | 344.0 | 0.0 | 344 | 6.6 | 79.0 | 0.2 | 0.3 |

**H**

| | Measure INFO/WEIGHT | per Measure KCAL | FAT | Nutrition Values per 100g / 100ml KCAL | PROT | CARB | FAT | FIBRE |
|---|---|---|---|---|---|---|---|---|
| **HARIBO*** | | | | | | | | |
| Jelly Babies, Haribo* | 1oz/28g | 97.0 | 0.0 | 348 | 4.5 | 82.1 | 0.2 | 0.5 |
| Jelly Beans, Haribo* | 1 Pack/100g | 379.0 | 0.0 | 379 | 0.6 | 93.8 | 0.2 | 0.1 |
| Kiddies Super Mix, Haribo* | 1 Pack/100g | 344.0 | 0.0 | 344 | 6.6 | 79.0 | 0.2 | 0.3 |
| Liquorice Cream Rock, Haribo* | 1oz/28g | 107.0 | 1.0 | 382 | 2.3 | 81.2 | 5.3 | 0.3 |
| Liquorice Favourite, Haribo* | 1oz/28g | 100.0 | 1.0 | 357 | 2.8 | 78.8 | 3.0 | 2.3 |
| Magic Mix, Haribo* | 1oz/28g | 102.0 | 1.0 | 366 | 5.4 | 82.0 | 1.9 | 0.3 |
| Maoam Stripes, Haribo* | 1 Chew/7g | 27.0 | 0.0 | 384 | 1.2 | 81.7 | 6.1 | 0.3 |
| Mega Roulette, Haribo* | 1oz/28g | 97.0 | 0.0 | 348 | 7.7 | 78.9 | 0.2 | 0.3 |
| Mega Roulette Sour, Haribo* | 1oz/28g | 95.0 | 0.0 | 340 | 6.3 | 78.3 | 0.2 | 0.5 |
| Micro Mix, Haribo* | 1oz/28g | 106.0 | 1.0 | 379 | 4.7 | 84.5 | 2.5 | 0.4 |
| Milky Mix, Haribo* | 1 Pack/175g | 607.0 | 0.0 | 347 | 7.1 | 79.6 | 0.2 | 0.4 |
| Mint Imperials, Haribo* | 1 Pack/175g | 695.0 | 1.0 | 397 | 0.4 | 98.8 | 0.5 | 0.1 |
| Peaches, Haribo* | 1oz/28g | 98.0 | 0.0 | 350 | 4.3 | 82.1 | 0.0 | 0.0 |
| Pontefract Cakes, Haribo* | 1 Pack/200g | 612.0 | 3.0 | 306 | 5.3 | 68.2 | 1.3 | 5.6 |
| Shrimps, Haribo* | 1oz/28g | 99.0 | 0.0 | 352 | 6.1 | 81.5 | 0.2 | 0.1 |
| Snakes, Haribo* | 1 Snake/8g | 28.0 | 0.0 | 348 | 7.7 | 78.9 | 0.2 | 0.3 |
| Starmix, Haribo* | 1 Pack/100g | 344.0 | 0.0 | 344 | 6.6 | 79.0 | 0.2 | 0.3 |
| Tangfastics, Haribo* | 1 Pack/100g | 359.0 | 2.0 | 359 | 6.3 | 78.3 | 2.3 | 0.5 |
| Tropifruit, Haribo* | 1oz/28g | 97.0 | 0.0 | 348 | 4.5 | 82.1 | 0.2 | 0.5 |
| **HASH** | | | | | | | | |
| Barbecue Beef, COU, M & S* | 1 Pack/400g | 360.0 | 2.0 | 90 | 7.0 | 14.0 | 0.4 | 1.4 |
| Corned Beef, Asda* | 1 Pack/400g | 416.0 | 14.0 | 104 | 6.0 | 12.0 | 3.6 | 1.1 |
| Corned Beef, Frozen, Tesco* | 1 Serving/400g | 348.0 | 10.0 | 87 | 5.7 | 10.3 | 2.6 | 0.7 |
| Corned Beef, M & S* | ½ Pack/321g | 385.0 | 20.0 | 120 | 8.1 | 7.4 | 6.3 | 1.3 |
| Corned Beef, Tesco* | 1 Serving/400g | 416.0 | 10.0 | 104 | 5.3 | 14.8 | 2.6 | 1.7 |
| Corned Beef, Value, Tesco* | 1 Pack/300g | 339.0 | 13.0 | 113 | 6.7 | 12.2 | 4.2 | 0.9 |
| Vegetable & Lentil, Asda* | 1 Pack/289g | 254.0 | 6.0 | 88 | 3.2 | 14.0 | 2.1 | 0.0 |
| **HASH BROWNS** | | | | | | | | |
| Birds Eye* | 1 Serving/63g | 126.0 | 7.0 | 200 | 2.0 | 21.9 | 11.6 | 1.6 |
| Oven Baked, Weighed Cooked, McCain* | 1 Piece/38g | 80.0 | 4.0 | 214 | 2.1 | 25.7 | 11.4 | 2.2 |
| Oven Baked, Weighed Frozen, McCain* | 1 Hash Brown/40g | 75.0 | 4.0 | 187 | 1.7 | 21.8 | 10.3 | 2.1 |
| Ross* | 1 Hash Brown/46g | 84.0 | 4.0 | 183 | 2.0 | 23.9 | 8.7 | 2.0 |
| Tesco* | 1oz/28g | 43.0 | 2.0 | 154 | 2.4 | 20.0 | 7.2 | 1.7 |
| **HAZELNUTS** | | | | | | | | |
| *Chopped, Average* | *1 Serving/10g* | *67.0* | *6.0* | *665* | *16.7* | *5.6* | *64.0* | *6.5* |
| Honey, Graze | 1 Pack/25g | 149.0 | 11.0 | 596 | 10.5 | 42.2 | 43.7 | 0.0 |
| Roasted, Graze* | 1 Pack/26g | 173.0 | 17.0 | 665 | 14.0 | 6.1 | 65.0 | 0.0 |
| *Whole, Average* | *10 Whole/10g* | *65.0* | *6.0* | *655* | *15.3* | *5.8* | *63.5* | *6.5* |
| **HEART** | | | | | | | | |
| *Lambs, Average* | *1 Heart/75g* | *91.0* | *4.0* | *122* | *16.0* | *1.0* | *6.0* | *0.0* |
| *Ox, Raw* | *1oz/28g* | *29.0* | *1.0* | *104* | *18.2* | *0.0* | *3.5* | *0.0* |
| *Ox, Stewed* | *1oz/28g* | *44.0* | *1.0* | *157* | *27.8* | *0.0* | *5.1* | *0.0* |
| *Pig, Raw* | *1oz/28g* | *27.0* | *1.0* | *97* | *17.1* | *0.0* | *3.2* | *0.0* |
| *Pig, Stewed* | *1oz/28g* | *45.0* | *2.0* | *162* | *25.1* | *0.0* | *6.8* | *0.0* |
| **HERMESETAS** | | | | | | | | |
| Powdered, Hermes* | 1 Tsp/0.78g | 3.0 | 0.0 | 387 | 1.0 | 96.8 | 0.0 | 0.0 |
| The Classic Sweetener, Hermes* | 1 Tablet/0.5g | 0.0 | 0.0 | 294 | 14.2 | 59.3 | 0.0 | 0.0 |
| **HEROES** | | | | | | | | |
| Dairy Milk, Whole Nut, Cadbury* | 1 Chocolate/11g | 60.0 | 4.0 | 545 | 9.1 | 48.2 | 35.2 | 0.0 |
| Fudge, Cadbury* | 1 Sweet/10g | 43.0 | 1.0 | 435 | 2.5 | 72.7 | 14.9 | 0.0 |
| **HERRING** | | | | | | | | |
| Canned, in Tomato Sauce, Average | 1oz/28g | 57.0 | 4.0 | 204 | 11.9 | 4.1 | 15.5 | 0.1 |
| *Dried, Salted, Average* | *1oz/28g* | *47.0* | *2.0* | *168* | *25.3* | *0.0* | *7.4* | *0.0* |

| | Measure INFO/WEIGHT | per Measure KCAL | per Measure FAT | Nutrition Values per 100g / 100ml KCAL | PROT | CARB | FAT | FIBRE |
|---|---|---|---|---|---|---|---|---|
| **HERRING** | | | | | | | | |
| Fillets, in Mustard & Dill Sauce, John West* | 1 Can/190g | 332.0 | 27.0 | 175 | 9.4 | 2.9 | 14.0 | 0.1 |
| Fillets, in Olive Oil, Succulent, Princes* | 1 Serving/50g | 107.0 | 7.0 | 215 | 20.0 | 0.0 | 15.0 | 0.0 |
| *Fillets, Raw, Average* | *1 Herring/100g* | *185.0* | *13.0* | *185* | *18.4* | *0.0* | *12.6* | *0.0* |
| *Grilled, Average* | *1oz/28g* | *51.0* | *3.0* | *181* | *20.1* | *0.0* | *11.2* | *0.0* |
| in Horseradish Sauce, John West* | 1oz/28g | 64.0 | 5.0 | 230 | 13.0 | 4.0 | 18.0 | 0.0 |
| Pickled, Average | 1oz/28g | 73.0 | 5.0 | 262 | 14.2 | 9.6 | 18.0 | 0.0 |
| Rollmop, with Onion, Asda* | 1 Rollmop/65g | 89.0 | 3.0 | 137 | 13.2 | 10.3 | 4.8 | 0.8 |
| Rollmops, Tesco* | 1 Rollmop/65g | 110.0 | 5.0 | 170 | 12.0 | 10.4 | 8.4 | 0.4 |
| Smoked, Pepper, in Oil, Glyngøre* | 1 Can/130g | 338.0 | 25.0 | 260 | 21.0 | 0.0 | 19.0 | 0.0 |
| **HIGH LIGHTS** | | | | | | | | |
| Choc Mint, Made Up, Cadbury* | 1 Serving/200ml | 40.0 | 1.0 | 20 | 1.0 | 2.5 | 0.7 | 0.3 |
| Chocolate Orange, Made Up, Cadbury* | 1 Serving/200ml | 40.0 | 1.0 | 20 | 1.0 | 2.3 | 0.7 | 0.3 |
| Dairy Fudge, Made Up, Cadbury* | 1 Serving/200ml | 40.0 | 1.0 | 20 | 1.0 | 2.8 | 0.5 | 0.2 |
| Dark Chocolate, Made Up, Cadbury* | 1 Serving/200ml | 35.0 | 1.0 | 17 | 1.2 | 2.0 | 0.4 | 0.0 |
| Espresso, Made Up, Cadbury* | 1 Serving/200ml | 35.0 | 1.0 | 17 | 1.2 | 1.9 | 0.4 | 0.0 |
| Fudge, Made Up, Cadbury* | 1 Serving/200ml | 40.0 | 1.0 | 20 | 0.9 | 2.5 | 0.5 | 0.0 |
| Hot Chocolate Drink, Instant, Made Up, Cadbury* | 1 Cup/200ml | 40.0 | 1.0 | 20 | 1.0 | 2.5 | 0.7 | 0.3 |
| Mint, Cadbury* | 1 Serving/200ml | 40.0 | 1.0 | 20 | 1.0 | 2.5 | 0.7 | 0.0 |
| Toffee Flavour, Made Up, Cadbury* | 1 Serving/200ml | 40.0 | 1.0 | 20 | 1.0 | 2.6 | 0.7 | 0.0 |
| **HOKI** | | | | | | | | |
| *Grilled* | *1oz/28g* | *34.0* | *1.0* | *121* | *24.1* | *0.0* | *2.7* | *0.0* |
| in Breadcrumbs, Average | 1 Piece/156g | 298.0 | 14.0 | 191 | 14.5 | 13.9 | 8.9 | 1.2 |
| *Raw* | *1oz/28g* | *24.0* | *1.0* | *85* | *16.9* | *0.0* | *1.9* | *0.0* |
| Steaks, in Batter, Crispy, Birds Eye* | 1 Steak/123g | 320.0 | 17.0 | 260 | 12.4 | 21.3 | 13.9 | 0.8 |
| **HONEY** | | | | | | | | |
| Acacia, Tesco* | 1 Tsp/4g | 12.0 | 0.0 | 307 | 0.4 | 76.4 | 0.0 | 0.0 |
| Australian Eucalyptus, Finest, Tesco* | 1 Tsp/4g | 12.0 | 0.0 | 307 | 0.4 | 76.4 | 0.0 | 0.0 |
| Canadian Clover, TTD, Sainsbury's* | 1 Tsp/5g | 17.0 | 0.0 | 339 | 0.1 | 84.7 | 0.1 | 0.3 |
| Clear, Basics, Sainsbury's* | 1 Tsp/15g | 46.0 | 0.0 | 307 | 0.4 | 76.4 | 0.1 | 0.0 |
| Clear, Runny, Sainsbury's* | 1 Serving/15g | 51.0 | 0.0 | 339 | 0.1 | 84.7 | 0.1 | 0.3 |
| Clear, Value, Tesco* | 1 Serving/27g | 86.0 | 0.0 | 320 | 1.0 | 78.0 | 0.0 | 0.0 |
| Florida Orange, Extra Special, Asda* | 1 Tbsp/15g | 50.0 | 0.0 | 334 | 0.5 | 83.0 | 0.0 | 0.0 |
| Greek, TTD, Sainsbury's* | 1 Tbsp/15g | 51.0 | 0.0 | 339 | 0.1 | 84.7 | 0.0 | 0.3 |
| Greek, Waitrose* | 1 Tsp/6g | 18.0 | 0.0 | 307 | 0.4 | 76.4 | 0.0 | 0.0 |
| Manuka Clear, TTD, Sainsbury's* | 1 Tsp/5g | 17.0 | 0.0 | 334 | 0.3 | 83.1 | 0.0 | 0.0 |
| Mexican, TTD, Sainsbury's* | 1 Tbsp/15g | 51.0 | 0.0 | 339 | 0.1 | 84.7 | 0.1 | 0.3 |
| *Pure, Clear, Average* | *1 Tbsp/20g* | *63.0* | *0.0* | *314* | *0.3* | *79.1* | *0.0* | *0.0* |
| *Pure, Set, Average* | *1 Tbsp/20g* | *62.0* | *0.0* | *312* | *0.4* | *77.6* | *0.0* | *0.0* |
| Scottish Heather, Waitrose* | 1 Serving/20g | 61.0 | 0.0 | 307 | 0.4 | 76.4 | 0.0 | 0.0 |
| Spanish Orange Blossom, Sainsbury's* | 1 Tbsp/15g | 51.0 | 0.0 | 339 | 0.1 | 84.7 | 0.0 | 0.3 |
| **HORLICKS** | | | | | | | | |
| Malted Drink, Chocolate, Extra Light, Dry Weight, Horlicks* | 1 Serving/32g | 95.0 | 2.0 | 296 | 9.2 | 47.0 | 7.8 | 17.3 |
| Malted Drink, Extra Light, Instant, Dry Weight, Horlicks* | 1 Serving/11g | 35.0 | 1.0 | 319 | 8.4 | 57.4 | 6.2 | 10.5 |
| Malted Drink, Light, Dry Weight, Horlicks* | 1 Serving/32g | 116.0 | 1.0 | 364 | 14.8 | 72.2 | 3.8 | 1.9 |
| Malted Drink, Light, Made Up, Horlicks* | 1 Mug/200ml | 116.0 | 1.0 | 58 | 2.3 | 11.5 | 0.6 | 0.3 |
| Powder, Made Up with Semi-Skimmed Milk | 1 Mug/227ml | 184.0 | 4.0 | 81 | 4.3 | 12.9 | 1.9 | 0.0 |
| Powder, Made Up with Skimmed Milk | 1 Mug/227ml | 159.0 | 1.0 | 70 | 4.3 | 12.9 | 0.5 | 0.0 |
| Powder, Made Up with Whole Milk | 1 Mug/227ml | 225.0 | 9.0 | 99 | 4.2 | 12.7 | 3.9 | 0.0 |
| Snoozoo, Chocolate, Horlicks* | 1 Sachet/20g | 74.0 | 1.0 | 370 | 8.6 | 74.2 | 4.3 | 4.3 |
| **HORSE** | | | | | | | | |
| *Meat, Raw, Average* | *1 Serving/110g* | *146.0* | *5.0* | *133* | *21.4* | *0.0* | *4.6* | *0.0* |
| **HORSERADISH** | | | | | | | | |
| *Prepared, Average* | *1 Tsp/5g* | *3.0* | *0.0* | *62* | *4.5* | *11.0* | *0.3* | *6.2* |

**H**

| | Measure INFO/WEIGHT | per Measure KCAL | FAT | Nutrition Values per 100g / 100ml KCAL | PROT | CARB | FAT | FIBRE |
|---|---|---|---|---|---|---|---|---|
| **HOT CHOCOLATE** | | | | | | | | |
| Cadbury* | 1 Serving/12g | 44.0 | 1.0 | 370 | 6.3 | 73.3 | 5.9 | 0.0 |
| Caramel, Whittards of Chelsea* | 1 Serving/20g | 71.0 | 1.0 | 355 | 7.5 | 64.5 | 7.5 | 13.0 |
| Caramel Flavoured, Instant, Dry, Aldi* | 1 Serving/11g | 40.0 | 2.0 | 363 | 18.5 | 40.6 | 14.1 | 8.5 |
| Chococino, Dulce Gusto, Nescafe* | 1 Serving/34g | 149.0 | 5.0 | 437 | 14.6 | 58.6 | 16.1 | 4.6 |
| Chocolate Break, Dry, Tesco* | 1 Serving/21g | 110.0 | 6.0 | 524 | 7.9 | 58.9 | 28.5 | 1.7 |
| Drink, Organic, Green & Black's* | 1 Tsp/4g | 13.0 | 0.0 | 374 | 9.1 | 63.5 | 9.3 | 0.1 |
| Dry Weight, Tassimo, Suchard* | 1 Cup/27g | 88.0 | 2.0 | 325 | 3.2 | 58.0 | 8.9 | 2.6 |
| From Coffee Shop, Waitrose* | 1 Serving/298ml | 217.0 | 6.0 | 73 | 3.6 | 10.9 | 2.0 | 0.0 |
| Galaxy, Mars* | 1 Sachet/28g | 115.0 | 3.0 | 411 | 7.0 | 68.7 | 12.1 | 0.0 |
| Horlicks* | 1 Serving/32g | 128.0 | 3.0 | 400 | 8.7 | 72.5 | 8.1 | 3.7 |
| Instant, BGTY, Made Up, Sainsbury's* | 1 Sachet/28g | 16.0 | 0.0 | 56 | 2.1 | 10.6 | 0.6 | 0.3 |
| Instant, GFY, Asda* | 1 Tsp/10g | 32.0 | 1.0 | 321 | 13.2 | 37.0 | 13.4 | 7.7 |
| Instant, Skinny Cow* | 1 Sachet/10g | 37.0 | 1.0 | 370 | 19.7 | 39.3 | 14.6 | 0.0 |
| Instant, Tesco* | 1 Serving/32g | 155.0 | 10.0 | 485 | 10.5 | 38.1 | 32.3 | 5.0 |
| Instant Break, Cadbury* | 1 Sachet/28g | 119.0 | 4.0 | 425 | 10.9 | 64.2 | 14.0 | 0.0 |
| Luxury, Skinny, Whittards of Chelsea* | 1 Serving/28g | 92.0 | 1.0 | 328 | 12.9 | 67.1 | 2.8 | 13.5 |
| Made Up, Tassimo, Suchard* | 1 Serving/280ml | 88.0 | 2.0 | 31 | 0.3 | 5.5 | 0.9 | 0.2 |
| Maltesers, Malt Drink, Instant, Made Up, Mars* | 1 Serving/220ml | 104.0 | 3.0 | 47 | 0.9 | 7.7 | 1.4 | 0.0 |
| Slim Fast* | 1 Serving/59g | 203.0 | 3.0 | 347 | 22.2 | 53.8 | 4.8 | 8.4 |
| Toffee Flavour, Good Intentions, Somerfield* | 1 Serving/34g | 130.0 | 2.0 | 381 | 7.4 | 77.0 | 4.8 | 2.6 |
| Value, Tesco* | 1 Serving/32g | 132.0 | 4.0 | 414 | 8.0 | 68.3 | 12.1 | 0.7 |
| Velvet, Cadbury* | 1 Serving/28g | 136.0 | 7.0 | 487 | 8.6 | 57.8 | 24.6 | 2.0 |
| **HOT DOG** | | | | | | | | |
| Feasters, Eat Well, M & S* | 1 Sausage/140g | 326.0 | 11.0 | 233 | 11.0 | 29.1 | 8.1 | 1.6 |
| Sausage, American Style, Average | 1 Sausage/75g | 180.0 | 14.0 | 241 | 11.6 | 6.2 | 19.0 | 0.0 |
| Sausage, Average | 1 Sausage/23g | 40.0 | 3.0 | 175 | 10.8 | 4.3 | 12.8 | 0.3 |
| **HOT DOG VEGETARIAN** | | | | | | | | |
| Meat Free, Sainsbury's* | 1 Sausage/30g | 71.0 | 5.0 | 237 | 18.0 | 7.6 | 15.0 | 1.0 |
| Tesco* | 1 Sausage/30g | 66.0 | 4.0 | 220 | 18.0 | 2.7 | 15.0 | 2.0 |
| **HOT POT** | | | | | | | | |
| Beef, Minced, Sainsbury's* | 1 Pack/450g | 463.0 | 22.0 | 103 | 5.3 | 9.5 | 4.9 | 2.2 |
| Beef, Ross* | 1 Pack/322g | 254.0 | 11.0 | 79 | 2.5 | 9.4 | 3.5 | 0.4 |
| Beef, Weight Watchers* | 1 Pack/320g | 209.0 | 7.0 | 65 | 3.5 | 8.1 | 2.1 | 1.3 |
| Beef & Vegetable, Weight Watchers* | 1 Pack/300g | 228.0 | 7.0 | 76 | 4.0 | 10.2 | 2.2 | 0.9 |
| Chicken, Chunky, Weight Watchers* | 1 Pack/320g | 275.0 | 9.0 | 86 | 4.7 | 10.4 | 2.8 | 0.6 |
| Chicken, Eat Smart, Morrisons* | 1 Pack/400g | 308.0 | 6.0 | 77 | 4.5 | 11.1 | 1.5 | 1.7 |
| Chicken, Frozen, Asda* | 1 Pack/400g | 300.0 | 6.0 | 75 | 5.5 | 9.9 | 1.5 | 0.8 |
| Chicken, GFY, Asda* | 1 Serving/400g | 256.0 | 5.0 | 64 | 4.8 | 8.2 | 1.3 | 1.4 |
| Chicken, Light Choices, Tesco* | 1 Pack/450g | 315.0 | 7.0 | 70 | 4.1 | 9.6 | 1.6 | 1.2 |
| Chicken, Sainsbury's* | 1 Pack/400g | 340.0 | 11.0 | 85 | 5.2 | 9.8 | 2.7 | 1.3 |
| Chicken & Cider, Ready Meals, Waitrose* | 1 Pack/400g | 500.0 | 20.0 | 125 | 6.8 | 12.9 | 5.1 | 1.1 |
| Chicken & Mushroom, HL, Tesco* | 1 Serving/450g | 369.0 | 7.0 | 82 | 6.3 | 11.8 | 1.5 | 0.5 |
| Chunky Vegetable & Tomato, Big Eat, Heinz* | 1 Pot/355g | 213.0 | 1.0 | 60 | 2.5 | 11.7 | 0.4 | 4.1 |
| Lamb, Heinz* | 1 Pack/340g | 337.0 | 11.0 | 99 | 4.9 | 12.7 | 3.1 | 1.7 |
| Lamb, Mini, Classics, Asda* | 1 Pack/300g | 223.0 | 10.0 | 74 | 5.3 | 5.4 | 3.5 | 3.3 |
| Lamb, Organic, Great Stuff, Asda* | 1 Pack/300g | 327.0 | 10.0 | 109 | 8.0 | 11.6 | 3.4 | 1.1 |
| Lamb & Vegetable, Asda* | 1 Pot/500g | 240.0 | 2.0 | 48 | 4.0 | 7.0 | 0.4 | 0.0 |
| Lamb Shank, Extra Special, Asda* | 1 Pack/450g | 508.0 | 20.0 | 113 | 10.2 | 7.8 | 4.5 | 1.3 |
| Lancashire, Asda* | 1 Pack/401g | 269.0 | 5.0 | 67 | 3.8 | 10.0 | 1.3 | 0.9 |
| Lancashire, M & S* | 1 Pack/454g | 431.0 | 15.0 | 95 | 10.1 | 6.7 | 3.3 | 1.0 |
| Lancashire, Sainsbury's* | ½ Pack/225g | 220.0 | 9.0 | 98 | 6.1 | 9.5 | 3.9 | 1.0 |
| Lancashire, Tesco* | ½ Pack/225g | 205.0 | 7.0 | 91 | 6.0 | 9.7 | 3.1 | 0.5 |
| Liver & Bacon, Tesco* | 1 Pack/550g | 693.0 | 31.0 | 126 | 6.4 | 12.3 | 5.7 | 1.5 |

**H**

| | Measure INFO/WEIGHT | per Measure KCAL | per Measure FAT | Nutrition Values per 100g / 100ml KCAL | PROT | CARB | FAT | FIBRE |
|---|---|---|---|---|---|---|---|---|
| **HOT POT** | | | | | | | | |
| Minced Beef, Asda* | 1 Pack/375g | 409.0 | 17.0 | 109 | 7.0 | 10.0 | 4.6 | 1.7 |
| Minced Beef, Frozen, Tesco* | 1 Pack/450g | 337.0 | 11.0 | 75 | 4.0 | 9.1 | 2.5 | 1.4 |
| Minced Beef, Mini Classic, Tesco* | 1 Pack/300g | 232.0 | 4.0 | 77 | 3.4 | 12.6 | 1.5 | 1.4 |
| Minced Beef, SmartPrice, Asda* | 1 Pack/300g | 199.0 | 4.0 | 66 | 3.7 | 10.0 | 1.3 | 0.4 |
| Minced Beef & Vegetable, COU, M & S* | 1 Pack/400g | 380.0 | 7.0 | 95 | 10.3 | 9.0 | 1.7 | 2.4 |
| Sausage, Aunt Bessie's* | ¼ Pack/200g | 212.0 | 9.0 | 106 | 3.6 | 12.6 | 4.6 | 1.9 |
| Sausage, SmartPrice, Asda* | 1 Pack/300g | 239.0 | 7.0 | 80 | 3.7 | 11.0 | 2.3 | 0.4 |
| Sausage with Baked Beans, Heinz* | 1 Can/340g | 354.0 | 11.0 | 104 | 4.6 | 14.3 | 3.2 | 2.4 |
| Vegetable, Gluten, Yeast & Dairy Free, Canned, GranoVita* | 1 Can/420g | 290.0 | 8.0 | 69 | 3.2 | 9.5 | 2.0 | 1.6 |
| Vegetable, Tesco* | 1 Serving/450g | 432.0 | 22.0 | 96 | 1.7 | 11.2 | 4.9 | 3.5 |
| Vegetable, Weight Watchers* | 1 Pack/335g | 228.0 | 6.0 | 68 | 2.6 | 9.9 | 1.9 | 1.5 |
| **HOUMOUS** | | | | | | | | |
| 30% Less Fat, Asda* | 1oz/28g | 73.0 | 5.0 | 259 | 9.0 | 13.0 | 19.0 | 3.8 |
| Balsamic Caramelised Red Onion, Extra Special, Asda* | ½ Pack/50g | 146.0 | 11.0 | 293 | 6.8 | 18.2 | 21.4 | 1.0 |
| Caramelised Onion, Tesco* | ¼ Pack/50g | 125.0 | 10.0 | 250 | 5.5 | 13.0 | 19.4 | 4.2 |
| Chilli & Red Pepper, Topped, Tesco* | ½ Pack/100g | 281.0 | 25.0 | 281 | 7.1 | 6.6 | 25.1 | 8.1 |
| Feta, Fresh, Sainsbury's* | 1 Serving/100g | 292.0 | 27.0 | 292 | 8.0 | 3.5 | 27.4 | 6.7 |
| Fresh, Sainsbury's* | 1 Serving/50g | 156.0 | 14.0 | 312 | 7.3 | 8.9 | 27.5 | 2.2 |
| Fresh, Waitrose* | 1 Serving/75g | 219.0 | 20.0 | 292 | 7.2 | 6.3 | 26.4 | 7.6 |
| Garlic & Pesto, Asda* | 1 Serving/34g | 107.0 | 9.0 | 314 | 8.0 | 12.0 | 26.0 | 0.0 |
| GFY, Asda* | 1 Serving/50g | 136.0 | 10.0 | 272 | 9.0 | 14.0 | 20.0 | 3.8 |
| Jalapeno, Asda* | 1 Serving/50g | 165.0 | 14.0 | 331 | 7.0 | 10.6 | 29.0 | 4.5 |
| Jalapeno, Sainsbury's* | ¼ Pot/50g | 148.0 | 13.0 | 296 | 6.4 | 7.2 | 26.8 | 5.7 |
| Jalapeno, Tesco* | ½ Pot/100g | 360.0 | 31.0 | 360 | 7.5 | 11.4 | 31.1 | 3.9 |
| Lemon & Coriander, GFY, Asda* | 1 Serving/50g | 129.0 | 10.0 | 259 | 8.3 | 12.0 | 19.8 | 5.1 |
| Lemon & Coriander, Reduced Fat, Tesco* | 1 Pot/60g | 135.0 | 9.0 | 225 | 7.4 | 13.8 | 15.3 | 4.7 |
| Lemon & Coriander, Sainsbury's* | ¼ Tub/50g | 145.0 | 13.0 | 291 | 7.0 | 9.1 | 25.1 | 6.0 |
| Lemon & Coriander, Tesco* | 1 Serving/50g | 170.0 | 14.0 | 340 | 7.0 | 12.7 | 29.0 | 2.1 |
| Light, Morrisons* | ½ Pack/85g | 200.0 | 15.0 | 235 | 7.4 | 10.9 | 18.0 | 0.0 |
| Mediterranean Deli, M & S* | ¼ Pack/70g | 203.0 | 18.0 | 290 | 7.8 | 8.0 | 25.3 | 6.5 |
| Mixed Olive, Sainsbury's* | ¼ Pot/50g | 134.0 | 12.0 | 268 | 6.7 | 8.4 | 23.1 | 7.7 |
| Moroccan, Tesco* | ¼ Pot/50g | 144.0 | 13.0 | 289 | 6.8 | 8.1 | 25.5 | 7.3 |
| Moroccan, With Corriander & Spices, Tesco* | ¼ Pot/50g | 131.0 | 10.0 | 262 | 9.4 | 11.6 | 19.8 | 5.2 |
| Moroccan Style, Sainsbury's* | ¼ Pot/50g | 113.0 | 10.0 | 227 | 5.5 | 7.3 | 19.5 | 6.6 |
| Olive & Sundried Tomato, Tesco* | 1 Serving/50g | 147.0 | 13.0 | 295 | 6.6 | 7.3 | 26.1 | 5.6 |
| Olive & Tomato, Mixed, Sainsbury's* | ¼ Tub/50g | 136.0 | 13.0 | 272 | 6.0 | 5.3 | 25.2 | 7.4 |
| Organic, M & S* | ¼ Pack/25g | 82.0 | 7.0 | 330 | 6.9 | 9.1 | 29.7 | 3.3 |
| Organic, Sainsbury's* | ¼ Pot/43g | 139.0 | 12.0 | 326 | 6.8 | 10.7 | 28.4 | 3.5 |
| Organic, Tesco* | ¼ Tub/42g | 134.0 | 11.0 | 320 | 6.5 | 12.3 | 27.2 | 2.4 |
| Red Pepper, Reduced Fat, Tesco* | 1 Pot/60g | 159.0 | 11.0 | 265 | 7.2 | 17.4 | 18.3 | 4.8 |
| Red Pepper Pesto, Tesco* | ¼ Pot/50g | 137.0 | 11.0 | 275 | 7.4 | 9.7 | 22.6 | 5.7 |
| Reduced Fat, Average | 1 Serving/30g | 72.0 | 5.0 | 241 | 9.2 | 13.3 | 16.8 | 3.6 |
| Reduced Fat, BGTY, Sainsbury's* | 1 Serving/50g | 76.0 | 4.0 | 153 | 6.6 | 11.7 | 8.9 | 6.1 |
| Reduced Fat, Eat Smart, Morrisons* | 1 Mini Pot/70g | 172.0 | 12.0 | 246 | 7.9 | 13.8 | 17.7 | 2.7 |
| Reduced Fat, Mediterranean Deli, M & S* | 1 Mini Pot/60g | 126.0 | 10.0 | 210 | 7.5 | 8.3 | 16.2 | 9.3 |
| Reduced Fat, Moroccan Style, Topped, M & S* | 1 Tub/170g | 374.0 | 26.0 | 220 | 6.6 | 13.2 | 15.3 | 9.2 |
| Reduced Fat, Snack Pots, Mini, BGTY, Sainsbury's* | 1 Mini Pot/60g | 85.0 | 5.0 | 142 | 5.3 | 10.0 | 8.9 | 6.6 |
| Reduced Fat, Tesco* | ¼ Sm Pot/50g | 120.0 | 8.0 | 241 | 9.2 | 13.3 | 16.8 | 3.6 |
| Reduced Fat, Waitrose* | 1 Serving/50g | 108.0 | 7.0 | 216 | 7.4 | 14.7 | 14.2 | 5.8 |
| Roasted Aubergine, M & S* | ½ Pot/85g | 132.0 | 10.0 | 155 | 4.9 | 6.9 | 12.1 | 5.1 |
| Roasted Red Pepper, 50% Less Fat, Tesco* | ½ Pot/85g | 156.0 | 11.0 | 184 | 7.3 | 10.9 | 12.4 | 9.5 |
| Roasted Red Pepper, BGTY, Sainsbury's* | ¼ Tub/50g | 84.0 | 5.0 | 169 | 6.5 | 14.4 | 9.5 | 6.2 |
| Roasted Red Pepper, Sainsbury's* | ½ Pot/85g | 253.0 | 23.0 | 297 | 7.0 | 7.4 | 26.6 | 3.5 |

H

|  | Measure INFO/WEIGHT | per Measure KCAL | FAT | Nutrition Values per 100g / 100ml KCAL | PROT | CARB | FAT | FIBRE |
|---|---|---|---|---|---|---|---|---|
| **HOUMOUS** | | | | | | | | |
| Roasted Red Pepper, Tesco* | 1 Serving/75g | 255.0 | 22.0 | 340 | 7.1 | 11.1 | 29.7 | 2.4 |
| Roasted Red Pepper, VLH Kitchens* | 1 Serving/17g | 31.0 | 1.4 | 183 | 6.5 | 15.6 | 8.4 | 6.2 |
| Roasted Vegetable, Fresh, Sainsbury's* | ¼ Pot/50g | 144.0 | 14.0 | 287 | 5.9 | 4.9 | 27.1 | 7.8 |
| Sea Salt & Cracked Black Pepper, Tesco* | ¼ Pot/50g | 147.0 | 14.0 | 295 | 7.0 | 4.8 | 27.2 | 9.5 |
| Spicy Red Pepper, With Crudite Dippers, M & S* | 1 Pack/130g | 123.0 | 8.0 | 95 | 3.3 | 7.1 | 6.1 | 3.4 |
| Sun Dried Tomato, Chunky, Tesco* | ½ Pot/95g | 322.0 | 27.0 | 339 | 6.7 | 14.0 | 28.4 | 3.3 |
| Sweet Chilli, Tesco* | ¼ Pot/50g | 145.0 | 11.0 | 290 | 8.1 | 15.0 | 21.9 | 5.1 |
| Three Bean, Reduced Fat, BGTY, Sainsbury's* | ¼ Tub/50g | 91.0 | 6.0 | 183 | 7.3 | 11.4 | 12.0 | 6.0 |
| with Extra Virgin Olive Oil, Tesco* | 1 Pack/190g | 564.0 | 46.0 | 297 | 7.9 | 11.7 | 24.3 | 5.1 |
| **HULA HOOPS** | | | | | | | | |
| Bacon & Ketchup Flavour, KP Snacks* | 1 Bag/27g | 140.0 | 8.0 | 517 | 3.4 | 56.3 | 30.9 | 2.0 |
| BBQ Beef, 55% Less Saturated Fat, KP Snacks* | 1 Pack/34g | 174.0 | 10.0 | 512 | 3.5 | 60.6 | 28.5 | 1.8 |
| Cheese & Onion 55% Less Saturated Fat, KP Snacks* | 1 Bag/34g | 175.0 | 10.0 | 515 | 3.6 | 61.0 | 28.5 | 1.9 |
| Chilli Salsa,Tortilla, KP Snacks* | 1 Bag /25g | 123.0 | 7.0 | 494 | 4.9 | 57.2 | 27.3 | 5.3 |
| Minis, Original, KP Snacks* | 1 Tub/140g | 752.0 | 49.0 | 537 | 3.0 | 52.9 | 34.8 | 1.7 |
| Multigrain, KP Snacks* | 1 Pack/23g | 113.0 | 6.0 | 491 | 5.6 | 60.0 | 25.6 | 4.3 |
| Original, 55% Less Saturated Fat, KP Snacks* | 1 Bag/34g | 175.0 | 10.0 | 515 | 3.2 | 61.6 | 28.4 | 1.8 |
| Original, KP Snacks* | 1 Bag/25g | 128.0 | 7.0 | 514 | 3.2 | 61.5 | 28.4 | 1.8 |
| Roast Chicken, 50% Less Saturated Fat, KP Snacks* | 1 Bag/34g | 175.0 | 10.0 | 514 | 3.4 | 61.0 | 28.5 | 1.7 |
| Salt & Vinegar, 50% Less Saturated Fat, KP Snacks* | 1 Pack/25g | 128.0 | 7.0 | 513 | 3.2 | 61.0 | 28.4 | 1.7 |
| Sizzling Bacon, KP Snacks* | 1 Bag/34g | 175.0 | 10.0 | 514 | 3.4 | 60.9 | 28.5 | 1.7 |
| **HUNGER BREAKS** | | | | | | | | |
| The Full Monty, Canned, Crosse & Blackwell* | 1 Can/410g | 332.0 | 16.0 | 81 | 5.6 | 7.2 | 3.8 | 1.3 |

**H**

# ICE CREAM

| | Measure INFO/WEIGHT | per Measure KCAL | FAT | KCAL | PROT | CARB | FAT | FIBRE |
|---|---|---|---|---|---|---|---|---|
| After Dinner, Mint, Dairy, Asda* | 1 Serving/100g | 182.0 | 8.0 | 182 | 3.4 | 24.0 | 8.0 | 0.4 |
| After Dinner Bites, Vanilla, Magnum, Wall's Ice Cream* | 1 Serving/29g | 100.0 | 7.0 | 344 | 3.4 | 31.0 | 23.0 | 1.4 |
| After Eight, Nestle* | 1 Serving/55g | 114.0 | 5.0 | 207 | 3.6 | 27.1 | 9.4 | 0.3 |
| Almond Indulgence, Sainsbury's* | 1 Serving/120g | 286.0 | 19.0 | 238 | 2.8 | 21.4 | 15.7 | 0.6 |
| Baked Alaska, Ben & Jerry's* | 1 Serving/100g | 260.0 | 15.0 | 260 | 4.0 | 29.0 | 15.0 | 0.1 |
| Bananas Foster, Haagen-Dazs* | 1 Serving/125ml | 260.0 | 15.0 | 208 | 3.2 | 22.4 | 12.0 | 0.0 |
| Banoffee, Haagen-Dazs* | 1 Serving/120ml | 274.0 | 16.0 | 228 | 4.0 | 23.0 | 13.0 | 0.0 |
| Banoffee Fudge, Sainsbury's* | 1/8 Pot/67g | 119.0 | 4.0 | 178 | 2.8 | 28.7 | 5.9 | 0.2 |
| Belgian Chocolate, Haagen-Dazs* | 1oz/28g | 89.0 | 6.0 | 318 | 4.6 | 28.4 | 20.7 | 0.0 |
| Bounty, Mars* | 1oz/28g | 77.0 | 5.0 | 274 | 3.3 | 23.8 | 18.3 | 0.0 |
| Bournville, Cadbury* | 1 Bar/120g | 258.0 | 14.0 | 215 | 3.5 | 26.0 | 11.6 | 0.0 |
| Brandy, Luxurious, M & S* | 1 Serving/100g | 228.0 | 13.0 | 228 | 3.8 | 19.1 | 13.3 | 0.2 |
| Cappuccino, Thorntons* | 1oz/28g | 61.0 | 4.0 | 218 | 4.4 | 20.7 | 12.9 | 0.0 |
| Caramel, Carte d'Or* | 2 Boules/50g | 106.0 | 4.0 | 212 | 2.6 | 30.8 | 8.7 | 0.0 |
| Caramel & Cinnamon Waffle, Carte d'Or* | 2 Scoops/55g | 121.0 | 6.0 | 220 | 3.0 | 27.0 | 11.0 | 0.0 |
| Caramel Chew Chew, Ben & Jerry's* | 1 Serving/100g | 270.0 | 16.0 | 270 | 3.0 | 29.0 | 16.0 | 0.0 |
| Caramel Craze, Organic, Tesco* | 1 Serving/100g | 253.0 | 15.0 | 253 | 3.3 | 25.5 | 15.3 | 0.0 |
| Cheeky Choc, Brownie, Skinny Cow* | 1 Tub/500ml | 590.0 | 5.0 | 118 | 3.0 | 23.9 | 1.1 | 4.1 |
| Cheesecake Brownie, Ben & Jerry's* | 1 Serving 100g | 260.0 | 16.0 | 260 | 4.0 | 26.0 | 16.0 | 0.0 |
| Cherry Garcia, Ben & Jerry's^ | 1 Serving/100g | 250.0 | 15.0 | 250 | 3.0 | 26.0 | 15.0 | 0.0 |
| Chilli Red, Purbeck* | 1 Serving/50g | 99.0 | 6.0 | 198 | 4.8 | 18.7 | 11.5 | 0.0 |
| Choc Chip, Cookie Dough, Haagen-Dazs* | 1oz/28g | 74.0 | 5.0 | 266 | 3.8 | 24.9 | 16.9 | 0.0 |
| Choc Chip, Haagen-Dazs* | 1oz/28g | 80.0 | 5.0 | 286 | 4.7 | 24.8 | 18.7 | 0.0 |
| Chocolate, COU, M & S^ | 1 Serving/140g | 231.0 | 4.0 | 165 | 3.9 | 35.0 | 2.9 | 0.8 |
| Chocolate, Haagen-Dazs* | 1 Serving/120ml | 269.0 | 18.0 | 224 | 4.0 | 19.0 | 15.0 | 0.0 |
| Chocolate, Organic, Green & Black's* | 1 Serving/125g | 310.0 | 18.0 | 248 | 5.0 | 25.3 | 14.1 | 1.1 |
| Chocolate, Organic, M & S* | 1oz/28g | 71.0 | 4.0 | 255 | 5.0 | 24.0 | 16.0 | 1.5 |
| Chocolate, Rich, Organic, Sainsbury's* | 1 Serving/100g | 213.0 | 12.0 | 213 | 4.4 | 22.6 | 11.7 | 1.2 |
| Chocolate, Soft Scoop, Tesco* | 1 Serving/50g | 93.0 | 4.0 | 186 | 3.2 | 25.1 | 8.1 | 0.3 |
| Chocolate, Swirl Pot, Skinny Cow* | 1 Pot/100ml | 98.0 | 1.0 | 98 | 2.9 | 20.2 | 0.6 | 2.7 |
| Chocolate, Weight Watchers* | 1 Serving/100ml | 140.0 | 1.0 | 140 | 4.3 | 28.7 | 1.2 | 0.0 |
| Chocolate & Marshmallow, Swirl, BGTY, Sainsbury's* | 1 Sm Scoop/40g | 69.0 | 1.0 | 173 | 3.9 | 33.8 | 2.5 | 2.8 |
| Chocolate & Orange, Organic, Green & Black's* | 1 Serving/100g | 248.0 | 14.0 | 248 | 5.0 | 25.3 | 14.1 | 0.1 |
| Chocolate Brownie with Walnuts, Haagen-Dazs* | 1 Cup/101g | 223.0 | 16.0 | 221 | 4.4 | 21.0 | 16.2 | 0.0 |
| Chocolate Chip, Baskin Robbins* | 1 Serving/75g | 170.0 | 10.0 | 227 | 4.0 | 24.0 | 13.3 | 0.0 |
| Chocolate Flavour, Soft Scoop, Sainsbury's* | 1 Serving/70g | 122.0 | 5.0 | 174 | 3.1 | 23.6 | 7.5 | 0.3 |
| Chocolate Fudge Brownie, Ben & Jerry's* | 1 Serving/50g | 130.0 | 6.0 | 260 | 4.0 | 32.0 | 13.0 | 1.5 |
| Chocolate Fudge Swirl, Haagen-Dazs* | 1oz/28g | 77.0 | 5.0 | 275 | 4.6 | 25.6 | 17.2 | 0.0 |
| Chocolate Honeycomb, COU, M & S* | 1 Serving/100ml | 150.0 | 3.0 | 150 | 3.5 | 31.5 | 2.6 | 0.7 |
| Chocolate Macadamia, Ben & Jerry's* | 1 Serving/100g | 260.0 | 18.0 | 260 | 4.0 | 22.0 | 18.0 | 0.8 |
| Chocolate Midnight Cookies, Haagen-Dazs* | 1oz/28g | 81.0 | 5.0 | 289 | 4.9 | 28.7 | 17.2 | 0.0 |
| Chocolate Ripple, Perfectly Balanced, Waitrose* | 1 Serving/125ml | 205.0 | 3.0 | 164 | 4.8 | 30.5 | 2.5 | 4.1 |
| Chocolate Trio, Thorntons* | 1 Bar/100g | 310.0 | 21.0 | 310 | 3.3 | 28.0 | 20.6 | 1.8 |
| Chocolatino, Tesco* | 1 Serving/56g | 115.0 | 4.0 | 205 | 3.4 | 31.4 | 6.8 | 1.8 |
| Chunky Monkey, Ben & Jerry's* | 1 Serving/100g | 290.0 | 17.0 | 290 | 4.0 | 27.0 | 17.0 | 1.0 |
| Chunky Monkey, Fairtrade, Ben & Jerry's* | 1 Serving/100g | 290.0 | 17.0 | 290 | 4.0 | 27.0 | 17.0 | 1.0 |
| Coconut, Carte d'Or* | 1 Serving/100ml | 125.0 | 7.0 | 125 | 1.8 | 14.0 | 7.1 | 0.5 |
| Coffee, Finest, Tesco* | ¼ Pot/93g | 236.0 | 15.0 | 254 | 4.9 | 22.5 | 16.0 | 0.0 |
| Coffee, Haagen-Dazs* | 1 Serving/120ml | 271.0 | 18.0 | 226 | 4.1 | 17.9 | 15.3 | 0.0 |
| Coffee, Waitrose* | ¼ Tub/125ml | 292.0 | 16.0 | 234 | 3.6 | 25.4 | 13.1 | 0.0 |
| Completely Mintal, Skinny Cow* | 1 Serving/100ml | 142.0 | 1.0 | 142 | 4.1 | 28.4 | 1.3 | 3.4 |
| Cookie Dough, Ben & Jerry's* | 1 Serving/100g | 270.0 | 14.0 | 270 | 4.0 | 31.0 | 14.0 | 0.0 |
| Cookies & Cream, Haagen-Dazs* | 1 Pot/100ml | 226.0 | 15.0 | 226 | 4.0 | 19.5 | 14.7 | 0.0 |

# ICE CREAM

| | Measure INFO/WEIGHT | per Measure KCAL | FAT | Nutrition Values per 100g / 100ml KCAL | PROT | CARB | FAT | FIBRE |
|---|---|---|---|---|---|---|---|---|
| Cornish, Asda* | 1 Serving/100ml | 100.0 | 5.0 | 100 | 1.8 | 12.0 | 5.0 | 0.0 |
| Cornish, Full Fat, Asda* | 1 Serving/100g | 204.0 | 12.0 | 204 | 3.5 | 21.4 | 11.6 | 0.1 |
| Cornish Clotted, M & S* | 1 Pot/90g | 207.0 | 13.0 | 230 | 2.8 | 21.8 | 14.5 | 0.1 |
| Cornish Vanilla, Soft Scoop, M & S* | 1oz/28g | 56.0 | 3.0 | 199 | 3.9 | 21.8 | 10.7 | 0.2 |
| Creamy Chocolate & Nut, Co-Op* | 1oz/28g | 66.0 | 4.0 | 235 | 4.0 | 25.0 | 13.0 | 0.5 |
| Crema Di Mascarpone, Carte d'Or* | 1 Serving/100g | 207.0 | 9.0 | 207 | 2.8 | 29.0 | 8.9 | 0.0 |
| Dairy, Flavoured | 1oz/28g | 50.0 | 2.0 | 179 | 3.5 | 24.7 | 8.0 | 0.0 |
| Dairy Milk, Orange, Cadbury* | 1 Serving/120ml | 259.0 | 14.0 | 216 | 3.5 | 26.0 | 11.6 | 0.0 |
| Dark Toffee, Organic, Green & Black's* | ¼ Pot/125ml | 192.0 | 10.0 | 154 | 2.8 | 18.1 | 7.9 | 0.1 |
| Date & Almond Cream, Haagen-Dazs* | 1 Serving/120ml | 254.0 | 16.0 | 212 | 5.0 | 19.0 | 13.0 | 0.0 |
| Demon Chocolate, M & S* | 1 Serving/79g | 208.0 | 9.0 | 263 | 3.7 | 37.1 | 11.1 | 0.6 |
| Double Chocolate, Nestle* | 1 Serving/78g | 248.0 | 14.0 | 320 | 4.8 | 33.7 | 18.4 | 0.0 |
| Dream, Cadbury* | 1 Bar/120ml | 264.0 | 14.0 | 220 | 3.6 | 26.0 | 11.9 | 0.0 |
| Dulce De Leche, Bar, Haagen-Dazs* | 1 Bar/105g | 370.0 | 24.0 | 352 | 3.8 | 32.3 | 22.9 | 0.0 |
| Fig & Orange Blossom Honey, Waitrose* | 1 Serving/100g | 219.0 | 12.0 | 219 | 3.9 | 24.3 | 11.8 | 0.4 |
| Fruit & Fresh Tropical, Carte d'Or* | 1 Serving/83g | 154.0 | 7.0 | 185 | 2.5 | 24.5 | 8.5 | 0.0 |
| Fun-Illa, Skinny Cow* | 1 Serving/100ml | 97.0 | 2.0 | 97 | 3.1 | 17.6 | 1.6 | 2.4 |
| Galaxy, Mars* | 1 Bar/60ml | 203.0 | 13.0 | 339 | 4.7 | 29.7 | 22.4 | 0.0 |
| Get Fruit, Tropical, Solero* | 1 Serving/125ml | 162.0 | 5.0 | 130 | 1.6 | 20.6 | 4.4 | 0.4 |
| Greek Yoghurt & Honey, Carte d'Or* | 1 Serving/55g | 114.0 | 5.0 | 207 | 2.7 | 29.0 | 8.8 | 0.0 |
| Half Baked, Ben & Jerry's* | 1 Serving/100g | 270.0 | 13.0 | 270 | 5.0 | 32.0 | 13.0 | 1.0 |
| Heavenly Vanilla, Cadbury* | 1 Serving/250ml | 355.0 | 23.0 | 142 | 2.5 | 12.8 | 9.3 | 0.0 |
| Honeycomb Harvest, Mackies* | 1 Serving/100g | 209.0 | 10.0 | 209 | 4.0 | 25.0 | 10.0 | 0.0 |
| Lavazza, Carte d'Or* | 1 Serving/55g | 120.0 | 5.0 | 218 | 3.5 | 29.0 | 9.9 | 0.0 |
| Lemon, Haagen-Dazs* | 1 Serving/120ml | 144.0 | 0.0 | 120 | 0.3 | 29.3 | 0.2 | 0.0 |
| Lemon & White Chocolate, Crackpots, Iceland* | 1 Serving/100g | 202.0 | 8.0 | 202 | 1.7 | 29.9 | 8.4 | 0.3 |
| Lemon Cream, Dairy, Sainsbury's* | 1 Serving/100g | 199.0 | 9.0 | 199 | 3.0 | 25.9 | 9.3 | 0.1 |
| Lemon Curd, Safeway* | 1 Serving/100g | 185.0 | 8.0 | 185 | 3.0 | 28.9 | 8.1 | 0.2 |
| Lemon Curd Swirl, Duchy Originals* | ¼ Pot/101g | 247.0 | 14.0 | 245 | 3.7 | 25.8 | 14.1 | 0.0 |
| Lemon Pie, Haagen-Dazs* | 1oz/28g | 73.0 | 5.0 | 261 | 3.9 | 24.5 | 16.3 | 0.0 |
| Less Than 5% Fat, Asda* | 1 Scoop/40g | 56.0 | 2.0 | 139 | 2.7 | 22.0 | 4.5 | 0.0 |
| Log, Mint Chocolate, Sainsbury's* | 1 Serving/51g | 100.0 | 5.0 | 197 | 3.0 | 23.8 | 10.0 | 0.2 |
| Luscious Mint Choc Chip, Morrisons* | 1 Serving/50g | 99.0 | 5.0 | 198 | 2.9 | 23.1 | 10.5 | 0.7 |
| Lychee Cream & Ginger, Haagen-Dazs* | 1 Serving/120ml | 258.0 | 13.0 | 215 | 3.6 | 26.1 | 10.6 | 0.0 |
| Macadamia Nut, Baskin Robbins* | 1 Serving/113g | 270.0 | 18.0 | 239 | 4.4 | 22.1 | 15.9 | 0.9 |
| Madly Deeply, Skinny Cow* | 1 Serving/100g | 149.0 | 2.0 | 149 | 4.2 | 28.3 | 2.2 | 3.4 |
| Magic Maple, M & S* | 1 Ice Cream/93g | 259.0 | 11.0 | 278 | 2.9 | 39.0 | 12.3 | 0.6 |
| Maple & Walnut, American, Sainsbury's* | 1/8 Pot/68g | 121.0 | 5.0 | 179 | 3.1 | 25.6 | 7.2 | 0.2 |
| Maple Brazil, Thorntons* | 1oz/28g | 66.0 | 4.0 | 236 | 4.1 | 24.4 | 13.6 | 0.0 |
| Marshallow, Weight Watchers* | ½ Tub/138g | 268.0 | 6.0 | 194 | 3.2 | 34.5 | 4.7 | 1.3 |
| Mint, Thorntons* | 1oz/28g | 66.0 | 4.0 | 237 | 4.0 | 25.0 | 13.4 | 0.0 |
| Mint & Chocolate, Sainsbury's* | 1 Serving/71g | 137.0 | 7.0 | 192 | 3.4 | 23.5 | 9.4 | 0.4 |
| Mint Choc Chip Soft Scoop, Asda* | 1 Serving/46g | 86.0 | 4.0 | 187 | 2.9 | 24.0 | 9.0 | 0.3 |
| Mint Chocolate Chip, Baskin Robbins* | 1 Scoop/113g | 270.0 | 16.0 | 239 | 4.4 | 24.8 | 14.2 | 0.9 |
| Mint Crisp, Nestle* | 1 Serving/75ml | 232.0 | 16.0 | 309 | 2.9 | 25.5 | 21.9 | 0.9 |
| Mint Crunch, Dairy Milk, Cadbury* | 1 Serving/60ml | 162.0 | 13.0 | 270 | 3.0 | 29.0 | 22.2 | 0.0 |
| Mocha Coffee Indulgence, Sainsbury's* | ¼ Pot/82g | 178.0 | 11.0 | 217 | 3.2 | 22.1 | 12.9 | 0.1 |
| Monster Mint, Sainsbury's* | 1/8 Pot/67g | 121.0 | 5.0 | 180 | 3.0 | 26.3 | 6.9 | 0.3 |
| Muddy Pigs, Wall's Ice Cream* | 1 Serving/150ml | 150.0 | 7.0 | 100 | 1.7 | 12.1 | 4.9 | 0.3 |
| Neapolitan, Brick, Tesco* | 1 Serving/50g | 81.0 | 3.0 | 163 | 3.3 | 21.9 | 6.9 | 0.4 |
| Neapolitan, Soft Scoop, Asda* | 1 Scoop/47g | 82.0 | 4.0 | 175 | 2.8 | 23.0 | 8.0 | 0.2 |
| Neapolitan, Soft Scoop, M & S* | 1/8 Tub/63g | 100.0 | 5.0 | 160 | 2.7 | 21.3 | 7.4 | 0.3 |
| Neopolitian, Soft Scoop, Tesco* | 1 Serving/43g | 70.0 | 3.0 | 163 | 3.3 | 21.9 | 6.9 | 0.4 |

# ICE CREAM

| Measure INFO/WEIGHT | per Measure KCAL | FAT | Nutrition Values per 100g / 100ml KCAL | PROT | CARB | FAT | FIBRE |
|---|---|---|---|---|---|---|---|

| | Measure INFO/WEIGHT | per Measure KCAL | FAT | KCAL | PROT | CARB | FAT | FIBRE |
|---|---|---|---|---|---|---|---|---|
| Non-Dairy, Mixes | 1oz/28g | 51.0 | 2.0 | 182 | 4.1 | 25.1 | 7.9 | 0.0 |
| Non-Dairy, Reduced Calorie | 1oz/28g | 33.0 | 2.0 | 119 | 3.4 | 13.7 | 6.0 | 0.0 |
| Panna Cotta, & Raspberry Swirl, Haagen-Dazs* | 1 Serving/120ml | 250.0 | 15.0 | 208 | 3.2 | 21.0 | 12.4 | 0.0 |
| Panna Cotta, Haagen-Dazs* | 1 Serving/120ml | 248.0 | 16.0 | 207 | 3.4 | 18.4 | 13.3 | 0.0 |
| Peach Melba, Soft Scoop, M & S* | 1oz/28g | 46.0 | 2.0 | 165 | 2.8 | 21.4 | 7.6 | 0.3 |
| Phish Food, Ben & Jerry's* | 1 Serving/100g | 260.0 | 13.0 | 260 | 3.5 | 35.0 | 13.0 | 0.1 |
| Picnic, Cadbury* | 1 Cone/125ml | 258.0 | 12.0 | 207 | 3.4 | 28.9 | 9.4 | 0.3 |
| Pistachio, Haagen-Dazs* | 1 Serving/120ml | 276.0 | 19.0 | 230 | 4.4 | 17.7 | 15.7 | 0.0 |
| Praline, Green & Black's* | 1 Sm Pot/100g | 191.0 | 11.0 | 191 | 3.5 | 20.0 | 10.8 | 0.9 |
| Praline & Chocolate, Thorntons* | 1oz/28g | 87.0 | 6.0 | 309 | 4.6 | 21.3 | 22.9 | 0.6 |
| Pralines & Cream, Haagen-Dazs* | 1 Pot/500ml | 1210.0 | 75.0 | 242 | 3.7 | 22.9 | 15.1 | 0.0 |
| Raspberries, Clotted Cream, Waitrose* | 1 Tub/500ml | 790.0 | 39.0 | 158 | 2.9 | 18.9 | 7.9 | 0.1 |
| Raspberry, Haagen-Dazs* | 1 Serving/120ml | 127.0 | 0.0 | 106 | 0.2 | 25.9 | 0.2 | 0.0 |
| Raspberry, Swirl Pot, Skinny Cow* | 1 Pot/100ml | 86.0 | 0.0 | 86 | 2.5 | 18.4 | 0.3 | 2.2 |
| Raspberry Ripple, Dairy, Waitrose* | 1 Serving/186ml | 195.0 | 10.0 | 105 | 1.9 | 12.3 | 5.4 | 0.0 |
| Raspberry Ripple, Soft Scoop, Sainsbury's* | 1 Serving/75g | 127.0 | 5.0 | 170 | 2.6 | 24.2 | 7.0 | 0.3 |
| Raspberry Ripple, Soft Scoop, Tesco* | 1 Scoop/25g | 39.0 | 2.0 | 157 | 2.5 | 23.0 | 6.1 | 0.2 |
| Raspberry Ripple Brick, Tesco* | 1 Serving/48g | 71.0 | 3.0 | 148 | 2.6 | 20.8 | 6.0 | 0.2 |
| Really Creamy After Dinner Mint, Asda* | 1 Serving/100g | 191.0 | 9.0 | 191 | 3.4 | 24.0 | 9.0 | 0.4 |
| Really Creamy Chocolate, Asda* | 1 Scrving/100g | 227.0 | 11.0 | 227 | 4.1 | 28.0 | 11.0 | 0.4 |
| Really Creamy Lemon Meringue, Asda* | 1 Serving/100ml | 100.0 | 5.0 | 100 | 1.8 | 12.0 | 5.0 | 0.1 |
| Really Creamy Toffee, Asda* | 1 Serving/120ml | 146.0 | 6.0 | 122 | 1.7 | 17.5 | 5.0 | 0.1 |
| Rocky Road, M & S* | 1 Tub/500g | 1475.0 | 88.0 | 295 | 4.2 | 29.5 | 17.7 | 1.2 |
| Rocky Road, Sainsbury's* | 1/8 Pot/67g | 137.0 | 5.0 | 205 | 3.8 | 30.9 | 7.3 | 1.0 |
| Rolo, Nestle* | ½ Tub/500ml | 1180.0 | 52.0 | 236 | 3.4 | 31.9 | 10.5 | 0.2 |
| Rum & Raisin, Haagen-Dazs* | 1 Serving/120ml | 264.0 | 18.0 | 220 | 3.4 | 18.6 | 14.7 | 0.0 |
| Smarties, Nestle* | 1 Serving/50g | 125.0 | 6.0 | 250 | 3.6 | 32.3 | 11.9 | 0.2 |
| Smarties Ice Cream Pot, Nestle* | 1 Pot/69g | 151.0 | 6.0 | 218 | 4.4 | 33.6 | 8.2 | 0.0 |
| Spagnola, Carte d'Or* | 1 Serving/100g | 187.0 | 6.0 | 187 | 2.0 | 32.0 | 5.7 | 0.0 |
| Stem Ginger with Belgian Chocolate, Waitrose* | 1 Lolly/110g | 255.0 | 14.0 | 232 | 2.9 | 25.5 | 13.1 | 1.7 |
| Strawberries & Cream, Deliciously Dairy, Co-Op* | 1oz/28g | 46.0 | 2.0 | 165 | 3.0 | 24.0 | 6.0 | 0.3 |
| Strawberry, Get Fruit, Solero* | 1 Serving/100ml | 120.0 | 4.0 | 120 | 1.5 | 18.8 | 4.5 | 1.3 |
| Strawberry, Haagen-Dazs* | 1oz/28g | 67.0 | 4.0 | 241 | 4.0 | 21.5 | 15.5 | 0.0 |
| Strawberry, Soft Scoop, Tesco* | 1 Serving/46g | 78.0 | 3.0 | 170 | 2.8 | 23.1 | 7.4 | 0.1 |
| Strawberry, Swirl Pot, Skinny Cow* | 1 Pot/100ml | 89.0 | 0.0 | 89 | 2.5 | 19.0 | 0.3 | 2.2 |
| Strawberry, Thorntons* | 1oz/28g | 52.0 | 3.0 | 185 | 3.2 | 22.5 | 9.3 | 0.1 |
| Strawberry, Weight Watchers* | 1 Pot/57g | 81.0 | 2.0 | 142 | 2.5 | 23.4 | 3.9 | 0.2 |
| Strawberry & Cream, Mivvi, Nestle* | 1 Serving/60g | 118.0 | 5.0 | 196 | 2.6 | 29.4 | 7.6 | 0.1 |
| Strawberry & Cream, Organic, Sainsbury's* | 1 Serving/100g | 193.0 | 10.0 | 193 | 3.6 | 22.6 | 9.8 | 0.4 |
| Strawberry Cheesecake, Ben & Jerry's* | 1 Serving 100g | 240.0 | 14.0 | 240 | 3.0 | 27.0 | 14.0 | 0.0 |
| Strawberry Cheesecake, Co-Op* | 1/6 Pot/86g | 163.0 | 6.0 | 190 | 3.0 | 29.0 | 7.0 | 0.2 |
| Tantilising Toffee, COU, M & S* | ¼ Pot/125ml | 125.0 | 3.0 | 100 | 0.6 | 18.0 | 2.8 | 0.0 |
| Taste Sensation, Mascarpone Forest Fruits, Aldi* | 1 Pot/73g | 159.0 | 7.0 | 217 | 1.8 | 29.6 | 10.1 | 0.6 |
| Terry's Chocolate Orange, Carte d'Or* | 1 Serving/100g | 182.0 | 7.0 | 182 | 2.8 | 27.0 | 7.1 | 0.0 |
| Tiramisu, COU, M & S* | ¼ Tub/86g | 120.0 | 2.0 | 140 | 2.1 | 26.4 | 2.9 | 3.0 |
| Tiramisu, Haagen-Dazs* | 1 Serving/120ml | 303.0 | 20.0 | 253 | 3.8 | 22.7 | 16.3 | 0.0 |
| Toblerone, Carte d'Or* | 1 Serving/100g | 211.0 | 9.0 | 211 | 3.7 | 29.0 | 9.1 | 0.0 |
| Toffee, Deliciously Dairy, Co-Op* | 1oz/28g | 45.0 | 2.0 | 160 | 3.0 | 21.0 | 7.0 | 0.2 |
| Toffee, Swirl Pot, Skinny Cow* | 1 Pot/66g | 92.0 | 0.0 | 140 | 3.8 | 29.8 | 0.6 | 4.5 |
| Toffee, Thorntons* | 1oz/28g | 61.0 | 3.0 | 218 | 4.1 | 24.5 | 11.6 | 0.0 |
| Toffee & Biscuit, Weight Watchers* | 1 Pot/100ml | 93.0 | 3.0 | 93 | 1.5 | 14.9 | 2.7 | 0.1 |
| Toffee & Vanilla, Sainsbury's* | 1 Serving/71g | 146.0 | 7.0 | 205 | 3.1 | 26.7 | 9.5 | 0.1 |
| Toffee Creme, Haagen-Dazs* | 1oz/28g | 74.0 | 4.0 | 265 | 4.5 | 26.7 | 15.6 | 0.0 |

I

# ICE CREAM

| | Measure INFO/WEIGHT | per Measure KCAL | FAT | Nutrition Values per 100g / 100ml KCAL | PROT | CARB | FAT | FIBRE |
|---|---|---|---|---|---|---|---|---|
| Toffee Crunch, Handmade Farmhouse, TTD, Sainsbury's* | ½ Pot/90g | 288.0 | 19.0 | 320 | 2.9 | 29.7 | 21.1 | 0.1 |
| Toffee Fudge, Soft Scoop, Asda* | 1 Serving/50g | 92.0 | 3.0 | 185 | 2.6 | 28.0 | 7.0 | 0.0 |
| Toffee Ripple, Tesco* | 1 Serving/100g | 173.0 | 7.0 | 173 | 2.7 | 24.4 | 7.2 | 0.1 |
| Toffee Vanilla, HE, Tesco* | 1 Serving/73g | 106.0 | 2.0 | 145 | 2.5 | 28.1 | 2.5 | 0.5 |
| Totally Toffee, Safeway* | 1 Serving/100ml | 136.0 | 5.0 | 136 | 1.3 | 21.1 | 5.1 | 0.1 |
| Traditional Cornish Blackberry, M & S* | 1oz/28g | 61.0 | 3.0 | 218 | 2.3 | 28.0 | 10.8 | 0.3 |
| Traditional Cornish Strawberry, M & S* | 1oz/28g | 64.0 | 3.0 | 229 | 2.3 | 29.7 | 11.2 | 0.2 |
| Triple Chocolate, Carte d'Or* | 1 Serving/58g | 122.0 | 6.0 | 210 | 3.7 | 27.0 | 9.8 | 0.0 |
| Triple Chocolate Centenary, Cadbury* | 1 Serving/100ml | 255.0 | 16.0 | 255 | 2.5 | 27.1 | 15.6 | 0.0 |
| Truffle Berry Fling, Skinny Cow* | 1 Serving/100g | 156.0 | 2.0 | 156 | 4.0 | 30.5 | 2.0 | 3.3 |
| Vanilla, Ben & Jerry's* | 1 Mini Tub/116g | 267.0 | 17.0 | 230 | 4.0 | 20.0 | 15.0 | 0.1 |
| Vanilla, Carte d'Or* | 1 Serving/50g | 105.0 | 5.0 | 210 | 3.0 | 26.0 | 9.5 | 0.0 |
| Vanilla, COU, M & S* | ¼ Pot/79g | 111.0 | 2.0 | 140 | 1.7 | 25.9 | 2.8 | 0.8 |
| Vanilla, Dairy, Average | 1 Scoop/40g | 80.0 | 4.0 | 201 | 3.5 | 23.6 | 11.0 | 0.7 |
| Vanilla, Dairy, Finest, Tesco* | 1 Serving/92g | 227.0 | 16.0 | 247 | 4.5 | 18.0 | 17.4 | 0.3 |
| Vanilla, Dairy, Organic, Yeo Valley* | 1 Serving/100g | 206.0 | 11.0 | 206 | 4.9 | 21.3 | 11.2 | 0.0 |
| Vanilla, Dairy Milk, Cadbury* | 1 Serving/120g | 259.0 | 14.0 | 216 | 3.5 | 26.0 | 11.6 | 0.1 |
| Vanilla, Deliciously Dairy, Co-Op* | 1oz/28g | 49.0 | 2.0 | 175 | 3.0 | 23.0 | 8.0 | 0.2 |
| Vanilla, Easy Serve, Co-Op* | 1oz/28g | 39.0 | 2.0 | 140 | 3.0 | 18.0 | 7.0 | 0.2 |
| Vanilla, Fairtrade, Ben & Jerry's* | 1 Serving/100g | 230.0 | 15.0 | 230 | 4.0 | 20.0 | 15.0 | 0.1 |
| Vanilla, Haagen-Dazs* | 1oz/28g | 70.0 | 5.0 | 250 | 4.5 | 19.7 | 17.1 | 0.0 |
| Vanilla, Handmade Farmhouse, TTD, Sainsbury's* | 1 Serving/100g | 252.0 | 20.0 | 252 | 4.2 | 14.4 | 19.7 | 0.0 |
| Vanilla, Light, Carte d'Or* | 1 Serving/100g | 136.0 | 4.0 | 136 | 2.4 | 22.0 | 4.4 | 4.0 |
| Vanilla, Light Soft Scoop, 25% Less Fat, Morrisons* | 1 Scoop/50g | 75.0 | 2.0 | 150 | 2.9 | 23.2 | 5.0 | 0.2 |
| Vanilla, Low Fat, Weight Watchers* | 1 Scoop/125ml | 75.0 | 2.0 | 60 | 1.1 | 9.7 | 1.7 | 0.1 |
| Vanilla, Non-Dairy, Average | 1 Serving/60g | 107.0 | 5.0 | 178 | 3.2 | 23.1 | 8.7 | 0.0 |
| Vanilla, Organic, Green & Black's* | 1 Sm Tub/100ml | 151.0 | 9.0 | 151 | 3.1 | 13.9 | 9.2 | 0.1 |
| Vanilla, Organic, Sainsbury's* | 1 Serving/85g | 176.0 | 10.0 | 207 | 4.3 | 20.5 | 12.0 | 0.1 |
| Vanilla, Organic, Tesco* | 1 Serving/100g | 237.0 | 17.0 | 237 | 3.7 | 16.8 | 17.2 | 0.0 |
| Vanilla, Pecan, Haagen-Dazs* | 1 Serving/120ml | 316.0 | 24.0 | 263 | 4.3 | 17.1 | 19.6 | 0.0 |
| Vanilla, Really Creamy, Asda* | 1 Serving/50g | 98.0 | 5.0 | 196 | 3.5 | 23.0 | 10.0 | 0.1 |
| Vanilla, Soft, Non Milk Fat, Waitrose* | 1 Serving/125ml | 77.0 | 3.0 | 62 | 1.3 | 8.0 | 2.7 | 0.1 |
| Vanilla, Soft Scoop, 25% Less Fat, Asda* | 1oz/28g | 42.0 | 1.0 | 149 | 2.9 | 23.0 | 5.0 | 0.0 |
| Vanilla, Soft Scoop, BGTY, Sainsbury's* | 1 Serving/75g | 88.0 | 1.0 | 117 | 3.1 | 22.2 | 1.7 | 0.2 |
| Vanilla, Soft Scoop, Tesco* | 1oz/28g | 46.0 | 2.0 | 164 | 3.1 | 21.8 | 7.1 | 0.1 |
| Vanilla, Soft Slice, Wall's Ice Cream* | 1 Serving/100ml | 90.0 | 4.0 | 90 | 1.4 | 11.2 | 4.4 | 0.1 |
| Vanilla, Thorntons* | 1oz/28g | 63.0 | 4.0 | 225 | 4.9 | 20.5 | 13.6 | 0.0 |
| Vanilla, Toffee Crunch, Ben & Jerry's* | 1 Tub/407g | 1099.0 | 65.0 | 270 | 4.0 | 29.0 | 16.0 | 0.5 |
| Vanilla, Too Good to Be True, Wall's Ice Cream* | 1 Serving/50ml | 35.0 | 0.0 | 70 | 2.0 | 14.9 | 0.4 | 0.1 |
| Vanilla, Value, Tesco* | 1 Serving/56g | 77.0 | 3.0 | 137 | 2.8 | 18.7 | 5.7 | 0.2 |
| Vanilla, with Vanilla Pods, Sainsbury's* | 1 Serving/100g | 195.0 | 10.0 | 195 | 3.5 | 22.5 | 10.1 | 0.1 |
| Vanilla & Chocolate Swirl, Safeway* | 1 Serving/125g | 250.0 | 11.0 | 200 | 3.3 | 26.2 | 9.1 | 0.1 |
| Vanilla & Cinnamon, Finest, Tesco* | 1 Serving/50g | 114.0 | 7.0 | 229 | 3.9 | 20.2 | 14.7 | 0.4 |
| Vanilla & Strawberry, Swirl, Safeway* | 1 Serving/100g | 190.0 | 7.0 | 190 | 2.9 | 27.0 | 7.5 | 0.2 |
| Vanilla & Strawberry, Weight Watchers* | 1 Serving/100ml | 81.0 | 2.0 | 81 | 1.4 | 13.3 | 2.2 | 0.1 |
| Vanilla Bean, Light, Deluxe* | 1 Serving/64g | 110.0 | 3.0 | 172 | 4.7 | 26.6 | 3.9 | 0.0 |
| Vanilla Bean, Purbeck* | 1 Serving/100g | 198.0 | 11.0 | 198 | 4.8 | 18.7 | 11.5 | 0.0 |
| Vanilla Caramel Brownie, Haagen-Dazs* | 1 Serving/150g | 410.0 | 25.0 | 273 | 4.5 | 26.8 | 16.5 | 0.0 |
| Vanilla Choc Fudge, Haagen-Dazs* | 1oz/28g | 75.0 | 5.0 | 267 | 4.3 | 23.5 | 17.2 | 0.0 |
| Vanilla Chocolate, Taste Sensation, Frosty's, Aldi* | 1 Pot/73g | 164.0 | 7.0 | 224 | 2.1 | 32.4 | 9.6 | 0.7 |
| Vanilla Flavour, Soft Scoop, Sainsbury's* | 1 Serving/71g | 96.0 | 4.0 | 136 | 2.9 | 18.8 | 5.5 | 0.2 |
| Vanilla Flavour, VLH Kitchens* | 1 Serving/100g | 235.0 | 15.6 | 235 | 4.0 | 22.1 | 15.0 | 0.2 |
| Vanilla with Strawberry Swirl, Mini Tub, Weight Watchers* | 1 Mini Tub/57g | 81.0 | 2.0 | 142 | 2.5 | 23.4 | 3.9 | 0.2 |

| | Measure INFO/WEIGHT | per Measure KCAL | FAT | Nutrition Values per 100g / 100ml KCAL | PROT | CARB | FAT | FIBRE |
|---|---|---|---|---|---|---|---|---|
| **ICE CREAM** | | | | | | | | |
| Viennetta, Biscuit Caramel, Wall's Ice Cream* | 1/6 Serving/58g | 183.0 | 12.0 | 315 | 3.3 | 27.8 | 20.9 | 0.0 |
| Viennetta, Cappuccino, Wall's Ice Cream* | 1 Serving/75g | 191.0 | 13.0 | 255 | 3.5 | 22.0 | 17.0 | 0.0 |
| Viennetta, Chocolate, Wall's Ice Cream* | ¼ Pot/80g | 200.0 | 12.0 | 250 | 4.1 | 24.0 | 15.2 | 0.0 |
| Viennetta, Forest Fruit, Wall's Ice Cream* | 1 Serving/98g | 265.0 | 16.0 | 270 | 3.4 | 27.2 | 16.2 | 0.0 |
| Viennetta, Mint, Wall's Ice Cream* | 1 Serving/80g | 204.0 | 13.0 | 255 | 3.4 | 23.0 | 16.6 | 0.0 |
| Viennetta, Selection Brownie, Wall's Ice Cream* | 1 Serving/70g | 194.0 | 11.0 | 277 | 4.2 | 28.5 | 16.2 | 0.0 |
| Viennetta, Strawberry, Wall's Ice Cream* | 1 Serving/80g | 204.0 | 13.0 | 255 | 3.4 | 22.1 | 16.8 | 0.0 |
| Viennetta, Vanilla, Wall's Ice Cream* | ¼ Bar/80g | 204.0 | 13.0 | 255 | 3.3 | 23.0 | 16.7 | 0.0 |
| Voluptuous Vanilla, COU, M & S* | 1 Pot/400g | 520.0 | 10.0 | 130 | 4.6 | 22.0 | 2.6 | 0.6 |
| Walnut & Maple, Waitrose* | 1 Serving/60g | 68.0 | 2.0 | 114 | 1.8 | 18.2 | 3.8 | 0.0 |
| White Vanilla, Soft Scoop, Tesco* | 1oz/28g | 46.0 | 2.0 | 164 | 3.1 | 21.8 | 7.1 | 0.1 |
| with Cherry Sauce, Tesco* | 1 Serving/58g | 121.0 | 3.0 | 210 | 2.8 | 37.0 | 5.6 | 0.2 |
| with Raspberry Sauce, Movenpick* | 1 Serving/50g | 130.0 | 7.0 | 260 | 4.0 | 27.0 | 14.0 | 0.2 |
| Zesty Lemon Meringue, COU, M & S* | ¼ Pot/73g | 120.0 | 2.0 | 165 | 2.6 | 33.0 | 2.5 | 0.5 |
| **ICE CREAM BAR** | | | | | | | | |
| Bailey's, Haagen-Dazs* | 1oz/28g | 86.0 | 6.0 | 307 | 4.1 | 24.8 | 21.2 | 0.0 |
| Bounty, 100 Ml Bar, Mars* | 1 Bar/100ml | 278.0 | 18.0 | 278 | 3.4 | 24.7 | 18.5 | 0.7 |
| Chunky Chocolate, Co-Op* | 1 Bar/60g | 204.0 | 12.0 | 340 | 5.0 | 35.0 | 20.0 | 1.0 |
| Chunky Toffee, Co-Op* | 1 Bar/60g | 204.0 | 13.0 | 340 | 4.0 | 34.0 | 21.0 | 1.0 |
| Dairy Milk, Caramel, Cadbury* | 1 Bar/60ml | 175.0 | 10.0 | 290 | 3.6 | 30.2 | 17.1 | 0.0 |
| Dairy Milk, Fruit & Nut, Cadbury* | 1 Bar/74g | 178.0 | 11.0 | 240 | 2.2 | 25.3 | 14.5 | 0.0 |
| Dairy Milk, Fudge, Cadbury* | 1 Bar/60g | 165.0 | 10.0 | 275 | 3.0 | 27.6 | 17.2 | 0.0 |
| Dream, Cadbury* | 1 Serving/118g | 260.0 | 14.0 | 220 | 3.6 | 26.0 | 11.9 | 0.0 |
| Galaxy, Mars* | 1 Bar/54g | 184.0 | 12.0 | 341 | 3.8 | 30.7 | 22.5 | 0.6 |
| Lion, Nestle* | 1 Bar/45g | 166.0 | 10.0 | 370 | 4.2 | 39.1 | 21.9 | 1.0 |
| Maltesers, Mars* | 1 Bar/45ml | 113.0 | 7.0 | 252 | 2.9 | 25.0 | 15.6 | 0.7 |
| Mars, Mars* | 1 Bar/63g | 177.0 | 10.0 | 283 | 3.6 | 30.1 | 16.4 | 0.0 |
| Red Fruits, Solero* | 1 Bar/80g | 99.0 | 2.0 | 124 | 1.6 | 25.0 | 2.7 | 0.0 |
| Snickers, Mars* | 1 Bar/67g | 250.0 | 15.0 | 373 | 6.0 | 37.3 | 22.4 | 0.0 |
| Toffee Crunch, English, Weight Watchers* | 1 Bar/40g | 110.0 | 6.0 | 275 | 2.5 | 32.5 | 15.0 | 5.0 |
| Yorkie, Nestle* | 1 Bar | 144.0 | 9.0 | 359 | 4.8 | 36.5 | 21.6 | 0.0 |
| **ICE CREAM CONE** | | | | | | | | |
| After Eight, Nestle* | 1 Cone/100ml | 174.0 | 8.0 | 174 | 2.4 | 23.0 | 8.0 | 0.9 |
| Average | 1 Cone/75g | 139.0 | 6.0 | 186 | 3.5 | 25.5 | 8.5 | 0.0 |
| Blackcurrant, GFY, Asda* | 1 Cone/67g | 162.0 | 6.0 | 241 | 3.0 | 37.0 | 9.0 | 0.1 |
| Carousel Wafer Company* | 1 Cone/5g | 19.0 | 0.0 | 392 | 9.8 | 78.6 | 4.2 | 0.0 |
| Chocolate, Mini, Cornetto, Wall's Ice Cream* | 1 Cone/19g | 69.0 | 4.0 | 363 | 4.2 | 34.2 | 23.2 | 0.0 |
| Chocolate, Vanilla & Hazelnut, Sainsbury's* | 1 Cone/62g | 190.0 | 10.0 | 306 | 4.5 | 33.9 | 16.9 | 0.6 |
| Chocolate & Caramel, Skinny Cow* | 1 Cone/110ml | 121.0 | 3.0 | 110 | 2.5 | 19.3 | 2.5 | 2.7 |
| Chocolate & Nut, Co-Op* | 1 Cone/110g | 307.0 | 17.0 | 279 | 3.9 | 31.0 | 15.5 | 0.6 |
| Chocolate & Vanilla, M & S* | 1oz/28g | 83.0 | 5.0 | 295 | 4.2 | 31.8 | 17.0 | 0.7 |
| Cornet, Wafer Cone, Askeys* | 1 Cone/4g | 13.0 | 0.0 | 376 | 10.7 | 77.6 | 2.5 | 0.0 |
| Cornetto, Classico, Mini, Wall's Ice Cream* | 1 Cone/19g | 67.0 | 4.0 | 353 | 4.2 | 32.6 | 23.2 | 0.0 |
| Cornetto, Classico, Wall's Ice Cream* | 1 Cone/98g | 200.0 | 13.0 | 205 | 2.7 | 19.7 | 12.9 | 0.0 |
| Cornetto, Flirt, Choc Chip, with Hazelnut, Wall's Ice Cream* | 1 Cone/70g | 223.0 | 11.0 | 320 | 4.0 | 40.0 | 16.0 | 0.0 |
| Cornetto, Frutti Disc, Wall's Ice Cream* | 1 Cone/80g | 200.0 | 9.0 | 250 | 2.5 | 35.0 | 11.0 | 0.0 |
| Cornetto, GFY, Asda* | 1 Cone/67g | 162.0 | 6.0 | 241 | 3.0 | 37.0 | 9.0 | 0.1 |
| Cornetto, Mint, Wall's Ice Cream* | 1 Cone/75g | 225.0 | 13.0 | 300 | 3.7 | 32.0 | 18.0 | 1.1 |
| Cornetto, Wall's Ice Cream* | 1 Cone/75g | 195.0 | 10.0 | 260 | 3.7 | 34.5 | 12.9 | 0.0 |
| Creme Egg, Cadbury* | 1 Cone/115ml | 270.0 | 13.0 | 235 | 2.9 | 29.3 | 11.6 | 0.0 |
| Cup Cornet, Wafer Cone, Askeys* | 1 Cone/4g | 13.0 | 0.0 | 376 | 10.7 | 77.6 | 2.5 | 0.0 |
| Dairy Milk, Mint, Cadbury* | 1 Cone/115mll | 190.0 | 9.0 | 165 | 2.4 | 21.5 | 7.7 | 0.0 |
| Flake 99, Cadbury* | 1 Cone/125ml | 244.0 | 12.0 | 195 | 2.6 | 23.2 | 10.0 | 0.0 |

| INFO/WEIGHT | per Measure KCAL | FAT | Nutrition Values per 100g / 100ml KCAL | PROT | CARB | FAT | FIBRE |
|---|---|---|---|---|---|---|---|

**ICE CREAM CONE**

| | Measure INFO/WEIGHT | per Measure KCAL | FAT | KCAL | PROT | CARB | FAT | FIBRE |
|---|---|---|---|---|---|---|---|---|
| Flake 99, Strawberry, Cadbury* | 1 Serving/125g | 250.0 | 11.0 | 200 | 2.6 | 27.3 | 8.7 | 0.0 |
| Mini, Sainsbury's* | 1 Cone/18g | 66.0 | 4.0 | 366 | 4.4 | 39.8 | 21.0 | 3.4 |
| Mini, Tesco* | 1 Cone/48g | 152.0 | 9.0 | 316 | 4.1 | 31.5 | 19.3 | 0.8 |
| Raspberry & Vanilla, Refreshing, Skinny Cow* | 1 Cone/110ml | 122.0 | 3.0 | 111 | 1.7 | 20.4 | 2.5 | 1.5 |
| Smarties, Nestle* | 1 Cone/100g | 177.0 | 8.0 | 177 | 2.4 | 23.6 | 8.1 | 0.7 |
| Strawberry, BGTY, Sainsbury's* | 1 Cone/69g | 151.0 | 4.0 | 219 | 2.6 | 37.5 | 6.5 | 1.3 |
| Strawberry, M & S* | 1oz/28g | 74.0 | 4.0 | 263 | 3.5 | 31.1 | 14.0 | 0.4 |
| Strawberry & Vanilla, Asda* | 1 Cone/115ml | 193.0 | 9.0 | 168 | 1.8 | 22.6 | 7.8 | 0.1 |
| Strawberry & Vanilla, HL, Tesco* | 1 Serving/69g | 149.0 | 4.0 | 216 | 3.4 | 36.4 | 6.3 | 1.4 |
| Strawberry & Vanilla, M & S* | 1oz/28g | 81.0 | 5.0 | 290 | 4.2 | 30.9 | 16.5 | 0.7 |
| Strawberry & Vanilla, Sainsbury's* | 1 Cone/70g | 171.0 | 7.0 | 243 | 3.4 | 35.6 | 9.7 | 1.0 |
| Strawberry & Vanilla, Tesco* | 1 Cone/70g | 194.0 | 9.0 | 277 | 3.0 | 35.9 | 13.5 | 0.3 |
| Toffee Flavoured, Somerfield* | 1 Cone/110ml | 320.0 | 15.0 | 291 | 4.0 | 39.0 | 14.0 | 0.0 |
| Tropical, GFY, Asda* | 1 Cone/100g | 135.0 | 5.0 | 135 | 2.6 | 20.0 | 5.0 | 0.3 |

**ICE CREAM ROLL**

| | | | | | | | | |
|---|---|---|---|---|---|---|---|---|
| Arctic, Average | 1 Serving/70g | 140.0 | 5.0 | 200 | 4.1 | 33.3 | 6.6 | 0.0 |
| Basics, Somerfield* | 1/6 Roll/110ml | 233.0 | 7.0 | 212 | 4.0 | 35.0 | 6.0 | 0.0 |
| M & S* | 1oz/28g | 60.0 | 2.0 | 215 | 3.6 | 35.2 | 6.7 | 0.0 |
| Mini, Cadbury* | 1 Roll/45ml | 99.0 | 6.0 | 220 | 3.4 | 24.3 | 13.1 | 0.0 |
| Tesco* | ¼ Roll/57g | 131.0 | 5.0 | 230 | 3.7 | 34.5 | 8.6 | 0.4 |

**ICE CREAM SANDWICH**

| | | | | | | | | |
|---|---|---|---|---|---|---|---|---|
| Mint, Skinny Cow* | 1 Sandwich/71g | 140.0 | 2.0 | 197 | 4.2 | 39.4 | 2.8 | 1.4 |
| Wich, Ben & Jerry's* | 1 Pack/117g | 398.0 | 20.0 | 340 | 4.0 | 44.0 | 17.0 | 1.0 |

**ICE LOLLY**

| | | | | | | | | |
|---|---|---|---|---|---|---|---|---|
| Assorted, Iceland* | 1 Lolly/51g | 33.0 | 0.0 | 65 | 0.0 | 16.2 | 0.0 | 0.0 |
| Assorted, Safeway* | 1 Lolly/31ml | 26.0 | 0.0 | 85 | 0.0 | 20.9 | 0.0 | 0.1 |
| Baby, Tesco* | 1 Lolly/32g | 26.0 | 0.0 | 80 | 0.1 | 20.0 | 0.0 | 0.1 |
| Berry Burst, Sainsbury's* | 1 Serving/90ml | 93.0 | 2.0 | 103 | 1.1 | 20.8 | 1.8 | 0.7 |
| Blackcurrant, Dairy Split, Sainsbury's* | 1 Lolly/73ml | 88.0 | 3.0 | 121 | 1.8 | 20.4 | 3.6 | 0.1 |
| Blackcurrant, Ribena* | 1 Lolly/55ml | 43.0 | 0.0 | 79 | 0.0 | 19.2 | 0.0 | 0.0 |
| Blackcurrant Split, Iceland* | 1 Lolly/75g | 61.0 | 2.0 | 81 | 1.1 | 12.0 | 3.2 | 0.1 |
| Bournville, Cadbury* | 1 Lolly/110g | 269.0 | 17.0 | 245 | 2.5 | 23.2 | 15.6 | 0.0 |
| Calippo, Lemon Lime, Mini, Wall's Ice Cream* | 1 Lolly/80g | 68.0 | 0.0 | 85 | 0.0 | 21.0 | 0.0 | 0.2 |
| Calippo, Orange, Mini, Wall's Ice Cream* | 1 Lolly/78g | 70.0 | 0.0 | 90 | 0.0 | 21.9 | 0.0 | 0.2 |
| Calippo, Strawberry Tropical, Wall's Ice Cream* | 1 Lolly/105g | 89.0 | 0.0 | 85 | 0.1 | 21.0 | 0.1 | 0.2 |
| Calippo Shots, Cool Lemon, Wall's Ice Cream* | 1oz/28g | 8.0 | 0.0 | 28 | 0.1 | 3.9 | 1.3 | 0.0 |
| Calippo Shots, Twisted Berry, Wall's Ice Cream* | 1oz/28g | 8.0 | 0.0 | 28 | 0.1 | 4.2 | 1.2 | 0.0 |
| Choc & Almond, Mini, Tesco* | 1 Lolly/31g | 103.0 | 7.0 | 331 | 4.4 | 24.8 | 23.8 | 0.9 |
| Choc Lime Split, Morrisons* | 1 Lolly/73ml | 120.0 | 6.0 | 164 | 1.6 | 20.4 | 8.4 | 0.1 |
| Chocolate, Mini Milk, Milk Time, Wall's Ice Cream* | 1 Lolly/23g | 31.0 | 1.0 | 135 | 4.3 | 22.0 | 3.1 | 1.0 |
| Chocolate, Plain, Mini, Tesco* | 1 Lolly/31g | 94.0 | 7.0 | 304 | 3.1 | 24.8 | 21.4 | 1.2 |
| Chocolate, Pooh Stick, Nestle* | 1 Lolly/40g | 36.0 | 1.0 | 89 | 2.1 | 12.9 | 3.6 | 0.0 |
| Chocolate & Vanilla, Sainsbury's* | 1 Lolly/40g | 143.0 | 10.0 | 357 | 3.7 | 28.7 | 25.3 | 2.2 |
| Cider Refresher, Treats* | 1 Lolly/70ml | 54.0 | 0.0 | 77 | 0.0 | 19.2 | 0.0 | 0.0 |
| Creamy Tropical Sorbet, Sticks, Waitrose* | 1 Lolly/85g | 100.0 | 2.0 | 118 | 1.9 | 22.9 | 2.1 | 0.8 |
| Elderflower, Tubes, Frozen, M & S* | 1oz/28g | 23.0 | 0.0 | 82 | 0.1 | 20.5 | 0.1 | 0.2 |
| Exotic Fruit, Mini, HL, Tesco* | 1 Lolly/31g | 41.0 | 1.0 | 131 | 1.0 | 26.4 | 2.0 | 1.0 |
| Exotic Fruit, Tesco* | 1 Lolly/32g | 41.0 | 1.0 | 131 | 1.8 | 26.4 | 2.0 | 0.6 |
| Exotic Split, Bars, M & S* | 1oz/28g | 36.0 | 1.0 | 127 | 2.5 | 25.0 | 1.9 | 0.4 |
| Fab, Nestle* | 1 Lolly/57g | 78.0 | 3.0 | 136 | 0.5 | 22.8 | 4.7 | 0.2 |
| Fab, Orange, Nestle* | 1 Lolly/58g | 81.0 | 3.0 | 140 | 0.6 | 24.0 | 4.7 | 0.0 |
| Feast, Chocolate, Mini, Wall's Ice Cream* | 1 Lolly/52g | 165.0 | 12.0 | 318 | 3.3 | 24.0 | 23.0 | 0.0 |
| Feast, Ice Cream, Original, Wall's Ice Cream* | 1 Lolly/92ml | 294.0 | 22.0 | 320 | 3.2 | 23.8 | 23.5 | 0.0 |

# ICE LOLLY

| | INFO/WEIGHT | KCAL | FAT | KCAL | PROT | CARB | FAT | FIBRE |
|---|---|---|---|---|---|---|---|---|
| Feast, Toffee, Mini, Wall's Ice Cream* | 1 Lolly/52g | 163.0 | 12.0 | 313 | 3.0 | 24.0 | 23.0 | 0.0 |
| Feast, Wall's Ice Cream* | 1 Lolly/92ml | 276.0 | 20.0 | 300 | 3.2 | 22.0 | 22.0 | 0.0 |
| Fruit, Red, Tesco* | 1 Lolly/32g | 40.0 | 1.0 | 128 | 1.8 | 25.6 | 2.0 | 0.6 |
| Fruit Ices, Made with Orange Juice, Del Monte* | 1 Lolly/75ml | 79.0 | 0.0 | 105 | 0.5 | 25.7 | 0.0 | 0.0 |
| Fruit Luxury, Mini, Co-Op* | 1 Lolly/45g | 58.0 | 3.0 | 130 | 2.0 | 18.0 | 6.0 | 0.2 |
| Fruit Pastilles, Rowntree's* | 1 Lolly/65ml | 61.0 | 0.0 | 94 | 0.1 | 23.2 | 0.0 | 0.0 |
| Fruit Split, Asda* | 1 Lolly/74g | 85.0 | 3.0 | 115 | 1.7 | 19.0 | 3.6 | 0.0 |
| Fruit Splits, Assorted, Somerfield* | 1 Lolly/73ml | 74.0 | 2.0 | 102 | 0.0 | 18.0 | 3.0 | 0.0 |
| Fruit Splits, Treats* | 1 Lolly/75ml | 77.0 | 3.0 | 103 | 1.4 | 17.6 | 4.1 | 0.0 |
| Fruity 'n' Freezy, Asda* | 1 Lolly/30ml | 24.0 | 0.0 | 80 | 0.1 | 20.0 | 0.0 | 0.0 |
| Funny Foot, Wall's Ice Cream* | 1 Lolly | 83.0 | 5.0 | 102 | 2.0 | 12.5 | 6.0 | 0.0 |
| Ice Lolly, Twister, Choc, Wall's Ice Cream* | 1 Mini Lolly/27g | 40.0 | 2.0 | 150 | 3.5 | 22.0 | 6.0 | 0.9 |
| Icicles, All Flavours, Freezepops, Calypso* | 1 Lolly/50ml | 1.0 | 0.0 | 1 | 0.0 | 0.3 | 0.0 | 0.0 |
| Kiwi Burst, Pineapple Sorbet in Kiwi Ice, Sainsbury's* | 1 Serving/90ml | 76.0 | 0.0 | 84 | 0.1 | 20.7 | 0.1 | 0.4 |
| Lemon & Lime, Mini Bar, M & S* | 1 Lolly/50g | 47.0 | 0.0 | 95 | 0.1 | 23.6 | 0.1 | 0.2 |
| Lemon & Lime, Tubes, Frozen, M & S* | 1oz/28g | 27.0 | 0.0 | 95 | 0.1 | 23.6 | 0.1 | 0.2 |
| Lemonade & Cola, Morrisons* | 1 Lolly/55ml | 36.0 | 0.0 | 65 | 0.0 | 16.2 | 0.0 | 0.0 |
| Lemonade Sparkle, Wall's Ice Cream* | 1 Lolly/55g | 40.0 | 0.0 | 73 | 0.0 | 18.2 | 0.0 | 0.0 |
| Mango & Lemon, BGTY, Sainsbury's* | 1 Lolly/72g | 84.0 | 0.0 | 116 | 0.3 | 28.1 | 0.3 | 0.5 |
| Mango & Passion Fruit, TTD, Sainsbury's* | 1 Lolly/73ml | 76.0 | 0.0 | 104 | 0.2 | 25.5 | 0.1 | 0.6 |
| Mango & Passion Fruit Smoothie, Waitrose* | 1 Lolly/73g | 60.0 | 0.0 | 82 | 0.7 | 18.9 | 0.4 | 0.7 |
| Mega Truffle, Nestle* | 1 Lolly/71g | 217.0 | 14.0 | 305 | 3.2 | 28.0 | 20.1 | 0.8 |
| Milk, Blue Parrot Cafe, Sainsbury's* | 1 Lolly/30ml | 34.0 | 1.0 | 113 | 2.7 | 18.0 | 3.3 | 0.3 |
| Milk Chocolate & Crisped Wheat, Co-Op* | 1 Lolly/110g | 258.0 | 13.0 | 235 | 3.0 | 28.0 | 12.0 | 0.7 |
| Mint Chocolate, Tesco* | 1 Lolly/70g | 234.0 | 14.0 | 334 | 3.6 | 35.4 | 19.8 | 1.2 |
| Nobbly Bobbly, Nestle* | 1 Lolly/70ml | 158.0 | 8.0 | 226 | 2.3 | 27.6 | 11.7 | 0.3 |
| Orange, Real Fruit Juice, Sainsbury's* | 1 Lolly/73ml | 49.0 | 0.0 | 67 | 0.2 | 16.5 | 0.1 | 0.1 |
| Orange, Real Juice, Sainsbury's* | 1 Lolly/72ml | 63.0 | 0.0 | 88 | 0.7 | 21.0 | 0.1 | 0.1 |
| Orange, Real Juice, Tesco* | 1 Lolly/32g | 25.0 | 0.0 | 78 | 0.6 | 18.7 | 0.0 | 0.3 |
| Orange, Ribena* | 1 Lolly/110ml | 95.0 | 0.0 | 86 | 0.1 | 21.4 | 0.0 | 0.0 |
| Orange, Tesco* | 1 Lolly/77g | 53.0 | 0.0 | 68 | 0.2 | 16.8 | 0.0 | 0.3 |
| Orange, Water, Iceland* | 1 Lolly/75g | 73.0 | 0.0 | 98 | 0.2 | 24.4 | 0.0 | 0.2 |
| Orange Juice, Asda* | 1 Lolly/70g | 58.0 | 0.0 | 83 | 0.7 | 20.0 | 0.0 | 0.0 |
| Orange Juice, Bar, M & S* | 1 Lolly/75g | 64.0 | 0.0 | 86 | 0.5 | 21.0 | 0.0 | 0.1 |
| Orange Juice, Freshly Squeezed, Finest, Tesco* | 1 Lolly/80ml | 89.0 | 0.0 | 111 | 0.7 | 27.0 | 0.0 | 0.0 |
| Orange Juice, Freshly Squeezed, Waitrose* | 1 Lolly/73g | 88.0 | 0.0 | 120 | 0.6 | 29.7 | 0.1 | 0.0 |
| Orange Juice, Morrisons* | 1 Lolly/55ml | 46.0 | 0.0 | 84 | 0.0 | 20.0 | 0.0 | 0.0 |
| Orange Juice, Tropicana* | 1 Lolly/50g | 42.0 | 0.0 | 85 | 0.5 | 20.7 | 0.0 | 0.0 |
| Orange Maid, Nestle* | 1 Lolly/73ml | 66.0 | 0.0 | 91 | 0.5 | 21.6 | 0.0 | 0.0 |
| Orange 'n' Cream, Tropicana* | 1 Lolly/65g | 83.0 | 3.0 | 129 | 1.4 | 20.5 | 4.5 | 0.3 |
| Pineapple, Dairy Split, Sainsbury's* | 1 Lolly/72ml | 84.0 | 3.0 | 116 | 1.8 | 19.0 | 3.6 | 0.1 |
| Pineapple, Real Fruit Juice, Sainsbury's* | 1 Lolly/73ml | 55.0 | 0.0 | 76 | 0.1 | 19.0 | 0.1 | 0.1 |
| Raspberry, Real Fruit Juice, Sainsbury's* | 1 Lolly/72g | 62.0 | 0.0 | 86 | 0.3 | 21.0 | 0.1 | 0.1 |
| Raspberry, Rocket Split, De Roma* | 1 Lolly/60ml | 65.0 | 3.0 | 108 | 1.0 | 16.2 | 4.3 | 0.2 |
| Raspberry, Smoothie, Iced, Del Monte* | 1 Lolly/90ml | 96.0 | 0.0 | 107 | 0.1 | 26.4 | 0.1 | 0.0 |
| Raspberry & Apple, Sainsbury's* | 1 Lolly/57ml | 39.0 | 0.0 | 68 | 0.1 | 17.1 | 0.1 | 0.1 |
| Real Fruit, Dairy Split, Sainsbury's* | 1 Lolly/73ml | 100.0 | 3.0 | 137 | 2.1 | 22.8 | 4.2 | 0.1 |
| Real Fruit Juice, Rocket, Blue Parrot Cafe, Sainsbury's* | 1 Lolly/58ml | 45.0 | 0.0 | 77 | 0.2 | 19.1 | 0.0 | 0.1 |
| Real Orange, Kids, Tesco* | 1 Lolly/32g | 25.0 | 0.0 | 78 | 0.6 | 18.7 | 0.0 | 0.3 |
| Refresher, Bassett's* | 1 Lolly/40g | 47.0 | 1.0 | 117 | 2.2 | 22.2 | 2.2 | 0.3 |
| Rocket, Sainsbury's* | 1 Lolly/58g | 42.0 | 0.0 | 72 | 0.1 | 17.8 | 0.1 | 0.1 |
| Rolo, Nestle* | 1 Lolly/75ml | 243.0 | 14.0 | 324 | 3.8 | 36.5 | 18.8 | 0.0 |
| Scooby-Doo, Freezepops, Calypso* | 1 Lolly/50ml | 14.0 | 0.0 | 28 | 0.0 | 7.0 | 0.0 | 0.0 |

| | Measure INFO/WEIGHT | per Measure KCAL | FAT | Nutrition Values per 100g / 100ml KCAL | PROT | CARB | FAT | FIBRE |
|---|---|---|---|---|---|---|---|---|
| **ICE LOLLY** | | | | | | | | |
| Solero, Exotic, Wall's Ice Cream* | 1 Lolly/82g | 99.0 | 2.0 | 121 | 1.6 | 21.9 | 2.8 | 0.5 |
| Solero, Orange Fresh, Wall's Ice Cream* | 1 Lolly/96g | 78.0 | 0.0 | 81 | 0.2 | 20.0 | 0.0 | 0.0 |
| Solero, Red Fruits, Wall's Ice Cream* | 1 Lolly/95g | 99.0 | 2.0 | 104 | 1.3 | 21.0 | 2.2 | 0.0 |
| Strawberries & Cream, Cadbury* | 1 Lolly/100ml | 225.0 | 12.0 | 225 | 2.9 | 27.0 | 11.7 | 0.0 |
| Strawberries 'n' Cream, Tropicana* | 1 Lolly/50g | 58.0 | 1.0 | 117 | 1.6 | 25.0 | 1.2 | 0.0 |
| Strawberry, Dairy Split, Sainsbury's* | 1 Lolly/73ml | 86.0 | 3.0 | 118 | 1.7 | 19.8 | 3.6 | 0.1 |
| Strawberry, Fruit Split, Iceland* | 1 Lolly/73g | 77.0 | 2.0 | 105 | 0.9 | 17.8 | 3.3 | 0.5 |
| Strawberry, Mini Milk, Milk Time, Wall's Ice Cream* | 1 Lolly/23g | 30.0 | 1.0 | 131 | 4.0 | 22.0 | 2.9 | 0.5 |
| Strawberry, Orange & Pineapple, Rocket, Iceland* | 1 Lolly/47g | 38.0 | 0.0 | 81 | 0.0 | 20.2 | 0.0 | 0.1 |
| Strawberry, So-Lo, Good Choice, Iceland* | 1 Lolly/66g | 85.0 | 1.0 | 128 | 2.4 | 25.6 | 1.8 | 0.1 |
| Strawberry & Banana, Smoothies, Sainsbury's* | 1 Lolly/60g | 100.0 | 3.0 | 166 | 1.5 | 28.0 | 5.3 | 0.2 |
| Strawberry & Vanilla, 99% Fat Free, So-Lo, Iceland* | 1 Lolly/92g | 98.0 | 0.0 | 107 | 2.3 | 23.5 | 0.4 | 2.2 |
| Strawberry Fruit, Double, Del Monte* | 1 Lolly/76g | 84.0 | 2.0 | 111 | 1.8 | 20.1 | 2.6 | 0.0 |
| Strawberry Split, Co-Op* | 1 Lolly/71ml | 75.0 | 2.0 | 105 | 1.0 | 17.0 | 3.0 | 0.1 |
| Tip Top, Calypso* | 1 Lolly/20ml | 6.0 | 0.0 | 30 | 0.1 | 7.1 | 0.1 | 0.0 |
| Traffic Light, Co-Op* | 1 Lolly/52g | 55.0 | 0.0 | 105 | 0.4 | 25.0 | 0.8 | 0.0 |
| Tropical, Mmmm, Tesco* | 1 Lolly/73g | 109.0 | 3.0 | 150 | 1.2 | 26.6 | 4.3 | 0.4 |
| Tropical Fruit, Starburst, Mars* | 1 Lolly/93ml | 94.0 | 0.0 | 101 | 0.3 | 24.8 | 0.1 | 0.0 |
| Tropical Fruit Sorbet, Waitrose* | 1 Lolly/110g | 90.0 | 2.0 | 82 | 1.5 | 14.5 | 2.0 | 0.2 |
| Twister, Wall's Ice Cream* | 1 Lolly/80ml | 76.0 | 2.0 | 95 | 0.6 | 18.4 | 1.9 | 0.0 |
| Vanilla, Mini Milk, Milk Time, Wall's Ice Cream* | 1 Lolly/23g | 29.0 | 1.0 | 127 | 3.8 | 21.0 | 2.9 | 0.3 |
| Vanilla, Pooh Stick, Nestle* | 1 Lolly/40g | 34.0 | 1.0 | 86 | 1.9 | 12.9 | 3.5 | 0.0 |
| Vimto* | 1 Lolly/73ml | 84.0 | 3.0 | 115 | 1.3 | 18.2 | 4.1 | 0.1 |
| Wonka Super Sour Tastic, Nestle* | 1 Lolly/60ml | 84.0 | 2.0 | 140 | 0.0 | 26.1 | 3.6 | 0.0 |
| Zoom, Nestle* | 1 Lolly/58ml | 54.0 | 0.0 | 93 | 0.9 | 20.6 | 0.7 | 0.0 |
| **ICED DESSERT** | | | | | | | | |
| Cafe Latte, BGTY, Sainsbury's* | 1 Serving/75g | 104.0 | 3.0 | 139 | 2.9 | 23.7 | 3.6 | 3.3 |
| Chocolate & Mallow, GFY, Asda* | 1 Pot/150ml | 142.0 | 2.0 | 95 | 2.0 | 19.0 | 1.2 | 2.3 |
| Chocolate & Marshmallow Swirls, BGTY, Sainsbury's* | ¼ Pot/75g | 130.0 | 2.0 | 173 | 3.9 | 33.8 | 2.5 | 2.8 |
| Chocolate Mint Crisp, COU, M & S* | ¼ Pot/85g | 115.0 | 2.0 | 135 | 5.4 | 21.9 | 2.9 | 1.0 |
| Summer Fruits, Yoghurt, BGTY, Sainsbury's* | ¼ Pot/85g | 105.0 | 1.0 | 124 | 3.3 | 25.6 | 0.9 | 0.5 |
| Toffee, 3% Fat, M & S* | 1oz/28g | 51.0 | 1.0 | 183 | 3.1 | 37.2 | 2.4 | 0.5 |
| Toffee & Walnut, Free From, Sainsbury's* | ¼ Tub/81g | 203.0 | 10.0 | 251 | 3.3 | 31.6 | 12.4 | 0.3 |
| Toffee Flavoured, Dairy, BGTY, Sainsbury's* | 1 Serving/70g | 103.0 | 3.0 | 147 | 2.7 | 24.0 | 4.5 | 0.2 |
| Vanilla, 3% Fat, M & S* | 1oz/28g | 40.0 | 1.0 | 143 | 3.5 | 25.9 | 2.8 | 0.7 |
| Vanilla, Dairy, Sainsbury's* | 1 Serving/65g | 77.0 | 2.0 | 119 | 3.0 | 19.9 | 3.0 | 3.7 |
| Vanilla, Non Dairy, Soft, Swedish Glace* | 1 Serving/100g | 200.0 | 10.0 | 200 | 2.5 | 25.0 | 10.0 | 1.0 |
| Vanilla & Chocolate, HL, Tesco* | 1 Pot/73g | 104.0 | 2.0 | 143 | 3.0 | 26.9 | 2.6 | 0.7 |
| Vanilla Flavour, HE, Tesco* | 1 Serving/50g | 67.0 | 1.0 | 134 | 3.9 | 24.1 | 2.4 | 4.6 |
| **INDIAN MEAL** | | | | | | | | |
| Banquet, for One, COU, M & S* | 1 Pack/500g | 400.0 | 6.0 | 80 | 6.7 | 10.2 | 1.2 | 3.1 |
| for One, Asda* | 1 Pack/550g | 834.0 | 25.0 | 152 | 6.7 | 20.9 | 4.6 | 1.4 |
| for One, Eat Smart, Safeway* | 1 Serving/600g | 690.0 | 16.0 | 115 | 6.5 | 16.2 | 2.6 | 2.0 |
| for One, GFY, Asda* | 1 Serving/495g | 643.0 | 23.0 | 130 | 8.0 | 14.0 | 4.7 | 1.0 |
| for One, HE, Tesco* | 1 Pack/420g | 437.0 | 9.0 | 104 | 7.4 | 14.0 | 2.1 | 1.4 |
| for One, Vegetarian, Asda* | 1 Pack/499g | 789.0 | 45.0 | 158 | 3.2 | 16.0 | 9.0 | 1.4 |
| for Two, Hot, Takeaway, Tesco* | 1 Pack/825g | 1215.0 | 61.0 | 147 | 6.6 | 13.6 | 7.3 | 1.9 |
| for Two, Menu, Tesco* | 1 Serving/537g | 811.0 | 34.0 | 151 | 6.3 | 17.0 | 6.4 | 0.8 |
| for Two, Peshwari Naan, Finest, Tesco* | ½ Pack/200g | 612.0 | 18.0 | 306 | 8.3 | 48.3 | 8.9 | 5.2 |
| **INSTANT WHIP** | | | | | | | | |
| Chocolate Flavour, Dry, Bird's* | 1oz/28g | 109.0 | 2.0 | 390 | 3.8 | 80.5 | 5.9 | 0.7 |
| Strawberry Flavour, Dry, Bird's* | 1oz/28g | 112.0 | 2.0 | 400 | 2.5 | 85.0 | 5.4 | 0.4 |

| | Measure INFO/WEIGHT | per Measure KCAL | FAT | Nutrition Values per 100g / 100ml KCAL | PROT | CARB | FAT | FIBRE |
|---|---|---|---|---|---|---|---|---|
| **JACKFRUIT** | | | | | | | | |
| *Raw, Average, Flesh Only* | 1 Portion/162g | 155.0 | 1.0 | 95 | 1.5 | 24.4 | 0.3 | 1.6 |
| *Raw, Average, Weighed with Skin & Seeds* | 1oz/28g | 26.0 | 0.0 | 94 | 1.5 | 24.0 | 0.3 | 1.6 |
| **JALFREZI** | | | | | | | | |
| Chicken, & Pilau Rice, Sainsbury's* | 1 Pack/500g | 600.0 | 20.0 | 120 | 6.9 | 13.9 | 4.1 | 1.5 |
| Chicken, & Pilau Rice, Takeaway, Asda* | 1 Pack/558g | 792.0 | 23.0 | 142 | 7.0 | 19.0 | 4.2 | 1.3 |
| Chicken, & Rice, Serves 1, Tesco* | 1 Serving/475g | 589.0 | 38.0 | 124 | 7.4 | 5.7 | 8.0 | 1.6 |
| Chicken, Asda* | 1 Pack/340g | 415.0 | 20.0 | 122 | 10.0 | 7.0 | 6.0 | 1.6 |
| Chicken, Finest, Tesco* | 1 Pack/350g | 402.0 | 16.0 | 115 | 10.4 | 6.9 | 4.7 | 1.2 |
| Chicken, GFY, Asda* | 1 Pack/350g | 238.0 | 3.0 | 68 | 9.0 | 6.0 | 0.9 | 1.8 |
| Chicken, Hot & Spicy, Sainsbury's* | ½ Pack/200g | 228.0 | 11.0 | 114 | 12.8 | 2.9 | 5.7 | 1.0 |
| Chicken, Medium, GFY, Asda* | 1 Pack/644g | 972.0 | 28.0 | 151 | 6.0 | 22.0 | 4.3 | 0.9 |
| Chicken, with Basmati Rice, Eat Smart, Safeway* | 1 Pack/400g | 300.0 | 4.0 | 75 | 6.8 | 8.5 | 1.0 | 1.7 |
| Chicken, with Basmati Rice, Weight Watchers* | 1 Pack/330g | 238.0 | 2.0 | 72 | 5.0 | 11.8 | 0.5 | 0.5 |
| Chicken, with Pilau Basmati Rice, Frozen, Patak's* | 1 Pack/400g | 556.0 | 18.0 | 139 | 9.8 | 14.7 | 4.6 | 0.9 |
| Chicken, with Pilau Rice, BGTY, Sainsbury's* | 1 Pack/400g | 337.0 | 4.0 | 84 | 7.1 | 11.5 | 1.1 | 1.9 |
| Chicken, with Pilau Rice, GFY, Asda* | 1 Pack/446g | 495.0 | 11.0 | 111 | 8.0 | 14.0 | 2.5 | 1.2 |
| Chicken, with Pilau Rice, Perfectly Balanced, Waitrose* | 1 Pack/400g | 388.0 | 4.0 | 97 | 8.0 | 14.0 | 1.0 | 2.4 |
| Chicken, with Pilau Rice, Tesco* | 1 Pack/460g | 506.0 | 17.0 | 110 | 5.3 | 13.6 | 3.8 | 0.9 |
| Chicken, with Rice, COU, M & S* | 1 Pack/400g | 320.0 | 4.0 | 80 | 9.2 | 8.3 | 1.1 | 1.2 |
| Chicken, with Rice, Morrisons* | 1 Pack/400g | 564.0 | 21.0 | 141 | 7.7 | 15.9 | 5.2 | 1.4 |
| Chicken, with Rice, Tesco* | 1 Pack/550g | 731.0 | 26.0 | 133 | 5.5 | 17.0 | 4.8 | 1.0 |
| Meal for One, M & S* | 1 Serving/500g | 700.0 | 35.0 | 140 | 6.1 | 13.4 | 7.0 | 3.0 |
| Vegetable, Take Away Menu for 1, BGTY, Sainsbury's* | 1 Pack/148g | 43.0 | 0.0 | 29 | 1.8 | 5.4 | 0.0 | 2.3 |
| Vegetable, Waitrose* | 1 Pack/400g | 256.0 | 16.0 | 64 | 2.2 | 4.7 | 4.0 | 3.7 |
| Vegetable, with Rice, Birds Eye* | 1 Pack/350g | 353.0 | 4.0 | 101 | 2.5 | 20.2 | 1.1 | 1.0 |
| **JAM** | | | | | | | | |
| *Apricot, Average* | 1 Tbsp/15g | 37.0 | 0.0 | 248 | 0.2 | 61.6 | 0.0 | 1.5 |
| *Apricot, Reduced Sugar, Average* | 1 Serving/20g | 37.0 | 0.0 | 186 | 0.4 | 46.0 | 0.3 | 0.4 |
| *Black Cherry, Average* | 1 Tbsp/15g | 37.0 | 0.0 | 247 | 0.4 | 61.2 | 0.3 | 0.4 |
| Blackberry, Extra Special, Asda* | 1 Tbsp/15g | 29.0 | 0.0 | 190 | 0.9 | 45.0 | 0.7 | 0.0 |
| *Blackcurrant, Average* | 1 Tbsp/15g | 38.0 | 0.0 | 250 | 0.2 | 62.3 | 0.0 | 1.0 |
| *Blackcurrant, Reduced Sugar, Average* | 1 Tsp/6g | 10.0 | 0.0 | 178 | 0.4 | 44.4 | 0.1 | 1.0 |
| Blueberry, Best, Hartley's* | 1 Tsp/20g | 49.0 | 0.0 | 244 | 0.3 | 60.6 | 0.1 | 0.0 |
| Blueberry, St Dalfour* | 1 Serving/20g | 46.0 | 0.0 | 228 | 0.5 | 56.0 | 0.2 | 2.2 |
| Blueberry & Blackberry, Baxters* | 1 Tsp/15g | 38.0 | 0.0 | 252 | 0.0 | 63.0 | 0.0 | 1.2 |
| Concorde Grape, Sugar Free, Smucker's* | 1 Serving/17g | 0.0 | 0.0 | 0 | 0.0 | 29.4 | 0.0 | 0.0 |
| Country Berries, Luxury, Baxters* | 1 Tsp/15g | 38.0 | 0.0 | 252 | 0.0 | 63.0 | 0.0 | 1.1 |
| Damson, Extra Fruit, Best, Hartley's* | 1 Tsp/5g | 12.0 | 0.0 | 244 | 0.2 | 60.8 | 0.0 | 0.0 |
| Kiwi & Goosberry, 66% Fruit, Asda* | 1 Serving/30g | 56.0 | 0.0 | 187 | 0.5 | 45.0 | 0.5 | 0.0 |
| *Mixed Fruit, Average* | 1 Tbsp/15g | 38.0 | 0.0 | 252 | 0.3 | 63.5 | 0.0 | 0.5 |
| Plum, Tesco* | 1 Serving/50g | 130.0 | 0.0 | 261 | 0.2 | 64.4 | 0.0 | 0.6 |
| *Rasberry, Reduced Sugar, Average* | 1 Tsp/6g | 10.0 | 0.0 | 160 | 0.5 | 39.3 | 0.2 | 0.6 |
| *Raspberry, Average* | 1 Tbsp/15g | 36.0 | 0.0 | 239 | 0.6 | 58.6 | 0.1 | 0.9 |
| *Raspberry, Seedless, Average* | 1 Tsp/10g | 26.0 | 0.0 | 257 | 0.4 | 63.6 | 0.0 | 0.3 |
| Rhubarb & Ginger, Baxters* | 1 Tsp/15g | 31.0 | 0.0 | 210 | 0.0 | 53.0 | 0.0 | 0.6 |
| *Strawberry, Average* | 1 Tsp/10g | 25.0 | 0.0 | 253 | 0.3 | 62.7 | 0.0 | 0.6 |
| *Strawberry, Reduced Sugar, Average* | 1 Tbsp/15g | 28.0 | 0.0 | 187 | 0.4 | 45.8 | 0.3 | 0.2 |
| Strawberry & Redcurrant, Reduced Sugar, Streamline* | 1 Tbsp/15g | 29.0 | 0.0 | 192 | 0.4 | 46.8 | 0.3 | 0.0 |
| Wild Blackberry Jelly, Baxters* | 1 Tsp/15g | 31.0 | 0.0 | 210 | 0.0 | 53.0 | 0.0 | 1.2 |
| **JAMBALAYA** | | | | | | | | |
| American Style, Tesco* | 1 Serving/275g | 432.0 | 19.0 | 157 | 7.7 | 16.0 | 7.0 | 0.5 |
| Cajun Chicken, BGTY, Sainsbury's* | 1 Pack/400g | 364.0 | 6.0 | 91 | 7.7 | 11.9 | 1.4 | 1.1 |
| Chicken, Spicy, Eat Smart, Morrisons* | 1 Pack/400g | 384.0 | 5.0 | 96 | 7.4 | 13.9 | 1.2 | 2.7 |

**J**

| | Measure INFO/WEIGHT | per Measure KCAL | FAT | Nutrition Values per 100g / 100ml KCAL | PROT | CARB | FAT | FIBRE |
|---|---|---|---|---|---|---|---|---|
| **JAMBALAYA** | | | | | | | | |
| COU, M & S* | 1 Pack/400g | 340.0 | 8.0 | 85 | 6.5 | 10.8 | 2.0 | 0.9 |
| GFY, Asda* | 1 Pack/450g | 387.0 | 3.0 | 86 | 6.0 | 14.0 | 0.7 | 2.7 |
| M & S* | 1 Pack/480g | 552.0 | 17.0 | 115 | 5.8 | 14.6 | 3.5 | 1.2 |
| Tesco* | 1 Pack/550g | 764.0 | 36.0 | 139 | 6.9 | 13.1 | 6.6 | 1.1 |
| **JELLY** | | | | | | | | |
| Apple & Watermelon, Low Calorie, Hartley's* | 1 Serving/175g | 5.0 | 0.0 | 3 | 0.0 | 0.3 | 0.0 | 0.3 |
| Blackberry, Unprepared, Morrisons* | 1 Serving/20g | 52.0 | 0.0 | 261 | 0.3 | 65.0 | 0.0 | 0.0 |
| Blackcurrant, Made Up, Rowntree's* | ¼ Jelly/140ml | 100.0 | 0.0 | 71 | 1.4 | 16.4 | 0.1 | 0.0 |
| Blackcurrant, Made Up, Sainsbury's* | ¼ Jelly/150g | 97.0 | 0.0 | 65 | 1.2 | 15.1 | 0.0 | 0.0 |
| Blackcurrant, Sugar Free, Unprepared, Rowntree's* | 1 Pack/24g | 73.0 | 0.0 | 305 | 50.0 | 25.0 | 0.0 | 25.0 |
| Blackcurrant, Tesco* | 1 Serving/100g | 84.0 | 0.0 | 84 | 0.2 | 20.5 | 0.1 | 0.4 |
| Bramble, Tesco* | 1 Serving/100g | 257.0 | 0.0 | 257 | 0.3 | 63.7 | 0.1 | 1.3 |
| Crystals, Orange, Sugar Free, Bird's* | 1 Sachet/12g | 39.0 | 0.0 | 335 | 62.5 | 6.4 | 0.9 | 0.0 |
| Crystals, Orange & Peach, Sugar Free, Weight Watchers* | ½ Pack/204g | 14.0 | 0.0 | 7 | 0.0 | 1.4 | 0.1 | 0.0 |
| Crystals, Strawberry, Made Up, Tesco* | 1 Serving/145g | 9.0 | 0.0 | 6 | 1.3 | 0.3 | 0.0 | 0.0 |
| Exotic Fruit, M & S* | 1 Pot/175g | 140.0 | 0.0 | 80 | 0.1 | 18.9 | 0.2 | 0.9 |
| Fresh Fruit, M & S* | 1 Pot/175g | 131.0 | 0.0 | 75 | 0.2 | 18.4 | 0.1 | 0.3 |
| Lemon & Lime, Sugar Free, Unprepared, Rowntree's* | 1oz/28g | 85.0 | 0.0 | 305 | 4.5 | 60.7 | 0.0 | 0.0 |
| Lime, Made Up, Rowntree's* | ¼ Jelly/140ml | 100.0 | 0.0 | 71 | 1.3 | 16.3 | 0.1 | 0.0 |
| Lime, Unprepared, Co-Op* | 1 Pack/135g | 397.0 | 0.0 | 294 | 5.5 | 68.1 | 0.0 | 1.0 |
| Lime, Unprepared, Somerfield* | 1 Pack/135g | 391.0 | 0.0 | 290 | 6.0 | 66.0 | 0.0 | 0.0 |
| Lime Flavour, Unprepared, Waitrose* | 1 Square/11g | 33.0 | 0.0 | 296 | 4.5 | 69.5 | 0.0 | 0.0 |
| *Made Up with Water, Average* | *1oz/28g* | *17.0* | *0.0* | *61* | *1.2* | *15.1* | *0.0* | *0.0* |
| Mandarin, Aroma, M & S* | 1oz/28g | 17.0 | 0.0 | 60 | 0.2 | 14.6 | 0.0 | 0.4 |
| Mandarin & Pineapple, Sainsbury's* | 1 Pot/125g | 95.0 | 0.0 | 76 | 0.2 | 18.9 | 0.1 | 1.2 |
| Orange, Quickset, Unprepared, Rowntree's* | 1oz/28g | 95.0 | 0.0 | 340 | 0.0 | 84.0 | 0.0 | 3.0 |
| Orange, Sugar Free, Crystals, Dry Weight, Hartley's* | 1 Pack/26g | 66.0 | 0.0 | 254 | 57.4 | 6.1 | 0.0 | 0.0 |
| Orange, Sugar Free, Rowntree's* | 1 Serving/140ml | 8.0 | 0.0 | 6 | 1.4 | 0.1 | 0.0 | 0.0 |
| Orange, Sugar Free, Unprepared, Asda* | 1 Serving/12g | 36.0 | 0.0 | 303 | 63.6 | 12.0 | 0.1 | 0.2 |
| Orange, Unprepared, Rowntree's* | 1 Square/11g | 33.0 | 0.0 | 296 | 4.4 | 69.6 | 0.0 | 0.0 |
| Pineapple, with Pineapple Pieces, Tesco* | 1 Serving/120g | 96.0 | 0.0 | 80 | 1.2 | 18.6 | 0.1 | 0.7 |
| Raspberry, Crystals, Vegetarian, Just Wholefoods* | 1 Packet/85g | 293.0 | 0.0 | 345 | 0.5 | 85.7 | 0.0 | 0.0 |
| Raspberry, Unprepared, Somerfield* | ¼ Serving/38g | 111.0 | 0.0 | 292 | 6.0 | 66.0 | 0.0 | 0.0 |
| Raspberry & Rose, Aroma, M & S* | 1oz/28g | 14.0 | 0.0 | 50 | 0.2 | 11.9 | 0.2 | 0.4 |
| Raspberry Flavour, Sugar Free, Made Up, Rowntree's* | 1 Serving/140ml | 9.0 | 0.0 | 6 | 1.4 | 0.1 | 0.0 | 0.0 |
| Raspberry Flavour, Tesco* | 1 Serving/34g | 22.0 | 0.0 | 64 | 1.0 | 15.0 | 0.0 | 0.1 |
| Raspberry Flavoured, with Raspberries, M & S* | 1 Sm Pot/175g | 105.0 | 1.0 | 60 | 0.2 | 14.0 | 0.3 | 1.5 |
| *Redcurrant, Average* | *1oz/28g* | *70.0* | *0.0* | *250* | *0.1* | *64.4* | *0.0* | *0.0* |
| Strawberry, No Added Sugar, Hartley's* | 1 Pot/115g | 3.0 | 0.0 | 3 | 0.0 | 0.4 | 0.0 | 0.3 |
| Strawberry, Sugar Free, Crystals, Dry Weight, Hartley's* | 1 Sachet/26g | 73.0 | 0.0 | 280 | 56.8 | 13.1 | 0.0 | 0.0 |
| Strawberry, Unprepared, Co-Op* | 1 Pack/135g | 402.0 | 0.0 | 298 | 5.5 | 69.1 | 0.0 | 0.0 |
| Strawberry & Raspberry, Sainsbury's* | ½ Pot/280g | 230.0 | 0.0 | 82 | 0.2 | 20.2 | 0.0 | 1.2 |
| Strawberry Flavour, Sugar Free, Made Up, Rowntree's* | 1 Serving/140ml | 10.0 | 0.0 | 7 | 1.5 | 0.1 | 0.0 | 0.0 |
| Strawberry Flavour, Sugar Free, Unprepared, Rowntree's* | 1oz/28g | 84.0 | 0.0 | 300 | 64.9 | 3.0 | 0.0 | 0.0 |
| Sugar Free, Dry, Tesco* | 1 Pack/13g | 36.0 | 0.0 | 285 | 55.4 | 15.6 | 0.0 | 0.2 |
| Sugar Free, Dry, Tesco* | 1 Pack/13g | 36.0 | 0.0 | 285 | 55.4 | 15.6 | 0.0 | 0.2 |
| **JELLY BABIES** | | | | | | | | |
| Bassett's* | 1 Baby/6g | 20.0 | 0.0 | 335 | 4.0 | 79.5 | 0.0 | 0.0 |
| Sainsbury's* | 1 Serving/70g | 247.0 | 0.0 | 353 | 4.1 | 82.5 | 0.7 | 0.3 |
| **JELLY BEANS** | | | | | | | | |
| Asda* | 1 Bag/100g | 364.0 | 0.0 | 364 | 0.1 | 90.0 | 0.4 | 0.2 |
| Jelly Belly* | 35 Beans/40g | 140.0 | 0.0 | 350 | 0.0 | 90.0 | 0.0 | 0.0 |
| M & S* | 1 Bag/113g | 407.0 | 0.0 | 360 | 0.1 | 89.6 | 0.0 | 0.0 |

**J**

| | Measure INFO/WEIGHT | per Measure KCAL | FAT | Nutrition Values per 100g / 100ml KCAL | PROT | CARB | FAT | FIBRE |
|---|---|---|---|---|---|---|---|---|
| **JELLY BEANS** | | | | | | | | |
| No Added Sugar, Jelly Belly* | 1 Serving/40g | 80.0 | 0.0 | 200 | 0.0 | 50.0 | 0.0 | 20.0 |
| Rowntree's* | 1 Pack/35g | 128.0 | 0.0 | 367 | 0.0 | 91.8 | 0.0 | 0.0 |
| **JELLY TOTS** | | | | | | | | |
| Rowntree's* | 1 Pack/42g | 145.0 | 0.0 | 346 | 0.1 | 86.5 | 0.0 | 0.0 |
| **JERKY** | | | | | | | | |
| Beef, Peppered, Jack Link's* | 1 Serving/28g | 80.0 | 1.0 | 286 | 53.6 | 14.3 | 1.8 | 0.0 |
| Shiitake Mushroom, Hot & Spicy, Primal Strips* | 1 Pack/28g | 108.0 | 4.0 | 386 | 21.4 | 42.9 | 14.3 | 21.4 |
| Soy, Cajun Chick'n, Vegan, Tasty Eats* | 1 Pack/28g | 90.0 | 3.0 | 321 | 42.9 | 14.3 | 10.7 | 7.1 |
| **JUICE** | | | | | | | | |
| 100% Vegetable, V8* | 1 Bottle/354ml | 57.0 | 0.0 | 16 | 0.7 | 3.3 | 0.0 | 0.8 |
| *Apple, Concentrate, Average* | *1 Tbsp/15ml* | *45.0* | *0.0* | *302* | *0.0* | *73.5* | *0.1* | *0.0* |
| Apple, English with Cherry, Cawston Vale* | 1 Can/250ml | 117.0 | 0.0 | 47 | 0.4 | 11.6 | 0.1 | 0.0 |
| *Apple, Pure, Average* | *1 Glass/100ml* | *47.0* | *0.0* | *47* | *0.1* | *11.2* | *0.0* | *0.0* |
| *Apple, Pure, Organic, Average* | *1 Serving/200ml* | *92.0* | *0.0* | *46* | *0.0* | *11.1* | *0.0* | *0.0* |
| Apple, Raspberry, & Grape, Pressed, Sainsbury's* | 1 Serving/200ml | 92.0 | 0.0 | 46 | 0.3 | 11.2 | 0.1 | 0.5 |
| Apple, Red Grape & Blueberry, Pure, Blends, Del Monte* | 1 Serving/250ml | 125.0 | 0.0 | 50 | 0.6 | 11.5 | 0.0 | 0.0 |
| Apple, with Calcium, Juice Plus, Tesco* | 1 Serving/250ml | 117.0 | 0.0 | 47 | 0.1 | 11.2 | 0.0 | 0.0 |
| *Apple & Cranberry, Average* | *1 Glass/250ml* | *114.0* | *0.0* | *45* | *0.1* | *10.1* | *0.0* | *0.0* |
| Apple & Elderflower, Copella* | 1 Glass/250ml | 107.0 | 0.0 | 43 | 0.4 | 10.2 | 0.1 | 0.0 |
| *Apple & Mango, Average* | *1 Glass/200ml* | *108.0* | *0.0* | *54* | *0.3* | *12.6* | *0.0* | *0.1* |
| Apple & Orange, Fresh Up* | 1 Serving/250ml | 105.0 | 0.0 | 42 | 0.0 | 10.3 | 0.0 | 0.0 |
| Apple & Pomegranate, Pommy, Sparky* | 1 Serving/250ml | 125.0 | 0.0 | 50 | 0.4 | 10.0 | 0.2 | 0.5 |
| *Apple & Raspberry, Average* | *1 Serving/200ml* | *89.0* | *0.0* | *44* | *0.4* | *10.1* | *0.0* | *0.1* |
| Apple & Rhubarb, Caxton Vale* | 1 Glass/250ml | 115.0 | 1.0 | 46 | 0.2 | 9.7 | 0.4 | 0.0 |
| Beetroot, Organic, James White* | 1 Glass/250ml | 105.0 | 0.0 | 42 | 0.9 | 9.3 | 0.1 | 0.0 |
| Breakfast, Sainsbury's* | 1 Serving/200ml | 94.0 | 0.0 | 47 | 0.7 | 11.3 | 0.1 | 0.3 |
| *Carrot, Average* | *1 Glass/200ml* | *46.0* | *0.0* | *23* | *0.6* | *5.2* | *0.0* | *0.1* |
| Citrus Fruit & Veg, V8* | 1 Serving/150ml | 55.0 | 0.0 | 37 | 0.3 | 8.4 | 0.2 | 0.0 |
| Clementine, Morrisons* | 1 Serving/100ml | 48.0 | 0.0 | 48 | 0.5 | 10.9 | 0.1 | 0.1 |
| Coconut, Foco* | 1 Can/520ml | 182.0 | 1.0 | 35 | 0.1 | 8.2 | 0.2 | 0.0 |
| *Cranberry, Average* | *1 Bottle/250ml* | *139.0* | *0.0* | *56* | *0.1* | *13.4* | *0.1* | *0.3* |
| *Cranberry, No Added Sugar, Average* | *1 Glass/200ml* | *11.0* | *0.0* | *5* | *0.1* | *0.8* | *0.0* | *0.0* |
| Exotic Fruit, Pure, Del Monte* | 1 Glass/200ml | 96.0 | 0.0 | 48 | 0.3 | 11.3 | 0.0 | 0.0 |
| Exotic Fruit, Waitrose* | 1 Glass/175ml | 87.0 | 0.0 | 50 | 0.4 | 11.6 | 0.0 | 0.0 |
| Fibre, Tropicana* | 1 Serving/200ml | 130.0 | 0.0 | 65 | 0.4 | 15.8 | 0.0 | 3.4 |
| Froot Refresh, Orange & Passion Fruit, Minute Maid* | 1 Bottle/330ml | 79.0 | 0.0 | 24 | 0.0 | 6.0 | 0.0 | 0.0 |
| Froot Refresh, Red Grape & Raspberry, Minute Maid* | 1 Bottle/330ml | 99.0 | 0.0 | 30 | 0.0 | 7.3 | 0.0 | 0.0 |
| Go!, Tropicana* | 1 Bottle/200ml | 80.0 | 0.0 | 40 | 0.3 | 9.7 | 0.0 | 0.0 |
| Gold Pineapple & Mango, Del Monte* | 1 Serving/200ml | 104.0 | 0.0 | 52 | 0.4 | 12.0 | 0.0 | 0.0 |
| Grape, Purple, Light, Welch's* | 1 Serving/100ml | 27.0 | 0.0 | 27 | 0.2 | 6.1 | 0.3 | 0.3 |
| Grape, Purple, Welch's* | 1 Serving/200ml | 136.0 | 0.0 | 68 | 0.1 | 16.5 | 0.0 | 0.0 |
| *Grape, Red, Average* | *1 Serving/100ml* | *62.0* | *0.0* | *62* | *0.1* | *15.1* | *0.0* | *0.0* |
| *Grape, White, Average* | *1 Can/160ml* | *95.0* | *0.0* | *59* | *0.2* | *14.3* | *0.1* | *0.1* |
| Grape & Peach, Don Simon* | 1 Serving/200ml | 94.0 | 0.0 | 47 | 0.4 | 11.3 | 0.0 | 0.0 |
| Grape & Raspberry, Pressed, M & S* | 1 Carton/330ml | 181.0 | 0.0 | 55 | 0.4 | 12.9 | 0.1 | 0.1 |
| *Grapefruit, Pink, Average* | *1 Glass/200ml* | *81.0* | *0.0* | *40* | *0.6* | *9.0* | *0.0* | *0.2* |
| *Grapefruit, Pure, Average* | *1 Glass/200ml* | *77.0* | *0.0* | *38* | *0.5* | *8.5* | *0.1* | *0.1* |
| *Lemon, Fresh, Average* | *1 Juiced/36ml* | *2.0* | *0.0* | *7* | *0.3* | *1.6* | *0.0* | *0.1* |
| *Lime, Fresh, Average* | *1 Tsp/5ml* | *0.0* | *0.0* | *9* | *0.4* | *1.6* | *0.1* | *0.1* |
| *Mango, Canned* | *1 Glass/200ml* | *78.0* | *0.0* | *39* | *0.1* | *9.8* | *0.2* | *0.0* |
| Mango, Peach, Papaya, Pure, Premium, Tropicana* | 1 Glass/200ml | 88.0 | 0.0 | 44 | 0.5 | 9.8 | 0.0 | 0.1 |
| Multivitamin, Fruit, Vitafit* | 1 Glass/200ml | 106.0 | 0.0 | 53 | 1.0 | 12.0 | 0.0 | 0.5 |
| Orange, Apple & Mango, Calypso* | 1 Carton/200ml | 92.0 | 0.0 | 46 | 0.0 | 11.0 | 0.2 | 0.1 |

**J**

| | Measure INFO/WEIGHT | per Measure KCAL | FAT | Nutrition Values per 100g / 100ml KCAL | PROT | CARB | FAT | FIBRE |
|---|---|---|---|---|---|---|---|---|
| **JUICE** | | | | | | | | |
| Orange, Mango & Passionfuit, Pure Squeezed, Waitrose* | 1 Serving/250ml | 130.0 | 1.0 | 52 | 0.6 | 10.9 | 0.3 | 0.3 |
| *Orange, Pure, Smooth, Average* | *1 Glass/200ml* | *88.0* | *0.0* | *44* | *0.7* | *9.8* | *0.0* | *0.2* |
| *Orange, Pure, with Bits, Average* | *1 Glass/200ml* | *90.0* | *0.0* | *45* | *0.6* | *10.2* | *0.1* | *0.1* |
| *Orange, Red, Average* | *1 Glass/250ml* | *115.0* | *0.0* | *46* | *0.4* | *10.7* | *0.0* | *0.2* |
| Orange, Sparkling, 55, Britvic* | 1 Bottle/275ml | 135.0 | 0.0 | 49 | 0.3 | 11.3 | 0.1 | 0.1 |
| Orange, with Raspberry & Zinc,100% Pure, Minute Maid* | ¼ Bottle/250ml | 82.0 | 0.0 | 33 | 0.5 | 8.2 | 0.0 | 0.0 |
| *Orange & Banana, Pure, Average* | *1 Glass/150ml* | *79.0* | *0.0* | *53* | *0.7* | *12.1* | *0.1* | *0.2* |
| *Orange & Grapefruit, Average* | *1 Serving/200g* | *84.0* | *0.0* | *42* | *0.7* | *9.2* | *0.1* | *0.4* |
| Orange & Kiwi Fruit, Tropicana* | 1 Serving/175ml | 90.0 | 0.0 | 51 | 0.5 | 12.0 | 0.0 | 0.0 |
| *Orange & Mango, Average* | *1 Bottle/375ml* | *176.0* | *0.0* | *47* | *0.5* | *10.7* | *0.1* | *0.2* |
| *Orange & Pineapple, Average* | *1 Glass/120ml* | *56.0* | *1.0* | *46* | *0.4* | *10.5* | *0.5* | *0.5* |
| *Orange & Raspberry, Average* | *1 fl oz/30ml* | *15.0* | *0.0* | *50* | *0.6* | *11.4* | *0.1* | *0.2* |
| *Orange & Strawberry, Average* | *1 Serving/125ml* | *64.0* | *0.0* | *51* | *0.6* | *10.9* | *0.4* | *0.8* |
| Orange Banana & Grapefruit, M & S* | 1 Serving/250ml | 125.0 | 0.0 | 50 | 0.8 | 11.5 | 0.2 | 0.3 |
| Orange with Carrot Puree, M & S* | 1 Bottle/500ml | 200.0 | 0.0 | 40 | 0.6 | 8.0 | 0.3 | 0.3 |
| Orange with Cranberry Juice, M & S* | 1 Bottle/250ml | 137.0 | 1.0 | 55 | 0.5 | 14.0 | 0.5 | 1.0 |
| *Passion Fruit, Average* | *1 Glass/200ml* | *94.0* | *0.0* | *47* | *0.8* | *10.7* | *0.1* | *0.0* |
| Peach, Mango & Passion Fruit, Sainsbury's* | 1 Glass/200ml | 92.0 | 0.0 | 46 | 0.3 | 10.3 | 0.1 | 0.5 |
| Pear, Pure, Heinz* | 1 Serving/100ml | 41.0 | 0.0 | 41 | 0.1 | 9.8 | 0.1 | 0.0 |
| Pear, with a Hint of Ginger, Pressed, M & S* | 1 Glass/250ml | 125.0 | 0.0 | 50 | 0.3 | 11.7 | 0.1 | 0.0 |
| *Pineapple, Average* | *1 Glass/200ml* | *100.0* | *0.0* | *50* | *0.3* | *11.7* | *0.1* | *0.1* |
| Pineapple & Coconut, Sainsbury's* | 1 Glass/250ml | 152.0 | 3.0 | 61 | 0.5 | 11.6 | 1.4 | 0.1 |
| Pineapple & Coconut, Tesco* | 1 Serving/250ml | 137.0 | 1.0 | 55 | 0.4 | 11.3 | 0.4 | 0.0 |
| Pineapple & Coconut, Waitrose* | 1 Serving/250ml | 125.0 | 1.0 | 50 | 0.2 | 11.5 | 0.3 | 0.2 |
| Pineapple and Guava, Tropicana* | 1 Glass/200ml | 106.0 | 0.0 | 53 | 0.3 | 12.3 | 0.0 | 1.2 |
| Pineapple Mango Crush, Just Juice* | 1 Glass/250ml | 107.0 | 0.0 | 43 | 0.0 | 10.6 | 0.0 | 0.0 |
| Pomegranate, Grape & Apple, Tropicana* | 1 Bottle/330ml | 211.0 | 0.0 | 64 | 0.2 | 15.5 | 0.0 | 0.6 |
| Pomegranate and Blueberry, Sainsbury's* | 1oz/28g | 14.0 | 0.0 | 49 | 0.0 | 11.7 | 0.0 | 0.1 |
| Pressed Apple, Strawberry & Lychee, M & S* | 1 Serving/250ml | 112.0 | 1.0 | 45 | 0.3 | 9.7 | 0.3 | 0.3 |
| Pressed Apple & Rhubarb, Cawston Vale* | 1 Glass/200ml | 92.0 | 1.0 | 46 | 0.2 | 9.7 | 0.4 | 0.0 |
| *Prune, Average* | *1 Serving/200ml* | *123.0* | *0.0* | *61* | *0.6* | *15.3* | *0.1* | *1.8* |
| Raspberry Cooler, with Mint, Sainsbury's* | 1 Serving/250ml | 62.0 | 0.0 | 25 | 0.1 | 6.0 | 0.1 | 0.1 |
| Red Grape, Raspberry & Cherry, Not Concentrate, Tesco* | 1 Glass/250ml | 131.0 | 0.0 | 52 | 0.3 | 12.5 | 0.1 | 1.3 |
| Red Grape & Yumberry, Tesco* | 1 Glass/150g | 84.0 | 0.0 | 56 | 0.3 | 13.6 | 0.0 | 0.1 |
| Sweet Carrot & Orange, Shapers, Boots* | 1 Serving/250ml | 100.0 | 0.0 | 40 | 0.9 | 8.8 | 0.2 | 0.4 |
| *Tomato, Average* | *1 Glass/200ml* | *40.0* | *0.0* | *20* | *0.7* | *4.0* | *0.0* | *0.4* |
| Tropical, Fruit & Vegetable, V8* | 1 Serving/150ml | 0.0 | 0.0 | 35 | 0.4 | 8.1 | 0.1 | 1.1 |
| Tropical, Pure, Sainsbury's* | 1 Glass/200ml | 104.0 | 0.0 | 52 | 0.5 | 12.0 | 0.1 | 0.1 |
| Tropical, Tropics, Tropicana* | 1 Serving/250ml | 112.0 | 0.0 | 45 | 0.4 | 11.0 | 0.0 | 0.0 |
| Tropical Fruit, Plenty* | 1 Glass/200ml | 120.0 | 0.0 | 60 | 0.5 | 13.7 | 0.1 | 0.0 |
| Vegetable, Organic, Evernat* | 1 Glass/200ml | 36.0 | 0.0 | 18 | 0.9 | 3.5 | 0.1 | 0.2 |
| White Apple & Ginger, James White* | 1 Glass/250ml | 122.0 | 0.0 | 49 | 0.1 | 11.8 | 0.0 | 0.0 |
| White Grape, Raspberry & Blackcurrant, Asda* | 1 Serving/200ml | 120.0 | 0.0 | 60 | 0.4 | 13.8 | 0.1 | 0.1 |
| White Grape & Peach, No Added Sugar, BGTY, Sainsbury's* | 1 Serving/200ml | 42.0 | 0.0 | 21 | 0.2 | 4.5 | 0.0 | 0.0 |
| **JUICE DRINK** | | | | | | | | |
| Apple, Cranberry, & Blueberry, Waitrose* | 1 Serving/150ml | 75.0 | 0.0 | 50 | 0.1 | 11.9 | 0.0 | 0.1 |
| Apple, Libby's* | 1 Serving/100ml | 43.0 | 0.0 | 43 | 0.0 | 10.3 | 0.0 | 0.0 |
| Apple, No Added Sugar, Asda* | 1 Glass/200ml | 10.0 | 0.0 | 5 | 0.0 | 1.0 | 0.0 | 0.0 |
| Apple & Blueberry, The Feel Good Drinks Co* | 1 Serving/375ml | 163.0 | 0.0 | 43 | 0.1 | 10.6 | 0.1 | 0.0 |
| Apple & Elderflower, Tesco* | 1 Serving/200ml | 76.0 | 0.0 | 38 | 0.0 | 9.4 | 0.0 | 0.0 |
| Apple & Raspberry, Dr Gillian McKeith* | 1 Bottle/200ml | 86.0 | 0.0 | 43 | 0.1 | 10.6 | 0.0 | 0.0 |
| Apple & Raspberry, Sainsbury's* | 1 Serving/200ml | 112.0 | 0.0 | 56 | 0.1 | 13.8 | 0.1 | 0.1 |
| Apple & Raspberry, Tesco* | 1 Serving/300ml | 138.0 | 0.0 | 46 | 0.0 | 11.2 | 0.0 | 0.0 |

J

| JUICE DRINK | Measure INFO/WEIGHT | per Measure KCAL | FAT | Nutrition Values per 100g / 100ml KCAL | PROT | CARB | FAT | FIBRE |
|---|---|---|---|---|---|---|---|---|
| Apple & Strawberry, Sainsbury's* | 1 Serving/250ml | 13.0 | 0.0 | 5 | 0.0 | 1.0 | 0.0 | 0.0 |
| Blackcurrant, 45% High, No Added Sugar, Asda* | 1 Serving/25ml | 2.0 | 0.0 | 7 | 0.0 | 1.4 | 0.0 | 0.0 |
| Blackcurrant, CVit* | 1 Glass/200ml | 4.0 | 0.0 | 2 | 0.0 | 0.2 | 0.0 | 0.0 |
| Blackcurrant, Kids, Tesco* | 1 Serving/250ml | 127.0 | 0.0 | 51 | 0.0 | 12.4 | 0.0 | 0.0 |
| Blackcurrant, Purity* | 1 Bottle/500ml | 265.0 | 0.0 | 53 | 0.0 | 13.2 | 0.0 | 0.0 |
| Blackcurrant & Apple, Oasis* | 1 Serving/500ml | 140.0 | 0.0 | 28 | 0.0 | 6.8 | 0.0 | 0.0 |
| Blackcurrant & Raspberry, with Soya, Adez* | 1 Glass/250ml | 82.0 | 1.0 | 33 | 1.1 | 6.3 | 0.4 | 0.3 |
| Blueberry, BGTY, Sainsbury's* | 1 Serving/250ml | 15.0 | 0.0 | 6 | 0.1 | 1.0 | 0.0 | 0.0 |
| Cherry, No Added Sugar, Sainsbury's* | 1 Carton/250ml | 25.0 | 0.0 | 10 | 0.2 | 1.9 | 0.0 | 0.0 |
| Citrus, Sainsbury's* | 1 Serving/200ml | 102.0 | 0.0 | 51 | 0.3 | 12.3 | 0.1 | 0.2 |
| Citrus Burst, 5 Alive* | 1 Carton/250ml | 125.0 | 0.0 | 50 | 0.0 | 12.8 | 0.0 | 0.0 |
| Cranberry, Classic, Ocean Spray* | 1 Bottle/500ml | 245.0 | 0.0 | 49 | 0.1 | 11.7 | 0.1 | 0.1 |
| Cranberry, Grape & Apple, Ocean Spray* | 1 Glass/200ml | 108.0 | 0.0 | 54 | 0.1 | 12.9 | 0.0 | 0.0 |
| Cranberry, Light, Classic, Ocean Spray* | 1 Glass/200ml | 16.0 | 0.0 | 8 | 0.0 | 1.4 | 0.0 | 0.0 |
| Cranberry, M & S* | 1 Serving/100ml | 60.0 | 0.0 | 60 | 0.1 | 14.3 | 0.0 | 0.0 |
| Cranberry, No Added Sugar, HL, Tesco* | 1 Glass/200ml | 8.0 | 0.0 | 4 | 0.0 | 1.1 | 0.0 | 0.0 |
| Cranberry, Organic, Sainsbury's* | 1 Serving/200ml | 100.0 | 0.0 | 50 | 0.0 | 11.9 | 0.0 | 0.0 |
| Cranberry, Original, Concentrated, Ocean Spray* | 1 Serving/15ml | 27.0 | 0.0 | 183 | 0.2 | 44.1 | 0.0 | 0.0 |
| Cranberry, Solevita* | 1 Serving/200ml | 98.0 | 0.0 | 49 | 0.5 | 11.7 | 0.0 | 0.0 |
| Cranberry, Tesco* | 1 Serving/330ml | 152.0 | 0.0 | 46 | 0.0 | 11.1 | 0.0 | 0.0 |
| Cranberry, Tropical, Ocean Spray* | 1 Glass/200ml | 96.0 | 0.0 | 48 | 0.1 | 11.5 | 0.0 | 0.0 |
| Cranberry, Waitrose* | 1 Serving/250ml | 145.0 | 0.0 | 58 | 0.1 | 13.9 | 0.0 | 0.1 |
| Cranberry & Apple, Ocean Spray* | 1 Glass/200ml | 92.0 | 0.0 | 46 | 0.0 | 11.1 | 0.0 | 0.0 |
| Cranberry & Blackberry, Ocean Spray* | 1 Glass/250ml | 120.0 | 0.0 | 48 | 0.1 | 11.3 | 0.1 | 0.2 |
| Cranberry & Blackcurrant, Ocean Spray* | 1 Bottle/500ml | 265.0 | 0.0 | 53 | 0.2 | 12.7 | 0.0 | 0.0 |
| Cranberry & Blueberry, Ocean Spray* | 1 Serving/100ml | 48.0 | 0.0 | 48 | 0.0 | 11.6 | 0.0 | 0.0 |
| Cranberry & Mango, Light, Ocean Spray* | 1 Glass/250ml | 22.0 | 0.0 | 9 | 0.0 | 2.0 | 0.0 | 0.1 |
| Cranberry & Orange, No Added Sugar, Sainsbury's* | 1 Glass/250ml | 15.0 | 0.0 | 6 | 0.1 | 1.2 | 0.1 | 0.1 |
| Cranberry & Pomegranate, Ocean Spray* | 1 Glass/250ml | 120.0 | 0.0 | 48 | 0.0 | 11.5 | 0.0 | 0.0 |
| Cranberry & Raspberry, Ocean Spray* | 1 Glass/200ml | 104.0 | 0.0 | 52 | 0.0 | 12.6 | 0.0 | 0.0 |
| Cranberry & Raspberry, Sainsbury's* | 1 Serving/250ml | 105.0 | 0.0 | 42 | 0.1 | 9.9 | 0.0 | 0.0 |
| Exotic, Tesco* | 1 Serving/250ml | 127.0 | 0.0 | 51 | 0.1 | 12.3 | 0.0 | 0.0 |
| Fruit Cocktail, Sainsbury's* | 1 Glass/200ml | 90.0 | 0.0 | 45 | 0.2 | 10.6 | 0.0 | 0.1 |
| Grape, Apple & Raspberry, Asda* | 1 Glass/200ml | 90.0 | 0.0 | 45 | 0.2 | 11.0 | 0.0 | 0.0 |
| Grape, Red, Sparkling, Schloer* | 1 Glass/200ml | 84.0 | 0.0 | 42 | 0.0 | 10.4 | 0.0 | 0.0 |
| Grape, White, Sparkling, Schloer* | 1 Serving/120ml | 50.0 | 0.0 | 42 | 0.0 | 10.5 | 0.0 | 0.0 |
| Grape & Elderflower, White, Sparkling, Schloer* | 1 Glass/200ml | 74.0 | 0.0 | 37 | 0.0 | 9.2 | 0.0 | 0.0 |
| Grapefruit & Cranberry, M & S* | 1 Serving/250ml | 125.0 | 0.0 | 50 | 0.2 | 11.9 | 0.1 | 0.0 |
| Grapefruit & Lime, Quest, M & S* | 1 Bottle/330ml | 53.0 | 0.0 | 16 | 0.0 | 4.0 | 0.0 | 0.0 |
| Guava Exotic, Rubicon* | 1 Carton/288ml | 150.0 | 0.0 | 52 | 0.2 | 12.8 | 0.1 | 0.0 |
| J20, Apple & Mango, Britvic* | 1 Bottle/275ml | 118.0 | 0.0 | 43 | 0.1 | 10.0 | 0.0 | 0.2 |
| J20, Apple & Raspberry, Britvic* | 1 Bottle/275ml | 146.0 | 0.0 | 53 | 0.1 | 12.0 | 0.1 | 0.0 |
| J20, Orange & Passion Fruit, Britvic* | 1 Bottle/275ml | 132.0 | 0.0 | 48 | 0.1 | 11.3 | 0.1 | 0.0 |
| Lemon, The Feel Good Drinks Co* | 1 Bottle/171ml | 78.0 | 0.0 | 46 | 0.1 | 10.8 | 0.1 | 0.0 |
| Lemon & Lime, Light, Oasis* | 1 Bottle/250ml | 6.0 | 0.0 | 3 | 0.0 | 0.2 | 0.0 | 0.0 |
| Lemon & Mandarin, Diet, Quest, M & S* | 1 Bottle/330ml | 13.0 | 0.0 | 4 | 0.0 | 1.0 | 0.0 | 0.0 |
| Mango, Rubicon* | 1 Serving/100ml | 54.0 | 0.0 | 54 | 0.1 | 13.1 | 0.1 | 0.0 |
| Mango, Sparkling, Rubicon* | 1 Can/330ml | 172.0 | 0.0 | 52 | 0.0 | 12.8 | 0.0 | 0.0 |
| Mango & Passionfruit, Shot, Big Shotz* | 1 Shot/120ml | 67.0 | 0.0 | 56 | 0.0 | 12.1 | 0.4 | 3.4 |
| Mango Madness, Snapple* | 1 Bottle/227ml | 104.0 | 0.0 | 46 | 0.0 | 12.0 | 0.0 | 0.0 |
| Mega Green, Smucker's* | 1 Serving/473ml | 236.0 | 0.0 | 50 | 0.0 | 12.5 | 0.0 | 0.0 |
| Orange, Juice Burst, Purity* | 1 Bottle/500ml | 220.0 | 0.0 | 44 | 1.0 | 10.2 | 0.0 | 0.0 |
| Orange, Mango & Lime, Fruit Crush, Shapers, Boots* | 1 Bottle/330ml | 150.0 | 1.0 | 45 | 0.4 | 10.6 | 0.2 | 0.4 |

J

|  | Measure INFO/WEIGHT | per Measure KCAL FAT | | Nutrition Values per 100g / 100ml | | | | |
|---|---|---|---|---|---|---|---|---|
|  |  | KCAL | FAT | KCAL | PROT | CARB | FAT | FIBRE |
| **JUICE DRINK** | | | | | | | | |
| Orange, Morrisons* | 1 Serving/250ml | 12.0 | 0.0 | 5 | 0.1 | 0.9 | 0.1 | 0.1 |
| Orange, Sainsbury's* | 1 Serving/250ml | 17.0 | 0.0 | 7 | 0.1 | 1.4 | 0.1 | 0.1 |
| Orange, Value, Tesco* | 1 Glass/250ml | 32.0 | 0.0 | 13 | 0.0 | 3.3 | 0.0 | 0.0 |
| Passion Fruit, Exotic, Rubicon* | 1 Serving/200ml | 110.0 | 0.0 | 55 | 0.1 | 13.6 | 0.0 | 0.0 |
| Peach, Passion Fruit, Extra Light, Oasis* | 1 Bottle/500ml | 17.0 | 0.0 | 3 | 0.0 | 0.6 | 0.0 | 0.0 |
| Peach & Passionfruit Fruit, Sunmagic* | 1 Serving/330ml | 172.0 | 0.0 | 52 | 0.3 | 13.0 | 0.0 | 0.1 |
| Pear, Prtially Made with Concentrate, Tesco* | 1 Glass/200ml | 110.0 | 0.0 | 55 | 0.0 | 12.4 | 0.0 | 0.2 |
| Pineapple, Mango & Passionfruit, Sainsbury's* | 1 Serving/200ml | 74.0 | 0.0 | 37 | 0.1 | 8.7 | 0.0 | 0.2 |
| Pineapple & Grapefruit, Shapers, Boots* | 1 Bottle/500ml | 10.0 | 0.0 | 2 | 0.1 | 0.2 | 0.1 | 0.0 |
| Pomegranate & Blueberry, Weight Watchers* | 1 Bottle/500ml | 15.0 | 0.0 | 3 | 0.0 | 0.5 | 0.0 | 0.0 |
| Pomegranate & Raspberry, Still, Shapers, Boots* | 1 Bottle/500ml | 45.0 | 0.0 | 9 | 0.0 | 2.0 | 0.0 | 0.0 |
| Raspberry & Pear, Tesco* | 1 Serving/250ml | 117.0 | 0.0 | 47 | 0.0 | 11.3 | 0.0 | 0.0 |
| Spirit, Lemon & Grapefruit, Tropicana* | 1 Bottle/400ml | 184.0 | 0.0 | 46 | 0.3 | 10.4 | 0.0 | 0.6 |
| Summer Fruits, Fresh, Tesco* | 1 Glass/250ml | 112.0 | 0.0 | 45 | 0.1 | 10.8 | 0.1 | 0.3 |
| Summer Fruits, Oasis* | 1 Bottle/500ml | 90.0 | 0.0 | 18 | 0.0 | 4.2 | 0.0 | 0.0 |
| Tropical Fruit, Tesco* | 1 Glass/250ml | 117.0 | 0.0 | 47 | 0.0 | 11.4 | 0.0 | 0.0 |
| Tropical Fruit, Waitrose* | 1 Glass/250ml | 117.0 | 0.0 | 47 | 0.2 | 11.2 | 0.0 | 0.0 |
| Tropical Hit, 5 Alive* | 1 Carton/250ml | 92.0 | 0.0 | 37 | 0.0 | 9.3 | 0.0 | 0.0 |
| White Cranberry & Grape, Oceanspay* | 1 Serving/100ml | 48.0 | 0.0 | 48 | 0.0 | 11.6 | 0.0 | 0.0 |
| White Cranberry & Lychee, Ocean Spray* | 1 Glass/200ml | 86.0 | 0.0 | 43 | 0.0 | 11.5 | 0.0 | 0.0 |
| White Grape & Peach, Sainsbury's* | 1 Glass/250ml | 95.0 | 0.0 | 38 | 0.2 | 9.0 | 0.1 | 0.1 |

**J**

| | Measure INFO/WEIGHT | per Measure KCAL | per Measure FAT | Nutrition Values per 100g / 100ml KCAL | PROT | CARB | FAT | FIBRE |
|---|---|---|---|---|---|---|---|---|

**KALE**

| | Measure INFO/WEIGHT | KCAL | FAT | KCAL | PROT | CARB | FAT | FIBRE |
|---|---|---|---|---|---|---|---|---|
| *Curly, Boiled in Salted Water, Average* | 1 Sm Serving/60g | 14.0 | 1.0 | 24 | 2.4 | 1.0 | 1.1 | 2.8 |
| *Curly, Raw, Average* | 1 Med Serving/90g | 30.0 | 1.0 | 33 | 3.4 | 1.4 | 1.6 | 3.1 |

**KANGAROO**

| | | | | | | | | |
|---|---|---|---|---|---|---|---|---|
| *Raw, Average* | 1 Serving/200g | 196.0 | 2.0 | 98 | 22.0 | 1.0 | 1.0 | 0.0 |
| *Steak, Grilled, Average** | 1 Steak/150g | 198.0 | 2.0 | 132 | 30.0 | 0.0 | 1.2 | 0.0 |

**KEBAB**

| | | | | | | | | |
|---|---|---|---|---|---|---|---|---|
| Beef, Hot & Spicy, Tesco* | 1 Kebab/41g | 111.0 | 8.0 | 270 | 15.7 | 4.4 | 20.6 | 1.6 |
| Beef, Kofta, Uncooked, Tesco* | 1 Kebab/73g | 163.0 | 13.0 | 225 | 14.0 | 3.2 | 17.3 | 1.2 |
| Beef & Pepper Kofta, Waitrose* | 1 Kebab/138g | 223.0 | 14.0 | 162 | 14.8 | 2.9 | 10.1 | 0.6 |
| Beef with Sweet Chilli Seasoning, Sainsbury's* | 1 Kebab/61g | 151.0 | 8.0 | 248 | 24.1 | 8.5 | 13.1 | 0.8 |
| Cajun Salmon, Tesco* | 1 Kebab/75g | 100.0 | 3.0 | 133 | 19.8 | 3.9 | 4.2 | 1.3 |
| Chicken, Barbecue, Sainsbury's* | 1 Pack/200g | 238.0 | 3.0 | 119 | 24.4 | 1.5 | 1.7 | 1.8 |
| Chicken, Breast, Mediterranean, Sainsbury's* | 1 Kebab/65g | 73.0 | 2.0 | 113 | 16.5 | 4.6 | 3.2 | 0.6 |
| Chicken, Breast, Salsa, Sainsbury's* | 1 Kebab/80g | 94.0 | 1.0 | 117 | 20.1 | 6.5 | 1.1 | 0.6 |
| Chicken, Breast, Sweet, Oriental, COU, M & S* | ½ Pack/200g | 220.0 | 2.0 | 110 | 20.8 | 4.3 | 1.0 | 0.1 |
| Chicken, Chilli & Lime, Breast Fillet, Sainsbury's* | 1 Kebab/77g | 120.0 | 1.0 | 156 | 29.9 | 6.2 | 0.9 | 0.3 |
| Chicken, Chinese, Mini, M & S* | 1 Kebab/11g | 24.0 | 1.0 | 215 | 19.5 | 5.1 | 12.9 | 0.6 |
| Chicken, Citrus Tikka, Mini, Sainsbury's* | 1 Serving/48g | 72.0 | 1.0 | 151 | 30.3 | 2.7 | 2.3 | 0.2 |
| Chicken, Fillet, Mini, with a Tikka Marinade, Sainsbury's* | 1 Kebab/25g | 41.0 | 1.0 | 164 | 33.4 | 0.6 | 3.1 | 0.1 |
| Chicken, Honey & Mustard, M & S* | 1oz/28g | 41.0 | 1.0 | 145 | 16.7 | 8.2 | 4.8 | 1.0 |
| Chicken, Mini Fillet, M & S* | 1 Serving/150g | 210.0 | 9.0 | 140 | 20.2 | 2.0 | 5.8 | 0.3 |
| Chicken, Red Pepper, Mini, Sainsbury's* | 1 Kebab/52g | 79.0 | 1.0 | 152 | 30.1 | 3.5 | 2.0 | 0.2 |
| Chicken, Shish, Average | 1 kebab/90g | 112.0 | 2.0 | 125 | 25.7 | 0.9 | 2.1 | 0.1 |
| Chicken, Sweet Chilli, Perfectly Balanced, Waitrose* | 1 Kebab/83g | 111.0 | 1.0 | 135 | 28.6 | 1.7 | 1.1 | 0.5 |
| Chicken, Thigh, Sticky Barbecue, M & S* | 1 Kebab/100g | 160.0 | 7.0 | 160 | 15.6 | 7.4 | 7.5 | 0.8 |
| Chicken, Thin Sliced, Heat 'n' Eat, Asda* | ½ Pack/50g | 92.0 | 6.0 | 184 | 15.0 | 3.9 | 12.0 | 1.1 |
| Chicken, with Sweet Chilli Sauce, Finest, Tesco* | ½ Pack/175g | 241.0 | 1.0 | 138 | 17.9 | 14.7 | 0.8 | 1.2 |
| Chicken, with Sweet Chilli Sauce, M & S* | 1 Serving/165g | 228.0 | 1.0 | 138 | 17.9 | 14.7 | 0.8 | 1.2 |
| Chicken & Sausage, with Teriyaki Sauce, Asda* | 1 Serving/110g | 257.0 | 15.0 | 234 | 17.0 | 10.0 | 14.0 | 1.0 |
| Chicken Tikka, with Red Pepper & Pineapple, Tesco* | 1 Kebab/80g | 92.0 | 2.0 | 115 | 16.5 | 6.7 | 2.4 | 0.5 |
| Citrus Tikka Chicken Breast, Sainsbury's* | 1 Kebab/61g | 79.0 | 0.0 | 129 | 25.6 | 5.4 | 0.5 | 0.9 |
| Doner, Heat 'n' Eat Thin Sliced, Asda* | 1 Pack/100g | 196.0 | 11.0 | 196 | 16.7 | 8.4 | 10.6 | 1.7 |
| Doner, Iceland* | 1 Serving/152g | 268.0 | 7.0 | 176 | 9.2 | 24.4 | 4.6 | 2.4 |
| Green Thai Chicken, Waitrose* | 1 Serving/180g | 223.0 | 7.0 | 124 | 20.5 | 1.4 | 4.0 | 1.4 |
| Halloumi & Vegetable, Waitrose* | 1 Kebab/127g | 235.0 | 22.0 | 185 | 5.6 | 2.2 | 17.0 | 2.4 |
| Honey & Mustard Chicken, Sainsbury's* | 1 Serving/50g | 65.0 | 1.0 | 131 | 24.5 | 4.3 | 1.8 | 0.0 |
| Lamb, Greek Style, Sainsbury's* | 1 Serving/70g | 196.0 | 15.0 | 282 | 16.1 | 4.9 | 22.0 | 1.8 |
| Lamb, Kofta, Citrus Tikka, Sainsbury's* | 1 Kebab/84g | 199.0 | 12.0 | 235 | 18.1 | 9.8 | 13.7 | 2.6 |
| Lamb, Kofta Kleftico, TTD, Sainsbury's* | 1 Pack/400g | 652.0 | 39.0 | 163 | 13.5 | 5.5 | 9.7 | 0.5 |
| Lamb, Shish, Sainsbury's* | 1 Kebab/85g | 178.0 | 11.0 | 210 | 19.7 | 2.8 | 13.3 | 0.7 |
| Lamb, Shish, Waitrose* | 1 Kebab/56g | 114.0 | 7.0 | 203 | 15.3 | 6.8 | 12.7 | 1.1 |
| Lamb, with Halloumi Cheese & Olives, Waitrose* | 1 Kebab/75g | 123.0 | 6.0 | 164 | 20.0 | 2.4 | 8.3 | 0.2 |
| Lamb, with Mint, Tesco* | 1 Serving/80g | 192.0 | 13.0 | 240 | 16.0 | 5.5 | 16.7 | 0.4 |
| Lamb Kofta, Indian Style, Waitrose* | 1 Kebab/125g | 266.0 | 20.0 | 213 | 12.3 | 5.5 | 15.8 | 1.6 |
| Lamb Shami with a Mint Raita Dip, M & S* | ½ Pack/90g | 189.0 | 12.0 | 210 | 12.8 | 9.7 | 13.4 | 3.5 |
| Lemon & Ginger Chicken, Delicatezze, Waitrose* | 1 Kebab/25g | 50.0 | 3.0 | 201 | 24.5 | 0.3 | 11.3 | 2.7 |
| Mango & Lime Chicken, Perfectly Balanced, Waitrose* | 1 Kebab/83g | 103.0 | 1.0 | 125 | 26.0 | 1.2 | 1.6 | 1.1 |
| Mango Salsa Chicken Breast, Sainsbury's* | 1 Kebab/60g | 85.0 | 1.0 | 142 | 26.3 | 5.5 | 1.6 | 0.6 |
| Pork & Pepper, BBQ, Sainsbury's* | 1 Kebab/41g | 65.0 | 2.0 | 158 | 24.1 | 3.1 | 5.4 | 1.9 |
| Pork Sausage, Mini, Grilled, Safeway* | 1 Serving/100g | 175.0 | 13.0 | 175 | 9.1 | 3.4 | 13.5 | 1.1 |
| Salmon, Hot & Spicy, Tesco* | 1 Kebab/75g | 88.0 | 2.0 | 118 | 22.0 | 1.1 | 2.9 | 0.0 |
| Shish in Pitta Bread with Salad | 1 Kebab/250g | 387.0 | 10.0 | 155 | 13.5 | 17.2 | 4.1 | 1.0 |
| Shish with Onions & Peppers | 1oz/28g | 59.0 | 5.0 | 212 | 12.9 | 3.9 | 16.2 | 1.2 |

**K**

| | Measure INFO/WEIGHT | per Measure KCAL | FAT | Nutrition Values per 100g / 100ml KCAL | PROT | CARB | FAT | FIBRE |
|---|---|---|---|---|---|---|---|---|
| **KEBAB** | | | | | | | | |
| Spicy Tomato Creole King Prawn, M & S* | 1 Pack/240g | 240.0 | 8.0 | 100 | 14.3 | 2.9 | 3.3 | 0.7 |
| Sweetcorn, Tesco* | 1 Kebab/130g | 74.0 | 1.0 | 57 | 2.0 | 9.9 | 1.0 | 0.9 |
| Tandoori, M & S* | 1oz/28g | 34.0 | 1.0 | 120 | 23.3 | 1.0 | 2.5 | 0.0 |
| Thai Style Chicken, Eat Smart, Safeway* | 1 Kebab/85g | 85.0 | 1.0 | 100 | 15.3 | 6.4 | 1.3 | 1.4 |
| Tiger Prawn, Asda* | 1oz/28g | 17.0 | 0.0 | 59 | 14.6 | 0.0 | 0.1 | 0.0 |
| Tikka, Mini, M & S* | 1 Kebab/11g | 23.0 | 1.0 | 205 | 18.4 | 4.0 | 12.7 | 0.6 |
| Turkey, with Chinese Style Dressing, Sainsbury's* | 1 Kebab/54g | 84.0 | 3.0 | 157 | 21.4 | 6.4 | 5.1 | 1.7 |
| Vegeatable, Mini, Sainsbury's* | 1 Kebab/36g | 22.0 | 1.0 | 61 | 2.5 | 7.4 | 2.3 | 2.4 |
| Vegetable, Sainsbury's* | 1 Kebab/100g | 36.0 | 0.0 | 36 | 1.5 | 6.4 | 0.5 | 1.2 |
| Vegetable, Tesco* | 1 Kebab/120g | 47.0 | 1.0 | 39 | 1.7 | 6.8 | 0.6 | 1.1 |
| **KEDGEREE** | | | | | | | | |
| Average | 1oz/28g | 48.0 | 2.0 | 171 | 15.9 | 7.8 | 8.7 | 0.1 |
| COU, M & S* | 1 Pack/370g | 388.0 | 8.0 | 105 | 7.6 | 13.7 | 2.2 | 2.1 |
| Seafood Masala, Perfectly Balanced, Waitrose* | 1 Pack/400g | 380.0 | 4.0 | 95 | 7.5 | 13.9 | 1.0 | 0.6 |
| Smoked Haddock, Big Dish, M & S* | 1 Pack/450g | 585.0 | 22.0 | 130 | 8.5 | 13.0 | 5.0 | 1.9 |
| **KETCHUP** | | | | | | | | |
| BBQ, Heinz* | 1 Serving/10g | 14.0 | 0.0 | 137 | 1.3 | 31.3 | 0.3 | 0.3 |
| Mild Chilli, Twisted, Heinz* | 1 Tbsp/15g | 16.0 | 0.0 | 108 | 1.0 | 24.9 | 0.2 | 0.7 |
| ***Tomato, Average*** | ***1 Tsp/5g*** | ***6.0*** | ***0.0*** | ***120*** | ***1.5*** | ***28.1*** | ***0.2*** | ***0.8*** |
| ***Tomato, Reduced Sugar, Average*** | ***1 Tbsp/10g*** | ***9.0*** | ***0.0*** | ***87*** | ***2.0*** | ***16.9*** | ***1.2*** | ***0.9*** |
| Wicked Orange, Heinz* | 1 Serving/11g | 12.0 | 0.0 | 108 | 1.0 | 24.7 | 0.1 | 0.6 |
| **KIDNEY** | | | | | | | | |
| ***Lamb, Raw, Average*** | ***1oz/28g*** | ***44.0*** | ***2.0*** | ***156*** | ***21.5*** | ***0.0*** | ***7.7*** | ***0.0*** |
| ***Ox, Raw*** | ***1oz/28g*** | ***25.0*** | ***1.0*** | ***88*** | ***17.2*** | ***0.0*** | ***2.1*** | ***0.0*** |
| ***Ox, Stewed*** | ***1oz/28g*** | ***39.0*** | ***1.0*** | ***138*** | ***24.5*** | ***0.0*** | ***4.4*** | ***0.0*** |
| ***Pig, Fried*** | ***1oz/28g*** | ***57.0*** | ***3.0*** | ***202*** | ***29.2*** | ***0.0*** | ***9.5*** | ***0.0*** |
| ***Pig, Raw*** | ***1oz/28g*** | ***24.0*** | ***1.0*** | ***86*** | ***15.5*** | ***0.0*** | ***2.7*** | ***0.0*** |
| ***Pig, Stewed*** | ***1oz/28g*** | ***43.0*** | ***2.0*** | ***153*** | ***24.4*** | ***0.0*** | ***6.1*** | ***0.0*** |
| **KIEV** | | | | | | | | |
| Cheese & Herb, Mini, Bernard Matthews* | 1 Kiev/23g | 46.0 | 2.0 | 199 | 15.7 | 12.1 | 9.8 | 0.0 |
| Chicken, Bernard Matthews* | 1 Kiev/125g | 374.0 | 28.0 | 299 | 10.6 | 13.9 | 22.3 | 2.7 |
| Chicken, BFY, Morrisons* | 1 Kiev/134g | 304.0 | 17.0 | 227 | 16.1 | 11.5 | 13.0 | 1.0 |
| Chicken, Breaded, Mini, Family, Bernard Matthews* | 1 Kiev/23g | 46.0 | 2.0 | 199 | 15.7 | 12.1 | 9.8 | 0.0 |
| Chicken, Breast, Hand Filled, Birds Eye* | 1 Kiev/172g | 330.0 | 17.0 | 192 | 15.5 | 9.9 | 10.0 | 2.0 |
| Chicken, Cheesy Bean, Asda* | 1 Kiev/94g | 202.0 | 10.0 | 215 | 12.0 | 17.0 | 11.0 | 1.9 |
| Chicken, COU, M & S* | 1 Kiev/150g | 187.0 | 3.0 | 125 | 15.8 | 10.8 | 1.8 | 0.5 |
| Chicken, Creamy Garlic, Chilled, Tesco* | ½ Pack/143g | 285.0 | 17.0 | 200 | 12.9 | 9.7 | 12.0 | 1.3 |
| Chicken, Creamy Peppercorn, Tesco* | 1 Kiev/130g | 312.0 | 21.0 | 240 | 11.5 | 12.0 | 15.8 | 1.4 |
| Chicken, Finest, Tesco* | 1 Kiev/249g | 411.0 | 13.0 | 165 | 18.3 | 11.5 | 5.1 | 4.0 |
| Chicken, Garlic, 25% Reduced Fat, Tesco* | 1 Kiev/130g | 299.0 | 19.0 | 230 | 13.7 | 11.5 | 14.3 | 0.7 |
| Chicken, Garlic, Fresh, Reduced Fat, Morrisons* | 1 Kiev/141g | 350.0 | 26.0 | 248 | 13.2 | 8.0 | 18.1 | 0.7 |
| Chicken, Garlic, M & S* | 1 Kiev/150g | 370.0 | 25.0 | 247 | 15.6 | 8.2 | 16.5 | 2.9 |
| Chicken, Garlic, Whole Breast, Asda* | 1 Pack/290g | 638.0 | 38.0 | 220 | 15.2 | 10.4 | 13.1 | 0.0 |
| Chicken, Garlic & Herb, Reduced Fat, Sainsbury's* | 1 Kiev/142g | 317.0 | 18.0 | 223 | 15.1 | 12.1 | 12.7 | 0.6 |
| Chicken, Garlic & Herb, Sainsbury's* | 1 Kiev/134g | 319.0 | 20.0 | 239 | 15.0 | 11.7 | 14.7 | 1.3 |
| Chicken, Garlic & Mushroom, Sainsbury's* | 1 Kiev/142g | 346.0 | 19.0 | 243 | 16.2 | 14.5 | 13.4 | 1.4 |
| Chicken, Garlic & Parsley, BGTY, Sainsbury's* | 1 Kiev/142g | 324.0 | 18.0 | 228 | 15.9 | 12.3 | 12.8 | 1.0 |
| Chicken, Garlic & Parsley, Sainsbury's* | 1 Kiev/120g | 365.0 | 26.0 | 304 | 11.1 | 17.1 | 21.3 | 0.8 |
| Chicken, Garlic Butter, HL, Tesco* | 1 Kiev/143g | 285.0 | 16.0 | 200 | 14.3 | 9.9 | 11.5 | 0.6 |
| Chicken, Ham, & Cheese, Tesco* | 1 Kiev/143g | 307.0 | 19.0 | 215 | 14.4 | 9.3 | 13.0 | 1.3 |
| Chicken, Ham & Cheese, BGTY, Sainsbury's* | 1 Kiev/132g | 264.0 | 10.0 | 200 | 13.2 | 19.5 | 7.7 | 0.8 |
| Chicken, in Crispy Breadcrumbs, Sainsbury's* | 1 Kiev/117g | 310.0 | 22.0 | 266 | 12.8 | 10.6 | 19.2 | 1.1 |
| Chicken, Italian Style, Sainsbury's* | 1 Kiev/135g | 341.0 | 22.0 | 253 | 14.3 | 12.8 | 16.1 | 1.3 |

| | Measure INFO/WEIGHT | per Measure KCAL | FAT | Nutrition Values per 100g / 100ml KCAL | PROT | CARB | FAT | FIBRE |
|---|---|---|---|---|---|---|---|---|
| **KIEV** | | | | | | | | |
| Chicken, Roast Garlic & Parsley, Sainsbury's* | 1 Kiev/143g | 369.0 | 21.0 | 258 | 14.5 | 16.5 | 14.9 | 0.8 |
| Chicken, Tomato & Mozzerella, Tesco* | 1 Kiev/143g | 285.0 | 17.0 | 200 | 13.4 | 9.0 | 12.2 | 1.4 |
| Chicken, Value, Tesco* | 1 Kiev/125g | 355.0 | 27.0 | 284 | 10.4 | 11.7 | 21.7 | 1.8 |
| Chicken, White Wine & Mushroom, Tesco* | 1 Kiev/145g | 281.0 | 14.0 | 194 | 16.7 | 10.3 | 9.5 | 0.5 |
| Chicken Breast, Garlic, Frozen, Tesco* | 1 Kiev/141g | 430.0 | 35.0 | 305 | 13.0 | 6.9 | 24.6 | 1.3 |
| Chicken Breast, Garlic Butter, Sun Valley* | 1 Kiev/141g | 436.0 | 33.0 | 309 | 13.2 | 11.8 | 23.2 | 0.9 |
| Cod & Parsley, Safeway* | 1 Kiev/160g | 310.0 | 15.0 | 194 | 10.6 | 17.0 | 9.2 | 0.0 |
| Garlic, Meat Free, Tesco* | 1 Kiev/125g | 244.0 | 11.0 | 195 | 15.0 | 12.5 | 9.0 | 2.6 |
| Garlic & Parsley, TTD, Sainsbury's* | 1 Kiev/150g | 370.0 | 23.0 | 247 | 15.7 | 11.1 | 15.6 | 0.8 |
| Salmon, Fillet, Tesco* | 1 Kiev/160g | 376.0 | 20.0 | 235 | 13.3 | 18.0 | 12.2 | 2.5 |
| Turkey, Mini, Baked, Bernard Matthews* | 1 Kiev/23g | 50.0 | 3.0 | 221 | 17.5 | 11.2 | 11.8 | 1.1 |
| **KIEV VEGETARIAN** | | | | | | | | |
| Cheesy Garlic, Meat Free, Sainsbury's* | 1 Kiev/123g | 263.0 | 14.0 | 214 | 17.3 | 10.6 | 11.4 | 3.0 |
| Garlic, Meat Free, Asda* | 1 Kiev/125g | 239.0 | 11.0 | 191 | 15.0 | 12.5 | 9.0 | 2.6 |
| Garlic Butter, Tivall* | 1 Kiev/125g | 366.0 | 26.0 | 293 | 15.1 | 10.8 | 21.0 | 2.6 |
| Vegetable, M & S* | 1 Kiev/155g | 325.0 | 21.0 | 210 | 4.6 | 17.8 | 13.4 | 2.5 |
| **KIPPER** | | | | | | | | |
| *Baked, Average* | *1oz/28g* | *57.0* | *3.0* | *205* | *25.5* | *0.0* | *11.4* | *0.0* |
| Fillets, in Brine, John West* | 1 Can/140g | 269.0 | 17.0 | 192 | 21.0 | 0.0 | 12.0 | 0.0 |
| Fillets, in Sunflower Oil, John West* | 1 Can/140g | 321.0 | 24.0 | 229 | 19.0 | 0.0 | 17.0 | 0.0 |
| *Fillets, Raw, Average* | *1 Serving/200g* | *451.0* | *34.0* | *226* | *17.0* | *0.0* | *17.1* | *0.0* |
| Fillets, Smoked, with Butter, Scottish, Boil in Bag, Tesco* | 1 Serving/100g | 225.0 | 17.0 | 225 | 17.0 | 0.0 | 17.2 | 0.0 |
| Fillets, with Butter, Scottish, Somerfield* | 1 Serving/100g | 178.0 | 12.0 | 178 | 16.5 | 0.0 | 12.4 | 0.0 |
| *Grilled, Average* | *1oz/28g* | *71.0* | *5.0* | *255* | *20.1* | *0.0* | *19.4* | *0.0* |
| *Smoked, Average* | *1 Serving/150g* | *322.0* | *23.0* | *214* | *18.9* | *0.0* | *15.3* | *0.0* |
| **KIT KAT** | | | | | | | | |
| 2 Finger, Nestle* | 2 Fingers/21g | 106.0 | 5.0 | 507 | 5.9 | 62.0 | 26.1 | 0.0 |
| 4 Finger, Nestle* | 4 Fingers/46g | 232.0 | 12.0 | 510 | 5.5 | 62.0 | 26.8 | 1.1 |
| Caramac, 4 Finger, Nestle* | 4 Fingers/49g | 259.0 | 14.0 | 532 | 5.9 | 61.9 | 29.0 | 0.6 |
| Chunky, Nestle* | 1 Bar/50hg | 259.0 | 14.0 | 518 | 5.2 | 60.9 | 28.2 | 1.0 |
| Chunky, Peanut, Nestle* | 1 Bar/50g | 268.0 | 16.0 | 537 | 8.4 | 54.9 | 31.5 | 0.0 |
| Chunky, Snack Size, Nestle* | 1 Bar/26g | 133.0 | 7.0 | 513 | 6.6 | 60.4 | 27.2 | 1.1 |
| Editions, Mango & Passionfruit, Nestle* | 1 Bar/45g | 225.0 | 11.0 | 499 | 4.7 | 69.0 | 23.4 | 0.0 |
| Editions, Red Berry, Chunky, Nestle* | 1 Bar/45g | 223.0 | 10.0 | 496 | 4.5 | 69.5 | 23.3 | 0.0 |
| Editions, Seville Orange, Nestle* | 1 Bar/45g | 223.0 | 10.0 | 496 | 4.6 | 69.3 | 23.0 | 0.8 |
| Kubes, Nestle* | 1 Pack/50g | 257.0 | 14.0 | 515 | 5.9 | 60.9 | 27.5 | 1.0 |
| Kubes, Orange, Nestle* | 4 Kubes/13g | 66.0 | 4.0 | 514 | 5.7 | 61.1 | 27.4 | 1.0 |
| Lemon & Yoghurt, Nestle* | 1 Pack/45g | 240.0 | 13.0 | 533 | 7.3 | 58.0 | 29.8 | 0.4 |
| Low Carb, 2 Finger, Nestle* | 2 Fingers/21g | 92.0 | 7.0 | 438 | 9.2 | 28.3 | 31.3 | 1.3 |
| Mini, Nestle* | 1 Bar/15g | 75.0 | 4.0 | 502 | 7.5 | 59.4 | 26.0 | 0.0 |
| Mint, 4 Finger, Nestle* | 4 Fingers/48g | 244.0 | 13.0 | 508 | 6.0 | 61.5 | 26.4 | 1.1 |
| Orange, 2 Finger, Nestle* | 2 Fingers/21g | 107.0 | 6.0 | 507 | 5.5 | 61.7 | 26.5 | 0.0 |
| Senses, Nestle* | 1 Bar/31g | 165.0 | 10.0 | 531 | 7.5 | 56.3 | 30.7 | 0.0 |
| White, Chunky, Nestle* | 1 Bar/53g | 276.0 | 15.0 | 521 | 8.3 | 60.3 | 27.5 | 0.7 |
| **KIWI FRUIT** | | | | | | | | |
| *Fresh, Raw, Average* | *1 Med Kiwi/60g* | *29.0* | *0.0* | *49* | *1.1* | *10.6* | *0.5* | *1.9* |
| *Weighed with Skin, Average* | *1 Kiwi/60g* | *25.0* | *0.0* | *42* | *1.0* | *9.1* | *0.4* | *1.6* |
| **KOHLRABI** | | | | | | | | |
| *Boiled in Salted Water* | *1oz/28g* | *5.0* | *0.0* | *18* | *1.2* | *3.1* | *0.2* | *1.9* |
| *Raw* | *1oz/28g* | *6.0* | *0.0* | *23* | *1.6* | *3.7* | *0.2* | *2.2* |
| **KORMA** | | | | | | | | |
| Chicken, & Basmati Rice, Tesco* | 1 Pot/350g | 588.0 | 33.0 | 168 | 4.3 | 16.9 | 9.3 | 2.3 |
| Chicken, & Pilau Rice, BGTY, Sainsbury's* | 1 Pack/400g | 404.0 | 5.0 | 101 | 8.0 | 14.3 | 1.3 | 0.6 |

K

| | Measure INFO/WEIGHT | per Measure KCAL | per Measure FAT | Nutrition Values per 100g / 100ml KCAL | PROT | CARB | FAT | FIBRE |
|---|---|---|---|---|---|---|---|---|
| **KORMA** | | | | | | | | |
| Chicken, & Pilau Rice, GFY, Asda* | 1 Pack/400g | 600.0 | 24.0 | 150 | 8.0 | 16.0 | 6.0 | 1.3 |
| Chicken, & Pilau Rice, Somerfield* | 1 Pack/340g | 687.0 | 37.0 | 202 | 9.0 | 16.0 | 11.0 | 0.0 |
| Chicken, & Rice, 95% Fat Free, Birds Eye* | 1 Pack/370g | 444.0 | 7.0 | 120 | 6.2 | 19.6 | 1.9 | 1.1 |
| Chicken, & Rice, Indian Meal for Two, Sainsbury's* | 1 Pack/500g | 785.0 | 40.0 | 157 | 6.8 | 14.3 | 8.1 | 3.1 |
| Chicken, & Rice, Light Choices, Tesco* | 1 Pack/450g | 495.0 | 9.0 | 110 | 7.2 | 16.0 | 2.0 | 0.8 |
| Chicken, & Rice, Organic, Tesco* | 1 Pack/450g | 922.0 | 48.0 | 205 | 6.0 | 21.5 | 10.6 | 0.4 |
| Chicken, & Rice, World Flavours* | 1 Pack/500g | 705.0 | 23.0 | 141 | 8.7 | 16.0 | 4.7 | 0.0 |
| Chicken, & White Rice, BGTY, Frozen, Sainsbury's* | 1 Pack/375g | 341.0 | 4.0 | 91 | 5.6 | 14.9 | 1.0 | 0.5 |
| Chicken, & Yellow Pilau Rice, Chilled, Tesco* | 1 Pack/550g | 698.0 | 21.0 | 127 | 8.2 | 15.0 | 3.8 | 1.2 |
| Chicken, Fresh, Chilled, Tesco* | 1 Pack/350g | 819.0 | 61.0 | 234 | 13.1 | 6.3 | 17.4 | 2.3 |
| Chicken, HL, Tesco* | 1 Pack/350g | 371.0 | 4.0 | 106 | 7.7 | 15.9 | 1.2 | 0.8 |
| Chicken, Indian, Take Away, Tesco* | ½ Pack/175g | 222.0 | 13.0 | 127 | 9.0 | 5.5 | 7.7 | 1.8 |
| Chicken, Indian Meal for 2, Finest, Tesco* | ½ Pack/200g | 348.0 | 24.0 | 174 | 10.3 | 6.2 | 12.0 | 2.5 |
| Chicken, Indian Takeaway for One, Sainsbury's* | 1 Serving/300g | 498.0 | 31.0 | 166 | 13.0 | 5.3 | 10.3 | 1.6 |
| Chicken, Less Than 3% Fat, Birds Eye* | 1 Pack/358g | 440.0 | 7.0 | 123 | 6.5 | 20.4 | 1.9 | 0.8 |
| Chicken, Less Than 3% Fat, Frozen, GFY, Asda* | 1 Pack/401g | 405.0 | 7.0 | 101 | 5.3 | 16.2 | 1.7 | 1.2 |
| Chicken, Morrisons* | 1 Pack/350g | 707.0 | 47.0 | 202 | 13.6 | 7.0 | 13.3 | 0.7 |
| Chicken, Safeway* | 1 Pack/350g | 647.0 | 37.0 | 185 | 14.1 | 8.4 | 10.6 | 2.0 |
| Chicken, Tesco* | 1 Pack/350g | 619.0 | 41.0 | 177 | 10.8 | 6.8 | 11.8 | 0.6 |
| Chicken, Tinned, Asda* | ½ Can/197g | 321.0 | 22.0 | 163 | 8.0 | 8.0 | 11.0 | 2.3 |
| Chicken, Waitrose* | 1 Pack/400g | 680.0 | 47.0 | 170 | 13.7 | 2.4 | 11.7 | 1.9 |
| Chicken, with Basmati Rice, Eat Smart, Safeway* | 1 Pack/380g | 399.0 | 7.0 | 105 | 7.0 | 13.8 | 1.9 | 1.5 |
| Chicken, with Coriander & Rice, Slim Fast* | 1 Pack/375g | 394.0 | 3.0 | 105 | 5.7 | 18.6 | 0.9 | 0.7 |
| Chicken, with Peshwari Coriander Rice, Finest, Tesco* | 1 Pack/550g | 907.0 | 48.0 | 165 | 7.5 | 13.9 | 8.8 | 0.9 |
| Chicken, with Pilau Rice, Perfectly Balanced, Waitrose* | 1 Pack/400g | 452.0 | 7.0 | 113 | 8.9 | 15.4 | 1.7 | 1.3 |
| Chicken, with Pilau Rice, Sharwood's* | 1 Pack/375g | 2186.0 | 80.0 | 583 | 21.1 | 76.5 | 21.4 | 4.1 |
| Chicken Breast, Chunks, Sainsbury's* | 1 Serving/227g | 354.0 | 9.0 | 156 | 28.0 | 1.7 | 4.1 | 0.8 |
| Vegetable, Ready to Cook, Fresh, Sainsbury's* | ½ Pack/255g | 263.0 | 17.0 | 103 | 2.8 | 7.7 | 6.8 | 2.1 |
| Vegetable, Sainsbury's* | 1 Serving/200g | 302.0 | 25.0 | 151 | 2.7 | 6.6 | 12.6 | 2.2 |
| Vegetable & Rice, Tesco* | 1 Pack/450g | 621.0 | 27.0 | 138 | 2.9 | 18.3 | 5.9 | 1.6 |
| **KRISPROLLS** | | | | | | | | |
| Cracked Wheat, Original, Pagen* | 1 Krisproll/13g | 47.0 | 1.0 | 380 | 12.0 | 67.0 | 7.0 | 9.0 |
| Golden, Swedish Toasts, Pagen* | 1 Krisproll/12g | 48.0 | 1.0 | 400 | 11.0 | 69.0 | 8.5 | 5.0 |
| Organic, Bio, Pagen* | 1 Krisproll/12g | 46.0 | 1.0 | 380 | 12.0 | 67.0 | 7.0 | 8.0 |
| **KULFI** | | | | | | | | |
| *Average* | *1oz/28g* | *119.0* | *11.0* | *424* | *5.4* | *11.8* | *39.9* | *0.6* |
| **KUMQUATS** | | | | | | | | |
| *Canned, in Syrup* | *1oz/28g* | *39.0* | *0.0* | *138* | *0.4* | *35.4* | *0.5* | *1.7* |
| *Raw* | *1oz/28g* | *12.0* | *0.0* | *43* | *0.9* | *9.3* | *0.5* | *3.8* |

**K**

| | Measure INFO/WEIGHT | per Measure KCAL | FAT | Nutrition Values per 100g / 100ml KCAL | PROT | CARB | FAT | FIBRE |
|---|---|---|---|---|---|---|---|---|
| **LACES** | | | | | | | | |
| Apple Flavour, Tesco* | 5 Laces/15g | 52.0 | 0.0 | 347 | 3.6 | 74.8 | 3.2 | 2.1 |
| Strawberry, Fizzy, Somerfield* | 1 Pack/100g | 380.0 | 2.0 | 380 | 3.0 | 86.0 | 2.0 | 0.0 |
| Strawberry, Sainsbury's* | 1 Serving/25g | 94.0 | 1.0 | 377 | 3.3 | 76.3 | 4.6 | 0.1 |
| Strawberry, Tesco* | 1 Serving/75g | 260.0 | 2.0 | 347 | 3.6 | 74.8 | 3.2 | 2.1 |
| **LAGER** | | | | | | | | |
| Alcohol Free, Becks* | 1 Serving/275ml | 55.0 | 0.0 | 20 | 0.7 | 5.0 | 0.0 | 0.0 |
| Amstel, Heineken N.V.* | 1 Pint/568ml | 227.0 | 0.0 | 40 | 0.5 | 3.0 | 0.0 | 0.0 |
| Average | 1 Pint/568ml | 233.0 | 0.0 | 41 | 0.3 | 3.1 | 0.0 | 0.0 |
| Becks* | 1 Can/275ml | 113.0 | 0.0 | 41 | 0.0 | 3.0 | 0.0 | 0.0 |
| Blanc, Kronenbourg* | ½ pt/284ml | 119.0 | 0.0 | 42 | 0.0 | 3.3 | 0.0 | 0.0 |
| C2, Carling* | ½ Pint/284ml | 80.0 | 0.0 | 28 | 0.0 | 3.5 | 0.0 | 0.0 |
| Draught, Carling* | 1 Pint/568ml | 189.0 | 0.0 | 33 | 0.0 | 1.4 | 0.0 | 0.0 |
| Edge, Carlsberg* | 1 Can/300ml | 126.0 | 0.0 | 42 | 0.0 | 4.3 | 0.0 | 0.0 |
| Export, Carlsberg* | 1 Can/440ml | 185.0 | 0.0 | 42 | 0.3 | 2.8 | 0.0 | 0.3 |
| Export, Foster's* | 1 Pint/568ml | 210.0 | 0.0 | 37 | 0.0 | 2.2 | 0.0 | 0.0 |
| Foster's* | 1 Pint/568ml | 227.0 | 0.0 | 40 | 0.0 | 3.1 | 0.0 | 0.0 |
| German, Low Alcohol, Sainsbury's* | 1 Bottle/330ml | 92.0 | 0.0 | 28 | 0.4 | 5.9 | 0.1 | 0.1 |
| Grolsch* | 1 Sm Can/330ml | 145.0 | 0.0 | 44 | 0.0 | 2.2 | 0.0 | 0.0 |
| Heineken, Heineken N.V.* | 1 Pint/568ml | 256.0 | 0.0 | 45 | 0.5 | 3.0 | 0.0 | 0.0 |
| 5%, Heineken N.V.* | 1 Bottle/250ml | 110.0 | 0.0 | 44 | 0.4 | 3.4 | 0.0 | 0.0 |
| Kaliber, Guinness* | 1 Can/440ml | 110.0 | 0.0 | 25 | 0.2 | 6.0 | 0.0 | 0.0 |
| Light, Coors* | 1 Pint/500ml | 160.0 | 0.0 | 32 | 0.3 | 1.7 | 0.0 | 0.0 |
| Light, Corona* | 1 Bottle/330ml | 105.0 | 0.0 | 32 | 1.5 | 0.0 | 0.0 | 0.0 |
| Light, Michelob* | 1 Serving/340ml | 113.0 | 0.0 | 33 | 0.3 | 2.0 | 0.0 | 0.0 |
| Low Alcohol | 1 Can/440ml | 44.0 | 0.0 | 10 | 0.2 | 1.5 | 0.0 | 0.0 |
| Organic, Tesco* | 1 Bottle/500ml | 215.0 | 0.0 | 43 | 0.2 | 3.5 | 0.0 | 0.0 |
| Pils, Holsten* | 1 Can/440ml | 167.0 | 0.0 | 38 | 0.3 | 2.4 | 0.0 | 0.0 |
| Premium | 1 Can/440ml | 260.0 | 0.0 | 59 | 0.3 | 2.4 | 0.0 | 0.0 |
| Premium, Co-Op* | 1 Can/440ml | 132.0 | 0.0 | 30 | 0.4 | 0.9 | 0.1 | 0.0 |
| Premium, French, Biere Speciale, Tesco* | 1 Serving/250ml | 105.0 | 0.0 | 42 | 0.3 | 3.3 | 0.0 | 0.0 |
| Premium, Tesco* | 1 Can/440ml | 229.0 | 0.0 | 52 | 0.4 | 4.0 | 0.0 | 0.0 |
| Shandy, Traditional Style, Asda* | 1 Serving/200ml | 44.0 | 0.0 | 22 | 0.0 | 4.6 | 0.0 | 0.0 |
| Ultra Low Carb, Michelob* | 1 Bottle/275ml | 88.0 | 0.0 | 32 | 0.2 | 0.9 | 0.0 | 0.0 |
| Value, Tesco* | 1 Can/440ml | 75.0 | 0.0 | 17 | 0.2 | 1.2 | 0.0 | 0.0 |
| **LAKSA** | | | | | | | | |
| Chicken, COU, M & S* | 1 Pack/450g | 360.0 | 10.0 | 80 | 7.5 | 7.0 | 2.2 | 1.1 |
| Thai Noodle, with Chicken, M & S* | 1 Pack/400g | 460.0 | 22.0 | 115 | 7.0 | 9.8 | 5.4 | 1.1 |
| **LAMB** | | | | | | | | |
| *Chops, Average* | *1oz/28g* | *65.0* | *5.0* | *231* | *20.5* | *0.4* | *16.3* | *0.0* |
| *Chops, Minted, Average* | *1 Chop/100g* | *260.0* | *15.0* | *260* | *25.9* | *5.1* | *15.1* | *0.3* |
| *Cutlets, Neck, Raw, Lean & Fat, Weighed with Bone* | *1 Pack 210g* | *485.0* | *43.0* | *231* | *11.9* | *0.0* | *20.4* | *0.0* |
| *Diced, From Supermarket, Healthy Range, Average* | *½ Pack/200g* | *277.0* | *9.0* | *138* | *24.6* | *0.1* | *4.5* | *0.0* |
| Escalope, Asda* | 1 Serving/100g | 173.0 | 5.0 | 173 | 32.0 | 0.0 | 5.0 | 0.0 |
| Escalope, British, HL, Tesco* | 1 Piece/95g | 104.0 | 3.0 | 110 | 20.1 | 0.0 | 3.3 | 0.0 |
| Fillet, Indian, Somerfield* | 1 Pack/300g | 570.0 | 36.0 | 190 | 17.0 | 4.0 | 12.0 | 0.0 |
| *Grill Steak, Average* | *1oz/28g* | *70.0* | *5.0* | *250* | *20.2* | *4.4* | *16.9* | *0.4* |
| *Grill Steak, Prime, Average* | *1 Steak/63g* | *197.0* | *16.0* | *312* | *18.5* | *2.0* | *25.5* | *0.1* |
| Grill Steak, Rosemary & Mint, Tesco* | 1 Steak/62g | 172.0 | 11.0 | 277 | 24.4 | 5.6 | 17.6 | 1.8 |
| *Leg, Joint, Raw, Average* | *1 Joint/510g* | *858.0* | *46.0* | *168* | *20.9* | *1.4* | *8.9* | *0.2* |
| *Leg, Roasted, Lean, Average* | *1oz/28g* | *58.0* | *3.0* | *206* | *29.9* | *0.0* | *9.6* | *0.0* |
| *Leg, Roasted, Lean & Fat, Average* | *1oz/28g* | *66.0* | *4.0* | *237* | *28.6* | *0.0* | *13.6* | *0.0* |
| *Mince, Average* | *1oz/28g* | *58.0* | *4.0* | *207* | *17.6* | *0.5* | *14.8* | *0.0* |
| Mince, Extra Lean, Sainsbury's* | 1 Serving/225g | 324.0 | 12.0 | 144 | 24.1 | 0.0 | 5.3 | 0.1 |

L

| | Measure INFO/WEIGHT | per Measure KCAL | FAT | Nutrition Values per 100g / 100ml KCAL | PROT | CARB | FAT | FIBRE |
|---|---|---|---|---|---|---|---|---|
| **LAMB** | | | | | | | | |
| *Rack, Raw, Lean & Fat* | *1oz/28g* | *79.0* | *7.0* | *283* | *17.3* | *0.0* | *23.8* | *0.0* |
| *Rack, Raw, Lean Only, Weighed with Bone* | *1 oz / 28g* | *48.0* | *3.0* | *169* | *20.0* | *0.0* | *9.2* | *0.0* |
| *Rack, Roasted, Lean* | *1oz/28g* | *63.0* | *4.0* | *225* | *27.1* | *0.0* | *13.0* | *0.0* |
| *Rack, Roasted, Lean & Fat* | *1oz/28g* | *102.0* | *8.0* | *363* | *23.0* | *0.0* | *30.1* | *0.0* |
| *Shoulder, Cooked, Lean & Fat* | *1oz/28g* | *84.0* | *6.0* | *301* | *24.4* | *0.0* | *22.5* | *0.0* |
| *Shoulder, Fillet, Average* | *1oz/28g* | *66.0* | *5.0* | *235* | *17.6* | *0.0* | *18.3* | *0.0* |
| *Shoulder, Raw, Average* | *1oz/28g* | *70.0* | *6.0* | *248* | *16.7* | *0.0* | *20.2* | *0.0* |
| *Shoulder, Roasted, Whole, Lean* | *1oz/28g* | *61.0* | *3.0* | *218* | *27.2* | *0.0* | *12.1* | *0.0* |
| *Steak, Leg, Raw, Average* | *1 Steak/150g* | *169.0* | *5.0* | *112* | *20.0* | *0.0* | *3.6* | *0.0* |
| *Steak, Minted, Average* | *1 Steak/125g* | *212.0* | *9.0* | *170* | *22.7* | *3.4* | *7.2* | *0.9* |
| *Steak, Raw, Average* | *1 Steak/140g* | *190.0* | *8.0* | *136* | *21.7* | *0.2* | *5.4* | *0.0* |
| *Stewing, Raw, Lean & Fat* | *1oz/28g* | *57.0* | *4.0* | *203* | *22.5* | *0.0* | *12.6* | *0.0* |
| *Stewing, Stewed, Lean* | *1oz/28g* | *67.0* | *4.0* | *240* | *26.6* | *0.0* | *14.8* | *0.0* |
| *Stewing, Stewed, Lean & Fat* | *1oz/28g* | *78.0* | *6.0* | *279* | *24.4* | *0.0* | *20.1* | *0.0* |
| **LAMB BRAISED** | | | | | | | | |
| & Mash, Tesco* | 1 Serving/450g | 413.0 | 12.0 | 92 | 6.1 | 10.7 | 2.7 | 0.8 |
| Shanks, with Chunky Vegetables, M & S* | ½ Pack/425g | 807.0 | 38.0 | 190 | 24.7 | 2.0 | 9.0 | 0.7 |
| **LAMB DINNER** | | | | | | | | |
| Roast, Birds Eye* | 1 Dinner/340g | 370.0 | 14.0 | 109 | 5.9 | 12.1 | 4.1 | 1.5 |
| **LAMB IN** | | | | | | | | |
| a Pot, Sainsbury's* | 1 Pack/450g | 553.0 | 17.0 | 123 | 7.6 | 14.6 | 3.8 | 0.7 |
| a Rich Balsamic Sauce, Shank, Safeway* | ½ Pack/705g | 1304.0 | 78.0 | 185 | 18.0 | 3.1 | 11.0 | 0.9 |
| Chops, Sweet Mint & Balsamic Sauce, Asda* | ½ Pack/160g | 381.0 | 24.0 | 238 | 24.2 | 1.2 | 15.1 | 0.9 |
| Garlic & Rosemary Gravy, Shank, Asda* | 1 Shank/280g | 451.0 | 23.0 | 161 | 19.8 | 1.7 | 8.3 | 0.5 |
| Gravy, Minted, Roast, M & S* | 1 Pack/200g | 140.0 | 3.0 | 70 | 6.8 | 6.6 | 1.5 | 0.9 |
| Gravy, Roast, Birds Eye* | 1 Pack/239g | 160.0 | 5.0 | 67 | 8.1 | 3.8 | 2.2 | 0.1 |
| Mint Gravy, Sliced, Sainsbury's* | 1 Pack/125g | 134.0 | 5.0 | 107 | 15.3 | 2.9 | 3.8 | 0.8 |
| Minted Gravy, Shank, Iceland* | 1 Shank/350g | 651.0 | 45.0 | 186 | 15.0 | 2.4 | 12.9 | 0.5 |
| Rich Minted Gravy, Shank, Morrisons* | 1 Pack/400g | 612.0 | 26.0 | 153 | 18.8 | 5.2 | 6.6 | 0.0 |
| **LAMB MEDITERRANEAN** | | | | | | | | |
| Shanks, Finest, Tesco* | 1 Serving/404g | 671.0 | 36.0 | 166 | 15.0 | 6.6 | 8.8 | 2.0 |
| **LAMB MOROCCAN** | | | | | | | | |
| with Cous Cous, Perfectly Balanced, Waitrose* | 1 Pack/400g | 390.0 | 5.0 | 97 | 7.7 | 13.6 | 1.3 | 2.2 |
| **LAMB TAGINE** | | | | | | | | |
| Moroccan Style, with Couscous, COU, M & S* | 1 Pack/400g | 340.0 | 6.0 | 85 | 8.9 | 8.3 | 1.4 | 1.6 |
| **LAMB WITH** | | | | | | | | |
| Carrot & Swede Mash, Braised, Eat Smart, Morrisons* | 1 Pack/400g | 304.0 | 9.0 | 76 | 5.2 | 8.2 | 2.3 | 1.5 |
| Cous Cous, Morrocan Style, Tesco* | 1 Pack/550g | 710.0 | 15.0 | 129 | 6.6 | 19.6 | 2.7 | 1.3 |
| Gravy, Joint, Tesco* | 1 Serving/225g | 277.0 | 13.0 | 123 | 14.9 | 2.8 | 5.8 | 0.0 |
| Mango & Mint, Shoulder Chops, Waitrose* | 1 Chop/250g | 555.0 | 40.0 | 222 | 16.7 | 2.3 | 16.2 | 0.5 |
| Mango & Mint Sauce, Boneless Joint, Asda* | 1 Serving/100g | 302.0 | 22.0 | 302 | 26.0 | 0.0 | 22.0 | 1.4 |
| Mint, Leg Chops, Morrisons* | 2 Chops/350g | 857.0 | 45.0 | 245 | 29.4 | 2.4 | 12.9 | 0.9 |
| Mint & Balsamic Vinegar Crust, Rump, Waitrose* | 1 Serving/166g | 259.0 | 12.0 | 156 | 18.1 | 5.0 | 7.1 | 0.0 |
| Mint Butter, Leg Steaks, Waitrose* | 1 Serving/155g | 270.0 | 16.0 | 174 | 19.6 | 0.4 | 10.5 | 0.0 |
| Mint Glaze & Redcurrant Sauce, Steaks, Leg, Asda* | ½ Pack/145g | 247.0 | 9.0 | 170 | 18.0 | 11.0 | 6.0 | 0.5 |
| Mint Gravy, Leg Chops, Tesco* | 1 Serving/175g | 213.0 | 10.0 | 122 | 15.0 | 3.2 | 5.6 | 1.7 |
| Mint Gravy, Shanks, Frozen, Tesco* | 1 Shank/200g | 420.0 | 26.0 | 210 | 20.1 | 1.6 | 13.2 | 0.7 |
| Redcurrant & Rosemary Sauce, Chops, Leg, Tesco* | 1 Pack/325g | 604.0 | 36.0 | 186 | 17.6 | 4.0 | 11.1 | 0.5 |
| Roasted Vegetables, Shank, M & S* | ½ Pack/420g | 660.0 | 31.0 | 157 | 14.9 | 8.3 | 7.3 | 0.7 |
| Rosemary, Joint, Tesco* | 1 Serving/125g | 250.0 | 18.0 | 200 | 17.5 | 0.8 | 14.1 | 0.5 |
| Rosemary Gravy, Shank, Sainsbury's* | 1 Serving/200g | 204.0 | 8.0 | 102 | 13.2 | 3.1 | 4.1 | 0.3 |
| Sticky Plum & Orange Glaze, Joint, Waitrose* | 1 Serving/100g | 164.0 | 8.0 | 164 | 13.4 | 9.8 | 7.9 | 3.1 |
| Sweet Mint Dressing, Joint, Tesco* | 1 Serving/50g | 96.0 | 6.0 | 193 | 19.9 | 1.8 | 11.8 | 0.6 |

**L**

| | Measure INFO/WEIGHT | per Measure KCAL | FAT | Nutrition Values per 100g / 100ml KCAL | PROT | CARB | FAT | FIBRE |
|---|---|---|---|---|---|---|---|---|
| **LARD** | | | | | | | | |
| *Average* | **1oz/28g** | **249.0** | **28.0** | **891** | **0.0** | **0.0** | **99.0** | **0.0** |
| **LASAGNE** | | | | | | | | |
| Al Forno, Beef, M & S* | 1 Pack/400g | 640.0 | 38.0 | 160 | 8.2 | 10.7 | 9.5 | 2.8 |
| Alla Bolognese, Weight Watchers* | 1 Pack/350g | 416.0 | 9.0 | 119 | 8.0 | 16.0 | 2.5 | 0.0 |
| Asda* | 1 Pack/398g | 502.0 | 24.0 | 126 | 7.3 | 10.6 | 6.0 | 1.1 |
| Asparagus, M & S* | 1 Pack/360g | 432.0 | 22.0 | 120 | 4.3 | 11.9 | 6.1 | 1.1 |
| Balsamic Onion & Chicken, M & S* | 1 Pack/375g | 562.0 | 25.0 | 150 | 9.5 | 12.5 | 6.7 | 1.5 |
| Basics, Sainsbury's* | 1 Pack/300g | 330.0 | 13.0 | 110 | 4.8 | 13.1 | 4.3 | 1.2 |
| Beef, BGTY, Sainsbury's* | 1 Pack/400g | 352.0 | 8.0 | 88 | 7.8 | 9.8 | 2.0 | 1.4 |
| Beef, Chilled, Safeway* | ½ Pack/325g | 452.0 | 19.0 | 139 | 7.5 | 11.8 | 5.9 | 1.2 |
| Beef, Eat Smart, Safeway* | 1 Pack/380g | 380.0 | 10.0 | 100 | 7.6 | 10.9 | 2.7 | 1.3 |
| Beef, Frozen, Eat Smart, Morrisons* | 1 Pack/380g | 331.0 | 10.0 | 87 | 6.1 | 9.5 | 2.7 | 1.3 |
| Beef, Frozen, GFY, Asda* | 1 Pack/400g | 380.0 | 10.0 | 95 | 6.0 | 12.0 | 2.6 | 0.7 |
| Beef, Frozen, Tesco* | 1 Pack/450g | 607.0 | 25.0 | 135 | 7.5 | 12.6 | 5.6 | 0.8 |
| Beef, Frozen, Weight Watchers* | 1 Pack/300g | 259.0 | 8.0 | 86 | 5.3 | 10.0 | 2.8 | 0.3 |
| Beef, GFY, Asda* | 1 Pack/350g | 385.0 | 7.0 | 110 | 9.0 | 14.0 | 2.0 | 1.0 |
| Beef, HL, Tesco* | 1 Pack/450g | 450.0 | 10.0 | 100 | 6.7 | 12.6 | 2.3 | 1.4 |
| Beef, Italian, Finest, Tesco* | ½ Pack/310g | 425.0 | 22.0 | 137 | 7.4 | 10.7 | 7.2 | 0.8 |
| Beef, Italian, Sainsbury's* | ½ Pack/350g | 493.0 | 27.0 | 141 | 7.5 | 10.3 | 7.7 | 2.0 |
| Beef, Less Than 5% Fat, Asda* | 1 Pack/400g | 460.0 | 17.0 | 115 | 5.0 | 14.0 | 4.3 | 0.6 |
| Beef, Ready Meals, Waitrose* | 1 Pack/ 400g | 444.0 | 21.0 | 111 | 5.8 | 10.4 | 5.1 | 0.8 |
| Beef, Taste of Italy, Somerfield* | ½ Pack/300g | 270.0 | 8.0 | 90 | 5.1 | 11.3 | 2.7 | 1.0 |
| Beef & Chunky Vegetable, HL, Tesco* | 1 Pack/340g | 354.0 | 10.0 | 104 | 5.9 | 13.8 | 2.8 | 1.2 |
| Beef & Red Wine, & Seasoned Wedges, Weight Watchers* | 1 Pack/400g | 400.0 | 13.0 | 100 | 5.1 | 12.5 | 3.3 | 0.2 |
| Bolognese, & Vegetable, Weight Watchers* | 1 Pack/300g | 279.0 | 8.0 | 93 | 5.0 | 12.4 | 2.6 | 0.0 |
| Bolognese, Co-Op* | 1 Pack/500g | 757.0 | 35.0 | 151 | 8.1 | 13.8 | 7.1 | 0.0 |
| Chicken, Italian, Sainsbury's* | 1 Pack/450g | 549.0 | 19.0 | 122 | 8.4 | 12.6 | 4.2 | 0.5 |
| Chicken, Italiano, Tesco* | 1 Serving/450g | 490.0 | 13.0 | 109 | 8.6 | 12.0 | 3.0 | 0.6 |
| Chicken, Light Choices, Tesco* | 1 Pack/400g | 344.0 | 7.0 | 86 | 7.1 | 10.5 | 1.7 | 1.8 |
| Chicken, Mushroom & Asparagus, Finest, Tesco* | ½ Pack/300g | 360.0 | 16.0 | 120 | 7.6 | 10.2 | 5.4 | 0.8 |
| Chicken, Ready Meals, Waitrose* | 1 Pack/300g | 411.0 | 20.0 | 137 | 6.3 | 13.0 | 6.6 | 0.9 |
| Chicken, Safeway* | 1 Pack/400g | 420.0 | 18.0 | 105 | 7.2 | 8.6 | 4.6 | 1.1 |
| Chilled, Somerfield* | 1 Pack/300g | 312.0 | 9.0 | 104 | 6.8 | 12.2 | 3.1 | 1.3 |
| Classic, Deep Filled, M & S* | 1 Pack/400g | 760.0 | 48.0 | 190 | 10.0 | 11.2 | 11.9 | 0.6 |
| Creamy Ricotta & Vegetable, HL, Tesco* | 1 Pack/384g | 407.0 | 11.0 | 106 | 5.5 | 14.6 | 2.8 | 3.6 |
| Extra Special, Asda* | ½ Pack/291g | 416.0 | 20.0 | 143 | 7.0 | 13.0 | 7.0 | 0.3 |
| Family, M & S* | ¼ Pack/225g | 281.0 | 14.0 | 125 | 10.3 | 6.9 | 6.2 | 1.1 |
| Finest, Tesco* | ½ Pack/310g | 425.0 | 22.0 | 137 | 7.4 | 10.7 | 7.2 | 0.8 |
| Fresh, Findus* | 1 Pack/350g | 402.0 | 16.0 | 115 | 6.2 | 11.7 | 4.5 | 0.0 |
| GFY, Asda* | 1 Pack/410g | 344.0 | 8.0 | 84 | 5.5 | 11.0 | 2.0 | 0.3 |
| Good Choice, Iceland* | 1 Pack/400g | 444.0 | 15.0 | 111 | 7.7 | 11.6 | 3.8 | 0.2 |
| HL, Tesco* | 1 Pack/430g | 426.0 | 11.0 | 99 | 6.4 | 12.5 | 2.6 | 0.7 |
| Iceland* | 1 Pack/400g | 548.0 | 22.0 | 137 | 7.5 | 14.3 | 5.5 | 0.9 |
| Italian, Fresh, Chilled, Sainsbury's* | 1 Pack/400g | 480.0 | 22.0 | 120 | 10.1 | 7.5 | 5.5 | 1.4 |
| Italian, Tesco* | 1 Sm Pack/400g | 540.0 | 29.0 | 135 | 6.3 | 11.1 | 7.2 | 1.5 |
| Layered, Asda* | 1 Pack/300g | 444.0 | 24.0 | 148 | 5.0 | 14.0 | 8.0 | 0.3 |
| Less Than 5% Fat, BFY, Morrisons* | ½ Pack/350g | 227.0 | 9.0 | 65 | 5.9 | 8.2 | 2.5 | 0.7 |
| Light Choices, Tesco* | 1 Pack/430g | 396.0 | 11.0 | 92 | 5.8 | 11.3 | 2.6 | 1.6 |
| Low Fat, Co-Op* | 1 Pack/300g | 255.0 | 9.0 | 85 | 6.0 | 10.0 | 3.0 | 1.0 |
| Low Saturated Fat, Waitrose* | 1 Pack/400g | 312.0 | 6.0 | 78 | 4.7 | 11.4 | 1.5 | 0.4 |
| M & S* | 1/3 Pack/333g | 466.0 | 25.0 | 140 | 8.5 | 10.4 | 7.4 | 0.9 |
| Made With Scottish Beef, TTD, Sainsbury's* | 1 Pack/400g | 596.0 | 31.0 | 149 | 10.1 | 9.6 | 7.8 | 2.2 |
| Mediterranean Vegetable, COU, M & S* | 1 Pack/360g | 306.0 | 10.0 | 85 | 3.4 | 11.5 | 2.7 | 1.4 |

L

| | Measure INFO/WEIGHT | per Measure KCAL | FAT | Nutrition Values per 100g / 100ml KCAL | PROT | CARB | FAT | FIBRE |
|---|---|---|---|---|---|---|---|---|
| **LASAGNE** | | | | | | | | |
| Mega, Value, Tesco* | 1 Pack/600g | 726.0 | 35.0 | 121 | 4.7 | 12.2 | 5.9 | 0.5 |
| Minced Beef, Great Stuff, Asda* | 1 Pack/300g | 333.0 | 13.0 | 111 | 6.2 | 11.7 | 4.4 | 1.3 |
| Roasted Mushrooms, Safeway* | 1 Serving/400g | 440.0 | 20.0 | 110 | 3.9 | 11.2 | 5.0 | 1.4 |
| Roasted Vegetable, GFY, Asda* | 1 Pack/425g | 306.0 | 7.0 | 72 | 3.3 | 10.9 | 1.7 | 1.6 |
| Salmon, King Prawn & Spinach, Finest, Tesco* | 1 Pack/400g | 600.0 | 30.0 | 150 | 10.6 | 9.6 | 7.4 | 0.8 |
| *Sheets, Boiled, Average* | *1 Sheet/20g* | *20.0* | *0.0* | *100* | *3.0* | *22.0* | *0.6* | *0.9* |
| *Sheets, Dry, Average* | *1 Sheet/20g* | *70.0* | *0.0* | *349* | *11.9* | *72.1* | *1.5* | *2.9* |
| *Sheets, Fresh, Dry, Average* | *1 Sheet/21g* | *56.0* | *0.0* | *271* | *10.9* | *52.7* | *2.1* | *1.9* |
| *Sheets, Verdi, Dry, Average* | *1 Sheet/20g* | *71.0* | *0.0* | *355* | *12.6* | *71.1* | *2.2* | *2.7* |
| Smoked Salmon & Asparagus, Sainsbury's* | 1 Pack/350g | 665.0 | 37.0 | 190 | 7.9 | 15.6 | 10.7 | 0.7 |
| Spinach & Cheese, Italian, Sainsbury's* | 1 Pack/450g | 666.0 | 31.0 | 148 | 6.0 | 15.5 | 6.8 | 0.5 |
| Spinach & Ricotta, Asda* | 1 Pack/400g | 488.0 | 24.0 | 122 | 4.9 | 12.0 | 6.0 | 1.5 |
| Spinach & Ricotta, Finest, Tesco* | 1 Pack/350g | 584.0 | 37.0 | 167 | 6.1 | 11.7 | 10.6 | 1.2 |
| Triangles with Chicken, COU, M & S* | 1 Pack/360g | 324.0 | 6.0 | 90 | 7.8 | 11.9 | 1.8 | 1.0 |
| Value, Tesco* | 1 Pack/300g | 330.0 | 15.0 | 110 | 3.3 | 12.9 | 5.0 | 0.8 |
| Vegetable, Average | 1oz/28g | 29.0 | 1.0 | 102 | 4.1 | 12.4 | 4.4 | 1.0 |
| Vegetable, BGTY, Sainsbury's* | 1 Pack/346g | 277.0 | 7.0 | 80 | 4.6 | 11.0 | 2.0 | 3.1 |
| Vegetable, Findus* | 1 Pack/330g | 313.0 | 8.0 | 95 | 4.0 | 13.0 | 2.5 | 0.0 |
| Vegetable, Italian, Frozen, Cooked, Sainsbury's* | 1 Pack/378g | 442.0 | 19.0 | 117 | 4.6 | 13.5 | 5.0 | 1.1 |
| Vegetable, Italian Roasted, Asda* | 1 Serving/200g | 234.0 | 14.0 | 117 | 2.6 | 11.0 | 7.0 | 0.7 |
| Vegetable, Italian Three Layer, Sainsbury's* | 1 Pack/450g | 553.0 | 23.0 | 123 | 4.8 | 14.3 | 5.2 | 0.5 |
| Vegetable, Italiano, Tesco* | 1 Pack/400g | 332.0 | 12.0 | 83 | 2.9 | 11.0 | 3.0 | 2.0 |
| Vegetable, Italiano, Tesco* | 1 Pack/425g | 382.0 | 14.0 | 90 | 2.7 | 11.7 | 3.3 | 1.2 |
| Vegetable, Light Choices, Tesco* | 1 Pack/400g | 320.0 | 6.0 | 80 | 4.0 | 12.1 | 1.6 | 1.9 |
| Vegetable, Low Fat, Co-Op* | 1 Pack/300g | 195.0 | 6.0 | 65 | 4.0 | 10.0 | 2.0 | 1.0 |
| Vegetable, Morrisons* | 1 Pack/400g | 464.0 | 23.0 | 116 | 3.8 | 12.3 | 5.7 | 0.7 |
| Vegetable, Ross* | 1 Pack/300g | 270.0 | 8.0 | 90 | 2.9 | 13.3 | 2.8 | 1.2 |
| Vegetable, Waitrose* | 1 Pack/400g | 440.0 | 23.0 | 110 | 3.1 | 11.3 | 5.8 | 1.2 |
| Vegetable, Weight Watchers* | 1 Pack/330g | 251.0 | 6.0 | 76 | 3.6 | 11.8 | 1.7 | 0.7 |
| **LASAGNE VEGETARIAN** | | | | | | | | |
| Linda McCartney* | 1 Pack/360g | 451.0 | 20.0 | 125 | 6.3 | 12.4 | 5.6 | 1.4 |
| Tesco* | 1 Pack/450g | 630.0 | 35.0 | 140 | 6.0 | 11.6 | 7.7 | 1.6 |
| **LAVERBREAD** | | | | | | | | |
| *Average* | *1oz/28g* | *15.0* | *1.0* | *52* | *3.2* | *1.6* | *3.7* | *0.0* |
| **LEEKS** | | | | | | | | |
| *Boiled, Average* | *1oz/28g* | *6.0* | *0.0* | *21* | *1.2* | *2.6* | *0.7* | *1.7* |
| Creamed, Frozen, Waitrose* | 1 Serving/225g | 115.0 | 5.0 | 51 | 1.8 | 5.5 | 2.4 | 0.0 |
| *Raw, Unprepared, Average* | *1oz/28g* | *7.0* | *0.0* | *25* | *1.7* | *3.7* | *0.4* | *2.4* |
| with Sage Butter, Steamer, TTD, Sainsbury's* | ½ Pack/140g | 104.0 | 7.0 | 74 | 1.2 | 5.9 | 5.0 | 2.8 |
| **LEMON** | | | | | | | | |
| *Fresh, Raw, Average* | *1 Slice/5g* | *0.0* | *0.0* | *7* | *0.3* | *1.6* | *0.0* | *1.7* |
| *Peel, Raw, Average* | *1 Tbsp/6g* | *3.0* | *0.0* | *47* | *1.5* | *16.0* | *0.3* | *10.6* |
| **LEMON CURD** | | | | | | | | |
| *Average* | *1 Tbsp/15g* | *44.0* | *1.0* | *294* | *0.7* | *62.9* | *4.7* | *0.1* |
| *Luxury, Average* | *1 Tsp/7g* | *23.0* | *1.0* | *326* | *2.8* | *59.7* | *8.4* | *0.1* |
| **LEMON SOLE** | | | | | | | | |
| *Fillets, Raw, Average* | *1 Serving/220g* | *180.0* | *3.0* | *82* | *17.3* | *0.2* | *1.3* | *0.3* |
| Goujons, Average | 1 Serving/150g | 359.0 | 18.0 | 239 | 13.9 | 18.5 | 12.2 | 1.0 |
| *Grilled, Average* | *1oz/28g* | *27.0* | *0.0* | *97* | *20.2* | *0.0* | *1.7* | *0.0* |
| in Breadcrumbs, Average | 1 Fillet/142g | 322.0 | 17.0 | 228 | 13.7 | 15.7 | 12.3 | 1.0 |
| Lemon Mayonnaise, Goujons, Finest, Tesco* | 1 Pack/230g | 713.0 | 52.0 | 310 | 10.6 | 15.6 | 22.8 | 1.0 |
| *Steamed, Average* | *1oz/28g* | *25.0* | *0.0* | *91* | *20.6* | *0.0* | *0.9* | *0.0* |
| White Wine, & Herb Butter, Fillets, M & S* | 1 Pack/220g | 385.0 | 28.0 | 175 | 15.1 | 0.1 | 12.6 | 0.0 |

**L**

| | INFO/WEIGHT | KCAL | FAT | KCAL | PROT | CARB | FAT | FIBRE |
|---|---|---|---|---|---|---|---|---|
| **LEMONADE** | | | | | | | | |
| 7-Up, Light, Britvic* | 1 Can/330ml | 4.0 | 0.0 | 1 | 0.1 | 0.2 | 0.0 | 0.0 |
| 7-Up, Zero, Britvic* | 1 Can/330ml | 6.0 | 0.0 | 2 | 0.1 | 0.1 | 0.0 | 0.0 |
| Asda* | 1 Glass/250ml | 82.0 | 0.0 | 33 | 0.0 | 8.0 | 0.0 | 0.0 |
| Average | 1 Glass/250ml | 52.0 | 0.0 | 21 | 0.1 | 5.0 | 0.1 | 0.1 |
| Cloudy, Diet, Sainsbury's* | 1 Can/330ml | 7.0 | 0.0 | 2 | 0.1 | 0.2 | 0.1 | 0.3 |
| Cloudy, Diet, Tesco* | 1 Serving/200ml | 6.0 | 0.0 | 3 | 0.0 | 0.8 | 0.0 | 0.0 |
| Cloudy, Sainsbury's* | 1 Glass/250ml | 117.0 | 0.0 | 47 | 0.1 | 12.0 | 0.1 | 0.1 |
| Cloudy, Shapers, Boots* | 1 Bottle/500ml | 15.0 | 0.0 | 3 | 0.0 | 0.3 | 0.0 | 0.0 |
| Cloudy, Waitrose* | 1 Glass/250ml | 125.0 | 0.0 | 50 | 0.0 | 12.2 | 0.0 | 0.0 |
| Diet, Amerista* | 1 Glass/200ml | 3.0 | 0.0 | 2 | 0.1 | 0.2 | 0.0 | 0.0 |
| Diet, Premium, Tesco* | 1 Glass/250ml | 7.0 | 0.0 | 3 | 0.0 | 0.4 | 0.0 | 0.0 |
| Diet, Traditional Style, Tesco* | 1 Glass/200ml | 6.0 | 0.0 | 3 | 0.0 | 0.8 | 0.0 | 0.0 |
| Lime, Safeway* | 1 Can/144ml | 63.0 | 0.0 | 44 | 0.0 | 10.6 | 0.0 | 0.0 |
| Low Calorie, SmartPrice, Asda* | 1 Glass/250ml | 1.0 | 0.0 | 0 | 0.0 | 0.1 | 0.0 | 0.0 |
| Minute Maid* | 1 Bottle/500ml | 10.0 | 0.0 | 2 | 0.0 | 0.6 | 0.0 | 0.0 |
| Organic, Tesco* | 1 Can/142ml | 61.0 | 0.0 | 43 | 0.0 | 10.6 | 0.0 | 0.0 |
| Premium, Freeway* | 1 Glass/250ml | 42.0 | 0.0 | 17 | 0.0 | 4.2 | 0.0 | 0.0 |
| R White* | 1 Glass/250ml | 65.0 | 0.0 | 26 | 0.1 | 6.2 | 0.0 | 0.0 |
| Sainsbury's* | 1 Glass/250ml | 52.0 | 0.0 | 21 | 0.1 | 4.9 | 0.1 | 0.1 |
| Schweppes* | 1 Glass/250ml | 45.0 | 0.0 | 18 | 0.0 | 4.2 | 0.0 | 0.0 |
| Sicilian, Sainsbury's* | 1 Glass/200ml | 98.0 | 0.0 | 49 | 0.1 | 11.5 | 0.1 | 0.1 |
| Sicilian, Traditional, TTD, Sainsbury's* | 1 Glass/250ml | 100.0 | 0.0 | 40 | 0.0 | 10.0 | 0.0 | 0.0 |
| Sparkling, Co-Op* | 1 Can/330ml | 25.0 | 0.0 | 8 | 0.0 | 1.5 | 0.0 | 0.0 |
| Sparkling, Morrisons* | 1 Glass/250ml | 63.0 | 0.0 | 25 | 0.0 | 6.1 | 0.0 | 0.0 |
| Sparkling, with Spanish Lemon Juice, Waitrose* | 1 Glass/250ml | 85.0 | 0.0 | 34 | 0.0 | 8.3 | 0.0 | 0.0 |
| Sprite* | 1 Bottle/500ml | 215.0 | 0.0 | 43 | 0.0 | 10.5 | 0.0 | 0.0 |
| Still, Freshly Squeezed, M & S* | ½ Bottle/250ml | 100.0 | 0.0 | 40 | 0.1 | 9.0 | 0.2 | 0.5 |
| SunJuice* | 1 Glass/250ml | 113.0 | 0.0 | 45 | 0.1 | 12.7 | 0.0 | 0.0 |
| Tesco* | 1 Glass/200ml | 30.0 | 0.0 | 15 | 0.0 | 3.6 | 0.0 | 0.0 |
| Traditional Style, Tesco* | 1 Glass/200ml | 100.0 | 0.0 | 50 | 0.0 | 12.3 | 0.0 | 0.0 |
| **LEMONCELLO** | | | | | | | | |
| Asda^ | 1 Serving/100g | 217.0 | 10.0 | 217 | 4.7 | 27.0 | 10.0 | 0.2 |
| **LEMONGRASS** | | | | | | | | |
| Stalks, Tesco* | 1 Stalk/13g | 12.0 | 0.0 | 99 | 1.8 | 25.3 | 0.5 | 0.0 |
| **LENTILS** | | | | | | | | |
| *Green & Brown, Dried, Boiled in Salted Water, Average* | *1 Tbsp/30g* | *31.0* | *0.0* | *105* | *8.8* | *16.9* | *0.7* | *3.8* |
| *Green Or Brown, Dried, Average* | *1 Serving/50g* | *150.0* | *1.0* | *301* | *22.8* | *49.8* | *1.5* | *9.6* |
| *Green Or Brown, in Water, Tinned, Average* | *½ Can/132g* | *131.0* | *1.0* | *99* | *8.1* | *15.4* | *0.6* | *3.8* |
| *Red, Boiled in Unsalted Water, Average* | *1oz/28g* | *28.0* | *0.0* | *101* | *7.6* | *17.5* | *0.4* | *2.6* |
| *Red, Dried, Average* | *1oz/28g* | *88.0* | *0.0* | *315* | *23.8* | *53.8* | *1.3* | *4.9* |
| **LETTUCE** | | | | | | | | |
| Cos, Sweet, Baby, Somerfield* | 1 Pack/600g | 90.0 | 3.0 | 15 | 0.8 | 1.7 | 0.5 | 0.9 |
| Crest, Sainsbury's* | 1 Serving/80g | 11.0 | 0.0 | 14 | 0.8 | 1.7 | 0.5 | 0.0 |
| Curly Leaf, Sainsbury's* | 1 Serving/80g | 11.0 | 0.0 | 14 | 0.8 | 1.7 | 0.5 | 0.0 |
| *Iceberg, Average* | *1 Serving/80g* | *11.0* | *0.0* | *13* | *0.8* | *1.8* | *0.3* | *0.5* |
| *Lamb's, Average* | *1 Serving/80g* | *12.0* | *0.0* | *14* | *1.3* | *1.5* | *0.2* | *0.9* |
| Leafy, Tesco* | 1 Serving/80g | 11.0 | 0.0 | 14 | 1.2 | 1.5 | 0.4 | 1.9 |
| *Radicchio, Red, Raw, Average* | *1 Med Head/220g* | *29.0* | *0.0* | *13* | *1.4* | *1.6* | *0.1* | *3.0* |
| *Romaine, Average* | *1 Serving/80g* | *12.0* | *0.0* | *15* | *0.9* | *1.7* | *0.5* | *0.7* |
| *Romaine, Hearts, Average* | *1 Serving/80g* | *12.0* | *0.0* | *15* | *0.9* | *1.7* | *0.5* | *1.0* |
| *Romaine, Sweet, Average* | *1 Serving/80g* | *12.0* | *0.0* | *15* | *0.9* | *1.6* | *0.5* | *0.8* |
| **LILT** | | | | | | | | |
| Fruit Crush, Coca-Cola* | 1 Can/330ml | 66.0 | 0.0 | 20 | 0.0 | 4.6 | 0.0 | 0.0 |

**L**

|  | Measure INFO/WEIGHT | per Measure KCAL | FAT | Nutrition Values per 100g / 100ml KCAL | PROT | CARB | FAT | FIBRE |
|---|---|---|---|---|---|---|---|---|
| **LILT** | | | | | | | | |
| Fruit Crush, Zero, Coca-Cola* | 1 Can/330ml | 12.0 | 0.0 | 3 | 0.0 | 0.3 | 0.0 | 0.0 |
| Z, Coca-Cola* | 1 Can/330ml | 10.0 | 0.0 | 3 | 0.0 | 0.4 | 0.0 | 0.0 |
| **LIME** | | | | | | | | |
| *Peel, Raw* | *1 Tbsp/6g* | *3.0* | *0.0* | *47* | *1.5* | *16.0* | *0.3* | *10.6* |
| *Raw, Flesh Only, Average* | *1 Lime/71g* | *18.0* | *0.0* | *25* | *0.6* | *8.8* | *0.2* | *2.3* |
| *Raw, Weighed with Peel & Seeds, Average* | *1 Lime/85g* | *25.0* | *0.0* | *30* | *0.7* | *10.5* | *0.2* | *2.8* |
| **LINGUINE** | | | | | | | | |
| Crab, Rocket & Chilli, Italian, Finest, Tesco* | 1 Pack/350g | 717.0 | 36.0 | 205 | 6.5 | 20.7 | 10.4 | 1.7 |
| Crab & Chilli, Waitrose* | 1 Pack/350g | 770.0 | 45.0 | 220 | 7.7 | 18.0 | 12.9 | 1.8 |
| *Dry, Average* | *1 Serving/100g* | *352.0* | *2.0* | *352* | *13.1* | *70.0* | *2.2* | *2.8* |
| *Fresh, Dry, Average* | *1 Pack/250g* | *681.0* | *6.0* | *272* | *12.3* | *51.7* | *2.6* | *4.0* |
| Garlic & Basil, Asda* | 1 Serving/75g | 108.0 | 0.0 | 144 | 5.4 | 29.5 | 0.5 | 2.5 |
| King Prawn, Asda* | 1 Pack/400g | 380.0 | 10.0 | 95 | 6.4 | 11.5 | 2.6 | 1.5 |
| King Prawn, FreshTastes, Asda* | 1 Serving/356g | 338.0 | 9.0 | 95 | 6.4 | 11.5 | 2.6 | 1.5 |
| King Prawn, Meal for One, M & S* | 1 Pack/400g | 380.0 | 7.0 | 95 | 6.6 | 13.1 | 1.7 | 2.2 |
| Pomodoro, M & S* | 1 Pack/300g | 360.0 | 10.0 | 120 | 4.1 | 17.6 | 3.5 | 1.2 |
| Prawn King & Roasted Garlic, Light Choices, Tesco* | 1 Pack/400g | 360.0 | 9.0 | 90 | 6.3 | 10.5 | 2.3 | 1.0 |
| Smoked Salmon, Sainsbury's* | 1 Serving/400g | 586.0 | 29.0 | 146 | 6.2 | 14.2 | 7.2 | 1.2 |
| Sun Dried Tomato & Chicken, Perfectly Balanced, Waitrose* | 1 Serving/400g | 316.0 | 8.0 | 79 | 7.5 | 8.0 | 1.9 | 3.5 |
| Sun Dried Tomato & Egg, Asda* | 1 Serving/200g | 324.0 | 5.0 | 162 | 7.0 | 28.0 | 2.4 | 3.9 |
| Tomato & Mushroom, Perfectly Balanced, Waitrose* | 1 Pack/350g | 294.0 | 13.0 | 84 | 2.2 | 10.6 | 3.8 | 1.0 |
| Vegetable & Ham, BGTY, Sainsbury's* | 1 Pack/450g | 409.0 | 13.0 | 91 | 4.4 | 11.7 | 3.0 | 0.9 |
| with Chicken & Basil Dressing, HL, Tesco* | 1 Pack/359g | 503.0 | 15.0 | 140 | 8.6 | 16.6 | 4.3 | 2.2 |
| with Prawns & Scallops, BGTY, Sainsbury's* | 1 Pack/400g | 320.0 | 2.0 | 80 | 6.2 | 12.7 | 0.5 | 0.8 |
| with Salmon, Hot Smoked, GFY, Asda* | 1 Pack/400g | 348.0 | 9.0 | 87 | 6.0 | 10.6 | 2.3 | 1.6 |
| **LINSEEDS** | | | | | | | | |
| *Average* | *1 Tsp/5g* | *23.0* | *2.0* | *464* | *21.7* | *18.5* | *33.5* | *26.3* |
| **LION BAR** | | | | | | | | |
| Mini, Nestle* | 1 Bar/16g | 80.0 | 4.0 | 486 | 4.6 | 67.7 | 21.7 | 0.0 |
| Nestle* | 1 Bar/43g | 206.0 | 9.0 | 478 | 6.5 | 64.6 | 21.6 | 0.0 |
| Peanut, Nestle* | 1 Bar/49g | 256.0 | 15.0 | 522 | 7.1 | 56.9 | 29.6 | 0.0 |
| **LIQUEURS** | | | | | | | | |
| *Amaretto, Average* | *1 Shot/25ml* | *97.0* | *0.0* | *388* | *0.0* | *60.0* | *0.0* | *0.0* |
| *Cream, Average* | *1 Shot/25ml* | *81.0* | *4.0* | *325* | *0.0* | *22.8* | *16.1* | *0.0* |
| *Grand Marnier** | *1 Shot/35ml* | *94.0* | *0.0* | *268* | *0.0* | *22.9* | *0.0* | *0.0* |
| *High Strength, Average* | *1 Shot/25ml* | *78.0* | *0.0* | *314* | *0.0* | *24.4* | *0.0* | *0.0* |
| *Kirsch, Average* | *1 Shot/25ml* | *67.0* | *0.0* | *267* | *0.0* | *20.0* | *0.0* | *0.0* |
| **LIQUORICE** | | | | | | | | |
| Allsorts, Average | 1 Sm Bag/56g | 195.0 | 3.0 | 349 | 3.7 | 76.7 | 5.2 | 2.0 |
| Allsorts, Bassett's* | 1 Pack/225g | 792.0 | 10.0 | 352 | 2.3 | 75.5 | 4.5 | 1.6 |
| Allsorts, Fruit, Bassett's* | 1 Serving/50g | 160.0 | 0.0 | 320 | 1.8 | 76.9 | 0.4 | 0.0 |
| Assorted, Filled, Panda* | 1 Sweet/4g | 15.0 | 0.0 | 385 | 3.7 | 68.0 | 11.0 | 0.0 |
| Bars, Panda* | 1 Bar/32g | 99.0 | 0.0 | 308 | 3.7 | 72.0 | 0.4 | 0.9 |
| Catherine Wheels, Barratt* | 1 Wheel/22g | 65.0 | 0.0 | 290 | 3.8 | 67.2 | 0.3 | 0.7 |
| Catherine Wheels, Sainsbury's* | 1 Wheel/17g | 49.0 | 0.0 | 286 | 3.8 | 67.2 | 0.3 | 0.7 |
| Comfits, M & S* | 1oz/28g | 100.0 | 0.0 | 357 | 2.4 | 86.2 | 0.3 | 0.7 |
| Log, Raspberry, Choc, RJ's Licorice Ltd* | 1 Log/45g | 178.0 | 5.0 | 395 | 3.9 | 74.0 | 10.0 | 0.9 |
| Organic, Laidback Liquorice* | 1 Bar/28g | 90.0 | 0.0 | 320 | 4.7 | 75.0 | 1.0 | 3.0 |
| Panda* | 1 Bar/32g | 109.0 | 0.0 | 340 | 3.8 | 78.0 | 0.5 | 0.0 |
| Piglets, Black or Red, Old Fashioned, Route 29 Napa Inc* | 1 Sweet/1.5g | 5.0 | 0.0 | 325 | 2.5 | 70.0 | 2.5 | 0.0 |
| Red, Fresh, 98% Fat Free, RJ's Licorice Ltd* | 1oz/28g | 96.0 | 0.0 | 342 | 3.0 | 75.0 | 1.7 | 0.0 |
| Shapes, Average | 1oz/28g | 78.0 | 0.0 | 278 | 5.5 | 65.0 | 1.4 | 1.9 |
| Soft Eating, Australia, Darrell Lea* | 1 Piece/20g | 68.0 | 0.0 | 338 | 2.8 | 76.1 | 1.9 | 0.0 |

L

| | INFO/WEIGHT | KCAL | FAT | KCAL | PROT | CARB | FAT | FIBRE |
|---|---|---|---|---|---|---|---|---|
| **LIQUORICE** | | | | | | | | |
| Twists, Tesco* | 1 Serving/63g | 186.0 | 0.0 | 297 | 2.7 | 71.0 | 0.3 | 0.7 |
| **LIVER** | | | | | | | | |
| *Calves, Fried* | *1oz/28g* | *49.0* | *3.0* | *176* | *22.3* | *0.0* | *9.6* | *0.0* |
| *Calves, Raw* | *1oz/28g* | *29.0* | *1.0* | *104* | *18.3* | *0.0* | *3.4* | *0.0* |
| Calves, with Fresh Sage Butter, M & S* | 1 Serving/117g | 210.0 | 12.0 | 180 | 12.8 | 10.1 | 10.7 | 1.5 |
| Calves, with Garlic Butter, M & S* | 1oz/28g | 56.0 | 4.0 | 200 | 13.3 | 7.3 | 13.5 | 0.4 |
| *Chicken, Cooked, Simmered, Average* | *1 Serving/100g* | *167.0* | *7.0* | *167* | *24.5* | *0.9* | *6.5* | *0.0* |
| *Chicken, Fried, Average* | *1oz/28g* | *47.0* | *3.0* | *169* | *22.1* | *0.0* | *8.9* | *0.0* |
| *Chicken, Raw, Average* | *1oz/28g* | *26.0* | *1.0* | *92* | *17.7* | *0.0* | *2.3* | *0.0* |
| *Lamb's, Braised, Average* | *1 Serving/100g* | *220.0* | *9.0* | *220* | *30.6* | *2.5* | *8.8* | *0.0* |
| *Lamb's, Fried, Average* | *1oz/28g* | *66.0* | *4.0* | *237* | *30.1* | *0.0* | *12.9* | *0.0* |
| *Lamb's, Raw, Average* | *1 Serving/125g* | *171.0* | *8.0* | *137* | *20.3* | *0.0* | *6.2* | *0.0* |
| Lamb's, with Jersey Butter Mash, Bacon, TTD, Sainsbury's* | 1 Pack/450g | 603.0 | 34.0 | 134 | 7.5 | 9.2 | 7.5 | 2.2 |
| Lamb's, with Onions, M & S* | 1oz/28g | 52.0 | 3.0 | 185 | 14.1 | 6.8 | 11.3 | 0.1 |
| *Ox, Raw* | *1oz/28g* | *43.0* | *2.0* | *155* | *21.1* | *0.0* | *7.8* | *0.0* |
| *Ox, Stewed* | *1oz/28g* | *55.0* | *3.0* | *198* | *24.8* | *3.6* | *9.5* | *0.0* |
| *Pig's, Raw* | *1oz/28g* | *32.0* | *1.0* | *113* | *21.3* | *0.0* | *3.1* | *0.0* |
| *Pig's, Stewed* | *1 Serving/70g* | *132.0* | *6.0* | *189* | *25.6* | *3.6* | *8.1* | *0.0* |
| **LIVER & BACON** | | | | | | | | |
| Meal for One, M & S* | 1 Pack/452g | 430.0 | 17.0 | 95 | 7.0 | 8.0 | 3.7 | 1.2 |
| with Creamy Mash, GFY, Asda* | 1 Pack/386g | 282.0 | 5.0 | 73 | 5.5 | 9.6 | 1.4 | 2.2 |
| with Fresh Mashed Potato, Waitrose* | 1 Pack/400g | 416.0 | 17.0 | 104 | 7.3 | 9.0 | 4.3 | 1.3 |
| with Mash, British Classics, Tesco* | 1 Pack/500g | 575.0 | 23.0 | 115 | 6.6 | 10.6 | 4.7 | 1.0 |
| **LIVER & ONIONS** | | | | | | | | |
| British Classics, Tesco* | 1 Pack/250g | 265.0 | 12.0 | 106 | 9.7 | 5.9 | 4.8 | 0.5 |
| Finest, Tesco* | ½ Pack/225g | 349.0 | 19.0 | 155 | 15.6 | 3.7 | 8.3 | 1.6 |
| M & S* | 1 Serving/200g | 250.0 | 12.0 | 125 | 7.6 | 10.5 | 6.0 | 0.9 |
| **LIVER SAUSAGE** | | | | | | | | |
| *Average* | *1 Slice/10g* | *22.0* | *2.0* | *216* | *15.3* | *4.4* | *15.2* | *0.2* |
| **LOBSTER** | | | | | | | | |
| *Boiled, Average* | *1oz/28g* | *29.0* | *0.0* | *103* | *22.1* | *0.0* | *1.6* | *0.0* |
| Breaded, Mini, Sainsbury's* | 1 Serving/100g | 204.0 | 10.0 | 204 | 8.7 | 18.8 | 10.1 | 1.4 |
| Breaded Squat, & Lemon Mayonnaise Dip, Finest, Tesco* | 1 Pack/210g | 380.0 | 19.0 | 181 | 6.3 | 18.4 | 9.1 | 0.1 |
| Dressed, John West* | 1 Can/43g | 45.0 | 2.0 | 105 | 13.0 | 2.0 | 5.0 | 0.0 |
| Dressed, M & S* | 1oz/28g | 76.0 | 7.0 | 273 | 14.3 | 0.8 | 23.6 | 0.1 |
| Half, M & S* | 1oz/28g | 66.0 | 5.0 | 235 | 12.1 | 2.4 | 19.6 | 0.2 |
| Thermidor, Finest, Tesco* | ½ Pack/140g | 381.0 | 25.0 | 272 | 15.3 | 12.1 | 18.0 | 1.0 |
| Thermidor, M & S* | 1 Serving/140g | 287.0 | 19.0 | 205 | 10.7 | 9.7 | 13.7 | 0.0 |
| **LOGANBERRIES** | | | | | | | | |
| *Raw* | *1oz/28g* | *5.0* | *0.0* | *17* | *1.1* | *3.4* | *0.0* | *2.5* |
| **LOLLIPOPS** | | | | | | | | |
| Assorted, Co-Op* | 1 Lolly/10g | 40.0 | 0.0 | 400 | 0.0 | 97.0 | 0.0 | 0.0 |
| Assorted Flavours, Asda* | 1 Lolly/7g | 27.0 | 0.0 | 380 | 0.0 | 95.0 | 0.0 | 0.0 |
| Blackcurrant, Sugar Free, Rowntree's* | 1 Lolly/15g | 35.0 | 0.0 | 233 | 0.1 | 89.4 | 0.0 | 0.0 |
| Chupa Chups* | 1 Lolly/18g | 44.0 | 0.0 | 247 | 0.0 | 96.5 | 1.3 | 0.0 |
| Cremosa, Sugar Free, Chupa Chups* | 1 Lolly/10g | 27.0 | 1.0 | 275 | 0.2 | 92.5 | 5.4 | 0.0 |
| Cuore Di Frutta, Chupa Chups* | 1 Lolly/10g | 25.0 | 0.0 | 247 | 0.0 | 96.5 | 1.3 | 0.0 |
| Orange, Sugar Free, Rowntree's* | 1 Lolly/15g | 35.0 | 0.0 | 235 | 0.1 | 89.5 | 0.0 | 0.6 |
| Refreshers, Bassett's* | 1 Lolly/6g | 25.0 | 0.0 | 417 | 0.0 | 108.3 | 0.0 | 0.0 |
| Sugar Free, Simpkins* | 1 Lolly/15g | 51.0 | 0.0 | 340 | 0.0 | 88.0 | 0.0 | 0.0 |
| Super Sour, Tesco* | 1 Lolly/8g | 32.0 | 0.0 | 385 | 0.1 | 95.6 | 0.2 | 0.5 |
| **LONGANS** | | | | | | | | |
| *Canned, in Syrup, Drained* | *1oz/28g* | *19.0* | *0.0* | *67* | *0.4* | *17.1* | *0.3* | *0.0* |

L

| | Measure INFO/WEIGHT | per Measure KCAL | FAT | Nutrition Values per 100g / 100ml KCAL | PROT | CARB | FAT | FIBRE |
|---|---|---|---|---|---|---|---|---|
| **LOQUATS** | | | | | | | | |
| *Raw* | *1oz/28g* | *8.0* | *0.0* | *28* | *0.7* | *6.3* | *0.2* | *0.0* |
| **LOZENGES** | | | | | | | | |
| Original, Victory V* | 1 Lozenge/3g | 9.0 | 0.0 | 350 | 0.0 | 91.0 | 0.0 | 0.0 |
| **LUCOZADE** | | | | | | | | |
| Citrus Clear, Energy, GlaxoSmithKline UK Limited* | 1 Bottle/380ml | 266.0 | 0.0 | 70 | 0.1 | 17.0 | 0.0 | 0.0 |
| Citrus Fruits, Hydro Active, Sport, Lucozade* | 1 Bottle/500ml | 50.0 | 0.0 | 10 | 0.0 | 2.0 | 0.0 | 0.0 |
| Orange Energy Drink, GlaxoSmithKline UK Limited* | 1 Bottle/500ml | 350.0 | 0.0 | 70 | 0.0 | 17.2 | 0.0 | 0.0 |
| Original, GlaxoSmithKline UK Limited* | 1 Bottle/345ml | 252.0 | 0.0 | 73 | 0.0 | 17.9 | 0.0 | 0.0 |
| Raspberry, GlaxoSmithKline UK Limited* | 1 Bottle/500ml | 140.0 | 0.0 | 28 | 0.0 | 6.4 | 0.0 | 0.0 |
| Tropical, GlaxoSmithKline UK Limited* | 1 Bottle/380ml | 266.0 | 0.0 | 70 | 0.0 | 17.2 | 0.0 | 0.0 |
| **LUNCHEON MEAT** | | | | | | | | |
| *Pork, Average* | *1oz/28g* | *81.0* | *7.0* | *288* | *13.3* | *4.0* | *24.3* | *0.0* |
| **LYCHEES** | | | | | | | | |
| *Fresh, Raw, Flesh Only* | *1oz/28g* | *16.0* | *0.0* | *58* | *0.9* | *14.3* | *0.1* | *0.7* |
| in Juice, Amoy* | 1oz/28g | 13.0 | 0.0 | 46 | 0.4 | 10.9 | 0.0 | 0.0 |
| *in Syrup, Average* | *1oz/28g* | *19.0* | *0.0* | *69* | *0.4* | *17.7* | *0.0* | *0.4* |
| *Raw, Weighed with Skin & Stone* | *1oz/28g* | *10.0* | *0.0* | *36* | *0.5* | *8.9* | *0.1* | *0.4* |

| | Measure | per Measure | | Nutrition Values per 100g / 100ml | | | | |
| --- | --- | --- | --- | --- | --- | --- | --- | --- |
| | INFO/WEIGHT | KCAL | FAT | KCAL | PROT | CARB | FAT | FIBRE |
| **M&M'S** | | | | | | | | |
| Mars* | 1 Pack/20g | 97.0 | 4.0 | 485 | 5.0 | 68.0 | 21.5 | 0.0 |
| Mini, Mars* | 1 Sm Pack/36g | 176.0 | 8.0 | 489 | 6.3 | 63.6 | 23.2 | 0.0 |
| Peanut, Mars* | 1 Pack/45g | 234.0 | 12.0 | 520 | 9.8 | 60.2 | 26.7 | 2.7 |
| Peanut Butter, Mars* | 1 Pack/42g | 230.0 | 12.0 | 548 | 9.5 | 57.1 | 28.6 | 4.8 |
| **MACADAMIA NUTS** | | | | | | | | |
| *Plain, Average* | *1 Pack/100g* | *750.0* | *78.0* | *750* | *7.9* | *4.8* | *77.6* | *5.3* |
| *Roasted, Salted, Average* | *6 Nuts/10g* | *75.0* | *8.0* | *748* | *7.9* | *4.8* | *77.6* | *5.3* |
| **MACARONI** | | | | | | | | |
| *Dry, Average* | *1oz/28g* | *99.0* | *0.0* | *354* | *11.9* | *73.5* | *1.7* | *2.6* |
| **MACARONI CHEESE** | | | | | | | | |
| & Spinach, TTD, Sainsbury's* | 1 Pack/500g | 1025.0 | 57.0 | 205 | 6.5 | 18.9 | 11.5 | 1.3 |
| Average | 1 Serving/300g | 534.0 | 32.0 | 178 | 7.3 | 13.6 | 10.8 | 0.5 |
| Bettabuy, Morrisons* | 1 Serving/205g | 229.0 | 12.0 | 112 | 4.3 | 10.8 | 5.7 | 0.4 |
| Birds Eye* | 1 Pack/300g | 470.0 | 15.0 | 157 | 5.7 | 22.3 | 5.0 | 0.8 |
| Canned, Sainsbury's* | 1 Can/400g | 480.0 | 24.0 | 120 | 4.4 | 12.0 | 6.0 | 0.3 |
| Chilled, GFY, Asda* | 1 Pack/443g | 469.0 | 13.0 | 106 | 6.0 | 14.0 | 2.9 | 1.6 |
| COU, M & S* | 1 Pack/360g | 360.0 | 9.0 | 100 | 5.8 | 13.9 | 2.4 | 1.2 |
| Finest, Tesco* | 1 Serving/500g | 1055.0 | 53.0 | 211 | 8.3 | 20.6 | 10.6 | 0.7 |
| Four Cheese, Extra Special, Asda* | 1 Pack/400g | 664.0 | 31.0 | 166 | 7.7 | 16.4 | 7.7 | 1.1 |
| HL, Tesco* | 1 Serving/385g | 443.0 | 5.0 | 115 | 9.3 | 15.9 | 1.2 | 1.0 |
| Italian, Sainsbury's* | ½ Pack/225g | 360.0 | 16.0 | 160 | 6.9 | 17.3 | 7.0 | 1.5 |
| Italian, Tesco* | 1 Pack/420g | 830.0 | 41.0 | 198 | 9.2 | 18.2 | 9.7 | 1.2 |
| Kids, Sainsbury's* | 1 Pack/300g | 336.0 | 7.0 | 112 | 4.6 | 17.9 | 2.4 | 1.7 |
| Light Choices, Tesco* | 1 Pack/385g | 465.0 | 7.0 | 121 | 7.0 | 18.7 | 1.9 | 1.5 |
| M & S* | 1 Pack/400g | 680.0 | 40.0 | 170 | 6.9 | 12.8 | 9.9 | 0.6 |
| Made With Fresh Pasta, Findus* | 1 Pack/360g | 360.0 | 7.0 | 100 | 5.0 | 16.0 | 2.0 | 0.5 |
| Morrisons, Canned, Morrisons* | 1 Can/410g | 279.0 | 6.0 | 68 | 5.1 | 8.8 | 1.4 | 1.0 |
| Red Leicester, Heinz* | 1 Can/400g | 332.0 | 11.0 | 83 | 3.5 | 11.1 | 2.7 | 0.3 |
| Ross* | 1 Pack/300g | 327.0 | 9.0 | 109 | 4.2 | 16.2 | 3.1 | 1.3 |
| SmartPrice, Asda* | 1 Can/410g | 291.0 | 6.0 | 71 | 2.6 | 11.8 | 1.5 | 0.4 |
| Value, Tesco* | 1 Pack/300g | 375.0 | 15.0 | 125 | 4.4 | 15.0 | 4.9 | 1.2 |
| Waitrose* | 1 Pack/350g | 465.0 | 33.0 | 133 | 6.8 | 5.2 | 9.4 | 0.0 |
| **MACAROONS** | | | | | | | | |
| Butterscotch, Picard* | 1 Macaroon/20g | 85.0 | 4.0 | 424 | 9.7 | 55.1 | 18.2 | 0.0 |
| Coconut, Sainsbury's* | 1 Macaroon/33g | 146.0 | 6.0 | 441 | 4.7 | 63.7 | 18.6 | 0.8 |
| Coconut, Tesco* | 1 Macaroon/33g | 140.0 | 6.0 | 425 | 4.4 | 59.0 | 18.6 | 5.7 |
| French, Average | 1 Serving/60g | 225.0 | 11.0 | 375 | 6.7 | 46.7 | 18.3 | 3.3 |
| **MACKEREL** | | | | | | | | |
| *Atlantic, Raw, Average* | *1 Fillet/75g* | *154.0* | *10.0* | *205* | *18.6* | *0.0* | *13.9* | *0.0* |
| Fillets, Honey Roast Smoked, Sainsbury's* | 1 Serving/100g | 349.0 | 27.0 | 349 | 21.5 | 4.5 | 27.3 | 12.4 |
| Fillets, in a Hot Chilli Dressing, Princes* | 1 Pack/125g | 370.0 | 34.0 | 296 | 13.3 | 0.0 | 27.0 | 0.0 |
| *Fillets, in Brine, Average* | *1 Can/88g* | *206.0* | *15.0* | *234* | *19.4* | *0.0* | *17.4* | *0.0* |
| Fillets, in Curry Sauce, John West* | 1 Can/125g | 275.0 | 21.0 | 220 | 14.2 | 3.5 | 16.6 | 0.2 |
| Fillets, in Green Peppercorn Sauce, John West* | 1 Can/125g | 329.0 | 26.0 | 263 | 14.0 | 4.5 | 21.0 | 0.1 |
| Fillets, in Hot Smoked Peppered, Asda* | 1 Fillet/100g | 341.0 | 28.0 | 341 | 19.0 | 3.3 | 28.0 | 0.6 |
| Fillets, in Mustard Sauce, Average | 1 Can/125g | 274.0 | 19.0 | 219 | 14.1 | 5.4 | 15.5 | 0.0 |
| Fillets, in Olive Oil, Average | 1 Serving/50g | 149.0 | 12.0 | 297 | 18.5 | 1.0 | 24.3 | 0.0 |
| Fillets, in Sunflower Oil, Average | 1 Can/94g | 262.0 | 21.0 | 279 | 20.2 | 0.2 | 21.9 | 0.2 |
| Fillets, in Tomato Sauce, Average | 1 Can/125g | 251.0 | 18.0 | 200 | 14.3 | 2.7 | 14.7 | 0.0 |
| Fillets, Red Pepper & Onion, Smoked, Asda* | 1 Serving/90g | 319.0 | 28.0 | 354 | 18.0 | 0.8 | 31.0 | 1.2 |
| *Fillets, Smoked, Average* | *1oz/28g* | *94.0* | *8.0* | *335* | *19.7* | *0.5* | *28.2* | *0.3* |
| *Fried in Blended Oil* | *1oz/28g* | *76.0* | *5.0* | *272* | *24.0* | *0.0* | *19.5* | *0.0* |
| *Grilled* | *1oz/28g* | *67.0* | *5.0* | *239* | *20.8* | *0.0* | *17.3* | *0.0* |

| | Measure INFO/WEIGHT | per Measure KCAL | FAT | Nutrition Values per 100g / 100ml KCAL | PROT | CARB | FAT | FIBRE |
|---|---|---|---|---|---|---|---|---|
| **MACKEREL** | | | | | | | | |
| *Raw, with Skin, Weighed with Bone, Average* | *1oz/28g* | *67.0* | *5.0* | *238* | *19.9* | *0.0* | *17.6* | *0.0* |
| Roasted, With Piri-piri, Tesco* | 1 Fillet/80g | 240.0 | 19.0 | 300 | 20.7 | 0.0 | 23.8 | 1.0 |
| Smoked, Lemon & Parsley, Morrisons* | ½ Pack/100g | 282.0 | 20.0 | 282 | 20.9 | 4.6 | 20.0 | 1.0 |
| *Smoked, Peppered, Average* | *1oz/28g* | *87.0* | *7.0* | *309* | *20.4* | *0.3* | *25.2* | *0.2* |
| **MADRAS** | | | | | | | | |
| Beef, Canned, BGTY, Sainsbury's* | 1 Can/400g | 344.0 | 14.0 | 86 | 9.5 | 4.0 | 3.6 | 0.9 |
| Beef, Tesco* | 1 Pack/460g | 616.0 | 38.0 | 134 | 10.6 | 4.5 | 8.2 | 1.2 |
| Beef, Weight Watchers* | 1 Pack/320g | 317.0 | 5.0 | 99 | 5.6 | 15.8 | 1.5 | 0.3 |
| Chicken, & Pilau Rice, Asda* | 1 Pack/400g | 588.0 | 28.0 | 147 | 8.0 | 13.0 | 7.0 | 1.7 |
| Chicken, & Pilau Rice, Somerfield* | 1 Pack/340g | 496.0 | 24.0 | 146 | 7.0 | 14.0 | 7.0 | 0.0 |
| Chicken, & Rice, Hot & Spicy, Sainsbury's* | 1 Pack/500g | 670.0 | 25.0 | 134 | 7.1 | 14.9 | 5.1 | 2.2 |
| Chicken, Asda* | 1 Serving/350g | 430.0 | 31.0 | 123 | 7.0 | 3.6 | 9.0 | 2.3 |
| Chicken, Frozen, GFY, Asda* | 1 Pack/400g | 448.0 | 5.0 | 112 | 5.6 | 19.4 | 1.3 | 1.2 |
| Chicken, Iceland* | 1 Pack/400g | 376.0 | 19.0 | 94 | 7.7 | 4.9 | 4.8 | 1.1 |
| Chicken, Indian, Tesco* | 1 Pack/350g | 518.0 | 31.0 | 148 | 11.3 | 5.6 | 8.9 | 1.9 |
| Chicken, Indian Take Away, Tesco* | 1 Serving/175g | 254.0 | 18.0 | 145 | 8.2 | 4.8 | 10.1 | 1.7 |
| Chicken, Morrisons* | 1 Pack/350g | 448.0 | 30.0 | 128 | 9.6 | 2.8 | 8.7 | 2.4 |
| Chicken, Safeway* | 1 Pack/350g | 469.0 | 25.0 | 134 | 13.4 | 4.0 | 7.2 | 1.8 |
| Chicken, Sainsbury's* | 1 Pack/400g | 468.0 | 27.0 | 117 | 11.7 | 2.2 | 6.8 | 2.8 |
| Chicken, Tesco* | 1 Pack/350g | 325.0 | 14.0 | 93 | 10.6 | 3.6 | 4.1 | 0.6 |
| Chicken, Waitrose* | 1 Pack/400g | 672.0 | 42.0 | 168 | 14.6 | 3.7 | 10.5 | 1.8 |
| **MAGNUM** | | | | | | | | |
| Almond, Wall's Ice Cream* | 1 Bar/86g | 275.0 | 18.0 | 320 | 5.0 | 30.0 | 21.0 | 0.0 |
| Caramel & Almond, Temptation, Wall's Ice Cream* | 1 Lolly/68g | 239.0 | 15.0 | 351 | 5.4 | 34.0 | 22.0 | 0.0 |
| Caramel & Nuts Bar, Wall's Ice Cream* | 1 Bar/60g | 132.0 | 9.0 | 220 | 4.0 | 19.0 | 15.0 | 0.0 |
| Classic, Mini, Wall's* | 1 Lolly/50g | 170.0 | 11.0 | 340 | 4.0 | 30.0 | 22.0 | 0.0 |
| Classic, Wall's Ice Cream* | 1 Lolly/86g | 261.0 | 16.0 | 303 | 3.8 | 29.0 | 19.0 | 0.0 |
| Double Chocolate, Wall's Ice Cream* | 1 Bar/92g | 346.0 | 22.0 | 378 | 4.5 | 36.0 | 24.0 | 0.0 |
| Gluttony, Wall's Ice Cream* | 1 Lolly/110ml | 425.0 | 29.0 | 386 | 4.5 | 32.7 | 26.4 | 0.0 |
| Greed, Wall's Ice Cream* | 1 Bar/110ml | 307.0 | 18.0 | 279 | 3.6 | 29.1 | 16.4 | 0.0 |
| White, Wall's Ice Cream* | 1 Lolly/87g | 256.0 | 15.0 | 296 | 3.8 | 32.0 | 17.0 | 0.0 |
| **MAKHANI** | | | | | | | | |
| Chicken, Sainsbury's* | ½ Pack/199g | 313.0 | 21.0 | 157 | 12.2 | 2.9 | 10.7 | 2.5 |
| King Prawns, Finest, Tesco* | 1 Pack/350g | 514.0 | 39.0 | 147 | 6.0 | 6.0 | 11.1 | 1.3 |
| **MALT DRINK** | | | | | | | | |
| Non-alcoholic, Supermalt* | 1 Bottle/330g | 210.0 | 0.0 | 64 | 0.8 | 15.1 | 0.0 | 0.0 |
| **MALTESERS** | | | | | | | | |
| Malteaster, Chocolate Bunny, Mars* | 1 Bunny/29g | 155.0 | 9.0 | 535 | 6.2 | 56.2 | 31.7 | 0.0 |
| Mars* | 1 Reg Bag/37g | 187.0 | 9.0 | 505 | 7.9 | 62.8 | 24.6 | 0.9 |
| White Chocolate, Mars* | 1 Pack/37g | 186.0 | 9.0 | 504 | 7.9 | 61.0 | 25.4 | 0.0 |
| **MANDARIN** | | | | | | | | |
| with Pineapple, in Juice, SPC Nature's Finest* | 1 Pot/220g | 110.0 | 0.0 | 50 | 0.4 | 12.9 | 0.1 | 0.3 |
| **MANDARIN ORANGES** | | | | | | | | |
| Broken, Segments in Fruit Juice, Basics, Sainsbury's* | ½ Can/149g | 51.0 | 0.0 | 34 | 0.7 | 7.7 | 0.0 | 0.3 |
| *in Juice, Average* | *1oz/28g* | *11.0* | *0.0* | *39* | *0.7* | *9.0* | *0.0* | *0.5* |
| *in Light Syrup, Average* | *1 Can/298g* | *201.0* | *0.0* | *67* | *0.5* | *15.9* | *0.0* | *0.1* |
| in Orange Gel, Del Monte* | 1 Can/128g | 60.0 | 0.0 | 47 | 0.0 | 10.9 | 0.0 | 0.0 |
| *Weighed with Peel, Average* | *1 Sm/50g* | *18.0* | *0.0* | *36* | *0.9* | *8.3* | *0.1* | *1.2* |
| **MANGE TOUT** | | | | | | | | |
| & Sugar Snap Peas, Tesco* | 1 Pack/150g | 102.0 | 1.0 | 68 | 7.0 | 9.2 | 0.4 | 3.8 |
| *Boiled in Salted Water* | *1oz/28g* | *7.0* | *0.0* | *26* | *3.2* | *3.3* | *0.1* | *2.2* |
| *Raw, Average* | *1 Serving/80g* | *26.0* | *0.0* | *32* | *3.6* | *4.2* | *0.2* | *1.1* |
| *Stir-Fried in Blended Oil* | *1oz/28g* | *20.0* | *1.0* | *71* | *3.8* | *3.5* | *4.8* | *2.4* |

| | Measure INFO/WEIGHT | per Measure KCAL | FAT | Nutrition Values per 100g / 100ml KCAL | PROT | CARB | FAT | FIBRE |
|---|---|---|---|---|---|---|---|---|
| **MANGO** | | | | | | | | |
| & Melon, Sliced, Shapers, Boots* | 1 Pack/80g | 33.0 | 0.0 | 41 | 0.7 | 9.2 | 0.2 | 1.8 |
| *Dried, Average* | *1 Serving/50g* | *173.0* | *0.0* | *347* | *1.4* | *83.1* | *1.0* | *4.9* |
| *in Syrup, Average* | *1oz/28g* | *22.0* | *0.0* | *80* | *0.3* | *20.5* | *0.0* | *0.9* |
| Pieces in Juice, Natures Finest* | 1 Pot/220g | 123.0 | 0.0 | 56 | 0.5 | 12.3 | 0.2 | 1.5 |
| Pineapple & Passionfruit, M & S* | 1 Pack/400g | 200.0 | 1.0 | 50 | 0.6 | 10.9 | 0.2 | 1.7 |
| *Ripe, Raw, Weighed with Skin & Stone, Average* | *1 Mango/225g* | *88.0* | *0.0* | *39* | *0.5* | *9.6* | *0.1* | *1.8* |
| *Ripe, Raw, Without Peel & Stone, Flesh Only, Average* | *1 Mango/207g* | *135.0* | *1.0* | *65* | *0.5* | *17.0* | *0.3* | *1.8* |
| **MANGOSTEEN** | | | | | | | | |
| *Canned, in Syrup, Drained, Average* | *1 Cup/196g* | *143.0* | *1.0* | *73* | *0.4* | *17.9* | *0.6* | *1.8* |
| *Raw, Fresh, Average** | *1 Serving/80g* | *50.0* | *0.0* | *63* | *0.6* | *15.6* | *0.6* | *5.1* |
| **MARBLE** | | | | | | | | |
| Cadbury* | 1 Bar/46g | 246.0 | 14.0 | 535 | 8.4 | 54.8 | 31.2 | 0.0 |
| **MARGARINE** | | | | | | | | |
| *Average* | *1 Thin Spread/7g* | *51.0* | *6.0* | *726* | *0.1* | *0.5* | *81.0* | *0.0* |
| *Butter Style, Average* | *1 Thin Spread/7g* | *44.0* | *5.0* | *627* | *0.7* | *1.1* | *68.9* | *0.0* |
| *for Baking, Average* | *1 Thin Spread/7g* | *42.0* | *5.0* | *607* | *0.2* | *0.4* | *67.2* | *0.0* |
| No Salt, Flora* | 1 Thin Spread/7g | 37.0 | 4.0 | 531 | 0.0 | 0.0 | 59.0 | 0.0 |
| Omega 3 Plus, Flora* | 1 Thin Spread/7g | 24.0 | 3.0 | 350 | 0.1 | 3.0 | 38.0 | 0.0 |
| Pro Activ, Extra Light, Flora* | 1 Thin Spread/7g | 15.0 | 2.0 | 218 | 0.1 | 2.9 | 23.0 | 0.2 |
| Pro Activ, Light, Flora* | 1 Thin Spread/7g | 23.0 | 2.0 | 331 | 0.1 | 4.0 | 35.0 | 0.0 |
| Pro Activ, with Olive Oil, Flora* | 1 Thin Spread/7g | 23.0 | 2.0 | 331 | 0.1 | 4.0 | 35.0 | 0.0 |
| *Reduced Fat, Average* | *1 Thin Spread/7g* | *25.0* | *3.0* | *356* | *0.5* | *3.0* | *38.0* | *0.0* |
| Soya, Granose* | 1 Thin Spread/7g | 52.0 | 6.0 | 745 | 0.1 | 0.1 | 82.0 | 0.0 |
| White, Flora* | 1 Thin Spread/7g | 60.0 | 7.0 | 855 | 0.0 | 0.0 | 95.0 | 0.0 |
| **MARINADE** | | | | | | | | |
| Barbecue, COU, M & S* | 1 Serving/35g | 52.0 | 0.0 | 150 | 1.2 | 35.5 | 0.2 | 1.0 |
| Barbecue, in Minutes, Knorr* | 1 Pack/110g | 337.0 | 1.0 | 306 | 6.2 | 66.4 | 1.3 | 3.4 |
| Hot & Spicy Barbecue, M & S* | 1 Serving/18g | 23.0 | 0.0 | 130 | 1.0 | 31.1 | 0.3 | 0.8 |
| Lemon & Rosemary, Nando's* | 1fl oz/30ml | 44.0 | 4.0 | 147 | 1.0 | 11.8 | 13.0 | 0.2 |
| Lime & Coriander with Peri Peri, Nando's* | 1 Tsp/5g | 9.0 | 1.0 | 182 | 0.0 | 13.1 | 16.6 | 0.2 |
| Sticky Barbecue, Tesco* | ¼ Jar/70g | 80.0 | 0.0 | 115 | 0.7 | 26.7 | 0.2 | 0.6 |
| Sun Dried Tomato & Basil with Peri-Peri, Nando's* | 1 Bottle/270g | 319.0 | 26.0 | 118 | 0.1 | 15.3 | 9.5 | 0.8 |
| Tequila Chilli Lime, M & S* | 1 Serving/75ml | 116.0 | 1.0 | 155 | 0.6 | 34.0 | 1.6 | 0.5 |
| Thai Coconut, Coriander & Lime, Lea & Perrins* | 1oz/28g | 45.0 | 2.0 | 159 | 1.3 | 25.7 | 6.1 | 0.0 |
| Tomato, Basil & Parmesan, M & S* | 1 Serving/50g | 37.0 | 1.0 | 75 | 2.1 | 10.1 | 2.5 | 1.5 |
| Tomato & Herb, Lea & Perrins* | 1oz/28g | 28.0 | 0.0 | 100 | 1.2 | 24.1 | 0.5 | 0.0 |
| White Wine, Garlic & Pepper, Lea & Perrins* | 1oz/28g | 28.0 | 0.0 | 99 | 0.0 | 23.7 | 0.7 | 0.0 |
| **MARJORAM** | | | | | | | | |
| *Dried* | *1 Tsp/1g* | *2.0* | *0.0* | *271* | *12.7* | *42.5* | *7.0* | *0.0* |
| **MARLIN** | | | | | | | | |
| Smoked, H. Forman & Son* | 1 Pack/200g | 240.0 | 0.0 | 120 | 29.8 | 0.0 | 0.1 | 0.0 |
| Steaks, Chargrilled, Sainsbury's* | 1 Steak/240g | 367.0 | 15.0 | 153 | 23.6 | 0.8 | 6.1 | 0.6 |
| Steaks, Raw, Sainsbury's* | 1 Steak/110g | 109.0 | 0.0 | 99 | 24.3 | 0.0 | 0.2 | 0.0 |
| **MARMALADE** | | | | | | | | |
| 3 Fruit, Thick Cut, Waitrose* | 1 Tsp/15g | 39.0 | 0.0 | 262 | 0.4 | 64.8 | 0.1 | 0.7 |
| Blood Orange, Grandessa* | 1 Serving/15g | 36.0 | 0.0 | 240 | 0.4 | 59.0 | 0.1 | 0.7 |
| Five Fruit, Tesco* | 1 Serving/10g | 28.0 | 0.0 | 278 | 0.2 | 68.2 | 0.1 | 0.9 |
| Four Citrus Fruits, Thin Cut, TTD, Sainsbury's* | 1 Serving/15g | 36.0 | 0.0 | 242 | 0.2 | 60.0 | 0.1 | 1.0 |
| Grapefruit, Fine Cut, Duerr's* | 1 Tsp/15g | 39.0 | 0.0 | 261 | 0.2 | 65.0 | 0.0 | 0.0 |
| Grapefruit & Cranberry, M & S* | 1 Tsp/15g | 36.0 | 0.0 | 240 | 0.3 | 60.3 | 0.0 | 1.5 |
| Lemon, Fine Cut, Tesco* | 1 Serving/15g | 39.0 | 0.0 | 257 | 0.2 | 64.0 | 0.0 | 0.5 |
| *Lemon, with Shred, Average* | *1 Serving/20g* | *49.0* | *0.0* | *247* | *0.1* | *61.6* | *0.0* | *0.6* |
| *Lemon & Lime, Average* | *1 Tbsp/20g* | *53.0* | *0.0* | *267* | *0.1* | *66.3* | *0.1* | *0.4* |

| INFO/WEIGHT | Measure | per Measure | | Nutrition Values per 100g / 100ml | | | | |
|---|---|---|---|---|---|---|---|---|
| | | KCAL | FAT | KCAL | PROT | CARB | FAT | FIBRE |

## MARMALADE

| | | | | | | | | |
|---|---|---|---|---|---|---|---|---|
| Lemon Jelly, No Peel, Tesco* | 1 Tsp/15g | 39.0 | 0.0 | 263 | 0.1 | 65.0 | 0.0 | 0.4 |
| *Lime, with Shred, Average* | *1 Tbsp/15g* | *39.0* | *0.0* | *261* | *0.1* | *65.0* | *0.1* | *0.3* |
| Orange, Lemon & Grapefruit, Baxters* | 1 Tsp/15g | 38.0 | 0.0 | 252 | 0.0 | 63.0 | 0.0 | 0.1 |
| *Orange, Reduced Sugar, Average* | *1 Tbsp/15g* | *26.0* | *0.0* | *170* | *0.4* | *42.0* | *0.1* | *0.6* |
| Orange, Reduced Sugar, Thin Cut, Streamline* | 1 Serving/10g | 18.0 | 0.0 | 178 | 0.5 | 43.0 | 0.3 | 0.0 |
| *Orange, Shredless, Average* | *1 Tsp/10g* | *26.0* | *0.0* | *261* | *0.2* | *65.0* | *0.0* | *0.1* |
| Orange, Thick Cut, with Drambuie, TTD, Sainsbury's* | 1 Serving/15g | 36.0 | 0.0 | 238 | 0.3 | 58.4 | 0.1 | 2.7 |
| Orange, with Drambuie, Finest, Tesco* | 1 Serving/10g | 33.0 | 0.0 | 329 | 0.3 | 82.0 | 0.0 | 0.7 |
| *Orange, with Shred, Average* | *1 Tbsp/15g* | *39.0* | *0.0* | *263* | *0.2* | *65.2* | *0.0* | *0.3* |
| *Orange & Ginger, Average* | *1 Tbsp/15g* | *40.0* | *0.0* | *264* | *0.2* | *65.7* | *0.1* | *0.3* |
| Orange & Tangerine, Tiptree, Wilkin & Sons* | 1 Tsp/15g | 40.0 | 0.0 | 268 | 0.0 | 67.0 | 0.0 | 0.3 |
| Orange Shred, Medium Cut, Tesco* | 1 Serving/15g | 39.0 | 0.0 | 260 | 0.3 | 64.7 | 0.0 | 0.5 |
| Pink Grapefruit, Thin Cut, Waitrose* | 1 Serving/10g | 26.0 | 0.0 | 261 | 0.2 | 65.0 | 0.0 | 0.4 |
| Three Fruit, Finest, Tesco* | 1 Serving/15g | 39.0 | 0.0 | 262 | 0.5 | 63.6 | 0.2 | 1.6 |
| Three Fruits, Fresh Fruit, Sainsbury's* | 1 Tsp/15g | 37.0 | 0.0 | 250 | 0.0 | 61.3 | 0.0 | 0.0 |

## MARMITE*

| | | | | | | | | |
|---|---|---|---|---|---|---|---|---|
| Yeast Extract, Marmite* | 1 Tsp/9g | 21.0 | 0.0 | 231 | 38.4 | 19.2 | 0.1 | 3.1 |

## MARROW

| | | | | | | | | |
|---|---|---|---|---|---|---|---|---|
| *Boiled, Average* | *1oz/28g* | *3.0* | *0.0* | *9* | *0.4* | *1.6* | *0.2* | *0.6* |
| *Raw* | *1oz/28g* | *3.0* | *0.0* | *12* | *0.5* | *2.2* | *0.2* | *0.5* |

## MARS

| | | | | | | | | |
|---|---|---|---|---|---|---|---|---|
| Bar, 5 Little Ones, Mars* | 1 Piece/8g | 38.0 | 1.0 | 477 | 4.5 | 73.6 | 18.3 | 0.0 |
| Bar, Duo, Mars* | 1 Bar/42g | 193.0 | 8.0 | 455 | 4.1 | 69.7 | 17.7 | 1.3 |
| Bar, Fun Size, Mars* | 1 Bar/20g | 89.0 | 3.0 | 444 | 3.7 | 69.7 | 16.8 | 1.1 |
| Bar, Mars* | 1 Std Bar/63g | 280.0 | 11.0 | 448 | 4.1 | 68.1 | 17.6 | 11.0 |
| Delight, Mars* | 1 Bar/20g | 110.0 | 7.0 | 552 | 4.5 | 57.8 | 33.6 | 1.3 |

## MARSHMALLOWS

| | | | | | | | | |
|---|---|---|---|---|---|---|---|---|
| Average | 1 Mallow/5g | 16.0 | 0.0 | 327 | 3.9 | 83.1 | 0.0 | 0.0 |
| Fat Free, Tesco* | 1 Mallow/7g | 24.0 | 0.0 | 339 | 3.4 | 80.8 | 0.2 | 0.5 |
| Haribo* | 1 Mallow/5g | 16.0 | 0.0 | 330 | 3.0 | 80.0 | 0.0 | 0.0 |
| Pascall* | 1 Mallow/5g | 15.0 | 0.0 | 335 | 2.6 | 80.0 | 0.0 | 0.0 |
| Pink & White, Co-Op* | 1 Mallow/7g | 24.0 | 0.0 | 340 | 3.0 | 82.0 | 0.0 | 0.0 |
| Princess* | 1 Mallow/5g | 16.0 | 0.0 | 314 | 3.4 | 80.0 | 0.0 | 0.0 |
| Raspberry & Cream, Sainsbury's* | 1 Mallow/7g | 23.0 | 0.0 | 330 | 4.1 | 78.5 | 0.0 | 0.5 |
| Sainsbury's* | 1 Mallow/7g | 23.0 | 0.0 | 330 | 4.1 | 78.5 | 0.0 | 0.5 |

## MARZIPAN

| | | | | | | | | |
|---|---|---|---|---|---|---|---|---|
| Bar, Chocolate, Plain, Thorntons* | 1 Bar/46g | 206.0 | 8.0 | 448 | 5.2 | 69.1 | 17.4 | 2.0 |
| Dark Chocolate, Thorntons* | 1 Serving/46g | 207.0 | 8.0 | 451 | 5.2 | 69.4 | 17.4 | 2.1 |
| *Plain, Average* | *1oz/28g* | *115.0* | *4.0* | *412* | *5.8* | *67.5* | *14.1* | *1.7* |

## MASALA

| | | | | | | | | |
|---|---|---|---|---|---|---|---|---|
| Chicken, Tandoori, M & S* | ½ Pack/175g | 210.0 | 12.0 | 120 | 11.3 | 4.3 | 6.6 | 4.5 |
| Prawn, & Rice, Tesco* | 1 Pack/475g | 655.0 | 25.0 | 138 | 5.2 | 17.9 | 5.2 | 1.2 |
| Prawn, King, Waitrose* | 1 Pack/350g | 385.0 | 26.0 | 110 | 7.1 | 3.8 | 7.4 | 1.8 |
| Vegetable, Sainsbury's* | 1 Pack/400g | 388.0 | 30.0 | 97 | 2.1 | 5.2 | 7.5 | 2.5 |
| Vegetable, Somerfield* | 1 Pack/350g | 406.0 | 24.0 | 116 | 2.7 | 11.0 | 6.8 | 3.0 |
| Vegetable, Waitrose* | 1 Serving/400g | 288.0 | 19.0 | 72 | 2.2 | 4.9 | 4.8 | 2.5 |

## MASH

| | | | | | | | | |
|---|---|---|---|---|---|---|---|---|
| Carrot & Parsnip, Direct Foods* | 1 Pack/380g | 201.0 | 9.0 | 53 | 1.0 | 7.6 | 2.3 | 3.2 |
| Davidstow Cheddar, Extra Special, Asda* | 1 Serving/225g | 292.0 | 17.0 | 130 | 5.3 | 10.4 | 7.5 | 2.6 |
| Parsnip & Parmesan, Finest, Tesco* | ½ Packet/250g | 245.0 | 12.0 | 98 | 1.6 | 11.9 | 4.9 | 2.4 |
| Potato, Carrot, Swede, Parsnip, Cream & Butter, Asda* | ½ Pack/200g | 94.0 | 3.0 | 47 | 1.0 | 7.2 | 1.5 | 3.3 |
| Root, Asda* | ½ Pack/200g | 142.0 | 8.0 | 71 | 0.7 | 8.0 | 4.0 | 3.1 |
| Root Vegetable, Finest, Tesco* | ½ Pack/250g | 225.0 | 12.0 | 90 | 1.1 | 9.1 | 5.0 | 3.4 |

| | Measure INFO/WEIGHT | per Measure KCAL | per Measure FAT | Nutrition Values per 100g / 100ml KCAL | PROT | CARB | FAT | FIBRE |
|---|---|---|---|---|---|---|---|---|
| **MASH** | | | | | | | | |
| Vegetables, Mousline, Maggi* | 1 Bag/39g | 127.0 | 1.0 | 328 | 8.2 | 67.0 | 3.0 | 10.4 |
| Winter Root, Sainsbury's* | 1 Serving/140g | 157.0 | 2.0 | 112 | 2.7 | 22.0 | 1.5 | 0.9 |
| **MAYONNAISE** | | | | | | | | |
| 50% Less Fat, GFY, Asda* | 1 Tbsp/10g | 32.0 | 3.0 | 322 | 0.8 | 10.0 | 31.0 | 0.0 |
| 60% Less Fat, BGTY, Sainsbury's* | 1 Tbsp/15ml | 42.0 | 4.0 | 277 | 0.4 | 7.3 | 27.3 | 0.0 |
| Aioli, Finest, Tesco* | 1 Tsp/5g | 20.0 | 2.0 | 408 | 0.8 | 8.5 | 41.2 | 0.0 |
| ***Average*** | *1 Tsp/11g* | *80.0* | *9.0* | *724* | *1.9* | *0.2* | *79.3* | *0.0* |
| Bramwells, Extra Light, Specially Selected, Aldi* | 1 Tbsp/33g | 40.0 | 3.0 | 121 | 1.1 | 7.2 | 9.7 | 2.4 |
| Deli, Caramelised Onion, Heinz* | 1 Serving/20g | 110.0 | 11.0 | 548 | 1.4 | 5.9 | 57.5 | 0.1 |
| Deli, Moroccan, Heinz* | 1 Tbsp/15g | 80.0 | 8.0 | 532 | 0.9 | 4.6 | 56.5 | 0.1 |
| Deli, Roasted Garlic, Heinz* | 1 Tbsp/15g | 81.0 | 8.0 | 537 | 1.1 | 5.5 | 56.6 | 0.0 |
| Deli, Sundried Tomato, Heinz* | 1 Tbsp/15g | 88.0 | 9.0 | 589 | 1.3 | 4.9 | 62.5 | 0.0 |
| Egg, Safeway* | 1 Serving/50g | 120.0 | 11.0 | 241 | 10.4 | 0.4 | 22.0 | 1.0 |
| Extra Light, Asda* | 1 Tbsp/10ml | 12.0 | 1.0 | 119 | 0.7 | 13.1 | 7.1 | 0.2 |
| Extra Light, Heinz* | 1 Tbsp/12ml | 9.0 | 0.0 | 75 | 0.6 | 11.4 | 3.0 | 0.6 |
| Extra Light, Now Only 3% Fat, Hellmann's* | 1 Serving/16g | 12.0 | 0.0 | 73 | 0.6 | 11.0 | 3.0 | 0.6 |
| Extra Light, Sainsbury's* | 1 Tbsp/15ml | 17.0 | 1.0 | 115 | 0.7 | 11.9 | 7.0 | 0.0 |
| Extra Light, Weight Watchers* | 1 Serving/15g | 15.0 | 1.0 | 97 | 1.1 | 9.6 | 5.9 | 3.2 |
| Finest, Tesco* | 1 Dtsp/22g | 155.0 | 17.0 | 703 | 1.1 | 1.5 | 77.0 | 0.0 |
| French, Light, Sainsbury's* | 1 Serving/15ml | 46.0 | 5.0 | 307 | 0.4 | 6.1 | 31.1 | 0.2 |
| French Style, BGTY, Sainsbury's* | 1 Tbsp/15ml | 55.0 | 6.0 | 366 | 0.6 | 7.5 | 36.9 | 0.0 |
| Garlic, Morrisons* | 1 Tbsp/15ml | 55.0 | 5.0 | 365 | 0.7 | 8.8 | 36.0 | 0.0 |
| Garlic, Waitrose* | 1 Tsp/6g | 21.0 | 2.0 | 346 | 0.6 | 8.6 | 34.3 | 0.0 |
| Garlic & Herb, M & S* | 1 Tsp/6g | 43.0 | 5.0 | 712 | 3.4 | 2.4 | 76.9 | 0.9 |
| Garlic & Herb, Reduced Calorie, Hellmann's* | 1 Serving/25ml | 58.0 | 5.0 | 233 | 0.7 | 13.1 | 19.3 | 0.4 |
| Heinz* | 1 Tbsp/15g | 99.0 | 11.0 | 663 | 0.9 | 3.0 | 71.8 | 0.0 |
| Lemon, Waitrose* | 1 Tsp/8ml | 56.0 | 6.0 | 694 | 1.2 | 1.3 | 76.0 | 5.4 |
| Light, BGTY, Sainsbury's* | 1 Tsp/11g | 33.0 | 3.0 | 296 | 0.5 | 7.2 | 29.3 | 0.0 |
| Light, Hellmann's* | 1 Serving/10g | 30.0 | 3.0 | 298 | 0.7 | 6.5 | 29.8 | 0.1 |
| Light, Kraft* | 1 Serving/25g | 61.0 | 5.0 | 245 | 0.6 | 15.0 | 20.0 | 0.0 |
| Light, Morrisons* | 1 Tsp/11g | 32.0 | 3.0 | 287 | 1.4 | 8.5 | 27.5 | 0.0 |
| Light, Reduced Fat, Heinz* | 1 Tbsp/15g | 42.0 | 4.0 | 279 | 1.1 | 7.7 | 26.8 | 0.5 |
| Light, Squeezable, Hellmann's* | 1 Tbsp/15g | 44.0 | 4.0 | 293 | 0.7 | 6.4 | 29.4 | 0.0 |
| Light, Tesco* | 1 Tbsp/15ml | 45.0 | 4.0 | 300 | 0.8 | 9.4 | 28.5 | 0.0 |
| Made with Free Range Eggs, M & S* | 1 Tbsp/15g | 108.0 | 12.0 | 720 | 1.1 | 1.2 | 78.5 | 0.0 |
| Organic, Evernat* | 1 Tsp/11g | 83.0 | 9.0 | 752 | 1.3 | 2.8 | 81.0 | 0.0 |
| Real, Asda* | 1 Serving/10g | 72.0 | 8.0 | 721 | 1.3 | 1.2 | 79.0 | 0.1 |
| Real, Best Foods* | 1 Tbsp/13g | 90.0 | 10.0 | 692 | 0.0 | 0.0 | 76.9 | 0.0 |
| Real, Hellmann's* | 1 Tsp/11g | 79.0 | 9.0 | 722 | 1.1 | 1.3 | 79.1 | 0.0 |
| Real, The Big Squeeze, Hellmann's* | 1 Tbsp/15ml | 101.0 | 11.0 | 676 | 1.0 | 1.2 | 74.0 | 0.0 |
| ***Reduced Calorie*** | *1 Tsp/11g* | *32.0* | *3.0* | *288* | *1.0* | *8.2* | *28.1* | *0.0* |
| Reduced Calorie, Tesco* | 1 Tbsp/15g | 49.0 | 5.0 | 326 | 0.8 | 9.8 | 31.5 | 0.0 |
| Reduced Calorie, Waitrose* | 1 Tsp/11g | 32.0 | 3.0 | 287 | 1.4 | 8.5 | 27.5 | 0.0 |
| Reduced Fat, Tesco* | 1 Tbsp/15ml | 44.0 | 4.0 | 292 | 0.8 | 7.9 | 28.6 | 0.0 |
| Sainsbury's* | 1 Tsp/11g | 75.0 | 8.0 | 686 | 0.4 | 1.2 | 75.4 | 0.0 |
| Value, Tesco* | 1 Tbsp/15g | 73.0 | 8.0 | 488 | 0.8 | 5.4 | 51.4 | 0.0 |
| Vegetarian, Tesco* | 1 Tsp/12g | 89.0 | 10.0 | 738 | 1.5 | 0.8 | 81.0 | 0.0 |
| Waitrose* | 1 Tbsp/15ml | 106.0 | 12.0 | 709 | 1.3 | 0.8 | 77.8 | 0.0 |
| with Dijon Mustard, Hellmann's* | 1 Tbsp/15ml | 31.0 | 3.0 | 210 | 2.9 | 5.1 | 19.7 | 0.0 |
| **MEAL REPLACEMENT** | | | | | | | | |
| Bars, Chocolate, Slim Fast* | 1 Bar/39g | 107.0 | 4.0 | 274 | 20.6 | 35.3 | 9.0 | 5.5 |
| Bars, Chocolate & Hazelnut, Tesco* | 1 Bar/65g | 250.0 | 7.0 | 385 | 24.2 | 41.0 | 11.0 | 6.3 |
| Bars, Toffee Delight, Slim Fast* | 1 Bar/78g | 248.0 | 7.0 | 318 | 20.6 | 45.3 | 9.6 | 5.9 |

| | Measure INFO/WEIGHT | per Measure KCAL | FAT | Nutrition Values per 100g / 100ml KCAL | PROT | CARB | FAT | FIBRE |
|---|---|---|---|---|---|---|---|---|
| **MEAL REPLACEMENT** | | | | | | | | |
| Shake, Chocolate, Advantage, Atkins* | 1 Serving/34g | 121.0 | 4.0 | 361 | 49.0 | 8.1 | 12.5 | 15.5 |
| Shake, Chocolate, Ready to Drink, Advantage, Atkins* | 1 Carton/330ml | 172.0 | 9.0 | 52 | 6.0 | 0.6 | 2.8 | 1.2 |
| Shake, Herbalife* | 1 Serving/250ml | 245.0 | 6.0 | 98 | 10.0 | 8.8 | 2.6 | 1.0 |
| Shake, Neways* | 1 Serving/39g | 142.0 | 4.0 | 364 | 46.0 | 34.0 | 9.0 | 15.4 |
| Shake, Vanilla, Ready to Drink, Advantage, Atkins* | 1 Carton/330ml | 175.0 | 9.0 | 53 | 6.2 | 0.6 | 2.7 | 0.9 |
| Ultra Slim, Ready to Drink, Strawberry, Tesco* | 1 Carton/330ml | 231.0 | 3.0 | 70 | 4.2 | 10.5 | 0.9 | 1.5 |
| Ultra Slim, Ready to Drink, Vanilla, Tesco* | 1 Carton/330ml | 224.0 | 3.0 | 68 | 4.2 | 10.5 | 0.9 | 1.5 |
| Ultra-Slim, Ready to Drink, Chocolate, Tesco* | 1 Carton/330ml | 215.0 | 4.0 | 65 | 3.9 | 9.8 | 1.1 | 1.3 |
| **MEAT LOAF** | | | | | | | | |
| Beef & Pork, Co-Op* | ¼ Loaf/114g | 313.0 | 25.0 | 275 | 13.0 | 7.0 | 22.0 | 1.0 |
| Iceland* | 1 Serving/150g | 331.0 | 24.0 | 221 | 10.8 | 9.3 | 15.7 | 0.9 |
| in Onion Gravy, M & S* | ¼ Pack/140g | 203.0 | 12.0 | 145 | 11.3 | 6.3 | 8.5 | 1.2 |
| Somerfield* | 1 Pack/454g | 867.0 | 59.0 | 191 | 10.0 | 8.0 | 13.0 | 0.0 |
| Turkey & Bacon, Tesco* | 1 Serving/225g | 400.0 | 22.0 | 178 | 14.7 | 7.4 | 9.9 | 1.1 |
| **MEATBALLS** | | | | | | | | |
| & Mashed Potato, Tesco* | 1 Pack/450g | 526.0 | 30.0 | 117 | 4.0 | 10.4 | 6.6 | 1.0 |
| & Pasta, Sainsbury's* | 1 Serving/300g | 333.0 | 9.0 | 111 | 5.3 | 15.5 | 3.1 | 1.9 |
| & Spaghetti, Asda* | 1 Pack/400g | 432.0 | 16.0 | 108 | 6.3 | 11.7 | 4.0 | 2.6 |
| Aberdeen Angus, Fresh, Chilled, Waitrose* | 1 Meatball/36g | 92.0 | 7.0 | 256 | 18.0 | 1.5 | 19.8 | 0.0 |
| Aberdeen Angus in Sauce, Perfectly Balanced, Waitrose* | ½ Pack/240g | 228.0 | 7.0 | 95 | 10.5 | 6.5 | 3.0 | 1.1 |
| Al Forno, Safeway* | 1 Pack/450g | 684.0 | 31.0 | 152 | 6.0 | 16.8 | 6.8 | 0.4 |
| Beef, Morrisons* | 3 Meatballs/85g | 213.0 | 14.0 | 251 | 23.1 | 3.1 | 16.2 | 0.9 |
| Beef, Sainsbury's* | 1 Meatball/29g | 75.0 | 5.0 | 257 | 21.7 | 3.4 | 17.4 | 0.8 |
| Beef, Tesco* | 3 Meatballs/53g | 140.0 | 11.0 | 265 | 15.0 | 2.9 | 21.5 | 0.9 |
| Chicken, in Tomato Sauce, Average | 1 Can/392g | 580.0 | 33.0 | 148 | 7.7 | 10.4 | 8.4 | 0.0 |
| Greek, M & S* | 1 Serving/350g | 402.0 | 19.0 | 115 | 7.7 | 9.1 | 5.4 | 1.5 |
| in Bolognese Sauce, Fray Bentos* | ½ Can/204g | 188.0 | 6.0 | 92 | 4.8 | 11.6 | 2.9 | 0.7 |
| in Bolognese Sauce, Somerfield* | 1 Pack/454g | 704.0 | 50.0 | 155 | 7.0 | 7.0 | 11.0 | 0.0 |
| in Gravy, Campbell's* | ½ Can/205g | 164.0 | 5.0 | 80 | 5.6 | 8.6 | 2.6 | 0.0 |
| in Gravy, Fray Bentos* | 1 Meatball/21g | 17.0 | 1.0 | 79 | 4.6 | 8.7 | 2.9 | 0.6 |
| in Onion Gravy, Tesco* | ½ Pack/200g | 310.0 | 17.0 | 155 | 8.4 | 11.3 | 8.5 | 0.8 |
| in Tomato Sauce, Canned, Average | 1 Can/410g | 387.0 | 15.0 | 94 | 5.6 | 9.8 | 3.7 | 0.0 |
| in Tomato Sauce, Fray Bentos* | ½ Can/206g | 183.0 | 6.0 | 89 | 4.7 | 11.1 | 2.9 | 0.7 |
| in Tomato Sauce, Tapas, Waitrose* | 1 Pack/185g | 285.0 | 17.0 | 154 | 10.8 | 7.2 | 9.1 | 1.3 |
| Italian Pork, Al Forno, Sainsbury's* | 1 Pack/450g | 643.0 | 24.0 | 143 | 6.1 | 17.6 | 5.3 | 1.4 |
| Lamb, Asda* | 1 Pack/340g | 928.0 | 71.0 | 273 | 16.0 | 5.1 | 21.0 | 0.6 |
| Pork & Beef, Swedish Style, Tesco* | 1 Meatball/14g | 34.0 | 2.0 | 245 | 14.3 | 6.5 | 17.7 | 2.0 |
| Roman-Style with Basil Mash, COU, M & S* | 1 Pack/430g | 344.0 | 9.0 | 80 | 3.7 | 10.9 | 2.2 | 1.9 |
| Spaghetti, Tesco* | 1 Pack/385g | 377.0 | 16.0 | 98 | 5.4 | 9.8 | 4.2 | 1.2 |
| Spicy, M & S* | 1 Pack/400g | 540.0 | 24.0 | 135 | 8.8 | 12.0 | 6.0 | 1.4 |
| Swedish, Average | ¼ Pack/88g | 198.0 | 14.0 | 224 | 14.0 | 7.4 | 15.7 | 1.3 |
| Turkey, GFY, Asda* | ½ Pack/330g | 333.0 | 12.0 | 101 | 10.0 | 7.0 | 3.7 | 0.0 |
| with Spicy Tomato Sauce, Just Cook, Sainsbury's* | ½ Pack/170g | 246.0 | 12.0 | 145 | 14.8 | 5.7 | 7.0 | 0.9 |
| **MEATBALLS VEGETARIAN** | | | | | | | | |
| Swedish Style, Sainsbury's* | 1 Ball/27g | 53.0 | 3.0 | 194 | 21.5 | 5.5 | 9.5 | 4.0 |
| with Penne, Tesco* | 1 Serving/460g | 414.0 | 11.0 | 90 | 5.9 | 11.4 | 2.3 | 2.1 |
| **MEDLAR** | | | | | | | | |
| *Raw, Flesh Only* | *1 Fruit/28g* | *11.0* | *0.0* | *40* | *0.5* | *10.6* | *0.4* | *10.0* |
| **MELBA TOAST** | | | | | | | | |
| Asda* | 1 Slice/3g | 13.0 | 0.0 | 395 | 12.0 | 76.0 | 4.8 | 4.6 |
| Average | 1 Serving/3g | 13.0 | 0.0 | 396 | 12.0 | 76.0 | 4.9 | 4.6 |
| Buitoni* | 1 Serving/33g | 130.0 | 2.0 | 395 | 12.1 | 75.5 | 4.9 | 4.6 |
| Dutch, Light Choices, Tesco* | 1 Pack/20g | 75.0 | 0.0 | 375 | 13.1 | 75.0 | 2.4 | 4.6 |

| | Measure INFO/WEIGHT | per Measure KCAL | per Measure FAT | Nutrition Values per 100g / 100ml KCAL | PROT | CARB | FAT | FIBRE |
|---|---|---|---|---|---|---|---|---|
| **MELON** | | | | | | | | |
| & Blueberry, Snack Pot, Great Stuff, Asda* | 1 Pack/80g | 25.0 | 0.0 | 31 | 0.6 | 6.8 | 0.1 | 1.2 |
| *Cantaloupe, Flesh Only, Average* | *½ Melon/255g* | *87.0* | *0.0* | *34* | *0.8* | *8.2* | *0.2* | *0.9* |
| *Cantaloupe, Weighed with Rind, Average* | *1 Slice/100g* | *35.0* | *0.0* | *35* | *0.8* | *8.3* | *0.3* | *0.8* |
| *Galia, Average* | *1 Serving/240g* | *60.0* | *0.0* | *25* | *0.7* | *5.7* | *0.0* | *0.2* |
| *Honeydew, Raw, Flesh Only, Average* | *1oz/28g* | *8.0* | *0.0* | *29* | *0.7* | *6.9* | *0.1* | *0.5* |
| Medley, Average | 1 Pack/240g | 66.0 | 0.0 | 27 | 0.6 | 6.0 | 0.1 | 0.5 |
| Pineapple & Strawberry, Fully Prepared, Sainsbury's* | 1 Serving/245g | 86.0 | 0.0 | 35 | 0.6 | 7.8 | 0.1 | 0.9 |
| **MELT** | | | | | | | | |
| Cheese, Chilli, Fresh, Asda* | 1 Melt/29g | 87.0 | 5.0 | 301 | 6.0 | 31.0 | 17.0 | 0.0 |
| Cheesy Fish, Youngs* | 1 Pack/340g | 418.0 | 22.0 | 123 | 7.6 | 8.3 | 6.6 | 0.9 |
| Chilli with Spicy Potato Wedges, Asda* | 1 Pack/450g | 540.0 | 20.0 | 120 | 8.0 | 12.0 | 4.4 | 1.2 |
| Salmon & Broccoli Wedge, From Heinz, Weight Watchers* | 1 Pack/320g | 298.0 | 11.0 | 93 | 5.1 | 10.6 | 3.3 | 1.1 |
| Tuna, Go Large, Asda* | 1 Melt/175g | 509.0 | 26.0 | 291 | 12.0 | 27.0 | 15.0 | 0.0 |
| Tuna, M & S* | 1 Pack/218g | 621.0 | 37.0 | 285 | 13.0 | 20.1 | 17.0 | 1.0 |
| Vegetable & Potato, Asda* | 1 Serving/100g | 451.0 | 23.0 | 451 | 17.0 | 44.0 | 23.0 | 6.2 |
| **MENTOS** | | | | | | | | |
| Cola, Mentos* | 1 Packet/38g | 146.0 | 1.0 | 390 | 0.0 | 93.0 | 2.0 | 0.0 |
| **MERINGUE** | | | | | | | | |
| *Average* | *1 Meringue/8g* | *30.0* | *0.0* | *379* | *5.3* | *95.4* | *0.0* | *0.0* |
| Belgian Chocolate, Mini, Extra Special, Asda* | 1 Meringue/6g | 28.0 | 1.0 | 459 | 6.0 | 75.0 | 15.0 | 0.7 |
| Chocolate, Waitrose* | 1 Meringue/77g | 341.0 | 11.0 | 444 | 2.6 | 75.3 | 14.7 | 0.5 |
| Coffee Fresh Cream, Asda* | 1 Meringue/28g | 109.0 | 5.0 | 396 | 3.8 | 57.0 | 17.0 | 0.3 |
| Cream, Fresh, Sainsbury's* | 1 Meringue/35g | 142.0 | 5.0 | 407 | 3.5 | 65.4 | 14.6 | 0.5 |
| Cream, M & S* | 1 Meringue/34g | 145.0 | 8.0 | 425 | 4.1 | 52.6 | 22.2 | 1.4 |
| Layered, Tesco* | 1/5 Meringue/52g | 146.0 | 1.0 | 280 | 3.5 | 63.2 | 1.5 | 1.4 |
| Lemon, Morrisons* | 1 Serving/120g | 295.0 | 14.0 | 246 | 2.5 | 32.0 | 12.0 | 0.5 |
| Mini, Extra Special, Asda* | 1 Meringue/4g | 14.0 | 0.0 | 394 | 5.0 | 93.0 | 0.2 | 0.5 |
| Mini, M & S* | 1 Meringue/4g | 15.0 | 0.0 | 395 | 6.1 | 91.6 | 0.0 | 0.2 |
| Nests, Asda* | 1 Nest/15g | 59.0 | 0.0 | 394 | 5.0 | 93.0 | 0.2 | 0.5 |
| Nests, M & S* | 1 Nest/12g | 47.0 | 0.0 | 390 | 6.1 | 91.6 | 0.0 | 0.0 |
| Nests, Morrisons* | 1 Nest/15g | 62.0 | 0.0 | 414 | 4.5 | 94.7 | 0.0 | 0.0 |
| Nests, Sainsbury's* | 1 Nest/13g | 52.0 | 0.0 | 392 | 4.2 | 93.6 | 0.1 | 0.1 |
| Shells, Sainsbury's* | 2 Shells/24g | 93.0 | 0.0 | 387 | 3.9 | 92.8 | 0.0 | 0.0 |
| Strawberry, COU, M & S* | 1 Meringue/5g | 20.0 | 0.0 | 385 | 6.4 | 90.0 | 0.1 | 1.4 |
| Summer Fruits, 90% Fat Free, Sara Lee* | 1 Meringue/135g | 308.0 | 11.0 | 228 | 2.5 | 35.7 | 8.5 | 2.2 |
| Toffee, M & S* | 1 Meringue/30g | 124.0 | 6.0 | 415 | 4.1 | 52.2 | 20.9 | 0.8 |
| **MESSICANI** | | | | | | | | |
| Egg, M & S* | 1 Serving/100g | 355.0 | 3.0 | 355 | 13.9 | 68.5 | 2.8 | 3.0 |
| **MIDGET GEMS** | | | | | | | | |
| M & S* | 1 Bag/113g | 367.0 | 0.0 | 325 | 6.3 | 75.1 | 0.1 | 0.0 |
| SmartPrice, Asda* | 1 Pack/178g | 586.0 | 0.0 | 329 | 6.0 | 76.0 | 0.1 | 0.0 |
| **MILK** | | | | | | | | |
| *Condensed, Semi Skimmed, Sweetened* | *1oz/28g* | *75.0* | *0.0* | *267* | *10.0* | *60.0* | *0.2* | *0.0* |
| *Condensed, Skimmed, Unsweetened, Average* | *1oz/28g* | *30.0* | *1.0* | *108* | *7.5* | *10.5* | *4.0* | *0.0* |
| *Condensed, Whole, Sweetened, Average* | *1oz/28g* | *93.0* | *3.0* | *333* | *8.5* | *55.5* | *10.1* | *0.0* |
| *Dried, Skimmed, Average* | *1oz/28g* | *99.0* | *0.0* | *355* | *35.4* | *52.3* | *0.9* | *0.0* |
| *Dried, Whole, Average* | *1oz/28g* | *137.0* | *7.0* | *490* | *26.3* | *39.4* | *26.3* | *0.0* |
| *Evaporated, Average* | *1 Serving/85g* | *136.0* | *8.0* | *160* | *8.2* | *11.6* | *9.0* | *0.0* |
| *Evaporated, Reduced Fat, Average* | *1oz/28g* | *33.0* | *1.0* | *118* | *7.4* | *10.5* | *5.2* | *0.0* |
| *Goats, Pasteurised* | *1 fl oz/30ml* | *18.0* | *1.0* | *60* | *3.1* | *4.4* | *3.5* | *0.0* |
| Goats, Semi-Skimmed, St Helen's Farm* | 1 Serving/250ml | 109.0 | 4.0 | 44 | 3.0 | 4.3 | 1.6 | 0.0 |
| Low Fat, Calcia Extra Calcium, Unigate* | 1 fl oz/30ml | 13.0 | 0.0 | 45 | 4.3 | 6.3 | 0.5 | 0.0 |
| Powder, Instant, Skimmed, Basics, Sainsbury's* | 1 Serving/60g | 209.0 | 0.0 | 349 | 35.6 | 50.4 | 0.6 | 0.0 |

# MILK

| | Measure INFO/WEIGHT | per Measure KCAL | FAT | Nutrition Values per 100g / 100ml KCAL | PROT | CARB | FAT | FIBRE |
|---|---|---|---|---|---|---|---|---|
| **MILK** | | | | | | | | |
| Semi Skimmed, Advance, with Omega 3, St Ivel* | 1 Glass/250ml | 122.0 | 4.0 | 49 | 3.4 | 5.0 | 1.7 | 0.0 |
| *Semi Skimmed, Average* | *1 fl oz/30ml* | *15.0* | *1.0* | *49* | *3.4* | *5.0* | *1.7* | *0.0* |
| *Semi Skimmed, Long Life, Average* | *1 fl oz/30ml* | *15.0* | *1.0* | *49* | *3.4* | *5.0* | *1.7* | *0.0* |
| Semi Skimmed, Low Lactose, Lactofree, Arla* | 1 Glass/125ml | 56.0 | 2.0 | 45 | 3.4 | 5.0 | 1.5 | 0.0 |
| *Skimmed, Average* | *1 fl oz/30ml* | *10.0* | *0.0* | *34* | *3.3* | *5.0* | *0.1* | *0.0* |
| *Skimmed, Uht, Average* | *1 fl oz/30ml* | *10.0* | *0.0* | *34* | *3.3* | *5.0* | *0.1* | *0.0* |
| Whole, Advance with Omega 3, St Ivel* | 1 Serving/250ml | 162.0 | 9.0 | 65 | 3.3 | 4.7 | 3.7 | 0.0 |
| *Whole, Average* | *1 Serving/200ml* | *134.0* | *8.0* | *67* | *3.3* | *4.7* | *3.9* | *0.0* |
| Whole, with Vitamin D, Oak Farms* | 1 Container/236ml | 150.0 | 8.0 | 64 | 3.4 | 4.7 | 3.4 | 0.0 |
| **MILK DRINK** | | | | | | | | |
| Banana Flavour, Sterilised, Low Fat, Gulp* | 1 Bottle/500ml | 315.0 | 5.0 | 63 | 3.8 | 9.7 | 1.0 | 0.0 |
| Chocolatte, Cafe Met* | 1 Bottle/290ml | 174.0 | 4.0 | 60 | 3.7 | 9.1 | 1.4 | 0.3 |
| Extra Choc, Mars* | 1 Bottle/330g | 280.0 | 7.0 | 85 | 3.1 | 13.7 | 2.0 | 0.0 |
| Family Fuel, Mars* | 1 Serving/200ml | 172.0 | 4.0 | 86 | 3.1 | 13.7 | 2.0 | 0.0 |
| No Added Sugar, Mars* | 1 Serving/200ml | 108.0 | 3.0 | 54 | 3.4 | 6.2 | 1.7 | 0.5 |
| Original, Mars* | 1 Serving/330g | 284.0 | 7.0 | 86 | 3.1 | 13.7 | 2.1 | 0.0 |
| Refuel, Mars* | 1 Bottle/388ml | 299.0 | 6.0 | 77 | 3.1 | 13.5 | 1.5 | 0.0 |
| Semi Skimmed, Cholesterol Lowering, Pro Activ, Flora* | 1 Serving/250ml | 125.0 | 4.0 | 50 | 3.6 | 4.8 | 1.8 | 0.0 |
| Strawberry Flavoured, Tesco* | 1 Serving/500ml | 370.0 | 8.0 | 74 | 4.4 | 10.4 | 1.6 | 0.3 |
| **MILK SHAKE** | | | | | | | | |
| Banana, Yazoo, Campina* | 1 Bottle/200ml | 130.0 | 3.0 | 65 | 3.1 | 10.3 | 1.3 | 0.0 |
| Banana Flavour, Frijj* | 1 Bottle/500ml | 310.0 | 4.0 | 62 | 3.4 | 10.1 | 0.8 | 0.0 |
| Banana Flavour, Shapers, Boots* | 1 Bottle/250ml | 201.0 | 2.0 | 80 | 5.6 | 12.8 | 0.8 | 1.9 |
| Chocolate, Asda* | 1 Serving/250ml | 197.0 | 9.0 | 79 | 4.4 | 7.0 | 3.7 | 0.4 |
| Chocolate Flavour, BGTY, Sainsbury's* | 1 Bottle/500ml | 290.0 | 2.0 | 58 | 5.3 | 8.0 | 0.5 | 0.9 |
| Chocolate Flavoured, Fresh, Thick, Frijj* | 1 Bottle/500ml | 350.0 | 5.0 | 70 | 3.5 | 11.7 | 1.0 | 0.0 |
| Powder, Made Up with Semi-Skimmed Milk | 1 Serving/250ml | 172.0 | 4.0 | 69 | 3.2 | 11.3 | 1.6 | 0.0 |
| Powder, Made Up with Whole Milk | 1 Serving/250ml | 217.0 | 9.0 | 87 | 3.1 | 11.1 | 3.7 | 0.0 |
| Strawberry, Yazoo, Campina* | 1 Bottle/500ml | 325.0 | 6.0 | 65 | 3.1 | 10.3 | 1.2 | 0.0 |
| Strawberry Flavour, Thick, Low Fat, Frijj* | 1 Bottle/250ml | 155.0 | 2.0 | 62 | 3.4 | 10.1 | 0.8 | 0.0 |
| Vanilla, Frijj* | 1 Bottle/500ml | 320.0 | 4.0 | 64 | 3.4 | 10.7 | 0.8 | 0.0 |
| Vanilla Flavour, BGTY, Sainsbury's* | 1 Bottle/500ml | 230.0 | 0.0 | 46 | 5.3 | 5.9 | 0.1 | 0.4 |
| **MILKY BAR** | | | | | | | | |
| Buttons, Nestle* | 1 Std Pack/30g | 164.0 | 10.0 | 547 | 7.3 | 58.4 | 31.7 | 0.0 |
| Chunky, Nestle* | ¼ Bar/38g | 207.0 | 12.0 | 547 | 7.3 | 58.4 | 31.7 | 0.0 |
| Crunchies, Nestle* | 1 Pack/30g | 168.0 | 10.0 | 560 | 7.0 | 54.9 | 34.7 | 0.0 |
| Eggs, Mini, Nestle* | 1 Pack/100g | 500.0 | 23.0 | 500 | 4.2 | 68.4 | 23.3 | 0.0 |
| Munchies, Nestle* | 1 Serving/70g | 392.0 | 24.0 | 560 | 7.0 | 54.9 | 34.7 | 0.1 |
| Nestle* | 1 Sm Bar/13g | 68.0 | 4.0 | 547 | 7.3 | 58.4 | 31.7 | 0.0 |
| **MILKY WAY** | | | | | | | | |
| Fun Size, Mars* | 1 Bar/17g | 75.0 | 3.0 | 447 | 3.8 | 71.6 | 16.2 | 0.0 |
| Magic Stars, Mars* | 1 Bag/33g | 184.0 | 11.0 | 559 | 6.3 | 55.3 | 34.7 | 0.0 |
| Mars* | 1 Single Bar/26g | 114.0 | 4.0 | 440 | 3.4 | 74.8 | 14.1 | 0.0 |
| **MINCEMEAT** | | | | | | | | |
| *Average* | *1oz/28g* | *77.0* | *1.0* | *274* | *0.6* | *62.1* | *4.3* | *1.3* |
| Organic, Waitrose* | 1oz/28g | 81.0 | 1.0 | 290 | 0.9 | 65.8 | 2.6 | 2.0 |
| Tesco* | 1 Serving/20g | 58.0 | 1.0 | 292 | 0.8 | 64.2 | 3.5 | 1.6 |
| Traditional, Robertson* | 1 Tbsp/17g | 49.0 | 1.0 | 286 | 0.6 | 62.5 | 3.4 | 2.5 |
| Traditional, Sainsbury's* | 1 Tbsp/23g | 65.0 | 1.0 | 282 | 0.9 | 62.4 | 3.2 | 1.4 |
| with Cherries, Almonds & Brandy, Tesco* | ¼ Jar/103g | 295.0 | 5.0 | 287 | 1.4 | 58.8 | 4.9 | 1.4 |
| **MINI BITES** | | | | | | | | |
| Apricot & Orange, COU, M & S* | 1 Bag/25g | 86.0 | 1.0 | 345 | 3.4 | 76.9 | 2.5 | 4.1 |
| Chocolate Caramel, M & S* | 1 Bite/21g | 95.0 | 5.0 | 460 | 5.6 | 53.5 | 24.6 | 1.6 |

| | Measure INFO/WEIGHT | per Measure KCAL | FAT | Nutrition Values per 100g / 100ml KCAL | PROT | CARB | FAT | FIBRE |
|---|---|---|---|---|---|---|---|---|
| **MINI BITES** | | | | | | | | |
| Chocolate Cornflake, M & S* | 1 Bite/12g | 55.0 | 2.0 | 470 | 6.2 | 66.3 | 20.1 | 3.6 |
| Chocolate Orange, M & S* | 1 Bite/22g | 95.0 | 5.0 | 430 | 5.5 | 54.6 | 21.6 | 1.8 |
| **MINSTRELS** | | | | | | | | |
| Galaxy, Mars* | 1 Serving/100g | 503.0 | 22.0 | 503 | 5.1 | 70.5 | 22.2 | 1.1 |
| **MINT** | | | | | | | | |
| *Dried, Average* | *1 Tsp/5g* | *14.0* | *0.0* | *279* | *24.8* | *34.6* | *4.6* | *0.0* |
| *Fresh, Average* | *2 Tbsp/3g* | *1.0* | *0.0* | *43* | *3.8* | *5.3* | *0.7* | *0.0* |
| **MINTOES** | | | | | | | | |
| Morrisons* | 1 Sweet/8g | 33.0 | 1.0 | 411 | 0.1 | 84.4 | 8.1 | 0.0 |
| **MINTS** | | | | | | | | |
| After Dinner, Sainsbury's* | 1 Mint/7g | 32.0 | 1.0 | 456 | 4.1 | 62.1 | 21.2 | 4.1 |
| After Eight, Dark Chocolate, Nestle* | 1 Sweet/7g | 32.0 | 1.0 | 461 | 5.0 | 63.0 | 12.9 | 2.0 |
| After Eight, Orange, Nestle* | 1 Sweet/7g | 29.0 | 1.0 | 417 | 2.5 | 72.6 | 12.9 | 1.1 |
| After Eight, Straws, Nestle* | 1 Sweet/5g | 24.0 | 1.0 | 526 | 5.1 | 56.6 | 31.0 | 4.0 |
| Butter Mintoes, M & S* | 1 Sweet/9g | 35.0 | 1.0 | 391 | 0.0 | 84.0 | 6.8 | 0.0 |
| Butter Mintoes, Tesco* | 1 Sweet/7g | 24.0 | 0.0 | 349 | 0.0 | 71.3 | 7.1 | 0.0 |
| Clear, Co-Op* | 1 Sweet/6g | 24.0 | 0.0 | 395 | 0.0 | 98.0 | 0.0 | 0.0 |
| Cream, Luxury, Thorntons* | 1 Sweet/13g | 62.0 | 3.0 | 477 | 4.2 | 62.3 | 23.8 | 2.3 |
| Creams, Bassett's* | 1 Sweet/11g | 40.0 | 0.0 | 365 | 0.0 | 91.8 | 0.0 | 0.0 |
| Everton, Co-Op* | 1 Sweet/6g | 25.0 | 0.0 | 410 | 0.6 | 92.0 | 4.0 | 0.0 |
| Extra Strong, Peppermint, Trebor* | 1 Roll/46g | 180.0 | 0.0 | 395 | 0.4 | 98.1 | 0.2 | 0.0 |
| Extra Strong, Spearmint, Trebor* | 1 Pack/44g | 174.0 | 0.0 | 395 | 0.4 | 98.7 | 0.0 | 0.0 |
| Glacier, Fox's* | 1 Sweet/5g | 19.0 | 0.0 | 386 | 0.0 | 96.4 | 0.0 | 0.0 |
| Humbugs, Co-Op* | 1 Sweet/8g | 34.0 | 1.0 | 425 | 0.6 | 89.9 | 7.0 | 0.0 |
| Humbugs, M & S* | 1 Sweet/9g | 37.0 | 0.0 | 407 | 0.6 | 91.1 | 4.4 | 0.0 |
| Humbugs, Thorntons* | 1 Sweet/9g | 31.0 | 0.0 | 340 | 1.0 | 87.8 | 4.4 | 0.0 |
| Imperials, Co-Op* | 1 Sweet/3g | 12.0 | 0.0 | 395 | 0.3 | 98.0 | 0.2 | 0.0 |
| Imperials, M & S* | 1 Sweet/3g | 12.0 | 0.0 | 391 | 0.0 | 97.8 | 0.0 | 0.0 |
| Imperials, Sainsbury's* | 1 Sweet/3g | 10.0 | 0.0 | 374 | 0.0 | 92.1 | 0.0 | 0.0 |
| Imperials, Tesco* | 1 Sweet/3g | 12.0 | 0.0 | 397 | 0.6 | 98.7 | 0.0 | 0.0 |
| Mento, Sugar Free, Mentos* | 1 Sweet/2g | 5.0 | 0.0 | 260 | 1.0 | 87.0 | 5.5 | 0.0 |
| Mint Assortment, M & S* | 1 Sweet/7g | 29.0 | 1.0 | 414 | 0.7 | 85.4 | 7.7 | 0.0 |
| Mint Favourites, Bassett's* | 1 Sweet/6g | 22.0 | 0.0 | 367 | 0.9 | 77.4 | 5.9 | 0.0 |
| Smooth, Weight Watchers* | 1 Tube/25g | 58.0 | 0.0 | 231 | 0.2 | 61.6 | 0.0 | 0.0 |
| Soft, Trebor* | 1 Pack/48g | 182.0 | 0.0 | 380 | 0.0 | 94.9 | 0.0 | 0.0 |
| Softmints, Peppermint, Trebor* | 1 Pack/48g | 170.0 | 0.0 | 355 | 0.0 | 88.9 | 0.0 | 0.0 |
| Softmints, Spearmint, Trebor* | 1 Pack/45g | 170.0 | 0.0 | 375 | 0.0 | 94.3 | 0.0 | 0.0 |
| **MISO** | | | | | | | | |
| *Average* | *1oz/28g* | *57.0* | *2.0* | *203* | *13.3* | *23.5* | *6.2* | *0.0* |
| **MIXED HERBS** | | | | | | | | |
| *Average* | *1 Tsp/5g* | *13.0* | *0.0* | *260* | *12.9* | *37.5* | *8.5* | *6.7* |
| Herbes De Provence, Dried, Schwartz* | 1 Tsp/2g | 7.0 | 0.0 | 364 | 12.9 | 65.0 | 5.8 | 0.0 |
| **MIXED SPICE** | | | | | | | | |
| Rub, Moroccan, Schwartz* | 1 Serving/3g | 9.0 | 0.0 | 309 | 15.0 | 36.4 | 11.4 | 19.5 |
| Schwartz* | 1 Tsp/2g | 8.0 | 0.0 | 390 | 10.4 | 65.8 | 9.5 | 2.0 |
| **MIXED VEGETABLES** | | | | | | | | |
| Baby, Iceland* | 1 Serving/100g | 20.0 | 0.0 | 20 | 1.2 | 3.9 | 0.0 | 2.7 |
| Baby, Steam, Fresh, Tesco* | 1 Pack/160g | 72.0 | 1.0 | 45 | 2.7 | 6.7 | 0.8 | 3.8 |
| Baby Corn, Mange Tout & Baby Carrots, Tesco* | 1 Pack/220g | 64.0 | 1.0 | 29 | 2.3 | 4.3 | 0.4 | 2.2 |
| Broccoli & Cauliflower Florets, Baby Carrots, Asda* | 1 Serving/113g | 28.0 | 1.0 | 25 | 2.2 | 2.6 | 0.6 | 2.4 |
| Canned, Drained, Sainsbury's* | 1 Can/200g | 114.0 | 1.0 | 57 | 3.0 | 10.6 | 0.3 | 2.3 |
| Carrot, Cauliflower, & Broccoli, Fresh, Tesco* | 1 Serving/80g | 26.0 | 0.0 | 32 | 2.6 | 3.9 | 0.2 | 2.8 |
| Carrot, Cauliflower & Fine Green Beans, Steam Veg, Tesco* | 1 Bag/160g | 37.0 | 0.0 | 23 | 1.4 | 3.6 | 0.3 | 2.9 |

# MIXED VEGETABLES

| | Measure INFO/WEIGHT | per Measure KCAL | FAT | Nutrition Values per 100g / 100ml KCAL | PROT | CARB | FAT | FIBRE |
|---|---|---|---|---|---|---|---|---|
| Carrot Batons, Cauliflower & Broccoli, Steamed, Asda* | 1 Bag/120g | 28.0 | 1.0 | 23 | 1.8 | 2.6 | 0.6 | 3.1 |
| Carrots, Broccoli & Sweetcorn, Easy Steam, Sainsbury's* | 1 Pack/120g | 67.0 | 1.0 | 56 | 2.6 | 8.7 | 1.2 | 2.0 |
| Carrots, Broccoli & Sweetcorn, Steam Veg, Tesco* | 1 Sachet/160g | 80.0 | 2.0 | 50 | 2.5 | 7.5 | 1.1 | 3.0 |
| Carrots, Cauliflower & Broccoli, Waitrose* | 1 Serving/100g | 35.0 | 1.0 | 35 | 2.4 | 4.9 | 0.6 | 2.9 |
| Carrots, Peas, Green Beans & Sweetcorn, Frozen, Tesco* | 1 Serving/80g | 38.0 | 1.0 | 48 | 3.1 | 7.3 | 0.7 | 3.9 |
| Casserole, Co-Op* | 1 Serving/100g | 40.0 | 0.0 | 40 | 1.2 | 7.5 | 0.3 | 2.1 |
| Casserole, Frozen, Tesco* | 1 Serving/100g | 26.0 | 0.0 | 26 | 0.8 | 4.8 | 0.4 | 2.0 |
| Casserole, Ready to Cook, Sainsbury's* | ½ Pack/240g | 74.0 | 1.0 | 31 | 0.9 | 6.2 | 0.3 | 1.4 |
| Casserole, Tesco* | 1 Pack/440g | 176.0 | 1.0 | 40 | 1.2 | 8.0 | 0.3 | 2.3 |
| Casserole, with Baby Potatoes, Fresh, M & S* | ½ Pack/350g | 140.0 | 1.0 | 40 | 1.2 | 7.8 | 0.3 | 2.1 |
| Cauliflower, Carrots, Green Beans, SteamFresh, Birds Eye* | 1 Bag/120g | 40.0 | 1.0 | 33 | 2.0 | 5.0 | 0.5 | 2.2 |
| Chef's Style, Ready Prepared, M & S* | 1 Pack/240g | 72.0 | 1.0 | 30 | 2.6 | 4.5 | 0.5 | 2.9 |
| Chunky, Frozen, Sainsbury's* | 1 Serving/85g | 31.0 | 1.0 | 37 | 2.9 | 4.7 | 0.7 | 3.1 |
| Country Selection, Budgens* | 1 Serving/113g | 27.0 | 0.0 | 24 | 1.6 | 3.6 | 0.4 | 2.9 |
| Crunchy, Tesco* | 1 Pack/210g | 63.0 | 1.0 | 30 | 1.7 | 5.0 | 0.4 | 2.4 |
| Farmhouse, Frozen, Waitrose* | 1 Serving/90g | 22.0 | 1.0 | 25 | 1.9 | 3.1 | 0.6 | 2.4 |
| Freshly Frozen, Asda* | 1 Serving/80g | 42.0 | 1.0 | 52 | 3.2 | 8.0 | 0.8 | 3.0 |
| Frozen, Safeway* | 1 Serving/120g | 70.0 | 1.0 | 58 | 3.0 | 9.4 | 0.9 | 3.4 |
| Frozen, Waitrose* | 1 Serving/80g | 43.0 | 1.0 | 54 | 3.1 | 8.7 | 0.8 | 3.5 |
| Frozen, Waitrose* | 1 Serving/80g | 44.0 | 1.0 | 55 | 3.3 | 8.2 | 1.0 | 3.7 |
| Green, Microwave, Aldi* | 1 Serving/300g | 189.0 | 9.0 | 63 | 3.5 | 5.6 | 3.0 | 4.1 |
| in Salt Water, Tesco* | 1/3 Can/65g | 34.0 | 0.0 | 53 | 2.6 | 9.2 | 0.6 | 2.7 |
| in Salted Water, Canned, Asda* | 1 Serving/65g | 31.0 | 0.0 | 48 | 2.6 | 9.0 | 0.2 | 1.7 |
| Organic, Waitrose* | 1oz/28g | 19.0 | 0.0 | 69 | 4.4 | 10.0 | 1.3 | 2.7 |
| Oriental, M & S* | 1 Serving/250g | 50.0 | 1.0 | 20 | 1.6 | 3.4 | 0.3 | 1.6 |
| Peas, Carrots, & Baby Leeks, Prepared, Tesco* | ½ Pack/130g | 57.0 | 1.0 | 44 | 3.1 | 5.8 | 0.9 | 3.5 |
| Potatoes, Broad Beans & Peas, M & S* | 1 Pack/245g | 147.0 | 3.0 | 60 | 2.9 | 12.9 | 1.3 | 3.4 |
| Premium, Frozen, Somerfield* | 1 Serving/100g | 53.0 | 1.0 | 53 | 3.2 | 7.9 | 1.0 | 2.7 |
| Ready to Roast, Asda* | ½ Pack/362g | 315.0 | 12.0 | 87 | 1.6 | 13.0 | 3.2 | 2.4 |
| Red Peppers & Courgette, Tesco* | 1 Pack/250g | 67.0 | 1.0 | 27 | 1.7 | 3.8 | 0.5 | 2.0 |
| Sainsbury's* | 1 Serving/230g | 55.0 | 1.0 | 24 | 2.1 | 2.5 | 0.6 | 0.0 |
| Seasonal Selection, Tesco* | 1 Serving/100g | 37.0 | 0.0 | 37 | 1.1 | 7.2 | 0.4 | 2.2 |
| Special, Freshly Frozen, Morrisons* | 1 Serving/100g | 48.0 | 1.0 | 48 | 3.2 | 7.2 | 0.8 | 0.0 |
| Special, Sainsbury's* | 1 Serving/120g | 68.0 | 1.0 | 57 | 3.2 | 8.9 | 1.0 | 2.9 |
| Summer, Tesco* | 1 Pack/167g | 55.0 | 1.0 | 33 | 2.6 | 4.5 | 0.5 | 2.8 |
| Supreme, Frozen, Somerfield* | 1 Serving/90g | 22.0 | 0.0 | 25 | 1.9 | 4.3 | 0.0 | 3.1 |

# MIXER

| | Measure INFO/WEIGHT | per Measure KCAL | FAT | Nutrition Values per 100g / 100ml KCAL | PROT | CARB | FAT | FIBRE |
|---|---|---|---|---|---|---|---|---|
| Russchian, Schweppes* | 1 Bottle/500ml | 125.0 | 0.0 | 25 | 0.0 | 6.0 | 0.0 | 0.0 |

# MOLASSES

| | Measure INFO/WEIGHT | per Measure KCAL | FAT | Nutrition Values per 100g / 100ml KCAL | PROT | CARB | FAT | FIBRE |
|---|---|---|---|---|---|---|---|---|
| *Average* | 1 Tbsp/20g | 53.0 | 0.0 | 266 | 0.0 | 68.8 | 0.1 | 0.0 |

# MONKEY NUTS

| | Measure INFO/WEIGHT | per Measure KCAL | FAT | Nutrition Values per 100g / 100ml KCAL | PROT | CARB | FAT | FIBRE |
|---|---|---|---|---|---|---|---|---|
| *Average* | 1oz/28g | 158.0 | 13.0 | 565 | 25.5 | 8.2 | 47.9 | 6.3 |

# MONKFISH

| | Measure INFO/WEIGHT | per Measure KCAL | FAT | Nutrition Values per 100g / 100ml KCAL | PROT | CARB | FAT | FIBRE |
|---|---|---|---|---|---|---|---|---|
| *Grilled* | 1oz/28g | 27.0 | 0.0 | 96 | 22.7 | 0.0 | 0.6 | 0.0 |
| *Raw* | 1oz/28g | 18.0 | 0.0 | 66 | 15.7 | 0.0 | 0.4 | 0.0 |

# MONSTER MUNCH

| | Measure INFO/WEIGHT | per Measure KCAL | FAT | Nutrition Values per 100g / 100ml KCAL | PROT | CARB | FAT | FIBRE |
|---|---|---|---|---|---|---|---|---|
| Flamin' Hot, Walkers* | 1 Std Bag/22g | 108.0 | 5.0 | 490 | 7.0 | 59.0 | 25.0 | 1.5 |
| Pickled Onion, Walkers* | 1 Std Bag/22g | 108.0 | 5.0 | 490 | 6.0 | 60.0 | 25.0 | 1.7 |
| Roast Beef, Walkers* | 1 Std Bag/22g | 108.0 | 5.0 | 490 | 7.0 | 59.0 | 25.0 | 1.7 |
| Spicy, Walkers* | 1 Std Bag/25g | 125.0 | 7.0 | 500 | 5.0 | 55.0 | 29.0 | 1.3 |

# MORNAY

| | Measure INFO/WEIGHT | per Measure KCAL | FAT | Nutrition Values per 100g / 100ml KCAL | PROT | CARB | FAT | FIBRE |
|---|---|---|---|---|---|---|---|---|
| Broccoli, Somerfield* | 1 Pack/400g | 372.0 | 25.0 | 93 | 3.5 | 5.9 | 6.2 | 0.5 |
| Cod, Nutritionally Balanced, M & S* | 1 Pack/400g | 320.0 | 10.0 | 80 | 6.8 | 7.2 | 2.6 | 1.6 |

| | Measure INFO/WEIGHT | per Measure KCAL | FAT | Nutrition Values per 100g / 100ml KCAL | PROT | CARB | FAT | FIBRE |
|---|---|---|---|---|---|---|---|---|
| **MORNAY** | | | | | | | | |
| Cod, Sainsbury's* | 1 Serving/180g | 277.0 | 17.0 | 154 | 15.2 | 2.2 | 9.4 | 0.9 |
| Haddock, COU, M & S* | ½ Pack/194g | 165.0 | 4.0 | 85 | 14.5 | 2.6 | 2.0 | 0.6 |
| Haddock, Perfectly Balanced, Waitrose* | 1 Pack/360g | 310.0 | 5.0 | 86 | 16.6 | 1.6 | 1.5 | 0.5 |
| Haddock, Youngs* | ½ Pack/190g | 236.0 | 15.0 | 124 | 12.1 | 1.3 | 7.8 | 0.6 |
| Salmon, with Broccoli, Weight Watchers* | 1 Pack/290g | 261.0 | 5.0 | 90 | 9.6 | 9.0 | 1.7 | 0.7 |
| Spinach, Waitrose* | ½ Pack/125g | 112.0 | 9.0 | 90 | 3.3 | 3.6 | 6.9 | 1.6 |
| **MOUSSAKA** | | | | | | | | |
| Aubergine & Lentil, Asda* | 1 Pack/451g | 370.0 | 17.0 | 82 | 3.9 | 8.1 | 3.8 | 2.9 |
| Beef, BGTY, Sainsbury's* | 1 Pack/400g | 300.0 | 10.0 | 75 | 6.1 | 6.8 | 2.6 | 1.2 |
| Beef, GFY, Asda* | 1 Pack/400g | 300.0 | 8.0 | 75 | 7.0 | 7.0 | 2.1 | 0.7 |
| Beef, HL, Tesco* | 1 Pack/450g | 396.0 | 12.0 | 88 | 5.0 | 10.9 | 2.7 | 0.8 |
| COU, M & S* | 1 Pack/340g | 272.0 | 10.0 | 80 | 5.3 | 8.5 | 2.9 | 1.4 |
| Lamb, Finest, Tesco* | 1 Pack/349g | 510.0 | 38.0 | 146 | 5.8 | 6.2 | 10.9 | 3.4 |
| Lamb, Light Choices, Tesco* | 1 Pack/350g | 259.0 | 7.0 | 74 | 5.3 | 8.5 | 2.1 | 2.6 |
| Lamb, Sainsbury's* | 1 Pack/329g | 497.0 | 32.0 | 151 | 8.4 | 7.2 | 9.8 | 1.0 |
| Low Saturated Fat, Waitrose* | 1 Pack/350g | 304.0 | 11.0 | 87 | 6.3 | 8.4 | 3.1 | 3.1 |
| Vegetable, Roasted, Safeway* | 1 Pack/365g | 365.0 | 21.0 | 100 | 3.7 | 7.9 | 5.7 | 2.9 |
| Vegetarian, COU, M & S* | 1 Pack/400g | 280.0 | 11.0 | 70 | 2.7 | 9.1 | 2.7 | 2.4 |
| Vegetarian, Tesco* | 1 Pack/300g | 489.0 | 31.0 | 163 | 6.4 | 11.0 | 10.4 | 0.9 |
| **MOUSSE** | | | | | | | | |
| Aero, Mint, Nestle* | 1 Pot/58g | 108.0 | 6.0 | 186 | 4.6 | 18.9 | 10.2 | 0.3 |
| Aero Chocolate, Nestle* | 1 Pot/58g | 101.0 | 3.0 | 174 | 4.8 | 27.3 | 5.1 | 1.1 |
| Aero Twist Cappuccino & Chocolate, Nestle* | 1 Pot/75g | 135.0 | 8.0 | 180 | 4.2 | 16.8 | 10.8 | 0.2 |
| Apricot, Lite, Onken* | 1 Pot/150g | 156.0 | 2.0 | 104 | 4.6 | 18.0 | 1.5 | 0.3 |
| Banoffee, COU, M & S^ | 1 Pot/70g | 101.0 | 1.0 | 145 | 2.9 | 28.8 | 2.1 | 1.5 |
| Belgian Chocolate, Finest, Tesco* | 1 Pot/120g | 360.0 | 23.0 | 300 | 5.1 | 26.6 | 18.9 | 1.1 |
| Belgian Chocolate & Vanilla, Weight Watchers* | 1 Pot/80g | 106.0 | 2.0 | 132 | 4.4 | 22.2 | 2.8 | 0.9 |
| Black Cherry, Lite, Onken* | 1 Pot/150g | 156.0 | 2.0 | 104 | 4.6 | 17.9 | 1.5 | 0.2 |
| Blackcurrant, HL, Tesco* | 1 Pot/113g | 80.0 | 3.0 | 71 | 3.7 | 8.3 | 2.6 | 1.8 |
| Blackcurrant, Onken* | 1 Pot/150g | 210.0 | 10.0 | 140 | 5.2 | 14.6 | 6.8 | 0.0 |
| Caramel, Meringue, Cadbury* | 1 Pot/65g | 181.0 | 7.0 | 277 | 4.6 | 42.4 | 10.3 | 1.0 |
| Caramelised Orange, COU, M & S* | 1 Pot/70g | 91.0 | 1.0 | 130 | 2.8 | 26.3 | 1.7 | 3.4 |
| Chocolate | 1 Pot/60g | 83.0 | 3.0 | 139 | 4.0 | 19.9 | 5.4 | 0.0 |
| Chocolate, Asda* | 1 Pot/61g | 134.0 | 6.0 | 219 | 3.7 | 26.0 | 10.0 | 1.0 |
| Chocolate, BGTY, Sainsbury's* | 1 Pot/63g | 83.0 | 2.0 | 133 | 4.9 | 21.8 | 2.9 | 0.5 |
| Chocolate, Cadbury* | 1 Pot/55g | 107.0 | 5.0 | 195 | 6.1 | 24.6 | 8.2 | 0.0 |
| Chocolate, COU, M & S* | 1 Pot/70g | 95.0 | 2.0 | 135 | 4.6 | 22.9 | 2.4 | 1.6 |
| Chocolate, GFY, Asda* | 1 Pot/60g | 70.0 | 2.0 | 117 | 4.8 | 17.9 | 2.9 | 3.5 |
| Chocolate, Light Choices, Light Choices, Tesco* | 1 Pot/63g | 91.0 | 2.0 | 145 | 4.3 | 25.3 | 2.7 | 0.5 |
| Chocolate, Low Fat, Danette, Danone* | 1 Pot/60g | 73.0 | 1.0 | 121 | 5.1 | 20.8 | 1.9 | 1.5 |
| Chocolate, Shapers, Boots* | 1 Pot/70g | 97.0 | 2.0 | 138 | 5.3 | 23.0 | 2.7 | 1.7 |
| Chocolate, Tesco* | 1 Pot/60g | 120.0 | 5.0 | 200 | 3.6 | 27.6 | 8.4 | 0.9 |
| Chocolate & Hazelnut, Onken* | 1 Pot/125g | 171.0 | 7.0 | 137 | 3.3 | 17.8 | 6.0 | 0.0 |
| Chocolate & Mint, COU, M & S* | 1 Pot/70g | 84.0 | 2.0 | 120 | 6.2 | 18.7 | 2.5 | 1.0 |
| Chocolate & Orange, COU, M & S* | 1 Pot/70g | 77.0 | 2.0 | 110 | 5.9 | 16.0 | 2.6 | 0.9 |
| Chocolate with Vanilla Layer, Cadbury* | 1 Pot/100g | 162.0 | 6.0 | 162 | 4.8 | 21.9 | 6.1 | 0.0 |
| Creamy Strawberry, Boots* | 1 Pot/90g | 59.0 | 3.0 | 66 | 3.9 | 6.4 | 2.8 | 0.3 |
| Lemon, Classic, Onken* | 1 Pot/150g | 210.0 | 9.0 | 140 | 5.1 | 15.8 | 6.3 | 0.0 |
| Lemon, COU, M & S* | 1 Pot/70g | 80.0 | 2.0 | 115 | 2.9 | 19.4 | 3.5 | 3.5 |
| Lemon, Dessert, Sainsbury's* | 1 Pot/63g | 114.0 | 6.0 | 182 | 3.6 | 20.7 | 9.4 | 0.6 |
| Lemon, GFY, Asda* | 1 Pot/63g | 57.0 | 2.0 | 92 | 3.6 | 13.0 | 2.8 | 1.7 |
| Lemon, Less Than 3% Fat, BGTY, Sainsbury's* | 1 Pot/62g | 70.0 | 2.0 | 113 | 4.5 | 17.6 | 2.8 | 0.3 |
| Lemon, Lite, Onken* | 1 Pot/150g | 156.0 | 2.0 | 104 | 4.6 | 17.2 | 1.5 | 0.1 |

# M

| MOUSSE | Measure INFO/WEIGHT | per Measure KCAL | per Measure FAT | Nutrition Values per 100g / 100ml KCAL | PROT | CARB | FAT | FIBRE |
|---|---|---|---|---|---|---|---|---|
| Lemon, Perfectly Balanced, Waitrose* | 1 Pot/95g | 150.0 | 3.0 | 158 | 3.1 | 30.2 | 2.7 | 0.1 |
| Lemon, Tesco* | 1 Pot/60g | 67.0 | 2.0 | 111 | 3.4 | 18.2 | 2.7 | 0.0 |
| Lemon Fruit Juice, Shape, Danone* | 1 Pot/100g | 116.0 | 3.0 | 116 | 3.5 | 18.6 | 2.8 | 0.0 |
| Orange, Mango & Lime, Onken* | 1 Pot/150g | 207.0 | 9.0 | 138 | 5.1 | 15.3 | 6.3 | 0.1 |
| Orange & Nectarine, Shape, Danone* | 1 Pot/100g | 47.0 | 2.0 | 47 | 3.0 | 4.9 | 1.9 | 0.0 |
| Peach, Onken* | 1 Pot/150g | 204.0 | 9.0 | 136 | 5.1 | 15.1 | 6.3 | 0.2 |
| Peach, Shape, Danone* | 1 Pot/100g | 43.0 | 2.0 | 43 | 3.0 | 3.9 | 1.8 | 0.1 |
| Peach & Passion Fruit, Perfectly Balanced, Waitrose* | 1 Pot/95g | 118.0 | 3.0 | 124 | 3.5 | 21.2 | 2.8 | 0.5 |
| Pineapple, COU, M & S* | 1 Pot/70g | 84.0 | 2.0 | 120 | 3.3 | 20.7 | 2.4 | 3.5 |
| Pineapple, Lite, Onken* | 1 Pot/150g | 162.0 | 2.0 | 108 | 4.6 | 19.0 | 1.5 | 0.2 |
| Pineapple, Shape, Danone* | 1 Pot/100g | 43.0 | 2.0 | 43 | 2.9 | 3.8 | 1.8 | 0.1 |
| Plain Chocolate, Low Fat, Nestle* | 1 Pot/120g | 71.0 | 1.0 | 59 | 2.4 | 10.4 | 0.7 | 0.0 |
| Raspberry, Lite, Onken* | 1 Pot/150g | 156.0 | 2.0 | 104 | 4.6 | 17.3 | 1.5 | 0.1 |
| Raspberry & Cranberry, Luxury, Weight Watchers* | 1 Pot/80g | 62.0 | 1.0 | 78 | 3.8 | 13.0 | 1.2 | 1.0 |
| Raspberry Ripple, Value, Tesco* | 1 Pot/47g | 70.0 | 3.0 | 149 | 2.1 | 21.3 | 6.1 | 0.1 |
| Rhubarb, COU, M & S* | 1 Pot/70g | 87.0 | 1.0 | 125 | 2.9 | 25.7 | 2.1 | 4.2 |
| Rhubarb, Lite, Onken* | 1 Pot/150g | 154.0 | 2.0 | 103 | 4.6 | 17.8 | 1.5 | 0.3 |
| Rhubarb & Vanilla, Onken* | 1 Pot/150g | 210.0 | 9.0 | 140 | 5.0 | 15.8 | 6.3 | 0.2 |
| Strawberry, Asda* | 1 Pot/64g | 107.0 | 6.0 | 167 | 3.5 | 18.0 | 9.0 | 0.2 |
| Strawberry, BGTY, Sainsbury's* | 1 Pot/63g | 63.0 | 2.0 | 101 | 3.4 | 15.0 | 2.8 | 0.2 |
| Strawberry, HL, Tesco* | 1 Pot/114g | 90.0 | 3.0 | 79 | 3.8 | 10.2 | 2.6 | 0.8 |
| Strawberry, Light, Muller* | 1 Pot/150g | 147.0 | 1.0 | 98 | 4.3 | 19.4 | 0.4 | 0.0 |
| Strawberry, Lite, Onken* | 1 Pot/150g | 151.0 | 2.0 | 101 | 4.6 | 17.2 | 1.5 | 0.1 |
| Strawberry, Low Fat, Waitrose* | 1 Pot/95g | 112.0 | 3.0 | 118 | 3.2 | 20.0 | 2.8 | 0.6 |
| Strawberry, Morrisons* | 1 Pot/63g | 106.0 | 6.0 | 170 | 3.5 | 17.6 | 9.5 | 0.2 |
| Strawberry, Sainsbury's* | 1 Pot/63g | 106.0 | 6.0 | 168 | 3.4 | 17.5 | 9.4 | 0.1 |
| Strawberry, Shape, Danone* | 1 Pot/100g | 44.0 | 2.0 | 44 | 3.0 | 4.0 | 1.8 | 0.0 |
| Strawberry, Tesco* | 1 Pot/63g | 106.0 | 6.0 | 169 | 3.5 | 17.9 | 9.3 | 0.2 |
| Strawberry & Vanilla, Weight Watchers* | 1 Pot/80g | 87.0 | 2.0 | 109 | 3.7 | 18.1 | 2.4 | 0.4 |
| Strawberry Fruity, Organic, Sainsbury's* | 1 Pot/125g | 129.0 | 4.0 | 103 | 6.2 | 15.7 | 3.0 | 3.6 |
| Summer Fruits, Light, Muller* | 1 Pot/149g | 143.0 | 1.0 | 96 | 4.3 | 18.7 | 0.4 | 0.0 |
| Toffee, M & S* | 1 Pot/90g | 180.0 | 7.0 | 200 | 4.5 | 27.6 | 8.0 | 0.6 |
| White Chocolate, Finest, Tesco* | 1 Pot/92g | 436.0 | 34.0 | 474 | 3.9 | 30.2 | 37.5 | 0.0 |
| **MUFFIN** | | | | | | | | |
| All Butter, M & S* | 1 Muffin/65g | 175.0 | 5.0 | 270 | 10.3 | 40.8 | 7.3 | 2.1 |
| All Butter, TTD, Sainsbury's* | 1 Muffin/70g | 183.0 | 5.0 | 261 | 10.7 | 40.0 | 6.5 | 2.7 |
| Apple, Sultana & Cinnamon, GFY, Asda* | 1 Muffin/50g | 134.0 | 2.0 | 268 | 6.0 | 53.0 | 3.5 | 3.9 |
| Berry Burst, Asda* | 1 Muffin/60g | 139.0 | 1.0 | 232 | 6.2 | 46.7 | 2.3 | 1.7 |
| Blueberry, & Redcurrant, BGTY, Sainsbury's* | 1 Muffin/65g | 159.0 | 2.0 | 245 | 5.0 | 50.0 | 2.5 | 3.1 |
| Blueberry, American Style, Sainsbury's* | 1 Muffin/72g | 256.0 | 13.0 | 355 | 5.1 | 42.7 | 18.2 | 1.9 |
| Blueberry, Big, Asda* | 1 Muffin/105g | 342.0 | 11.0 | 326 | 7.5 | 49.8 | 10.7 | 2.3 |
| Blueberry, GFY, Asda* | 1 Muffin/59g | 146.0 | 1.0 | 249 | 6.0 | 51.0 | 2.3 | 3.0 |
| Blueberry, M & S* | 1 Muffin/75g | 255.0 | 13.0 | 340 | 4.9 | 41.9 | 16.8 | 1.3 |
| Blueberry, Mini, Sainsbury's* | 1 Muffin/28g | 82.0 | 2.0 | 293 | 6.3 | 48.9 | 8.1 | 1.9 |
| Blueberry, Mini, Tesco* | 1 Muffin/28g | 104.0 | 5.0 | 370 | 5.6 | 43.5 | 19.3 | 1.2 |
| Blueberry, Perfectly Balanced, Waitrose* | 1 Muffin/100g | 225.0 | 2.0 | 225 | 4.6 | 46.5 | 2.2 | 1.8 |
| Blueberry, Tesco* | 1 Muffin/73g | 248.0 | 12.0 | 340 | 4.7 | 41.0 | 17.1 | 1.9 |
| Blueberry, Waitrose* | 1 Muffin/65g | 239.0 | 9.0 | 367 | 4.7 | 55.2 | 14.2 | 1.7 |
| Blueberry, Weight Watchers* | 1 Muffin/65g | 172.0 | 4.0 | 265 | 6.4 | 46.9 | 5.7 | 2.6 |
| Bran, Average | 1 Muffin/57g | 155.0 | 4.0 | 272 | 7.8 | 45.6 | 7.7 | 7.7 |
| Bran & Sultana, Weight Watchers* | 1 Muffin/60g | 144.0 | 1.0 | 240 | 4.5 | 50.7 | 2.1 | 2.3 |
| Choc Chip, Mini, Weight Watchers* | 1 Muffin/15g | 47.0 | 1.0 | 312 | 6.6 | 52.1 | 8.6 | 3.1 |
| Chocolate, Galaxy, McVitie's* | 1 Muffin/88g | 319.0 | 17.0 | 364 | 5.0 | 44.5 | 19.5 | 0.0 |

| | Measure INFO/WEIGHT | per Measure KCAL | per Measure FAT | Nutrition Values per 100g / 100ml KCAL | PROT | CARB | FAT | FIBRE |
|---|---|---|---|---|---|---|---|---|
| **MUFFIN** | | | | | | | | |
| Chocolate, HL, Tesco* | 1 Muffin/71g | 204.0 | 6.0 | 288 | 5.5 | 46.9 | 8.7 | 5.5 |
| Chocolate Chip, American Style, Sainsbury's* | 1 Muffin/72g | 284.0 | 14.0 | 395 | 5.0 | 48.8 | 20.0 | 2.1 |
| Chocolate Chip, BGTY, Sainsbury's* | 1 Muffin/75g | 282.0 | 12.0 | 376 | 5.2 | 51.8 | 16.4 | 1.6 |
| Chocolate Chip, Mini, Asda* | 1 Muffin/22g | 77.0 | 3.0 | 349 | 7.0 | 51.0 | 13.0 | 2.1 |
| Chocolate Chip, Mini, BGTY, Sainsbury's* | 1 Muffin/28g | 91.0 | 2.0 | 324 | 6.5 | 55.1 | 8.7 | 1.6 |
| Chocolate Chip, Plain, Tesco* | 1 Muffin/72g | 270.0 | 13.0 | 375 | 5.0 | 48.1 | 17.6 | 1.4 |
| Chocolate Indulgence, McVitie's* | 1 Muffin/75g | 253.0 | 7.0 | 338 | 5.8 | 57.9 | 9.2 | 1.3 |
| Chunky Chocolate Chip, McVitie's* | 1 Muffin/94g | 393.0 | 20.0 | 418 | 5.3 | 50.6 | 21.6 | 0.8 |
| Cinnamon & Sultana, Morrisons* | 1 Muffin/75g | 169.0 | 1.0 | 226 | 8.7 | 44.1 | 1.6 | 4.5 |
| Cranberry & White Chocolate, Sainsbury's* | 1 Muffin/72g | 253.0 | 13.0 | 352 | 5.7 | 40.7 | 18.5 | 1.5 |
| Deeply Fruity, Belgian Chocolate & Forest Fruits, Waitrose* | 1 Muffin/125g | 451.0 | 23.0 | 361 | 5.4 | 43.3 | 18.4 | 0.5 |
| Double Choc Chip, Weight Watchers* | 1 Muffin/65g | 189.0 | 5.0 | 291 | 6.8 | 47.2 | 8.3 | 3.6 |
| Double Chocolate, Chocolate Chip, Mini, Tesco* | 1 Muffin/28g | 116.0 | 6.0 | 414 | 4.6 | 45.7 | 23.0 | 1.4 |
| Double Chocolate, Free From, Tesco* | 1 Muffin/70g | 281.0 | 13.0 | 402 | 4.7 | 54.8 | 18.2 | 1.7 |
| Double Chocolate, Mini, M & S* | 1 Muffin/32g | 133.0 | 7.0 | 416 | 5.4 | 49.8 | 21.7 | 1.1 |
| Double Chocolate Chip, American Style, Sainsbury's* | 1 Muffin/72g | 276.0 | 15.0 | 384 | 5.2 | 45.0 | 20.3 | 2.9 |
| Double Chocolate Chip, Mini, Asda* | 1 Muffin/19g | 76.0 | 4.0 | 400 | 7.4 | 48.5 | 19.6 | 2.7 |
| Double Chocolate Chip, Mini, Weight Watchers* | 1 Muffin/15g | 45.0 | 1.0 | 300 | 7.0 | 48.5 | 8.7 | 3.5 |
| Double Chocolate Chip, Tesco* | 1 Muffin/100g | 360.0 | 18.0 | 360 | 6.1 | 44.9 | 17.9 | 5.4 |
| English | 1 Muffin/57g | 120.0 | 1.0 | 211 | 7.0 | 43.9 | 1.8 | 1.8 |
| English, Kingsmill* | 1 Muffin/75g | 168.0 | 1.0 | 224 | 9.8 | 42.3 | 1.7 | 2.2 |
| English, M & S* | 1 Muffin/60g | 135.0 | 1.0 | 225 | 11.2 | 43.7 | 1.9 | 2.9 |
| English, Tesco* | 1 Muffin/72g | 171.0 | 2.0 | 237 | 11.2 | 41.7 | 3.2 | 2.8 |
| Lemon & Blueberry, Tesco* | 1 Muffin/110g | 411.0 | 23.0 | 374 | 4.0 | 42.4 | 20.9 | 1.1 |
| Lemon & Poppy Seed, M & S* | 1 Muffin/72g | 281.0 | 14.0 | 390 | 6.3 | 46.1 | 19.8 | 1.5 |
| Lemon & Sultana, BGTY, Sainsbury's* | 1 Muffin/75g | 211.0 | 3.0 | 281 | 4.5 | 55.6 | 4.5 | 1.4 |
| Mini, Tesco* | 1 Muffin/28g | 120.0 | 6.0 | 428 | 6.4 | 50.0 | 22.6 | 1.2 |
| Plain, Morrisons* | 1 Muffin/70g | 140.0 | 1.0 | 200 | 8.0 | 41.4 | 1.1 | 0.0 |
| Plain, Prepared From Recipe, Average | 1 Sm Muffin/57g | 169.0 | 6.0 | 296 | 6.9 | 41.4 | 11.4 | 2.7 |
| Raspberry, Perfectly Balanced, Waitrose* | 1 Muffin/101g | 220.0 | 2.0 | 219 | 4.7 | 45.4 | 2.1 | 3.7 |
| Raspberry Cream, Sainsbury's* | 1 Muffin/90g | 314.0 | 20.0 | 349 | 3.9 | 33.8 | 22.0 | 1.3 |
| Rolo, Nestle* | 1 Muffin/80g | 289.0 | 14.0 | 361 | 5.4 | 44.3 | 18.0 | 0.8 |
| Sausage, Egg & Cheese, American Style, Tesco* | 1 Muffin/155g | 383.0 | 20.0 | 247 | 12.2 | 19.9 | 13.2 | 1.0 |
| Spiced Fruit, Co-Op* | 1 Muffin/60g | 159.0 | 1.0 | 265 | 11.0 | 52.0 | 2.0 | 3.0 |
| Spiced Fruit, TTD, Sainsbury's* | 1 Muffin/70g | 181.0 | 4.0 | 259 | 10.1 | 43.1 | 5.1 | 2.3 |
| Sunblest* | 1 Muffin/72g | 166.0 | 1.0 | 230 | 9.6 | 43.9 | 1.8 | 2.2 |
| Toffee, The Handmade Flapjack Company* | 1 Muffin/135g | 533.0 | 32.0 | 395 | 4.4 | 41.2 | 23.4 | 0.0 |
| Toffee & Pecan, Finest, Tesco* | 1 Muffin/127g | 551.0 | 29.0 | 434 | 5.4 | 51.8 | 22.8 | 0.9 |
| Toffee Choo Choo, Tesco* | 1 Muffin/95g | 402.0 | 21.0 | 423 | 6.4 | 49.1 | 22.4 | 1.0 |
| Toffee Temptation, McVitie's* | 1 Muffin/86g | 297.0 | 8.0 | 347 | 4.7 | 60.8 | 9.5 | 0.8 |
| Vanilla & Choc Chip, GFY, Asda* | 1 Muffin/59g | 152.0 | 1.0 | 260 | 7.0 | 53.0 | 2.2 | 1.6 |
| White, All Butter, Sainsbury's* | 1 Muffin/67g | 173.0 | 4.0 | 258 | 10.6 | 39.6 | 6.3 | 3.6 |
| White, Asda* | 1 Muffin/67g | 148.0 | 1.0 | 222 | 11.0 | 40.0 | 2.0 | 2.5 |
| White, Finest, Tesco* | 1 Muffin/70g | 159.0 | 1.0 | 227 | 8.4 | 45.7 | 1.2 | 2.1 |
| White, M & S* | 1 Muffin/60g | 135.0 | 1.0 | 225 | 11.2 | 43.7 | 1.9 | 2.9 |
| White, Tesco* | 1 Muffin/72g | 173.0 | 2.0 | 240 | 11.3 | 41.6 | 3.2 | 2.8 |
| Wholemeal, Tesco* | 1 Muffin/65g | 130.0 | 1.0 | 200 | 12.6 | 32.9 | 2.0 | 5.7 |
| **MUFFIN MIX** | | | | | | | | |
| Banana Nut, Betty Crocker* | 1 Serving/30g | 130.0 | 5.0 | 433 | 6.7 | 70.0 | 16.7 | 0.0 |
| **MULBERRIES** | | | | | | | | |
| *Raw* | *1oz/28g* | *10.0* | *0.0* | *36* | *1.3* | *8.1* | *0.0* | *0.0* |
| **MULLET** | | | | | | | | |
| *Grey, Grilled* | *1oz/28g* | *42.0* | *1.0* | *150* | *25.7* | *0.0* | *5.2* | *0.0* |

# MULLET

| INFO/WEIGHT | Measure KCAL | per Measure FAT | KCAL | PROT | CARB | FAT | FIBRE |
|---|---|---|---|---|---|---|---|
| | | | Nutrition Values per 100g / 100ml | | | | |

## MULLET

| | INFO/WEIGHT | KCAL | FAT | KCAL | PROT | CARB | FAT | FIBRE |
|---|---|---|---|---|---|---|---|---|
| *Grey, Raw* | *1oz/28g* | *32.0* | *1.0* | *115* | *19.8* | *0.0* | *4.0* | *0.0* |
| *Red, Grilled* | *1oz/28g* | *34.0* | *1.0* | *121* | *20.4* | *0.0* | *4.4* | *0.0* |
| *Red, Raw, Weighed Whole* | *1oz/28g* | *31.0* | *1.0* | *109* | *18.7* | *0.0* | *3.8* | *0.0* |

## MUNCHIES

| | INFO/WEIGHT | KCAL | FAT | KCAL | PROT | CARB | FAT | FIBRE |
|---|---|---|---|---|---|---|---|---|
| Mint, Nestle* | 1 Pack/62g | 267.0 | 10.0 | 432 | 3.8 | 67.5 | 16.4 | 0.0 |
| Original, Tube, Nestle* | 1 Pack/55g | 272.0 | 13.0 | 498 | 4.1 | 65.6 | 24.4 | 0.5 |

## MUSHROOMS

| | INFO/WEIGHT | KCAL | FAT | KCAL | PROT | CARB | FAT | FIBRE |
|---|---|---|---|---|---|---|---|---|
| *Breaded, Average* | *1oz/28g* | *42.0* | *2.0* | *151* | *4.3* | *20.8* | *5.7* | *0.6* |
| Breaded, Garlic, Average | 1 Serving/50g | 92.0 | 5.0 | 183 | 5.2 | 18.7 | 9.7 | 1.7 |
| Buna Shimeji, Livesey Brothers* | ½ Pack/75g | 29.0 | 0.0 | 39 | 2.7 | 5.9 | 0.4 | 1.2 |
| *Button, Average* | *1 Serving/50g* | *7.0* | *0.0* | *15* | *2.3* | *0.5* | *0.4* | *1.2* |
| Chargrilled & Truffle Sauce, The Best, Safeway* | 1 Pot/350g | 385.0 | 27.0 | 110 | 3.4 | 5.8 | 7.6 | 0.8 |
| Cheesey, Stuffed, Asda* | 1 Serving/290g | 322.0 | 17.0 | 111 | 4.3 | 10.0 | 6.0 | 0.0 |
| *Chestnut, Average* | *1 Med/5g* | *1.0* | *0.0* | *13* | *1.8* | *0.4* | *0.5* | *0.5* |
| *Chinese, Dried, Raw* | *1oz/28g* | *80.0* | *1.0* | *284* | *10.0* | *59.9* | *1.8* | *0.0* |
| *Closed Cup, Average* | *1oz/28g* | *5.0* | *0.0* | *18* | *2.9* | *0.4* | *0.5* | *0.5* |
| *Common, Boiled in Salted Water, Average* | *1oz/28g* | *3.0* | *0.0* | *11* | *1.8* | *0.4* | *0.3* | *1.1* |
| *Common, Fried, Average* | *1oz/28g* | *44.0* | *5.0* | *157* | *2.4* | *0.3* | *16.2* | *1.5* |
| *Common, Raw, Average* | *1 Serving/80g* | *10.0* | *0.0* | *13* | *1.9* | *0.3* | *0.5* | *1.1* |
| *Creamed, Average* | *1oz/28g* | *23.0* | *2.0* | *82* | *1.3* | *6.8* | *5.5* | *0.5* |
| Crispy, M & S* | 1 Serving/130g | 390.0 | 33.0 | 300 | 4.2 | 12.5 | 25.7 | 1.8 |
| *Dried* | *1oz/28g* | *45.0* | *2.0* | *159* | *21.8* | *4.8* | *6.0* | *13.3* |
| *Enoki, Average* | *1 Serving/80g* | *34.0* | *0.0* | *42* | *3.0* | *7.0* | *0.0* | *3.0* |
| *Flat, Large, Average* | *1 Mushroom/52g* | *10.0* | *0.0* | *19* | *3.3* | *0.5* | *0.5* | *0.7* |
| Garlic, Average | ½ Pack/150g | 159.0 | 14.0 | 106 | 2.1 | 3.7 | 9.3 | 1.7 |
| Giant, with Tomatoes & Mozzarella, M & S* | 1 Serving/145g | 217.0 | 16.0 | 150 | 6.3 | 7.1 | 10.9 | 5.5 |
| Medley, Asda* | ½ Pack/100g | 89.0 | 8.0 | 89 | 3.2 | 1.4 | 7.8 | 2.8 |
| *Oyster, Average* | *1 Serving/80g* | *12.0* | *0.0* | *15* | *1.6* | *1.6* | *0.2* | *1.3* |
| Porcini, Dried, Asda* | 1 Bag/25g | 65.0 | 1.0 | 260 | 30.4 | 24.1 | 4.7 | 17.5 |
| Porcini, Wild, Dried, Merchant Gourmet* | 1 Pack/25g | 85.0 | 1.0 | 340 | 27.6 | 52.0 | 2.4 | 0.0 |
| *Shiitake, Cooked* | *1oz/28g* | *15.0* | *0.0* | *55* | *1.6* | *12.3* | *0.2* | *0.0* |
| *Shiitake, Dried, Raw* | *1oz/28g* | *83.0* | *0.0* | *296* | *9.6* | *63.9* | *1.0* | *0.0* |
| *Sliced, Average* | *1oz/28g* | *3.0* | *0.0* | *12* | *1.8* | *0.4* | *0.3* | *1.1* |
| *Straw, Canned, Drained* | *1oz/28g* | *4.0* | *0.0* | *15* | *2.1* | *1.2* | *0.2* | *0.0* |

## MUSSELS

| | INFO/WEIGHT | KCAL | FAT | KCAL | PROT | CARB | FAT | FIBRE |
|---|---|---|---|---|---|---|---|---|
| Boiled, Average | 1 Mussel/7g | 7.0 | 0.0 | 104 | 16.7 | 3.5 | 2.7 | 0.0 |
| *Pickled, Drained, Average* | *1oz/28g* | *31.0* | *1.0* | *112* | *20.0* | *1.5* | *2.2* | *0.0* |
| *Raw, Average* | *1oz/28g* | *24.0* | *1.0* | *87* | *12.7* | *3.6* | *2.5* | *0.2* |

## MUSSELS IN

| | INFO/WEIGHT | KCAL | FAT | KCAL | PROT | CARB | FAT | FIBRE |
|---|---|---|---|---|---|---|---|---|
| Creamy Garlic Butter Sauce, Bantry Bay* | 1 Serving/225g | 198.0 | 8.0 | 88 | 9.0 | 5.2 | 3.5 | 0.6 |
| Garlic Butter Sauce, Average | ½ Pack/225g | 179.0 | 11.0 | 79 | 6.3 | 1.9 | 5.1 | 0.1 |
| Thai Sauce, Scottish, Waitrose* | 1 Serving/250g | 135.0 | 6.0 | 54 | 5.4 | 2.6 | 2.5 | 0.6 |
| White Wine, Cream, Shallot & Garlic Sauce, COOK!, M & S* | 1 Pack/450g | 360.0 | 13.0 | 80 | 11.7 | 1.6 | 2.8 | 2.1 |
| White Wine Cream Sauce, Cooked, Scottish, Morrisons* | ½ Pack/250g | 222.0 | 9.0 | 89 | 8.0 | 5.8 | 3.7 | 0.0 |
| White Wine Sauce, Sainsbury's* | ½ Pack/250g | 221.0 | 9.0 | 88 | 8.0 | 5.8 | 3.7 | 0.0 |

## MUSSELS WITH

| | INFO/WEIGHT | KCAL | FAT | KCAL | PROT | CARB | FAT | FIBRE |
|---|---|---|---|---|---|---|---|---|
| Tomato & Garlic, Fresh, M & S* | 1 Serving/650g | 455.0 | 10.0 | 70 | 7.9 | 6.5 | 1.6 | 0.1 |

## MUSTARD

| | INFO/WEIGHT | KCAL | FAT | KCAL | PROT | CARB | FAT | FIBRE |
|---|---|---|---|---|---|---|---|---|
| *American, Average* | *1 Tsp/5g* | *5.0* | *0.0* | *102* | *4.4* | *10.5* | *5.0* | *2.5* |
| Cajun, Colman's* | 1 Tsp/6g | 11.0 | 0.0 | 187 | 7.0 | 23.0 | 6.5 | 2.7 |
| *Coarse Grain, Average* | *1 Tsp/5g* | *7.0* | *0.0* | *141* | *7.7* | *8.4* | *8.3* | *5.9* |
| *Dijon, Average* | *1 Tsp/5g* | *8.0* | *1.0* | *163* | *7.4* | *7.7* | *11.3* | *1.1* |
| *English, Average* | *1 Tsp/5g* | *9.0* | *0.0* | *173* | *6.8* | *19.2* | *7.6* | *1.2* |

| | Measure INFO/WEIGHT | per Measure KCAL | FAT | Nutrition Values per 100g / 100ml KCAL | PROT | CARB | FAT | FIBRE |
|---|---|---|---|---|---|---|---|---|
| **MUSTARD** | | | | | | | | |
| *French, Average* | *1 Tsp/5g* | *5.0* | *0.0* | *105* | *5.4* | *8.1* | *5.6* | *1.8* |
| German Style, Sainsbury's* | 1 Serving/10g | 9.0 | 1.0 | 92 | 5.5 | 2.8 | 6.5 | 0.0 |
| *Powder, Average* | *1 Tsp/3g* | *15.0* | *1.0* | *452* | *28.9* | *20.7* | *28.7* | *0.0* |
| *Powder, Made Up, Average* | *1oz/28g* | *63.0* | *4.0* | *226* | *14.5* | *10.4* | *14.4* | *0.0* |
| *Smooth, Average* | *1 Tsp/8g* | *11.0* | *1.0* | *139* | *7.1* | *9.7* | *8.2* | *0.0* |
| *Smooth, Average* | *1 Tsp/8g* | *11.0* | *1.0* | *139* | *7.1* | *9.7* | *8.2* | *0.0* |
| *Whole Grain, Average* | *1 Tsp/8g* | *11.0* | *1.0* | *140* | *8.2* | *4.2* | *10.2* | *4.9* |
| **MUSTARD CRESS** | | | | | | | | |
| *Raw* | *1oz/28g* | *4.0* | *0.0* | *13* | *1.6* | *0.4* | *0.6* | *1.1* |

| | Measure INFO/WEIGHT | per Measure KCAL | FAT | Nutrition Values per 100g / 100ml KCAL | PROT | CARB | FAT | FIBRE |
|---|---|---|---|---|---|---|---|---|
| **NACHOS** | | | | | | | | |
| American Chilli Beef, Asda* | 1 Serving/200g | 208.0 | 10.0 | 104 | 10.0 | 4.7 | 5.0 | 0.8 |
| Cheesy, with Salsa & Soured Cream, Sainsbury's* | ½ Pack/170g | 449.0 | 27.0 | 264 | 8.8 | 21.5 | 15.8 | 1.4 |
| Chilli, Sainsbury's* | ½ Pack/250g | 695.0 | 32.0 | 278 | 10.9 | 29.5 | 12.9 | 1.3 |
| Kit, Old El Paso* | ½ Pack/260g | 598.0 | 26.0 | 230 | 4.0 | 31.0 | 10.0 | 0.0 |
| **NASI GORENG** | | | | | | | | |
| Indonesian, Asda* | 1 Pack/360g | 778.0 | 23.0 | 216 | 7.4 | 32.3 | 6.3 | 1.3 |
| **NECTARINES** | | | | | | | | |
| **Weighed with Stone, Fresh, Raw, Average** | **1 Med/140g** | **53.0** | **0.0** | **38** | **1.3** | **8.5** | **0.1** | **1.1** |
| **NESQUIK** | | | | | | | | |
| Chocolate Flavour, Powder, Dry Weight, Nesquik, Nestle* | 1 Serving/15g | 56.0 | 0.0 | 372 | 3.0 | 82.9 | 3.1 | 6.5 |
| Strawberry Flavour, Powder, Dry Weight, Nesquik, Nestle* | 1 Serving/15g | 59.0 | 0.0 | 393 | 0.0 | 98.1 | 0.0 | 0.0 |
| **NIK NAKS** | | | | | | | | |
| Cream 'n' Cheesy, Golden Wonder* | 1 Bag/34g | 195.0 | 13.0 | 575 | 5.2 | 52.7 | 38.1 | 0.2 |
| Nice 'n' Spicy, Golden Wonder* | 1 Bag/30g | 168.0 | 11.0 | 561 | 4.7 | 49.6 | 38.3 | 3.0 |
| Rib 'n' Saucy, Golden Wonder* | 1 Bag/34g | 194.0 | 13.0 | 571 | 4.5 | 53.7 | 37.6 | 0.5 |
| Scampi 'n' Lemon, Golden Wonder* | 1 Bag/34g | 195.0 | 13.0 | 573 | 4.9 | 53.1 | 37.5 | 0.1 |
| **NOODLE BOWL** | | | | | | | | |
| Chilli Beef, HL, Tesco* | 1 Pack/400g | 368.0 | 6.0 | 92 | 4.5 | 15.4 | 1.4 | 1.1 |
| Chow Mein, Chicken, Uncle Ben's* | 1 Pack/330g | 307.0 | 5.0 | 93 | 6.1 | 13.5 | 1.4 | 0.0 |
| Coconut & Coriander Chicken, Oriental, Finest, Tesco* | 1 Pack/450g | 562.0 | 23.0 | 125 | 8.3 | 10.8 | 5.2 | 2.1 |
| King Prawn, Hot & Sour, Finest, Tesco* | 1 Pack/400g | 260.0 | 6.0 | 65 | 4.4 | 8.6 | 1.4 | 1.7 |
| Szechuan Style Prawn, Tesco* | 1 Pack/400g | 376.0 | 1.0 | 94 | 5.5 | 17.3 | 0.3 | 0.9 |
| **NOODLE BOX** | | | | | | | | |
| Cantonese Chow Mein, Sharwood's* | 1 Pack/350g | 465.0 | 10.0 | 133 | 3.8 | 22.9 | 2.9 | 1.5 |
| Hong Kong Sweet & Sour, Sharwood's* | 1 Pack/350g | 409.0 | 5.0 | 117 | 3.7 | 22.6 | 1.3 | 1.8 |
| Thai Red Curry, Sharwood's* | 1 Pack/350g | 444.0 | 11.0 | 127 | 3.9 | 20.9 | 3.1 | 1.6 |
| **NOODLES** | | | | | | | | |
| Barbecue Beef, Instant, Asda* | 1 Pack/333g | 420.0 | 16.0 | 126 | 2.6 | 18.0 | 4.8 | 0.0 |
| Beef, Oriental, GFY, Asda* | 1 Pack/400g | 372.0 | 7.0 | 93 | 7.4 | 12.1 | 1.7 | 1.7 |
| Beef Flavour, Instant, Prepared, Heinz* | 1 Pack/384g | 257.0 | 0.0 | 67 | 2.1 | 14.4 | 0.1 | 0.6 |
| Chicken, Chinese Style, GFY, Asda* | 1 Pack/393g | 295.0 | 7.0 | 75 | 6.0 | 9.0 | 1.7 | 0.6 |
| Chicken, Dry Weight, Heinz* | 1 Pack/85g | 257.0 | 0.0 | 302 | 9.5 | 65.3 | 0.4 | 2.7 |
| Chicken, Instant, Less Than 1% Fat, Prepared, Heinz* | 1 Pack/385g | 258.0 | 0.0 | 67 | 2.1 | 14.4 | 0.1 | 0.6 |
| Chicken, Instant, Weight Watchers* | 1 Pack/385g | 269.0 | 0.0 | 70 | 2.3 | 14.9 | 0.1 | 0.6 |
| Chicken Curry Flavour, Instant, Sainsbury's* | 1 Pack/85g | 167.0 | 6.0 | 196 | 4.6 | 27.9 | 7.3 | 0.8 |
| Chicken Flavour, Dry, Princes* | 1 Pack/85g | 395.0 | 16.0 | 465 | 10.0 | 63.8 | 18.8 | 0.0 |
| Chicken Flavour, Instant, Made Up, Tesco* | ½ Pack/168g | 285.0 | 11.0 | 170 | 4.1 | 23.7 | 6.3 | 1.5 |
| Chicken Flavour, Instant, Sainsbury's* | 1 Pack/335g | 549.0 | 21.0 | 164 | 4.4 | 22.3 | 6.4 | 1.3 |
| Chicken Flavour, Value, Made Up, Tesco* | 1 Serving/265g | 450.0 | 17.0 | 170 | 4.1 | 23.7 | 6.3 | 1.5 |
| Chilli Beef, Finest, Tesco* | 1 Pack/450g | 486.0 | 9.0 | 108 | 7.7 | 15.2 | 1.9 | 0.9 |
| Chilli Chicken, GFY, Asda* | 1 Pack/415g | 461.0 | 3.0 | 111 | 6.0 | 20.0 | 0.8 | 1.0 |
| Chilli Infused, Blue Dragon* | 1 Serving/150g | 286.0 | 1.0 | 191 | 6.1 | 33.6 | 0.7 | 0.3 |
| Chinese, Stir Fry, Sainsbury's* | 1 Serving/100g | 185.0 | 5.0 | 185 | 6.0 | 29.5 | 4.8 | 1.5 |
| Chow Mein, Dry Weight, Snack in a Pot, HL, Tesco* | 1 Pot/56g | 202.0 | 1.0 | 360 | 13.4 | 72.2 | 1.4 | 5.0 |
| Chow Mein, Instant, Made Up, Tesco* | 1 Pack/168g | 255.0 | 8.0 | 152 | 3.8 | 23.0 | 5.0 | 1.2 |
| Chow Mein, Sainsbury's* | 1 Pack/125g | 136.0 | 2.0 | 109 | 3.9 | 19.2 | 1.8 | 0.8 |
| Chow Mein, Stir Fry, Tesco* | 1 Serving/200g | 116.0 | 2.0 | 58 | 2.1 | 9.7 | 1.2 | 1.0 |
| Chow Mein Flavour, Dry, Princes* | 1 Pack/85g | 396.0 | 16.0 | 466 | 10.1 | 64.6 | 18.6 | 0.0 |
| Chow Mein Flavour, Instant, Morrisons* | 1 Pack/85g | 162.0 | 6.0 | 191 | 4.8 | 29.9 | 6.5 | 1.6 |
| Crispy, Dry, Blue Dragon* | 1 Box/125g | 437.0 | 1.0 | 350 | 2.4 | 84.0 | 0.5 | 0.0 |
| Curry, Instant, Dry, Heinz* | 1 Serving/85g | 261.0 | 0.0 | 307 | 9.5 | 66.4 | 0.4 | 2.7 |
| Curry Flavour, Instant, Dry, Asda* | 1 Serving/65g | 415.0 | 11.0 | 638 | 20.0 | 101.5 | 16.9 | 0.9 |
| Curry Flavour, Instant, From Heinz, Weight Watchers* | 1 Pack/385g | 266.0 | 0.0 | 69 | 2.2 | 14.8 | 0.1 | 0.6 |

## NOODLES

| | Measure INFO/WEIGHT | per Measure KCAL | FAT | Nutrition Values per 100g / 100ml KCAL | PROT | CARB | FAT | FIBRE |
|---|---|---|---|---|---|---|---|---|
| Curry Flavour, Instant, Sainsbury's* | 1 Pack/335g | 412.0 | 15.0 | 123 | 2.6 | 17.8 | 4.6 | 0.1 |
| Egg, & Bean Sprouts, Cooked, Tesco* | 1 Pack/250g | 237.0 | 5.0 | 95 | 4.4 | 14.6 | 2.1 | 1.5 |
| Egg, Asda* | 1 Pack/184g | 213.0 | 13.0 | 116 | 2.3 | 11.0 | 7.0 | 0.6 |
| *Egg, Boiled* | *1oz/28g* | *17.0* | *0.0* | *62* | *2.2* | *13.0* | *0.5* | *0.6* |
| Egg, Cooked, Somerfield* | ½ Pack/150g | 189.0 | 8.0 | 126 | 3.2 | 16.0 | 5.5 | 0.6 |
| *Egg, Dry* | *1 Block/63g* | *244.0* | *5.0* | *391* | *12.1* | *71.7* | *8.2* | *2.9* |
| Egg, Fine, Blue Dragon* | 1 Serving/100g | 171.0 | 1.0 | 171 | 5.5 | 35.0 | 0.9 | 0.0 |
| Egg, Fine, Dry Weight, Sharwood's* | 1 Block/63g | 216.0 | 1.0 | 346 | 12.0 | 70.0 | 2.1 | 2.5 |
| Egg, Fine, Fresh, M & S* | 1 Pack/275g | 330.0 | 6.0 | 120 | 4.4 | 20.7 | 2.2 | 1.5 |
| Egg, Fine, Waitrose* | ¼ Pack/63g | 221.0 | 2.0 | 353 | 15.0 | 67.3 | 2.6 | 3.8 |
| Egg, Fine Thread, Dry, M & S* | 1 Serving/63g | 220.0 | 1.0 | 350 | 14.3 | 71.6 | 0.9 | 5.1 |
| Egg, Free Range, Asda* | 1 Serving/125g | 205.0 | 5.0 | 164 | 5.1 | 27.0 | 3.9 | 1.8 |
| Egg, Fresh, Just Stir Fry, Sainsbury's* | ½ Pack/192g | 314.0 | 7.0 | 163 | 5.0 | 28.1 | 3.4 | 1.8 |
| Egg, Fresh, Tesco* | 1 Serving/150g | 102.0 | 2.0 | 68 | 2.8 | 11.8 | 1.3 | 0.6 |
| Egg, M & S* | ½ Pack/110g | 165.0 | 2.0 | 150 | 4.9 | 28.3 | 1.7 | 2.8 |
| Egg, Medium, Asda* | 1 Serving/83g | 125.0 | 1.0 | 150 | 4.8 | 31.0 | 0.8 | 1.3 |
| Egg, Medium, Dry, Blue Dragon* | 1 Serving/81g | 288.0 | 1.0 | 356 | 13.8 | 70.0 | 1.7 | 3.4 |
| Egg, Medium, Dry, Sharwood's* | 1 Serving/63g | 216.0 | 1.0 | 346 | 12.0 | 70.0 | 2.1 | 2.5 |
| Egg, Medium, Sainsbury's* | 1 Serving/122g | 168.0 | 1.0 | 138 | 5.7 | 26.9 | 0.8 | 1.0 |
| Egg, Tossed in Sesame Oil, Asda* | ½ Pack/150g | 174.0 | 10.0 | 116 | 2.3 | 11.0 | 7.0 | 0.6 |
| *Fried, Average* | *1oz/28g* | *43.0* | *3.0* | *153* | *1.9* | *11.3* | *11.5* | *0.5* |
| Garlic, Chilli & Ginger, Tesco* | 1 Serving/350g | 507.0 | 11.0 | 145 | 4.8 | 24.1 | 3.2 | 2.6 |
| Instant, Dry, Sainsbury's* | 1 Pack/100g | 392.0 | 14.0 | 392 | 9.4 | 57.0 | 14.0 | 0.2 |
| Instant, Express, Dry, Blue Dragon* | 1 Serving/75g | 337.0 | 13.0 | 450 | 10.0 | 65.0 | 17.0 | 2.0 |
| Oriental, Snack Pot, Dry, HL, Tesco* | 1 Pot/57g | 210.0 | 1.0 | 369 | 14.0 | 74.4 | 1.7 | 2.0 |
| Oriental, Snack Pot, Made Up, HL, Tesco* | 1 Serving/238g | 221.0 | 1.0 | 93 | 3.1 | 19.4 | 0.3 | 0.6 |
| Pasta, 100% Hard Durum Wheat, Dry, Goody* | 1 Serving/100g | 362.0 | 2.0 | 362 | 12.5 | 73.0 | 1.7 | 0.0 |
| Peking Duck, Shapers, Boots* | 1 Pack/280g | 395.0 | 4.0 | 141 | 7.2 | 25.0 | 1.4 | 1.8 |
| *Plain, Boiled* | *1oz/28g* | *17.0* | *0.0* | *62* | *2.4* | *13.0* | *0.4* | *0.7* |
| *Plain, Dry* | *1oz/28g* | *109.0* | *2.0* | *388* | *11.7* | *76.1* | *6.2* | *2.9* |
| Prawn, Instant, Made Up, Tesco* | 1 Serving/168g | 251.0 | 9.0 | 150 | 3.8 | 21.9 | 5.2 | 1.3 |
| Prawn Satay, Safeway* | 1 Serving/400g | 460.0 | 18.0 | 115 | 5.3 | 12.4 | 4.6 | 1.8 |
| Ramen, with Chilli Beef, M & S* | 1 Pack/484g | 532.0 | 17.0 | 110 | 8.1 | 11.9 | 3.6 | 0.8 |
| Ramen, with Wakame, The Original Noodle Company* | ½ Pack/124g | 304.0 | 1.0 | 245 | 7.4 | 51.8 | 0.8 | 1.8 |
| Rice, Cooked, Sharwood's* | 1 Serving/200g | 239.0 | 1.0 | 119 | 2.0 | 27.1 | 0.3 | 0.7 |
| Rice, Dry, Blue Dragon* | 1 Serving/30g | 113.0 | 0.0 | 376 | 7.0 | 84.0 | 0.0 | 0.0 |
| Rice, Medium, Blue Dragon* | 1 Serving/63g | 235.0 | 0.0 | 376 | 7.0 | 84.0 | 0.0 | 0.0 |
| Rice, Oriental, Thai, Stir Fry, Dry Weight, Sharwood's* | 1 Serving/63g | 226.0 | 1.0 | 361 | 6.5 | 86.8 | 1.0 | 2.4 |
| Rice, Stir Fry, Tesco* | ½ Pack/190g | 304.0 | 11.0 | 160 | 2.0 | 24.8 | 5.7 | 1.0 |
| Savoury Vegetable, COU, M & S* | 1 Pack/450g | 270.0 | 3.0 | 60 | 2.9 | 11.5 | 0.6 | 1.2 |
| Singapore, Light Choices, Tesco* | 1 Pack/450g | 337.0 | 8.0 | 75 | 4.8 | 9.8 | 1.7 | 1.2 |
| Singapore, Morrisons* | 1 Serving/400g | 480.0 | 27.0 | 120 | 4.8 | 11.6 | 6.7 | 1.6 |
| Singapore, Sainsbury's* | 1 Pack/400g | 432.0 | 16.0 | 108 | 6.5 | 11.7 | 3.9 | 2.8 |
| Singapore, Somerfield* | 1 Pot/300g | 261.0 | 3.0 | 87 | 5.0 | 15.0 | 1.0 | 0.0 |
| Singapore, Waitrose* | 1 Pack/400g | 476.0 | 18.0 | 119 | 7.3 | 12.6 | 4.4 | 2.1 |
| Singapore Spicy, Safeway* | 1 Serving/225g | 270.0 | 10.0 | 120 | 6.0 | 14.2 | 4.3 | 1.7 |
| Singapore Style, Asda* | 1 Pack/400g | 688.0 | 32.0 | 172 | 7.0 | 18.0 | 8.0 | 1.0 |
| Spicy, Sainsbury's* | 1 Serving/180g | 182.0 | 8.0 | 101 | 10.4 | 4.5 | 4.6 | 0.9 |
| Spicy Thai, Instant, Heinz* | 1 Pack/385g | 262.0 | 0.0 | 68 | 2.1 | 14.6 | 0.1 | 0.6 |
| Stir Fry, Tesco* | 1 Serving/150g | 202.0 | 4.0 | 135 | 5.3 | 23.0 | 2.4 | 1.5 |
| Straight to Wok, Medium, Amoy* | 1 Pack/150g | 240.0 | 2.0 | 160 | 5.8 | 31.7 | 1.5 | 0.0 |
| Straight to Wok, Rice, Amoy* | 1 Pack/150g | 174.0 | 0.0 | 116 | 1.6 | 27.4 | 0.1 | 0.0 |
| Straight to Wok, Singapore, Amoy* | 1 Serving/150g | 232.0 | 4.0 | 155 | 4.8 | 28.4 | 2.8 | 0.0 |

| | Measure INFO/WEIGHT | per Measure KCAL | FAT | Nutrition Values per 100g / 100ml KCAL | PROT | CARB | FAT | FIBRE |
|---|---|---|---|---|---|---|---|---|
| **NOODLES** | | | | | | | | |
| Straight to Wok, Thread, Fine, Amoy* | 1 Pack/150g | 237.0 | 4.0 | 158 | 5.0 | 28.7 | 2.6 | 0.0 |
| Straight to Wok, Udon, Amoy* | 1 Pack/150g | 211.0 | 2.0 | 141 | 4.4 | 28.8 | 1.3 | 0.0 |
| Super, Barbecue Beef, Made Up, Batchelors* | 1 Serving/100g | 156.0 | 7.0 | 156 | 3.2 | 20.9 | 6.7 | 1.1 |
| Super, Barbecue Beef, to Go, 98% Fat Free, Batchelors* | 1 Pack/380g | 308.0 | 1.0 | 81 | 2.4 | 17.5 | 0.2 | 0.6 |
| Super, Chicken & Herb, Low Fat, Made Up, Batchelors* | 1 Pack/170g | 322.0 | 2.0 | 189 | 6.1 | 39.2 | 0.9 | 1.2 |
| Super, Chicken Flavour, Made Up, Batchelors* | 1 Serving/100g | 170.0 | 7.0 | 170 | 3.3 | 22.9 | 7.3 | 0.9 |
| Super, Chow Mein Flavour, Made Up, Batchelors* | ½ Pack/150g | 262.0 | 12.0 | 175 | 3.0 | 23.0 | 7.9 | 0.4 |
| Super, Mild Curry Flavour, Made Up, Batchelors* | 1 Serving/100g | 157.0 | 7.0 | 157 | 3.2 | 20.9 | 6.7 | 1.0 |
| Super, Mushroom Flavour, Made Up, Batchelors* | 1 Serving/100g | 157.0 | 7.0 | 157 | 3.2 | 20.9 | 6.8 | 1.0 |
| Super, Roast Chicken, to Go, 98% Fat Free, Batchelors* | 1 Serving/380g | 308.0 | 1.0 | 81 | 2.6 | 17.2 | 0.2 | 0.5 |
| Super, Southern Fried Chicken, Made Up, Batchelors* | 1 Serving/100g | 171.0 | 7.0 | 171 | 3.3 | 23.2 | 7.2 | 0.5 |
| Super, Spicy Balti, Made Up, Batchelors* | 1 Serving/100g | 166.0 | 7.0 | 166 | 3.0 | 21.5 | 7.5 | 1.1 |
| Super, Spicy Salsa, Dry Weight, Batchelors* | 1 Pack/105g | 474.0 | 20.0 | 451 | 7.0 | 63.8 | 18.6 | 1.7 |
| Super, Sweet Thai Chilli, Dry Weight, Batchelors* | 1 Pack/85g | 292.0 | 1.0 | 343 | 10.6 | 72.5 | 1.2 | 3.0 |
| Super, Sweet Thai Chilli Flavour, 98% Fat Free, Batchelors* | 1 Pack/270g | 292.0 | 1.0 | 108 | 3.3 | 22.8 | 0.4 | 0.9 |
| **NOUGAT** | | | | | | | | |
| Almond & Cherry, M & S* | 1 Sweet/7g | 28.0 | 1.0 | 405 | 4.5 | 76.0 | 9.1 | 1.1 |
| Average | 1 Sm Bar/28g | 108.0 | 2.0 | 384 | 4.4 | 77.3 | 8.5 | 0.9 |
| Bassetts & Beyond, Cadbury* | 1oz/28g | 105.0 | 1.0 | 375 | 4.0 | 82.0 | 4.0 | 0.0 |
| Raspberry & Orange Hazelnut, Thorntons* | 1 Sweet/9g | 39.0 | 2.0 | 433 | 4.8 | 60.0 | 20.0 | 2.2 |
| Soft, Bar, Bassett's* | 1 Bar/25g | 94.0 | 1.0 | 375 | 4.0 | 82.0 | 4.0 | 0.0 |
| **NUT ROAST** | | | | | | | | |
| Asda* | 1 Roast/230g | 389.0 | 16.0 | 169 | 8.7 | 23.2 | 7.1 | 5.6 |
| Average | 1 Serving/200g | 704.0 | 51.0 | 352 | 13.3 | 18.3 | 25.7 | 4.2 |
| *Lentil, Average* | *1oz/28g* | *62.0* | *3.0* | *222* | *10.6* | *18.8* | *12.1* | *3.8* |
| Tomato & Courgette, Vegetarian, Organic, Waitrose* | ½ Pack/142g | 295.0 | 17.0 | 208 | 11.7 | 12.5 | 12.3 | 4.9 |
| **NUTMEG** | | | | | | | | |
| *Ground, Average* | *1 Tsp/3g* | *16.0* | *1.0* | *525* | *5.8* | *45.3* | *36.3* | *0.0* |
| **NUTS** | | | | | | | | |
| Clusters, Sweet Tomato Salsa, Sensations, Walkers* | 1 Serving/35g | 187.0 | 13.0 | 535 | 14.0 | 36.0 | 37.0 | 5.0 |
| Lemon & Chilli Flavour, Mix, TTD, Sainsbury's* | 1 Serving/50g | 320.0 | 29.0 | 641 | 20.0 | 11.2 | 57.3 | 5.7 |
| Luxury Assortment, Tesco* | 1 Serving/10g | 68.0 | 6.0 | 676 | 17.5 | 6.1 | 64.6 | 5.0 |
| Mixed | 1 Pack/40g | 243.0 | 22.0 | 607 | 22.9 | 7.9 | 54.1 | 6.0 |
| Mixed, Chopped, Sainsbury's* | 1 Serving/100g | 605.0 | 51.0 | 605 | 27.1 | 9.6 | 50.9 | 6.0 |
| Mixed, Chopped, Tesco* | 1 Serving/25g | 149.0 | 13.0 | 595 | 23.5 | 10.5 | 50.6 | 6.0 |
| Mixed, Delicious, Boots* | 1 Pack/38g | 235.0 | 22.0 | 628 | 18.0 | 6.1 | 59.0 | 10.0 |
| Mixed, Honey Roasted, Waitrose* | 1 Serving/50g | 291.0 | 22.0 | 583 | 17.1 | 27.5 | 45.0 | 5.3 |
| Mixed, Natural, Asda* | 1 Snack/30g | 197.0 | 19.0 | 656 | 18.0 | 4.3 | 62.7 | 7.4 |
| Mixed, Roasted, Salted, Waitrose* | 1 Pack/200g | 1252.0 | 117.0 | 626 | 13.7 | 11.3 | 58.4 | 4.4 |
| Mixed, Roasted, Waitrose* | 1 Serving/25g | 165.0 | 16.0 | 662 | 15.2 | 6.2 | 64.0 | 8.2 |
| Mixed, Unsalted, Sainsbury's* | 1 Serving/50g | 311.0 | 29.0 | 622 | 18.5 | 7.2 | 57.7 | 8.7 |
| Natural, Mixed, Waitrose* | 1 Serving/50g | 324.0 | 31.0 | 648 | 17.7 | 6.8 | 61.1 | 8.2 |
| Natural Assortment, Tesco* | 1 Serving/50g | 338.0 | 32.0 | 676 | 17.5 | 6.1 | 64.6 | 5.0 |
| Oak Smoke Flavour Selection, Finest, Tesco* | 1 Serving/25g | 158.0 | 14.0 | 633 | 21.4 | 11.2 | 55.8 | 6.3 |
| Peanuts & Cashews, Honey Roast, Tesco* | 1 Serving/25g | 145.0 | 11.0 | 579 | 21.6 | 26.6 | 42.9 | 4.2 |
| Peri-Peri, Nando's* | 1 Serving/75g | 193.0 | 18.0 | 257 | 8.0 | 4.0 | 24.0 | 0.0 |
| Pine, Tesco* | 1 Pack/100g | 699.0 | 69.0 | 699 | 16.5 | 4.0 | 68.6 | 1.9 |
| Roasted, Salted, Assortment, Luxury, Tesco* | 1 Serving/25g | 161.0 | 14.0 | 643 | 21.1 | 9.4 | 57.9 | 8.1 |
| Salted, Selection, Sainsbury's* | 1 Serving/30g | 190.0 | 17.0 | 634 | 20.6 | 9.7 | 56.9 | 8.2 |
| Salted, Selection, TTD, Sainsbury's* | 1 Pack/75g | 508.0 | 48.0 | 678 | 16.3 | 8.9 | 64.2 | 7.2 |
| Soya, Dry Roasted, The Food Doctor* | 1 Serving/50g | 203.0 | 11.0 | 406 | 37.5 | 15.9 | 21.4 | 16.1 |
| Unsalted, Selection, Sainsbury's* | 1 Serving/75g | 491.0 | 48.0 | 655 | 14.7 | 5.0 | 64.0 | 6.7 |

| | Measure INFO/WEIGHT | per Measure KCAL | FAT | Nutrition Values per 100g / 100ml KCAL | PROT | CARB | FAT | FIBRE |
|---|---|---|---|---|---|---|---|---|
| **OAT BAKES** | | | | | | | | |
| Cheese, Nairn's* | 1 Bag/30g | 127.0 | 4.0 | 423 | 14.7 | 60.7 | 13.7 | 6.3 |
| Mediterranean Tomato and Herb, Nairn's* | 1 Bag/30g | 129.0 | 5.0 | 431 | 8.1 | 64.2 | 15.8 | 8.3 |
| Sweet Chilli, Nairn's* | 1 Bag/30g | 128.0 | 4.0 | 426 | 8.1 | 68.4 | 13.3 | 7.2 |
| **OAT CAKES** | | | | | | | | |
| Bran, Paterson's* | 1 Cake/13g | 52.0 | 2.0 | 416 | 10.0 | 58.5 | 15.8 | 9.5 |
| Cheese, Nairn's* | 1 Cake/9g | 42.0 | 2.0 | 471 | 13.2 | 43.3 | 27.2 | 6.8 |
| Fine Milled, Nairn's* | 1 Cake/8g | 35.0 | 2.0 | 449 | 10.5 | 52.6 | 21.8 | 8.6 |
| Herb and Pumpkin Seed, Nairn's* | 1 Cake/10g | 43.0 | 2.0 | 426 | 12.2 | 46.8 | 21.1 | 13.0 |
| Highland, Organic, Sainsbury's* | 1 Cake/13g | 57.0 | 2.0 | 456 | 10.2 | 59.8 | 19.5 | 5.5 |
| Highland, Walkers* | 1 Cake/12g | 54.0 | 2.0 | 451 | 10.3 | 56.0 | 20.6 | 6.7 |
| Oatmeal, Rough, Nairn's* | 1 Cake/11g | 45.0 | 2.0 | 421 | 10.6 | 52.8 | 18.6 | 10.5 |
| Oatmeal, Rough, Organic, Nairn's* | 1 Cake/10g | 43.0 | 2.0 | 418 | 10.2 | 57.7 | 16.3 | 7.5 |
| Retail, Average | 1 Cake/13g | 57.0 | 2.0 | 441 | 10.0 | 63.0 | 18.3 | 0.0 |
| Rough, Sainsbury's* | 1 Cake/11g | 45.0 | 2.0 | 426 | 11.7 | 65.2 | 16.9 | 8.6 |
| Rough, Scottish, Tesco* | 1 Cake/10g | 45.0 | 2.0 | 435 | 11.4 | 55.3 | 18.4 | 8.0 |
| Rough Scottish, Sainsbury's* | 1 Cake/11g | 51.0 | 2.0 | 462 | 12.3 | 59.9 | 19.3 | 6.5 |
| Scottish, Organic, Waitrose* | 1 Cake/13g | 58.0 | 3.0 | 447 | 11.2 | 57.0 | 19.4 | 6.6 |
| Scottish, Rough, Waitrose* | 1 Cake/13g | 55.0 | 2.0 | 438 | 10.4 | 57.4 | 18.5 | 8.0 |
| Traditional, M & S* | 1 Cake/11g | 49.0 | 2.0 | 445 | 11.0 | 59.3 | 18.3 | 6.6 |
| with Cracked Black Pepper, Walkers* | 1 Cake/10g | 41.0 | 2.0 | 433 | 10.4 | 55.0 | 19.0 | 8.5 |
| **OAT DRINK** | | | | | | | | |
| Healthy Oat, Enriched, Oatly* | 1 Serving/250ml | 112.0 | 4.0 | 45 | 1.0 | 6.5 | 1.5 | 0.8 |
| Healthy Oat, Organic, Oatly* | 1 Serving/250ml | 87.0 | 2.0 | 35 | 1.0 | 6.5 | 0.7 | 0.8 |
| **OATMEAL** | | | | | | | | |
| *Raw* | *1oz/28g* | *112.0* | *2.0* | *401* | *12.4* | *72.8* | *8.7* | *6.8* |
| **OCEAN** | | | | | | | | |
| Pinks, Asda* | 1oz/28g | 24.0 | 0.0 | 86 | 10.0 | 10.0 | 0.7 | 0.2 |
| Prawnies, Mini, Asda* | 1 Prawnie/11g | 9.0 | 0.0 | 84 | 11.0 | 8.0 | 0.9 | 0.5 |
| Snacks, Sainsbury's* | 1 Stick/16g | 18.0 | 0.0 | 113 | 7.0 | 21.0 | 0.1 | 0.1 |
| Sticks, Average | 1 Stick/16g | 17.0 | 0.0 | 109 | 7.1 | 19.8 | 0.1 | 0.1 |
| **OCTOPUS** | | | | | | | | |
| Chunks, in Olive Oil, Palacio De Oriente* | 1 Can/111g | 148.0 | 4.0 | 133 | 21.6 | 4.5 | 3.6 | 0.0 |
| *Raw* | *1oz/28g* | *23.0* | *0.0* | *83* | *17.9* | *0.0* | *1.3* | *0.0* |
| **OIL** | | | | | | | | |
| Again & Again, No Cholesterol, Anglia* | 1 Tbsp/15ml | 124.0 | 14.0 | 828 | 0.0 | 0.0 | 92.0 | 0.0 |
| Avocado, Olivado* | 1 Tsp/5ml | 40.0 | 4.0 | 802 | 0.0 | 0.0 | 88.0 | 0.0 |
| Black Truffle, Grapeseed, Cuisine Perel* | 1 Tsp/5ml | 43.0 | 5.0 | 857 | 0.0 | 7.1 | 100.0 | 0.0 |
| *Chilli, Average* | *1 Tsp/5ml* | *41.0* | *5.0* | *823* | *0.0* | *0.0* | *91.5* | *0.0* |
| Chinese Stir Fry, Asda* | 1 Tbsp/15ml | 123.0 | 14.0 | 823 | 0.0 | 0.0 | 91.4 | 0.0 |
| *Coconut, Average* | *1 Tsp/5ml* | *45.0* | *5.0* | *899* | *0.0* | *0.0* | *99.9* | *0.0* |
| *Cod Liver, Average* | *1 Capsule/1g* | *9.0* | *1.0* | *900* | *0.0* | *0.0* | *100.0* | *0.0* |
| *Corn, Average* | *1 Tsp/5ml* | *43.0* | *5.0* | *864* | *0.0* | *0.0* | *95.9* | *0.0* |
| Dipping, Herb, Italian Style, Finest, Tesco* | 1 Serving/5g | 44.0 | 5.0 | 877 | 0.4 | 0.9 | 96.9 | 0.4 |
| Dipping, with Balsamic Vinegar, Finest, Tesco* | 1 Tsp/5ml | 33.0 | 4.0 | 668 | 0.0 | 4.4 | 71.7 | 0.0 |
| *Evening Primrose, Average* | *1 Serving/1g* | *9.0* | *1.0* | *900* | *0.0* | *0.0* | *100.0* | *0.0* |
| *Fish, Average* | *1 Serving/1g* | *9.0* | *1.0* | *900* | *0.0* | *0.0* | *100.0* | *0.0* |
| *Flax Seed, Average* | *1 Tbsp/15ml* | *124.0* | *14.0* | *829* | *0.0* | *0.0* | *92.5* | *0.0* |
| Fry Light, Bodyline* | 1 Spray/0.25ml | 1.0 | 0.0 | 522 | 0.0 | 0.0 | 55.2 | 0.0 |
| *Grapeseed, Average* | *1 Tsp/5ml* | *43.0* | *5.0* | *865* | *0.0* | *0.0* | *96.1* | *0.0* |
| *Groundnut, Average* | *1 Serving/25ml* | *206.0* | *23.0* | *824* | *0.0* | *0.0* | *91.8* | *0.0* |
| *Hazelnut, Average* | *1 Tsp/5ml* | *45.0* | *5.0* | *899* | *0.0* | *0.0* | *99.9* | *0.0* |
| Linseed, Organic, Biona* | 1 Serving/10ml | 84.0 | 9.0 | 837 | 0.0 | 0.0 | 93.0 | 0.0 |
| Macadamia Nut, Oz Tukka* | 1 Tsp/5ml | 40.0 | 5.0 | 805 | 0.0 | 0.0 | 91.0 | 0.0 |

**O**

| | Measure INFO/WEIGHT | per Measure KCAL | FAT | Nutrition Values per 100g / 100ml KCAL | PROT | CARB | FAT | FIBRE |
|---|---|---|---|---|---|---|---|---|
| **OIL** | | | | | | | | |
| *Olive, Average* | *1 Tsp/5ml* | *43.0* | *5.0* | *855* | *0.0* | *0.0* | *94.9* | *0.0* |
| Olive, Basil Infused, Tesco* | 1 Serving/20ml | 180.0 | 20.0 | 900 | 0.0 | 0.0 | 100.0 | 0.0 |
| *Olive, Extra Virgin, Average* | *1 Tsp/5ml* | *42.0* | *5.0* | *848* | *0.0* | *0.0* | *94.5* | *0.0* |
| Olive, Extra Virgin, Only 1 Cal, Spray, Fry Light* | 1 Spray/0.2ml | 1.0 | 0.0 | 498 | 0.0 | 0.0 | 55.2 | 0.0 |
| *Olive, Garlic, Average* | *1 Tbsp/15ml* | *127.0* | *14.0* | *848* | *0.0* | *0.0* | *94.3* | *0.0* |
| Olive, Lemon Flavoured, Sainsbury's* | 1 Tbsp/15ml | 123.0 | 14.0 | 823 | 0.1 | 0.0 | 91.4 | 0.1 |
| *Olive, Mild, Average* | *1 Tbsp/15mll* | *129.0* | *14.0* | *861* | *0.0* | *0.0* | *95.7* | *0.0* |
| Omega, Organic, Clearspring* | 1 Tbsp/15ml | 124.0 | 14.0 | 828 | 0.0 | 0.0 | 92.0 | 0.0 |
| *Palm, Average* | *1 Tsp/5ml* | *45.0* | *5.0* | *899* | *0.0* | *0.0* | *99.9* | *0.0* |
| *Peanut, Average* | *1 Tsp/5ml* | *45.0* | *5.0* | *899* | *0.0* | *0.0* | *99.9* | *0.0* |
| *Rapeseed, Average* | *1 Tbsp/15ml* | *130.0* | *14.0* | *863* | *0.0* | *0.0* | *95.9* | *0.0* |
| Red Palm & Canola, Carotino* | 1 Tsp/5ml | 41.0 | 5.0 | 812 | 0.0 | 0.0 | 92.0 | 0.0 |
| *Safflower, Average* | *1 Tsp/5ml* | *45.0* | *5.0* | *899* | *0.0* | *0.0* | *99.9* | *0.0* |
| *Sesame, Average* | *1 Tsp/5ml* | *45.0* | *5.0* | *892* | *0.1* | *0.0* | *99.9* | *0.0* |
| *Soya, Average* | *1 Tsp/5ml* | *45.0* | *5.0* | *899* | *0.0* | *0.0* | *99.9* | *0.0* |
| *Sunflower, Average* | *1 Tsp/5ml* | *43.0* | *5.0* | *869* | *0.0* | *0.0* | *96.6* | *0.0* |
| Sunflower, Spray, Fry Light* | 1 Spray/0.2ml | 1.0 | 0.0 | 522 | 0.0 | 0.0 | 55.2 | 0.0 |
| *Vegetable, Average* | *1 Tbsp/15ml* | *129.0* | *14.0* | *858* | *0.0* | *0.0* | *95.3* | *0.0* |
| *Walnut, Average* | *1 Tsp/5ml* | *45.0* | *5.0* | *899* | *0.0* | *0.0* | *99.9* | *0.0* |
| *Wheatgerm, Average* | *1 Tsp/5ml* | *45.0* | *5.0* | *899* | *0.0* | *0.0* | *99.9* | *0.0* |
| **OKRA** | | | | | | | | |
| *Boiled in Unsalted Water, Average* | *1 Serving/80g* | *22.0* | *1.0* | *28* | *2.5* | *2.7* | *0.9* | *3.6* |
| *Canned, Drained, Average* | *1 Serving/80g* | *17.0* | *1.0* | *21* | *1.4* | *2.5* | *0.7* | *2.6* |
| *Raw, Average* | *1 Serving/80g* | *25.0* | *1.0* | *31* | *2.8* | *3.0* | *1.0* | *4.0* |
| *Stir-Fried in Corn Oil, Average* | *1 Serving/80g* | *215.0* | *21.0* | *269* | *4.3* | *4.4* | *26.1* | *6.3* |
| **OLIVES** | | | | | | | | |
| *Black, Pitted, Average* | *½ Jar/82g* | *135.0* | *13.0* | *164* | *1.0* | *3.5* | *16.2* | *3.1* |
| Black & Green, with Greek Feta Cheese, Tesco* | 1 Pot/100g | 200.0 | 20.0 | 200 | 3.4 | 0.3 | 20.1 | 4.6 |
| Green, Garlic Stuffed, Asda* | 1 Olive/3g | 6.0 | 1.0 | 174 | 1.8 | 3.5 | 17.0 | 0.0 |
| Green, Pimiento Stuffed, Somerfield* | 1 Olive/3g | 4.0 | 0.0 | 126 | 1.0 | 4.0 | 12.0 | 0.0 |
| *Green, Pitted, Average* | *1 Olive/3g* | *4.0* | *0.0* | *129* | *1.1* | *0.9* | *13.3* | *2.5* |
| Green, Pitted, Stuffed with Anchovies, Sainsbury's* | 1 Serving/50g | 77.0 | 8.0 | 155 | 1.8 | 0.6 | 16.1 | 3.2 |
| Green, Pitted & Stuffed with Minced Pimiento, Sainsbury's* | 1 Olive/5g | 8.0 | 1.0 | 147 | 1.2 | 3.9 | 14.1 | 2.0 |
| Green, Stuffed with Almonds, Pitted, Waitrose* | 1 Serving/50g | 90.0 | 8.0 | 180 | 3.8 | 3.2 | 16.9 | 2.5 |
| *Kalamata* | *1 Olive/3g* | *9.0* | *1.0* | *300* | *1.0* | *6.7* | *30.0* | *0.0* |
| Marinated, Selection, M & S* | 4 Olives/20g | 44.0 | 4.0 | 225 | 1.4 | 3.9 | 22.6 | 2.1 |
| Mixed, Chilli & Garlic, Asda* | 1 Serving/30g | 43.0 | 5.0 | 144 | 0.9 | 0.0 | 15.6 | 6.1 |
| Mixed, Marinated, Anti Pasti, Asda* | 1 Serving/100g | 215.0 | 22.0 | 215 | 1.8 | 0.7 | 22.0 | 3.1 |
| Mixed, Marinated, with Feta & Red Peppers, Asda* | 1 Pot/120g | 233.0 | 22.0 | 194 | 5.8 | 2.2 | 18.0 | 1.7 |
| Pimento Stuffed, in Brine, Tesco* | 1 Serving/25g | 38.0 | 4.0 | 153 | 0.8 | 0.1 | 16.4 | 2.1 |
| Pitted, with Anchovy Paste, Safeway* | 1/3 Can/50g | 69.0 | 7.0 | 139 | 2.7 | 0.1 | 14.2 | 2.0 |
| **OMELETTE** | | | | | | | | |
| Cheese, 2 Egg, Average | 1 Omelette/180g | 479.0 | 41.0 | 266 | 15.9 | 0.0 | 22.6 | 0.0 |
| Cheese, Asda* | 1 Omelette/119g | 268.0 | 23.0 | 225 | 12.0 | 1.5 | 19.0 | 0.0 |
| Cheese, Findus* | 1 Serving/200g | 400.0 | 26.0 | 200 | 9.5 | 14.0 | 13.0 | 0.0 |
| Ham & Mushroom, Farmfoods* | 1 Omelette/120g | 200.0 | 17.0 | 167 | 8.7 | 1.8 | 13.9 | 0.1 |
| Mushroom & Cheese, Tesco* | 1 Omelette/120g | 248.0 | 21.0 | 207 | 9.8 | 1.6 | 17.9 | 0.2 |
| Plain, 2 Egg | 1 Omelette/120g | 229.0 | 20.0 | 191 | 10.9 | 0.0 | 16.4 | 0.0 |
| Spanish | 1oz/28g | 34.0 | 2.0 | 120 | 5.7 | 6.2 | 8.3 | 1.4 |
| **ONION RINGS** | | | | | | | | |
| Battered, Asda* | 1 Serving/100g | 343.0 | 23.0 | 343 | 3.8 | 31.0 | 22.7 | 1.7 |
| Battered, Sainsbury's* | 1 Ring/12g | 26.0 | 1.0 | 219 | 3.9 | 28.4 | 10.0 | 3.5 |
| Breadcrumbs, Tesco* | 1 Serving/100g | 294.0 | 16.0 | 294 | 4.3 | 34.1 | 15.6 | 2.3 |

O

| | Measure INFO/WEIGHT | per Measure KCAL | FAT | Nutrition Values per 100g / 100ml KCAL | PROT | CARB | FAT | FIBRE |
|---|---|---|---|---|---|---|---|---|
| **ONION RINGS** | | | | | | | | |
| Breaded, Asda* | 1 Serving/10g | 29.0 | 1.0 | 289 | 4.4 | 34.0 | 15.0 | 2.7 |
| Breaded, Sainsbury's* | 1 Serving/100g | 280.0 | 12.0 | 280 | 4.6 | 37.6 | 12.4 | 4.1 |
| Oven Crisp Batter, Tesco* | 1 Ring/17g | 40.0 | 2.0 | 236 | 4.2 | 24.8 | 13.3 | 2.5 |
| **ONIONS** | | | | | | | | |
| *Baked* | *1oz/28g* | *29.0* | *0.0* | *103* | *3.5* | *22.3* | *0.6* | *3.9* |
| *Boiled in Unsalted Water* | *1oz/28g* | *5.0* | *0.0* | *17* | *0.6* | *3.7* | *0.1* | *0.7* |
| Borettane, Char-Grilled, Sacla* | 1 Serving/100g | 90.0 | 6.0 | 90 | 0.9 | 8.9 | 5.6 | 2.5 |
| *Dried, Raw, Average* | *1oz/28g* | *88.0* | *0.0* | *313* | *10.2* | *68.6* | *1.7* | *12.1* |
| *Fried, Average* | *1oz/28g* | *46.0* | *3.0* | *164* | *2.3* | *14.1* | *11.2* | *3.1* |
| *Pickled, Average* | *1 Onion/15g* | *3.0* | *0.0* | *23* | *0.8* | *4.9* | *0.1* | *0.7* |
| *Raw, Average* | *1 Med/180g* | *55.0* | *0.0* | *31* | *1.3* | *6.0* | *0.2* | *1.4* |
| *Red, Raw, Average* | *1 Med/180g* | *66.0* | *0.0* | *37* | *1.2* | *7.9* | *0.2* | *1.5* |
| *Spring Or Scallion, Raw, Average* | *1 Med/15g* | *5.0* | *0.0* | *33* | *1.8* | *7.3* | *0.2* | *2.6* |
| **OPTIONS** | | | | | | | | |
| Belgian Chocolate Drink, Ovaltine* | 1 Sachet/11g | 37.0 | 1.0 | 336 | 11.8 | 52.7 | 8.2 | 0.0 |
| Choca Mocha Drink, Ovaltine* | 1 Sachet/11g | 39.0 | 1.0 | 359 | 14.1 | 50.1 | 11.4 | 7.0 |
| Chocolate Au Lait, Ovaltine* | 1 Sachet/10g | 35.0 | 1.0 | 355 | 11.8 | 54.5 | 10.0 | 7.3 |
| Cracking Hazelnut, Ovaltine* | 1 Sachet/11g | 40.0 | 1.0 | 361 | 16.0 | 57.0 | 11.0 | 0.0 |
| Irish Cream, Ovaltine* | 1 Sachet/11g | 39.0 | 1.0 | 357 | 13.9 | 50.0 | 11.3 | 8.1 |
| Mint Madness, Ovaltine* | 1 Serving/11g | 40.0 | 1.0 | 365 | 15.0 | 50.6 | 11.4 | 0.0 |
| Outrageous Orange, Ovaltine* | 1 Serving/11g | 32.0 | 1.0 | 289 | 11.7 | 43.3 | 7.7 | 18.0 |
| Tempting Toffee, Ovaltine* | 1 Sachet/11g | 43.0 | 1.0 | 391 | 13.6 | 66.4 | 9.1 | 0.0 |
| Wicked White Chocolate, Ovaltine* | 1 Sachet/11g | 46.0 | 1.0 | 414 | 10.3 | 68.1 | 11.1 | 0.5 |
| **ORANGES** | | | | | | | | |
| *Blood, Average* | *1 Orange/140g* | *82.0* | *0.0* | *58* | *0.8* | *13.3* | *0.0* | *2.5* |
| Cherry, Graze* | 1 Pack /120g | 56.0 | 0.0 | 47 | 0.9 | 11.8 | 0.1 | 0.0 |
| *Fresh, Weighed with Peel, Average* | *1 Med/185g* | *115.0* | *0.0* | *62* | *1.0* | *15.6* | *0.3* | *3.2* |
| *Fresh, without Peel, Average* | *1 Med/145g* | *90.0* | *0.0* | *62* | *1.0* | *15.6* | *0.3* | *3.2* |
| *Peel Only, Raw, Average* | *1 Tbsp/6g* | *6.0* | *0.0* | *97* | *1.5* | *25.0* | *0.2* | *10.6* |
| Ruby Red, Tesco* | 1 Med/130g | 51.0 | 0.0 | 39 | 1.1 | 8.5 | 0.1 | 1.7 |
| **OREGANO** | | | | | | | | |
| *Dried,* | *1 Tsp/1g* | *3.0* | *0.0* | *306* | *11.0* | *49.5* | *10.3* | *0.0* |
| *Fresh* | *1oz/28g* | *18.0* | *1.0* | *66* | *2.2* | *9.7* | *2.0* | *0.0* |
| **OVALTINE*** | | | | | | | | |
| Hi Malt, Light, Instant Drink, Ovaltine* | 1 Sachet/20g | 72.0 | 1.0 | 358 | 9.1 | 67.1 | 5.9 | 2.8 |
| Powder, Made Up with Semi-Skimmed Milk, Ovaltine* | 1 Mug/227ml | 179.0 | 4.0 | 79 | 3.9 | 13.0 | 1.7 | 0.0 |
| Powder, Made Up with Whole Milk, Ovaltine* | 1 Mug/227ml | 220.0 | 9.0 | 97 | 3.8 | 12.9 | 3.8 | 0.0 |
| **OXTAIL** | | | | | | | | |
| *Raw* | *1oz/28g* | *48.0* | *3.0* | *171* | *20.0* | *0.0* | *10.1* | *0.0* |
| *Stewed* | *1oz/28g* | *68.0* | *4.0* | *243* | *30.5* | *0.0* | *13.4* | *0.0* |
| **OYSTERS** | | | | | | | | |
| in Vegetable Oil, Smoked, John West* | 1oz/28g | 64.0 | 4.0 | 230 | 16.0 | 10.0 | 14.0 | 0.0 |
| *Raw* | *1oz/28g* | *18.0* | *0.0* | *65* | *10.8* | *2.7* | *1.3* | *0.0* |

**O**

|  | Measure | per Measure | | Nutrition Values per 100g / 100ml | | | | |
|---|---|---|---|---|---|---|---|---|
|  | INFO/WEIGHT | KCAL | FAT | KCAL | PROT | CARB | FAT | FIBRE |
| **PAELLA** | | | | | | | | |
| Bistro, Waitrose* | 1 Serving/300g | 534.0 | 20.0 | 178 | 7.4 | 22.2 | 6.6 | 0.7 |
| Chicken, Chorizo & King Prawn, Finest, Tesco* | ½ Pack/400g | 520.0 | 20.0 | 130 | 7.0 | 14.2 | 4.9 | 1.2 |
| Chicken, HL, Tesco* | 1 Pack/400g | 432.0 | 2.0 | 108 | 6.7 | 19.2 | 0.5 | 1.7 |
| Chicken, King Prawns, British, Sainsbury's* | 1 Pack/400g | 380.0 | 5.0 | 95 | 7.6 | 13.3 | 1.2 | 0.9 |
| Chicken, Tesco* | 1 Serving/475g | 575.0 | 14.0 | 121 | 7.9 | 15.7 | 3.0 | 1.6 |
| Chicken & Chorizo, Asda* | 1 Pack/390g | 484.0 | 9.0 | 124 | 10.0 | 16.0 | 2.2 | 2.6 |
| Chicken & Chorizo, Big Dish, M & S* | 1 Pack/450g | 630.0 | 18.0 | 140 | 7.9 | 18.4 | 3.9 | 1.6 |
| Chicken & King Prawn, HL, Tesco* | 1 Pack/385g | 346.0 | 6.0 | 90 | 5.3 | 12.7 | 1.6 | 2.0 |
| Chicken & Prawn, Asda* | 1 Pack/400g | 352.0 | 4.0 | 88 | 5.8 | 13.7 | 1.1 | 1.4 |
| Chicken & Vegetable, HL, Tesco* | 1 Pack/450g | 441.0 | 6.0 | 98 | 9.7 | 11.8 | 1.3 | 1.1 |
| Enjoy, Birds Eye* | 1 Pack/500g | 620.0 | 16.0 | 124 | 7.7 | 16.2 | 3.2 | 0.6 |
| Seafood, Finest, Tesco* | 1 Pack/400g | 756.0 | 24.0 | 189 | 6.8 | 27.2 | 5.9 | 1.0 |
| Seafood, M & S* | 1 Pack/450g | 517.0 | 17.0 | 115 | 6.4 | 13.7 | 3.8 | 3.2 |
| Seafood, Sainsbury's* | 1 Pack/400g | 504.0 | 5.0 | 126 | 8.3 | 20.3 | 1.3 | 0.6 |
| Spanish, TTD, Sainsbury's* | ½ Pack/350g | 448.0 | 13.0 | 128 | 7.9 | 15.9 | 3.6 | 0.2 |
| Tesco* | 1 Serving/460g | 584.0 | 17.0 | 127 | 4.6 | 18.9 | 3.7 | 1.0 |
| Vegetable, Waitrose* | 1 Serving/174g | 202.0 | 3.0 | 116 | 2.2 | 22.7 | 1.8 | 1.5 |
| with Prawns, Chicken, Cod & Salmon, Sainsbury's* | 1 Pack/750g | 772.0 | 1.0 | 103 | 8.3 | 16.9 | 0.2 | 3.1 |
| **PAIN AU CHOCOLAT** | | | | | | | | |
| Asda* | 1 Serving/58g | 244.0 | 14.0 | 420 | 8.0 | 43.0 | 24.0 | 3.3 |
| M & S* | 1 Pastry/60g | 210.0 | 12.0 | 350 | 5.9 | 38.0 | 19.2 | 1.6 |
| Mini, Asda* | 1 Pastry/23g | 96.0 | 5.0 | 420 | 8.0 | 43.0 | 24.0 | 3.3 |
| Mini, Cafe Simple* | 1 Pastry/27g | 122.0 | 7.0 | 452 | 10.2 | 42.8 | 26.7 | 2.5 |
| Sainsbury's* | 1 Serving/58g | 241.0 | 14.0 | 415 | 7.9 | 42.5 | 23.7 | 3.3 |
| Small, Asda* | 1 Serving/23g | 106.0 | 6.0 | 462 | 8.0 | 49.0 | 26.0 | 0.0 |
| Waitrose* | 1 Pastry/53g | 230.0 | 13.0 | 435 | 8.8 | 45.5 | 23.9 | 3.7 |
| **PAIN AU RAISIN** | | | | | | | | |
| Twist, Extra Special, Asda* | 1 Pastry/110g | 421.0 | 21.0 | 383 | 7.0 | 46.0 | 19.0 | 2.5 |
| **PAK CHOI** | | | | | | | | |
| *Raw, Average* | *1 Leaf/14g* | *2.0* | *0.0* | *13* | *1.5* | *2.2* | *0.2* | *1.0* |
| **PAKORA** | | | | | | | | |
| Chicken, Tikka, Asda* | 1 Pack/350g | 696.0 | 38.0 | 199 | 16.0 | 9.0 | 11.0 | 1.1 |
| Potato & Spinach, Waitrose* | 1 Pakora/50g | 120.0 | 8.0 | 240 | 5.5 | 17.3 | 16.5 | 4.7 |
| Prawn, Indian Appetisers, Waitrose* | 1 Pakora/21g | 35.0 | 2.0 | 165 | 16.8 | 5.9 | 8.2 | 1.5 |
| Sainsbury's* | 1 Pakora/55g | 166.0 | 10.0 | 302 | 7.3 | 26.8 | 18.3 | 1.1 |
| Spinach, Sainsbury's* | 1 Pakora/18g | 35.0 | 2.0 | 195 | 5.1 | 19.4 | 10.8 | 3.8 |
| Vegetable, Indian Selection, Party, Co-Op* | 1 Pakora/23g | 47.0 | 2.0 | 205 | 6.0 | 28.0 | 7.0 | 4.0 |
| Vegetable, Indian Starter Selection, M & S* | 1 Pakora/23g | 61.0 | 4.0 | 265 | 6.3 | 19.6 | 18.1 | 2.9 |
| Vegetable, Mini, Indian Snack Collection, Tesco* | 1 Pakora/21g | 36.0 | 2.0 | 173 | 6.0 | 16.8 | 9.1 | 4.9 |
| Vegetable, Somerfield* | 1 Pakora/15g | 46.0 | 3.0 | 305 | 7.0 | 19.0 | 23.0 | 0.0 |
| **PANCAKE** | | | | | | | | |
| Apple, GFY, Asda* | 1 Pancake/74g | 100.0 | 2.0 | 135 | 4.2 | 24.0 | 2.5 | 1.0 |
| Apple & Sultana, M & S* | 1 Serving/80g | 160.0 | 6.0 | 200 | 2.2 | 30.2 | 7.9 | 1.2 |
| Asda* | 1 Pancake/23g | 59.0 | 2.0 | 254 | 4.8 | 43.0 | 7.0 | 4.0 |
| Bramley Apple, Sainsbury's* | 1 Pancake/85g | 114.0 | 2.0 | 134 | 4.2 | 23.6 | 2.5 | 1.0 |
| Cherry, GFY, Asda* | 1 Serving/206g | 206.0 | 4.0 | 100 | 1.9 | 18.9 | 1.8 | 1.8 |
| Chinatown, Asda* | 1 Pancake/10g | 33.0 | 1.0 | 335 | 10.9 | 51.7 | 9.2 | 2.4 |
| Chinese Roll, Farmfoods* | 1 Pancake/88g | 125.0 | 4.0 | 142 | 4.3 | 21.6 | 4.3 | 1.0 |
| Chinese Style, Cherry Valley* | 1 Pancake/8g | 25.0 | 0.0 | 310 | 9.2 | 54.7 | 6.0 | 0.0 |
| Chocolate, M & S* | 1 Pancake/80g | 125.0 | 5.0 | 156 | 3.1 | 22.1 | 6.1 | 0.2 |
| for Duck, Sainsbury's* | 1 Pancake/10g | 33.0 | 1.0 | 333 | 10.9 | 51.7 | 9.3 | 2.4 |
| HL, Tesco* | 1 Pancake/25g | 60.0 | 0.0 | 240 | 5.8 | 48.8 | 2.0 | 1.9 |
| Lemon, M & S* | 1 Pancake/38g | 90.0 | 3.0 | 235 | 4.5 | 38.5 | 7.2 | 2.8 |

| | Measure INFO/WEIGHT | per Measure KCAL | FAT | Nutrition Values per 100g / 100ml KCAL | PROT | CARB | FAT | FIBRE |
|---|---|---|---|---|---|---|---|---|
| **PANCAKE** | | | | | | | | |
| Light Choices, Tesco* | 1 Pancake/27g | 66.0 | 1.0 | 243 | 6.9 | 47.7 | 2.6 | 0.0 |
| Maple & Raisin, M & S* | 1 Pancake/33g | 88.0 | 2.0 | 269 | 6.5 | 49.7 | 5.4 | 2.2 |
| Mini, for, Kids, Tesco* | 1 Pancake/16g | 45.0 | 1.0 | 283 | 6.6 | 51.7 | 5.5 | 1.3 |
| Mini, Scotch, Tesco* | 1 Pancake/16g | 44.0 | 1.0 | 277 | 6.7 | 50.0 | 5.6 | 1.4 |
| Morrisons* | 1 Pancake/60g | 133.0 | 3.0 | 221 | 8.4 | 37.3 | 5.0 | 1.5 |
| Perfect, Kingsmill* | 1 Pancake/27g | 71.0 | 1.0 | 264 | 6.2 | 49.7 | 4.5 | 1.2 |
| Plain, Sainsbury's* | 1 Pancake/46g | 102.0 | 2.0 | 221 | 6.9 | 36.1 | 5.3 | 1.2 |
| Raisin & Lemon, Asda* | 1 Serving/30g | 92.0 | 2.0 | 304 | 6.0 | 52.0 | 8.0 | 1.4 |
| Raisin & Lemon, Sainsbury's* | 1 Pancake/35g | 95.0 | 2.0 | 272 | 6.3 | 51.8 | 4.4 | 2.2 |
| Savoury, Made with Skimmed Milk, Average | 1 6"/77g | 192.0 | 11.0 | 249 | 6.4 | 24.1 | 14.7 | 0.8 |
| Savoury, Made with Whole Milk, Average | 1 6"/77g | 210.0 | 13.0 | 273 | 6.3 | 24.0 | 17.5 | 0.8 |
| Scotch | 1 Pancake/50g | 146.0 | 6.0 | 292 | 5.8 | 43.6 | 11.7 | 1.4 |
| Scotch, BGTY, Sainsbury's* | 1 Pancake/30g | 76.0 | 1.0 | 252 | 5.3 | 48.5 | 4.1 | 1.3 |
| Scotch, Low Fat, Asda* | 1 Pancake/32g | 87.0 | 1.0 | 272 | 6.0 | 57.0 | 2.2 | 1.3 |
| Scotch, M & S* | 1 Pancake/34g | 95.0 | 1.0 | 280 | 6.5 | 54.5 | 4.0 | 1.6 |
| Sultana & Syrup, Asda* | 1 Pancake/34g | 89.0 | 2.0 | 263 | 5.9 | 43.7 | 7.2 | 1.5 |
| Sultana & Syrup Scotch, Sainsbury's* | 1 Pancake/35g | 113.0 | 3.0 | 322 | 6.7 | 55.2 | 8.3 | 1.7 |
| Sweet, Made with Skimmed Milk | 1oz/28g | 78.0 | 4.0 | 280 | 6.0 | 35.1 | 13.8 | 0.8 |
| Sweet, Made with Whole Milk | 1oz/28g | 84.0 | 5.0 | 301 | 5.9 | 35.0 | 16.2 | 0.8 |
| Sweet, Raspberry Ripple Sauce, Findus* | 1 Pancake/38g | 80.0 | 2.0 | 210 | 3.9 | 37.1 | 4.7 | 0.9 |
| Syrup, Tesco* | 1 Pancake/30g | 79.0 | 2.0 | 265 | 4.7 | 42.1 | 8.2 | 1.5 |
| Traditional, Aunt Bessie's* | 1 Pancake/60g | 90.0 | 2.0 | 150 | 6.1 | 24.6 | 3.1 | 1.1 |
| Traditional, Tesco* | 1 Pancake/62g | 137.0 | 3.0 | 221 | 8.4 | 35.6 | 5.0 | 1.5 |
| Warburton's* | 1 Pancake/35g | 84.0 | 2.0 | 239 | 7.6 | 37.7 | 6.4 | 2.4 |
| **PANCAKE MIX** | | | | | | | | |
| Fresh, M & S* | 1 Pancake/38g | 90.0 | 5.0 | 235 | 7.5 | 22.4 | 13.1 | 0.5 |
| Glutano* | 1 Tbs/15g | 57.0 | 0.0 | 378 | 8.9 | 75.6 | 2.2 | 0.0 |
| Traditional, Asda* | 1 Pack/256g | 545.0 | 23.0 | 213 | 6.0 | 27.0 | 9.0 | 1.8 |
| **PANCETTA** | | | | | | | | |
| *Average* | *½ Pack/65g* | *212.0* | *19.0* | *326* | *17.0* | *0.1* | *28.7* | *0.0* |
| Cubes, Tesco* | 1 Serving/38g | 135.0 | 12.0 | 355 | 17.5 | 0.5 | 32.2 | 0.0 |
| **PANINI** | | | | | | | | |
| Bacon, British Midland* | 1 Serving/150g | 273.0 | 10.0 | 182 | 9.1 | 21.6 | 6.6 | 0.0 |
| Cheese, Tesco* | 1 Panini/100g | 249.0 | 9.0 | 249 | 10.5 | 31.3 | 9.1 | 3.1 |
| Mozzarella & Tomato, M & S* | 1 Serving/176g | 484.0 | 29.0 | 275 | 11.3 | 21.3 | 16.2 | 2.1 |
| Tuna & Sweetcorn, Tesco* | 1 Serving/250g | 559.0 | 16.0 | 224 | 12.0 | 29.3 | 6.6 | 1.4 |
| **PANNA COTTA** | | | | | | | | |
| BGTY, Sainsbury's* | 1 Pot/150g | 150.0 | 3.0 | 100 | 2.4 | 18.2 | 1.9 | 1.4 |
| Caramel, Sainsbury's* | 1 Pot/120g | 335.0 | 16.0 | 279 | 2.5 | 34.6 | 13.1 | 3.3 |
| Sainsbury's* | 1 Pot/100g | 304.0 | 16.0 | 304 | 3.0 | 41.5 | 15.7 | 4.0 |
| Strawberry, COU, M & S* | 1 Pot/145g | 145.0 | 4.0 | 100 | 2.6 | 15.7 | 2.6 | 0.8 |
| **PAPAYA** | | | | | | | | |
| Dried, Pieces, Nature's Harvest* | 1 Serving/50g | 177.0 | 0.0 | 355 | 0.2 | 85.4 | 0.0 | 2.6 |
| Dried, Strips, Tropical Wholefoods* | 1 Strip/10g | 31.0 | 0.0 | 310 | 3.9 | 71.4 | 0.9 | 1.5 |
| Dried, Sweetened, Tesco* | 4 Pieces/25g | 59.0 | 0.0 | 235 | 0.4 | 56.3 | 0.9 | 2.9 |
| *Raw, Flesh Only, Average* | *1 Serving/140g* | *37.0* | *0.0* | *26* | *0.4* | *6.6* | *0.1* | *1.2* |
| *Raw, Weighed with Seeds & Skin* | *1 Cup, cubes / 140g* | *55.0* | *0.0* | *39* | *0.6* | *9.8* | *0.1* | *1.8* |
| *Unripe, Raw, Weighed with Seeds & Skin* | *1oz/28g* | *8.0* | *0.0* | *27* | *0.9* | *5.5* | *0.1* | *1.5* |
| **PAPPADS** | | | | | | | | |
| Green Chilli & Garlic, Sharwood's* | 1 Pappad/14g | 38.0 | 0.0 | 268 | 23.2 | 39.4 | 1.9 | 14.6 |
| **PAPPARDELLE** | | | | | | | | |
| Basil, Fresh, Sainsbury's* | 1 Serving/240g | 281.0 | 3.0 | 117 | 5.0 | 21.2 | 1.4 | 2.0 |
| Buitoni* | 1 Serving/65g | 242.0 | 3.0 | 373 | 15.0 | 67.5 | 4.8 | 0.0 |

**P**

| | Measure INFO/WEIGHT | per Measure KCAL | FAT | Nutrition Values per 100g / 100ml KCAL | PROT | CARB | FAT | FIBRE |
|---|---|---|---|---|---|---|---|---|
| **PAPPARDELLE** | | | | | | | | |
| Chilli, Fresh, Sainsbury's* | 1 Serving/250g | 302.0 | 4.0 | 121 | 5.7 | 20.7 | 1.7 | 2.0 |
| *Egg, Dry, Average* | *1 Serving/100g* | *364.0* | *4.0* | *364* | *14.1* | *68.5* | *3.7* | *2.1* |
| Egg, Fresh, Waitrose* | ¼ Pack/125g | 350.0 | 3.0 | 280 | 12.9 | 51.0 | 2.7 | 1.9 |
| Egg & Spinach, Extra Special, Asda* | ½ Pack/200g | 328.0 | 4.0 | 164 | 6.5 | 30.5 | 1.8 | 1.4 |
| Saffron, Eat Well, M & S* | 1 Serving/100g | 360.0 | 2.0 | 360 | 14.0 | 69.0 | 2.5 | 3.2 |
| The Best Fresh, Morrisons* | ¼ Pack/240g | 353.0 | 4.0 | 147 | 6.3 | 26.9 | 1.6 | 1.9 |
| with Salmon, COU, M & S* | 1 Pack/358g | 340.0 | 7.0 | 95 | 6.3 | 13.0 | 1.9 | 0.8 |
| **PAPRIKA** | | | | | | | | |
| *Average* | *1 Tsp/2g* | *6.0* | *0.0* | *289* | *14.8* | *34.9* | *13.0* | *0.0* |
| **PARATHA** | | | | | | | | |
| *Average* | *1 Paratha/80g* | *258.0* | *11.0* | *322* | *8.0* | *43.2* | *14.3* | *4.0* |
| Lachha, Waitrose* | 1 Paratha/75g | 322.0 | 18.0 | 429 | 7.8 | 46.0 | 23.8 | 1.8 |
| Roti, Plain, Crown Farms* | 1 Slice/80g | 250.0 | 10.0 | 312 | 5.0 | 46.2 | 12.5 | 1.2 |
| **PARCELS** | | | | | | | | |
| Basil & Parmesan, Fresh, Sainsbury's* | 1 Pack/250g | 550.0 | 21.0 | 220 | 10.0 | 26.4 | 8.3 | 3.3 |
| Beef Steak, Sainsbury's* | ½ Pack/226g | 488.0 | 35.0 | 216 | 12.2 | 6.6 | 15.6 | 1.0 |
| Cheese & Ham, Sainsbury's* | 1 Pack/250g | 445.0 | 19.0 | 178 | 7.4 | 19.9 | 7.6 | 1.5 |
| Chilli Beef, Tex Mex Feast, Asda* | 1 Parcel/25g | 67.0 | 3.0 | 270 | 9.0 | 27.0 | 14.0 | 2.1 |
| Filo, Brie & Cranberry, Tesco* | 1 Parcel/22g | 82.0 | 5.0 | 373 | 9.5 | 29.3 | 24.2 | 1.5 |
| Filo, Mushroom Leek & Gruyere, Finest, Tesco* | 1 Serving/160g | 440.0 | 34.0 | 275 | 6.9 | 20.5 | 21.0 | 1.5 |
| Pasta, Salmon with Mango Dressing, HL, Tesco* | 1 Pack/350g | 227.0 | 6.0 | 65 | 3.1 | 9.0 | 1.7 | 1.5 |
| Salmon, in Lemon Sauce, M & S* | 1 Serving/185g | 350.0 | 28.0 | 189 | 12.1 | 1.4 | 15.1 | 0.5 |
| Smoked Salmon, Sainsbury's* | 1 Pack/115g | 269.0 | 20.0 | 234 | 15.8 | 3.5 | 17.6 | 0.2 |
| Smoked Salmon, with Soft Cheese & Herb, Waitrose* | 1 Pack/100g | 246.0 | 20.0 | 246 | 14.6 | 1.2 | 20.2 | 0.0 |
| Turkey Breast, with Cheddar Cheese & Chive, Asda* | 1 Parcel/140g | 242.0 | 10.0 | 173 | 23.0 | 4.6 | 7.0 | 0.9 |
| **PARSLEY** | | | | | | | | |
| *Dried* | *1 Tsp/1g* | *2.0* | *0.0* | *181* | *15.8* | *14.5* | *7.0* | *26.9* |
| *Fresh, Average* | *1 Tbsp/4g* | *1.0* | *0.0* | *34* | *3.0* | *2.7* | *1.3* | *5.0* |
| **PARSNIP** | | | | | | | | |
| *Boiled, Average* | *1 Serving/80g* | *53.0* | *1.0* | *66* | *1.6* | *12.9* | *1.2* | *4.7* |
| Fragrant, Tesco* | 1 Serving/50g | 33.0 | 1.0 | 67 | 1.8 | 12.5 | 1.1 | 4.6 |
| Honey Glazed, Roasting, Cooked, Betty Smith's* | 1 Serving/100g | 144.0 | 7.0 | 144 | 2.6 | 23.4 | 7.2 | 6.3 |
| Honey Roasted, Tesco* | 1 Serving/125g | 202.0 | 10.0 | 162 | 1.9 | 20.0 | 8.2 | 2.2 |
| *Raw, Unprepared, Average* | *1oz/28g* | *19.0* | *0.0* | *66* | *1.8* | *12.5* | *1.1* | *4.6* |
| Roast, Honey Glazed, Baked, Aunt Bessie's* | 1 Serving/125g | 162.0 | 9.0 | 130 | 1.7 | 14.0 | 7.5 | 4.1 |
| **PARTRIDGE** | | | | | | | | |
| *Meat Only, Roasted* | *1oz/28g* | *59.0* | *2.0* | *212* | *36.7* | *0.0* | *7.2* | *0.0* |
| **PASANDA** | | | | | | | | |
| Chicken, M & S* | ½ Pack/150g | 240.0 | 16.0 | 160 | 11.3 | 3.8 | 10.9 | 1.3 |
| Chicken, Sainsbury's* | 1 Serving/200g | 368.0 | 25.0 | 184 | 14.7 | 3.4 | 12.4 | 2.3 |
| Chicken, with Pilau Rice, HL, Tesco* | 1 Pack/440g | 466.0 | 11.0 | 106 | 5.7 | 15.2 | 2.5 | 0.9 |
| **PASSATA** | | | | | | | | |
| Basil, Del Monte* | 1 Jar/500g | 160.0 | 1.0 | 32 | 1.4 | 5.9 | 0.2 | 0.0 |
| Napolina* | 1 Bottle/690g | 172.0 | 1.0 | 25 | 1.4 | 4.5 | 0.1 | 0.0 |
| SmartPrice, Asda* | 1 Serving/100g | 25.0 | 0.0 | 25 | 1.4 | 4.5 | 0.1 | 0.2 |
| So Organic, Sainsbury's* | ¼ Jar/175g | 38.0 | 1.0 | 22 | 0.9 | 3.8 | 0.4 | 0.9 |
| with Fresh Leaf Basil, Waitrose* | ¼ Jar/170g | 44.0 | 0.0 | 26 | 1.0 | 5.2 | 0.1 | 0.8 |
| with Garlic & Herbs, Roughly Chopped, Tesco* | 1 Serving/200g | 56.0 | 0.0 | 28 | 1.4 | 5.5 | 0.0 | 1.0 |
| with Garlic & Italian Herbs, Tesco* | 1 Serving/165g | 53.0 | 0.0 | 32 | 1.2 | 6.4 | 0.2 | 1.1 |
| **PASSION FRUIT** | | | | | | | | |
| *Raw, Fresh* | *1 Fruit/30g* | *18.0* | *0.0* | *60* | *0.7* | *14.4* | *0.2* | *0.2* |
| *Weighed with Skin* | *1oz/28g* | *6.0* | *0.0* | *22* | *1.7* | *3.5* | *0.2* | *2.0* |

| | Measure INFO/WEIGHT | per Measure KCAL | per Measure FAT | Nutrition Values per 100g / 100ml KCAL | PROT | CARB | FAT | FIBRE |
|---|---|---|---|---|---|---|---|---|
| **PASTA** | | | | | | | | |
| Bean & Tuna, BGTY, Sainsbury's* | 1 Serving/200g | 176.0 | 2.0 | 88 | 7.3 | 12.6 | 0.9 | 2.8 |
| Blue Cheese, Bacon & Spinach, M & S* | 1 Pack/400g | 640.0 | 34.0 | 160 | 6.5 | 13.8 | 8.5 | 0.7 |
| Cajun Chicken, GFY, Asda* | 1 Serving/297g | 312.0 | 8.0 | 105 | 8.0 | 12.0 | 2.8 | 2.1 |
| Carbonara, with Cheese & Bacon, Slim Fast* | 1 Serving/70g | 240.0 | 4.0 | 343 | 22.7 | 48.9 | 6.3 | 5.7 |
| Chargrilled Chicken, Asda* | 1 Serving/250g | 537.0 | 27.0 | 215 | 7.0 | 22.0 | 11.0 | 1.7 |
| Chargrilled Chicken & Bacon, Tesco* | 1 Pack/200g | 420.0 | 24.0 | 210 | 6.7 | 18.8 | 11.8 | 1.3 |
| Cheese, Tomato, & Pesto, Boots* | 1 Pack/250g | 355.0 | 11.0 | 142 | 5.9 | 20.0 | 4.4 | 2.0 |
| Cheese & Broccoli, Light Choices, Tesco* | 1 Pack/348g | 435.0 | 8.0 | 125 | 4.4 | 21.2 | 2.3 | 2.4 |
| Cheese & Broccoli, Tubes, Tesco* | 1 Serving/202g | 319.0 | 14.0 | 158 | 5.0 | 19.1 | 6.9 | 2.3 |
| Cheese & Ham, Shapers, Boots* | 1 Pack/76g | 220.0 | 5.0 | 289 | 23.7 | 34.2 | 6.4 | 6.4 |
| Chicken, Tomato & Basil, GFY, Asda* | 1 Pack/400g | 404.0 | 9.0 | 101 | 6.4 | 13.6 | 2.3 | 1.4 |
| Chicken, Tomato & Basil, HL, Tesco* | 1 Pack/400g | 264.0 | 2.0 | 66 | 7.9 | 7.5 | 0.5 | 1.1 |
| Chicken, Tomato & Herb, Easy Steam, Tesco* | 1 Serving/400g | 528.0 | 25.0 | 132 | 8.9 | 10.2 | 6.2 | 1.3 |
| Chicken, Tomato & Mascarpone, Easy Steam, Tesco* | 1 Pack/400g | 468.0 | 16.0 | 117 | 9.7 | 10.3 | 4.1 | 0.9 |
| Chicken, Tomato & Mascarpone, Heathly Living, Tesco* | 1 Pack/450g | 504.0 | 11.0 | 112 | 7.5 | 14.8 | 2.5 | 1.1 |
| Chicken & Asparagus, GFY, Asda* | 1 Pack/400g | 388.0 | 9.0 | 97 | 10.9 | 8.5 | 2.2 | 1.5 |
| Chicken & Green Pesto, HL, Tesco* | 1 Serving/376g | 440.0 | 5.0 | 117 | 8.3 | 18.5 | 1.2 | 1.4 |
| Chicken & Ham, Easy Steam, Tesco* | 1 Pack/400g | 572.0 | 26.0 | 143 | 9.8 | 11.2 | 6.6 | 0.6 |
| Chicken & Mushroom, Big Eat, Heinz* | 1 Pot/350g | 339.0 | 16.0 | 97 | 4.8 | 9.2 | 4.5 | 0.5 |
| Chicken & Mushroom, Pasta & Sauce, Dry, Tesco* | 1 Pack/120g | 427.0 | 4.0 | 356 | 16.0 | 65.0 | 3.6 | 3.9 |
| Chicken & Pineapple, Shapers, Boots* | 1 Pack/221g | 210.0 | 3.0 | 95 | 5.4 | 15.0 | 1.5 | 0.9 |
| Chicken & Roasted Tomato, HL, Tesco* | 1 Serving/374g | 426.0 | 7.0 | 114 | 7.4 | 16.7 | 1.9 | 1.3 |
| Chicken & Tomato, Classic, Mini, Tesco* | 1 Pack/300g | 165.0 | 7.0 | 55 | 6.6 | 1.7 | 2.4 | 1.7 |
| Chicken & Vegetable, Mediterranean, Waitrose* | 1 Serving/400g | 375.0 | 9.0 | 94 | 7.5 | 10.5 | 2.3 | 2.2 |
| Creamy Cheese, Big Eat, Heinz* | 1 Pot/350g | 437.0 | 32.0 | 125 | 3.7 | 7.0 | 9.2 | 1.8 |
| Creamy Mushroom, Light Choices, Tesco* | 1 Pack/350g | 455.0 | 5.0 | 130 | 4.3 | 25.0 | 1.4 | 1.3 |
| Creamy Mushroom, Sainsbury's* | 1 Serving/63g | 148.0 | 9.0 | 237 | 4.5 | 21.7 | 14.6 | 1.2 |
| Creamy Vegetable, Meal in 5, Ainsley Harriott* | 1 Pot/387g | 414.0 | 10.0 | 107 | 2.8 | 18.1 | 2.6 | 0.8 |
| Feta & Black Olive Girasole, Extra Special, Asda* | ½ Pack/150g | 360.0 | 15.0 | 240 | 8.3 | 28.4 | 10.3 | 0.0 |
| Fiorelli, Egg, M & S* | 1 Serving/100g | 355.0 | 3.0 | 355 | 13.9 | 68.5 | 2.8 | 3.0 |
| Fiorelli, Mozzarella, Tomato & Basil, Waitrose* | 1 Serving/125g | 352.0 | 12.0 | 282 | 10.8 | 38.9 | 9.3 | 1.7 |
| Garlic Mushroom Filled, Extra Special, Asda* | 1 Serving/125g | 224.0 | 9.0 | 179 | 8.0 | 21.0 | 7.0 | 2.5 |
| Girasole, Filled with Red Pepper & Goats Cheese, Asda* | ½ Pack/150g | 261.0 | 10.0 | 174 | 7.2 | 21.4 | 6.6 | 1.8 |
| Honey & Mustard Chicken, Light Choices, Tesco* | 1 Pack/375g | 881.0 | 48.0 | 235 | 6.7 | 22.0 | 12.9 | 1.2 |
| Hot Smoked Salmon, Tesco* | 1 Pack/275g | 426.0 | 17.0 | 155 | 7.1 | 16.6 | 6.2 | 4.1 |
| King Prawn & Pesto, Asda* | 1 Pack/400g | 488.0 | 18.0 | 122 | 7.6 | 12.9 | 4.4 | 1.2 |
| Lumache, Tesco* | 1 Serving/100g | 345.0 | 2.0 | 345 | 13.2 | 68.5 | 2.0 | 2.9 |
| Meat Feast, Italian, Sainsbury's* | 1 Pack/450g | 508.0 | 18.0 | 113 | 7.4 | 11.8 | 4.0 | 0.6 |
| Medaglioni, Bolognese, Rich Red Wine, Waitrose* | ½ Pack/125g | 266.0 | 7.0 | 213 | 12.5 | 28.1 | 5.6 | 2.6 |
| Mediterranean Vegetable, Weight Watchers* | 1 Pack/400g | 262.0 | 3.0 | 65 | 2.6 | 12.0 | 0.8 | 1.6 |
| Mini Spirals, in Cheese Sauce, Heinz* | 1 Can/154g | 120.0 | 4.0 | 78 | 3.9 | 10.4 | 2.3 | 0.3 |
| Organic, Gluten Free, Doves Farm Organic* | 1 Serving/100g | 338.0 | 1.0 | 338 | 7.9 | 70.3 | 1.5 | 4.1 |
| Orzo, with British Chicken, Tomato & Basil, Eat Well, M & S* | 1 Pack/300g | 390.0 | 11.0 | 130 | 7.9 | 16.5 | 3.7 | 1.9 |
| Penne, Creamy Mushroom, Prepared, Tesco* | ½ Pack/200g | 288.0 | 13.0 | 144 | 4.5 | 17.4 | 6.4 | 3.3 |
| Penne, Mediterranean, HL, Tesco* | 1 Pack/400g | 296.0 | 11.0 | 74 | 2.9 | 9.6 | 2.7 | 1.5 |
| Pepper & Tomato, Asda* | 1 Serving/250g | 340.0 | 17.0 | 136 | 3.2 | 15.0 | 7.0 | 2.4 |
| Pomodoro, with Tomato & Herbs, Slim Fast* | 1 Serving/71g | 235.0 | 3.0 | 331 | 21.5 | 51.5 | 4.3 | 6.0 |
| Quadrotti, Asparagus, TTD, Sainsbury's* | 1 Pack/250g | 315.0 | 8.0 | 126 | 7.0 | 17.4 | 3.1 | 2.7 |
| Quadrotti, Pumpkin, TTD, Sainsbury's* | ½ Pack/125g | 167.0 | 4.0 | 134 | 6.1 | 20.7 | 3.0 | 2.8 |
| Raviolini, Gorgonzola & Walnut, M & S* | ½ Pack/125g | 381.0 | 16.0 | 305 | 12.6 | 33.6 | 13.2 | 2.0 |
| Riccioli, Dry Weight, Buitoni* | 1 Serving/75g | 264.0 | 1.0 | 352 | 11.2 | 72.6 | 1.9 | 0.0 |
| Sausage & Tomato, Italiano, Tesco* | 1 Serving/450g | 679.0 | 27.0 | 151 | 5.7 | 18.8 | 5.9 | 1.6 |
| Spicy Tomato, Meal in 5, Ainsley Harriott* | 1 Pot/387g | 369.0 | 2.0 | 95 | 2.6 | 19.9 | 0.5 | 1.5 |

| | Measure INFO/WEIGHT | per Measure KCAL | per Measure FAT | Nutrition Values per 100g / 100ml KCAL | PROT | CARB | FAT | FIBRE |
|---|---|---|---|---|---|---|---|---|
| **PASTA** | | | | | | | | |
| Spinach & Pine Nut, Finest, Tesco* | 1 Pack/195g | 546.0 | 35.0 | 280 | 6.4 | 23.1 | 17.9 | 1.5 |
| Stuffed Mushroom & Emmental, Sainsbury's* | 1 Pack/250g | 650.0 | 23.0 | 260 | 11.3 | 33.5 | 9.2 | 3.7 |
| Sundried Tomato, Sainsbury's* | 1 Serving/50g | 196.0 | 18.0 | 393 | 4.5 | 13.4 | 35.7 | 6.2 |
| Tomato & Bacon, Value, Tesco* | 1 Pack/300g | 300.0 | 4.0 | 100 | 4.0 | 17.8 | 1.4 | 1.1 |
| Tomato & Basil Chicken, Boots* | 1 Serving/320g | 621.0 | 29.0 | 194 | 9.0 | 19.0 | 9.0 | 1.4 |
| Tomato & Chicken Spiralli, HL, Tesco* | 1 Pack/350g | 402.0 | 5.0 | 115 | 7.8 | 17.3 | 1.5 | 1.6 |
| Tomato & Mascarpone, GFY, Asda* | ½ Can/200g | 128.0 | 4.0 | 64 | 2.1 | 9.0 | 2.2 | 0.0 |
| Tomato & Onion, Shells, Tesco* | 1 Serving/193g | 643.0 | 3.0 | 333 | 12.5 | 67.1 | 1.6 | 6.3 |
| Tomato & Pepper, GFY, Asda* | 1 Pack/400g | 344.0 | 8.0 | 86 | 3.1 | 14.0 | 1.9 | 1.1 |
| Twists, Quick Cook, Morrisons* | 1 Serving/75g | 265.0 | 1.0 | 353 | 12.0 | 72.0 | 2.0 | 3.1 |
| Twists, with Tuna, Italian, Weight Watchers* | 1 Can/385g | 239.0 | 5.0 | 62 | 4.3 | 8.2 | 1.4 | 0.6 |
| Vegetable, Creamy, BGTY, Sainsbury's* | 1 Pack/400g | 348.0 | 6.0 | 87 | 4.0 | 14.3 | 1.5 | 1.9 |
| Vegetable, Mediterranean, Sainsbury's* | 1 Pack/400g | 504.0 | 12.0 | 126 | 4.0 | 20.9 | 2.9 | 1.8 |
| Whole Wheat, Penne, Asda* | 1 Serving/100g | 333.0 | 2.0 | 333 | 12.1 | 66.3 | 2.1 | 6.9 |
| Wholewheat, Cooked, Tesco* | 1 Serving/200g | 284.0 | 2.0 | 142 | 5.7 | 27.9 | 0.9 | 4.5 |
| **PASTA BAKE** | | | | | | | | |
| Aberdeen Angus Meatball, Waitrose* | ½ Pack/350g | 501.0 | 28.0 | 143 | 5.2 | 12.5 | 8.0 | 0.9 |
| Bacon & Leek, Sainsbury's* | 1 Pack/400g | 660.0 | 28.0 | 165 | 7.3 | 18.5 | 6.9 | 1.8 |
| Bacon & Leek, Tesco* | 1 Pack/450g | 774.0 | 37.0 | 172 | 8.1 | 16.1 | 8.3 | 2.0 |
| Bolgnese, GFY, Asda* | 1 Pack/400g | 376.0 | 8.0 | 94 | 5.8 | 13.1 | 2.1 | 0.9 |
| Bolognese, Finest, Tesco* | 1 Serving/250g | 375.0 | 16.0 | 150 | 7.3 | 16.1 | 6.3 | 1.1 |
| Bolognese, Weight Watchers* | 1 Pack/400g | 324.0 | 8.0 | 81 | 6.1 | 9.6 | 2.0 | 1.3 |
| Cheese & Bacon, Asda* | 1 Serving/120g | 168.0 | 14.0 | 140 | 2.9 | 5.2 | 12.0 | 0.3 |
| Cheese & Bacon, Fresh Italian, Asda* | 1 Serving/250g | 265.0 | 20.0 | 106 | 6.0 | 2.6 | 8.0 | 0.5 |
| Cheese & Tomato, Italiano, Tesco* | 1 Bake/300g | 354.0 | 13.0 | 118 | 3.9 | 16.1 | 4.2 | 1.0 |
| Cheese & Tomato, Tesco* | 1 Pack/400g | 388.0 | 6.0 | 97 | 3.4 | 17.8 | 1.4 | 1.2 |
| Chicken, Light Choices, Tesco* | 1 Pack/400g | 340.0 | 3.0 | 85 | 6.1 | 13.1 | 0.8 | 1.4 |
| Chicken, Morrisons* | 1 Pack/402g | 442.0 | 14.0 | 110 | 4.6 | 14.8 | 3.6 | 0.9 |
| Chicken, Mozzarella & Tomato, Birds Eye* | 1 Pack/360g | 468.0 | 7.0 | 130 | 7.1 | 14.3 | 1.9 | 0.3 |
| Chicken & Bacon, Asda* | ¼ Pack/374g | 610.0 | 26.0 | 163 | 9.0 | 16.0 | 7.0 | 4.1 |
| Chicken & Bacon, Asda* | 1 Pack/400g | 592.0 | 25.0 | 148 | 8.6 | 14.2 | 6.3 | 3.0 |
| Chicken & Broccoli, Morrisons* | 1 Pack/400g | 452.0 | 16.0 | 113 | 6.1 | 13.3 | 4.0 | 0.6 |
| Chicken & Broccoli, Weight Watchers* | 1 Bake/305g | 290.0 | 5.0 | 95 | 6.0 | 14.2 | 1.5 | 0.9 |
| Chicken & Courgette, Asda* | ½ Pack/387g | 519.0 | 23.0 | 134 | 6.0 | 14.0 | 6.0 | 0.6 |
| Chicken & Leek, HL, Tesco* | 1 Pack/400g | 460.0 | 8.0 | 115 | 10.8 | 13.1 | 1.9 | 1.6 |
| Chicken & Mushroom, Waitrose* | 1 Pack/400g | 532.0 | 31.0 | 133 | 6.7 | 9.1 | 7.7 | 0.8 |
| Chicken & Roast Mushroom, HL, Tesco* | 1 Pack/390g | 413.0 | 0.0 | 106 | 8.6 | 17.6 | 0.1 | 1.3 |
| Chicken & Spinach, GFY, Asda* | 1 Pack/400g | 374.0 | 6.0 | 93 | 5.0 | 15.0 | 1.5 | 1.2 |
| Chicken & Spinach, Sainsbury's* | 1 Pack/340g | 286.0 | 9.0 | 84 | 4.9 | 10.0 | 2.7 | 0.6 |
| Chilli & Cheese, American Style, Tesco* | 1 Pack/425g | 637.0 | 17.0 | 150 | 6.8 | 21.8 | 3.9 | 1.5 |
| Chilli Beef, Asda* | 1 Pack/1500g | 2010.0 | 90.0 | 134 | 7.0 | 13.0 | 6.0 | 1.2 |
| Creamy Tomato, Dolmio* | 1 Serving/125g | 141.0 | 9.0 | 113 | 2.3 | 8.4 | 7.2 | 0.0 |
| Findus* | 1 Pack/320g | 448.0 | 22.0 | 140 | 7.5 | 12.0 | 7.0 | 0.0 |
| Ham & Broccoli, Asda* | 1 Pack/340g | 309.0 | 14.0 | 91 | 3.4 | 10.0 | 4.1 | 0.5 |
| Italian Creamy Tomato & Bacon, Asda* | 1 Serving/125g | 131.0 | 11.0 | 105 | 2.0 | 3.9 | 9.0 | 0.6 |
| King Prawn & Salmon, GFY, Asda* | 1 Pack/400g | 420.0 | 12.0 | 105 | 6.9 | 12.7 | 2.9 | 1.2 |
| Leek & Bacon, Morrisons* | 1 Pack/401g | 553.0 | 36.0 | 138 | 4.8 | 9.9 | 9.0 | 0.2 |
| Meatball, Tesco* | 1 Pack/400g | 576.0 | 19.0 | 144 | 5.9 | 19.3 | 4.8 | 0.5 |
| Meatfeast, Italian, Tesco* | 1 Serving/500g | 675.0 | 19.0 | 135 | 6.4 | 17.8 | 3.8 | 2.3 |
| Mediterranean, Weight Watchers* | 1 Pack/397g | 262.0 | 3.0 | 66 | 2.6 | 12.0 | 0.8 | 1.6 |
| Mediterranean Style, Tesco* | 1 Pack/450g | 423.0 | 2.0 | 94 | 2.9 | 19.6 | 0.4 | 2.0 |
| Mix, Tuna, Colman's* | 1 Sachet/45g | 145.0 | 2.0 | 323 | 9.2 | 60.0 | 5.2 | 4.7 |
| Mushroom, Creamy, Asda* | ¼ Jar/118g | 204.0 | 20.0 | 173 | 1.8 | 3.3 | 17.0 | 0.5 |

| | Measure INFO/WEIGHT | per Measure KCAL | per Measure FAT | Nutrition Values per 100g / 100ml KCAL | PROT | CARB | FAT | FIBRE |
|---|---|---|---|---|---|---|---|---|
| **PASTA BAKE** | | | | | | | | |
| Penne Mozzarella, Tesco* | 1 Pack/340g | 408.0 | 8.0 | 120 | 4.7 | 19.7 | 2.5 | 0.6 |
| Penne Pasta, with Tomato & Mozzarella, Sainsbury's* | 1 Pack/400g | 536.0 | 19.0 | 134 | 5.4 | 17.6 | 4.7 | 2.8 |
| Pepperoni & Ham, Tesco* | ½ Pack/425g | 501.0 | 3.0 | 118 | 8.9 | 19.3 | 0.6 | 2.5 |
| Spicy Tomato & Pepperoni, Asda* | 1 Pack/440g | 431.0 | 26.0 | 98 | 1.1 | 10.0 | 6.0 | 1.2 |
| Three Bean, Asda* | ¼ Jar/125g | 187.0 | 15.0 | 150 | 2.4 | 8.0 | 12.0 | 1.3 |
| Tomato & Herb, Asda* | 1 Jar/436g | 715.0 | 57.0 | 164 | 1.8 | 10.0 | 13.0 | 1.2 |
| Tomato & Mozzarella, Light Choices, Tesco* | 1 Pack/400g | 368.0 | 8.0 | 92 | 3.7 | 14.8 | 2.0 | 1.5 |
| Tomato & Red Pepper, with Crunch Topping, Homepride* | 1 Jar/535g | 417.0 | 9.0 | 78 | 1.8 | 14.1 | 1.6 | 0.9 |
| Tuna, Co-Op* | 1 Serving/340g | 306.0 | 7.0 | 90 | 7.0 | 12.0 | 2.0 | 1.0 |
| Tuna, COU, M & S* | 1 Pack/360g | 432.0 | 15.0 | 120 | 8.0 | 11.9 | 4.3 | 0.8 |
| Tuna, Lean Cuisine* | 1 Pack/346g | 380.0 | 9.0 | 110 | 5.0 | 16.0 | 2.5 | 1.5 |
| Tuna, Light Choices, Tesco* | 1 Pack/400g | 380.0 | 5.0 | 95 | 10.8 | 10.0 | 1.3 | 2.2 |
| Tuna, Weight Watchers* | 1 Pack/400g | 292.0 | 3.0 | 73 | 7.0 | 9.4 | 0.8 | 1.4 |
| Tuna & Sweetcorn, Asda* | 1 Serving/250g | 332.0 | 22.0 | 133 | 5.0 | 8.0 | 9.0 | 0.9 |
| Tuna & Tomato, BGTY, Sainsbury's* | 1 Pack/450g | 553.0 | 19.0 | 123 | 8.7 | 12.6 | 4.2 | 0.4 |
| Tuna Conchiglie, M & S* | 1 Pack/400g | 360.0 | 13.0 | 90 | 8.4 | 6.7 | 3.3 | 1.0 |
| Vegetable, Asda* | 1 Serving/300g | 231.0 | 10.0 | 77 | 2.4 | 9.0 | 3.5 | 0.8 |
| Vegetable, Findus* | 1 Pack/331g | 430.0 | 22.0 | 130 | 6.0 | 13.0 | 6.5 | 0.0 |
| Vegetable, M & S* | 1 Pack/350g | 455.0 | 20.0 | 130 | 4.8 | 14.6 | 5.7 | 1.6 |
| Vegetable, Mediterranean, HL, Tesco* | 1 Serving/450g | 373.0 | 4.0 | 83 | 2.9 | 16.0 | 0.8 | 1.5 |
| Vegetable, Mediterranean, Tesco* | 1 Serving/450g | 495.0 | 21.0 | 110 | 4.3 | 12.9 | 4.6 | 1.3 |
| **PASTA IN** | | | | | | | | |
| a Rich Tomato & Mushroom Sauce, Spirals, Tesco* | 1 Serving/217g | 326.0 | 14.0 | 150 | 4.6 | 18.8 | 6.3 | 2.5 |
| **PASTA 'N' SAUCE** | | | | | | | | |
| Bolognese Flavour, Dry, Batchelors* | ½ Pack/65g | 228.0 | 2.0 | 353 | 15.1 | 67.2 | 2.6 | 3.9 |
| Bolognese Flavour, Dry, Batchelors* | ½ Pack/65g | 228.0 | 2.0 | 353 | 15.1 | 67.2 | 2.6 | 3.9 |
| Carbonara Flavour, Dry, Batchelors* | 1 Pack/120g | 463.0 | 6.0 | 386 | 14.3 | 71.0 | 5.0 | 3.1 |
| Carbonara Flavour, Dry, Batchelors* | 1 Pack/120g | 463.0 | 6.0 | 386 | 14.3 | 71.0 | 5.0 | 3.1 |
| Cheese, Leek & Ham, Batchelors* | 1 Pack/120g | 454.0 | 6.0 | 378 | 16.1 | 67.0 | 5.1 | 2.0 |
| Cheese, Leek & Ham, Batchelors* | 1 Pack/120g | 454.0 | 6.0 | 378 | 16.1 | 67.0 | 5.1 | 2.0 |
| Cheese & Broccoli Sauce Mix, Made Up, Sainsbury's* | 1 Pack/120g | 164.0 | 7.0 | 137 | 4.2 | 17.2 | 5.7 | 1.1 |
| Cheese & Broccoli Sauce Mix, Made Up, Sainsbury's* | 1 Pack/120g | 164.0 | 7.0 | 137 | 4.2 | 17.2 | 5.7 | 1.1 |
| Chicken & Mushroom, Batchelors* | ½ Pack/63g | 227.0 | 1.0 | 361 | 14.1 | 72.3 | 1.7 | 2.8 |
| Chicken & Mushroom, Batchelors* | ½ Pack/63g | 227.0 | 1.0 | 361 | 14.1 | 72.3 | 1.7 | 2.8 |
| Chicken & Mushroom, Made Up, Morrisons* | 1 Pack/110g | 166.0 | 6.0 | 151 | 5.0 | 20.3 | 5.6 | 2.1 |
| Chicken & Mushroom, Made Up, Morrisons* | 1 Pack/110g | 166.0 | 6.0 | 151 | 5.0 | 20.3 | 5.6 | 2.1 |
| Chicken & Mushroom, Made Up, SmartPrice, Asda* | 1 Pack/110g | 183.0 | 7.0 | 166 | 5.0 | 23.0 | 6.0 | 2.2 |
| Chicken & Roasted Garlic Flavour, Dry, Batchelors* | ½ Pack/60g | 223.0 | 2.0 | 372 | 12.6 | 73.8 | 2.9 | 3.4 |
| Chicken & Roasted Garlic Flavour, Dry, Batchelors* | ½ Pack/60g | 223.0 | 2.0 | 372 | 12.6 | 73.8 | 2.9 | 3.4 |
| Creamy Tomato & Mushroom, Dry, Batchelors* | 1 Pack/125g | 457.0 | 4.0 | 366 | 13.0 | 71.0 | 3.3 | 3.2 |
| Creamy Tomato & Mushroom, Dry, Batchelors* | 1 Pack/125g | 457.0 | 4.0 | 366 | 13.0 | 71.0 | 3.3 | 3.2 |
| Macaroni Cheese, Dry, Batchelors* | 1 Pack/108g | 402.0 | 5.0 | 372 | 17.2 | 65.2 | 4.7 | 2.7 |
| Macaroni Cheese, Dry, Batchelors* | 1 Pack/108g | 402.0 | 5.0 | 372 | 17.2 | 65.2 | 4.7 | 2.7 |
| Mild Cheese & Broccoli, Batchelors* | ½ Pack/61g | 221.0 | 2.0 | 363 | 15.0 | 67.0 | 3.9 | 4.0 |
| Mild Cheese & Broccoli, Batchelors* | ½ Pack/61g | 221.0 | 2.0 | 363 | 15.0 | 67.0 | 3.9 | 4.0 |
| Mushroom & Wine, Batchelors* | ½ Pack/50g | 242.0 | 3.0 | 483 | 18.5 | 89.9 | 5.5 | 4.4 |
| Mushroom & Wine, Batchelors* | ½ Pack/50g | 242.0 | 3.0 | 483 | 18.5 | 89.9 | 5.5 | 4.4 |
| Mushroom & Wine, Dry, Batchelors* | 1 Pack/132g | 498.0 | 6.0 | 377 | 12.0 | 71.3 | 4.9 | 2.5 |
| Mushroom & Wine, Dry, Batchelors* | 1 Pack/132g | 498.0 | 6.0 | 377 | 12.0 | 71.3 | 4.9 | 2.5 |
| Tomato, Onion & Herb, Made Up, Morrisons* | 1 Serving/110g | 141.0 | 5.0 | 128 | 3.2 | 18.7 | 4.5 | 2.3 |
| Tomato, Onion & Herb, Made Up, Morrisons* | 1 Serving/110g | 141.0 | 5.0 | 128 | 3.2 | 18.7 | 4.5 | 2.3 |
| Tomato, Onion & Herbs, Dry, Batchelors* | 1 Pack/135g | 470.0 | 3.0 | 348 | 13.8 | 68.8 | 2.0 | 4.0 |
| Tomato, Onion & Herbs, Dry, Batchelors* | 1 Pack/135g | 470.0 | 3.0 | 348 | 13.8 | 68.8 | 2.0 | 4.0 |

P

| | Measure INFO/WEIGHT | per Measure | | Nutrition Values per 100g / 100ml | | | | |
|---|---|---|---|---|---|---|---|---|
| | | KCAL | FAT | KCAL | PROT | CARB | FAT | FIBRE |
| **PASTA 'N' SAUCE** | | | | | | | | |
| Tomato & Bacon Flavour, Dry, Batchelors* | 1 Pack/134g | 476.0 | 3.0 | 355 | 13.0 | 70.0 | 2.6 | 3.0 |
| Tomato & Bacon Flavour, Dry, Batchelors* | 1 Pack/134g | 476.0 | 3.0 | 355 | 13.0 | 70.0 | 2.6 | 3.0 |
| Tomato & Mascarpone, BGTY, Sainsbury's* | 1 Pack/380g | 555.0 | 7.0 | 146 | 6.6 | 25.6 | 1.9 | 1.3 |
| Tomato & Mascarpone, BGTY, Sainsbury's* | 1 Pack/380g | 555.0 | 7.0 | 146 | 6.6 | 25.6 | 1.9 | 1.3 |
| **PASTA QUILLS** | | | | | | | | |
| *Dry, Average* | *1 Serving/75g* | *256.0* | *1.0* | *342* | *12.0* | *72.3* | *1.2* | *2.0* |
| Gluten Free, Salute* | 1 Serving/75g | 269.0 | 1.0 | 359 | 7.5 | 78.0 | 1.9 | 0.0 |
| **PASTA SALAD** | | | | | | | | |
| Caesar, Chicken, Shapers, Boots* | 1 Pack/218g | 288.0 | 8.0 | 132 | 6.7 | 18.0 | 3.8 | 1.8 |
| Caesar & Santa Tomatoes, M & S* | 1 Serving/220g | 495.0 | 34.0 | 225 | 5.2 | 15.9 | 15.3 | 0.8 |
| Chargrilled Chicken, Italian Style, Fresh, Asda* | 1 Pack/200g | 318.0 | 14.0 | 159 | 7.0 | 17.0 | 7.0 | 0.4 |
| Chargrilled Chicken, M & S* | 1 Serving/190g | 285.0 | 6.0 | 150 | 9.6 | 23.6 | 2.9 | 1.6 |
| Chargrilled Chicken & Pesto Pasta, Sainsbury's* | 1 Pack/240g | 454.0 | 22.0 | 189 | 7.2 | 19.4 | 9.2 | 0.0 |
| Chargrilled Chicken & Red Pepper, Tesco* | 1 Pack/270g | 553.0 | 24.0 | 205 | 9.8 | 20.3 | 8.9 | 3.1 |
| Chargrilled Red Pepper & Sunblush Tomato, Finest, Tesco* | 1 Serving/100g | 165.0 | 4.0 | 165 | 4.9 | 26.0 | 4.3 | 3.3 |
| Chargrilled Vegetables & Tomato, Shapers, Boots* | 1 Pack/175g | 187.0 | 5.0 | 107 | 2.8 | 17.0 | 3.1 | 1.5 |
| Cheddar Cheese, Tesco* | 1 Pot/215g | 546.0 | 44.0 | 254 | 5.7 | 12.0 | 20.4 | 0.8 |
| Cheese, Asda* | 1 Serving/40g | 118.0 | 9.0 | 296 | 6.5 | 16.6 | 22.6 | 0.5 |
| Cheese, Layered, Asda* | 1 Pack/440g | 647.0 | 41.0 | 147 | 4.5 | 11.4 | 9.3 | 0.0 |
| Cheese, Morrisons* | ½ Pot/125g | 341.0 | 27.0 | 273 | 5.7 | 14.7 | 21.3 | 1.0 |
| Cheese, with Mayonnaise & Vinaigrette, Sainsbury's* | ¼ Pot/50g | 124.0 | 9.0 | 249 | 6.1 | 17.0 | 17.3 | 1.7 |
| Cherry Tomato & Rocket, HE, Tesco* | 1 Pack/225g | 223.0 | 6.0 | 99 | 3.2 | 15.8 | 2.5 | 1.0 |
| Chicken, Asda* | 1 Pot/250g | 322.0 | 12.0 | 129 | 5.8 | 15.5 | 4.9 | 1.3 |
| Chicken & Bacon, Tesco* | ½ Pack/200g | 450.0 | 29.0 | 225 | 6.3 | 16.8 | 14.5 | 3.2 |
| Chicken & Smoked Bacon, M & S* | 1 Pack/380g | 817.0 | 47.0 | 215 | 7.5 | 19.0 | 12.3 | 1.9 |
| Chicken & Sweetcorn, Eat Smart, Safeway* | 1 Serving/200g | 230.0 | 4.0 | 115 | 7.5 | 16.3 | 1.8 | 1.0 |
| Chicken Caesar, Asda* | 1 Pack/297g | 683.0 | 41.0 | 230 | 9.6 | 16.6 | 13.9 | 2.5 |
| Chicken Caesar, Ginsters* | 1 Pack/220g | 504.0 | 35.0 | 229 | 7.5 | 13.6 | 16.1 | 0.0 |
| Chilli & Cheese, Sainsbury's* | 1 Serving/300g | 384.0 | 17.0 | 128 | 4.3 | 15.5 | 5.6 | 0.3 |
| Goats Cheese, & Mixed Pepper, Sainsbury's* | 1 Pack/200g | 366.0 | 19.0 | 183 | 6.4 | 18.2 | 9.4 | 1.5 |
| Ham, Sainsbury's* | 1 Pot/250g | 610.0 | 48.0 | 244 | 4.1 | 13.4 | 19.3 | 0.8 |
| Hot Smoked Salmon, No Mayonnaise, Tesco* | 1 Pack/275g | 426.0 | 17.0 | 155 | 7.1 | 16.6 | 6.2 | 4.1 |
| Italian, Tesco* | ½ Pack/225g | 315.0 | 8.0 | 140 | 3.5 | 22.6 | 3.7 | 2.3 |
| Italian Style, Sainsbury's* | 1/3 Pot/84g | 129.0 | 5.0 | 153 | 3.5 | 20.5 | 6.3 | 1.4 |
| Italian Style, Snack, Asda* | 1 Pack/150g | 141.0 | 6.0 | 94 | 3.4 | 11.0 | 4.0 | 4.1 |
| Lime & Coriander Chicken, M & S* | 1 Serving/190g | 370.0 | 23.0 | 195 | 7.6 | 14.4 | 12.2 | 0.6 |
| Mediterranean Style, Layered, Waitrose* | 1 Pot/275g | 190.0 | 4.0 | 69 | 2.6 | 11.8 | 1.3 | 1.0 |
| Mediterranean Tuna, Shapers, Boots* | 1 Serving/239g | 232.0 | 3.0 | 97 | 6.2 | 15.0 | 1.3 | 0.9 |
| Mediterranean Vegetable & Bean, BGTY, Sainsbury's* | 1 Serving/66g | 53.0 | 1.0 | 80 | 3.2 | 12.5 | 1.9 | 2.8 |
| Pepper, HE, Tesco* | 1 Salad/210g | 139.0 | 1.0 | 66 | 2.4 | 13.3 | 0.4 | 1.0 |
| Pepper, Side, Tesco* | 1 Serving/46g | 56.0 | 3.0 | 122 | 2.4 | 13.0 | 6.5 | 1.3 |
| Pepper & Tomato, Fire Roasted, Finest, Tesco* | 1 Pack/200g | 260.0 | 8.0 | 130 | 3.7 | 19.4 | 4.1 | 2.5 |
| Poached Salmon, M & S* | 1 Serving/200g | 340.0 | 17.0 | 170 | 7.8 | 16.2 | 8.4 | 1.4 |
| Poached Salmon, Sainsbury's* | 1 Serving/200g | 472.0 | 31.0 | 236 | 6.7 | 17.9 | 15.3 | 12.0 |
| Prawn, Layered, Asda* | ½ Pack/220g | 205.0 | 6.0 | 93 | 4.2 | 12.8 | 2.8 | 2.0 |
| Prawn, Shapers, Boots* | 1 Pot/250g | 250.0 | 8.0 | 100 | 4.1 | 14.0 | 3.1 | 0.4 |
| Prawn, Tesco* | ½ Pack/250g | 487.0 | 28.0 | 195 | 4.9 | 18.9 | 11.1 | 2.0 |
| Prawn Cocktail, Shapers, Boots* | 1 Pack/248g | 255.0 | 7.0 | 103 | 5.0 | 15.0 | 2.7 | 1.6 |
| Roast Garlic Mushroom, TTD, Sainsbury's* | 1 Pot/200g | 358.0 | 18.0 | 179 | 5.1 | 19.8 | 8.8 | 0.0 |
| Roasted Mushroom, Spinach & Tarragon, Tesco* | 1 Pot/200g | 216.0 | 5.0 | 108 | 4.3 | 17.2 | 2.4 | 0.8 |
| Roasted Vegetable, Waitrose* | 1 Pack/190g | 270.0 | 9.0 | 142 | 6.8 | 18.2 | 4.6 | 1.1 |
| Sainsbury's* | ½ Pack/160g | 235.0 | 10.0 | 147 | 3.2 | 20.0 | 6.0 | 1.5 |
| Salmon, M & S* | 1 Serving/380g | 817.0 | 58.0 | 215 | 6.8 | 12.7 | 15.2 | 0.7 |

P

|  | Measure INFO/WEIGHT | per Measure | | Nutrition Values per 100g / 100ml | | | | |
|---|---|---|---|---|---|---|---|---|
|  |  | KCAL | FAT | KCAL | PROT | CARB | FAT | FIBRE |
| **PASTA SALAD** | | | | | | | | |
| Spicy Chicken, Geo Adams* | 1 Pack/230g | 580.0 | 44.0 | 252 | 5.1 | 14.9 | 19.1 | 2.9 |
| Spicy Chilli Pesto, Sainsbury's* | ¼ Pot/63g | 170.0 | 12.0 | 272 | 3.8 | 20.1 | 19.6 | 1.6 |
| Sun Dried Tomato Dressing, Sainsbury's* | 1 Pack/320g | 442.0 | 14.0 | 138 | 3.7 | 20.8 | 4.4 | 3.6 |
| Sweetcorn & Pepper, GFY, Asda* | 1 Serving/175g | 68.0 | 1.0 | 39 | 1.9 | 7.0 | 0.4 | 0.0 |
| Three Cheese, Tesco* | 1 Serving/300g | 633.0 | 41.0 | 211 | 7.5 | 14.4 | 13.7 | 2.8 |
| Tomato, Aldi* | 1 Serving/50g | 58.0 | 2.0 | 117 | 3.9 | 18.6 | 3.6 | 0.0 |
| Tomato, Bacon & Cheese, Ginsters* | 1 Pack/220g | 381.0 | 20.0 | 173 | 7.4 | 15.6 | 9.0 | 0.0 |
| Tomato & Basil, Perfectly Balanced, Waitrose* | 1 Serving/100g | 97.0 | 2.0 | 97 | 3.7 | 16.8 | 1.7 | 0.0 |
| Tomato & Basil, Sainsbury's* | 1 Serving/62g | 87.0 | 4.0 | 141 | 3.2 | 16.4 | 6.9 | 3.8 |
| Tomato & Basil Chicken, M & S* | 1 Serving/279g | 446.0 | 22.0 | 160 | 7.0 | 14.8 | 7.9 | 1.8 |
| Tomato & Chargrilled Vegetable, Tesco* | 1 Serving/200g | 248.0 | 8.0 | 124 | 3.7 | 18.6 | 3.9 | 1.4 |
| Tomato & Mozzarella, Leaf, Shapers, Boots* | 1 Pack/185g | 356.0 | 22.0 | 192 | 5.1 | 16.0 | 12.0 | 2.5 |
| Tomato & Mozzarella, Sainsbury's* | 1 Pack/200g | 440.0 | 23.0 | 220 | 7.5 | 22.2 | 11.3 | 1.3 |
| Tomato & Mozzarella, Waitrose* | 1 Pack/225g | 380.0 | 28.0 | 169 | 4.3 | 10.0 | 12.4 | 0.6 |
| Tomato & Pepper, HL, Tesco* | 1 Serving/200g | 162.0 | 3.0 | 81 | 2.6 | 13.9 | 1.6 | 1.4 |
| Tomato & Tuna, Snack, Sainsbury's* | 1 Serving/200g | 238.0 | 2.0 | 119 | 5.3 | 21.7 | 1.2 | 0.0 |
| Tuna, Arrabiatta, BGTY, Sainsbury's* | 1 Serving/200g | 196.0 | 3.0 | 98 | 6.8 | 14.7 | 1.3 | 0.0 |
| Tuna, Perfectly Balanced, Waitrose* | 1 Tub/190g | 180.0 | 4.0 | 95 | 7.0 | 11.5 | 2.3 | 1.1 |
| Tuna, Tesco* | 1 Pot/300g | 399.0 | 22.0 | 133 | 6.2 | 10.5 | 7.3 | 0.0 |
| Tuna & Spinach, COU, M & S* | 1 Pack/270g | 256.0 | 5.0 | 95 | 6.8 | 14.3 | 1.8 | 3.8 |
| Tuna & Sweetcorn, COU, M & S* | 1 Pack/200g | 210.0 | 2.0 | 105 | 7.1 | 18.3 | 0.9 | 1.2 |
| Tuna & Sweetcorn, Sainsbury's* | 1 Serving/100g | 111.0 | 1.0 | 111 | 7.1 | 18.3 | 1.2 | 1.2 |
| Tuna Crunch, Shapers, Boots* | 1 Pack/250g | 352.0 | 7.0 | 141 | 9.8 | 19.0 | 2.7 | 2.8 |
| Tuna Nicoise, Waitrose* | 1 Pot/190g | 306.0 | 17.0 | 161 | 5.1 | 14.9 | 9.0 | 1.1 |
| **PASTA SAUCE** | | | | | | | | |
| Amatriciana, Asda* | 1 Jar/320g | 496.0 | 42.0 | 155 | 4.4 | 5.0 | 13.0 | 1.0 |
| Amatriciana, Italiano, Tesco* | ½ Pot/175g | 124.0 | 7.0 | 71 | 4.1 | 5.3 | 3.8 | 0.9 |
| Amatriciana, M & S* | 1 Jar/340g | 425.0 | 32.0 | 125 | 3.4 | 6.3 | 9.5 | 2.9 |
| Amatriciana, Morrisons* | 1 Tub/350g | 157.0 | 6.0 | 45 | 3.7 | 4.6 | 1.6 | 0.5 |
| Arrabbiata, Fresh, Co-Op* | ½ Pot/150g | 82.0 | 4.0 | 55 | 1.0 | 5.0 | 3.0 | 1.0 |
| Arrabbiata, GFY, Asda* | 1 Serving/350g | 133.0 | 4.0 | 38 | 1.1 | 6.0 | 1.1 | 0.0 |
| Arrabbiata, Italian, Waitrose* | 1 Jar/320g | 115.0 | 3.0 | 36 | 1.5 | 6.7 | 1.0 | 1.4 |
| Arrabbiata, M & S* | 1 Jar/320g | 240.0 | 17.0 | 75 | 1.2 | 6.2 | 5.3 | 0.8 |
| Arrabbiata, Red Pepper, Sainsbury's* | ½ Pot/175g | 79.0 | 5.0 | 45 | 1.4 | 3.3 | 2.9 | 1.6 |
| Arrabbiata, Stir in, BGTY, Sainsbury's* | 1 Serving/75g | 53.0 | 3.0 | 71 | 1.3 | 7.6 | 3.9 | 0.7 |
| Basil & Oregano, Ragu, Knorr* | 1 Jar/500g | 215.0 | 0.0 | 43 | 1.3 | 9.4 | 0.0 | 1.1 |
| Bolognese, Dolmio* | 1 Serving/100g | 56.0 | 1.0 | 56 | 1.5 | 9.4 | 1.5 | 1.1 |
| Bolognese, Finest, Tesco* | 1 Serving/175g | 170.0 | 11.0 | 97 | 7.0 | 3.8 | 6.1 | 0.5 |
| Bolognese, Fresh, Sainsbury's* | ½ Pot/150g | 120.0 | 6.0 | 80 | 6.0 | 4.7 | 4.1 | 1.2 |
| Bolognese, Light, Original, Ragu, Knorr* | 1 Jar/515g | 196.0 | 1.0 | 38 | 1.4 | 8.2 | 0.1 | 1.2 |
| Bolognese, Mediterranean Vegetable, Chunky, Dolmio* | ½ Jar/250g | 137.0 | 4.0 | 55 | 1.3 | 8.8 | 1.6 | 0.0 |
| Bolognese, SmartPrice, Asda* | ½ Jar/226g | 88.0 | 2.0 | 39 | 0.9 | 7.0 | 0.8 | 0.6 |
| Bolognese, VLH Kitchens* | 1 Serving/380g | 316.0 | 15.6 | 83 | 6.0 | 4.7 | 4.1 | 1.2 |
| Bolognese with Beef, Tesco* | ½ Can/213g | 179.0 | 10.0 | 84 | 4.9 | 5.5 | 4.7 | 0.0 |
| Carbonara, Fresh, Chilled, Finest, Tesco* | ½ Tub/175g | 297.0 | 25.0 | 170 | 5.5 | 4.2 | 14.2 | 0.0 |
| Carbonara, Fresh, TTD, Sainsbury's* | 1 Tub/300g | 606.0 | 52.0 | 202 | 7.4 | 4.1 | 17.3 | 0.5 |
| Carbonara, Italian, Asda* | ½ Pack/175g | 359.0 | 30.0 | 205 | 7.0 | 6.0 | 17.0 | 0.1 |
| Carbonara, Reduced Fat, BFY, Morrisons* | ½ Pot/175g | 135.0 | 6.0 | 77 | 6.6 | 5.1 | 3.3 | 0.5 |
| Carbonara, with Pancetta, Loyd Grossman* | ½ Pack/170g | 209.0 | 15.0 | 123 | 2.8 | 7.5 | 9.1 | 0.1 |
| Chargrilled Vegetable with Extra Virgin Olive Oil, Bertolli* | ½ Jar/250g | 150.0 | 5.0 | 60 | 2.1 | 8.7 | 1.9 | 2.4 |
| Cheese, Fresh, Perfectly Balanced, Waitrose* | ½ Pot/175g | 143.0 | 5.0 | 82 | 6.1 | 7.9 | 2.9 | 0.5 |
| Cheese & Tuna, Safeway* | 1 Serving/175g | 175.0 | 10.0 | 100 | 6.9 | 4.8 | 5.7 | 0.6 |
| Cherry Tomato & Basil, Sacla* | 1 Serving/96g | 90.0 | 7.0 | 94 | 1.2 | 5.3 | 7.4 | 0.0 |

## PASTA SAUCE

| | Measure INFO/WEIGHT | per Measure KCAL | FAT | Nutrition Values per 100g / 100ml KCAL | PROT | CARB | FAT | FIBRE |
|---|---|---|---|---|---|---|---|---|
| Chilli with Jalapeno Peppers, Seeds of Change* | 1 Jar/350g | 322.0 | 5.0 | 92 | 3.6 | 16.0 | 1.5 | 2.2 |
| Chunky Vegetable, Asda* | 1 Serving/250g | 122.0 | 4.0 | 49 | 1.4 | 7.0 | 1.7 | 1.2 |
| Creamy Mushroom, Dolmio* | 1 Pack/150g | 166.0 | 15.0 | 111 | 1.3 | 3.7 | 10.0 | 0.0 |
| Creamy Tomato, Carb Check, Heinz* | 1 Serving/150g | 91.0 | 6.0 | 61 | 2.0 | 4.2 | 4.0 | 0.5 |
| Creamy Tomato & Basil, BGTY, Sainsbury's* | ½ Jar/250g | 172.0 | 9.0 | 69 | 1.7 | 7.6 | 3.6 | 1.0 |
| Five Cheese, Italiano, Tesco* | ½ Tub/175g | 271.0 | 20.0 | 155 | 6.8 | 6.0 | 11.5 | 0.0 |
| Four Cheese, Asda* | ½ Jar/155g | 242.0 | 22.0 | 156 | 3.5 | 3.9 | 14.0 | 0.1 |
| Four Cheese, BGTY, Sainsbury's* | 1 Serving/150g | 103.0 | 6.0 | 69 | 2.9 | 5.5 | 4.0 | 0.1 |
| Four Cheese, Fresh, Asda* | ½ Pot/162g | 309.0 | 29.0 | 191 | 5.4 | 2.2 | 17.8 | 0.5 |
| Four Cheese, Loyd Grossman* | 1 Jar/350g | 476.0 | 42.0 | 136 | 2.6 | 4.6 | 11.9 | 0.0 |
| Garlic, Perfectly Balanced, Waitrose* | 1 Jar/440g | 330.0 | 7.0 | 75 | 2.3 | 12.7 | 1.7 | 2.3 |
| Garlic & Chilli, Slow Roasted, Seeds of Change* | ½ Jar/175g | 157.0 | 9.0 | 90 | 1.7 | 8.7 | 5.3 | 2.0 |
| Garlic & Onion, Finest, Tesco* | 1 Serving/126g | 43.0 | 1.0 | 34 | 0.8 | 6.9 | 0.4 | 1.3 |
| Grilled Vegetable with Extra Virgin Olive Oil, Bertolli* | ½ Jar/250g | 150.0 | 5.0 | 60 | 2.1 | 8.7 | 1.9 | 2.4 |
| Ham & Mushroom, Creamy, Stir & Serve, Homepride* | 1 Serving/92g | 124.0 | 11.0 | 135 | 1.8 | 5.5 | 11.7 | 0.0 |
| Hot, Heinz* | 1 Serving/200g | 120.0 | 7.0 | 60 | 1.2 | 5.7 | 3.6 | 0.9 |
| Hot & Spicy, Morrisons* | 1 Serving/130g | 81.0 | 3.0 | 62 | 1.4 | 8.5 | 2.4 | 1.1 |
| Hot Pepper & Mozzarella, Stir Through, Sacla* | ½ Jar/95g | 229.0 | 20.0 | 241 | 4.7 | 7.2 | 21.5 | 0.0 |
| Italian Cheese, Finest, Tesco* | ½ Pot/175g | 171.0 | 9.0 | 98 | 4.8 | 8.4 | 5.1 | 0.0 |
| Italian Mushroom, Sainsbury's* | 1 Serving/85g | 56.0 | 2.0 | 66 | 2.0 | 9.8 | 2.1 | 1.7 |
| Italian Tomato & Herb, for Pasta, Sainsbury's* | ½ Jar/146g | 102.0 | 3.0 | 70 | 2.0 | 11.1 | 2.0 | 1.4 |
| Italian Tomato & Smoked Bacon, Stir-In, Safeway* | ½ Jar/75g | 152.0 | 13.0 | 203 | 2.9 | 7.3 | 18.0 | 1.2 |
| Layered Tomato & Mozzarella, Finest, Tesco* | 1 Jar/160g | 232.0 | 16.0 | 145 | 6.6 | 6.9 | 10.1 | 0.7 |
| Leek & Bacon, Safeway* | ½ Pot/171g | 145.0 | 8.0 | 85 | 4.0 | 5.7 | 4.9 | 0.5 |
| Mediterrainean Vegetable Pasta, Tesco* | 1 Serving/166g | 95.0 | 3.0 | 57 | 1.4 | 9.0 | 1.7 | 1.2 |
| Mediterranean, Fresh, Waitrose* | 1 Pot/350g | 213.0 | 14.0 | 61 | 1.4 | 5.0 | 3.9 | 2.4 |
| Mediterranean Tomato, Asda* | 1 Jar/500g | 285.0 | 6.0 | 57 | 1.5 | 10.0 | 1.2 | 0.0 |
| Mediterranean Vegetable, Rustico, Bertolli* | ½ Jar/160g | 141.0 | 12.0 | 88 | 1.7 | 4.1 | 7.2 | 0.7 |
| Mushroom, Co-Op* | ¼ Jar/125g | 75.0 | 2.0 | 60 | 2.0 | 9.0 | 2.0 | 1.0 |
| Mushroom, GFY, Asda* | 1 Serving/175g | 112.0 | 5.0 | 64 | 2.7 | 7.0 | 2.8 | 0.0 |
| Mushroom, Microwaveable, Dolmio* | 1 Serving/150g | 160.0 | 14.0 | 107 | 1.4 | 3.8 | 9.6 | 0.0 |
| Mushroom, Morrisons* | 1 Serving/128g | 76.0 | 3.0 | 59 | 1.6 | 7.9 | 2.3 | 1.1 |
| Mushroom, Perfectly Balanced, Waitrose* | 1 Jar/440g | 330.0 | 8.0 | 75 | 2.6 | 11.8 | 1.9 | 2.2 |
| Mushroom, Sainsbury's* | 1 Serving/100g | 66.0 | 2.0 | 66 | 2.0 | 9.8 | 2.1 | 1.7 |
| Mushroom, Tesco* | ¼ Jar/188g | 90.0 | 3.0 | 48 | 1.4 | 6.8 | 1.7 | 1.0 |
| Mushroom & Garlic, 98% Fat Free, Homepride* | 1 Jar/450g | 229.0 | 6.0 | 51 | 1.1 | 8.9 | 1.4 | 0.5 |
| Mushroom & Garlic, Deliciously Good, Homepride* | 1/3 Jar/147g | 109.0 | 7.0 | 74 | 0.9 | 6.9 | 4.8 | 0.3 |
| Mushroom & Mascarpone, Morrisons* | ½ Pot/175g | 199.0 | 17.0 | 114 | 2.3 | 4.3 | 9.7 | 0.0 |
| Napoletana, BGTY, Sainsbury's* | ½ Pot/151g | 71.0 | 4.0 | 47 | 1.2 | 5.0 | 2.5 | 1.3 |
| Napoletana, Buitoni* | ½ Jar/200g | 146.0 | 8.0 | 73 | 1.6 | 7.3 | 4.1 | 2.2 |
| Napoletana, GFY, Asda* | 1 Serving/175g | 58.0 | 2.0 | 33 | 1.0 | 5.0 | 1.0 | 0.0 |
| Napoletana, Morrisons* | 1 Serving/175g | 82.0 | 3.0 | 47 | 2.6 | 6.7 | 1.5 | 0.0 |
| Napoletana, Sainsbury's* | ½ Pot/150g | 126.0 | 8.0 | 84 | 1.9 | 6.6 | 5.6 | 0.9 |
| Onion & Garlic, Co-Op* | 1 Serving/125g | 106.0 | 4.0 | 85 | 2.0 | 12.0 | 3.0 | 0.7 |
| Onion & Garlic, Tesco* | 1 Serving/125g | 35.0 | 0.0 | 28 | 1.2 | 5.6 | 0.1 | 2.6 |
| Onion & Roasted Garlic, Knorr* | 1 Jar/500g | 210.0 | 0.0 | 42 | 1.3 | 9.2 | 0.0 | 1.1 |
| Original, BFY, Morrisons* | 1/3 Jar/200g | 100.0 | 0.0 | 50 | 1.6 | 10.6 | 0.1 | 1.2 |
| Original, Tesco* | 1 Jar/300g | 123.0 | 4.0 | 41 | 1.0 | 6.1 | 1.4 | 2.3 |
| Parmesan & Pesto, Weight Watchers* | ½ Jar/175g | 86.0 | 3.0 | 49 | 1.8 | 6.7 | 1.6 | 1.0 |
| Pepper & Tomato, M & S* | 1 Jar/320g | 224.0 | 13.0 | 70 | 1.6 | 6.1 | 4.2 | 0.9 |
| Porcini Mushroom & Pepperoni, Asda* | ½ Jar/140g | 158.0 | 8.0 | 113 | 3.8 | 11.0 | 6.0 | 0.0 |
| Porcini Mushroom Stir in, BGTY, Sainsbury's* | ½ Jar/75g | 57.0 | 3.0 | 76 | 3.8 | 5.7 | 4.2 | 1.9 |
| Primavera, Fresh, Morrisons* | ½ Pot/175g | 152.0 | 10.0 | 87 | 2.4 | 6.1 | 5.9 | 0.0 |

## PASTA SAUCE

| INFO/WEIGHT | Measure KCAL | FAT | KCAL | PROT | CARB | FAT | FIBRE |
|---|---|---|---|---|---|---|---|
| Primavera, Loyd Grossman* | 1 Jar/350g | 343.0 26.0 | 98 | 1.4 | 6.3 | 7.4 | 0.9 |
| Puttanesca, Loyd Grossman* | 1 Jar/350g | 315.0 22.0 | 90 | 1.7 | 6.8 | 6.2 | 0.9 |
| Puttanesca, M & S* | 1 Jar/320g | 256.0 18.0 | 80 | 1.5 | 6.2 | 5.5 | 1.9 |
| Puttanesca, Sainsbury's* | 1 Serving/110g | 132.0 10.0 | 120 | 2.0 | 8.1 | 8.8 | 0.0 |
| Rich Tomato with Basil Pesto, Express, Dolmio* | 1 Pack/170g | 146.0 10.0 | 86 | 2.0 | 6.2 | 5.9 | 0.0 |
| Roasted Garlic, Weight Watchers* | ½ Jar/177g | 60.0 1.0 | 34 | 1.3 | 6.4 | 0.4 | 1.2 |
| Roasted Red Pepper & Tomato, Finest, Tesco* | 1 Serving/145g | 117.0 8.0 | 81 | 1.2 | 6.8 | 5.4 | 2.2 |
| Roasted Vegetable, & Olive, TTD, Sainsbury's* | ½ Pot/150g | 84.0 4.0 | 56 | 1.7 | 6.9 | 2.4 | 2.0 |
| Roasted Vegetable, GFY, Asda* | ½ Pot/175g | 84.0 3.0 | 48 | 1.3 | 7.0 | 1.6 | 0.5 |
| Roasted Vegetable, Microwaveable, Dolmio* | ½ Pack/190g | 103.0 4.0 | 54 | 1.4 | 7.6 | 2.0 | 0.0 |
| Roasted Vegetable, Sainsbury's* | ½ Pot/151g | 103.0 6.0 | 68 | 1.6 | 6.7 | 3.9 | 0.4 |
| Roasted Vegetable, Tesco* | 1 Pack/175g | 114.0 5.0 | 65 | 1.5 | 8.0 | 3.0 | 0.8 |
| Roasted Vegetables & Tuna, BGTY, Sainsbury's* | ½ Pot/150g | 73.0 3.0 | 49 | 3.5 | 4.5 | 1.9 | 3.1 |
| Rustico Sweet Chilli & Red Onion, Bertolli* | ½ Jar/160g | 146.0 12.0 | 91 | 1.7 | 4.9 | 7.2 | 0.7 |
| Siciliana, Sainsbury's* | 1/3 Jar/113g | 168.0 15.0 | 149 | 1.8 | 6.2 | 13.0 | 0.0 |
| Sliced Mushroom, Tesco* | 1 Jar/460g | 161.0 1.0 | 35 | 1.3 | 7.0 | 0.2 | 0.8 |
| Smoky Bacon, Loyd Grossman* | 1 Jar/350g | 343.0 25.0 | 98 | 3.1 | 5.4 | 7.2 | 0.7 |
| Spicy Italian Chilli, Express, Dolmio* | 1 Serving/170g | 87.0 3.0 | 51 | 1.5 | 7.5 | 1.6 | 0.0 |
| Spicy Pepper, Tesco* | 1 Jar/500g | 245.0 5.0 | 49 | 1.7 | 8.4 | 1.0 | 1.0 |
| Spicy Pepper & Tomato, Sacla* | ½ Jar/95g | 132.0 11.0 | 139 | 1.4 | 6.8 | 11.8 | 0.0 |
| Spicy Roasted Garlic, Seeds of Change* | 1 Serving/195g | 123.0 4.0 | 63 | 1.5 | 9.7 | 2.0 | 1.2 |
| Spicy Tomato, Asda* | 1 Serving/155g | 76.0 2.0 | 49 | 1.5 | 8.0 | 1.2 | 1.0 |
| Spicy with Peppers, Tesco* | 1 Jar/455g | 177.0 1.0 | 39 | 1.2 | 7.9 | 0.3 | 1.1 |
| Spinach & Ricotta, Asda* | ½ Pot/175g | 175.0 12.0 | 100 | 3.2 | 6.0 | 7.0 | 0.5 |
| Spinach & Ricotta, BGTY, Sainsbury's* | 1 Serving/150g | 73.0 4.0 | 49 | 2.7 | 3.4 | 2.7 | 2.2 |
| Spinach & Ricotta, Fresh, Perfectly Balanced, Waitrose* | ½ Pot/175g | 96.0 4.0 | 55 | 3.3 | 5.7 | 2.1 | 0.9 |
| Spinach & Ricotta, Stir Through, Sacla* | ½ Jar/95g | 196.0 19.0 | 206 | 3.7 | 3.7 | 19.6 | 0.0 |
| Stir & Serve, Homepride* | 1 Bottle/480g | 187.0 6.0 | 39 | 1.2 | 6.0 | 1.2 | 0.0 |
| Sun Dried Tomato, Asda* | ½ Jar/159g | 165.0 13.0 | 104 | 1.9 | 6.0 | 8.0 | 1.5 |
| Sun Dried Tomato, Garlic & Basil, Finest, Tesco* | 1 Jar/340g | 493.0 39.0 | 145 | 1.8 | 7.7 | 11.5 | 2.3 |
| Sun Dried Tomato, Stir In, Light, Dolmio* | 1 Serving/75g | 62.0 4.0 | 83 | 1.7 | 9.8 | 4.7 | 0.0 |
| Sun Dried Tomato & Basil, Free From, Sainsbury's* | ½ Jar/172g | 124.0 5.0 | 72 | 2.9 | 8.7 | 2.8 | 1.5 |
| Sun Dried Tomato & Garlic, Sacla* | 1 Serving/95g | 177.0 14.0 | 186 | 3.0 | 10.3 | 14.7 | 0.0 |
| Sun Ripened Tomato & Basil, Dolmio* | 1 Serving/150g | 117.0 7.0 | 78 | 1.3 | 7.9 | 4.6 | 0.0 |
| Sun Ripened Tomato & Basil, Express, Dolmio* | 1 Pouch/170g | 88.0 3.0 | 52 | 1.5 | 7.9 | 1.6 | 0.0 |
| Sundried Tomato, Heinz* | ½ Jar/150g | 55.0 0.0 | 37 | 1.5 | 7.3 | 0.2 | 1.1 |
| Sundried Tomato & Basil ,Organic, Seeds of Change* | ½ Jar/100g | 155.0 13.0 | 155 | 1.6 | 7.7 | 13.1 | 0.0 |
| Sundried Tomato & Garlic, M & S* | ½ Jar/95g | 147.0 13.0 | 155 | 2.9 | 4.4 | 13.7 | 0.8 |
| Sweet Pepper, Dolmio* | 1 Serving/150g | 238.0 20.0 | 159 | 1.6 | 8.8 | 13.4 | 0.0 |
| Sweet Red Pepper, Loyd Grossman* | 1 Jar/350g | 304.0 20.0 | 87 | 1.7 | 7.3 | 5.6 | 1.2 |
| Three Cheeses, Co-Op* | 1 Pack/300g | 405.0 27.0 | 135 | 6.0 | 6.0 | 9.0 | 0.1 |
| Tomato, Bacon & Mushroom, Asda* | ½ Pot/50g | 33.0 2.0 | 66 | 2.5 | 6.0 | 3.6 | 0.0 |
| Tomato, Chilli & Onion, Bertolli* | 1 Serving/100g | 49.0 2.0 | 49 | 1.8 | 6.7 | 1.7 | 1.8 |
| Tomato, Garlic & Chilli, Finest, Tesco* | 1 Serving/145g | 199.0 16.0 | 137 | 2.0 | 7.1 | 11.2 | 3.4 |
| Tomato, Ginger & Basil, Cranks* | ½ Jar/175g | 129.0 8.0 | 74 | 1.7 | 6.3 | 4.7 | 1.1 |
| Tomato, Low Price, Sainsbury's* | 1 Jar/440g | 220.0 3.0 | 50 | 0.6 | 10.1 | 0.7 | 0.4 |
| Tomato, Mushroom & Roasted Garlic, Bertolli* | 1 Jar/500g | 235.0 9.0 | 47 | 1.9 | 5.3 | 1.9 | 0.0 |
| Tomato, Pecorino Romano Cheese & Garlic, Bertolli* | 1 Serving/125g | 76.0 3.0 | 61 | 2.3 | 6.5 | 2.8 | 0.9 |
| Tomato, Pepper & Herb, Somerfield* | 1 Serving/186g | 232.0 9.0 | 125 | 3.0 | 17.4 | 4.8 | 0.8 |
| Tomato, Red Pepper and Chilli, Slow Cooked, Dress Italian* | 1 Jar/350g | 318.0 22.0 | 91 | 1.9 | 6.6 | 6.4 | 1.3 |
| Tomato, Red Wine, Shallots, Bertolli* | ½ Jar/250g | 112.0 4.0 | 45 | 1.7 | 7.2 | 1.7 | 1.5 |
| Tomato & Aubergine, TTD, Sainsbury's* | 1 Serving/150g | 106.0 5.0 | 71 | 2.1 | 7.7 | 3.5 | 2.0 |
| Tomato & Basil, Bertolli* | 1 Jar/500g | 215.0 5.0 | 43 | 1.2 | 7.3 | 1.0 | 0.4 |

| | Measure<br>INFO/WEIGHT | per Measure<br>KCAL | FAT | Nutrition Values per 100g / 100ml<br>KCAL | PROT | CARB | FAT | FIBRE |
|---|---|---|---|---|---|---|---|---|
| **PASTA SAUCE** | | | | | | | | |
| Tomato & Basil, Carb Check, Heinz* | 1 Serving/150g | 84.0 | 5.0 | 56 | 1.5 | 4.4 | 3.6 | 0.6 |
| Tomato & Basil, Dolmio* | 1 Serving/170g | 95.0 | 4.0 | 56 | 1.4 | 7.9 | 2.1 | 0.0 |
| Tomato & Basil, Loyd Grossman* | ½ Jar/175g | 157.0 | 10.0 | 90 | 1.7 | 7.9 | 5.7 | 0.8 |
| Tomato & Black Olive, Carb Control, Tesco* | 1 Serving/110g | 74.0 | 5.0 | 67 | 1.3 | 6.0 | 4.3 | 2.3 |
| Tomato & Chargrilled Vegetable, Loyd Grossman* | 1 Serving/150g | 133.0 | 8.0 | 89 | 1.8 | 7.9 | 5.6 | 0.9 |
| Tomato & Chilli, Loyd Grossman* | ½ Jar/175g | 154.0 | 10.0 | 88 | 1.7 | 7.3 | 5.7 | 0.9 |
| Tomato & Chilli, Pour Over, M & S* | 1 Jar/330g | 231.0 | 13.0 | 70 | 1.3 | 7.6 | 3.8 | 1.8 |
| Tomato & Chunky Mushroom, Dolmio* | 1 Pack/475g | 323.0 | 18.0 | 68 | 1.2 | 7.6 | 3.7 | 0.0 |
| Tomato & Creme Fraiche, Perfectly Balanced, Waitrose* | ½ Pot/177g | 85.0 | 2.0 | 48 | 1.8 | 7.1 | 1.3 | 2.0 |
| Tomato & Herb, M & S* | 1 Jar/500g | 400.0 | 15.0 | 80 | 2.6 | 10.1 | 3.1 | 1.7 |
| Tomato & Herb, Organic, Sainsbury's* | 1 Serving/75g | 38.0 | 1.0 | 51 | 1.2 | 6.6 | 2.0 | 0.5 |
| Tomato & Herb, Perfectly Balanced, Waitrose* | ½ Tub/176g | 65.0 | 2.0 | 37 | 1.3 | 5.3 | 1.2 | 2.3 |
| Tomato & Herb, with Extra Garlic, Sainsbury's* | ½ Pot/150g | 61.0 | 2.0 | 41 | 1.4 | 6.3 | 1.1 | 1.6 |
| Tomato & Mascarpone, Finest, Tesco* | 1 Serving/175g | 135.0 | 9.0 | 77 | 2.7 | 5.4 | 5.0 | 0.8 |
| Tomato & Mascarpone, Fresh, Sainsbury's* | 1 Serving/150g | 177.0 | 15.0 | 118 | 2.2 | 4.2 | 10.3 | 1.1 |
| Tomato & Mascarpone, Sacla* | ½ Jar/95g | 161.0 | 14.0 | 169 | 2.2 | 6.2 | 15.0 | 0.0 |
| Tomato & Mascarpone, Sainsbury's* | ½ Pot/150g | 137.0 | 10.0 | 91 | 2.1 | 5.9 | 6.6 | 1.2 |
| Tomato & Mascarpone, So Organic, Sainsbury's* | 1/3 Jar/146g | 180.0 | 13.0 | 123 | 1.9 | 8.7 | 9.0 | 2.8 |
| Tomato & Mascarpone, Tesco* | 1 Serving/175g | 194.0 | 15.0 | 111 | 2.8 | 5.4 | 8.7 | 0.6 |
| Tomato & Mascarpone, Waitrose* | ½ Pot/175g | 184.0 | 15.0 | 105 | 1.9 | 5.5 | 8.4 | 1.1 |
| Tomato & Mushroom, Organic, Sainsbury's* | 1 Serving/150g | 87.0 | 4.0 | 58 | 1.6 | 7.1 | 2.6 | 1.5 |
| Tomato & Olives, La Doria* | 1 Jar/90g | 76.0 | 6.0 | 84 | 1.2 | 5.0 | 6.6 | 0.0 |
| Tomato & Parmesan, Seeds of Change* | 1 Serving/150g | 100.0 | 4.0 | 67 | 2.5 | 7.8 | 2.9 | 1.1 |
| Tomato & Pesto, Planet Cook, Heinz* | 1 Jar/300g | 237.0 | 17.0 | 79 | 1.7 | 5.2 | 5.7 | 1.0 |
| Tomato & Ricotta, Italian, Sainsbury's* | 1 Pack/390g | 238.0 | 12.0 | 61 | 2.5 | 6.1 | 3.0 | 1.2 |
| Tomato & Roasted Garlic, Loyd Grossman* | ½ Jar/175g | 161.0 | 10.0 | 92 | 2.0 | 8.8 | 5.5 | 0.8 |
| Tomato & Smokey Bacon, Dolmio* | 1 Pot/150g | 240.0 | 20.0 | 160 | 5.5 | 5.8 | 13.1 | 0.0 |
| Tomato Bacon, Stir & Serve, Homepride* | 1 Serving/96g | 81.0 | 4.0 | 84 | 2.7 | 8.1 | 4.5 | 0.0 |
| **PASTA SHAPES** | | | | | | | | |
| Alphabetti, in Tomato Sauce, Heinz* | 1 Can/200g | 118.0 | 1.0 | 59 | 1.8 | 11.7 | 0.5 | 1.5 |
| Bob The Builder, in Tomato Sauce, Heinz* | 1 Can/205g | 111.0 | 1.0 | 54 | 1.7 | 11.3 | 0.3 | 1.5 |
| Cooked, Tesco* | 1 Serving/260g | 356.0 | 2.0 | 137 | 5.1 | 26.3 | 0.8 | 1.1 |
| Disney Princess, in Tomato Sauce, Heinz* | 1 Can/200g | 114.0 | 1.0 | 57 | 1.8 | 11.9 | 0.3 | 1.5 |
| Dried, Tesco* | 1 Serving/100g | 345.0 | 2.0 | 345 | 13.2 | 68.5 | 2.0 | 2.9 |
| Durum Wheat, Dry, Basics, Sainsbury's* | 1 Serving/75g | 259.0 | 1.0 | 346 | 12.0 | 70.0 | 2.0 | 4.0 |
| Funky Fish, in Tomato Sauce, Heinz* | 1 Can/200g | 108.0 | 1.0 | 54 | 1.4 | 11.6 | 0.3 | 0.4 |
| Pirates of the Caribbean, with Cannon Balls, Heinz* | 1 Can/200g | 182.0 | 7.0 | 91 | 4.2 | 10.9 | 3.3 | 1.5 |
| Postman Pat, HP* | 1 Can/410g | 279.0 | 2.0 | 68 | 1.8 | 14.3 | 0.4 | 0.7 |
| Scooby Doo, HP* | 1 Can/410g | 279.0 | 2.0 | 68 | 1.8 | 14.3 | 0.4 | 0.7 |
| Shrek, Multigrain, in Tomato Sauce, with Omega 3, Heinz* | 1 Can/200g | 120.0 | 1.0 | 60 | 1.9 | 12.0 | 0.5 | 1.5 |
| Spiderman, in Tomato Sauce, Heinz* | ½ Can/200g | 114.0 | 1.0 | 57 | 1.7 | 11.4 | 0.5 | 1.5 |
| Spiderman, with Mini Sausages, in Tomato Sauce, Heinz* | 1 Can/200g | 178.0 | 6.0 | 89 | 3.6 | 11.6 | 3.1 | 0.5 |
| Teletubbies, in Tomato Sauce, Heinz* | 1 Can/400g | 244.0 | 2.0 | 61 | 2.0 | 12.3 | 0.4 | 0.6 |
| Thomas Tank Engine, in Tomato Sauce, Heinz* | 1 Can/205g | 109.0 | 0.0 | 53 | 1.7 | 11.0 | 0.2 | 0.5 |
| Tweenies, in Tomato Sauce, Heinz* | 1 Can/205g | 121.0 | 1.0 | 59 | 1.8 | 11.7 | 0.5 | 1.5 |
| **PASTA SHELLS** | | | | | | | | |
| *Dry, Average* | *1 Serving/75g* | *265.0* | *1.0* | *353* | *11.1* | *71.8* | *2.0* | *2.0* |
| *Egg, Fresh, Average* | *1 Serving/125g* | *344.0* | *4.0* | *275* | *11.5* | *49.7* | *2.8* | *3.4* |
| *Fresh, Dry, Average* | *1 Serving/125g* | *216.0* | *2.0* | *173* | *7.4* | *32.0* | *1.6* | *1.5* |
| Wholewheat, Healthy Living, Co-Op* | 1 Serving/75g | 232.0 | 1.0 | 310 | 11.0 | 64.0 | 1.0 | 12.0 |
| **PASTA SNACK** | | | | | | | | |
| Cheese & Ham, Pot, Tesco* | 1 Serving/208g | 254.0 | 8.0 | 122 | 3.4 | 17.9 | 4.1 | 1.5 |
| Cheese & Ham, Tubes, Made Up, Tesco* | 1 Serving/214g | 312.0 | 12.0 | 146 | 4.9 | 19.5 | 5.4 | 2.6 |

| | Measure INFO/WEIGHT | per Measure KCAL | per Measure FAT | Nutrition Values per 100g / 100ml KCAL | PROT | CARB | FAT | FIBRE |
|---|---|---|---|---|---|---|---|---|
| **PASTA SNACK** | | | | | | | | |
| Chicken, Morrisons* | 1 Pack/250g | 285.0 | 7.0 | 114 | 3.3 | 19.3 | 2.7 | 0.0 |
| Chicken, with Sweetcorn & Mushroom, Pot, Tesco* | 1 Pot/216g | 238.0 | 6.0 | 110 | 3.0 | 18.5 | 2.7 | 0.7 |
| Chicken & Smoked Bacon, Sainsbury's* | 1 Pack/190g | 490.0 | 36.0 | 258 | 7.2 | 14.1 | 19.2 | 0.0 |
| Creamy Cheese, Mug Shot, Asda* | 1 Serving/250g | 272.0 | 6.0 | 109 | 2.5 | 19.0 | 2.5 | 1.8 |
| Ham & Mushroom, Tesco* | 1 Pack/300g | 618.0 | 43.0 | 206 | 4.2 | 15.0 | 14.3 | 1.1 |
| Tomato & Herb, in a Pot, Dry, Tesco* | 1 Pot/59g | 207.0 | 1.0 | 352 | 11.8 | 70.7 | 2.4 | 2.6 |
| Tomato & Herb, Morrisons* | 1 Pot/247g | 247.0 | 3.0 | 100 | 3.1 | 19.5 | 1.1 | 0.0 |
| Tomato 'n' Herb, Mug Shot* | 1 Sachet/257g | 265.0 | 2.0 | 103 | 2.3 | 21.6 | 0.8 | 1.2 |
| **PASTA SPIRALS** | | | | | | | | |
| Co-Op* | 1 Serving/100g | 350.0 | 1.0 | 350 | 12.0 | 73.0 | 1.0 | 3.0 |
| Glutenfree, Glutano* | 1oz/28g | 100.0 | 0.0 | 357 | 4.0 | 83.0 | 1.0 | 0.0 |
| **PASTA TWIRLS** | | | | | | | | |
| Dry, Asda* | 1 Serving/50g | 173.0 | 1.0 | 346 | 12.0 | 71.0 | 1.5 | 3.0 |
| Tri-Colour, Sainsbury's* | 1 Serving/75g | 268.0 | 1.0 | 357 | 12.3 | 73.1 | 1.7 | 2.5 |
| **PASTA TWISTS** | | | | | | | | |
| *Dry, Average* | *1oz/28g* | *99.0* | *0.0* | *354* | *12.2* | *71.8* | *1.5* | *2.2* |
| Wheat & Gluten Free, Glutafin* | 1 Serving/75g | 262.0 | 1.0 | 350 | 8.0 | 75.0 | 2.0 | 0.1 |
| **PASTE** | | | | | | | | |
| Bacon & Tomato, Tesco* | 1 Serving/20g | 46.0 | 4.0 | 232 | 14.0 | 3.4 | 18.0 | 0.1 |
| BBQ Bean, Princes* | 1 Serving/33g | 35.0 | 0.0 | 106 | 5.7 | 19.8 | 0.4 | 0.0 |
| Beef, Asda* | 1 Serving/37g | 72.0 | 5.0 | 194 | 17.0 | 0.1 | 14.0 | 0.0 |
| Beef, Princes* | 1 Serving/18g | 40.0 | 3.0 | 220 | 14.4 | 5.2 | 15.8 | 0.0 |
| Beef, Sainsbury's* | 1 Jar/75g | 142.0 | 10.0 | 189 | 16.0 | 1.5 | 13.2 | 1.4 |
| Chicken, Asda* | 1 Thin Spread/7g | 13.0 | 1.0 | 184 | 16.0 | 0.8 | 13.0 | 0.0 |
| Chicken, Princes* | 1 Thin Spread/9g | 22.0 | 2.0 | 240 | 12.6 | 5.6 | 18.5 | 0.0 |
| Chicken, Tesco* | 1 Serving/12g | 30.0 | 2.0 | 248 | 14.8 | 2.3 | 20.0 | 0.1 |
| Chicken, Value, Tesco* | 1 Thin Spread/9g | 18.0 | 1.0 | 196 | 15.1 | 1.8 | 14.3 | 0.1 |
| Chicken & Ham, Sainsbury's* | 1 Thin Spread/9g | 14.0 | 1.0 | 158 | 16.0 | 1.1 | 10.0 | 1.1 |
| Chicken & Ham, Tesco* | 1 Serving/19g | 44.0 | 4.0 | 231 | 12.5 | 1.4 | 19.5 | 0.0 |
| Chicken & Mushroom, Princes* | 1 Serving/50g | 93.0 | 5.0 | 187 | 17.1 | 5.0 | 11.0 | 0.0 |
| Chicken & Stuffing, Asda* | ½ Jar/35g | 71.0 | 5.0 | 203 | 16.0 | 3.3 | 14.0 | 0.0 |
| Chicken & Stuffing, Princes* | 1 Jar/100g | 229.0 | 17.0 | 229 | 15.7 | 3.3 | 17.0 | 0.0 |
| Crab, Princes* | 1 Pot/35g | 36.0 | 1.0 | 104 | 13.4 | 4.8 | 3.5 | 0.0 |
| Crab, Tesco* | 1 Jar/75g | 116.0 | 6.0 | 155 | 14.4 | 4.6 | 8.4 | 0.1 |
| Salmon, Asda* | 1 Serving/53g | 76.0 | 4.0 | 143 | 15.0 | 5.0 | 7.0 | 0.0 |
| Salmon, Princes* | 1 Serving/30g | 58.0 | 4.0 | 195 | 13.5 | 6.5 | 12.8 | 0.0 |
| Salmon, Value, Tesco* | 1 Serving/10g | 16.0 | 1.0 | 165 | 14.0 | 4.6 | 10.1 | 0.8 |
| Salmon & Shrimp, Tesco* | 1 Jar/75g | 83.0 | 3.0 | 111 | 15.1 | 5.0 | 3.4 | 0.1 |
| Sardine & Tomato, Asda* | 1 Thin Spread/9g | 11.0 | 1.0 | 123 | 14.0 | 3.3 | 6.0 | 0.0 |
| Sardine & Tomato, Co-Op* | 1 Serving/25g | 34.0 | 1.0 | 135 | 16.0 | 3.0 | 6.0 | 2.0 |
| Sardine & Tomato, Princes* | 1 Jar/75g | 109.0 | 5.0 | 146 | 15.4 | 5.0 | 7.2 | 0.0 |
| Sardine & Tomato, Sainsbury's* | 1 Mini Pot/35g | 59.0 | 4.0 | 170 | 16.9 | 1.2 | 10.8 | 1.3 |
| Sardine & Tomato, Tesco* | 1 Jar/75g | 97.0 | 4.0 | 130 | 14.6 | 4.8 | 5.8 | 0.1 |
| Smokey Bacon, Princes* | 1 Serving/30g | 60.0 | 4.0 | 199 | 17.3 | 5.4 | 12.0 | 0.0 |
| Tuna & Mayonnaise, Princes* | 1 Pot/75g | 86.0 | 12.0 | 115 | 16.8 | 3.8 | 16.4 | 0.0 |
| Tuna & Mayonnaise, Sainsbury's* | 1 Tbsp/17g | 41.0 | 3.0 | 242 | 19.2 | 0.6 | 18.1 | 1.6 |
| Tuna & Mayonnaise, Tesco* | 1 Serving/15g | 31.0 | 2.0 | 209 | 14.9 | 2.1 | 15.7 | 0.1 |
| Vegetable, Sainsbury's* | 1 Serving/17g | 26.0 | 2.0 | 154 | 7.4 | 5.9 | 11.2 | 3.4 |
| **PASTILLES** | | | | | | | | |
| Blackcurrant, Rowntree's* | 1 Tube/53g | 188.0 | 0.0 | 353 | 4.4 | 84.0 | 0.0 | 0.0 |
| Fruit, Average | 1 Tube/33g | 108.0 | 0.0 | 327 | 2.8 | 84.2 | 0.0 | 0.0 |
| Fruit, Co-Op* | 1 Sweet/6g | 20.0 | 0.0 | 337 | 2.8 | 81.5 | 0.0 | 0.0 |
| Fruit, Rowntree's* | 1 Tube/53g | 186.0 | 0.0 | 351 | 4.4 | 83.7 | 0.0 | 0.0 |

**P**

| | Measure INFO/WEIGHT | per Measure KCAL | FAT | Nutrition Values per 100g / 100ml KCAL | PROT | CARB | FAT | FIBRE |
|---|---|---|---|---|---|---|---|---|
| **PASTILLES** | | | | | | | | |
| Fruit, Sainsbury's* | 1 Sweet/7g | 23.0 | 0.0 | 332 | 3.4 | 78.7 | 0.1 | 0.1 |
| **PASTRAMI** | | | | | | | | |
| *Beef, Average* | *1 Serving/40g* | *51.0* | *1.0* | *128* | *23.1* | *1.1* | *3.6* | *0.2* |
| *Turkey, Average* | *½ Packet/35g* | *38.0* | *1.0* | *107* | *21.8* | *1.7* | *1.5* | *0.5* |
| **PASTRY** | | | | | | | | |
| *Case, From Supermarket, Average* | *1 Case/230g* | *1081.0* | *59.0* | *470* | *5.8* | *55.9* | *25.6* | *1.2* |
| *Choux, Cooked, Average* | *1oz/28g* | *91.0* | *6.0* | *325* | *8.5* | *29.8* | *19.8* | *1.2* |
| *Choux, Raw, Average* | *1oz/28g* | *59.0* | *4.0* | *211* | *5.5* | *19.4* | *12.9* | *0.8* |
| *Filo, Average* | *1 Sheet/45g* | *137.0* | *1.0* | *304* | *9.0* | *61.4* | *2.7* | *0.9* |
| Filo, Frozen, Jus-Rol* | 1 Sheet/45g | 105.0 | 1.0 | 234 | 8.1 | 52.1 | 2.7 | 2.1 |
| *Flaky, Chinese, Average* | *1oz/28g* | *110.0* | *5.0* | *392* | *5.4* | *59.3* | *16.4* | *0.0* |
| *Flaky, Cooked, Average* | *1oz/28g* | *157.0* | *11.0* | *560* | *5.6* | *45.9* | *40.6* | *1.8* |
| *Flaky, Raw, Average* | *1oz/28g* | *119.0* | *9.0* | *424* | *4.2* | *34.8* | *30.7* | *1.4* |
| *Flan Case, Average* | *1 Case/113g* | *615.0* | *38.0* | *544* | *7.1* | *56.7* | *33.6* | *1.8* |
| *Greek, Average* | *1oz/28g* | *90.0* | *5.0* | *322* | *4.7* | *40.0* | *17.0* | *0.0* |
| Puff, Fresh, Sainsbury's* | ½ Pack/250g | 1112.0 | 86.0 | 445 | 5.4 | 28.8 | 34.3 | 1.3 |
| *Puff, Frozen, Average* | *1 Serving/47g* | *188.0* | *12.0* | *400* | *5.0* | *29.2* | *25.6* | *0.0* |
| *Shortcrust, Cooked, Average* | *1oz/28g* | *146.0* | *9.0* | *521* | *6.6* | *54.2* | *32.3* | *2.2* |
| *Shortcrust, Raw, Average* | *1oz/28g* | *127.0* | *8.0* | *453* | *5.6* | *44.0* | *29.1* | *1.3* |
| Spring Roll Wrapper, TYJ Food Manufacturing* | 1 Lge Sheet/18g | 54.0 | 0.0 | 300 | 0.0 | 73.0 | 0.0 | 0.0 |
| *Wholemeal, Cooked, Average* | *1oz/28g* | *140.0* | *9.0* | *499* | *8.9* | *44.6* | *32.9* | *6.3* |
| *Wholemeal, Raw, Average* | *1oz/28g* | *121.0* | *8.0* | *431* | *7.7* | *38.5* | *28.4* | *5.4* |
| **PASTY** | | | | | | | | |
| Cheddar & Onion, Hand Crimped, Waitrose* | 1 Pasty/200g | 546.0 | 42.0 | 273 | 8.8 | 22.5 | 21.1 | 2.2 |
| Cheese & Onion, Co-Op* | 1 Pasty/75g | 235.0 | 15.0 | 313 | 9.2 | 24.5 | 19.8 | 1.7 |
| Cheese & Onion, Farmfoods* | 1 Pasty/191g | 485.0 | 27.0 | 254 | 6.6 | 25.5 | 14.0 | 2.0 |
| Cheese & Onion, Freshbake* | 1 Pastry/135g | 368.0 | 22.0 | 272 | 5.6 | 25.5 | 16.6 | 1.1 |
| Cheese & Onion, Geo Adams* | 1 Pasty/150g | 420.0 | 23.0 | 280 | 6.9 | 27.9 | 15.6 | 1.1 |
| Cheese & Onion, Somerfield* | 1 Pasty/145g | 419.0 | 26.0 | 289 | 7.0 | 24.0 | 18.0 | 0.0 |
| Cheese & Onion, Tesco* | 1 Pasty/150g | 415.0 | 26.0 | 277 | 5.9 | 23.7 | 17.6 | 2.2 |
| Chicken, Port Royal* | 1 Pattie/130g | 289.0 | 11.0 | 222 | 5.5 | 31.2 | 8.4 | 0.0 |
| Chicken & Vegetable, Proper Cornish Ltd* | 1 Pasty/255g | 671.0 | 35.0 | 263 | 7.4 | 30.2 | 13.6 | 2.4 |
| Cornish, Asda* | 1 Pasty/100g | 287.0 | 19.0 | 287 | 7.0 | 22.0 | 19.0 | 1.2 |
| Cornish, BGTY, Sainsbury's* | 1 Pasty/135g | 308.0 | 13.0 | 228 | 7.7 | 28.2 | 9.4 | 1.6 |
| Cornish, Cheese & Onion, Ginsters* | 1 Pasty/130g | 511.0 | 33.0 | 393 | 10.4 | 30.7 | 25.4 | 2.3 |
| Cornish, Chicken & Bacon, Ginsters* | 1 Pasty/227g | 574.0 | 35.0 | 253 | 6.9 | 22.2 | 15.2 | 0.8 |
| Cornish, Co-Op* | 1 Pasty/75g | 200.0 | 12.0 | 267 | 6.4 | 23.4 | 16.4 | 1.6 |
| Cornish, Ginsters* | 1 Pasty/227g | 549.0 | 32.0 | 242 | 5.3 | 23.2 | 14.2 | 3.1 |
| Cornish, Mini, M & S* | 1 Pasty/75g | 244.0 | 18.0 | 325 | 7.3 | 21.9 | 23.4 | 1.8 |
| Cornish, Mini, Sainsbury's* | 1 Pasty/70g | 280.0 | 20.0 | 400 | 7.3 | 28.1 | 28.7 | 1.5 |
| Cornish, Mini, Tesco* | 1 Pasty/24g | 66.0 | 4.0 | 274 | 5.6 | 23.2 | 17.7 | 0.5 |
| Cornish, Pork Farms* | 1 Pasty/250g | 672.0 | 41.0 | 269 | 7.7 | 22.8 | 16.3 | 0.0 |
| Cornish, Safeway* | 1 Pasty/170g | 490.0 | 32.0 | 288 | 7.5 | 22.6 | 18.6 | 1.5 |
| Cornish, Sainsbury's* | 1 Pasty/150g | 489.0 | 32.0 | 326 | 6.7 | 26.6 | 21.4 | 2.0 |
| Cornish, SmartPrice, Asda* | 1 Pasty/94g | 286.0 | 15.0 | 304 | 8.0 | 32.0 | 16.0 | 1.7 |
| Cornish, Tesco* | 1 Pasty/150g | 466.0 | 33.0 | 311 | 6.8 | 21.9 | 21.8 | 1.6 |
| Cornish, Traditional Style, Geo Adams* | 1 Pasty/165g | 488.0 | 30.0 | 296 | 7.1 | 25.4 | 18.4 | 1.3 |
| Cornish, Value, Tesco* | 1 Pasty/150g | 425.0 | 27.0 | 283 | 6.7 | 24.2 | 17.7 | 2.2 |
| Cornish Roaster, Ginsters* | 1 Pasty/130g | 417.0 | 24.0 | 321 | 8.5 | 29.9 | 18.6 | 1.3 |
| Lamb, Port Royal* | 1 Pattie/130g | 352.0 | 17.0 | 271 | 7.2 | 30.5 | 13.4 | 0.0 |
| Salt Fish, Port Royal* | 1 Pattie/130g | 300.0 | 13.0 | 231 | 6.8 | 27.8 | 10.3 | 0.0 |
| Tandoori & Vegetable, Holland & Barrett* | 1 Pack/110g | 232.0 | 9.0 | 211 | 4.3 | 29.4 | 8.5 | 1.8 |
| Vegetable, Hand Crimped, Waitrose* | 1 Pasty/200g | 454.0 | 23.0 | 227 | 4.5 | 26.8 | 11.3 | 2.2 |

| | Measure INFO/WEIGHT | per Measure KCAL | FAT | Nutrition Values per 100g / 100ml KCAL | PROT | CARB | FAT | FIBRE |
|---|---|---|---|---|---|---|---|---|

## PASTY

| | | | | | | | | |
|---|---|---|---|---|---|---|---|---|
| Vegetarian, Country Slice, Linda McCartney* | 1 Pasty/150g | 373.0 | 20.0 | 249 | 5.6 | 26.5 | 13.5 | 2.9 |
| Vegetarian, Port Royal* | 1 Pattie/130g | 315.0 | 14.0 | 242 | 12.5 | 24.1 | 10.6 | 0.0 |

## PATE

| | | | | | | | | |
|---|---|---|---|---|---|---|---|---|
| Apricot, Asda* | 1 Serving/50g | 156.0 | 14.0 | 312 | 12.0 | 3.0 | 28.0 | 0.0 |
| Ardennes, Asda* | 1 Serving/50g | 143.0 | 12.0 | 286 | 13.9 | 3.6 | 24.0 | 1.3 |
| Ardennes, BGTY, Sainsbury's* | ¼ Pack/50g | 90.0 | 6.0 | 180 | 16.6 | 2.9 | 11.4 | 0.0 |
| Ardennes, HL, Tesco* | ½ Pack/88g | 154.0 | 11.0 | 176 | 12.1 | 3.6 | 12.6 | 1.8 |
| Ardennes, Iceland* | 1 Serving/70g | 223.0 | 20.0 | 318 | 12.0 | 3.4 | 28.5 | 0.5 |
| Ardennes, Reduced Fat, Safeway* | 1 Serving/50g | 97.0 | 6.0 | 194 | 18.5 | 3.1 | 11.9 | 0.1 |
| Ardennes, Reduced Fat, Waitrose* | ¼ Pack/42g | 94.0 | 7.0 | 224 | 15.4 | 2.6 | 16.9 | 0.5 |
| Ardennes, Tesco* | 1 Tbsp/15g | 53.0 | 5.0 | 354 | 13.3 | 0.5 | 33.2 | 1.2 |
| Ardennes, with Bacon, Tesco* | ½ Pack/85g | 241.0 | 21.0 | 284 | 11.4 | 5.1 | 24.2 | 1.1 |
| Asparagus, Sainsbury's* | ½ Pot/58g | 88.0 | 8.0 | 153 | 3.4 | 5.4 | 13.1 | 1.0 |
| Bean Feast, Redwood* | 1 Serving/60g | 161.0 | 10.0 | 268 | 7.3 | 21.1 | 17.0 | 3.8 |
| Breton, Country, with Apricots, Coarse, Sainsbury's* | 1 Serving/21g | 60.0 | 5.0 | 285 | 13.5 | 7.0 | 22.5 | 0.5 |
| Brie & Cranberry, M & S* | 1 Serving/55g | 192.0 | 18.0 | 350 | 6.0 | 7.3 | 33.3 | 1.5 |
| Brussels, & Garlic, Reduced Fat, Tesco* | 1 Serving/65g | 135.0 | 8.0 | 208 | 16.2 | 8.1 | 12.3 | 0.6 |
| Brussels, & Garlic, Tesco* | 1 Serving/40g | 145.0 | 14.0 | 363 | 8.7 | 6.0 | 33.8 | 0.0 |
| Brussels, & Mushroom, Mini, GFY, Asda* | 1 Pack/40g | 67.0 | 4.0 | 167 | 14.7 | 2.3 | 11.0 | 3.9 |
| Brussels, 25% Less Fat, Morrisons* | ¼ Pack/43g | 106.0 | 9.0 | 249 | 14.2 | 0.7 | 20.6 | 0.0 |
| Brussels, BGTY, 50% Less Fat, Sainsbury's* | 1 Serving/100g | 223.0 | 16.0 | 223 | 14.6 | 5.1 | 16.0 | 0.1 |
| Brussels, Finest, Tesco* | ½ Pack/85g | 306.0 | 29.0 | 360 | 8.6 | 5.2 | 33.8 | 0.8 |
| Brussels, HL, Tesco* | 1 Serving/29g | 66.0 | 4.0 | 229 | 14.4 | 8.4 | 15.3 | 1.8 |
| Brussels, M & S* | 1 Pot/170g | 518.0 | 45.0 | 305 | 13.3 | 2.8 | 26.6 | 1.0 |
| Brussels, Sainsbury's* | 1 Pack/170g | 663.0 | 65.0 | 390 | 10.6 | 1.1 | 38.2 | 0.1 |
| Brussels, Smooth, 50% Less Fat, Tesco* | 1 Pack/175g | 350.0 | 27.0 | 200 | 14.1 | 1.2 | 15.3 | 1.8 |
| Brussels, Smooth, Reduced Fat, Tesco* | 1 Serving/15g | 30.0 | 2.0 | 200 | 14.1 | 1.2 | 15.3 | 1.8 |
| Brussels, Smooth, Spreadable, Sainsbury's* | 1 Serving/30g | 97.0 | 9.0 | 323 | 10.7 | 4.7 | 29.0 | 0.0 |
| Brussels, Tesco* | 1 Serving/28g | 92.0 | 9.0 | 330 | 11.0 | 3.0 | 30.5 | 1.1 |
| Brussels, with Forest Mushroom, Co-Op* | 1 Serving/57g | 180.0 | 17.0 | 315 | 12.0 | 2.0 | 29.0 | 1.0 |
| Brussels, with Garlic, Asda* | 1 Serving/50g | 170.0 | 16.0 | 340 | 10.7 | 4.0 | 31.3 | 2.5 |
| Brussels, with Herbs, Tesco* | 1 Serving/25g | 87.0 | 8.0 | 347 | 8.4 | 6.4 | 32.6 | 1.5 |
| Carrot, Ginger & Spring Onion, M & S* | 1 Serving/50g | 72.0 | 5.0 | 145 | 1.5 | 9.6 | 11.0 | 0.9 |
| Celery, Stilton & Walnut, Waitrose* | 1 Pot/115g | 294.0 | 26.0 | 256 | 9.0 | 3.2 | 23.0 | 2.2 |
| Chargrilled Vegetable, BGTY, Sainsbury's* | ½ Pot/57g | 43.0 | 1.0 | 75 | 4.9 | 10.8 | 1.3 | 2.7 |
| Chick Pea & Black Olive, Cauldron Foods* | 1 Pot/113g | 193.0 | 12.0 | 171 | 7.6 | 11.4 | 10.5 | 6.6 |
| Chicken & Brandy, Morrisons* | 1 Serving/44g | 133.0 | 12.0 | 303 | 10.8 | 4.3 | 26.9 | 0.8 |
| Chicken Liver, & Brandy, Asda* | 1 Serving/50g | 176.0 | 16.0 | 353 | 9.0 | 5.5 | 32.8 | 3.2 |
| Chicken Liver, & Garlic, Smooth, Asda* | 1 Serving/31g | 119.0 | 11.0 | 388 | 9.0 | 7.0 | 36.0 | 3.2 |
| Chicken Liver, Asda* | 1 Serving/65g | 131.0 | 10.0 | 202 | 13.0 | 4.0 | 16.0 | 0.8 |
| Chicken Liver, BGTY, Sainsbury's* | 1 Serving/30g | 64.0 | 5.0 | 214 | 11.5 | 6.0 | 16.0 | 0.5 |
| Chicken Liver, Organic, Waitrose* | ½ Tub/88g | 204.0 | 16.0 | 233 | 12.6 | 1.8 | 18.4 | 1.4 |
| Chicken Liver Parfait, TTD, Sainsbury's* | 1 Serving/20g | 72.0 | 7.0 | 359 | 8.0 | 2.0 | 35.0 | 0.5 |
| Coarse Farmhouse, Organic, Sainsbury's* | 1 Serving/56g | 138.0 | 11.0 | 246 | 13.3 | 3.7 | 19.7 | 0.8 |
| Coarse Pork Liver with Garlic, Asda* | 1 Pack/40g | 130.0 | 12.0 | 326 | 13.0 | 1.0 | 30.0 | 0.0 |
| De Campagne, Sainsbury's* | 1 Serving/55g | 129.0 | 10.0 | 235 | 16.3 | 1.4 | 18.2 | 0.0 |
| Duck & Orange, Asda* | 1 Serving/40g | 94.0 | 7.0 | 235 | 16.0 | 2.2 | 18.0 | 0.0 |
| Duck & Orange, Smooth, Tesco* | 1 Serving/50g | 188.0 | 18.0 | 377 | 10.5 | 4.0 | 35.4 | 0.5 |
| Duck & Truffle, Medallions, M & S* | 1 Serving/25g | 91.0 | 9.0 | 365 | 9.0 | 4.8 | 35.0 | 1.4 |
| Duck Liver with Champagne & Truffles, TTD, Sainsbury's* | 1 Serving/50g | 211.0 | 21.0 | 423 | 8.2 | 2.5 | 42.2 | 0.0 |
| Farmhouse Mushroom, Asda* | 1 Serving/50g | 126.0 | 10.0 | 252 | 13.0 | 5.0 | 20.0 | 0.7 |
| Farmhouse Style, Finest, Tesco* | 1 Serving/28g | 83.0 | 7.0 | 295 | 11.9 | 3.6 | 25.9 | 1.0 |
| Farmhouse Style, M & S* | ¼ Pack/42g | 90.0 | 7.0 | 215 | 14.4 | 1.9 | 16.9 | 1.2 |

| | Measure INFO/WEIGHT | per Measure KCAL | FAT | Nutrition Values per 100g / 100ml KCAL | PROT | CARB | FAT | FIBRE |
|---|---|---|---|---|---|---|---|---|
| **PATE** | | | | | | | | |
| Farmhouse Style, Weight Watchers* | 1 Serving/37g | 49.0 | 2.0 | 133 | 14.8 | 5.5 | 5.7 | 0.5 |
| Farmhouse with Herbes De Provence, Tesco* | 1 Serving/50g | 136.0 | 11.0 | 273 | 13.9 | 5.4 | 21.6 | 1.0 |
| Farmhouse with Mushrooms & Garlic, Tesco* | 1 Serving/90g | 256.0 | 23.0 | 285 | 13.8 | 0.6 | 25.3 | 1.3 |
| Forestiere, M & S* | 1 Serving/20g | 61.0 | 5.0 | 305 | 11.5 | 4.2 | 26.6 | 1.4 |
| Herb, Organic, Suma* | 1 Serving/25g | 58.0 | 4.0 | 234 | 12.0 | 6.0 | 18.0 | 0.0 |
| Isle of Skye Smoked Salmon, TTD, Sainsbury's* | ½ Pot/58g | 161.0 | 13.0 | 277 | 16.5 | 0.8 | 23.1 | 0.1 |
| Kipper, Waitrose* | ¼ Tub/28g | 105.0 | 9.0 | 370 | 16.8 | 2.0 | 32.7 | 0.6 |
| Liver, Value, Tesco* | 1 Serving/50g | 151.0 | 13.0 | 302 | 13.0 | 4.1 | 26.0 | 0.5 |
| Liver & Bacon, Tesco* | 1 Serving/10g | 28.0 | 2.0 | 276 | 12.9 | 4.3 | 23.0 | 0.4 |
| Liver & Pork, HE, Tesco* | 1 Serving/28g | 64.0 | 4.0 | 229 | 14.4 | 8.4 | 15.3 | 1.3 |
| Mackerel, Tesco* | 1 Serving/29g | 102.0 | 9.0 | 353 | 14.3 | 0.5 | 32.6 | 0.0 |
| Mediterranean Roast Vegetable, Tesco* | 1 Serving/28g | 31.0 | 3.0 | 112 | 2.4 | 4.3 | 9.4 | 1.2 |
| Mushroom, BGTY, Sainsbury's* | ½ Pot/58g | 29.0 | 0.0 | 50 | 4.6 | 6.7 | 0.5 | 3.0 |
| Mushroom, M & S* | 1 Pot/115g | 224.0 | 20.0 | 195 | 4.2 | 4.8 | 17.5 | 1.5 |
| Mushroom, Roast, Tesco* | 1 Serving/25g | 36.0 | 3.0 | 145 | 3.6 | 3.6 | 12.9 | 4.5 |
| Mushroom, Sainsbury's* | ½ Pot/58g | 89.0 | 7.0 | 153 | 3.3 | 7.8 | 12.1 | 2.1 |
| Mushroom & Tarragon, Cauldron Foods* | 1 Pot/113g | 118.0 | 9.0 | 104 | 2.7 | 5.9 | 8.3 | 1.2 |
| Pheasant, TTD, Sainsbury's* | 1/6 Pack/28g | 59.0 | 4.0 | 212 | 15.4 | 3.9 | 15.0 | 0.8 |
| Pork, with Apple & Cider, Sainsbury's* | 1 Serving/50g | 151.0 | 13.0 | 303 | 12.5 | 6.3 | 25.3 | 1.1 |
| Pork, with Peppercorns, Tesco* | 1 Serving/28g | 84.0 | 8.0 | 300 | 12.9 | 1.4 | 26.8 | 0.7 |
| Pork with Port & Cranberry, Tesco* | 1 Serving/28g | 83.0 | 7.0 | 296 | 12.1 | 4.3 | 25.6 | 0.6 |
| Ricotta, Subdried Tomato & Basil, Princes* | 1 Jar/110g | 343.0 | 32.0 | 312 | 5.2 | 8.3 | 28.7 | 0.0 |
| Roasted Red Pepper, Princes* | 1 Serving/35g | 47.0 | 2.0 | 135 | 4.8 | 17.6 | 5.0 | 0.0 |
| Roasted Red Pepper & Houmous, Princes* | ¼ Jar/27g | 32.0 | 2.0 | 120 | 4.6 | 12.4 | 5.8 | 0.0 |
| Roasted Vegetable, COU, M & S* | 1 Pot/115g | 86.0 | 2.0 | 75 | 6.2 | 9.1 | 1.5 | 1.4 |
| Roasted Vegetable & Feta, Cauldron Foods* | 1 Pot/115g | 148.0 | 8.0 | 129 | 4.3 | 10.0 | 7.1 | 2.1 |
| Salmon, John West* | 1 Serving/50g | 136.0 | 12.0 | 272 | 14.9 | 0.0 | 23.5 | 0.2 |
| Salmon Dill, Princes* | 1 Serving/70g | 124.0 | 8.0 | 177 | 15.4 | 4.0 | 11.1 | 0.5 |
| Salsa, Princes* | 1 Serving/25g | 21.0 | 0.0 | 84 | 3.6 | 16.7 | 0.3 | 0.0 |
| Scottish Smoked Salmon, M & S* | 1 Serving/30g | 81.0 | 7.0 | 270 | 17.0 | 0.2 | 22.3 | 0.0 |
| Smoked Duck, with Cranberry Coulis, TTD, Sainsbury's* | 1 Serving/62g | 174.0 | 14.0 | 280 | 10.7 | 9.3 | 22.2 | 1.0 |
| Smoked Mackerel, Sainsbury's* | ½ Pot/57g | 215.0 | 20.0 | 378 | 14.2 | 0.8 | 35.3 | 0.0 |
| Smoked Mackerel, Scottish, M & S* | ½ Pot/58g | 158.0 | 13.0 | 275 | 15.9 | 0.6 | 23.2 | 0.1 |
| Smoked Salmon, Luxury, Morrisons* | ½ Pot/57g | 150.0 | 12.0 | 266 | 16.0 | 0.9 | 22.0 | 0.5 |
| Smoked Salmon, Organic, Waitrose* | 1oz/28g | 83.0 | 7.0 | 296 | 13.9 | 2.4 | 25.6 | 0.0 |
| Smoked Salmon, Tesco* | 1 Pack/115g | 282.0 | 22.0 | 245 | 15.0 | 3.0 | 19.1 | 1.0 |
| Smoked Salmon, Waitrose* | ½ Pot/57g | 120.0 | 9.0 | 212 | 17.1 | 0.5 | 15.7 | 0.6 |
| Smoked Trout, Waitrose* | ½ Pot/56g | 130.0 | 10.0 | 232 | 15.8 | 0.9 | 18.4 | 0.6 |
| Spiced Parsnip & Carrot, Organic, Asda* | ½ Pot/58g | 63.0 | 3.0 | 109 | 3.7 | 10.0 | 6.0 | 2.6 |
| Spicy Bean, BGTY, Sainsbury's* | ½ Pot/58g | 56.0 | 1.0 | 97 | 5.0 | 15.1 | 1.9 | 5.4 |
| Spicy Bean, Princes* | ½ Pot/55g | 46.0 | 0.0 | 84 | 3.6 | 16.7 | 0.3 | 0.0 |
| Spicy Bean, Weight Watchers* | 1 Serving/37g | 33.0 | 1.0 | 89 | 5.7 | 12.9 | 1.6 | 4.2 |
| Spicy Mexican, Organic, Waitrose* | 1 Serving/50g | 57.0 | 3.0 | 115 | 6.2 | 8.6 | 6.2 | 3.5 |
| **PAVLOVA** | | | | | | | | |
| Bucks Fizz Mini Champagne, Co-Op* | 1 Pavlova/19g | 62.0 | 3.0 | 325 | 3.0 | 38.0 | 18.0 | 0.5 |
| Mandarin, Mini, Iceland* | 1 Pavlova/22g | 59.0 | 3.0 | 268 | 2.1 | 37.9 | 12.0 | 1.7 |
| Raspberry, Co-Op* | 1/6 Pavlova/49g | 147.0 | 6.0 | 300 | 3.2 | 44.8 | 12.0 | 1.1 |
| Raspberry, Individual, M & S* | 1 Pavlova/65g | 133.0 | 2.0 | 205 | 4.0 | 41.8 | 2.4 | 0.2 |
| Raspberry, M & S* | 1 Serving/84g | 193.0 | 8.0 | 230 | 2.3 | 33.3 | 9.6 | 0.3 |
| Raspberry, Mini, Co-Op* | 1 Pavlova/19g | 61.0 | 2.0 | 320 | 3.0 | 56.0 | 9.0 | 0.6 |
| Raspberry, Sara Lee* | 1/6 Pavlova/55g | 168.0 | 8.0 | 303 | 2.7 | 38.5 | 15.3 | 1.1 |
| Raspberry, Tesco* | 1 Serving/65g | 191.0 | 8.0 | 294 | 2.7 | 41.8 | 12.9 | 1.1 |
| Raspberry & Lemon, Asda* | 1 Serving/43g | 102.0 | 2.0 | 235 | 2.8 | 46.0 | 4.4 | 0.5 |

| | Measure INFO/WEIGHT | per Measure KCAL | FAT | Nutrition Values per 100g / 100ml KCAL | PROT | CARB | FAT | FIBRE |
|---|---|---|---|---|---|---|---|---|
| **PAVLOVA** | | | | | | | | |
| Sticky Toffee, Sainsbury's* | 1/6 Pavlova/60g | 249.0 | 10.0 | 415 | 3.7 | 63.1 | 16.4 | 0.9 |
| Strawberry, Co-Op* | 1 Serving/52g | 177.0 | 7.0 | 340 | 3.0 | 50.0 | 14.0 | 0.4 |
| Strawberry, Farmfoods* | 1/6 Pavlova/52g | 152.0 | 8.0 | 292 | 2.3 | 36.9 | 15.0 | 2.2 |
| Strawberry & Champagne, Mini, Co-Op* | 1 Pavlova/19g | 65.0 | 4.0 | 340 | 3.0 | 40.0 | 19.0 | 0.8 |
| Toffee, Co-Op* | 1/6 Pavlova/53g | 193.0 | 8.0 | 365 | 3.0 | 52.0 | 16.0 | 0.6 |
| Toffee, Mini, Iceland* | 1 Pavlova/19g | 68.0 | 3.0 | 353 | 3.0 | 51.5 | 15.0 | 1.9 |
| **PAW-PAW** | | | | | | | | |
| *Raw, Fresh* | *1oz/28g* | *10.0* | *0.0* | *36* | *0.5* | *8.8* | *0.1* | *2.2* |
| *Raw, Weighed with Skin & Pips* | *1oz/28g* | *8.0* | *0.0* | *27* | *0.4* | *6.6* | *0.1* | *1.7* |
| **PEACH** | | | | | | | | |
| *Dried, Average* | *1 Pack/250g* | *472.0* | *2.0* | *189* | *2.5* | *44.9* | *0.6* | *6.9* |
| *in Fruit Juice, Average* | *1oz/28g* | *13.0* | *0.0* | *47* | *0.5* | *11.2* | *0.0* | *0.7* |
| *in Syrup, Average* | *1oz/28g* | *19.0* | *0.0* | *67* | *0.4* | *16.3* | *0.1* | *0.4* |
| Pieces in Strawberry Jelly, Fruitini, Del Monte* | 1 Can/140g | 91.0 | 0.0 | 65 | 0.3 | 15.3 | 0.1 | 0.0 |
| *Raw, Average* | *1 Peach/125g* | *39.0* | *0.0* | *31* | *0.9* | *7.2* | *0.1* | *1.4* |
| Raw, Stoned | 1oz/28g | 11.0 | 0.0 | 39 | 0.9 | 9.5 | 0.2 | 1.5 |
| **PEANUT BRITTLE** | | | | | | | | |
| Thorntons* | 2 Pieces/32g | 163.0 | 9.0 | 509 | 12.4 | 54.3 | 26.9 | 2.6 |
| **PEANUT BUTTER** | | | | | | | | |
| Creamy, Smooth, Sun Pat* | 1 Serving/15g | 93.0 | 8.0 | 620 | 24.0 | 17.5 | 50.2 | 6.1 |
| Crunchy, Asda* | 1 Serving/10g | 61.0 | 5.0 | 611 | 28.0 | 12.0 | 51.0 | 6.0 |
| Crunchy, Bettabuy, Morrisons* | 1 Serving/10g | 61.0 | 5.0 | 606 | 22.5 | 17.3 | 52.2 | 5.7 |
| Crunchy, Organic, No Added Sugar, Waitrose* | 1 Serving/12g | 71.0 | 6.0 | 595 | 14.6 | 9.9 | 50.8 | 7.1 |
| Crunchy, Organic, Tesco* | 1 Serving/25g | 149.0 | 12.0 | 595 | 23.6 | 12.5 | 49.7 | 6.9 |
| Crunchy, Original Style, Whole Earth* | 1 Serving/20g | 118.0 | 10.0 | 592 | 24.9 | 10.1 | 50.2 | 7.3 |
| Crunchy, Sainsbury's* | 1 Serving/10g | 59.0 | 5.0 | 594 | 23.2 | 12.4 | 50.2 | 6.7 |
| Crunchy, Tesco* | 1 Serving/20g | 123.0 | 10.0 | 614 | 27.8 | 12.0 | 50.5 | 6.5 |
| Crunchy, Whole Nut, Organic, Meridian Foods* | 1 Serving/28g | 171.0 | 14.0 | 612 | 31.2 | 12.2 | 48.7 | 6.5 |
| Extra Crunchy, Sun Pat* | 1 Serving/20g | 119.0 | 10.0 | 597 | 21.9 | 12.6 | 51.0 | 7.3 |
| SmartPrice, Asda* | 1 Serving/15g | 87.0 | 7.0 | 582 | 23.0 | 10.0 | 50.0 | 6.0 |
| Smooth, 25% Less Fat, Tesco* | 1 Serving/15g | 85.0 | 6.0 | 555 | 20.5 | 31.0 | 38.7 | 5.5 |
| Smooth, 33% Less Fat, BGTY, Sainsbury's* | 1 Serving/10g | 53.0 | 4.0 | 533 | 22.6 | 31.7 | 35.1 | 6.7 |
| Smooth, Average | 1 Serving/20g | 125.0 | 11.0 | 623 | 22.6 | 13.1 | 53.7 | 5.4 |
| Smooth, Kraft* | 1 Serving/20g | 127.0 | 11.0 | 636 | 23.1 | 17.6 | 53.5 | 0.0 |
| Smooth, Light, Kraft* | 1 Serving/20g | 114.0 | 8.0 | 571 | 16.3 | 40.1 | 38.6 | 0.0 |
| Smooth, Morrisons* | 1 Serving/10g | 60.0 | 5.0 | 596 | 23.3 | 12.4 | 50.3 | 0.0 |
| Smooth, No Added Sugar, Organic, Whole Earth* | 1 Serving/20g | 119.0 | 10.0 | 595 | 24.5 | 9.9 | 50.8 | 7.1 |
| Smooth, Organic, Meridian Foods* | 1 Serving/10g | 61.0 | 5.0 | 612 | 31.2 | 12.2 | 48.7 | 6.5 |
| Smooth, Organic, Waitrose* | 1 Serving/12g | 71.0 | 6.0 | 595 | 24.6 | 9.9 | 50.8 | 7.1 |
| Smooth, Sun Pat* | 1 Serving/20g | 120.0 | 10.0 | 601 | 25.0 | 15.2 | 48.9 | 6.7 |
| Smooth, Tesco* | 1 Serving/20g | 123.0 | 10.0 | 614 | 27.8 | 12.0 | 50.5 | 6.5 |
| Stripy, Sun Pat* | 1 Tsp/10g | 62.0 | 5.0 | 617 | 13.0 | 35.0 | 47.0 | 3.0 |
| Whole Nut, Crunchy, Average | 1 Tsp/10g | 61.0 | 5.0 | 606 | 24.9 | 7.7 | 53.1 | 6.0 |
| Wholenut, Sainsbury's* | 1 Serving/15g | 90.0 | 8.0 | 598 | 24.2 | 9.8 | 51.3 | 7.0 |
| Wholenut, Tesco* | 1 Tbsp/15g | 95.0 | 8.0 | 620 | 24.0 | 12.9 | 52.1 | 6.9 |
| **PEANUT SHOOTS** | | | | | | | | |
| Cooked with Oil, Sainsbury's* | 1 Pack/80g | 177.0 | 14.0 | 221 | 10.6 | 4.1 | 16.9 | 2.5 |
| Raw, without Oil, Sainsbury's* | 1 Serving/80g | 48.0 | 0.0 | 60 | 10.6 | 4.1 | 0.0 | 2.5 |
| **PEANUTS** | | | | | | | | |
| Chilli, Average | ½ Pack/50g | 303.0 | 25.0 | 605 | 28.2 | 9.3 | 50.6 | 6.8 |
| Dry Roasted, Average | 1 Serving/20g | 117.0 | 10.0 | 587 | 25.7 | 11.5 | 48.8 | 6.5 |
| Honey Roasted, Average | 1oz/28g | 169.0 | 13.0 | 605 | 26.8 | 23.5 | 47.0 | 5.5 |
| Hot Chilli, Holland & Barrett* | 1 Pack/100g | 523.0 | 31.0 | 523 | 14.0 | 47.0 | 31.0 | 5.5 |

| | Measure INFO/WEIGHT | per Measure KCAL | FAT | Nutrition Values per 100g / 100ml KCAL | PROT | CARB | FAT | FIBRE |
|---|---|---|---|---|---|---|---|---|
| **PEANUTS** | | | | | | | | |
| Milk Chocolate Coated, Graze* | 1 Pack/35g | 187.0 | 13.0 | 533 | 14.6 | 34.9 | 37.3 | 0.0 |
| *Plain, Average* | *10 Whole/10g* | *59.0* | *5.0* | *592* | *24.7* | *11.0* | *50.0* | *6.3* |
| Roast, Salted, Average | 10 Nuts/12g | 74.0 | 6.0 | 614 | 27.8 | 7.9 | 52.4 | 4.9 |
| Salted, Average | 10 Peanuts/6g | 37.0 | 3.0 | 609 | 27.0 | 8.3 | 52.0 | 5.4 |
| White Chocolate Coated, Graze* | 1 Pack/30g | 166.0 | 12.0 | 553 | 14.7 | 37.8 | 39.3 | 0.0 |
| Yoghurt Coated, Graze* | 1 Pack/35g | 189.0 | 12.0 | 540 | 9.9 | 48.1 | 35.1 | 0.0 |
| **PEARL BARLEY** | | | | | | | | |
| *Boiled* | *1oz/28g* | *34.0* | *0.0* | *123* | *2.3* | *28.2* | *0.4* | *0.0* |
| *Raw, Average* | *1oz/28g* | *99.0* | *0.0* | *352* | *9.9* | *77.7* | *1.2* | *15.6* |
| **PEARS** | | | | | | | | |
| *Abate Fetel, Average* | *1 Med/133g* | *48.0* | *0.0* | *36* | *0.4* | *8.3* | *0.1* | *2.2* |
| *Asian, Nashi, Raw, Average* | *1 Large/209g* | *88.0* | *0.0* | *42* | *0.5* | *10.6* | *0.2* | *3.6* |
| Blush, Morrisons* | 1 Sm/148g | 86.0 | 0.0 | 58 | 0.4 | 15.5 | 0.1 | 3.1 |
| Cape, Quartered, Tesco* | 1 Serving/100g | 35.0 | 0.0 | 35 | 0.3 | 8.5 | 0.0 | 1.4 |
| *Comice, Raw, Weighed with Core* | *1 Med/170g* | *56.0* | *0.0* | *33* | *0.3* | *8.5* | *0.0* | *2.0* |
| *Conference, Average* | *1 Lge/209g* | *102.0* | *0.0* | *49* | *0.3* | *11.6* | *0.2* | *2.3* |
| Dessert, Green, Sainsbury's* | 1 Sm/135g | 53.0 | 0.0 | 39 | 0.3 | 9.2 | 0.1 | 2.0 |
| *Dried, Average* | *1 Pear Half/16g* | *33.0* | *0.0* | *204* | *1.9* | *48.4* | *0.5* | *9.7* |
| *in Fruit Juice, Average* | *1 Serving/225g* | *102.0* | *0.0* | *45* | *0.3* | *10.9* | *0.0* | *1.2* |
| *in Syrup, Average* | *1oz/28g* | *16.0* | *0.0* | *58* | *0.2* | *14.4* | *0.1* | *1.4* |
| *Prickly, Raw, Fresh* | *1oz/28g* | *14.0* | *0.0* | *49* | *0.7* | *11.5* | *0.3* | *0.0* |
| *Raw, Weighed with Core, Average* | *1 Lge/209g* | *78.0* | *0.0* | *37* | *0.3* | *9.1* | *0.1* | *1.4* |
| Red, Tesco* | 1 Med/180g | 65.0 | 0.0 | 36 | 0.4 | 8.3 | 0.1 | 2.2 |
| *William, Raw, Average* | *1 Med/170g* | *58.0* | *0.0* | *34* | *0.4* | *8.3* | *0.1* | *2.2* |
| **PEAS** | | | | | | | | |
| *Dried, Boiled in Unsalted Water, Average* | *1oz/28g* | *31.0* | *0.0* | *109* | *6.9* | *19.9* | *0.8* | *5.5* |
| *Dried, Raw, Average* | *1oz/28g* | *85.0* | *1.0* | *303* | *21.6* | *52.0* | *2.4* | *13.0* |
| *Edible Podded, Whole, Raw* | *1 Cup/63g* | *26.0* | *0.0* | *42* | *2.8* | *7.6* | *0.2* | *2.6* |
| *Frozen, Average* | *1 Serving/85g* | *55.0* | *1.0* | *64* | *5.4* | *9.0* | *0.8* | *4.9* |
| *Frozen, Boiled, Average* | *1 Serving/75g* | *51.0* | *1.0* | *68* | *6.0* | *9.4* | *0.9* | *5.1* |
| *Garden, Canned, No Sugar Or Salt, Average* | *1 Can/80g* | *36.0* | *0.0* | *45* | *4.4* | *6.0* | *0.4* | *2.8* |
| *Garden, Canned, with Sugar & Salt, Average* | *1 Serving/90g* | *59.0* | *1.0* | *66* | *5.3* | *9.3* | *0.7* | *5.1* |
| *Garden, Frozen, Average* | *1 Serving/90g* | *66.0* | *1.0* | *74* | *6.3* | *9.7* | *1.1* | *3.3* |
| *Garden, Minted, Average* | *1 Serving/80g* | *59.0* | *1.0* | *74* | *6.3* | *9.7* | *1.1* | *5.9* |
| Hand Shelled, & Baby Leeks, Sainsbury's* | 1 Serving/120g | 59.0 | 1.0 | 49 | 4.0 | 5.8 | 1.2 | 3.3 |
| *Marrowfat, Average* | *1 Sm Can/160g* | *140.0* | *1.0* | *88* | *6.4* | *14.3* | *0.6* | *3.9* |
| *Mushy, Average* | *1 Can/200g* | *173.0* | *1.0* | *86* | *6.2* | *14.3* | *0.5* | *2.2* |
| *Processed, Canned, Average* | *1 Sm Can/220g* | *176.0* | *2.0* | *80* | *6.1* | *12.3* | *0.8* | *3.6* |
| *Snow* | *1 Serving/80g* | *24.0* | *0.0* | *29* | *3.3* | *3.9* | *0.2* | *2.1* |
| *Sugar Snap, Average* | *1 Serving/80g* | *27.0* | *0.0* | *34* | *3.3* | *4.9* | *0.2* | *1.4* |
| **PEASE PUDDING** | | | | | | | | |
| Canned, Re-Heated, Drained | 1oz/28g | 26.0 | 0.0 | 93 | 6.8 | 16.1 | 0.6 | 1.8 |
| **PECAN NUTS** | | | | | | | | |
| *Average* | *3 Nuts/18g* | *125.0* | *13.0* | *692* | *10.0* | *5.6* | *70.1* | *4.7* |
| Honey, Graze* | 1 Pack/26g | 160.0 | 14.0 | 614 | 6.7 | 39.4 | 52.0 | 0.0 |
| **PENNE** | | | | | | | | |
| *Cooked, Average* | *1 Serving/185g* | *244.0* | *1.0* | *132* | *4.7* | *26.7* | *0.7* | *1.1* |
| Corn, Free From, Dry Weight, Sainsbury's* | 1 Serving/100g | 348.0 | 2.0 | 348 | 7.6 | 74.2 | 2.3 | 5.2 |
| *Dry, Average* | *1 Serving/100g* | *352.0* | *2.0* | *352* | *12.4* | *71.3* | *1.9* | *2.7* |
| *Egg, Fresh, Average* | *1 Serving/125g* | *352.0* | *4.0* | *282* | *11.1* | *52.2* | *3.2* | *2.0* |
| Free From, Tesco* | 1 Serving/100g | 340.0 | 2.0 | 340 | 8.0 | 72.5 | 2.0 | 2.5 |
| *Fresh, Dry, Average* | *1 Serving/125g* | *222.0* | *2.0* | *178* | *7.3* | *32.2* | *1.9* | *1.6* |
| *Organic, Dry, Average* | *1 Serving/100g* | *352.0* | *2.0* | *352* | *12.4* | *71.6* | *1.8* | *1.9* |

| | Measure INFO/WEIGHT | KCAL | FAT | KCAL | PROT | CARB | FAT | FIBRE |
|---|---|---|---|---|---|---|---|---|
| **PENNE** | | | | | | | | |
| *Rigate, Dry Weight, Average* | *1 Serving/90g* | *318.0* | *2.0* | *353* | *12.3* | *72.1* | *1.8* | *1.8* |
| Wholewheat, Authentic, Italiano, Tesco* | 1 Cooked Portion/75g | 244.0 | 2.0 | 325 | 12.5 | 62.5 | 2.5 | 9.0 |
| **PEPERAMI*** | | | | | | | | |
| Firestick, Peperami* | 1 Stick/25g | 127.0 | 11.0 | 508 | 24.5 | 3.5 | 44.0 | 1.2 |
| Hot, Peperami* | 1 Stick/25g | 126.0 | 11.0 | 504 | 24.5 | 2.5 | 44.0 | 1.2 |
| Mini, 30% Less Fat, Peperami* | 1 Stick/10g | 38.0 | 3.0 | 379 | 25.0 | 1.5 | 30.0 | 3.0 |
| Original, Peperami* | 1 Stick/25g | 126.0 | 11.0 | 504 | 24.0 | 2.5 | 44.0 | 0.1 |
| **PEPPER** | | | | | | | | |
| *Black, Freshly Ground, Average* | *1 Tsp/2g* | *5.0* | *0.0* | *255* | *10.9* | *64.8* | *3.3* | *26.5* |
| *Cayenne, Ground* | *1 Tsp/2g* | *6.0* | *0.0* | *318* | *12.0* | *31.7* | *17.3* | *0.0* |
| *White* | *½ Tsp/1g* | *3.0* | *0.0* | *296* | *10.4* | *68.6* | *2.1* | *26.2* |
| **PEPPERONATA** | | | | | | | | |
| Salmon, BGTY, Sainsbury's* | 1 Pack/380g | 300.0 | 9.0 | 79 | 5.8 | 8.8 | 2.3 | 0.9 |
| **PEPPERS** | | | | | | | | |
| *Capsicum, Green, Boiled in Salted Water* | *1oz/28g* | *5.0* | *0.0* | *18* | *1.0* | *2.6* | *0.5* | *1.8* |
| *Capsicum, Green, Raw, Unprepared, Average* | *1 Med/160g* | *24.0* | *0.0* | *15* | *0.8* | *2.6* | *0.3* | *1.6* |
| *Capsicum, Red, Boiled in Salted Water* | *1oz/28g* | *10.0* | *0.0* | *34* | *1.1* | *7.0* | *0.4* | *1.7* |
| *Capsicum, Red, Raw, Unprepared, Average* | *1 Med/160g* | *51.0* | *1.0* | *32* | *1.0* | *6.4* | *0.4* | *1.6* |
| *Capsicum, Sweet, Raw, Average* | *1 Serving/100g* | *16.0* | *0.0* | *16* | *0.8* | *2.6* | *0.3* | *1.6* |
| *Capsicum, Yellow, Raw, Unprepared, Average* | *1 Med/160g* | *42.0* | *0.0* | *26* | *1.2* | *5.3* | *0.2* | *1.7* |
| Chilli, Chopped, Stir Fry, Schwartz* | 1 Tbsp/19g | 24.0 | 1.0 | 130 | 2.2 | 15.6 | 6.5 | 0.0 |
| Chilli, Crushed, Schwartz* | 1 Tsp/0.5g | 2.0 | 0.0 | 321 | 12.0 | 29.0 | 17.0 | 27.0 |
| Chilli, Dried, Whole, Red, Schwartz* | 1 Tsp/0.5g | 2.0 | 0.0 | 425 | 15.9 | 56.4 | 15.1 | 0.0 |
| *Chilli, Green, Raw, Unprepared, Average* | *1 Med/13g* | *5.0* | *0.0* | *40* | *2.0* | *9.5* | *0.2* | *1.5* |
| Chilli, Green, Very Lazy, The English Provender Co.* | 1 Serving/10g | 11.0 | 0.0 | 114 | 4.2 | 15.3 | 4.0 | 0.5 |
| *Chilli, Red, Raw, Unprepared, Average* | *1 Sm Pepper/13g* | *5.0* | *0.0* | *40* | *2.0* | *9.5* | *0.2* | *1.5* |
| Chilli, Red, Very Lazy, The English Provender Co.* | 1 Serving/15g | 17.0 | 1.0 | 114 | 4.2 | 15.3 | 4.0 | 0.5 |
| Flame Seared, with Greek Feta, M & S* | ½ Tub/85g | 106.0 | 8.0 | 125 | 3.6 | 5.4 | 9.7 | 1.8 |
| Green, Filled, Tesco* | 1 Pepper/150g | 117.0 | 5.0 | 78 | 2.6 | 9.0 | 3.5 | 0.7 |
| Italian Style, Sainsbury's* | 1 Serving/150g | 160.0 | 7.0 | 107 | 3.5 | 14.1 | 5.0 | 2.1 |
| Jalapeno, Crushed, Schwartz* | 1 Tsp/0.5g | 1.0 | 0.0 | 136 | 15.9 | 56.4 | 15.1 | 0.0 |
| *Jalapeno, Raw* | *1 Cup, sliced / 90g* | *27.0* | *1.0* | *30* | *1.3* | *5.9* | *0.6* | *2.8* |
| *Mixed Bag, From Supermarket, Average* | *1oz/28g* | *7.0* | *0.0* | *25* | *1.0* | *4.4* | *0.4* | *1.7* |
| Pickled, Hot, Turkish, Melis | 1 Serving/25g | 9.0 | 0.0 | 35 | 1.0 | 7.9 | 0.0 | 1.0 |
| Ramiro, Red, Sainsbury's* | 1 Serving/100g | 30.0 | 0.0 | 30 | 1.6 | 5.1 | 0.3 | 2.2 |
| Red, Filled with Feta, COU, M & S* | 1 Pepper/154g | 200.0 | 11.0 | 130 | 4.1 | 12.4 | 7.2 | 0.6 |
| Red, Roasted, Melis* | 1 Serving/100g | 90.0 | 1.0 | 90 | 1.1 | 18.8 | 1.0 | 0.2 |
| *Sweet, Orange, Raw, Average* | *1oz/28g* | *8.0* | *0.0* | *30* | *1.8* | *5.0* | *0.3* | *1.5* |
| Sweet, Tinned, Sainsbury's* | ½ Can/125g | 45.0 | 0.0 | 36 | 1.1 | 7.0 | 0.4 | 1.7 |
| **PERCH** | | | | | | | | |
| *Raw, Atlantic* | *1oz/28g* | *26.0* | *0.0* | *94* | *18.6* | *0.0* | *1.6* | *0.0* |
| **PERNOD*** | | | | | | | | |
| *19% Volume, Pernod** | *1 Shot/35ml* | *45.0* | *0.0* | *130* | *0.0* | *0.0* | *0.0* | *0.0* |
| **PESTO** | | | | | | | | |
| Chargrilled Aubergine, Sacla* | 1 Serving/30g | 102.0 | 10.0 | 339 | 2.4 | 3.8 | 34.9 | 0.0 |
| Green, Alla Genovese, Finest, Tesco* | 1 Serving/65g | 188.0 | 26.0 | 290 | 5.7 | 1.5 | 39.6 | 2.8 |
| Green, Asda* | 2 Dtsp/25g | 93.0 | 10.0 | 374 | 5.0 | 0.8 | 39.0 | 5.0 |
| Green, Classic, Sacla* | 1 Serving/40g | 185.0 | 19.0 | 462 | 5.2 | 7.6 | 46.5 | 0.0 |
| Green, Free From, Meridian Foods* | 1 Tsp/5g | 26.0 | 3.0 | 519 | 5.9 | 5.2 | 52.6 | 2.2 |
| Green, GFY, Asda* | 1 Jar/190g | 376.0 | 35.0 | 198 | 3.4 | 4.3 | 18.6 | 2.9 |
| Green, Verde, Bertolli* | ¼ Jar/46g | 266.0 | 28.0 | 575 | 5.7 | 4.3 | 59.5 | 0.0 |
| Red, Rosso, Bertolli* | 1 Jar/185g | 703.0 | 65.0 | 380 | 6.8 | 9.5 | 35.0 | 2.0 |
| Roasted Red Pepper, Sacla* | 1 Serving/30g | 72.0 | 7.0 | 241 | 4.3 | 4.6 | 22.8 | 5.3 |

P

| | Measure INFO/WEIGHT | per Measure KCAL | FAT | Nutrition Values per 100g / 100ml KCAL | PROT | CARB | FAT | FIBRE |
|---|---|---|---|---|---|---|---|---|
| **PESTO** | | | | | | | | |
| Spinach & Parmesan, Sainsbury's* | ¼ Jar/46g | 162.0 | 16.0 | 349 | 4.6 | 5.3 | 34.4 | 2.5 |
| Sun Dried Tomato, Sacla* | 1 Serving/30g | 87.0 | 8.0 | 289 | 4.2 | 5.2 | 27.9 | 0.0 |
| Tomato, Organic, Sacla* | 1 Serving/30g | 95.0 | 9.0 | 317 | 3.9 | 4.3 | 31.6 | 0.0 |
| Wild Rocket, Sacla* | 1 Serving/30g | 127.0 | 13.0 | 425 | 5.2 | 3.2 | 43.5 | 4.5 |
| **PETIT FOURS** | | | | | | | | |
| Milk Chocolate, Belgian, Safeway* | 1 Cake/11g | 55.0 | 3.0 | 525 | 6.2 | 49.9 | 33.2 | 1.8 |
| **PETIT POIS** | | | | | | | | |
| & Baby Carrots, Tesco* | ½ Drained Jar/110g | 37.0 | 1.0 | 34 | 3.0 | 4.4 | 0.5 | 4.2 |
| *Average* | *1 Serving/65g* | *34.0* | *0.0* | *53* | *5.0* | *6.8* | *0.7* | *3.5* |
| Freshly Frozen, Boiled, Asda* | 1 Serving/80g | 39.0 | 1.0 | 49 | 5.0 | 5.5 | 0.9 | 4.5 |
| Frozen, M & S* | 1 Serving/80g | 56.0 | 1.0 | 70 | 5.0 | 5.5 | 0.9 | 4.5 |
| in Water, Sugar & Salt Added, Sainsbury's* | ½ Tin/140g | 81.0 | 1.0 | 58 | 4.0 | 9.4 | 0.5 | 2.0 |
| **PHEASANT** | | | | | | | | |
| *Meat Only, Roasted* | *1oz/28g* | *62.0* | *3.0* | *220* | *27.9* | *0.0* | *12.0* | *0.0* |
| *Meat Only, Roasted, Weighed with Bone* | *1oz/28g* | *32.0* | *2.0* | *114* | *14.5* | *0.0* | *6.2* | *0.0* |
| Stuffed, Easy Carve, Finest, Tesco* | 1 Serving/200g | 540.0 | 37.0 | 270 | 23.2 | 2.2 | 18.7 | 0.9 |
| **PHYSALIS** | | | | | | | | |
| *Raw, without Husk, Average* | *5 Fruits/30g* | *16.0* | *0.0* | *53* | *1.9* | *11.2* | *0.7* | *0.4* |
| **PICCALILLI** | | | | | | | | |
| Dijon, Sainsbury's* | 1 Dtsp/15g | 14.0 | 0.0 | 91 | 1.8 | 19.0 | 0.9 | 0.7 |
| Haywards* | 1 Serving/28g | 18.0 | 0.0 | 66 | 1.4 | 13.9 | 0.5 | 0.0 |
| Heinz* | 1 Serving/10g | 11.0 | 0.0 | 107 | 1.7 | 21.6 | 0.7 | 0.6 |
| Morrisons* | 1 Serving/50g | 37.0 | 0.0 | 75 | 1.6 | 15.0 | 0.7 | 0.6 |
| Sainsbury's* | 1 Dtsp/15g | 9.0 | 0.0 | 60 | 1.8 | 11.9 | 0.6 | 0.7 |
| Sandwich, Tesco* | 1 Serving/20g | 16.0 | 0.0 | 80 | 0.4 | 18.5 | 0.0 | 1.6 |
| Sweet, Asda* | 1 Tbsp/15g | 17.0 | 0.0 | 112 | 0.5 | 27.0 | 0.2 | 0.6 |
| Tesco* | 1 Serving/50g | 51.0 | 2.0 | 102 | 0.5 | 17.8 | 3.6 | 2.0 |
| **PICKLE** | | | | | | | | |
| Branston, Crosse & Blackwell* | 1 Tsp/10g | 11.0 | 0.0 | 109 | 0.8 | 26.1 | 0.2 | 1.1 |
| Brinjal, Patak's* | 1 Tsp/16g | 59.0 | 4.0 | 367 | 2.2 | 34.6 | 24.4 | 0.9 |
| Chilli, Branston* | 1 Tsp/16g | 21.0 | 0.0 | 130 | 0.7 | 30.0 | 0.7 | 1.5 |
| Chilli, Patak's* | 1 Tsp/16g | 52.0 | 5.0 | 325 | 4.3 | 1.3 | 33.7 | 0.0 |
| Garlic, Patak's* | 1 Tsp/16g | 42.0 | 3.0 | 261 | 3.6 | 20.0 | 18.5 | 1.6 |
| Lime, Hot, Asda* | 1 Dtsp/10g | 12.0 | 1.0 | 123 | 2.2 | 6.0 | 10.0 | 1.0 |
| Lime, Hot, Patak's* | 1 Tsp/16g | 31.0 | 3.0 | 194 | 2.2 | 4.0 | 18.7 | 0.4 |
| Lime, M & S* | 1 Tsp/16g | 34.0 | 1.0 | 215 | 0.8 | 42.5 | 4.8 | 2.4 |
| *Lime, Oily* | *1oz/28g* | *50.0* | *4.0* | *178* | *1.9* | *8.3* | *15.5* | *0.0* |
| Lime, Sharwood's* | 1 Tsp/16g | 24.0 | 1.0 | 152 | 2.2 | 15.0 | 9.3 | 2.9 |
| Mango, Hot, Patak's* | 1 Tsp/16g | 43.0 | 4.0 | 270 | 2.3 | 7.4 | 25.7 | 1.9 |
| Mild Mustard, Heinz* | 1 Tbsp/10g | 13.0 | 0.0 | 129 | 2.2 | 25.7 | 1.3 | 0.9 |
| Mixed, Haywards* | ½ Jar/120g | 22.0 | 0.0 | 18 | 1.4 | 2.4 | 0.3 | 0.0 |
| Mixed, Patak's* | 1 Serving/30g | 78.0 | 8.0 | 259 | 2.3 | 4.7 | 25.7 | 0.8 |
| Sandwich, Branston* | 1 Tsp/10g | 14.0 | 0.0 | 140 | 0.7 | 34.2 | 0.3 | 1.3 |
| Sandwich, Tesco* | 1 Serving/5g | 7.0 | 0.0 | 138 | 1.0 | 33.1 | 0.2 | 1.0 |
| Small Chunk, Branston* | 1 Serving/20g | 22.0 | 0.0 | 109 | 0.8 | 26.1 | 0.2 | 1.1 |
| Spicy, Branston* | 1 Tsp/15g | 21.0 | 0.0 | 140 | 0.7 | 34.7 | 0.3 | 1.3 |
| *Sweet* | *1 Tsp/10g* | *14.0* | *0.0* | *141* | *0.6* | *36.0* | *0.1* | *1.2* |
| Sweet, Branston* | 1 Serving/30g | 33.0 | 0.0 | 109 | 0.8 | 26.1 | 0.2 | 1.1 |
| Sweet, Country, Morrisons* | 1 Tbsp/15g | 19.0 | 0.0 | 130 | 0.9 | 31.1 | 0.2 | 0.0 |
| Sweet, Frank Cooper* | 1 Pot/20g | 21.0 | 0.0 | 104 | 0.5 | 25.3 | 0.1 | 0.8 |
| Sweet, Hartley's* | 1 Tsp/16g | 22.0 | 0.0 | 140 | 0.5 | 36.2 | 0.0 | 0.0 |
| Sweet, Value, Tesco* | 1 Serving/10g | 10.0 | 0.0 | 96 | 0.6 | 23.0 | 0.2 | 0.7 |
| Sweet Harvest, Asda* | 1 Serving/25g | 38.0 | 0.0 | 154 | 0.8 | 37.0 | 0.3 | 0.8 |

| | Measure INFO/WEIGHT | per Measure KCAL | FAT | Nutrition Values per 100g / 100ml KCAL | PROT | CARB | FAT | FIBRE |
|---|---|---|---|---|---|---|---|---|
| **PICKLE** | | | | | | | | |
| Tangy, Sandwich, Heinz* | 1 Tsp/10g | 13.0 | 0.0 | 134 | 0.7 | 31.4 | 0.2 | 0.9 |
| Tomato, Tangy, Heinz* | 1 Tsp/10g | 10.0 | 0.0 | 102 | 2.0 | 22.0 | 0.3 | 1.5 |
| **PICKLES** | | | | | | | | |
| Cornichons, in Sweet & Sour Vinegar, Waitrose* | 1 Serving/10g | 3.0 | 0.0 | 28 | 0.6 | 6.1 | 0.1 | 0.6 |
| Red Cabbage, Asda* | 1 Serving/50g | 16.0 | 0.0 | 32 | 1.6 | 6.0 | 0.1 | 0.0 |
| **PICNIC** | | | | | | | | |
| Cadbury* | 1 Bar/48g | 228.0 | 11.0 | 475 | 7.5 | 58.3 | 23.6 | 0.0 |
| **PIE** | | | | | | | | |
| Admiral's, Frozen, Youngs* | 1 Pie/360g | 378.0 | 18.0 | 105 | 4.6 | 10.7 | 4.9 | 0.7 |
| Admiral's, Ross* | 1 Pie/340g | 357.0 | 16.0 | 105 | 4.8 | 10.9 | 4.6 | 0.7 |
| Apple, & Blackberry, Fruit, Finest, Tesco* | 1 Pie/95g | 265.0 | 11.0 | 279 | 13.7 | 29.3 | 11.9 | 2.8 |
| Apple, American, Iceland* | 1 Portion/92g | 258.0 | 11.0 | 280 | 4.8 | 39.2 | 11.6 | 2.2 |
| Apple, Asda* | ¼ Pack/107g | 287.0 | 12.0 | 269 | 3.6 | 39.0 | 11.0 | 1.7 |
| Apple, Bramley, Aunt Bessie's* | ¼ Pie/138g | 351.0 | 15.0 | 255 | 2.8 | 36.2 | 11.0 | 1.2 |
| Apple, Bramley, Free From, Tesco* | 1 Pie/60g | 185.0 | 5.0 | 309 | 2.5 | 55.4 | 8.6 | 1.4 |
| Apple, Bramley, Individual, Sainsbury's* | 1 Pie/54g | 165.0 | 5.0 | 307 | 3.6 | 52.2 | 9.3 | 1.3 |
| Apple, Bramley, Individual, Tesco* | 1 Pie/61g | 210.0 | 8.0 | 344 | 3.4 | 53.1 | 13.0 | 1.5 |
| Apple, Bramley, Large, Tesco* | 1/8 Pie/87g | 311.0 | 13.0 | 358 | 3.9 | 51.9 | 15.0 | 1.9 |
| Apple, Deep Filled, Iceland* | 1 Portion/116g | 332.0 | 15.0 | 286 | 2.5 | 39.2 | 13.2 | 1.1 |
| Apple, Deep Filled, Sainsbury's* | ¼ Pie/137g | 374.0 | 18.0 | 273 | 3.8 | 35.6 | 12.8 | 1.6 |
| Apple, Family, Asda* | 1/6 Pie/119g | 314.0 | 13.0 | 265 | 3.6 | 38.0 | 11.0 | 2.9 |
| Apple, Family, Morrisons* | 1/6 Pie/116g | 326.0 | 14.0 | 281 | 3.1 | 39.9 | 12.1 | 3.1 |
| Apple, Lattice, Tesco* | 1 Serving/145g | 325.0 | 13.0 | 224 | 2.2 | 33.2 | 9.2 | 1.4 |
| Apple, McVitie's* | 1 Serving/117g | 316.0 | 13.0 | 270 | 3.0 | 39.0 | 11.0 | 2.0 |
| Apple, Puff Pastry, M & S* | 1 Pie/135g | 337.0 | 17.0 | 250 | 2.4 | 31.3 | 12.7 | 1.0 |
| Apple, Ready Baked, Sara Lee* | 1/6 Pie/90g | 249.0 | 12.0 | 277 | 2.8 | 35.4 | 13.8 | 1.2 |
| Apple, Ready to Bake, TTD, Sainsbury's* | 1/6 Pie/125g | 352.0 | 16.0 | 282 | 3.2 | 38.2 | 12.9 | 0.7 |
| Apple, Sainsbury's* | 1/6 Pie/118g | 314.0 | 14.0 | 266 | 3.4 | 37.1 | 11.5 | 0.6 |
| Apple, Sultana & Cinnamon, Finest, Tesco* | 1 Slice/83g | 193.0 | 7.0 | 233 | 2.8 | 35.6 | 8.8 | 5.0 |
| Apple, Tesco* | 1 Pie/47g | 191.0 | 8.0 | 406 | 3.3 | 59.4 | 17.2 | 1.5 |
| Apple, VLH Kitchens* | 1 Slice/50g | 136.0 | 5.6 | 272 | 3.7 | 40.0 | 11.2 | 1.7 |
| Apple & Blackberry, Co-Op* | 1 Serving/138g | 338.0 | 15.0 | 245 | 3.0 | 33.0 | 11.0 | 2.0 |
| Apple & Blackberry, Lattice Topped, BGTY, Sainsbury's* | ¼ Serving/100g | 256.0 | 7.0 | 256 | 2.8 | 44.4 | 7.5 | 3.1 |
| Apple & Blackberry, Shortcrust, M & S* | 1 Serving/142g | 469.0 | 18.0 | 330 | 4.3 | 50.2 | 12.5 | 1.1 |
| Apple & Blackberry, Tesco* | 1 Serving/106g | 287.0 | 12.0 | 271 | 4.2 | 38.4 | 11.2 | 1.7 |
| Apple & Blackcurrant, Mr Kipling* | 1 Pie/66g | 211.0 | 8.0 | 320 | 3.3 | 47.9 | 12.8 | 1.2 |
| Apricot, Weight Watchers* | 1 Serving 40g | 123.0 | 0.0 | 308 | 4.6 | 56.4 | 0.9 | 14.6 |
| Apricot Fruit, GFY, Asda* | 1 Serving/52g | 162.0 | 5.0 | 311 | 3.3 | 52.0 | 10.0 | 0.0 |
| Banoffee, Individual, Sainsbury's* | 1 Pie/104g | 365.0 | 21.0 | 351 | 3.2 | 39.2 | 20.2 | 2.2 |
| Banoffee, Tesco* | 1/6 Pie/94g | 365.0 | 20.0 | 390 | 3.9 | 45.8 | 21.1 | 1.5 |
| Banoffee Cream, American Dream, McVitie's* | 1 Portion/70g | 277.0 | 18.0 | 396 | 4.3 | 36.7 | 25.5 | 0.8 |
| Beef, Lean, BGTY, Sainsbury's* | 1 Serving/212g | 280.0 | 13.0 | 132 | 7.3 | 12.2 | 6.0 | 1.5 |
| Beef, Minced, Aberdeen Angus, Shortcrust, M & S* | 1 Pie/171g | 435.0 | 27.0 | 255 | 9.3 | 19.3 | 15.6 | 3.0 |
| Beef, Sainsbury's* | 1 Pie/210g | 535.0 | 30.0 | 255 | 10.3 | 21.2 | 14.3 | 2.0 |
| Beef & Vegetable, Macdougalls, McDougalls* | ¼ Pie/114g | 292.0 | 19.0 | 256 | 5.3 | 20.6 | 16.9 | 0.3 |
| Beef Steak, Aberdeen Angus, Top Crust, Waitrose* | ½ Pie/280g | 476.0 | 24.0 | 170 | 10.0 | 13.4 | 8.6 | 4.1 |
| Blackcurrant, Deep Filled, Sainsbury's* | 1 Slice/137g | 440.0 | 19.0 | 321 | 5.8 | 42.6 | 14.1 | 2.2 |
| Blackcurrant, Shortcrust, M & S* | 1 Pie/142g | 412.0 | 14.0 | 290 | 3.9 | 45.6 | 10.1 | 1.3 |
| Bramley Apple, M & S* | 1 Pie/55g | 184.0 | 6.0 | 335 | 2.9 | 57.6 | 11.7 | 1.6 |
| Cheese & Onion, Hollands* | 1 Pie/200g | 516.0 | 24.0 | 258 | 6.3 | 30.9 | 12.2 | 0.0 |
| Cheese & Potato, Aunt Bessie's* | ¼ Portion/200g | 288.0 | 19.0 | 144 | 4.6 | 11.7 | 9.4 | 1.5 |
| Cherry, Asda* | 1/6 Pie/117g | 337.0 | 14.0 | 289 | 3.1 | 41.2 | 12.4 | 1.8 |
| Cherry, Deep Filled, Somerfield* | 1/6 Pie/90g | 259.0 | 11.0 | 288 | 3.0 | 41.0 | 12.0 | 0.0 |

P

# PIE

| | Measure INFO/WEIGHT | per Measure KCAL | FAT | Nutrition Values per 100g / 100ml KCAL | PROT | CARB | FAT | FIBRE |
|---|---|---|---|---|---|---|---|---|
| Cherry, Sainsbury's* | 1 Serving/117g | 325.0 | 14.0 | 278 | 3.9 | 39.6 | 11.6 | 1.7 |
| Cherry, Tesco* | 1 Serving/106g | 294.0 | 13.0 | 277 | 4.0 | 38.3 | 12.0 | 1.8 |
| Cherry Bakewell Meringue, Sara Lee* | 1 Slice/70g | 228.0 | 8.0 | 326 | 4.1 | 51.9 | 11.3 | 1.4 |
| Chicken, Aunt Bessie's* | ¼ Pie/200g | 474.0 | 24.0 | 237 | 10.6 | 21.4 | 12.1 | 2.1 |
| Chicken, Bacon & Cheddar Cheese, Lattice, Birds Eye* | 1 Pie/155g | 454.0 | 27.0 | 293 | 13.4 | 21.0 | 17.3 | 1.5 |
| Chicken, Broccoli & White Wine, Waitrose* | 1 Serving/200g | 605.0 | 40.0 | 302 | 12.5 | 17.7 | 20.2 | 2.3 |
| Chicken, Cheese & Bacon, HL, Tesco* | 1 Pack/450g | 382.0 | 10.0 | 85 | 5.9 | 9.4 | 2.2 | 1.6 |
| Chicken, Cheese & Broccoli Lattice, Birds Eye* | 1 Pie/155g | 446.0 | 25.0 | 288 | 12.6 | 22.7 | 16.3 | 1.1 |
| Chicken, Cheese & Leek Lattice, Sun Valley* | 1 Lattice/125g | 315.0 | 22.0 | 252 | 15.2 | 8.6 | 17.5 | 1.0 |
| Chicken, Cottage, Frozen, Tesco* | 1 Pack/450g | 292.0 | 2.0 | 65 | 2.8 | 11.7 | 0.5 | 1.0 |
| Chicken, Deep Filled, Puff Pastry, Sainsbury's* | 1 Pie/210g | 538.0 | 32.0 | 256 | 10.0 | 19.9 | 15.2 | 3.1 |
| Chicken, Finest, Tesco* | 1 Pie/250g | 615.0 | 32.0 | 246 | 10.7 | 21.9 | 12.9 | 1.2 |
| Chicken, Individual, Made with 100% Breast, Birds Eye* | 1 Pie/154g | 455.0 | 28.0 | 296 | 7.9 | 25.0 | 18.3 | 1.0 |
| Chicken, Individual Shortcrust, Asda* | 1 Pie/175g | 534.0 | 30.0 | 305 | 10.0 | 28.0 | 17.0 | 1.0 |
| Chicken, Leek & Bacon Filo, Willow Farm, Finest, Tesco* | ½ Pie/225g | 574.0 | 33.0 | 255 | 11.1 | 18.5 | 14.7 | 1.4 |
| Chicken, Leek & Ham, Morrisons* | 1 Serving/113g | 305.0 | 17.0 | 270 | 8.8 | 25.7 | 14.7 | 1.1 |
| Chicken, Puff Pastry, Tesco* | ¼ Pie/114g | 250.0 | 13.0 | 220 | 8.6 | 21.3 | 11.2 | 1.4 |
| Chicken, Roast, In Gravy, Deep Fill, Tesco* | 1 Pie/800g | 1640.0 | 78.0 | 205 | 9.3 | 20.2 | 9.7 | 3.0 |
| Chicken, Roast, Puff Pastry, Deep Fill, Asda* | ½ Pie/259g | 739.0 | 44.0 | 285 | 10.0 | 23.0 | 17.0 | 0.8 |
| Chicken, Roast, Sainsbury's* | 1/3 Pie/173g | 538.0 | 31.0 | 311 | 10.5 | 27.2 | 17.8 | 0.9 |
| Chicken, Roast, Shortcrust, Sainsbury's* | 1 Pie/200g | 1012.0 | 56.0 | 506 | 19.2 | 44.4 | 28.0 | 2.4 |
| Chicken, Short Crust, M & S* | 1 Pie/170g | 510.0 | 30.0 | 300 | 9.7 | 26.2 | 17.4 | 1.7 |
| Chicken & Asparagus, Lattice, Waitrose* | 1 Serving/100g | 295.0 | 20.0 | 295 | 7.4 | 22.3 | 19.6 | 1.8 |
| Chicken & Asparagus, McDougalls* | 1 Serving/170g | 394.0 | 22.0 | 232 | 7.4 | 21.6 | 12.9 | 1.5 |
| Chicken & Asparagus, Tesco* | 1 Serving/170g | 467.0 | 29.0 | 275 | 8.3 | 22.4 | 16.9 | 0.8 |
| Chicken & Bacon, Filo Pastry, Finest, Tesco* | 1 Serving/160g | 362.0 | 19.0 | 226 | 11.3 | 18.9 | 11.7 | 1.7 |
| Chicken & Bacon, Puff Pastry, Deep Fill, Sainsbury's* | 1/3 Pie/200g | 532.0 | 34.0 | 266 | 9.1 | 19.1 | 17.0 | 1.3 |
| Chicken & Bacon, with Cheese Sauce, Tesco* | 1 Serving/200g | 540.0 | 34.0 | 270 | 12.0 | 17.6 | 16.8 | 0.8 |
| Chicken & Broccoli, BGTY, Sainsbury's* | 1 Pack/450g | 297.0 | 4.0 | 66 | 5.9 | 8.9 | 0.8 | 1.8 |
| Chicken & Broccoli, COU, M & S* | 1 Serving/320g | 272.0 | 6.0 | 85 | 8.1 | 8.8 | 1.9 | 1.3 |
| Chicken & Broccoli, Lattice, Tesco* | ½ Pie/200g | 496.0 | 31.0 | 248 | 8.5 | 18.9 | 15.4 | 2.1 |
| Chicken & Broccoli, Light Choices, Tesco* | 1 Pack/450g | 337.0 | 9.0 | 75 | 6.6 | 6.8 | 1.9 | 1.7 |
| Chicken & Broccoli Lattice, Sainsbury's* | ½ Pie/192g | 520.0 | 31.0 | 271 | 9.3 | 22.4 | 16.0 | 0.9 |
| Chicken & Broccoli Potato, Top, Asda* | 1 Pack/400g | 319.0 | 7.0 | 80 | 5.2 | 10.7 | 1.7 | 0.6 |
| Chicken & Gravy, Deep Fill, Asda* | 1 Serving/130g | 370.0 | 22.0 | 285 | 10.0 | 23.0 | 17.0 | 0.8 |
| Chicken & Gravy, Light Choices, Tesco* | 1 Pack/450g | 337.0 | 7.0 | 75 | 5.4 | 9.4 | 1.6 | 1.2 |
| Chicken & Gravy, Puff Pastry, Deep Fill, Sainsbury's* | 1 Pie/250g | 575.0 | 31.0 | 230 | 9.1 | 20.9 | 12.3 | 1.9 |
| Chicken & Gravy, Shortcrust Pastry, Large, Tesco* | 1 Pie/600g | 1578.0 | 91.0 | 263 | 8.2 | 23.4 | 15.2 | 1.0 |
| Chicken & Gravy, Shortcrust Pastry, Sainsbury's* | 1 Serving/250g | 637.0 | 35.0 | 255 | 8.0 | 24.1 | 14.1 | 1.0 |
| Chicken & Ham, Deep Filled, Sainsbury's* | 1 Pie/210g | 594.0 | 37.0 | 283 | 8.0 | 23.0 | 17.7 | 1.0 |
| Chicken & Ham, Morrisons* | ¼ Pie/115g | 267.0 | 14.0 | 232 | 8.7 | 22.5 | 11.9 | 0.8 |
| Chicken & Ham, Sainsbury's* | 1 Pie/128g | 461.0 | 29.0 | 360 | 11.0 | 28.5 | 22.4 | 2.0 |
| Chicken & Ham, Tesco* | 1 Serving/113g | 293.0 | 18.0 | 259 | 9.4 | 20.2 | 15.6 | 1.2 |
| Chicken & Leek, Deep Filled, Puff Pastry, Sainsbury's* | 1/3 Pie/451g | 1109.0 | 65.0 | 246 | 10.1 | 18.7 | 14.5 | 1.5 |
| Chicken & Leek, Light Choices, Tesco* | 1 Pie/350g | 297.0 | 6.0 | 85 | 6.6 | 10.3 | 1.6 | 1.3 |
| Chicken & Mushroom, Asda* | 1 Pie/ 150g | 384.0 | 24.0 | 256 | 9.0 | 19.0 | 16.0 | 1.0 |
| Chicken & Mushroom, Co-Op* | 1 Pie/150g | 442.0 | 27.0 | 295 | 8.0 | 27.0 | 18.0 | 0.8 |
| Chicken & Mushroom, Deep Filled, Frozen, Tesco* | ¼ Pie/198g | 465.0 | 22.0 | 235 | 9.0 | 23.8 | 11.2 | 1.2 |
| Chicken & Mushroom, Dietary Specials* | 1 Pie/140g | 300.0 | 14.0 | 214 | 6.3 | 24.7 | 10.0 | 0.9 |
| Chicken & Mushroom, Fray Bentos* | 1 Pie/425g | 684.0 | 40.0 | 161 | 6.7 | 11.5 | 9.5 | 0.0 |
| Chicken & Mushroom, Luxury, M & S* | ½ Pie/275g | 880.0 | 62.0 | 320 | 9.9 | 20.0 | 22.5 | 1.0 |
| Chicken & Mushroom, Morrisons* | 1 Serving/100g | 261.0 | 15.0 | 261 | 7.6 | 22.9 | 15.4 | 0.9 |
| Chicken & Mushroom, Puff Pastry, Sainsbury's* | 1 Pie/150g | 450.0 | 25.0 | 300 | 7.8 | 29.6 | 16.7 | 0.9 |

| PIE | Measure INFO/WEIGHT | per Measure KCAL | per Measure FAT | Nutrition Values per 100g / 100ml KCAL | PROT | CARB | FAT | FIBRE |
|---|---|---|---|---|---|---|---|---|
| Chicken & Vegetable, Kids, Tesco* | 1 Serving/235g | 235.0 | 11.0 | 100 | 5.9 | 9.1 | 4.5 | 0.7 |
| Chicken & Vegetable, Microbake, Freshbake* | 1 Pie/100g | 348.0 | 16.0 | 348 | 10.2 | 40.8 | 16.1 | 1.8 |
| Chicken & Vegetable, Perfectly Balanced, Waitrose* | 1 Serving/375g | 285.0 | 5.0 | 76 | 5.1 | 10.8 | 1.4 | 1.3 |
| Chicken & Vegetable, Potato Topped, Somerfield* | 1 Pack/350g | 270.0 | 10.0 | 77 | 3.7 | 8.8 | 3.0 | 2.0 |
| Chicken & Vegetable, Value, Tesco* | 1 Pie/150g | 378.0 | 22.0 | 252 | 8.0 | 21.9 | 14.7 | 1.3 |
| Chicken & Wiltshire Ham, Finest, Tesco* | 1 Pie/250g | 687.0 | 37.0 | 275 | 11.6 | 22.7 | 14.9 | 1.1 |
| Chicken Curry, Iceland* | 1 Pie/156g | 440.0 | 24.0 | 282 | 10.2 | 26.2 | 15.2 | 2.0 |
| Cod & Smoked Haddock, COU, M & S* | 1 Pack/400g | 320.0 | 10.0 | 80 | 6.1 | 9.0 | 2.4 | 1.2 |
| Cottage, Asda* | 1 Pack/400g | 360.0 | 10.0 | 90 | 6.5 | 10.6 | 2.4 | 1.0 |
| Cottage, Aunt Bessie's* | 1 Pack/350g | 413.0 | 18.0 | 118 | 4.8 | 12.1 | 5.2 | 1.0 |
| Cottage, British Pies, Chilled, Tesco* | 1 Pack/500g | 450.0 | 14.0 | 90 | 4.6 | 10.3 | 2.8 | 1.5 |
| Cottage, Chicken, Tesco* | 1 Pack/400g | 340.0 | 3.0 | 85 | 6.0 | 12.8 | 0.7 | 1.7 |
| Cottage, Classics, Asda* | ½ Pack/450g | 531.0 | 27.0 | 118 | 7.0 | 9.0 | 6.0 | 1.0 |
| Cottage, Family, Iceland* | ¼ Pack/259g | 262.0 | 11.0 | 101 | 4.2 | 11.8 | 4.1 | 0.8 |
| Cottage, Fresh, M & S* | 1 Pie/400g | 460.0 | 22.0 | 115 | 6.8 | 9.9 | 5.6 | 0.6 |
| Cottage, Healthy Living, Co-Op* | 1 Pack/400g | 320.0 | 6.0 | 80 | 5.0 | 11.0 | 1.6 | 2.0 |
| Cottage, Individual, SmartPrice, Asda* | 1 Pie/159g | 149.0 | 6.0 | 94 | 3.1 | 12.0 | 3.7 | 0.7 |
| Cottage, Light Choices, Tesco* | 1 Pack/500g | 400.0 | 8.0 | 80 | 4.5 | 11.4 | 1.7 | 1.7 |
| Cottage, Sainsbury's* | 1 Pack/300g | 297.0 | 10.0 | 99 | 6.4 | 10.7 | 3.4 | 1.1 |
| Cottage, Salmon, Sainsbury's* | 1 Serving/299g | 218.0 | 4.0 | 73 | 4.6 | 10.4 | 1.4 | 1.3 |
| Cottage, Vegetarian, Sainsbury's* | 1 Pack/450g | 328.0 | 10.0 | 73 | 3.0 | 10.2 | 2.2 | 1.8 |
| Cottage, Vegetarian, Tesco* | 1 Pie/448g | 345.0 | 13.0 | 77 | 3.6 | 8.9 | 3.0 | 1.9 |
| Cottage, Waitrose* | 1 Pack/400g | 424.0 | 20.0 | 106 | 3.4 | 12.1 | 4.9 | 1.2 |
| Cottage, Weight Watchers* | 1 Pack/300g | 186.0 | 4.0 | 62 | 3.6 | 9.0 | 1.3 | 0.3 |
| Cumberland, Asda* | 1 Pack/400g | 504.0 | 22.0 | 126 | 6.3 | 12.7 | 5.6 | 1.5 |
| Cumberland, BGTY, Sainsbury's* | 1 Pack/450g | 360.0 | 9.0 | 80 | 5.3 | 10.1 | 2.0 | 1.6 |
| Cumberland, Cod & Prawn, Tesco* | 1 Pack/450g | 427.0 | 11.0 | 95 | 7.9 | 9.5 | 2.5 | 1.3 |
| Cumberland, GFY, Asda* | 1 Pack/451g | 469.0 | 10.0 | 104 | 11.4 | 11.4 | 2.2 | 2.1 |
| Cumberland, HL, Tesco* | 1 Pie/500g | 430.0 | 13.0 | 86 | 4.5 | 10.8 | 2.7 | 1.2 |
| Cumberland, M & S* | 1 Pie/195g | 312.0 | 20.0 | 160 | 6.9 | 10.1 | 10.4 | 1.1 |
| Fish | 1 Serving/250g | 262.0 | 7.0 | 105 | 8.0 | 12.3 | 3.0 | 0.7 |
| Fish, Asda* | 1 Pack/450g | 558.0 | 28.0 | 124 | 7.3 | 9.5 | 6.3 | 1.0 |
| Fish, BFY, Morrisons* | 1 Pack/350g | 301.0 | 10.0 | 86 | 5.0 | 10.0 | 2.9 | 0.9 |
| Fish, Chilled, GFY, Asda* | 1 Pie/450g | 405.0 | 13.0 | 90 | 6.8 | 9.3 | 2.8 | 1.4 |
| Fish, Co-Op* | 1 Pack/400g | 380.0 | 16.0 | 95 | 4.0 | 12.0 | 4.0 | 0.9 |
| Fish, Creamy, Classics, Small, Tesco* | 1 Pack/400g | 520.0 | 28.0 | 130 | 8.7 | 7.7 | 7.0 | 0.7 |
| Fish, Frozen, GFY, Asda* | 1 Pack/360g | 342.0 | 9.0 | 95 | 5.8 | 12.5 | 2.4 | 0.9 |
| Fish, HL, Tesco* | 1 Pack/400g | 316.0 | 9.0 | 79 | 4.0 | 10.8 | 2.2 | 1.7 |
| Fish, Kids, Great Stuff, Asda* | 1 Pack/300g | 276.0 | 9.0 | 92 | 7.8 | 8.4 | 3.0 | 1.4 |
| Fish, Luxury, Cafe Culture, M & S* | 1 Pack/660g | 627.0 | 26.0 | 95 | 7.1 | 7.8 | 4.0 | 1.1 |
| Fish, Mix, Tesco* | 1 Pack/320g | 480.0 | 26.0 | 150 | 19.3 | 0.0 | 8.0 | 0.0 |
| Fish, Seasonal, Mix, Sainsbury's* | 1 Pack/320g | 480.0 | 28.0 | 150 | 17.7 | 0.0 | 8.8 | 0.0 |
| Fish, with Cheddar & Parsley Sauce, Go Cook, Asda* | ½ Pack/450g | 427.0 | 16.0 | 95 | 7.8 | 7.9 | 3.6 | 0.8 |
| Fish & Prawn, Perfectly Balanced, Waitrose* | 1 Serving/375g | 379.0 | 13.0 | 101 | 6.8 | 10.4 | 3.6 | 0.7 |
| Fish with Cheese, Ross* | 1 Pack/300g | 321.0 | 13.0 | 107 | 4.7 | 12.0 | 4.5 | 0.8 |
| Fish with Vegetables, Ross* | 1 Pack/300g | 255.0 | 9.0 | 85 | 4.4 | 10.2 | 2.9 | 1.3 |
| Fisherman's, Asda* | 1 Serving/300g | 429.0 | 21.0 | 143 | 7.0 | 13.0 | 7.0 | 0.0 |
| Fisherman's, Famous, Chilled, Youngs* | 1 Pack/400g | 448.0 | 23.0 | 112 | 7.6 | 7.6 | 5.7 | 0.9 |
| Fisherman's, Healthy Options, Asda* | 1 Pie/406g | 337.0 | 10.0 | 83 | 5.0 | 10.0 | 2.5 | 0.9 |
| Fisherman's, M & S* | 1 Pie/248g | 335.0 | 16.0 | 135 | 9.3 | 9.8 | 6.4 | 0.3 |
| Fisherman's, Morrisons* | 1 Serving/300g | 246.0 | 10.0 | 82 | 3.8 | 9.5 | 3.3 | 1.0 |
| Fishermans, Perfectly Balanced, Waitrose* | 1 Serving/400g | 436.0 | 11.0 | 109 | 8.1 | 12.8 | 2.8 | 0.9 |
| Fisherman's, Sainsbury's* | 1 Pack/300g | 195.0 | 4.0 | 65 | 3.9 | 9.7 | 1.2 | 1.2 |

P

# PIE

| | Measure INFO/WEIGHT | per Measure KCAL | FAT | Nutrition Values per 100g / 100ml KCAL | PROT | CARB | FAT | FIBRE |
|---|---|---|---|---|---|---|---|---|
| Fisherman's, Tesco* | 1 Pie/400g | 400.0 | 20.0 | 100 | 4.2 | 9.8 | 4.9 | 1.1 |
| Fruit, Pastry Top & Bottom | 1oz/28g | 73.0 | 4.0 | 260 | 3.0 | 34.0 | 13.3 | 1.8 |
| Fruit, Selection, Mr Kipling* | 1 Pie/66g | 232.0 | 9.0 | 350 | 3.5 | 53.5 | 13.6 | 1.3 |
| Gala, Tesco* | 1 Serving/70g | 241.0 | 18.0 | 344 | 10.6 | 24.5 | 25.2 | 0.0 |
| Haddock & Broccoli, M & S* | 1 Serving/250g | 262.0 | 10.0 | 105 | 8.1 | 9.3 | 4.0 | 0.5 |
| Key Lime, Sainsbury's* | ¼ Pie/80g | 280.0 | 11.0 | 350 | 4.2 | 51.8 | 14.0 | 0.7 |
| Lamb & Mint, Shortcrust Pasty, Tesco* | ¼ Pack/150g | 412.0 | 26.0 | 275 | 5.9 | 23.6 | 17.4 | 1.6 |
| Lemon Meringue | 1oz/28g | 89.0 | 4.0 | 319 | 4.5 | 45.9 | 14.4 | 0.7 |
| Lemon Meringue, 90% Fat Free, Sara Lee* | 1/6 Slice/75g | 204.0 | 7.0 | 272 | 2.4 | 46.1 | 8.9 | 0.9 |
| Lemon Meringue, Mini, Asda* | 1 Pie/26g | 101.0 | 3.0 | 396 | 3.7 | 66.0 | 13.0 | 1.8 |
| Lemon Meringue, Mr Kipling* | 1 Cake/51g | 184.0 | 6.0 | 360 | 2.9 | 59.9 | 12.1 | 3.0 |
| Lemon Meringue, Ready to Bake, Aunt Bessie's* | ¼ Pie/106g | 305.0 | 9.0 | 288 | 3.8 | 49.8 | 8.2 | 2.0 |
| Lemon Meringue, Sainsbury's* | ¼ Pie/110g | 351.0 | 10.0 | 319 | 2.3 | 57.3 | 9.0 | 0.5 |
| Lemon Meringue, Tesco* | 1 Pie/385g | 989.0 | 28.0 | 257 | 4.0 | 43.7 | 7.3 | 0.5 |
| Lemon Meringue, Weight Watchers* | 1 Serving/85g | 161.0 | 0.0 | 189 | 2.4 | 43.1 | 0.5 | 0.6 |
| Mariner's, Ross* | 1 Pie/340g | 435.0 | 20.0 | 128 | 5.0 | 13.9 | 5.9 | 1.0 |
| Meat & Potato, Shortcrust, Co-Op* | ¼ Pie/137g | 403.0 | 26.0 | 294 | 7.3 | 23.3 | 19.1 | 1.4 |
| Meat & Potato, Tesco* | 1 Serving/150g | 414.0 | 27.0 | 276 | 5.1 | 23.6 | 17.9 | 1.6 |
| Meat & Potato, Value, Tesco* | 1 Pie/95g | 274.0 | 17.0 | 288 | 6.9 | 23.8 | 18.4 | 3.5 |
| Mediteranean Vegetable, Cheesy, COU, M & S* | 1 Pack/400g | 280.0 | 8.0 | 70 | 2.1 | 10.6 | 2.1 | 2.1 |
| Mince, Asda* | 1 Pie/53g | 204.0 | 8.0 | 382 | 3.8 | 58.0 | 15.0 | 1.5 |
| Mince, Brandy Rich, Mini, TTD, Sainsbury's* | 1 Pie/25g | 97.0 | 4.0 | 390 | 3.1 | 60.4 | 14.6 | 2.0 |
| Mince, Christmas, Sainsbury's* | 1 Pie/37g | 147.0 | 6.0 | 397 | 4.5 | 58.0 | 16.3 | 2.6 |
| Mince, Deep, Morrisons* | 1 Pie/65g | 243.0 | 9.0 | 371 | 3.7 | 57.8 | 13.9 | 1.5 |
| Mince, Dusted, Mini, Finest, Tesco* | 1 Pie/20g | 76.0 | 2.0 | 379 | 7.3 | 62.9 | 12.2 | 5.0 |
| Mince, Extra Special, Asda* | 1 Pie/60g | 225.0 | 8.0 | 378 | 3.9 | 59.0 | 14.0 | 2.2 |
| Mince, Finest, Tesco* | 1 Pie/61g | 234.0 | 9.0 | 384 | 4.3 | 59.9 | 14.1 | 2.7 |
| Mince, Iced Top, Asda* | 1 Pie/57g | 214.0 | 7.0 | 375 | 2.8 | 61.0 | 12.0 | 1.1 |
| Mince, Iced Top, Tesco* | 1 Serving/52g | 202.0 | 7.0 | 387 | 2.8 | 65.7 | 12.5 | 1.1 |
| Mince, Individual, Average | 1 Pie/48g | 203.0 | 10.0 | 423 | 4.3 | 59.0 | 20.4 | 2.1 |
| Mince, Individual, Mr Kipling* | 1 Pie/67g | 250.0 | 9.0 | 376 | 3.7 | 59.0 | 13.9 | 1.5 |
| Mince, Lattice, Classics, M & S* | 1 Pie/53g | 210.0 | 8.0 | 400 | 4.0 | 61.7 | 15.2 | 2.4 |
| Mince, Luxury, Deep Filled, M & S* | 1 Pie/65g | 234.0 | 9.0 | 360 | 4.3 | 55.0 | 13.8 | 3.8 |
| Mince, Mini, M & S* | 1 Pie/28g | 105.0 | 4.0 | 380 | 4.3 | 57.8 | 14.6 | 4.0 |
| Mince, Organic, Sainsbury's* | 1 Pie/46g | 177.0 | 7.0 | 384 | 5.0 | 54.5 | 16.2 | 5.6 |
| Mince, Rowan Hill Bakery* | 1 Pie/55g | 202.0 | 8.0 | 370 | 3.8 | 54.8 | 15.1 | 0.0 |
| Mince, Shortcrust, Waitrose* | 1 Pie/55g | 210.0 | 8.0 | 385 | 3.6 | 60.0 | 14.6 | 20.9 |
| Mince, Tesco* | 1 Pie/47g | 180.0 | 8.0 | 383 | 3.9 | 54.7 | 16.5 | 1.5 |
| Mince, Topped with Nibbed Almonds, Mini, Finest, Tesco* | 1 Pie/20g | 77.0 | 3.0 | 383 | 4.9 | 59.0 | 14.1 | 3.4 |
| Mince, Value, Tesco* | 1 Pie/45g | 184.0 | 8.0 | 410 | 4.3 | 58.4 | 17.7 | 1.6 |
| Minced Beef & Onion, Birds Eye* | 1 Pie/145g | 419.0 | 25.0 | 289 | 7.1 | 26.3 | 17.3 | 0.7 |
| Minced Beef & Onion, Tesco* | 1 Pie/150g | 454.0 | 28.0 | 303 | 5.7 | 27.4 | 19.0 | 1.7 |
| Minced Beef & Vegetable, Pot, M & S* | 1/3 Pie/183g | 366.0 | 27.0 | 200 | 7.8 | 9.1 | 14.5 | 7.1 |
| Minced Steak & Onion, Puff Pastry, Individual, Sainsbury's* | 1 Pie/150g | 477.0 | 29.0 | 318 | 8.9 | 27.0 | 19.4 | 0.9 |
| Mississippi Mud, Tesco* | 1 Serving/104g | 399.0 | 27.0 | 384 | 5.3 | 33.1 | 25.6 | 1.8 |
| Mushroom & Parsley Potato, Waitrose* | 1 Pack/350g | 346.0 | 17.0 | 99 | 2.5 | 10.9 | 5.0 | 1.2 |
| Ocean, Basics, Sainsbury's* | 1 Serving/302g | 196.0 | 4.0 | 65 | 3.9 | 9.7 | 1.2 | 1.2 |
| Ocean, Frozen, BGTY, Sainsbury's* | 1 Pack/350g | 318.0 | 5.0 | 91 | 7.0 | 12.4 | 1.5 | 0.9 |
| Ocean, M & S* | 1 Pie/650g | 617.0 | 23.0 | 95 | 8.2 | 7.6 | 3.5 | 0.9 |
| Ocean, Original, Frozen, Youngs* | 1 Pack/375g | 420.0 | 21.0 | 112 | 7.6 | 7.6 | 5.7 | 0.9 |
| Ocean, Weight Watchers* | 1 Pack/300g | 207.0 | 4.0 | 69 | 4.5 | 9.5 | 1.4 | 0.2 |
| Pork, & Egg, M & S* | ¼ Pie/108g | 379.0 | 28.0 | 351 | 9.7 | 19.8 | 25.9 | 0.8 |
| Pork, & Pickle, Bowyers* | 1 Pie/150g | 576.0 | 41.0 | 384 | 10.0 | 26.3 | 27.3 | 0.0 |

| | Measure INFO/WEIGHT | per Measure KCAL | FAT | Nutrition Values per 100g / 100ml KCAL | PROT | CARB | FAT | FIBRE |
|---|---|---|---|---|---|---|---|---|
| **PIE** | | | | | | | | |
| Pork, Buffet, Bowyers* | 1 Pie/60g | 217.0 | 15.0 | 362 | 10.4 | 24.9 | 24.5 | 0.0 |
| Pork, Cheese & Pickle, Mini, Tesco* | 1 Pie/49g | 191.0 | 13.0 | 389 | 9.2 | 29.3 | 26.1 | 1.2 |
| Pork, Crusty Bake, Mini, Sainsbury's* | 1 Pie/43g | 165.0 | 11.0 | 384 | 11.5 | 26.0 | 26.0 | 1.5 |
| Pork, Crusty Bake, Sainsbury's* | 1 Pie/75g | 292.0 | 20.0 | 390 | 10.5 | 27.0 | 26.7 | 1.0 |
| Pork, Geo Adams* | 1 Pie/125g | 487.0 | 35.0 | 390 | 11.8 | 23.1 | 27.8 | 0.9 |
| Pork, Medium, Pork Farms* | 1 Pie/200g | 744.0 | 53.0 | 372 | 9.5 | 23.6 | 26.5 | 1.7 |
| Pork, Melton Mowbray, Ginsters* | 1 Pie/75g | 317.0 | 23.0 | 423 | 12.3 | 25.2 | 30.3 | 0.9 |
| Pork, Melton Mowbray, Individual, Sainsbury's* | 1 Pie/75g | 296.0 | 21.0 | 395 | 10.2 | 26.1 | 27.7 | 2.4 |
| Pork, Melton Mowbray, Lattice, Sainsbury's* | 1 Serving/100g | 342.0 | 24.0 | 342 | 10.8 | 21.7 | 23.6 | 1.2 |
| Pork, Melton Mowbray, Mini, Finest, Tesco* | 1 Pie/50g | 179.0 | 11.0 | 359 | 12.1 | 26.6 | 22.7 | 0.9 |
| Pork, Melton Mowbray, Mini, Morrisons* | 1 Pie/50g | 197.0 | 12.0 | 393 | 10.9 | 31.3 | 24.9 | 0.9 |
| Pork, Melton Mowbray, Mini, Tesco* | 1 Pie/50g | 196.0 | 14.0 | 392 | 12.6 | 20.8 | 28.7 | 2.9 |
| Pork, Melton Mowbray, Tesco* | 1 Sm Pie/148g | 679.0 | 50.0 | 459 | 10.0 | 29.0 | 33.7 | 1.3 |
| Pork, Mini, Tesco* | 1 Pie/45g | 162.0 | 11.0 | 359 | 10.2 | 25.9 | 23.8 | 1.0 |
| Pork, VLH Kitchens* | 1 Pie/36g | 168.0 | 13.0 | 466 | 11.0 | 26.0 | 36.0 | 0.0 |
| Pork, with Cheese & Pickle, Waitrose* | 1 Pack/150g | 568.0 | 37.0 | 379 | 10.3 | 29.1 | 24.6 | 2.7 |
| Potato & Meat, Farmfoods* | 1 Pie/158g | 416.0 | 27.0 | 263 | 5.4 | 22.0 | 17.0 | 1.0 |
| Rhubarb, Sara Lee* | 1 Serving/90g | 224.0 | 12.0 | 250 | 2.9 | 28.7 | 13.8 | 1.3 |
| Roast Chicken, COU, M & S* | 1 Pack/320g | 272.0 | 3.0 | 85 | 9.4 | 9.7 | 1.0 | 0.8 |
| Roast Chicken & Vegetable, Pot, M & S* | 1/3 Pie/183g | 366.0 | 23.0 | 200 | 7.7 | 13.5 | 12.5 | 4.5 |
| Salmon, Value, Tesco* | 1 Pack/300g | 312.0 | 13.0 | 104 | 4.5 | 11.3 | 4.5 | 1.0 |
| Salmon & Broccoli, Birds Eye* | 1 Pie/351g | 449.0 | 22.0 | 128 | 6.6 | 11.4 | 6.2 | 0.7 |
| Salmon & Broccoli, Filo Pastry, Finest, Tesco* | 1 Pie/170g | 386.0 | 23.0 | 227 | 7.9 | 18.9 | 13.3 | 2.1 |
| Salmon & Broccoli, Light Choices, Tesco* | 1 Pack/400g | 320.0 | 8.0 | 80 | 6.4 | 8.9 | 2.0 | 1.4 |
| Salmon & Broccoli Lattice Bar, Asda* | 1/3 Bar/133g | 360.0 | 20.0 | 271 | 6.0 | 28.0 | 15.0 | 0.8 |
| Sausage & Onion, Lattice, Puff Pastry, Tesco* | 1/3 Pie/133g | 480.0 | 22.0 | 361 | 9.1 | 20.6 | 16.9 | 4.6 |
| Sausage & Onion, Tesco* | 1 Pack/300g | 333.0 | 18.0 | 111 | 2.3 | 11.7 | 6.1 | 0.5 |
| Scotch, Co-Op* | 1 Pie/132g | 408.0 | 25.0 | 309 | 7.3 | 27.3 | 18.9 | 1.5 |
| Scotch, Farmfoods* | 1 Pie/151g | 430.0 | 25.0 | 285 | 7.8 | 26.8 | 16.3 | 1.2 |
| Shepherd's, Asda* | 1 Pie/153g | 193.0 | 9.0 | 126 | 5.0 | 13.0 | 6.0 | 0.8 |
| Shepherd's, Average | 1oz/28g | 31.0 | 2.0 | 112 | 6.0 | 9.3 | 5.9 | 0.7 |
| **Shepherd's, Baked Bean Cuisine, Heinz*** | **1 Pie/340g** | **299.0** | **10.0** | **88** | **4.1** | **11.6** | **2.8** | **1.5** |
| Shepherd's, BGTY, Sainsbury's* | 1 Pack/300g | 225.0 | 7.0 | 75 | 3.6 | 10.2 | 2.2 | 1.7 |
| Shepherd's, British Classics, Chilled, Tesco* | 1 Pack/500g | 500.0 | 20.0 | 100 | 4.8 | 10.6 | 4.1 | 1.2 |
| Shepherd's, Classic British, Sainsbury's* | 1 Pack/450g | 499.0 | 21.0 | 111 | 6.6 | 10.8 | 4.6 | 0.7 |
| Shepherds, Classics, Asda* | 1 Pack/455g | 459.0 | 23.0 | 101 | 5.0 | 9.0 | 5.0 | 1.1 |
| Shepherd's, COU, M & S* | 1 Pack/300g | 210.0 | 4.0 | 70 | 5.2 | 8.6 | 1.3 | 1.6 |
| Shepherd's, Frozen, Tesco* | 1 Pack/400g | 508.0 | 28.0 | 127 | 4.2 | 11.7 | 7.1 | 1.0 |
| Shepherd's, GFY, Asda* | 1 Pack/399g | 339.0 | 11.0 | 85 | 4.0 | 11.1 | 2.7 | 1.4 |
| Shepherd's, Iceland* | 1 Serving/170g | 224.0 | 10.0 | 132 | 5.4 | 14.7 | 5.6 | 0.8 |
| Shepherd's, Sainsbury's* | 1 Pie/300g | 225.0 | 7.0 | 75 | 3.6 | 10.2 | 2.2 | 1.7 |
| Shepherd's, Weight Watchers* | 1 Pack/400g | 300.0 | 7.0 | 75 | 2.4 | 12.5 | 1.7 | 0.9 |
| Shepherd's, Welsh Hill Lamb, Gastropub, M & S* | ½ Pack/330g | 313.0 | 12.0 | 95 | 5.4 | 10.2 | 3.5 | 1.5 |
| Smoked Haddock, Eat Smart, Safeway* | 1 Pack/400g | 376.0 | 10.0 | 94 | 8.1 | 10.1 | 2.4 | 1.2 |
| Steak, Au Gratin, Tesco* | 1 Pack/450g | 594.0 | 27.0 | 132 | 8.7 | 10.7 | 6.0 | 1.1 |
| Steak, Braised, Shortcrust Pastry, Asda* | ½ Pack/260g | 785.0 | 47.0 | 302 | 9.0 | 26.0 | 18.0 | 0.9 |
| Steak, Dietary Specials* | 1 Pie/140g | 328.0 | 14.0 | 234 | 9.8 | 25.7 | 10.3 | 0.4 |
| Steak, in Rich Gravy, Aunt Bessie's* | ¼ Pie/200g | 440.0 | 21.0 | 220 | 9.6 | 22.0 | 10.3 | 1.5 |
| Steak, in Rich Gravy, Shortcrust Pastry, Large, Sainsbury's* | 1/3 Pie/200g | 528.0 | 30.0 | 264 | 12.0 | 19.6 | 15.2 | 3.6 |
| Steak, Individual, British Classics, Tesco* | 1 Pie/150g | 450.0 | 28.0 | 300 | 9.1 | 23.3 | 18.4 | 2.5 |
| Steak, Mini, Asda* | 1 Serving/67g | 117.0 | 5.0 | 176 | 9.0 | 17.0 | 8.0 | 0.9 |
| Steak, Mushroom & Ale, Topcrust, Waitrose* | 1 Pie/250g | 500.0 | 29.0 | 200 | 11.1 | 12.2 | 11.8 | 1.1 |
| Steak, Safeway* | ¼ Pie/130g | 381.0 | 21.0 | 293 | 9.4 | 27.4 | 16.2 | 1.1 |

P

| | INFO/WEIGHT | KCAL | FAT | KCAL | PROT | CARB | FAT | FIBRE |
|---|---|---|---|---|---|---|---|---|
| **PIE** | | | | | | | | |
| Steak, Scotch, Bell's Bakery* | 1 Serving/150g | 378.0 | 20.0 | 252 | 13.6 | 18.6 | 13.5 | 0.7 |
| Steak, Tesco* | 1 Serving/205g | 556.0 | 34.0 | 271 | 7.2 | 23.3 | 16.5 | 1.4 |
| Steak & Ale, Fray Bentos* | 1 Pie/425g | 697.0 | 39.0 | 164 | 7.6 | 13.0 | 9.1 | 0.0 |
| Steak & Ale, Pub Style, Co-Op* | 1 Pie/250g | 537.0 | 30.0 | 215 | 9.0 | 17.0 | 12.0 | 2.0 |
| Steak & Ale, Sainsbury's* | 1 Serving/190g | 445.0 | 23.0 | 234 | 8.3 | 22.6 | 12.3 | 0.9 |
| Steak & Guinness, Sainsbury's* | ¼ Pie/137g | 399.0 | 25.0 | 291 | 8.7 | 22.2 | 18.6 | 1.0 |
| Steak & Kidney, Birds Eye* | 1 Pie/146g | 447.0 | 28.0 | 306 | 9.0 | 23.7 | 19.5 | 2.3 |
| Steak & Kidney, Family, Co-Op* | 1/6 Pie/87g | 278.0 | 17.0 | 320 | 9.0 | 26.0 | 20.0 | 0.9 |
| Steak & Kidney, Premium, Tesco* | 1 Serving/170g | 428.0 | 26.0 | 252 | 9.9 | 18.3 | 15.5 | 1.2 |
| Steak & Kidney, Princes* | ½ Pack/212g | 379.0 | 20.0 | 179 | 8.8 | 14.8 | 9.4 | 0.0 |
| Steak & Kidney, Puff Pastry, Sainsbury's* | 1 Pie/150g | 423.0 | 24.0 | 282 | 8.2 | 26.9 | 15.7 | 0.9 |
| Steak & Kidney, Tinned, Fray Bentos* | ½ Pie/212g | 346.0 | 19.0 | 163 | 8.2 | 12.9 | 8.8 | 0.0 |
| Steak & Mushroom, Asda* | 1 Pie/130g | 350.0 | 18.0 | 270 | 9.0 | 27.0 | 14.0 | 1.4 |
| Steak & Mushroom, Co-Op* | 1 Pie/454g | 1158.0 | 68.0 | 255 | 9.0 | 20.0 | 15.0 | 1.0 |
| Steak & Mushroom, Deep Fill, Asda* | 1/3 Pie/175g | 476.0 | 28.0 | 272 | 11.0 | 21.0 | 16.0 | 1.1 |
| Steak & Mushroom, Family, Iceland* | ¼ Pie/164g | 366.0 | 22.0 | 223 | 10.5 | 15.4 | 13.3 | 2.9 |
| Steak & Mushroom, Finest, Tesco* | 1 Pie/250g | 640.0 | 36.0 | 256 | 9.2 | 21.9 | 14.6 | 1.1 |
| Steak & Mushroom, Individual, Birds Eye* | 1 Pie/142g | 389.0 | 24.0 | 274 | 7.5 | 22.7 | 17.0 | 2.0 |
| Steak & Mushroom, Sainsbury's* | ¼ Pie/130g | 372.0 | 21.0 | 286 | 8.6 | 26.0 | 16.4 | 1.0 |
| Steak & Onion, Minced, Aberdeen Angus, Tesco* | ½ Pie/300g | 897.0 | 58.0 | 299 | 9.4 | 22.1 | 19.2 | 0.7 |
| Steak & Potato, Asda* | 1/3 Pie/173g | 442.0 | 26.0 | 255 | 6.9 | 23.1 | 15.0 | 0.9 |
| Summer Fruits, Orchard Tree* | 1/8 Pie/75g | 242.0 | 10.0 | 323 | 3.0 | 46.6 | 13.8 | 1.2 |
| Teviot, Minced Beef, Morrisons* | ½ Pie/250g | 382.0 | 17.0 | 153 | 8.0 | 14.5 | 6.9 | 1.6 |
| Tuna & Sweetcorn, HL, Tesco* | 1 Pack/450g | 391.0 | 12.0 | 87 | 7.1 | 8.6 | 2.7 | 2.0 |
| Turkey & Ham, Shortcrust, M & S* | 1/3 Pie/183g | 494.0 | 29.0 | 270 | 11.9 | 19.5 | 15.9 | 1.0 |
| Vegetable | 1oz/28g | 42.0 | 2.0 | 151 | 3.0 | 18.9 | 7.6 | 1.5 |
| Vegetable & Cheddar Cheese, Waitrose* | 1 Pie/210g | 475.0 | 31.0 | 226 | 4.9 | 17.8 | 15.0 | 1.2 |
| Vegetable & Cheese, Asda* | 1 Pie/141g | 330.0 | 16.0 | 234 | 5.8 | 26.9 | 11.5 | 1.0 |
| Welsh Lamb, Sainsbury's* | ¼ Pie/120g | 290.0 | 17.0 | 242 | 9.1 | 19.2 | 14.3 | 0.8 |
| West Country Chicken, Sainsbury's* | 1 Serving/240g | 614.0 | 37.0 | 256 | 11.9 | 17.1 | 15.6 | 2.1 |
| **PIE FILLING** | | | | | | | | |
| Apple, Sainsbury's* | 1 Serving/75g | 67.0 | 0.0 | 89 | 0.1 | 22.1 | 0.1 | 1.0 |
| Black Cherry, Fruit, Sainsbury's* | 1 Serving/100g | 73.0 | 0.0 | 73 | 0.3 | 17.7 | 0.1 | 0.3 |
| Blackcurrant, Fruit, Sainsbury's* | 1 Serving/100g | 82.0 | 0.0 | 82 | 0.4 | 20.0 | 0.1 | 1.6 |
| Cherry | 1oz/28g | 23.0 | 0.0 | 82 | 0.4 | 21.5 | 0.0 | 0.4 |
| Fruit | 1oz/28g | 22.0 | 0.0 | 77 | 0.4 | 20.1 | 0.0 | 1.0 |
| Lemon, Sainsbury's* | 1 Sachet/280g | 218.0 | 1.0 | 78 | 0.1 | 18.6 | 0.4 | 0.0 |
| Summer Fruits, Fruit, Tesco* | 1 Can/385g | 377.0 | 0.0 | 98 | 0.4 | 24.1 | 0.0 | 0.9 |
| **PIGEON** | | | | | | | | |
| *Meat Only, Roasted, Average* | *1 Pigeon/115g* | *215.0* | *9.0* | *187* | *29.0* | *0.0* | *7.9* | *0.0* |
| *Meat Only, Roasted, Weighed with Bone, Average* | *1oz/28g* | *25.0* | *1.0* | *88* | *13.6* | *0.0* | *3.7* | *0.0* |
| **PIKELETS** | | | | | | | | |
| Classics, M & S* | 1 Pikelet/35g | 70.0 | 0.0 | 200 | 7.3 | 39.1 | 1.3 | 1.6 |
| Free From, Tesco* | 1 Pikelet/30g | 58.0 | 1.0 | 194 | 2.8 | 36.2 | 4.3 | 1.4 |
| Tesco* | 1 Pikelet/35g | 68.0 | 0.0 | 193 | 5.8 | 40.9 | 0.7 | 1.7 |
| **PILAF** | | | | | | | | |
| Bulgar Wheat, Sainsbury's* | 1 Pack/381g | 347.0 | 11.0 | 91 | 3.9 | 12.3 | 2.9 | 6.3 |
| Forest Mushroom & Pine Nut, Bistro, Waitrose* | 1 Serving/225g | 337.0 | 15.0 | 150 | 7.0 | 15.8 | 6.5 | 1.5 |
| with Tomato, Average | 1oz/28g | 40.0 | 1.0 | 144 | 2.5 | 28.0 | 3.3 | 0.4 |
| **PILCHARDS** | | | | | | | | |
| Fillets, in Tomato Sauce, Average | 1 Can/120g | 158.0 | 8.0 | 132 | 16.2 | 2.2 | 6.5 | 0.1 |
| Fillets, in Virgin Olive Oil, Glenryck* | 1 Serving/92g | 223.0 | 14.0 | 242 | 23.3 | 2.0 | 15.7 | 0.0 |
| *in Brine, Average* | *½ Can/77g* | *114.0* | *6.0* | *148* | *20.8* | *0.0* | *7.3* | *0.0* |

| | Measure INFO/WEIGHT | per Measure KCAL | FAT | Nutrition Values per 100g / 100ml KCAL | PROT | CARB | FAT | FIBRE |
|---|---|---|---|---|---|---|---|---|
| **PIMMS*** | | | | | | | | |
| & Lemonade, Premixed, Canned, Pimms* | 1 Can/250ml | 85.0 | 0.0 | 34 | 0.0 | 8.0 | 0.0 | 0.0 |
| *25% Volume, Pimms** | *1 Serving/25ml* | *40.0* | *0.0* | *160* | *0.0* | *5.0* | *0.0* | *0.0* |
| **PINE NUTS** | | | | | | | | |
| *Average* | *1oz/28g* | *195.0* | *19.0* | *695* | *15.7* | *3.9* | *68.6* | *1.9* |
| **PINEAPPLE** | | | | | | | | |
| & Papaya, Dried, Garden Gang, Asda* | 1 Pack/50g | 141.0 | 1.0 | 283 | 2.8 | 64.0 | 1.7 | 8.0 |
| Dried, Sweetened, Ready to Eat, Tesco* | 1/5 Pack/50g | 117.0 | 1.0 | 235 | 0.4 | 52.9 | 1.9 | 1.7 |
| Dried, Tropical Wholefoods* | 1 Slice/10g | 35.0 | 0.0 | 355 | 1.8 | 84.2 | 1.2 | 8.6 |
| Dried, Unsweetened, Sainsbury's* | 1 Bag/75g | 255.0 | 1.0 | 340 | 1.7 | 84.7 | 2.0 | 6.0 |
| *in Juice, Average* | *1 Can/106g* | *57.0* | *0.0* | *53* | *0.3* | *12.9* | *0.0* | *0.6* |
| *in Syrup, Average* | *1 Can/240g* | *158.0* | *0.0* | *66* | *0.3* | *16.1* | *0.0* | *0.8* |
| Pieces, Yoghurt Coated, Holland & Barrett* | 1 Pack/100g | 344.0 | 19.0 | 344 | 2.1 | 46.8 | 19.3 | 0.6 |
| *Raw, Average* | *1 Pineapple/472g* | *233.0* | *1.0* | *49* | *0.4* | *11.6* | *0.1* | *0.9* |
| **PISTACHIO NUTS** | | | | | | | | |
| Roasted, Graze* | 1 Pack/50g | 166.0 | 15.0 | 333 | 9.9 | 4.6 | 31.0 | 0.0 |
| *Roasted & Salted, Average* | *1 Serving/25g* | *152.0* | *14.0* | *608* | *19.6* | *9.9* | *54.5* | *6.1* |
| **PIZZA** | | | | | | | | |
| American Hot, 12 Inch, Pizza Express* | ½ Pizza/264g | 562.0 | 20.0 | 213 | 10.5 | 25.9 | 7.5 | 2.6 |
| American Hot, Chicago Town* | 1 Pizza/170g | 445.0 | 20.0 | 262 | 8.2 | 30.8 | 11.8 | 0.9 |
| Bacon & Mushroom, Stone Bake, M & S* | 1 Pizza/375g | 750.0 | 24.0 | 200 | 9.9 | 27.2 | 6.4 | 1.6 |
| Bacon & Mushroom, Stonebaked, Tesco* | 1 Serving/157g | 352.0 | 15.0 | 224 | 10.5 | 24.3 | 9.4 | 3.3 |
| Bacon & Mushroom, Thin & Crispy, Sainsbury's* | ½ Pizza/150g | 396.0 | 16.0 | 264 | 12.9 | 29.2 | 10.6 | 1.7 |
| Balsamic Roast Vegetable & Mozzarella, Sainsbury's* | ½ Pizza/200g | 444.0 | 16.0 | 222 | 8.5 | 29.4 | 7.8 | 2.4 |
| BBQ Chicken, M & S* | ½ Pizza/210g | 430.0 | 12.0 | 205 | 11.6 | 27.5 | 5.6 | 1.8 |
| BBQ Chicken, Thin & Crispy, Sainsbury's* | ½ Pizza/147g | 384.0 | 12.0 | 261 | 13.8 | 33.1 | 8.2 | 1.6 |
| BBQ Chicken, Thin & Crispy, Tesco* | 1 Serving/165g | 355.0 | 7.0 | 215 | 11.9 | 31.6 | 4.5 | 1.2 |
| BBQ Chicken, Weight Watchers* | 1 Pizza/224g | 412.0 | 8.0 | 184 | 11.5 | 26.5 | 3.5 | 2.7 |
| BBQ Chicken Stuffed Crust, Asda* | ½ Pizza/245g | 612.0 | 24.0 | 250 | 13.0 | 27.0 | 10.0 | 2.7 |
| Bianca, Bistro, Waitrose* | ½ Pizza/207g | 618.0 | 33.0 | 298 | 12.9 | 26.2 | 15.7 | 2.3 |
| Big American, Dr Oetker* | 1 Serving/225g | 571.0 | 25.0 | 254 | 9.7 | 28.9 | 11.0 | 0.0 |
| Bistro Salami & Pepperoni, Waitrose* | ½ Pizza/190g | 492.0 | 19.0 | 259 | 12.9 | 28.8 | 10.2 | 1.5 |
| Buffalo Mozzarella, Rustic Tomato, Tuscan, Finest, Tesco* | ½ Pizza/172g | 354.0 | 11.0 | 206 | 6.8 | 29.8 | 6.6 | 1.9 |
| Cajun Chicken, BGTY, Sainsbury's* | ½ Pizza/165g | 363.0 | 6.0 | 220 | 11.0 | 36.0 | 3.6 | 1.7 |
| Cajun Chicken, Sainsbury's* | ½ Pizza/146g | 285.0 | 3.0 | 195 | 12.9 | 31.8 | 1.8 | 2.6 |
| Cajun Style Chicken, Stonebaked, Tesco* | 1 Pizza/561g | 1318.0 | 55.0 | 235 | 11.9 | 24.8 | 9.8 | 1.4 |
| Calzone Speciale, Ristorante, Dr Oetker* | ½ Pizza/145g | 378.0 | 23.0 | 261 | 11.5 | 22.1 | 16.0 | 0.0 |
| Capricciosa, Pizza Express* | 1 Serving/300g | 753.0 | 29.0 | 251 | 13.6 | 29.0 | 9.8 | 0.0 |
| Caprina, Pizza Express* | 1 Pizza/300g | 635.0 | 22.0 | 212 | 8.0 | 31.0 | 7.3 | 0.0 |
| Charged Up Chilli Beef, Goodfella's* | ½ Pizza/357g | 857.0 | 33.0 | 240 | 12.8 | 26.4 | 9.2 | 1.6 |
| Chargrilled Chicken, Thin & Crispy, Asda* | 1 Pizza/373g | 780.0 | 19.0 | 209 | 9.0 | 32.0 | 5.0 | 1.6 |
| Chargrilled Chicken & Vegetable, GFY, Asda* | ½ Pizza/166g | 355.0 | 3.0 | 214 | 13.0 | 36.0 | 2.0 | 2.0 |
| Chargrilled Vegetable, Frozen, BGTY, Sainsbury's* | 1 Pizza/290g | 548.0 | 13.0 | 189 | 10.2 | 26.7 | 4.6 | 3.0 |
| Chargrilled Vegetable, Thin & Crispy, GFY, Asda* | 1 Serving/188g | 290.0 | 4.0 | 154 | 6.0 | 28.0 | 2.0 | 3.1 |
| Cheese, Deep Pan, Tesco* | ½ Pizza/455g | 990.0 | 26.0 | 218 | 11.4 | 29.8 | 5.8 | 3.1 |
| Cheese, Onion & Garlic, Pizzeria, Waitrose* | ½ Pizza/245g | 684.0 | 29.0 | 279 | 10.8 | 29.8 | 11.8 | 2.5 |
| Cheese, Stuffed, Crust, Sainsbury's* | 1 Pizza/525g | 1428.0 | 52.0 | 272 | 14.0 | 31.5 | 10.0 | 2.0 |
| Cheese, Three, Slice, Microwaveable, Tesco* | 1 Slice/160g | 486.0 | 19.0 | 304 | 13.3 | 36.7 | 11.7 | 1.6 |
| Cheese & Onion, Tesco* | 1 Serving/22g | 56.0 | 2.0 | 255 | 10.5 | 32.7 | 9.1 | 2.7 |
| Cheese & Tomato, Average | 1 Serving/300g | 711.0 | 35.0 | 237 | 9.1 | 25.2 | 11.8 | 1.4 |
| Cheese & Tomato, Big Value, Ross* | 1 Pizza/716g | 1446.0 | 34.0 | 202 | 7.8 | 32.2 | 4.7 | 2.7 |
| Cheese & Tomato, Bistro, Waitrose* | ½ Pizza/205g | 488.0 | 20.0 | 238 | 10.0 | 27.6 | 9.7 | 1.2 |
| Cheese & Tomato, Blue Parrot Cafe, Sainsbury's* | ¼ Pizza/88g | 217.0 | 8.0 | 248 | 12.7 | 29.5 | 8.8 | 1.2 |
| Cheese & Tomato, Deep Pan, Goodfella's* | ¼ Pizza/102g | 259.0 | 11.0 | 253 | 11.5 | 29.6 | 10.5 | 3.7 |

P

## PIZZA

| INFO/WEIGHT | Measure | per Measure KCAL | per Measure FAT | KCAL | PROT | CARB | FAT | FIBRE |
|---|---|---|---|---|---|---|---|---|
| Cheese & Tomato, Deep Pan, Sainsbury's* | 1 Pizza/182g | 470.0 | 16.0 | 258 | 11.7 | 33.1 | 8.7 | 1.9 |
| Cheese & Tomato, Economy, Sainsbury's* | 1 Pizza/60g | 142.0 | 4.0 | 237 | 11.2 | 34.1 | 6.2 | 1.8 |
| Cheese & Tomato, French Bread, Co-Op* | 1 Pizza/135g | 270.0 | 8.0 | 200 | 9.0 | 27.0 | 6.0 | 2.0 |
| Cheese & Tomato, Frozen, Sainsbury's* | 1 Serving/122g | 300.0 | 11.0 | 246 | 13.7 | 28.0 | 8.8 | 3.0 |
| Cheese & Tomato, Kids, Tesco* | 1 Pizza/95g | 219.0 | 5.0 | 231 | 11.5 | 33.9 | 5.5 | 1.9 |
| Cheese & Tomato, Micro, McCain* | 1 Pizza/122g | 319.0 | 12.0 | 262 | 13.4 | 29.7 | 10.0 | 2.4 |
| Cheese & Tomato, Mini, M & S* | 1 Pizza/95g | 233.0 | 6.0 | 245 | 10.0 | 38.7 | 5.8 | 1.6 |
| Cheese & Tomato, Piccadella, Tesco* | 1 Pizza/295g | 684.0 | 31.0 | 232 | 9.1 | 24.8 | 10.6 | 1.5 |
| Cheese & Tomato, Sainsbury's* | 1 Pizza/247g | 706.0 | 24.0 | 286 | 13.7 | 35.4 | 9.9 | 2.4 |
| Cheese & Tomato, SmartPrice, Asda* | 1 Pizza/151g | 393.0 | 8.0 | 260 | 4.7 | 27.0 | 5.0 | 1.6 |
| Cheese & Tomato, Value, Tesco* | 1 Serving/140g | 388.0 | 14.0 | 277 | 11.4 | 36.0 | 9.7 | 1.8 |
| Cheese & Tomato Slice, Ross* | 1 Slice/77g | 148.0 | 7.0 | 192 | 6.5 | 22.2 | 8.6 | 2.0 |
| Cheese & Tomato Thin & Crispy, Stonebaked, Tesco* | 1 Pizza/155g | 355.0 | 12.0 | 229 | 11.6 | 28.1 | 7.8 | 1.3 |
| Cheese Feast, Deep Pan, Asda* | ½ Pizza/210g | 422.0 | 19.0 | 201 | 13.0 | 17.0 | 9.0 | 2.3 |
| Cheese Feast, Thin Crust, Chilled, Tesco* | ½ Pizza/175g | 467.0 | 22.0 | 267 | 14.7 | 23.4 | 12.8 | 2.5 |
| Cheese Supreme, New Recipe, Goodfella's* | ¼ Pizza/102g | 269.0 | 10.0 | 264 | 12.3 | 31.2 | 10.0 | 2.2 |
| Cheesefeast, Deep & Crispy 12", Takeaway, Iceland* | 1 Slice/132g | 342.0 | 11.0 | 259 | 13.1 | 32.8 | 8.4 | 1.5 |
| Chesse & Tomato, Kids Crew, Iceland* | 1 Pizza/90g | 204.0 | 6.0 | 227 | 9.6 | 32.4 | 6.5 | 1.2 |
| Chicken, Thin & Crispy, Iceland* | ½ Pizza/157g | 469.0 | 20.0 | 299 | 13.0 | 33.2 | 12.7 | 3.1 |
| Chicken & Bacon, Pizzeria, Italian, Sainsbury's* | ½ Pizza/170g | 508.0 | 24.0 | 300 | 13.6 | 29.4 | 14.2 | 2.7 |
| Chicken & Bacon Carbonara, Thin Crust, Italian, Asda* | 1 Pizza/492g | 1156.0 | 34.0 | 235 | 12.0 | 31.0 | 7.0 | 3.4 |
| Chicken & Maple Bacon Carbonara, Asda* | ½ Pizza/195g | 484.0 | 16.0 | 248 | 11.0 | 33.0 | 8.0 | 2.2 |
| Chicken & Pesto, Californian Style, Asda* | ½ Pizza/235g | 533.0 | 16.0 | 227 | 10.0 | 31.0 | 7.0 | 2.0 |
| Chicken & Pesto, with Red Peppers, Italian, Sainsbury's* | ½ Pizza/192g | 471.0 | 19.0 | 245 | 12.0 | 27.3 | 9.7 | 2.7 |
| Chicken & Red Pepper, HE, Tesco* | 1 Pizza/260g | 608.0 | 6.0 | 234 | 12.7 | 40.1 | 2.5 | 0.7 |
| Chicken & Spinach, Eat Smart, Safeway* | 1 Pizza/165g | 322.0 | 3.0 | 195 | 19.0 | 24.0 | 2.1 | 2.5 |
| Chicken & Sweetfire Red Pepper, Stonebaked, GFY, Asda* | ½ Pizza/167g | 363.0 | 8.0 | 217 | 10.0 | 34.0 | 4.6 | 1.6 |
| Chicken & Vegetable, Chargrill, Italiano, Tesco* | ½ Pizza/184g | 383.0 | 15.0 | 208 | 10.6 | 23.3 | 8.0 | 2.4 |
| Chicken & Vegetable, Stone Baked, GFY, Asda* | ½ Pizza/161g | 349.0 | 4.0 | 217 | 13.0 | 36.0 | 2.3 | 1.7 |
| Chicken Alfredo, Chicago Town* | 1 Pizza/265g | 583.0 | 25.0 | 220 | 11.9 | 21.9 | 9.4 | 1.8 |
| Chicken Arrabbiata, M & S* | 1 Pizza/325g | 617.0 | 14.0 | 190 | 11.6 | 26.5 | 4.2 | 1.1 |
| Chicken Arrabiata, Sainsbury's* | ½ Pizza/191g | 444.0 | 12.0 | 232 | 12.1 | 31.4 | 6.4 | 1.7 |
| Chicken Provencal, Goodfella's* | ½ Pizza/143g | 388.0 | 18.0 | 272 | 13.7 | 25.9 | 12.6 | 2.1 |
| Chicken Salsa, HL, Tesco* | ½ Pizza/169g | 269.0 | 4.0 | 159 | 11.1 | 24.0 | 2.1 | 2.2 |
| Chicken Salsa, Thin Crust, Healthy Selection, Budgens* | ½ Pizza/163g | 295.0 | 3.0 | 181 | 10.5 | 30.5 | 1.9 | 1.4 |
| Chilli Beef, Stone Bake, M & S* | 1 Pizza/395g | 790.0 | 23.0 | 200 | 9.6 | 26.7 | 5.8 | 1.9 |
| Chorizo & Cherrybell Peppers, TTD, Sainsbury's* | ½ Pizza/195g | 588.0 | 25.0 | 302 | 13.8 | 33.0 | 12.8 | 2.2 |
| Cream Cheese & Pepperonata, Calzone, Waitrose* | ½ Pizza/165g | 383.0 | 16.0 | 232 | 7.0 | 29.4 | 9.6 | 1.5 |
| Deep South, Chicago Town* | 1 Pizza/171g | 363.0 | 12.0 | 212 | 6.9 | 30.0 | 7.1 | 0.0 |
| Delicata Four Season Ultra Thin, TTD, Sainsbury's* | ½ Pizza/168g | 445.0 | 22.0 | 265 | 13.3 | 24.3 | 12.9 | 2.3 |
| Diavolo, Pizza Express* | ½ Pizza/164g | 322.0 | 11.0 | 197 | 9.4 | 24.6 | 6.7 | 2.1 |
| Double Cheese, Chicago Town* | 1 Pizza/405g | 931.0 | 27.0 | 230 | 11.7 | 30.6 | 6.7 | 0.0 |
| Double Cheese, Square Snacks, Food Explorer, Waitrose* | 1 Pizza/146g | 416.0 | 11.0 | 286 | 12.4 | 40.2 | 7.5 | 1.9 |
| Easy Cheesy, Deep Pan, Chicago Town* | ½ Pizza/547g | 1455.0 | 59.0 | 266 | 11.4 | 30.9 | 10.8 | 1.7 |
| Fajita Chicken, COU, M & S* | 1 Pizza/255g | 433.0 | 6.0 | 170 | 9.9 | 25.5 | 2.4 | 1.2 |
| Fajita Vegetable, BGTY, Sainsbury's* | 1 Pizza/214g | 366.0 | 3.0 | 171 | 8.9 | 30.8 | 1.4 | 2.9 |
| Farmhouse, Tesco* | ½ Pizza/190g | 353.0 | 14.0 | 186 | 9.7 | 20.3 | 7.4 | 2.7 |
| Fingers, Oven Baked, McCain* | 1 Finger/30g | 78.0 | 2.0 | 261 | 12.6 | 34.8 | 7.9 | 2.4 |
| Fire Roasted Pepper, Sainsbury's* | 1 Pizza/344g | 605.0 | 5.0 | 176 | 5.3 | 35.3 | 1.5 | 1.6 |
| Fire Roasted Peppers & Vegetables, Waitrose* | ½ Pizza/235g | 442.0 | 17.0 | 188 | 9.8 | 21.3 | 7.1 | 2.7 |
| Five Cheese & Pepperoni, Deep & Crispy, Waitrose* | 1/3 Pizza/200g | 560.0 | 23.0 | 280 | 11.7 | 32.3 | 11.6 | 1.3 |
| Flamed Chicken & Vegetables, BGTY, Sainsbury's* | 1 Pizza/260g | 660.0 | 11.0 | 254 | 14.2 | 39.3 | 4.4 | 2.3 |
| Flamin' Hot, Deep Dish, Chicago Town* | 1 Pizza/170g | 454.0 | 20.0 | 267 | 8.6 | 31.1 | 12.0 | 0.0 |

| | Measure INFO/WEIGHT | per Measure KCAL | FAT | Nutrition Values per 100g / 100ml KCAL | PROT | CARB | FAT | FIBRE |
|---|---|---|---|---|---|---|---|---|

## PIZZA

| | Measure INFO/WEIGHT | KCAL | FAT | KCAL | PROT | CARB | FAT | FIBRE |
|---|---|---|---|---|---|---|---|---|
| Focaccia Tomato & Black Olive, TTD, Sainsbury's* | ½ Pizza/222g | 515.0 | 20.0 | 232 | 9.3 | 28.7 | 8.9 | 2.9 |
| Four Cheese, Finest, Tesco* | ½ Pizza/230g | 575.0 | 21.0 | 250 | 12.1 | 29.8 | 9.2 | 1.3 |
| Four Cheese, Stuffed Crust, Takeaway, Chicago Town* | ¼ Pizza/149g | 410.0 | 16.0 | 275 | 12.6 | 31.4 | 11.0 | 2.2 |
| Four Cheese, Thin & Crispy, Sainsbury's* | 1 Pizza/265g | 729.0 | 33.0 | 275 | 11.8 | 29.3 | 12.3 | 3.5 |
| Four Cheese, Thin Crust, Tesco* | ½ Pizza/142g | 386.0 | 14.0 | 272 | 14.5 | 31.8 | 9.6 | 1.8 |
| Four Cheese, Weight Watchers* | 1 Pizza/186g | 400.0 | 7.0 | 215 | 10.7 | 34.9 | 3.8 | 1.6 |
| French Bread, Blue Parrot Cafe, Sainsbury's* | 1 Pizza/132g | 271.0 | 6.0 | 205 | 10.7 | 30.8 | 4.3 | 1.3 |
| Frutti Di Mare, Express, Pizza Express* | 1 Pizza/373g | 500.0 | 10.0 | 134 | 9.1 | 20.1 | 2.6 | 0.0 |
| Funghi, Pizzaroma, Safeway* | ½ Pizza/205g | 506.0 | 20.0 | 247 | 10.8 | 29.3 | 9.6 | 2.9 |
| Funghi, Ristorante, Dr Oetker* | 1 Pizza/365g | 865.0 | 43.0 | 237 | 7.9 | 22.5 | 11.9 | 0.0 |
| Garden Style, Hot Stuff* | 1 Slice/188g | 370.0 | 21.0 | 197 | 0.0 | 21.3 | 11.2 | 1.6 |
| Garlic & Mushroom, Asda* | ½ Pizza/241g | 696.0 | 41.0 | 289 | 10.0 | 24.0 | 17.0 | 1.6 |
| Garlic & Mushroom, Thin & Crispy, Sainsbury's* | 1 Pizza/260g | 829.0 | 43.0 | 319 | 11.1 | 31.2 | 16.6 | 1.7 |
| Garlic Chicken, Deep Pan, Sainsbury's* | ½ Pizza/214g | 464.0 | 14.0 | 217 | 11.2 | 28.3 | 6.5 | 3.3 |
| Garlic Chicken, Thin & Crispy, Stonebake, Sainsbury's* | ½ Pizza/160g | 386.0 | 17.0 | 241 | 10.7 | 25.2 | 10.8 | 3.5 |
| Garlic Chicken & Spinach, Perfectly Balanced, Waitrose* | ½ Pizza/172g | 351.0 | 5.0 | 204 | 13.3 | 30.8 | 3.1 | 2.3 |
| Garlic Mushroom, BGTY, Sainsbury's* | ½ Pizza/123g | 262.0 | 2.0 | 213 | 11.6 | 37.2 | 2.0 | 2.7 |
| Garlic Mushroom, Ciabatta Style, Stonebake, Goodfella's* | ½ Pizza/187g | 474.0 | 23.0 | 254 | 10.0 | 27.9 | 12.3 | 2.2 |
| Garlic Mushroom, Tesco* | 1 Pizza/425g | 829.0 | 34.0 | 195 | 9.3 | 21.6 | 8.0 | 5.3 |
| Giardiniera, From Supermarket, Pizza Express* | ½ Pizza/144g | 291.0 | 11.0 | 202 | 8.6 | 25.5 | 7.3 | 2.1 |
| Grilled Pepper, Weight Watchers* | 1 Pizza/220g | 392.0 | 5.0 | 178 | 10.0 | 29.3 | 2.3 | 1.8 |
| Ham, Mushroom & Gruyere, Sainsbury's* | ¼ Pizza/169g | 404.0 | 14.0 | 239 | 10.2 | 31.3 | 8.1 | 3.7 |
| Ham, Mushroom & Tomato, BGTY, Sainsbury's* | ½ Pizza/150g | 309.0 | 6.0 | 206 | 11.8 | 30.4 | 4.1 | 1.2 |
| Ham, Pepperoni & Milano, M & S* | 1 Pizza/290g | 696.0 | 28.0 | 240 | 14.0 | 23.3 | 9.8 | 1.1 |
| Ham & Cheese, Chunky, Asda* | 1 Serving/90g | 211.0 | 3.0 | 234 | 12.0 | 39.0 | 3.3 | 4.7 |
| Ham & Mushroom, Deep Pan, Asda* | ½ Pizza/223g | 444.0 | 16.0 | 199 | 9.0 | 25.0 | 7.0 | 1.2 |
| Ham & Mushroom, Deep Pan, Waitrose* | ½ Pizza/220g | 453.0 | 14.0 | 206 | 10.9 | 26.6 | 6.2 | 1.0 |
| Ham & Mushroom, Finest, Tesco* | ½ Pizza/240g | 576.0 | 26.0 | 240 | 9.5 | 25.9 | 11.0 | 2.2 |
| Ham & Mushroom, Thin & Crispy, Tesco* | 1 Serving/166g | 349.0 | 11.0 | 210 | 13.0 | 23.9 | 6.9 | 2.4 |
| Ham & Mushroom Calzone, Waitrose* | ½ Pizza/145g | 362.0 | 13.0 | 250 | 10.0 | 31.6 | 9.3 | 1.6 |
| Ham & Onion, Tesco* | 1 Serving/181g | 452.0 | 17.0 | 250 | 11.8 | 29.0 | 9.6 | 2.2 |
| Ham & Pineapple, American Deep Pan, Sainsbury's* | 1 Pizza/412g | 1001.0 | 32.0 | 243 | 10.5 | 32.6 | 7.8 | 1.7 |
| Ham & Pineapple, Chicago Town* | 1 Pizza/435g | 866.0 | 20.0 | 199 | 10.0 | 29.7 | 4.5 | 0.0 |
| Ham & Pineapple, Deep Dish, Individual, Chicago Town* | 1 Pizza/170g | 410.0 | 15.0 | 241 | 9.9 | 30.4 | 8.9 | 1.6 |
| Ham & Pineapple, Deep Pan, Ciabatta, Iceland* | ½ Pizza/185g | 440.0 | 14.0 | 238 | 11.6 | 30.3 | 7.8 | 0.8 |
| Ham & Pineapple, Deep Pan, Tesco* | 1 Pizza/237g | 437.0 | 7.0 | 184 | 9.8 | 29.8 | 2.9 | 1.9 |
| Ham & Pineapple, HL, Tesco* | ¼ Pizza/105g | 170.0 | 2.0 | 162 | 10.0 | 25.9 | 2.1 | 2.4 |
| Ham & Pineapple, Loaded, Tesco* | ½ Pizza/265g | 556.0 | 15.0 | 210 | 11.3 | 28.7 | 5.5 | 1.4 |
| Ham & Pineapple, Pizzerai, Simply Italian, Sainsbury's* | ½ Pizza/178g | 434.0 | 15.0 | 244 | 11.5 | 30.4 | 8.5 | 2.4 |
| Ham & Pineapple, Stone Bake, M & S* | 1 Pizza/345g | 690.0 | 20.0 | 200 | 10.1 | 28.3 | 5.7 | 1.6 |
| Ham & Pineapple, Tesco* | 1/6 Pizza/56g | 134.0 | 5.0 | 240 | 10.4 | 30.9 | 8.3 | 2.1 |
| Hawaiian, San Marco* | ¼ Pizza/90g | 208.0 | 8.0 | 231 | 8.9 | 29.7 | 9.2 | 1.5 |
| Hawaiian, Thin Crust, Tesco* | ½ Pizza/192g | 365.0 | 9.0 | 190 | 10.3 | 25.6 | 4.9 | 1.8 |
| Hickory Steak, M & S* | 1 Pizza/400g | 820.0 | 27.0 | 205 | 9.9 | 25.7 | 6.7 | 1.4 |
| Hot & Spicy, Deep Dish, Chicago Town* | 1 Pizza/177g | 434.0 | 18.0 | 245 | 8.6 | 30.4 | 9.9 | 0.9 |
| Hot & Spicy, Deep Dish, Schwan's* | 1 Pizza/170g | 423.0 | 19.0 | 249 | 9.1 | 27.6 | 11.4 | 0.0 |
| Hot & Spicy, Pizzeria Style, Sainsbury's* | 1 Pizza/376g | 986.0 | 46.0 | 262 | 12.5 | 25.5 | 12.3 | 2.4 |
| Hot & Spicy Chicken, Deep Pan, Morrisons* | ½ Pizza/233g | 521.0 | 13.0 | 224 | 10.5 | 32.9 | 5.6 | 1.0 |
| Hot & Spicy Chicken, Deep Pan, Tesco* | ½ Pizza/222g | 423.0 | 7.0 | 191 | 10.5 | 30.0 | 3.3 | 2.1 |
| Hot Chicken, Stone Bake, M & S* | 1 Pizza/380g | 798.0 | 26.0 | 210 | 11.5 | 25.1 | 6.8 | 1.3 |
| Hot Dog, Kids, Tesco* | 1 Pizza/95g | 233.0 | 6.0 | 245 | 9.8 | 36.6 | 6.6 | 2.0 |
| Italian Cheese & Ham, The Little Big Food Company* | 1 Pizza/95g | 236.0 | 6.0 | 248 | 10.9 | 36.2 | 6.5 | 1.0 |
| Italian Meat, So Good, Somerfield* | ½ Pizza/200g | 468.0 | 11.0 | 234 | 14.0 | 32.4 | 5.4 | 2.4 |

P

# PIZZA

| INFO/WEIGHT | Measure | per Measure | | Nutrition Values per 100g / 100ml | | | | |
|---|---|---|---|---|---|---|---|---|
| | | KCAL | FAT | KCAL | PROT | CARB | FAT | FIBRE |
| Italian Meat Feast, Thin & Crispy, Waitrose* | 1 Pizza/182g | 477.0 | 23.0 | 262 | 10.7 | 26.5 | 12.6 | 1.8 |
| Italian Meats, Finest, Tesco* | ½ Pizza/217g | 449.0 | 8.0 | 207 | 13.6 | 29.4 | 3.9 | 1.3 |
| Italian Meats, TTD, Sainsbury's* | ½ Pizza/224g | 586.0 | 27.0 | 262 | 12.8 | 25.6 | 12.0 | 2.4 |
| Italian Mozzarella & Black Forest Ham, Asda* | ¼ Pizza/110g | 227.0 | 7.0 | 206 | 10.0 | 28.0 | 6.0 | 2.7 |
| Italian Sausage & Roasted Peppers, Finest, Tesco* | 1 Pizza/325g | 650.0 | 14.0 | 200 | 7.8 | 31.7 | 4.2 | 1.9 |
| Kids Smart, Morrisons* | 1 Pizza/91g | 203.0 | 4.0 | 223 | 8.8 | 36.9 | 4.4 | 3.1 |
| Le Reine, 8 Inch, Supermarket, Pizza Express* | 1 Pizza/283g | 546.0 | 16.0 | 193 | 10.2 | 25.0 | 5.8 | 2.7 |
| Leggera, Dr Oetker* | ½ Pizza/175g | 317.0 | 10.0 | 181 | 8.8 | 23.1 | 5.8 | 2.7 |
| Loaded Cheese, Goodfella's* | 1 Pizza/410g | 1115.0 | 50.0 | 272 | 11.4 | 29.4 | 12.1 | 1.7 |
| Margherita, 12 Inch, Supermarket, Pizza Express* | ½ Pizza/247g | 513.0 | 15.0 | 208 | 10.1 | 28.5 | 6.0 | 2.4 |
| Margherita, Cheese & Tomato, San Marco* | ½ Pizza/200g | 454.0 | 14.0 | 227 | 10.7 | 29.8 | 7.2 | 1.2 |
| Margherita, HL, Tesco* | ½ Pizza/125g | 222.0 | 2.0 | 178 | 10.8 | 29.3 | 2.0 | 2.5 |
| Margherita, Italiano, Tesco* | ½ Pizza/168g | 395.0 | 12.0 | 235 | 11.7 | 29.9 | 7.2 | 1.2 |
| Margherita, Light Choices, Tesco* | 1 Pizza/200g | 410.0 | 5.0 | 205 | 11.0 | 33.8 | 2.5 | 1.7 |
| Margherita, Morrisons* | ½ Pizza/163g | 416.0 | 18.0 | 256 | 12.9 | 26.1 | 11.1 | 2.3 |
| Margherita, Pizzeria, Italian, Sainsbury's* | ½ Pizza/169g | 426.0 | 17.0 | 253 | 12.2 | 27.9 | 10.3 | 2.5 |
| Margherita, Primafresco, Tesco* | ½ Pizza/204g | 500.0 | 20.0 | 245 | 10.7 | 27.4 | 10.0 | 2.4 |
| Margherita, Stone Baked, GFY, Asda* | ¼ Pizza/73g | 158.0 | 1.0 | 217 | 11.0 | 39.0 | 1.9 | 1.8 |
| Margherita, Stonebaked Ciabatta, Goodfella's* | ½ Pizza/150g | 404.0 | 17.0 | 270 | 11.3 | 32.8 | 11.5 | 2.6 |
| Margherita, Thin & Crispy, Iceland* | ½ Pizza/170g | 391.0 | 14.0 | 230 | 12.7 | 25.9 | 8.5 | 2.8 |
| Margherita, Thin Crust, Tesco* | 1 Serving/170g | 354.0 | 13.0 | 208 | 10.1 | 24.1 | 7.9 | 3.6 |
| Meat, Mediterranean Style, Pizzeria, Waitrose* | ¼ Pizza/174g | 395.0 | 15.0 | 227 | 11.1 | 25.8 | 8.8 | 2.0 |
| Meat Feast, American Style, Sainsbury's* | ½ Pizza/263g | 642.0 | 26.0 | 244 | 12.6 | 26.2 | 9.9 | 2.9 |
| Meat Feast, Deep & Crispy, Iceland* | 1/6 Pizza/136g | 345.0 | 11.0 | 254 | 11.2 | 33.7 | 8.3 | 2.0 |
| Meat Feast, Deep & Loaded, Sainsbury's* | ½ Pizza/298g | 818.0 | 30.0 | 275 | 13.2 | 32.7 | 10.1 | 2.6 |
| Meat Feast, Deep Pan, Co-Op* | 1 Pizza/450g | 1102.0 | 45.0 | 245 | 11.0 | 28.0 | 10.0 | 2.0 |
| Meat Feast, Hot & Spicy, Thin & Crispy, Sainsbury's* | ½ Pizza/170g | 462.0 | 22.0 | 272 | 13.0 | 26.5 | 12.7 | 3.2 |
| Meat Feast, Large, Tesco* | 1 Pizza/735g | 1904.0 | 69.0 | 259 | 10.9 | 32.6 | 9.4 | 2.0 |
| Meat Feast, Loaded, Deep Pan, Large, Tesco* | ½ Pizza/282g | 775.0 | 38.0 | 275 | 12.0 | 26.1 | 13.6 | 1.9 |
| Meat Feast, Mega, Asda* | ½ Pizza/428g | 1044.0 | 34.0 | 244 | 9.5 | 33.6 | 7.9 | 3.2 |
| Meat Feast, Stuffed Crust, Asda* | ½ Pizza/238g | 597.0 | 24.0 | 251 | 14.6 | 25.5 | 10.1 | 3.1 |
| Meat Feast, Thin & Crispy, Asda* | ½ Pizza/183g | 410.0 | 15.0 | 224 | 11.0 | 27.0 | 8.0 | 1.4 |
| Meat Feast, Thin & Crispy, Safeway* | ½ Pizza/179g | 430.0 | 16.0 | 240 | 12.0 | 27.2 | 9.2 | 4.8 |
| Meat Feast, Thin Crust, Tesco* | ½ Pizza/178g | 430.0 | 20.0 | 242 | 13.6 | 21.3 | 11.4 | 2.3 |
| Meat Mayhem, Goodfella's* | 1 Pizza/437g | 1100.0 | 42.0 | 252 | 10.6 | 30.9 | 9.6 | 2.5 |
| Mediterranean, Delicia, Goodfella's* | ½ Pizza/150g | 371.0 | 18.0 | 247 | 9.1 | 25.3 | 12.2 | 2.1 |
| Mediterranean Madness, Goodfella's* | ¼ Pizza/109g | 235.0 | 9.0 | 216 | 9.1 | 27.0 | 8.0 | 3.9 |
| Mediterranean Vegetable, Stonebaked, Sainsbury's* | ½ Pizza/260g | 622.0 | 16.0 | 239 | 9.8 | 35.7 | 6.3 | 3.1 |
| Mexican Style, Morrisons* | ½ Pizza/180g | 437.0 | 17.0 | 243 | 13.7 | 26.0 | 9.4 | 2.0 |
| Mini, Party, Tesco* | 1 Pizza/11g | 26.0 | 1.0 | 248 | 11.4 | 28.6 | 10.5 | 1.9 |
| Mozzarella & Cherry Tomato, Stonebaked, Safeway* | ½ Pizza/263g | 617.0 | 20.0 | 235 | 10.6 | 30.3 | 7.8 | 3.5 |
| Mozzarella & Tomato, Asda* | 1 Pizza/360g | 824.0 | 32.0 | 229 | 12.0 | 25.0 | 9.0 | 2.4 |
| Mozzarella & Tomato, Gluten Free | 1 Pizza/320g | 646.0 | 15.0 | 202 | 6.7 | 33.1 | 4.7 | 1.3 |
| Mozzarella E Provolone, La Bottega, Goodfella's* | ½ Pizza/156g | 372.0 | 15.0 | 238 | 10.1 | 27.9 | 9.6 | 2.4 |
| Mushroom & Roasted Onion, Waitrose* | ½ Pizza/187g | 403.0 | 13.0 | 215 | 9.8 | 28.9 | 6.7 | 1.3 |
| Napoletana, Sainsbury's* | ½ Pizza/186g | 424.0 | 14.0 | 228 | 9.7 | 29.9 | 7.7 | 3.1 |
| Napoletana, TTD, Sainsbury's* | 1 Pizza/374g | 1070.0 | 46.0 | 286 | 11.1 | 28.5 | 12.2 | 2.0 |
| Napoli, Tesco* | ½ Pizza/184g | 431.0 | 12.0 | 235 | 11.9 | 32.6 | 6.3 | 1.4 |
| Napoli Ham & Mushroom, San Marco* | ½ Pizza/219g | 449.0 | 13.0 | 205 | 10.0 | 27.5 | 6.1 | 2.8 |
| Oval, Ham & Pineapple, Weight Watchers* | 1 Pizza/130g | 220.0 | 2.0 | 169 | 11.6 | 26.7 | 1.8 | 3.0 |
| Pasta, Ristorante, Dr Oetker* | ½ Pizza/205g | 449.0 | 18.0 | 219 | 8.0 | 26.6 | 8.9 | 0.0 |
| Pepperonata, Delicata, Sainsbury's* | 1 Pizza/330g | 917.0 | 48.0 | 278 | 12.9 | 24.3 | 14.4 | 2.6 |
| Pepperoni, American Style Deep Pan, Co-Op* | 1 Pizza/395g | 987.0 | 39.0 | 250 | 12.0 | 28.0 | 10.0 | 1.0 |

| PIZZA | Measure INFO/WEIGHT | per Measure KCAL | FAT | Nutrition Values per 100g / 100ml KCAL | PROT | CARB | FAT | FIBRE |
|---|---|---|---|---|---|---|---|---|
| Pepperoni, Asda* | ½ Pizza/150g | 385.0 | 13.0 | 257 | 10.0 | 34.0 | 9.0 | 2.7 |
| Pepperoni, Chicago Town* | 1 Sm Pizza/170g | 471.0 | 22.0 | 277 | 11.5 | 28.8 | 12.9 | 0.0 |
| Pepperoni, Deep & Crispy, Somerfield* | ¼ Slice/101g | 236.0 | 7.0 | 234 | 10.7 | 31.6 | 7.2 | 1.6 |
| Pepperoni, Deep Pan, Frozen, Tesco* | ½ Pizza/215g | 527.0 | 17.0 | 245 | 11.9 | 31.1 | 8.1 | 2.6 |
| Pepperoni, Deep Pan, Goodfella's* | ¼ Slice/109g | 294.0 | 13.0 | 270 | 12.7 | 28.9 | 11.6 | 1.6 |
| Pepperoni, Deep Pan, Sainsbury's* | ½ Pizza/191g | 477.0 | 21.0 | 250 | 9.9 | 28.3 | 10.8 | 3.2 |
| Pepperoni, Double, Italian, Chilled, Tesco* | ½ Pizza/160g | 455.0 | 23.0 | 285 | 12.4 | 25.6 | 14.6 | 2.4 |
| Pepperoni, Extra, Chicago Town* | 1 Pizza/460g | 994.0 | 34.0 | 216 | 9.6 | 27.7 | 7.4 | 0.0 |
| Pepperoni, Feast, Deep Dish, Schwan's* | 1 Pizza/435g | 1188.0 | 62.0 | 273 | 9.9 | 26.3 | 14.2 | 0.0 |
| Pepperoni, Freschetta, Schwan's* | 1 Pizza/310g | 846.0 | 36.0 | 273 | 10.8 | 31.6 | 11.5 | 0.0 |
| Pepperoni, Goodfella's* | 1 Pizza/337g | 900.0 | 43.0 | 267 | 13.2 | 26.3 | 12.9 | 1.7 |
| Pepperoni, Hot & Spicy, Stuffed Crust, Asda* | 1 Pizza/245g | 666.0 | 30.0 | 272 | 13.9 | 26.5 | 12.2 | 2.4 |
| Pepperoni, Italian, Tesco* | ½ Pizza/186g | 484.0 | 21.0 | 260 | 11.4 | 28.0 | 11.1 | 1.1 |
| Pepperoni, Italian Stonebaked, Asda* | ¼ Pizza/132g | 329.0 | 13.0 | 250 | 12.0 | 28.0 | 10.0 | 2.8 |
| Pepperoni, Pizzeria, Sainsbury's* | ½ Pizza/197g | 559.0 | 26.0 | 284 | 13.4 | 28.3 | 13.1 | 2.4 |
| Pepperoni, Speciale, Sainsbury's* | ½ Pizza/179g | 447.0 | 20.0 | 250 | 11.9 | 26.6 | 10.9 | 2.3 |
| Pepperoni, Stone Baked, Carlos* | 1 Pizza/330g | 832.0 | 40.0 | 252 | 13.0 | 23.0 | 12.0 | 0.0 |
| Pepperoni, Stonebake, 10", Asda* | ½ Pizza/170g | 435.0 | 19.0 | 256 | 12.9 | 25.9 | 11.2 | 2.5 |
| Pepperoni, Thin & Crispy, Co-Op* | 1 Pizza/270g | 688.0 | 30.0 | 255 | 11.0 | 26.0 | 11.0 | 1.0 |
| Pepperoni, Thin & Crispy, Goodfella's* | 1 Pizza/593g | 1595.0 | 70.0 | 269 | 13.8 | 26.9 | 11.8 | 2.3 |
| Pepperoni, TTD, Sainsbury's* | 1/3 Pizza/171g | 461.0 | 18.0 | 270 | 14.2 | 29.3 | 10.7 | 2.3 |
| Pepperoni, XXX Hot, Deep & Crispy, Chilled, Tesco* | ½ Pizza/263g | 656.0 | 27.0 | 250 | 9.1 | 30.1 | 10.3 | 2.0 |
| Pepperoni & Cheese, Asda* | ½ Pizza/150g | 385.0 | 13.0 | 257 | 10.0 | 34.0 | 9.0 | 2.7 |
| Pepperoni & Onion, 9", Sainsbury's* | ½ Pizza/207g | 615.0 | 27.0 | 297 | 13.4 | 31.7 | 13.0 | 1.9 |
| Pleasure with Fire Roasted Vegetables, Heinz* | ½ Pizza/200g | 418.0 | 16.0 | 209 | 9.5 | 24.8 | 8.0 | 2.4 |
| Pollo, Ristorante, Dr Oetker* | ½ Pizza/178g | 383.0 | 17.0 | 216 | 8.9 | 23.4 | 9.5 | 0.0 |
| Pollo Ad Astra, Pizza Express* | 1 Pizza/317g | 602.0 | 15.0 | 190 | 11.6 | 25.2 | 4.7 | 2.7 |
| Prosciutto, Classico, Tesco* | ½ Pizza/205g | 461.0 | 10.0 | 225 | 11.7 | 33.6 | 4.9 | 2.5 |
| Prosciutto, Italian Style, Co-Op* | ½ Pizza/183g | 421.0 | 13.0 | 230 | 13.0 | 29.0 | 7.0 | 3.0 |
| Prosciutto, Pizzaria, Sainsbury's* | 1 Pizza/325g | 806.0 | 23.0 | 248 | 11.4 | 34.7 | 7.1 | 3.2 |
| Prosciutto, Ristorante, Dr Oetker* | 1 Pizza/330g | 752.0 | 32.0 | 228 | 10.3 | 24.6 | 9.8 | 0.0 |
| Prosciutto & Fresh Rocket, TTD, Sainsbury's* | ½ Pizza/164g | 542.0 | 22.0 | 330 | 11.9 | 39.9 | 13.6 | 2.5 |
| Prosciutto & Mascarpone, Safeway* | ½ Pizza/200g | 522.0 | 21.0 | 261 | 12.3 | 29.8 | 10.3 | 2.2 |
| Quattro Formaggio, Tesco* | ½ Pizza/219g | 583.0 | 27.0 | 266 | 13.3 | 25.1 | 12.5 | 1.8 |
| Roasted Tomato & Mozzarella, BGTY, Sainsbury's* | 1 Pizza/204g | 526.0 | 16.0 | 258 | 17.8 | 28.6 | 8.0 | 6.0 |
| Roasted Vegetable, for One, GFY, Asda* | 1 Pizza/96g | 190.0 | 4.0 | 198 | 9.0 | 32.0 | 3.8 | 1.5 |
| Salame, Ristorante, Dr Oetker* | ½ Pizza/160g | 455.0 | 24.0 | 285 | 10.4 | 26.3 | 15.3 | 0.0 |
| Salami & Ham, Pizzeria, Waitrose* | ½ Pizza/205g | 443.0 | 14.0 | 216 | 10.1 | 28.7 | 6.7 | 1.8 |
| Salami & Pepperoni, Waitrose* | ½ Pizza/190g | 578.0 | 31.0 | 304 | 13.4 | 29.3 | 16.2 | 2.1 |
| Salami Con Mozarella, Lidl* | ½ Pizza/200g | 534.0 | 22.0 | 267 | 9.9 | 31.5 | 11.2 | 0.0 |
| Sicilian, Premium, Co-Op* | 1 Pizza/600g | 1320.0 | 48.0 | 220 | 9.0 | 27.0 | 8.0 | 2.0 |
| Spicy Chicken, Foccacia, Sainsbury's* | ½ Pizza/245g | 581.0 | 19.0 | 237 | 12.0 | 30.3 | 7.6 | 2.5 |
| Spicy Chicken, HL, Tesco* | 1 Serving/252g | 418.0 | 4.0 | 166 | 10.9 | 27.1 | 1.6 | 2.7 |
| Spicy Chicken, Iceland* | 1 Pizza/345g | 797.0 | 23.0 | 231 | 13.4 | 29.9 | 6.6 | 1.5 |
| Spicy Chicken, Micro, McCain* | 1 Pizza/133g | 388.0 | 20.0 | 292 | 12.4 | 26.9 | 15.0 | 0.0 |
| Spicy Chorizo, Red Pepper & Chilli, Classico, Tesco* | 1 Serving/218g | 474.0 | 17.0 | 218 | 10.3 | 26.4 | 8.0 | 2.5 |
| Spicy Vegetable, Low Fat, Bertorelli* | 1 Pizza/180g | 243.0 | 4.0 | 135 | 6.0 | 23.4 | 2.4 | 1.9 |
| Spicy Vegetable Nacho, GFY, Asda* | 1 Pizza/283g | 636.0 | 13.0 | 225 | 10.0 | 36.0 | 4.5 | 3.3 |
| Spinach & Bacon, Thin & Crispy, M & S* | 1 Pizza/290g | 739.0 | 35.0 | 255 | 10.6 | 26.8 | 12.1 | 1.0 |
| Spinach & Ricotta, BGTY, Sainsbury's* | 1 Pizza/265g | 535.0 | 7.0 | 202 | 10.4 | 34.4 | 2.5 | 2.6 |
| Spinach & Ricotta, Extra Special, Asda* | 1 Pizza/400g | 940.0 | 28.0 | 235 | 9.0 | 34.0 | 7.0 | 1.9 |
| Spinach & Ricotta, GFY, Asda* | 1 Pizza/160g | 375.0 | 7.0 | 234 | 8.7 | 40.0 | 4.4 | 1.8 |
| Spinach & Ricotta, Italian, Chilled, Sainsbury's* | 1 Pizza/361g | 859.0 | 35.0 | 238 | 9.3 | 28.7 | 9.6 | 2.3 |

| | Measure INFO/WEIGHT | per Measure KCAL | FAT | Nutrition Values per 100g / 100ml KCAL | PROT | CARB | FAT | FIBRE |
|---|---|---|---|---|---|---|---|---|
| **PIZZA** | | | | | | | | |
| Spinach & Ricotta, Perfectly Balanced, Waitrose* | ½ Pizza/165g | 272.0 | 3.0 | 165 | 9.7 | 27.7 | 1.7 | 2.6 |
| Spinach & Ricotta, Pizzaria, Waitrose* | ½ Pizza/238g | 501.0 | 21.0 | 211 | 10.7 | 21.9 | 8.9 | 2.6 |
| Spinach & Ricotta, Thin Crust, Italian, Tesco* | ½ Pizza/190g | 365.0 | 17.0 | 192 | 9.6 | 18.7 | 8.8 | 1.9 |
| Spinach with Bacon & Mushroom, GFY, Asda* | 1 Serving/270g | 618.0 | 12.0 | 229 | 13.0 | 34.0 | 4.5 | 2.6 |
| Steak, Stone Bake, M & S* | 1 Pizza/400g | 820.0 | 27.0 | 205 | 9.9 | 25.7 | 6.7 | 1.4 |
| Sunblushed Tomato & Mascarpone, Pizzadella, Tesco* | 1 Serving/275g | 894.0 | 44.0 | 325 | 8.5 | 36.7 | 16.0 | 1.5 |
| Super Supreme, Family, Chicago Town* | ¼ Pizza/225g | 526.0 | 24.0 | 234 | 9.6 | 24.5 | 10.8 | 0.0 |
| Supreme, Deep Dish, Individual, Chicago Town* | 1 Pizza/170g | 456.0 | 20.0 | 268 | 9.2 | 30.8 | 12.0 | 1.0 |
| Supreme, McCain* | 1 Serving/125g | 267.0 | 9.0 | 214 | 10.9 | 27.0 | 6.9 | 0.0 |
| Sweet & Sour Chicken, Thin Crust, Tesco* | ½ Pizza/186g | 366.0 | 13.0 | 197 | 11.9 | 21.9 | 6.9 | 2.3 |
| Sweet Chilli Chicken, BGTY, Sainsbury's* | ½ Pizza/138g | 276.0 | 2.0 | 200 | 13.0 | 33.2 | 1.7 | 2.1 |
| Sweet Chilli Chicken, Stonebaked, Goodfella's* | ½ Pizza/170g | 423.0 | 21.0 | 249 | 12.9 | 22.3 | 12.1 | 3.0 |
| Tomato | 1oz/28g | 54.0 | 3.0 | 193 | 3.3 | 22.6 | 10.6 | 1.4 |
| Triple Cheese, Deep Dish, Chicago Town* | 1 Serving/170g | 418.0 | 18.0 | 246 | 9.9 | 27.6 | 10.7 | 0.0 |
| Triple Cheese, Deep Pan, Morrisons* | 1/6 Pizza/75g | 198.0 | 9.0 | 265 | 10.4 | 28.2 | 12.3 | 1.9 |
| Tuna & Caramelised Red Onion, COU, M & S* | 1 Pizza/245g | 429.0 | 6.0 | 175 | 9.6 | 26.7 | 2.3 | 1.2 |
| Tuna Sweetcorn, BGTY, Sainsbury's* | 1 Pizza/304g | 602.0 | 6.0 | 198 | 13.5 | 31.7 | 1.9 | 2.7 |
| Tuscan Vegetable & Mozzarella, Way to Five, Sainsbury's* | 1 Pizza/317g | 552.0 | 16.0 | 174 | 5.7 | 26.6 | 5.0 | 2.3 |
| Ultimate Meat Feast, Sainsbury's* | 1 Pizza/465g | 1302.0 | 48.0 | 280 | 13.5 | 35.1 | 10.3 | 1.7 |
| Vegetable, COU, M & S* | 1 Pizza/294g | 397.0 | 7.0 | 135 | 6.4 | 23.2 | 2.4 | 1.9 |
| Vegetable, Deep & Crispy, Somerfield* | ½ Pizza/212g | 477.0 | 16.0 | 225 | 9.7 | 29.2 | 7.7 | 1.5 |
| Vegetable, Deep Pan, Co-Op* | 1 Pizza/425g | 829.0 | 30.0 | 195 | 8.0 | 25.0 | 7.0 | 2.0 |
| Vegetable, Frozen, HL, Tesco* | 1 Pizza/400g | 604.0 | 11.0 | 151 | 8.1 | 23.5 | 2.7 | 4.4 |
| Vegetable, GFY, Asda* | ¼ Pizza/94g | 141.0 | 3.0 | 150 | 7.0 | 24.0 | 2.9 | 3.7 |
| Vegetable, Stonebake, Thin & Crispy, Sainsbury's* | ½ Pizza/156g | 329.0 | 13.0 | 211 | 8.3 | 25.5 | 8.6 | 3.5 |
| Vegetable Supreme, Safeway* | ¼ Pizza/170g | 352.0 | 12.0 | 207 | 10.4 | 25.9 | 6.9 | 2.9 |
| Vegetale, Ristorante, Dr Oetker* | ½ Pizza/185g | 386.0 | 17.0 | 209 | 8.1 | 23.9 | 9.0 | 0.0 |
| **PIZZA BASE** | | | | | | | | |
| Deep Pan, Italian, Sainsbury's* | 1 Base/220g | 684.0 | 11.0 | 311 | 7.0 | 59.5 | 5.0 | 1.4 |
| Deep Pan, Napolina* | 1 Base/260g | 757.0 | 8.0 | 291 | 7.9 | 58.0 | 3.0 | 0.2 |
| Gluten & Wheat Free, Glutafin* | 1 Base/110g | 309.0 | 5.0 | 281 | 3.0 | 56.0 | 5.0 | 6.0 |
| Gluten Free, Glutafin* | 1 Base/110g | 278.0 | 5.0 | 253 | 3.0 | 49.0 | 5.0 | 4.5 |
| Italian, Classic, Sainsbury's* | 1 Base/150g | 451.0 | 7.0 | 301 | 7.6 | 57.0 | 4.8 | 1.5 |
| Italian, The Pizza Compny* | 1 Base/260g | 624.0 | 7.0 | 240 | 7.6 | 46.5 | 2.6 | 0.0 |
| Italiana, Parmalat* | 1 Base/150g | 450.0 | 7.0 | 300 | 9.0 | 55.0 | 4.9 | 0.0 |
| Light & Crispy, Napolina* | 1 Base/150g | 436.0 | 4.0 | 291 | 7.9 | 58.0 | 3.0 | 0.2 |
| Mini, Napolina* | 1 Base/75g | 218.0 | 2.0 | 291 | 7.9 | 58.0 | 3.0 | 0.2 |
| Thin & Crispy, Sainsbury's* | 1 Base/135g | 338.0 | 4.0 | 251 | 8.4 | 47.3 | 3.1 | 4.4 |
| Trufree* | 1 Base/110g | 345.0 | 7.0 | 314 | 3.0 | 63.0 | 6.0 | 4.0 |
| Value, Tesco* | 1 Base/150g | 432.0 | 5.0 | 288 | 8.1 | 56.2 | 3.4 | 3.2 |
| **PIZZA BASE MIX** | | | | | | | | |
| Morrisons* | 1 Serving/77g | 313.0 | 4.0 | 407 | 12.7 | 77.9 | 5.0 | 3.6 |
| Sainsbury's* | 1 Pack/145g | 486.0 | 6.0 | 335 | 12.8 | 62.3 | 3.8 | 2.9 |
| Tesco* | 1 Serving/36g | 99.0 | 2.0 | 272 | 10.2 | 43.0 | 6.6 | 3.8 |
| **PLAICE** | | | | | | | | |
| Fillets, in Breadcrumbs, Average | 1 Serving/150g | 331.0 | 18.0 | 221 | 12.8 | 15.5 | 11.9 | 0.8 |
| Fillets, Lightly Dusted, Average | 1 Fillet/113g | 188.0 | 9.0 | 166 | 12.9 | 10.4 | 8.1 | 0.6 |
| *Fillets, Raw, Average* | *1oz/28g* | *24.0* | *0.0* | *87* | *18.2* | *0.0* | *1.5* | *0.0* |
| Goujons, Baked | 1oz/28g | 85.0 | 5.0 | 304 | 8.8 | 27.7 | 18.3 | 0.0 |
| Goujons, Fried in Blended Oil | 1oz/28g | 119.0 | 9.0 | 426 | 8.5 | 27.0 | 32.3 | 0.0 |
| *Grilled* | *1oz/28g* | *27.0* | *0.0* | *96* | *20.1* | *0.0* | *1.7* | *0.0* |
| in Batter, Fried in Blended Oil | 1oz/28g | 72.0 | 5.0 | 257 | 15.2 | 12.0 | 16.8 | 0.5 |
| *Steamed* | *1oz/28g* | *26.0* | *1.0* | *93* | *18.9* | *0.0* | *1.9* | *0.0* |

P

| | Measure INFO/WEIGHT | per Measure KCAL | FAT | Nutrition Values per 100g / 100ml KCAL | PROT | CARB | FAT | FIBRE |
|---|---|---|---|---|---|---|---|---|
| **PLAICE WITH** | | | | | | | | |
| Mushrooms, Filled, Somerfield* | 1 Serving/170g | 338.0 | 18.0 | 199 | 10.2 | 15.7 | 10.6 | 1.2 |
| Mushrooms & Prawns, Sainsbury's* | 1 Serving/170g | 354.0 | 18.0 | 208 | 12.0 | 15.9 | 10.7 | 1.7 |
| Prawns & Garlic, Filled, Somerfield* | 1 Serving/171g | 366.0 | 20.0 | 214 | 12.0 | 14.8 | 11.9 | 0.7 |
| Spinach & Cheddar Cheese, Fillets, Sainsbury's* | 1 Serving/154g | 222.0 | 13.0 | 144 | 13.6 | 3.1 | 8.6 | 0.8 |
| Spinach & Ricotta Cheese, Whole, Sainsbury's* | 1 Serving/159g | 334.0 | 17.0 | 210 | 11.6 | 17.2 | 10.5 | 0.8 |
| **PLANTAIN** | | | | | | | | |
| *Boiled in Unsalted Water* | *1oz/28g* | *31.0* | *0.0* | *112* | *0.8* | *28.5* | *0.2* | *1.2* |
| *Raw, Average* | *1 Med/179g* | *218.0* | *1.0* | *122* | *1.3* | *31.9* | *0.4* | *2.3* |
| *Ripe, Fried in Vegetable Oil* | *1oz/28g* | *75.0* | *3.0* | *267* | *1.5* | *47.5* | *9.2* | *2.3* |
| **PLUMS** | | | | | | | | |
| *Average, Stewed without Sugar* | *1oz/28g* | *8.0* | *0.0* | *30* | *0.5* | *7.3* | *0.1* | *1.3* |
| Soft Dried, Blue Parrot Cafe, Sainsbury's* | 1 Pack/50g | 118.0 | 0.0 | 237 | 2.6 | 55.6 | 0.5 | 7.1 |
| *Weighed with Stone, Average* | *1 Plum/90g* | *32.0* | *0.0* | *36* | *0.6* | *8.6* | *0.1* | *1.6* |
| Whole, Dried, Graze* | 1 Pack/60g | 143.0 | 0.0 | 239 | 2.6 | 56.0 | 0.5 | 0.0 |
| Yellow, Waitrose* | 1 Plum/50g | 19.0 | 0.0 | 39 | 0.6 | 8.8 | 0.1 | 1.5 |
| **POLENTA** | | | | | | | | |
| Merchant Gourmet* | 1 Serving/65g | 232.0 | 1.0 | 357 | 7.4 | 78.8 | 1.4 | 1.3 |
| Organic, Kallo* | 1 Serving/150g | 543.0 | 3.0 | 362 | 8.5 | 78.0 | 1.8 | 0.0 |
| **POLLOCK** | | | | | | | | |
| Breaded, Asda* | 1 Serving/97g | 200.0 | 10.0 | 206 | 12.0 | 17.0 | 10.0 | 1.0 |
| **POLO** | | | | | | | | |
| Citrus Sharp, Nestle* | 1 Tube/34g | 134.0 | 0.0 | 393 | 0.0 | 96.6 | 1.0 | 0.0 |
| Fruits, Nestle* | 1 Tube/37g | 142.0 | 0.0 | 383 | 0.0 | 96.0 | 0.0 | 0.0 |
| Mints, Clear Ice, Nestle* | 1 Sweet/4g | 16.0 | 0.0 | 390 | 0.0 | 97.5 | 0.0 | 0.0 |
| Mints, Original, Nestle* | 1 Sweet/2g | 8.0 | 0.0 | 404 | 0.0 | 98.9 | 1.1 | 0.0 |
| Smoothies, Nestle* | 1 Sweet/4g | 16.0 | 0.0 | 408 | 0.1 | 86.9 | 6.8 | 0.0 |
| Spearmint, Nestle* | 1 Tube/35g | 141.0 | 0.0 | 402 | 0.0 | 98.2 | 1.1 | 0.0 |
| **POMEGRANATE** | | | | | | | | |
| *Raw, Fresh, Flesh Only, Average* | *1 Sm Fruit/86g* | *59.0* | *0.0* | *68* | *0.9* | *17.2* | *0.3* | *0.6* |
| *Raw, Weighed with Rind & Skin, Average* | *1 Sm Fruit/154g* | *105.0* | *0.0* | *68* | *0.9* | *17.2* | *0.3* | *0.1* |
| **POMELO** | | | | | | | | |
| *Fresh, Raw, Weighed with Skin & Seeds* | *100 Grams/100g* | *38.0* | *0.0* | *38* | *0.8* | *9.6* | *0.0* | *1.0* |
| **POP TARTS** | | | | | | | | |
| Bustin' Berry, Kellogg's* | 1 Tart/50g | 200.0 | 6.0 | 400 | 4.0 | 69.0 | 12.0 | 2.0 |
| Chocomallow, Kellogg's* | 1 Tart/50g | 198.0 | 6.0 | 396 | 6.0 | 66.0 | 12.0 | 2.5 |
| Cookies 'n' Creme, Kellogg's* | 1 Tart/50g | 197.0 | 5.0 | 394 | 4.0 | 72.0 | 10.0 | 1.5 |
| Cream Cheese & Cherry Swirl, Kellogg's* | 1 Tart/62g | 250.0 | 11.0 | 403 | 3.2 | 59.7 | 17.7 | 1.0 |
| Frosted Brown Sugar Cinnamon, Kellogg's* | 1 Tart/50g | 210.0 | 7.0 | 420 | 6.0 | 68.0 | 14.0 | 2.0 |
| Strawberry Sensation, Kellogg's* | 1 Tart/50g | 197.0 | 5.0 | 395 | 4.0 | 70.0 | 11.0 | 2.0 |
| **POPCORN** | | | | | | | | |
| 94% Fat Free, Orville Redenbacher's* | 1 Bag/76g | 220.0 | 0.0 | 289 | 13.2 | 65.8 | 0.0 | 0.0 |
| Air Popped, Plain, Average | 1oz/28g | 110.0 | 1.0 | 387 | 12.9 | 77.9 | 4.5 | 14.5 |
| Butter, 6% Fat, Orville Redenbacher's* | 1 Portion/21g | 86.0 | 1.0 | 410 | 11.9 | 77.6 | 5.7 | 14.3 |
| Butter Flavour, Microwave, Popz* | 1 Serving/100g | 504.0 | 30.0 | 504 | 7.0 | 51.5 | 30.0 | 9.2 |
| Butter Toffee, Tesco* | 1 Pack/350g | 1417.0 | 27.0 | 405 | 2.2 | 81.7 | 7.7 | 4.3 |
| Butter Toffee, Yummy* | 1 Serving/50g | 227.0 | 6.0 | 455 | 2.5 | 82.4 | 12.8 | 3.1 |
| Plain, Oil Popped, Average | 1 Bag/74g | 439.0 | 32.0 | 593 | 6.2 | 48.7 | 42.8 | 0.0 |
| Ready Salted, Microwave, Popz* | 1 Serving/20g | 101.0 | 6.0 | 504 | 7.0 | 51.5 | 30.0 | 9.2 |
| Salted, Blockbuster* | 1 Bowl/25g | 99.0 | 3.0 | 397 | 10.6 | 62.2 | 11.7 | 8.6 |
| Salted, Sold At Cinema, Playtime Popcorn* | 1 Av Sm/74g | 384.0 | 25.0 | 519 | 8.3 | 45.9 | 33.6 | 0.0 |
| Super, Perri* | 1 Packet/30g | 139.0 | 7.0 | 464 | 8.4 | 55.5 | 23.2 | 8.5 |
| Sweet, Best-In* | 1 Serving/34g | 161.0 | 6.0 | 473 | 7.3 | 72.6 | 17.0 | 0.0 |
| Sweet, Butterkist, Butterkist* | 1 Pack/120g | 612.0 | 30.0 | 510 | 2.8 | 68.5 | 24.8 | 5.6 |

**P**

| | Measure INFO/WEIGHT | per Measure KCAL | FAT | Nutrition Values per 100g / 100ml KCAL | PROT | CARB | FAT | FIBRE |
|---|---|---|---|---|---|---|---|---|
| **POPCORN** | | | | | | | | |
| Sweet, Cinema Style, Butterkist* | 1 Serving/100g | 391.0 | 7.0 | 391 | 4.9 | 76.2 | 7.4 | 0.0 |
| Sweet, Microwave, Cinema, Popz* | 1 Bag/85g | 420.0 | 22.0 | 494 | 6.0 | 60.0 | 25.5 | 8.2 |
| Sweet, Vanilla & Sugar, Microwave, Act II* | 1 Pack75g | 369.0 | 18.0 | 492 | 7.9 | 60.8 | 24.1 | 10.4 |
| Toffee, 90% Fat Free, Butterkist* | 1 Pack/35g | 142.0 | 3.0 | 406 | 2.8 | 77.7 | 9.3 | 0.0 |
| Toffee, Butterkist* | 1 Serving/35g | 135.0 | 3.0 | 385 | 1.8 | 76.4 | 8.0 | 3.5 |
| Toffee, Chicago Joes* | 1 Serving/10g | 31.0 | 0.0 | 314 | 3.1 | 84.6 | 4.8 | 0.0 |
| Toffee, Milk Chocolate Coated, Sainsbury's* | ¼ Bag/25g | 130.0 | 7.0 | 520 | 6.5 | 64.1 | 26.4 | 1.3 |
| Toffee, Sainsbury's* | 1 Serving/50g | 207.0 | 6.0 | 415 | 1.8 | 73.8 | 12.7 | 3.3 |
| Vanilla, Cinema Sweet Microwave, Act II* | ½ Pack/50g | 234.0 | 8.0 | 468 | 9.0 | 71.0 | 16.0 | 12.0 |
| **POPCORN CAKES** | | | | | | | | |
| Caramel, Orville Redenbacher's* | 1 Cake/12g | 47.0 | 0.0 | 392 | 7.2 | 89.0 | 0.9 | 6.0 |
| **POPPADOM BITES** | | | | | | | | |
| Lime & Coriander Chutney, Sensations, Walkers* | 1 Serving/18g | 83.0 | 4.0 | 460 | 7.0 | 59.0 | 22.0 | 4.5 |
| Spicy Tandoori Masala, Sensations, Walkers* | 1 Sm Bag/18g | 88.0 | 4.0 | 490 | 7.5 | 59.0 | 25.0 | 4.0 |
| **POPPADOMS** | | | | | | | | |
| Fried in Vegetable Oil, Average | 1 Poppadom/10g | 37.0 | 2.0 | 369 | 17.5 | 39.1 | 16.9 | 0.0 |
| Indian, Asda* | 1 Pack/45g | 232.0 | 16.0 | 516 | 14.5 | 36.2 | 34.8 | 7.8 |
| Mercifully Mild, Phileas Fogg* | 1 Serving/30g | 150.0 | 10.0 | 499 | 14.8 | 36.8 | 32.6 | 6.0 |
| Mini, Sainsbury's* | ½ Pack/50g | 249.0 | 16.0 | 498 | 14.9 | 36.9 | 32.3 | 7.6 |
| Plain, Asda* | 1 Poppadom/9g | 44.0 | 3.0 | 484 | 18.0 | 40.0 | 28.0 | 0.0 |
| Plain, Indian to Go, Sainsbury's* | 1 Poppadom/8g | 34.0 | 1.0 | 405 | 18.4 | 43.4 | 17.5 | 9.0 |
| Plain, Tesco* | 1 Serving/9g | 41.0 | 2.0 | 439 | 17.8 | 44.4 | 21.1 | 4.6 |
| Plain, Waitrose* | 1 Serving/9g | 37.0 | 2.0 | 408 | 21.0 | 39.3 | 18.6 | 9.1 |
| Spicy, COU, M & S* | 1 Pack/26g | 84.0 | 1.0 | 325 | 23.5 | 51.9 | 2.4 | 8.1 |
| **POPPETS*** | | | | | | | | |
| Chocolate Raisins, Poppets* | 1 Pack/35g | 140.0 | 5.0 | 401 | 4.9 | 65.4 | 13.3 | 0.0 |
| Peanut, Poppets* | 1 Box/100g | 544.0 | 37.0 | 544 | 16.4 | 37.0 | 37.0 | 0.0 |
| Toffee, Milk Chocolate, Poppets* | 1 Box/100g | 491.0 | 23.0 | 491 | 5.3 | 68.0 | 23.0 | 0.0 |
| **POPPING CORN** | | | | | | | | |
| Average | 1 Serving/30g | 112.0 | 1.0 | 375 | 10.9 | 73.1 | 4.3 | 12.7 |
| **PORK** | | | | | | | | |
| Belly, Roasted, Lean & Fat | 1oz/28g | 82.0 | 6.0 | 293 | 25.1 | 0.0 | 21.4 | 0.0 |
| *Chop, Lean & Fat, Raw, Average* | *1oz/28g* | *67.0* | *4.0* | *240* | *29.2* | *0.0* | *13.7* | *0.0* |
| *Diced, Lean, Average* | *1oz/28g* | *31.0* | *0.0* | *109* | *22.0* | *0.0* | *1.7* | *0.0* |
| *Escalope, Average* | *1 Escalope/75g* | *108.0* | *2.0* | *144* | *31.0* | *0.0* | *2.2* | *0.0* |
| *Escalope, Lean, Healthy Range, Average* | *1 Escalope/75g* | *80.0* | *2.0* | *106* | *22.0* | *0.0* | *2.0* | *0.0* |
| *Joint, Ready to Roast, Average* | *½ Joint/254g* | *375.0* | *18.0* | *147* | *19.2* | *2.3* | *7.1* | *0.1* |
| *Joint, with Crackling, Ready to Roast, Average* | *1 Joint/567g* | *1283.0* | *80.0* | *226* | *24.2* | *0.8* | *14.1* | *0.0* |
| *Leg, Joint, Healthy Range, Average* | *1 Serving/200g* | *206.0* | *4.0* | *103* | *20.0* | *0.6* | *2.2* | *0.0* |
| Loin, Applewood Smoked, Asda* | 1 Slice/15g | 18.0 | 1.0 | 122 | 21.8 | 0.5 | 3.6 | 0.0 |
| *Loin, Chops, Boneless, Grilled, Average* | *1oz/28g* | *90.0* | *4.0* | *320* | *29.0* | *0.0* | *15.7* | *0.0* |
| *Loin, Chops, Grilled, Lean* | *1oz/28g* | *52.0* | *2.0* | *184* | *31.6* | *0.0* | *6.4* | *0.0* |
| *Loin, Joint, Roast, Lean* | *1oz/28g* | *51.0* | *2.0* | *182* | *30.1* | *0.0* | *6.8* | *0.0* |
| *Loin, Joint, Roasted, Lean & Fat* | *1oz/28g* | *71.0* | *4.0* | *253* | *26.3* | *0.0* | *15.3* | *0.0* |
| Loin, Roasted, with Rosemary, Arista, Sainsbury's* | 1 Slice/17g | 24.0 | 1.0 | 144 | 20.8 | 0.1 | 6.8 | 0.7 |
| *Loin, Steak, Fried, Lean* | *1oz/28g* | *53.0* | *2.0* | *191* | *31.5* | *0.0* | *7.2* | *0.0* |
| *Loin, Steak, Fried, Lean & Fat* | *1oz/28g* | *77.0* | *5.0* | *276* | *27.5* | *0.0* | *18.4* | *0.0* |
| Loin, Steak, Lean, Raw, Average | 1 Serving/175g | 345.0 | 20.0 | 197 | 22.7 | 1.8 | 11.2 | 0.4 |
| Loin, Stuffed, Roast, M & S* | 1 Slice/12g | 22.0 | 1.0 | 180 | 24.4 | 2.4 | 7.9 | 0.0 |
| *Medallions, Average* | *1 Pack/220g* | *359.0* | *5.0* | *163* | *35.1* | *0.0* | *2.5* | *0.4* |
| *Mince, Lean, Healthy Range, Average* | *1 Pack/400g* | *504.0* | *20.0* | *126* | *19.7* | *0.4* | *5.0* | *0.3* |
| *Mince, Raw* | *1oz/28g* | *46.0* | *3.0* | *164* | *19.2* | *0.0* | *9.7* | *0.0* |
| *Mince, Stewed* | *1oz/28g* | *53.0* | *3.0* | *191* | *24.4* | *0.0* | *10.4* | *0.0* |

| | Measure INFO/WEIGHT | per Measure KCAL | per Measure FAT | Nutrition Values per 100g / 100ml KCAL | PROT | CARB | FAT | FIBRE |
|---|---|---|---|---|---|---|---|---|
| **PORK** | | | | | | | | |
| *Raw, Lean, Average* | *1oz/28g* | *42.0* | *1.0* | *151* | *28.6* | *0.0* | *4.1* | *0.0* |
| *Roast, Lean Only, Average* | *1oz/28g* | *34.0* | *1.0* | *121* | *22.7* | *0.3* | *3.3* | *0.0* |
| *Roast, Slices, Average* | *1 Slice/30g* | *40.0* | *1.0* | *133* | *22.7* | *0.4* | *4.5* | *0.0* |
| *Shoulder, Slices, Cured* | *1oz/28g* | *29.0* | *1.0* | *103* | *16.9* | *0.9* | *3.6* | *0.0* |
| *Shoulder, Whole, Lean & Fat, Raw, Average* | *100g* | *236.0* | *18.0* | *236* | *17.2* | *0.0* | *18.0* | *0.0* |
| *Steak, Lean, Stewed* | *1oz/28g* | *49.0* | *1.0* | *176* | *33.6* | *0.0* | *4.6* | *0.0* |
| *Steak, Lean & Fat, Average* | *1oz/28g* | *61.0* | *4.0* | *219* | *23.8* | *0.0* | *13.7* | *0.1* |
| *Stir Fry Strips, Lean, Healthy Range, Average* | *¼ Pack/113g* | *118.0* | *2.0* | *104* | *21.3* | *0.0* | *2.0* | *0.0* |
| Tenderloin, Roulade, Waitrose* | 1 Pack/171g | 282.0 | 13.0 | 165 | 18.4 | 5.9 | 7.5 | 1.8 |
| **PORK &** | | | | | | | | |
| Apricots, Aromatic, Cafe Culture, M & S* | ½ Pack/420g | 672.0 | 31.0 | 160 | 10.3 | 12.5 | 7.4 | 2.1 |
| **PORK CHAR SUI** | | | | | | | | |
| Chinese, Tesco* | 1 Pack/400g | 520.0 | 17.0 | 130 | 7.2 | 15.7 | 4.3 | 0.6 |
| in Cantonese Sauce, Asda* | 1 Pack/360g | 623.0 | 8.0 | 173 | 9.8 | 28.4 | 2.2 | 0.5 |
| Takeaway, Iceland* | 1 Pack/400g | 412.0 | 10.0 | 103 | 7.9 | 12.5 | 2.4 | 1.2 |
| with Chicken, & Egg Fried Rice, Tesco* | 1 Serving/450g | 602.0 | 16.0 | 134 | 7.1 | 18.3 | 3.6 | 0.9 |
| **PORK CHINESE** | | | | | | | | |
| Sliced, M & S* | 1 Serving/140g | 224.0 | 4.0 | 160 | 26.4 | 6.1 | 3.1 | 0.0 |
| Style, GFY, Asda* | 1 Serving/170g | 286.0 | 6.0 | 168 | 18.8 | 15.3 | 3.5 | 0.4 |
| with Noodles, Tesco* | 1 Serving/450g | 612.0 | 26.0 | 136 | 7.0 | 14.2 | 5.7 | 1.1 |
| **PORK DINNER** | | | | | | | | |
| Roast, Birds Eye* | 1 Pack/340g | 410.0 | 12.0 | 121 | 7.6 | 14.7 | 3.5 | 1.6 |
| **PORK IN** | | | | | | | | |
| Kentish Cider, With Bramley Apple Mash, Tesco* | 1 Pack/450g | 495.0 | 22.0 | 110 | 5.6 | 10.6 | 4.8 | 1.1 |
| Light Mustard Sauce, Fillet, COU, M & S* | 1 Pack/390g | 312.0 | 9.0 | 80 | 10.9 | 3.5 | 2.4 | 0.7 |
| Rich Sage & Onion Gravy, Steaks, Tesco* | 1 Serving/160g | 218.0 | 10.0 | 136 | 16.0 | 3.2 | 6.5 | 1.5 |
| **PORK SCRATCHINGS** | | | | | | | | |
| Crunch, Mr Porky* | 1 Pack/30g | 159.0 | 10.0 | 531 | 60.4 | 0.5 | 31.9 | 4.6 |
| KP Snacks* | 1 Pack/20g | 125.0 | 10.0 | 624 | 47.3 | 0.5 | 48.1 | 0.5 |
| Tavern Snacks* | 1 Pack/30g | 187.0 | 14.0 | 624 | 47.3 | 0.5 | 48.1 | 0.5 |
| **PORK WITH** | | | | | | | | |
| Apricot & Orange Stuffing, Joint, Sainsbury's* | ¼ Joint/200g | 566.0 | 36.0 | 283 | 29.0 | 0.9 | 18.1 | 1.4 |
| Cheese & Pineapple, Loin Steaks, M & S* | 1 Steak/141g | 240.0 | 14.0 | 170 | 14.0 | 6.3 | 9.9 | 0.0 |
| Herbes De Provence, Joint, Sainsbury's* | ¼ Joint/200g | 302.0 | 16.0 | 151 | 19.2 | 0.1 | 8.2 | 0.6 |
| Honey & Mustard Sauce, Steaks, Tesco* | ½ Pack/160g | 258.0 | 12.0 | 161 | 16.3 | 8.7 | 7.4 | 1.4 |
| Honey & Soy, Sainsbury's* | 1 Serving/260g | 260.0 | 7.0 | 100 | 12.3 | 6.2 | 2.9 | 0.3 |
| Leek & Bacon Stuffing, Roast, Shoulder, Sainsbury's* | 1 Serving/150g | 237.0 | 12.0 | 158 | 18.8 | 2.4 | 8.3 | 0.5 |
| Leek & Cheese Stuffing, Joint, Sainsbury's* | 1 Serving/100g | 231.0 | 10.0 | 231 | 31.0 | 3.0 | 10.5 | 1.1 |
| Medallions, with Bramley Apple, M & S* | 1 Serving/380g | 418.0 | 13.0 | 110 | 17.7 | 2.5 | 3.4 | 0.5 |
| Peppers, Marinated, Tapas, Waitrose* | 1 Serving/105g | 181.0 | 7.0 | 172 | 26.3 | 2.2 | 6.4 | 0.3 |
| Roasted Rosemary Potatoes, Porchetta, Finest, Tesco* | ½ Pack/370g | 455.0 | 32.0 | 123 | 6.9 | 4.6 | 8.6 | 0.5 |
| Sage, Onion & Lemon Stuffing, Joint, Sainsbury's* | 1 Serving/260g | 699.0 | 43.0 | 269 | 27.4 | 2.2 | 16.7 | 1.4 |
| Sage & Onion Stuffing, Joint, BGTY, Sainsbury's* | 1 Serving/150g | 246.0 | 5.0 | 164 | 29.5 | 3.3 | 3.6 | 1.3 |
| Sage & Onion Stuffing, Joint, Tesco* | 1 Serving/200g | 208.0 | 6.0 | 104 | 17.1 | 2.7 | 2.8 | 0.0 |
| Stuffing, Belly, Norfolk Outdoor Reared, Finest, Tesco* | 1 Serving/180g | 524.0 | 45.0 | 291 | 14.9 | 1.7 | 24.9 | 0.0 |
| **PORT** | | | | | | | | |
| *Average* | *1 Serving/50ml* | *78.0* | *0.0* | *157* | *0.1* | *12.0* | *0.0* | *0.0* |
| **POT NOODLE*** | | | | | | | | |
| Balti Curry, Made Up, Pot Noodle* | 1 Pot/301g | 268.0 | 2.0 | 89 | 3.1 | 17.8 | 0.5 | 0.5 |
| Beef & Tomato, Made Up, Pot Noodle* | 1 Pot/300g | 378.0 | 14.0 | 126 | 3.1 | 18.1 | 4.7 | 1.1 |
| Beef & Tomato, Mini, Pot Noodle* | 1 Pot/190g | 254.0 | 9.0 | 134 | 3.5 | 18.7 | 5.0 | 1.7 |
| Bombay Bad Boy, Made Up, Pot Noodle* | 1 Pot/305g | 384.0 | 14.0 | 126 | 3.1 | 17.9 | 4.6 | 1.1 |
| Chicken & Mushroom, King, Pot Noodle* | 1 Pack/401g | 513.0 | 19.0 | 128 | 3.2 | 18.1 | 4.8 | 1.1 |

**P**

| | Measure INFO/WEIGHT | per Measure | | Nutrition Values per 100g / 100ml | | | | |
|---|---|---|---|---|---|---|---|---|
| | | KCAL | FAT | KCAL | PROT | CARB | FAT | FIBRE |
| **POT NOODLE*** | | | | | | | | |
| Chicken & Mushroom, Made Up, Pot Noodle* | 1 Pot/300g | 384.0 | 14.0 | 128 | 3.2 | 18.0 | 4.7 | 1.1 |
| Chicken & Mushroom, Mini, Made Up, Pot Noodle* | 1 Pot/190g | 243.0 | 9.0 | 128 | 3.8 | 18.2 | 4.5 | 1.4 |
| Chicken Curry, Hot, Made Up, Pot Noodle* | 1 Pot/300g | 384.0 | 14.0 | 128 | 2.8 | 18.7 | 4.7 | 1.1 |
| Hot, Made Up, Pot Noodle* | 1 Pot/300g | 378.0 | 16.0 | 126 | 3.0 | 16.9 | 5.2 | 1.1 |
| Hot Dog & Ketchup, Fun Pots, Made Up, Pot Noodle* | 1 Pot/190g | 243.0 | 9.0 | 128 | 3.6 | 18.3 | 4.5 | 1.5 |
| Korma Curry, Made Up, Pot Noodle* | 1 Pot/300g | 273.0 | 3.0 | 91 | 2.9 | 17.4 | 1.1 | 0.4 |
| Nice & Spicy, Made Up, Pot Noodle* | 1 Pot/300g | 381.0 | 14.0 | 127 | 2.8 | 18.3 | 4.7 | 1.1 |
| Seedy Sanchez, Made Up, Pot Noodle* | 1 Pot/300g | 396.0 | 14.0 | 132 | 3.1 | 19.1 | 4.8 | 1.1 |
| Spicy Chilli, Posh, Made Up, Pot Noodle* | 1 Pot/301g | 328.0 | 18.0 | 109 | 2.5 | 11.7 | 5.9 | 1.0 |
| Spicy Curry, Made Up, Pot Noodle* | 1 Pot/300g | 393.0 | 14.0 | 131 | 2.9 | 19.1 | 4.8 | 1.1 |
| Sweet & Sour, Dry, Pot Noodle* | 1 Pot/86g | 376.0 | 14.0 | 437 | 12.1 | 60.9 | 16.1 | 3.1 |
| Sweet & Sour, King, Dry, Pot Noodle* | 1 Pot/105g | 473.0 | 20.0 | 450 | 8.8 | 60.0 | 19.1 | 4.8 |
| Sweet & Sour, Oriental, Posh, Pot Noodle* | 1 Pot/300g | 375.0 | 14.0 | 125 | 1.7 | 19.2 | 4.6 | 0.5 |
| **POT RICE*** | | | | | | | | |
| Chicken & Sweetcorn, Dry, Pot Rice* | 1 Pot/68g | 243.0 | 3.0 | 357 | 13.1 | 65.8 | 4.6 | 4.0 |
| Chicken Curry, Dry, Pot Rice* | 1 Pot/74g | 253.0 | 2.0 | 342 | 11.0 | 67.2 | 2.3 | 3.3 |
| **POTATO** | | | | | | | | |
| Mash, Jersey Butter, Luxury, TTD, Sainsbury's* | 1 Pack/450g | 490.0 | 29.0 | 109 | 1.3 | 11.4 | 6.5 | 2.8 |
| Mashed, Ready to Eat, Sainsbury's* | ½ Pack/200g | 142.0 | 4.0 | 71 | 1.4 | 12.1 | 1.9 | 2.0 |
| Rings, Value, Tesco* | 1 Pack/20g | 95.0 | 4.0 | 475 | 3.8 | 74.1 | 18.0 | 2.4 |
| **POTATO BITES** | | | | | | | | |
| Barbecue, Baked, COU, M & S* | 1 Pack/26g | 92.0 | 1.0 | 355 | 7.1 | 76.7 | 2.4 | 4.2 |
| Butter & Chive, Baked, COU, M & S* | 1 Serving/26g | 92.0 | 1.0 | 355 | 7.6 | 77.2 | 2.0 | 4.7 |
| Crispy, Morrisons* | 1 Serving/115g | 240.0 | 8.0 | 209 | 3.5 | 32.6 | 7.2 | 2.2 |
| **POTATO BOMBAY** | | | | | | | | |
| Average | 1oz/28g | 33.0 | 2.0 | 117 | 2.0 | 13.7 | 6.8 | 1.2 |
| Canned, Tesco* | 1 Can/400g | 380.0 | 12.0 | 95 | 2.5 | 13.5 | 2.9 | 2.3 |
| Flavours of India, Canned, Sainsbury's* | ½ Can/200g | 160.0 | 4.0 | 80 | 2.4 | 13.3 | 1.9 | 1.8 |
| Indian Meal for Two, Sainsbury's* | ½ Pack/151g | 154.0 | 8.0 | 102 | 1.6 | 11.4 | 5.6 | 3.1 |
| M & S* | 1 Pack/300g | 300.0 | 14.0 | 100 | 1.5 | 12.1 | 4.8 | 1.6 |
| Meal Solutions, Co-Op* | 1 Pack/300g | 210.0 | 12.0 | 70 | 1.0 | 8.0 | 4.0 | 2.0 |
| Morrisons* | 1 Serving/175g | 180.0 | 9.0 | 103 | 1.5 | 13.0 | 5.0 | 1.7 |
| Sainsbury's* | 1 Pack/300g | 285.0 | 15.0 | 95 | 1.8 | 10.8 | 4.9 | 2.5 |
| Tesco* | 1 Pack/300g | 240.0 | 13.0 | 80 | 1.3 | 9.3 | 4.2 | 2.1 |
| Waitrose* | 1 Pack/300g | 246.0 | 13.0 | 82 | 1.6 | 9.3 | 4.3 | 2.2 |
| **POTATO CAKES** | | | | | | | | |
| Average | 1 Cake/70g | 127.0 | 1.0 | 180 | 3.8 | 37.5 | 1.7 | 2.4 |
| Fried, Average | 1oz/28g | 66.0 | 3.0 | 237 | 4.9 | 35.0 | 9.0 | 0.8 |
| **POTATO CHIPS** | | | | | | | | |
| Beef & Horseradish, Tyrells* | ¼ Pack/37g | 177.0 | 9.0 | 473 | 9.0 | 58.6 | 24.8 | 2.4 |
| Hand Fried Mature Cheddar, Burts* | 1 Serving/40g | 202.0 | 11.0 | 504 | 6.4 | 57.4 | 27.7 | 0.0 |
| Lightly Sea Salted, Tyrells* | 1 Pack/150g | 739.0 | 38.0 | 493 | 7.7 | 58.9 | 25.4 | 2.6 |
| Mature Cheese & Chives, Tyrells* | 1 Bag/50g | 261.0 | 14.0 | 522 | 6.1 | 56.5 | 27.9 | 0.0 |
| Ready Salted, Sainsbury's* | ¼ Pack/33g | 174.0 | 11.0 | 526 | 5.6 | 51.7 | 33.0 | 3.8 |
| Sweet Chilli & Red Pepper, Tyrells* | ¼ Pack/37g | 180.0 | 9.0 | 481 | 7.9 | 59.7 | 24.5 | 2.4 |
| Worcester Sauce, with Sun Dried Tomato, Tyrells* | 1 Bag/50g | 241.0 | 12.0 | 482 | 7.6 | 60.1 | 24.8 | 2.5 |
| **POTATO CREAMED** | | | | | | | | |
| with Cabbage, Asda* | 1 Pack/350g | 255.0 | 9.0 | 73 | 1.3 | 11.0 | 2.6 | 0.0 |
| **POTATO CRUNCHIES** | | | | | | | | |
| Oven Crunchies, Ross* | 1 Serving/100g | 240.0 | 12.0 | 240 | 3.6 | 30.0 | 11.7 | 2.4 |
| **POTATO FRIED** | | | | | | | | |
| Crispy, M & S* | 1 Pack/400g | 660.0 | 28.0 | 165 | 2.0 | 22.6 | 7.1 | 1.4 |

| | Measure INFO/WEIGHT | per Measure KCAL | FAT | Nutrition Values per 100g / 100ml KCAL | PROT | CARB | FAT | FIBRE |
|---|---|---|---|---|---|---|---|---|
| **POTATO FRITTERS** | | | | | | | | |
| Crispy, Oven Baked, Birds Eye* | 1 Fritter/20g | 29.0 | 2.0 | 145 | 2.0 | 16.3 | 8.0 | 1.2 |
| with Sweetcorn, M & S* | 1 Pack/135g | 304.0 | 17.0 | 225 | 4.4 | 24.1 | 12.6 | 2.3 |
| **POTATO MASH** | | | | | | | | |
| Bacon & Cheese, Tesco* | 1 Serving/200g | 252.0 | 13.0 | 126 | 3.1 | 13.9 | 6.4 | 1.3 |
| Bacon & Spring Onion, Finest, Tesco* | ½ Pack/200g | 214.0 | 10.0 | 107 | 4.3 | 10.8 | 5.2 | 1.6 |
| Cheddar, Irish, Finest, Tesco* | ½ Pack/250g | 350.0 | 20.0 | 140 | 6.3 | 10.2 | 7.9 | 1.4 |
| Cheddar Cheese, TTD, Sainsbury's* | ½ Pack/225g | 157.0 | 5.0 | 70 | 2.1 | 9.9 | 2.4 | 2.9 |
| Cheese & Onion, Eat Smart, Morrisons* | 1 Pack/400g | 340.0 | 6.0 | 85 | 4.4 | 13.2 | 1.6 | 1.3 |
| Cheese & Onion, Tesco* | 1 Serving/200g | 210.0 | 9.0 | 105 | 3.2 | 12.6 | 4.7 | 1.0 |
| Leek & Bacon, Tesco* | 1 Serving/400g | 356.0 | 14.0 | 89 | 3.0 | 11.1 | 3.6 | 1.9 |
| Leek & Cheese, COU, M & S* | ½ Pack/225g | 180.0 | 5.0 | 80 | 3.0 | 12.0 | 2.1 | 1.3 |
| Mustard, with Caramelised Onions, Finest, Tesco* | 1 Serving/200g | 232.0 | 9.0 | 116 | 2.6 | 16.0 | 4.6 | 1.8 |
| Roast Onion, Snack in a Pot, Tesco* | 1 Pot/218g | 257.0 | 13.0 | 118 | 1.6 | 14.7 | 5.9 | 0.6 |
| Savoy Cabbage & Spring Onion, M & S* | 1 Serving/225g | 250.0 | 16.0 | 111 | 2.0 | 10.2 | 6.9 | 1.3 |
| Sun Dried Tomato & Basil, COU, M & S* | 1 Serving/170g | 127.0 | 3.0 | 75 | 1.0 | 14.4 | 1.5 | 1.2 |
| with Cracked Pepper & Sea Salt, Luxury, Sainsbury's* | ½ Pack/225g | 389.0 | 28.0 | 173 | 1.6 | 13.2 | 12.6 | 1.0 |
| with Sweetcorn & Flaked Tuna, Quick, Sainsbury's* | 1 Pot/224g | 240.0 | 9.0 | 107 | 2.4 | 15.0 | 4.1 | 2.1 |
| with Vegetables, GFY, Asda* | 1 Pack/290g | 186.0 | 3.0 | 64 | 1.6 | 12.0 | 1.1 | 2.3 |
| with Vegetables, Sainsbury's* | ½ Pack/229g | 142.0 | 2.0 | 62 | 1.8 | 11.4 | 1.0 | 3.1 |
| **POTATO RINGS** | | | | | | | | |
| Mature Cheddar & Red Onion, GFY, Asda* | 1 Pack/10g | 36.0 | 0.0 | 360 | 5.2 | 81.6 | 1.5 | 2.9 |
| Ready Salted, M & S* | 1 Serving/75g | 375.0 | 21.0 | 500 | 3.5 | 58.9 | 28.1 | 2.6 |
| Ready Salted, Sainsbury's* | 1 Serving/50g | 257.0 | 14.0 | 514 | 3.2 | 61.5 | 28.4 | 1.8 |
| Salt Vinegar, Sainsbury's* | 1 Pack/25g | 114.0 | 5.0 | 456 | 3.6 | 65.6 | 19.6 | 2.8 |
| **POTATO SKINS** | | | | | | | | |
| American Style, Loaded, Asda* | 1 Serving/78g | 294.0 | 18.0 | 375 | 15.0 | 27.0 | 23.0 | 2.4 |
| American Style, Loaded, Tesco* | 1 Serving/340g | 388.0 | 8.0 | 114 | 6.8 | 16.3 | 2.4 | 3.3 |
| Cheese & Bacon, Loaded, Asda* | ½ Pack/125g | 275.0 | 15.0 | 220 | 13.0 | 15.0 | 12.0 | 3.3 |
| Cheese & Bacon, Loaded, Sour Cream & Chive Dip, Tesco* | ½ Pack/210g | 622.0 | 33.0 | 296 | 3.1 | 4.1 | 15.5 | 1.7 |
| Cheese & Bacon, Sainsbury's* | 1 Serving/140g | 349.0 | 22.0 | 249 | 10.3 | 17.3 | 15.4 | 2.5 |
| Cheese & Bacon, Waitrose* | 1 Serving/75g | 146.0 | 9.0 | 195 | 7.3 | 13.1 | 12.6 | 3.5 |
| Cheese & Chive, Sainsbury's* | 2 Skins/150g | 286.0 | 18.0 | 191 | 7.7 | 13.3 | 11.9 | 2.8 |
| Cheese & Ham, Iceland* | 2 Skins/108g | 155.0 | 5.0 | 143 | 6.3 | 19.3 | 4.5 | 2.0 |
| Cheese & Onion, Loaded, Sour Cream & Chive Dip, Tesco* | 1 Skin/60g | 114.0 | 6.0 | 190 | 5.8 | 17.6 | 10.8 | 1.4 |
| Soured Cream, Loaded, M & S* | ½ Pack/150g | 307.0 | 18.0 | 205 | 9.1 | 15.8 | 11.9 | 0.9 |
| **POTATO SMILES** | | | | | | | | |
| Weighed Baked, McCain* | 1 Serving/100g | 237.0 | 10.0 | 237 | 3.4 | 33.4 | 10.1 | 3.1 |
| Weighed Frozen, McCain* | 1 Serving/100g | 191.0 | 8.0 | 191 | 2.6 | 27.0 | 8.0 | 2.7 |
| **POTATO SUMTHINGS** | | | | | | | | |
| Weighed Baked, McCain* | 1 Serving/100g | 220.0 | 9.0 | 220 | 3.4 | 31.3 | 9.0 | 2.8 |
| Weighed Frozen, McCain* | 1 Serving/100g | 187.0 | 8.0 | 187 | 2.9 | 26.2 | 7.9 | 2.4 |
| **POTATO TWIRLS** | | | | | | | | |
| Sainsbury's* | 1 Serving/50g | 217.0 | 7.0 | 435 | 3.0 | 72.8 | 14.6 | 3.1 |
| **POTATO WAFFLES** | | | | | | | | |
| Birds Eye* | 1 Waffle/60g | 105.0 | 5.0 | 175 | 2.5 | 21.6 | 8.7 | 1.5 |
| Frozen, Cooked | 1oz/28g | 56.0 | 2.0 | 200 | 3.2 | 30.3 | 8.2 | 2.3 |
| Frozen, Grilled, Asda* | 1 Waffle/57g | 104.0 | 6.0 | 183 | 2.0 | 21.0 | 10.1 | 1.7 |
| Mini, Sainsbury's* | 1 Waffle/11g | 27.0 | 2.0 | 242 | 2.8 | 20.1 | 16.7 | 1.0 |
| Sainsbury's* | 1 Waffle/56g | 108.0 | 6.0 | 194 | 2.9 | 22.8 | 10.1 | 1.1 |
| Southern Fried, Asda* | 1 Waffle/51g | 107.0 | 5.0 | 209 | 2.8 | 27.0 | 10.0 | 2.1 |
| **POTATO WEDGES** | | | | | | | | |
| & Dip, M & S* | 1 Pack/450g | 697.0 | 33.0 | 155 | 2.5 | 20.4 | 7.4 | 1.8 |
| Aldi* | 1 Serving/100g | 150.0 | 7.0 | 150 | 2.1 | 20.2 | 6.8 | 0.0 |

**P**

| | Measure INFO/WEIGHT | per Measure KCAL | FAT | Nutrition Values per 100g / 100ml KCAL | PROT | CARB | FAT | FIBRE |
|---|---|---|---|---|---|---|---|---|
| **POTATO WEDGES** | | | | | | | | |
| Asda* | 1 Wedge/40g | 57.0 | 2.0 | 142 | 3.4 | 21.0 | 4.9 | 1.7 |
| Baked, GFY, Asda* | 1 Pack/450g | 616.0 | 12.0 | 137 | 3.4 | 25.0 | 2.6 | 3.4 |
| BBQ Chicken Spicy, Good Intentions, Somerfield* | 1 Pack/400g | 380.0 | 5.0 | 95 | 7.4 | 13.6 | 1.2 | 1.4 |
| BBQ Flavour, Asda* | 1 Serving/100g | 185.0 | 9.0 | 185 | 2.9 | 23.0 | 9.0 | 1.7 |
| BGTY, Sainsbury's* | ½ Pack/190g | 179.0 | 3.0 | 94 | 3.0 | 16.4 | 1.8 | 3.4 |
| Bombay, with Yoghurt & Mint Dip, HL, Tesco* | 1 Serving/170g | 139.0 | 4.0 | 82 | 1.3 | 14.5 | 2.1 | 0.9 |
| Crispy, M & S* | 1 Serving/200g | 340.0 | 14.0 | 170 | 1.3 | 25.3 | 7.1 | 1.7 |
| Four Cheese & Red Onion, Chicago Town* | 1 Serving/150g | 210.0 | 8.0 | 140 | 2.1 | 21.0 | 5.3 | 2.4 |
| Garlic & Herb, COU, M & S* | 1 Pack/300g | 300.0 | 8.0 | 100 | 2.3 | 16.4 | 2.6 | 3.2 |
| Garlic & Herb Crusted, Chicago Town* | 1 Serving/150g | 216.0 | 6.0 | 144 | 1.9 | 24.4 | 4.3 | 2.2 |
| Jumbo, Finest, Tesco* | 1 Serving/126g | 145.0 | 3.0 | 115 | 1.4 | 22.7 | 2.1 | 1.7 |
| Mexican, Inspire, Asda* | 1 Pack/500g | 525.0 | 17.0 | 105 | 2.2 | 16.5 | 3.4 | 1.8 |
| Only 5% Fat, Weighed Baked, McCain* | 1 Serving/100g | 173.0 | 4.0 | 173 | 3.3 | 30.2 | 4.3 | 2.8 |
| Only 5% Fat, Weighed Frozen, McCain* | 1 Serving/100g | 123.0 | 3.0 | 123 | 2.2 | 21.8 | 3.0 | 1.9 |
| Perfectly Balanced, Waitrose* | 1 Serving/275g | 278.0 | 5.0 | 101 | 2.5 | 19.0 | 1.7 | 3.5 |
| Savoury, Waitrose* | 1/3 Bag/250g | 350.0 | 11.0 | 140 | 2.3 | 22.9 | 4.3 | 1.9 |
| Sour Cream & Chives, McCain* | 1 Serving/100g | 132.0 | 4.0 | 132 | 2.4 | 24.0 | 4.1 | 0.0 |
| Southern Fried, Asda* | 1 Serving/100g | 157.0 | 4.0 | 157 | 3.0 | 26.0 | 4.5 | 3.5 |
| Southern Fried Style, Tesco* | 1 Serving/155g | 232.0 | 14.0 | 150 | 3.0 | 14.1 | 9.1 | 2.0 |
| Spicy, & Garlic Dip, Linda McCartney* | 1 Pack/300g | 366.0 | 17.0 | 122 | 2.6 | 15.3 | 5.6 | 3.1 |
| Spicy, Asda* | 1 Serving/100g | 145.0 | 6.0 | 145 | 1.8 | 21.8 | 5.7 | 2.1 |
| Spicy, M & S* | ½ Pack/225g | 349.0 | 15.0 | 155 | 2.4 | 21.8 | 6.5 | 1.3 |
| Spicy, Occasions, Sainsbury's* | 1 Serving/100g | 144.0 | 4.0 | 144 | 2.5 | 23.7 | 4.3 | 0.4 |
| Spicy, Simple Solutions, Tesco* | 1 Serving/150g | 141.0 | 4.0 | 94 | 4.6 | 12.2 | 3.0 | 1.4 |
| with Broccoli & Mozzarella Cheese, Weight Watchers* | 1 Pack/320g | 294.0 | 10.0 | 92 | 3.1 | 13.3 | 3.0 | 1.0 |
| with Chilli, COU, M & S* | 1 Pack/400g | 380.0 | 11.0 | 95 | 5.2 | 13.7 | 2.7 | 2.3 |
| with Olive Oil & Parsley Dressing, Inspire, Asda* | ½ Pack/300g | 219.0 | 7.0 | 73 | 0.1 | 12.7 | 2.4 | 2.1 |
| **POTATOES** | | | | | | | | |
| Alphabites, Captain Birds Eye, Birds Eye* | 9 Bites/56g | 75.0 | 3.0 | 134 | 2.0 | 19.5 | 5.3 | 1.4 |
| Anya, Boiled in Unsalted Water, TTD, Sainsbury's* | 1 Serving/80g | 60.0 | 0.0 | 75 | 1.5 | 17.8 | 0.3 | 1.1 |
| Baby, Dressed with Garlic & Rosemary, M & S* | 1 Serving/185g | 129.0 | 5.0 | 70 | 2.0 | 9.0 | 2.8 | 2.4 |
| Baby, Garlic & Sea Salt Roasted, Finest, Tesco* | 1 Serving/200g | 192.0 | 7.0 | 96 | 3.1 | 13.5 | 3.3 | 1.0 |
| Baby, New, with Butter, Mint & Parsley, Organic, Asda* | 1 Pack/360g | 414.0 | 10.0 | 115 | 1.7 | 20.4 | 2.9 | 2.5 |
| Baby, Oven Bake, Aunt Bessie's* | 1 Serving/120g | 103.0 | 2.0 | 86 | 2.2 | 16.3 | 1.4 | 3.0 |
| Baby, Roasted & Garlic, TTD, Sainsbury's* | ½ Pack/200g | 174.0 | 3.0 | 87 | 2.6 | 15.9 | 1.4 | 3.4 |
| Baby, with Butter & Herbs, Sainsbury's* | ¼ Pack/143g | 107.0 | 2.0 | 75 | 1.3 | 14.7 | 1.2 | 2.1 |
| Baby, with Herb Butter, Safeway* | 1 Serving/200g | 158.0 | 2.0 | 79 | 1.4 | 15.6 | 1.2 | 1.4 |
| *Baked, Flesh & Skin, Average* | *1 Med/200g* | *218.0* | *0.0* | *109* | *2.3* | *25.2* | *0.1* | *2.4* |
| *Baked, Flesh Only, Weighed with Skin, Average* | *1oz/28g* | *26.0* | *0.0* | *93* | *2.0* | *21.6* | *0.1* | *1.5* |
| *Baked, in Microwave, Flesh & Skin, Average* | *1oz/28g* | *29.0* | *0.0* | *105* | *2.4* | *24.1* | *0.1* | *2.3* |
| *Baked, in Microwave, Flesh Only, Average* | *1oz/28g* | *28.0* | *0.0* | *100* | *2.1* | *23.3* | *0.1* | *1.6* |
| *Baked, in Microwave, Skin Only, Average* | *1oz/28g* | *37.0* | *0.0* | *132* | *4.4* | *29.6* | *0.1* | *5.5* |
| Baked, Jacket, Baby, Veg, COOK!, M & S* | 1 Pack/675g | 776.0 | 38.0 | 115 | 2.1 | 14.3 | 5.6 | 2.3 |
| Baked, Jacket, Beef Chilli Filled, GFY, Asda* | 1 Serving/300g | 261.0 | 1.0 | 87 | 4.6 | 16.0 | 0.5 | 3.2 |
| Baked, Jacket, Cheddar Cheese, COU, M & S* | 1 Potato/164g | 164.0 | 3.0 | 100 | 2.9 | 17.3 | 1.9 | 2.0 |
| Baked, Jacket, Cheese & Beans, Somerfield* | 1 Pack/340g | 306.0 | 7.0 | 90 | 4.1 | 13.8 | 2.0 | 2.2 |
| Baked, Jacket, Cheesy, GFY, Asda* | 1 Serving/155g | 129.0 | 2.0 | 83 | 2.6 | 16.0 | 1.0 | 2.1 |
| Baked, Jacket, Chicken Tikka, COU, M & S* | 1 Serving/300g | 240.0 | 5.0 | 80 | 5.4 | 10.9 | 1.6 | 1.3 |
| Baked, Jacket, Chilli, BGTY, Sainsbury's* | 1 Pack/350g | 318.0 | 5.0 | 91 | 5.3 | 14.3 | 1.4 | 1.2 |
| Baked, Jacket, Chilli Con Carne, COU, M & S* | 1 Pack/300g | 270.0 | 6.0 | 90 | 6.0 | 11.1 | 2.1 | 1.2 |
| Baked, Jacket, Creamy Mushroom, Asda* | 1 Serving/100g | 124.0 | 2.0 | 124 | 3.5 | 22.0 | 2.4 | 1.7 |
| Baked, Jacket, Garlic, Mini, Asda* | 1 Serving/65g | 59.0 | 2.0 | 91 | 2.2 | 13.0 | 3.3 | 0.0 |
| Baked, Jacket, Garlic Butter Filling, Morrisons* | 1 Potato/210g | 239.0 | 12.0 | 114 | 1.7 | 13.6 | 5.9 | 0.9 |

P

## POTATOES

| | Measure INFO/WEIGHT | per Measure KCAL | FAT | Nutrition Values per 100g / 100ml KCAL | PROT | CARB | FAT | FIBRE |
|---|---|---|---|---|---|---|---|---|
| Baked, Jacket, Garlic Mushrooms, BGTY, Sainsbury's* | 1 Pack/350g | 262.0 | 3.0 | 75 | 2.3 | 14.4 | 0.9 | 1.2 |
| Baked, Jacket, Halves, M & S* | 1 Serving/250g | 187.0 | 3.0 | 75 | 2.0 | 14.2 | 1.1 | 1.7 |
| Baked, Jacket, Ham & Cheddar Cheese, Asda* | 1 Pack/300g | 435.0 | 11.0 | 145 | 7.0 | 21.0 | 3.7 | 1.6 |
| Baked, Jacket, Herb & Rock Salt Seasoning, M & S* | 1 Pack/500g | 375.0 | 5.0 | 75 | 2.0 | 14.2 | 1.1 | 1.7 |
| Baked, Jacket, Leek & Cheese, M & S* | 1 Serving/206g | 206.0 | 6.0 | 100 | 3.8 | 13.4 | 3.1 | 3.2 |
| Baked, Jacket, Mature Cheddar Cheese, Finest, Tesco* | 1 Potato/245g | 360.0 | 18.0 | 147 | 5.4 | 14.6 | 7.5 | 2.3 |
| Baked, Jacket, Mature Cheddar Cheese, M & S* | ½ Pack/206g | 225.0 | 7.0 | 109 | 3.6 | 16.9 | 3.2 | 1.0 |
| Baked, Jacket, Stuffed, Garlic & Herb Butter, Tesco* | 1 Pack/435g | 570.0 | 33.0 | 131 | 1.3 | 14.6 | 7.5 | 1.0 |
| Baked, Jacket, Tuna & Sweetcorn, Average | 1 Serving/300g | 273.0 | 7.0 | 91 | 5.0 | 12.5 | 2.2 | 0.9 |
| Baked, Jacket, Tuna & Sweetcorn, BGTY, Sainsbury's* | 1 Pack/350g | 360.0 | 9.0 | 103 | 6.5 | 13.2 | 2.7 | 1.3 |
| Baked, Jacket, Tuna & Sweetcorn, COU, M & S* | 1 Pack/300g | 270.0 | 5.0 | 90 | 5.1 | 12.8 | 1.8 | 1.4 |
| Baked, Jacket, with Baked Bean & Sausage, Asda* | 1 Pack/300g | 447.0 | 10.0 | 149 | 5.0 | 25.0 | 3.2 | 2.7 |
| Baked, Jacket, with Beef Chilli, Asda* | 1 Pack/300g | 381.0 | 8.0 | 127 | 5.0 | 21.0 | 2.6 | 2.0 |
| Baked, Jacket, with Beef Chilli, M & S* | 1 Pack/360g | 288.0 | 7.0 | 80 | 5.9 | 9.6 | 2.0 | 0.9 |
| Baked, Jacket, with Cheese, Freshly Prepared, Tesco* | ½ Pack/215g | 150.0 | 3.0 | 70 | 3.9 | 9.7 | 1.4 | 2.8 |
| Baked, Jacket, with Cheese, HL, Tesco* | 1 Potato/225g | 202.0 | 5.0 | 90 | 4.5 | 13.0 | 2.2 | 1.8 |
| Baked, Jacket, with Cheese & Bacon, Finest, Tesco* | 1 Potato/245g | 360.0 | 20.0 | 147 | 6.0 | 12.6 | 8.0 | 2.5 |
| Baked, Jacket, with Cheese & Butter, Tesco* | 1 Potato/225g | 263.0 | 11.0 | 117 | 3.1 | 14.9 | 5.0 | 2.3 |
| Baked, Jacket, with Cheese & Vegetarian Bacon, Tesco* | ½ Pack/225g | 279.0 | 11.0 | 124 | 4.7 | 15.5 | 4.8 | 1.3 |
| Baked, Jacket, with Cheese Mash, GFY, Asda* | 1 Potato/200g | 192.0 | 6.0 | 96 | 4.8 | 13.0 | 2.8 | 2.2 |
| Baked, Jacket, with Smoked Bacon, Finest, Tesco* | ½ Pack/200g | 200.0 | 8.0 | 100 | 3.5 | 12.1 | 4.0 | 2.5 |
| *Baked, Skin Only, Average* | *1oz/28g* | *55.0* | *0.0* | *198* | *4.3* | *46.1* | *0.1* | *7.9* |
| *Baking, Raw, Average* | *1 Med/250g* | *197.0* | *0.0* | *79* | *2.1* | *18.0* | *0.1* | *1.6* |
| *Boiled, Average* | *1 Serving/120g* | *86.0* | *0.0* | *72* | *1.8* | *17.0* | *0.1* | *1.2* |
| *Boiled, with Skin* | *1 Potato/125g* | *97.0* | *0.0* | *78* | *2.9* | *17.2* | *0.1* | *3.3* |
| Boulangere, M & S* | ½ Pack/225g | 180.0 | 2.0 | 80 | 2.8 | 15.9 | 0.9 | 0.9 |
| *Charlotte, Average* | *1 Serving/184g* | *139.0* | *0.0* | *76* | *1.6* | *17.4* | *0.2* | *3.3* |
| Crispy Bites, Weighed Frozen, McCain* | 1 Serving/100g | 141.0 | 4.0 | 141 | 2.5 | 20.4 | 4.4 | 1.5 |
| Crispy Slices, Weighed Baked, McCain* | 1 Serving/100g | 240.0 | 11.0 | 240 | 3.2 | 32.1 | 11.0 | 2.1 |
| Crispy Slices, Weighed Frozen, McCain* | 1 Portion/100g | 163.0 | 7.0 | 163 | 2.1 | 21.9 | 7.4 | 1.4 |
| *Dauphinoise, Average* | *1 Serving/200g* | *335.0* | *24.0* | *167* | *2.2* | *12.7* | *11.9* | *1.5* |
| *Desiree, Average* | *1 Serving/200g* | *152.0* | *0.0* | *76* | *2.1* | *16.3* | *0.2* | *0.6* |
| Garlic, Tapas Selection, Sainsbury's* | 1 Serving/22g | 49.0 | 4.0 | 224 | 2.6 | 10.4 | 19.1 | 0.7 |
| *Hasselback, Average* | *1 Serving/175g* | *182.0* | *2.0* | *104* | *1.9* | *22.0* | *0.9* | *2.9* |
| Italian Style, & Vegetables, Waitrose* | 1 Serving/126g | 138.0 | 4.0 | 110 | 2.0 | 19.2 | 2.8 | 3.4 |
| *Jersey Royal, Canned, Average* | *1 Can/186g* | *116.0* | *0.0* | *62* | *1.4* | *14.0* | *0.1* | *1.2* |
| *Jersey Royal, New, Raw, Average* | *1oz/28g* | *21.0* | *0.0* | *75* | *1.6* | *17.2* | *0.2* | *1.5* |
| Jersey Royal with Mint Butter, Extra Special, Asda* | ½ Pack/172g | 148.0 | 5.0 | 86 | 1.6 | 13.0 | 3.1 | 1.5 |
| Juliette, Sainsbury's* | 1 Serving/250g | 200.0 | 0.0 | 80 | 1.4 | 19.7 | 0.1 | 1.0 |
| King Edward, Tesco* | 1 Serving/100g | 77.0 | 0.0 | 77 | 2.1 | 16.8 | 0.2 | 1.3 |
| Lemon & Rosemary, Finest, Tesco* | ½ Pack/200g | 200.0 | 7.0 | 100 | 2.1 | 14.7 | 3.7 | 2.0 |
| *Maris Piper, Raw, Average* | *1 Serving/200g* | *151.0* | *0.0* | *75* | *2.0* | *16.5* | *0.2* | *1.4* |
| Mashed, Colcannon, Sainsbury's* | ½ Pack/300g | 192.0 | 12.0 | 64 | 0.4 | 6.7 | 4.0 | 1.4 |
| Mashed, Colcannon, Tesco* | 1 Serving/250g | 225.0 | 13.0 | 90 | 1.6 | 8.4 | 5.4 | 1.8 |
| Mashed, Colcannon, Waitrose* | ½ Pack/150g | 138.0 | 6.0 | 92 | 1.7 | 12.8 | 3.8 | 1.4 |
| Mashed, Fresh Mash, Light Choices, Tesco* | 1 Pack/450g | 292.0 | 10.0 | 65 | 2.0 | 9.3 | 2.2 | 1.6 |
| Mashed, From Supermarket, Average | ½ Pack/200g | 197.0 | 8.0 | 98 | 1.8 | 13.3 | 4.1 | 1.5 |
| Mashed, From Supermarket, Healthy Range, Average | 1 Serving/200g | 160.0 | 3.0 | 80 | 1.8 | 14.6 | 1.6 | 1.3 |
| Mashed, From Supermarket, Premium, Average | 1 Serving/225g | 305.0 | 18.0 | 136 | 1.7 | 14.4 | 7.9 | 1.1 |
| Mashed, Maris Piper, Tesco* | ½ Pack/228g | 182.0 | 4.0 | 80 | 1.5 | 14.0 | 1.7 | 0.9 |
| Mashed, Maris Piper, with Cream & Butter, M & S* | ½ Pack/200g | 180.0 | 7.0 | 90 | 1.1 | 12.9 | 3.6 | 0.4 |
| Mashed, Vintage Cheddar Cheese, M & S* | ½ Pack/225g | 247.0 | 12.0 | 110 | 4.6 | 12.6 | 5.3 | 1.0 |
| Mashed, with Carrot & Swede, M & S* | 1 Serving/225g | 214.0 | 14.0 | 95 | 1.6 | 8.3 | 6.4 | 1.4 |

| | Measure INFO/WEIGHT | per Measure | | Nutrition Values per 100g / 100ml | | | | |
|---|---|---|---|---|---|---|---|---|
| | | KCAL | FAT | KCAL | PROT | CARB | FAT | FIBRE |
| **POTATOES** | | | | | | | | |
| Mashed, with Carrot & Swede, Sainsbury's* | ½ Pack/226g | 230.0 | 12.0 | 102 | 1.9 | 11.7 | 5.3 | 1.5 |
| Mashed, with Creme Fraiche & Seasoning, Waitrose* | ½ Pack/225g | 189.0 | 6.0 | 84 | 2.0 | 12.7 | 2.8 | 1.4 |
| Mashed, with Leeks, Creamy, Birds Eye* | 1 Pack/300g | 300.0 | 21.0 | 100 | 2.0 | 7.3 | 7.0 | 0.8 |
| Mashed, with Spring Onion, Weight Watchers* | 1 Serving/100g | 79.0 | 2.0 | 79 | 2.0 | 11.2 | 2.4 | 1.1 |
| *New, Average* | *1 Serving/100g* | *75.0* | *0.0* | *75* | *1.5* | *17.8* | *0.3* | *1.1* |
| *New, Baby, Average* | *1 Serving/180g* | *135.0* | *0.0* | *75* | *1.7* | *17.1* | *0.3* | *1.6* |
| *New, Baby, Canned, Average* | *1 Can/120g* | *70.0* | *0.0* | *59* | *1.4* | *13.2* | *0.2* | *1.4* |
| New, Baby, with Herb Dressing & Seasoned Butter, Tesco* | ½ Pack/160g | 112.0 | 4.0 | 70 | 1.5 | 10.2 | 2.6 | 2.6 |
| New, Garlic, Herb & Parsley Butter, Co-Op* | 1 Serving/100g | 115.0 | 5.0 | 115 | 1.0 | 15.0 | 5.0 | 2.0 |
| New, in a Herb Marinade, Tesco* | ¼ Pack/150g | 151.0 | 7.0 | 101 | 1.3 | 13.0 | 4.9 | 1.5 |
| New, with Butter, Chives & Mint, M & S* | ¼ Pack/145g | 116.0 | 2.0 | 80 | 1.1 | 16.2 | 1.4 | 2.3 |
| New, with English Churned Butter, M & S* | 1 Pack/180g | 261.0 | 4.0 | 145 | 1.3 | 29.5 | 2.2 | 2.1 |
| New, with Herbs & Butter, Waitrose* | 1 Serving/385g | 443.0 | 23.0 | 115 | 1.7 | 13.8 | 5.9 | 1.2 |
| New, with Parsley Butter, TTD, Sainsbury's* | 1 Serving/150g | 126.0 | 4.0 | 84 | 2.2 | 13.3 | 2.4 | 1.0 |
| New, with Sunblush Tomato, M & S* | 1 Pack/385g | 346.0 | 7.0 | 90 | 1.6 | 17.2 | 1.8 | 1.3 |
| Pan Fried, Aldi* | 1 Serving/250g | 182.0 | 2.0 | 73 | 2.7 | 13.7 | 0.8 | 0.0 |
| *Red, Flesh Only, Average* | *1 Serving/300g* | *217.0* | *0.0* | *72* | *1.9* | *16.3* | *0.1* | *1.2* |
| Roast, Basted in Beef Dripping, Waitrose* | 1 Serving/165g | 213.0 | 9.0 | 129 | 2.2 | 18.0 | 5.4 | 1.9 |
| Roast, Extra Crispy, Oven Baked, Aunt Bessie's* | 1 Serving/100g | 223.0 | 12.0 | 223 | 2.9 | 26.1 | 11.8 | 3.6 |
| Roast, Frozen, Average | 1 Potato/70g | 105.0 | 3.0 | 149 | 2.6 | 23.5 | 5.0 | 1.4 |
| Roast, Frozen, Healthy Range, Average | 1 Potato/70g | 70.0 | 2.0 | 100 | 2.5 | 18.1 | 2.4 | 2.1 |
| Roast, Garlic, Sainsbury's* | ½ Pack/225g | 358.0 | 22.0 | 159 | 3.2 | 14.6 | 9.7 | 1.4 |
| *Roast, in Lard, Average* | *1oz/28g* | *42.0* | *1.0* | *149* | *2.9* | *25.9* | *4.5* | *1.8* |
| *Roast, in Oil, Average* | *1oz/28g* | *42.0* | *1.0* | *149* | *2.9* | *25.9* | *4.5* | *1.8* |
| Roast, New, Rosemary, Ainsley Harriott* | 1 Serving/150g | 133.0 | 4.0 | 89 | 2.0 | 16.0 | 2.7 | 1.3 |
| Roast, Oven Baked, Aunt Bessie's* | 1 Serving/165g | 305.0 | 15.0 | 185 | 2.3 | 22.9 | 9.3 | 1.8 |
| Roast, Seasoned, Butter Basted, Tesco* | ½ Pack/225g | 337.0 | 13.0 | 150 | 2.3 | 21.9 | 5.7 | 2.4 |
| Roast, with Caramelised Onions, Finest, Tesco* | ½ Pack/200g | 500.0 | 16.0 | 250 | 5.5 | 38.6 | 8.2 | 2.9 |
| Roast, with Goose Fat, TTD, Sainsbury's* | 1 Serving/100g | 149.0 | 7.0 | 149 | 2.2 | 19.3 | 7.0 | 1.9 |
| *Roasting, Average* | *1 Serving/150g* | *202.0* | *5.0* | *135* | *2.5* | *23.3* | *3.5* | *1.6* |
| Salad, Value, Tesco* | 1 Serving/150g | 111.0 | 0.0 | 74 | 1.7 | 16.1 | 0.3 | 1.0 |
| Saute, Deep Fried, McCain* | 1oz/28g | 47.0 | 2.0 | 167 | 2.6 | 23.3 | 7.0 | 0.0 |
| Saute, Oven Baked, McCain* | 1oz/28g | 56.0 | 1.0 | 199 | 4.4 | 36.9 | 3.8 | 0.0 |
| Saute, with Onion, & Bacon, Country Supper, Waitrose* | ¼ Pack/100g | 112.0 | 4.0 | 112 | 1.9 | 16.4 | 4.3 | 1.3 |
| Slices, in Batter, Crispy, Ready To Bake, Waitrose* | 1 Pack/475g | 860.0 | 45.0 | 181 | 2.5 | 21.4 | 9.5 | 3.1 |
| Slices, in Rich Crispy Batter, Crispy, Chilled, Sainsbury's* | ½ Pack/238g | 591.0 | 37.0 | 249 | 2.4 | 24.8 | 15.6 | 2.8 |
| Slices, Spicy Coated, Safeway* | ½ Pack/150g | 305.0 | 19.0 | 203 | 2.5 | 19.7 | 12.4 | 2.5 |
| Spicy, with Chorizo, Tapas, Waitrose* | 1 Serving/260g | 512.0 | 36.0 | 197 | 6.7 | 11.8 | 13.7 | 1.1 |
| Vivaldi, Boiled in Unsalted Water, Sainsbury's* | 1 Serving/200g | 144.0 | 0.0 | 72 | 1.8 | 17.0 | 0.1 | 1.2 |
| *White, Raw, Weighed with Skin, Flesh Only, Average* | *1 Med/213g* | *160.0* | *0.0* | *75* | *2.0* | *16.8* | *0.2* | *1.3* |
| with Garlic & Parsley Butter, Herb Oil Dressed, Co-Op* | 1 Serving/178g | 205.0 | 9.0 | 115 | 1.0 | 15.0 | 5.0 | 2.0 |
| with Seafood & Seasoned Butter, Tapas, Waitrose* | Pack/170g | 330.0 | 19.0 | 194 | 6.2 | 16.7 | 11.4 | 2.1 |
| **POTATOES INSTANT** | | | | | | | | |
| Mashed, Dry, Tesco* | 1 Serving/70g | 225.0 | 0.0 | 321 | 7.7 | 72.0 | 0.2 | 7.1 |
| Mashed, Dry, Value, Tesco* | 1/6 Pack/42g | 157.0 | 0.0 | 373 | 7.0 | 84.0 | 1.0 | 6.9 |
| Mashed, Made Up with Water, Average | 1 Serving/180g | 118.0 | 0.0 | 66 | 1.7 | 14.5 | 0.2 | 1.3 |
| Mashed, Original, Dry Weight, Smash* | 1 Serving/30g | 107.0 | 1.0 | 358 | 10.7 | 68.1 | 4.8 | 3.4 |
| Mashed, with Fried Onion, Smash* | ½ Pack/269g | 191.0 | 3.0 | 71 | 1.6 | 13.4 | 1.3 | 0.7 |
| Mashed, with Smoked Bacon, Smash* | 1 Serving/169g | 137.0 | 4.0 | 81 | 1.7 | 13.6 | 2.2 | 0.6 |
| **POUSSIN** | | | | | | | | |
| *Meat & Skin, Raw, Average* | *1oz/28g* | *57.0* | *4.0* | *202* | *19.1* | *0.0* | *13.9* | *0.0* |
| Spatchcock, British, Waitrose* | ½ Poussin/225g | 364.0 | 20.0 | 162 | 19.0 | 1.2 | 9.0 | 0.0 |
| Spatchcock, with Garlic & Herbs, Finest, Tesco* | ½ Poussin/235g | 348.0 | 17.0 | 148 | 19.7 | 1.0 | 7.3 | 0.5 |

| | Measure INFO/WEIGHT | per Measure KCAL | FAT | KCAL | PROT | CARB | FAT | FIBRE |
|---|---|---|---|---|---|---|---|---|
| **POWERADE** | | | | | | | | |
| Berry & Tropical Fruit, Coca-Cola* | 1 Bottle/500ml | 120.0 | 0.0 | 24 | 0.0 | 5.6 | 0.0 | 0.0 |
| Citrus Charge, Coca-Cola* | 1 Bottle/500ml | 120.0 | 0.0 | 24 | 0.0 | 6.0 | 0.0 | 0.0 |
| Gold Rush, Coca-Cola* | 1 Bottle/500ml | 120.0 | 0.0 | 24 | 0.0 | 6.0 | 0.0 | 0.0 |
| Ice Storm, Coca-Cola* | 1 Bottle/500ml | 120.0 | 0.0 | 24 | 0.0 | 6.0 | 0.0 | 0.0 |
| Isotonic, Sports Drink, Coca-Cola* | 1 Bottle/500ml | 120.0 | 0.0 | 24 | 0.0 | 5.6 | 0.0 | 0.0 |
| Lemon & Grapefruit, Coca-Cola* | 1 Bottle/500ml | 120.0 | 0.0 | 24 | 0.0 | 6.0 | 0.0 | 0.0 |
| **PRAWN COCKTAIL** | | | | | | | | |
| 20% More Prawns, M & S* | ½ Pack/100g | 330.0 | 32.0 | 330 | 8.9 | 2.2 | 31.6 | 0.2 |
| BFY, Morrisons* | 1 Serving/100g | 149.0 | 10.0 | 149 | 4.7 | 9.7 | 10.3 | 0.1 |
| Delicious, Boots* | 1 Pack/250g | 285.0 | 6.0 | 114 | 5.5 | 17.0 | 2.6 | 1.2 |
| Half Fat, Safeway* | 1 Serving/200g | 362.0 | 28.0 | 181 | 8.0 | 6.4 | 13.8 | 0.6 |
| HL, Tesco* | 1 Serving/200g | 276.0 | 23.0 | 138 | 6.8 | 2.3 | 11.3 | 0.6 |
| Light Choices, Tesco* | 1 Pot/140g | 210.0 | 16.0 | 150 | 7.5 | 4.3 | 11.4 | 1.3 |
| Reduced Fat, M & S* | 1 Pack/200g | 260.0 | 15.0 | 130 | 11.9 | 3.2 | 7.5 | 0.7 |
| Reduced Fat, Tesco* | 1 Serving/200g | 304.0 | 21.0 | 152 | 7.6 | 6.5 | 10.6 | 0.4 |
| Sainsbury's* | 1 Serving/200g | 706.0 | 69.0 | 353 | 7.9 | 2.7 | 34.5 | 0.5 |
| Tesco* | 1 Tub/200g | 834.0 | 83.0 | 417 | 7.3 | 3.5 | 41.5 | 0.1 |
| **PRAWN CRACKERS** | | | | | | | | |
| Asda* | 1 Serving/25g | 134.0 | 9.0 | 535 | 2.0 | 53.0 | 35.0 | 0.0 |
| Cooked in Sunflower Oil, Sharwood's* | 1 Cracker/2g | 10.0 | 0.0 | 479 | 0.7 | 68.3 | 22.6 | 0.8 |
| Food to Go, Sainsbury's* | 1 Bag/40g | 214.0 | 13.0 | 534 | 2.9 | 60.2 | 31.3 | 0.4 |
| Green Thai Curry, M & S* | 1 Pack/50g | 250.0 | 13.0 | 500 | 3.2 | 62.2 | 25.8 | 1.6 |
| M & S* | 1 Bag/50g | 262.0 | 16.0 | 525 | 2.8 | 57.4 | 31.3 | 0.8 |
| Ready to Eat, Sharwood's* | 1 Bag/60g | 316.0 | 18.0 | 527 | 0.5 | 62.0 | 30.8 | 1.2 |
| Red Mill* | 1 Bag/50g | 281.0 | 19.0 | 563 | 2.8 | 53.1 | 37.7 | 0.7 |
| Sainsbury's* | 1 Cracker/3g | 16.0 | 1.0 | 537 | 2.4 | 60.4 | 31.7 | 0.8 |
| Tesco* | 1/3 Pack/20g | 114.0 | 7.0 | 570 | 2.5 | 56.5 | 37.1 | 0.9 |
| Uncooked, Sharwood's* | 1oz/28g | 136.0 | 8.0 | 487 | 0.7 | 52.7 | 29.7 | 1.7 |
| Waitrose* | 1 Pack/50g | 266.0 | 16.0 | 533 | 2.4 | 58.6 | 32.1 | 1.6 |
| **PRAWN CREOLE** | | | | | | | | |
| with Rice, Perfectly Balanced, Waitrose* | 1 Serving/404g | 275.0 | 4.0 | 68 | 4.2 | 10.3 | 1.1 | 2.9 |
| **PRAWN TOAST** | | | | | | | | |
| Chinese Selection, Tesco* | 1 Toast/10g | 36.0 | 3.0 | 362 | 8.2 | 20.7 | 27.5 | 1.7 |
| Chinese Snack Selection, Morrisons* | 1 Toast/13g | 41.0 | 3.0 | 328 | 11.3 | 23.1 | 21.2 | 6.6 |
| Dim Sum Selection, Sainsbury's* | 1 Toast/8g | 23.0 | 1.0 | 283 | 9.9 | 19.2 | 18.5 | 2.0 |
| Mini, Oriental Selection, Party, Iceland* | 1 Toast/15g | 52.0 | 4.0 | 345 | 10.5 | 22.0 | 23.9 | 2.1 |
| Oriental Selection, Waitrose* | 1 Toast/14g | 38.0 | 2.0 | 272 | 11.1 | 18.3 | 17.2 | 2.1 |
| Sesame, Occasions, Sainsbury's* | 1 Toast/12g | 34.0 | 2.0 | 283 | 9.9 | 19.2 | 18.5 | 2.0 |
| Sesame, Oriental Snack Selection, Sainsbury's* | 1 Toast/12g | 40.0 | 3.0 | 335 | 9.3 | 23.0 | 22.9 | 5.1 |
| Sesame Prawn, Toasted Triangles, M & S* | 1 Pack/220g | 616.0 | 40.0 | 280 | 12.4 | 17.3 | 18.0 | 2.0 |
| Waitrose* | 1 Toast/21g | 47.0 | 4.0 | 223 | 9.7 | 7.4 | 17.2 | 5.8 |
| **PRAWNS** | | | | | | | | |
| Batter Crisp, Lyons* | 1 Pack/160g | 350.0 | 20.0 | 219 | 8.0 | 18.2 | 12.7 | 1.1 |
| ***Boiled*** | ***1 Prawn/3g*** | ***3.0*** | ***0.0*** | ***99*** | ***22.6*** | ***0.0*** | ***0.9*** | ***0.0*** |
| Brine, John West* | ½ Can/60g | 58.0 | 1.0 | 97 | 21.0 | 1.0 | 1.0 | 0.0 |
| ***Cooked & Peeled, Average*** | ***1oz/28g*** | ***21.0*** | ***0.0*** | ***77*** | ***17.6*** | ***0.2*** | ***0.6*** | ***0.0*** |
| Crevettes, Asda* | 1oz/28g | 11.0 | 0.0 | 41 | 8.6 | 0.0 | 0.7 | 0.0 |
| ***Dried, Average*** | ***1 Prawn/3g*** | ***8.0*** | ***0.0*** | ***281*** | ***62.4*** | ***0.0*** | ***3.5*** | ***0.0*** |
| Filo Wrapped & Breaded, M & S* | 1 Serving/19g | 45.0 | 2.0 | 235 | 9.5 | 20.4 | 13.0 | 1.4 |
| Honduran, & Cocktail Sauce Dipper, M & S* | 1 Pack/120g | 258.0 | 22.0 | 215 | 13.6 | 0.0 | 18.0 | 1.1 |
| Hot & Spicy, Average | 1 Serving/170g | 461.0 | 27.0 | 271 | 9.4 | 22.8 | 15.8 | 2.1 |
| ***Icelandic, Raw, Average*** | ***1oz/28g*** | ***30.0*** | ***0.0*** | ***105*** | ***22.7*** | ***0.0*** | ***1.5*** | ***0.0*** |
| King, Crevettes, Sainsbury's* | 1 Pack/225g | 205.0 | 1.0 | 91 | 21.8 | 0.1 | 0.5 | 0.3 |

| | Measure INFO/WEIGHT | per Measure KCAL | FAT | Nutrition Values per 100g / 100ml KCAL | PROT | CARB | FAT | FIBRE |
|---|---|---|---|---|---|---|---|---|
| **PRAWNS** | | | | | | | | |
| King, in Filo, Finest, Tesco* | 1 Prawn/20g | 38.0 | 1.0 | 189 | 13.0 | 27.8 | 2.9 | 1.6 |
| King, in Sweet Chilli Sauce, with Noodles, COU, M & S* | 1 Pack/400g | 260.0 | 2.0 | 65 | 4.8 | 10.3 | 0.4 | 1.5 |
| *King, Raw, Average* | *1 Bag/200g* | *145.0* | *2.0* | *72* | *15.8* | *0.2* | *0.9* | *0.1* |
| King, Sizzler, with Rice Noodles, BGTY, Sainsbury's* | 1 Pack/400g | 276.0 | 5.0 | 69 | 3.8 | 10.6 | 1.3 | 1.6 |
| King, Tandoori, Average | 1 Prawn/59g | 33.0 | 1.0 | 55 | 5.7 | 5.9 | 1.1 | 0.7 |
| King, with Garlic, Parsley & Lemon Butter, COOK!, M & S* | ½ Pack/110g | 160.0 | 11.0 | 145 | 12.9 | 0.8 | 10.2 | 0.5 |
| King, with Garlic Butter, M & S* | 1 Serving/100g | 165.0 | 9.0 | 165 | 12.5 | 9.1 | 9.0 | 0.5 |
| King, with Ginger & Spring Onion, Waitrose* | 1 Pack/300g | 130.0 | 2.0 | 43 | 5.3 | 3.6 | 0.7 | 0.8 |
| *North Atlantic, Peeled, Cooked, Average* | *1oz/28g* | *22.0* | *0.0* | *80* | *17.5* | *0.0* | *1.1* | *0.0* |
| *North Atlantic, Raw, Average* | *1oz/28g* | *17.0* | *0.0* | *61* | *14.4* | *0.0* | *0.4* | *0.0* |
| *Raw, Average* | *1oz/28g* | *22.0* | *0.0* | *79* | *17.8* | *0.2* | *0.7* | *0.0* |
| Sweet Chilli, Skewers, Tesco* | 1 Skewer/22g | 26.0 | 0.0 | 120 | 20.4 | 6.9 | 0.9 | 0.5 |
| *Tiger, Cooked & Peeled, Average* | *1 Pack/180g* | *151.0* | *2.0* | *84* | *18.4* | *0.1* | *1.1* | *0.0* |
| *Tiger, Jumbo, Average* | *1 Serving/50g* | *39.0* | *0.0* | *78* | *18.2* | *0.3* | *0.5* | *0.0* |
| *Tiger, Raw, Average* | *1oz/28g* | *18.0* | *0.0* | *64* | *14.2* | *0.0* | *0.7* | *0.0* |
| Tiger, Vegetarian, Crispy, Tkc* | ½ Pack/150g | 225.0 | 6.0 | 150 | 12.0 | 17.0 | 4.0 | 5.0 |
| Tiger, Wrapped, M & S* | 1 Pack/190g | 477.0 | 26.0 | 251 | 11.3 | 20.7 | 13.6 | 1.3 |
| **PRAWNS CHILLI** | | | | | | | | |
| & Coriander, King, Honduran, M & S* | ½ Pack/70g | 70.0 | 2.0 | 100 | 17.2 | 0.1 | 3.2 | 0.4 |
| Battered, Cantonese, King, Sainsbury's* | 1 Pack/300g | 570.0 | 23.0 | 190 | 10.0 | 20.2 | 7.7 | 0.8 |
| Battered, M & S* | 1oz/28g | 63.0 | 3.0 | 225 | 7.2 | 23.8 | 11.5 | 0.5 |
| Sweet, Crispy, Dipping Sauce, M & S* | 1 Pack/240g | 515.0 | 28.0 | 215 | 7.5 | 19.9 | 11.6 | 2.3 |
| Sweet, Thai, King, Sainsbury's* | 1 Serving/150g | 177.0 | 6.0 | 118 | 6.4 | 13.9 | 4.1 | 1.9 |
| with Spicy Chilli Dip, King, Sainsbury's* | ½ Pack/150g | 282.0 | 11.0 | 188 | 8.6 | 22.2 | 7.2 | 1.0 |
| **PRAWNS CREOLE** | | | | | | | | |
| GFY, Asda* | 1 Serving/300g | 222.0 | 3.0 | 74 | 3.2 | 13.0 | 1.0 | 1.4 |
| Spicy, BGTY, Sainsbury's* | 1 Pack/350g | 357.0 | 8.0 | 102 | 4.8 | 15.6 | 2.4 | 0.4 |
| with Vegetable Rice, King, COU, M & S* | 1 Pack/400g | 300.0 | 2.0 | 75 | 4.5 | 13.3 | 0.6 | 0.7 |
| **PRAWNS GULNARI** | | | | | | | | |
| with Rice, COU, M & S* | 1 Pack/400g | 400.0 | 3.0 | 100 | 4.0 | 18.7 | 0.8 | 1.6 |
| **PRAWNS IN** | | | | | | | | |
| Creamy Garlic Sauce, Youngs* | 1 Serving/158g | 261.0 | 23.0 | 165 | 8.5 | 0.3 | 14.5 | 0.0 |
| Sweet Chilli Sauce, Asda* | 1 Pack/360g | 500.0 | 25.0 | 139 | 4.1 | 15.0 | 6.9 | 0.3 |
| **PRAWNS ORIENTAL** | | | | | | | | |
| M & S* | 1 Pack/200g | 440.0 | 23.0 | 220 | 11.9 | 16.9 | 11.7 | 0.9 |
| **PRAWNS SZECHUAN** | | | | | | | | |
| Spicy, COU, M & S* | 1 Pack/400g | 380.0 | 4.0 | 95 | 4.5 | 16.9 | 0.9 | 1.5 |
| **PRAWNS WITH** | | | | | | | | |
| a Spicy Cajun Dip, King, Sainsbury's* | 1 Pack/240g | 254.0 | 4.0 | 106 | 14.8 | 9.1 | 1.8 | 1.4 |
| Caribbean Style Sauce, GFY, Asda* | 1 Serving/400g | 408.0 | 7.0 | 102 | 4.7 | 17.0 | 1.7 | 2.1 |
| Chilli, Coriander & Lime, King, Waitrose* | 1 Pack/140g | 143.0 | 3.0 | 102 | 19.9 | 0.5 | 2.3 | 0.6 |
| Garlic & Herb Butter, King, Fresh, M & S* | 1 Serving/200g | 330.0 | 18.0 | 165 | 12.5 | 9.1 | 9.0 | 0.5 |
| Ginger & Spring Onion, Sainsbury's* | 1 Pack/300g | 198.0 | 9.0 | 66 | 4.7 | 4.7 | 3.1 | 0.3 |
| Green Thai Sauce, Tiger, Waitrose* | ½ Pack/117g | 108.0 | 3.0 | 92 | 16.1 | 0.8 | 2.3 | 0.1 |
| Lemon & Pepper, Honduran, King, M & S* | 1 Pack/140g | 133.0 | 4.0 | 95 | 17.4 | 0.4 | 2.6 | 0.7 |
| Rice, Sweet Chilli, Tesco* | 1 Pack/460g | 488.0 | 10.0 | 106 | 2.4 | 19.2 | 2.2 | 0.5 |
| **PRETZELS** | | | | | | | | |
| American Style, Salted, Sainsbury's* | 1 Serving/50g | 201.0 | 2.0 | 403 | 10.8 | 79.7 | 4.5 | 1.8 |
| Cheddar Cheese, Penn State Pretzels* | 1 Sm Bag/30g | 124.0 | 3.0 | 412 | 10.0 | 71.6 | 9.3 | 3.8 |
| Giant, Penn State Pretzels* | 1 Pretzel/18g | 66.0 | 1.0 | 374 | 10.5 | 74.7 | 3.7 | 4.1 |
| Jumbo, Tesco* | 1 Serving/50g | 194.0 | 3.0 | 388 | 9.7 | 71.9 | 6.8 | 5.4 |
| Lightly Salted, Tesco* | 1 Serving/25g | 99.0 | 2.0 | 395 | 9.3 | 73.4 | 7.1 | 5.5 |
| Mini, 99% Fat Free, Free Natural* | 1 Serving/50g | 188.0 | 0.0 | 376 | 10.1 | 81.7 | 1.0 | 0.0 |

| | INFO/WEIGHT | KCAL | FAT | KCAL | PROT | CARB | FAT | FIBRE |
|---|---|---|---|---|---|---|---|---|
| **PRETZELS** | | | | | | | | |
| Mini, M & S* | 1 Pack/45g | 193.0 | 6.0 | 430 | 10.4 | 66.6 | 13.4 | 4.9 |
| New York Style, Salted, Mini, Shapers, Boots* | 1 Bag/25g | 94.0 | 1.0 | 375 | 10.0 | 79.0 | 2.1 | 4.2 |
| Salt & Cracked Black Pepper, COU, M & S* | 1 Pack/25g | 95.0 | 1.0 | 380 | 9.7 | 83.3 | 2.4 | 2.7 |
| Salted, Average | 1 Serving/30g | 114.0 | 1.0 | 380 | 10.3 | 79.8 | 2.6 | 3.0 |
| Salted, Mini, M & S* | 1 Pack/25g | 94.0 | 1.0 | 375 | 10.0 | 79.0 | 2.1 | 4.2 |
| Salted, Sainsbury's* | 1 Serving/50g | 200.0 | 2.0 | 401 | 9.8 | 82.4 | 3.6 | 3.4 |
| Salted, Stars, Tesco* | 1oz/28g | 104.0 | 1.0 | 371 | 8.2 | 73.7 | 4.8 | 3.1 |
| Sea Salt & Black Pepper, Penn State Pretzels* | 1 Serving/25g | 94.0 | 1.0 | 375 | 10.4 | 73.7 | 4.2 | 4.7 |
| Sea Salt & Black Pepper, Tesco* | 1 Serving/50g | 189.0 | 1.0 | 379 | 10.0 | 79.0 | 2.6 | 4.1 |
| Selection Tray, M & S* | 1oz/28g | 112.0 | 2.0 | 401 | 9.7 | 75.5 | 6.7 | 3.4 |
| Snacks, Fabulous Bakin' Boys* | 1 Pack/24g | 96.0 | 1.0 | 401 | 9.0 | 79.5 | 4.9 | 2.5 |
| Soft, Garlic, Auntie Anne's* | 1 Pretzel/74g | 320.0 | 1.0 | 432 | 12.2 | 89.2 | 1.3 | 2.7 |
| Soft, Jalapeno, Auntie Anne's* | 1 Pretzel/74g | 270.0 | 1.0 | 365 | 10.8 | 78.4 | 1.3 | 2.7 |
| Soft, Jalapeno, with Butter, Auntie Anne's* | 1 Pretzel/74g | 310.0 | 4.0 | 419 | 10.8 | 79.7 | 6.1 | 2.7 |
| Soft, Salted, with Butter, Original, Auntie Anne's* | 1 Pretzel/74g | 370.0 | 4.0 | 500 | 13.5 | 97.3 | 5.4 | 4.0 |
| Soft, Sour Cream & Onion, Auntie Anne's* | 1 Pretzel/74g | 310.0 | 1.0 | 419 | 12.2 | 89.2 | 1.3 | 2.7 |
| Soft, Whole Wheat, Auntie Anne's* | 1 Pretzel/74g | 350.0 | 2.0 | 473 | 14.9 | 97.3 | 2.0 | 9.5 |
| Sour Cream & Chive, Hoops, BGTY, Sainsbury's* | 1 Bag/25g | 98.0 | 1.0 | 391 | 10.4 | 80.9 | 2.3 | 1.6 |
| Sour Cream & Chive, Mini, HL, Tesco* | 1 Pack/25g | 92.0 | 1.0 | 369 | 10.9 | 76.3 | 2.2 | 4.6 |
| Sour Cream & Chive, Penn State Pretzels* | 1 Serving/25g | 102.0 | 2.0 | 410 | 9.8 | 72.8 | 8.8 | 3.9 |
| Sour Cream & Onion, M & S* | 1 Serving/30g | 136.0 | 4.0 | 455 | 11.0 | 70.9 | 14.5 | 0.7 |
| Sour Cream & Onion, Tesco* | 1 Serving/25g | 114.0 | 4.0 | 457 | 8.4 | 67.7 | 17.0 | 2.3 |
| Spicy Salsa, Penn State Pretzels* | 1 Serving/25g | 105.0 | 3.0 | 420 | 9.5 | 72.4 | 10.4 | 1.3 |
| Sweet Thai Chilli Twists, Penn State Pretzels* | 1 Serving/25g | 98.0 | 2.0 | 393 | 9.8 | 70.1 | 8.2 | 6.8 |
| Wheat, Gluten Free, Trufree* | 1 Bag/60g | 282.0 | 12.0 | 470 | 2.4 | 70.0 | 20.0 | 1.0 |
| **PRINGLES*** | | | | | | | | |
| Barbecue, Pringles* | 1 Serving/50g | 266.0 | 18.0 | 533 | 4.9 | 48.0 | 36.0 | 5.1 |
| BBQ Spare Rib, Rice Infusions, Pringles* | 1 Pack/23g | 108.0 | 5.0 | 469 | 5.1 | 60.0 | 23.0 | 2.6 |
| Cheese & Onion, Pringles* | 1 Serving/25g | 132.0 | 8.0 | 528 | 4.1 | 50.0 | 34.0 | 3.4 |
| Hot & Spicy, Pringles* | 1 Serving/25g | 132.0 | 8.0 | 530 | 4.6 | 49.0 | 34.0 | 3.7 |
| Light, Aromas, Greek Cheese & Avocado Oil, Pringles* | 1 Serving/25g | 122.0 | 6.0 | 488 | 4.6 | 57.0 | 25.0 | 3.6 |
| Light, Original, Pringles* | 1 Serving/25g | 121.0 | 6.0 | 484 | 4.3 | 59.0 | 25.0 | 3.6 |
| Light, Sour Cream & Onion, Pringles* | 1 Serving/25g | 122.0 | 6.0 | 487 | 4.7 | 57.0 | 25.0 | 3.6 |
| Minis, Original, Pringles* | 1 Pack/23g | 118.0 | 7.0 | 514 | 5.1 | 55.0 | 30.0 | 3.7 |
| Minis, Salt & Vinegar, Pringles* | 1 Pack/23g | 115.0 | 6.0 | 502 | 4.5 | 55.0 | 28.0 | 3.6 |
| Minis, Sour Cream & Onion, Pringles* | 1 Pack/23g | 118.0 | 7.0 | 511 | 5.2 | 56.0 | 29.0 | 3.5 |
| Minis, Texas BBQ Sauce, Pringles* | 1 Pack/23g | 116.0 | 6.0 | 504 | 5.0 | 56.0 | 28.0 | 3.8 |
| Original, Pringles* | 1 Serving/25g | 135.0 | 9.0 | 540 | 4.1 | 49.0 | 36.0 | 3.6 |
| Paprika, Pringles* | 1 Serving/25g | 132.0 | 8.0 | 529 | 4.9 | 49.0 | 34.0 | 6.5 |
| Salt & Vinegar, Pringles* | 1 Serving/25g | 132.0 | 8.0 | 527 | 3.9 | 50.0 | 34.0 | 3.4 |
| Sour Cream & Onion, Pringles* | 1 Serving/25g | 133.0 | 9.0 | 531 | 4.5 | 49.0 | 35.0 | 3.6 |
| Texas BBQ Sauce, Pringles* | 1 Serving/25g | 132.0 | 8.0 | 527 | 4.2 | 50.0 | 34.0 | 3.5 |
| **PROBIOTIC DRINK** | | | | | | | | |
| Cranberry & Raspberry, Dairy, Asda* | 1 Bottle/100ml | 64.0 | 1.0 | 64 | 2.3 | 12.0 | 0.8 | 2.4 |
| Orange, Health, Tesco* | 1 Serving/100g | 67.0 | 1.0 | 67 | 1.5 | 13.4 | 0.9 | 1.3 |
| Peach, Dairy, Asda* | 1 Bottle/100ml | 68.0 | 1.0 | 68 | 2.3 | 13.0 | 0.8 | 2.3 |
| Strawberry, Dairy, Asda* | 1 Bottle/100ml | 64.0 | 1.0 | 64 | 2.3 | 12.0 | 0.8 | 2.3 |
| Yoghurt, Original, Tesco* | 1 Bottle/100g | 68.0 | 1.0 | 68 | 1.7 | 13.1 | 1.0 | 1.4 |
| **PROFITEROLES** | | | | | | | | |
| Asda* | 1 Serving/64g | 218.0 | 17.0 | 343 | 5.0 | 20.0 | 27.0 | 0.0 |
| Chocolate, Co-Op* | 1Pot/91g | 260.0 | 14.0 | 285 | 6.0 | 33.0 | 15.0 | 3.0 |
| Chocolate, Sainsbury's* | 1/6 Pot/95g | 192.0 | 8.0 | 202 | 5.4 | 25.1 | 8.9 | 0.8 |
| Chocolate, Stack, Sainsbury's* | ¼ Pack/76g | 311.0 | 19.0 | 409 | 5.3 | 39.3 | 25.6 | 2.0 |

**P**

| | Measure INFO/WEIGHT | per Measure KCAL | FAT | Nutrition Values per 100g / 100ml KCAL | PROT | CARB | FAT | FIBRE |
|---|---|---|---|---|---|---|---|---|
| **PROFITEROLES** | | | | | | | | |
| Chocolate, Tesco* | 1 Serving/76g | 293.0 | 22.0 | 386 | 5.1 | 26.9 | 28.7 | 0.5 |
| Choux & Chocolate Sauce, Tesco* | 1 Serving/77g | 295.0 | 22.0 | 386 | 5.1 | 26.9 | 28.7 | 0.5 |
| Classic French, Sainsbury's* | 1 Serving/90g | 284.0 | 15.0 | 316 | 6.6 | 33.7 | 17.2 | 0.1 |
| Dairy Cream, Co-Op* | ¼ Pack/70g | 241.0 | 17.0 | 345 | 6.0 | 24.0 | 25.0 | 0.5 |
| Filled with Cream, Stack, Fresh, M & S* | 1 Serving/75g | 281.0 | 21.0 | 375 | 5.3 | 23.6 | 28.5 | 1.9 |
| in a Pot, Waitrose* | 1 Pot/80g | 207.0 | 11.0 | 259 | 6.3 | 25.6 | 14.1 | 2.9 |
| Waitrose* | 4 Profiteroles/75g | 269.0 | 18.0 | 359 | 4.8 | 31.1 | 23.9 | 0.7 |
| **PROVENCALE** | | | | | | | | |
| Cabillaud à la, Weight Watchers* | 1 Pack/380g | 327.0 | 10.0 | 86 | 5.1 | 10.3 | 2.7 | 0.0 |
| Chicken, M & S* | 1 Pack/430g | 365.0 | 12.0 | 85 | 13.2 | 2.3 | 2.7 | 0.6 |
| Chicken, Steam Cuisine, M & S* | 1oz/28g | 34.0 | 1.0 | 120 | 9.6 | 12.7 | 3.8 | 1.4 |
| King Prawn & Mushroom, M & S* | ½ Pack/185g | 120.0 | 5.0 | 65 | 7.2 | 3.9 | 2.5 | 0.9 |
| Mushroom, Fresh, COU, M & S* | ½ Pack/150g | 60.0 | 2.0 | 40 | 2.6 | 4.1 | 1.5 | 1.8 |
| Prawn & Mushroom with Pasta, COU, M & S* | 1 Pack/400g | 360.0 | 2.0 | 90 | 5.9 | 15.7 | 0.5 | 0.0 |
| Ratatouille, Asda* | ½ Can/195g | 97.0 | 4.0 | 50 | 1.0 | 7.0 | 2.0 | 1.0 |
| **PRUNES** | | | | | | | | |
| *Dried, Average* | *1 Serving/50g* | *79.0* | *0.0* | *157* | *2.5* | *36.4* | *0.4* | *5.8* |
| *in Apple Juice, Average* | *1 Serving/90g* | *76.0* | *0.0* | *84* | *0.8* | *19.8* | *0.1* | *1.4* |
| *in Fruit Juice, Average* | *1oz/28g* | *25.0* | *0.0* | *88* | *0.9* | *21.4* | *0.2* | *3.0* |
| *in Syrup, Average* | *1oz/28g* | *26.0* | *0.0* | *92* | *1.0* | *22.1* | *0.2* | *2.6* |
| *Stewed with Sugar* | *1oz/28g* | *29.0* | *0.0* | *103* | *1.3* | *25.5* | *0.2* | *3.1* |
| *Stewed without Sugar* | *1oz/28g* | *23.0* | *0.0* | *81* | *1.4* | *19.5* | *0.3* | *3.3* |
| **PUDDING** | | | | | | | | |
| Apple & Blackberry Crumble, Custard Style, Somerfield* | 1oz/28g | 34.0 | 1.0 | 123 | 3.0 | 17.0 | 5.0 | 0.0 |
| Apple & Custard, Sainsbury's* | 1 Serving/115g | 132.0 | 2.0 | 115 | 5.4 | 19.0 | 1.9 | 0.1 |
| Banana Fudge Crunch, Bird's* | 1oz/28g | 125.0 | 4.0 | 445 | 5.4 | 75.0 | 14.0 | 0.8 |
| Blackberry & Bramley Apple, M & S* | ¼ Pudding/152g | 365.0 | 12.0 | 240 | 3.3 | 38.2 | 8.2 | 2.0 |
| Butterscotch, Instant, Fat Free, Jell-O* | 1 Serving/8g | 25.0 | 0.0 | 333 | 1.3 | 78.7 | 1.3 | 0.0 |
| Cherry Cobbler, GFY, Asda* | 1 Pudding/100g | 158.0 | 2.0 | 158 | 2.1 | 33.0 | 2.0 | 0.9 |
| Chocolate, M & S* | ¼ Pudding/76g | 265.0 | 12.0 | 350 | 4.1 | 48.0 | 15.8 | 2.1 |
| Chocolate, Melting Middle, M & S* | 1 Pudding/155g | 510.0 | 28.0 | 330 | 5.8 | 36.2 | 18.0 | 3.1 |
| Chocolate, Perfectly Balanced, Waitrose* | 1 Pot/105g | 196.0 | 3.0 | 187 | 3.8 | 36.0 | 3.1 | 0.8 |
| Chocolate, Tesco* | 1 Serving/110g | 348.0 | 21.0 | 316 | 3.1 | 32.9 | 19.1 | 1.9 |
| Chocolate, with Chocolate Sauce, Ration Pack, Wayfayrer* | 1 Pack/200g | 426.0 | 19.0 | 213 | 2.8 | 29.6 | 9.3 | 0.4 |
| Chocolate with Cream, Delice, Campina* | 1 Pot/100g | 136.0 | 5.0 | 136 | 2.5 | 18.9 | 5.4 | 0.0 |
| Creamed Sago, Ambrosia* | 1 Serving/200g | 158.0 | 3.0 | 79 | 2.5 | 13.6 | 1.6 | 0.2 |
| Creme Aux Oeufs a la Vanille, Weight Watchers* | 1 Pot/100g | 116.0 | 3.0 | 116 | 4.8 | 17.0 | 3.2 | 0.0 |
| Creme Aux Oeufs Au Chocolat, Weight Watchers* | 1 Pot/100g | 136.0 | 4.0 | 136 | 4.7 | 19.7 | 4.3 | 0.0 |
| Eve's, Average | 1oz/28g | 67.0 | 4.0 | 241 | 3.5 | 28.9 | 13.1 | 1.4 |
| Eve's, BGTY, Sainsbury's* | 1 Pudding/145g | 164.0 | 2.0 | 113 | 2.2 | 23.4 | 1.2 | 0.7 |
| Eve's, with Custard, Less Than 5% Fat, M & S* | 1 Pudding/205g | 318.0 | 9.0 | 155 | 3.4 | 24.7 | 4.6 | 0.7 |
| Jam Roly Poly & Custard, Co-Op* | 1 Serving/105g | 262.0 | 7.0 | 250 | 3.0 | 44.0 | 7.0 | 0.8 |
| Lemon, BGTY, Sainsbury's* | 1 Serving/100g | 151.0 | 2.0 | 151 | 2.9 | 31.0 | 1.9 | 0.5 |
| Lemon, M & S* | 1 Pudding/105g | 328.0 | 16.0 | 312 | 4.3 | 39.4 | 15.2 | 2.3 |
| Lemon, Perfectly Balanced, Waitrose* | 1 Serving/105g | 212.0 | 3.0 | 202 | 3.4 | 41.7 | 2.4 | 0.6 |
| Lemon Crunch, Bird's* | 1oz/28g | 125.0 | 4.0 | 445 | 5.5 | 74.0 | 14.0 | 0.7 |
| Low Fat Chocolate Pudding, Good Intentions, Somerfield* | 1 Pudding/110g | 200.0 | 2.0 | 182 | 3.0 | 37.6 | 2.2 | 2.4 |
| Plum, Spiced, Safeway* | 1 Pudding/125g | 275.0 | 3.0 | 220 | 2.7 | 45.7 | 2.5 | 0.9 |
| Queen of Puddings | 1oz/28g | 60.0 | 2.0 | 213 | 4.8 | 33.1 | 7.8 | 0.2 |
| Rhubarb & Custard, BGTY, Sainsbury's* | 1 Pudding/140g | 137.0 | 3.0 | 98 | 2.0 | 18.4 | 2.0 | 1.4 |
| Rhubarb Crumble, Custard Style, Somerfield* | 1oz/28g | 33.0 | 1.0 | 119 | 3.0 | 16.0 | 5.0 | 0.0 |
| Rich Chocolate, Tryton Foods* | 1oz/28g | 76.0 | 3.0 | 273 | 4.7 | 41.7 | 9.5 | 1.8 |
| Sticky Toffee, Co-Op* | ¼ Pudding/100g | 355.0 | 20.0 | 355 | 3.0 | 40.0 | 20.0 | 0.7 |

**P**

| | Measure INFO/WEIGHT | per Measure | | Nutrition Values per 100g / 100ml | | | | |
|---|---|---|---|---|---|---|---|---|
| | | KCAL | FAT | KCAL | PROT | CARB | FAT | FIBRE |
| **PUDDING** | | | | | | | | |
| Sticky Toffee, Extra Special, Asda* | ¼ Pudding/100g | 378.0 | 18.0 | 378 | 1.9 | 52.0 | 18.0 | 1.8 |
| Sticky Toffee, HL, Tesco* | 1 Pack/125g | 245.0 | 6.0 | 196 | 4.0 | 34.9 | 4.5 | 0.6 |
| Sticky Toffee, Tesco* | 1 Serving/110g | 287.0 | 15.0 | 261 | 3.3 | 31.8 | 13.4 | 0.7 |
| Sticky Toffee, with Custard, Somerfield* | 1 Pack/245g | 576.0 | 20.0 | 235 | 3.0 | 38.0 | 8.0 | 0.0 |
| Sticky Toffee & Sticky Toffee Sauce, BGTY, Sainsbury's* | 1 Serving/130g | 318.0 | 5.0 | 245 | 5.0 | 49.3 | 4.1 | 2.2 |
| Strawberry Jam with Custard, Farmfoods* | 1 Serving/145g | 525.0 | 35.0 | 362 | 3.2 | 35.5 | 23.9 | 0.9 |
| Summer Fruits, Co-Op* | 1 Pack/260g | 273.0 | 1.0 | 105 | 1.0 | 25.0 | 0.2 | 1.0 |
| Summer Fruits, Eat Well, M & S* | 1 Pudding/135g | 128.0 | 1.0 | 95 | 1.7 | 20.8 | 0.5 | 3.0 |
| Summer Pudding, BGTY, Sainsbury's* | 1 Pot/110g | 223.0 | 5.0 | 203 | 3.2 | 40.9 | 4.6 | 2.4 |
| Summer Pudding, Waitrose* | 1 Pot/120g | 125.0 | 0.0 | 104 | 2.0 | 23.1 | 0.4 | 1.4 |
| Syrup, Individual, Co-Op* | 1 Pudding/170g | 603.0 | 36.0 | 355 | 3.0 | 38.0 | 21.0 | 1.0 |
| Syrup, M & S* | 1 Serving/105g | 370.0 | 10.0 | 352 | 3.9 | 61.7 | 10.0 | 0.8 |
| **PULSES** | | | | | | | | |
| Mixed, in Water, Sainsbury's* | ½ Can/120g | 131.0 | 3.0 | 109 | 8.7 | 13.6 | 2.2 | 4.6 |
| **PUMPKIN** | | | | | | | | |
| ***Boiled in Salted Water*** | ***1oz/28g*** | ***4.0*** | ***0.0*** | ***13*** | ***0.6*** | ***2.1*** | ***0.3*** | ***1.1*** |
| Kabocha, Tesco* | 1 Serving 50g | 19.0 | 0.0 | 39 | 1.1 | 8.3 | 0.1 | 1.6 |
| Solid Pack, 100% Pure, Canned, Libby's* | 1 Can/425g | 139.0 | 2.0 | 33 | 1.6 | 7.4 | 0.4 | 4.1 |
| **PUPPODUMS** | | | | | | | | |
| Cracked Black Pepper, Ready to Eat, Sharwood's* | 1 Puppodum/9g | 41.0 | 2.0 | 461 | 16.7 | 37.2 | 27.3 | 7.3 |
| Garlic & Coriander, Ready to Eat, Sharwood's* | 1 Puppodum/9g | 39.0 | 2.0 | 438 | 18.4 | 43.0 | 21.4 | 6.5 |
| Plain, Cook to Eat, Sharwood's* | 1 Puppodum/12g | 32.0 | 0.0 | 273 | 21.9 | 45.7 | 1.0 | 10.1 |
| Plain, Mini, Cook to Eat, Sharwood's* | 1 Puppodum/4g | 11.0 | 0.0 | 273 | 21.9 | 45.7 | 0.3 | 10.1 |
| Plain, Ready to Eat, Sharwood's* | 1 Puppodum/9g | 41.0 | 2.0 | 461 | 17.0 | 40.6 | 25.6 | 0.0 |
| Spicy, Cook to Eat, Sharwood's* | 1 Puppodum/12g | 30.0 | 0.0 | 257 | 20.2 | 43.0 | 0.5 | 13.0 |

P

| | Measure INFO/WEIGHT | per Measure KCAL | FAT | Nutrition Values per 100g / 100ml KCAL | PROT | CARB | FAT | FIBRE |
|---|---|---|---|---|---|---|---|---|
| **QUADRELLI** | | | | | | | | |
| Organic, M & S* | 1 Serving/75g | 262.0 | 1.0 | 350 | 13.4 | 71.1 | 1.4 | 3.0 |
| **QUAVERS** | | | | | | | | |
| Cheese, Walkers* | 1 Bag/16g | 87.0 | 5.0 | 530 | 2.5 | 62.0 | 30.0 | 1.1 |
| Prawn Cocktail, Walkers* | 1 Bag/16g | 90.0 | 5.0 | 550 | 1.9 | 63.7 | 31.9 | 1.2 |
| Salt & Vinegar, Walkers* | 1 Bag/16g | 86.0 | 5.0 | 525 | 1.9 | 62.0 | 30.0 | 1.2 |
| **QUICHE** | | | | | | | | |
| Asparagus & Cheese, Safeway* | ¼ Quiche/100g | 260.0 | 17.0 | 260 | 7.5 | 18.2 | 17.4 | 1.4 |
| Asparagus & Mushroom, Tesco* | ½ Quiche/200g | 474.0 | 33.0 | 237 | 5.1 | 17.2 | 16.4 | 1.2 |
| Baby Spinach & Gruyere, Sainsbury's* | ¼ Quiche/93g | 228.0 | 16.0 | 245 | 7.4 | 15.1 | 17.2 | 1.0 |
| Bacon, Leek, & Cheese, Weight Watchers* | 1 Quiche/165g | 307.0 | 13.0 | 186 | 7.4 | 21.0 | 8.1 | 1.8 |
| Bacon, Leek & Mushroom, M & S* | ¼ Quiche/100g | 245.0 | 16.0 | 245 | 6.9 | 17.2 | 16.4 | 1.3 |
| Bacon, Mushroom & Tomato, Somerfield* | ¼ Quiche/100g | 264.0 | 17.0 | 264 | 7.6 | 19.6 | 17.2 | 1.0 |
| Bacon & Cheese, Pork Farms* | 1 Pack/120g | 378.0 | 24.0 | 315 | 11.1 | 20.8 | 20.0 | 0.0 |
| Bacon & Cheese, Sainsbury's* | ¼ Quiche/100g | 237.0 | 15.0 | 237 | 7.0 | 18.6 | 15.0 | 0.7 |
| Bacon & Leek, Asda* | ¼ Quiche/100g | 252.0 | 16.0 | 252 | 8.4 | 18.9 | 15.9 | 1.5 |
| Bacon & Leek, Individual, Tesco* | 1 Quiche/175g | 485.0 | 32.0 | 277 | 8.3 | 19.4 | 18.5 | 0.9 |
| Bacon & Leek, Tesco* | ¼ Quiche/100g | 260.0 | 18.0 | 260 | 6.9 | 17.5 | 18.0 | 1.2 |
| Bacon & Tomato, Asda* | 1 Serving/107g | 201.0 | 9.0 | 188 | 8.0 | 21.0 | 8.0 | 1.1 |
| Bacon & Tomato, Safeway* | ¼ Quiche/100g | 287.0 | 19.0 | 287 | 8.6 | 20.3 | 19.0 | 1.4 |
| Brie & Smoked Bacon, Asda* | ¼ Quiche/90g | 249.0 | 17.0 | 277 | 8.9 | 17.8 | 18.9 | 1.0 |
| Broccoli, Extra, Value, Tesco* | 1 Serving/125g | 341.0 | 24.0 | 273 | 10.0 | 15.1 | 19.2 | 0.8 |
| Broccoli, Tesco* | 1 Serving/100g | 249.0 | 17.0 | 249 | 6.0 | 17.6 | 17.2 | 1.4 |
| Broccoli, Tomato & Cheese, BGTY, Sainsbury's* | 1 Quiche/390g | 632.0 | 32.0 | 162 | 6.4 | 15.7 | 8.2 | 1.3 |
| Broccoli, Tomato & Cheese, Deep Filled, Sainsbury's* | ¼ Quiche/100g | 203.0 | 13.0 | 203 | 5.2 | 16.9 | 12.9 | 2.3 |
| Broccoli & Cheddar Cheese, Safeway* | 1 Pack/300g | 813.0 | 54.0 | 271 | 7.7 | 19.8 | 17.9 | 1.9 |
| Broccoli & Gruyere Cheese, Waitrose* | 1 Serving/100g | 241.0 | 18.0 | 241 | 7.3 | 13.0 | 17.8 | 2.9 |
| Broccoli & Stilton, Mini, Sainsbury's* | 1 Quiche/14g | 52.0 | 3.0 | 369 | 8.8 | 35.2 | 21.4 | 3.3 |
| Cheddar Cheese, & Onion, Safeway* | ¼ Quiche/100g | 293.0 | 19.0 | 293 | 8.3 | 21.6 | 19.3 | 1.5 |
| Cheese, Onion & Chive, SmartPrice, Asda* | ¼ Quiche/83g | 213.0 | 14.0 | 257 | 6.0 | 20.0 | 17.0 | 0.7 |
| Cheese, Onion & Chive, Tesco* | 1oz/28g | 90.0 | 7.0 | 320 | 10.6 | 15.5 | 24.0 | 0.6 |
| Cheese & Bacon, SmartPrice, Asda* | ¼ Quiche/82g | 211.0 | 14.0 | 257 | 6.0 | 20.0 | 17.0 | 0.7 |
| Cheese & Bacon, Tesco* | ¼ Quiche/100g | 255.0 | 16.0 | 255 | 8.1 | 17.9 | 16.3 | 0.7 |
| Cheese & Chive, HE, Tesco* | 1 Serving/86g | 169.0 | 6.0 | 197 | 10.4 | 22.1 | 7.4 | 1.2 |
| Cheese & Egg | 1oz/28g | 88.0 | 6.0 | 314 | 12.5 | 17.3 | 22.2 | 0.6 |
| Cheese & Ham, Sainsbury's* | 1 Serving/100g | 266.0 | 19.0 | 266 | 9.3 | 14.4 | 19.0 | 1.2 |
| Cheese & Ham, Somerfield* | 1 Quiche/325g | 835.0 | 58.0 | 257 | 7.0 | 18.0 | 18.0 | 0.0 |
| Cheese & Mushroom, Budgens* | ½ Quiche/170g | 474.0 | 33.0 | 279 | 7.8 | 18.4 | 19.3 | 1.4 |
| Cheese & Onion, 25% Reduced Fat, Asda* | ½ Quiche/78g | 163.0 | 7.0 | 209 | 11.0 | 21.0 | 9.0 | 2.4 |
| Cheese & Onion, Asda* | ½ Quiche/200g | 578.0 | 40.0 | 289 | 9.0 | 18.6 | 19.8 | 1.5 |
| Cheese & Onion, Co-Op* | ¼ Quiche/88g | 262.0 | 19.0 | 300 | 10.0 | 17.0 | 22.0 | 1.0 |
| Cheese & Onion, Crustless, Asda* | 1 Quiche/160g | 277.0 | 15.0 | 173 | 7.6 | 14.3 | 9.5 | 1.3 |
| Cheese & Onion, Deep Filled, Sainsbury's* | ¼ Quiche/100g | 254.0 | 17.0 | 254 | 7.3 | 17.2 | 17.2 | 2.2 |
| Cheese & Onion, Finest, Tesco* | 1 Serving/130g | 346.0 | 24.0 | 266 | 9.1 | 15.3 | 18.7 | 2.5 |
| Cheese & Onion, HL, Tesco* | 1 Quarter/100g | 180.0 | 8.0 | 180 | 9.4 | 17.6 | 7.8 | 1.8 |
| Cheese & Onion, Individual, Sainsbury's* | 1 Quiche/180g | 542.0 | 35.0 | 301 | 9.9 | 21.6 | 19.4 | 1.5 |
| Cheese & Onion, M & S* | 1 Slice/100g | 250.0 | 17.0 | 250 | 8.2 | 16.1 | 17.2 | 1.5 |
| Cheese & Onion, Mini, Somerfield* | 1oz/28g | 110.0 | 8.0 | 394 | 9.0 | 27.0 | 28.0 | 0.0 |
| Cheese & Onion, Safeway* | 1 Serving/310g | 797.0 | 44.0 | 257 | 7.2 | 25.2 | 14.2 | 0.0 |
| Cheese & Onion, Sainsbury's* | 1oz/28g | 67.0 | 4.0 | 241 | 6.8 | 18.3 | 15.6 | 2.6 |
| Cheese & Onion, Snack, Tasty Pastry* | 1 Quiche/50g | 137.0 | 9.0 | 274 | 4.9 | 24.9 | 17.2 | 1.2 |
| Cheese & Onion, Value, Tesco* | ½ Quiche/200g | 526.0 | 36.0 | 263 | 8.6 | 16.1 | 18.2 | 0.7 |
| Cheese & Onion, VLH Kitchens* | 1 Serving/80g | 133.6 | 4.8 | 167 | 9.6 | 18.1 | 6.0 | 1.8 |
| Cheese & Onion, Weight Watchers* | 1 Quiche/165g | 325.0 | 15.0 | 197 | 7.0 | 21.2 | 9.3 | 1.6 |

Q

| | Measure<br>INFO/WEIGHT | per Measure<br>KCAL FAT | | Nutrition Values per 100g / 100ml<br>KCAL PROT CARB FAT FIBRE | | | | |
|---|---|---|---|---|---|---|---|---|

## QUICHE

| | Measure INFO/WEIGHT | per Measure KCAL | FAT | KCAL | PROT | CARB | FAT | FIBRE |
|---|---|---|---|---|---|---|---|---|
| Cheese & Tomato, Asda* | ¼ Quiche/105g | 274.0 | 18.0 | 261 | 8.0 | 19.0 | 17.0 | 0.9 |
| Cheese & Tomato, M & S* | 1 Serving/100g | 230.0 | 16.0 | 230 | 7.7 | 15.1 | 15.6 | 1.6 |
| Cheese & Tomato, Morrisons* | ½ Quiche/64g | 195.0 | 13.0 | 304 | 7.3 | 22.8 | 20.5 | 1.0 |
| Cherry Tomato, Mozzarella & Pesto, TTD, Sainsbury's* | 1 Quiche/475g | 1111.0 | 77.0 | 234 | 5.5 | 16.5 | 16.2 | 2.1 |
| Chicken, Garlic & Herb, Asda* | 1/8 Quiche/52g | 137.0 | 8.0 | 264 | 10.0 | 20.0 | 16.0 | 1.2 |
| Chicken & Basil, Finest, Tesco* | 1 Serving/134g | 381.0 | 25.0 | 284 | 9.3 | 19.8 | 18.6 | 1.3 |
| Chicken & Mushroom, Somerfield* | 1oz/28g | 90.0 | 6.0 | 320 | 12.0 | 22.0 | 21.0 | 0.0 |
| Crustless, Green Vegetable, Light Choices, Tesco* | 1 Quiche/160g | 200.0 | 9.0 | 125 | 6.0 | 11.9 | 5.8 | 4.7 |
| Cumberland Sausage & Onion, Sainsbury's* | 1 Serving/180g | 486.0 | 33.0 | 270 | 7.0 | 18.8 | 18.5 | 1.3 |
| Davidstow Cheddar Cheese & Caramelised Onion, Asda* | 1/3 Quiche/117g | 367.0 | 27.0 | 315 | 7.0 | 20.0 | 23.0 | 1.0 |
| Farmhouse Cheddar & Onion, Waitrose* | ¼ Quiche/100g | 257.0 | 18.0 | 257 | 8.1 | 15.4 | 18.1 | 1.3 |
| Gammon, Leek & Cheddar Cheese, Somerfield* | ¼ Quiche/95g | 251.0 | 16.0 | 264 | 7.6 | 19.9 | 17.1 | 0.9 |
| Gammon, Leek & Mustard, Weight Watchers* | 1 Quiche/165g | 305.0 | 15.0 | 185 | 5.7 | 20.7 | 8.8 | 3.4 |
| Garlic Mushroom, Asda* | ¼ Quiche/105g | 273.0 | 17.0 | 260 | 7.0 | 22.0 | 16.0 | 0.7 |
| Goats Cheese & Red Pepper, Finest, Tesco* | 1 Serving/200g | 600.0 | 45.0 | 300 | 5.9 | 18.5 | 22.5 | 1.5 |
| Ham, Cheese & Chive, GFY, Asda* | 1 Serving/78g | 173.0 | 8.0 | 222 | 9.0 | 24.0 | 10.0 | 1.5 |
| Ham & Mustard, GFY, Asda* | 1 Quiche/155g | 327.0 | 17.0 | 211 | 9.0 | 19.0 | 11.0 | 3.9 |
| Ham & Soft Cheese, Tesco* | ¼ Quiche/100g | 280.0 | 20.0 | 280 | 7.4 | 17.5 | 20.1 | 1.9 |
| Ham & Tomato, M & S* | ½ Pack/200g | 440.0 | 31.0 | 220 | 8.1 | 12.4 | 15.5 | 2.9 |
| Leek, Cheese & Chive, Sainsbury's* | 1/3 Quiche/125g | 292.0 | 20.0 | 234 | 7.1 | 14.9 | 16.2 | 1.3 |
| Leek & Sweet Potato, Waitrose* | ½ Quiche/200g | 440.0 | 29.0 | 220 | 5.3 | 17.0 | 14.5 | 2.3 |
| Lorraine, Asda* | ¼ Quiche/100g | 246.0 | 16.0 | 246 | 6.6 | 18.5 | 16.2 | 4.2 |
| Lorraine, Average | 1oz/28g | 109.0 | 8.0 | 391 | 16.1 | 19.8 | 28.1 | 0.7 |
| Lorraine, BGTY, Sainsbury's* | 1 Serving/128g | 273.0 | 14.0 | 213 | 10.9 | 17.7 | 10.9 | 0.7 |
| Lorraine, Crustless, Asda* | 1 Quiche/160g | 259.0 | 13.0 | 162 | 9.3 | 13.5 | 7.9 | 1.1 |
| Lorraine, Crustless, Light Choices, Tesco* | 1 Pack/160g | 280.0 | 13.0 | 175 | 12.6 | 11.8 | 8.4 | 2.5 |
| Lorraine, Extra Special, Asda* | ¼ Quiche/100g | 270.0 | 18.0 | 270 | 8.0 | 19.0 | 18.0 | 2.3 |
| Lorraine, Finest, Tesco* | 1 Serving/100g | 330.0 | 25.0 | 330 | 8.4 | 17.5 | 25.1 | 1.5 |
| Lorraine, Half Fat, Waitrose* | ¼ Quiche/100g | 189.0 | 9.0 | 189 | 8.1 | 19.0 | 8.9 | 1.4 |
| Lorraine, Light Choices, Tesco* | ¼ Pack/100g | 170.0 | 6.0 | 170 | 12.3 | 15.5 | 6.4 | 3.2 |
| Lorraine, Meat Free, Tesco* | 1 Quiche/140g | 335.0 | 19.0 | 240 | 9.4 | 19.1 | 13.8 | 2.8 |
| Lorraine, Mini, M & S* | 1oz/28g | 95.0 | 7.0 | 340 | 11.6 | 21.0 | 23.6 | 1.6 |
| Lorraine, Quiche Selection, M & S* | 1 Slice/56g | 160.0 | 12.0 | 285 | 12.8 | 12.3 | 20.6 | 2.1 |
| Lorraine, Reduced Fat, Eat Smart, Morrisons* | ¼ Quiche/100g | 209.0 | 10.0 | 209 | 9.4 | 17.8 | 9.8 | 0.5 |
| Lorraine, Sainsbury's* | ½ Quiche/200g | 598.0 | 42.0 | 299 | 10.6 | 16.3 | 21.2 | 0.9 |
| Lorraine, Small, Waitrose* | 1 Pack/170g | 507.0 | 35.0 | 298 | 9.8 | 18.4 | 20.6 | 2.3 |
| Lorraine, Smoked Bacon & Cheese, M & S* | ¼ Quiche/100g | 270.0 | 18.0 | 270 | 9.7 | 16.4 | 18.4 | 1.6 |
| Lorraine, Snack, Morrisons* | 1 Serving/50g | 142.0 | 9.0 | 285 | 10.2 | 19.0 | 18.7 | 2.0 |
| Lorraine, Tesco* | 1 Serving/81g | 215.0 | 13.0 | 265 | 8.9 | 20.0 | 16.6 | 0.8 |
| Lorraine, TTD, Sainsbury's* | 1/3 Quiche/158g | 482.0 | 36.0 | 305 | 10.2 | 15.1 | 22.7 | 0.9 |
| Lorraine, Weight Watchers* | 1 Quiche/165g | 292.0 | 13.0 | 177 | 8.7 | 17.5 | 8.0 | 3.2 |
| Meat Feast, Tesco* | 1 ¼ /100g | 265.0 | 19.0 | 265 | 6.2 | 17.2 | 19.0 | 2.5 |
| Mediterranean, GFY, Asda* | 1 Serving/25g | 54.0 | 2.0 | 217 | 9.0 | 25.0 | 9.0 | 2.4 |
| Mediterranean, M & S* | 1oz/28g | 64.0 | 4.0 | 230 | 6.6 | 16.6 | 15.3 | 0.9 |
| Mediterranean Pepper, Good Intentions, Somerfield* | 1/3 Quiche/130g | 264.0 | 12.0 | 203 | 7.9 | 22.2 | 9.2 | 1.3 |
| Mediterranean Vegetable, BGTY, Sainsbury's* | ½ Quiche/90g | 160.0 | 7.0 | 178 | 7.3 | 19.2 | 8.0 | 1.7 |
| Mediterranean Vegetable, Mini, M & S* | 1oz/28g | 78.0 | 5.0 | 280 | 6.8 | 23.9 | 17.5 | 1.6 |
| Mediterranean Vegetable, Weight Watchers* | 1 Quiche/165g | 285.0 | 14.0 | 173 | 3.8 | 21.1 | 8.2 | 4.0 |
| Mushroom | 1oz/28g | 80.0 | 5.0 | 284 | 10.0 | 18.3 | 19.5 | 0.9 |
| Mushroom, M & S* | ¼ Quiche/100g | 235.0 | 17.0 | 235 | 6.1 | 14.6 | 16.7 | 2.8 |
| Mushroom, Tesco* | ¼ Quiche/100g | 250.0 | 17.0 | 250 | 5.6 | 17.4 | 17.5 | 1.0 |
| Mushroom Medley, Waitrose* | ¼ Quiche/100g | 222.0 | 15.0 | 222 | 6.4 | 15.0 | 15.2 | 2.9 |
| Mushroom Medley & Gruyere, TTD, Sainsbury's* | 1/3 Quiche/158g | 426.0 | 30.0 | 269 | 6.3 | 18.0 | 19.1 | 1.4 |

Q

| | Measure INFO/WEIGHT | per Measure KCAL | FAT | Nutrition Values per 100g / 100ml KCAL | PROT | CARB | FAT | FIBRE |
|---|---|---|---|---|---|---|---|---|
| **QUICHE** | | | | | | | | |
| Red Pepper, Goats Cheese & Spinach, Waitrose* | 1 Serving/100g | 218.0 | 14.0 | 218 | 6.5 | 15.8 | 14.3 | 2.6 |
| Red Pepper, Rocket & Parmesan, Waitrose* | 1 Serving/100g | 236.0 | 17.0 | 236 | 6.1 | 14.8 | 16.9 | 1.9 |
| Roast Sweet Potato, Carrot & Coriander, Asda* | ½ Quiche/208g | 523.0 | 33.0 | 252 | 7.0 | 20.0 | 16.0 | 1.0 |
| Salmon & Asparagus, HE, Tesco* | 1 Quiche/345g | 621.0 | 27.0 | 180 | 7.5 | 20.2 | 7.7 | 1.2 |
| Salmon & Broccoli, Asda* | ¼ Quiche/106g | 289.0 | 18.0 | 273 | 10.0 | 20.0 | 17.0 | 2.6 |
| Salmon & Broccoli, Sainsbury's* | 1 Serving | 346.0 | 23.0 | 260 | 7.9 | 18.5 | 17.1 | 0.8 |
| Salmon & Broccoli, Tesco* | 1 Serving/133g | 311.0 | 20.0 | 234 | 7.9 | 16.6 | 15.1 | 0.9 |
| Salmon & Spinach, Sainsbury's* | 1/3 Quiche/125g | 318.0 | 22.0 | 254 | 8.2 | 15.9 | 17.5 | 1.0 |
| Sausage & Onion, Sainsbury's* | 1 Serving/100g | 287.0 | 20.0 | 287 | 7.1 | 19.7 | 20.0 | 1.2 |
| Spinach, Ricotta & Gruyere Slice, Somerfield* | 1 Serving/130g | 348.0 | 26.0 | 268 | 7.0 | 15.0 | 20.0 | 0.0 |
| Spinach & Gruyere, Mini, Somerfield* | 1oz/28g | 108.0 | 8.0 | 384 | 11.0 | 25.0 | 27.0 | 0.0 |
| Spinach & Gruyere, Sainsbury's* | ¼ Quiche/100g | 258.0 | 19.0 | 258 | 7.7 | 13.9 | 19.1 | 1.0 |
| Spinach & Ricotta, M & S* | 1oz/28g | 73.0 | 5.0 | 260 | 8.0 | 14.9 | 18.8 | 1.7 |
| Spinach & Ricotta, Tesco* | ¼ Quiche/100g | 237.0 | 15.0 | 237 | 5.8 | 19.9 | 14.9 | 1.0 |
| Sunblush Tomato, Basil & Mozzarella, Somerfield* | ¼ Quiche/88g | 221.0 | 15.0 | 251 | 7.7 | 17.9 | 16.5 | 1.0 |
| Sweet Cherry Pepper & Fontal Cheese, Finest, Tesco* | ¼ Quiche/100g | 293.0 | 22.0 | 293 | 6.7 | 16.9 | 22.1 | 0.9 |
| Sweetfire Pepper, Feta & Olive, Waitrose* | ¼ Quiche/100g | 238.0 | 17.0 | 238 | 5.7 | 15.7 | 16.9 | 1.4 |
| Three Cheese & Onion, GFY, Asda* | 1 Serving/73g | 188.0 | 10.0 | 258 | 10.0 | 23.0 | 14.0 | 3.1 |
| Tomato, Cheese & Courgette, Asda* | 1 Quiche/100g | 333.0 | 17.0 | 333 | 11.0 | 34.0 | 17.0 | 5.0 |
| Tomato, GFY, Asda* | ¼ Quiche/50g | 94.0 | 4.0 | 188 | 8.0 | 21.0 | 8.0 | 0.8 |
| Tomato, Mozzarella, & Basil, Weight Watchers* | 1 Quiche/165g | 300.0 | 12.0 | 182 | 6.1 | 22.8 | 7.4 | 1.3 |
| Tomato, Mushroom & Bacon, Sainsbury's* | 1 Serving/187g | 447.0 | 31.0 | 239 | 7.5 | 15.2 | 16.5 | 1.1 |
| Tomato Cheese & Courgette, GFY, Asda* | 1 Serving/155g | 333.0 | 17.0 | 215 | 7.0 | 22.0 | 11.0 | 3.3 |
| Tuna, Tomato & Basil, Asda* | 1 Serving/125g | 305.0 | 20.0 | 244 | 9.0 | 16.0 | 16.0 | 1.5 |
| Vegetable, Tesco* | 1 Serving/100g | 257.0 | 18.0 | 257 | 6.9 | 17.5 | 17.7 | 1.5 |
| **QUICK SNACK** | | | | | | | | |
| Mash, Roasted Onion, Sainsbury's* | 1 Pot/58g | 75.0 | 4.0 | 130 | 1.8 | 14.8 | 7.1 | 0.0 |
| Rice, Chilli, Sainsbury's* | 1 Pack/280g | 241.0 | 1.0 | 86 | 2.5 | 18.6 | 0.2 | 0.0 |
| Rice, Sweet & Sour, Sainsbury's* | 1 Serving/237g | 230.0 | 1.0 | 97 | 2.5 | 20.5 | 0.5 | 0.0 |
| **QUINCE** | | | | | | | | |
| *Average* | *1oz/28g* | *7.0* | *0.0* | *26* | *0.3* | *6.3* | *0.1* | *0.0* |
| **QUINOA** | | | | | | | | |
| *Boiled, Average* | *1 Serving/100g* | *77.0* | *1.0* | *77* | *3.5* | *13.9* | *1.3* | *2.2* |
| *Dry Weight, Average* | *1 Serving/70g* | *262.0* | *4.0* | *374* | *13.1* | *68.9* | *5.8* | *5.9* |
| **QUORN*** | | | | | | | | |
| Bacon Style, Rashers, Streaky, Frozen, Quorn* | ¼ Pack/3 Strips | 74.0 | 6.0 | 198 | 11.0 | 3.5 | 15.5 | 5.0 |
| Bacon Style, Slices, Smoky, Frozen, Quorn* | ¼ Pack/38g | 75.0 | 6.0 | 199 | 11.8 | 3.0 | 15.5 | 5.0 |
| Balls, Al Forno, Quorn* | 1 Serving/400g | 348.0 | 7.0 | 87 | 4.7 | 13.1 | 1.8 | 1.8 |
| Balls, Swedish Style, Quorn* | 1 Pack/300g | 354.0 | 6.0 | 118 | 17.0 | 8.0 | 2.0 | 2.0 |
| Beef Style Pieces, Quorn* | ½ Pack/75g | 69.0 | 2.0 | 92 | 13.5 | 4.5 | 2.2 | 5.0 |
| Bites, BBQ, Quorn* | 1 Pack/140g | 147.0 | 3.0 | 105 | 13.5 | 7.0 | 2.5 | 5.5 |
| Bites, Indian, Quorn* | 1 Bite/15g | 34.0 | 2.0 | 222 | 6.0 | 27.0 | 10.0 | 3.0 |
| Burgers, Chicken Style, Quorn* | 1 Burger/70g | 136.0 | 7.0 | 194 | 11.0 | 16.0 | 9.6 | 4.6 |
| Burgers, Original, Quorn* | 1 Burger/50g | 73.0 | 2.0 | 146 | 18.9 | 6.7 | 4.8 | 3.0 |
| Burgers, Premium, Quorn* | 1 Burger/82g | 88.0 | 3.0 | 107 | 11.3 | 6.5 | 4.0 | 3.5 |
| Burgers, Quarter Pounder, Quorn* | 1 Burger/114g | 158.0 | 5.0 | 139 | 18.0 | 6.5 | 4.5 | 4.5 |
| Burgers, Southern Style, Quorn* | 1 Burger/63g | 119.0 | 6.0 | 189 | 10.7 | 14.5 | 9.8 | 3.1 |
| Casserole, Quorn* | 1oz/28g | 46.0 | 3.0 | 165 | 11.9 | 5.1 | 10.9 | 0.9 |
| Casserole, with Dumplings, Quorn* | 1oz/28g | 36.0 | 2.0 | 127 | 4.5 | 14.2 | 5.8 | 1.7 |
| Chicken Style Dippers, Quorn* | 1 Dipper/19g | 32.0 | 2.0 | 167 | 11.0 | 7.2 | 10.5 | 4.0 |
| Chicken Style Pieces, Frozen Or Chilled, Quorn* | 1 Serving/87g | 90.0 | 2.0 | 103 | 14.0 | 5.8 | 2.6 | 5.5 |
| Chilli, Quorn* | 1oz/28g | 23.0 | 1.0 | 81 | 4.7 | 6.9 | 4.2 | 2.5 |
| Cottage Pie, Quorn* | 1 Lg Pack/500g | 295.0 | 7.0 | 59 | 2.5 | 9.0 | 1.4 | 2.6 |

| | Measure INFO/WEIGHT | per Measure KCAL | per Measure FAT | Nutrition Values per 100g / 100ml KCAL | PROT | CARB | FAT | FIBRE |
|---|---|---|---|---|---|---|---|---|
| **QUORN\*** | | | | | | | | |
| Curry, Red Thai, Quorn\* | 1 Pack/400g | 464.0 | 16.0 | 116 | 4.6 | 15.5 | 3.9 | 4.0 |
| Curry & Rice, Quorn\* | 1 Pack/400g | 412.0 | 8.0 | 103 | 3.8 | 17.5 | 2.0 | 1.5 |
| Eggs, Picnic, Quorn\* | 1 Egg/20g | 50.0 | 2.0 | 248 | 15.0 | 21.0 | 11.5 | 4.6 |
| En Croute, Cheddar Cheese & Ham Style, Quorn\* | 1 Pastry/200g | 486.0 | 28.0 | 243 | 7.2 | 22.0 | 14.0 | 3.0 |
| En Croute, Creamy Mushroom & Garlic, Quorn\* | 1 Pastry/200g | 460.0 | 29.0 | 230 | 5.9 | 19.0 | 14.5 | 3.2 |
| Enchiladas, Quorn\* | 1 Pack/401g | 405.0 | 15.0 | 101 | 5.3 | 11.7 | 3.7 | 1.9 |
| Escalopes, Creamy Garlic & Mushroom, Quorn\* | 1 Escalope/120g | 266.0 | 15.0 | 222 | 7.9 | 19.4 | 12.5 | 3.1 |
| Escalopes, Creamy Peppercorn, Quorn\* | 1 Escalope/120g | 252.0 | 15.0 | 210 | 7.8 | 16.0 | 12.7 | 4.0 |
| Escalopes, Feta & Tomato, Quorn\* | 1 Escalope/120g | 257.0 | 15.0 | 214 | 8.0 | 18.0 | 12.2 | 4.0 |
| Escalopes, Garlic & Herb, Quorn\* | 1 Escalope/140g | 293.0 | 17.0 | 209 | 8.9 | 16.9 | 11.8 | 3.8 |
| Escalopes, Korma, Quorn\* | 1 Escalope/120g | 270.0 | 16.0 | 225 | 7.0 | 20.0 | 13.0 | 3.0 |
| Escalopes, Mature Cheddar & Broccoli, Quorn\* | 1 Escalope/120g | 244.0 | 14.0 | 203 | 8.7 | 16.5 | 11.4 | 2.9 |
| Fajita, Strips, Quorn\* | ½ New Pack/70g | 69.0 | 1.0 | 98 | 14.0 | 7.0 | 1.5 | 5.0 |
| Fajita Meal Kit, Quorn\* | ½ Pack/214g | 268.0 | 5.0 | 125 | 7.0 | 18.5 | 2.5 | 3.5 |
| Fillets, Chargrilled Tikka Style, Mini, Quorn\* | ½ Pack/85g | 110.0 | 2.0 | 129 | 12.5 | 14.4 | 2.4 | 5.0 |
| Fillets, Chinese Style Chargrilled, Mini, Quorn\* | 1 Serving/85g | 115.0 | 2.0 | 135 | 12.1 | 15.6 | 2.7 | 4.7 |
| Fillets, Crispy, Quorn\* | 1 Fillet/100g | 197.0 | 10.0 | 197 | 13.0 | 14.2 | 9.8 | 4.0 |
| Fillets, Garlic & Herb, Quorn\* | 1 Fillet/100g | 208.0 | 10.0 | 208 | 13.9 | 16.1 | 9.8 | 4.1 |
| Fillets, Plain, Quorn\* | 1 Fillet/52g | 47.0 | 1.0 | 90 | 12.6 | 5.9 | 1.8 | 4.7 |
| Fillets, Thai, Quorn\* | 1 Serving/79g | 96.0 | 4.0 | 121 | 11.0 | 9.0 | 4.5 | 4.0 |
| Goujons, Quorn\* | 1 Goujon/31g | 57.0 | 3.0 | 187 | 10.2 | 15.0 | 9.6 | 4.5 |
| Goujons, with Chunky Salsa Dip, Quorn\* | 1oz/28g | 57.0 | 3.0 | 204 | 10.4 | 17.0 | 10.5 | 3.0 |
| Grills, Lamb Style, Quorn\* | 1 Grill/89g | 97.0 | 3.0 | 109 | 11.2 | 7.6 | 3.7 | 4.3 |
| Kievs, Mini, Quorn\* | 1 Kiev/20g | 41.0 | 2.0 | 207 | 14.0 | 13.0 | 11.0 | 6.5 |
| Lasagne, Quorn\* | 1 Pack/400g | 332.0 | 12.0 | 83 | 3.7 | 10.6 | 2.9 | 1.8 |
| Mince, Frozen Or Chilled, Quorn\* | 1 Serving/87g | 82.0 | 2.0 | 94 | 14.5 | 4.5 | 2.0 | 5.5 |
| Moussaka, Quorn\* | 1 Pack/400g | 364.0 | 16.0 | 91 | 3.6 | 9.8 | 4.1 | 1.2 |
| Pasty, Cornish Style, Quorn\* | 1 Pasty/150g | 399.0 | 24.0 | 266 | 5.5 | 25.0 | 16.0 | 3.0 |
| Pate, Brussels Style, Deli, Quorn\* | 1/3 Pack/43g | 55.0 | 2.0 | 128 | 11.3 | 8.5 | 5.4 | 4.0 |
| Pie, & Vegetable, Quorn\* | 1oz/28g | 52.0 | 3.0 | 186 | 6.9 | 14.7 | 11.5 | 2.0 |
| Pie, Creamy Mushroom, Quorn\* | 1 Pie/142g | 359.0 | 21.0 | 253 | 4.5 | 26.0 | 14.5 | 2.0 |
| Pie, Mince & Onion, Quorn\* | 1 Pie/142g | 360.0 | 20.0 | 254 | 5.0 | 27.0 | 14.0 | 1.5 |
| Pork Style Ribsters, Quorn\* | 2 Ribsters/85g | 105.0 | 3.0 | 124 | 15.9 | 6.3 | 3.9 | 2.1 |
| Satay Sticks, Quorn\* | ½ Pack/90g | 149.0 | 8.0 | 165 | 13.0 | 7.1 | 9.4 | 3.2 |
| Sausage Roll, Chilled, Quorn\* | 1 Roll/75g | 194.0 | 10.0 | 258 | 12.0 | 24.0 | 12.7 | 4.0 |
| Sausages, Cumberland, Quorn\* | 1 Sausage/50g | 60.0 | 2.0 | 120 | 13.1 | 7.0 | 4.4 | 2.4 |
| Sausages, Frozen, Quorn\* | 1 Sausage/50g | 56.0 | 2.0 | 113 | 14.9 | 4.9 | 3.7 | 3.3 |
| Sausages, Leek & Pork Style, Quorn\* | 1 Sausage/44g | 56.0 | 2.0 | 127 | 15.1 | 5.5 | 4.9 | 4.3 |
| Sausages, Pork & Apple Style, Quorn\* | 1 Sausage/50g | 58.0 | 2.0 | 117 | 11.5 | 7.5 | 4.6 | 3.0 |
| Sausages, Quorn\* | 1 Sausage/43g | 48.0 | 2.0 | 113 | 14.9 | 4.9 | 3.7 | 3.3 |
| Sausages, Spinach & Cheese, Quorn\* | 1 Sausage/50g | 60.0 | 2.0 | 120 | 15.1 | 6.0 | 4.0 | 2.8 |
| Sausages, Tomato & Basil, Quorn\* | 1 Sausage/50g | 51.0 | 1.0 | 102 | 14.3 | 6.0 | 2.3 | 2.8 |
| Slices, Chicken Style, Deli, Quorn\* | ½ Pack/50g | 53.0 | 1.0 | 107 | 16.3 | 4.5 | 2.6 | 6.0 |
| Slices, Chicken Style, Wafer Thin, Deli, Quorn\* | 1/3 Pack/60g | 64.0 | 2.0 | 107 | 16.3 | 4.5 | 2.6 | 5.9 |
| Slices, Ham Style, Deli, Quorn\* | ½ Pack/50g | 55.0 | 1.0 | 110 | 16.0 | 6.5 | 2.2 | 5.8 |
| Slices, Ham Style, Wafer Thin, Deli, Quorn\* | 1/3 Pack/60g | 66.0 | 1.0 | 110 | 16.0 | 6.5 | 2.2 | 5.8 |
| Slices, Peppered Beef Style, Quorn\* | ½ Pack/50g | 53.0 | 1.0 | 107 | 14.5 | 7.6 | 2.1 | 4.0 |
| Slices, Turkey Style & Cranberry, Quorn\* | ½ Pack/50g | 56.0 | 1.0 | 113 | 14.5 | 8.0 | 2.5 | 4.0 |
| Spaghetti Bolognese, Quorn\* | 1 Pack/400g | 240.0 | 4.0 | 60 | 3.7 | 9.2 | 0.9 | 1.6 |
| Spaghetti Carbonara, Quorn\* | 1 Pack/400g | 460.0 | 26.0 | 115 | 5.0 | 9.1 | 6.5 | 1.1 |
| Steaks, Peppered, Quorn\* | 1 Steak/98g | 107.0 | 4.0 | 109 | 11.4 | 7.4 | 3.8 | 4.0 |
| Tandoori Pieces, Quorn\* | ½ Pack/70g | 93.0 | 3.0 | 133 | 12.0 | 11.0 | 4.5 | 5.0 |

Q

| | Measure<br>INFO/WEIGHT | per Measure<br>KCAL | FAT | Nutrition Values per 100g / 100ml<br>KCAL | PROT | CARB | FAT | FIBRE |
|---|---|---|---|---|---|---|---|---|
| **RABBIT** | | | | | | | | |
| *Meat Only, Raw* | *1oz/28g* | *38.0* | *2.0* | *137* | *21.9* | *0.0* | *5.5* | *0.0* |
| *Meat Only, Stewed* | *1oz/28g* | *32.0* | *1.0* | *114* | *21.2* | *0.0* | *3.2* | *0.0* |
| *Meat Only, Stewed, Weighed with Bone* | *1oz/28g* | *19.0* | *1.0* | *68* | *12.7* | *0.0* | *1.9* | *0.0* |
| **RADDICCIO** | | | | | | | | |
| *Raw* | *1oz/28g* | *4.0* | *0.0* | *14* | *1.4* | *1.7* | *0.2* | *1.8* |
| **RADISH** | | | | | | | | |
| *Red, Unprepared, Average* | *1 Radish/8g* | *1.0* | *0.0* | *12* | *0.7* | *1.9* | *0.2* | *0.9* |
| *White, Mooli, Raw* | *1oz/28g* | *4.0* | *0.0* | *15* | *0.8* | *2.9* | *0.1* | *0.0* |
| **RAISINS** | | | | | | | | |
| & Apricot, The Fruit Factory* | 1 Box/14g | 41.0 | 0.0 | 290 | 3.5 | 67.9 | 0.5 | 6.3 |
| & Cranberries, Waitrose* | 1 Serving/30g | 94.0 | 0.0 | 312 | 1.5 | 75.7 | 0.3 | 3.4 |
| & Sultanas, Jumbo, M & S* | 1 Serving/80g | 212.0 | 0.0 | 265 | 2.4 | 62.4 | 0.5 | 2.6 |
| & Sultanas, Jumbo, Safeway* | 1 Pack/250g | 772.0 | 2.0 | 309 | 2.4 | 73.1 | 0.8 | 5.7 |
| Blueberry Yoghurt Covered Raisins, Boots* | 1 Pack/75g | 322.0 | 13.0 | 429 | 2.7 | 64.0 | 18.0 | 0.7 |
| *Seedless, Average* | *1 Serving/75g* | *215.0* | *0.0* | *287* | *2.2* | *68.5* | *0.5* | *3.1* |
| **RAITA** | | | | | | | | |
| Cucumber & Mint, Patak's* | 1oz/28g | 18.0 | 1.0 | 64 | 3.4 | 8.4 | 1.8 | 0.0 |
| Plain | 1oz/28g | 46.0 | 4.0 | 166 | 2.6 | 5.5 | 15.3 | 0.0 |
| **RASPBERRIES** | | | | | | | | |
| *Fresh, Raw, Average* | *1 Serving/80g* | *21.0* | *0.0* | *26* | *1.3* | *4.7* | *0.3* | *6.5* |
| *in Fruit Juice, Average* | *1oz/28g* | *9.0* | *0.0* | *31* | *0.8* | *6.7* | *0.1* | *1.7* |
| *in Syrup, Canned* | *1oz/28g* | *25.0* | *0.0* | *88* | *0.6* | *22.5* | *0.1* | *1.5* |
| **RATATOUILLE** | | | | | | | | |
| Average | 1oz/28g | 23.0 | 2.0 | 82 | 1.3 | 3.8 | 7.0 | 1.8 |
| Chicken, Finest, Tesco* | 1 Pack/550g | 407.0 | 12.0 | 74 | 7.8 | 5.9 | 2.1 | 0.0 |
| Princes* | 1 Can/360g | 86.0 | 1.0 | 24 | 1.0 | 4.2 | 0.4 | 0.0 |
| Roasted Vegetable, Sainsbury's* | 1 Pack/300g | 134.0 | 3.0 | 45 | 1.4 | 7.5 | 1.0 | 2.3 |
| Sainsbury's* | 1 Pack/300g | 99.0 | 2.0 | 33 | 1.5 | 5.5 | 0.6 | 1.6 |
| **RAVIOLI** | | | | | | | | |
| Amatriciana, TTD, Sainsbury's* | 1 Serving/125g | 390.0 | 16.0 | 312 | 16.6 | 33.3 | 12.5 | 3.5 |
| Asparagus & Ham, HE, Tesco* | ½ Pack/125g | 202.0 | 3.0 | 162 | 8.2 | 26.5 | 2.6 | 0.6 |
| Basil & Parmesan, Organic, Sainsbury's* | ½ Pack/192g | 290.0 | 10.0 | 151 | 7.4 | 21.1 | 5.2 | 2.1 |
| Beef, GFY, Asda* | ½ Pack/150g | 288.0 | 5.0 | 192 | 7.0 | 33.9 | 3.2 | 1.9 |
| Beef, Tesco* | 1 Serving/194g | 175.0 | 5.0 | 90 | 4.3 | 12.3 | 2.6 | 1.5 |
| Beef & Red Wine, Italiano, Tesco* | ½ Pack/150g | 315.0 | 10.0 | 210 | 7.3 | 30.0 | 6.5 | 2.3 |
| Beef & Shiraz, Finest, Tesco* | ½ Pack/200g | 358.0 | 9.0 | 179 | 8.4 | 26.1 | 4.5 | 1.8 |
| Beef in Tomato Sauce, Canned, Asda* | 1 Can/400g | 352.0 | 8.0 | 88 | 3.6 | 14.0 | 2.0 | 3.0 |
| Cheese, Garlic, & Herb, Fresh, Organic, Tesco* | 1 Serving/125g | 382.0 | 19.0 | 306 | 11.3 | 30.1 | 15.6 | 0.9 |
| Cheese, in Tomato Sauce, Canned, Tesco* | 1 Can/410g | 328.0 | 8.0 | 80 | 2.5 | 13.0 | 2.0 | 0.5 |
| Cheese & Asparagus, Waitrose* | 1 Serving/100g | 242.0 | 7.0 | 242 | 12.6 | 31.7 | 7.2 | 2.4 |
| Cheese & Tomato, Fresh, Organic, Tesco* | 1 Serving/125g | 342.0 | 14.0 | 274 | 12.5 | 30.8 | 11.2 | 1.1 |
| Cheese & Tomato, Heinz* | 1 Can/400g | 340.0 | 8.0 | 85 | 2.4 | 13.9 | 2.1 | 0.9 |
| Cherry Tomato & Mushroom, Somerfield* | 1 Pack/400g | 436.0 | 25.0 | 109 | 3.5 | 9.8 | 6.2 | 1.2 |
| Chicken & Bacon, Sainsbury's* | ½ Pack/150g | 238.0 | 8.0 | 159 | 5.5 | 22.2 | 5.4 | 2.0 |
| Chicken & Mushroom, Finest, Tesco* | ½ Pack/125g | 267.0 | 9.0 | 214 | 11.6 | 25.8 | 7.1 | 1.1 |
| Chicken & Rosemary, Perfectly Balanced, Waitrose* | ½ Pack/125g | 266.0 | 4.0 | 213 | 14.9 | 30.4 | 3.5 | 2.1 |
| Chicken & Tomato, Perfectly Balanced, Waitrose* | 1 Serving/125g | 265.0 | 3.0 | 212 | 13.5 | 33.4 | 2.7 | 2.8 |
| Feta Cheese, M & S* | 1 Serving/100g | 195.0 | 8.0 | 195 | 9.1 | 20.5 | 8.5 | 1.3 |
| Five Cheese, Weight Watchers* | 1 Pack/330g | 271.0 | 9.0 | 82 | 3.2 | 11.1 | 2.8 | 0.8 |
| Florentine, Weight Watchers* | 1 Serving/241g | 220.0 | 5.0 | 91 | 3.7 | 14.1 | 2.1 | 1.2 |
| Four Cheese, Italian Choice, Asda* | 1 Pack/449g | 467.0 | 27.0 | 104 | 3.4 | 9.0 | 6.0 | 2.1 |
| Fresh, Pasta Reale* | 1 Serving/150g | 459.0 | 9.0 | 306 | 13.1 | 53.3 | 5.9 | 0.0 |
| Garlic & Herb, Italiano, Tesco* | 1 Serving/100g | 318.0 | 13.0 | 318 | 11.1 | 39.1 | 13.0 | 2.6 |

| | Measure INFO/WEIGHT | per Measure KCAL | FAT | Nutrition Values per 100g / 100ml KCAL | PROT | CARB | FAT | FIBRE |
|---|---|---|---|---|---|---|---|---|
| **RAVIOLI** | | | | | | | | |
| Garlic Mushroom, Finest, Tesco* | 1 Serving/250g | 552.0 | 18.0 | 221 | 8.9 | 30.0 | 7.3 | 2.0 |
| Goat's Cheese & Pesto, Asda* | ½ Pack/150g | 204.0 | 5.0 | 136 | 6.0 | 20.0 | 3.6 | 0.0 |
| Goats Cheese & Roasted Red Pepper, Finest, Tesco* | ½ Pack/125g | 307.0 | 10.0 | 246 | 11.4 | 32.8 | 7.7 | 1.8 |
| Grana Padano & Rocket, Finest, Tesco* | ½ Pack/150g | 270.0 | 7.0 | 180 | 7.5 | 26.0 | 5.0 | 1.8 |
| in Tomato Sauce, Canned, Sainsbury's* | ½ Can/200g | 166.0 | 2.0 | 83 | 3.1 | 15.5 | 1.0 | 0.5 |
| in Tomato Sauce, Heinz* | 1 Can/400g | 308.0 | 7.0 | 77 | 2.4 | 13.2 | 1.7 | 0.9 |
| in Tomato Sauce, Meat Free, Heinz* | 1 Can/410g | 307.0 | 3.0 | 75 | 2.4 | 14.4 | 0.8 | 0.5 |
| Meat, Italian, Fresh, Asda* | ½ Pack/150g | 261.0 | 6.0 | 174 | 8.0 | 26.0 | 4.2 | 0.0 |
| Mozzarella Tomato & Basil, Tesco* | 1 Serving/125g | 304.0 | 13.0 | 243 | 13.6 | 24.1 | 10.2 | 0.5 |
| Mushroom, Fresh, Sainsbury's* | ½ Pack/125g | 196.0 | 5.0 | 157 | 7.4 | 22.6 | 4.1 | 1.9 |
| Mushroom, Italiano, Tesco* | 1 Serving/125g | 332.0 | 16.0 | 266 | 10.4 | 27.0 | 12.9 | 3.0 |
| Mushroom, Ready Meals, M & S* | 1oz/28g | 38.0 | 1.0 | 135 | 8.1 | 22.0 | 1.9 | 2.2 |
| Mushroom, Wild, Finest, Tesco* | 1 Serving/200g | 472.0 | 12.0 | 236 | 10.8 | 34.4 | 6.1 | 1.9 |
| Mushroomi, Tesco* | ½ Pack/125g | 332.0 | 16.0 | 266 | 10.4 | 27.0 | 12.9 | 3.0 |
| Pancetta & Mozzarella, Finest, Tesco* | 1 Serving/125g | 344.0 | 13.0 | 275 | 12.2 | 32.8 | 10.6 | 1.8 |
| Pork, in Tomato Sauce, Low Fat, Morrisons* | 1oz/28g | 23.0 | 0.0 | 81 | 2.7 | 15.5 | 0.9 | 1.3 |
| Red Onion & Brunello Wine, TTD, Sainsbury's* | 1 Serving/125g | 235.0 | 9.0 | 188 | 7.5 | 23.0 | 7.3 | 2.5 |
| Red Pepper, Basil & Chilli, Waitrose* | ½ Pack/125g | 312.0 | 10.0 | 250 | 11.6 | 32.0 | 8.4 | 1.7 |
| Roast Garlic & Herb, Tesco* | ½ Pack/125g | 342.0 | 14.0 | 274 | 12.8 | 31.1 | 10.9 | 1.1 |
| Roasted Pepper, M & S* | 1 Pack/400g | 540.0 | 31.0 | 135 | 5.4 | 11.0 | 7.7 | 1.1 |
| Roasted Vegetable, Asda* | ½ Pack/150g | 217.0 | 1.0 | 145 | 6.0 | 29.0 | 0.5 | 0.0 |
| Salmon & Dill, Sainsbury's* | 1 Pack/300g | 615.0 | 21.0 | 205 | 8.7 | 26.5 | 7.1 | 3.0 |
| Smoked Ham, Bacon & Tomato, Italiano, Tesco* | 1 Can/125g | 302.0 | 10.0 | 242 | 10.8 | 32.3 | 7.7 | 2.9 |
| Smoked Salmon & Dill, Sainsbury's* | 1 Serving/125g | 256.0 | 9.0 | 205 | 8.7 | 26.5 | 7.1 | 0.7 |
| Spinach & Ricotta, Waitrose* | 1 Serving/125g | 309.0 | 9.0 | 247 | 10.5 | 35.0 | 7.2 | 1.9 |
| Sweet Pepper & Chilli, Tesco* | ½ Pack/125g | 324.0 | 14.0 | 259 | 12.5 | 27.1 | 11.2 | 2.7 |
| Vegetable, Canned, Sainsbury's* | 1 Can/400g | 328.0 | 3.0 | 82 | 2.6 | 16.3 | 0.7 | 0.7 |
| Vegetable, Morrisons* | 1 Can/400g | 276.0 | 2.0 | 69 | 2.4 | 13.9 | 0.4 | 0.0 |
| Vegetable, Tesco* | ½ Can/200g | 164.0 | 1.0 | 82 | 2.6 | 16.3 | 0.7 | 0.7 |
| Vegetable, with Omega 3, Heinz* | 1 Can/200g | 144.0 | 3.0 | 72 | 2.2 | 12.2 | 1.6 | 0.6 |
| Vegetable in Tomato Sauce, Italiana, Weight Watchers* | 1 Can/385g | 266.0 | 8.0 | 69 | 1.7 | 11.0 | 2.1 | 0.5 |
| **RED BULL*** | | | | | | | | |
| Regular, Red Bull* | 1 Can/250ml | 112.0 | 0.0 | 45 | 0.0 | 11.3 | 0.0 | 0.0 |
| **REDCURRANTS** | | | | | | | | |
| *Raw, Average* | *1oz/28g* | *6.0* | *0.0* | *21* | *1.1* | *4.4* | *0.0* | *3.4* |
| **REEF*** | | | | | | | | |
| Orange & Passionfruit, Reef* | 1 Bottle/275ml | 179.0 | 0.0 | 65 | 0.0 | 9.5 | 0.0 | 0.0 |
| **REFRESHERS** | | | | | | | | |
| Bassett's* | 1oz/28g | 106.0 | 0.0 | 377 | 4.3 | 78.1 | 0.0 | 0.0 |
| **RELISH** | | | | | | | | |
| Barbeque, Sainsbury's* | 1 Serving/50g | 50.0 | 1.0 | 100 | 1.0 | 19.3 | 2.1 | 1.1 |
| Burger, Juicy, Asda* | 1 Tbsp/15g | 17.0 | 0.0 | 113 | 1.2 | 25.4 | 0.7 | 0.7 |
| Caramelised Onion & Chilli, M & S* | 1 Serving/20g | 47.0 | 0.0 | 235 | 1.4 | 55.1 | 1.1 | 1.0 |
| Caramelised Red Onion, Tesco* | 1 Serving/10g | 28.0 | 0.0 | 280 | 0.6 | 69.1 | 0.1 | 0.7 |
| Onion, M & S* | 1oz/28g | 46.0 | 1.0 | 165 | 1.0 | 32.1 | 3.0 | 1.1 |
| Onion, Sainsbury's* | 1 Serving/15g | 23.0 | 0.0 | 151 | 0.9 | 36.0 | 0.4 | 0.7 |
| Onion, Sweet, Heinz* | 1 Tbsp/38g | 38.0 | 0.0 | 102 | 1.0 | 23.5 | 0.4 | 0.6 |
| Onion & Garlic, Spicy, Waitrose* | 1 Tbsp/15g | 35.0 | 0.0 | 232 | 0.8 | 54.2 | 1.1 | 1.7 |
| Sweet Onion, Branston* | 1 Serving/10g | 14.0 | 0.0 | 145 | 1.0 | 34.2 | 0.4 | 0.6 |
| Sweetcorn, American Style, Maryland, Tesco* | 1 Serving/15g | 15.0 | 0.0 | 101 | 1.1 | 23.9 | 0.1 | 0.9 |
| Sweetcorn, Bick's* | 1 Tbsp/22g | 23.0 | 0.0 | 103 | 1.3 | 24.3 | 0.2 | 0.0 |
| Tomato, M & S* | 1oz/28g | 36.0 | 0.0 | 130 | 1.8 | 30.2 | 0.3 | 1.5 |
| Tomato, Sweet, Heinz* | 1 Serving/25g | 34.0 | 0.0 | 136 | 0.9 | 32.6 | 0.2 | 0.9 |

R

| | Measure INFO/WEIGHT | per Measure KCAL | per Measure FAT | Nutrition Values per 100g / 100ml KCAL | PROT | CARB | FAT | FIBRE |
|---|---|---|---|---|---|---|---|---|
| **RELISH** | | | | | | | | |
| Tomato & Chilli Texan Style, Tesco* | 1 Tbsp/14g | 20.0 | 0.0 | 140 | 1.7 | 32.0 | 0.1 | 1.1 |
| Tomato Spicy, Bick's* | 1 Serving/28g | 28.0 | 0.0 | 99 | 1.3 | 23.2 | 0.2 | 0.0 |
| **REVELS** | | | | | | | | |
| Mars* | 1 Packet/35g | 168.0 | 7.0 | 480 | 5.1 | 68.0 | 20.9 | 0.0 |
| **RHUBARB** | | | | | | | | |
| *Raw, Average* | *1 Stalk/51g* | *11.0* | *0.0* | *21* | *0.9* | *4.5* | *0.2* | *1.8* |
| *Stewed with Sugar, Average* | *1oz/28g* | *32.0* | *0.0* | *116* | *0.4* | *31.2* | *0.0* | *2.0* |
| **RIBENA*** | | | | | | | | |
| Apple Juice Drink, Ribena* | 1 Carton/287ml | 132.0 | 0.0 | 46 | 0.0 | 11.1 | 0.0 | 0.0 |
| Blackcurrant, Diluted with Water, Ribena* | 1 Serving/180ml | 81.0 | 0.0 | 45 | 0.0 | 11.0 | 0.0 | 0.0 |
| Blackcurrant, Really Light, No Added Sugar, Ribena* | 1 Carton/250ml | 7.0 | 0.0 | 3 | 0.0 | 0.7 | 0.0 | 0.0 |
| Blackcurrant & Cranberry, Ribena* | 1 Bottle/500ml | 205.0 | 0.0 | 41 | 0.0 | 9.9 | 0.0 | 0.0 |
| Blackcurrant Juice Drink, Ribena* | 1 Carton/288ml | 147.0 | 0.0 | 51 | 0.0 | 12.6 | 0.0 | 0.0 |
| Light, Ribena* | 1 Carton/288ml | 26.0 | 0.0 | 9 | 0.1 | 2.1 | 0.0 | 0.0 |
| Orange, Juice Drink, Ribena* | 1 Serving/288ml | 98.0 | 0.0 | 34 | 0.1 | 8.1 | 0.0 | 0.0 |
| Really Light, Undiluted, Ribena* | 1 Serving/25ml | 4.0 | 0.0 | 15 | 0.0 | 2.5 | 0.0 | 0.0 |
| Strawberry Juice Drink, Ribena* | 1 Carton/288ml | 138.0 | 0.0 | 48 | 0.0 | 11.8 | 0.0 | 0.0 |
| **RIBS** | | | | | | | | |
| Loin, BBQ, Sainsbury's* | 1 Rib/42g | 104.0 | 6.0 | 247 | 24.7 | 7.3 | 13.2 | 0.9 |
| Loin, Chinese, Sainsbury's* | 1 Rib/42g | 103.0 | 5.0 | 246 | 27.2 | 7.2 | 12.0 | 0.9 |
| Pork, Barbecue, Average | 1 Serving/100g | 275.0 | 18.0 | 275 | 21.4 | 7.2 | 17.9 | 0.3 |
| Pork, Chinese Style, Average | 1 Serving/300g | 736.0 | 45.0 | 245 | 17.9 | 10.0 | 14.9 | 0.7 |
| Pork, Full Rack, Sainsbury's* | 1 Serving/225g | 567.0 | 39.0 | 252 | 18.0 | 6.5 | 17.2 | 0.9 |
| Pork, Raw, Average | 1oz/28g | 47.0 | 3.0 | 169 | 18.6 | 1.8 | 9.9 | 0.2 |
| Spare, Chinese Style, Meal Solutions, Co-Op* | 1 Serving/165g | 214.0 | 15.0 | 130 | 8.0 | 4.0 | 9.0 | 0.2 |
| Spare, Chinese Style, Summer Eating, Asda* | 1 Serving/116g | 334.0 | 19.0 | 288 | 32.0 | 4.1 | 16.0 | 0.8 |
| Spare, Sweet, Sticky, Mini, M & S* | 1 Pack/300g | 615.0 | 34.0 | 205 | 16.6 | 8.6 | 11.5 | 0.2 |
| **RIBSTEAKS** | | | | | | | | |
| Smokey Barbecue Style, Dalepak* | 1 Serving/75g | 164.0 | 10.0 | 219 | 16.1 | 8.8 | 13.1 | 0.8 |
| **RICE** | | | | | | | | |
| *Arborio, Dry, Average* | *1 Serving/80g* | *279.0* | *1.0* | *348* | *7.1* | *78.3* | *0.8* | *0.8* |
| Basmati, & Wild, Cooked, Sainsbury's* | ½ Pack/125g | 150.0 | 1.0 | 120 | 3.1 | 25.7 | 0.6 | 1.3 |
| Basmati, & Wild, Dry Weight, Tilda* | 1 Serving/70g | 244.0 | 0.0 | 349 | 9.4 | 77.0 | 0.5 | 1.0 |
| Basmati, Boil in the Bag, Dry, Average | 1 Serving/50g | 176.0 | 0.0 | 352 | 8.4 | 77.8 | 0.8 | 0.4 |
| *Basmati, Brown, Dry, Average* | *1 Serving/50g* | *177.0* | *2.0* | *353* | *9.5* | *71.8* | *3.0* | *2.2* |
| *Basmati, Cooked, Average* | *1 Serving/140g* | *189.0* | *2.0* | *135* | *3.6* | *26.0* | *1.8* | *0.7* |
| *Basmati, Dry Weight, Average* | *1 Serving/60g* | *212.0* | *1.0* | *353* | *8.1* | *77.9* | *1.0* | *0.6* |
| *Basmati, Indian, Dry, Average* | *1 Serving/75g* | *260.0* | *1.0* | *346* | *8.4* | *76.1* | *0.9* | *0.1* |
| Basmati, Microwave, Cooked, Average | 1 Serving/125g | 182.0 | 2.0 | 145 | 2.7 | 30.0 | 1.8 | 0.0 |
| Basmati, Microwaveable, Tesco* | ½ Pack/125g | 212.0 | 2.0 | 170 | 4.0 | 34.1 | 1.8 | 0.5 |
| *Basmati, White, Dry, Average* | *1 Serving/75g* | *262.0* | *0.0* | *349* | *8.1* | *77.1* | *0.6* | *2.2* |
| Basmati, Wholegrain, Cooked, Tilda* | 1 Serving/60g | 68.0 | 1.0 | 113 | 3.3 | 23.0 | 0.9 | 3.2 |
| BBQ & Spicy, M & S* | 1 Pack/250g | 462.0 | 18.0 | 185 | 6.1 | 23.7 | 7.2 | 1.2 |
| Black, Artemide, Eat Well, M & S* | 1 Serving/75g | 251.0 | 2.0 | 335 | 8.5 | 73.3 | 2.6 | 4.0 |
| *Brown, Cooked, Average* | *1 Serving/140g* | *173.0* | *1.0* | *123* | *2.6* | *26.6* | *1.1* | *0.9* |
| *Brown, Dry, Average* | *1 Serving/75g* | *266.0* | *2.0* | *355* | *7.5* | *76.2* | *3.0* | *1.4* |
| *Brown, Long Grain, Dry, Average* | *1 Serving/50g* | *182.0* | *1.0* | *363* | *7.6* | *76.8* | *2.8* | *2.0* |
| *Brown, Short Grain, Dry, Average* | *1 Serving/50g* | *175.0* | *1.0* | *351* | *6.8* | *77.6* | *2.8* | *0.9* |
| *Brown, Whole Grain, Cooked, Average* | *1 Serving/170g* | *223.0* | *2.0* | *131* | *2.6* | *27.8* | *1.1* | *1.2* |
| *Brown, Whole Grain, Dry, Average* | *1 Serving/40g* | *138.0* | *1.0* | *344* | *7.4* | *71.6* | *2.9* | *3.0* |
| Chicken, Savoury, Batchelors* | 1 Pack/124g | 455.0 | 2.0 | 367 | 8.9 | 79.4 | 1.5 | 2.6 |
| Chicken, Savoury, SmartPrice, Asda* | ½ Pack/168g | 210.0 | 2.0 | 125 | 3.2 | 26.0 | 0.9 | 2.4 |
| Chicken, Savoury, Tesco* | 1 Serving/87g | 177.0 | 2.0 | 204 | 6.4 | 39.4 | 2.2 | 6.7 |

## RICE

| | Measure INFO/WEIGHT | per Measure KCAL | FAT | Nutrition Values per 100g / 100ml KCAL | PROT | CARB | FAT | FIBRE |
|---|---|---|---|---|---|---|---|---|
| Chicken & Sweetcorn, Savoury, Asda* | ½ Pack/60g | 195.0 | 2.0 | 325 | 10.0 | 65.0 | 2.8 | 10.0 |
| Chinese Savoury, Batchelors* | 1 Serving/50g | 177.0 | 1.0 | 354 | 9.9 | 73.1 | 2.4 | 2.8 |
| Chinese Style, Express, Uncle Ben's* | 1 Pack/250g | 392.0 | 5.0 | 157 | 3.4 | 30.9 | 2.2 | 0.4 |
| Coconut, M & S* | ½ Pack/124g | 217.0 | 5.0 | 175 | 3.1 | 31.8 | 4.0 | 0.3 |
| Coconut, Thai, Sainsbury's* | ½ Pack/100g | 178.0 | 9.0 | 178 | 2.6 | 21.3 | 9.1 | 1.9 |
| Coconut & Lime, Asda* | 1 Pack/360g | 695.0 | 18.0 | 193 | 4.5 | 32.7 | 4.9 | 0.9 |
| Coriander & Herb, Packet, Cooked, Sainsbury's* | ¼ Pack/150g | 204.0 | 1.0 | 136 | 2.5 | 30.4 | 0.5 | 1.5 |
| Coriander & Herbs, Batchelors* | 1/3 Pack/76g | 280.0 | 3.0 | 369 | 7.9 | 79.6 | 3.5 | 5.0 |
| Curry, Savoury, Somerfield* | ½ Pack/160g | 194.0 | 1.0 | 121 | 2.2 | 26.0 | 0.9 | 1.3 |
| Egg, Fried, 2 Minute Meals, Sainsbury's* | 1 Pack/250g | 342.0 | 1.0 | 137 | 3.8 | 29.2 | 0.6 | 0.8 |
| Egg Fried, Average | 1 Serving/300g | 624.0 | 32.0 | 208 | 4.2 | 25.7 | 10.6 | 0.4 |
| Egg Fried, Chinese Style, Tesco* | 1 Portion/250g | 417.0 | 10.0 | 167 | 4.4 | 27.9 | 4.2 | 0.7 |
| Egg Fried, Express, Uncle Ben's* | ½ Pack/125g | 216.0 | 5.0 | 173 | 4.0 | 29.9 | 4.2 | 0.3 |
| Egg Fried, M & S* | ½ Pack/150g | 315.0 | 10.0 | 210 | 4.2 | 32.4 | 7.0 | 0.3 |
| Egg Fried, Micro, Tesco* | 1 Pack/250g | 312.0 | 9.0 | 125 | 4.6 | 18.3 | 3.7 | 6.4 |
| Egg Fried, Sainsbury's* | 1 Pack/250g | 432.0 | 9.0 | 173 | 4.5 | 30.3 | 3.8 | 0.8 |
| Fried, Duck, Chicken & Pork Celebration, Sainsbury's* | 1 Pack/450g | 544.0 | 16.0 | 121 | 7.9 | 14.2 | 3.6 | 1.5 |
| Garlic & Butter Flavoured, Batchelors* | 1 Serving/50g | 175.0 | 1.0 | 350 | 8.0 | 79.8 | 2.8 | 5.0 |
| Garlic & Coriander Flavoured, Patak's* | 1 Serving/125g | 186.0 | 3.0 | 149 | 2.6 | 28.9 | 2.2 | 0.0 |
| Golden Savoury, Dry Weight, Batchelors* | 1 Pack/120g | 437.0 | 3.0 | 364 | 10.1 | 74.7 | 2.8 | 2.4 |
| Golden Vegetable, Freshly Frozen, Asda* | 1 Sachet/200g | 238.0 | 3.0 | 119 | 3.2 | 23.6 | 1.3 | 1.3 |
| Golden Vegetable, Savoury, Morrisons* | 1 Serving/50g | 70.0 | 0.0 | 141 | 3.4 | 30.1 | 0.8 | 1.1 |
| Golden Vegetable, Savoury, Sainsbury's* | ¼ Pack/100g | 122.0 | 1.0 | 122 | 2.9 | 25.4 | 1.0 | 0.3 |
| *Long Grain, & Wild, Dry, Average* | *1 Serving/75g* | *254.0* | *1.0* | *338* | *7.6* | *72.6* | *2.0* | *1.7* |
| *Long Grain, American, Cooked, Average* | *1 Serving/160g* | *229.0* | *3.0* | *143* | *3.0* | *28.7* | *1.7* | *0.2* |
| *Long Grain, American, Dry, Average* | *1 Serving/50g* | *175.0* | *1.0* | *350* | *7.1* | *77.8* | *1.1* | *0.6* |
| *Long Grain, Dry, Average* | *1 Serving/50g* | *169.0* | *0.0* | *337* | *7.4* | *75.5* | *1.0* | *1.7* |
| Long Grain, Microwavable, Cooked, Average | 1 Serving/150g | 180.0 | 1.0 | 120 | 2.7 | 25.8 | 0.6 | 0.7 |
| Mexican Style, Cooked, Express, Uncle Ben's* | 1 Pack/250g | 385.0 | 5.0 | 154 | 3.2 | 31.1 | 1.9 | 0.7 |
| Mexican Style, Old El Paso* | 1 Serving/75g | 268.0 | 1.0 | 357 | 9.0 | 78.0 | 1.0 | 0.0 |
| Mild Curry, Cooked, Tesco* | 1 Serving/154g | 217.0 | 2.0 | 141 | 3.1 | 29.7 | 1.1 | 2.1 |
| Mixed Vegetable, Savoury, Dry Weight, Tesco* | 1 Pack/120g | 450.0 | 3.0 | 375 | 7.8 | 79.1 | 2.7 | 2.9 |
| Mushroom, Savoury, Somerfield* | ½ Pack/160g | 144.0 | 1.0 | 90 | 2.1 | 18.8 | 0.7 | 1.5 |
| Mushroom & Coconut, Organic, Waitrose* | 1 Pack/300g | 474.0 | 15.0 | 158 | 3.7 | 24.5 | 5.0 | 1.4 |
| Mushroom & Pepper, Savoury, Cooked, Morrisons* | 1 Serving/200g | 204.0 | 2.0 | 102 | 2.3 | 21.5 | 0.8 | 0.0 |
| Mushroom Pilau, Bombay Brasserie, Sainsbury's* | 1 Pack/400g | 672.0 | 17.0 | 168 | 3.7 | 28.6 | 4.3 | 0.7 |
| Mushroom Savoury, Batchelors* | ½ Pack/61g | 217.0 | 1.0 | 356 | 10.7 | 73.6 | 2.1 | 2.8 |
| Mushroom Savoury, Bettabuy, Morrisons* | 1 Serving/128g | 131.0 | 1.0 | 102 | 2.3 | 21.5 | 0.8 | 0.0 |
| Paella, Savoury, Tesco* | 1 Serving/60g | 220.0 | 3.0 | 367 | 8.4 | 72.7 | 4.7 | 4.5 |
| *Pilau, Cooked, Average* | *1 Serving/140g* | *244.0* | *6.0* | *174* | *3.5* | *30.3* | *4.4* | *0.8* |
| *Pilau, Dry, Average* | *1oz/28g* | *101.0* | *1.0* | *361* | *8.4* | *78.2* | *2.3* | *3.4* |
| Pilau, Indian Mushroom, Sainsbury's* | 1 Serving/100g | 119.0 | 2.0 | 119 | 3.0 | 21.3 | 2.4 | 1.9 |
| Pilau, Mushroom, Sainsbury's* | 1 Pack/250g | 400.0 | 14.0 | 160 | 3.4 | 24.1 | 5.5 | 2.4 |
| Pilau, Spinach, Bombay Brasserie, Sainsbury's* | 1 Pack/401g | 642.0 | 17.0 | 160 | 3.5 | 26.9 | 4.3 | 0.8 |
| Pilau, Spinach & Carrot, Waitrose* | 1 Pack/350g | 465.0 | 8.0 | 133 | 3.1 | 24.8 | 2.4 | 1.2 |
| Pudding, Dry Weight, Average | 1 Serving/100g | 355.0 | 1.0 | 355 | 6.9 | 82.0 | 1.1 | 0.3 |
| *Risotto, Dry, Average* | *1 Serving/50g* | *174.0* | *1.0* | *348* | *7.8* | *76.2* | *1.3* | *2.4* |
| *Saffron, Cooked, Average* | *1 Serving/150g* | *208.0* | *5.0* | *139* | *2.5* | *25.3* | *3.1* | *0.5* |
| Spanish Style Savoury, Safeway* | 1 Pack/394g | 449.0 | 4.0 | 114 | 2.7 | 23.7 | 0.9 | 1.4 |
| Special Fried, Asda* | 1oz/28g | 42.0 | 1.0 | 149 | 5.4 | 21.0 | 4.9 | 1.5 |
| Special Fried, M & S* | 1 Pack/450g | 922.0 | 35.0 | 205 | 6.2 | 27.2 | 7.8 | 0.5 |
| Special Fried, Sainsbury's* | 1 Serving/166g | 272.0 | 8.0 | 164 | 5.1 | 25.5 | 4.6 | 0.7 |
| Spicy Mexican Style, Savoury, Made Up, Tesco* | 1 Serving/164g | 213.0 | 3.0 | 130 | 2.9 | 26.3 | 1.5 | 2.4 |

R

| | Measure INFO/WEIGHT | KCAL | FAT | KCAL | PROT | CARB | FAT | FIBRE |
|---|---|---|---|---|---|---|---|---|
| **RICE** | | | | | | | | |
| Sticky Thai, Safeway* | 1 Pack/200g | 260.0 | 4.0 | 130 | 2.5 | 25.6 | 1.8 | 1.4 |
| Stir Fry, Oriental Style, Oriental Express* | 1 Serving/150g | 216.0 | 5.0 | 144 | 4.2 | 24.1 | 3.4 | 1.9 |
| Sweet & Sour, Rice Bowl, Uncle Ben's* | 1 Pack/350g | 364.0 | 2.0 | 104 | 5.2 | 19.5 | 0.6 | 0.0 |
| Sweet & Sour, Savoury, Batchelors* | 1 Serving/135g | 418.0 | 3.0 | 310 | 9.4 | 75.6 | 2.1 | 3.1 |
| Sweet & Sour Savoury, Cooked, Asda* | ½ Pack/126g | 154.0 | 1.0 | 122 | 2.5 | 26.0 | 0.9 | 3.0 |
| Sweet & Spicy, Express, Uncle Ben's* | 1 Pack/250g | 417.0 | 10.0 | 167 | 2.7 | 30.1 | 4.0 | 0.0 |
| Tandoori, Savoury, Batchelors* | 1 Serving/120g | 430.0 | 3.0 | 358 | 10.3 | 73.5 | 2.5 | 3.0 |
| **Thai, Cooked, Average** | **1 Serving/100g** | **135.0** | **2.0** | **135** | **2.5** | **27.4** | **1.7** | **0.3** |
| **Thai, Dry, Average** | **1 Serving/50g** | **174.0** | **0.0** | **348** | **7.1** | **78.9** | **0.4** | **0.9** |
| **Thai, Fragrant, Dry, Average** | **1 Serving/75g** | **272.0** | **1.0** | **363** | **7.2** | **82.0** | **0.7** | **0.3** |
| Thai Sticky, Tesco* | 1 Serving/250g | 357.0 | 6.0 | 143 | 2.5 | 27.6 | 2.5 | 0.4 |
| Thai Style Lemon Chicken, Made Up, Tesco* | ½ Pack/138g | 192.0 | 2.0 | 139 | 3.4 | 27.5 | 1.7 | 2.1 |
| **White, Cooked, Average** | **1 Serving/140g** | **182.0** | **1.0** | **130** | **2.6** | **28.7** | **0.8** | **0.1** |
| **White, Cooked, Frozen, Average** | **1 Serving/150g** | **168.0** | **1.0** | **112** | **2.9** | **23.8** | **0.5** | **1.1** |
| **White, Flaked, Dry Weight, Average** | **1oz/28g** | **97.0** | **0.0** | **346** | **6.6** | **77.5** | **1.2** | **0.0** |
| White, Fried | 1oz/28g | 37.0 | 1.0 | 131 | 2.2 | 25.0 | 3.2 | 0.6 |
| **White, Long Grain, Dry Weight, Average** | **1 Serving/50g** | **181.0** | **1.0** | **362** | **7.1** | **79.1** | **1.9** | **0.4** |
| White, Microwave, Cooked, Average | 1 Serving/150g | 157.0 | 1.0 | 105 | 2.7 | 22.4 | 0.5 | 1.1 |
| **Whole Grain, Dry, Average** | **1 Serving/50g** | **171.0** | **1.0** | **341** | **8.2** | **72.0** | **2.3** | **4.0** |
| Wild, Coronation, Sainsbury's* | ¼ Pot/75g | 139.0 | 5.0 | 186 | 3.1 | 29.1 | 6.4 | 0.9 |
| Wild, Giant Canadian, Dry Weight, Tilda* | 1 Serving/75g | 262.0 | 1.0 | 350 | 11.5 | 74.2 | 0.8 | 1.9 |
| with Brocolli, Sweetcorn & Peas, SteamFresh, Birds Eye* | 1 Bag/170g | 192.0 | 6.0 | 113 | 3.5 | 17.3 | 3.3 | 2.1 |
| with Red Kidney Beans, Average | 1oz/28g | 49.0 | 1.0 | 175 | 5.6 | 32.4 | 3.5 | 2.5 |
| Yellow, Ready Cooked, Tesco* | 1oz/28g | 32.0 | 0.0 | 113 | 2.7 | 27.1 | 1.3 | 0.1 |
| **RICE BITES** | | | | | | | | |
| Cheese & Onion Flavour, Asda* | 1 Pack/30g | 137.0 | 5.0 | 456 | 7.0 | 71.0 | 16.0 | 0.2 |
| **RICE BOWL** | | | | | | | | |
| Beef with Black Bean Sauce, Uncle Ben's* | 1 Pack/350g | 367.0 | 5.0 | 105 | 5.6 | 17.4 | 1.4 | 0.0 |
| Chicken Tikka Masala, Uncle Ben's* | 1 Pack/350g | 381.0 | 8.0 | 109 | 5.9 | 15.9 | 2.4 | 0.0 |
| Free From, Sainsbury's* | 1 Serving/182g | 146.0 | 1.0 | 80 | 1.6 | 17.1 | 0.6 | 1.4 |
| Honey BBQ Chicken, Uncle Ben's* | 1 Pack/350g | 420.0 | 2.0 | 120 | 5.4 | 23.1 | 0.6 | 0.0 |
| Sweet 'n' Sour, Sharwood's* | 1 Bowl/350g | 437.0 | 12.0 | 125 | 4.8 | 18.6 | 3.5 | 0.8 |
| Thai Green, Sharwood's* | 1 Bowl/350g | 549.0 | 27.0 | 157 | 4.8 | 17.3 | 7.6 | 0.9 |
| Thai Red, Sharwood's* | 1 Bowl/350g | 486.0 | 19.0 | 139 | 4.7 | 18.1 | 5.3 | 1.0 |
| **RICE CAKES** | | | | | | | | |
| Apple & Cinnamon Flavour, Kallo* | 1 Cake/11g | 41.0 | 0.0 | 376 | 6.2 | 83.1 | 2.2 | 3.9 |
| Asda* | 1 Cake/8g | 31.0 | 0.0 | 386 | 8.7 | 81.1 | 3.0 | 2.8 |
| Bacon, Asda* | 1 Cake/9g | 42.0 | 2.0 | 462 | 8.0 | 67.0 | 18.0 | 0.0 |
| Barbeque, Tesco* | 1 Cake/9g | 28.0 | 0.0 | 328 | 9.6 | 66.8 | 2.5 | 6.2 |
| Black & White Sesame, Clearspring* | 1 Cake/8g | 31.0 | 0.0 | 385 | 7.4 | 82.2 | 2.9 | 0.0 |
| Caramel, Jumbo, Tesco* | 1 Cake/10g | 34.0 | 0.0 | 340 | 7.0 | 74.0 | 3.0 | 5.0 |
| Caramel, Less Than 3% Fat, Sainsbury's* | 1 Pack/35g | 134.0 | 1.0 | 382 | 5.6 | 86.4 | 1.6 | 1.8 |
| Caramel, Snack Size, Tesco* | 1 Pack/35g | 133.0 | 1.0 | 379 | 5.5 | 82.7 | 2.9 | 0.9 |
| Caramel, Tesco* | 1 Serving/2g | 9.0 | 0.0 | 379 | 5.5 | 98.2 | 2.9 | 0.9 |
| Caramel Flavour, Kallo* | 1 Cake/10g | 38.0 | 0.0 | 383 | 6.2 | 78.9 | 4.8 | 3.9 |
| Chocolate, Fabulous Bakin' Boys* | 1 Biscuit/17g | 83.0 | 4.0 | 490 | 6.4 | 66.7 | 22.0 | 1.6 |
| Co-Op* | 1 Cake/20g | 80.0 | 1.0 | 402 | 8.0 | 84.0 | 3.1 | 0.0 |
| Dark Chocolate, Organic, Kallo* | 1 Cake/12g | 57.0 | 3.0 | 471 | 6.8 | 57.2 | 24.1 | 7.4 |
| Five Grain, Finncrisp* | 1 Cake/10g | 36.0 | 0.0 | 356 | 9.8 | 73.9 | 1.7 | 9.7 |
| High Fibre, Oat & Rice, Slightly Salted, Thick Slice, Kallo* | 1 Cake/8g | 27.0 | 0.0 | 356 | 10.6 | 75.0 | 5.5 | 9.0 |
| Honey, Kallo* | 1 Cake/10g | 40.0 | 0.0 | 388 | 5.4 | 86.6 | 2.2 | 1.6 |
| Japanese, Black Sesame, Clearspring* | 1 Cake/8g | 29.0 | 0.0 | 385 | 7.4 | 82.2 | 2.9 | 0.0 |
| Lightly Salted, Perfectly Balanced, Waitrose* | 1 Cake/8g | 31.0 | 0.0 | 387 | 8.3 | 82.4 | 2.7 | 2.1 |

R

| | Measure INFO/WEIGHT | KCAL | FAT | KCAL | PROT | CARB | FAT | FIBRE |
|---|---|---|---|---|---|---|---|---|
| | | per Measure | | Nutrition Values per 100g / 100ml | | | | |

## RICE CAKES

| | Measure INFO/WEIGHT | per Measure KCAL | FAT | KCAL | PROT | CARB | FAT | FIBRE |
|---|---|---|---|---|---|---|---|---|
| Lightly Salted, Thick Slice, Low Fat, Kallo* | 1 Cake/8g | 28.0 | 0.0 | 372 | 8.0 | 78.7 | 2.8 | 5.1 |
| Milk Chocolate, Organic, Kallo* | 1 Rice Cake/11g | 57.0 | 3.0 | 509 | 6.5 | 56.2 | 28.7 | 3.5 |
| Multigrain, Ryvita* | 3 Cakes/11g | 43.0 | 1.0 | 384 | 9.1 | 76.2 | 4.7 | 5.3 |
| Organic, Tesco* | 1 Cake/8g | 29.0 | 0.0 | 380 | 7.2 | 80.7 | 2.9 | 3.4 |
| Plain, Finger Foods, Organic, Organix* | 3 Cakes/6g | 22.0 | 0.0 | 370 | 6.5 | 82.9 | 1.4 | 3.2 |
| Rice Crunchies, Safeway* | 1 Small Pack/25g | 94.0 | 0.0 | 378 | 7.4 | 84.2 | 1.3 | 1.5 |
| Salt & Vinegar, Jumbo, Tesco* | 1 Cake/9g | 31.0 | 0.0 | 347 | 8.4 | 72.7 | 2.5 | 6.0 |
| Salt & Vinegar, Sainsbury's* | 1 Pack/30g | 121.0 | 2.0 | 403 | 8.3 | 73.3 | 8.3 | 2.7 |
| Salt & Vinegar, Snack, Tesco* | 1 Pack/35g | 116.0 | 1.0 | 332 | 7.5 | 71.5 | 1.8 | 1.1 |
| Savoury, Jumbo, HL, Tesco* | 1 Cake/8g | 31.0 | 0.0 | 369 | 11.9 | 75.0 | 2.4 | 3.6 |
| Sesame, No Added Salt, Thick Sliced, Organic, Kallo* | 1 Cake/10g | 37.0 | 0.0 | 373 | 8.0 | 78.0 | 3.2 | 5.4 |
| Sesame, Slightly Salted, Thick Slice, Organic, Kallo* | 1 Cake/8g | 28.0 | 0.0 | 373 | 8.0 | 78.0 | 3.2 | 5.4 |
| Sesame Garlic, Clearspring* | 1 Serving/8g | 29.0 | 0.0 | 382 | 7.8 | 82.3 | 2.4 | 0.0 |
| Sesame Teriyaki, Clearspring* | 1 Cake/7g | 28.0 | 0.0 | 377 | 6.5 | 82.8 | 2.2 | 0.0 |
| Slightly Salted, with Cracked Pepper, Snack Size, Kallo* | 1 Cake/2g | 8.0 | 0.0 | 372 | 8.0 | 78.7 | 2.8 | 5.1 |
| Sour Cream & Chive Flavour, Sainsbury's* | 1 Pack/30g | 119.0 | 3.0 | 396 | 7.9 | 72.0 | 8.5 | 2.9 |
| Toasted Sesame, Ryvita* | 1 Pack/11g | 43.0 | 1.0 | 391 | 8.4 | 78.4 | 4.9 | 3.5 |
| Whole Grain, No Added Salt, Thick Slice, Organic, Kallo* | 1 Cake/9g | 33.0 | 0.0 | 365 | 7.6 | 80.0 | 3.1 | 3.4 |
| Wholegrain, No Added Salt, BGTY, Sainsbury's* | 1 Cake/8g | 30.0 | 0.0 | 372 | 8.0 | 78.7 | 2.8 | 5.1 |
| Wholegrain, Salt & Vinegar, Tesco* | 1 Cake/9g | 28.0 | 0.0 | 314 | 8.4 | 61.9 | 2.6 | 6.0 |

## RICE CRACKERS

| | Measure INFO/WEIGHT | per Measure KCAL | FAT | KCAL | PROT | CARB | FAT | FIBRE |
|---|---|---|---|---|---|---|---|---|
| Barbecue, Sakata* | ½ Pack/50g | 203.0 | 1.0 | 407 | 7.3 | 85.2 | 2.6 | 1.6 |
| Barbecue Flavour, Tesco* | 1 Pack/25g | 102.0 | 2.0 | 409 | 6.7 | 78.8 | 7.4 | 1.7 |
| Brown, Wakama* | 1 Cracker/5g | 19.0 | 0.0 | 375 | 8.0 | 84.8 | 0.4 | 0.0 |
| Cheese, Tesco* | 1 Serving/25g | 104.0 | 2.0 | 416 | 7.9 | 78.1 | 8.0 | 1.8 |
| Chilli, Temptations, Tesco* | 1 Serving/25g | 128.0 | 7.0 | 512 | 4.4 | 58.0 | 28.8 | 0.0 |
| Cracked Pepper, Sakata* | ½ Pack/50g | 200.0 | 1.0 | 400 | 7.3 | 84.4 | 3.0 | 2.0 |
| Crispy, Chilli & Lime, Go Ahead, McVitie's* | 1 Serving/25g | 101.0 | 1.0 | 405 | 7.1 | 83.6 | 3.6 | 2.1 |
| Crispy, Sea Salt & Vinegar, Go Ahead, McVitie's* | 1 Serving/25g | 102.0 | 1.0 | 408 | 6.6 | 80.6 | 5.4 | 1.8 |
| Crispy, Sour Cream & Herbs, Go Ahead, McVitie's* | 1 Serving/25g | 105.0 | 2.0 | 422 | 7.1 | 78.2 | 8.0 | 1.8 |
| Japanese, Apollo* | 1 Pack/75g | 297.0 | 4.0 | 396 | 9.6 | 78.8 | 4.7 | 0.9 |
| Japanese, Julian Graves* | 1 Serving/25g | 92.0 | 0.0 | 369 | 8.8 | 79.5 | 1.7 | 3.8 |
| Japanese, Mini, Sunrise* | 1 Serving/50g | 180.0 | 0.0 | 360 | 7.0 | 83.0 | 0.0 | 7.0 |
| Japanese Style, Tesco* | 1 Serving/25g | 101.0 | 2.0 | 405 | 11.7 | 75.2 | 6.1 | 3.3 |
| Korean Chilli, Graze* | 1 Box/26g | 135.0 | 7.0 | 519 | 5.0 | 64.0 | 27.0 | 0.0 |
| Mix, M & S* | ½ Pack/63g | 225.0 | 0.0 | 360 | 6.5 | 82.9 | 0.1 | 1.6 |
| Sainsbury's* | 1 Serving/20g | 87.0 | 2.0 | 433 | 11.2 | 74.3 | 9.4 | 1.0 |
| Salt & Pepper, Asda* | 1 Cracker/5g | 19.0 | 0.0 | 385 | 7.0 | 87.0 | 1.0 | 2.2 |
| Salt & Vinegar, Namchow* | 1 Serving/38g | 139.0 | 1.0 | 370 | 6.7 | 77.5 | 3.7 | 0.0 |
| Sour Cream & Chive, Sakata* | 1 Serving/25g | 107.0 | 2.0 | 430 | 7.8 | 80.6 | 7.9 | 0.0 |
| Spicy Mix, Asda* | 1 Serving/25g | 115.0 | 4.0 | 461 | 6.4 | 71.2 | 16.7 | 0.2 |
| Thai, M & S* | 1 Serving/55g | 209.0 | 2.0 | 380 | 7.0 | 80.2 | 3.3 | 1.2 |
| Thai, Sesame & Soy Sauce, M & S* | 1 Pack/55g | 210.0 | 3.0 | 385 | 7.6 | 77.8 | 4.8 | 1.4 |
| Thai Chilli, Nature's Harvest* | 1 Pack/75g | 401.0 | 22.0 | 535 | 4.6 | 61.5 | 29.7 | 4.2 |
| Thin, Blue Dragon* | 3 Crackers/5g | 20.0 | 0.0 | 395 | 6.1 | 84.4 | 3.7 | 0.0 |

## RICE MILK

| | Measure INFO/WEIGHT | per Measure KCAL | FAT | KCAL | PROT | CARB | FAT | FIBRE |
|---|---|---|---|---|---|---|---|---|
| Organic, Provamel* | 1 Serving/250ml | 122.0 | 4.0 | 49 | 0.1 | 9.5 | 1.5 | 0.0 |
| Original, Rice Dream* | 1 Serving/150ml | 70.0 | 1.0 | 47 | 0.1 | 9.4 | 1.0 | 0.1 |

## RICE PUDDING

| | Measure INFO/WEIGHT | per Measure KCAL | FAT | KCAL | PROT | CARB | FAT | FIBRE |
|---|---|---|---|---|---|---|---|---|
| & Conserve, M & S* | 1oz/28g | 53.0 | 3.0 | 190 | 2.3 | 17.4 | 12.5 | 0.3 |
| 50% Less Fat, Asda* | ½ Can/212g | 180.0 | 2.0 | 85 | 3.3 | 16.2 | 0.8 | 0.2 |
| Apple, Mullerrice, Muller* | 1 Pot/200g | 224.0 | 4.0 | 112 | 3.2 | 19.8 | 2.2 | 0.4 |
| Banana, Ambrosia* | 1 Pot/150g | 153.0 | 4.0 | 102 | 3.2 | 16.6 | 2.5 | 0.0 |

R

| | Measure INFO/WEIGHT | per Measure | | Nutrition Values per 100g / 100ml | | | | |
|---|---|---|---|---|---|---|---|---|
| | | KCAL | FAT | KCAL | PROT | CARB | FAT | FIBRE |

## RICE PUDDING

| | | | | | | | | |
|---|---|---|---|---|---|---|---|---|
| Canned, Average | 1oz/28g | 25.0 | 1.0 | 89 | 3.4 | 14.0 | 2.5 | 0.2 |
| Canned, Basics, Sainsbury's* | ½ Can/213g | 176.0 | 2.0 | 83 | 3.1 | 15.5 | 0.9 | 0.1 |
| Canned, BGTY, Sainsbury's* | 1 Can/425g | 348.0 | 3.0 | 82 | 3.1 | 15.7 | 0.8 | 0.1 |
| Caramel, Ambrosia* | 1 Pot/150g | 149.0 | 4.0 | 99 | 3.1 | 16.1 | 2.5 | 0.0 |
| Clotted Cream, Cornish, Waitrose* | 1 Serving/150g | 304.0 | 20.0 | 203 | 3.0 | 17.6 | 13.4 | 0.5 |
| Clotted Cream, M & S* | 1 Pudding/185g | 431.0 | 31.0 | 233 | 3.0 | 19.2 | 16.6 | 0.2 |
| Co-Op* | 1oz/28g | 49.0 | 3.0 | 175 | 5.0 | 20.0 | 9.0 | 2.0 |
| COU, M & S* | 1 Pot/171g | 145.0 | 3.0 | 85 | 2.4 | 15.5 | 1.7 | 0.5 |
| Creamed, Asda* | 1 Serving/215g | 196.0 | 3.0 | 91 | 3.2 | 16.0 | 1.6 | 0.0 |
| Creamed, Canned, Ambrosia* | 1 Can/425g | 382.0 | 8.0 | 90 | 3.1 | 15.2 | 1.9 | 0.0 |
| Creamed, Canned, Sainsbury's* | ½ Can/212g | 195.0 | 3.0 | 92 | 3.1 | 16.2 | 1.6 | 0.1 |
| Creamed, HL, Tesco* | 1 Can/425g | 340.0 | 3.0 | 80 | 3.0 | 15.1 | 0.6 | 0.2 |
| Creamed, Low Fat, Ambrosia* | 1 Serving/150g | 129.0 | 1.0 | 86 | 3.3 | 16.1 | 0.9 | 0.0 |
| Creamed, Luxury, with Added Cream, Canned, Sainsbury's* | ½ Can/213g | 272.0 | 12.0 | 128 | 3.3 | 15.9 | 5.7 | 0.0 |
| Creamed, Value, Tesco* | 1 Can/425g | 361.0 | 3.0 | 85 | 3.1 | 16.0 | 0.8 | 0.1 |
| Creamed, Weight Watchers* | 1 Pot/130g | 108.0 | 1.0 | 83 | 3.2 | 16.0 | 0.7 | 0.3 |
| Creamed with Sultanas & Nutmeg, Ambrosia* | ½ Can/200g | 210.0 | 6.0 | 105 | 3.2 | 16.6 | 2.9 | 0.1 |
| Creamy, Delicious, Taste of Home, Heinz* | ½ Can/212g | 225.0 | 4.0 | 106 | 3.4 | 18.6 | 1.9 | 0.2 |
| Creamy Rice, Shape, Danone* | 1 Serving/175g | 149.0 | 2.0 | 85 | 3.5 | 15.4 | 1.0 | 0.4 |
| Creamy Rice with Tropical Crunch, Ambrosia* | 1 Pack/210g | 307.0 | 9.0 | 146 | 3.6 | 23.4 | 4.2 | 0.6 |
| Creamy with Strawberry Crunch, Ambrosia* | 1 Pack/205g | 297.0 | 9.0 | 145 | 3.9 | 23.0 | 4.2 | 0.7 |
| GFY, Asda* | 1 Pudding/119g | 115.0 | 2.0 | 97 | 4.2 | 17.0 | 1.4 | 0.5 |
| Libby's* | 1 Serving/200g | 180.0 | 3.0 | 90 | 3.3 | 16.2 | 1.6 | 0.2 |
| Light, Creamy, Delicious, Taste of Home, Heinz* | ½ Can/213g | 194.0 | 1.0 | 91 | 3.4 | 18.0 | 0.6 | 0.2 |
| Low Fat, Ambrosia* | ½ Can/212g | 176.0 | 2.0 | 83 | 3.2 | 15.7 | 0.8 | 0.0 |
| Low Fat, Co-Op* | 1 Sm Can/170g | 144.0 | 1.0 | 85 | 3.0 | 16.0 | 0.8 | 0.0 |
| Low Fat, Good Intentions, Somerfield* | ½ Can/212g | 164.0 | 1.0 | 77 | 3.0 | 15.1 | 0.6 | 0.2 |
| Low Fat, No Added Sugar, Canned, Weight Watchers* | ½ Can/212g | 155.0 | 3.0 | 73 | 3.7 | 11.4 | 1.5 | 0.0 |
| Organic, Ambrosia* | 1 Can/425g | 455.0 | 16.0 | 107 | 3.4 | 15.1 | 3.7 | 0.0 |
| Organic, Co-Op* | 1 Can/425g | 446.0 | 13.0 | 105 | 3.0 | 16.0 | 3.0 | 0.2 |
| Organic, Evernat* | 1oz/28g | 39.0 | 1.0 | 141 | 5.5 | 22.9 | 3.0 | 0.0 |
| Original, Muller Rice, Muller* | 1 Pot/200g | 212.0 | 5.0 | 106 | 3.7 | 16.9 | 2.6 | 0.3 |
| Perfectly Balanced, Waitrose* | 1 Serving/154g | 140.0 | 2.0 | 91 | 3.4 | 15.7 | 1.6 | 1.2 |
| Raspberry, BGTY, Sainsbury's* | 1 Pot/135g | 126.0 | 2.0 | 93 | 3.2 | 17.2 | 1.2 | 1.3 |
| Raspberry, Muller Rice, Muller* | 1 Std Pot/200g | 218.0 | 4.0 | 109 | 3.2 | 19.1 | 2.2 | 0.6 |
| Rhubarb, Muller* | 1 Pot/200g | 226.0 | 4.0 | 113 | 3.2 | 20.0 | 2.2 | 0.0 |
| Strawberry, Muller Rice, Muller* | 1 Pot/200g | 220.0 | 4.0 | 110 | 3.2 | 19.3 | 2.2 | 0.4 |
| Thick & Creamy, Co-Op* | 1 Can/425g | 531.0 | 25.0 | 125 | 3.0 | 16.0 | 6.0 | 0.0 |
| Thick & Creamy, Nestle* | 1 Can/425g | 527.0 | 24.0 | 124 | 3.1 | 15.4 | 5.6 | 0.2 |
| Vanilla Custard, Muller Rice, Muller* | 1 Pot/200g | 230.0 | 5.0 | 115 | 3.4 | 19.8 | 2.5 | 0.3 |

## RICE SALAD

| | | | | | | | | |
|---|---|---|---|---|---|---|---|---|
| Chicken Tikka, COU, M & S* | 1 Pack/390g | 409.0 | 4.0 | 105 | 5.1 | 18.7 | 1.0 | 0.6 |
| Hot Smoked Salmon, Deli Meal, M & S* | 1 Pack/380g | 570.0 | 26.0 | 150 | 6.5 | 15.1 | 6.9 | 0.2 |
| Indian Style, with Chickpeas & Yoghurt Dressing, M & S* | 1 Pack/220g | 264.0 | 7.0 | 120 | 3.7 | 19.3 | 3.2 | 3.4 |
| Mexican, with Beans, COU, M & S* | 1 Serving/250g | 250.0 | 3.0 | 100 | 6.0 | 15.6 | 1.4 | 1.2 |
| Rainbow, M & S* | 1 Serving/262g | 340.0 | 8.0 | 130 | 2.5 | 23.3 | 3.2 | 1.5 |
| Red, with Feta, M & S* | 1 Pack/244g | 440.0 | 21.0 | 180 | 4.8 | 21.0 | 8.5 | 1.3 |
| Spanish Style, with Chicken, M & S* | 1 Serving/220g | 319.0 | 13.0 | 145 | 5.8 | 17.4 | 5.8 | 0.5 |

## RICE STICKS

| | | | | | | | | |
|---|---|---|---|---|---|---|---|---|
| Chakri, Cofresh* | 1 Serving/100g | 480.0 | 20.0 | 480 | 7.7 | 66.1 | 20.5 | 0.0 |
| Mediterranean Tomato, Weight Watchers* | 1 Bag/20g | 72.0 | 0.0 | 360 | 7.3 | 77.7 | 2.2 | 2.8 |
| Salt & Vinegar, Weight Watchers* | 1 Serving/20g | 73.0 | 0.0 | 365 | 7.7 | 79.7 | 1.7 | 2.4 |
| Thai Sweet Chilli Flavour, Weight Watchers* | 1 Serving/20g | 73.0 | 0.0 | 363 | 7.6 | 79.5 | 1.6 | 2.2 |

R

| | Measure INFO/WEIGHT | per Measure KCAL | per Measure FAT | Nutrition Values per 100g / 100ml KCAL | PROT | CARB | FAT | FIBRE |
|---|---|---|---|---|---|---|---|---|
| **RICE WINE** | | | | | | | | |
| *Sake, Average* | *1oz/28g* | *38.0* | *0.0* | *134* | *0.5* | *5.0* | *0.0* | *0.0* |
| **RIGATONI** | | | | | | | | |
| Carbonara, Tesco* | 1 Serving/205g | 236.0 | 12.0 | 115 | 5.2 | 10.6 | 5.8 | 1.2 |
| *Dry, Average* | *1 Serving/80g* | *272.0* | *1.0* | *339* | *11.4* | *68.4* | *1.5* | *2.7* |
| Tomato & Cheese, Perfectly Balanced, Waitrose* | 1 Pack/400g | 664.0 | 9.0 | 166 | 7.6 | 28.6 | 2.3 | 2.3 |
| **RISOTTO** | | | | | | | | |
| Balls, Mushroom, Occasions, Sainsbury's* | 1 Ball/25g | 76.0 | 3.0 | 304 | 3.8 | 41.2 | 13.8 | 1.7 |
| Balls, Sun Dried Tomato, Occasions, Sainsbury's* | 1 Ball/25g | 71.0 | 4.0 | 285 | 6.8 | 30.8 | 15.0 | 2.9 |
| Beef, Vesta* | 1 Serving/100g | 346.0 | 6.0 | 346 | 15.3 | 57.8 | 5.9 | 5.6 |
| Butternut, Pearl Barely, Veg Pot, Innocent* | 1 Pot/390g | 285.0 | 5.0 | 73 | 2.9 | 12.6 | 1.3 | 3.8 |
| Butternut Squash, TTD, Sainsbury's* | 1 Pack/450g | 630.0 | 29.0 | 140 | 3.5 | 17.2 | 6.4 | 0.3 |
| Caramelised Onion & Gruyere Cheese, M & S* | 1 Pack/200g | 350.0 | 21.0 | 175 | 3.0 | 17.8 | 10.3 | 1.7 |
| Chargrilled Chicken, Ready Meal, M & S* | 1 Pack/365g | 493.0 | 25.0 | 135 | 6.4 | 11.6 | 6.9 | 0.7 |
| Cheese Flavour, Made Up, Ainsley Harriott* | 1 Sachet/140g | 565.0 | 15.0 | 404 | 7.8 | 69.6 | 10.4 | 9.1 |
| Cherry Tomato, COU, M & S* | 1 Pack/360g | 324.0 | 8.0 | 90 | 2.0 | 15.4 | 2.3 | 1.8 |
| Chicken, BGTY, Sainsbury's* | 1 Pack/327g | 356.0 | 6.0 | 109 | 7.5 | 15.5 | 1.9 | 1.0 |
| Chicken, Enjoy, Birds Eye* | 1 Pack/500g | 735.0 | 31.0 | 147 | 8.5 | 14.0 | 6.3 | 0.5 |
| Chicken, Lemon & Wild Rocket, Sainsbury's* | 1 Pack/360g | 683.0 | 41.0 | 190 | 16.2 | 5.6 | 11.4 | 0.1 |
| Chicken, Ready Meal, M & S* | 1 Pack/360g | 450.0 | 16.0 | 125 | 6.7 | 14.4 | 4.4 | 0.9 |
| Chicken, Tomato & Mozzarella, GFY, Asda* | 1 Pack/400g | 356.0 | 4.0 | 89 | 8.1 | 11.9 | 1.0 | 1.2 |
| Chicken & Bacon, Italiano, Tesco* | 1 Pack/450g | 652.0 | 20.0 | 145 | 5.9 | 20.2 | 4.5 | 1.5 |
| Chicken & Lemon, Weight Watchers* | 1 Pack/330g | 330.0 | 9.0 | 100 | 5.9 | 13.0 | 2.7 | 0.4 |
| Chicken & Mushroom, Finest, Tesco* | 1 Pack/400g | 496.0 | 11.0 | 124 | 7.4 | 17.2 | 2.8 | 0.5 |
| Chicken & Mushroom, Weight Watchers* | 1 Pack/320g | 323.0 | 8.0 | 101 | 5.7 | 13.8 | 2.5 | 0.3 |
| Chicken & Sun Dried Tomato, Waitrose* | 1 Pack/350g | 385.0 | 22.0 | 110 | 6.0 | 7.2 | 6.3 | 0.3 |
| Green Bean, Asparagus & Pecorino, Finest, Tesco* | 1 Pack/400g | 460.0 | 16.0 | 115 | 4.4 | 15.0 | 3.9 | 1.5 |
| Hot Smoked Salmon & Spinach, M & S* | ½ Pack/300g | 420.0 | 24.0 | 140 | 6.4 | 11.0 | 8.0 | 0.6 |
| Italian Red Wine with Creamed Spinach, Sainsbury's* | 1 Pack/400g | 596.0 | 28.0 | 149 | 2.4 | 19.3 | 6.9 | 0.4 |
| Lemon & Mint, Perfectly Balanced, Waitrose* | 1 Pack/350g | 462.0 | 13.0 | 132 | 3.9 | 20.7 | 3.7 | 1.0 |
| Mushroom, Asda* | 1 Pack/340g | 340.0 | 12.0 | 100 | 2.3 | 15.0 | 3.4 | 0.6 |
| Mushroom, BGTY, Sainsbury's* | 1 Pack/400g | 320.0 | 3.0 | 80 | 2.6 | 15.6 | 0.8 | 0.6 |
| Mushroom, HL, Tesco* | 1 Pack/400g | 320.0 | 3.0 | 80 | 2.6 | 15.6 | 0.8 | 0.6 |
| Mushroom, Perfectly Balanced, Waitrose* | 1 Pack/400g | 384.0 | 6.0 | 96 | 4.3 | 16.1 | 1.6 | 2.1 |
| Roasted Red Pepper & Italian Cheese, M & S* | 1 Pack/400g | 500.0 | 13.0 | 125 | 2.9 | 20.4 | 3.3 | 1.0 |
| Roasted Vegetable, Made Up, Ainsley Harriott* | 1 Sachet/140g | 766.0 | 18.0 | 547 | 11.0 | 96.5 | 13.0 | 15.5 |
| Roasted Vegetable & Sunblush Tomato, Finest, Tesco* | ½ Pack/200g | 306.0 | 18.0 | 153 | 3.7 | 14.5 | 9.0 | 1.4 |
| Roasted Vegetables, Stir-In, Uncle Ben's* | ½ Pack/75g | 86.0 | 7.0 | 115 | 1.7 | 5.0 | 9.7 | 0.0 |
| Salmon & Prawn, Eat Smart, Morrisons* | 1 Pack/381g | 339.0 | 5.0 | 89 | 4.9 | 14.1 | 1.4 | 0.8 |
| Seafood, HL, Tesco* | 1 Pack/365g | 328.0 | 4.0 | 90 | 5.3 | 14.1 | 1.0 | 0.9 |
| Seafood, Youngs* | 1 Pack/350g | 423.0 | 13.0 | 121 | 4.5 | 17.4 | 3.7 | 0.1 |
| Spring Vegetable, M & S* | 1 Serving/330g | 330.0 | 13.0 | 100 | 2.0 | 14.2 | 4.0 | 0.9 |
| Vegetable, Average | 1oz/28g | 41.0 | 2.0 | 147 | 4.2 | 19.2 | 6.5 | 2.2 |
| Vegetable, Brown Rice, Average | 1oz/28g | 40.0 | 2.0 | 143 | 4.1 | 18.6 | 6.4 | 2.4 |
| Vegetable, Great Stuff, Asda* | 1 Pack/300g | 315.0 | 6.0 | 105 | 4.3 | 17.6 | 1.9 | 1.3 |
| Wild Mushroom, Made Up, Ainsley Harriott* | 1 Sachet/140g | 785.0 | 22.0 | 561 | 12.0 | 93.3 | 15.5 | 14.7 |
| **RISSOLES** | | | | | | | | |
| Lentil, Fried in Vegetable Oil, Average | 1oz/28g | 59.0 | 3.0 | 211 | 8.9 | 22.0 | 10.5 | 3.6 |
| **RIVELLA*** | | | | | | | | |
| Blue, Rivella* | 1 Can/330ml | 16.0 | 0.0 | 5 | 0.0 | 1.2 | 0.0 | 0.0 |
| **ROCK SALMON** | | | | | | | | |
| *Raw, Flesh Only, Average* | *1oz/28g* | *43.0* | *3.0* | *154* | *16.6* | *0.0* | *9.7* | *0.0* |
| **ROCKET** | | | | | | | | |
| *Fresh, Raw, Average* | *1 Serving/80g* | *20.0* | *1.0* | *25* | *2.6* | *3.6* | *0.7* | *1.6* |

R

| | Measure INFO/WEIGHT | per Measure KCAL | per Measure FAT | Nutrition Values per 100g / 100ml KCAL | PROT | CARB | FAT | FIBRE |
|---|---|---|---|---|---|---|---|---|
| **ROE** | | | | | | | | |
| *Cod, Average* | **1 Can/100g** | **96.0** | **3.0** | **96** | **17.1** | **0.5** | **2.8** | **0.0** |
| Cod, Hard, Coated in Batter, Fried | 1oz/28g | 53.0 | 3.0 | 189 | 12.4 | 8.9 | 11.8 | 0.2 |
| Cod, Hard, Fried in Blended Oil | 1oz/28g | 57.0 | 3.0 | 202 | 20.9 | 3.0 | 11.9 | 0.1 |
| Herring, Soft, Fried in Blended Oil | 1oz/28g | 74.0 | 4.0 | 265 | 26.3 | 4.7 | 15.8 | 0.2 |
| *Herring, Soft, Raw* | **1oz/28g** | **25.0** | **1.0** | **91** | **16.8** | **0.0** | **2.6** | **0.0** |
| **ROGAN JOSH** | | | | | | | | |
| Chicken & Rice, Sainsbury's* | 1 Pack/500g | 675.0 | 27.0 | 135 | 6.7 | 14.1 | 5.4 | 2.4 |
| Chicken Breast, Chunks, Hot, Sainsbury's* | ½ Pack/114g | 143.0 | 2.0 | 126 | 23.6 | 3.9 | 1.8 | 1.0 |
| Lamb, & Pilau Rice, Indian Takeaway, Asda* | 1 Pack/569g | 888.0 | 28.0 | 156 | 7.0 | 21.0 | 4.9 | 1.7 |
| Lamb, & Pilau Rice, Tesco* | 1 Pack/550g | 770.0 | 29.0 | 140 | 6.0 | 16.9 | 5.3 | 1.0 |
| Lamb, Asda* | 1 Pack/450g | 688.0 | 40.0 | 153 | 13.0 | 5.0 | 9.0 | 3.1 |
| Lamb, Sainsbury's* | 1 Pack/400g | 660.0 | 44.0 | 165 | 11.3 | 4.9 | 11.1 | 1.9 |
| Lamb, Tesco* | 1 Pack/350g | 402.0 | 20.0 | 115 | 10.2 | 5.0 | 5.8 | 1.3 |
| Lamb, Waitrose* | 1 Serving/60g | 79.0 | 5.0 | 131 | 12.3 | 3.0 | 7.8 | 1.3 |
| Lamb with Basmati Rice, Eat Smart, Safeway* | 1 Pack/380g | 380.0 | 6.0 | 100 | 6.9 | 14.0 | 1.5 | 1.9 |
| Prawn, COU, M & S* | 1 Pack/400g | 360.0 | 2.0 | 90 | 4.9 | 16.2 | 0.6 | 0.8 |
| Prawn & Pilau Rice, BGTY, Sainsbury's* | 1 Pack/401g | 353.0 | 3.0 | 88 | 4.8 | 15.3 | 0.8 | 1.9 |
| **ROLL** | | | | | | | | |
| All Day Breakfast, Asda* | 1 Roll/220g | 581.0 | 26.0 | 264 | 10.0 | 29.0 | 12.0 | 0.0 |
| Bacon & Sausage, M & S* | 1oz/28g | 88.0 | 8.0 | 315 | 13.3 | 3.4 | 27.7 | 0.7 |
| Beef, Weight Watchers* | 1 Roll/174g | 276.0 | 4.0 | 159 | 10.8 | 23.1 | 2.5 | 1.0 |
| Brie & Grapes, M & S* | 1 Roll/57g | 174.0 | 10.0 | 306 | 11.1 | 24.5 | 18.2 | 1.4 |
| Cheese & Chutney, M & S* | 1 Roll/165g | 256.0 | 1.0 | 155 | 13.9 | 23.1 | 0.7 | 1.2 |
| Cheese & Onion, Asda* | 1 Serving/67g | 199.0 | 12.0 | 298 | 7.0 | 27.0 | 18.0 | 2.0 |
| Cheese & Onion, M & S* | 1 Roll/25g | 80.0 | 5.0 | 320 | 9.6 | 24.7 | 20.5 | 1.3 |
| Cheese & Onion, Sainsbury's* | 1 Roll/67g | 205.0 | 14.0 | 306 | 8.0 | 22.9 | 20.3 | 1.9 |
| Cheese & Onion, Tesco* | 1 Roll/67g | 203.0 | 12.0 | 305 | 7.3 | 28.0 | 18.1 | 1.9 |
| Cheese & Pickle, Sainsbury's* | 1 Roll/136g | 359.0 | 14.0 | 264 | 10.6 | 35.1 | 10.0 | 0.0 |
| Cheese Ploughman's, Malted Wheat, BGTY, Sainsbury's* | 1 Roll/172g | 309.0 | 4.0 | 180 | 10.9 | 29.3 | 2.1 | 3.8 |
| Chicken, Salad, Mini, Selection Pack, British, M & S* | 1 Roll/61g | 134.0 | 4.0 | 220 | 11.9 | 28.1 | 6.8 | 2.1 |
| Chicken & Beef Duo, M & S* | 1 Serving/147g | 235.0 | 4.0 | 160 | 12.0 | 22.1 | 2.6 | 2.7 |
| Chicken & Herb, Shapers, Boots* | 1 Roll/168g | 290.0 | 5.0 | 173 | 12.0 | 25.0 | 2.8 | 1.7 |
| Chicken & Stuffing, Tesco* | 1 Roll/323g | 1043.0 | 59.0 | 323 | 10.4 | 29.4 | 18.2 | 1.0 |
| Chicken & Sun Dried Tomato, Weight Watchers* | 1 Pack/170g | 272.0 | 3.0 | 160 | 12.9 | 22.7 | 1.9 | 1.2 |
| Chicken & Sweetcorn, Sainsbury's* | 1 Serving/170g | 462.0 | 24.0 | 272 | 12.5 | 24.2 | 13.9 | 0.0 |
| Chicken Salad, HL, Tesco* | 1 Serving/100g | 149.0 | 2.0 | 149 | 10.6 | 22.3 | 2.0 | 1.2 |
| Chicken Salsa, BGTY, Sainsbury's* | 1 Pack/197g | 323.0 | 5.0 | 164 | 11.1 | 24.8 | 2.3 | 0.0 |
| Chunky Cheese & Mustard, Finest, Tesco* | 1 Roll/88g | 260.0 | 9.0 | 295 | 10.9 | 40.0 | 10.2 | 2.4 |
| Chunky Herbes De Provence, Finest, Tesco* | 1 Roll/82g | 196.0 | 3.0 | 239 | 7.4 | 45.2 | 3.2 | 2.6 |
| Cornish, in Pastry, Pork Farms* | 1 Roll/75g | 226.0 | 15.0 | 301 | 6.6 | 24.5 | 20.1 | 0.0 |
| Egg & Bacon, Sub, Shapers, Boots* | 1 Serving/169g | 320.0 | 7.0 | 189 | 11.0 | 27.0 | 4.3 | 1.3 |
| Egg & Cress, HL, Tesco* | 1 Pack/175g | 322.0 | 7.0 | 184 | 9.6 | 27.7 | 3.9 | 1.2 |
| Egg & Tomato, Shapers, Boots* | 1 Roll/166g | 301.0 | 5.0 | 181 | 8.0 | 30.0 | 3.2 | 2.6 |
| Egg Mayonnaise & Cress, Sub, Delicious, Boots* | 1 Pack/205g | 399.0 | 14.0 | 195 | 10.0 | 23.0 | 6.9 | 2.4 |
| Ham & Cheese, in Pastry, Pork Farms* | 1 Roll/70g | 216.0 | 13.0 | 308 | 8.0 | 28.8 | 17.9 | 0.0 |
| Ham Salad, BGTY, Sainsbury's* | 1 Roll/178g | 292.0 | 3.0 | 164 | 10.8 | 25.9 | 1.9 | 0.0 |
| Ham Salad, HL, Tesco* | 1 Roll/203g | 284.0 | 5.0 | 140 | 9.8 | 19.3 | 2.6 | 0.0 |
| Mushroom & Bacon, Crusty, M & S* | 1 Roll/160g | 424.0 | 20.0 | 265 | 8.7 | 29.0 | 12.6 | 2.3 |
| Oak Smoked Salmon, M & S* | 1 Roll/55g | 139.0 | 6.0 | 252 | 14.6 | 23.1 | 11.3 | 1.2 |
| Roast Chicken & Mayonnaise, Big, Sainsbury's* | 1 Pack/185g | 479.0 | 27.0 | 259 | 9.6 | 21.8 | 14.8 | 0.0 |
| Roast Chicken & Sweetcure Bacon, Boots* | 1 Pack/245g | 690.0 | 34.0 | 282 | 13.0 | 26.0 | 14.0 | 1.6 |
| Roast Chicken Salad, Improved, Shapers, Boots* | 1 Pack/188g | 302.0 | 4.0 | 161 | 11.0 | 25.0 | 1.9 | 1.6 |
| Roast Pork, Stuffing & Apple Sauce, Boots* | 1 Roll/218g | 602.0 | 26.0 | 276 | 10.0 | 32.0 | 12.0 | 1.8 |

**R**

| | Measure INFO/WEIGHT | per Measure KCAL | FAT | Nutrition Values per 100g / 100ml KCAL | PROT | CARB | FAT | FIBRE |
|---|---|---|---|---|---|---|---|---|
| **ROLL** | | | | | | | | |
| Spicy Chicken, Crusty, M & S* | 1 Roll/150g | 382.0 | 17.0 | 255 | 12.8 | 25.8 | 11.1 | 2.0 |
| Steak & Onion, M & S* | 1 Serving/150g | 307.0 | 10.0 | 205 | 11.0 | 24.5 | 7.0 | 3.8 |
| Tomato & Basil, Sub, COU, M & S* | 1 Roll/35g | 93.0 | 1.0 | 265 | 11.0 | 48.7 | 2.7 | 2.4 |
| Tuna Cheese Melt, Boots* | 1 Roll/199g | 612.0 | 36.0 | 308 | 13.0 | 23.0 | 18.0 | 1.2 |
| Turkey, Stuffed, GFY, Asda* | ½ Pack/225g | 319.0 | 9.0 | 142 | 14.0 | 12.0 | 4.2 | 0.8 |
| **ROLO** | | | | | | | | |
| Giant, Nestle* | 1 Sweet/9g | 42.0 | 2.0 | 470 | 3.1 | 70.1 | 19.7 | 0.3 |
| Little, Nestle* | 1 Pack/40g | 196.0 | 9.0 | 491 | 4.0 | 65.5 | 23.5 | 0.5 |
| Nestle* | 1 Sweet/5g | 24.0 | 1.0 | 471 | 3.2 | 68.5 | 20.5 | 0.3 |
| **ROLY POLY** | | | | | | | | |
| Frozen, Tesco* | 1 Serving/81g | 287.0 | 11.0 | 354 | 4.4 | 52.7 | 14.0 | 0.5 |
| Jam, & Custard, Co-Op* | ¼ Pack/100g | 235.0 | 8.0 | 235 | 4.0 | 36.0 | 8.0 | 0.7 |
| Jam, Aunt Bessie's* | 1 Serving/100g | 384.0 | 16.0 | 384 | 5.4 | 53.9 | 16.3 | 1.7 |
| Jam, Sainsbury's* | ¼ Pack/81g | 291.0 | 12.0 | 359 | 4.4 | 53.3 | 14.2 | 0.5 |
| Jam, Tesco* | 1 Serving/82g | 307.0 | 14.0 | 375 | 4.7 | 51.5 | 16.7 | 1.2 |
| Jam & Custard, Safeway* | 1 Serving/112g | 299.0 | 10.0 | 267 | 3.8 | 43.0 | 8.9 | 0.8 |
| **ROOT BEER** | | | | | | | | |
| Average | 1 Can/330ml | 135.0 | 0.0 | 41 | 0.0 | 10.6 | 0.0 | 0.0 |
| **ROSE WATER** | | | | | | | | |
| English Provender* | 1 Tsp/5g | 0.0 | 0.0 | 2 | 0.1 | 0.6 | 0.1 | 0.1 |
| **ROSEMARY** | | | | | | | | |
| *Dried* | *1 Tsp/1g* | *3.0* | *0.0* | *331* | *4.9* | *46.4* | *15.2* | *0.0* |
| *Fresh* | *1oz/28g* | *28.0* | *1.0* | *99* | *1.4* | *13.5* | *4.4* | *0.0* |
| **ROSTI** | | | | | | | | |
| Garlic & Mushroom, Finest, Tesco* | 1 Serving/200g | 346.0 | 20.0 | 173 | 5.7 | 15.4 | 9.8 | 1.7 |
| Honey & Parsnip, Tesco* | 1 Rosti/75g | 79.0 | 2.0 | 105 | 1.8 | 17.0 | 3.2 | 3.9 |
| Oven Baked, McCain* | 1 Rosti/100g | 194.0 | 9.0 | 194 | 2.6 | 25.0 | 9.3 | 2.3 |
| Peppered Steak, British Classics, Tesco* | 1 Pack/450g | 598.0 | 28.0 | 133 | 9.0 | 10.7 | 6.2 | 1.7 |
| Potato, Chicken & Sweetcorn Bake, Asda* | 1 Serving/400g | 440.0 | 19.0 | 110 | 7.0 | 10.0 | 4.7 | 0.6 |
| Potato, McCain* | 1 Rosti/95g | 161.0 | 9.0 | 169 | 2.2 | 19.6 | 9.1 | 0.0 |
| Potato, Mini, Party Bites, Sainsbury's* | 1 Serving/100g | 218.0 | 11.0 | 218 | 2.5 | 26.2 | 11.5 | 3.0 |
| Potato, Mini, Party Range, Tesco* | 1 Rosti/17g | 32.0 | 2.0 | 193 | 2.1 | 20.6 | 11.4 | 3.3 |
| Potato, Onion & Gruyere, Finest, Tesco* | ½ Pack/200g | 206.0 | 11.0 | 103 | 3.2 | 10.5 | 5.3 | 2.0 |
| Potato & Leek, Sainsbury's* | ½ Pack/190g | 296.0 | 21.0 | 156 | 4.5 | 9.8 | 11.0 | 0.3 |
| Potato & Root Vegetable, COU, M & S* | 1 Rosti/100g | 85.0 | 3.0 | 85 | 1.6 | 13.3 | 2.7 | 1.5 |
| Potato Cakes, Baby, M & S* | 1 Rosti/23g | 40.0 | 2.0 | 175 | 3.5 | 25.1 | 6.7 | 1.6 |
| Spinach & Mozzarella, Vegetarian, Tesco* | 1 Rosti/140g | 245.0 | 14.0 | 175 | 4.8 | 17.0 | 9.7 | 2.3 |
| Vegetable, Waitrose* | 1 Pack/400g | 248.0 | 9.0 | 62 | 1.4 | 8.8 | 2.3 | 1.3 |
| Waitrose* | 1 Rosti/45g | 112.0 | 7.0 | 248 | 3.8 | 22.5 | 15.9 | 2.7 |
| **ROUGHY** | | | | | | | | |
| *Orange, Raw* | *1oz/28g* | *35.0* | *2.0* | *126* | *14.7* | *0.0* | *7.0* | *0.0* |
| **RUM** | | | | | | | | |
| *21% Volume, Malibu** | *1 Shot/35ml* | *70.0* | *0.0* | *200* | *0.0* | *29.0* | *0.0* | *0.0* |
| *37.5% Volume* | *1 Shot/35ml* | *72.0* | *0.0* | *207* | *0.0* | *0.0* | *0.0* | *0.0* |
| *40% Volume* | *1 Shot/35ml* | *78.0* | *0.0* | *222* | *0.0* | *0.0* | *0.0* | *0.0* |
| *White* | *1 Shot/35ml* | *72.0* | *0.0* | *207* | *0.0* | *0.0* | *0.0* | *0.0* |
| **RUSKS** | | | | | | | | |
| Banana, Farleys* | 1 Serving/17g | 70.0 | 2.0 | 409 | 7.3 | 75.1 | 8.8 | 2.9 |
| Mini, Farleys* | 1 Serving/30g | 121.0 | 2.0 | 405 | 7.0 | 77.7 | 7.3 | 2.1 |
| Original, Farleys* | 1 Rusk/17g | 69.0 | 1.0 | 406 | 7.1 | 77.6 | 7.1 | 2.3 |

R

| | Measure INFO/WEIGHT | per Measure | | Nutrition Values per 100g / 100ml | | | | |
|---|---|---|---|---|---|---|---|---|
| | | KCAL | FAT | KCAL | PROT | CARB | FAT | FIBRE |
| **SAAG** | | | | | | | | |
| Aloo, Canned, Tesco* | ½ Can/200g | 124.0 | 4.0 | 62 | 1.8 | 9.3 | 1.9 | 2.0 |
| Aloo, Fresh, Sainsbury's* | 1 Pack/400g | 388.0 | 13.0 | 97 | 2.0 | 14.7 | 3.3 | 4.8 |
| Aloo, Jar, Sainsbury's* | ½ Jar/135g | 121.0 | 6.0 | 90 | 1.6 | 11.0 | 4.3 | 1.7 |
| Aloo, Packet, Sainsbury's* | ½ Pack/150g | 184.0 | 12.0 | 123 | 2.1 | 9.9 | 8.3 | 2.7 |
| Aloo, Sainsbury's* | 1 Pack/300g | 441.0 | 32.0 | 147 | 2.1 | 10.7 | 10.6 | 3.5 |
| Aloo, Tesco* | 1 Serving/200g | 144.0 | 7.0 | 72 | 2.1 | 8.0 | 3.5 | 2.0 |
| Aloo Gobi, Waitrose* | 1 Pack/300g | 240.0 | 14.0 | 80 | 2.6 | 7.1 | 4.6 | 2.9 |
| Gobi Aloo, Indian, Tesco* | 1 Pack/225g | 225.0 | 16.0 | 100 | 2.1 | 6.5 | 7.3 | 1.8 |
| Gobi Aloo, Indian Takeaway, Sainsbury's* | 1 Pack/334g | 164.0 | 4.0 | 49 | 1.7 | 8.0 | 1.1 | 1.5 |
| Gobi Aloo, M & S* | 1 Pack/225g | 270.0 | 19.0 | 120 | 1.9 | 9.3 | 8.5 | 2.4 |
| Gobi Aloo, Tesco* | 1 Serving/175g | 166.0 | 9.0 | 95 | 2.1 | 9.5 | 5.1 | 1.9 |
| **SAFFRON** | | | | | | | | |
| *Average* | *1 Tsp/1g* | *2.0* | *0.0* | *310* | *11.4* | *61.5* | *5.9* | *0.0* |
| **SAGE** | | | | | | | | |
| *Dried, Ground* | *1 Tsp/1g* | *3.0* | *0.0* | *315* | *10.6* | *42.7* | *12.7* | *0.0* |
| *Fresh* | *1oz/28g* | *33.0* | *1.0* | *119* | *3.9* | *15.6* | *4.6* | *0.0* |
| **SAGO** | | | | | | | | |
| *Raw* | *1oz/28g* | *99.0* | *0.0* | *355* | *0.2* | *94.0* | *0.2* | *0.5* |
| **SALAD** | | | | | | | | |
| 3 Bean, Sainsbury's* | 1 Tub/270g | 281.0 | 6.0 | 104 | 7.1 | 13.6 | 2.3 | 5.9 |
| Alfresco Style, Tesco* | 1 Serving/200g | 40.0 | 1.0 | 20 | 0.9 | 3.3 | 0.3 | 2.1 |
| All Seasons, Sainsbury's* | 1oz/28g | 3.0 | 0.0 | 12 | 1.0 | 1.5 | 0.2 | 1.2 |
| American Ranch, Asda* | 1 Serving/220g | 253.0 | 20.0 | 115 | 2.5 | 6.0 | 9.0 | 2.0 |
| American Style, Morrisons* | 1 Serving/25g | 5.0 | 0.0 | 22 | 1.1 | 3.9 | 0.3 | 2.3 |
| Aromatic Herb, Waitrose* | ¼ Pack/27g | 4.0 | 0.0 | 15 | 0.9 | 1.7 | 0.5 | 1.0 |
| Assorted, Asda* | 1 Serving/100g | 22.0 | 1.0 | 22 | 2.4 | 1.7 | 0.6 | 0.0 |
| Avocado & Feta, Gourmet To Go, M & S* | 1 Pack/320g | 512.0 | 32.0 | 160 | 5.4 | 12.1 | 10.0 | 3.1 |
| Baby Leaf, Florette* | 1 Serving/40g | 5.0 | 0.0 | 12 | 2.0 | 0.4 | 0.3 | 1.0 |
| Baby Leaf, Italian Style, M & S* | 1 Serving/55g | 11.0 | 0.0 | 20 | 1.3 | 2.3 | 0.5 | 1.3 |
| Baby Leaf, M & S* | 1 Pack/100g | 20.0 | 0.0 | 20 | 3.0 | 1.7 | 0.2 | 0.5 |
| Baby Leaf, Organic, Sainsbury's* | 1 Serving/20g | 3.0 | 0.0 | 14 | 1.5 | 1.4 | 0.3 | 1.1 |
| Baby Leaf, Sainsbury's* | 1 Serving/60g | 12.0 | 1.0 | 20 | 2.8 | 1.1 | 1.9 | 1.9 |
| Baby Leaf & Herb, Asda* | 1 Serving/50g | 7.0 | 0.0 | 14 | 2.3 | 0.7 | 0.2 | 2.4 |
| Baby Plum & Sundried Tomato Salad, Waitrose* | 1 Serving/200g | 226.0 | 18.0 | 113 | 1.3 | 6.8 | 8.9 | 0.8 |
| Baby Spinach & Red Mustard, M & S* | 1 Pack/170g | 263.0 | 27.0 | 155 | 1.7 | 1.1 | 15.7 | 0.1 |
| Baby Tomato, Tesco* | 1 Pack/205g | 35.0 | 1.0 | 17 | 0.8 | 2.8 | 0.3 | 0.9 |
| Bacon Caesar, M & S* | 1oz/28g | 48.0 | 4.0 | 170 | 5.5 | 5.7 | 14.0 | 1.2 |
| Bacon Caesar, Sainsbury's* | 1 Pack/256g | 415.0 | 33.0 | 162 | 4.7 | 12.0 | 12.7 | 1.4 |
| Bean, Mixed, Vinaigrette, Tesco* | 1 Can/400g | 280.0 | 2.0 | 70 | 3.2 | 13.1 | 0.5 | 1.9 |
| Bean, Retail | 1oz/28g | 41.0 | 3.0 | 147 | 4.2 | 12.8 | 9.3 | 3.0 |
| Bean & Sweetcorn, Side, M & S* | 1 Serving/125g | 131.0 | 9.0 | 105 | 2.5 | 7.0 | 7.2 | 1.3 |
| Beetroot | 1oz/28g | 28.0 | 2.0 | 100 | 2.0 | 8.4 | 6.8 | 1.7 |
| Beetroot, 1% Fat, M & S* | 1 Serving/225g | 130.0 | 6.0 | 58 | 1.1 | 7.7 | 2.7 | 1.7 |
| Beetroot, Asda* | 1 Carton/270g | 119.0 | 1.0 | 44 | 1.3 | 8.8 | 0.4 | 2.4 |
| Beetroot, Co-Op* | 1 Pack/250g | 100.0 | 1.0 | 40 | 0.9 | 8.0 | 0.3 | 2.0 |
| Beetroot, Freshly Prepared, Tesco* | 1 Pack/240g | 58.0 | 1.0 | 24 | 1.9 | 3.3 | 0.3 | 2.7 |
| Beetroot, M & S* | 1 Serving/225g | 124.0 | 1.0 | 55 | 1.0 | 12.0 | 0.3 | 3.0 |
| Beetroot, Organic, M & S* | 1oz/28g | 20.0 | 1.0 | 73 | 1.5 | 9.1 | 3.4 | 1.9 |
| Beetroot, Sainsbury's* | 1 Tub/200g | 148.0 | 2.0 | 74 | 1.7 | 14.1 | 1.2 | 1.7 |
| Beetroot & Cherry Tomato, & Lemon Dressing, M & S* | 1 Pack/215g | 129.0 | 8.0 | 60 | 1.3 | 5.2 | 3.8 | 1.5 |
| Beetroot & Lettuce, Asda* | 1 Serving/30g | 5.0 | 0.0 | 16 | 1.4 | 2.7 | 0.0 | 2.5 |
| Bistro, Asda* | 1 Serving/180g | 29.0 | 0.0 | 16 | 1.4 | 2.7 | 0.0 | 2.5 |
| Bistro, Sainsbury's* | 1 Pack/150g | 25.0 | 0.0 | 17 | 1.9 | 2.0 | 0.2 | 2.0 |

S

| | Measure INFO/WEIGHT | per Measure KCAL | per Measure FAT | Nutrition Values per 100g / 100ml KCAL | PROT | CARB | FAT | FIBRE |
|---|---|---|---|---|---|---|---|---|
| **SALAD** | | | | | | | | |
| Bistro, Washed Ready to Eat, Tesco* | 1 Pack/140g | 22.0 | 1.0 | 16 | 1.1 | 1.7 | 0.5 | 1.0 |
| British Ham & Free Range Egg, M & S* | 1 Pack/280g | 182.0 | 6.0 | 65 | 6.1 | 5.3 | 2.3 | 1.0 |
| Brown Rice, Tossed UK* | 1 Pack/200g | 335.0 | 2.0 | 167 | 13.3 | 19.9 | 0.9 | 0.0 |
| Cabbage & Leek, Crunchy Mix, Sainsbury's* | ½ Pack/126g | 24.0 | 1.0 | 19 | 1.2 | 2.1 | 0.6 | 1.9 |
| Caesar, & New Potatoes with Asparagus, M & S* | 1 Pack/200g | 270.0 | 15.0 | 135 | 3.1 | 13.8 | 7.6 | 1.7 |
| Caesar, Bacon, M & S* | 1 Serving/250g | 400.0 | 31.0 | 160 | 7.1 | 4.1 | 12.5 | 1.3 |
| Caesar, Chicken & Bacon, Tesco* | 1 Pack/200g | 506.0 | 40.0 | 253 | 6.6 | 11.4 | 20.1 | 1.0 |
| Caesar, Finest, Tesco* | 1 Bowl/220g | 374.0 | 31.0 | 170 | 4.9 | 5.1 | 13.9 | 1.6 |
| Caesar, Florette* | 1 Serving/100g | 163.0 | 12.0 | 163 | 2.7 | 10.2 | 12.4 | 1.8 |
| Caesar, GFY, Asda* | ½ Pack/87g | 76.0 | 3.0 | 87 | 8.0 | 7.0 | 3.0 | 1.5 |
| Caesar, M & S* | 1 Pack/268g | 510.0 | 41.0 | 190 | 5.7 | 8.3 | 15.1 | 1.3 |
| Caesar, Morrisons* | 1 Serving/115g | 194.0 | 18.0 | 169 | 3.6 | 5.9 | 15.7 | 0.3 |
| Caesar, Sainsbury's* | ½ Bag/128g | 227.0 | 19.0 | 177 | 3.6 | 6.7 | 15.1 | 1.0 |
| Caesar, with Dressing, Croutons & Parmesan, M & S* | 1 Serving/115g | 190.0 | 16.0 | 165 | 4.3 | 6.4 | 13.5 | 1.4 |
| Caesar, with Parmigiano Reggiano, Tesco* | 1 Bag/275g | 552.0 | 49.0 | 201 | 4.1 | 5.8 | 17.8 | 1.3 |
| Caesar, with Romaine Lettuce, Kit, BGTY, Sainsbury's* | ½ Pack/130g | 139.0 | 8.0 | 107 | 3.7 | 9.2 | 6.1 | 1.4 |
| Cajun Chicken, David Lloyd Leisure* | 1 Pack/300g | 429.0 | 10.0 | 143 | 11.7 | 17.7 | 3.3 | 1.0 |
| Cannelini Bean & Chorizo, Sainsbury's* | 1 Pack/250g | 227.0 | 8.0 | 91 | 5.3 | 10.2 | 3.2 | 1.6 |
| Cannellini Bean & Chicken, M & S* | 1 Serving/225g | 250.0 | 15.0 | 111 | 5.9 | 7.4 | 6.5 | 3.1 |
| Cannellini Bean & Tuna, M & S* | 1 Serving/255g | 215.0 | 12.0 | 84 | 5.3 | 5.4 | 4.5 | 2.1 |
| Caponata, Organic, Florentin* | 1 Serving/100g | 111.0 | 12.0 | 111 | 1.5 | 3.7 | 12.3 | 0.0 |
| Caribbean Chicken, Shapers, Boots* | 1 Pack/220g | 222.0 | 5.0 | 101 | 5.8 | 14.0 | 2.3 | 1.2 |
| Carrot, M & S* | 1 Pack/215g | 280.0 | 7.0 | 130 | 3.1 | 22.4 | 3.4 | 2.7 |
| Carrot, Peanut & Sultana, Asda* | 1 Serving/20g | 54.0 | 4.0 | 272 | 8.0 | 15.0 | 20.0 | 4.5 |
| Carrot, with Fresh Coriander Vinaigrette, M & S* | ½ Pack/105g | 136.0 | 4.0 | 130 | 2.8 | 21.9 | 3.4 | 3.5 |
| Carrot & Nut, with French Dressing, Average | 1oz/28g | 61.0 | 5.0 | 218 | 2.1 | 13.7 | 17.6 | 2.4 |
| Carrot & Sultana, BGTY, Sainsbury's* | ½ Pack/100g | 55.0 | 0.0 | 55 | 0.6 | 12.4 | 0.3 | 0.0 |
| Carrot & Sultana, HL, Tesco* | 1 Tub/225g | 142.0 | 1.0 | 63 | 1.2 | 13.2 | 0.6 | 2.5 |
| Celery, Nut & Sultana, Waitrose* | 1oz/28g | 54.0 | 5.0 | 192 | 2.8 | 8.4 | 16.4 | 1.0 |
| Chargrilled Chicken, Tesco* | 1 Serving/300g | 384.0 | 14.0 | 128 | 6.1 | 15.0 | 4.8 | 2.4 |
| Chargrilled Chicken, Weight Watchers* | 1 Pack/182g | 265.0 | 4.0 | 146 | 11.7 | 20.0 | 2.1 | 2.2 |
| Chargrilled Chicken & Bacon, Tesco* | 1 Pack/300g | 657.0 | 38.0 | 219 | 7.8 | 18.7 | 12.6 | 0.9 |
| Chargrilled Chicken & Pesto, Sainsbury's* | 1 Pack/250g | 375.0 | 15.0 | 150 | 7.9 | 15.8 | 6.1 | 1.3 |
| Chargrilled Chicken & Quinoa, Shapers, Boots* | 1 Pack/185g | 139.0 | 2.0 | 75 | 6.2 | 10.0 | 1.0 | 1.8 |
| Chargrilled Pepper with Cous Cous, Asda* | 1 Pack/325g | 426.0 | 11.0 | 131 | 4.3 | 21.0 | 3.3 | 0.0 |
| Chargrilled Vegetable, M & S* | 1 Tub/165g | 91.0 | 5.0 | 55 | 1.4 | 5.3 | 3.3 | 2.6 |
| Cheese, Layered, Sainsbury's* | 1 Pack/235g | 367.0 | 26.0 | 156 | 4.3 | 10.1 | 10.9 | 2.0 |
| Cheese, Layered, Tesco* | 1 Serving/225g | 437.0 | 32.0 | 194 | 5.8 | 10.8 | 14.2 | 0.8 |
| Cheese, Ploughmans, Asda* | 1 Bowl/300g | 246.0 | 11.0 | 82 | 3.6 | 8.9 | 3.6 | 1.0 |
| Cheese & Coleslaw, Tesco* | 1 Serving/125g | 135.0 | 11.0 | 108 | 3.4 | 3.4 | 8.7 | 1.1 |
| Cheese Layered, M & S* | 1 Pack/450g | 922.0 | 76.0 | 205 | 4.3 | 9.0 | 17.0 | 0.7 |
| Cherry Tomato, Fresh, Safeway* | 1 Pack/170g | 31.0 | 1.0 | 18 | 0.8 | 2.9 | 0.3 | 0.9 |
| Cherry Tomato, Tesco* | 1 Pack/210g | 136.0 | 9.0 | 65 | 0.9 | 4.2 | 4.5 | 1.1 |
| Chick Pea & Cous Cous, Tesco* | 1 Serving/250g | 245.0 | 6.0 | 98 | 3.2 | 15.5 | 2.6 | 0.0 |
| Chick Pea & Spinach, M & S* | 1 Serving/260g | 299.0 | 11.0 | 115 | 7.3 | 12.5 | 4.1 | 2.7 |
| Chicken, Avacado & Bacon, M & S* | 1 Serving/235g | 235.0 | 14.0 | 100 | 8.5 | 2.8 | 5.8 | 2.8 |
| Chicken, Italian Style, Snack Pot, Carb Check, Heinz* | 1 Pot/218g | 131.0 | 4.0 | 60 | 5.9 | 4.3 | 2.0 | 1.0 |
| Chicken, Layer, HE, Tesco* | 1 Pack/400g | 268.0 | 4.0 | 67 | 5.8 | 8.4 | 1.1 | 2.1 |
| Chicken, Roast, & Coleslaw, Boots* | 1 Serving/245g | 392.0 | 34.0 | 160 | 4.5 | 3.9 | 14.0 | 1.3 |
| Chicken, Roast, 93 Cals, Shapers, Boots* | 1 Pack/233g | 93.0 | 1.0 | 40 | 8.6 | 0.6 | 0.4 | 1.8 |
| Chicken, Safeway* | 1 Serving/200g | 279.0 | 7.0 | 139 | 8.9 | 17.9 | 3.6 | 1.4 |
| Chicken, Sweet Chilli, BGTY, Sainsbury's* | 1 Serving/200g | 206.0 | 1.0 | 103 | 6.0 | 18.7 | 0.4 | 0.0 |
| Chicken, Sweetcorn & Pasta, Safeway* | 1 Serving/200g | 230.0 | 4.0 | 115 | 7.5 | 16.3 | 1.8 | 1.0 |

S

| | Measure INFO/WEIGHT | per Measure KCAL | FAT | Nutrition Values per 100g / 100ml KCAL | PROT | CARB | FAT | FIBRE |
|---|---|---|---|---|---|---|---|---|
| **SALAD** | | | | | | | | |
| Chicken, Tesco* | 1 Serving/300g | 348.0 | 22.0 | 116 | 5.3 | 7.0 | 7.4 | 1.0 |
| Chicken, Tomato, & Basil, Safeway* | 1 Serving/200g | 330.0 | 18.0 | 165 | 6.9 | 14.2 | 8.9 | 0.6 |
| Chicken, Tomato Chilli, & Rice, COU, M & S* | 1 Pack/340g | 357.0 | 5.0 | 105 | 6.8 | 16.0 | 1.5 | 0.9 |
| Chicken & Bacon, Asda* | 1 Pack/381g | 480.0 | 23.0 | 126 | 7.0 | 11.0 | 6.0 | 0.0 |
| Chicken & Bacon, Carb Control, Tesco* | 1 Serving/188g | 244.0 | 15.0 | 130 | 13.2 | 1.7 | 7.8 | 0.5 |
| Chicken & Bacon, Layered, Asda* | 1 Serving/375g | 472.0 | 22.0 | 126 | 7.0 | 11.0 | 6.0 | 1.6 |
| Chicken & Bacon, Layered, Tesco* | 1 Bowl/380g | 475.0 | 28.0 | 125 | 4.8 | 9.1 | 7.5 | 2.7 |
| Chicken Caesar, Asda* | 1 Pack/273g | 535.0 | 44.0 | 196 | 10.0 | 3.0 | 16.0 | 1.9 |
| Chicken Caesar, Eat Well, M & S* | 1 Pack/397g | 595.0 | 25.0 | 150 | 9.9 | 18.7 | 6.2 | 2.1 |
| Chicken Caesar, TTD, Sainsbury's* | 1 Serving/190g | 308.0 | 23.0 | 162 | 11.1 | 1.6 | 12.3 | 1.5 |
| Chicken Fajita, Shapers, Boots* | 1 Pack/258g | 181.0 | 3.0 | 70 | 7.0 | 7.4 | 1.3 | 2.7 |
| Chicken Noodle, Thai Style, Sainsbury's* | 1 Pack/260g | 283.0 | 8.0 | 109 | 6.6 | 14.2 | 2.9 | 1.3 |
| Chicken Noodle & Sweet Chilli, Shapers, Boots* | 1 Pack/197g | 266.0 | 5.0 | 135 | 12.0 | 16.0 | 2.6 | 0.9 |
| Chicken with Mayonnaise, Waitrose* | 1 Pack/208g | 406.0 | 20.0 | 195 | 10.3 | 17.1 | 9.5 | 2.5 |
| Chilli, Tomato, Chick Pea & Butterbean, Tesco* | 1 Pack/130g | 146.0 | 6.0 | 112 | 3.4 | 14.3 | 4.6 | 0.5 |
| Chilli Chicken & Spicy Cous Cous, HE, Tesco* | 1 Serving/190g | 251.0 | 5.0 | 132 | 6.5 | 21.1 | 2.4 | 1.5 |
| Coleslaw, Classics, M & S* | 1 Pot/190g | 123.0 | 4.0 | 65 | 1.9 | 8.8 | 2.3 | 1.3 |
| Coleslaw, Layered, Fresh Tastes, Asda* | 1oz/28g | 17.0 | 1.0 | 59 | 1.1 | 3.4 | 4.5 | 1.6 |
| Coleslaw & Potato, 3% Fat, M & S* | 1oz/28g | 20.0 | 1.0 | 72 | 2.7 | 7.7 | 3.4 | 1.5 |
| Coleslaw Layered, Fresh, Asda* | 1 Tub/197g | 209.0 | 18.0 | 106 | 1.2 | 5.0 | 9.0 | 1.5 |
| Complete Hot Greek, Sainsbury's* | 1 Pack/299g | 287.0 | 22.0 | 96 | 4.3 | 2.9 | 7.5 | 1.7 |
| Continental, Co-Op* | 1 Serving/80g | 12.0 | 0.0 | 15 | 1.0 | 2.0 | 0.4 | 1.0 |
| Continental Four Leaf, Sainsbury's* | ½ Pack/100g | 13.0 | 0.0 | 13 | 1.2 | 1.7 | 0.2 | 1.9 |
| Continental Leaf, Asda* | 1oz/28g | 4.0 | 0.0 | 16 | 1.4 | 1.4 | 0.5 | 1.4 |
| Continental Style, Co-Op* | 1 Bag/100g | 15.0 | 0.0 | 15 | 1.0 | 2.0 | 0.3 | 0.5 |
| Coronation Chicken, Salad Bar, Asda* | 1oz/28g | 82.0 | 6.0 | 293 | 5.7 | 16.4 | 22.7 | 0.7 |
| Coronation Chicken & Rice, Asda* | 1oz/28g | 67.0 | 5.0 | 241 | 6.7 | 15.2 | 17.0 | 0.4 |
| Coronation Rice, Tesco* | 1 Serving/50g | 103.0 | 8.0 | 207 | 2.0 | 15.9 | 15.1 | 0.8 |
| Cosmopolitan, Fresh, Sainsbury's* | 1 Bag/135g | 20.0 | 1.0 | 15 | 1.2 | 1.6 | 0.4 | 1.9 |
| Country Style, Co-Op* | ½ Pack/100g | 20.0 | 0.0 | 20 | 1.0 | 3.0 | 0.4 | 2.0 |
| Cous Cous, & Roasted Vegetable, Waitrose* | 1 Pack/220g | 396.0 | 13.0 | 180 | 5.1 | 26.1 | 6.1 | 1.2 |
| Cous Cous, BFY, Morrisons* | ½ Pot/113g | 164.0 | 4.0 | 145 | 4.6 | 23.8 | 3.5 | 0.5 |
| Cous Cous, BGTY, Sainsbury's* | 1 Pot/200g | 236.0 | 4.0 | 118 | 4.7 | 19.7 | 2.2 | 2.8 |
| Cous Cous, Tesco* | 1 Serving/25g | 35.0 | 0.0 | 141 | 4.8 | 26.9 | 1.6 | 0.6 |
| Cous Cous, Waitrose* | 1 Pot/200g | 344.0 | 10.0 | 172 | 4.9 | 26.9 | 5.0 | 1.4 |
| Cous Cous, with Mixed Peppers & Cucumber, GFY, Asda* | ¼ Pot/56g | 66.0 | 0.0 | 117 | 3.9 | 25.0 | 0.2 | 1.5 |
| Cous Cous & Roast Vegetable, GFY, Asda* | 1 Serving/100g | 120.0 | 2.0 | 120 | 3.5 | 23.0 | 1.6 | 2.7 |
| Crisp, Mixed, Morrisons* | 1 Pack/230g | 39.0 | 1.0 | 17 | 1.0 | 2.8 | 0.3 | 0.0 |
| Crisp & Crunchy, Asda* | 1 Pack/250g | 55.0 | 1.0 | 22 | 0.8 | 3.3 | 0.6 | 1.4 |
| Crisp & Crunchy with French Dressing, GFY, Asda* | 1/3 Pack/116g | 26.0 | 1.0 | 22 | 0.8 | 3.3 | 0.6 | 1.4 |
| Crisp & Light, M & S* | 1 Serving/170g | 51.0 | 1.0 | 30 | 0.5 | 5.4 | 0.8 | 1.0 |
| Crisp & Sweet Lettuce Leaves, Florette* | ¼ Pack/70g | 10.0 | 0.0 | 14 | 0.8 | 1.7 | 0.5 | 0.9 |
| Crisp Mixed, Tesco* | 1 Pack/200g | 40.0 | 1.0 | 20 | 1.1 | 3.2 | 0.3 | 2.0 |
| Crispy, Florette* | 1 Portion/100g | 22.0 | 0.0 | 22 | 1.5 | 3.4 | 0.3 | 3.0 |
| Crispy, Tesco* | 1oz/28g | 6.0 | 0.0 | 20 | 1.2 | 3.0 | 0.3 | 1.6 |
| Crispy Green, Sainsbury's* | 1 Serving/70g | 8.0 | 0.0 | 12 | 0.9 | 1.6 | 0.2 | 0.8 |
| Crispy Leaf, Sainsbury's* | ½ Pack/68g | 9.0 | 0.0 | 14 | 1.0 | 1.7 | 0.4 | 1.7 |
| Crispy Medley, Waitrose* | 1 Serving/50g | 7.0 | 0.0 | 15 | 0.8 | 1.7 | 0.5 | 0.9 |
| Crunchy, Basics, Sainsbury's* | 1 Pack/200g | 40.0 | 0.0 | 20 | 1.3 | 3.4 | 0.2 | 2.2 |
| Crunchy, Fully Prepared, Sainsbury's* | ½ Pack/150g | 24.0 | 0.0 | 16 | 1.1 | 3.0 | 0.1 | 1.7 |
| Crunchy, Simple, M & S* | 1 Serving/50g | 7.0 | 0.0 | 15 | 1.0 | 1.6 | 0.5 | 1.8 |
| Crunchy, Value, Tesco* | 1 Serving/56g | 11.0 | 0.0 | 19 | 1.2 | 2.8 | 0.3 | 2.1 |
| Crunchy, Waitrose* | ½ Pack100g | 18.0 | 0.0 | 18 | 1.0 | 2.6 | 0.4 | 1.5 |

| SALAD | Measure INFO/WEIGHT | per Measure KCAL | FAT | Nutrition Values per 100g / 100ml KCAL | PROT | CARB | FAT | FIBRE |
|---|---|---|---|---|---|---|---|---|
| Crunchy Layered, Tesco* | 1 Serving/54g | 15.0 | 0.0 | 27 | 1.1 | 4.9 | 0.3 | 1.7 |
| Edamame & Butterbean, TTD, Sainsbury's* | 1 Pack/185g | 179.0 | 5.0 | 97 | 6.6 | 11.8 | 2.6 | 3.2 |
| Edamame Bean, Oriental Style, Asda* | 1 Pack/220g | 183.0 | 8.0 | 83 | 4.8 | 7.3 | 3.8 | 4.0 |
| Egg & Baby Spinach, Waitrose* | 1 Pack/215g | 167.0 | 13.0 | 78 | 3.5 | 1.8 | 6.3 | 1.0 |
| Egg & Coleslaw, Boots* | 1 Pot/233g | 405.0 | 37.0 | 174 | 3.0 | 4.6 | 16.0 | 1.0 |
| Egg & Ham, With Salad Cream Dressing, M & S* | 1 Pack/240g | 168.0 | 8.0 | 70 | 5.2 | 4.0 | 3.5 | 0.6 |
| Egg & Potato, Fresh, M & S* | 1 Serving/250g | 150.0 | 7.0 | 60 | 3.0 | 4.6 | 2.9 | 0.9 |
| Endive & Radicchio, Somerfield* | 1 Pack/150g | 19.0 | 0.0 | 13 | 2.0 | 1.0 | 0.0 | 0.0 |
| English Garden, Tesco* | 1 Serving/180g | 22.0 | 0.0 | 12 | 0.7 | 1.8 | 0.2 | 0.7 |
| Exotic, with Mango & Chilli Dressing, Co-Op* | ½ Pack/65g | 25.0 | 0.0 | 38 | 0.6 | 7.7 | 0.6 | 0.8 |
| Family, Florette* | 1 Serving/50g | 14.0 | 0.0 | 29 | 1.1 | 5.5 | 0.2 | 3.0 |
| Feta Cheese & Sunblushed Tomato, M & S* | 1 Serving/190g | 361.0 | 21.0 | 190 | 5.5 | 17.2 | 11.1 | 2.1 |
| Florida, Retail, Average | 1oz/28g | 63.0 | 6.0 | 224 | 0.9 | 9.7 | 20.5 | 1.0 |
| Four Bean, Finest, Tesco* | 1 Pack/225g | 259.0 | 9.0 | 115 | 5.0 | 14.2 | 4.2 | 4.6 |
| Four Leaf, M & S* | 1 Serving/130g | 19.0 | 0.0 | 15 | 0.9 | 2.0 | 0.3 | 1.4 |
| Four Leaf, Tesco* | 1oz/28g | 4.0 | 0.0 | 15 | 0.8 | 1.8 | 0.5 | 0.9 |
| French Goat's Cheese, Extra Fine, Asda* | 1 Pack/185g | 462.0 | 35.0 | 250 | 8.4 | 11.4 | 19.0 | 0.8 |
| French Style, M & S* | 1 Pack/140g | 140.0 | 14.0 | 100 | 1.0 | 2.5 | 9.7 | 0.9 |
| French Style, Waitrose* | ½ Pack/82g | 149.0 | 12.0 | 182 | 5.1 | 7.2 | 14.8 | 1.8 |
| Fusion, Fully Prepared, Sainsbury's* | ½ Pack/63g | 15.0 | 0.0 | 24 | 3.7 | 0.3 | 0.8 | 3.4 |
| Garden, Classic, Morrisons* | 1 Tray/175g | 33.0 | 1.0 | 19 | 0.8 | 3.2 | 0.3 | 2.8 |
| Garden, Side, Asda* | 1 Pack/175g | 31.0 | 1.0 | 18 | 0.9 | 2.8 | 0.3 | 1.3 |
| Garden, Sweet & Crispy, Tesco* | 1 Bag/225g | 54.0 | 1.0 | 24 | 1.0 | 4.2 | 0.4 | 1.4 |
| Garden, Tesco* | 1 Serving/225g | 34.0 | 1.0 | 15 | 1.0 | 2.0 | 0.3 | 0.9 |
| Garden, Tray, Asda* | ½ Pack/88g | 16.0 | 0.0 | 18 | 0.7 | 3.1 | 0.3 | 1.6 |
| Garden, Value, Tesco* | ¼ Pack/50g | 9.0 | 0.0 | 18 | 1.0 | 2.9 | 0.3 | 2.1 |
| Garden with Watercress, M & S* | 1 Salad/80g | 10.0 | 0.0 | 12 | 1.5 | 1.4 | 0.1 | 1.4 |
| Garden with Yoghurt & Mint Dressing, GFY, Asda* | 1 Serving/195g | 51.0 | 2.0 | 26 | 1.1 | 3.2 | 1.0 | 0.0 |
| Gourmet Chargrilled Chicken & Bacon, Atkins* | 1 Pack/245g | 311.0 | 20.0 | 127 | 12.0 | 2.5 | 8.2 | 1.0 |
| Gourmet Continental, Waitrose* | 1 Serving/150g | 22.0 | 1.0 | 15 | 0.8 | 1.7 | 0.5 | 0.9 |
| Greek | 1oz/28g | 36.0 | 3.0 | 130 | 2.7 | 1.9 | 12.5 | 0.8 |
| Greek, BGTY, Sainsbury's* | 1 Serving/199g | 133.0 | 5.0 | 67 | 2.0 | 9.0 | 2.5 | 0.8 |
| Greek, Side, Waitrose* | 1 Pack/150g | 156.0 | 12.0 | 104 | 3.2 | 4.6 | 8.1 | 0.9 |
| Greek, Tesco* | 1 Serving/200g | 188.0 | 14.0 | 94 | 3.2 | 4.3 | 7.1 | 0.9 |
| Greek Style, Fresh, Food Counter, Sainsbury's* | 1 Serving/166g | 247.0 | 23.0 | 149 | 1.9 | 2.7 | 14.0 | 0.0 |
| Greek Style, Waitrose* | ½ Pack/125g | 54.0 | 3.0 | 43 | 1.9 | 4.0 | 2.2 | 1.2 |
| Greek Style, with Herb Dressing, Tesco* | 1 Pack/240g | 305.0 | 28.0 | 127 | 3.2 | 2.0 | 11.8 | 1.0 |
| Greek Style, with Houmous Dip, & Pitta, Sainsbury's* | 1 Bowl/195g | 296.0 | 17.0 | 152 | 5.4 | 12.5 | 8.9 | 2.6 |
| Greek Style, with White Wine Vinaigrette, Tesco* | 1 Pack/235g | 256.0 | 22.0 | 109 | 3.5 | 2.3 | 9.5 | 1.5 |
| Greek Style Feta, Tip & Mix, M & S* | 1 Pack/195g | 214.0 | 18.0 | 110 | 4.0 | 2.5 | 9.4 | 1.6 |
| Greek Style Layered, Perfectly Balanced, Waitrose* | 1 Pack/280g | 134.0 | 8.0 | 48 | 2.4 | 3.2 | 2.8 | 0.7 |
| Green, Average | 1oz/28g | 4.0 | 0.0 | 13 | 0.8 | 1.8 | 0.3 | 0.9 |
| Green, Complete, Sainsbury's* | 1/3 Pack/55g | 92.0 | 7.0 | 168 | 4.2 | 10.3 | 12.2 | 1.4 |
| Green, Fresh, Safeway* | ½ Pack/98g | 14.0 | 0.0 | 14 | 0.9 | 1.9 | 0.3 | 0.8 |
| Green, M & S* | 1oz/28g | 4.0 | 0.0 | 13 | 0.8 | 1.7 | 0.3 | 0.9 |
| Green, Mixed, Average | 1oz/28g | 3.0 | 0.0 | 12 | 0.7 | 1.8 | 0.3 | 1.0 |
| Green Side, M & S* | 1 Serving/200g | 30.0 | 0.0 | 15 | 0.9 | 2.5 | 0.2 | 0.0 |
| Green Side, Sainsbury's* | 1 Pack/200g | 28.0 | 0.0 | 14 | 1.2 | 2.1 | 0.1 | 1.4 |
| Green Side, Tesco* | 1 Serving/100g | 12.0 | 0.0 | 12 | 0.7 | 1.6 | 0.3 | 1.3 |
| Green with Chives, Tesco* | ½ Pack/90g | 13.0 | 0.0 | 14 | 1.0 | 1.6 | 0.4 | 1.7 |
| Ham, Antony Worrall Thompson's* | 1 Pack/202g | 257.0 | 3.0 | 127 | 9.8 | 19.1 | 1.3 | 2.7 |
| Ham & Free Range Egg, Fresh Tastes, Asda* | 1 Bowl/265g | 167.0 | 9.0 | 63 | 5.7 | 2.2 | 3.5 | 0.8 |
| Ham Hock, Waitrose* | 1 Pack/350g | 245.0 | 9.0 | 70 | 6.6 | 4.8 | 2.7 | 2.0 |

| | Measure INFO/WEIGHT | per Measure KCAL | per Measure FAT | Nutrition Values per 100g / 100ml KCAL | PROT | CARB | FAT | FIBRE |
|---|---|---|---|---|---|---|---|---|

## SALAD

| | Measure INFO/WEIGHT | KCAL | FAT | KCAL | PROT | CARB | FAT | FIBRE |
|---|---|---|---|---|---|---|---|---|
| Herb, M & S* | 1 Pack/100g | 20.0 | 0.0 | 20 | 2.9 | 1.4 | 0.4 | 1.9 |
| Herb, Organic, Sainsbury's* | 1 Serving/100g | 17.0 | 0.0 | 17 | 1.8 | 1.3 | 0.5 | 1.8 |
| Herb, Sainsbury's* | 1 Pack/120g | 22.0 | 1.0 | 18 | 2.7 | 0.8 | 0.5 | 2.2 |
| Herb, Tesco* | 1oz/28g | 4.0 | 0.0 | 16 | 1.1 | 1.8 | 0.5 | 0.9 |
| Herb Garden, Morrisons* | 1 Serving/28g | 4.0 | 0.0 | 14 | 0.9 | 1.7 | 0.5 | 0.0 |
| Honey Smoked Salmon & New Potato, M & S* | 1 Pack/270g | 270.0 | 14.0 | 100 | 5.5 | 7.5 | 5.3 | 1.5 |
| Houmous, Delicious, Boots* | 1 Pack/230g | 154.0 | 4.0 | 67 | 5.3 | 7.4 | 1.9 | 3.1 |
| Iceberg & Cabbage, Asda* | ½ Pack/125g | 24.0 | 0.0 | 19 | 1.0 | 3.1 | 0.3 | 1.5 |
| Italian, Complete, Sainsbury's* | 1 Pack/160g | 237.0 | 14.0 | 148 | 5.4 | 11.4 | 9.0 | 1.6 |
| Italian Style, Asda* | 1 Serving/20g | 3.0 | 0.0 | 15 | 1.1 | 1.6 | 0.5 | 1.2 |
| Italian Style, Organic, Waitrose* | ½ Pack/45g | 7.0 | 0.0 | 15 | 0.8 | 1.7 | 0.5 | 0.9 |
| Italian Style, Tesco* | 1/3 Pack/40g | 6.0 | 0.0 | 16 | 1.0 | 1.9 | 0.5 | 1.2 |
| Italian Wild Rocket & Parmesan, Sainsbury's* | 1 Serving/50g | 88.0 | 7.0 | 177 | 7.5 | 3.4 | 14.8 | 0.5 |
| Jardin, Tesco* | 1 Serving/50g | 7.0 | 0.0 | 14 | 0.8 | 1.8 | 0.6 | 1.4 |
| King Prawn, GFY, Asda* | 1 Serving/175g | 112.0 | 3.0 | 64 | 4.7 | 8.0 | 1.5 | 1.3 |
| King Prawn, Thai Style, M & S* | 1 Pack/295g | 265.0 | 7.0 | 90 | 4.4 | 12.6 | 2.5 | 1.3 |
| King Prawn & New Potato, COU, M & S* | 1 Pack/300g | 180.0 | 7.0 | 60 | 3.0 | 6.9 | 2.3 | 0.8 |
| King Prawn & Pasta, COU, M & S* | 1 Pack/270g | 283.0 | 6.0 | 105 | 5.9 | 15.1 | 2.4 | 2.7 |
| Layered with Egg, Somerfield* | 1 Pot/300g | 543.0 | 54.0 | 181 | 3.0 | 3.0 | 18.0 | 0.0 |
| Layered with Tuna, Somerfield* | 1 Pot/255g | 599.0 | 56.0 | 235 | 5.0 | 5.0 | 22.0 | 0.0 |
| Leafy, Organic, Sainsbury's* | ½ Pack/50g | 7.0 | 0.0 | 15 | 1.7 | 1.3 | 0.3 | 1.8 |
| Leafy, Tesco* | 1oz/28g | 4.0 | 0.0 | 14 | 1.2 | 1.5 | 0.4 | 1.9 |
| Leafy, with Tatsoi, Sainsbury's* | 1 Bag/ 115g | 17.0 | 0.0 | 15 | 1.0 | 1.6 | 0.3 | 1.7 |
| Leafy, with Tatsoi, Tesco* | 1 Serving/42g | 6.0 | 0.0 | 14 | 1.2 | 1.5 | 0.4 | 1.9 |
| Leaves, Oriental Mix, Waitrose* | 1 Bag/100g | 18.0 | 1.0 | 18 | 1.5 | 1.7 | 0.6 | 1.9 |
| Lentil & Wild Rice, TTD, Sainsbury's* | 1 Serving/100g | 181.0 | 8.0 | 181 | 4.7 | 23.6 | 7.6 | 2.5 |
| Mediterranean, Side, Sainsbury's* | 1 Pack/170g | 44.0 | 2.0 | 26 | 0.9 | 2.7 | 1.3 | 1.3 |
| Mediterranean Style, Asda* | ½ Pack/135g | 22.0 | 0.0 | 16 | 1.0 | 3.0 | 0.0 | 0.0 |
| Mediterranean Style, Morrisons* | 1 Serving/90g | 13.0 | 0.0 | 14 | 1.5 | 1.9 | 0.2 | 0.0 |
| Mexican Style Bean & Cheese, M & S* | ½ Pot/150g | 150.0 | 5.0 | 100 | 6.1 | 11.2 | 3.5 | 4.8 |
| Mixed, Florette* | 1 Serving/100g | 20.0 | 0.0 | 20 | 1.3 | 3.4 | 0.2 | 3.0 |
| Mixed, Sainsbury's* | 1 Serving/100g | 21.0 | 0.0 | 21 | 1.4 | 3.4 | 0.2 | 2.1 |
| Mixed, Tesco* | 1 Serving/100g | 24.0 | 0.0 | 24 | 1.0 | 4.2 | 0.3 | 2.0 |
| Mixed Bean, Asda* | ½ Can/145g | 126.0 | 4.0 | 87 | 5.0 | 11.0 | 2.5 | 6.0 |
| Mixed Bean, Morrisons* | 1 Serving/145g | 129.0 | 2.0 | 89 | 5.8 | 13.7 | 1.2 | 0.0 |
| Mixed Bean, Sainsbury's* | 1 Can/270g | 227.0 | 2.0 | 84 | 5.4 | 13.5 | 0.9 | 3.8 |
| Mixed Bean, Tesco* | 1 Serving/70g | 49.0 | 0.0 | 70 | 3.2 | 13.1 | 0.5 | 1.9 |
| Mixed Leaf, Asda* | 1 Serving/100g | 21.0 | 0.0 | 21 | 1.5 | 3.2 | 0.2 | 2.1 |
| Mixed Leaf, Tomato, Feta, Boots* | 1 Pack/179g | 218.0 | 17.0 | 122 | 3.7 | 5.4 | 9.5 | 1.0 |
| Mixed Leaf Medley, Waitrose* | 1 Serving/25g | 4.0 | 0.0 | 15 | 0.8 | 1.7 | 0.5 | 1.4 |
| Mixed Leaf Tomato & Olive, Tesco* | 1 Serving/170g | 150.0 | 13.0 | 88 | 1.0 | 3.4 | 7.8 | 2.0 |
| Mixed Leaf with Olive Oil Dressing, Pizza Express* | 1 Pack/240g | 326.0 | 34.0 | 136 | 0.9 | 2.1 | 14.1 | 0.7 |
| Mixed Leaves, Bondelle* | 1 Serving/50g | 10.0 | 0.0 | 21 | 1.4 | 3.3 | 0.2 | 0.0 |
| Mixed Pepper, Asda* | ½ Pack/100g | 24.0 | 0.0 | 24 | 1.0 | 4.3 | 0.3 | 1.7 |
| Mixed Vegetable, Aldi* | 1 Serving/200g | 120.0 | 4.0 | 60 | 0.6 | 10.0 | 2.0 | 0.0 |
| Mixed with Peppers & Iceberg Lettuce, Somerfield* | 1 Pack/200g | 50.0 | 0.0 | 25 | 1.0 | 5.0 | 0.0 | 0.0 |
| Moroccan Styles, COU, M & S* | ½ Pack/100g | 160.0 | 1.0 | 160 | 5.0 | 32.8 | 1.2 | 4.8 |
| Mozzarella & Cherry Tomato, Shapers, Boots* | 1 Bowl/194g | 184.0 | 14.0 | 95 | 4.1 | 3.3 | 7.3 | 0.9 |
| Mozerella & Tomato, M & S* | 1 Serving/310g | 400.0 | 15.0 | 129 | 5.5 | 15.5 | 4.8 | 0.9 |
| Mozzarella & Rocket, Asda* | 1 Serving/265g | 435.0 | 32.0 | 164 | 7.0 | 7.0 | 12.0 | 1.5 |
| Mozzarella & Sunkissed Tomato, Tesco* | 1 Bag/160g | 270.0 | 23.0 | 169 | 4.6 | 4.3 | 14.3 | 2.1 |
| New Potato, Co-Op* | 1 Serving/50g | 97.0 | 8.0 | 195 | 1.0 | 10.0 | 16.0 | 2.0 |
| New Potato, Less Than 5% Fat, M & S* | 1 Serving/110g | 88.0 | 3.0 | 80 | 1.3 | 12.1 | 3.1 | 1.5 |

S

## SALAD

| Item | Measure INFO/WEIGHT | per Measure KCAL | FAT | KCAL | PROT | CARB | FAT | FIBRE |
|---|---|---|---|---|---|---|---|---|
| New Potato, Luxury, Morrisons* | ½ Tub/125g | 341.0 | 31.0 | 273 | 1.7 | 11.2 | 24.6 | 0.0 |
| New Potato, M & S* | 1 Serving/60g | 114.0 | 10.0 | 190 | 0.9 | 9.9 | 16.3 | 1.3 |
| New Potato, Tomato, Egg, with Salad Cream, M & S* | 1 Pack/305g | 152.0 | 7.0 | 50 | 2.9 | 7.1 | 2.2 | 1.9 |
| New Potato, Tuna & Egg, M & S* | 1 Pack/340g | 255.0 | 13.0 | 75 | 3.8 | 6.7 | 3.8 | 0.7 |
| New Potato & Free Range Egg, M & S* | 1 Pack/305g | 213.0 | 12.0 | 70 | 2.5 | 7.0 | 3.8 | 0.8 |
| New Potato & Free Range Egg, Side, Sainsbury's* | 1 Pack/290g | 174.0 | 12.0 | 60 | 2.5 | 3.1 | 4.2 | 1.4 |
| New Potato & King Prawn, M & S* | 1 Pack/210g | 220.0 | 9.0 | 105 | 5.6 | 10.2 | 4.5 | 1.7 |
| New Potato & Sweet Chilli Prawn, M & S* | 1 Pack/210g | 147.0 | 1.0 | 70 | 2.8 | 14.0 | 0.5 | 0.7 |
| New Potato & Tuna Sweetcorn, Eat Well, M & S* | 1 Pack/190g | 133.0 | 3.0 | 70 | 5.4 | 8.4 | 1.8 | 1.9 |
| New World, Finest, Tesco* | 1 Bag/125g | 24.0 | 1.0 | 19 | 1.7 | 1.9 | 0.5 | 1.1 |
| Nicoise, Tesco* | 1 Pack/260g | 286.0 | 22.0 | 110 | 3.2 | 5.3 | 8.4 | 1.4 |
| Nicoise Style, Layered, Waitrose* | 1 Bowl/275g | 129.0 | 4.0 | 47 | 2.7 | 5.8 | 1.4 | 1.0 |
| Noodle, Sweet Chilli Chicken, Shapers, Boots* | 1 Serving/197g | 256.0 | 4.0 | 130 | 11.0 | 17.0 | 2.1 | 1.1 |
| Noodle, Thai Style, BGTY, Sainsbury's* | 1 Pack/185g | 150.0 | 4.0 | 81 | 2.7 | 13.5 | 1.9 | 0.0 |
| Noodle & King Prawn, Perfectly Balanced, Waitrose* | 1 Pack/225g | 223.0 | 2.0 | 99 | 5.0 | 17.4 | 1.0 | 1.0 |
| Orchard, Panera* | 1 Serving/132g | 210.0 | 12.0 | 159 | 3.8 | 11.4 | 9.1 | 1.5 |
| Orzo, Pea & Spinach, TTD, Sainsbury's* | 1 Pot/200g | 326.0 | 13.0 | 163 | 6.6 | 20.0 | 6.3 | 2.3 |
| Orzo & Sunbaked Tomato, BGTY, Sainsbury's* | 1 Tub/276g | 292.0 | 6.0 | 106 | 3.1 | 18.5 | 2.2 | 2.5 |
| Pasta & Cheese, Asda* | 1 Serving/125g | 319.0 | 24.0 | 255 | 6.0 | 15.0 | 19.0 | 1.2 |
| Pasta & Garlic, Iceland* | 1 Serving/75g | 149.0 | 11.0 | 199 | 2.2 | 15.4 | 14.3 | 1.6 |
| Pasta & Ham, Safeway* | 1 Pot/225g | 283.0 | 10.0 | 126 | 4.5 | 16.9 | 4.5 | 0.3 |
| Pasta & Mushroom, Waitrose* | 1 Pack/200g | 320.0 | 19.0 | 160 | 4.1 | 14.0 | 9.7 | 0.6 |
| Pasta & Pepper Side, Tesco* | 1 Pack/230g | 278.0 | 15.0 | 121 | 2.4 | 13.0 | 6.6 | 1.3 |
| Pasta & Sweetcorn, Less Than 3% Fat, M & S* | ½ Pack/100g | 85.0 | 1.0 | 85 | 2.8 | 14.7 | 1.4 | 1.5 |
| Pasta & Tomato, GFY, Asda* | 1 Pack/300g | 348.0 | 9.0 | 116 | 3.0 | 19.0 | 3.1 | 1.6 |
| Pea Leaf, with Baby Mint, TTD, Sainsbury's* | 1 Serving/80g | 11.0 | 0.0 | 14 | 1.5 | 1.8 | 0.1 | 1.7 |
| Pea Shoot, Baby Cos & Batavia Lettuce, Bagged, M & S* | 1 Bag/120g | 24.0 | 1.0 | 20 | 2.6 | 0.8 | 0.5 | 2.3 |
| Potato, 30% Less Fat, BGTY, Sainsbury's* | 1 Serving/60g | 64.0 | 4.0 | 106 | 1.7 | 11.1 | 6.1 | 1.1 |
| Potato, Asda* | ¼ Pot/57g | 67.0 | 4.0 | 117 | 0.9 | 12.5 | 7.0 | 1.1 |
| Potato, Chunky, Somerfield* | 1oz/28g | 59.0 | 6.0 | 212 | 1.0 | 3.0 | 22.0 | 0.0 |
| Potato, Creamy, Asda* | 1oz/28g | 61.0 | 5.0 | 219 | 1.0 | 11.9 | 18.6 | 0.7 |
| Potato, Creamy, Waitrose* | 1 Serving/100g | 163.0 | 12.0 | 163 | 1.3 | 12.7 | 11.9 | 1.1 |
| Potato, Finest, Tesco* | 1 Tub/250g | 587.0 | 51.0 | 235 | 2.4 | 9.7 | 20.6 | 1.2 |
| Potato, GFY, Asda* | ½ Pack/125g | 145.0 | 9.0 | 116 | 1.3 | 12.0 | 7.0 | 0.0 |
| Potato, Heinz* | ½ Can/97g | 137.0 | 8.0 | 141 | 1.4 | 14.8 | 8.5 | 0.8 |
| Potato, HL, Tesco* | 1 Tub/250g | 287.0 | 12.0 | 115 | 1.7 | 15.4 | 4.8 | 1.2 |
| Potato, Less Than 4% Fat, Safeway* | 1 Serving/250g | 212.0 | 7.0 | 85 | 2.1 | 13.1 | 2.7 | 0.9 |
| Potato, Light Choices, Tesco* | 1 Pack/100g | 110.0 | 6.0 | 110 | 1.3 | 12.5 | 5.9 | 0.9 |
| Potato, Luxury, Asda* | 1 Serving/50g | 118.0 | 10.0 | 237 | 1.0 | 11.0 | 21.0 | 0.0 |
| Potato, M & S* | 1oz/28g | 55.0 | 5.0 | 195 | 1.2 | 8.5 | 17.3 | 1.3 |
| Potato, Perfectly Balanced, Waitrose* | ½ Pot/125g | 99.0 | 4.0 | 79 | 2.4 | 10.5 | 3.0 | 1.0 |
| Potato, Salad Bar, Asda* | 1oz/28g | 52.0 | 4.0 | 187 | 0.6 | 11.6 | 15.4 | 1.1 |
| Potato, Side, Waitrose* | 1 Pack/250g | 181.0 | 11.0 | 72 | 3.0 | 5.2 | 4.4 | 1.0 |
| Potato, Tesco* | 1 Serving/100g | 165.0 | 13.0 | 165 | 1.3 | 9.5 | 13.5 | 1.3 |
| Potato, with Onions & Chives, Co-Op* | 1 Serving/50g | 80.0 | 6.0 | 160 | 1.0 | 12.0 | 12.0 | 1.0 |
| Potato & Cheese, Sainsbury's* | 1 Serving/125g | 200.0 | 16.0 | 160 | 2.7 | 7.9 | 13.1 | 3.4 |
| Potato & Egg, Fresh, Safeway* | 1 Serving/105g | 84.0 | 4.0 | 80 | 8.4 | 3.0 | 3.6 | 1.6 |
| Potato & Egg, with Mayonnaise, Tesco* | ½ Tub/150g | 115.0 | 9.0 | 77 | 2.9 | 3.1 | 5.7 | 1.2 |
| Potato Baby, with Mint, TTD, Sainsbury's* | 1 Serving/100g | 204.0 | 17.0 | 204 | 2.0 | 10.8 | 17.0 | 0.7 |
| Potato Layered, Tesco* | 1 Pack/350g | 283.0 | 17.0 | 81 | 1.3 | 7.8 | 4.9 | 1.3 |
| Potato with Mayonnaise, Retail | 1oz/28g | 80.0 | 7.0 | 287 | 1.5 | 11.4 | 26.5 | 0.8 |
| Potato with Reduced Calorie Dressing, Retail | 1oz/28g | 27.0 | 1.0 | 97 | 1.3 | 14.8 | 4.1 | 0.8 |
| Prawn, King, with Noodles, Delicious, Boots* | 1 Pack/228g | 251.0 | 4.0 | 110 | 6.3 | 18.0 | 1.6 | 1.8 |

| | Measure INFO/WEIGHT | per Measure KCAL | per Measure FAT | Nutrition Values per 100g / 100ml KCAL | PROT | CARB | FAT | FIBRE |
|---|---|---|---|---|---|---|---|---|
| **SALAD** | | | | | | | | |
| Prawn, King & Rice Noodle, M & S* | 1 Pack/320g | 208.0 | 3.0 | 65 | 2.9 | 11.6 | 0.8 | 0.9 |
| Prawn, Layered, Sainsbury's* | 1 Pack/275g | 355.0 | 21.0 | 129 | 3.6 | 11.2 | 7.7 | 1.1 |
| Prawn, Layered, Single Size, Asda* | 1 Serving/197g | 217.0 | 10.0 | 110 | 4.3 | 12.0 | 5.0 | 1.0 |
| Prawn, Tesco* | 1 Pack/280g | 314.0 | 14.0 | 112 | 4.7 | 12.0 | 5.0 | 0.9 |
| Prawn & Avocado, M & S* | 1 Serving/220g | 176.0 | 15.0 | 80 | 3.0 | 2.0 | 6.8 | 3.1 |
| Prawn Cocktail, HL, Tesco* | 1 Serving/300g | 279.0 | 3.0 | 93 | 5.7 | 15.3 | 1.0 | 2.0 |
| Prawn Cocktail, Shapers, Boots* | 1 Pack/245g | 120.0 | 6.0 | 49 | 4.7 | 2.2 | 2.4 | 0.7 |
| Prawn Cocktail, Tesco* | 1 Pack/300g | 360.0 | 18.0 | 120 | 5.7 | 10.9 | 6.0 | 0.8 |
| Prawn Layer, M & S* | 1 Pack/220g | 143.0 | 5.0 | 65 | 4.3 | 6.9 | 2.1 | 1.4 |
| Prawn Satay & Noodle, Tesco* | 1 Serving/250g | 320.0 | 17.0 | 128 | 7.1 | 9.5 | 6.8 | 1.2 |
| Primavera, Finest, Tesco* | 1 Pack/100g | 25.0 | 1.0 | 25 | 2.4 | 2.4 | 0.6 | 2.6 |
| Rainbow, Sainsbury's* | 1 Pack/215g | 300.0 | 15.0 | 140 | 5.5 | 13.8 | 6.9 | 3.9 |
| Red Hot, Very Special, Asda* | 1 Serving/85g | 9.0 | 0.0 | 11 | 1.9 | 0.9 | 0.0 | 1.4 |
| Ribbon, M & S* | 1oz/28g | 5.0 | 0.0 | 17 | 0.8 | 3.2 | 0.2 | 1.7 |
| Rice, Courgette & Pine Nut, BGTY, Sainsbury's* | 1/3 Pot/65g | 68.0 | 1.0 | 105 | 2.7 | 20.0 | 1.6 | 1.5 |
| Rocket, Leafy, Asda* | 1 Serving/75g | 10.0 | 0.0 | 13 | 1.5 | 1.4 | 0.1 | 1.8 |
| Rocket, Morrisons* | 1 Serving/100g | 14.0 | 0.0 | 14 | 0.8 | 1.7 | 0.5 | 0.0 |
| Rocket, Tesco* | 1oz/28g | 4.0 | 0.0 | 14 | 0.8 | 1.7 | 0.5 | 0.9 |
| Rocket, Wild, Safeway* | 1 Serving/25g | 6.0 | 0.0 | 25 | 3.3 | 2.3 | 0.3 | 1.7 |
| Ruby, Tesco* | 1 Serving/48g | 12.0 | 0.0 | 25 | 1.4 | 4.1 | 0.4 | 2.2 |
| Salad, Bistro, Somerfield* | ½ Pack/50g | 7.0 | 0.0 | 14 | 0.8 | 1.6 | 0.5 | 1.4 |
| Santa Plum Tomato with Dressing, M & S* | 1 Pack/225g | 135.0 | 11.0 | 60 | 0.9 | 3.1 | 4.8 | 0.9 |
| Santa Tomato, Side, M & S* | 1 Pack/225g | 146.0 | 12.0 | 65 | 0.8 | 3.3 | 5.5 | 0.9 |
| Seafood, Marinated, M & S* | 1 Serving/90g | 108.0 | 6.0 | 120 | 13.4 | 2.3 | 6.4 | 0.8 |
| Seafood, Marinated, Waitrose* | 1 Tub/160g | 235.0 | 11.0 | 147 | 16.3 | 5.5 | 6.6 | 0.0 |
| Seasonal, Organic, Waitrose* | ¼ Pack/25g | 4.0 | 0.0 | 15 | 0.8 | 1.7 | 0.5 | 0.9 |
| Selection, Fresh, M & S* | 1 Pack/230g | 32.0 | 1.0 | 14 | 0.7 | 2.1 | 0.3 | 0.9 |
| Selection, Side, M & S* | 1 Serving/255g | 153.0 | 13.0 | 60 | 1.1 | 2.5 | 5.0 | 1.3 |
| Shredded Beetroot, Asda* | 1 Serving/140g | 29.0 | 0.0 | 21 | 1.1 | 3.5 | 0.3 | 1.5 |
| Simply Chicken, Ginsters* | 1 Pack/187g | 317.0 | 7.0 | 170 | 11.4 | 22.7 | 3.7 | 0.0 |
| Skipjack Tuna, John West* | 1 Can/192g | 190.0 | 12.0 | 99 | 7.3 | 3.7 | 6.1 | 0.0 |
| Smoked Ham, Weight Watchers* | 1 Pack/181g | 233.0 | 4.0 | 129 | 11.0 | 16.6 | 2.0 | 3.0 |
| Spicy Bean, Tesco* | 1 Serving/125g | 111.0 | 3.0 | 89 | 4.9 | 12.1 | 2.3 | 2.5 |
| Spicy Chickpea, BGTY, Sainsbury's* | ½ Pack/125g | 119.0 | 2.0 | 95 | 4.7 | 15.3 | 1.7 | 5.5 |
| Spicy Chickpea & Halloumi, Cranks* | 1 Pack/238g | 295.0 | 11.0 | 124 | 5.0 | 15.5 | 4.7 | 2.6 |
| Spicy Rice, Waitrose* | 1 Serving/200g | 318.0 | 13.0 | 159 | 3.2 | 21.7 | 6.6 | 0.9 |
| Spinach, Rocket, & Watercress, Asda* | 1 Serving/100g | 21.0 | 1.0 | 21 | 2.8 | 1.2 | 0.6 | 1.9 |
| Spinach, Waitrose* | 1 Pack/100g | 25.0 | 1.0 | 25 | 2.8 | 1.6 | 0.8 | 2.1 |
| Spinach, Watercress & Rocket, Safeway* | 1 Serving/60g | 14.0 | 0.0 | 24 | 3.0 | 1.5 | 0.7 | 1.8 |
| Spring, American Style, M & S* | 1 Serving/60g | 9.0 | 0.0 | 15 | 1.9 | 1.4 | 0.2 | 1.3 |
| Sugar Plum Tomato, Fresh, Safeway* | 1 Serving/160g | 46.0 | 2.0 | 29 | 1.1 | 3.2 | 1.3 | 1.2 |
| Summer, M & S* | 1oz/28g | 6.0 | 0.0 | 20 | 0.8 | 3.6 | 0.4 | 1.2 |
| Sweet, Crunchy, Mixed, Co-Op* | 1 Serving/100g | 30.0 | 0.0 | 30 | 1.0 | 6.0 | 0.2 | 2.0 |
| Sweet, Layered, Tesco* | 1 Serving/285g | 80.0 | 1.0 | 28 | 1.1 | 5.0 | 0.4 | 1.6 |
| Sweet, Shredded, Tesco* | 1 Serving/100g | 20.0 | 0.0 | 20 | 1.1 | 2.9 | 0.4 | 1.9 |
| Sweet & Crispy, M & S* | 1 Serving/140g | 49.0 | 1.0 | 35 | 1.7 | 4.7 | 1.0 | 1.6 |
| Sweet & Crispy, Side, Sainsbury's* | ¼ Bag/93g | 23.0 | 0.0 | 25 | 1.3 | 4.4 | 0.2 | 2.2 |
| Sweet & Crunchy, Co-Op* | 1 Serving/100g | 20.0 | 0.0 | 20 | 1.0 | 3.0 | 0.5 | 1.0 |
| Sweet & Crunchy, Sainsbury's* | 1 Pack/150g | 22.0 | 0.0 | 15 | 0.9 | 2.6 | 0.1 | 1.8 |
| Sweet & Crunchy, Tesco* | 1 Pack/285g | 54.0 | 1.0 | 19 | 0.8 | 3.3 | 0.4 | 1.9 |
| Sweet & Sour Prawn Noodle, HE, Tesco* | 1 Pack/190g | 122.0 | 1.0 | 64 | 5.0 | 9.4 | 0.7 | 0.4 |
| Sweet Carrot, 3% Fat, M & S* | 1oz/28g | 21.0 | 0.0 | 75 | 1.3 | 16.7 | 1.2 | 1.4 |
| Sweet Leaf, Fully Prepared, Fresh, Sainsbury's* | ¼ Pack/75g | 12.0 | 0.0 | 16 | 0.8 | 3.0 | 0.1 | 2.1 |

S

| | Measure INFO/WEIGHT | per Measure KCAL | FAT | Nutrition Values per 100g / 100ml KCAL | PROT | CARB | FAT | FIBRE |
|---|---|---|---|---|---|---|---|---|
| **SALAD** | | | | | | | | |
| Sweet Leaf, M & S* | 1 Pack/110g | 38.0 | 1.0 | 35 | 1.5 | 5.3 | 0.8 | 2.1 |
| Sweet Leaf, Sainsbury's* | 1 Serving/100g | 21.0 | 0.0 | 21 | 0.8 | 3.2 | 0.5 | 1.5 |
| Sweet Leaf & Carrot, Asda* | ½ Pack/164g | 34.0 | 0.0 | 21 | 0.9 | 3.6 | 0.3 | 1.4 |
| Sweet Leafy, Organic, Tesco* | 1 Serving/250g | 45.0 | 1.0 | 18 | 0.8 | 2.7 | 0.4 | 1.9 |
| Sweet Pepper, Medley, Waitrose* | ½ Pack/100g | 22.0 | 0.0 | 22 | 0.9 | 3.8 | 0.4 | 1.5 |
| Sweet Pepper Side, Tesco* | 1 Serving/54g | 22.0 | 0.0 | 41 | 1.3 | 8.0 | 0.4 | 2.1 |
| Sweet Pepper with Corn, Tesco* | 1 Pack/270g | 103.0 | 1.0 | 38 | 1.3 | 7.2 | 0.5 | 1.5 |
| Tabbouleh, HL, Tesco* | 1 Serving/200g | 194.0 | 4.0 | 97 | 3.5 | 16.8 | 1.8 | 1.3 |
| Tabbouleh & Feta, Tesco* | 1 Pack/225g | 301.0 | 11.0 | 134 | 5.4 | 16.7 | 5.0 | 0.6 |
| Tabbouleh Feta, Finest, Tesco* | 1 Pack/225g | 265.0 | 12.0 | 118 | 4.2 | 13.7 | 5.2 | 0.6 |
| Tabbouleh Style, Perfectly Balanced, Waitrose* | 1 Pack/225g | 234.0 | 9.0 | 104 | 2.8 | 14.3 | 3.9 | 2.6 |
| Tenderleaf, Waitrose* | 1 Serving/200g | 30.0 | 1.0 | 15 | 0.9 | 1.6 | 0.5 | 1.1 |
| Tenderleaf, with Mizuna, Sainsbury's* | 1 Serving/50g | 10.0 | 0.0 | 20 | 3.6 | 0.2 | 0.6 | 2.2 |
| Three Bean, Pot, Tesco* | 1 Pot/210g | 204.0 | 9.0 | 97 | 4.1 | 10.2 | 4.4 | 2.3 |
| Three Bean, with Mint Vinaigrette, M & S* | 1 Pack/250g | 175.0 | 6.0 | 70 | 5.9 | 6.4 | 2.4 | 13.0 |
| Three Bean & Mint, Finest, Tesco* | ½ Pot/115g | 150.0 | 6.0 | 130 | 7.9 | 12.6 | 5.2 | 5.0 |
| Three Leaf Blend, Sainsbury's* | 1 Pack/50g | 9.0 | 0.0 | 19 | 1.7 | 1.8 | 0.6 | 1.2 |
| Tiger Prawn & Pasta, GFY, Asda* | 1 Serving/200g | 250.0 | 6.0 | 125 | 4.6 | 20.0 | 2.9 | 2.0 |
| Tomato, Lettuce & Cucumber, Classics, M & S* | 1 Serving/275g | 151.0 | 12.0 | 55 | 0.9 | 3.3 | 4.2 | 1.6 |
| Tomato & Onion | 1oz/28g | 20.0 | 2.0 | 72 | 0.8 | 4.0 | 6.1 | 1.0 |
| Tuna, Breton Style, Snack Pot, Carb Check, Heinz* | 1 Pot/219g | 239.0 | 14.0 | 109 | 8.4 | 4.6 | 6.3 | 1.5 |
| Tuna, HE, Tesco* | 1 Serving/300g | 399.0 | 22.0 | 133 | 6.2 | 10.5 | 7.3 | 0.9 |
| Tuna, Layered, Tesco* | 1 Serving/370g | 466.0 | 29.0 | 126 | 4.4 | 9.4 | 7.9 | 1.0 |
| Tuna, with Lemon Dressing, Tesco* | 1 Serving/300g | 282.0 | 24.0 | 94 | 4.2 | 1.4 | 8.0 | 1.0 |
| Tuna & Three Bean, Healthily Balanced, M & S* | 1 Serving/350g | 332.0 | 10.0 | 95 | 8.7 | 8.8 | 2.9 | 4.6 |
| Tuna & Tomato, Boots* | 1 Pack/171g | 150.0 | 10.0 | 88 | 6.5 | 2.0 | 6.0 | 1.0 |
| Tuna & Vegetable, Tesco* | ½ Can/140g | 189.0 | 10.0 | 135 | 9.0 | 8.5 | 7.2 | 3.3 |
| Tuna Nicoise, BGTY, Sainsbury's* | 1 Pack/300g | 315.0 | 6.0 | 105 | 6.3 | 15.5 | 2.0 | 2.5 |
| Tuna Nicoise, Finest, Tesco* | 1 Serving/250g | 430.0 | 23.0 | 172 | 8.5 | 13.3 | 9.4 | 0.8 |
| Tuna Nicoise, No Mayonnaise, Shapers, Boots* | 1 Pack/276g | 133.0 | 4.0 | 48 | 4.0 | 5.0 | 1.3 | 0.8 |
| Tuscan Style Bean & Sunblush Tomato, Waitrose* | 1 Pot/225g | 308.0 | 11.0 | 137 | 5.6 | 17.9 | 4.8 | 1.0 |
| Vegetable, Canned | 1oz/28g | 40.0 | 3.0 | 143 | 1.6 | 13.0 | 9.8 | 1.2 |
| Vegetable, Heinz* | 1 Can/195g | 259.0 | 17.0 | 133 | 1.5 | 12.6 | 8.5 | 1.3 |
| Waldorf, Average | 1 Serving/100g | 193.0 | 18.0 | 193 | 1.4 | 7.5 | 17.7 | 1.3 |
| Watercress, Baby Spinach & Rocket, Somerfield* | 1 Serving/100g | 25.0 | 1.0 | 25 | 3.0 | 1.2 | 0.9 | 1.7 |
| Watercress, Morrisons* | 1 Bag/100g | 17.0 | 1.0 | 17 | 1.7 | 1.2 | 0.7 | 0.0 |
| Watercress, Mustard Leaf & Mizuna, M & S* | ½ Pack/60g | 9.0 | 0.0 | 15 | 2.4 | 0.4 | 0.3 | 3.0 |
| Watercress, Spinach & Rocket, Tesco* | 1 Serving/30g | 7.0 | 0.0 | 22 | 3.0 | 0.8 | 0.8 | 1.9 |
| Watercress, Spinach & Rocket, Waitrose* | 1 Bag/145g | 30.0 | 1.0 | 21 | 2.2 | 1.2 | 0.8 | 1.5 |
| Watercress & Spinach, Asda* | 1 Serving/50g | 10.0 | 0.0 | 21 | 2.8 | 1.2 | 0.6 | 1.9 |
| Wild Rocket & Chard, Waitrose* | ½ Bag/53g | 8.0 | 0.0 | 15 | 0.8 | 1.7 | 0.5 | 1.4 |
| **SALAD BOWL** | | | | | | | | |
| Chicken & Bacon, Layered, Tesco* | 1 Serving/350g | 437.0 | 23.0 | 125 | 5.3 | 10.2 | 6.7 | 1.8 |
| Coleslaw, M & S* | 1 Pack/325g | 292.0 | 24.0 | 90 | 1.3 | 4.9 | 7.4 | 1.3 |
| Coleslaw, Tesco* | 1 Bowl/300g | 327.0 | 30.0 | 109 | 1.0 | 3.4 | 10.1 | 1.3 |
| Egg Layered, Tesco* | 1 Pack/410g | 726.0 | 58.0 | 177 | 4.2 | 8.4 | 14.1 | 1.3 |
| French Style, Way to Five, Sainsbury's* | 1 Pack/264g | 103.0 | 6.0 | 39 | 0.7 | 4.2 | 2.2 | 2.2 |
| Goats Cheese, Sainsbury's* | 1 Serving/100g | 161.0 | 12.0 | 161 | 5.8 | 7.6 | 11.9 | 1.3 |
| Greek Style, M & S* | 1 Bowl/255g | 242.0 | 21.0 | 95 | 2.5 | 2.4 | 8.2 | 0.7 |
| Greek Style, Somerfield* | 1 Bowl/225g | 178.0 | 14.0 | 79 | 2.2 | 3.5 | 6.2 | 1.1 |
| Honey & Mustard Chicken, Fresh, Sainsbury's* | 1 Serving/300g | 408.0 | 24.0 | 136 | 5.9 | 10.3 | 7.9 | 1.7 |
| Italian Avocado & Tomato, Sainsbury's* | 1 Bowl/180g | 97.0 | 5.0 | 54 | 1.0 | 6.7 | 2.6 | 1.3 |
| Mushrooms in Tomato Sauce, Sainsbury's* | 1 Serving/100g | 72.0 | 5.0 | 72 | 2.5 | 3.3 | 4.8 | 0.5 |

S

| | Measure INFO/WEIGHT | per Measure KCAL | FAT | Nutrition Values per 100g / 100ml KCAL | PROT | CARB | FAT | FIBRE |
|---|---|---|---|---|---|---|---|---|
| **SALAD BOWL** | | | | | | | | |
| Prawn, Sainsbury's* | 1 Bowl/400g | 632.0 | 47.0 | 158 | 3.7 | 9.4 | 11.7 | 1.2 |
| Red Cheddar & Edam, Way to Five, Sainsbury's* | ½ Pack/224g | 240.0 | 9.0 | 107 | 4.4 | 12.8 | 4.2 | 1.1 |
| Tomato, Sainsbury's* | ½ Bowl/150g | 93.0 | 7.0 | 62 | 0.9 | 4.4 | 4.5 | 1.6 |
| Tomato, Way to Five, Sainsbury's* | 1 Bowl/300g | 174.0 | 12.0 | 58 | 0.8 | 4.5 | 4.1 | 2.8 |
| Tomato & Basil, M & S* | 1 Serving/225g | 225.0 | 23.0 | 100 | 0.8 | 3.7 | 10.1 | 1.1 |
| Tuna, BGTY, Sainsbury's* | ½ Pack/175g | 180.0 | 3.0 | 103 | 7.0 | 15.4 | 1.5 | 1.7 |
| Tuna, Fresh, Asda* | 1 Serving/160g | 184.0 | 11.0 | 115 | 8.0 | 5.0 | 7.0 | 0.0 |
| Tuna, Sainsbury's* | 1 Serving/200g | 336.0 | 21.0 | 168 | 6.1 | 11.7 | 10.7 | 1.5 |
| with Crunchy Coleslaw, M & S* | 1 Pack/325g | 455.0 | 45.0 | 140 | 1.0 | 2.5 | 13.8 | 2.0 |
| **SALAD CREAM** | | | | | | | | |
| *Average* | *1 Tsp/5g* | *17.0* | *1.0* | *335* | *1.7* | *18.6* | *27.8* | *0.1* |
| *Reduced Calorie, Average* | *1 Tsp/5g* | *6.0* | *0.0* | *130* | *1.0* | *12.9* | *7.9* | *0.1* |
| **SALAD KIT** | | | | | | | | |
| Caesar, Asda* | ½ Pack/113g | 154.0 | 9.0 | 136 | 5.0 | 11.0 | 8.0 | 1.4 |
| Caesar, HL, Tesco* | ½ Pack/133g | 148.0 | 11.0 | 112 | 3.3 | 5.9 | 8.3 | 1.4 |
| Caesar, New Improved, Tesco* | ½ Pack/138g | 279.0 | 25.0 | 202 | 4.7 | 4.5 | 18.3 | 1.3 |
| Caesar, Waitrose* | 1 Bag/250g | 445.0 | 39.0 | 178 | 5.0 | 4.2 | 15.7 | 1.1 |
| Ranch, HL, Tesco* | 1 Serving/115g | 69.0 | 3.0 | 60 | 4.4 | 5.0 | 2.5 | 1.8 |
| **SALAD SEASONING** | | | | | | | | |
| Sesame Seed, Coriander & Cumin, Schwartz* | 1 Tsp/4g | 13.0 | 0.0 | 314 | 16.5 | 38.5 | 10.4 | 11.4 |
| **SALAD SNACK** | | | | | | | | |
| Chargrilled Chicken, Tesco* | 1 Pot/300g | 384.0 | 14.0 | 128 | 6.1 | 15.0 | 4.8 | 2.4 |
| Cheese & Tomato, Tesco* | 1 Pot/300g | 519.0 | 20.0 | 173 | 6.3 | 21.7 | 6.8 | 2.2 |
| Cheese Layered, Sainsbury's* | 1 Pack/190g | 397.0 | 29.0 | 209 | 5.4 | 12.4 | 15.3 | 0.0 |
| Chicken & Bacon, Tesco* | 1 Pack/300g | 501.0 | 31.0 | 167 | 7.2 | 10.9 | 10.5 | 3.2 |
| Chicken Caesar, Sainsbury's* | 1 Pack/182g | 164.0 | 9.0 | 90 | 5.9 | 5.3 | 5.0 | 1.0 |
| Chicken Caesar, Tesco* | 1 Serving/300g | 420.0 | 20.0 | 140 | 8.2 | 11.4 | 6.8 | 1.7 |
| Chicken Noodle, Sainsbury's* | 1 Snack/240g | 278.0 | 12.0 | 116 | 5.2 | 12.4 | 5.1 | 1.4 |
| Ham & Mushroom, Tesco* | 1 Pot/300g | 600.0 | 32.0 | 200 | 4.7 | 21.2 | 10.7 | 1.4 |
| Hoi Sin Chicken & Noodle, TTD, Sainsbury's* | 1 Pack/230g | 214.0 | 3.0 | 93 | 4.7 | 15.2 | 1.5 | 1.8 |
| Pasta, Cheese, Somerfield* | 1 Salad/200g | 422.0 | 28.0 | 211 | 8.0 | 14.0 | 14.0 | 0.0 |
| Pasta, Egg Mayo, Asda* | 1 Serving/180g | 364.0 | 27.0 | 202 | 4.0 | 12.8 | 15.0 | 0.3 |
| Pasta, Tuna, Asda* | 1 Serving/180g | 196.0 | 7.0 | 109 | 5.5 | 13.2 | 3.8 | 0.9 |
| Pasta, Tuna, Sainsbury's* | 1 Pot/260g | 218.0 | 4.0 | 84 | 6.0 | 11.5 | 1.6 | 2.3 |
| Pasta & Tuna, BGTY, Sainsbury's* | 1 Pack/260g | 218.0 | 4.0 | 84 | 6.0 | 11.5 | 1.6 | 2.3 |
| Roast Chicken, Tesco* | 1 Pack/300g | 324.0 | 22.0 | 108 | 6.0 | 4.8 | 7.2 | 1.9 |
| Salmon & Dill, Tesco* | 1 Pack/300g | 600.0 | 38.0 | 200 | 7.7 | 13.4 | 12.8 | 0.8 |
| Sausage & Tomato, Tesco* | 1 Serving/300g | 529.0 | 27.0 | 176 | 4.5 | 19.1 | 9.1 | 4.0 |
| Thai Prawn, Good Intentions, Somerfield* | 1 Serving/215g | 230.0 | 4.0 | 107 | 5.0 | 17.9 | 1.7 | 1.1 |
| Tuna, HL, Tesco* | 1 Serving/300g | 237.0 | 3.0 | 79 | 7.2 | 10.1 | 1.1 | 1.7 |
| Tuna & Pasta, BGTY, Sainsbury's* | 1 Pack/260g | 255.0 | 6.0 | 98 | 5.7 | 13.9 | 2.2 | 1.3 |
| Tuna & Sweetcorn, Tesco* | 1 Pack/300g | 540.0 | 18.0 | 180 | 7.3 | 23.9 | 6.1 | 0.7 |
| **SALAMI** | | | | | | | | |
| Ardennes Pepper, Waitrose* | 1 Serving/7g | 30.0 | 3.0 | 429 | 18.6 | 1.9 | 38.5 | 1.1 |
| *Average* | *1 Slice/5g* | *18.0* | *1.0* | *360* | *28.4* | *1.8* | *26.1* | *0.0* |
| *Danish, Average* | *1 Serving/17g* | *89.0* | *9.0* | *524* | *13.2* | *1.3* | *51.7* | *0.0* |
| Emiliano, Sainsbury's* | 1 Serving/70g | 209.0 | 14.0 | 298 | 28.8 | 0.1 | 20.3 | 0.0 |
| *German, Average* | *1 Serving/60g* | *200.0* | *16.0* | *333* | *20.3* | *1.6* | *27.3* | *0.1* |
| *German, Peppered, Average* | *3 Slices/25g* | *86.0* | *7.0* | *342* | *22.2* | *2.5* | *27.1* | *0.2* |
| *Healthy Range, Average* | *4 Slices/25g* | *55.0* | *4.0* | *220* | *22.3* | *0.6* | *14.3* | *0.0* |
| *Milano, Average* | *1 Serving/70g* | *278.0* | *23.0* | *397* | *25.9* | *0.9* | *32.2* | *0.0* |
| *Napoli, Average* | *1 Slice/5g* | *17.0* | *1.0* | *341* | *27.1* | *0.7* | *25.5* | *0.0* |
| Pepperoni, Italian, Morrisons* | 1 Slice/6g | 23.0 | 2.0 | 406 | 24.0 | 0.9 | 34.0 | 0.0 |

| | Measure INFO/WEIGHT | per Measure KCAL | per Measure FAT | Nutrition Values per 100g / 100ml KCAL | PROT | CARB | FAT | FIBRE |
|---|---|---|---|---|---|---|---|---|
| **SALAMI** | | | | | | | | |
| Spanish, Wafer Thin, Tesco* | 1 Pack/80g | 273.0 | 19.0 | 341 | 25.5 | 6.8 | 23.5 | 0.0 |
| Ungherese, Tesco* | 1 Serving/35g | 136.0 | 11.0 | 388 | 24.5 | 0.5 | 32.0 | 0.0 |
| **SALBA** | | | | | | | | |
| Grain, Salba* | 1 Tbsp/12g | 46.0 | 4.0 | 383 | 25.0 | 33.3 | 33.3 | 33.3 |
| **SALMON** | | | | | | | | |
| Crunchies, Tesco* | 1 Serving/112g | 211.0 | 11.0 | 188 | 9.0 | 15.9 | 9.8 | 1.3 |
| Fillets, A Malted Wholegrain Crumb, Simply, Birds Eye* | 1 Fillet/130g | 195.0 | 8.0 | 150 | 16.8 | 6.4 | 6.3 | 0.5 |
| Fillets, Cajun, Waitrose* | 1 Serving/150g | 214.0 | 10.0 | 143 | 20.6 | 0.4 | 6.5 | 0.0 |
| Fillets, Chargrilled, Sainsbury's* | 1 Serving/270 g | 270.0 | 20.0 | 243 | 20.9 | 0.2 | 17.6 | 0.0 |
| Fillets, Chilli & Lemon Pink, Northern Catch* | 1 Fillet/140g | 260.0 | 10.0 | 186 | 16.9 | 12.9 | 7.4 | 0.7 |
| Fillets, Honey Roast, Co-Op* | 1 Fillet/100g | 250.0 | 14.0 | 250 | 26.7 | 4.7 | 13.8 | 0.1 |
| Fillets, Lime & Coriander, Tesco* | 1 Pack/250g | 282.0 | 5.0 | 113 | 18.2 | 5.4 | 2.1 | 0.0 |
| Fillets, Lime & Coriander Marinade, Pacific, Sainsbury's* | 1 Serving/100g | 139.0 | 4.0 | 139 | 24.4 | 1.3 | 4.1 | 0.9 |
| *Fillets, Raw, Average* | *1 Fillet/79g* | *149.0* | *9.0* | *189* | *20.9* | *0.1* | *11.7* | *0.1* |
| Fillets, with Lemon & Herb Butter, Asda* | 1 Fillet/125g | 305.0 | 22.0 | 244 | 20.0 | 0.4 | 18.0 | 0.2 |
| Fillets, with Orange & Dill Dressing, Tesco* | 1 Serving/300g | 540.0 | 31.0 | 180 | 17.7 | 4.1 | 10.3 | 0.7 |
| Fillets, with Sea Salt & Black Pepper Butter, Safeway* | 1 Fillet/115g | 287.0 | 22.0 | 250 | 20.4 | 0.1 | 18.7 | 0.0 |
| Fillets, with Sicilian Citrus Glaze, Sainsbury's* | 1 Fillet/145g | 371.0 | 26.0 | 256 | 21.9 | 2.3 | 17.8 | 0.0 |
| *Flakes, Honey Roast, Average* | *1oz/28g* | *56.0* | *3.0* | *198* | *24.0* | *1.9* | *10.7* | *0.2* |
| Goujons, Average | 1 Pack/150g | 321.0 | 16.0 | 214 | 16.4 | 12.4 | 10.9 | 1.1 |
| Gravadlax, Finest, Tesco* | 1 Serving/70g | 125.0 | 7.0 | 178 | 22.1 | 0.2 | 9.9 | 0.0 |
| Gravadlax, M & S* | 1 Serving/140g | 294.0 | 16.0 | 210 | 18.4 | 5.3 | 11.4 | 0.5 |
| Gravadlax, Scottish, M & S* | 1 Serving/70g | 147.0 | 8.0 | 210 | 18.4 | 5.3 | 11.4 | 0.5 |
| Gravadlax, TTD, Sainsbury's* | ¼ Pack/35g | 64.0 | 3.0 | 182 | 22.9 | 1.1 | 9.5 | 0.6 |
| Gravadlax, with Mustard Sauce, Waitrose* | 1 Serving/100g | 191.0 | 11.0 | 191 | 21.8 | 1.0 | 11.1 | 0.4 |
| *Grilled* | *1oz/28g* | *60.0* | *4.0* | *215* | *24.2* | *0.0* | *13.1* | *0.0* |
| *Hot Smoked, Average* | *1 Serving/62g* | *103.0* | *4.0* | *166* | *24.0* | *0.9* | *7.2* | *0.1* |
| Lemon & Rosemary, Easy Steam, BGTY, Sainsbury's* | 1 Pack/350g | 329.0 | 13.0 | 94 | 6.4 | 9.0 | 3.6 | 1.3 |
| Lime & Coriander, Tesco* | 1 Serving/120g | 176.0 | 4.0 | 147 | 21.4 | 7.0 | 3.7 | 0.7 |
| *Mild Oak Smoked, Average* | *1 Slice/25g* | *45.0* | *3.0* | *182* | *22.6* | *0.1* | *10.2* | *0.0* |
| Moroccan Style, Light Lunch, John West* | 1 Pack/240g | 199.0 | 1.0 | 83 | 5.5 | 14.0 | 0.6 | 3.1 |
| Mousse, Tesco* | 1 Mousse/57g | 100.0 | 7.0 | 177 | 13.5 | 2.9 | 12.4 | 0.2 |
| Oak Smoked, TTD, Sainsbury's* | ½ Pack/60g | 132.0 | 8.0 | 220 | 23.3 | 0.1 | 14.0 | 0.1 |
| *Pink, Average* | *1 Serving/125g* | *162.0* | *7.0* | *130* | *19.5* | *0.1* | *5.8* | *0.1* |
| *Pink, in Brine, Average* | *1oz/28g* | *43.0* | *2.0* | *153* | *23.5* | *0.0* | *6.6* | *0.0* |
| *Poached, Average* | *1 Serving/90g* | *176.0* | *10.0* | *195* | *22.5* | *0.2* | *11.7* | *0.3* |
| Potted, M & S* | 1 Serving/75g | 184.0 | 15.0 | 245 | 17.1 | 0.5 | 19.4 | 1.2 |
| *Red, Average* | *½ Can/90g* | *141.0* | *7.0* | *156* | *20.4* | *0.1* | *8.2* | *0.1* |
| *Red, in Brine, Average* | *1oz/28g* | *47.0* | *2.0* | *169* | *22.4* | *0.0* | *8.9* | *0.0* |
| Rillettes, John West* | ½ Can/62g | 169.0 | 15.0 | 272 | 14.9 | 0.1 | 23.5 | 0.0 |
| Roasted. Slices, Tesco* | 1 Slice/33g | 71.0 | 3.0 | 215 | 26.7 | 2.7 | 10.5 | 1.9 |
| Roasties, Lemon & Pepper, Hot Smoked, Scottish, Asda* | 1 Pack/100g | 195.0 | 8.0 | 195 | 26.0 | 5.5 | 7.7 | 0.5 |
| Scottish Lochmuir Sashimi Smoked, M & S* | 1 Pack/130g | 214.0 | 11.0 | 165 | 18.6 | 3.3 | 8.5 | 0.5 |
| Slices, Stuffed, Hot Smoked, TTD, Sainsbury's* | ½ Pack/60g | 110.0 | 6.0 | 183 | 20.3 | 2.6 | 10.2 | 0.8 |
| Smoked, Appetisers, Tesco* | 1/3 Pack/33g | 80.0 | 6.0 | 240 | 16.3 | 1.1 | 18.5 | 0.0 |
| *Smoked, Average* | *1 Serving/70g* | *126.0* | *7.0* | *179* | *21.9* | *0.5* | *10.0* | *0.1* |
| Smoked, Birch & Juniper, Sainsbury's* | ½ Pack/30g | 47.0 | 2.0 | 156 | 24.7 | 0.3 | 6.4 | 0.0 |
| *Smoked, Trimmings, Average* | *1 Serving/55g* | *101.0* | *6.0* | *184* | *22.8* | *0.2* | *10.3* | *0.0* |
| *Steaks* | *1 Serving/100g* | *180.0* | *11.0* | *180* | *20.2* | *0.0* | *11.0* | *0.0* |
| *Steamed* | *1oz/28g* | *55.0* | *4.0* | *197* | *20.1* | *0.0* | *13.0* | *0.0* |
| Tail Joint, Lemon & Herb Butter, M & S* | 1 Pack/480g | 864.0 | 55.0 | 180 | 18.8 | 0.8 | 11.4 | 0.2 |
| Zesty, with Baby New Potatoes, GFY, Asda* | 1 Pack/400g | 264.0 | 7.0 | 66 | 6.8 | 5.9 | 1.7 | 2.0 |

**S**

| | Measure INFO/WEIGHT | per Measure KCAL | per Measure FAT | Nutrition Values per 100g / 100ml KCAL | PROT | CARB | FAT | FIBRE |
|---|---|---|---|---|---|---|---|---|
| **SALMON &** | | | | | | | | |
| Spinach, Roulade, Tesco* | 1 Serving/60g | 155.0 | 14.0 | 258 | 9.5 | 1.7 | 23.7 | 0.2 |
| Vegetables, M & S* | 1 Serving/200g | 220.0 | 14.0 | 110 | 6.0 | 5.2 | 6.9 | 0.8 |
| **SALMON DINNER** | | | | | | | | |
| Fillet, Youngs* | 1 Box/395g | 332.0 | 11.0 | 84 | 6.7 | 7.9 | 2.8 | 1.6 |
| **SALMON EN CROUTE** | | | | | | | | |
| Chilled, Youngs* | 1 Pastry/200g | 531.0 | 37.0 | 265 | 9.6 | 14.8 | 18.6 | 2.3 |
| Frozen, Tesco* | 1 Serving/166g | 365.0 | 18.0 | 220 | 10.1 | 19.1 | 11.1 | 1.1 |
| Frozen, Youngs* | 1 Pastry/185g | 542.0 | 38.0 | 293 | 10.2 | 16.5 | 20.7 | 1.0 |
| Iceland* | 1 Serving/170g | 476.0 | 31.0 | 280 | 8.5 | 20.1 | 18.4 | 1.0 |
| Luxury, M & S* | 1oz/28g | 59.0 | 4.0 | 210 | 11.9 | 9.4 | 13.7 | 2.2 |
| M & S* | ½ Pack/185g | 573.0 | 41.0 | 310 | 10.4 | 17.3 | 21.9 | 0.6 |
| Retail, Average | 1oz/28g | 81.0 | 5.0 | 288 | 11.8 | 18.0 | 19.1 | 0.0 |
| **SALMON IN** | | | | | | | | |
| Dill Sauce, Youngs* | 1 Pack/435g | 265.0 | 10.0 | 61 | 6.1 | 4.2 | 2.3 | 0.1 |
| Lemon Mayonnaise, From Heinz, Weight Watchers* | 1 Can/80g | 130.0 | 8.0 | 163 | 10.2 | 6.4 | 10.6 | 0.1 |
| Lime & Coriander, Fillets, Good Choice, Iceland* | ½ Pack/150g | 189.0 | 4.0 | 126 | 19.8 | 5.1 | 2.9 | 0.8 |
| Pancetta, Wrapped, Finest, Tesco* | 1 Serving/150g | 328.0 | 26.0 | 219 | 14.9 | 1.0 | 17.2 | 0.1 |
| Tomato & Mascarpone Sauce, Fillets, Asda* | ½ Pack/181g | 279.0 | 20.0 | 154 | 13.0 | 0.8 | 11.0 | 0.6 |
| Watercress Sauce, Pink, Wild Alaskan, Sainsbury's* | ½ Pack/180g | 194.0 | 10.0 | 108 | 13.9 | 0.9 | 5.4 | 0.8 |
| Watercress Sauce, Waitrose* | ½ Pack/150g | 264.0 | 19.0 | 176 | 13.7 | 1.2 | 12.9 | 0.1 |
| White Wine & Cream Sauce, Tesco* | 1 Serving/170g | 279.0 | 19.0 | 164 | 13.5 | 2.0 | 11.3 | 1.2 |
| White Wine & Parsley Dressing, Fillets, Tesco* | 1 Fillet/150g | 291.0 | 20.0 | 194 | 17.5 | 0.3 | 13.6 | 0.6 |
| **SALMON LUNCHBOX** | | | | | | | | |
| COU, M & S* | 1 Pack/235g | 200.0 | 3.0 | 85 | 5.1 | 13.1 | 1.4 | 0.9 |
| **SALMON MEDITERRANEAN** | | | | | | | | |
| Style, Crusted, Sainsbury's* | 1 Serving/166g | 322.0 | 19.0 | 194 | 18.0 | 5.3 | 11.5 | 0.8 |
| **SALMON MOROCCAN** | | | | | | | | |
| Style, Fillets, Asda* | 1 Serving/240g | 454.0 | 29.0 | 189 | 19.0 | 1.3 | 12.0 | 0.0 |
| **SALMON PARCELS** | | | | | | | | |
| & Garlic Butter, Finest, Tesco* | 1 Serving/164g | 321.0 | 23.0 | 196 | 16.8 | 0.6 | 14.1 | 0.5 |
| Smoked, Tesco* | 1 Serving/50g | 146.0 | 13.0 | 293 | 16.4 | 0.0 | 25.3 | 0.2 |
| with Light Creamy Mousse Filling, Smoked, Tesco* | 1 Parcel/57g | 100.0 | 6.0 | 177 | 17.5 | 1.7 | 11.1 | 0.1 |
| **SALMON PLATTER** | | | | | | | | |
| GFY, Asda* | 1 Pack/400g | 376.0 | 15.0 | 94 | 7.0 | 8.0 | 3.8 | 1.4 |
| **SALMON WITH** | | | | | | | | |
| a Cream Sauce, Scottish Fillets, M & S* | 1 Serving/200g | 360.0 | 26.0 | 180 | 13.8 | 1.0 | 13.0 | 0.1 |
| Asparagus & Rice, Fillets, Perfectly Balanced, Waitrose* | 1 Serving/400g | 348.0 | 4.0 | 87 | 8.2 | 11.4 | 1.0 | 0.9 |
| Coriander & Lime, Pacific, Asda* | 1 Serving/113g | 154.0 | 3.0 | 137 | 27.0 | 0.5 | 3.0 | 0.0 |
| Garlic & Herb Butter, Tesco* | 1 Fillet/112g | 291.0 | 23.0 | 260 | 17.6 | 0.0 | 20.6 | 0.0 |
| Herb Vegetables, HE, Tesco* | 1 Pack/350g | 227.0 | 9.0 | 65 | 6.6 | 3.8 | 2.6 | 0.9 |
| Mozzarella & Tomato Crust, Just Cook, Sainsbury's* | ½ Pack/171g | 220.0 | 9.0 | 129 | 15.0 | 5.2 | 5.4 | 0.4 |
| New Potatoes, Honey Roast, Naturally Good Food, Tesco* | 1 Pack/390g | 351.0 | 14.0 | 90 | 6.8 | 7.6 | 3.5 | 1.9 |
| Pasta, Frozen, Youngs* | ½ Bag/175g | 234.0 | 8.0 | 134 | 7.4 | 16.3 | 4.4 | 1.2 |
| Penne Pasta & Dill Sauce, SteamFresh, Birds Eye* | 1 Pack/424g | 335.0 | 6.0 | 79 | 6.4 | 9.9 | 1.5 | 1.1 |
| Prawns, & Fusilli Pasta, Frozen, Youngs* | 1 Pack/375g | 439.0 | 28.0 | 117 | 5.6 | 7.0 | 7.4 | 1.1 |
| Rice, Oriental Style, M & S* | 1 Pot/210g | 252.0 | 7.0 | 120 | 5.9 | 16.5 | 3.3 | 3.3 |
| Sweet Chilli, Hot Smoked, Scottish, Tesco* | 1 Fillet/120g | 252.0 | 13.0 | 210 | 26.1 | 1.7 | 10.6 | 0.6 |
| Sweet Chilli Lime & Ginger, Simply Fish, Tesco* | ½ Pack/98g | 235.0 | 17.0 | 240 | 17.4 | 3.2 | 17.5 | 0.0 |
| Sweet Soy Sauce, Fillets, Inspired To Cook, Sainsbury's* | 1 Fillet/142g | 278.0 | 16.0 | 196 | 17.5 | 5.3 | 11.6 | 0.4 |
| **SALSA** | | | | | | | | |
| Bottled, M & S* | ½ Jar/136g | 95.0 | 3.0 | 70 | 1.2 | 12.0 | 2.4 | 1.5 |
| Chunky, Sainsbury's* | ½ Pot/84g | 43.0 | 1.0 | 51 | 1.1 | 7.8 | 1.7 | 1.2 |
| Cool, Sainsbury's* | 1 Serving/100g | 31.0 | 0.0 | 31 | 1.0 | 6.1 | 0.3 | 1.2 |

S

| | Measure INFO/WEIGHT | per Measure KCAL | per Measure FAT | Nutrition Values per 100g / 100ml KCAL | PROT | CARB | FAT | FIBRE |
|---|---|---|---|---|---|---|---|---|
| **SALSA** | | | | | | | | |
| Extra Hot, Fresh, Somerfield* | 1oz/28g | 13.0 | 0.0 | 47 | 1.0 | 8.0 | 1.0 | 0.0 |
| Fire Roasted Pepper, Somerfield* | 1 Pot/120g | 50.0 | 1.0 | 42 | 1.2 | 8.1 | 0.5 | 1.3 |
| Fresh, Asda* | 1oz/28g | 10.0 | 0.0 | 35 | 1.2 | 6.2 | 0.6 | 2.0 |
| Fresh, Sainsbury's* | 1oz/28g | 15.0 | 1.0 | 54 | 1.7 | 7.0 | 2.1 | 0.9 |
| GFY, Asda* | ½ Pot/236g | 85.0 | 1.0 | 36 | 1.1 | 7.0 | 0.4 | 0.7 |
| Hot, Fresh, Chilled, Tesco* | 1 Tub/200g | 120.0 | 5.0 | 60 | 1.4 | 7.5 | 2.4 | 1.2 |
| Hot, Primula* | 1oz/28g | 10.0 | 0.0 | 35 | 1.8 | 6.6 | 0.2 | 1.0 |
| Medium Hot, Discovery* | 1 Serving/30g | 17.0 | 0.0 | 56 | 1.4 | 11.7 | 0.4 | 0.8 |
| Mild, Heinz* | 1 Serving/20g | 16.0 | 0.0 | 79 | 1.2 | 17.9 | 0.1 | 0.8 |
| Original, From Dinner Kit, Old El Paso* | 1 Jar/226g | 71.0 | 1.0 | 32 | 1.2 | 6.0 | 0.3 | 0.0 |
| Prawn & Tomato, Fresh, Anti Pasti, Asda* | 1 Pot/150g | 100.0 | 4.0 | 67 | 8.0 | 3.1 | 2.5 | 1.3 |
| Red Onion & Tomato, Tapas Selection, Sainsbury's* | 1 Serving/22g | 17.0 | 1.0 | 77 | 3.0 | 6.0 | 4.5 | 0.9 |
| Red Pepper, Sainsbury's* | 1 Serving/85g | 31.0 | 1.0 | 37 | 1.7 | 3.8 | 1.7 | 1.5 |
| Smokey BBQ, Weight Watchers* | 1 Serving/56g | 20.0 | 0.0 | 36 | 1.1 | 7.6 | 0.1 | 2.3 |
| Spiced Mango, Ginger & Chilli, Weight Watchers* | ½ Pot/50g | 42.0 | 0.0 | 85 | 1.0 | 19.9 | 0.2 | 2.6 |
| Spicy, Less Than 3% Fat, M & S* | ½ Pot/85g | 30.0 | 1.0 | 35 | 1.3 | 5.6 | 0.8 | 0.8 |
| Spicy Mango & Lime, Morrisons* | ½ Pot/85g | 62.0 | 0.0 | 73 | 1.0 | 15.9 | 0.4 | 1.3 |
| Spicy Red Pepper, Fresh, Waitrose* | ½ Pot/85g | 27.0 | 1.0 | 32 | 1.9 | 4.1 | 0.9 | 1.6 |
| Spicy Red Pepper, Sainsbury's* | 1 Pot/170g | 54.0 | 2.0 | 32 | 1.4 | 3.2 | 1.4 | 1.3 |
| Sweetcorn, Fresh, Sainsbury's* | ¼ Pot/51g | 32.0 | 1.0 | 63 | 1.1 | 10.5 | 1.8 | 1.3 |
| Tomato, Chunky, Tesco* | 1 Pot/170g | 68.0 | 2.0 | 40 | 1.1 | 5.9 | 1.3 | 1.1 |
| Tomato, Chunky, Tex Mex, Tesco* | 1 Serving/50g | 26.0 | 1.0 | 52 | 1.0 | 6.4 | 2.5 | 1.0 |
| Tomato, Mexican Style, Dip, Morrisons* | ½ Pack/50g | 25.0 | 1.0 | 51 | 1.2 | 7.6 | 1.8 | 0.8 |
| Tomato, Onion, Coriander & Chilli, Fresh, Waitrose* | 1 Tub/170g | 110.0 | 5.0 | 65 | 1.3 | 8.0 | 3.1 | 1.2 |
| Tomato, Reduced Fat, Waitrose* | 1 Serving/1g | 0.0 | 0.0 | 27 | 1.5 | 4.7 | 0.2 | 1.4 |
| Tomato, Spicy, Worldwide Sauces* | 1 Serving/25g | 7.0 | 0.0 | 30 | 1.2 | 5.9 | 0.2 | 1.2 |
| Tomato, Vine Ripened, Tesco* | ½ Tub/100g | 47.0 | 2.0 | 47 | 1.0 | 6.7 | 1.8 | 1.1 |
| Tomato & Avocado, Chunky, COU, M & S* | ½ Pack/86g | 30.0 | 1.0 | 35 | 0.8 | 5.4 | 1.4 | 1.4 |
| Vine Ripened Tomato & Jalapeno, Sainsbury's* | ¼ Tub/50g | 34.0 | 2.0 | 68 | 1.1 | 8.0 | 3.5 | 1.2 |
| **SALT** | | | | | | | | |
| Alternative, Reduced Sodium, Losalt* | 10g | 0.0 | 0.0 | 0 | 0.0 | 0.0 | 0.0 | 0.0 |
| Sea, Organic, M & S* | 1oz/28g | 132.0 | 7.0 | 472 | 5.3 | 54.2 | 24.0 | 7.0 |
| Seasoning, Magic, Chef Paul* | ¼ Tsp/1g | 0.0 | 0.0 | 0 | 0.0 | 0.0 | 0.0 | 0.0 |
| *Table, Average* | *1 Tsp/5g* | *0.0* | *0.0* | *0* | *0.0* | *0.0* | *0.0* | *0.0* |
| **SAMBUCA** | | | | | | | | |
| *Average* | *1 Shot/35ml* | *122.0* | *0.0* | *348* | *0.0* | *37.2* | *0.0* | *0.0* |
| **SAMOSAS** | | | | | | | | |
| Chicken Tikka, Sainsbury's* | 1 Samosa/50g | 119.0 | 6.0 | 239 | 8.3 | 22.5 | 12.9 | 3.1 |
| Co-Op* | 1oz/28g | 70.0 | 3.0 | 250 | 6.0 | 34.0 | 10.0 | 2.0 |
| Dim Sum Selection, Sainsbury's* | 1 Samosa/12g | 24.0 | 1.0 | 196 | 3.4 | 28.6 | 7.6 | 2.8 |
| Indian Style Selection, Co-Op* | 1 Samosa/21g | 50.0 | 3.0 | 240 | 5.0 | 27.0 | 13.0 | 3.0 |
| Lamb, Morrisons* | 1 Samosa/50g | 144.0 | 8.0 | 288 | 9.8 | 27.0 | 15.7 | 1.5 |
| Lamb, Waitrose* | 1oz/28g | 87.0 | 6.0 | 310 | 8.5 | 18.1 | 22.6 | 0.8 |
| Vegetable, Indian Starter Selection, M & S* | 1 Samosa/21g | 60.0 | 3.0 | 290 | 5.0 | 29.0 | 16.9 | 3.3 |
| Vegetable, Large, Individual, Sainsbury's* | 1 Samosa/110g | 254.0 | 16.0 | 231 | 3.3 | 20.7 | 15.0 | 2.1 |
| Vegetable, Large, Tesco* | 1 Samosa/64g | 148.0 | 8.0 | 231 | 4.8 | 25.2 | 12.4 | 3.4 |
| Vegetable, M & S* | 1 Samosa/45g | 115.0 | 7.0 | 255 | 5.1 | 24.8 | 15.3 | 2.8 |
| Vegetable, Mini, Asda* | 1 Samosa/23g | 52.0 | 2.0 | 233 | 6.0 | 32.0 | 9.0 | 2.6 |
| Vegetable, Mini, Indian Snack Selection, Sainsbury's* | 1 Samosa/25g | 70.0 | 4.0 | 280 | 4.7 | 29.8 | 15.8 | 3.2 |
| Vegetable, Mini, Indian Snack Selection, Tesco* | 1 Samosa/32g | 76.0 | 4.0 | 238 | 4.7 | 25.5 | 13.0 | 3.3 |
| Vegetable, Mini, Waitrose* | 1 Samosa/29g | 70.0 | 4.0 | 242 | 3.6 | 27.1 | 13.2 | 3.1 |
| Vegetable, Morrisons* | 1 Samosa/60g | 101.0 | 3.0 | 169 | 4.9 | 24.1 | 5.8 | 2.0 |
| Vegetable, Retail, Average | 1 Samosa/110g | 239.0 | 10.0 | 217 | 5.1 | 30.0 | 9.3 | 2.5 |

**S**

| | Measure INFO/WEIGHT | per Measure KCAL | FAT | Nutrition Values per 100g / 100ml KCAL | PROT | CARB | FAT | FIBRE |
|---|---|---|---|---|---|---|---|---|
| **SAMOSAS** | | | | | | | | |
| Vegetable, Waitrose* | 1 Samosa/50g | 118.0 | 7.0 | 236 | 3.7 | 23.1 | 14.3 | 2.7 |
| Vegetable Lightly Spiced, Sainsbury's* | 1 Samosa/50g | 112.0 | 6.0 | 223 | 4.0 | 23.5 | 12.5 | 1.2 |
| **SANDWICH** | | | | | | | | |
| All Day Breakfast, BGTY, Sainsbury's* | 1 Pack/188g | 294.0 | 5.0 | 156 | 9.6 | 22.7 | 2.4 | 0.0 |
| All Day Breakfast, Finest, Tesco* | 1 Pack/275g | 660.0 | 42.0 | 240 | 9.7 | 16.4 | 15.1 | 1.6 |
| All Day Breakfast, Ginsters* | 1 Pack/241g | 538.0 | 27.0 | 223 | 10.8 | 20.3 | 11.0 | 0.0 |
| All Day Breakfast, HL, Tesco* | 1 Pack/223g | 328.0 | 8.0 | 147 | 11.9 | 16.8 | 3.6 | 2.7 |
| All Day Breakfast, Shapers, Boots* | 1 Pack/207g | 323.0 | 5.0 | 156 | 11.0 | 23.0 | 2.5 | 2.2 |
| All Day Breakfast, Wall's* | 1 Pack/225g | 610.0 | 35.0 | 271 | 9.2 | 24.3 | 15.4 | 1.4 |
| All Day Breakfast, Weight Watchers* | 1 Pack/158g | 298.0 | 4.0 | 189 | 11.0 | 30.2 | 2.7 | 1.9 |
| Avocado, & Spinach, M & S* | 1 Pack/242g | 580.0 | 27.0 | 240 | 4.0 | 21.0 | 11.3 | 4.8 |
| Avocado, Mozzarella & Tomato, M & S* | 1 Pack/273g | 655.0 | 36.0 | 240 | 8.8 | 21.7 | 13.2 | 2.3 |
| Bacon, & Brie, Asda* | 1 Pack/181g | 603.0 | 38.0 | 333 | 13.3 | 22.9 | 21.1 | 1.3 |
| Bacon, & Brie, Finest, Tesco* | 1 Pack/201g | 571.0 | 34.0 | 284 | 14.1 | 19.4 | 16.7 | 2.1 |
| Bacon, & Egg, Boots* | 1 Pack/179g | 480.0 | 29.0 | 268 | 12.0 | 19.0 | 16.0 | 1.4 |
| Bacon, & Egg, Co-Op* | 1 Pack/188g | 536.0 | 32.0 | 285 | 13.0 | 20.0 | 17.0 | 2.0 |
| Bacon, & Egg, Deep Fill, Ginsters* | 1 Pack/210g | 590.0 | 38.0 | 281 | 11.5 | 18.8 | 18.2 | 0.0 |
| Bacon, & Egg, Ginsters* | 1 Pack/210g | 523.0 | 24.0 | 249 | 13.2 | 22.0 | 11.6 | 0.0 |
| Bacon, & Egg, HL, Tesco* | 1 Serving/178g | 328.0 | 9.0 | 184 | 11.5 | 22.7 | 5.2 | 1.7 |
| Bacon, & Egg, Sainsbury's* | 1 Pack/215g | 535.0 | 26.0 | 249 | 12.3 | 23.2 | 11.9 | 0.0 |
| Bacon, & Egg, Tesco* | 1 Pack/188g | 481.0 | 24.0 | 256 | 14.1 | 21.0 | 12.9 | 1.9 |
| Bacon, & Tomato, COU, M & S* | 1 Pack/169g | 270.0 | 5.0 | 160 | 9.5 | 25.6 | 2.7 | 2.5 |
| Bacon, Brie, & Mango Chutney, Daily Bread* | 1 Serving/213g | 555.0 | 23.0 | 261 | 12.7 | 28.6 | 10.7 | 0.0 |
| Bacon, Cheese & Chicken, Triple, BGTY, Sainsbury's* | 1 Serving/266g | 506.0 | 17.0 | 190 | 12.7 | 20.7 | 6.3 | 2.6 |
| Bacon, Lettuce & Tomato, Weight Watchers* | 1 Pack/153g | 237.0 | 2.0 | 155 | 9.4 | 25.8 | 1.6 | 2.4 |
| Bap, Chicken, & Sweetcorn, Sainsbury's* | 1 Serving/170g | 462.0 | 24.0 | 272 | 12.5 | 24.2 | 13.9 | 0.0 |
| Bap, Chicken, Chargrilled, Malted, Co-Op* | 1 Bap/201g | 492.0 | 26.0 | 245 | 9.0 | 23.0 | 13.0 | 2.0 |
| Bap, Ham, & Salad, Co-Op* | 1 Bap/164g | 295.0 | 5.0 | 180 | 8.0 | 30.0 | 3.0 | 2.0 |
| Bap, Tuna, & Sweetcorn, Malted, Co-Op* | 1 Bap/212g | 530.0 | 28.0 | 250 | 9.0 | 24.0 | 13.0 | 2.0 |
| Beef, & Horseradish, Deep Filled, BGTY, Sainsbury's* | 1 Pack/202g | 313.0 | 5.0 | 155 | 11.4 | 22.0 | 2.4 | 2.4 |
| Beef, & Horseradish, Sainsbury's* | 1 Pack/187g | 389.0 | 13.0 | 208 | 12.0 | 24.1 | 7.1 | 0.0 |
| Beef, & Horseradish, Shapers, Boots* | 1 Pack/156g | 276.0 | 3.0 | 177 | 12.0 | 28.0 | 1.7 | 1.8 |
| Beef, & Horseradish Mayonnaise, Roast, Rare, Waitrose* | 1 Pack/197g | 415.0 | 15.0 | 211 | 12.2 | 23.1 | 7.8 | 2.0 |
| Beef, & Onion, Co-Op* | 1 Pack/221g | 530.0 | 24.0 | 240 | 11.0 | 24.0 | 11.0 | 1.0 |
| Beef, & Onion, Roast, Deep Filled, Asda* | 1 Pack/258g | 550.0 | 28.0 | 213 | 11.3 | 22.6 | 10.8 | 1.1 |
| Beef, & Onion, Roast, HL, Tesco* | 1 Pack/185g | 278.0 | 4.0 | 150 | 13.3 | 20.0 | 1.9 | 2.7 |
| Beef, & Pate, M & S* | 1 Pack/188g | 310.0 | 7.0 | 165 | 11.2 | 21.6 | 3.9 | 2.4 |
| Beef, Roast, Daily Bread* | 1 Pack/199g | 281.0 | 5.0 | 141 | 8.7 | 20.0 | 2.7 | 0.0 |
| Beef, Roast, Finest, Tesco* | 1 Sandwich/222g | 455.0 | 15.0 | 205 | 13.2 | 22.3 | 6.8 | 2.5 |
| Beef, Roast, Handmade, Tesco* | 1 Pack/223g | 439.0 | 16.0 | 197 | 12.5 | 20.7 | 7.1 | 1.6 |
| Beef, Roast, Plain, From Restaurant, Average | 1 Sandwich/139g | 346.0 | 14.0 | 249 | 15.5 | 24.1 | 9.9 | 0.0 |
| Beef, Roast, Sainsbury's* | 1 Pack/174g | 426.0 | 17.0 | 245 | 9.4 | 29.3 | 10.0 | 0.0 |
| Beef, Salt, with Gherkins, & Mustard Mayo, Sainsbury's* | 1 Pack/242g | 486.0 | 18.0 | 201 | 9.3 | 24.1 | 7.5 | 3.1 |
| Beef, Tomato & Horseradish, Asda* | 1 Pack/169g | 255.0 | 4.0 | 151 | 10.0 | 22.0 | 2.6 | 2.7 |
| Beef, Topside, Deli* | 1 Serving/191g | 447.0 | 21.0 | 234 | 15.4 | 18.3 | 11.0 | 0.0 |
| Big Breakfast, with Ketchup, Flora Light, Flora* | 1 Pack/206g | 546.0 | 28.0 | 265 | 11.1 | 25.0 | 13.4 | 1.0 |
| BLT, Asda* | 1 Sandwich/172g | 325.0 | 12.0 | 189 | 9.9 | 21.8 | 6.9 | 4.6 |
| BLT, BGTY, Sainsbury's* | 1 Pack/196g | 331.0 | 4.0 | 169 | 10.4 | 27.0 | 2.2 | 0.0 |
| BLT, Classic, Somerfield* | 1 Pack/160g | 338.0 | 6.0 | 211 | 11.2 | 33.6 | 3.5 | 3.9 |
| BLT, Classic, Taste!* | 1 Serving/150g | 345.0 | 15.0 | 230 | 9.3 | 25.2 | 9.9 | 0.0 |
| BLT, COU, M & S* | 1 Pack/174g | 278.0 | 5.0 | 160 | 9.5 | 25.6 | 2.7 | 2.5 |
| BLT, Daily Bread* | 1 Pack/171g | 344.0 | 19.0 | 201 | 9.1 | 21.6 | 11.0 | 0.0 |
| BLT, Deep Fill, Safeway* | 1 Pack/202g | 565.0 | 24.0 | 280 | 14.0 | 29.2 | 12.0 | 2.2 |

S

| | Measure INFO/WEIGHT | per Measure KCAL | per Measure FAT | Nutrition Values per 100g / 100ml KCAL | PROT | CARB | FAT | FIBRE |
|---|---|---|---|---|---|---|---|---|

## SANDWICH

| | Measure INFO/WEIGHT | KCAL | FAT | KCAL | PROT | CARB | FAT | FIBRE |
|---|---|---|---|---|---|---|---|---|
| BLT, GFY, Asda* | 1 Pack/171g | 294.0 | 6.0 | 172 | 9.0 | 26.0 | 3.5 | 1.6 |
| BLT, Ginsters* | 1 Pack/192g | 516.0 | 30.0 | 269 | 15.6 | 21.2 | 15.6 | 0.0 |
| BLT, Healthy Selection, Somerfield* | 1 Pack/150g | 217.0 | 3.0 | 145 | 9.4 | 22.2 | 2.1 | 2.5 |
| BLT, HL, Tesco* | 1 Pack/190g | 287.0 | 3.0 | 151 | 10.1 | 24.5 | 1.4 | 1.6 |
| BLT, M & S* | 1 Serving/181g | 381.0 | 15.0 | 210 | 10.7 | 23.8 | 8.1 | 1.8 |
| BLT, Salt Controlled, Shapers, Boots* | 1 Pack/180g | 290.0 | 6.0 | 161 | 9.3 | 23.0 | 3.4 | 3.0 |
| BLT, Shapers, Boots* | 1 Pack/169g | 254.0 | 6.0 | 150 | 10.7 | 18.9 | 3.7 | 5.9 |
| BLT, Tesco* | 1 Pack/203g | 520.0 | 29.0 | 256 | 11.9 | 19.5 | 14.4 | 1.5 |
| BLT, Waitrose* | 1 Pack/210g | 577.0 | 31.0 | 275 | 9.3 | 25.6 | 15.0 | 2.3 |
| Breakfast, Mega Triple, Co-Op* | 1 Pack/267g | 750.0 | 40.0 | 281 | 11.6 | 25.5 | 15.0 | 3.4 |
| Brie, & Grape, Finest, Tesco* | 1 Pack/209g | 527.0 | 32.0 | 252 | 8.5 | 20.6 | 15.1 | 1.5 |
| Brie, with Apple & Grapes, Sainsbury's* | 1 Pack/220g | 473.0 | 24.0 | 215 | 8.2 | 20.8 | 11.0 | 0.0 |
| Brunch, Eat Smart, Safeway* | 1 Pack/250g | 362.0 | 5.0 | 145 | 9.4 | 21.6 | 1.9 | 2.9 |
| Brunch, St Ivel* | 1 Pack/225g | 580.0 | 28.0 | 258 | 10.2 | 26.0 | 12.6 | 0.0 |
| Cheddar, & Celery, M & S* | 1 Pack/200g | 540.0 | 32.0 | 270 | 9.7 | 22.4 | 15.9 | 1.5 |
| Cheddar, & Coleslaw, Simply, Boots* | 1 Pack/185g | 538.0 | 33.0 | 291 | 9.2 | 23.0 | 18.0 | 1.8 |
| Cheddar, & Ham, British, M & S* | 1 Serving/165g | 395.0 | 19.0 | 240 | 15.1 | 20.0 | 11.3 | 1.7 |
| Cheddar, & Ham, M & S* | 1 Pack/165g | 396.0 | 19.0 | 240 | 15.1 | 20.0 | 11.3 | 1.7 |
| Cheddar, & Ham, Smoked, Deep Filled, Tesco* | 1 Serving/203g | 573.0 | 33.0 | 282 | 14.3 | 19.5 | 16.3 | 1.2 |
| Cheddar, & Ham, with Pickle, Smoked, Finest, Tesco* | 1 Pack/217g | 532.0 | 25.0 | 245 | 11.9 | 23.7 | 11.4 | 3.9 |
| Cheddar, & Pickle, Mature, Sainsbury's* | 1 Pack/171g | 588.0 | 27.0 | 344 | 14.3 | 38.7 | 15.8 | 7.0 |
| Cheddar, & Salad, Mature, Upper Crust* | 1 Pack/225g | 466.0 | 22.0 | 207 | .9.5 | 20.3 | 9.8 | 0.0 |
| Cheddar, & Tomato, Mature, Big, Sainsbury's* | 1 Pack/233g | 596.0 | 26.0 | 256 | 12.9 | 26.3 | 11.0 | 0.0 |
| Cheddar, & Tomato, Red, Tesco* | 1 Pack/182g | 526.0 | 32.0 | 289 | 9.2 | 24.0 | 17.4 | 1.1 |
| Cheddar, Red Leicester, & Onion, Tesco* | 1 Pack/182g | 604.0 | 39.0 | 332 | 11.0 | 23.8 | 21.4 | 2.5 |
| Cheese, & Apple, & Celery, Asda* | 1 Pack/173g | 244.0 | 5.0 | 141 | 8.0 | 21.0 | 2.8 | 2.7 |
| Cheese, & Apple & Grape, COU, M & S* | 1 Pack/186g | 270.0 | 2.0 | 145 | 8.5 | 24.9 | 1.2 | 2.0 |
| Cheese, & Celery, Shapers, Boots* | 1 Pack/181g | 288.0 | 4.0 | 159 | 11.0 | 24.0 | 2.3 | 3.0 |
| Cheese, & Coleslaw, Asda* | 1 Pack/262g | 799.0 | 51.0 | 305 | 10.1 | 22.1 | 19.6 | 3.3 |
| Cheese, & Coleslaw, Eat Smart, Safeway* | 1 Pack/169g | 245.0 | 4.0 | 145 | 10.1 | 20.7 | 2.2 | 4.0 |
| Cheese, & Coleslaw, M & S* | 1 Pack/186g | 498.0 | 32.0 | 268 | 10.2 | 17.6 | 17.4 | 3.2 |
| Cheese, & Coleslaw, Shapers, Boots* | 1 Pack/224g | 338.0 | 5.0 | 151 | 11.0 | 22.0 | 2.1 | 3.2 |
| Cheese, & Ham, & Pickle, HL, Tesco* | 1 Pack/201g | 312.0 | 4.0 | 155 | 13.1 | 21.0 | 2.1 | 1.7 |
| Cheese, & Ham, & Pickle, Shapers, Boots* | 1 Pack/184g | 318.0 | 8.0 | 173 | 13.0 | 20.0 | 4.6 | 2.5 |
| Cheese, & Ham, & Pickle, Tesco* | 1 Serving/215g | 497.0 | 25.0 | 231 | 11.7 | 20.3 | 11.5 | 1.8 |
| Cheese, & Onion, Deep Fill, Tesco* | 1 Pack/212g | 742.0 | 52.0 | 350 | 12.3 | 20.2 | 24.5 | 1.3 |
| Cheese, & Onion, GFY, Asda* | 1 Pack/156g | 317.0 | 4.0 | 203 | 14.0 | 31.0 | 2.6 | 2.7 |
| Cheese, & Onion, Light Choices, Tesco* | 1 Pack/144g | 310.0 | 9.0 | 215 | 12.7 | 26.5 | 6.5 | 3.6 |
| Cheese, & Onion, M & S* | 1 Serving/188g | 460.0 | 24.0 | 245 | 11.2 | 21.3 | 12.9 | 2.9 |
| Cheese, & Onion, Morrisons* | 1 Pack/142g | 260.0 | 2.0 | 183 | 14.1 | 27.8 | 1.7 | 2.9 |
| Cheese, & Onion, Tesco* | 1 Pack/178g | 573.0 | 38.0 | 322 | 11.6 | 21.0 | 21.3 | 3.5 |
| Cheese, & Onion, Triple, Tesco* | 1 Pack/273g | 906.0 | 58.0 | 332 | 11.0 | 23.8 | 21.4 | 2.5 |
| Cheese, & Onion, Waitrose* | 1 Pack/176g | 579.0 | 39.0 | 329 | 12.5 | 20.2 | 22.0 | 2.8 |
| Cheese, & Pickle, & Tomato, Somerfield* | 1 Pack/167g | 318.0 | 7.0 | 191 | 12.5 | 25.6 | 4.3 | 3.5 |
| Cheese, & Pickle, Heinz* | 1 Pack/178g | 543.0 | 27.0 | 305 | 13.8 | 28.4 | 15.1 | 3.8 |
| Cheese, & Pickle, Shapers, Boots* | 1 Pack/165g | 342.0 | 8.0 | 207 | 9.8 | 31.0 | 4.9 | 2.3 |
| Cheese, & Pickle, Tesco* | 1 Pack/140g | 400.0 | 19.0 | 286 | 12.7 | 27.8 | 13.8 | 1.4 |
| Cheese, & Pickle, Virgin Trains* | 1 Pack/158g | 444.0 | 20.0 | 281 | 11.5 | 31.1 | 12.4 | 0.0 |
| Cheese, & Salad, & Reduced Fat Mayonnaise, Waitrose* | 1 Pack/180g | 301.0 | 9.0 | 167 | 9.8 | 20.8 | 5.0 | 3.1 |
| Cheese, & Salad, COU, M & S* | 1 Pack/188g | 244.0 | 3.0 | 130 | 12.1 | 17.0 | 1.6 | 2.4 |
| Cheese, & Salad, Shapers, Boots* | 1 Pack/205g | 307.0 | 5.0 | 150 | 9.7 | 22.0 | 2.5 | 2.2 |
| Cheese, & Salad, Tesco* | 1 Serving/188g | 429.0 | 22.0 | 228 | 10.1 | 20.2 | 11.9 | 2.1 |
| Cheese, & Spring Onion, Asda* | 1 Pack/160g | 576.0 | 40.0 | 361 | 13.0 | 21.0 | 25.0 | 1.9 |

S

# SANDWICH

| | Measure INFO/WEIGHT | per Measure KCAL | FAT | Nutrition Values per 100g / 100ml KCAL | PROT | CARB | FAT | FIBRE |
|---|---|---|---|---|---|---|---|---|
| Cheese, & Spring Onion, Mixed, Scottish Slimmers* | 1 Pack/139g | 298.0 | 9.0 | 214 | 12.4 | 26.5 | 6.5 | 2.1 |
| Cheese, & Spring Onion, Sainsbury's* | 1 Serving/177g | 605.0 | 39.0 | 342 | 11.4 | 24.0 | 22.3 | 1.1 |
| Cheese, & Tomato, Asda* | 1 Pack/154g | 388.0 | 20.0 | 252 | 11.0 | 23.2 | 12.8 | 3.7 |
| Cheese, & Tomato, Organic, M & S* | 1 Pack/165g | 559.0 | 35.0 | 339 | 11.8 | 24.8 | 21.4 | 1.9 |
| Cheese, & Tomato, Sainsbury's* | 1 Pack/216g | 542.0 | 26.0 | 251 | 12.9 | 22.8 | 12.2 | 0.0 |
| Cheese, & Tomato, Tesco* | 1 Pack/182g | 582.0 | 39.0 | 320 | 9.2 | 22.6 | 21.4 | 1.1 |
| Cheese, Asda* | 1 Pack/262g | 618.0 | 31.0 | 236 | 12.2 | 20.3 | 12.0 | 3.0 |
| Cheese, Crunch, Scottish Slimmers* | 1 Pack/137g | 292.0 | 9.0 | 213 | 11.0 | 27.6 | 6.6 | 2.3 |
| Cheese, Ham, BLT, Triple Pack, Asda* | 1 Pack/260g | 614.0 | 31.0 | 236 | 12.2 | 20.3 | 12.0 | 3.0 |
| Chicken, & Avocado, Tesco* | 1 Serving/219g | 559.0 | 32.0 | 255 | 11.9 | 19.5 | 14.4 | 2.4 |
| Chicken, & Bacon, & Salad, Big, Sainsbury's* | 1 Pack/249g | 610.0 | 32.0 | 245 | 11.1 | 21.7 | 12.7 | 0.0 |
| Chicken, & Bacon, Antony Worrall Thompson's* | 1 Pack/191g | 577.0 | 27.0 | 302 | 16.0 | 25.9 | 14.3 | 2.1 |
| Chicken, & Bacon, Baton, Tesco* | 1 Pack/201g | 511.0 | 26.0 | 254 | 9.4 | 24.7 | 13.1 | 1.7 |
| Chicken, & Bacon, BGTY, Sainsbury's* | 1 Pack/211g | 315.0 | 5.0 | 149 | 11.7 | 20.8 | 2.3 | 0.0 |
| Chicken, & Bacon, Big Fill, Somerfield* | 1 Pack/210g | 566.0 | 28.0 | 270 | 12.0 | 25.0 | 13.5 | 2.3 |
| Chicken, & Bacon, COU, M & S* | 1 Pack/179g | 250.0 | 4.0 | 140 | 13.5 | 15.8 | 2.0 | 3.8 |
| Chicken, & Bacon, Deep Filled, Ginsters* | 1 Pack/200g | 540.0 | 32.0 | 270 | 13.1 | 18.3 | 16.1 | 0.0 |
| Chicken, & Bacon, HL, Tesco* | 1 Pack/193g | 318.0 | 6.0 | 165 | 13.5 | 19.5 | 3.2 | 2.7 |
| Chicken, & Bacon, M & S* | 1 Pack/185g | 509.0 | 27.0 | 275 | 15.9 | 20.2 | 14.7 | 2.1 |
| Chicken, & Bacon, Shapers, Boots* | 1 Pack/179g | 317.0 | 9.0 | 177 | 14.0 | 19.0 | 5.0 | 3.1 |
| Chicken, & Bacon, Tesco* | 1 Pack/195g | 486.0 | 24.0 | 249 | 14.3 | 20.0 | 12.4 | 2.7 |
| Chicken, & Bacon, Waitrose* | 1 Serving/191g | 495.0 | 24.0 | 259 | 11.8 | 25.3 | 12.3 | 2.2 |
| Chicken, & Coleslaw, Tesco* | 1 Pack/160g | 305.0 | 7.0 | 191 | 12.0 | 25.7 | 4.4 | 2.4 |
| Chicken, & Coriander, Taste!* | 1 Serving/159g | 228.0 | 5.0 | 143 | 5.6 | 23.3 | 2.9 | 0.0 |
| Chicken, & Coriander, with Lime, BGTY, Sainsbury's* | 1 Pack/168g | 282.0 | 6.0 | 168 | 10.6 | 23.5 | 3.5 | 0.0 |
| Chicken, & Ham, HL, Tesco* | 1 Serving/244g | 327.0 | 3.0 | 134 | 13.2 | 17.9 | 1.1 | 1.3 |
| Chicken, & Ham, Oak Smoked, Big, Sainsbury's* | 1 Pack/244g | 461.0 | 18.0 | 189 | 12.3 | 18.8 | 7.2 | 0.0 |
| Chicken, & Ham, Roast, Ginsters* | 1 Pack/180g | 425.0 | 24.0 | 236 | 11.2 | 18.5 | 13.6 | 0.0 |
| Chicken, & Ham, Roast, Tesco* | 1 Pack/228g | 561.0 | 32.0 | 246 | 13.3 | 16.6 | 14.0 | 1.2 |
| Chicken, & Lemon, with Mint, Delilite* | 1 Pack/179g | 325.0 | 6.0 | 182 | 12.3 | 23.1 | 3.6 | 1.7 |
| Chicken, & Mayo, The Sandwich Company* | 1 Pack/72g | 251.0 | 11.0 | 348 | 17.8 | 35.9 | 14.8 | 0.0 |
| Chicken, & Mayonnaise, Country Harvest* | 1 Pack/120g | 268.0 | 9.0 | 223 | 13.1 | 27.6 | 7.5 | 0.0 |
| Chicken, & Mayonnaise, Simply, Oldfields* | 1 Pack/128g | 357.0 | 16.0 | 279 | 12.8 | 30.2 | 12.8 | 2.1 |
| Chicken, & Pepperonata, COU, M & S* | 1 Pack/171g | 240.0 | 3.0 | 140 | 10.4 | 20.9 | 1.7 | 1.3 |
| Chicken, & Pesto, Shapers, Boots* | 1 Pack/181g | 311.0 | 4.0 | 172 | 12.0 | 26.0 | 2.3 | 1.7 |
| Chicken, & Pesto Salad, Bells* | 1 Pack/196g | 430.0 | 23.0 | 220 | 12.0 | 16.6 | 11.7 | 0.0 |
| Chicken, & Salad, COU, M & S* | 1 Pack/194g | 262.0 | 4.0 | 135 | 9.8 | 19.0 | 1.9 | 1.6 |
| Chicken, & Salad, Daily Bread* | 1 Serving/187g | 270.0 | 15.0 | 144 | 9.6 | 13.4 | 8.2 | 0.0 |
| Chicken, & Salad, Deep Filled, Asda* | 1 Pack/247g | 551.0 | 18.0 | 223 | 18.1 | 22.2 | 7.4 | 1.3 |
| Chicken, & Salad, Deep Filled, Tesco* | 1 Pack/238g | 440.0 | 19.0 | 185 | 13.1 | 14.6 | 8.2 | 2.8 |
| Chicken, & Salad, GFY, Asda* | 1 Pack/194g | 252.0 | 3.0 | 130 | 12.0 | 17.0 | 1.5 | 2.6 |
| Chicken, & Salad, Ham & Cheese, Twin, Tesco* | 1 Pack/189g | 434.0 | 22.0 | 230 | 10.8 | 21.1 | 11.4 | 2.3 |
| Chicken, & Salad, Healthy Choice, Ginsters* | 1 Serving/100g | 257.0 | 5.0 | 257 | 18.3 | 33.8 | 4.7 | 0.0 |
| Chicken, & Salad, Heinz* | 1 Pack/166g | 331.0 | 16.0 | 200 | 8.6 | 19.9 | 9.6 | 2.0 |
| Chicken, & Salad, HL, Tesco* | 1 Pack/207g | 290.0 | 4.0 | 140 | 13.9 | 16.8 | 1.9 | 2.7 |
| Chicken, & Salad, Low Fat, Heinz* | 1 Pack/166g | 246.0 | 2.0 | 148 | 11.8 | 22.3 | 1.3 | 5.3 |
| Chicken, & Salad, Low Fat, Waitrose* | 1 Pack/188g | 291.0 | 8.0 | 155 | 10.4 | 18.6 | 4.3 | 2.1 |
| Chicken, & Salad, Sainsbury's* | 1 Pack/240g | 425.0 | 14.0 | 177 | 12.1 | 18.8 | 5.9 | 0.0 |
| Chicken, & Salad, Scottish Slimmers* | 1 Pack/169g | 275.0 | 6.0 | 163 | 9.5 | 22.8 | 3.8 | 1.8 |
| Chicken, & Salad, Tesco* | 1 Pack/193g | 386.0 | 18.0 | 200 | 11.9 | 17.6 | 9.1 | 1.5 |
| Chicken, & Salad, Waitrose* | 1 Pack/208g | 406.0 | 20.0 | 195 | 10.3 | 17.1 | 9.5 | 2.5 |
| Chicken, & Salad, with Mayo, BGTY, Sainsbury's* | 1 Serving/200g | 314.0 | 5.0 | 157 | 12.0 | 21.9 | 2.4 | 0.0 |
| Chicken, & Salad, with Mayo, Yummy Food Company* | 1 Pack/154g | 275.0 | 10.0 | 178 | 11.9 | 17.8 | 6.6 | 0.0 |

| | Measure INFO/WEIGHT | per Measure | | Nutrition Values per 100g / 100ml | | | | |
|---|---|---|---|---|---|---|---|---|
| | | KCAL | FAT | KCAL | PROT | CARB | FAT | FIBRE |

## SANDWICH

| | Measure INFO/WEIGHT | per Measure KCAL | per Measure FAT | KCAL | PROT | CARB | FAT | FIBRE |
|---|---|---|---|---|---|---|---|---|
| Chicken, & Salad with Mayo, Roast, Big, Sainsbury's* | 1 Pack/269g | 559.0 | 24.0 | 208 | 11.0 | 20.9 | 8.9 | 9.0 |
| Chicken, & Stuffing, Antony Worrall Thompson's* | 1 Pack/198g | 485.0 | 28.0 | 245 | 16.0 | 13.1 | 14.3 | 2.8 |
| Chicken, & Stuffing, Light Choices, Tesco* | 1 Pack/172g | 275.0 | 5.0 | 160 | 14.4 | 18.7 | 2.8 | 6.9 |
| Chicken, & Stuffing, M & S* | 1 Pack/166g | 398.0 | 17.0 | 240 | 13.9 | 23.1 | 10.3 | 5.6 |
| Chicken, & Stuffing, Roast, Deep Fill, Tesco* | 1 Serving/220g | 532.0 | 27.0 | 242 | 14.0 | 19.0 | 12.2 | 1.3 |
| Chicken, & Stuffing, Roast, Shapers, Boots* | 1 Pack/186g | 324.0 | 4.0 | 174 | 14.0 | 25.0 | 2.1 | 3.1 |
| Chicken, & Stuffing, Roast, Tesco* | 1 Sandwich/200g | 450.0 | 14.0 | 225 | 15.0 | 24.8 | 7.2 | 1.9 |
| Chicken, & Stuffing, Roast, Weight Watchers* | 1 Pack/159g | 283.0 | 4.0 | 178 | 14.1 | 24.2 | 2.8 | 3.1 |
| Chicken, & Stuffing, Tesco* | 1 Pack/323g | 1043.0 | 59.0 | 323 | 10.4 | 29.4 | 18.2 | 1.0 |
| Chicken, & Stuffing, Waitrose* | 1 Pack/183g | 450.0 | 19.0 | 246 | 12.8 | 25.6 | 10.3 | 1.5 |
| Chicken, & Sweet Chilli, Flora Light, Flora* | 1 Pack/154g | 296.0 | 6.0 | 192 | 13.1 | 27.0 | 3.7 | 1.9 |
| Chicken, & Sweetcorn, Scottish Slimmers* | 1 Pack/147g | 289.0 | 7.0 | 197 | 11.1 | 27.4 | 4.9 | 2.2 |
| Chicken, & Sweetcorn, Shapers, Boots* | 1 Pack/180g | 324.0 | 6.0 | 180 | 12.0 | 25.0 | 3.5 | 2.0 |
| Chicken, & Sweetcorn, with Mayo, Benedicts* | 1 Pack/185g | 437.0 | 20.0 | 236 | 12.2 | 20.6 | 10.7 | 0.0 |
| Chicken, & Tomato Relish, Chargrilled, Shapers, Boots* | 1 Pack/190g | 294.0 | 6.0 | 155 | 12.0 | 20.0 | 3.0 | 3.1 |
| Chicken, & Tomato Salsa, Chargrilled, BGTY, Sainsbury's* | 1 Pack/225g | 218.0 | 4.0 | 97 | 1.5 | 15.9 | 1.8 | 2.9 |
| Chicken, & Watercress, Chargrilled, BGTY, Sainsbury's* | 1 Pack/172g | 318.0 | 6.0 | 185 | 14.5 | 24.1 | 3.4 | 0.0 |
| Chicken, & Watercress, Chargrilled, M & S* | 1 Pack/173g | 285.0 | 3.0 | 165 | 12.8 | 23.9 | 1.7 | 2.1 |
| Chicken, & Watercress, COU, M & S* | 1 Pack/164g | 266.0 | 3.0 | 162 | 12.8 | 23.9 | 1.7 | 2.1 |
| Chicken, Asian, Shapers, Boots* | 1 Pack/190g | 273.0 | 5.0 | 144 | 12.0 | 19.0 | 2.4 | 2.9 |
| Chicken, Bacon, & Avocado, M & S* | 1 Pack/242g | 508.0 | 28.0 | 210 | 10.7 | 15.8 | 11.7 | 3.2 |
| Chicken, Bacon & Lettuce, No Mayo, Light Choices, Tesco* | 1 Pack/186g | 325.0 | 7.0 | 175 | 15.2 | 19.6 | 3.7 | 2.5 |
| Chicken, Bacon & Sweet Chilli, Feel Good, Shell* | 1 Pack/174g | 366.0 | 9.0 | 211 | 14.1 | 29.2 | 5.0 | 0.0 |
| Chicken, Bacon & Tomato, BGTY, Sainsbury's* | 1 Pack/190g | 270.0 | 4.0 | 142 | 11.4 | 19.0 | 2.3 | 0.0 |
| Chicken, Beef, & Ham, Triple Pack, Tesco* | 1 Serving/272g | 583.0 | 21.0 | 214 | 12.1 | 24.3 | 7.6 | 2.0 |
| Chicken, BLT, Daily Bread* | 1 Pack/187g | 322.0 | 13.0 | 172 | 9.0 | 19.5 | 7.0 | 0.0 |
| Chicken, BLT, Deli* | 1 Pack/224g | 509.0 | 27.0 | 227 | 12.4 | 17.3 | 12.0 | 0.0 |
| Chicken, BLT, Taste!* | 1 Pack/239g | 458.0 | 20.0 | 192 | 10.3 | 19.0 | 8.3 | 0.0 |
| Chicken, Breast, BGTY, Sainsbury's* | 1 Pack/165g | 251.0 | 1.0 | 152 | 12.2 | 24.7 | 0.5 | 0.0 |
| Chicken, Breast, Millers* | 1 Pack/162g | 343.0 | 14.0 | 212 | 13.8 | 19.3 | 8.9 | 0.0 |
| Chicken, Breast, Oldfields* | 1 Pack/193g | 311.0 | 8.0 | 161 | 11.7 | 19.8 | 4.2 | 3.0 |
| Chicken, Caesar, & Bacon, Club, TTD, Sainsbury's* | 1 Pack/247g | 661.0 | 35.0 | 268 | 14.0 | 21.2 | 14.1 | 0.0 |
| Chicken, Caesar, & Salad, GFY, Asda* | 1 Pack/163g | 289.0 | 5.0 | 177 | 11.0 | 27.0 | 2.8 | 2.1 |
| Chicken, Caesar, & Salad, Sainsbury's* | 1 Pack/186g | 299.0 | 7.0 | 161 | 11.2 | 20.4 | 3.8 | 0.0 |
| Chicken, Caesar, Boots* | 1 Pack/226g | 531.0 | 27.0 | 235 | 9.8 | 22.0 | 12.0 | 1.7 |
| Chicken, Caesar, Chargrilled, Big, Sainsbury's* | 1 Pack/216g | 657.0 | 37.0 | 304 | 12.2 | 25.3 | 17.1 | 0.0 |
| Chicken, Caesar, COU, M & S* | 1 Pack/181g | 244.0 | 4.0 | 135 | 12.2 | 19.9 | 2.4 | 4.3 |
| Chicken, Caesar, Finest, Tesco* | 1 Pack/199g | 454.0 | 20.0 | 228 | 15.4 | 19.2 | 10.0 | 1.4 |
| Chicken, Chargrilled, Ginsters* | 1 Pack/209g | 431.0 | 17.0 | 206 | 11.3 | 21.6 | 8.3 | 0.0 |
| Chicken, Chargrilled, Go Foods Ltd* | 1 Pack/331g | 695.0 | 14.0 | 210 | 14.5 | 29.0 | 4.1 | 0.0 |
| Chicken, Chargrilled, No Mayo, Rustlers* | 1 Pack/150g | 228.0 | 1.0 | 152 | 16.0 | 20.1 | 0.8 | 0.0 |
| Chicken, Chargrilled, Pitta Pocket, M & S* | 1 Pack/208g | 279.0 | 7.0 | 134 | 11.2 | 14.5 | 3.5 | 1.6 |
| Chicken, Chargrilled, with Salad, Weight Watchers* | 1 Pack/181g | 264.0 | 4.0 | 146 | 11.7 | 20.0 | 2.1 | 2.2 |
| Chicken, Cheese, Bacon, Big, Sainsbury's* | 1 Pack/254g | 734.0 | 45.0 | 289 | 11.7 | 18.0 | 17.9 | 0.0 |
| Chicken, Chilli, Taste!* | 1 Pack/196g | 317.0 | 6.0 | 162 | 11.5 | 22.6 | 2.9 | 0.0 |
| Chicken, Chinese, Low Calorie, Tesco* | 1 Pack/169g | 270.0 | 4.0 | 160 | 11.8 | 22.6 | 2.5 | 2.0 |
| Chicken, Chinese, Malted Brown Bread, Waitrose* | 1 Pack/164g | 333.0 | 11.0 | 203 | 13.5 | 21.9 | 6.8 | 3.3 |
| Chicken, Chinese, Snack & Shop, Esso* | 1 Pack/178g | 409.0 | 16.0 | 230 | 13.0 | 22.8 | 9.0 | 4.0 |
| Chicken, Coronation, Indulgence, Taste!* | 1 Pack/159g | 396.0 | 19.0 | 249 | 9.1 | 26.5 | 11.8 | 0.0 |
| Chicken, Coronation, M & S* | 1 Pack/210g | 420.0 | 20.0 | 200 | 11.2 | 20.2 | 9.7 | 3.1 |
| Chicken, Coronation, Taste!* | 1 Pack/178g | 367.0 | 13.0 | 206 | 10.6 | 24.0 | 7.5 | 0.0 |
| Chicken, Creole, & Italian Leaves, Northern Bites* | 1 Pack/190g | 298.0 | 5.0 | 157 | 13.1 | 22.1 | 2.4 | 2.4 |
| Chicken, Flame Grilled, Rustlers* | 1 Pack/150g | 346.0 | 14.0 | 231 | 16.3 | 20.1 | 9.5 | 0.0 |

| SANDWICH | Measure INFO/WEIGHT | per Measure KCAL | FAT | Nutrition Values per 100g / 100ml KCAL | PROT | CARB | FAT | FIBRE |
|---|---|---|---|---|---|---|---|---|
| Chicken, Ham, & Prawn, Triple, Weight Watchers* | 1 Pack/250g | 337.0 | 4.0 | 135 | 9.8 | 20.5 | 1.5 | 2.6 |
| Chicken, Ham, Prawn, Triple Pack, HL, Tesco* | 1 Pack/247g | 350.0 | 5.0 | 142 | 10.7 | 20.2 | 2.1 | 2.2 |
| Chicken, Ham & Pepperoni, Meat Feast, Tesco* | 1 Pack/196g | 470.0 | 23.0 | 240 | 14.7 | 19.4 | 11.5 | 1.5 |
| Chicken, Healthier Choice, Ginsters* | 1 Pack/183g | 247.0 | 3.0 | 135 | 10.2 | 20.5 | 1.4 | 0.0 |
| Chicken, Honey & Mustard, BGTY, Sainsbury's* | 1 Pack/171g | 296.0 | 5.0 | 173 | 13.1 | 24.0 | 2.7 | 0.0 |
| Chicken, Honey & Mustard, on Softgrain Bread, Tasties* | 1 Pack/152g | 304.0 | 5.0 | 200 | 14.4 | 28.5 | 3.3 | 0.0 |
| Chicken, Honey & Mustard, Safeway* | 1 Pack/167g | 399.0 | 17.0 | 239 | 12.7 | 23.6 | 10.4 | 2.5 |
| Chicken, Kashmir, French Cuisiniers* | 1 Pack/145g | 204.0 | 2.0 | 141 | 12.9 | 20.3 | 1.6 | 2.9 |
| Chicken, Lemon, & Mint, Brambles* | 1 Pack/161g | 338.0 | 9.0 | 210 | 13.4 | 24.6 | 5.4 | 3.2 |
| Chicken, Lemon, & Relish, Perfectly Balanced, Waitrose* | 1 Pack/151g | 243.0 | 4.0 | 161 | 12.3 | 21.4 | 2.9 | 3.5 |
| Chicken, Lime & Coriander, BP* | 1 Pack/155g | 292.0 | 6.0 | 189 | 12.5 | 25.2 | 4.2 | 0.0 |
| Chicken, Mexican, Healthy Choices, Shell* | 1 Serving/168g | 376.0 | 12.0 | 224 | 12.2 | 28.1 | 7.0 | 0.0 |
| Chicken, Moroccan, Sainsbury's* | ½ Pack/100g | 185.0 | 4.0 | 186 | 10.6 | 27.9 | 3.6 | 0.0 |
| Chicken, No Mayonnaise, Waitrose* | 1 Pack/173g | 332.0 | 10.0 | 192 | 11.6 | 24.0 | 5.5 | 2.1 |
| Chicken, Oriental, Triple, Shapers, Boots* | 1 Pack/215g | 398.0 | 12.0 | 185 | 12.0 | 22.0 | 5.4 | 2.6 |
| Chicken, Red Thai, BGTY, Sainsbury's* | 1 Pack/195g | 326.0 | 4.0 | 167 | 11.3 | 26.4 | 1.9 | 0.0 |
| Chicken, Red Thai, Taste!* | 1 Pack/164g | 335.0 | 10.0 | 204 | 11.5 | 26.1 | 6.0 | 0.0 |
| Chicken, Rustlers* | 1 Pack/150g | 346.0 | 14.0 | 231 | 16.3 | 20.1 | 9.5 | 0.0 |
| Chicken, Salad, M & S* | 1 Pack/226g | 350.0 | 9.0 | 155 | 10.6 | 18.8 | 4.1 | 3.0 |
| Chicken, Salad, On Malted Bread, BGTY, Sainsbury's* | 1 Pack/216g | 346.0 | 7.0 | 160 | 12.7 | 19.7 | 3.4 | 2.7 |
| Chicken, Shell* | 1 Pack/121g | 334.0 | 16.0 | 276 | 13.9 | 25.9 | 13.0 | 0.0 |
| Chicken, Simply, Brambles* | 1 Pack/136g | 283.0 | 4.0 | 208 | 14.0 | 31.0 | 3.1 | 1.3 |
| Chicken, Smokey, BGTY, Sainsbury's* | 1 Pack/178g | 276.0 | 2.0 | 155 | 11.1 | 25.6 | 1.0 | 0.0 |
| Chicken, Southern Fried, Rustlers* | 1 Serving/145g | 436.0 | 21.0 | 301 | 11.7 | 30.6 | 14.7 | 0.0 |
| Chicken, Southern Spiced, M & S* | 1 Pack/179g | 421.0 | 23.0 | 235 | 11.2 | 21.7 | 13.0 | 3.1 |
| Chicken, Spicy, Deep Filled, Co-Op* | 1 Pack/216g | 421.0 | 15.0 | 195 | 10.0 | 24.0 | 7.0 | 3.0 |
| Chicken, Sundried Tomato & Herb, Bells* | 1 Pack/198g | 400.0 | 19.0 | 202 | 10.2 | 18.9 | 9.5 | 0.0 |
| Chicken, Sutherland* | 1 Pack/220g | 465.0 | 19.0 | 211 | 10.4 | 22.9 | 8.7 | 0.0 |
| Chicken, Tandoori, Finest, Tesco* | 1 Pack/224g | 421.0 | 17.0 | 188 | 10.8 | 19.2 | 7.5 | 1.4 |
| Chicken, Tandoori, Waitrose* | 1 Pack/181g | 302.0 | 6.0 | 167 | 11.6 | 23.0 | 3.1 | 4.1 |
| Chicken, Tangy Lime & Ginger, Shapers, Boots* | 1 Pack/168g | 319.0 | 11.0 | 190 | 12.0 | 21.0 | 6.4 | 5.1 |
| Chicken, Thai, BGTY, Sainsbury's* | 1 Pack/196g | 280.0 | 5.0 | 143 | 10.2 | 19.6 | 2.6 | 0.6 |
| Chicken, Thai, Tesco* | 1 Pack/244g | 634.0 | 38.0 | 260 | 8.5 | 21.1 | 15.7 | 1.5 |
| Chicken, Tikka, Asda* | 1 Pack/186g | 316.0 | 9.0 | 170 | 11.0 | 21.0 | 4.7 | 1.5 |
| Chicken, Tikka, COU, M & S* | 1 Pack/185g | 268.0 | 3.0 | 145 | 12.1 | 20.5 | 1.8 | 3.2 |
| Chicken, Tikka, Garlic & Herb Bread Pocket, Somerfield* | 1 Pack/168g | 341.0 | 7.0 | 203 | 11.0 | 30.0 | 4.3 | 2.0 |
| Chicken, Tikka, M & S* | 1 Pack/180g | 391.0 | 20.0 | 217 | 10.4 | 19.5 | 10.9 | 2.0 |
| Chicken, Tikka, on Pepper Chilli Bread, Shapers, Boots* | 1 Pack/172g | 296.0 | 4.0 | 172 | 13.0 | 25.0 | 2.6 | 2.5 |
| Chicken, Tikka, Weight Watchers* | 1 Pack/158g | 250.0 | 2.0 | 158 | 13.1 | 23.2 | 1.4 | 2.9 |
| Chicken, Working Lunch* | 1 Pack/169g | 298.0 | 8.0 | 176 | 14.0 | 19.9 | 4.5 | 1.8 |
| Chicken Salad, Choice* | 1 Pack/174g | 285.0 | 5.0 | 164 | 11.5 | 22.9 | 2.9 | 1.7 |
| Chicken Salad, HL, Tesco* | 1 Serving/190g | 247.0 | 3.0 | 130 | 12.3 | 15.8 | 1.8 | 4.5 |
| Chicken Salad, Light Choices, Tesco* | 1 Pack/207g | 290.0 | 4.0 | 140 | 13.9 | 16.8 | 1.9 | 2.7 |
| Christmas Special, Ginsters* | 1 Pack/220g | 583.0 | 34.0 | 265 | 9.5 | 23.2 | 15.6 | 0.0 |
| Classic, Triple Pack, Somerfield* | 1 Serving/250g | 652.0 | 36.0 | 261 | 10.2 | 22.1 | 14.6 | 2.5 |
| Classic Feast, M & S* | 1 Serving/295g | 841.0 | 52.0 | 285 | 10.6 | 21.3 | 17.5 | 4.7 |
| Club, New York Style, Sainsbury's* | 1 Serving/212g | 608.0 | 33.0 | 287 | 13.3 | 22.8 | 15.8 | 2.7 |
| Corned Beef, & Tomato, & Onion, Salad Garden* | 1 Pack/137g | 338.0 | 15.0 | 247 | 14.2 | 23.0 | 10.8 | 0.0 |
| Corned Beef, on White, Simply, Brambles* | 1 Pack/126g | 325.0 | 11.0 | 258 | 14.2 | 30.8 | 8.6 | 1.4 |
| Crab, Marie Rose, Brown Bread, Royal London Hospital* | 1 Pack/158g | 293.0 | 11.0 | 185 | 9.7 | 22.0 | 7.1 | 0.0 |
| Crayfish, & Lemon Mayonnaise, Daily Bread* | 1 Pack/173g | 391.0 | 11.0 | 226 | 9.5 | 31.0 | 6.6 | 0.0 |
| Crayfish, & Rocket, Bistro, Waitrose* | 1 Pack/193g | 422.0 | 19.0 | 219 | 11.5 | 20.4 | 10.1 | 2.4 |
| Crayfish, & Rocket, Foo-Go* | 1 Pack/199g | 425.0 | 15.0 | 214 | 9.6 | 26.7 | 7.6 | 3.0 |

S

| | Measure INFO/WEIGHT | per Measure KCAL | FAT | Nutrition Values per 100g / 100ml KCAL | PROT | CARB | FAT | FIBRE |
|---|---|---|---|---|---|---|---|---|
| **SANDWICH** | | | | | | | | |
| Crayfish, & Rocket, Go Eat* | 1 Pack/163g | 289.0 | 7.0 | 177 | 10.6 | 24.6 | 4.3 | 1.9 |
| Crayfish, & Rocket, Shapers, Boots* | 1 Pack/172g | 291.0 | 4.0 | 169 | 11.0 | 26.0 | 2.2 | 2.5 |
| Crayfish & Rocket, Bells* | 1 Pack/144g | 276.0 | 12.0 | 192 | 11.2 | 18.4 | 8.2 | 2.0 |
| Crayfish & Rocket, Finest, Tesco* | 1 Pack/178g | 365.0 | 11.0 | 205 | 9.8 | 27.5 | 5.9 | 2.1 |
| Cream Cheese, & Ham, Tesco* | 1 Pack/212g | 655.0 | 37.0 | 309 | 11.0 | 27.2 | 17.3 | 1.2 |
| Cream Cheese, & Peppers, Taste!* | 1 Pack/154g | 296.0 | 10.0 | 192 | 7.3 | 25.5 | 6.8 | 0.0 |
| Cream Cheese, & Salad, Choice* | 1 Serving/156g | 294.0 | 7.0 | 188 | 7.8 | 28.1 | 4.7 | 0.0 |
| Cream Cheese, & Salad, Sandwich Box* | 1 Pack/138g | 250.0 | 8.0 | 181 | 5.6 | 26.3 | 5.8 | 0.0 |
| Cream Cheese, Red Pepper & Spinach, Daily Bread* | 1 Pack/156g | 273.0 | 8.0 | 175 | 7.4 | 24.0 | 5.2 | 0.0 |
| Duck, Peking, No Mayo, Boots* | 1 Pack/222g | 399.0 | 10.0 | 180 | 7.7 | 27.0 | 4.6 | 1.7 |
| Edam, & Tomato, & Spring Onion, BHS* | 1 Serving/184g | 313.0 | 9.0 | 170 | 8.6 | 22.5 | 5.1 | 3.2 |
| Edam, & Tomato, Low Fat, Oldfields* | 1 Pack/173g | 306.0 | 6.0 | 177 | 9.6 | 26.3 | 3.7 | 2.7 |
| Edam, Oldfields* | 1 Pack/175g | 326.0 | 10.0 | 186 | 9.8 | 23.9 | 5.7 | 0.0 |
| Egg, & Bacon, & Lincolnshire Sausage, Waitrose* | 1 Pack/249g | 655.0 | 33.0 | 263 | 11.3 | 24.7 | 13.2 | 0.9 |
| Egg, & Bacon, Weight Watchers* | 1 Pack/139g | 246.0 | 5.0 | 177 | 10.1 | 26.1 | 3.6 | 1.9 |
| Egg, & Cress, BGTY, Sainsbury's* | 1 Pack/166g | 281.0 | 7.0 | 169 | 9.7 | 23.1 | 4.2 | 3.8 |
| Egg, & Cress, COU, M & S* | 1 Pack/192g | 240.0 | 5.0 | 125 | 9.8 | 15.5 | 2.7 | 2.8 |
| Egg, & Cress, Free Range, Co-Op* | 1 Pack/154g | 370.0 | 19.0 | 240 | 8.0 | 25.0 | 12.0 | 3.0 |
| Egg, & Cress, M & S* | 1 Pack/182g | 331.0 | 18.0 | 182 | 10.1 | 13.6 | 9.7 | 3.2 |
| Egg, & Cress, Organic, M & S* | 1 Pack/185g | 444.0 | 26.0 | 240 | 9.6 | 18.0 | 14.2 | 3.6 |
| Egg, & Cress, Reduced Fat, Waitrose* | 1 Pack/162g | 262.0 | 10.0 | 162 | 9.7 | 16.5 | 6.4 | 6.4 |
| Egg, & Cress, Sainsbury's* | 1 Pack/170g | 384.0 | 20.0 | 226 | 10.6 | 19.8 | 11.6 | 0.0 |
| Egg, & Cress, White Batton, Sandwich King* | 1 Sandwich/155g | 387.0 | 21.0 | 250 | 8.0 | 25.3 | 13.7 | 0.0 |
| Egg, & Gammon, Safeway* | 1 Pack/233g | 490.0 | 19.0 | 210 | 12.9 | 20.4 | 8.0 | 0.0 |
| Egg, & Ham, Asda* | 1 Pack/262g | 589.0 | 34.0 | 225 | 10.4 | 16.8 | 12.8 | 2.1 |
| Egg, & Salad, Deep Filled, Asda* | 1 Pack/231g | 395.0 | 16.0 | 171 | 8.0 | 19.0 | 7.0 | 1.0 |
| Egg, & Salad, Free Range, Sainsbury's* | 1 Pack/225g | 449.0 | 17.0 | 200 | 8.5 | 24.5 | 7.5 | 0.0 |
| Egg, & Salad, Free Range, Waitrose* | 1 Pack/180g | 281.0 | 12.0 | 156 | 7.6 | 16.9 | 6.4 | 3.3 |
| Egg, & Salad, GFY, Asda* | 1 Pack/157g | 229.0 | 5.0 | 146 | 8.0 | 22.0 | 2.9 | 2.9 |
| Egg, & Salad, Shapers, Boots* | 1 Pack/184g | 304.0 | 8.0 | 165 | 6.9 | 24.0 | 4.6 | 1.1 |
| Egg, & Salad, Weight Watchers* | 1 Pack/172g | 237.0 | 5.0 | 138 | 7.1 | 21.3 | 2.7 | 2.2 |
| Egg, & Salad, with Mayonnaise, Wholemeal, Waitrose* | 1 Pack/180g | 257.0 | 9.0 | 143 | 8.3 | 16.5 | 4.9 | 3.6 |
| Egg, & Tomato, Tesco* | 1 Pack/172g | 311.0 | 11.0 | 181 | 8.5 | 22.6 | 6.3 | 2.3 |
| Egg, & Tomato, with Salad Cream, Big, Sainsbury's* | 1 Pack/266g | 463.0 | 15.0 | 174 | 9.1 | 21.3 | 5.8 | 0.0 |
| Egg, Delilite* | 1 Pack/180g | 336.0 | 13.0 | 187 | 8.0 | 22.0 | 7.2 | 3.0 |
| Egg Mayo, Free Range, Asda* | 1 Sandwich/178g | 311.0 | 10.0 | 175 | 9.3 | 21.5 | 5.7 | 2.1 |
| Egg Mayonaise, & Cress, Co-Op* | 1 Serving/159g | 405.0 | 24.0 | 255 | 9.0 | 21.0 | 15.0 | 2.0 |
| Egg Mayonaise, & Iceburg Lettuce, Northern Bites* | 1 Serving/152g | 333.0 | 17.0 | 219 | 7.7 | 20.9 | 11.3 | 0.0 |
| Egg Mayonnaise, & Bacon, Boots* | 1 Serving/200g | 426.0 | 14.0 | 213 | 13.5 | 23.5 | 7.0 | 2.8 |
| Egg Mayonnaise, & Cress, Co-Op* | 1 Pack/159g | 405.0 | 24.0 | 255 | 8.8 | 20.8 | 15.1 | 1.9 |
| Egg Mayonnaise, & Cress, Go Simple, Asda* | 1 Pack/169g | 370.0 | 19.0 | 219 | 10.0 | 20.0 | 11.0 | 1.7 |
| Egg Mayonnaise, & Cress, Millers* | 1 Pack/166g | 369.0 | 20.0 | 222 | 9.4 | 18.8 | 12.2 | 0.0 |
| Egg Mayonnaise, & Cress, Reduced Fat, Waitrose* | 1 Pack/162g | 300.0 | 13.0 | 185 | 10.4 | 18.1 | 7.9 | 3.4 |
| Egg Mayonnaise, & Cress, Shapers, Boots* | 1 Pack/156g | 292.0 | 8.0 | 187 | 11.0 | 25.0 | 4.9 | 2.6 |
| Egg Mayonnaise, & Cress, Wheatgerm Bread, Asda* | 1 Pack/158g | 371.0 | 20.0 | 235 | 9.7 | 21.3 | 12.4 | 1.9 |
| Egg Mayonnaise, Free Range, Finest, Tesco* | 1 Pack/217g | 412.0 | 19.0 | 190 | 10.9 | 16.8 | 8.8 | 2.3 |
| Egg Mayonnaise, HL, Tesco* | 1 Pack/162g | 253.0 | 6.0 | 156 | 9.3 | 21.4 | 3.7 | 2.8 |
| Egg Mayonnaise, on Hi Bran Bread, Ginsters* | 1 Pack/143g | 343.0 | 22.0 | 240 | 10.7 | 17.6 | 15.2 | 0.0 |
| Egg Mayonnaise, Simply, Boots* | 1 Pack/181g | 449.0 | 27.0 | 248 | 9.2 | 19.0 | 15.0 | 2.9 |
| Egg Mayonnaise, Waitrose* | 1 Pack/180g | 396.0 | 21.0 | 220 | 10.1 | 19.1 | 11.4 | 3.4 |
| Egg Salad, Light Choices, Tesco* | 1 Pack/270g | 364.0 | 6.0 | 135 | 7.4 | 20.8 | 2.1 | 2.6 |
| Feta Cheese, & Salad, Tastte* | 1 Pack/178g | 367.0 | 13.0 | 206 | 10.6 | 24.0 | 7.5 | 0.0 |
| Feta Cheese, Bells* | 1 Pack/223g | 468.0 | 26.0 | 210 | 7.1 | 18.8 | 11.8 | 0.0 |

| | Measure INFO/WEIGHT | per Measure KCAL | FAT | Nutrition Values per 100g / 100ml KCAL | PROT | CARB | FAT | FIBRE |
|---|---|---|---|---|---|---|---|---|

## SANDWICH

| | Measure INFO/WEIGHT | KCAL | FAT | KCAL | PROT | CARB | FAT | FIBRE |
|---|---|---|---|---|---|---|---|---|
| Fish, Triple, Co-Op* | 1 Serving/233g | 420.0 | 9.0 | 180 | 10.0 | 26.0 | 4.0 | 3.0 |
| Gammon, & Salad, Tasties* | 1 Pack/172g | 261.0 | 6.0 | 152 | 9.6 | 20.6 | 3.5 | 0.0 |
| Goat's Cheese, & Cranberry, Shapers, Boots* | 1 Pack/150g | 323.0 | 6.0 | 216 | 8.4 | 36.0 | 4.2 | 2.6 |
| Goat's Cheese, & Sunblush Tomato, Pesto Mayo, Deli* | 1 Pack/179g | 480.0 | 29.0 | 268 | 9.5 | 20.5 | 16.4 | 0.0 |
| Goat's Chesse, & Chargrilled Vegetables, Finest, Tesco* | 1 Pack/214g | 481.0 | 20.0 | 225 | 7.7 | 27.8 | 9.2 | 1.4 |
| Greek Salad, Classic, Cafe, Primo* | 1 Serving/216g | 513.0 | 27.0 | 238 | 8.6 | 23.1 | 12.5 | 1.8 |
| Ham, & Cheese, Light Choices, Tesco* | 1 Pack/158g | 284.0 | 5.0 | 180 | 14.5 | 22.8 | 3.2 | 5.0 |
| Ham, & Cheese, Morrisons* | 1 Serving/183g | 273.0 | 5.0 | 149 | 12.5 | 19.2 | 2.5 | 4.1 |
| Ham, & Coleslaw, Smoked, Brambles* | 1 Pack/166g | 283.0 | 4.0 | 171 | 8.2 | 28.8 | 2.5 | 1.8 |
| Ham, & Mustard, Heinz* | 1 Pack/180g | 460.0 | 21.0 | 255 | 11.8 | 25.6 | 11.5 | 5.0 |
| Ham, & Mustard, Salad, BGTY, Sainsbury's* | 1 Pack/183g | 261.0 | 4.0 | 143 | 8.7 | 22.4 | 2.1 | 2.6 |
| Ham, & Mustard, Simply, Ginsters* | 1 Pack/157g | 399.0 | 20.0 | 254 | 11.7 | 23.5 | 12.6 | 0.0 |
| Ham, & Mustard, Tesco* | 1 Pack/147g | 437.0 | 28.0 | 297 | 10.6 | 20.8 | 19.0 | 1.2 |
| Ham, & Philadelphia Light, Dry Cured, Boots* | 1 Pack/172g | 339.0 | 9.0 | 197 | 12.8 | 24.4 | 5.4 | 2.5 |
| Ham, & Pineapple Salsa, Maple Flavoured, Waitrose* | 1 Pack/194g | 329.0 | 9.0 | 170 | 8.4 | 23.8 | 4.6 | 3.1 |
| Ham, & Salad, & Mustard, Darwins Deli* | 1 Serving/180g | 574.0 | 14.0 | 319 | 14.0 | 48.5 | 7.6 | 0.0 |
| Ham, & Salad, Brambles* | 1 Serving/173g | 289.0 | 7.0 | 167 | 10.1 | 23.2 | 3.9 | 1.2 |
| Ham, & Salad, Foo-Go* | 1 Pack/178g | 297.0 | 7.0 | 167 | 9.8 | 22.9 | 4.0 | 0.0 |
| Ham, & Salad, Fulfilled* | 1 Serving/183g | 288.0 | 6.0 | 157 | 11.8 | 19.9 | 3.5 | 0.0 |
| Ham, & Salad, Ginsters* | 1 Pack/179g | 287.0 | 6.0 | 160 | 8.8 | 23.5 | 3.4 | 0.0 |
| Ham, & Salad, Healthy Options, Oldfields* | 1 Pack/156g | 229.0 | 3.0 | 147 | 8.7 | 24.0 | 1.9 | 0.0 |
| Ham, & Salad, Leicester, Waitrose* | 1 Serving/187g | 325.0 | 9.0 | 174 | 8.6 | 24.0 | 4.8 | 1.6 |
| Ham, & Salad, Select* | 1 Serving/180g | 266.0 | 5.0 | 148 | 8.0 | 23.2 | 2.6 | 0.0 |
| Ham, & Salad, Shapers, Boots* | 1 Pack/195g | 269.0 | 3.0 | 138 | 9.4 | 22.0 | 1.4 | 1.8 |
| Ham, & Salad, Smoked, Ainsley Harriott* | 1 Pack/218g | 307.0 | 6.0 | 141 | 8.9 | 19.9 | 2.9 | 0.0 |
| Ham, & Salad, Smoked, Taste!* | 1 Serving/188g | 309.0 | 10.0 | 164 | 9.8 | 19.8 | 5.2 | 0.0 |
| Ham, & Salad, Snack & Shop, Esso* | 1 Pack/191g | 304.0 | 7.0 | 159 | 9.2 | 22.9 | 3.4 | 5.0 |
| Ham, & Salad, Wild Bean Cafe* | 1 Pack/212g | 301.0 | 6.0 | 142 | 10.7 | 18.8 | 2.6 | 2.0 |
| Ham, & Salad, with Mustard, Finest, Tesco* | 1 Pack/200g | 466.0 | 21.0 | 233 | 15.3 | 19.3 | 10.5 | 1.3 |
| Ham, & Soft Cheese, Tesco* | 1 Serving/164g | 333.0 | 12.0 | 203 | 11.6 | 22.5 | 7.4 | 2.2 |
| Ham, & Swiss Cheese, Big, Sainsbury's* | 1 Pack/218g | 652.0 | 36.0 | 299 | 11.6 | 25.4 | 16.7 | 0.5 |
| Ham, & Swiss Cheese, M & S* | 1 Pack/159g | 393.0 | 20.0 | 247 | 14.7 | 18.9 | 12.6 | 3.3 |
| Ham, & Tomato, Brambles* | 1 Pack/159g | 288.0 | 7.0 | 181 | 11.1 | 24.1 | 4.6 | 3.3 |
| Ham, & Tomato, GFY, Asda* | 1 Pack/173g | 254.0 | 3.0 | 147 | 10.0 | 23.0 | 1.7 | 1.4 |
| Ham, & Tomato, Honey Roast, Feel Good, Shell* | 1 Pack/171g | 388.0 | 19.0 | 227 | 9.8 | 22.1 | 11.0 | 0.0 |
| Ham, & Turkey, & Salad, Sutherland* | 1 Pack/185g | 303.0 | 5.0 | 164 | 9.8 | 25.2 | 2.6 | 0.0 |
| Ham, & Turkey, Asda* | 1 Pack/190g | 393.0 | 19.0 | 207 | 12.9 | 15.8 | 10.2 | 2.3 |
| Ham, & Turkey, Healthy, Felix Van Den Berghe* | 1 Pack/149g | 263.0 | 6.0 | 177 | 9.4 | 26.2 | 4.0 | 0.0 |
| Ham, & Turkey, with Salad, Co-Op* | 1 Pack/188g | 263.0 | 6.0 | 140 | 9.0 | 21.0 | 3.0 | 2.0 |
| Ham, Asda* | 1 Pack/262g | 618.0 | 31.0 | 236 | 12.2 | 20.3 | 12.0 | 3.0 |
| Ham, Cheese, & Pickle, BGTY, Sainsbury's* | 1 Sandwich/198g | 325.0 | 5.0 | 164 | 14.0 | 21.3 | 2.5 | 2.1 |
| Ham, Cheese, & Pickle, Heinz* | 1 Pack/188g | 466.0 | 24.0 | 248 | 11.3 | 21.7 | 12.9 | 4.8 |
| Ham, Cheese, & Pickle, Leicester, Waitrose* | 1 Pack/205g | 512.0 | 24.0 | 250 | 11.9 | 23.7 | 11.9 | 2.1 |
| Ham, Cheese, & Pickle, Platter, M & S* | 1 Sandwich/224g | 582.0 | 33.0 | 260 | 11.9 | 19.3 | 14.9 | 5.3 |
| Ham, Cheese, Pickle & Lettuce, No Mayo, Tesco* | 1 Pack/207g | 435.0 | 16.0 | 210 | 12.2 | 23.0 | 7.8 | 2.7 |
| Ham, Cheese & Pickle, Deep Fill, Tesco* | 1 Pack/225g | 495.0 | 21.0 | 220 | 14.6 | 19.4 | 9.2 | 2.4 |
| Ham, M & S* | 1 Pack/200g | 220.0 | 5.0 | 110 | 17.2 | 3.2 | 2.6 | 0.0 |
| Ham, Smoked, & Mustard, on Oatmeal Bread, Sainsbury's* | 1 Pack/154g | 275.0 | 8.0 | 179 | 11.9 | 20.8 | 5.3 | 3.0 |
| Ham, Smoked, Fresh, Taste!* | 1 Pack/187g | 286.0 | 9.0 | 153 | 9.1 | 18.4 | 4.8 | 0.0 |
| Ham, Tomato, & Lettuce, Oldfields* | 1 Pack/216g | 393.0 | 17.0 | 182 | 12.3 | 19.0 | 8.1 | 3.5 |
| Houmous, & Crunchy Salad, Oldfields* | 1 Pack/180g | 256.0 | 8.0 | 142 | 6.3 | 20.0 | 4.2 | 0.0 |
| Houmous, Tomato, & Red Onion, Daily Bread* | 1 Serving/184g | 367.0 | 18.0 | 199 | 6.9 | 22.7 | 9.6 | 0.0 |
| Houmous & Carrot, Shapers, Boots* | 1 Pack/204g | 323.0 | 10.0 | 158 | 7.5 | 21.0 | 5.0 | 5.2 |

S

# SANDWICH

| | INFO/WEIGHT | KCAL | FAT | KCAL | PROT | CARB | FAT | FIBRE |
|---|---|---|---|---|---|---|---|---|
| Houmous Salad, in Flatbread, Greek Inspired, Sainsbury's* | 1 Pack/177g | 313.0 | 11.0 | 177 | 5.5 | 24.7 | 6.2 | 3.3 |
| Indian Triple, Sainsbury's* | 1 Serving/265g | 549.0 | 16.0 | 207 | 12.8 | 25.2 | 6.1 | 0.0 |
| Just Chicken, No Mayo, Tesco* | 1 Pack/120g | 246.0 | 4.0 | 205 | 15.9 | 28.1 | 3.2 | 3.8 |
| Just Ham, No Mayo, Tesco* | 1 Pack/122g | 250.0 | 5.0 | 205 | 11.6 | 30.4 | 4.0 | 2.1 |
| King Prawn, & Wild Rocket, Honduran, M & S* | 1 Serving/196g | 450.0 | 24.0 | 230 | 9.4 | 20.3 | 12.2 | 1.4 |
| King Prawn, Sainsbury's* | 1 Pack/204g | 424.0 | 16.0 | 208 | 11.6 | 22.3 | 8.0 | 0.0 |
| Lemon Chicken & Mangetout Salad, COU, M & S* | 1 Pack/186g | 260.0 | 5.0 | 140 | 10.6 | 19.0 | 2.7 | 3.7 |
| Mediterranean Style, Triple, GFY, Asda* | 1 Pack/211g | 352.0 | 4.0 | 167 | 11.0 | 26.0 | 2.1 | 2.3 |
| Mixed Peppers, Houmous & Baby Spinach, Waitrose* | 1 Pack/170g | 269.0 | 7.0 | 158 | 7.1 | 23.5 | 3.9 | 3.3 |
| Mozzarella, & Pepperoni, Sainsbury's* | 1 Pack/171g | 380.0 | 12.0 | 222 | 10.5 | 29.0 | 7.1 | 0.0 |
| Mozzarella, & Roast Vegetables, Felix Van Den Berghe* | 1 Pack/158g | 330.0 | 13.0 | 209 | 9.5 | 23.8 | 8.4 | 0.0 |
| Mozzarella, & Tomato, Waitrose* | 1 Pack/193g | 359.0 | 18.0 | 186 | 9.7 | 15.7 | 9.4 | 2.3 |
| Mozzarella, Italian Style, Taste!* | 1 Pack/183g | 390.0 | 19.0 | 213 | 9.2 | 20.1 | 10.6 | 2.0 |
| Mozzarella, Pesto & Pine Nuts, Sainsbury's* | 1 Pack/180g | 423.0 | 17.0 | 235 | 10.2 | 26.8 | 9.7 | 2.8 |
| Mozzarella, Tomato, & Basil, Healthy Options, Oldfields* | 1 Pack/175g | 285.0 | 8.0 | 163 | 8.1 | 22.1 | 4.8 | 3.3 |
| New York Deli, Boots* | 1 Pack/245g | 397.0 | 12.0 | 162 | 10.0 | 19.0 | 5.1 | 1.7 |
| New York Deli, Extra Special, Asda* | 1 Pack/200g | 403.0 | 15.0 | 201 | 12.4 | 20.6 | 7.7 | 3.8 |
| Philadelphia Salad, The Classic Sandwich Co* | 1 Pack/135g | 264.0 | 12.0 | 196 | 6.2 | 22.1 | 9.1 | 0.0 |
| Pitta, Falafel, Houmous & Salad, Benedicts* | 1 Pack/220g | 405.0 | 13.0 | 184 | 6.8 | 26.1 | 5.9 | 0.0 |
| Ploughman's, Cheddar, Heinz* | 1 Pack/208g | 552.0 | 28.0 | 265 | 9.3 | 27.1 | 13.3 | 2.4 |
| Ploughman's, Cheddar, Mature Vintage, Sainsbury's* | 1 Pack/204g | 439.0 | 20.0 | 215 | 9.3 | 22.3 | 9.9 | 0.0 |
| Ploughman's, Cheese, 50% Less Fat, BGTY, Sainsbury's* | 1 Pack/204g | 335.0 | 6.0 | 164 | 10.7 | 23.3 | 3.1 | 3.1 |
| Ploughman's, Cheese, BGTY, Sainsbury's* | 1 Pack/193g | 326.0 | 8.0 | 169 | 9.8 | 22.8 | 4.2 | 3.6 |
| Ploughman's, Deep Fill, Ginsters* | 1 Pack/232g | 636.0 | 41.0 | 274 | 9.6 | 20.8 | 17.6 | 0.0 |
| Ploughman's, Deep Fill, Tesco* | 1 Pack/245g | 551.0 | 27.0 | 225 | 10.9 | 20.2 | 11.2 | 1.4 |
| Ploughman's, Deep Filled, Asda* | 1 Pack/254g | 650.0 | 37.0 | 256 | 10.3 | 21.3 | 14.5 | 2.9 |
| Ploughmans, Light Choices, Tesco* | 1 Pack/178g | 320.0 | 7.0 | 180 | 12.2 | 22.9 | 4.2 | 3.3 |
| Poached Salmon, & Watercress, Lochmuir, M & S* | 1 Pack/192g | 355.0 | 12.0 | 185 | 10.3 | 22.3 | 6.1 | 1.6 |
| Pork, & Apple Sauce, Bells* | 1 Pack/180g | 341.0 | 8.0 | 190 | 11.5 | 26.1 | 4.5 | 0.0 |
| Prawn, & Coriander, M & S* | 1 Serving/213g | 575.0 | 35.0 | 270 | 9.5 | 20.6 | 16.6 | 3.7 |
| Prawn, & Salmon, Waitrose* | 1 Pack/154g | 345.0 | 15.0 | 224 | 12.5 | 22.0 | 9.5 | 2.8 |
| Prawn, & Smoked Salmon, M & S* | 1 Pack/445g | 1135.0 | 64.0 | 255 | 11.7 | 19.3 | 14.3 | 1.4 |
| Prawn, & Thai Dressing, Tiger, Waitrose* | 1 Pack/200g | 342.0 | 9.0 | 171 | 9.6 | 23.6 | 4.3 | 2.2 |
| Prawn, Egg & Chicken, Triple, Weight Watchers* | 1 Pack/224g | 367.0 | 6.0 | 164 | 10.2 | 24.8 | 2.7 | 2.9 |
| Prawn, Marie Rose, Waitrose* | 1 Pack/164g | 226.0 | 6.0 | 138 | 8.8 | 18.0 | 3.4 | 1.9 |
| Prawn, Salad, COU, M & S* | 1 Pack/200g | 230.0 | 4.0 | 115 | 8.0 | 16.6 | 1.8 | 3.8 |
| Prawn, Thai Style, Ginsters* | 1 Pack/183g | 313.0 | 9.0 | 171 | 9.2 | 22.5 | 4.9 | 0.0 |
| Prawn Cocktail, Classic, Heinz* | 1 Pack/193g | 409.0 | 17.0 | 212 | 8.4 | 25.0 | 8.7 | 2.5 |
| Prawn Cocktail, Jumbo Tiger, Benedicts* | 1 Serving/225g | 349.0 | 11.0 | 155 | 7.4 | 20.4 | 4.8 | 0.0 |
| Prawn Cocktail, Platter, M & S* | 1 Sandwich/200g | 460.0 | 26.0 | 230 | 8.1 | 22.3 | 12.8 | 2.2 |
| Prawn Cocktail, Waitrose* | 1 Pack/196g | 300.0 | 8.0 | 153 | 8.3 | 20.7 | 4.1 | 2.5 |
| Prawn Cocktail, Weight Watchers* | 1 Pack/168g | 252.0 | 8.0 | 150 | 8.9 | 18.1 | 4.6 | 2.8 |
| Prawn Mayonnaise, COU, M & S* | 1 Pack/155g | 240.0 | 4.0 | 155 | 10.2 | 22.9 | 2.3 | 2.8 |
| Prawn Mayonnaise, Eat Smart, Morrisons* | 1 Pack/166g | 245.0 | 4.0 | 148 | 9.5 | 22.2 | 2.3 | 3.5 |
| Prawn Mayonnaise, GFY, Asda* | 1 Pack/160g | 251.0 | 4.0 | 157 | 10.0 | 23.0 | 2.8 | 2.8 |
| Prawn Mayonnaise, Ginsters* | 1 Pack/152g | 415.0 | 27.0 | 273 | 12.4 | 17.8 | 17.8 | 0.0 |
| Prawn Mayonnaise, Heinz* | 1 Pack/180g | 493.0 | 28.0 | 274 | 8.9 | 24.0 | 15.8 | 2.5 |
| Prawn Mayonnaise, Light Choices, HL, Tesco* | 1 Pack/157g | 243.0 | 5.0 | 155 | 10.7 | 20.1 | 3.5 | 2.1 |
| Prawn Mayonnaise, M & S* | 1 Pack/156g | 328.0 | 12.0 | 210 | 10.0 | 24.7 | 7.7 | 2.2 |
| Prawn Mayonnaise, Nutritionally Balanced, M & S* | 1 Pack/162g | 300.0 | 11.0 | 185 | 10.2 | 21.2 | 6.6 | 1.9 |
| Prawn Mayonnaise, Oatmeal Bread, Waitrose* | 1 Pack/180g | 463.0 | 27.0 | 257 | 10.2 | 20.4 | 15.0 | 3.2 |
| Prawn Mayonnaise, on Oatmeal Bread, Weight Watchers* | 1 Pack/148g | 235.0 | 4.0 | 159 | 9.7 | 24.3 | 2.5 | 2.2 |
| Prawn Mayonnaise, Sainsbury's* | 1 Pack/151g | 323.0 | 14.0 | 214 | 11.6 | 20.9 | 9.3 | 0.0 |

# SANDWICH

| INFO/WEIGHT | Measure | per Measure KCAL | FAT | KCAL | PROT | CARB | FAT | FIBRE |
|---|---|---|---|---|---|---|---|---|
| Prawn Mayonnaise, Shapers, Boots* | 1 Pack/161g | 254.0 | 4.0 | 158 | 9.0 | 25.0 | 2.5 | 1.8 |
| Prawn Mayonnaise, Tesco* | 1 Pack/143g | 300.0 | 10.0 | 210 | 11.6 | 25.3 | 6.8 | 1.8 |
| Prawn Mayonnaise, Triple, Asda* | 1 Pack/248g | 635.0 | 40.0 | 256 | 9.0 | 19.0 | 16.0 | 3.4 |
| Prawn Mayonnaise, Triple, Tesco* | 1 Pack/231g | 603.0 | 33.0 | 261 | 9.5 | 23.5 | 14.3 | 1.6 |
| Prawn Mayonnaise, Upper Crust* | 1 Pack/208g | 343.0 | 10.0 | 165 | 9.2 | 20.9 | 5.0 | 0.0 |
| Rib, BBQ, Rustlers* | 1 Pack/170g | 444.0 | 20.0 | 261 | 14.6 | 23.8 | 11.9 | 0.0 |
| Salad, & Salad Cream, Fulfilled* | 1 Pack/172g | 244.0 | 7.0 | 142 | 4.9 | 21.5 | 4.1 | 0.0 |
| Salad, Healthy, Cambridge University Catering* | 1 Pack/156g | 246.0 | 4.0 | 158 | 5.9 | 27.4 | 2.8 | 0.0 |
| Salad, Northern Bites* | 1 Pack/210g | 193.0 | 4.0 | 92 | 4.1 | 15.3 | 2.0 | 3.0 |
| Salad, Serious About Sandwiches* | 1 Pack/237g | 322.0 | 12.0 | 136 | 5.8 | 17.1 | 4.9 | 0.8 |
| Salad, Simply, Brambles* | 1 Serving/151g | 242.0 | 6.0 | 160 | 5.8 | 25.2 | 4.0 | 3.6 |
| Salad, Simply, Shapers, Boots* | 1 Pack/216g | 300.0 | 6.0 | 139 | 5.2 | 23.0 | 2.9 | 1.8 |
| Salad, Taste!* | 1 Serving/200g | 246.0 | 6.0 | 123 | 4.4 | 18.9 | 3.2 | 0.0 |
| Salmon, & Black Pepper, Smoked, Fulfilled* | 1 Pack/120g | 293.0 | 10.0 | 244 | 13.8 | 29.0 | 8.6 | 0.0 |
| Salmon, & Cucumber, Brown Bread, Waitrose* | 1 Pack/150g | 295.0 | 11.0 | 197 | 10.5 | 22.7 | 7.1 | 1.4 |
| Salmon, & Cucumber, M & S* | 1 Pack/168g | 329.0 | 14.0 | 196 | 11.0 | 19.5 | 8.3 | 2.6 |
| Salmon, & Cucumber, Red, BGTY, Sainsbury's* | 1 Pack/192g | 278.0 | 4.0 | 145 | 9.4 | 21.7 | 2.3 | 2.4 |
| Salmon, & Cucumber, Red, Healthy Choice, Asda* | 1 Pack/149g | 285.0 | 11.0 | 191 | 10.6 | 19.9 | 7.7 | 2.1 |
| Salmon, & Cucumber, Red, Tesco* | 1 Pack/144g | 284.0 | 9.0 | 197 | 11.1 | 23.8 | 6.4 | 1.9 |
| Salmon, & Cucumber, White Bread, Waitrose* | 1 Pack/161g | 305.0 | 9.0 | 189 | 9.8 | 25.5 | 5.3 | 1.7 |
| Salmon, & Lemon, & Black Pepper, Smoked, Deli* | 1 Pack/116g | 282.0 | 10.0 | 244 | 12.9 | 29.5 | 8.3 | 0.0 |
| Salmon, & Rocket, Poached, M & S* | 1 Pack/180g | 495.0 | 27.0 | 275 | 13.5 | 21.2 | 14.9 | 2.1 |
| Salmon, & Soft Cheese, Feel Good, Shell* | 1 Pack/174g | 404.0 | 13.0 | 232 | 13.5 | 28.0 | 7.4 | 1.0 |
| Salmon, & Soft Cheese, Smoked, Waitrose* | 1 Pack/154g | 300.0 | 10.0 | 195 | 14.8 | 19.2 | 6.5 | 4.2 |
| Salmon, & Spinach, Poached, Shapers, Boots* | 1 Pack/168g | 284.0 | 8.0 | 169 | 9.2 | 23.0 | 4.5 | 3.1 |
| Salmon, Poached, Prawn & Rocket, Waitrose* | 1 Pack/166g | 308.0 | 9.0 | 186 | 11.2 | 23.5 | 5.2 | 2.1 |
| Salmon, Smoked, Daily Bread* | 1 Pack/122g | 296.0 | 11.0 | 243 | 13.5 | 28.0 | 8.7 | 0.0 |
| Salmon, Smoked, Felix Van Den Berghe* | 1 Pack/119g | 291.0 | 7.0 | 245 | 13.9 | 29.4 | 6.2 | 0.0 |
| Salmon, Smoked & Cream Cheese, M & S* | 1 Pack/184g | 450.0 | 22.0 | 245 | 12.7 | 20.8 | 12.2 | 1.8 |
| Salmon & Cucumber, on Malted Bread, BGTY, Sainsbury's* | 1 Pack/189g | 305.0 | 6.0 | 161 | 9.2 | 24.3 | 3.0 | 2.3 |
| Salsa Chicken, HL, Tesco* | 1 Pack/182g | 300.0 | 3.0 | 165 | 13.4 | 23.6 | 1.8 | 1.9 |
| Sausage, Caramelised Onion Chutney & Stuffing, Tesco* | 1 Pack/216g | 530.0 | 22.0 | 245 | 9.2 | 29.0 | 10.2 | 0.7 |
| Sausage, Egg & Bacon, Boots* | 1 Pack/325g | 887.0 | 52.0 | 273 | 9.3 | 23.0 | 16.0 | 2.2 |
| Sausage, Speedy Snacks* | 1 Serving/93g | 258.0 | 9.0 | 279 | 11.6 | 35.2 | 10.2 | 0.0 |
| Sausage, Triple Pack, GFY, Asda* | 1 Pack/215g | 424.0 | 10.0 | 197 | 9.0 | 30.0 | 4.5 | 2.3 |
| Seafood, Mixed, Tesco* | 1 Pack/184g | 502.0 | 31.0 | 273 | 7.3 | 23.2 | 16.8 | 0.8 |
| Seafood Cocktail, Asda* | 1 Pack/190g | 486.0 | 30.0 | 256 | 6.7 | 21.3 | 15.8 | 1.6 |
| Seafood Cocktail, Waitrose* | 1 Pack/210g | 267.0 | 6.0 | 127 | 7.3 | 17.6 | 3.0 | 8.1 |
| Seafood Medley, M & S* | 1 Pack/227g | 468.0 | 28.0 | 206 | 7.2 | 16.3 | 12.4 | 3.5 |
| Soft Cheese, & Roasted Pepper, Weight Watchers* | 1 Pack/158g | 289.0 | 6.0 | 183 | 9.4 | 27.7 | 3.8 | 1.5 |
| Spicy Falafel, & Houmous Salad, Delifresh* | 1 Pack/209g | 429.0 | 20.0 | 205 | 6.1 | 24.0 | 9.4 | 2.6 |
| Steak, Hot, M & S* | 1 Roll/190g | 513.0 | 15.0 | 270 | 11.9 | 37.0 | 8.0 | 3.2 |
| Sub, Beef, & Onion, M & S* | 1 Pack/207g | 611.0 | 32.0 | 295 | 13.3 | 25.6 | 15.3 | 1.5 |
| Sub, Beef, & Onion, Roast, Sainsbury's* | 1 Serving/174g | 426.0 | 17.0 | 245 | 9.4 | 29.3 | 10.0 | 0.0 |
| Sub, Chicken, & Salad, Asda* | 1 Sub/200g | 460.0 | 27.0 | 230 | 9.4 | 17.4 | 13.6 | 0.9 |
| Sub, Chicken, & Stuffing, Safeway* | 1 Roll/275g | 605.0 | 29.0 | 220 | 10.3 | 21.3 | 10.4 | 4.2 |
| Sub, Chicken, & Stuffing, Shell* | 1 Serving/183g | 437.0 | 12.0 | 239 | 13.3 | 32.0 | 6.4 | 0.0 |
| Sub, Chicken, Caesar, Chargrilled, Sainsbury's* | 1 Pack/216g | 611.0 | 30.0 | 283 | 13.4 | 25.6 | 14.1 | 0.0 |
| Sub, Chicken, Nacho Style, Global, Somerfield* | 1 Roll/226g | 513.0 | 19.0 | 227 | 7.4 | 30.8 | 8.3 | 4.2 |
| Sub, Chicken & Bacon, Sainsbury's* | 1 Pack/190g | 554.0 | 27.0 | 291 | 13.4 | 27.4 | 14.2 | 0.8 |
| Sub, Chicken Caesar, Sainsbury's* | 1 Roll/210g | 590.0 | 34.0 | 281 | 11.3 | 22.1 | 16.4 | 1.9 |
| Sub, Egg Mayonnaise, Daily Bread* | 1 Pack/165g | 441.0 | 22.0 | 267 | 9.6 | 29.6 | 13.5 | 0.0 |
| Sub, Ham, & Tomato Salad, Shapers, Boots* | 1 Pack/170g | 286.0 | 4.0 | 168 | 9.2 | 28.0 | 2.3 | 1.4 |

S

| | Measure INFO/WEIGHT | per Measure KCAL | FAT | Nutrition Values per 100g / 100ml KCAL | PROT | CARB | FAT | FIBRE |
|---|---|---|---|---|---|---|---|---|

## SANDWICH

| | Measure INFO/WEIGHT | KCAL | FAT | KCAL | PROT | CARB | FAT | FIBRE |
|---|---|---|---|---|---|---|---|---|
| Three Cheese & Onion, on White Bread, Weight Watchers* | 1 Pack/158g | 283.0 | 3.0 | 179 | 12.4 | 28.4 | 1.8 | 1.5 |
| Tuna, & Celery, Perfectly Balanced, Waitrose* | 1 Pack/172g | 272.0 | 6.0 | 158 | 11.7 | 20.5 | 3.2 | 3.9 |
| Tuna, & Chargrilled Vegetables, BGTY, Sainsbury's* | 1 Pack/196g | 329.0 | 9.0 | 168 | 10.7 | 21.5 | 4.4 | 0.0 |
| Tuna, & Cucumber, & Red Onion, Brambles* | 1 Pack/161g | 264.0 | 4.0 | 164 | 11.3 | 24.3 | 2.4 | 1.6 |
| Tuna, & Cucumber, Antony Worrall Thompson's* | 1 Pack/188g | 284.0 | 4.0 | 151 | 11.6 | 21.0 | 2.3 | 2.9 |
| Tuna, & Cucumber, BGTY, Sainsbury's* | 1 Pack/178g | 268.0 | 3.0 | 151 | 11.3 | 22.3 | 1.8 | 3.1 |
| Tuna, & Cucumber, Healthy Living, Co-Op* | 1 Pack/192g | 250.0 | 3.0 | 130 | 10.9 | 17.9 | 1.8 | 3.0 |
| Tuna, & Cucumber, Low Fat, Heinz* | 1 Serving/183g | 277.0 | 3.0 | 151 | 12.3 | 21.6 | 1.6 | 6.8 |
| Tuna, & Cucumber, on Malted Wheatgrain, Ginsters* | 1 Pack/175g | 318.0 | 8.0 | 182 | 14.1 | 21.8 | 4.3 | 0.0 |
| Tuna, & Cucumber, Perfectly Balanced, Waitrose* | 1 Pack/178g | 240.0 | 4.0 | 135 | 11.0 | 18.3 | 2.0 | 3.6 |
| Tuna, & Cucumber, Shapers, Boots* | 1 Pack/186g | 285.0 | 5.0 | 153 | 11.0 | 22.0 | 2.5 | 2.2 |
| Tuna, & Cucumber, Shell* | 1 Pack/188g | 431.0 | 19.0 | 229 | 12.3 | 21.9 | 10.2 | 0.0 |
| Tuna, & Cucumber, Weight Watchers* | 1 Pack/173g | 279.0 | 3.0 | 161 | 11.4 | 25.1 | 1.7 | 1.4 |
| Tuna, & Green Pesto, BGTY, Sainsbury's* | 1 Pack/211g | 279.0 | 5.0 | 132 | 11.0 | 17.0 | 2.2 | 0.0 |
| Tuna, & Lemon Mayo, Shapers, Boots* | 1 Pack/206g | 318.0 | 10.0 | 154 | 10.0 | 18.0 | 4.7 | 1.7 |
| Tuna, & Pepper & Sweetcorn Salad, Shapers, Boots* | 1 Pack/204g | 345.0 | 8.0 | 169 | 9.2 | 24.0 | 4.0 | 1.9 |
| Tuna, & Salad, Bloomer, M & S* | 1 Pack/231g | 600.0 | 37.0 | 260 | 11.8 | 17.8 | 16.0 | 2.6 |
| Tuna, & Salad, M & S* | 1 Pack/250g | 575.0 | 31.0 | 230 | 12.5 | 16.8 | 12.6 | 2.1 |
| Tuna, & Salad, Tesco* | 1 Pack/197g | 339.0 | 15.0 | 172 | 9.9 | 16.5 | 7.4 | 2.8 |
| Tuna, & Sweetcorn, & Red Onion, Co-Op* | 1 Pack/256g | 614.0 | 28.0 | 240 | 11.0 | 23.0 | 11.0 | 4.0 |
| Tuna, & Sweetcorn, COU, M & S* | 1 Pack/180g | 270.0 | 4.0 | 150 | 12.6 | 19.0 | 2.4 | 3.8 |
| Tuna, & Sweetcorn, Ginsters* | 1 Pack/163g | 307.0 | 8.0 | 188 | 10.5 | 25.2 | 5.0 | 0.0 |
| Tuna, & Sweetcorn, Heinz* | 1 Pack/208g | 528.0 | 27.0 | 254 | 10.4 | 23.5 | 13.2 | 1.6 |
| Tuna, & Sweetcorn, Light Choices, HL, Tesco* | 1 Pack/168g | 285.0 | 3.0 | 170 | 11.2 | 25.9 | 1.9 | 2.8 |
| Tuna, & Sweetcorn, Sainsbury's* | 1 Pack/183g | 392.0 | 16.0 | 214 | 12.1 | 22.3 | 8.5 | 0.0 |
| Tuna, & Sweetcorn, Shapers, Boots* | 1 Pack/170g | 295.0 | 4.0 | 174 | 12.4 | 25.3 | 2.6 | 2.0 |
| Tuna, & Tomato, & Onion, COU, M & S* | 1 Pack/177g | 250.0 | 4.0 | 141 | 11.1 | 18.8 | 2.4 | 2.2 |
| Tuna, Crunch, HL, Tesco* | 1 Pack/180g | 261.0 | 4.0 | 145 | 11.0 | 19.9 | 2.4 | 0.5 |
| Tuna, Crunch, Shapers, Boots* | 1 Pack/200g | 290.0 | 6.0 | 145 | 9.1 | 20.0 | 3.2 | 3.2 |
| Tuna, Heinz* | 1 Serving/183g | 277.0 | 3.0 | 151 | 12.3 | 21.6 | 1.6 | 6.8 |
| Tuna, Mayonnaise & Cucumber, Finest, Tesco* | 1 Pack/225g | 484.0 | 19.0 | 215 | 11.6 | 23.1 | 8.5 | 1.7 |
| Tuna, Mediterranean, COU, M & S* | 1 Pack/260g | 364.0 | 6.0 | 140 | 10.3 | 19.6 | 2.2 | 1.6 |
| Tuna, Mediterranean, Scottish Slimmers* | 1 Pack/147g | 259.0 | 5.0 | 176 | 8.5 | 27.8 | 3.6 | 3.2 |
| Tuna, Melt, Swedish Bread, Shapers, Boots* | 1 Pack/163g | 254.0 | 4.0 | 156 | 14.0 | 20.0 | 2.2 | 2.1 |
| Tuna, Nicoise, Taste!* | 1 Pack/218g | 404.0 | 14.0 | 185 | 11.3 | 20.1 | 6.6 | 0.0 |
| Tuna, Simply, Ginsters* | 1 Pack/167g | 466.0 | 25.0 | 279 | 12.8 | 22.9 | 15.1 | 0.0 |
| Tuna Mayonnaise, & Cucumber, Classic* | 1 Serving/185g | 429.0 | 23.0 | 232 | 10.6 | 19.8 | 12.3 | 0.0 |
| Tuna Mayonnaise, & Cucumber, Daily Bread* | 1 Pack/190g | 392.0 | 17.0 | 206 | 12.1 | 19.8 | 8.7 | 0.0 |
| Tuna Mayonnaise, & Cucumber, Simply, Boots* | 1 Pack/200g | 498.0 | 26.0 | 249 | 12.0 | 21.0 | 13.0 | 2.4 |
| Tuna Mayonnaise, & Salad, Serious About Sandwiches* | 1 Pack/192g | 305.0 | 9.0 | 159 | 8.6 | 20.5 | 4.7 | 2.9 |
| Tuna Mayonnaise, on White Bread, Oldfields* | 1 Pack/142g | 394.0 | 18.0 | 278 | 15.2 | 27.4 | 12.8 | 2.0 |
| Tuna Savoury, Bells* | 1 Pack/149g | 295.0 | 10.0 | 198 | 11.8 | 22.5 | 6.7 | 1.0 |
| Turkey, & Bacon, COU, M & S* | 1 Pack/165g | 256.0 | 4.0 | 155 | 12.0 | 21.0 | 2.4 | 1.7 |
| Turkey, & Cranberry, COU, M & S* | 1 Pack/180g | 279.0 | 3.0 | 155 | 12.1 | 22.8 | 1.7 | 2.9 |
| Turkey, & Cranberry Salad, Fullfillers* | 1 Serving/180g | 319.0 | 6.0 | 177 | 13.0 | 23.3 | 3.2 | 0.0 |
| Turkey, & Lettuce & Tomato, Shapers, Boots* | 1 Pack/217g | 310.0 | 5.0 | 143 | 9.8 | 21.0 | 2.2 | 2.9 |
| Turkey, & Sage, & Mayonnaise, Bells* | 1 Pack/164g | 414.0 | 22.0 | 253 | 11.6 | 21.2 | 13.5 | 0.0 |
| Turkey, & Salad, Brambles* | 1 Pack/170g | 248.0 | 2.0 | 146 | 9.3 | 24.5 | 1.2 | 2.0 |
| Turkey, & Salad, Fullfillers* | 1 Serving/218g | 320.0 | 7.0 | 147 | 10.3 | 18.6 | 3.2 | 0.0 |
| Turkey, & Stuffing, M & S* | 1 Pack/190g | 351.0 | 9.0 | 185 | 12.3 | 23.1 | 4.9 | 1.9 |
| Turkey, & Sun Dried Tomato, Festive Feast, Taste!* | 1 Pack/159g | 401.0 | 22.0 | 252 | 8.8 | 23.0 | 13.9 | 0.0 |
| Turkey, Gibsons* | 1 Pack/138g | 260.0 | 5.0 | 188 | 12.5 | 26.0 | 3.8 | 0.0 |
| Turkey, Just Turkey, White Bread, Sandwich King* | 1 Serving/135g | 317.0 | 7.0 | 235 | 17.3 | 29.7 | 5.2 | 0.0 |

**S**

| | Measure INFO/WEIGHT | per Measure KCAL | FAT | Nutrition Values per 100g / 100ml KCAL | PROT | CARB | FAT | FIBRE |
|---|---|---|---|---|---|---|---|---|
| **SANDWICH** | | | | | | | | |
| Turkey, Northern Bites* | 1 Pack/200g | 354.0 | 9.0 | 177 | 11.9 | 22.8 | 4.3 | 0.0 |
| Turkey, Pork Sausage, & Stuffing, Somerfield* | 1 Pack/209g | 475.0 | 19.0 | 227 | 11.6 | 24.3 | 9.3 | 2.1 |
| Turkey, Stuffing & Cranberry, Boots Shapers* | 1 Pack/192g | 328.0 | 2.0 | 171 | 12.0 | 28.0 | 1.1 | 2.5 |
| Vegetable, & Chilli Bean, Roasted, M & S* | 1 Pack/200g | 340.0 | 11.0 | 170 | 5.2 | 24.5 | 5.7 | 2.1 |
| Vegetable, Chargrilled, Eat Smart, Safeway* | 1 Pack/183g | 265.0 | 4.0 | 145 | 7.4 | 23.4 | 2.3 | 2.8 |
| Vegetable, M & S* | 1 Serving/180g | 252.0 | 4.0 | 140 | 6.1 | 23.5 | 2.3 | 2.1 |
| Vegetable, Roasted, Open, COU, M & S* | 1 Pack/150g | 260.0 | 2.0 | 173 | 8.4 | 31.3 | 1.5 | 4.4 |
| Vegetable, Spicy Cajun, Sandwich King* | 1 Pack/141g | 288.0 | 9.0 | 205 | 6.0 | 30.3 | 6.7 | 0.0 |
| Wedge, Chicken, & Salad, Tesco* | 1 Serving/257g | 599.0 | 24.0 | 233 | 11.3 | 25.3 | 9.5 | 1.2 |
| Wedge, Sausage, & Egg, Tesco* | 1 Pack/269g | 699.0 | 39.0 | 260 | 9.1 | 23.6 | 14.4 | 1.1 |
| Wedge, Tuna, & Salad, Tesco* | 1 Pack/205g | 291.0 | 3.0 | 142 | 8.1 | 23.9 | 1.5 | 0.8 |
| Wensleydale, & Carrot, M & S* | 1 Pack/183g | 430.0 | 23.0 | 235 | 9.9 | 21.4 | 12.3 | 2.8 |
| **SANDWICH FILLER** | | | | | | | | |
| Beef & Onion, Deli, Asda* | 1 Serving/50g | 78.0 | 6.0 | 157 | 10.0 | 0.1 | 13.0 | 1.1 |
| Big Breakfast, Asda* | 1 Serving/125g | 314.0 | 26.0 | 251 | 12.0 | 3.5 | 21.0 | 0.5 |
| Cajun Chicken, Sainsbury's* | 1 Serving/60g | 109.0 | 8.0 | 182 | 13.4 | 1.8 | 13.5 | 1.8 |
| Chargrilled Vegetable, Sainsbury's* | ½ Pot/85g | 192.0 | 19.0 | 226 | 3.4 | 2.2 | 22.7 | 0.6 |
| Cheese & Bacon, Tesco* | 1 Serving/50g | 199.0 | 19.0 | 398 | 12.2 | 2.6 | 37.6 | 1.2 |
| Cheese & Celery, Sainsbury's* | 1 Tub/250g | 397.0 | 35.0 | 159 | 5.7 | 2.1 | 14.2 | 3.0 |
| Cheese & Ham, Sainsbury's* | 1 Serving/25g | 124.0 | 12.0 | 497 | 12.4 | 0.8 | 49.3 | 0.3 |
| Cheese & Onion, Deli, Asda* | 1 Serving/57g | 217.0 | 21.0 | 381 | 10.0 | 2.0 | 37.0 | 2.0 |
| Cheese & Onion, Sainsbury's* | 1 Tub/200g | 632.0 | 60.0 | 316 | 8.7 | 3.2 | 29.8 | 2.2 |
| Cheese & Onion, Tesco* | 1 Pack/170g | 721.0 | 72.0 | 424 | 10.0 | 0.2 | 42.6 | 1.5 |
| Cheese & Spring Onion, M & S* | 1 Serving/56g | 199.0 | 19.0 | 355 | 8.5 | 5.0 | 33.6 | 0.2 |
| Chicken, Bacon & Sweetcorn, BGTY, Sainsbury's* | 1 Tub/300g | 399.0 | 18.0 | 133 | 14.0 | 5.5 | 6.1 | 0.5 |
| Chicken, Stuffing & Bacon, COU, M & S* | 1 Pack/170g | 170.0 | 4.0 | 100 | 13.1 | 6.2 | 2.2 | 1.3 |
| Chicken, Sweetcorn & Bacon, Tesco* | 1 Serving/50g | 167.0 | 15.0 | 334 | 12.3 | 4.3 | 29.7 | 1.6 |
| Chicken, Tomato & Sweetcure Bacon, M & S* | 1 Pot/170g | 501.0 | 45.0 | 295 | 11.4 | 2.8 | 26.4 | 0.7 |
| Chicken & Bacon with Sweetcorn, Sainsbury's* | 1 Serving/60g | 123.0 | 9.0 | 205 | 12.0 | 4.0 | 15.7 | 0.9 |
| Chicken & Stuffing, Sainsbury's* | ½ Tub/120g | 397.0 | 38.0 | 331 | 6.5 | 5.3 | 31.5 | 1.7 |
| Chicken & Sweetcorn, Sainsbury's* | 1 Tub/170g | 396.0 | 34.0 | 233 | 11.0 | 2.7 | 19.8 | 1.9 |
| Chicken Caesar, BGTY, Sainsbury's* | ½ Jar/85g | 117.0 | 6.0 | 137 | 15.6 | 2.5 | 7.2 | 2.2 |
| Chicken Fajita, Tesco* | 1 Serving/50g | 77.0 | 4.0 | 155 | 13.8 | 5.9 | 8.5 | 1.4 |
| Chicken Tikka, BGTY, Sainsbury's* | ½ Pot/85g | 99.0 | 3.0 | 117 | 16.5 | 6.0 | 3.0 | 1.0 |
| Chicken Tikka, Mild, Heinz* | 1 Serving/52g | 102.0 | 7.0 | 196 | 5.2 | 12.3 | 14.0 | 0.7 |
| Chicken Tikka & Citrus Raita, COU, M & S* | ½ Pot/85g | 76.0 | 2.0 | 90 | 12.6 | 4.9 | 2.0 | 0.9 |
| Chicken with Salad Vegetables, Heinz* | 1 Serving/56g | 114.0 | 8.0 | 203 | 5.1 | 11.7 | 15.1 | 0.5 |
| Chickpea, Moroccan Style, Sainsbury's* | ½ Tub/120g | 160.0 | 9.0 | 133 | 4.1 | 11.7 | 7.8 | 4.2 |
| Chunky Egg & Smoked Ham, Tesco* | 1 Serving/100g | 234.0 | 21.0 | 234 | 11.8 | 0.2 | 20.7 | 0.3 |
| Chunky Seafood Cocktail, Tesco* | 1 Serving/100g | 308.0 | 28.0 | 308 | 6.0 | 8.3 | 27.8 | 2.0 |
| Corned Beef & Onion, Deli, Asda* | 1 Serving/50g | 170.0 | 15.0 | 340 | 12.0 | 3.3 | 31.0 | 0.7 |
| Coronation Chicken, BGTY, Sainsbury's* | 1 Portion/50g | 73.0 | 3.0 | 146 | 11.9 | 8.9 | 7.0 | 1.4 |
| Coronation Chicken, Sainsbury's* | ¼ Tub/60g | 183.0 | 15.0 | 305 | 12.1 | 8.9 | 24.6 | 1.2 |
| Coronation Chicken, Tesco* | 1 Tbsp/30g | 84.0 | 7.0 | 279 | 14.7 | 6.1 | 21.8 | 0.7 |
| Coronation Chicken, Waitrose* | 1 Pack/170g | 554.0 | 43.0 | 326 | 11.1 | 13.2 | 25.4 | 2.0 |
| Egg & Bacon, Fresh, Tesco* | 1 Serving/45g | 112.0 | 9.0 | 248 | 12.7 | 4.2 | 20.1 | 0.6 |
| Egg & Smoked Bacon, BGTY, Sainsbury's* | ½ Pot/120g | 187.0 | 14.0 | 156 | 9.7 | 3.8 | 11.3 | 0.5 |
| Egg Mayonaise, BFY, Morrisons* | 1 Serving/50g | 71.0 | 5.0 | 142 | 10.0 | 1.7 | 10.6 | 0.0 |
| Egg Mayonnaise, BGTY, Sainsbury's* | ½ Tub/120g | 134.0 | 8.0 | 112 | 9.7 | 3.6 | 6.5 | 0.5 |
| Egg Mayonnaise, Chunky Free Range, Tesco* | 1 Serving/50g | 104.0 | 9.0 | 209 | 11.3 | 0.9 | 17.8 | 1.6 |
| Egg Mayonnaise, Deli, Asda* | 1 Serving/50g | 113.0 | 10.0 | 227 | 11.0 | 0.8 | 20.0 | 0.3 |
| Egg Mayonnaise, M & S* | 1oz/28g | 62.0 | 6.0 | 220 | 10.1 | 0.8 | 19.7 | 1.1 |
| Egg Mayonnaise, Sainsbury's* | 1 Serving/60g | 129.0 | 11.0 | 215 | 10.4 | 2.0 | 18.4 | 0.5 |

|  | Measure INFO/WEIGHT | per Measure KCAL | FAT | Nutrition Values per 100g / 100ml KCAL | PROT | CARB | FAT | FIBRE |
|---|---|---|---|---|---|---|---|---|
| **SANDWICH FILLER** | | | | | | | | |
| Egg Mayonnaise, Tesco* | 1 Serving/50g | 114.0 | 10.0 | 228 | 10.2 | 1.9 | 20.0 | 0.5 |
| Ham & Salad Vegetables, Heinz* | 1oz/28g | 57.0 | 4.0 | 204 | 5.3 | 10.0 | 15.9 | 0.4 |
| Poached Salmon & Cucumber, Deli, M & S* | 1 Pot/170g | 348.0 | 28.0 | 205 | 14.0 | 1.0 | 16.3 | 0.5 |
| Prawn Marie Rose, Sainsbury's* | 1 Serving/60g | 121.0 | 11.0 | 201 | 8.1 | 2.5 | 17.6 | 0.9 |
| Prawn Mayonnaise, GFY, Asda* | 1 Serving/57g | 101.0 | 7.0 | 177 | 12.0 | 3.0 | 13.0 | 0.1 |
| Prawn Mayonnaise, M & S* | ½ Pack/170g | 501.0 | 48.0 | 295 | 10.6 | 0.6 | 28.0 | 0.3 |
| Prawn Mayonnaise, Waitrose* | 1 Pot/170g | 537.0 | 53.0 | 316 | 8.9 | 0.2 | 31.1 | 0.0 |
| Roast Beef, Onion & Horseradish, Sainsbury's* | 1 Serving/100g | 372.0 | 37.0 | 372 | 6.4 | 3.7 | 36.8 | 1.2 |
| Roast Chicken & Stuffing, Sainsbury's* | 1 Serving/100g | 424.0 | 41.0 | 424 | 10.8 | 1.9 | 41.5 | 1.2 |
| Seafood, BGTY, Sainsbury's* | 1oz/28g | 36.0 | 2.0 | 128 | 8.7 | 7.6 | 7.0 | 0.5 |
| Seafood Cocktail, M & S* | 1oz/28g | 76.0 | 7.0 | 272 | 6.4 | 8.2 | 23.8 | 0.2 |
| Seafood Cocktail, Sainsbury's* | ½ Tub/120g | 314.0 | 28.0 | 262 | 5.7 | 8.1 | 23.0 | 1.0 |
| Smoked Ham, Roasted Onion & Mustard, Sainsbury's* | 1 Serving/100g | 343.0 | 33.0 | 343 | 7.3 | 3.4 | 33.4 | 0.0 |
| Smoked Salmon & Soft Cheese, M & S* | 1 Pack/170g | 450.0 | 41.0 | 265 | 11.1 | 4.9 | 23.9 | 0.0 |
| Tex-Mex Chicken, Tesco* | 1 Pack/250g | 255.0 | 2.0 | 102 | 12.3 | 11.2 | 0.9 | 1.2 |
| Tuna, Carb Check, Heinz* | 1 Serving/52g | 84.0 | 6.0 | 161 | 6.6 | 6.3 | 12.0 | 0.7 |
| Tuna, Tomato & Black Olive, BGTY, Sainsbury's* | 1 Pack/100g | 88.0 | 2.0 | 88 | 12.6 | 5.9 | 1.6 | 1.2 |
| Tuna & Sweetcorn, COU, M & S* | ½ Pot/85g | 76.0 | 2.0 | 90 | 11.6 | 5.7 | 2.0 | 1.3 |
| Tuna & Sweetcorn, GFY, Asda* | 1/3 Pot/57g | 71.0 | 2.0 | 125 | 12.0 | 10.0 | 4.1 | 0.8 |
| Tuna & Sweetcorn, HL, Tesco* | 1 Serving/60g | 69.0 | 3.0 | 115 | 11.2 | 5.0 | 5.3 | 1.4 |
| Tuna & Sweetcorn, M & S* | 1oz/28g | 70.0 | 6.0 | 250 | 14.2 | 2.3 | 20.7 | 1.3 |
| Tuna & Sweetcorn, Morrisons* | 1 Tub/170g | 382.0 | 28.0 | 225 | 15.3 | 7.0 | 16.7 | 3.4 |
| Tuna & Sweetcorn with Salad Vegetables, Heinz* | 1oz/28g | 53.0 | 4.0 | 191 | 5.8 | 12.1 | 13.2 | 0.7 |
| Tuna Mayonnaise, & Cucumber, Choice, Tesco* | 1 Serving/200g | 463.0 | 23.0 | 231 | 12.8 | 23.2 | 11.4 | 1.5 |
| Tuna Mayonnaise, BGTY, Sainsbury's* | 1 Serving/100g | 114.0 | 3.0 | 114 | 17.6 | 3.5 | 3.4 | 0.1 |
| **SANDWICH SPREAD** | | | | | | | | |
| Beef, Classic, Shippam's* | 1 Pot/75g | 133.0 | 9.0 | 177 | 15.5 | 2.2 | 11.8 | 0.0 |
| Chicken, Classic, Shippam's* | 1 Serving/35g | 64.0 | 4.0 | 182 | 15.5 | 1.8 | 12.5 | 0.0 |
| Chicken & Bacon, Asda* | ¼ Jar/43g | 153.0 | 13.0 | 359 | 18.0 | 2.0 | 31.0 | 1.0 |
| Crab, Classic, Shippam's* | 1 Jar/35g | 59.0 | 4.0 | 170 | 13.1 | 4.6 | 10.9 | 0.0 |
| Cucumber, Heinz* | 1oz/28g | 46.0 | 3.0 | 164 | 1.7 | 12.7 | 11.6 | 0.6 |
| Peppered Mackerel, Creamy, Shippam's* | 1 Serving/15g | 27.0 | 0.0 | 177 | 7.8 | 6.5 | 0.0 | 0.0 |
| Salmon, Classic, Shippam's* | 1 Serving/35g | 70.0 | 5.0 | 200 | 14.7 | 4.2 | 14.1 | 0.0 |
| Tuna & Mayonnaise, Shippam's* | 1 Pot/75g | 189.0 | 14.0 | 252 | 18.3 | 3.1 | 18.5 | 0.0 |
| **SARDINES** | | | | | | | | |
| Boneless, in Tomato Sauce, John West* | 1 Can/120g | 197.0 | 12.0 | 164 | 17.0 | 1.5 | 10.0 | 0.0 |
| *Grilled* | *1oz/28g* | *55.0* | *3.0* | *195* | *25.3* | *0.0* | *10.4* | *0.0* |
| in Barbecue Sauce, Princes* | 1 Can/120g | 182.0 | 10.0 | 152 | 15.1 | 5.0 | 8.0 | 0.0 |
| *in Brine, Canned, Drained* | *1oz/28g* | *48.0* | *3.0* | *172* | *21.5* | *0.0* | *9.6* | *0.0* |
| *in Oil, Canned, Drained* | *1oz/28g* | *62.0* | *4.0* | *220* | *23.3* | *0.0* | *14.1* | *0.0* |
| in Smoky Barbecue Sauce, Princes* | 1 Can/120g | 182.0 | 10.0 | 152 | 15.1 | 5.0 | 8.0 | 0.0 |
| in Spring Water, Portuguese, Sainsbury's* | 1 Can/90g | 165.0 | 9.0 | 183 | 22.4 | 0.0 | 10.3 | 0.0 |
| in Tomato Sauce, Canned | 1oz/28g | 45.0 | 3.0 | 162 | 17.0 | 1.4 | 9.9 | 0.0 |
| Piccanti, in Olive Oil, Drained, Canned, Waitrose* | 1 Can/88g | 265.0 | 22.0 | 301 | 17.9 | 0.3 | 25.4 | 0.0 |
| *Raw* | *1oz/28g* | *46.0* | *3.0* | *165* | *20.6* | *0.0* | *9.2* | *0.0* |
| **SATAY** | | | | | | | | |
| Chicken, Breast, Iceland* | 1 Satay/10g | 15.0 | 0.0 | 155 | 34.1 | 2.7 | 0.9 | 0.1 |
| Chicken, Breast, Party Bites, Sainsbury's* | 1 Stick/10g | 16.0 | 0.0 | 157 | 34.1 | 2.7 | 0.9 | 0.1 |
| Chicken, Indonesian, Mini, Sainsbury's* | 1 Stick/10g | 17.0 | 1.0 | 171 | 23.0 | 4.0 | 7.0 | 0.7 |
| Chicken, M & S* | 1 Satay/43g | 90.0 | 5.0 | 210 | 19.1 | 4.4 | 12.7 | 0.7 |
| Chicken, Mini, Iceland* | 1 Satay/8g | 19.0 | 1.0 | 236 | 23.0 | 4.5 | 14.0 | 0.7 |
| Chicken, Morrisons* | 1 Satay/10g | 17.0 | 1.0 | 171 | 23.5 | 3.5 | 7.0 | 0.7 |
| Chicken, Occasions, Sainsbury's* | 1 Satay/10g | 15.0 | 1.0 | 150 | 22.0 | 2.0 | 6.0 | 0.7 |

**S**

| | Measure INFO/WEIGHT | per Measure KCAL | FAT | Nutrition Values per 100g / 100ml KCAL | PROT | CARB | FAT | FIBRE |
|---|---|---|---|---|---|---|---|---|
| **SATAY** | | | | | | | | |
| Chicken, Oriental, Tesco* | 1 Serving/100g | 160.0 | 5.0 | 160 | 23.6 | 5.1 | 5.0 | 0.4 |
| Chicken, Party, Mini, Tesco* | 1 Satay/10g | 13.0 | 0.0 | 133 | 23.7 | 3.4 | 2.8 | 1.0 |
| Chicken, Sticks, Asda* | 1 Stick/20g | 43.0 | 3.0 | 216 | 18.0 | 4.5 | 14.0 | 0.0 |
| Chicken, Stuffed, Asda* | ½ Pack/168g | 242.0 | 6.0 | 144 | 22.0 | 6.0 | 3.6 | 0.8 |
| Chicken, Taste Original* | 1 Stick/20g | 33.0 | 1.0 | 164 | 23.0 | 2.5 | 6.5 | 0.7 |
| Chicken, with Peanut Sauce, Waitrose* | 1 Pack/250g | 492.0 | 27.0 | 197 | 18.9 | 6.0 | 10.8 | 0.5 |
| Chicken & Turkey, Morrisons* | 1 Stick/20g | 39.0 | 2.0 | 197 | 20.3 | 1.0 | 12.4 | 2.3 |
| Chicken & Turkey, Sainsbury's* | 1 Stick/20g | 44.0 | 3.0 | 222 | 20.0 | 4.0 | 14.0 | 1.9 |
| Szechuan Style, Occasions, Sainsbury's* | 1 Satay/10g | 20.0 | 1.0 | 196 | 22.8 | 6.4 | 8.8 | 0.5 |
| **SATSUMAS** | | | | | | | | |
| *Fresh, Raw, Flesh Only, Average* | *1 Sm/56g* | *30.0* | *0.0* | *53* | *0.8* | *13.3* | *0.3* | *1.8* |
| *Weighed with Peel, Average* | *1 Med/80g* | *21.0* | *0.0* | *26* | *0.6* | *6.0* | *0.1* | *0.9* |
| **SAUCE** | | | | | | | | |
| Apple, Baxters* | 1 Tsp/15g | 7.0 | 0.0 | 49 | 0.1 | 11.1 | 0.4 | 0.7 |
| Apple, Bramley, Sainsbury's* | 1 Tsp/15g | 17.0 | 0.0 | 111 | 0.2 | 27.2 | 0.1 | 1.8 |
| Apple, Heinz* | 1 Tsp/15g | 8.0 | 0.0 | 56 | 0.3 | 13.4 | 0.2 | 1.5 |
| Apple, SmartPrice, Asda* | 1 Tsp/5g | 5.0 | 0.0 | 101 | 0.3 | 25.0 | 0.0 | 0.9 |
| Apple, Value, Tesco* | 1 Serving/50g | 29.0 | 0.0 | 58 | 0.1 | 14.4 | 0.0 | 0.5 |
| Apple & Brandy, Asda* | 1 Serving/125g | 56.0 | 0.0 | 45 | 0.2 | 11.0 | 0.0 | 0.0 |
| Apricot & Almond Tagine, Sainsbury's* | 1/3 Jar/120g | 98.0 | 2.0 | 82 | 2.0 | 17.9 | 1.6 | 2.5 |
| Aromatic Cantonese, Express, Uncle Ben's* | 1 Serving/170g | 172.0 | 0.0 | 101 | 0.6 | 24.6 | 0.1 | 0.0 |
| Arrabbiata, Italian, Tesco* | ½ Pot/175g | 72.0 | 1.0 | 41 | 1.3 | 8.3 | 0.3 | 1.1 |
| Arrabbiata, Lazio, Sainsbury's* | 1/3 Jar/113g | 154.0 | 12.0 | 136 | 2.2 | 7.2 | 10.9 | 0.0 |
| Arrabbiata, Weight Watchers* | ½ Pot/150g | 43.0 | 1.0 | 29 | 1.1 | 5.0 | 0.5 | 1.7 |
| Arrabiatta, Fresh, Waitrose* | 1 Serving/100g | 52.0 | 2.0 | 52 | 1.4 | 5.9 | 2.5 | 2.0 |
| Au Poivre, TTD, Sainsbury's* | 1 Serving/150g | 300.0 | 28.0 | 200 | 2.5 | 6.2 | 18.4 | 0.6 |
| Balti, 97% Fat Free, Homepride* | 1 Serving/230g | 133.0 | 4.0 | 58 | 1.1 | 9.1 | 1.9 | 1.8 |
| Balti, Cooking, BGTY, Sainsbury's* | ¼ Jar/129g | 98.0 | 4.0 | 76 | 1.1 | 10.9 | 3.1 | 0.6 |
| Balti, Cooking, Indian Inspired, Asda* | 1 Jar/320g | 243.0 | 11.0 | 76 | 0.9 | 10.5 | 3.4 | 1.8 |
| Balti, Cooking, Organic, Perfectly Balanced, Waitrose* | 1 Jar/450g | 301.0 | 6.0 | 67 | 1.6 | 12.1 | 1.3 | 3.1 |
| Balti, Cooking, Organic, Sainsbury's* | 1 Serving/225g | 157.0 | 5.0 | 70 | 2.2 | 10.0 | 2.3 | 0.5 |
| Balti, Cooking, Sharwood's* | 1/3 Jar/140g | 105.0 | 5.0 | 75 | 1.6 | 9.4 | 3.5 | 3.0 |
| Balti, Cooking, Tesco* | 1 Serving/500g | 395.0 | 20.0 | 79 | 1.5 | 9.2 | 4.0 | 2.2 |
| Balti, Deliciously Good, Homepride* | 1/3 Jar/153g | 89.0 | 3.0 | 58 | 1.1 | 9.1 | 1.9 | 0.6 |
| Balti, Indian Style, Iceland* | 1 Serving/220g | 154.0 | 6.0 | 70 | 1.6 | 10.1 | 2.6 | 0.5 |
| Balti, Reduced Fat, Healthy Living, Cook in, Co-Op* | ½ Jar/225g | 135.0 | 5.0 | 60 | 2.0 | 7.5 | 2.4 | 2.3 |
| Balti, Tomato & Coriander, Canned, Patak's* | 1 Can/283g | 235.0 | 17.0 | 83 | 0.8 | 6.5 | 6.0 | 1.2 |
| Balti Curry, Tesco* | 1 Serving/200g | 126.0 | 9.0 | 63 | 1.7 | 4.3 | 4.6 | 1.7 |
| Balti Indian, M & S* | 1oz/28g | 25.0 | 2.0 | 90 | 1.6 | 5.6 | 6.7 | 1.8 |
| Barbecue, Asda* | 1 Serving/135g | 128.0 | 0.0 | 95 | 1.2 | 22.0 | 0.2 | 0.6 |
| Barbecue, Chicken Tonight, Knorr* | ¼ Jar/125g | 76.0 | 0.0 | 61 | 2.0 | 12.4 | 0.4 | 0.9 |
| Barbecue, Cooking, BGTY, Sainsbury's* | ¼ Jar/124g | 46.0 | 0.0 | 37 | 0.4 | 8.4 | 0.2 | 0.7 |
| Barbecue, Original, Sainsbury's* | 1 Tbsp/15g | 19.0 | 0.0 | 127 | 0.9 | 29.6 | 0.1 | 0.3 |
| Barbecue, Smoky, Ainsley Harriott* | 1 Serving/10g | 15.0 | 0.0 | 153 | 0.8 | 36.4 | 0.1 | 0.0 |
| Barbeque, Cook in, Homepride* | 1 Can/500g | 375.0 | 7.0 | 75 | 0.7 | 14.6 | 1.5 | 0.6 |
| Barbeque, Simply Sausages Ranch, Colman's* | 1 Serving/130g | 96.0 | 0.0 | 74 | 1.8 | 16.6 | 0.1 | 1.1 |
| Basil & Pesto, M & S* | 1 Serving/65g | 348.0 | 30.0 | 535 | 7.5 | 20.7 | 46.9 | 1.4 |
| BBQ, Heinz* | 1 Serving/20g | 29.0 | 0.0 | 143 | 1.1 | 32.9 | 0.3 | 0.5 |
| BBQ, Hellmann's* | 1 Serving/10g | 12.0 | 0.0 | 125 | 0.8 | 27.7 | 0.7 | 0.0 |
| BBQ, HP* | 1 Serving/20ml | 29.0 | 0.0 | 143 | 0.8 | 33.1 | 0.2 | 0.0 |
| Bearnaise, Sainsbury's* | 1 Tbsp/15g | 59.0 | 6.0 | 393 | 0.6 | 5.0 | 41.0 | 0.0 |
| Bechamel, for Lasagne, Loyd Grossman* | 1 Jar/400g | 396.0 | 33.0 | 99 | 0.6 | 5.4 | 8.3 | 0.1 |
| Beef Bolognese, Weight Watchers* | 1 Pot/300g | 171.0 | 8.0 | 57 | 4.3 | 3.6 | 2.8 | 1.4 |

| | Measure INFO/WEIGHT | per Measure KCAL | FAT | Nutrition Values per 100g / 100ml KCAL | PROT | CARB | FAT | FIBRE |
|---|---|---|---|---|---|---|---|---|
| **SAUCE** | | | | | | | | |
| Beef in Ale, Cooking, Asda* | 1 Jar/500g | 160.0 | 1.0 | 32 | 1.6 | 6.0 | 0.2 | 0.0 |
| Bhuna, Cooking, Sharwood's* | 1/3 Jar/140g | 116.0 | 8.0 | 83 | 1.2 | 7.6 | 5.4 | 1.6 |
| Black Bean, Asda* | 1 Serving/55g | 55.0 | 1.0 | 100 | 2.9 | 19.0 | 1.4 | 0.0 |
| Black Bean, Canton, Stir Fry, Blue Dragon* | ½ Pack/60g | 53.0 | 1.0 | 88 | 2.8 | 14.8 | 2.0 | 1.5 |
| Black Bean, Cooking, Tesco* | 1 Tbsp/15g | 13.0 | 0.0 | 90 | 2.5 | 14.9 | 2.0 | 0.6 |
| Black Bean, Crushed, Stir Fry Sensations, Amoy* | 1 Pouch/150g | 150.0 | 4.0 | 100 | 2.4 | 16.9 | 2.9 | 1.0 |
| Black Bean, Finest, Tesco* | 1 Jar/350g | 252.0 | 2.0 | 72 | 0.8 | 16.1 | 0.5 | 0.8 |
| Black Bean, Fresh, Sainsbury's* | 1 Sachet/50ml | 78.0 | 1.0 | 156 | 6.7 | 27.5 | 2.6 | 1.7 |
| Black Bean, Loyd Grossman* | 1 Serving/175g | 177.0 | 8.0 | 101 | 2.4 | 12.6 | 4.5 | 0.7 |
| Black Bean, Ready to Stir Fry, M & S* | 1 Sachet/120g | 78.0 | 1.0 | 65 | 2.5 | 11.5 | 0.9 | 1.4 |
| Black Bean, Stir Fry, Fresh, M & S* | 1 Pot/120g | 120.0 | 1.0 | 100 | 2.6 | 20.3 | 0.6 | 1.4 |
| Black Bean, Stir Fry, Fresh Ideas, Tesco* | ½ Sachet/25g | 33.0 | 1.0 | 132 | 4.2 | 22.6 | 2.8 | 0.8 |
| Black Bean, Stir Fry, Sainsbury's* | ½ Pack/75ml | 91.0 | 3.0 | 121 | 3.3 | 17.6 | 4.3 | 1.7 |
| Black Bean, Stir Fry, Sharwood's* | 1 Jar/195g | 191.0 | 3.0 | 98 | 2.2 | 18.8 | 1.5 | 0.6 |
| Black Bean, Stir Fry Additions, Tesco* | 1 Sachet/50g | 69.0 | 1.0 | 138 | 4.1 | 23.6 | 3.0 | 0.0 |
| Black Bean, Uncle Ben's* | 1 Serving/125g | 89.0 | 2.0 | 71 | 2.0 | 12.8 | 1.3 | 0.0 |
| Black Bean & Chillli, Stir Fry, Asda* | ½ Jar/97g | 158.0 | 12.0 | 163 | 3.7 | 10.0 | 12.0 | 0.8 |
| Black Bean & Green Pepper, Stir Fry, Sharwood's* | 1 Serving/150g | 82.0 | 0.0 | 55 | 2.0 | 11.0 | 0.3 | 0.5 |
| Black Bean & Red Pepper, Sharwood's* | ½ Jar/213g | 132.0 | 3.0 | 62 | 1.9 | 10.5 | 1.4 | 1.2 |
| Black Pepper, Stir Fry, Blue Dragon* | ½ Sachet/60g | 47.0 | 3.0 | 79 | 1.6 | 8.4 | 4.4 | 0.1 |
| Bolognese, Emilia Romagna, Fresh, Sainsbury's* | ½ Pot/150g | 99.0 | 5.0 | 66 | 5.9 | 3.4 | 3.2 | 1.7 |
| Bolognese, for Beef, Tesco* | ½ Pack/175g | 177.0 | 10.0 | 101 | 5.4 | 6.9 | 5.8 | 0.8 |
| Bolognese, Italiano, Tesco* | 1 Serving/175g | 194.0 | 13.0 | 111 | 5.9 | 4.8 | 7.5 | 0.8 |
| Bolognese, Loyd Grossman* | ¼ Jar/106g | 79.0 | 3.0 | 75 | 2.0 | 10.2 | 2.9 | 1.4 |
| Bolognese, Original, Deliciously Good, Homepride* | ¼ Jar/112g | 39.0 | 0.0 | 35 | 1.3 | 7.1 | 0.2 | 0.8 |
| Bolognese, Tinned, Sainsbury's* | 1/3 Can/141g | 86.0 | 3.0 | 61 | 4.5 | 5.7 | 2.2 | 1.0 |
| Bolognese, Waitrose* | 1 Serving/175g | 150.0 | 9.0 | 86 | 5.4 | 5.3 | 4.9 | 2.0 |
| Bourguignon, Beef Tonight, Knorr* | ¼ Jar/125g | 71.0 | 3.0 | 57 | 0.6 | 7.6 | 2.6 | 0.4 |
| Branston Smooth, Crosse & Blackwell* | 1 Serving/25g | 35.0 | 0.0 | 139 | 0.6 | 34.0 | 0.1 | 1.4 |
| Brazilian Chicken, Chicken Tonight, Knorr* | ¼ Jar/125g | 49.0 | 1.0 | 39 | 1.2 | 7.0 | 0.7 | 1.3 |
| Bread, Luxury, M & S* | 1 Serving/115g | 195.0 | 16.0 | 170 | 3.2 | 8.1 | 14.1 | 2.2 |
| Bread, M & S* | 1 Serving/85g | 153.0 | 12.0 | 180 | 3.1 | 8.7 | 14.6 | 0.2 |
| Bread, Made with Semi-Skimmed Milk | 1 Serving/45g | 42.0 | 1.0 | 93 | 4.3 | 12.8 | 3.1 | 0.3 |
| Brown, Asda* | 1 Serving/10g | 10.0 | 0.0 | 97 | 0.7 | 23.0 | 0.2 | 0.4 |
| Brown, Bottled | 1 Tsp/6g | 6.0 | 0.0 | 99 | 1.1 | 25.2 | 0.0 | 0.7 |
| Brown, Iceland* | 1 Serving/20g | 16.0 | 0.0 | 82 | 0.7 | 19.3 | 0.2 | 1.1 |
| Brown, Tesco* | 1 Tsp/10g | 10.0 | 0.0 | 104 | 0.7 | 25.1 | 0.1 | 0.6 |
| Burger, Hellmann's* | 1 Tbsp/15g | 36.0 | 3.0 | 240 | 1.1 | 12.0 | 21.0 | 0.0 |
| Butter & Tarragon, Chicken Tonigh, Knorr* | ¼ Jar/125g | 132.0 | 13.0 | 106 | 1.0 | 2.1 | 10.4 | 0.7 |
| Cajun, Sizzle & Stir, Chicken Tonight, Knorr* | 1/3 Jar/150g | 189.0 | 12.0 | 126 | 0.8 | 12.0 | 8.3 | 0.0 |
| Cantonese, Sizzling, Uncle Ben's* | ½ Jar/270g | 416.0 | 16.0 | 154 | 0.7 | 24.0 | 6.1 | 0.0 |
| Cantonese Chow Mein Stir Fry, Sainsbury's* | ½ Jar/100g | 67.0 | 2.0 | 67 | 0.4 | 12.1 | 1.9 | 0.8 |
| Caramelised Onion & Red Wine, M & S* | 1 Serving/52g | 31.0 | 2.0 | 60 | 1.9 | 6.7 | 3.1 | 0.6 |
| Carbonara, HE, Tesco* | 1 Serving/175g | 121.0 | 5.0 | 69 | 5.2 | 6.2 | 2.6 | 0.0 |
| Carbonara, Less Than 5% Fat, GFY, Asda* | ½ Tub/150g | 121.0 | 7.0 | 81 | 5.0 | 5.0 | 4.5 | 0.5 |
| Chasseur, Classic, Chicken Tonight, Knorr* | ¼ Jar/125g | 61.0 | 4.0 | 49 | 0.6 | 5.3 | 2.9 | 0.7 |
| Chasseur, Cook in, Homepride* | 1 Can/390g | 160.0 | 0.0 | 41 | 0.7 | 9.2 | 0.1 | 0.4 |
| Cheddar Cheese, Colemans* | 1 Serving/85ml | 348.0 | 13.0 | 410 | 19.2 | 48.5 | 15.4 | 1.9 |
| Cheddar Cheese, Dry, Knorr* | 1 Serving/10g | 47.0 | 3.0 | 469 | 7.8 | 38.0 | 31.8 | 0.3 |
| Cheese, Basics, Sainsbury's* | ¼ Pot/124g | 71.0 | 3.0 | 57 | 2.5 | 6.1 | 2.5 | 0.5 |
| Cheese, Dry, Asda* | 1 Serving/27g | 101.0 | 3.0 | 373 | 4.4 | 64.0 | 11.0 | 7.0 |
| Cheese, Fresh, Italiano, Tesco* | ½ Tub/175g | 236.0 | 16.0 | 135 | 6.8 | 6.2 | 9.2 | 0.0 |
| Cheese, Fresh, Waitrose* | 1 Pot/350g | 458.0 | 34.0 | 131 | 5.1 | 5.7 | 9.8 | 0.0 |

S

# SAUCE

| Measure INFO/WEIGHT | per Measure KCAL | FAT | Nutrition Values per 100g / 100ml KCAL | PROT | CARB | FAT | FIBRE |
|---|---|---|---|---|---|---|---|
| Cheese, Instant, Morrisons* | 1 Serving/14g | 38.0 | 3.0 | 272 | 7.9 | 14.3 | 20.3 | 0.0 |
| Cheese, Italian, Tesco* | ½ Carton/175g | 238.0 | 16.0 | 136 | 5.8 | 8.3 | 8.9 | 0.0 |
| Cheese, Italian Style, Finest, Tesco* | ½ Pot/175g | 355.0 | 21.0 | 203 | 10.1 | 14.0 | 11.9 | 0.0 |
| Cheese, Italiano, Tesco* | 1 Pot/350g | 367.0 | 20.0 | 105 | 5.3 | 8.0 | 5.7 | 0.0 |
| Cheese, Made with Semi-Skimmed Milk | 1 Serving/60g | 107.0 | 8.0 | 179 | 8.1 | 9.1 | 12.6 | 0.2 |
| Cheese, Made with Whole Milk | 1 Serving/60g | 118.0 | 9.0 | 197 | 8.0 | 9.0 | 14.6 | 0.2 |
| Cheese, Sainsbury's* | 1 Serving/125g | 140.0 | 9.0 | 112 | 5.0 | 6.1 | 7.5 | 1.2 |
| Cherry Tomato, Finest, Tesco* | ½ Pot/171g | 120.0 | 4.0 | 70 | 1.5 | 9.4 | 2.6 | 1.1 |
| Cherry Tomato & Fresh Basil, M & S* | 1 Serving/175g | 131.0 | 9.0 | 75 | 1.2 | 5.5 | 5.3 | 1.1 |
| Chicken, Sizzling, Dolmio* | 1 Serving/100g | 102.0 | 7.0 | 102 | 1.2 | 7.5 | 7.5 | 0.0 |
| Chicken Jalfrezi, Sizzle & Stir, Knorr* | 1 Jar/455g | 514.0 | 46.0 | 113 | 1.1 | 4.4 | 10.1 | 2.4 |
| Chilli, Amoy* | 1 Tsp/6g | 1.0 | 0.0 | 25 | 1.0 | 5.2 | 0.0 | 1.0 |
| Chilli, Hot, Asda* | 1 Jar/570g | 445.0 | 3.0 | 78 | 3.7 | 14.4 | 0.6 | 3.2 |
| Chilli, Hot, Blue Dragon* | 1 Tbsp/15ml | 14.0 | 0.0 | 96 | 0.5 | 23.0 | 0.2 | 0.0 |
| Chilli, Hot, Co-Op* | 1 Jar/440g | 242.0 | 2.0 | 55 | 2.0 | 10.0 | 0.5 | 2.0 |
| Chilli, Hot, Heinz* | 1 Portion/10g | 8.0 | 0.0 | 80 | 1.4 | 18.0 | 0.0 | 0.0 |
| Chilli, Hot, Mexican, Morrisons* | ¼ Jar/125g | 72.0 | 1.0 | 58 | 2.2 | 11.2 | 0.5 | 2.0 |
| Chilli, HP* | 1 Tsp/6g | 8.0 | 0.0 | 134 | 1.2 | 32.3 | 0.0 | 0.0 |
| Chilli, Iceland* | 1 Serving/115g | 75.0 | 1.0 | 65 | 2.7 | 12.0 | 0.7 | 1.6 |
| Chilli, Medium, Deliciously Good, Homepride* | 1 Jar/460g | 258.0 | 2.0 | 56 | 2.3 | 10.4 | 0.5 | 1.2 |
| Chilli, Medium, Somerfield* | ¼ Jar/110g | 57.0 | 0.0 | 52 | 2.4 | 9.6 | 0.4 | 2.1 |
| Chilli, Mild, Healthy Eating, Asda* | ½ Jar/250g | 172.0 | 6.0 | 69 | 2.1 | 10.0 | 2.3 | 1.7 |
| Chilli, Mild, Safeway* | 1 Serving/250g | 187.0 | 5.0 | 75 | 2.4 | 11.3 | 2.2 | 1.2 |
| Chilli, Sweet, Thai, Dipping, Original, Blue Dragon* | 1 Serving/30ml | 69.0 | 0.0 | 229 | 0.6 | 55.1 | 0.7 | 1.6 |
| Chilli, Tesco* | 1 Tsp/5ml | 4.0 | 0.0 | 90 | 1.3 | 14.0 | 3.2 | 1.1 |
| *Chilli, Tomato Based, Bottled, Average* | *1 Tbsp/15g* | *16.0* | *0.0* | *104* | *2.5* | *19.8* | *0.3* | *5.9* |
| Chilli, with Kidney Beans, Old El Paso* | 1 Serving/115g | 92.0 | 1.0 | 80 | 4.3 | 14.8 | 0.4 | 0.0 |
| Chilli & Garlic, Blue Dragon* | 1 Serving/30ml | 25.0 | 0.0 | 85 | 1.1 | 19.7 | 0.2 | 0.0 |
| Chilli & Garlic, Lea & Perrins* | 1 Tsp/6g | 4.0 | 0.0 | 60 | 1.0 | 14.9 | 0.0 | 0.0 |
| Chilli & Garlic, Stir Fry, M & S* | 1 Serving/83g | 120.0 | 1.0 | 145 | 0.7 | 32.4 | 1.2 | 1.1 |
| Chilli Con Carne, Asda* | 1 Lge Jar/570g | 370.0 | 4.0 | 65 | 2.6 | 12.0 | 0.7 | 0.0 |
| Chilli Con Carne, Cook in, BGTY, Sainsbury's* | ¼ Jar/125g | 69.0 | 1.0 | 55 | 1.7 | 11.0 | 0.5 | 2.5 |
| Chilli Con Carne, Cook in, Homepride* | 1 Can/390g | 234.0 | 2.0 | 60 | 2.5 | 11.2 | 0.6 | 0.0 |
| Chilli Con Carne, Hot, Sainsbury's* | 1 Serving/116g | 66.0 | 0.0 | 57 | 2.4 | 11.3 | 0.2 | 1.6 |
| Chilli Con Carne, Hot, Uncle Ben's* | 1 Jar/500g | 295.0 | 3.0 | 59 | 2.3 | 10.9 | 0.6 | 1.7 |
| Chilli Con Carne, Sizzle & Stir, Knorr* | 1 Jar/455g | 505.0 | 32.0 | 111 | 2.7 | 9.1 | 7.1 | 2.7 |
| Chilli Con Carne, Weight Watchers* | ½ Jar/175g | 84.0 | 0.0 | 48 | 1.8 | 9.7 | 0.2 | 2.0 |
| Chilli Soy, Amoy* | 1 Tbsp/15g | 8.0 | 0.0 | 55 | 4.6 | 9.1 | 0.0 | 0.0 |
| Chinese, Stir Fry, Sachet, Fresh, Sainsbury's* | ½ Sachet/51ml | 83.0 | 6.0 | 163 | 1.7 | 14.1 | 11.1 | 1.8 |
| Chinese 5 Spice, Stir It Up, Chicken Tonight, Knorr* | 1 Jar/80g | 478.0 | 40.0 | 597 | 2.4 | 34.1 | 50.1 | 6.6 |
| Chinese Orange, Honey & Ginger, Cooking, Sainsbury's* | 1 Serving/125g | 91.0 | 0.0 | 73 | 0.3 | 17.2 | 0.3 | 0.3 |
| Chinese Stir Fry, Sainsbury's* | ½ Sachet/75g | 61.0 | 2.0 | 81 | 0.4 | 14.1 | 2.5 | 1.0 |
| Chinese Style, Stir Fry, Fresh, Asda* | ½ Sachet/50ml | 93.0 | 6.0 | 186 | 1.5 | 18.0 | 12.0 | 0.0 |
| Chip Shop Curry, Knorr* | 1 Sachet/150ml | 145.0 | 7.0 | 97 | 1.7 | 12.4 | 4.6 | 0.7 |
| Chocolate, Dry, Sainsbury's* | 1 Serving/30g | 108.0 | 3.0 | 360 | 1.3 | 62.8 | 11.6 | 0.9 |
| Chocolate, Sainsbury's* | 1 Serving/25g | 81.0 | 2.0 | 323 | 1.8 | 64.7 | 6.3 | 2.7 |
| Chop Suey, Blue Dragon* | ½ Sachet/60g | 34.0 | 1.0 | 57 | 0.5 | 8.3 | 2.4 | 0.5 |
| Chop Suey, Cantonese, Sharwood's* | 1 Serving/200g | 146.0 | 3.0 | 73 | 0.6 | 14.4 | 1.4 | 0.4 |
| Chop Suey, Stir Fry, Sharwood's* | 1 Jar/160g | 120.0 | 2.0 | 75 | 0.7 | 14.6 | 1.5 | 0.2 |
| Chow Mein, Sainsbury's* | 1 Serving/50g | 35.0 | 1.0 | 71 | 1.8 | 10.5 | 2.4 | 0.0 |
| Chow Mein, Stir Fry, Asda* | ½ Jar/98g | 97.0 | 1.0 | 99 | 1.6 | 21.0 | 1.0 | 0.1 |
| Chow Mein, Stir Fry, Blue Dragon* | 1 Sachet/120g | 110.0 | 3.0 | 92 | 1.1 | 15.4 | 2.9 | 0.4 |
| Chow Mein Stir Fry, Morrisons* | ½ Sachet/50g | 85.0 | 3.0 | 170 | 1.3 | 29.0 | 5.1 | 0.7 |

| | Measure INFO/WEIGHT | per Measure KCAL | FAT | Nutrition Values per 100g / 100ml KCAL | PROT | CARB | FAT | FIBRE |
|---|---|---|---|---|---|---|---|---|
| **SAUCE** | | | | | | | | |
| Coconut, Chilli & Lime, Cook-In, Homepride* | 1 Serving/115g | 110.0 | 9.0 | 96 | 1.1 | 5.9 | 7.5 | 0.0 |
| Coconut, Thai Style, Stir Fry, Waitrose* | ½ Pack/50ml | 52.0 | 4.0 | 105 | 1.5 | 5.5 | 8.6 | 1.8 |
| Coconut & Red Chilli, Noodle Sauce, Tesco* | 1/3 Jar/110g | 88.0 | 7.0 | 80 | 1.7 | 3.8 | 6.4 | 0.7 |
| Cooking, Balti, Extra Special, Asda* | 1 Jar/120g | 180.0 | 10.0 | 150 | 2.0 | 17.0 | 8.0 | 1.0 |
| Cooking, Honey & Mustard, Light Choices, Tesco* | 1 Serving/124g | 93.0 | 2.0 | 75 | 1.4 | 13.0 | 1.6 | 1.2 |
| Cooking, Korma, Light Choices, Tesco* | ¼ Jar/125g | 100.0 | 4.0 | 80 | 1.6 | 10.2 | 3.2 | 1.6 |
| Coronation, Heinz* | 1 Tbsp/10g | 33.0 | 3.0 | 334 | 0.8 | 13.1 | 31.0 | 0.9 |
| Coronation Chicken, Cook in, Homepride* | 1 Serving/250g | 232.0 | 10.0 | 93 | 0.8 | 13.2 | 4.2 | 0.0 |
| Country French, Chicken Tonigh, Knorr* | ¼ Jar/125g | 112.0 | 10.0 | 90 | 0.5 | 4.1 | 8.0 | 0.7 |
| Country French, Low Fat, Chicken Tonight, Knorr* | ¼ Jar/125g | 56.0 | 4.0 | 45 | 0.4 | 4.4 | 2.9 | 0.7 |
| Cranberry, Safeway* | 1 Tsp/15g | 25.0 | 0.0 | 168 | 0.2 | 41.0 | 0.3 | 1.3 |
| Cranberry, Sainsbury's* | 1 Tsp/15g | 23.0 | 0.0 | 154 | 0.8 | 37.1 | 0.3 | 1.3 |
| Cranberry, Tesco* | 1 Tsp/15g | 23.0 | 0.0 | 156 | 0.1 | 38.8 | 0.0 | 0.9 |
| Cranberry, Waitrose* | 1 Tbsp/20g | 31.0 | 0.0 | 156 | 0.2 | 38.5 | 0.2 | 14.0 |
| Cranberry, with Brandy & Orange Zest, Finest, Tesco* | 1 Serving/10g | 23.0 | 0.0 | 235 | 0.3 | 57.2 | 0.6 | 1.3 |
| Cranberry & Port, M & S* | 1 Serving/75g | 71.0 | 0.0 | 95 | 2.3 | 20.2 | 0.4 | 2.1 |
| Cranberry Jelly, Baxters* | 1 Tsp/15g | 40.0 | 0.0 | 268 | 0.0 | 67.0 | 0.0 | 0.0 |
| Cranberry Jelly, Morrisons* | 1 Tsp/12g | 23.0 | 0.0 | 189 | 0.2 | 47.0 | 0.0 | 0.1 |
| Creamy, Curry, BGTY, Sainsbury's* | ¼ Jar/125g | 84.0 | 5.0 | 67 | 1.4 | 6.8 | 3.8 | 0.5 |
| Creamy Ham, Knorr* | 1 Pouch/100ml | 163.0 | 16.0 | 163 | 0.3 | 4.0 | 16.0 | 0.3 |
| Creamy Horseradish with Garlic, So Good, Somerfield* | 1 Tsp/6g | 19.0 | 1.0 | 317 | 4.1 | 25.0 | 22.3 | 0.0 |
| Creamy Mushroom, Cooking, M & S* | 1 Jar/510g | 663.0 | 58.0 | 130 | 1.3 | 5.4 | 11.3 | 0.5 |
| Creamy Mushroom, Knorr* | 1 Serving/125g | 111.0 | 10.0 | 89 | 0.4 | 4.5 | 7.7 | 0.4 |
| Creamy Peppercorn & Whisky, Baxters* | 1 Pack/320g | 422.0 | 35.0 | 132 | 1.9 | 6.7 | 10.8 | 0.2 |
| Creole, Soulful, Sauce & Spice Mix, Two Step, Discovery* | 1 Jar/370g | 314.0 | 7.0 | 85 | 1.7 | 18.0 | 1.8 | 3.3 |
| Cumberland Sausage, Colman's* | ¼ Jar/126g | 43.0 | 0.0 | 34 | 0.7 | 7.4 | 0.2 | 0.8 |
| Curry, 98% Fat Free, Homepride* | 1oz/28g | 16.0 | 1.0 | 56 | 1.1 | 8.6 | 1.9 | 0.5 |
| Curry, Cook in, Homepride* | ½ Can/250g | 140.0 | 5.0 | 56 | 1.1 | 8.6 | 1.9 | 0.5 |
| Curry, Creamy, Chicken Tonight, Knorr* | ½ Jar/250g | 207.0 | 18.0 | 83 | 0.6 | 3.6 | 7.4 | 0.8 |
| Curry, Creamy, Cooking, BGTY, Sainsbury's* | ¼ Jar/125g | 94.0 | 4.0 | 75 | 1.8 | 10.1 | 3.0 | 1.0 |
| Curry, Deliciously Good, Homepride* | 1/3 Jar/149g | 91.0 | 3.0 | 61 | 1.1 | 10.0 | 1.8 | 0.5 |
| Curry, Green Thai, BGTY, Sainsbury's* | ¼ Jar/125g | 61.0 | 3.0 | 49 | 0.6 | 5.7 | 2.6 | 1.4 |
| Curry, Green Thai, Finest, Tesco* | 1 Serving/350g | 420.0 | 37.0 | 120 | 1.4 | 4.8 | 10.6 | 0.7 |
| Curry, Green Thai, Sharwood's* | 1 Serving/403g | 431.0 | 31.0 | 107 | 1.1 | 8.4 | 7.6 | 0.1 |
| Curry, Mild, Tesco* | 1 Jar/500g | 420.0 | 14.0 | 84 | 1.1 | 13.4 | 2.8 | 0.8 |
| Curry, Red Thai, BGTY, Sainsbury's* | 1 Serving/124g | 77.0 | 5.0 | 62 | 0.6 | 6.0 | 3.9 | 1.4 |
| Curry, Red Thai, Finest, Tesco* | 1 Jar/350g | 388.0 | 31.0 | 111 | 1.3 | 6.2 | 9.0 | 0.9 |
| Curry, Red Thai, Sainsbury's* | ½ Pouch/250g | 390.0 | 36.0 | 156 | 1.7 | 5.0 | 14.3 | 1.5 |
| Curry, Red Thai, Sharwood's* | 1 Serving/138g | 150.0 | 11.0 | 109 | 1.2 | 7.9 | 8.0 | 0.2 |
| Curry, Red Thai, Sizzle & Stir, Chicken Tonight, Knorr* | 1 Jar/485g | 873.0 | 84.0 | 180 | 1.5 | 4.5 | 17.3 | 1.7 |
| Curry, Thai Coconut, Uncle Ben's* | 1 Serving/125g | 127.0 | 6.0 | 102 | 1.4 | 13.2 | 4.8 | 0.0 |
| Curry, Value, Tesco* | 1 Can/390g | 355.0 | 18.0 | 91 | 1.6 | 11.0 | 4.5 | 1.3 |
| Curry, Yellow Thai, Cooking, Sainsbury's* | 1 Jar/500g | 785.0 | 70.0 | 157 | 2.3 | 5.4 | 14.0 | 2.3 |
| Dark Soy, Sesame & Ginger, for Fish, Schwartz* | 1 Pack/300g | 279.0 | 4.0 | 93 | 1.3 | 18.8 | 1.4 | 0.5 |
| Dhansak, Medium, Sharwood's* | 1 Jar/420g | 370.0 | 13.0 | 88 | 3.6 | 11.1 | 3.2 | 1.0 |
| Dhansak, Sharwood's* | 1 Jar/445g | 667.0 | 35.0 | 150 | 4.7 | 15.2 | 7.8 | 1.4 |
| Dill & Lemon, Delicate, for Fish, Schwartz* | 1 Pack/300g | 387.0 | 34.0 | 129 | 1.1 | 5.6 | 11.4 | 0.5 |
| Dill & Mustard, for Gravadlax, Dry, Waitrose* | 1 Sachet/35g | 123.0 | 9.0 | 352 | 2.5 | 27.8 | 25.7 | 0.6 |
| Dipping for Dim Sum, Amoy* | 1 Tbsp/15ml | 28.0 | 0.0 | 190 | 0.0 | 48.0 | 0.0 | 0.0 |
| Dopiaza, Cooking, Tesco* | 1 Serving/166g | 176.0 | 11.0 | 106 | 2.2 | 9.4 | 6.6 | 1.9 |
| Dopiaza, Tomato & Onion, Original, in Glass Jar, Patak's* | 1 Jar/540g | 605.0 | 39.0 | 112 | 1.6 | 9.8 | 7.3 | 1.2 |
| Dopiaza, medium, Cook in, Sharwood's* | ½ Bottle/210g | 193.0 | 11.0 | 92 | 1.4 | 10.2 | 5.1 | 0.6 |
| Enchilada, Medium, Old El Paso* | 1 Can/270g | 92.0 | 5.0 | 34 | 0.0 | 5.0 | 1.7 | 0.0 |

**S**

## SAUCE

| | Measure INFO/WEIGHT | per Measure KCAL | FAT | KCAL | PROT | CARB | FAT | FIBRE |
|---|---|---|---|---|---|---|---|---|
| Exotic Curry, Heinz* | 1 Serving/15ml | 41.0 | 3.0 | 271 | 0.7 | 15.3 | 22.8 | 0.6 |
| Fajita, Asda* | ¼ Jar/125g | 79.0 | 5.0 | 63 | 1.0 | 5.0 | 4.3 | 1.0 |
| Fajita, M & S* | 1oz/28g | 24.0 | 2.0 | 85 | 1.3 | 6.4 | 6.1 | 2.2 |
| Fish, Nuoc Mam, Thai, Blue Dragon* | 1 Tsp/5ml | 7.0 | 0.0 | 145 | 5.9 | 30.9 | 0.1 | 0.0 |
| Florentina, Italiano, Tesco* | ½ Tub/175g | 128.0 | 10.0 | 73 | 2.1 | 3.8 | 5.5 | 0.6 |
| Flour, Dry, Sainsbury's* | 1 Serving/20g | 69.0 | 0.0 | 343 | 9.8 | 73.0 | 1.3 | 3.0 |
| for Fajitas, Original Smoky BBQ, Cooking, Old El Paso* | 1 Jar/395g | 222.0 | 5.0 | 56 | 1.5 | 9.6 | 1.3 | 0.0 |
| for Lasagne, White, Tesco* | 1 Jar/460g | 506.0 | 41.0 | 110 | 1.9 | 5.3 | 9.0 | 0.6 |
| Four Cheese, Asda* | ½ Jar/155g | 242.0 | 22.0 | 156 | 3.5 | 3.9 | 14.0 | 0.1 |
| Four Cheese, Reduced Fat, Morrisons* | ½ Tub/175g | 161.0 | 9.0 | 92 | 6.1 | 4.8 | 5.4 | 0.5 |
| Fruity, HP* | 1 Tsp/6g | 8.0 | 0.0 | 141 | 1.2 | 35.1 | 0.1 | 0.0 |
| Garlic, Heinz* | 1 Serving/10ml | 32.0 | 3.0 | 323 | 1.0 | 12.1 | 29.9 | 1.2 |
| Garlic, Lea & Perrins* | 1 Tsp/6g | 20.0 | 2.0 | 337 | 1.8 | 17.8 | 29.0 | 0.0 |
| Garlic & Chive, Heinz* | 1 Serving/10ml | 35.0 | 3.0 | 350 | 1.0 | 11.3 | 33.2 | 0.1 |
| Green Peppercorn, Dry, Sainsbury's* | 1 Tbsp/15ml | 68.0 | 7.0 | 455 | 0.4 | 3.8 | 48.5 | 0.1 |
| Green Tandoori, M & S* | 1 Jar/385g | 500.0 | 38.0 | 130 | 3.6 | 6.8 | 9.9 | 1.5 |
| Green Thai, Cooking, Perfectly Balanced, Waitrose* | ½ Jar/215g | 112.0 | 7.0 | 52 | 0.8 | 4.9 | 3.2 | 1.5 |
| Green Thai, Loyd Grossman* | ½ Jar/175g | 182.0 | 11.0 | 104 | 1.6 | 10.0 | 6.4 | 0.8 |
| Green Thai, So Good, Somerfield* | 1 Jar/350g | 413.0 | 33.0 | 118 | 1.2 | 7.0 | 9.5 | 0.5 |
| Green Thai, Stir Fry, Additions, Tesco* | 1 Pack/100g | 173.0 | 16.0 | 173 | 2.1 | 6.1 | 15.6 | 0.5 |
| Green Thai, Stir Fry, Asda* | 1 Pack/180ml | 344.0 | 27.0 | 191 | 2.4 | 11.1 | 15.2 | 1.0 |
| Green Thai, Stir Fry, Fresh Ideas, Tesco* | 1 Pack/50g | 91.0 | 8.0 | 182 | 2.1 | 6.2 | 16.6 | 0.1 |
| Green Thai, Stir Fry, Safeway* | 1 Serving/75ml | 259.0 | 24.0 | 345 | 1.2 | 12.2 | 32.0 | 2.1 |
| Green Thai, Stir Fry, Sainsbury's* | ½ Pack/75g | 112.0 | 8.0 | 149 | 1.2 | 11.9 | 10.7 | 1.0 |
| Hoi Sin, M & S* | ½ Pot/50ml | 80.0 | 1.0 | 160 | 3.2 | 31.8 | 2.0 | 2.2 |
| Hoi Sin, Sharwood's* | 1 Tbsp/15g | 32.0 | 0.0 | 211 | 2.7 | 49.5 | 0.3 | 0.1 |
| Hoi Sin, Stir Fry, Asda* | 1 Serving/100g | 165.0 | 1.0 | 165 | 2.6 | 36.9 | 0.8 | 1.0 |
| Hoi Sin & Garlic, Blue Dragon* | 1 Serving/60g | 80.0 | 2.0 | 133 | 1.2 | 26.1 | 2.6 | 0.0 |
| Hoi Sin & Plum, Chinatown, Knorr* | ¼ Jar/131g | 96.0 | 1.0 | 73 | 0.8 | 15.8 | 0.7 | 1.2 |
| Hoi Sin & Plum, Sweet & Fruity, Stir Fry, Sharwood's* | 1 Serving/136g | 128.0 | 2.0 | 94 | 0.7 | 19.9 | 1.3 | 0.9 |
| Hoi Sin & Spring Onion, Stir Fry, Sharwood's* | 1 Jar/165g | 196.0 | 2.0 | 119 | 1.3 | 26.5 | 0.9 | 0.8 |
| Hollandaise, Classic, for Fish, Schwartz* | 1 Sachet/300g | 456.0 | 49.0 | 152 | 0.7 | 0.4 | 16.4 | 2.0 |
| Hollandaise, Classic, Knorr* | 1 Serving/100ml | 202.0 | 20.0 | 202 | 0.6 | 3.9 | 20.5 | 0.4 |
| Hollandaise, Dry, M & S* | 1oz/28g | 115.0 | 12.0 | 410 | 0.9 | 3.6 | 43.6 | 0.5 |
| Hollandaise, Finest, Tesco* | 1 Serving/98g | 473.0 | 44.0 | 485 | 1.4 | 17.2 | 45.6 | 0.3 |
| Hollandaise, Full Fat, Dry, M & S* | 1 Tbsp/20g | 67.0 | 7.0 | 336 | 1.1 | 4.5 | 34.9 | 0.1 |
| Hollandaise, Homemade, Average | 1oz/28g | 198.0 | 21.0 | 707 | 4.8 | 0.0 | 76.2 | 0.0 |
| Hollandaise, M & S* | 1 Serving/10g | 41.0 | 4.0 | 410 | 0.9 | 3.6 | 43.6 | 0.5 |
| Hollandaise, Pour Over, Knorr* | 1oz/28g | 44.0 | 4.0 | 158 | 0.0 | 7.0 | 14.0 | 0.0 |
| Hollandaise, Sainsbury's* | 1 Tbsp/15g | 72.0 | 8.0 | 478 | 0.2 | 5.9 | 50.4 | 0.4 |
| Honey & Coriander, Stir Fry, Blue Dragon* | 1 Pack/120g | 115.0 | 1.0 | 96 | 0.5 | 22.1 | 0.6 | 0.3 |
| Honey & Mustard, COU, M & S* | ½ Jar/160g | 112.0 | 5.0 | 70 | 2.3 | 9.2 | 2.9 | 0.7 |
| Honey & Mustard, for Cooking, Asda* | 1 Serving/200g | 234.0 | 14.0 | 117 | 0.6 | 13.0 | 7.0 | 0.0 |
| Honey & Mustard, Low Fat, Chicken Tonight, Knorr* | ¼ Jar/131g | 105.0 | 3.0 | 80 | 1.0 | 13.8 | 2.3 | 0.8 |
| Hong Kong Curry, Loyd Grossman* | 1 Jar/350g | 371.0 | 27.0 | 106 | 1.3 | 7.8 | 7.7 | 0.8 |
| Horseradish, Asda* | 1oz/28g | 38.0 | 2.0 | 135 | 2.2 | 14.0 | 7.0 | 2.0 |
| Horseradish, Colman's* | 1 Tbsp/15ml | 17.0 | 1.0 | 112 | 1.9 | 9.8 | 6.2 | 2.6 |
| Horseradish, Creamed, Colman's* | 1 Tsp/16g | 37.0 | 2.0 | 229 | 4.3 | 21.4 | 13.3 | 0.0 |
| Horseradish, Creamy, Sainsbury's* | 1 Tsp/5g | 11.0 | 1.0 | 223 | 2.8 | 28.9 | 11.8 | 1.6 |
| Horseradish, Hot, Tesco* | 1 Tsp/5g | 9.0 | 1.0 | 185 | 2.3 | 19.7 | 10.6 | 2.3 |
| Horseradish, Mustard, Sainsbury's* | 1 Tsp/5g | 8.0 | 0.0 | 163 | 7.9 | 18.2 | 6.6 | 3.5 |
| Horseradish, Sainsbury's* | 1 Dtsp/10g | 14.0 | 1.0 | 145 | 1.5 | 17.8 | 6.6 | 2.4 |
| Horseradish Cream, Tesco* | 1 Serving/15g | 29.0 | 2.0 | 195 | 2.3 | 18.7 | 11.9 | 2.1 |

S

| | Measure INFO/WEIGHT | per Measure KCAL | FAT | Nutrition Values per 100g / 100ml KCAL | PROT | CARB | FAT | FIBRE |
|---|---|---|---|---|---|---|---|---|
| **SAUCE** | | | | | | | | |
| Hot Chilli, Deliciously Good, Homepride* | 1 Serving/120g | 62.0 | 1.0 | 52 | 1.3 | 10.6 | 0.5 | 1.1 |
| Hot Chilli, Sharwood's* | 1 fl oz/30ml | 36.0 | 0.0 | 120 | 0.5 | 29.4 | 0.6 | 1.3 |
| Hot Onion, Sainsbury's* | 1 Serving/10g | 17.0 | 0.0 | 167 | 0.2 | 41.0 | 0.1 | 0.1 |
| Hot Pepper | 1oz/28g | 7.0 | 0.0 | 26 | 1.6 | 1.7 | 1.5 | 0.0 |
| HP* | 1 Tbsp/15g | 18.0 | 0.0 | 119 | 1.1 | 27.1 | 0.2 | 1.3 |
| Indian Tikka, Chicken Tonight, Knorr* | 1 Serving/250g | 320.0 | 23.0 | 128 | 1.3 | 10.0 | 9.2 | 1.2 |
| Italian Hot Chilli, Dolmio* | ½ Pack/150g | 103.0 | 6.0 | 69 | 1.3 | 7.1 | 3.9 | 0.0 |
| Italian Onion & Garlic, Sainsbury's* | 1 Jar/500g | 375.0 | 10.0 | 75 | 2.2 | 12.1 | 2.0 | 1.7 |
| Italian Tomato & Herb, for Pasta, BGTY, Sainsbury's* | ½ Jar/250g | 137.0 | 1.0 | 55 | 2.1 | 10.9 | 0.3 | 0.0 |
| Italian Tomato & Herb, Sainsbury's* | ¼ Jar/126g | 88.0 | 3.0 | 70 | 2.0 | 11.1 | 2.0 | 1.4 |
| Italian Tomato & Mascarpone, Sainsbury's* | ½ Tub/175g | 157.0 | 10.0 | 90 | 2.6 | 6.8 | 5.8 | 1.2 |
| Jalfrezi, Cooking, Asda* | 1 Jar/570g | 519.0 | 36.0 | 91 | 1.2 | 7.4 | 6.3 | 1.7 |
| Jalfrezi, Cooking, Sainsbury's* | 1 Serving/250g | 160.0 | 6.0 | 64 | 1.0 | 9.6 | 2.4 | 1.7 |
| Jalfrezi, Stir Fry, Patak's* | 1 Jar/250g | 260.0 | 19.0 | 104 | 1.4 | 7.6 | 7.5 | 1.4 |
| Jalfrezi, Sweet Pepper & Coconut, in Glass Jar, Patak's* | 1 Jar/540g | 626.0 | 38.0 | 116 | 1.7 | 11.3 | 7.0 | 1.4 |
| Jamaican Jerk, Stir It Up, Chicken Tonight, Knorr* | 1 Jar/80g | 506.0 | 43.0 | 633 | 3.9 | 20.9 | 53.9 | 5.4 |
| Jambalaya, Cajun, Seasoned Pioneers* | 1 Pack/400g | 248.0 | 20.0 | 62 | 0.8 | 3.2 | 5.1 | 1.0 |
| Kaffir Lime Chilli & Basil, Stir Fry, Sainsbury's* | 1 Serving/150g | 157.0 | 10.0 | 105 | 1.2 | 10.6 | 6.4 | 1.0 |
| Kashmiri, Chilli & Peppers, Patak's* | ½ Jar/212g | 159.0 | 9.0 | 75 | 1.3 | 7.7 | 4.4 | 1.1 |
| Kashmiri, Sharwood's* | ½ Bottle/210g | 231.0 | 11.0 | 110 | 3.0 | 13.0 | 5.1 | 1.5 |
| Kashmiri Moglai, TTD, Sainsbury's* | ½ Jar/175g | 184.0 | 13.0 | 105 | 1.7 | 8.1 | 7.3 | 1.6 |
| Korma, Asda* | 1 Serving/225g | 434.0 | 34.0 | 193 | 2.5 | 12.0 | 15.0 | 2.2 |
| Korma, Authentic, VLH Kitchens* | 1/3 Jar/118g | 180.1 | 15.3 | 153 | 1.9 | 6.7 | 13.0 | 0.8 |
| Korma, Cooking, BGTY, Sainsbury's* | ¼ Jar/125g | 100.0 | 3.0 | 80 | 1.1 | 12.9 | 2.7 | 1.2 |
| Korma, Cooking, GFY, Asda* | ¼ Jar/143g | 110.0 | 4.0 | 77 | 2.0 | 10.2 | 3.1 | 0.6 |
| Korma, Deliciously Good, Homepride* | 1 Jar/450g | 396.0 | 20.0 | 88 | 1.4 | 10.6 | 4.4 | 1.4 |
| Korma, Free From, Sainsbury's* | ½ Jar/175g | 191.0 | 14.0 | 109 | 1.9 | 7.6 | 7.9 | 1.2 |
| Korma, GFY, Asda* | 1 Serving/240g | 336.0 | 22.0 | 140 | 1.7 | 13.0 | 9.0 | 1.5 |
| Korma, Homepride* | 1 Serving/160g | 110.0 | 3.0 | 69 | 1.3 | 11.6 | 2.0 | 0.0 |
| Korma, Indian, M & S* | 1oz/28g | 60.0 | 5.0 | 215 | 3.8 | 11.7 | 17.3 | 0.9 |
| Korma, Sharwood's* | 1 Serving/105g | 150.0 | 10.0 | 143 | 1.4 | 12.2 | 9.8 | 1.8 |
| Korma, Sizzle & Stir, Knorr* | 1 Jar/455g | 1092.0 | 96.0 | 240 | 1.2 | 11.2 | 21.2 | 2.7 |
| Korma, Tesco* | ¼ Jar/125g | 192.0 | 15.0 | 154 | 2.4 | 9.9 | 11.7 | 1.3 |
| Laksa, Finest, Tesco* | 1/3 Jar/111g | 105.0 | 8.0 | 95 | 1.3 | 5.5 | 7.4 | 1.8 |
| Lamb Hot Pot, for Cooking, Dry, Asda* | 1 Pack/42g | 147.0 | 3.0 | 351 | 7.0 | 65.0 | 7.0 | 3.3 |
| Lemon, Amoy* | 1 Tsp/5ml | 5.0 | 0.0 | 104 | 0.0 | 26.0 | 0.0 | 0.0 |
| Lemon, Stir Fry, Straight to Wok, Amoy* | ½ Sachet/50g | 81.0 | 0.0 | 162 | 0.3 | 40.0 | 0.2 | 0.0 |
| Lemon, Stir Fry, Tesco* | 1 Jar/450g | 369.0 | 1.0 | 82 | 0.1 | 19.3 | 0.2 | 0.1 |
| Lemon & Ginger, Stir Fry, Finest, Tesco* | ¼ Jar/85g | 144.0 | 0.0 | 169 | 0.2 | 41.7 | 0.2 | 0.2 |
| Lemon & Sesame, Stir Fry, Sharwood's* | 1 Serving/100g | 125.0 | 0.0 | 125 | 0.1 | 30.9 | 0.1 | 0.1 |
| Lemon Pepper, Californian Style, Stir It Up, Knorr* | 1 Jar/80g | 527.0 | 47.0 | 659 | 5.2 | 26.1 | 59.3 | 2.7 |
| Lime & Coriander, Tangy, for Fish, Schwartz* | 1 Pack/300g | 381.0 | 37.0 | 127 | 1.1 | 2.7 | 12.4 | 1.3 |
| Lime Honey & Ginger, Stir Fry, Sharwood's* | 1 Serving/50g | 34.0 | 0.0 | 69 | 0.3 | 16.6 | 0.1 | 0.2 |
| Madras, Cooking, HL, Tesco* | 1 Serving/128g | 55.0 | 3.0 | 43 | 1.6 | 4.8 | 2.0 | 2.3 |
| Mango, Kashmiri Style, Finest, Tesco* | ½ Jar/175g | 285.0 | 24.0 | 163 | 2.4 | 7.7 | 13.6 | 0.9 |
| Mediterranean Tomato, Spread & Bake, Heinz* | ¼ Jar/70g | 56.0 | 2.0 | 80 | 1.3 | 13.8 | 2.5 | 1.9 |
| Mediterranean Vegetable, M & S* | 1 Pot/350g | 227.0 | 12.0 | 65 | 1.7 | 6.8 | 3.3 | 2.0 |
| Mexican, Cooking, BGTY, Sainsbury's* | ¼ Jar/124g | 51.0 | 0.0 | 41 | 0.7 | 9.2 | 0.2 | 0.8 |
| Mexican Mild Chilli, Asda* | 1 Serving/100g | 55.0 | 0.0 | 55 | 2.0 | 10.8 | 0.4 | 1.8 |
| Mint, Sainsbury's* | 1 Dtsp/10g | 13.0 | 0.0 | 126 | 2.5 | 28.7 | 0.1 | 4.0 |
| Mint, SmartPrice, Asda* | 1 Serving/5g | 3.0 | 0.0 | 52 | 0.1 | 13.0 | 0.0 | 1.2 |
| Mint Garden, Fresh, Tesco* | 1 Tsp/5g | 2.0 | 0.0 | 40 | 2.6 | 3.6 | 0.4 | 1.5 |
| Moglai, Tomato & Fennel, Cooking, Patak's* | 1 Jar/283g | 374.0 | 25.0 | 132 | 3.1 | 9.7 | 8.9 | 1.8 |

**S**

| | Measure INFO/WEIGHT | per Measure KCAL | per Measure FAT | Nutrition Values per 100g / 100ml KCAL | PROT | CARB | FAT | FIBRE |
|---|---|---|---|---|---|---|---|---|
| **SAUCE** | | | | | | | | |
| Mornay, Cheese, Asda* | ¼ Pot/71g | 114.0 | 9.0 | 161 | 6.8 | 6.6 | 12.7 | 0.4 |
| Moroccan, Spread & Bake, Heinz* | ¼ Jar/70g | 64.0 | 2.0 | 91 | 1.7 | 15.8 | 2.3 | 2.1 |
| Moroccan Seven Vegetable Cous Cous, Sainsbury's* | 1 Serving/50g | 89.0 | 8.0 | 178 | 2.6 | 5.9 | 16.0 | 0.0 |
| Mushroom, Creamy, Asda* | 1 Serving/125g | 76.0 | 5.0 | 61 | 0.8 | 6.0 | 3.7 | 0.5 |
| Mushroom, Creamy, Chicken Tonight, Knorr* | ¼ Jar/125g | 101.0 | 8.0 | 81 | 0.8 | 5.4 | 6.3 | 0.3 |
| Mushroom, Creamy, Low Fat, Chicken Tonight, Knorr* | ¼ Jar/125g | 59.0 | 4.0 | 47 | 0.8 | 7.3 | 2.9 | 0.4 |
| Mushroom, Creamy, Tesco* | ½ Pot/175g | 142.0 | 10.0 | 81 | 1.5 | 5.6 | 5.8 | 0.4 |
| Mushroom, Not Just for Pasta, Sainsbury's* | ½ Pot/150g | 91.0 | 7.0 | 61 | 1.7 | 3.6 | 4.4 | 0.9 |
| Mushroom, Schwartz* | 1 Pack/170g | 207.0 | 19.0 | 122 | 1.2 | 3.9 | 11.3 | 0.5 |
| Mushroom, TTD, Sainsbury's* | 1 Serving/150g | 250.0 | 24.0 | 167 | 2.6 | 3.5 | 15.8 | 1.4 |
| Mushroom & Garlic, 95% Fat Free, Homepride* | 1 Serving/220g | 154.0 | 9.0 | 70 | 0.9 | 7.0 | 4.2 | 0.3 |
| Mushroom & Herb, Cooking, BGTY, Sainsbury's* | ¼ Jar/125g | 67.0 | 3.0 | 54 | 1.8 | 6.6 | 2.3 | 0.5 |
| Mushroom & White Wine, Knorr* | 1 Serving/100ml | 99.0 | 8.0 | 99 | 1.0 | 4.0 | 8.0 | 0.6 |
| Napoletana, Fresh, Sainsbury's* | ½ Pot/150g | 94.0 | 4.0 | 63 | 1.7 | 7.3 | 3.0 | 2.3 |
| Napoletana, Italian, Tesco* | 1 Pot/350g | 178.0 | 4.0 | 51 | 1.5 | 8.5 | 1.2 | 1.0 |
| Napoletana, Organic, Tesco* | ½ Pot/175g | 70.0 | 1.0 | 40 | 1.3 | 7.3 | 0.6 | 1.0 |
| Napoletana, Waitrose* | 1 Pot/600g | 252.0 | 8.0 | 42 | 1.8 | 5.5 | 1.4 | 1.7 |
| Onion, Made with Semi-Skimmed Milk | 1 Serving/60g | 52.0 | 3.0 | 86 | 2.9 | 8.4 | 5.0 | 0.4 |
| Onion, Made with Skimmed Milk | 1 Serving/60g | 46.0 | 2.0 | 77 | 2.9 | 8.4 | 4.0 | 0.4 |
| Orange & Dill Sauce, for Fish, Zesty, Schwartz* | 1 Pack/300g | 180.0 | 1.0 | 60 | 0.4 | 13.5 | 0.5 | 0.5 |
| Orange & Green Ginger, Blue Dragon* | 1 Pack/120g | 118.0 | 2.0 | 98 | 0.5 | 20.4 | 1.6 | 0.5 |
| Oriental Orange & Ginger, Homepride* | 1 Serving/100g | 68.0 | 0.0 | 68 | 0.7 | 15.9 | 0.1 | 0.0 |
| Oriental Sweet & Sour, Express, Uncle Ben's* | 1 Serving/170g | 221.0 | 3.0 | 130 | 0.8 | 27.5 | 1.9 | 0.0 |
| Oyster, Blue Dragon* | 1 Tsp/5ml | 6.0 | 0.0 | 121 | 3.4 | 26.9 | 0.0 | 0.0 |
| Oyster, Stir Fry, Sainsbury's* | 1 Tbsp/15g | 9.0 | 0.0 | 61 | 1.6 | 13.3 | 0.1 | 0.2 |
| Oyster & Garlic, Stir Fry, Straight to Wok, Amoy* | ½ Pack/50g | 97.0 | 1.0 | 195 | 4.9 | 37.0 | 3.0 | 0.0 |
| Oyster & Spring Onion, Stir Fry, Blue Dragon* | 1 Sachet/120g | 110.0 | 1.0 | 92 | 1.6 | 19.9 | 0.7 | 1.1 |
| Oyster Flavoured, Amoy* | 1 Tsp/5ml | 5.0 | 0.0 | 108 | 2.0 | 25.0 | 0.0 | 0.0 |
| Paprika Chicken, Chicken Tonight, Knorr* | ½ Jar/250g | 240.0 | 22.0 | 96 | 0.9 | 3.5 | 8.7 | 1.4 |
| Parsley, Fresh, Sainsbury's* | ½ Pot/150g | 117.0 | 8.0 | 78 | 2.0 | 5.9 | 5.1 | 0.5 |
| Parsley, Instant, Dry, Asda* | 1 Serving/23g | 82.0 | 2.0 | 355 | 7.0 | 66.0 | 7.0 | 4.4 |
| Parsley, Instant, Made Up, Semi Skim Milk, Sainsbury's* | ¼ Sachet/51ml | 34.0 | 1.0 | 67 | 3.5 | 8.6 | 2.1 | 0.1 |
| Parsley, Tesco* | ½ Pack/89g | 85.0 | 5.0 | 95 | 2.8 | 8.1 | 5.7 | 1.1 |
| Peanut, Sainsbury's* | 1 Sachet/70g | 185.0 | 9.0 | 264 | 1.9 | 34.7 | 13.1 | 1.6 |
| Peking, Sizzle & Stir, Chicken Tonight, Knorr* | 1 Jar/510g | 617.0 | 45.0 | 121 | 0.8 | 9.4 | 8.9 | 1.6 |
| Peking Lemon, Stir Fry, Blue Dragon* | 1 Serving/35g | 58.0 | 1.0 | 166 | 0.3 | 36.8 | 1.9 | 0.1 |
| Pepper, Creamy, Schwartz* | 1 Pack/170g | 116.0 | 9.0 | 68 | 1.5 | 3.4 | 5.4 | 1.0 |
| Pepper, Creamy, Tesco* | 1 Serving/85ml | 128.0 | 11.0 | 151 | 1.2 | 6.4 | 13.4 | 0.5 |
| Pepper & Tomato, Spicy, Stir Through, M & S* | ½ Jar/95g | 166.0 | 15.0 | 175 | 1.6 | 7.5 | 15.4 | 0.0 |
| Peppercorn, Creamy, Asda* | ¼ Jar/137g | 137.0 | 11.0 | 100 | 1.1 | 6.0 | 8.0 | 0.2 |
| Peppercorn, Creamy, Chicken Tonight, Knorr* | ¼ Jar/125g | 110.0 | 10.0 | 88 | 0.3 | 3.8 | 7.8 | 0.4 |
| Peri-Peri, Extra Hot, Nando's* | 1 Serving/5g | 3.0 | 0.0 | 58 | 0.0 | 5.6 | 3.8 | 0.2 |
| Peri-Peri, Hot, Nando's* | 1 Serving/5g | 3.0 | 0.0 | 65 | 0.0 | 5.2 | 4.8 | 0.6 |
| Peri-Peri, Sweet, Nando's* | 1 Tbsp/25g | 35.0 | 1.0 | 142 | 0.5 | 30.7 | 2.1 | 0.0 |
| Pesto, Basil, M & S* | 1 Serving/65g | 348.0 | 30.0 | 535 | 7.5 | 20.7 | 46.9 | 1.4 |
| Pesto, Green, Asda* | 1 Tsp/5g | 21.0 | 2.0 | 429 | 4.7 | 3.5 | 44.0 | 1.4 |
| Pesto, Green, Half the Fat, Grandissimo* | 1 Serving/48g | 85.0 | 8.0 | 177 | 4.4 | 2.2 | 16.7 | 0.0 |
| Pesto, Green, Italiano, Tesco* | 1 Serving/50g | 251.0 | 24.0 | 502 | 9.6 | 5.6 | 49.0 | 1.2 |
| Pesto, Green, Less Than 60% Fat, BGTY, Sainsbury's* | ¼ Jar/48g | 61.0 | 5.0 | 128 | 4.2 | 2.6 | 11.2 | 0.0 |
| Pesto, Green, Morrisons* | 1 Serving/50g | 255.0 | 25.0 | 510 | 10.7 | 4.7 | 49.8 | 0.0 |
| Pesto, Green, Tesco* | ¼ Jar/48g | 192.0 | 20.0 | 405 | 5.6 | 0.6 | 42.2 | 4.4 |
| Pesto, Green Basil, Stir-In, Fresh, Chilled, Waitrose* | ½ Pot/73g | 324.0 | 31.0 | 447 | 8.8 | 5.2 | 43.4 | 1.2 |
| Pesto, Knorr* | 1 Serving/100g | 216.0 | 21.0 | 216 | 2.7 | 3.8 | 21.1 | 0.0 |

**S**

| SAUCE | Measure INFO/WEIGHT | per Measure KCAL | per Measure FAT | Nutrition Values per 100g / 100ml KCAL | PROT | CARB | FAT | FIBRE |
|---|---|---|---|---|---|---|---|---|
| Pesto, Red, M & S* | 1oz/28g | 93.0 | 9.0 | 331 | 3.6 | 6.9 | 33.2 | 3.5 |
| Pesto, Red, Morrisons* | 1 Tbsp/15g | 47.0 | 4.0 | 311 | 5.7 | 6.6 | 29.0 | 5.9 |
| Pesto, Red, Tesco* | ¼ Jar/50g | 162.0 | 15.0 | 325 | 5.6 | 6.3 | 30.3 | 6.0 |
| Pesto, with Basil, Napolina* | 1 Tsp/5g | 20.0 | 2.0 | 409 | 5.5 | 5.5 | 40.5 | 0.0 |
| Piquant Pepper Coriander & Lime, Sainsbury's* | 1/3 Pot/100g | 43.0 | 0.0 | 43 | 1.2 | 8.4 | 0.5 | 0.8 |
| Plum, Spiced, Heinz* | 1 Serving/25g | 32.0 | 0.0 | 128 | 0.5 | 31.1 | 0.1 | 1.0 |
| Plum & Ginger, Stir Fry, Asda* | ½ Jar/97g | 94.0 | 1.0 | 97 | 0.7 | 22.0 | 0.7 | 0.3 |
| Plum & Sesame, Stir Fry, M & S* | ½ Jar/115g | 138.0 | 0.0 | 120 | 0.9 | 29.0 | 0.1 | 1.8 |
| Puttanesca, Fresh, Waitrose* | ½ Pot/176g | 118.0 | 8.0 | 67 | 1.8 | 6.2 | 4.4 | 1.2 |
| Red & Yellow Pepper, Roasted, Sacla* | 1 Serving/290g | 232.0 | 17.0 | 80 | 1.1 | 5.5 | 5.9 | 0.0 |
| Red Pepper, Fresh, Asda* | ¼ Pot/82g | 35.0 | 1.0 | 43 | 1.4 | 6.8 | 1.2 | 1.1 |
| Red Pepper, GFY, Asda* | 1 Serving/100g | 43.0 | 1.0 | 43 | 1.2 | 7.0 | 1.1 | 0.0 |
| Red Pepper, Sainsbury's* | 1 Serving/37g | 118.0 | 12.0 | 320 | 4.3 | 5.0 | 31.4 | 0.0 |
| Red Thai, Cooking, Perfectly Balanced, Waitrose* | 1 Jar/430g | 267.0 | 15.0 | 62 | 1.1 | 6.2 | 3.6 | 1.6 |
| Red Wine, Cook in, Homepride* | ¼ Can/98g | 47.0 | 1.0 | 48 | 0.5 | 10.1 | 0.6 | 0.0 |
| Red Wine, Cooking, BGTY, Sainsbury's* | 1 Serving/125g | 52.0 | 1.0 | 42 | 0.5 | 8.8 | 0.5 | 0.8 |
| Red Wine, Cooking, Homepride* | 1 Serving/250ml | 115.0 | 1.0 | 46 | 0.4 | 9.8 | 0.6 | 0.0 |
| Red Wine, Cooking, Iceland* | 1 Serving/100g | 33.0 | 0.0 | 33 | 0.8 | 7.2 | 0.2 | 0.2 |
| Red Wine & Onion, Rich, Simply Sausages, Colman's* | ¼ Jar/125g | 49.0 | 0.0 | 39 | 0.9 | 8.5 | 0.2 | 1.3 |
| Redcurrant, Colman's* | 1 Tsp/12g | 44.0 | 0.0 | 368 | 0.7 | 90.0 | 0.0 | 0.0 |
| Risotto, Mushroom & White Wine, Sacla* | 1 Serving/95g | 151.0 | 12.0 | 159 | 3.7 | 6.9 | 13.0 | 0.0 |
| Roast Vegetable with Basil & Tomato, M & S* | 1 Serving/100g | 85.0 | 4.0 | 85 | 2.0 | 9.5 | 4.1 | 1.2 |
| Roasted Peanut Satay, Stir Fry Sensations, Amoy* | 1 Pouch/160g | 354.0 | 20.0 | 221 | 4.7 | 21.9 | 12.4 | 1.0 |
| Roasted Vegetable, Finest, Tesco* | 1 Serving/175g | 101.0 | 4.0 | 58 | 1.4 | 7.8 | 2.4 | 1.0 |
| Rogan Josh, 99% Fat Free, Homepride* | 1/3 Jar/153g | 92.0 | 1.0 | 60 | 1.8 | 11.6 | 0.7 | 2.0 |
| Rogan Josh, Asda* | ¼ Jar/125g | 135.0 | 10.0 | 108 | 0.9 | 8.0 | 8.0 | 0.6 |
| Rogan Josh, Cooking, Light Choices, Tesco* | ¼ Jar/125g | 57.0 | 3.0 | 46 | 1.4 | 4.8 | 2.4 | 2.5 |
| Rogan Josh, Medium, Sharwood's* | ½ Jar/210g | 151.0 | 8.0 | 72 | 1.4 | 8.6 | 3.6 | 0.5 |
| Rogan Josh, Sharwood's* | ½ Jar/210g | 220.0 | 17.0 | 105 | 1.2 | 7.0 | 8.0 | 1.5 |
| Rogan Josh, Tesco* | ½ Can/220g | 156.0 | 10.0 | 71 | 1.3 | 5.9 | 4.7 | 1.4 |
| Rogan Josh, VLH Kitchens* | 1 Jar/460g | 374.0 | 24.4 | 82 | 1.4 | 6.1 | 5.3 | 1.4 |
| Royal Korma, Tilda* | 1 Pack/400ml | 824.0 | 73.0 | 206 | 1.9 | 8.4 | 18.3 | 0.7 |
| Satay, Stir Fry & Dipping, Finest, Tesco* | 1 Tsp/5g | 22.0 | 2.0 | 432 | 9.0 | 20.7 | 34.8 | 2.7 |
| Sausage Casserole, Cook in, Homepride* | ½ Jar/250g | 92.0 | 0.0 | 37 | 0.7 | 8.0 | 0.2 | 0.6 |
| Seafood, 25% Less Fat, Tesco* | 1 Tsp/5g | 17.0 | 1.0 | 344 | 2.7 | 18.2 | 28.5 | 0.3 |
| Seafood, Asda* | 1 Serving/10g | 45.0 | 4.0 | 448 | 1.6 | 16.0 | 42.0 | 0.2 |
| Seafood, Baxters* | 1oz/28g | 149.0 | 15.0 | 533 | 1.5 | 9.9 | 54.2 | 0.7 |
| Seafood, Colman's* | 1 Tbsp/15ml | 44.0 | 3.0 | 296 | 0.9 | 21.5 | 22.9 | 0.4 |
| Seafood, GFY, Asda* | 1 Dstp/10ml | 31.0 | 3.0 | 313 | 0.6 | 17.0 | 27.0 | 0.0 |
| Seafood, Sainsbury's* | 1 Tbsp/15g | 49.0 | 4.0 | 330 | 0.7 | 17.6 | 28.2 | 0.1 |
| Sichuan, M & S* | 1 Serving/120g | 192.0 | 1.0 | 160 | 1.6 | 36.8 | 0.5 | 0.5 |
| Sizzling Szechuan, Uncle Ben's* | 1 Serving/260g | 289.0 | 18.0 | 111 | 0.9 | 10.8 | 7.1 | 0.0 |
| Smoked Bacon & Tomato, Stir in, Dolmio* | ½ Tub/75g | 73.0 | 4.0 | 98 | 4.6 | 7.2 | 5.6 | 1.3 |
| Smoked Paprika & Tomato, M & S* | 1 Serving/300g | 135.0 | 5.0 | 45 | 1.3 | 6.1 | 1.7 | 0.9 |
| Soy, Average | 1 Tsp/5ml | 3.0 | 0.0 | 64 | 8.7 | 8.3 | 0.0 | 0.0 |
| Soy, Dark, Amoy* | 1 Tsp/5ml | 5.0 | 0.0 | 106 | 0.9 | 25.6 | 0.0 | 0.0 |
| Soy, Dark, Asda* | 1oz/28g | 26.0 | 0.0 | 92 | 2.0 | 21.0 | 0.0 | 0.4 |
| Soy, Light, Amoy* | 1 Tbsp/15g | 8.0 | 0.0 | 52 | 2.5 | 10.5 | 0.0 | 0.0 |
| Soy, Light, Asda* | 1 Tbsp/15ml | 7.0 | 0.0 | 47 | 0.8 | 11.0 | 0.0 | 0.0 |
| Soy, Light, Sharwood's* | 1 Tsp/5ml | 2.0 | 0.0 | 37 | 2.7 | 6.4 | 0.2 | 0.0 |
| Soy, Naturally Brewed, Kikkoman* | 1 Tbsp/15g | 11.0 | 0.0 | 74 | 10.3 | 8.1 | 0.0 | 0.0 |
| Soy, Premium, Light, Heinz* | 1 Serving/15g | 11.0 | 0.0 | 71 | 7.4 | 9.1 | 0.5 | 0.0 |
| Soy, Reduced Salt, Amoy* | 1 Tsp/5ml | 3.0 | 0.0 | 56 | 4.0 | 10.0 | 0.0 | 0.0 |

S

| | Measure INFO/WEIGHT | per Measure | | Nutrition Values per 100g / 100ml | | | | |
|---|---|---|---|---|---|---|---|---|
| | | KCAL | FAT | KCAL | PROT | CARB | FAT | FIBRE |
| **SAUCE** | | | | | | | | |
| Soy, Rich, Sharwood's* | 1 Tsp/5ml | 4.0 | 0.0 | 79 | 3.1 | 16.6 | 0.4 | 0.0 |
| Soy, Wasabi & Lemon Grass, Stir Fry, Finest, Tesco* | 1 Pack/125g | 119.0 | 3.0 | 95 | 1.5 | 16.3 | 2.2 | 0.9 |
| Soy & Garlic, Stir Fry, Fresh Tastes, Asda* | 1 Pack/180g | 175.0 | 7.0 | 97 | 1.7 | 14.1 | 3.7 | 0.5 |
| Soya, Japanese, Waitrose* | 1 Tbsp/15ml | 11.0 | 0.0 | 74 | 7.7 | 9.4 | 0.6 | 0.8 |
| Spanish Chicken, Chicken Tonight, Knorr* | ½ Jar/250g | 115.0 | 3.0 | 46 | 1.5 | 7.0 | 1.4 | 0.6 |
| Spanish Style, Cooking, Light Choices, Tesco* | 1 Jar/485g | 131.0 | 1.0 | 27 | 1.0 | 5.0 | 0.3 | 1.4 |
| Spicy Peanut, Sharwood's* | 1oz/28g | 29.0 | 1.0 | 103 | 2.5 | 12.1 | 5.0 | 0.6 |
| Spicy Sweet & Sour, Sharwood's* | 1 Serving/138g | 142.0 | 1.0 | 103 | 0.7 | 23.8 | 0.5 | 0.4 |
| Spicy Szechuan, Safe To Eat* | 1 Pouch/400g | 124.0 | 2.0 | 31 | 1.0 | 4.8 | 0.6 | 0.3 |
| Spicy Tikka, Cooking, Sharwood's* | 1oz/28g | 27.0 | 2.0 | 95 | 1.3 | 9.4 | 5.9 | 0.8 |
| Sri Lankan, Seasoned Pioneers* | 1 Pouch/400g | 388.0 | 34.0 | 97 | 1.8 | 3.4 | 8.4 | 0.8 |
| Sticky BBQ, Spread & Bake, Heinz* | ¼ Jar/78g | 131.0 | 0.0 | 168 | 1.0 | 39.6 | 0.6 | 1.2 |
| Sticky Plum, Stir Fry, Blue Dragon* | 1 Serving/60g | 145.0 | 0.0 | 242 | 0.1 | 35.6 | 0.3 | 0.0 |
| Sticky Ribz, Ainsley Harriott* | 1 Serving/50g | 107.0 | 0.0 | 214 | 0.4 | 52.2 | 0.1 | 0.0 |
| Stir Fry, Chinese, with Soy, Ginger & Garlic, Tesco* | 1 Pack/150g | 180.0 | 8.0 | 120 | 2.1 | 14.2 | 5.6 | 0.8 |
| Stir Fry, Chow Mein, Safeway* | 1 Serving/105g | 79.0 | 1.0 | 75 | 1.1 | 16.2 | 0.6 | 1.3 |
| Stir Fry, Fragrant Sichuan, M & S* | 1 Jar/155g | 194.0 | 4.0 | 125 | 0.7 | 24.4 | 2.9 | 0.3 |
| Stir Fry, Laksa, Cook Asian, M & S* | ½ Pack/75g | 82.0 | 6.0 | 110 | 0.9 | 8.9 | 8.0 | 1.0 |
| Stir Fry, Pad Thai, Tesco* | 1 Pack/125g | 112.0 | 3.0 | 90 | 1.3 | 15.8 | 2.3 | 0.8 |
| Stroganoff, Asda* | 1 Serving/285g | 305.0 | 26.0 | 107 | 1.5 | 5.0 | 9.0 | 0.3 |
| Stroganoff, M & S* | 1oz/28g | 30.0 | 2.0 | 107 | 3.8 | 4.9 | 8.0 | 0.6 |
| Stroganoff, Tesco* | 1 Serving/100g | 89.0 | 7.0 | 89 | 0.7 | 5.3 | 7.3 | 0.4 |
| Succulent Szechuan Tomato, Stir Fry Sensations, Amoy* | 1 Serving/64g | 71.0 | 1.0 | 111 | 1.4 | 23.7 | 1.0 | 1.6 |
| Sun Dried Tomato, Heinz* | 1 Serving/10ml | 7.0 | 0.0 | 73 | 1.5 | 14.9 | 0.6 | 0.9 |
| Sun Dried Tomato & Basil, Free From, Sainsbury's* | 1 Serving/175g | 126.0 | 5.0 | 72 | 2.9 | 8.7 | 2.8 | 1.5 |
| Swedish Mustard & Dill, Safeway* | 1 Serving/20g | 32.0 | 2.0 | 162 | 17.1 | 1.5 | 9.8 | 0.2 |
| Sweet & Sour, Basics, Sainsbury's* | ¼ Jar/110g | 59.0 | 0.0 | 54 | 0.3 | 12.4 | 0.3 | 0.4 |
| Sweet & Sour, Classic, Canned, Homepride* | 1 Can/500g | 440.0 | 0.0 | 88 | 0.3 | 21.5 | 0.1 | 0.5 |
| Sweet & Sour, Cook In, Glass Jar, Homepride* | 1 Jar/500g | 335.0 | 0.0 | 67 | 0.3 | 16.2 | 0.1 | 0.5 |
| Sweet & Sour, Cooking, Light Choices, Tesco* | 1 Jar/510g | 138.0 | 1.0 | 27 | 1.1 | 5.1 | 0.2 | 3.9 |
| Sweet & Sour, Cooking, Organic, Sainsbury's* | 1/3 Jar/150g | 150.0 | 1.0 | 100 | 0.8 | 22.1 | 0.9 | 0.5 |
| Sweet & Sour, Extra Pineapple, Chinatown, Knorr* | 1 Jar/525g | 441.0 | 1.0 | 84 | 0.4 | 20.4 | 0.1 | 0.6 |
| Sweet & Sour, Extra Pineapple, Uncle Ben's* | 1 Serving/165g | 144.0 | 0.0 | 87 | 0.3 | 21.4 | 0.0 | 0.0 |
| Sweet & Sour, Fresh, Sainsbury's* | 1 Sachet/50ml | 102.0 | 4.0 | 205 | 0.8 | 31.2 | 8.6 | 0.3 |
| Sweet & Sour, Fresh Ideas, Tesco* | 1 Serving/50ml | 77.0 | 1.0 | 154 | 1.1 | 34.3 | 1.4 | 0.5 |
| Sweet & Sour, GFY, Asda* | ½ Jar/164g | 77.0 | 0.0 | 47 | 0.4 | 11.0 | 0.2 | 0.3 |
| Sweet & Sour, Oriental, Chicken Tonight, Knorr* | ½ Jar/262g | 217.0 | 3.0 | 83 | 0.4 | 20.8 | 1.0 | 0.5 |
| Sweet & Sour, Original, Uncle Ben's* | 1 Pack/300g | 264.0 | 0.0 | 88 | 0.5 | 21.7 | 0.0 | 0.0 |
| Sweet & Sour, Perfectly Balanced, Waitrose* | 1 Serving/175g | 140.0 | 0.0 | 80 | 0.6 | 18.9 | 0.2 | 1.1 |
| Sweet & Sour, Sizzle & Stir, Knorr* | 1 Serving/460g | 676.0 | 41.0 | 147 | 0.6 | 15.6 | 9.0 | 0.2 |
| Sweet & Sour, Sizzling, Uncle Ben's* | ½ Jar/270g | 375.0 | 18.0 | 139 | 0.6 | 19.2 | 6.7 | 0.0 |
| Sweet & Sour, Spicy, Uncle Ben's* | 1 Jar/400g | 364.0 | 0.0 | 91 | 0.6 | 22.1 | 0.1 | 0.0 |
| Sweet & Sour, Stir Fry, Asda* | 1 Serving/63g | 146.0 | 3.0 | 232 | 0.8 | 46.0 | 5.0 | 0.0 |
| Sweet & Sour, Stir Fry, Blue Dragon* | 1 Sachet/120g | 137.0 | 1.0 | 114 | 0.6 | 25.6 | 1.1 | 0.6 |
| Sweet & Sour, Stir Fry, GFY, Asda* | ½ Pack/51ml | 43.0 | 2.0 | 85 | 0.9 | 11.0 | 4.1 | 3.4 |
| Sweet & Sour, Stir Fry, M & S* | 1 Pack/120g | 150.0 | 0.0 | 125 | 0.7 | 29.8 | 0.4 | 1.3 |
| Sweet & Sour, Stir Fry, Sharwood's* | 1 Jar 160g | 168.0 | 1.0 | 105 | 0.6 | 24.5 | 0.5 | 0.8 |
| Sweet & Sour, Stir Fry, Tesco* | ½ Jar/222g | 164.0 | 0.0 | 74 | 0.6 | 17.0 | 0.2 | 0.4 |
| Sweet & Sour, Stir Fry, Waitrose* | 1 Serving/50ml | 93.0 | 2.0 | 187 | 1.2 | 35.6 | 4.4 | 1.8 |
| Sweet & Sour, Stir Fry Additions, Tesco* | 1 Sachet/50g | 83.0 | 0.0 | 167 | 0.8 | 38.7 | 1.0 | 0.5 |
| Sweet & Sour, Take-Away | 1oz/28g | 44.0 | 1.0 | 157 | 0.2 | 32.8 | 3.4 | 0.0 |
| Sweet & Sour, Two Stage, Uncle Ben's* | ½ Jar/200g | 314.0 | 18.0 | 157 | 1.0 | 18.1 | 9.1 | 0.0 |
| Sweet & Sour, Weight Watchers* | ½ Jar/125g | 61.0 | 0.0 | 49 | 0.6 | 11.5 | 0.1 | 0.2 |

**S**

| | Measure INFO/WEIGHT | per Measure KCAL | FAT | Nutrition Values per 100g / 100ml KCAL | PROT | CARB | FAT | FIBRE |
|---|---|---|---|---|---|---|---|---|
| **SAUCE** | | | | | | | | |
| Sweet & Sour, with Mango, Sharwood's* | 1/3 Jar/138g | 134.0 | 0.0 | 97 | 0.7 | 23.3 | 0.1 | 1.3 |
| Sweet Chilli, Dipping, M & S* | 1 Tbsp/15g | 34.0 | 0.0 | 225 | 0.9 | 53.2 | 0.7 | 0.6 |
| Sweet Chilli, Garlic, Stir Fry, Blue Dragon* | 1 Pack/120g | 192.0 | 0.0 | 160 | 0.1 | 22.8 | 0.3 | 0.2 |
| Sweet Chilli, Heinz* | 1 Serving/25g | 37.0 | 0.0 | 150 | 0.3 | 36.5 | 0.4 | 6.4 |
| Sweet Chilli, Sharwood's* | 1 Bottle/150ml | 325.0 | 1.0 | 217 | 0.7 | 52.8 | 0.4 | 1.7 |
| Sweet Chilli & Coriander, Sharwood's* | 1 Pack/370g | 407.0 | 4.0 | 110 | 0.3 | 24.4 | 1.2 | 0.1 |
| Sweet Chilli & Coriander, Sizzling, Homepride* | 1 Serving/100g | 51.0 | 0.0 | 51 | 0.7 | 11.5 | 0.2 | 0.0 |
| Sweet Chilli & Lemon Grass, Stir Fry, Sharwood's* | 1 Serving/155g | 127.0 | 0.0 | 82 | 0.3 | 19.7 | 0.1 | 0.3 |
| Sweet Chilli & Lime, Chinatown, Knorr* | 1 Jar/525g | 635.0 | 17.0 | 121 | 0.6 | 22.0 | 3.3 | 0.5 |
| Sweet Pepper, Stir in, Dolmio* | ½ Pot/75g | 103.0 | 8.0 | 137 | 1.5 | 9.7 | 10.3 | 0.0 |
| Sweet Soy & Sesame, Uncle Ben's* | 1 Serving/100g | 110.0 | 2.0 | 110 | 0.7 | 23.0 | 1.7 | 0.0 |
| Sweet Soy & Spring Onion, Stir Fry Sensations, Amoy* | 1 Pouch/160g | 312.0 | 10.0 | 195 | 2.0 | 31.5 | 6.5 | 0.6 |
| Szechuan, Spicy Tomato, Stir Fry, Blue Dragon* | 1 Sachet/120g | 151.0 | 7.0 | 126 | 1.3 | 17.6 | 5.6 | 2.0 |
| Szechuan, Stir Fry, Sharwood's* | 1 Jar/150g | 126.0 | 2.0 | 84 | 3.0 | 15.5 | 1.1 | 0.4 |
| Szechuan Style, Stir Fry, Fresh Ideas, Tesco* | 1 Sachet/50g | 114.0 | 5.0 | 228 | 1.9 | 33.4 | 9.7 | 0.1 |
| Tabasco | 1 Tsp/5ml | 1.0 | 0.0 | 12 | 1.3 | 0.8 | 0.8 | 0.6 |
| Tagine, Cooking, Perfectly Balanced, Waitrose* | 1 Jar/430g | 258.0 | 9.0 | 60 | 1.0 | 9.6 | 2.0 | 1.5 |
| Tamarind & Lime, Stir Fry, Sainsbury's* | 1 Serving/75g | 88.0 | 6.0 | 117 | 1.1 | 11.4 | 7.4 | 0.8 |
| Tartare | 1oz/28g | 84.0 | 7.0 | 299 | 1.3 | 17.9 | 24.6 | 0.0 |
| Tartare, Rich, Colman's* | 1 Tsp/5ml | 14.0 | 1.0 | 284 | 1.2 | 17.0 | 23.0 | 0.6 |
| Tartare, Sainsbury's* | 1 Serving/20ml | 94.0 | 10.0 | 469 | 0.4 | 5.8 | 49.0 | 1.0 |
| Tartare, Tesco* | 1 Tbsp/15g | 43.0 | 3.0 | 287 | 1.5 | 19.6 | 21.8 | 0.3 |
| Teriyaki, Asda* | 1 Serving/98g | 99.0 | 0.0 | 101 | 2.1 | 23.0 | 0.1 | 0.0 |
| Teriyaki, Stir Fry, Blue Dragon* | 1 Sachet/120g | 208.0 | 0.0 | 173 | 2.0 | 28.6 | 0.0 | 0.0 |
| Teriyaki, Stir Fry, Fresh Ideas, Tesco* | 1 Serving/25g | 33.0 | 1.0 | 133 | 1.1 | 26.9 | 2.3 | 0.0 |
| Teriyaki, Stir Fry, Sharwood's* | 1 Jar/150g | 144.0 | 0.0 | 96 | 0.9 | 22.5 | 0.3 | 0.3 |
| Texan Barbecue, Stir It Up, Chicken Tonight, Knorr* | 1 Jar/80g | 482.0 | 42.0 | 602 | 4.4 | 33.8 | 52.5 | 5.8 |
| Texan Honey & Hickory, Safeway* | 1 Serving/110g | 173.0 | 10.0 | 157 | 1.7 | 17.7 | 8.8 | 1.3 |
| Thai, Lemongrass, Lime, & Chili, Stir Fry, Sainsbury's* | 1 Serving/50ml | 145.0 | 13.0 | 290 | 4.0 | 10.2 | 26.5 | 3.5 |
| Thai Curry, Yellow, Loyd Grossman* | 1 Serving/100g | 111.0 | 7.0 | 111 | 1.7 | 9.1 | 7.5 | 1.0 |
| Thai Green, Sainsbury's* | ¼ Pack/125g | 170.0 | 12.0 | 136 | 1.8 | 10.8 | 9.5 | 2.1 |
| Thai Panang, Sainsbury's* | 1/3 Pack/166g | 229.0 | 20.0 | 138 | 1.4 | 6.6 | 11.8 | 1.4 |
| Thai Sweet Chilli, Sizzle & Stir, Chicken Tonight, Knorr* | 1 Jar/510g | 694.0 | 58.0 | 136 | 0.6 | 7.5 | 11.4 | 2.9 |
| Tikka, BFY, Morrisons* | ½ Jar/238g | 259.0 | 8.0 | 109 | 2.3 | 17.2 | 3.4 | 1.3 |
| Tikka, Cooking, BGTY, Sainsbury's* | 1 Jar/500g | 370.0 | 9.0 | 74 | 1.2 | 12.9 | 1.9 | 0.3 |
| Tikka Bhuna, Sizzle & Stir, Chicken Tonight, Knorr* | ½ Jar/230g | 267.0 | 22.0 | 116 | 1.2 | 6.7 | 9.4 | 1.1 |
| Tikka Masala, Deliciously Good, Homepride* | ¼ Jar/149g | 121.0 | 5.0 | 81 | 2.1 | 10.0 | 3.6 | 1.5 |
| Tikka Masala, GFY, Asda* | ½ Jar/250g | 190.0 | 8.0 | 76 | 2.9 | 9.0 | 3.2 | 0.5 |
| Tikka Masala, Jar, Sharwood's* | 1 Jar/435g | 492.0 | 33.0 | 113 | 1.4 | 9.6 | 7.6 | 1.4 |
| Tikka Masala, Lemon & Coriander, Canned, Patak's* | 1 Can/283g | 487.0 | 37.0 | 172 | 2.5 | 11.0 | 13.0 | 1.1 |
| Tikka Masala, Light Choices, Tesco* | ¼ Jar/125g | 87.0 | 4.0 | 70 | 2.6 | 8.2 | 3.0 | 1.2 |
| Tikka Masala, Perfectly Balanced, Waitrose* | ½ Jar/175g | 107.0 | 1.0 | 61 | 2.7 | 10.7 | 0.8 | 1.5 |
| Tikka Masala, Sizzle & Stir, Chicken Tonight, Knorr* | 1/3 Jar/168g | 336.0 | 29.0 | 200 | 2.0 | 8.4 | 17.3 | 2.6 |
| Tikka Masala, Spicy, Sharwood's* | 1 Jar/420g | 449.0 | 30.0 | 107 | 1.2 | 9.6 | 7.1 | 0.1 |
| Tikka Masala, Weight Watchers* | 1 Jar/350g | 259.0 | 7.0 | 74 | 2.6 | 11.2 | 2.1 | 0.7 |
| Toffee, GFY, Asda* | 1 Serving/5g | 15.0 | 0.0 | 306 | 2.2 | 68.0 | 2.8 | 0.0 |
| Toffee Fudge, Sainsbury's* | 1 Serving/40g | 134.0 | 1.0 | 336 | 1.9 | 73.9 | 3.7 | 0.4 |
| Tomato, Heinz* | 1 Tbsp/17g | 18.0 | 0.0 | 103 | 0.9 | 24.1 | 0.1 | 0.7 |
| Tomato, Mozzarella & Wild Rocket, Bistro, Waitrose* | ½ Pot/175g | 96.0 | 5.0 | 55 | 1.6 | 7.0 | 2.9 | 1.5 |
| Tomato, Olive & Rosemary, for Fish, Chunky, Schwartz* | 1 Pack/300g | 147.0 | 8.0 | 49 | 1.9 | 4.2 | 2.7 | 0.5 |
| Tomato, Organic, Heinz* | 1 Tsp/5g | 5.0 | 0.0 | 105 | 1.3 | 24.0 | 0.1 | 0.9 |
| Tomato, Parmesan & Dill, Tesco* | 1 Serving/70g | 80.0 | 6.0 | 115 | 3.1 | 4.8 | 9.2 | 0.7 |
| Tomato, Pizza Topping, Napolina* | 1 Serving/70g | 34.0 | 2.0 | 49 | 0.9 | 6.3 | 2.2 | 0.6 |

S

| | Measure INFO/WEIGHT | per Measure KCAL | FAT | Nutrition Values per 100g / 100ml KCAL | PROT | CARB | FAT | FIBRE |
|---|---|---|---|---|---|---|---|---|

**SAUCE**

| | Measure INFO/WEIGHT | KCAL | FAT | KCAL | PROT | CARB | FAT | FIBRE |
|---|---|---|---|---|---|---|---|---|
| Tomato & Basil, Cooking, BGTY, Sainsbury's* | 1 Jar/500g | 335.0 | 6.0 | 67 | 2.6 | 11.3 | 1.3 | 0.7 |
| Tomato & Basil, Cooking, M & S* | 1 Serving/130g | 78.0 | 4.0 | 60 | 1.4 | 5.7 | 3.4 | 1.2 |
| Tomato & Basil, Fresh, Asda* | ½ Tub/175g | 100.0 | 4.0 | 57 | 1.5 | 7.9 | 2.1 | 0.5 |
| Tomato & Basil, Fresh, Organic, Waitrose* | ¼ Pot/175g | 77.0 | 3.0 | 44 | 1.0 | 6.2 | 1.7 | 0.8 |
| Tomato & Basil, Italian, Sainsbury's* | ½ Pot/175g | 80.0 | 4.0 | 46 | 1.6 | 5.1 | 2.1 | 2.5 |
| Tomato & Basil, Tesco* | ½ Jar/175g | 84.0 | 6.0 | 48 | 0.7 | 3.8 | 3.3 | 0.8 |
| Tomato & Chilli, Waitrose* | 1 Pot/350g | 182.0 | 9.0 | 52 | 10.0 | 6.2 | 2.6 | 3.2 |
| Tomato & Creme Fraiche, Less Than 3% Fat, Asda* | 1 Pot/300g | 168.0 | 8.0 | 56 | 0.7 | 7.0 | 2.8 | 0.5 |
| Tomato & Creme Fraiche, Perfectly Balanaced, Waitrose* | ½ Pot/175g | 84.0 | 2.0 | 48 | 1.8 | 7.1 | 1.3 | 2.0 |
| Tomato & Marscapone, Italiano, Tesco* | 1 Serving/175g | 194.0 | 15.0 | 111 | 2.8 | 5.4 | 8.7 | 0.6 |
| Tomato & Mascarpone, Fresh, Sainsbury's* | 1/3 Pot/100g | 91.0 | 7.0 | 91 | 2.1 | 5.9 | 6.6 | 1.2 |
| Tomato & Mascarpone, Fresh, Tesco* | ½ Pot/175g | 206.0 | 15.0 | 118 | 2.8 | 7.1 | 8.7 | 0.6 |
| Tomato & Mascarpone, Light Choices, Tesco* | ½ Pot/175g | 77.0 | 3.0 | 44 | 1.6 | 4.9 | 2.0 | 0.8 |
| Tomato & Mozzarella, Finest, Tesco* | 1 Serving/175g | 89.0 | 6.0 | 51 | 1.6 | 4.1 | 3.2 | 0.6 |
| Tomato & Onion, Cook in, Homepride* | 1 Can/390g | 183.0 | 2.0 | 47 | 0.9 | 9.8 | 0.5 | 0.0 |
| Tomato & Roasted Garlic, Stir in, Dolmio* | ½ Pack/75g | 94.0 | 8.0 | 125 | 1.2 | 7.7 | 10.2 | 0.0 |
| Tomato & Smoked Bacon, Italiano, Tesco* | ½ Pot/175g | 96.0 | 4.0 | 55 | 3.0 | 4.7 | 2.5 | 1.0 |
| Tomato & Wild Mushroom, Organic, Fresh, Sainsbury's* | 1 Serving/152g | 102.0 | 7.0 | 67 | 1.9 | 3.9 | 4.9 | 1.7 |
| Tomato & Worcester, Table, Lea & Perrins* | 1 Serving/10g | 10.0 | 0.0 | 102 | 0.8 | 23.0 | 0.5 | 0.7 |
| Vegetable, Chunky, Tesco* | 1 Can/455g | 155.0 | 1.0 | 34 | 1.2 | 7.0 | 0.2 | 1.0 |
| Vegetables, Hoi Sin & Plum, Stir Fry, Sharwood's* | 1 Pack/360g | 367.0 | 5.0 | 102 | 1.1 | 21.4 | 1.3 | 0.2 |
| Vine Ripened Tomato & Aromatic Basil, Discovery* | 1 Serving/125g | 161.0 | 9.0 | 129 | 1.8 | 14.3 | 7.2 | 0.0 |
| Vine Ripened Tomato & Mascarpone, Stir Through, Sacla* | ½ Jar/100g | 171.0 | 16.0 | 171 | 1.4 | 5.9 | 15.8 | 0.0 |
| Vodka & Chilli, Finest, Tesco* | 1 Serving/350g | 343.0 | 20.0 | 98 | 2.2 | 9.4 | 5.7 | 2.1 |
| Vongole, Sainsbury's* | ½ Pot/150g | 106.0 | 4.0 | 71 | 3.1 | 7.8 | 3.0 | 1.9 |
| Watercress, & Stilton, Creamy, for Fish, Schwartz* | 1 Pack/300g | 141.0 | 12.0 | 47 | 0.6 | 2.0 | 4.1 | 0.7 |
| Watercress, TTD, Sainsbury's* | 1 Serving/100g | 82.0 | 7.0 | 82 | 2.3 | 2.7 | 6.9 | 4.4 |
| Watercress & Creme Fraiche, COU, M & S* | ½ Pack/154g | 100.0 | 3.0 | 65 | 3.2 | 9.2 | 1.8 | 0.5 |
| White, for Lasagne, Dolmio* | 1 Jar/470g | 451.0 | 34.0 | 96 | 0.6 | 7.0 | 7.3 | 0.0 |
| White, Savoury, Made with Semi-Skimmed Milk | 1oz/28g | 36.0 | 2.0 | 128 | 4.2 | 11.1 | 7.8 | 0.2 |
| White, Savoury, Made with Whole Milk | 1oz/28g | 42.0 | 3.0 | 150 | 4.1 | 10.9 | 10.3 | 0.2 |
| White Granules, Sauce in Seconds, Dry, Asda* | 1 Pack/57g | 237.0 | 7.0 | 415 | 3.7 | 73.0 | 12.0 | 0.9 |
| White Wine, Chardonnay, M & S* | 1 Serving/160ml | 184.0 | 16.0 | 115 | 1.4 | 4.6 | 10.0 | 0.9 |
| White Wine, Dry, Alcohol Boiled Off | 1 Serving/125ml | 3.0 | 0.0 | 3 | 0.1 | 0.6 | 0.0 | 0.0 |
| White Wine & Mushroom, BGTY, Sainsbury's* | ¼ Jar/125g | 81.0 | 2.0 | 65 | 2.8 | 9.0 | 2.0 | 0.3 |
| White Wine & Tarragon, French, for Fish, Schwartz* | 1 Pack/300g | 372.0 | 33.0 | 124 | 1.1 | 5.0 | 11.1 | 0.8 |
| White Wine and Cream, Cook in Sauce, Homepride* | ¼ Can/125g | 101.0 | 5.0 | 81 | 1.0 | 8.0 | 4.1 | 0.4 |
| White Wine Mushroom & Herb, 98% Fat Free, Homepride* | 1 Jar/450g | 180.0 | 5.0 | 40 | 0.8 | 7.0 | 1.2 | 0.5 |
| Whole Cherry Tomato & Chilli, Finest, Tesco* | 1 Jar/340g | 255.0 | 16.0 | 75 | 1.7 | 6.8 | 4.6 | 2.3 |
| Wild Mushroom, Finest, Tesco* | ½ Pack/175g | 157.0 | 12.0 | 90 | 1.9 | 5.2 | 6.8 | 0.4 |
| *Worcestershire, Average* | *1 Tsp/5g* | *3.0* | *0.0* | *65* | *1.4* | *15.5* | *0.1* | *0.0* |
| Worcestershire, Lea & Perrins* | 1 Tsp/5ml | 4.0 | 0.0 | 88 | 1.1 | 22.0 | 0.0 | 0.0 |
| Worcestershire, Special Edition, Lea & Perrins* | 1 Serving/10ml | 13.0 | 0.0 | 130 | 1.3 | 28.8 | 0.2 | 0.1 |
| Yellow Bean & Cashew, Tesco* | ½ Jar/210g | 170.0 | 6.0 | 81 | 1.6 | 11.9 | 2.9 | 0.3 |
| Yellow Bean & Ginger, Stir Fry, Finest, Tesco* | 1 Jar/350g | 318.0 | 3.0 | 91 | 2.1 | 18.3 | 1.0 | 1.1 |

**SAUCE MIX**

| | Measure INFO/WEIGHT | KCAL | FAT | KCAL | PROT | CARB | FAT | FIBRE |
|---|---|---|---|---|---|---|---|---|
| Bacon & Mushroom Tagliatelle, Schwartz* | 1 Pack/33g | 110.0 | 1.0 | 333 | 7.5 | 69.2 | 2.9 | 8.3 |
| Beef Bourguignon, Colman's* | 1 Pack/40g | 123.0 | 1.0 | 308 | 4.9 | 68.6 | 1.6 | 2.2 |
| Beef Stroganoff, Colman's* | 1 Pack/40g | 140.0 | 4.0 | 350 | 11.6 | 56.1 | 8.9 | 2.7 |
| Bombay Potatoes, Schwartz* | 1 Pack/33g | 84.0 | 4.0 | 254 | 16.1 | 20.1 | 12.1 | 31.1 |
| Bread, Colman's* | 1 Pack/40g | 131.0 | 0.0 | 327 | 11.4 | 67.9 | 1.1 | 3.2 |
| Bread, Knorr* | ½ Pint/40g | 177.0 | 9.0 | 442 | 7.9 | 49.9 | 23.3 | 2.1 |
| Bread, Luxury, Schwartz* | 1 Pack/40g | 142.0 | 3.0 | 355 | 12.9 | 61.5 | 6.4 | 6.5 |

**S**

## SAUCE MIX

| | INFO/WEIGHT | KCAL | FAT | KCAL | PROT | CARB | FAT | FIBRE |
|---|---|---|---|---|---|---|---|---|
| Cajun Chicken, Schwartz* | 1 Pack/38g | 108.0 | 0.0 | 285 | 6.4 | 61.9 | 1.3 | 0.5 |
| Cheddar Cheese, Colman's* | 1 Pack/40g | 163.0 | 6.0 | 407 | 18.3 | 48.8 | 15.4 | 1.2 |
| Cheddar Cheese, Schwartz* | 1 Pack/40g | 144.0 | 3.0 | 361 | 18.4 | 55.1 | 7.4 | 2.3 |
| Cheese, Knorr* | 1 Pack/58g | 132.0 | 3.0 | 227 | 7.8 | 38.0 | 4.9 | 1.8 |
| Cheese, Made Up, Crosse & Blackwell* | 1 Pack/30g | 26.0 | 1.0 | 86 | 5.1 | 9.2 | 3.2 | 0.7 |
| Cheese, Made Up with Skimmed Milk | 1 Serving/60g | 47.0 | 1.0 | 78 | 5.4 | 9.5 | 2.3 | 0.0 |
| Chicken Chasseur, Colman's* | 1 Pack/45g | 128.0 | 1.0 | 284 | 8.0 | 59.2 | 1.6 | 3.8 |
| Chicken Chasseur, Schwartz* | 1 Pack/40g | 126.0 | 2.0 | 316 | 9.6 | 59.1 | 4.6 | 6.8 |
| Chicken Korma, Colman's* | ½ Pack/50g | 229.0 | 15.0 | 459 | 6.6 | 38.8 | 30.8 | 13.2 |
| Chicken Korma, Schwartz* | 1 Pack/40g | 154.0 | 4.0 | 385 | 3.5 | 70.5 | 9.9 | 4.3 |
| Chicken Supreme, Colman's* | 1 Pack/40g | 143.0 | 4.0 | 358 | 12.1 | 56.7 | 9.2 | 2.4 |
| Chilli Con Carne, Asda* | 1 Sachet/50g | 157.0 | 1.0 | 314 | 7.0 | 68.0 | 1.6 | 2.5 |
| Chilli Con Carne, Hot, Colman's* | 1 Pack/40g | 127.0 | 1.0 | 317 | 10.4 | 62.4 | 2.9 | 7.0 |
| Chilli Con Carne, Schwartz* | 1 Pack/41g | 120.0 | 1.0 | 293 | 7.9 | 57.2 | 3.6 | 9.5 |
| Creamy Chicken Curry, Colman's* | 1 Sachet/50g | 192.0 | 9.0 | 385 | 11.0 | 46.4 | 17.3 | 7.9 |
| Creamy Pepper & Mushroom, Colman's* | 1 Pack/25g | 83.0 | 1.0 | 332 | 9.6 | 64.6 | 3.8 | 3.0 |
| Curry, Batchelors* | 1 Serving/100g | 359.0 | 8.0 | 359 | 7.1 | 63.9 | 8.3 | 3.9 |
| for Garlic Mushrooms, Creamy, Schwartz* | 1 Pack/35g | 109.0 | 2.0 | 311 | 7.6 | 59.7 | 4.7 | 4.2 |
| Four Cheese, Colman's* | 1 Pack/35g | 127.0 | 4.0 | 362 | 17.1 | 48.4 | 11.1 | 1.8 |
| Hollandaise, Colman's* | 1 Pack/28g | 104.0 | 3.0 | 372 | 6.4 | 61.6 | 11.1 | 1.8 |
| Hollandaise, Schwartz* | 1 Pack/25g | 98.0 | 3.0 | 394 | 10.6 | 59.2 | 12.8 | 3.7 |
| Lamb Hotpot, Colman's* | 1 Pack/40g | 119.0 | 1.0 | 297 | 6.9 | 63.3 | 1.7 | 2.1 |
| Lasagne, Mediterranean Vegetable, Schwartz* | 1 Pack/30g | 79.0 | 1.0 | 263 | 9.3 | 46.0 | 4.4 | 15.2 |
| Lasagne, Schwartz* | 1 Pack/36g | 106.0 | 1.0 | 294 | 7.0 | 63.4 | 1.4 | 7.0 |
| Lemon Butter, for Fish, Schwartz* | 1 Pack/38g | 136.0 | 3.0 | 357 | 6.1 | 65.3 | 8.0 | 5.8 |
| Mexican Chilli Chicken, Schwartz* | 1 Pack/35g | 105.0 | 2.0 | 299 | 7.0 | 55.1 | 5.6 | 12.0 |
| Moussaka, Schwartz* | 1 Pack/35g | 101.0 | 1.0 | 288 | 8.8 | 58.6 | 2.0 | 9.0 |
| Mustard & Sweet Dill, TTD, Sainsbury's* | ¼ Sachet/10g | 25.0 | 1.0 | 248 | 2.8 | 25.8 | 14.9 | 2.6 |
| Onion, Colman's* | ½ Pack/17g | 55.0 | 0.0 | 325 | 9.1 | 69.4 | 1.3 | 4.8 |
| Onion, Creamy, Schwartz* | 1 Pack/25g | 90.0 | 2.0 | 362 | 10.1 | 59.6 | 9.2 | 5.3 |
| Paprika Chicken, Creamy, Schwartz* | 1 Pack/34g | 116.0 | 3.0 | 342 | 9.7 | 53.9 | 9.8 | 9.5 |
| Parsley, Colman's* | 1 Pack/20g | 63.0 | 0.0 | 314 | 7.2 | 67.9 | 1.5 | 3.7 |
| Parsley, Knorr* | 1 Sachet/48g | 210.0 | 12.0 | 437 | 4.2 | 50.6 | 24.2 | 0.8 |
| Parsley & Chive, for Fish, Schwartz* | 1 Pack/38g | 132.0 | 3.0 | 348 | 9.0 | 58.9 | 8.5 | 7.7 |
| Pepper, Creamy, Colman's* | 1 Pack/25g | 88.0 | 3.0 | 352 | 13.0 | 50.0 | 11.0 | 0.0 |
| Pepper, Creamy, Schwartz* | 1 Pack/25g | 85.0 | 2.0 | 342 | 17.9 | 52.0 | 6.9 | 7.0 |
| Pork & Mushroom, Creamy, Schwartz* | 1 Pack/40g | 116.0 | 2.0 | 289 | 8.6 | 54.7 | 4.0 | 12.1 |
| Savoury Mince, Schwartz* | 1 Pack/35g | 108.0 | 1.0 | 310 | 14.6 | 58.3 | 2.0 | 1.8 |
| Shepherd's Pie, Schwartz* | 1 Pack/38g | 104.0 | 1.0 | 273 | 7.9 | 54.4 | 2.6 | 11.1 |
| Spaghetti Bolognese, Colman's* | 1 Pack/40g | 120.0 | 0.0 | 300 | 8.9 | 64.1 | 0.9 | 5.2 |
| Spaghetti Bolognese, Schwartz* | 1 Pack/40g | 114.0 | 1.0 | 285 | 9.2 | 59.0 | 1.6 | 7.0 |
| Spaghetti Bolognese, with Mushrooms, Colman's* | 1 Pack/45g | 138.0 | 0.0 | 307 | 7.8 | 66.8 | 0.9 | 4.7 |
| Spaghetti Carbonara, Schwartz* | 1 Pack/32g | 135.0 | 6.0 | 421 | 10.4 | 49.4 | 20.1 | 7.2 |
| Stroganoff, Beef, Schwartz* | 1 Pack/35g | 125.0 | 4.0 | 358 | 15.6 | 50.8 | 10.3 | 4.4 |
| Stroganoff, Mushroom, Schwartz* | 1 Pack/35g | 113.0 | 2.0 | 324 | 10.0 | 59.2 | 5.3 | 9.6 |
| Sweet & Sour, Colman's* | 1 Pack/40g | 133.0 | 0.0 | 333 | 2.6 | 79.9 | 0.4 | 2.2 |
| Thai Green Curry, Schwartz* | 1 Pack/41g | 137.0 | 3.0 | 333 | 7.6 | 57.6 | 8.1 | 13.0 |
| Thai Red Curry, Schwartz* | 1 Pack/35g | 120.0 | 2.0 | 342 | 5.9 | 63.5 | 7.1 | 7.6 |
| Three Cheese, for Vegetables, Schwartz* | 1 Pack/40g | 168.0 | 8.0 | 421 | 17.4 | 41.7 | 20.5 | 4.8 |
| Tikka Masala, Creamy, Schwartz* | 1 Pack/31g | 100.0 | 4.0 | 324 | 11.9 | 43.5 | 11.4 | 18.1 |
| Tuna & Mushroom Pasta Melt, Schwartz* | 1 Pack/40g | 122.0 | 3.0 | 304 | 10.2 | 49.7 | 7.1 | 7.7 |
| Tuna & Pasta Bake, Colman's* | 1 Pack/45g | 144.0 | 2.0 | 319 | 10.4 | 57.1 | 5.4 | 5.2 |
| Tuna Napolitana, Schwartz* | 1 Pack/30g | 107.0 | 4.0 | 357 | 10.3 | 49.6 | 13.1 | 0.5 |

**S**

| | Measure INFO/WEIGHT | per Measure KCAL | FAT | Nutrition Values per 100g / 100ml KCAL | PROT | CARB | FAT | FIBRE |
|---|---|---|---|---|---|---|---|---|
| **SAUCE MIX** | | | | | | | | |
| White, Dry Weight, Bisto* | 1 Dtsp/9g | 45.0 | 3.0 | 496 | 3.2 | 57.4 | 28.2 | 0.4 |
| White, Instant, Made Up, Sainsbury's* | 1 Serving/90ml | 65.0 | 3.0 | 72 | 0.8 | 10.9 | 2.8 | 0.1 |
| White, Made Up with Semi-Skimmed Milk | 1oz/28g | 20.0 | 1.0 | 73 | 4.0 | 9.6 | 2.4 | 0.0 |
| White, Made Up with Skimmed Milk | 1oz/28g | 17.0 | 0.0 | 59 | 4.0 | 9.6 | 0.9 | 0.0 |
| White, Savoury, Colman's* | 1 Pack/25g | 84.0 | 1.0 | 335 | 10.7 | 66.5 | 2.9 | 2.6 |
| White, Savoury, Knorr* | ½ Pack/16g | 46.0 | 1.0 | 290 | 7.8 | 52.2 | 5.6 | 5.2 |
| White, Savoury, Schwartz* | 1 Pack/25g | 108.0 | 6.0 | 434 | 11.5 | 45.6 | 22.9 | 5.9 |
| White Wine, with Herbs, Creamy, Schwartz* | 1 Pack/26g | 86.0 | 2.0 | 330 | 8.0 | 60.0 | 6.5 | 9.1 |
| Wholegrain Mustard, Creamy, Schwartz* | 1 Pack/25g | 92.0 | 3.0 | 370 | 12.9 | 54.4 | 11.2 | 7.5 |
| **SAUERKRAUT** | | | | | | | | |
| *Average* | *1oz/28g* | *4.0* | *0.0* | *13* | *1.3* | *1.9* | *0.0* | *1.1* |
| **SAUSAGE** | | | | | | | | |
| BBQ Hotdog, M & S* | 1 Sausage/100g | 300.0 | 25.0 | 300 | 12.1 | 5.4 | 25.3 | 2.0 |
| *Beef, Average* | *1 Sausage/60g* | *151.0* | *11.0* | *252* | *14.5* | *7.0* | *18.5* | *0.6* |
| Beef, with Onion & Red Wine, Finest, Tesco* | 1 Sausage/63g | 117.0 | 7.0 | 185 | 13.2 | 8.5 | 10.9 | 1.2 |
| Billy Bear, Kids, Tesco* | 1 Slice/20g | 37.0 | 2.0 | 185 | 13.7 | 7.5 | 11.2 | 0.4 |
| ***Bockwurst, Average*** | *1 Sausage/45g* | *114.0* | *10.0* | *253* | *10.7* | *0.7* | *23.0* | *0.0* |
| Bratwurst, Frozen, Lidl* | 1 Sausage/80g | 235.0 | 21.0 | 294 | 12.8 | 0.5 | 26.8 | 0.0 |
| Cambridge Gluten Free, Waitrose* | 1 Sausage/57g | 121.0 | 9.0 | 213 | 14.6 | 1.9 | 16.3 | 1.3 |
| Cheese & Leek, Tesco* | 1 Sausage/55g | 135.0 | 7.0 | 246 | 6.9 | 24.0 | 13.6 | 1.7 |
| Chicken, Manor Farm* | 1 Sausage/65g | 126.0 | 8.0 | 194 | 13.7 | 6.6 | 12.5 | 1.2 |
| Chicken & Tarragon, Butchers Choice, Sainsbury's* | 1 Sausage/47g | 106.0 | 7.0 | 225 | 18.1 | 5.8 | 14.4 | 0.2 |
| Chicken & Turkey, Morrisons* | 1 Sausage/57g | 86.0 | 4.0 | 152 | 16.0 | 5.8 | 7.2 | 1.1 |
| Chilli Beef, Boston Style, Waitrose* | 1 Sausage/67g | 135.0 | 10.0 | 203 | 14.7 | 3.4 | 14.6 | 0.9 |
| *Chipolata, Average* | *1 Sausage/28g* | *81.0* | *6.0* | *291* | *12.1* | *8.7* | *23.1* | *0.7* |
| Chipolata, Chicken & Sweet Chilli, TTD, Sainsbury's* | 1 Sausage/38g | 77.0 | 5.0 | 206 | 18.4 | 5.4 | 13.3 | 1.2 |
| Chipolata, Lamb & Rosemary, Tesco* | 1 Sausage/32g | 69.0 | 5.0 | 218 | 11.3 | 8.3 | 15.5 | 0.0 |
| Chipolata, Pork, Extra Lean, BGTY, Sainsbury's* | 1 Sausage/24g | 46.0 | 2.0 | 189 | 16.9 | 10.9 | 8.6 | 0.5 |
| Chipolata, Pork & Tomato, Organic, Tesco* | 1 Sausage/28g | 79.0 | 7.0 | 283 | 12.2 | 4.3 | 24.1 | 0.9 |
| *Chipolata, Premium, Average* | *1 Serving/80g* | *187.0* | *14.0* | *233* | *14.8* | *4.7* | *17.3* | *1.2* |
| *Chorizo, Average* | *1 Serving/80g* | *250.0* | *19.0* | *313* | *21.1* | *2.6* | *24.2* | *0.2* |
| *Chorizo, Lean, Average* | *1 Sausage/67g* | *131.0* | *9.0* | *195* | *15.7* | *2.3* | *13.7* | *0.8* |
| *Cocktail, Average* | *1oz/28g* | *90.0* | *7.0* | *323* | *12.1* | *8.6* | *26.7* | *0.9* |
| *Cumberland, Average* | *1 Sausage/57g* | *167.0* | *13.0* | *293* | *13.8* | *8.5* | *22.7* | *0.8* |
| *Cumberland, Healthy Range, Average* | *1 Sausage/53g* | *75.0* | *2.0* | *142* | *17.4* | *9.0* | *4.0* | *0.9* |
| Cumberland, Quorn* | 1 Sausage/50g | 60.0 | 2.0 | 120 | 12.3 | 7.0 | 4.8 | 4.0 |
| Cumberland, with Cracked Black Pepper & Herbs, Asda* | 1 Sausage/56g | 127.0 | 8.0 | 225 | 13.6 | 10.8 | 14.2 | 2.2 |
| Duck & Orange, TTD, Sainsbury's* | 1 Sausage/41g | 123.0 | 11.0 | 301 | 13.8 | 3.2 | 25.9 | 0.9 |
| Extrawurst, German, Waitrose* | 1 Slice/28g | 80.0 | 7.0 | 281 | 13.0 | 1.0 | 25.0 | 0.0 |
| Free From Wheat & Gulten, Sainsbury's* | 1 Serving/23g | 61.0 | 5.0 | 268 | 15.2 | 4.5 | 21.0 | 1.8 |
| French Saucisson, Tesco* | 1 Slice/5g | 19.0 | 1.0 | 379 | 26.7 | 4.1 | 28.4 | 0.0 |
| *Garlic, Average* | *1 Slice/11g* | *25.0* | *2.0* | *227* | *15.7* | *0.8* | *18.2* | *0.0* |
| German, Bierwurst, Selection, Sainsbury's* | 1 Slice/4g | 8.0 | 1.0 | 224 | 15.0 | 1.0 | 17.8 | 0.1 |
| German, Extrawurst, Selection, Sainsbury's* | 1 Slice/3g | 9.0 | 1.0 | 279 | 13.1 | 0.5 | 25.0 | 0.1 |
| Hot & Spicy Pork Cocktail, Cooked, Asda* | 1 Sausage/10g | 31.0 | 2.0 | 312 | 13.0 | 11.0 | 24.0 | 1.3 |
| Hot Mustard Porker, Tesco* | 1 Sausage/52g | 143.0 | 10.0 | 275 | 16.1 | 8.1 | 19.8 | 3.1 |
| *Irish, Average* | *1 Sausage/40g* | *119.0* | *8.0* | *297* | *10.7* | *17.2* | *20.7* | *0.7* |
| *Lincolnshire, Average* | *1 Sausage/42g* | *122.0* | *9.0* | *291* | *14.6* | *9.2* | *21.8* | *0.6* |
| *Lincolnshire, Healthy Range, Average* | *1 Sausage/50g* | *89.0* | *4.0* | *177* | *15.8* | *9.0* | *8.6* | *0.8* |
| *Lorne, Average* | *1 Sausage/25g* | *78.0* | *6.0* | *312* | *10.8* | *16.0* | *23.1* | *0.6* |
| Mediterranean Style, 95% Fat Free, Bowyers* | 1 Sausage/50g | 60.0 | 2.0 | 120 | 13.9 | 8.9 | 3.2 | 0.0 |
| Mediterranean Style Paprika, Waitrose* | 1 Sausage/67g | 190.0 | 16.0 | 283 | 12.1 | 4.6 | 24.0 | 1.9 |
| Mortadella, Sainsbury's* | 1 Slice/13g | 34.0 | 3.0 | 261 | 17.3 | 0.1 | 21.2 | 0.1 |

| | Measure INFO/WEIGHT | per Measure KCAL | FAT | Nutrition Values per 100g / 100ml KCAL | PROT | CARB | FAT | FIBRE |
|---|---|---|---|---|---|---|---|---|
| **SAUSAGE** | | | | | | | | |
| Polish Kabanos, Sainsbury's* | 1 Sausage/25g | 92.0 | 8.0 | 366 | 23.0 | 0.1 | 30.4 | 0.1 |
| Polony, Slicing, Value, Tesco* | 1 Serving/40g | 92.0 | 7.0 | 229 | 10.0 | 10.0 | 16.5 | 1.0 |
| Pork, & Sweet Chilli, Waitrose* | 1 Sausage/67g | 146.0 | 10.0 | 219 | 15.6 | 4.6 | 15.3 | 0.8 |
| Pork, Apricot & Herb, Waitrose* | 1 Sausage/67g | 165.0 | 11.0 | 246 | 11.2 | 12.9 | 16.6 | 1.3 |
| *Pork, Average* | *1 Sausage/50g* | *152.0* | *12.0* | *305* | *12.8* | *9.8* | *23.8* | *0.7* |
| Pork, Bacon & Cheese, Asda* | ¼ Pack/114g | 329.0 | 24.0 | 289 | 18.0 | 7.0 | 21.0 | 0.4 |
| *Pork, Extra Lean, Average* | *1 Sausage/54g* | *84.0* | *4.0* | *155* | *17.3* | *6.1* | *6.8* | *0.8* |
| Pork, Free From, Tesco* | 1 Sausage/57g | 124.0 | 9.0 | 218 | 12.1 | 8.5 | 15.0 | 2.2 |
| *Pork, Frozen, Fried* | *1oz/28g* | *88.0* | *7.0* | *316* | *13.8* | *10.0* | *24.8* | *0.0* |
| *Pork, Frozen, Grilled* | *1oz/28g* | *81.0* | *6.0* | *289* | *14.8* | *10.5* | *21.2* | *0.0* |
| *Pork, Garlic & Herb, Average* | *1 Sausage/76g* | *203.0* | *17.0* | *268* | *12.0* | *5.9* | *21.8* | *1.1* |
| Pork, Ham & Asparagus, Tesco* | 1 Sausage/76g | 173.0 | 13.0 | 228 | 14.9 | 3.8 | 17.0 | 1.1 |
| *Pork, Premium, Average* | *1 Sausage/74g* | *191.0* | *14.0* | *258* | *14.9* | *8.3* | *18.4* | *1.0* |
| *Pork, Reduced Fat, Chilled, Grilled* | *1oz/28g* | *64.0* | *4.0* | *230* | *16.2* | *10.8* | *13.8* | *1.5* |
| *Pork, Reduced Fat, Chilled, Raw* | *1oz/28g* | *50.0* | *3.0* | *180* | *13.0* | *8.7* | *10.6* | *1.2* |
| *Pork, Reduced Fat, Healthy Range, Average* | *1 Sausage/57g* | *86.0* | *3.0* | *151* | *15.6* | *9.0* | *6.0* | *0.9* |
| *Pork, Skinless, Average* | *1oz/28g* | *81.0* | *7.0* | *291* | *11.7* | *8.2* | *23.6* | *0.6* |
| Pork, Smoked Bacon, & Garlic, Finest, Tesco* | 1 Sausage/67g | 115.0 | 8.0 | 173 | 14.7 | 0.2 | 12.6 | 0.4 |
| *Pork, Thick, Average* | *1 Sausage/39g* | *115.0* | *9.0* | *296* | *13.3* | *10.0* | *22.4* | *1.0* |
| *Pork, Thick, Reduced Fat, Healthy Range, Average* | *1 Sausage/52g* | *90.0* | *4.0* | *172* | *14.0* | *12.3* | *7.4* | *0.8* |
| *Pork & Apple, Average* | *1 Sausage/57g* | *146.0* | *11.0* | *255* | *14.5* | *7.5* | *18.8* | *1.9* |
| *Pork & Beef, Average* | *1 Sausage/45g* | *133.0* | *10.0* | *295* | *8.7* | *13.6* | *22.7* | *0.5* |
| Pork & Chilli, Tesco* | 1 Sausage/67g | 124.0 | 8.0 | 186 | 16.4 | 3.2 | 12.0 | 1.1 |
| *Pork & Herb, Average* | *1 Sausage/75g* | *231.0* | *19.0* | *308* | *13.1* | *5.4* | *25.9* | *0.3* |
| *Pork & Herb, Healthy Range, Average* | *1 Sausage/59g* | *75.0* | *1.0* | *126* | *16.0* | *10.7* | *2.4* | *1.1* |
| *Pork & Leek, Average* | *1oz/28g* | *73.0* | *6.0* | *262* | *14.6* | *6.0* | *19.9* | *1.1* |
| Pork & Onion, Gluten Free, Asda* | 1 Sausage/41g | 105.0 | 7.0 | 257 | 20.0 | 6.0 | 17.0 | 1.8 |
| *Pork & Stilton, Average* | *1 Sausage/57g* | *180.0* | *15.0* | *316* | *13.2* | *5.8* | *26.7* | *0.3* |
| *Pork & Tomato, Grilled, Average* | *1 Sausage/47g* | *127.0* | *10.0* | *273* | *13.9* | *7.5* | *20.8* | *0.4* |
| Pork with Mozzarella, Italian Style, Tesco* | 1 Sausage/76g | 205.0 | 15.0 | 271 | 12.0 | 10.1 | 20.3 | 1.0 |
| *Premium, Chilled, Fried* | *1oz/28g* | *77.0* | *6.0* | *275* | *15.8* | *6.7* | *20.7* | *0.0* |
| *Premium, Chilled, Grilled* | *1oz/28g* | *82.0* | *6.0* | *292* | *16.8* | *6.3* | *22.4* | *0.0* |
| Rich Venison & Redcurrant, Grilled, TTD, Sainsbury's* | 1 Sausage/46g | 138.0 | 10.0 | 299 | 21.2 | 3.0 | 22.5 | 1.8 |
| Round, Breakfast Pack, Healthy Choice, Asda* | 1 Sausage/53g | 85.0 | 3.0 | 160 | 23.0 | 6.0 | 4.9 | 0.0 |
| *Smoked, Average* | *1 Sausage/174g* | *588.0* | *52.0* | *338* | *13.0* | *4.0* | *30.0* | *0.0* |
| Smoky Cajun, TTD, Sainsbury's* | 1 Sausage/46g | 116.0 | 8.0 | 250 | 24.2 | 1.6 | 16.3 | 0.9 |
| Spanish, Wafer Thin, Asda* | 1 Slice/4g | 12.0 | 1.0 | 298 | 25.4 | 4.1 | 20.0 | 0.0 |
| Spicy, Pork, Polenta & Sun Dried Tomato, Waitrose* | 1 Sausage/67g | 165.0 | 12.0 | 247 | 11.8 | 9.8 | 17.8 | 0.9 |
| Spicy Pork & Pepper, Summer Selection, Sainsbury's* | 1 Sausage/33g | 86.0 | 6.0 | 260 | 20.1 | 6.0 | 17.3 | 1.6 |
| Toulouse, M & S* | 1 Sausage/57g | 123.0 | 9.0 | 215 | 12.4 | 5.8 | 15.6 | 1.3 |
| Toulouse, TTD, Sainsbury's* | 1 Sausage/67g | 186.0 | 14.0 | 277 | 22.0 | 0.3 | 20.9 | 1.2 |
| Tuna, Mediterranean Style, Sainsbury's* | 1 Serving/50g | 102.0 | 5.0 | 204 | 15.1 | 14.7 | 9.5 | 1.2 |
| Tuna & Herb, Sainsbury's* | 1 Sausage/47g | 109.0 | 6.0 | 231 | 19.6 | 10.0 | 12.5 | 1.5 |
| *Turkey, Average* | *1 Sausage/57g* | *90.0* | *5.0* | *157* | *15.7* | *6.3* | *8.0* | *0.0* |
| *Turkey & Chicken, Average* | *1 Sausage/57g* | *126.0* | *8.0* | *221* | *14.4* | *8.2* | *14.5* | *1.7* |
| Turkey & Ham, Tesco* | 1 Sausage/57g | 101.0 | 6.0 | 178 | 13.8 | 8.3 | 10.0 | 1.0 |
| Tuscan, M & S* | 1 Sausage/66g | 145.0 | 11.0 | 220 | 14.9 | 4.6 | 16.0 | 0.6 |
| Venison, & Red Wine, TTD, Sainsbury's* | 1 Sausage/66g | 150.0 | 9.0 | 226 | 19.7 | 6.8 | 13.3 | 1.7 |
| Venison, Grilled, Finest, Tesco* | 1 Sausage/40g | 56.0 | 2.0 | 140 | 18.6 | 5.3 | 4.5 | 1.1 |
| Venison, Oisin, M & S* | 1 Serving/25g | 41.0 | 2.0 | 165 | 16.8 | 3.8 | 9.3 | 0.7 |
| Wiejska, Polish, Sainsbury's* | 1/8 Pack/50g | 78.0 | 4.0 | 157 | 18.7 | 0.4 | 9.0 | 0.5 |
| **SAUSAGE & MASH** | | | | | | | | |
| British Classic, Tesco* | 1 Pack/450g | 675.0 | 43.0 | 150 | 5.1 | 11.1 | 9.5 | 0.9 |

S

| | Measure INFO/WEIGHT | per Measure KCAL | FAT | Nutrition Values per 100g / 100ml KCAL | PROT | CARB | FAT | FIBRE |
|---|---|---|---|---|---|---|---|---|
| **SAUSAGE & MASH** | | | | | | | | |
| GFY, Asda* | 1 Pack/400g | 330.0 | 10.0 | 82 | 4.2 | 10.7 | 2.5 | 1.7 |
| Light Choices, HE, Tesco* | 1 Pack/450g | 405.0 | 10.0 | 90 | 4.4 | 12.3 | 2.3 | 1.1 |
| Onion, M & S* | 1 Pack/300g | 315.0 | 17.0 | 105 | 4.1 | 9.0 | 5.7 | 1.5 |
| Vegetarian, GFY, Asda* | 1 Pack/400g | 292.0 | 9.0 | 73 | 4.2 | 9.0 | 2.2 | 2.1 |
| Vegetarian, Tesco* | 1 Pack/410g | 398.0 | 16.0 | 97 | 4.6 | 11.1 | 3.8 | 2.0 |
| Waitrose* | 1 Pack/420g | 517.0 | 31.0 | 123 | 4.2 | 9.9 | 7.4 | 0.1 |
| with Onion Gravy, Tesco* | 1 Pack/500g | 525.0 | 27.0 | 105 | 3.0 | 11.1 | 5.4 | 1.6 |
| with Red Wine & Onion Gravy, BGTY, Sainsbury's* | 1 Pack/380g | 315.0 | 7.0 | 83 | 5.0 | 11.4 | 1.9 | 2.0 |
| **SAUSAGE MEAT** | | | | | | | | |
| **Pork, Average** | **1oz/28g** | **96.0** | **8.0** | **344** | **9.9** | **10.1** | **29.4** | **0.6** |
| **SAUSAGE MEAT FREE** | | | | | | | | |
| Cheese & Sundried Tomato, Tesco* | 1 Sausage/50g | 82.0 | 3.0 | 165 | 17.4 | 7.7 | 6.8 | 6.5 |
| **SAUSAGE ROLL** | | | | | | | | |
| Asda* | 1 Roll/64g | 216.0 | 16.0 | 337 | 7.0 | 21.0 | 25.0 | 0.8 |
| BGTY, Sainsbury's* | 1 Roll/65g | 200.0 | 11.0 | 308 | 9.6 | 27.9 | 17.6 | 1.4 |
| Buffet, HE, Tesco* | 1 Roll/30g | 83.0 | 4.0 | 278 | 9.6 | 31.2 | 12.8 | 1.5 |
| Cocktail, M & S* | 1 Roll/14g | 50.0 | 3.0 | 350 | 10.4 | 26.4 | 22.3 | 2.2 |
| Cocktail, Mini, Sainsbury's* | 1 Roll/15g | 54.0 | 4.0 | 361 | 9.0 | 27.6 | 23.8 | 2.6 |
| Co-Op* | 1 Roll/66g | 244.0 | 18.0 | 370 | 8.0 | 25.0 | 27.0 | 2.0 |
| Jumbo, Sainsbury's* | 1 Roll/145g | 492.0 | 34.0 | 339 | 8.2 | 23.2 | 23.7 | 1.5 |
| Kingsize, Pork Farms* | ½ Roll/50g | 241.0 | 16.0 | 483 | 10.5 | 39.9 | 31.8 | 0.0 |
| Large, Frozen, Tesco* | 1 Roll/50g | 182.0 | 12.0 | 365 | 6.0 | 31.0 | 23.8 | 0.9 |
| Lincolnshire, Geo Adams* | 1 Roll/130g | 474.0 | 32.0 | 365 | 8.3 | 28.2 | 24.3 | 1.1 |
| Mini, Tesco* | 1 Roll/15g | 53.0 | 4.0 | 356 | 9.0 | 23.9 | 24.9 | 1.5 |
| Mini, Waitrose* | 1 Roll/35g | 124.0 | 9.0 | 353 | 13.0 | 16.1 | 26.3 | 1.0 |
| Party, Sainsbury's* | 1 Roll/13g | 54.0 | 4.0 | 422 | 8.7 | 26.7 | 31.1 | 1.2 |
| Party, Value, Tesco* | 1 Roll/12g | 33.0 | 1.0 | 274 | 6.8 | 35.9 | 11.5 | 0.6 |
| Pork, Morrisons* | 1 Roll/70g | 195.0 | 9.0 | 278 | 9.6 | 31.2 | 12.8 | 1.5 |
| Pork Farms* | 1 Roll/54g | 196.0 | 13.0 | 363 | 7.9 | 30.0 | 23.9 | 0.0 |
| Puff Pastry, Sainsbury's* | 1 Roll/65g | 250.0 | 18.0 | 384 | 8.3 | 25.0 | 27.9 | 0.9 |
| Reduced Fat, Sainsbury's* | 1 Roll/66g | 191.0 | 9.0 | 289 | 10.5 | 29.8 | 14.2 | 1.8 |
| Sainsbury's* | 1 Roll/67g | 244.0 | 16.0 | 367 | 9.5 | 27.8 | 24.2 | 2.7 |
| Snack, GFY, Asda* | 1 Roll/34g | 112.0 | 7.0 | 329 | 9.4 | 26.5 | 20.6 | 0.9 |
| Snack, Sainsbury's* | 1 Roll/34g | 130.0 | 8.0 | 383 | 9.7 | 29.9 | 25.0 | 2.1 |
| Snack Size, Tesco* | 1 Roll/32g | 118.0 | 9.0 | 369 | 9.1 | 21.7 | 27.4 | 2.3 |
| Tesco* | 1 Roll/67g | 241.0 | 18.0 | 360 | 8.1 | 21.3 | 26.4 | 2.3 |
| Value, Tesco* | 1 Roll/64g | 211.0 | 13.0 | 330 | 6.8 | 29.1 | 20.7 | 4.1 |
| Waitrose* | 1 Roll/75g | 287.0 | 20.0 | 383 | 10.1 | 27.0 | 26.1 | 1.3 |
| **SAUSAGE ROLL VEGETARIAN** | | | | | | | | |
| Linda McCartney* | 1 Roll/52g | 142.0 | 7.0 | 273 | 9.7 | 28.2 | 13.5 | 2.5 |
| **SAUSAGE VEGETARIAN** | | | | | | | | |
| Asda* | 1 Sausage/43g | 81.0 | 4.0 | 189 | 20.0 | 7.0 | 9.0 | 2.9 |
| Cumberland, Waitrose* | 1 Sausage/50g | 80.0 | 3.0 | 160 | 12.6 | 12.3 | 6.7 | 2.4 |
| Glamorgan, Asda* | 1 Sausage/50g | 100.0 | 5.0 | 199 | 4.6 | 22.4 | 10.1 | 2.0 |
| Glamorgan, Organic, Waitrose* | 1 Sausage/42g | 81.0 | 4.0 | 194 | 14.5 | 11.2 | 10.1 | 1.7 |
| Glamorgan Leek & Cheese, Sainsbury's* | 1 Sausage/50g | 98.0 | 5.0 | 197 | 4.3 | 21.3 | 10.5 | 2.7 |
| Glamorgan Leek & Cheese, TTD, Sainsbury's* | 1 Sausage/53g | 171.0 | 14.0 | 323 | 18.9 | 3.3 | 26.0 | 0.6 |
| Lincolnshire, Asda* | 1 Sausage/56g | 96.0 | 4.0 | 172 | 17.0 | 8.0 | 8.0 | 1.4 |
| Lincolnshire, Chilled, Cauldron Foods* | 1 Sausage/50g | 83.0 | 5.0 | 166 | 10.0 | 9.5 | 9.8 | 7.0 |
| Lincolnshire, Frozen, Tesco* | 1 Sausage/50g | 77.0 | 2.0 | 155 | 15.5 | 10.8 | 5.0 | 3.0 |
| Linda McCartney* | 1 Sausage/50g | 101.0 | 4.0 | 202 | 22.6 | 8.2 | 8.8 | 1.6 |
| Morrisons* | 1 Serving/90g | 149.0 | 9.0 | 165 | 17.2 | 2.0 | 9.8 | 8.1 |
| Mushroom & Herb, Waitrose* | 1 Sausage/50g | 61.0 | 3.0 | 123 | 10.2 | 8.1 | 5.4 | 0.5 |

S

| | Measure INFO/WEIGHT | per Measure KCAL | per Measure FAT | Nutrition Values per 100g / 100ml KCAL | PROT | CARB | FAT | FIBRE |
|---|---|---|---|---|---|---|---|---|
| **SAUSAGE VEGETARIAN** | | | | | | | | |
| Realeat* | 1 Sausage/40g | 66.0 | 4.0 | 165 | 17.2 | 2.0 | 9.8 | 8.1 |
| Roasted Garlic & Oregano, Cauldron Foods* | 1 Sausage/50g | 89.0 | 5.0 | 179 | 13.1 | 9.0 | 10.1 | 2.1 |
| Smoked Paprika & Chilli, Cauldron Foods* | 1 Sausage/50g | 76.0 | 4.0 | 152 | 7.8 | 11.8 | 8.2 | 2.6 |
| Spinach, Leek & Cheese, Gourmet, Wicken Fen* | 1 Sausage/46g | 92.0 | 5.0 | 201 | 10.3 | 17.0 | 10.2 | 1.9 |
| Sun Dried Tomato & Black Olive, Cauldron Foods* | 1 Sausage/50g | 71.0 | 4.0 | 142 | 8.7 | 9.4 | 7.7 | 2.6 |
| Sun Dried Tomato & Herb, Linda McCartney* | 1 Sausage/35g | 93.0 | 5.0 | 266 | 21.8 | 10.1 | 15.4 | 1.7 |
| **SAVOURY EGGS** | | | | | | | | |
| Bites, Sainsbury's* | 1 Egg/20g | 55.0 | 4.0 | 277 | 9.6 | 18.8 | 18.2 | 2.1 |
| Mini, Iceland* | 1 Egg/20g | 66.0 | 5.0 | 327 | 11.0 | 17.5 | 23.7 | 1.1 |
| Mini, Tesco* | 1 Egg/20g | 55.0 | 3.0 | 274 | 9.2 | 20.2 | 17.4 | 2.3 |
| Snack, Tesco* | 1 Egg/45g | 133.0 | 9.0 | 295 | 9.0 | 19.6 | 19.7 | 1.8 |
| **SCALLOPS** | | | | | | | | |
| Asda* | 1oz/28g | 33.0 | 0.0 | 118 | 23.2 | 1.4 | 1.4 | 0.0 |
| Breaded, Thai Style with Plum Sauce, Finest, Tesco* | 1 Serving/210g | 401.0 | 15.0 | 191 | 11.5 | 20.6 | 7.0 | 0.8 |
| Breaded, with Plum & Chilli Dipping Sauce, Tesco* | 1 Pack/210g | 441.0 | 15.0 | 210 | 10.6 | 25.6 | 7.2 | 0.8 |
| Canadian, Finest, Tesco* | ½ Pack/100g | 80.0 | 0.0 | 80 | 16.4 | 2.6 | 0.2 | 0.1 |
| Hotbake Shells, Sainsbury's* | 1 Serving/140g | 241.0 | 16.0 | 172 | 9.5 | 8.4 | 11.2 | 0.8 |
| Lemon & Pepper, TTD, Sainsbury's* | 1 Serving/100g | 213.0 | 8.0 | 213 | 13.8 | 20.6 | 8.4 | 1.7 |
| Lemon Grass & Ginger, Tesco* | ½ Pack/112g | 90.0 | 1.0 | 80 | 15.2 | 2.5 | 1.0 | 0.6 |
| *Raw, Bay Or Sea, with Roe, Average* | *1 Lge Scallop/15g* | *13.0* | *0.0* | *88* | *16.8* | *2.4* | *0.8* | *0.0* |
| Steamed, Average | 1oz/28g | 33.0 | 0.0 | 118 | 23.2 | 3.4 | 1.4 | 0.0 |
| with Roasted Garlic Butter, Finest, Tesco* | 1 Serving/100g | 201.0 | 14.0 | 201 | 16.2 | 1.8 | 14.3 | 0.4 |
| **SCAMPI** | | | | | | | | |
| Breaded, Average | ½ Pack/255g | 565.0 | 27.0 | 222 | 10.7 | 20.5 | 10.7 | 1.0 |
| Wholetail, Premium, Youngs* | 1 Serving/125g | 256.0 | 11.0 | 205 | 29.5 | 21.6 | 9.1 | 2.1 |
| Wholetails, in Crunchy Crumb, Morrisons* | 1 Pack/250g | 507.0 | 22.0 | 203 | 9.6 | 19.9 | 8.7 | 1.7 |
| **SCONE** | | | | | | | | |
| 3% Fat, M & S* | 1 Scone/65g | 179.0 | 2.0 | 275 | 7.2 | 55.1 | 2.5 | 2.3 |
| All Butter, Tesco* | 1 Scone/41g | 126.0 | 3.0 | 308 | 7.2 | 52.3 | 7.8 | 1.6 |
| Cheese, Average | 1 Scone/40g | 145.0 | 7.0 | 363 | 10.1 | 43.2 | 17.8 | 1.6 |
| Cheese, Sainsbury's* | 1 Scone/70g | 250.0 | 13.0 | 357 | 10.6 | 36.9 | 18.6 | 2.0 |
| Cheese & Black Pepper, Mini, M & S* | 1 Scone/18g | 67.0 | 3.0 | 370 | 10.2 | 41.1 | 18.3 | 1.7 |
| Cherry, M & S* | 1 Scone/60g | 202.0 | 7.0 | 337 | 6.9 | 49.7 | 12.2 | 1.9 |
| Cream, Sainsbury's* | 1 Scone/50g | 172.0 | 9.0 | 345 | 4.6 | 42.5 | 17.4 | 3.1 |
| Derby, Asda* | 1 Scone/59g | 202.0 | 6.0 | 342 | 7.0 | 56.0 | 10.0 | 0.0 |
| Derby, Tesco* | 1 Scone/60g | 201.0 | 6.0 | 335 | 7.2 | 53.7 | 10.2 | 2.0 |
| Devon, M & S* | 1 Scone/59g | 225.0 | 10.0 | 380 | 7.1 | 50.8 | 16.2 | 1.5 |
| Devon, Sainsbury's* | 1 Scone/54g | 201.0 | 8.0 | 372 | 7.1 | 51.1 | 15.5 | 1.6 |
| Devon, Waitrose* | 1 Scone/72g | 268.0 | 9.0 | 373 | 7.5 | 56.0 | 13.2 | 2.3 |
| Fresh Cream, Finest, Tesco* | 1 Serving/133g | 469.0 | 23.0 | 354 | 4.6 | 44.5 | 17.5 | 1.7 |
| Fresh Cream, Tesco* | 1 Scone/80g | 242.0 | 10.0 | 304 | 15.8 | 32.3 | 12.5 | 0.9 |
| Fresh Cream, TTD, Sainsbury's* | 1 Serving/110g | 379.0 | 16.0 | 346 | 5.8 | 48.1 | 14.5 | 2.6 |
| Fresh Cream with Strawberry Jam, Tesco* | 1 Scone/83g | 290.0 | 16.0 | 352 | 4.7 | 40.7 | 18.9 | 1.1 |
| Fruit, Average | 1 Scone/40g | 126.0 | 4.0 | 316 | 7.3 | 52.9 | 9.8 | 0.0 |
| Fruit, SmartPrice, Asda* | 1 Scone/41g | 139.0 | 4.0 | 338 | 7.0 | 55.0 | 10.0 | 3.0 |
| Fruit, Waitrose* | 1 Scone/59g | 190.0 | 5.0 | 325 | 6.3 | 56.5 | 8.2 | 2.2 |
| Luxury, Hovis* | 1 Scone/85g | 267.0 | 8.0 | 314 | 5.6 | 51.8 | 9.3 | 2.2 |
| Plain, Average | 1 Scone/40g | 145.0 | 6.0 | 362 | 7.2 | 53.8 | 14.6 | 1.9 |
| Potato, Average | 1 Scone/40g | 118.0 | 6.0 | 296 | 5.1 | 39.1 | 14.3 | 1.6 |
| Strawberry, Fresh Cream, BGTY, Sainsbury's* | 1 Scone/50g | 154.0 | 6.0 | 309 | 5.1 | 47.0 | 11.2 | 1.1 |
| Strawberry, Fresh Cream, Sainsbury's* | 1 Scone/60g | 218.0 | 11.0 | 363 | 6.5 | 42.5 | 18.6 | 1.4 |
| Sultana, BGTY, Sainsbury's* | 1 Scone/63g | 178.0 | 2.0 | 283 | 7.7 | 56.7 | 2.8 | 2.4 |
| Sultana, GFY, Asda* | 1 Scone/59g | 192.0 | 3.0 | 324 | 7.0 | 64.0 | 4.4 | 2.0 |

**S**

| | Measure INFO/WEIGHT | per Measure KCAL | FAT | Nutrition Values per 100g / 100ml KCAL | PROT | CARB | FAT | FIBRE |
|---|---|---|---|---|---|---|---|---|
| **SCONE** | | | | | | | | |
| Sultana, M & S* | 1 Scone/66g | 231.0 | 8.0 | 350 | 6.5 | 53.0 | 12.5 | 2.0 |
| Sultana, Reduced Fat, Waitrose* | 1 Scone/65g | 187.0 | 3.0 | 287 | 6.6 | 53.2 | 5.3 | 2.6 |
| Sultana, Sainsbury's* | 1 Scone/54g | 176.0 | 6.0 | 327 | 6.9 | 50.2 | 11.0 | 6.5 |
| Sultana, Tesco* | 1 Scone/60g | 189.0 | 5.0 | 315 | 7.1 | 52.5 | 8.4 | 2.6 |
| Sultana, Value, Tesco* | 1 Scone/40g | 134.0 | 4.0 | 335 | 6.5 | 53.8 | 10.1 | 2.7 |
| Wholemeal | 1 Scone/40g | 130.0 | 6.0 | 326 | 8.7 | 43.1 | 14.4 | 5.2 |
| Wholemeal, Fruit | 1 Scone/40g | 130.0 | 5.0 | 324 | 8.1 | 47.2 | 12.8 | 4.9 |
| **SCONE MIX** | | | | | | | | |
| Fruit, Asda* | 1 Scone/48g | 143.0 | 2.0 | 301 | 7.0 | 57.0 | 5.0 | 3.7 |
| **SCOTCH EGGS** | | | | | | | | |
| Asda* | 1 Egg/114g | 286.0 | 19.0 | 251 | 11.2 | 13.7 | 16.8 | 1.4 |
| Budgens* | 1 Egg/113g | 294.0 | 20.0 | 260 | 11.4 | 13.8 | 17.6 | 0.0 |
| Finest, Tesco* | 1 Egg/114g | 280.0 | 20.0 | 247 | 11.6 | 10.4 | 17.7 | 1.1 |
| Ginsters* | 1 Egg/95g | 228.0 | 15.0 | 240 | 15.3 | 9.7 | 15.9 | 0.6 |
| Morrisons* | 1 Egg/114g | 286.0 | 19.0 | 251 | 11.2 | 13.7 | 16.8 | 1.4 |
| Retail | 1 Egg/120g | 301.0 | 21.0 | 251 | 12.0 | 13.1 | 17.1 | 0.0 |
| Sainsbury's* | 1 Egg/113g | 311.0 | 22.0 | 275 | 11.1 | 14.2 | 19.3 | 0.9 |
| Savoury, M & S* | 1 Egg/21g | 63.0 | 5.0 | 305 | 11.0 | 15.7 | 21.8 | 1.3 |
| **SEA BASS** | | | | | | | | |
| *Cooked, Dry Heat, Average* | *1 Fillet/101g* | *125.0* | *3.0* | *124* | *23.6* | *0.0* | *2.6* | *0.0* |
| *Raw, Average* | *1oz/28g* | *32.0* | *1.0* | *113* | *20.3* | *0.0* | *3.5* | *0.1* |
| With Roasted Fennel & Orange Butter, TTD, Sainsbury's* | ½ Pack/115g | 238.0 | 17.0 | 207 | 17.0 | 0.6 | 15.2 | 0.8 |
| **SEA BREAM** | | | | | | | | |
| *Fillets, Raw, Average* | *1oz/28g* | *27.0* | *1.0* | *96* | *17.5* | *0.0* | *2.9* | *0.0* |
| **SEAFOOD COCKTAIL** | | | | | | | | |
| Asda* | 1oz/28g | 26.0 | 0.0 | 92 | 14.0 | 5.7 | 1.5 | 0.1 |
| Average | 1oz/28g | 24.0 | 0.0 | 87 | 15.6 | 2.9 | 1.5 | 0.0 |
| Somerfield* | 1oz/28g | 23.0 | 1.0 | 81 | 14.0 | 2.0 | 2.0 | 0.0 |
| **SEAFOOD MEDLEY** | | | | | | | | |
| Sainsbury's* | ½ Pack/175g | 157.0 | 3.0 | 90 | 14.3 | 4.0 | 1.9 | 0.5 |
| Steam Cuisine, M & S* | 1 Pack/400g | 320.0 | 12.0 | 80 | 8.5 | 4.5 | 3.1 | 1.3 |
| **SEAFOOD MIX** | | | | | | | | |
| Asda* | 1 Serving/213g | 175.0 | 2.0 | 82 | 12.0 | 6.0 | 1.1 | 0.0 |
| **SEAFOOD SELECTION** | | | | | | | | |
| Fresh, Tesco* | 1 Pack/234g | 187.0 | 2.0 | 80 | 17.7 | 0.1 | 1.0 | 0.0 |
| Luxury, Safeway* | 1 Pack/250g | 215.0 | 5.0 | 86 | 13.8 | 3.1 | 2.0 | 0.0 |
| M & S* | 1 Serving/200g | 170.0 | 2.0 | 85 | 17.4 | 1.6 | 1.0 | 0.5 |
| Sainsbury's* | ½ Pack/125g | 85.0 | 1.0 | 68 | 14.6 | 0.8 | 1.0 | 2.5 |
| Somerfield* | 1 Serving/200g | 170.0 | 3.0 | 85 | 15.9 | 1.7 | 1.6 | 0.4 |
| **SEAFOOD STICKS** | | | | | | | | |
| Average | 1 Stick/15g | 16.0 | 0.0 | 106 | 8.0 | 18.4 | 0.2 | 0.2 |
| Low Price, Sainsbury's* | 1 Stick/16g | 16.0 | 0.0 | 101 | 7.3 | 16.0 | 0.9 | 0.6 |
| with Cocktail Dip, Asda* | 1 Pot/95g | 126.0 | 5.0 | 133 | 6.0 | 16.0 | 5.0 | 0.1 |
| **SEASONING** | | | | | | | | |
| Aromat, Knorr* | 1oz/28g | 46.0 | 1.0 | 164 | 12.4 | 20.5 | 3.6 | 1.0 |
| Sushi, Mitsukan* | 2 Tbsp/30ml | 50.0 | 1.0 | 167 | 0.0 | 36.7 | 3.3 | 0.0 |
| **SEASONING CUBES** | | | | | | | | |
| for Potato, Mint, Perfect Potato, Knorr* | 1 Cube/10g | 56.0 | 5.0 | 560 | 5.1 | 21.2 | 50.5 | 1.8 |
| for Rice, Pilau, Knorr* | 1 Cube/10g | 30.0 | 2.0 | 305 | 11.4 | 13.9 | 22.6 | 1.4 |
| for Rice, Saffron, Knorr* | 1 Cube/10g | 29.0 | 2.0 | 291 | 13.8 | 17.5 | 18.4 | 2.2 |
| for Stir Fry, Oriental Spices, Knorr* | 1 Cube/10g | 41.0 | 3.0 | 414 | 9.7 | 25.0 | 30.6 | 1.1 |
| Oriental Spice, Knorr* | 1 Cube/10g | 41.0 | 3.0 | 409 | 9.5 | 23.7 | 30.7 | 0.0 |
| Perfect Pasta, Knorr* | 1 Cube/10g | 28.0 | 2.0 | 278 | 10.3 | 5.2 | 24.0 | 0.0 |

**S**

| | Measure INFO/WEIGHT | per Measure KCAL | FAT | KCAL | PROT | CARB | FAT | FIBRE |
|---|---|---|---|---|---|---|---|---|
| **SEASONING CUBES** | | | | | | | | |
| Wild Mushroom, Knorr* | 1 Cube/10g | 36.0 | 3.0 | 365 | 10.3 | 21.3 | 26.5 | 0.2 |
| **SEASONING MIX** | | | | | | | | |
| Balti, Aromatic, Schwartz* | 1 Serving/10g | 34.0 | 1.0 | 340 | 13.7 | 56.6 | 6.8 | 0.0 |
| Beef Taco, Colman's* | 1 Pack/30g | 76.0 | 4.0 | 252 | 9.1 | 26.9 | 12.0 | 14.0 |
| Cajun, Sizzle & Grill, Schwartz* | 1 Tsp/4g | 7.0 | 0.0 | 182 | 9.8 | 23.0 | 5.6 | 24.4 |
| Chicken, Chargrilled, Grill & Sizzle, Schwartz* | 1 Tsp/5g | 12.0 | 0.0 | 232 | 8.2 | 40.8 | 4.0 | 13.1 |
| Chicken Fajitas, Schwartz* | 1 Pack/35g | 99.0 | 1.0 | 283 | 10.9 | 54.1 | 2.5 | 10.8 |
| Chilli, Old El Paso* | 1 Pack/39g | 117.0 | 2.0 | 301 | 7.0 | 57.0 | 5.0 | 0.0 |
| Fajita, Chicken, Colman's* | 1 Pack/40g | 138.0 | 3.0 | 344 | 9.4 | 62.5 | 6.3 | 4.8 |
| Fish, Schwartz* | 1 Tsp/4g | 9.0 | 0.0 | 222 | 6.5 | 55.5 | 2.3 | 11.6 |
| Italian Herb, Schwartz* | 1 Tsp/1g | 3.0 | 0.0 | 338 | 11.0 | 64.5 | 4.0 | 0.0 |
| Mediterranean Roasted Vegetable, Schwartz* | 1 Pack/30g | 86.0 | 1.0 | 288 | 6.9 | 56.1 | 4.0 | 10.3 |
| Moroccan Spiced Vegetables, Schwartz* | 1 Pack/40g | 99.0 | 2.0 | 247 | 12.2 | 38.4 | 4.9 | 22.0 |
| Potato Roasties, Rosemary & Garlic, Crispy, Schwartz* | 1 Pack/33g | 88.0 | 3.0 | 267 | 13.0 | 36.1 | 7.8 | 21.1 |
| Potato Roasties, Southern Fried, Crispy, Schwartz* | 1 Pack/35g | 78.0 | 2.0 | 222 | 9.2 | 36.2 | 4.4 | 25.1 |
| Potato Wedges, Cajun, Schwartz* | 1 Pack/38g | 112.0 | 3.0 | 295 | 9.1 | 47.6 | 7.6 | 14.3 |
| Potato Wedges, Garlic & Herb, Schwartz* | 1 Pack/38g | 106.0 | 2.0 | 278 | 11.4 | 47.1 | 4.9 | 11.7 |
| Potato Wedges, Nacho Cheese, Schwartz* | 1 Pack/38g | 114.0 | 4.0 | 299 | 13.6 | 39.3 | 9.7 | 7.7 |
| Potato Wedges, Onion & Chive, Schwartz* | 1 Pack/38g | 113.0 | 1.0 | 297 | 10.9 | 59.4 | 1.8 | 6.5 |
| Season-All, Schwartz* | 1 Tsp/6g | 4.0 | 0.0 | 72 | 2.3 | 11.6 | 1.8 | 0.0 |
| Shepherd's Pie, Colman's* | 1 Pack/50g | 141.0 | 1.0 | 282 | 12.5 | 54.7 | 1.4 | 4.3 |
| Shotz, Cajun Chicken Seasoning, Schwartz* | 1 Pack/3g | 8.0 | 0.0 | 268 | 9.9 | 45.6 | 5.2 | 0.0 |
| Shotz, Chargrilled Chicken Seasoning, Schwartz* | 1 Pack/3g | 8.0 | 0.0 | 283 | 7.5 | 52.0 | 4.9 | 0.0 |
| Shotz, Garlic Pepper Steak Seasoning, Schwartz* | 1 Pack/3g | 11.0 | 0.0 | 370 | 14.0 | 67.0 | 5.0 | 0.0 |
| Shotz, Moroccan Chicken Seasoning, Schwartz* | 1 Pack/3g | 9.0 | 0.0 | 312 | 9.7 | 56.7 | 5.2 | 0.0 |
| Shotz, Seven Pepper Steak Seasoning, Schwartz* | 1 Pack/3g | 7.0 | 0.0 | 246 | 8.2 | 47.8 | 2.4 | 0.0 |
| Spanish Roasted Vegetables, Schwartz* | 1 Pack/15g | 22.0 | 1.0 | 147 | 9.1 | 14.1 | 6.0 | 22.6 |
| Taco, Old El Paso* | ¼ Pack/9g | 30.0 | 0.0 | 334 | 5.5 | 69.0 | 4.0 | 0.0 |
| **SEAWEED** | | | | | | | | |
| *Crispy, Average* | *1oz/28g* | *182.0* | *17.0* | *651* | *7.5* | *15.6* | *61.9* | *7.0* |
| *Irish Moss, Raw* | *1oz/28g* | *2.0* | *0.0* | *8* | *1.5* | *0.0* | *0.2* | *12.3* |
| *Kombu, Dried, Raw* | *1oz/28g* | *12.0* | *0.0* | *43* | *7.1* | *0.0* | *1.6* | *58.7* |
| *Nori, Dried, Raw* | *1oz/28g* | *38.0* | *0.0* | *136* | *30.7* | *0.0* | *1.5* | *44.4* |
| *Wakame, Dried, Raw* | *1oz/28g* | *20.0* | *1.0* | *71* | *12.4* | *0.0* | *2.4* | *47.1* |
| **SEED MIX** | | | | | | | | |
| Cajun, Graze* | 1 Sm Pack/43g | 246.0 | 21.0 | 573 | 26.5 | 18.1 | 49.0 | 11.5 |
| Chilli, Graze* | 1 Pack/25g | 151.0 | 12.0 | 606 | 30.4 | 6.1 | 47.2 | 5.2 |
| Granola, Graze* | 1 Pack/25g | 122.0 | 7.0 | 490 | 12.0 | 43.7 | 29.7 | 0.0 |
| Naked, Graze* | 1 Pack/25g | 151.0 | 13.0 | 604 | 11.9 | 26.3 | 50.1 | 0.0 |
| Omega, Graze* | 1 Pack/25g | 153.0 | 12.0 | 613 | 28.4 | 13.1 | 49.7 | 0.0 |
| Omega, Morrisons* | ¼ Pack/25g | 138.0 | 11.0 | 554 | 20.9 | 15.0 | 45.6 | 6.4 |
| Omega, Munchy Seeds* | 1 Bag/30g | 184.0 | 15.0 | 613 | 28.4 | 13.1 | 49.7 | 2.2 |
| Original, The Food Doctor* | 1 Serving/30g | 157.0 | 13.0 | 522 | 28.2 | 3.7 | 44.4 | 17.7 |
| Roasted, Graze* | 1 Pack/25g | 160.0 | 13.0 | 640 | 27.1 | 4.8 | 51.5 | 0.0 |
| Salad Sprinkle, Nature's Harvest* | 1 Serving/8g | 48.0 | 4.0 | 598 | 20.0 | 14.6 | 51.1 | 4.9 |
| Toasted, Asda* | 1 Serving/28g | 132.0 | 9.0 | 470 | 34.4 | 10.6 | 32.2 | 11.6 |
| **SEEDS** | | | | | | | | |
| *Fenugreek, Average* | *1 Tsp/4g* | *12.0* | *0.0* | *323* | *23.0* | *58.3* | *6.4* | *24.6* |
| *Melon, Average* | *1 Tbsp/15g* | *87.0* | *7.0* | *583* | *28.5* | *9.9* | *47.7* | *0.0* |
| *Mustard, Average* | *1 Tsp/3g* | *15.0* | *1.0* | *469* | *34.9* | *34.9* | *28.8* | *14.7* |
| *Nigella, Average* | *1oz/28g* | *110.0* | *9.0* | *392* | *21.3* | *1.9* | *33.3* | *8.4* |
| *Poppy, Average* | *1 Tbsp/9g* | *47.0* | *4.0* | *533* | *18.0* | *23.7* | *44.7* | *10.0* |
| *Pumpkin, Average* | *1 Tbsp/10g* | *57.0* | *5.0* | *568* | *27.9* | *13.0* | *45.9* | *3.8* |

**S**

| | Measure<br>INFO/WEIGHT | per Measure<br>KCAL | FAT | Nutrition Values per 100g / 100ml<br>KCAL | PROT | CARB | FAT | FIBRE |
|---|---|---|---|---|---|---|---|---|
| **SEEDS** | | | | | | | | |
| *Pumpkin, Whole, Roasted, Salted, Average* | *1 Serving/50g* | *261.0* | *21.0* | *522* | *33.0* | *13.4* | *42.1* | *3.9* |
| *Sesame, Average* | *1oz/28g* | *171.0* | *16.0* | *610* | *22.3* | *3.6* | *56.4* | *7.7* |
| Sesame, Tesco* | 1 Tsp/4g | 24.0 | 2.0 | 598 | 18.2 | 0.9 | 58.0 | 7.9 |
| *Sunflower, Average* | *1 Tbsp/10g* | *59.0* | *5.0* | *585* | *23.4* | *15.0* | *48.7* | *5.7* |
| **SEMOLINA** | | | | | | | | |
| *Average* | *1oz/28g* | *98.0* | *1.0* | *348* | *11.0* | *75.2* | *1.8* | *2.1* |
| Pudding, Creamed, Ambrosia* | 1 Can/425g | 344.0 | 7.0 | 81 | 3.3 | 13.1 | 1.7 | 0.2 |
| Pudding, Creamed, Co-Op* | 1 Can/425g | 382.0 | 8.0 | 90 | 4.0 | 15.0 | 2.0 | 0.0 |
| **SHALLOTS** | | | | | | | | |
| Pickled, in Hot & Spicy Vinegar, Tesco* | 1 Onion/18g | 14.0 | 0.0 | 77 | 1.0 | 18.0 | 0.1 | 1.9 |
| *Raw, Average* | *1 Serving/80g* | *16.0* | *0.0* | *20* | *1.5* | *3.3* | *0.2* | *1.4* |
| **SHANDY** | | | | | | | | |
| Bitter, Original, Ben Shaws* | 1 Can/330ml | 89.0 | 0.0 | 27 | 0.0 | 6.0 | 0.0 | 0.0 |
| Homemade, Average | 1 Pint/568ml | 148.0 | 0.0 | 26 | 0.2 | 2.9 | 0.0 | 0.0 |
| Lemonade, Schweppes* | 1 Can/330ml | 76.0 | 0.0 | 23 | 0.0 | 5.1 | 0.0 | 0.0 |
| Lemonade, Traditional Style, Tesco* | 1 Can/330ml | 63.0 | 0.0 | 19 | 0.0 | 4.7 | 0.0 | 0.0 |
| **SHARK** | | | | | | | | |
| *Raw* | *1oz/28g* | *29.0* | *0.0* | *102* | *23.0* | *0.0* | *1.1* | *0.0* |
| **SHARON FRUIT** | | | | | | | | |
| *Average* | *1oz/28g* | *20.0* | *0.0* | *73* | *0.8* | *18.6* | *0.0* | *1.6* |
| **SHERBET LEMONS** | | | | | | | | |
| M & S* | 1oz/28g | 107.0 | 0.0 | 382 | 0.0 | 93.9 | 0.0 | 0.0 |
| **SHERRY** | | | | | | | | |
| *Dry, Average* | *1 Std Glass/120ml* | *139.0* | *0.0* | *116* | *0.2* | *1.4* | *0.0* | *0.0* |
| *Medium* | *1 Serving/50ml* | *58.0* | *0.0* | *116* | *0.1* | *5.9* | *0.0* | *0.0* |
| *Sweet* | *1 Serving/50ml* | *68.0* | *0.0* | *136* | *0.3* | *6.9* | *0.0* | *0.0* |
| **SHORTBREAD** | | | | | | | | |
| All Butter, Deans* | 1 Biscuit/15g | 77.0 | 4.0 | 511 | 4.9 | 65.7 | 25.4 | 1.2 |
| All Butter, Petticoat Tails, Co-Op* | 1 Biscuit/13g | 68.0 | 4.0 | 520 | 5.0 | 60.0 | 29.0 | 2.0 |
| All Butter, Petticoat Tails, Gardiners of Scotland* | 1 Biscuit/12g | 64.0 | 3.0 | 514 | 5.2 | 62.1 | 27.2 | 0.0 |
| All Butter, Round, Luxury, M & S* | 1 Biscuit/20g | 105.0 | 6.0 | 525 | 6.2 | 60.0 | 29.0 | 2.0 |
| All Butter, Royal Edinburgh, Asda* | 1 Biscuit/18g | 93.0 | 5.0 | 519 | 5.8 | 60.3 | 28.3 | 1.8 |
| All Butter, Thins, M & S* | 1 Biscuit/10g | 50.0 | 2.0 | 485 | 5.8 | 68.4 | 21.1 | 3.5 |
| Assortment, Parkside* | 1 Serving/30g | 155.0 | 9.0 | 517 | 5.4 | 59.8 | 28.5 | 2.0 |
| Average | 1oz/28g | 139.0 | 7.0 | 498 | 5.9 | 63.9 | 26.1 | 1.9 |
| Belgian Chocolate Chunk, Asda* | 1 Biscuit/20g | 106.0 | 6.0 | 531 | 7.0 | 56.0 | 31.0 | 1.8 |
| Choc Chip, Fair Trade, Co-Op* | 1 Biscuit/19g | 100.0 | 6.0 | 526 | 5.3 | 57.9 | 31.6 | 2.6 |
| Chocolate Chip, Jacob's* | 1 Biscuit/17g | 87.0 | 5.0 | 513 | 5.2 | 61.2 | 27.5 | 1.8 |
| Clotted Cream, Finest, Tesco* | 1 Biscuit/20g | 109.0 | 6.0 | 543 | 5.2 | 58.0 | 32.2 | 1.7 |
| Crawfords* | 1 Biscuit/13g | 67.0 | 3.0 | 533 | 6.6 | 65.0 | 27.4 | 2.0 |
| Dutch, M & S* | 1 Biscuit/17g | 90.0 | 5.0 | 530 | 5.7 | 58.2 | 30.6 | 0.9 |
| Farmhouse, TTD, Sainsbury's* | 1 Finger/20g | 106.0 | 6.0 | 528 | 5.1 | 61.6 | 29.0 | 1.7 |
| Fingers, All Butter, Co-Op* | 1 Finger/16g | 85.0 | 5.0 | 520 | 6.0 | 58.0 | 30.0 | 2.0 |
| Fingers, All Butter, McVitie's* | 1 Finger/20g | 106.0 | 5.0 | 530 | 6.5 | 64.7 | 27.2 | 0.0 |
| Fingers, All Butter, Scottish, M & S* | 1 Finger/18g | 90.0 | 5.0 | 510 | 5.7 | 58.9 | 27.8 | 4.7 |
| Fingers, All Butter, Tesco* | 1 Finger/13g | 67.0 | 4.0 | 519 | 5.8 | 60.3 | 28.3 | 1.8 |
| Fingers, All Butter, Traditional, Scottish, Tesco* | 1 Finger/18g | 93.0 | 5.0 | 520 | 6.0 | 58.5 | 29.1 | 1.8 |
| Fingers, Asda* | 1 Finger/18g | 93.0 | 5.0 | 519 | 5.8 | 60.3 | 28.3 | 18.0 |
| Fingers, Deans* | 1 Finger/24g | 115.0 | 6.0 | 488 | 5.1 | 60.1 | 24.8 | 1.4 |
| Fingers, Light & Buttery, TTD, Sainsbury's* | 1 Finger/20g | 105.0 | 6.0 | 528 | 5.1 | 61.6 | 29.0 | 0.7 |
| Free From, Sainsbury's* | 1 Biscuit/20g | 98.0 | 5.0 | 490 | 6.0 | 58.0 | 26.0 | 6.0 |
| Hearts, with Milk Chocolate, M & S* | 1 Biscuit/25g | 125.0 | 6.0 | 500 | 7.2 | 59.5 | 25.8 | 3.0 |
| Highland, Organic, Duchy Originals* | 1 Biscuit/16g | 80.0 | 4.0 | 515 | 5.2 | 61.8 | 27.4 | 1.7 |

| | Measure INFO/WEIGHT | per Measure KCAL | per Measure FAT | Nutrition Values per 100g / 100ml KCAL | PROT | CARB | FAT | FIBRE |
|---|---|---|---|---|---|---|---|---|
| **SHORTBREAD** | | | | | | | | |
| Highland, Petticoat Tails, Sainsbury's* | 1 Biscuit/13g | 65.0 | 3.0 | 518 | 5.7 | 60.8 | 28.0 | 1.8 |
| Highland Demerara Rounds, Sainsbury's* | 1 Biscuit/20g | 113.0 | 6.0 | 565 | 5.5 | 70.5 | 29.0 | 2.0 |
| Honey & Oatmeal, Walkers* | 1 Biscuit/34g | 158.0 | 8.0 | 465 | 6.7 | 64.1 | 22.4 | 3.8 |
| Mini Bites, Co-Op* | 1 Biscuit/10g | 53.0 | 3.0 | 530 | 7.0 | 59.0 | 30.0 | 2.0 |
| Mini Bites, Country Table* | 1 Biscuit/10g | 52.0 | 3.0 | 525 | 7.1 | 59.3 | 29.5 | 1.5 |
| Orange Marmalade & Oatflake, Deans* | 1 Biscuit/20g | 105.0 | 6.0 | 524 | 6.7 | 59.3 | 29.6 | 3.2 |
| Organic, Waitrose* | 1 Biscuit/13g | 62.0 | 3.0 | 495 | 5.8 | 63.0 | 24.4 | 1.8 |
| Pecan All Butter, Sainsbury's* | 1 Biscuit/18g | 99.0 | 7.0 | 548 | 5.3 | 49.9 | 36.3 | 2.5 |
| Pure Butter, Jacob's* | 1 Biscuit/20g | 105.0 | 6.0 | 525 | 5.7 | 58.6 | 29.7 | 1.8 |
| Raspberry & Oatmeal, Deans* | 1 Biscuit/20g | 103.0 | 6.0 | 514 | 4.7 | 63.1 | 28.6 | 1.4 |
| Reduced Sugar, Tesco* | 1 Biscuit/17g | 86.0 | 5.0 | 519 | 6.7 | 57.1 | 29.4 | 2.1 |
| Rings, Handbaked, Border* | 1 Biscuit/17g | 86.0 | 5.0 | 520 | 6.2 | 61.2 | 29.5 | 0.0 |
| Rounds, Safeway* | 1 Biscuit/20g | 107.0 | 6.0 | 538 | 5.4 | 59.2 | 31.1 | 1.6 |
| Stem Ginger, Waitrose* | 1 Biscuit/15g | 71.0 | 3.0 | 487 | 4.7 | 66.0 | 22.7 | 1.6 |
| Wheat & Gluten Free, Free From Range, Tesco* | 1 Biscuit/20g | 98.0 | 5.0 | 490 | 6.0 | 58.0 | 26.0 | 6.0 |
| **SHRIMP** | | | | | | | | |
| *Boiled, Average* | *1 Serving/60g* | *70.0* | *1.0* | *117* | *23.8* | *0.0* | *2.4* | *0.0* |
| *Dried, Average* | *1oz/28g* | *69.0* | *1.0* | *245* | *55.8* | *0.0* | *2.4* | *0.0* |
| *Frozen, Average* | *1oz/28g* | *20.0* | *0.0* | *73* | *16.5* | *0.0* | *0.8* | *0.0* |
| *in Brine, Canned, Drained, Average* | *1oz/28g* | *26.0* | *0.0* | *94* | *20.8* | *0.0* | *1.2* | *0.0* |
| **SKATE** | | | | | | | | |
| *Grilled* | *1oz/28g* | *22.0* | *0.0* | *79* | *18.9* | *0.0* | *0.5* | *0.0* |
| in Batter, Fried in Blended Oil | 1oz/28g | 47.0 | 3.0 | 168 | 14.7 | 4.9 | 10.1 | 0.2 |
| *Raw* | *1oz/28g* | *18.0* | *0.0* | *64* | *15.1* | *0.0* | *0.4* | *0.0* |
| **SKIPS** | | | | | | | | |
| Bacon, KP Snacks* | 1 Bag/17g | 81.0 | 4.0 | 474 | 6.5 | 62.1 | 22.2 | 2.3 |
| Cheesy, KP Snacks* | 1 Bag/17g | 89.0 | 5.0 | 524 | 6.2 | 58.5 | 29.5 | 1.0 |
| Pickled Onion, KP Snacks* | 1 Bag/13g | 67.0 | 4.0 | 512 | 3.4 | 56.4 | 30.3 | 1.4 |
| Prawn Cocktail, KP Snacks* | 1 Bag/17g | 89.0 | 5.0 | 523 | 3.1 | 60.6 | 29.9 | 1.4 |
| Tangy Tomato, KP Snacks* | 1 Bag/17g | 88.0 | 5.0 | 517 | 3.2 | 59.6 | 29.5 | 1.2 |
| **SKITTLES** | | | | | | | | |
| Mars* | 1 Pack/55g | 223.0 | 2.0 | 406 | 0.0 | 90.6 | 4.4 | 0.0 |
| **SLICES** | | | | | | | | |
| Bacon & Cheese, Pastry, Tesco* | 1 Slice/165g | 480.0 | 32.0 | 291 | 7.4 | 21.7 | 19.4 | 1.0 |
| Bacon & Cheese, Savoury, Pastry, Somerfield* | 1 Slice/165g | 490.0 | 33.0 | 297 | 7.4 | 21.2 | 20.3 | 1.5 |
| Beef, Minced, Morrisons* | 1 Slice/143g | 457.0 | 30.0 | 320 | 8.8 | 24.6 | 20.7 | 1.0 |
| Beef, Minced Steak & Onion, Tesco* | 1 Slice/150g | 424.0 | 27.0 | 283 | 8.7 | 21.3 | 18.1 | 1.6 |
| Beef, Minced with Onion, Sainsbury's* | 1 Slice/120g | 328.0 | 20.0 | 273 | 6.8 | 24.5 | 16.4 | 1.1 |
| Belgian Chocolate, Weight Watchers* | 1 Slice/30g | 99.0 | 2.0 | 329 | 5.9 | 61.6 | 6.7 | 2.3 |
| Cheddar Cheese & Onion, Ginsters* | 1 Slice/180g | 583.0 | 41.0 | 324 | 7.1 | 22.8 | 22.7 | 1.0 |
| Cheese, Potato & Onion, Pastry, Taste!* | 1 Slice/155g | 501.0 | 30.0 | 323 | 8.6 | 28.1 | 19.6 | 0.0 |
| Cheese & Ham, Pastry, Sainsbury's* | 1 Slice/118g | 352.0 | 23.0 | 298 | 7.8 | 22.5 | 19.7 | 1.8 |
| Cheese & Onion, Pastry, Tesco* | 1 Slice/150g | 502.0 | 37.0 | 335 | 8.0 | 20.1 | 24.7 | 1.4 |
| Chicken, Spicy, Deep Fill, Ginsters* | 1 Slice/180g | 499.0 | 31.0 | 277 | 9.2 | 21.8 | 17.0 | 1.4 |
| Chicken & Ham, Taste!* | 1 Slice/155g | 356.0 | 15.0 | 230 | 10.8 | 24.2 | 9.9 | 0.0 |
| Chicken & Leek, Taste!* | 1 Slice/155g | 406.0 | 19.0 | 262 | 10.1 | 27.6 | 12.3 | 0.0 |
| Chicken & Mushroom, Asda* | 1 Slice/128g | 354.0 | 22.0 | 277 | 7.0 | 24.0 | 17.0 | 2.1 |
| Chicken & Mushroom, Ginsters* | 1 Slice/155g | 420.0 | 27.0 | 271 | 6.6 | 21.8 | 17.5 | 1.7 |
| Chicken & Mushroom, Sainsbury's* | 1 Slice/164g | 427.0 | 27.0 | 259 | 7.3 | 21.3 | 16.1 | 1.0 |
| Chicken & Mushroom, Tesco* | 1 Slice/165g | 457.0 | 29.0 | 277 | 9.2 | 20.6 | 17.5 | 0.9 |
| Custard, Pastry, Tesco* | 1 Slice/108g | 275.0 | 11.0 | 255 | 2.8 | 37.2 | 10.3 | 1.3 |
| Fresh Cream, Tesco* | 1 Slice/75g | 311.0 | 21.0 | 414 | 3.5 | 37.4 | 27.9 | 1.0 |
| Ham & Cheese, Pastry, Ginsters* | 1 Slice/155g | 625.0 | 44.0 | 403 | 9.8 | 31.9 | 28.2 | 4.2 |

**S**

| | Measure INFO/WEIGHT | per Measure KCAL | FAT | Nutrition Values per 100g / 100ml KCAL | PROT | CARB | FAT | FIBRE |
|---|---|---|---|---|---|---|---|---|
| **SLICES** | | | | | | | | |
| Minced Steak & Onion, Sainsbury's* | 1 Slice/165g | 475.0 | 30.0 | 288 | 15.2 | 16.0 | 18.1 | 2.5 |
| Peppered Steak, Asda* | 1 Slice/164g | 483.0 | 31.0 | 295 | 9.0 | 22.0 | 19.0 | 1.2 |
| Prawn & Avocado, Plait, Extra Special, Asda* | 1 Serving/198g | 331.0 | 7.0 | 167 | 11.0 | 23.0 | 3.4 | 1.3 |
| Salmon, & Watercress, Honey Roast, Plait, Asda* | 1 Plait/166g | 421.0 | 17.0 | 254 | 13.0 | 28.0 | 10.0 | 0.4 |
| Spinach & Ricotta, Sainsbury's* | 1 Slice/165g | 500.0 | 35.0 | 303 | 6.5 | 21.1 | 21.4 | 2.9 |
| Steak, Peppered, Deep Fill, Ginsters* | 1 Slice/180g | 513.0 | 36.0 | 285 | 9.4 | 16.1 | 20.1 | 3.1 |
| Steak, Peppered, Ginsters* | 1 Slice/155g | 415.0 | 24.0 | 268 | 9.9 | 21.5 | 15.8 | 1.9 |
| Steak & Onion, Aberdeen Angus, Tesco* | 1 Slice/165g | 444.0 | 28.0 | 269 | 8.7 | 20.7 | 16.8 | 1.3 |
| **SLIMFAST*** | | | | | | | | |
| Meal Bar, Chocolate Crunch, Slim Fast* | 1 Bar/60g | 206.0 | 6.0 | 343 | 23.9 | 42.8 | 9.9 | 7.7 |
| Meal Bar, Fruits of the Forest, Slim Fast* | 1 Bar/60g | 211.0 | 6.0 | 351 | 23.7 | 42.1 | 10.1 | 7.3 |
| Meal Bar, Yoghurt & Muesli, Slim Fast* | 1 Bar/60g | 208.0 | 6.0 | 347 | 23.9 | 42.2 | 10.8 | 7.4 |
| Milk Shake, Banana, Canned, Slim Fast* | 1 Can/325ml | 214.0 | 8.0 | 66 | 4.2 | 10.6 | 2.6 | 4.9 |
| Milk Shake, Chocolate, Powder, Dry, Slim Fast* | 2 Scoops/38g | 136.0 | 3.0 | 363 | 13.9 | 59.0 | 7.5 | 10.9 |
| Milk Shake, Chocolate, Ready to Drink, Slim Fast* | 1 Bottle/325ml | 211.0 | 5.0 | 65 | 4.6 | 8.0 | 1.6 | 1.5 |
| Milk Shake, Peach, Canned, Slim Fast* | 1 Can/325ml | 214.0 | 3.0 | 66 | 4.2 | 10.6 | 0.8 | 1.5 |
| Milk Shake, Summer Strawberry, Ready to Drink, Slim Fast* | 1 Bottle/325ml | 211.0 | 6.0 | 65 | 4.4 | 7.4 | 2.0 | 1.4 |
| Milk Shake, Vanilla, Powder, Dry, Slim Fast* | 2 Scoops/37g | 131.0 | 2.0 | 360 | 13.4 | 60.9 | 6.5 | 11.0 |
| **SMARTIES** | | | | | | | | |
| Biscuits, Nestle* | 1 Biscuit/5g | 26.0 | 1.0 | 519 | 7.7 | 57.6 | 28.6 | 0.0 |
| Giants, Nestle* | 1 Pack/186g | 882.0 | 36.0 | 474 | 4.6 | 70.4 | 19.3 | 0.7 |
| Mini Cones, Nestle* | 1 Serving/44g | 145.0 | 6.0 | 330 | 4.5 | 45.0 | 13.1 | 0.0 |
| Mini Eggs, Nestle* | 1 Lge Bag/112g | 535.0 | 22.0 | 478 | 4.8 | 69.6 | 20.0 | 0.7 |
| Nestle* | 1 Tube/40g | 184.0 | 7.0 | 461 | 4.0 | 73.6 | 16.6 | 0.6 |
| Tree Decoration, Nestle* | 1 Chocolate/18g | 95.0 | 5.0 | 529 | 5.6 | 58.9 | 30.1 | 0.8 |
| **SMIRNOFF*** | | | | | | | | |
| Ice, Smirnoff* | 1 Bottle/275ml | 188.0 | 0.0 | 68 | 1.8 | 12.0 | 0.0 | 0.0 |
| **SMOOTHIE** | | | | | | | | |
| Apple, Grapes & Blackcurrant, PJ Smoothies* | 1 Bottle/250ml | 125.0 | 1.0 | 50 | 0.8 | 11.1 | 0.3 | 0.7 |
| Apple, Kiwi & Lime, SunJuice* | 1 Bottle/250ml | 132.0 | 0.0 | 53 | 0.5 | 13.4 | 0.1 | 0.8 |
| Apple, Strawberry, Cherry & Banana, M & S* | 1 Bottle/250ml | 125.0 | 1.0 | 50 | 0.5 | 11.2 | 0.3 | 0.6 |
| Apricot & Peach, COU, M & S* | 1 Bottle/250ml | 100.0 | 1.0 | 40 | 0.9 | 8.3 | 0.4 | 0.4 |
| Banana, Dairy, Probiotic, Boots* | 1 Bottle/250ml | 147.0 | 1.0 | 59 | 1.6 | 12.0 | 0.5 | 1.0 |
| Banana, Dairy, Tesco* | 1 Bottle/250ml | 165.0 | 1.0 | 66 | 1.6 | 14.0 | 0.4 | 0.4 |
| Banana, M & S* | 1 Bottle/500ml | 400.0 | 2.0 | 80 | 1.8 | 16.8 | 0.4 | 1.2 |
| Banana & Mango, Juice, Calypso* | 1 Carton/200ml | 106.0 | 0.0 | 53 | 0.0 | 12.8 | 0.0 | 1.0 |
| Blackberries & Blueberries, Innocent* | 1 Bottle/250ml | 120.0 | 0.0 | 48 | 0.5 | 12.0 | 0.1 | 2.1 |
| Blackcurrant & Apple, for Kids, Innocent* | 1 Carton/180ml | 112.0 | 0.0 | 62 | 0.4 | 14.5 | 0.2 | 0.8 |
| Blackcurrants & Gooseberries, for Autumn, Innocent* | 1 Bottle/250ml | 117.0 | 0.0 | 47 | 0.5 | 12.5 | 0.1 | 0.0 |
| Blueberry, Blackberry & Strawberry, COU, M & S* | 1 Bottle/250ml | 150.0 | 1.0 | 60 | 0.8 | 13.1 | 0.3 | 0.3 |
| Blueberry & Pear, COU, M & S* | 1 Bottle/250ml | 112.0 | 1.0 | 45 | 0.3 | 10.4 | 0.3 | 0.3 |
| Boysenberry & Raspberry, Fruit, TTD, Sainsbury's* | 1 Bottle/250ml | 107.0 | 0.0 | 43 | 0.7 | 10.0 | 0.1 | 1.6 |
| Cherries & Strawberries, Innocent* | 1 Bottle/250ml | 122.0 | 0.0 | 49 | 0.6 | 12.6 | 0.1 | 0.0 |
| Cranberries & Raspberries, Innocent* | 1 Bottle/250ml | 112.0 | 0.0 | 45 | 0.5 | 12.0 | 0.0 | 2.3 |
| Cranberries & Strawberries, Innocent* | 1 Bottle/250ml | 102.0 | 0.0 | 41 | 0.5 | 9.5 | 0.2 | 0.0 |
| Fruit Kick, Orange, Mango & Pineapple, PJ Smoothies* | 1 Carton/100ml | 54.0 | 0.0 | 54 | 0.6 | 12.2 | 0.0 | 0.0 |
| Ginseng & Ace Vitamins, M & S* | 1 Bottle/250ml | 137.0 | 0.0 | 55 | 0.7 | 13.0 | 0.2 | 0.9 |
| Guavas, Mangoes & Goji Berries, Innocent* | 1 Bottle/250ml | 112.0 | 0.0 | 45 | 0.6 | 12.0 | 0.1 | 2.1 |
| It's Alive, PJ Smoothies* | 1 Bottle/250ml | 150.0 | 1.0 | 60 | 0.7 | 13.6 | 0.3 | 0.0 |
| Kiwi, Apples & Limes, Innocent* | 1 Bottle/250ml | 130.0 | 0.0 | 52 | 0.3 | 11.7 | 0.1 | 1.4 |
| Mango & West Indian Cherry, Plus, Tesco* | 1 Serving/250ml | 133.0 | 1.0 | 53 | 0.6 | 12.2 | 0.2 | 0.5 |
| Mangoes, Coconuts & Lemongrass, Innocent* | 1 Bottle/250ml | 172.0 | 3.0 | 69 | 0.6 | 12.9 | 1.4 | 1.2 |
| Mangoes & Passion Fruits, Pure Fruit, Innocent* | 1 Bottle/250ml | 140.0 | 0.0 | 56 | 0.6 | 14.7 | 0.2 | 2.0 |

S

| | Measure INFO/WEIGHT | per Measure | | Nutrition Values per 100g / 100ml | | | | |
|---|---|---|---|---|---|---|---|---|
| | | KCAL | FAT | KCAL | PROT | CARB | FAT | FIBRE |
| **SMOOTHIE** | | | | | | | | |
| Orange, Banana & Pineapple, Innocent* | 1 Bottle/250ml | 120.0 | 1.0 | 48 | 0.6 | 10.8 | 0.4 | 0.0 |
| Orange, Mandarin & Guava, PJ Smoothies* | 1 Bottle/250ml | 122.0 | 0.0 | 49 | 0.7 | 10.9 | 0.0 | 1.6 |
| Orange & Mango, Fruit, Morrisons* | 1 Bottle/250ml | 145.0 | 0.0 | 58 | 0.5 | 14.0 | 0.0 | 0.7 |
| Orange & Mango, Safeway* | 1 Bottle/250ml | 130.0 | 0.0 | 52 | 0.5 | 12.1 | 0.2 | 0.7 |
| Oranges, Bananas & Pineapples, Innocent* | 1 Bottle/250ml | 142.0 | 0.0 | 57 | 0.6 | 14.1 | 0.1 | 0.0 |
| Passionfruit Lychee, SunJuice* | 1 Bottle/250ml | 145.0 | 0.0 | 58 | 0.5 | 13.5 | 0.2 | 0.8 |
| Peach, Mild & Fruity, Campina* | 1 Bottle/330ml | 211.0 | 0.0 | 64 | 2.7 | 13.1 | 0.0 | 0.0 |
| Pineapple, Banana & Pear, Asda* | 1 Bottle/250ml | 147.0 | 0.0 | 59 | 0.5 | 13.6 | 0.1 | 0.3 |
| Pineapple, Mango & Passionfruit, 100% Fruit, Sainsbury's* | 1 Bottle/250ml | 162.0 | 0.0 | 65 | 0.7 | 15.2 | 0.1 | 1.0 |
| Pineapple, Strawberries & Passion Fruit, PJ Smoothies* | 1 Bottle/330ml | 152.0 | 0.0 | 46 | 0.6 | 10.8 | 0.1 | 1.3 |
| Pineapples, Bananas & Coconuts, Innocent* | 1 Bottle/250ml | 182.0 | 3.0 | 73 | 0.7 | 15.3 | 1.2 | 1.0 |
| Pomegranate, Raspberry & Cranberry, PJ Smoothies* | 1 Bottle/250ml | 132.0 | 0.0 | 53 | 1.1 | 11.6 | 0.2 | 0.0 |
| Pomegranates & Raspberries, Innocent* | 1 Bottle/250ml | 150.0 | 0.0 | 60 | 0.6 | 15.4 | 0.1 | 2.0 |
| Raspberry, Banana & Peach, Sainsbury's* | 1 Bottle/251ml | 138.0 | 0.0 | 55 | 0.8 | 12.8 | 0.1 | 1.5 |
| Raspberry, M & S* | 1 Bottle/250ml | 137.0 | 1.0 | 55 | 1.7 | 12.2 | 0.6 | 1.9 |
| Raspberry & Blueberry, Plus, Tesco* | 1 Serving/100ml | 59.0 | 0.0 | 59 | 2.6 | 11.6 | 0.3 | 0.5 |
| Raspberry & Boysenberry, Shapers, Boots* | 1 Bottle/248ml | 109.0 | 0.0 | 44 | 0.7 | 10.0 | 0.0 | 1.6 |
| Strawberries, Blackberries, Raspberries, Kids, Innocent* | 1 Carton/180ml | 88.0 | 0.0 | 49 | 0.5 | 11.2 | 0.1 | 1.2 |
| Strawberries & Bananas, PJ Smoothies* | 1 Bottle/250ml | 117.0 | 0.0 | 47 | 0.4 | 11.0 | 0.1 | 0.0 |
| Strawberries & Bananas, Pure Fruit, Innocent* | 1 Bottle/250ml | 142.0 | 0.0 | 57 | 0.5 | 14.4 | 0.1 | 1.3 |
| Strawberries & Raspberries, Squeezie, Innocent* | 1 Squeezie/40g | 16.0 | 0.0 | 39 | 0.3 | 8.5 | 0.0 | 2.1 |
| Strawberry, Dairy, Finest, Tesco* | 1 Bottle/250ml | 162.0 | 0.0 | 65 | 2.9 | 13.2 | 0.1 | 0.1 |
| Strawberry, Raspberry, Apple & Banana, PJ Smoothies* | 1 Bottle/250ml | 132.0 | 1.0 | 53 | 0.8 | 11.9 | 0.3 | 0.7 |
| Strawberry, Raspberry & Banana, Waitrose* | 1 Bottle/250ml | 122.0 | 0.0 | 49 | 0.7 | 10.8 | 0.1 | 0.8 |
| Strawberry & Banana, Fruit, Finest, Tesco* | 1 Bottle/250ml | 135.0 | 1.0 | 54 | 0.3 | 12.5 | 0.3 | 0.5 |
| Strawberry & Banana, Juice, Calypso* | 1 Carton/200ml | 100.0 | 0.0 | 50 | 0.0 | 11.9 | 0.0 | 0.0 |
| Strawberry & Cherry, Organic, M & S* | 1 Bottle/250ml | 137.0 | 1.0 | 55 | 0.8 | 12.3 | 0.3 | 0.4 |
| Strawberry & Raspberry, Fruity, Sainsbury's* | 1 Glass/200ml | 106.0 | 0.0 | 53 | 0.6 | 11.9 | 0.0 | 2.4 |
| Strawberry & Raspberry, Rhapsody, M & S* | 1 Glass/200ml | 90.0 | 0.0 | 45 | 0.6 | 9.4 | 0.1 | 0.9 |
| Strawberry & Raspberry, Shapers, Boots* | 1 Bottle/250ml | 122.0 | 0.0 | 49 | 0.3 | 12.0 | 0.2 | 0.6 |
| Strawberry & White Chocolate, M & S* | 1 Bottle/250ml | 100.0 | 2.0 | 40 | 2.5 | 5.5 | 1.0 | 0.1 |
| Strawberry Dairy, Shapers, Boots* | 1 Bottle/250ml | 120.0 | 1.0 | 48 | 1.7 | 9.7 | 0.3 | 0.5 |
| Tangy Apple & Blackcurrant, Sainsbury's* | 1 Bottle/250ml | 160.0 | 0.0 | 64 | 0.5 | 14.6 | 0.0 | 1.5 |
| Vanilla & Honey, Sainsbury's* | 1 Bottle/250ml | 237.0 | 6.0 | 95 | 3.2 | 14.8 | 2.4 | 0.3 |
| Vanilla Bean, M & S* | 1 Bottle/500ml | 450.0 | 13.0 | 90 | 3.3 | 13.9 | 2.6 | 0.0 |
| Yoghurt, Vanilla Bean & Honey, Thickie, Innocent* | 1 Bottle/250g | 235.0 | 6.0 | 94 | 3.5 | 14.5 | 2.6 | 0.0 |
| **SMOOTHIE MIX** | | | | | | | | |
| Strawberry & Banana, Asda* | 1 Tbsp/20g | 9.0 | 0.0 | 46 | 0.7 | 10.4 | 0.2 | 1.7 |
| **SNACK MIX** | | | | | | | | |
| Bowl, Bombay, Tesco* | ¼ Bowl/131g | 626.0 | 35.0 | 477 | 19.5 | 40.0 | 26.6 | 3.6 |
| Bowl, Oriental Style, Tesco* | ¼ Bowl/80g | 298.0 | 1.0 | 373 | 7.2 | 84.2 | 0.8 | 1.0 |
| Roasted, Organic, Clearspring* | 1 Bag/60g | 271.0 | 17.0 | 451 | 37.5 | 11.1 | 28.5 | 14.4 |
| **SNACK PACK** | | | | | | | | |
| Cheesestring & Ham Wrap, Attack-A-Snack, Golden Vale* | 1 Pack/100g | 240.0 | 9.0 | 240 | 15.0 | 23.0 | 9.0 | 1.3 |
| Philadelphia, Light, with Italian Breadsticks, Kraft* | 1 Pack/50g | 117.0 | 6.0 | 235 | 8.8 | 23.5 | 11.5 | 2.0 |
| **SNACK POT** | | | | | | | | |
| Chicken & Sweetcorn Noodles, Morrisons* | 1 Pot/247g | 249.0 | 1.0 | 101 | 4.1 | 19.8 | 0.6 | 1.6 |
| Potato & Vegetable, Quick Snack, Made Up, Tru Free* | 1 Pack/246g | 236.0 | 7.0 | 96 | 1.0 | 15.0 | 3.0 | 1.0 |
| Potato & Vegetable, Wheat & Gluten Free, Trufree* | 1 Pot/245g | 225.0 | 9.0 | 92 | 1.3 | 13.8 | 3.5 | 1.1 |
| Rice & Lentil, Quick Snack, Made Up, Tru Free* | 1 Pack/270g | 291.0 | 5.0 | 108 | 3.0 | 20.4 | 1.8 | 0.6 |
| **SNACK SALAD** | | | | | | | | |
| Prawn, Lime & Chilli, Good Intentions, Somerfield* | 1 Pack/226g | 276.0 | 9.0 | 122 | 4.1 | 17.3 | 4.1 | 1.8 |

**S**

| | Measure INFO/WEIGHT | per Measure KCAL | FAT | Nutrition Values per 100g / 100ml KCAL | PROT | CARB | FAT | FIBRE |
|---|---|---|---|---|---|---|---|---|
| **SNACK STOP** | | | | | | | | |
| Bolognese Style, Big, Made Up, Crosse & Blackwell* | 1 Pot/407g | 403.0 | 4.0 | 99 | 2.8 | 19.5 | 1.1 | 0.0 |
| Cheese & Pepperoni, Made Up, Crosse & Blackwell* | 1 Pot/237g | 237.0 | 10.0 | 100 | 2.9 | 13.3 | 4.1 | 0.0 |
| Chicken & Mushroom Flavour Pasta, Crosse & Blackwell* | 1 Pot/60g | 251.0 | 5.0 | 418 | 10.3 | 74.3 | 8.8 | 0.0 |
| Creamy Cheese Pasta, Made Up, Crosse & Blackwell* | 1 Pot/218g | 251.0 | 6.0 | 115 | 3.0 | 19.2 | 2.9 | 0.0 |
| Creamy Chicken Pasta, Made Up, Crosse & Blackwell* | 1 Pot/247g | 210.0 | 4.0 | 85 | 2.7 | 15.7 | 1.6 | 0.0 |
| Macaroni Cheese, Light, Made Up, Crosse & Blackwell* | 1 Pot/248g | 260.0 | 7.0 | 105 | 3.2 | 16.4 | 3.0 | 0.9 |
| Mushroom Pasta Twirls, Made Up, Crosse & Blackwell* | 1 Pot/248g | 248.0 | 7.0 | 100 | 3.1 | 15.9 | 2.7 | 0.9 |
| Roast Onion & Potato, Made Up, Crosse & Blackwell* | 1 Pot/210g | 210.0 | 8.0 | 100 | 1.7 | 14.4 | 3.7 | 0.0 |
| Roast Parsnip & Potato, Made Up, Crosse & Blackwell* | 1 Pot/210g | 199.0 | 8.0 | 95 | 1.7 | 13.6 | 3.6 | 0.0 |
| Spicy Tomato Pasta, Made Up, Crosse & Blackwell* | 1 Pot/412g | 358.0 | 6.0 | 87 | 2.4 | 15.9 | 1.5 | 0.0 |
| **SNACK-A-JACKS** | | | | | | | | |
| Apple Danish, Jumbo, Quaker* | 1 Cake/10g | 39.0 | 0.0 | 390 | 5.0 | 87.0 | 2.5 | 1.0 |
| Barbecue, Jumbo, Quaker* | 1 Cake/10g | 38.0 | 0.0 | 380 | 8.0 | 83.0 | 2.0 | 1.7 |
| Barbecue, Snack, Quaker* | 1 Bag/30g | 123.0 | 2.0 | 410 | 7.5 | 81.0 | 6.0 | 1.0 |
| Caramel, Jumbo, Quaker* | 1 Cake/13g | 51.0 | 0.0 | 390 | 5.5 | 87.0 | 2.1 | 1.4 |
| Caramel, Snack, Quaker* | 1 Bag/35g | 142.0 | 1.0 | 405 | 6.0 | 88.0 | 3.0 | 0.8 |
| Cheese, Jumbo, Quaker* | 1 Cake/10g | 38.0 | 0.0 | 380 | 8.5 | 81.0 | 2.5 | 1.7 |
| Cheese, Snack, Quaker* | 1 Bag/30g | 124.0 | 2.0 | 415 | 8.5 | 77.0 | 8.0 | 0.9 |
| Cheese & Onion, Snack, Quaker* | 1 Bag/30g | 120.0 | 2.0 | 400 | 6.7 | 77.0 | 7.5 | 1.5 |
| Chocolate & Caramel, Delights, Quaker* | 1 Cake/15g | 62.0 | 1.0 | 415 | 6.0 | 83.0 | 6.0 | 1.6 |
| Chocolate & Orange, Delights, Quaker* | 1 Cake/15g | 59.0 | 1.0 | 394 | 5.5 | 83.0 | 4.5 | 1.0 |
| Chocolate Chip, Delights, Quaker* | 1 Cake/15g | 61.0 | 1.0 | 410 | 6.0 | 81.0 | 7.0 | 1.7 |
| Mini Bites, Mature Cheese & Red Onion, Quaker* | 1 Bag/28g | 116.0 | 3.0 | 415 | 7.5 | 76.0 | 9.0 | 2.0 |
| Mini Bites, Smoked Ham, Quaker* | 1 Bag/28g | 114.0 | 2.0 | 408 | 6.5 | 78.3 | 7.5 | 2.0 |
| Mini Bites, Sour Cream & Sweet Chilli, Quaker* | 1 Bag/28g | 115.0 | 2.0 | 410 | 6.5 | 78.0 | 8.0 | 2.0 |
| Mini Breadsticks, Cheese & Onion, Quaker* | 1 Bag/35g | 145.0 | 3.0 | 414 | 12.9 | 71.1 | 8.9 | 3.7 |
| Prawn Cocktail, Snack, Quaker* | 1 Bag/30g | 123.0 | 2.0 | 410 | 7.0 | 78.0 | 7.5 | 0.8 |
| Roast Chicken, Snack, Quaker* | 1 Bag/30g | 124.0 | 2.0 | 415 | 7.0 | 77.5 | 8.0 | 1.0 |
| Salt & Vinegar, Snack, Quaker* | 1 Bag/30g | 123.0 | 2.0 | 410 | 7.0 | 79.0 | 7.5 | 0.9 |
| Sour Cream & Chive, Snack, Quaker* | 1 Bag/30g | 124.0 | 2.0 | 415 | 8.0 | 79.0 | 7.5 | 1.3 |
| **SNAPPER** | | | | | | | | |
| *Red, Fried in Blended Oil* | *1oz/28g* | *35.0* | *1.0* | *126* | *24.5* | *0.0* | *3.1* | *0.0* |
| *Red, Weighed with Bone, Raw* | *1oz/28g* | *25.0* | *0.0* | *90* | *19.6* | *0.0* | *1.3* | *0.0* |
| **SNICKERS** | | | | | | | | |
| Cruncher, Mars* | 1 Bar/40g | 209.0 | 12.0 | 523 | 9.0 | 57.0 | 30.0 | 2.3 |
| Mars* | 1 Std Bar/63g | 313.0 | 18.0 | 501 | 9.3 | 52.9 | 28.1 | 0.0 |
| **SORBET** | | | | | | | | |
| Blackcurrant, Iceland* | ¼ Pot/100g | 100.0 | 0.0 | 100 | 0.0 | 25.0 | 0.0 | 0.0 |
| Exotic Fruit, Sainsbury's* | 1 Serving/75g | 90.0 | 1.0 | 120 | 1.2 | 24.1 | 2.0 | 0.0 |
| Jamaican Me Crazy, Ben & Jerry's* | 1 Serving/100g | 130.0 | 0.0 | 130 | 0.2 | 32.0 | 0.0 | 0.4 |
| Lemon, Asda* | 1 Serving/100g | 120.0 | 0.0 | 120 | 0.0 | 30.0 | 0.0 | 0.0 |
| Lemon, Del Monte* | 1 Sorbet/500g | 570.0 | 0.0 | 114 | 0.1 | 29.2 | 0.1 | 0.0 |
| Lemon, Sainsbury's* | ¼ Pot/89g | 100.0 | 0.0 | 112 | 0.0 | 28.1 | 0.0 | 0.1 |
| Lemon, Sticks, Haagen-Dazs* | 1oz/28g | 67.0 | 3.0 | 238 | 1.5 | 32.5 | 11.3 | 0.0 |
| Lemon, Tesco* | 1 Serving/75g | 79.0 | 0.0 | 106 | 0.0 | 26.2 | 0.0 | 0.4 |
| Lemon, The Real Ice Company* | 1 Serving/100g | 117.0 | 0.0 | 117 | 0.1 | 29.1 | 0.1 | 0.4 |
| Lemon, Zesty, Haagen-Dazs* | 1 Serving/125ml | 120.0 | 0.0 | 96 | 0.0 | 24.8 | 0.0 | 1.0 |
| Mango, Del Monte* | 1 Sorbet/500g | 575.0 | 0.0 | 115 | 0.2 | 29.6 | 0.1 | 0.0 |
| Mango, Organic, M & S* | 1 Serving/100g | 99.0 | 0.0 | 99 | 0.3 | 24.1 | 0.1 | 0.9 |
| Mango, Tesco* | 1 Serving/100g | 107.0 | 0.0 | 107 | 0.1 | 26.5 | 0.0 | 0.3 |
| Mango, Tropicale, Haagen-Dazs* | 1oz/28g | 32.0 | 0.0 | 116 | 0.2 | 28.6 | 0.1 | 0.0 |
| Mango, Waitrose* | 1 Pot/100g | 90.0 | 0.0 | 90 | 0.1 | 22.1 | 0.0 | 0.6 |
| Mango Berry Swirl, Ben & Jerry's* | 1 Serving/100g | 100.0 | 0.0 | 100 | 0.2 | 25.0 | 0.0 | 1.5 |

S

| | Measure INFO/WEIGHT | per Measure KCAL | FAT | Nutrition Values per 100g / 100ml KCAL | PROT | CARB | FAT | FIBRE |
|---|---|---|---|---|---|---|---|---|

## SORBET

| | Measure INFO/WEIGHT | KCAL | FAT | KCAL | PROT | CARB | FAT | FIBRE |
|---|---|---|---|---|---|---|---|---|
| Mango Lemon, Fruit Ice, BGTY, Sainsbury's* | 1 Lolly/72g | 84.0 | 0.0 | 116 | 0.3 | 28.1 | 0.3 | 0.5 |
| Orange, Del Monte* | 1 Sorbet/500g | 625.0 | 0.0 | 125 | 0.2 | 32.1 | 0.1 | 0.0 |
| Passion Fruit, Fat Free, M & S* | 1 Sorbet/125g | 129.0 | 0.0 | 103 | 0.4 | 25.0 | 0.0 | 0.4 |
| Peach & Strawberry, Haagen-Dazs* | 1oz/28g | 30.0 | 0.0 | 108 | 0.0 | 27.0 | 0.0 | 0.0 |
| Peach & Vanilla Fruit Swirl, HL, Tesco* | 1 Pot/73g | 93.0 | 1.0 | 127 | 1.1 | 28.9 | 0.8 | 0.5 |
| Pear, Organic, Evernat* | 1oz/28g | 33.0 | 0.0 | 119 | 0.0 | 28.3 | 0.6 | 0.0 |
| Pineapple, Del Monte* | 1 Sorbet/500g | 600.0 | 0.0 | 120 | 0.3 | 30.6 | 0.1 | 0.0 |
| Raspberry, Haagen-Dazs* | ½ Cup/105g | 120.0 | 0.0 | 114 | 0.0 | 28.6 | 0.0 | 1.9 |
| Raspberry, Sticks, Haagen-Dazs* | 1oz/28g | 28.0 | 0.0 | 99 | 0.2 | 24.2 | 0.1 | 0.0 |
| Raspberry, Tesco* | 1 Serving/70ml | 97.0 | 0.0 | 138 | 0.5 | 34.0 | 0.0 | 0.0 |
| Raspberry, Waitrose* | 1 Pot/750ml | 690.0 | 1.0 | 92 | 0.5 | 22.2 | 0.1 | 1.1 |
| Raspberry & Blackberry, Fat Free, M & S* | 1 Sorbet/125g | 140.0 | 0.0 | 112 | 0.4 | 27.5 | 0.0 | 0.6 |
| Strawberry, M & S* | 1oz/28g | 27.0 | 0.0 | 95 | 0.3 | 23.4 | 0.1 | 0.5 |
| Strawberry & Champagne, Sainsbury's* | ¼ Pot/89g | 95.0 | 0.0 | 107 | 0.2 | 25.5 | 0.0 | 0.6 |
| Summer Berry, Swirl, Asda* | ¼ Pack/89g | 97.0 | 0.0 | 109 | 3.0 | 26.0 | 0.4 | 0.0 |

## SOUFFLE

| | Measure INFO/WEIGHT | KCAL | FAT | KCAL | PROT | CARB | FAT | FIBRE |
|---|---|---|---|---|---|---|---|---|
| Cheese | 1oz/28g | 71.0 | 5.0 | 253 | 11.4 | 9.3 | 19.2 | 0.3 |
| Cheese, Mini, Waitrose* | 1 Souffle/14g | 32.0 | 2.0 | 232 | 16.0 | 2.9 | 17.4 | 2.4 |
| Chocolate, Gu* | 1 Pot/70g | 307.0 | 25.0 | 439 | 6.3 | 24.4 | 35.6 | 2.9 |
| Chocolate & Toffee, Gu* | 1 Pot/95g | 353.0 | 16.0 | 372 | 4.6 | 46.4 | 16.6 | 2.5 |
| Lemon, Finest, Tesco* | 1 Pot/80g | 270.0 | 20.0 | 338 | 2.9 | 24.1 | 25.6 | 0.2 |
| Plain | 1oz/28g | 56.0 | 4.0 | 201 | 7.6 | 10.4 | 14.7 | 0.3 |
| Raspberry & Amaretto, M & S* | 1oz/28g | 83.0 | 5.0 | 298 | 2.8 | 33.1 | 16.7 | 0.1 |
| Ricotta & Spinach, M & S* | 1 Serving/120g | 186.0 | 13.0 | 155 | 8.0 | 6.2 | 11.1 | 2.1 |
| Strawberry, M & S* | 1 Serving/95g | 171.0 | 10.0 | 180 | 1.6 | 19.5 | 10.6 | 0.9 |

## SOUP

| | Measure INFO/WEIGHT | KCAL | FAT | KCAL | PROT | CARB | FAT | FIBRE |
|---|---|---|---|---|---|---|---|---|
| Asparagus, Batchelors* | 1 Serving/223g | 143.0 | 6.0 | 64 | 0.5 | 9.2 | 2.8 | 0.4 |
| Asparagus, Fresh, Finest, Tesco* | ½ Pot/300g | 153.0 | 8.0 | 51 | 1.6 | 5.0 | 2.7 | 1.0 |
| Asparagus, Fresh, M & S* | 1 Serving/300g | 135.0 | 11.0 | 45 | 1.1 | 2.5 | 3.6 | 0.9 |
| Asparagus, Hi Taste Low Cal, Cup Soup, Ainsley Harriott* | 1 Sachet/22g | 36.0 | 1.0 | 164 | 2.3 | 29.1 | 4.1 | 2.3 |
| Asparagus, M & S* | 1 Serving/300g | 180.0 | 13.0 | 60 | 1.1 | 3.3 | 4.5 | 0.7 |
| Asparagus, New Covent Garden Food Co* | ½ Carton/300g | 132.0 | 7.0 | 44 | 1.5 | 4.1 | 2.4 | 0.9 |
| Asparagus, Simmer & Serve, Dried, Sainsbury's* | 1/3 Pack/200ml | 70.0 | 3.0 | 35 | 0.4 | 4.8 | 1.6 | 0.3 |
| Asparagus, Slimline, Cup, Waitrose* | 1 Sachet/204ml | 51.0 | 1.0 | 25 | 0.4 | 4.3 | 0.7 | 0.7 |
| Asparagus, Waitrose* | 1 Serving/300g | 60.0 | 4.0 | 20 | 0.9 | 1.5 | 1.2 | 0.9 |
| Asparagus & Chicken, Waitrose* | 1 Can/415g | 166.0 | 5.0 | 40 | 2.1 | 5.3 | 1.1 | 0.7 |
| Asparagus & Creme Fraiche, Morrisons* | ½ Pot/300g | 186.0 | 12.0 | 62 | 1.3 | 5.4 | 3.9 | 0.5 |
| Autumn Vegetable, Vie, Knorr* | 1 Pack/500ml | 190.0 | 10.0 | 38 | 0.7 | 4.3 | 2.0 | 0.7 |
| Autumn Vegetable & Lentil, Heinz* | 1 Can/400g | 184.0 | 1.0 | 46 | 2.3 | 8.6 | 0.3 | 1.0 |
| Bean, Italian Style, Tesco* | 1 Can/300g | 153.0 | 4.0 | 51 | 2.8 | 7.3 | 1.2 | 1.1 |
| Beef, Mushroom & Red Wine, Farmers Market, Heinz* | 1 Can/515g | 263.0 | 9.0 | 51 | 2.4 | 6.4 | 1.8 | 0.7 |
| Beef, Tripe, In Broth, Flaki, Asda* | 1 Jar/520ml | 192.0 | 6.0 | 37 | 5.9 | 1.3 | 1.2 | 0.0 |
| Beef & Mushroom, Big Soup, Heinz* | 1 Can/515g | 216.0 | 3.0 | 42 | 2.3 | 7.0 | 0.5 | 0.7 |
| Beef & Tomato, Cup a Soup, Batchelors* | 1 Serving/252g | 83.0 | 2.0 | 33 | 0.6 | 6.3 | 0.6 | 0.4 |
| Beef & Tomato, in a Cup, Sainsbury's* | 1 Serving/210ml | 61.0 | 1.0 | 29 | 0.6 | 5.6 | 0.5 | 0.2 |
| Beef & Vegetable, Big Soup, Heinz* | 1 Can/400g | 212.0 | 4.0 | 53 | 3.5 | 7.5 | 1.0 | 0.9 |
| Beef & Vegetable, Chunky, Canned, Sainsbury's* | 1 Can/400g | 188.0 | 3.0 | 47 | 3.2 | 6.7 | 0.8 | 1.3 |
| Beef & Vegetable, Chunky, Meal, Tesco* | 1 Can/400g | 344.0 | 19.0 | 86 | 7.0 | 5.3 | 4.8 | 0.6 |
| Beef & Vegetable, for One, Fresh, Tesco* | 1 Pot/300g | 102.0 | 3.0 | 34 | 2.9 | 3.3 | 1.0 | 1.1 |
| Beef & Vegetable, Fresh, New Covent Garden Food Co* | ½ Carton/300g | 177.0 | 7.0 | 59 | 4.5 | 5.4 | 2.2 | 0.7 |
| Beef & Vegetable, Ten Calorie, Gourmet Cuisine* | 1 Sachet/200g | 10.0 | 0.0 | 5 | 0.3 | 1.0 | 0.0 | 0.1 |
| Beef & Vegetable Broth, Chunky, Canned, M & S* | 1 Can/415g | 166.0 | 3.0 | 40 | 1.9 | 6.4 | 0.8 | 0.6 |
| Beef & Winter Vegetable, Favourites, Baxters* | 1 Can/415g | 195.0 | 5.0 | 47 | 2.3 | 6.9 | 1.1 | 0.4 |

S

| | Measure INFO/WEIGHT | per Measure | | Nutrition Values per 100g / 100ml | | | | |
|---|---|---|---|---|---|---|---|---|
| | | KCAL | FAT | KCAL | PROT | CARB | FAT | FIBRE |

## SOUP

| | Measure INFO/WEIGHT | KCAL | FAT | KCAL | PROT | CARB | FAT | FIBRE |
|---|---|---|---|---|---|---|---|---|
| Beef Broth, Classic, Heinz* | 1 Can/400g | 180.0 | 3.0 | 45 | 2.2 | 7.2 | 0.7 | 0.8 |
| Beef Stew & Dumplings, Taste of Home, Heinz* | 1 Pot/430g | 335.0 | 13.0 | 78 | 3.1 | 9.4 | 3.1 | 0.8 |
| Beijing, Vitasia* | 1 Can/400ml | 168.0 | 4.0 | 42 | 1.1 | 7.2 | 1.0 | 0.0 |
| Big Red Tomato, Heinz* | ½ Can/210g | 63.0 | 1.0 | 30 | 0.5 | 6.4 | 0.4 | 0.0 |
| Blended Autumn Vegetable, Heinz* | ½ Can/200g | 114.0 | 6.0 | 57 | 1.2 | 6.4 | 3.0 | 0.7 |
| Blended Leek & Bacon, Heinz* | ½ Can/200g | 108.0 | 6.0 | 54 | 1.9 | 5.0 | 2.9 | 0.5 |
| Blended Sweetcorn & Yellow Pepper, Heinz* | ½ Can/200g | 98.0 | 4.0 | 49 | 0.9 | 6.6 | 2.1 | 0.6 |
| Bloody Mary, Fresh, Sainsbury's* | ½ Carton/300g | 65.0 | 1.0 | 22 | 0.4 | 4.3 | 0.3 | 0.9 |
| Boston Bean & Ham, New Covent Garden Food Co* | ½ Carton/300g | 171.0 | 1.0 | 57 | 2.4 | 7.8 | 0.2 | 1.6 |
| British Mushroom, With Scottish Ceps, TTD, Sainsbury's* | 1 Pot/300g | 102.0 | 5.0 | 34 | 1.1 | 3.3 | 1.8 | 1.4 |
| Broccoli, Baxters* | 1 Can/425g | 191.0 | 8.0 | 45 | 1.3 | 5.9 | 1.8 | 0.4 |
| Broccoli & Cauliflower, Cup, BFY, Morrisons* | 1 Sachet/15g | 56.0 | 2.0 | 376 | 4.9 | 57.2 | 14.2 | 4.9 |
| Broccoli & Cheddar, Heinz* | 1 Can/430g | 340.0 | 24.0 | 79 | 2.6 | 4.4 | 5.6 | 0.6 |
| Broccoli & Potato, Organic, Baxters* | 1 Can/425g | 161.0 | 3.0 | 38 | 1.5 | 6.2 | 0.8 | 0.7 |
| Broccoli & Stilton, Canned, Sainsbury's* | ½ Can/200g | 108.0 | 7.0 | 54 | 2.0 | 3.7 | 3.5 | 0.6 |
| Broccoli & Stilton, Canned, Tesco* | 1 Can/400g | 240.0 | 14.0 | 60 | 1.7 | 5.0 | 3.5 | 0.4 |
| Broccoli & Stilton, Classics, Fresh, Tesco* | ½ Pot/300g | 180.0 | 8.0 | 60 | 2.9 | 5.8 | 2.8 | 1.1 |
| Broccoli & Stilton, Cup Soup, Ainsley Harriott* | 1 Satchet/229ml | 87.0 | 2.0 | 38 | 1.0 | 7.0 | 0.8 | 1.3 |
| Broccoli & Stilton, Fresh, Sainsbury's* | ½ Pot/300ml | 141.0 | 10.0 | 47 | 2.7 | 1.8 | 3.3 | 1.5 |
| Broccoli & Stilton, New Covent Garden Food Co* | 1 Carton/600ml | 336.0 | 26.0 | 56 | 2.3 | 1.8 | 4.4 | 0.7 |
| Broccoli & Stilton, Tesco* | 1 Can/400g | 192.0 | 10.0 | 48 | 1.9 | 4.2 | 2.6 | 1.2 |
| Broccoli with Mustard, New Covent Garden Food Co* | 1 Carton/568g | 204.0 | 11.0 | 36 | 1.3 | 3.3 | 1.9 | 1.2 |
| Brocoli & Stilton, Fresh, Safeway* | 1 Serving/500g | 290.0 | 14.0 | 58 | 3.5 | 4.8 | 2.8 | 0.7 |
| Butternut Squash, Creamy, New Covent Garden Food Co* | ½ Carton/300g | 153.0 | 7.0 | 51 | 0.8 | 6.4 | 2.5 | 0.9 |
| Butternut Squash, Fresh, Waitrose* | ½ Pot/300g | 153.0 | 9.0 | 51 | 0.5 | 5.8 | 2.9 | 0.8 |
| Butternut Squash & Red Pepper, Baxters* | 1 Can/415g | 158.0 | 4.0 | 38 | 0.7 | 6.5 | 1.0 | 0.6 |
| Cantonese Hot & Sour Noodle, Baxters* | 1 Serving/215g | 133.0 | 3.0 | 62 | 1.4 | 11.1 | 1.3 | 0.5 |
| Carrot, Eat Smart, Safeway* | ½ Pot/225g | 79.0 | 3.0 | 35 | 0.6 | 5.5 | 1.3 | 0.4 |
| Carrot, Onion & Chick Pea, Healthy Choice, Baxters* | 1 Can/415ml | 170.0 | 1.0 | 41 | 1.9 | 8.0 | 0.2 | 1.2 |
| Carrot, Orange & Coriander, COU, M & S* | 1 Pack/415g | 145.0 | 2.0 | 35 | 0.6 | 6.9 | 0.6 | 1.2 |
| Carrot, Orange & Ginger, Go Organic* | 1 Jar/495g | 119.0 | 4.0 | 24 | 0.5 | 3.6 | 0.8 | 1.4 |
| Carrot, Parsnip & Nutmeg, Organic, Baxters* | 1 Can/425g | 144.0 | 2.0 | 34 | 0.7 | 6.6 | 0.5 | 1.1 |
| Carrot, Parsnip & Sweet Potato, Classic, Baxters* | 1 Carton/600g | 348.0 | 17.0 | 58 | 0.9 | 7.2 | 2.8 | 1.3 |
| Carrot, Potato & Coriander, Weight Watchers* | 1 Can/295g | 74.0 | 0.0 | 25 | 0.5 | 5.5 | 0.1 | 0.6 |
| Carrot & Butter Bean, Baxters* | ½ Can/207g | 112.0 | 4.0 | 54 | 1.6 | 7.7 | 1.9 | 1.7 |
| Carrot & Coriander, Baxters* | 1 Can/415g | 170.0 | 6.0 | 41 | 0.8 | 6.0 | 1.5 | 0.8 |
| Carrot & Coriander, Blended, Heinz* | ½ Can/200g | 104.0 | 5.0 | 52 | 0.7 | 6.2 | 2.7 | 0.6 |
| Carrot & Coriander, Canned, BGTY, Sainsbury's* | ½ Can/200g | 62.0 | 2.0 | 31 | 0.8 | 4.8 | 1.0 | 0.9 |
| Carrot & Coriander, Canned, Tesco* | 1 Can/400g | 220.0 | 12.0 | 55 | 0.7 | 5.7 | 2.9 | 0.8 |
| Carrot & Coriander, Carton, Campbell's* | 1 Serving/250ml | 110.0 | 5.0 | 44 | 0.7 | 5.4 | 2.2 | 0.0 |
| Carrot & Coriander, Classic Homestyle, M & S* | 1 Can/425g | 170.0 | 8.0 | 40 | 0.6 | 5.6 | 2.0 | 0.7 |
| Carrot & Coriander, Fresh, M & S* | ½ Pot/300g | 90.0 | 4.0 | 30 | 0.4 | 4.2 | 1.5 | 0.5 |
| Carrot & Coriander, Fresh, New Covent Garden Food Co* | ½ Carton/300g | 129.0 | 7.0 | 43 | 0.6 | 5.2 | 2.2 | 1.2 |
| Carrot & Coriander, Fresh, Organic, Simply Organic* | 1 Pot/600g | 276.0 | 18.0 | 46 | 0.5 | 4.5 | 3.0 | 1.3 |
| Carrot & Coriander, Fresh, Waitrose* | ½ Pot/300g | 150.0 | 10.0 | 50 | 0.5 | 4.4 | 3.4 | 0.9 |
| Carrot & Coriander, GFY, Asda* | 1 Carton/600g | 132.0 | 4.0 | 22 | 0.5 | 3.3 | 0.7 | 1.2 |
| Carrot & Coriander, Heinz* | 1 Can/400g | 196.0 | 11.0 | 49 | 0.5 | 5.6 | 2.7 | 1.0 |
| Carrot & Coriander, Less Than 5% Fat, Asda* | 1 Serving/300g | 96.0 | 1.0 | 32 | 1.0 | 6.0 | 0.3 | 0.8 |
| Carrot & Coriander, Perfectly Balanced, Waitrose* | ½ Can/208g | 33.0 | 0.0 | 16 | 0.5 | 3.1 | 0.2 | 1.0 |
| Carrot & Coriander, Selection, Campbell's* | 1 Carton/500ml | 185.0 | 5.0 | 37 | 0.6 | 6.4 | 1.0 | 0.6 |
| Carrot & Coriander, Soup in a Mug, HL, Tesco* | 1 Serving/21g | 81.0 | 2.0 | 385 | 4.8 | 66.4 | 10.7 | 5.1 |
| Carrot & Coriander, Soup-A-Cup, Asda* | 1 Serving/26g | 102.0 | 4.0 | 392 | 4.6 | 62.0 | 14.0 | 4.5 |
| Carrot & Coriander, Tesco* | 1 Carton/600g | 234.0 | 14.0 | 39 | 0.7 | 3.9 | 2.3 | 1.5 |

S

| | Measure INFO/WEIGHT | per Measure | | Nutrition Values per 100g / 100ml | | | | |
|---|---|---|---|---|---|---|---|---|
| | | KCAL | FAT | KCAL | PROT | CARB | FAT | FIBRE |
| **SOUP** | | | | | | | | |
| Carrot & Coriander, Vie, Knorr* | 1 Pack/500ml | 190.0 | 11.0 | 38 | 0.6 | 3.9 | 2.2 | 1.0 |
| Carrot & Coriander, Waistline, Crosse & Blackwell* | 1 Sachet/300g | 111.0 | 2.0 | 37 | 0.7 | 6.8 | 0.8 | 1.0 |
| Carrot & Coriander, with Creme Fraiche, Heinz* | 1 Can/515g | 232.0 | 9.0 | 45 | 0.7 | 6.6 | 1.8 | 0.9 |
| Carrot & Coriander Soup, Low Fat, Fresh, Sainsbury's* | 1 Tub/600g | 114.0 | 4.0 | 19 | 0.2 | 3.2 | 0.6 | 1.9 |
| Carrot & Ginger, Fresh, Sainsbury's* | 1 Pot/600g | 150.0 | 5.0 | 25 | 0.4 | 3.9 | 0.9 | 1.0 |
| Carrot & Ginger, Perfectly Balanced, Waitrose* | ½ Pot/300g | 66.0 | 3.0 | 22 | 0.4 | 3.1 | 0.9 | 1.0 |
| Carrot & Lentil, Microwave, Heinz* | 1 Can/303g | 94.0 | 0.0 | 31 | 1.5 | 6.1 | 0.1 | 0.8 |
| Carrot & Lentil, Weight Watchers* | 1 Can/295g | 86.0 | 0.0 | 29 | 1.3 | 5.7 | 0.1 | 0.7 |
| Carrot & Orange | 1oz/28g | 6.0 | 0.0 | 20 | 0.4 | 3.7 | 0.5 | 1.0 |
| Carrot & Orange, Baxters* | 1 Can/415g | 174.0 | 2.0 | 42 | 1.0 | 8.3 | 0.5 | 0.4 |
| Carrot & Orange, Fresh, Finest, Tesco* | ½ Tub/300g | 150.0 | 6.0 | 50 | 0.7 | 7.5 | 1.9 | 1.1 |
| Carrot & Orange, Pouch, Heinz* | ½ Pack/300g | 165.0 | 7.0 | 55 | 0.6 | 8.3 | 2.2 | 1.0 |
| Carrot with Creme Fraiche, Baxters* | 1 Can/415g | 170.0 | 7.0 | 41 | 0.5 | 5.9 | 1.7 | 0.7 |
| Celeriac & Truffle, New Covent Garden Food Co* | 1 Serving/300g | 225.0 | 18.0 | 75 | 1.1 | 4.3 | 5.9 | 0.7 |
| Chantenay Carrot & Parsnip, Fresh, Extra Special, Asda* | ½ Pot/300g | 114.0 | 6.0 | 38 | 0.6 | 4.2 | 2.1 | 0.8 |
| Cheese, Leek & Bacon, Somerfield* | 1 Carton/300g | 441.0 | 36.0 | 147 | 5.0 | 5.0 | 12.0 | 0.0 |
| Cheese & Bacon, with Pasta, Meal in a Mug, Tesco* | 1 Serving/37g | 142.0 | 3.0 | 383 | 9.1 | 69.5 | 7.6 | 2.8 |
| Chicken, & Barley, Broth, Heinz* | 1 Can/400g | 128.0 | 1.0 | 32 | 1.3 | 5.9 | 0.3 | 0.8 |
| Chicken, Campbell's* | 1 Can/295g | 142.0 | 11.0 | 48 | 1.1 | 3.5 | 3.6 | 0.0 |
| Chicken, Coconut & Lemon Grass, Fresh, Waitrose* | ½ Pot/300g | 303.0 | 25.0 | 101 | 2.6 | 4.1 | 8.3 | 0.8 |
| Chicken, Condensed, 99% Fat Free, Campbell's* | 1 Can/295g | 77.0 | 2.0 | 26 | 1.0 | 3.8 | 0.7 | 0.1 |
| Chicken, Cream Of, Canned | 1oz/28g | 16.0 | 1.0 | 58 | 1.7 | 4.5 | 3.8 | 0.0 |
| Chicken, Cream Of, Canned, Tesco* | 1 Can/400g | 260.0 | 15.0 | 65 | 1.2 | 5.5 | 3.8 | 0.0 |
| Chicken, Fresh, Sainsbury's* | ½ Carton/300g | 126.0 | 6.0 | 42 | 2.2 | 4.0 | 1.9 | 0.3 |
| Chicken, Green Thai, Sainsbury's* | 1 Pot/600g | 366.0 | 20.0 | 61 | 1.9 | 5.8 | 3.3 | 0.3 |
| Chicken, in a Cup, Sainsbury's* | 1 Serving/221ml | 86.0 | 4.0 | 39 | 0.7 | 5.3 | 1.7 | 0.1 |
| Chicken, Jamaican Jerk & Pumpkin, Sainsbury's* | ½ Pot/300g | 141.0 | 5.0 | 47 | 2.7 | 5.1 | 1.7 | 0.2 |
| Chicken, Leek & Potato, Weight Watchers* | 1 Can/400g | 136.0 | 4.0 | 34 | 1.2 | 5.3 | 0.9 | 0.3 |
| Chicken, Leek & White Wine, Fresh, Finest, Tesco* | 1 Pack/300g | 216.0 | 13.0 | 72 | 2.8 | 5.7 | 4.2 | 0.3 |
| Chicken, M & S* | 1 Pack/213g | 196.0 | 15.0 | 92 | 1.6 | 5.5 | 7.2 | 0.2 |
| Chicken, Moroccan Inspired, Sainsbury's* | 1 Bowl/342g | 202.0 | 3.0 | 59 | 2.6 | 10.2 | 0.9 | 7.5 |
| Chicken, Mulligatawny, Finest, Tesco* | ½ Pot/300g | 240.0 | 12.0 | 80 | 4.0 | 7.0 | 4.0 | 0.8 |
| Chicken, Mushroom, & Potato, Big Soup, Heinz* | ½ Can/200g | 132.0 | 5.0 | 66 | 3.4 | 8.1 | 2.3 | 0.4 |
| Chicken, Mushroom & Rice, Chilled, M & S* | ½ Pot/300g | 225.0 | 10.0 | 75 | 3.2 | 7.3 | 3.4 | 1.8 |
| Chicken, New Covent Garden Food Co* | 1 Carton/600g | 510.0 | 32.0 | 85 | 3.8 | 5.4 | 5.4 | 0.6 |
| Chicken, Packet, Knorr* | 1 Packet/85g | 423.0 | 27.0 | 498 | 7.7 | 44.3 | 32.3 | 0.2 |
| Chicken, Potato, & Lentil, Weight Watchers* | 1 Can/400g | 136.0 | 4.0 | 34 | 1.2 | 5.3 | 0.9 | 0.3 |
| Chicken, Potato & Bacon, Big Soup, Heinz* | 1 Can/515g | 278.0 | 10.0 | 54 | 3.1 | 6.2 | 1.9 | 0.5 |
| Chicken, Red Thai, Chunky, Fresh, Sainsbury's* | ½ Pot/300g | 165.0 | 10.0 | 55 | 0.9 | 5.4 | 3.3 | 0.9 |
| Chicken, Red Thai, Waitrose* | 1 Pot/600g | 348.0 | 19.0 | 58 | 3.5 | 4.1 | 3.1 | 1.1 |
| Chicken, Roasted, Canned, Tesco* | 1 Can/400g | 220.0 | 11.0 | 55 | 1.0 | 6.6 | 2.7 | 0.3 |
| Chicken, Sweetcorn & Potato, Heinz* | 1 Can/400g | 204.0 | 11.0 | 51 | 1.2 | 5.4 | 2.8 | 0.3 |
| Chicken, Thai, Fresh, Finest, Tesco* | ½ Tub/300g | 255.0 | 16.0 | 85 | 4.1 | 4.2 | 5.4 | 1.1 |
| Chicken, Thai, GFY, Asda* | 1 Serving/200g | 85.0 | 3.0 | 42 | 1.7 | 5.5 | 1.5 | 0.5 |
| Chicken, Thai, Noodle, Baxters* | 1 Serving/430g | 400.0 | 32.0 | 93 | 1.6 | 4.8 | 7.5 | 0.3 |
| Chicken, Thai, Spicy, Baxters* | 1 Can/415g | 278.0 | 15.0 | 67 | 1.8 | 7.1 | 3.5 | 0.3 |
| Chicken, Thai & Coconut, Safeway* | 1 Serving/300g | 235.0 | 16.0 | 78 | 3.4 | 4.6 | 5.2 | 0.9 |
| Chicken, Thai Blend, Baxters* | ½ Pot/300g | 282.0 | 22.0 | 94 | 1.7 | 5.3 | 7.3 | 0.4 |
| Chicken, Thai Style, Canned, Sainsbury's* | ½ Can/200g | 106.0 | 4.0 | 53 | 2.9 | 5.5 | 2.1 | 0.7 |
| Chicken, Thai Style, Canned, Soupreme* | 1 Can/400g | 200.0 | 11.0 | 50 | 2.5 | 3.8 | 2.7 | 1.1 |
| Chicken, Thai Style, Morrisons* | 1 Serving/250g | 240.0 | 15.0 | 96 | 4.6 | 5.5 | 6.2 | 1.2 |
| Chicken, Thai Style, Thick & Creamy, in a Mug, Tesco* | 1 Sachet/28g | 107.0 | 4.0 | 390 | 3.7 | 61.3 | 14.5 | 5.1 |
| Chicken, Tomato & Red Pepper, Italian, Big Soup, Heinz* | ½ Can/200g | 78.0 | 2.0 | 39 | 1.6 | 6.2 | 0.9 | 0.7 |

S

## SOUP

| | Measure INFO/WEIGHT | per Measure KCAL | per Measure FAT | Nutrition Values per 100g / 100ml KCAL | PROT | CARB | FAT | FIBRE |
|---|---|---|---|---|---|---|---|---|
| Chicken, Weight Watchers* | 1 Can/300g | 97.0 | 3.0 | 32 | 1.6 | 4.1 | 1.0 | 0.0 |
| Chicken & Bacon, with Pasta, Meal in a Mug, Tesco* | 1 Sachet/37g | 142.0 | 3.0 | 384 | 9.2 | 69.5 | 7.6 | 2.7 |
| Chicken & Broccoli, Soup a Cups, GFY, Asda* | 1 Cup/226ml | 52.0 | 1.0 | 23 | 0.5 | 4.0 | 0.6 | 0.4 |
| Chicken & Broccoli, Soup-A-Slim, Asda* | 1 Sachet/16g | 55.0 | 1.0 | 341 | 7.0 | 58.0 | 9.0 | 6.0 |
| Chicken & Broccoli Cup a Soup, Asda* | 1 Serving/16g | 55.0 | 1.0 | 341 | 7.0 | 58.0 | 9.0 | 6.0 |
| Chicken & Country Vegetable, Farmers Market, Heinz* | 1 Can/342g | 229.0 | 11.0 | 67 | 3.2 | 6.0 | 3.3 | 0.5 |
| Chicken & Country Vegetable, Soupfulls, Batchelors* | 1 Serving/400g | 164.0 | 4.0 | 41 | 5.1 | 3.0 | 0.9 | 1.3 |
| Chicken & Ham, Big, Heinz* | ½ Can/200g | 92.0 | 2.0 | 46 | 2.3 | 6.9 | 1.0 | 0.7 |
| Chicken & Ham, Chunky, Canned, Sainsbury's* | ½ Can/200g | 80.0 | 1.0 | 40 | 2.7 | 6.0 | 0.6 | 0.9 |
| Chicken & Herb, Farmers Market, Heinz* | ½ Carton/300g | 183.0 | 7.0 | 61 | 2.2 | 7.8 | 2.3 | 0.5 |
| Chicken & King Prawn, Noodle, Fresh, Tesco* | 1 Pot/400g | 180.0 | 2.0 | 45 | 4.7 | 5.5 | 0.4 | 0.4 |
| Chicken & Leek, Big Soup, Heinz* | ½ Can/258g | 162.0 | 5.0 | 63 | 3.0 | 8.2 | 2.0 | 0.6 |
| Chicken & Leek, Cup a Soup, Made Up, Batchelors* | 1 Serving/259g | 96.0 | 5.0 | 37 | 0.5 | 4.7 | 1.8 | 0.7 |
| Chicken & Leek, Fresh, TTD, Sainsbury's* | ½ Pot/300ml | 177.0 | 10.0 | 59 | 4.7 | 2.1 | 3.5 | 0.3 |
| Chicken & Leek, Simmer & Serve, Dried, Sainsbury's* | 1/3 Sachet/200ml | 62.0 | 2.0 | 31 | 0.4 | 5.2 | 0.9 | 0.3 |
| Chicken & Leek, Soup in a Cup, Made Up, Sainsbury's* | 1 Serving/200ml | 82.0 | 3.0 | 41 | 0.4 | 6.1 | 1.6 | 0.1 |
| Chicken & Mushroom, BFY, Dry, Morrisons* | 1 Serving/14g | 47.0 | 1.0 | 337 | 16.0 | 54.8 | 6.1 | 2.5 |
| Chicken & Mushroom, Canned, Tesco* | ½ Can/200g | 130.0 | 8.0 | 65 | 1.4 | 5.6 | 3.8 | 0.1 |
| Chicken & Mushroom, Extra, Slim a Soup, Batchelors* | 1 Serving/257g | 90.0 | 2.0 | 35 | 1.4 | 5.9 | 0.6 | 0.3 |
| Chicken & Mushroom, Meal in a Mug, Tesco* | 1 Sachet/40g | 146.0 | 3.0 | 366 | 10.8 | 65.3 | 6.8 | 5.1 |
| Chicken & Mushroom, Soup-A-Slim, Asda* | 1 Sachet/14g | 51.0 | 1.0 | 362 | 10.0 | 58.0 | 10.0 | 4.2 |
| Chicken & Mushroom in a Cup, Sainsbury's* | 1 Sachet/223ml | 107.0 | 4.0 | 48 | 0.7 | 7.1 | 1.9 | 0.1 |
| Chicken & Pasta Big, Heinz* | ½ Can/200g | 68.0 | 1.0 | 34 | 1.8 | 5.9 | 0.4 | 0.8 |
| Chicken & Red Pepper Noodle, Fresh, Tesco* | 1 Serving/400ml | 200.0 | 1.0 | 50 | 3.6 | 8.5 | 0.3 | 0.4 |
| Chicken & Sweetcorn, Asda* | 1 Pot/600g | 246.0 | 8.0 | 41 | 2.2 | 4.9 | 1.4 | 1.6 |
| Chicken & Sweetcorn, Baxters* | 1 Can/425g | 166.0 | 4.0 | 39 | 1.6 | 6.2 | 0.9 | 0.6 |
| Chicken & Sweetcorn, Canned, BGTY, Sainsbury's* | ½ Can/200g | 56.0 | 1.0 | 28 | 1.5 | 4.5 | 0.4 | 0.2 |
| Chicken & Sweetcorn, Canned, Tesco* | 1 Can/400ml | 240.0 | 6.0 | 60 | 1.6 | 8.2 | 1.5 | 0.7 |
| Chicken & Sweetcorn, Cantonese, Fresh, Sainsbury's* | ½ Pot/300ml | 135.0 | 1.0 | 45 | 2.1 | 7.9 | 0.5 | 0.5 |
| Chicken & Sweetcorn, Cup, Morrisons* | 1 Serving/14g | 52.0 | 2.0 | 375 | 8.4 | 51.2 | 15.2 | 0.0 |
| Chicken & Sweetcorn, Fresh, Asda* | 1 Pack/500g | 260.0 | 9.0 | 52 | 2.6 | 6.0 | 1.9 | 0.0 |
| Chicken & Sweetcorn, Fresh, Sainsbury's* | ½ Carton/300ml | 156.0 | 6.0 | 52 | 2.8 | 5.4 | 2.1 | 1.2 |
| Chicken & Sweetcorn, GFY, Asda* | 1 Can/400g | 108.0 | 2.0 | 27 | 1.5 | 4.2 | 0.5 | 0.2 |
| Chicken & Sweetcorn, in a Mug, Tesco* | 1 Sachet/28g | 122.0 | 5.0 | 434 | 4.8 | 63.4 | 17.9 | 1.1 |
| Chicken & Sweetcorn, Light Choice, Tesco* | ½ Can 200g | 84.0 | 1.0 | 42 | 1.7 | 7.9 | 0.4 | 0.2 |
| Chicken & Sweetcorn, New Covent Garden Food Co* | 1 Carton/600g | 282.0 | 5.0 | 47 | 1.0 | 8.7 | 0.9 | 0.5 |
| Chicken & Tarragon, Thick & Creamy, Batchelors* | 1 Sachet/281g | 118.0 | 6.0 | 42 | 0.8 | 5.7 | 2.3 | 0.3 |
| Chicken & Vegetable, Big Soup, Heinz* | ½ Can/200g | 104.0 | 3.0 | 52 | 3.3 | 6.7 | 1.4 | 0.8 |
| Chicken & Vegetable, Chunky, Canned, Eat Well, M & S* | ½ Can/213g | 138.0 | 4.0 | 65 | 4.6 | 6.9 | 1.9 | 1.0 |
| Chicken & Vegetable, Chunky, Canned, Sainsbury's* | ½ Can/200g | 94.0 | 2.0 | 47 | 4.0 | 6.0 | 0.8 | 1.6 |
| Chicken & Vegetable, Classic, Heinz* | 1 Can/400g | 132.0 | 2.0 | 33 | 1.1 | 6.2 | 0.4 | 0.6 |
| Chicken & Vegetable, Healthy Choice, Canned, Baxters* | 1 Can/415g | 162.0 | 2.0 | 39 | 1.9 | 6.8 | 0.5 | 1.7 |
| Chicken & Vegetable, Loyd Grossman* | 1 Pack/400g | 272.0 | 15.0 | 68 | 0.5 | 8.0 | 3.8 | 0.6 |
| Chicken & Vegetable, Micro, Tesco* | 1 Pot/330g | 139.0 | 5.0 | 42 | 2.1 | 5.0 | 1.5 | 0.6 |
| Chicken & Vegetable, Mighty, Asda* | 1 Can/410g | 176.0 | 5.0 | 43 | 2.5 | 6.8 | 1.3 | 0.7 |
| Chicken & Vegetable, Soup in a Mug, Value, Tesco* | 1 Serving/19g | 75.0 | 3.0 | 395 | 4.4 | 64.1 | 13.4 | 1.6 |
| Chicken & Vegetable, with Croutons, in a Cup, Sainsbury's* | 1 Serving/24g | 102.0 | 4.0 | 425 | 7.5 | 58.3 | 17.9 | 2.5 |
| Chicken & Vegetable Broth, Canned, BFY, Morrisons* | ½ Can/205g | 50.0 | 0.0 | 24 | 1.2 | 4.5 | 0.2 | 0.5 |
| Chicken & Vegetable with Pasta, Select, Campbell's* | 1 Can/480ml | 220.0 | 1.0 | 46 | 2.9 | 7.9 | 0.2 | 0.8 |
| Chicken & White Wine, Campbell's* | 1 Serving/295g | 145.0 | 10.0 | 49 | 1.0 | 4.0 | 3.3 | 0.0 |
| Chicken Broth, Baxters* | 1 Can/415g | 129.0 | 2.0 | 31 | 1.5 | 5.4 | 0.4 | 0.6 |
| Chicken Curry, Mild, Indian, Soups of the World, Heinz* | 1 Can/515g | 381.0 | 21.0 | 74 | 3.6 | 5.9 | 4.1 | 0.3 |
| Chicken Mulligatawny, Asda* | 1 Serving/300g | 150.0 | 2.0 | 50 | 3.8 | 7.0 | 0.8 | 0.8 |

S

## SOUP

| | Measure INFO/WEIGHT | per Measure KCAL | per Measure FAT | KCAL | PROT | CARB | FAT | FIBRE |
|---|---|---|---|---|---|---|---|---|
| Chicken Mulligatawny, Chunky, Meal, Weight Watchers* | 1 Pack/340g | 163.0 | 4.0 | 48 | 2.2 | 6.8 | 1.3 | 1.5 |
| Chicken Mulligatawny, Perfectly Balanced, Waitrose* | 1 Serving/300g | 138.0 | 6.0 | 46 | 1.7 | 5.3 | 2.0 | 0.4 |
| Chicken Noodle, Batchelors* | 1 Pack/284g | 71.0 | 1.0 | 25 | 1.6 | 4.2 | 0.2 | 0.3 |
| Chicken Noodle, Canned, Sainsbury's* | ½ Can/217g | 78.0 | 1.0 | 36 | 1.7 | 7.4 | 0.3 | 0.7 |
| Chicken Noodle, Chunky, Campbell's* | ½ Can/200g | 86.0 | 1.0 | 43 | 2.8 | 6.5 | 0.6 | 0.0 |
| Chicken Noodle, Classic, Heinz* | 1 Can/400g | 124.0 | 1.0 | 31 | 1.2 | 6.0 | 0.3 | 0.2 |
| Chicken Noodle, Clear, Weight Watchers* | 1 Can/295g | 50.0 | 0.0 | 17 | 0.7 | 3.1 | 0.1 | 0.2 |
| Chicken Noodle, Cup Soup, Dry, Heinz* | 1 Sachet/15g | 48.0 | 0.0 | 320 | 10.7 | 61.3 | 3.3 | 2.0 |
| Chicken Noodle, Cup Soup, Eat Smart, Morrisons* | 1 Sachet /216g | 41.0 | 0.0 | 19 | 0.6 | 4.1 | 0.1 | 0.2 |
| Chicken Noodle, Cup Soup, Made Up, Heinz* | 1 Serving/218ml | 48.0 | 0.0 | 22 | 0.7 | 4.3 | 0.2 | 0.1 |
| Chicken Noodle, Simmer & Serve, Dried, Sainsbury's* | 1 Pack/600ml | 102.0 | 1.0 | 17 | 0.8 | 2.9 | 0.2 | 0.0 |
| Chicken Noodle, Soup in a Cup, Made Up, Sainsbury's* | 1 Serving/200ml | 44.0 | 0.0 | 22 | 0.7 | 4.7 | 0.1 | 0.2 |
| Chicken Noodle, with Sweetcorn, Baxters* | 1 Can/415g | 141.0 | 2.0 | 34 | 1.4 | 5.8 | 0.6 | 0.2 |
| Chicken Noodle & Vegetable, Slim a Soup, Batchelors* | 1 Serving/203g | 55.0 | 1.0 | 27 | 0.8 | 4.8 | 0.5 | 0.6 |
| Chicken,Noodle, Canned, Asda* | 1 Can/400g | 148.0 | 4.0 | 37 | 1.7 | 5.1 | 1.1 | 0.7 |
| Chilli, Meal, Chunky, Canned, Tesco* | ½ Can/200g | 120.0 | 2.0 | 60 | 5.0 | 6.3 | 1.2 | 1.6 |
| Chilli Bean, M & S* | ½ Carton/300g | 150.0 | 7.0 | 50 | 2.5 | 4.7 | 2.5 | 2.7 |
| Chilli Beef, Mighty, Asda* | 1 Can/400g | 236.0 | 6.0 | 59 | 4.9 | 6.8 | 1.4 | 1.2 |
| Chilli Con Carne, Chunky, Sainsbury's* | ½ Can/200g | 110.0 | 2.0 | 55 | 3.6 | 8.0 | 0.9 | 1.5 |
| Chilli Pumpkin, Fresh, Sainsbury's* | ½ Carton/300g | 120.0 | 7.0 | 40 | 0.6 | 4.0 | 2.4 | 1.3 |
| Chilli Tomato & Pasta, COU, M & S* | 1 Serving/300g | 150.0 | 6.0 | 50 | 1.3 | 7.2 | 1.9 | 0.9 |
| Chinese Chicken & Sweetcorn, Soups of the World, Heinz* | ½ Can/260g | 117.0 | 4.0 | 45 | 1.9 | 6.2 | 1.4 | 0.3 |
| Chinese Chicken Noodle, Dry, Knorr* | 1 Pack/45g | 138.0 | 2.0 | 307 | 15.1 | 51.8 | 4.4 | 2.9 |
| Chinese Chicken Noodle, Slim a Soup Extra, Batchelors* | 1 Sachet/246g | 69.0 | 1.0 | 28 | 1.0 | 5.3 | 0.3 | 0.4 |
| Chorizo & Tomato with Vegetables, Canned, Sainsbury's* | ½ Can/200g | 114.0 | 6.0 | 57 | 2.6 | 4.9 | 3.0 | 0.3 |
| Chowder, Bacon & Corn, M & S* | ½ Pot/300g | 195.0 | 11.0 | 65 | 2.5 | 6.0 | 3.6 | 1.8 |
| Chowder, Clam, New England, Select, Campbell's* | 1 Cup/240ml | 221.0 | 14.0 | 92 | 2.5 | 6.0 | 6.0 | 0.8 |
| Chowder, Haddock, Smoked, Asda* | 1 Serving/300g | 462.0 | 12.0 | 154 | 1.6 | 28.0 | 4.0 | 0.5 |
| Chowder, Prawn, Manhattan, Fresh, Sainsbury's* | 1 Serving/300g | 177.0 | 7.0 | 59 | 1.6 | 7.9 | 2.3 | 0.1 |
| Chowder, Seafood, Baxters* | ½ Can/213g | 160.0 | 10.0 | 75 | 3.3 | 5.4 | 4.5 | 0.4 |
| Chowder, Smoked Haddock, Canned, Sainsbury's* | ½ Can/200g | 128.0 | 8.0 | 64 | 1.6 | 5.3 | 4.0 | 0.3 |
| Chowder, Sweetcorn & Chicken, Heinz* | 1 Serving/200g | 148.0 | 6.0 | 74 | 3.3 | 9.1 | 2.8 | 0.6 |
| Chunky Chicken Hotpot, Big Soup, Heinz* | ½ Can/258g | 126.0 | 3.0 | 49 | 2.3 | 7.4 | 1.2 | 0.8 |
| Cock-A-Leekie, Traditional, Baxters* | 1 Can/425g | 98.0 | 2.0 | 23 | 1.0 | 3.7 | 0.5 | 0.3 |
| Country Mushroom, Baxters* | 1 Pot/600g | 378.0 | 25.0 | 63 | 0.9 | 5.5 | 4.1 | 0.1 |
| Country Mushroom, Selection, Campbell's* | 1 Serving/250ml | 80.0 | 4.0 | 32 | 0.6 | 3.4 | 1.8 | 0.5 |
| Country Vegetable, Asda* | 1 Serving/125g | 59.0 | 4.0 | 47 | 0.6 | 4.5 | 2.9 | 0.8 |
| Country Vegetable, Chunky, Asda* | ½ Pot/300g | 138.0 | 2.0 | 46 | 2.0 | 8.2 | 0.6 | 0.5 |
| Country Vegetable, Chunky, Healthy Choice, Baxters* | 1 Pot/274g | 126.0 | 1.0 | 46 | 2.0 | 8.8 | 0.3 | 1.7 |
| Country Vegetable, Fresh, Chilled, M & S* | 1 Pot/600g | 210.0 | 13.0 | 35 | 0.5 | 3.2 | 2.1 | 1.0 |
| Country Vegetable, Fresh, Sainsbury's* | ½ Pot/300g | 123.0 | 3.0 | 41 | 1.6 | 6.6 | 0.9 | 2.5 |
| Country Vegetable, Knorr* | 1 Pack/500ml | 160.0 | 3.0 | 32 | 0.9 | 5.5 | 0.7 | 1.2 |
| Country Vegetable, M & S* | ½ Pot/300g | 135.0 | 6.0 | 45 | 1.0 | 5.2 | 2.0 | 1.4 |
| Country Vegetable, Weight Watchers* | 1 Can/297g | 92.0 | 1.0 | 31 | 1.1 | 6.1 | 0.2 | 1.0 |
| Country Vegetable & Herb, Farmers Market, Heinz* | ½ Carton/300g | 114.0 | 4.0 | 38 | 1.2 | 5.7 | 1.2 | 0.9 |
| Country Vegetable Casserole, Taste of Home, Heinz* | 1 Pot/430g | 206.0 | 6.0 | 48 | 1.3 | 7.6 | 1.4 | 1.3 |
| Courgette, Parmesan & Bacon, Somerfield* | 1 Pack/500g | 255.0 | 20.0 | 51 | 2.0 | 2.0 | 4.0 | 0.0 |
| Courgette & Parmesan, Fresh, Sainsbury's* | 1 Pack/300ml | 198.0 | 17.0 | 66 | 1.5 | 2.5 | 5.6 | 0.4 |
| Cream of Asparagus, Baxters* | 1 Can/415g | 278.0 | 18.0 | 67 | 1.1 | 6.0 | 4.3 | 0.2 |
| Cream of Asparagus, Cup a Soup, Batchelors* | 1 Sachet/223g | 143.0 | 6.0 | 64 | 0.5 | 9.2 | 2.8 | 0.4 |
| Cream of Asparagus, in a Cup, Sainsbury's* | 1 Serving/230ml | 129.0 | 5.0 | 56 | 0.7 | 8.2 | 2.3 | 0.1 |
| Cream of Asparagus, in Seconds, Dry, Knorr* | 1 Pack/61g | 320.0 | 22.0 | 524 | 6.5 | 42.2 | 36.6 | 1.1 |
| Cream of Asparagus, Soup-A-Cup, Asda* | 1 Pack/112g | 491.0 | 25.0 | 438 | 6.0 | 54.0 | 22.0 | 4.1 |

S

## SOUP

| | Measure INFO/WEIGHT | per Measure KCAL | per Measure FAT | KCAL | PROT | CARB | FAT | FIBRE |
|---|---|---|---|---|---|---|---|---|
| Cream of Celery, Asda* | 1 Can/410g | 189.0 | 11.0 | 46 | 0.6 | 4.8 | 2.7 | 0.2 |
| Cream of Celery, Campbell's* | 1 Serving/150g | 70.0 | 5.0 | 47 | 0.6 | 3.2 | 3.4 | 0.0 |
| Cream of Chicken, Asda* | 1 Can/410g | 209.0 | 14.0 | 51 | 1.2 | 4.0 | 3.4 | 0.1 |
| Cream of Chicken, Batchelors* | 1 Pack/289g | 165.0 | 10.0 | 57 | 1.1 | 5.6 | 3.3 | 0.3 |
| Cream of Chicken, Baxters* | ½ Can/209g | 144.0 | 9.0 | 69 | 1.8 | 6.1 | 4.2 | 0.1 |
| Cream of Chicken, Campbell's* | 1 Can/590g | 283.0 | 21.0 | 48 | 1.1 | 3.5 | 3.6 | 0.0 |
| Cream of Chicken, Canned, Sainsbury's* | ½ Can/200g | 96.0 | 5.0 | 48 | 2.3 | 3.7 | 2.7 | 0.2 |
| Cream of Chicken, Classic, Heinz* | 1 Can/400g | 208.0 | 12.0 | 52 | 1.7 | 4.7 | 3.0 | 0.1 |
| Cream of Chicken, for One, Heinz* | 1 Can/290g | 142.0 | 8.0 | 49 | 1.5 | 4.5 | 2.7 | 0.1 |
| Cream of Chicken, Fresh, Waitrose* | 1 Serving/300g | 180.0 | 12.0 | 60 | 2.6 | 3.7 | 3.9 | 0.2 |
| Cream of Chicken, Homepride* | ¼ Bottle/250ml | 112.0 | 7.0 | 45 | 1.3 | 4.0 | 2.9 | 0.0 |
| Cream of Chicken, in Seconds, Dry, Knorr* | 1 Pack/58g | 300.0 | 21.0 | 518 | 11.2 | 36.0 | 36.6 | 0.3 |
| Cream of Chicken, Simmer & Serve, Dried, Sainsbury's* | 1 Pack/500ml | 181.0 | 7.0 | 36 | 0.8 | 4.9 | 1.5 | 0.8 |
| Cream of Chicken & Mushroom, Campbell's* | 1 Can/250g | 140.0 | 11.0 | 56 | 0.9 | 3.5 | 4.4 | 0.0 |
| Cream of Chicken & Mushroom, Canned, Sainsbury's* | 1 Can/400g | 248.0 | 17.0 | 62 | 1.8 | 4.0 | 4.3 | 0.4 |
| Cream of Chicken & Mushroom, Heinz* | ½ Can/200g | 98.0 | 6.0 | 49 | 1.3 | 4.6 | 2.9 | 0.1 |
| Cream of Leek, Baxters* | 1 Can/415g | 237.0 | 17.0 | 57 | 1.1 | 3.8 | 4.2 | 0.7 |
| Cream of Leek in Seconds, Dry, Knorr* | 1 Pack/64g | 326.0 | 22.0 | 509 | 5.9 | 45.2 | 33.8 | 1.4 |
| Cream of Mushroom, Asda* | 1 Can/400g | 168.0 | 10.0 | 42 | 1.2 | 3.5 | 2.6 | 0.3 |
| Cream of Mushroom, Canned, Sainsbury's* | 1 Can/400g | 220.0 | 21.0 | 55 | 0.6 | 1.4 | 5.2 | 0.1 |
| Cream of Mushroom, Classics, Heinz* | 1 Can/400g | 208.0 | 11.0 | 52 | 1.5 | 5.2 | 2.8 | 0.1 |
| Cream of Mushroom, Cup a Soup, Batchelors* | 1 Serving/219g | 125.0 | 6.0 | 57 | 0.6 | 7.5 | 2.8 | 0.4 |
| Cream of Mushroom, Dry, Knorr* | 1 Serving/25g | 125.0 | 8.0 | 500 | 5.2 | 47.8 | 31.8 | 1.0 |
| Cream of Mushroom, GFY, Asda* | 1 Serving/250g | 92.0 | 1.0 | 37 | 2.1 | 6.0 | 0.5 | 0.3 |
| Cream of Mushroom, Packet, Knorr* | 1 Pack/75g | 388.0 | 26.0 | 518 | 5.2 | 44.8 | 35.3 | 0.9 |
| Cream of Mushroom in a Bottle, Homepride* | ¼ Bottle/250ml | 110.0 | 8.0 | 44 | 0.5 | 3.5 | 3.1 | 0.0 |
| Cream of Potato & Leek, Canned, Sainsbury's* | ½ Can/200g | 80.0 | 3.0 | 40 | 0.6 | 6.1 | 1.5 | 0.0 |
| Cream of Sweetcorn, Campbell's* | 1 Serving/80g | 41.0 | 2.0 | 51 | 0.6 | 6.2 | 2.7 | 0.5 |
| Cream of Vegatable, Cup Soup, Soupreme* | 1 Serving/27g | 95.0 | 3.0 | 352 | 4.8 | 59.6 | 10.5 | 6.3 |
| Creamed Asparagus, Dry, Asda* | 1 Sachet/30g | 135.0 | 7.0 | 451 | 6.0 | 55.0 | 23.0 | 1.1 |
| Creamed Vegetable, in a Mug, Safeway* | 1 Sachet/29g | 117.0 | 5.0 | 405 | 5.6 | 57.9 | 16.8 | 3.2 |
| Creamy Chicken & Mushroom, Baxters* | 1 Can/415g | 216.0 | 11.0 | 52 | 1.6 | 5.3 | 2.7 | 0.1 |
| Creamy Chicken & Mushroom, Very Special, Heinz* | 1 Serving/260g | 130.0 | 6.0 | 50 | 1.9 | 5.3 | 2.4 | 0.0 |
| Creamy Leek, with Croutons, in a Cup, Sainsbury's* | 1 Serving/228g | 130.0 | 6.0 | 57 | 1.1 | 7.2 | 2.6 | 0.1 |
| Creamy Mushroom, Asda* | 1 Pot/500g | 228.0 | 14.0 | 46 | 1.1 | 4.0 | 2.8 | 1.3 |
| Creamy Mushroom, Fresh, Asda* | 1 Serving/250g | 110.0 | 7.0 | 44 | 1.1 | 3.8 | 2.7 | 1.3 |
| Creamy Potato, Bacon & Onion, Cup a Soup, Batchelors* | 1 Sachet/280ml | 106.0 | 3.0 | 38 | 0.9 | 7.3 | 1.0 | 0.5 |
| Creamy Potato & Leek, Cup a Soup, Batchelors* | 1 Sachet/280ml | 132.0 | 4.0 | 47 | 0.8 | 7.4 | 1.5 | 1.1 |
| Creamy Tomato, Very Special, Heinz* | 1 Serving/290g | 148.0 | 6.0 | 51 | 0.7 | 6.5 | 2.2 | 0.0 |
| Cullen Skink, Baxters* | 1 Can/415g | 357.0 | 14.0 | 86 | 6.4 | 7.7 | 3.3 | 0.4 |
| Cumberland Sausage & Vegetable, Big Soup, Heinz* | 1 Can/515g | 211.0 | 4.0 | 41 | 2.1 | 6.7 | 0.7 | 0.8 |
| Farmhouse Chicken Leek, Dry, Knorr* | 1 Pack/54g | 248.0 | 16.0 | 459 | 10.3 | 39.3 | 29.0 | 1.5 |
| Farmhouse Vegetable, Canned, BGTY, Sainsbury's* | ½ Can/200ml | 52.0 | 2.0 | 26 | 0.5 | 4.4 | 0.8 | 0.9 |
| Farmhouse Vegetable, Soup-A-Cup, GFY, Asda* | 1 Sachet/219ml | 59.0 | 1.0 | 27 | 0.6 | 4.9 | 0.5 | 0.4 |
| Fire Roasted Tomato & Red Pepper, Asda* | ½ Tub/265g | 114.0 | 7.0 | 43 | 0.7 | 4.1 | 2.6 | 1.0 |
| Flame Roasted Red Pepper & Tomato, Baxters* | ½ Can/207g | 116.0 | 6.0 | 56 | 0.9 | 6.8 | 2.8 | 0.6 |
| Florentine Pea, The Best, Safeway* | ½ Pot/300g | 165.0 | 7.0 | 55 | 2.5 | 4.9 | 2.5 | 1.4 |
| Florida Spring Vegetable, Dry, Knorr* | 1 Pack/36g | 104.0 | 2.0 | 290 | 7.8 | 52.2 | 5.6 | 5.2 |
| Four Mushroom, Loyd Grossman* | 1 Pack/420g | 202.0 | 16.0 | 48 | 0.8 | 2.5 | 3.9 | 0.2 |
| French Onion | 1oz/28g | 11.0 | 1.0 | 40 | 0.2 | 5.7 | 2.1 | 1.0 |
| French Onion, Chilled, M & S* | ½ Pot/300g | 150.0 | 4.0 | 50 | 2.0 | 7.2 | 1.5 | 1.0 |
| French Onion, Favourites, Baxters* | ½ Can/208g | 56.0 | 0.0 | 27 | 0.9 | 5.5 | 0.1 | 0.7 |
| French Onion, Fresh, Morrisons* | 1 Serving/500g | 155.0 | 4.0 | 31 | 0.8 | 5.0 | 0.9 | 0.5 |

# SOUP

| Measure INFO/WEIGHT | per Measure KCAL | FAT | Nutrition Values per 100g / 100ml KCAL | PROT | CARB | FAT | FIBRE |
|---|---|---|---|---|---|---|---|

| | Measure INFO/WEIGHT | per Measure KCAL | FAT | KCAL | PROT | CARB | FAT | FIBRE |
|---|---|---|---|---|---|---|---|---|
| French Onion, GFY, Asda* | ½ Pot/253g | 91.0 | 1.0 | 36 | 1.9 | 6.0 | 0.5 | 0.4 |
| French Onion, Heinz* | 1 Pack/400g | 100.0 | 0.0 | 25 | 0.5 | 5.7 | 0.1 | 0.4 |
| French Onion, Knorr* | 1 Pack/40g | 118.0 | 1.0 | 296 | 6.0 | 62.5 | 2.5 | 6.6 |
| French Onion & Cider, Waitrose* | 1 Can/425g | 93.0 | 0.0 | 22 | 0.5 | 4.8 | 0.1 | 0.4 |
| French Onion & Croutons, Dry, Tesco* | 1 Serving/30g | 106.0 | 2.0 | 353 | 7.3 | 63.7 | 7.7 | 2.0 |
| French Onion & Gruyere Cheese, Fresh, Finest, Tesco* | ½ Pot/300g | 210.0 | 15.0 | 70 | 1.4 | 4.7 | 5.1 | 0.5 |
| Garden Pea & Wiltshire Cured Ham, Finest, Tesco* | ½ Pot/300g | 195.0 | 8.0 | 65 | 3.4 | 5.9 | 2.7 | 1.6 |
| Garden Vegetable, Baxters* | 1 Serving/200g | 70.0 | 1.0 | 35 | 0.9 | 6.6 | 0.6 | 0.8 |
| Garden Vegetable, Dry, Slim Fast* | 1 Serving/60g | 224.0 | 6.0 | 373 | 23.8 | 45.0 | 10.3 | 7.0 |
| Garden Vegetable, Heinz* | 1 Can/400g | 160.0 | 3.0 | 40 | 0.9 | 7.2 | 0.8 | 0.9 |
| Gazpacho, Canned, Average | 1 Can/400g | 76.0 | 0.0 | 19 | 2.9 | 1.8 | 0.1 | 0.2 |
| Goats Cheese & Rocket, Fresh, Sainsbury's* | ½ Carton/300g | 180.0 | 13.0 | 60 | 2.0 | 3.2 | 4.4 | 0.3 |
| Golden Vegetable, Asda* | 1 Pack/300g | 150.0 | 6.0 | 50 | 1.9 | 6.0 | 2.0 | 0.0 |
| Golden Vegetable, Cup, Calorie Counter, Co-Op* | 1 Sachet/11g | 35.0 | 1.0 | 320 | 7.0 | 50.0 | 10.0 | 9.0 |
| Golden Vegetable, Dry, Knorr* | 1 Pack/76g | 299.0 | 14.0 | 394 | 10.4 | 45.4 | 19.0 | 3.3 |
| Golden Vegetable, Slim a Soup, Batchelors* | 1 Sachet/207g | 58.0 | 2.0 | 28 | 0.5 | 4.7 | 0.8 | 0.7 |
| Golden Vegetable, Soup-A-Slim, Asda* | 1 Sachet/15g | 50.0 | 1.0 | 336 | 6.0 | 60.0 | 8.0 | 1.9 |
| Golden Vegetable with Croutons, Instant, Dry, Morrisons* | 1 Sachet/27g | 118.0 | 5.0 | 438 | 5.3 | 60.7 | 19.3 | 0.0 |
| Green Split Pea & Ham Soup, TTD, Sainsbury's* | ½ Pot/300g | 204.0 | 7.0 | 68 | 4.3 | 7.4 | 2.3 | 2.2 |
| Green Vegetables & Lentil, Lima* | 1 Serving/300g | 96.0 | 4.0 | 32 | 1.6 | 3.7 | 1.2 | 0.5 |
| Gumbo, Spicy, Fresh, Sainsbury's* | ½ Pot/300g | 120.0 | 5.0 | 40 | 1.5 | 4.5 | 1.8 | 0.9 |
| Haddock, Smoked, Fresh, Finest, Tesco* | 1 Pot/550g | 302.0 | 14.0 | 55 | 2.7 | 5.1 | 2.5 | 0.8 |
| Haggis Broth, Baxters* | 1 Can/415g | 187.0 | 6.0 | 45 | 1.8 | 6.1 | 1.5 | 0.6 |
| Harvest Carrot & Lima Bean, Heinz* | 1oz/28g | 11.0 | 0.0 | 40 | 0.8 | 6.9 | 1.0 | 1.3 |
| Harvest Vegetable, with Croutons, in a Cup, Sainsbury's* | 1 Sachet/226ml | 86.0 | 3.0 | 38 | 1.0 | 5.9 | 1.2 | 0.9 |
| Hearty Vegetable, 99% Fat Free, Prepared, Campbell's* | 1 Can/295g | 91.0 | 1.0 | 31 | 0.8 | 6.1 | 0.4 | 0.0 |
| Hearty Vegetable Broth, Weight Watchers, Heinz* | 1 Can/295g | 127.0 | 1.0 | 43 | 2.0 | 8.2 | 0.2 | 1.4 |
| Highlander's Broth, Baxters* | ½ Can/206g | 97.0 | 3.0 | 47 | 1.8 | 6.5 | 1.5 | 0.6 |
| Hot & Sour, Szechuan, Cup Soup, Ainsley Harriott* | 1 Sachet /219ml | 57.0 | 0.0 | 26 | 0.5 | 5.9 | 0.0 | 1.1 |
| Hot Sweet Piquante Pepper & Carrot, Choices, Baxters* | 1 Pouch/300g | 135.0 | 3.0 | 45 | 0.8 | 8.2 | 1.0 | 0.6 |
| Indian Chicken, Glorious!* | ½ Pot/300g | 201.0 | 7.0 | 67 | 3.4 | 7.6 | 2.5 | 0.7 |
| Italian, Chunky, New Covent Garden Food Co* | ½ Carton/300g | 111.0 | 4.0 | 37 | 1.5 | 4.7 | 1.4 | 0.9 |
| Italian Bean & Pasta, Baxters* | 1 Can/415g | 180.0 | 1.0 | 43 | 2.0 | 7.9 | 0.3 | 1.1 |
| Italian Bean & Pasta, Healthy Choice, Baxters* | 1 Can/415g | 170.0 | 1.0 | 41 | 1.7 | 8.2 | 0.2 | 1.3 |
| Italian Chicken Broth, Healthy Choice, Baxters* | ½ Can/210g | 84.0 | 2.0 | 40 | 1.5 | 6.6 | 0.8 | 0.8 |
| Italian Meatball & Tomato, Soups of the World, Heinz* | 1 Can/515g | 319.0 | 15.0 | 62 | 2.5 | 6.4 | 2.9 | 1.8 |
| Italian Minestrone, Dry, Knorr* | 1 Pack/62g | 193.0 | 3.0 | 311 | 11.5 | 57.1 | 4.1 | 7.8 |
| Italian Minestrone, M & S* | 1 Can/425g | 191.0 | 2.0 | 45 | 2.2 | 9.0 | 0.5 | 0.8 |
| Italian Plum Tomato & Basil, Perfectly Balanced, Waitrose* | ½ Pot/300g | 69.0 | 1.0 | 23 | 0.9 | 3.8 | 0.5 | 0.9 |
| Italian Tomato & Basil, Go Organic* | 1 Jar/495g | 183.0 | 10.0 | 37 | 1.2 | 3.3 | 2.1 | 0.8 |
| Lamb & Cous Cous, M & S* | ½ Can/208g | 100.0 | 4.0 | 48 | 2.1 | 6.2 | 1.8 | 0.9 |
| Lamb & Vegetable, Big Soup, Heinz* | ½ Can/200g | 120.0 | 3.0 | 60 | 3.0 | 9.1 | 1.3 | 1.3 |
| Lamb & Vegetable, Mega, Morrisons* | 1 Pack/410g | 172.0 | 4.0 | 42 | 1.9 | 6.3 | 1.0 | 0.8 |
| Lancashire Lamb Hotpot, Taste of Home, Heinz* | 1 Pot/430g | 279.0 | 9.0 | 65 | 2.9 | 8.8 | 2.0 | 1.1 |
| Leek & Chicken, Knorr* | 1 Serving/300ml | 82.0 | 5.0 | 27 | 0.6 | 2.4 | 1.7 | 0.1 |
| Leek & Maris Piper Potato, Chilled, M & S* | 1 Serving/300g | 165.0 | 11.0 | 55 | 0.6 | 4.5 | 3.8 | 0.9 |
| Leek & Potato, Chunky, Meal, Canned, Tesco* | ½ Can/200g | 60.0 | 3.0 | 30 | 1.0 | 3.5 | 1.3 | 1.0 |
| Leek & Potato, Cup a Soup, Batchelors* | 1 Sachet/28g | 121.0 | 5.0 | 432 | 5.2 | 63.2 | 17.6 | 1.8 |
| Leek & Potato, Fresh, Sainsbury's* | ½ Pot/300ml | 141.0 | 7.0 | 47 | 1.0 | 5.3 | 2.4 | 0.4 |
| Leek & Potato, Fresh, Tesco* | ½ Tub/300g | 171.0 | 10.0 | 57 | 1.0 | 5.3 | 3.5 | 0.7 |
| Leek & Potato, in a Cup, BGTY, Sainsbury's* | 1 Serving/218ml | 59.0 | 2.0 | 27 | 0.4 | 4.9 | 0.7 | 0.2 |
| Leek & Potato, In A Mug, Light Choices, Tesco* | 1 Sachet/220g | 55.0 | 1.0 | 25 | 0.5 | 4.9 | 0.4 | 0.6 |
| Leek & Potato, Slim a Soup, Batchelors* | 1 Serving/204g | 57.0 | 1.0 | 28 | 0.4 | 5.0 | 0.7 | 0.2 |

## SOUP

| | Measure INFO/WEIGHT | per Measure KCAL | per Measure FAT | Nutrition Values per 100g / 100ml KCAL | PROT | CARB | FAT | FIBRE |
|---|---|---|---|---|---|---|---|---|
| Leek & Potato, Smooth, Vie, Knorr* | 1 Pack/500ml | 155.0 | 4.0 | 31 | 0.9 | 4.8 | 0.9 | 1.0 |
| Leek & Potato, Soup in a Cup, Made Up, Waitrose* | 1 Sachet/204ml | 47.0 | 1.0 | 23 | 0.3 | 4.3 | 0.5 | 0.5 |
| Leek & Potato, Thick & Creamy, Soup in a Mug, Tesco* | 1 Serving/25g | 94.0 | 2.0 | 378 | 4.2 | 68.5 | 9.7 | 4.9 |
| Leek & Potato, Weight Watchers* | 1 Sachet/215ml | 58.0 | 1.0 | 27 | 0.5 | 5.1 | 0.5 | 0.1 |
| Leek with Croutons in a Cup, Sainsbury's* | 1 Sachet/24g | 91.0 | 5.0 | 379 | 6.7 | 42.9 | 20.0 | 12.1 |
| Lenti, Asda* | 1 Can /400g | 192.0 | 1.0 | 48 | 1.4 | 10.2 | 0.2 | 1.2 |
| Lentil, & Potato, Spiced, Heinz* | 1 Can/295g | 118.0 | 1.0 | 40 | 2.0 | 7.7 | 0.2 | 0.7 |
| Lentil, Asda* | ½ Can/202g | 89.0 | 0.0 | 44 | 2.6 | 8.0 | 0.2 | 0.7 |
| Lentil, Average | 1 Serving/220g | 218.0 | 8.0 | 99 | 4.4 | 12.7 | 3.8 | 1.1 |
| Lentil, Bacon & Mixed Bean, Low Fat, Aldi* | 1 Serving/400g | 260.0 | 4.0 | 65 | 4.7 | 9.5 | 0.9 | 1.6 |
| Lentil, Campbell's* | 1 Can/295g | 139.0 | 2.0 | 47 | 2.6 | 7.7 | 0.6 | 0.0 |
| Lentil, Canned | 1 Serving/220g | 86.0 | 0.0 | 39 | 3.1 | 6.5 | 0.2 | 1.2 |
| Lentil, Carrot & Cumin, Canned, BGTY, Sainsbury's* | 1 Can/400g | 204.0 | 4.0 | 51 | 2.3 | 8.4 | 0.9 | 0.1 |
| Lentil, Classic, Heinz* | 1 Can/400g | 168.0 | 1.0 | 42 | 2.3 | 7.7 | 0.2 | 1.0 |
| Lentil, Tomato & Vegetable, M & S* | 1 Can/415g | 170.0 | 3.0 | 41 | 2.0 | 6.3 | 0.8 | 1.4 |
| Lentil & Bacon, Baxters* | 1 Can/425g | 221.0 | 4.0 | 52 | 3.2 | 7.7 | 0.9 | 0.7 |
| Lentil & Bacon, Canned, Tesco* | 1 Serving/200g | 96.0 | 1.0 | 48 | 3.2 | 7.2 | 0.7 | 0.5 |
| Lentil & Bacon, Chunky, Fresh, Sainsbury's* | ½ Pot/300g | 117.0 | 2.0 | 39 | 2.3 | 5.7 | 0.8 | 2.0 |
| Lentil & Bacon, Gluten Free, Baxters* | 1 Can/207g | 114.0 | 3.0 | 55 | 2.9 | 7.8 | 1.3 | 0.8 |
| Lentil & Bean, Spicy, Canned, Organic, Asda* | 1 Can/400g | 212.0 | 3.0 | 53 | 2.8 | 8.6 | 0.8 | 3.0 |
| Lentil & Chick Pea, Fresh, Organic, Tesco* | 1 Serving/300ml | 117.0 | 2.0 | 39 | 1.9 | 6.1 | 0.8 | 0.5 |
| Lentil & Pancetta, Tesco* | ½ Can/192g | 115.0 | 2.0 | 60 | 3.1 | 8.0 | 1.3 | 1.6 |
| Lentil & Parsley, Simply Organic* | 1 Pot/600g | 390.0 | 2.0 | 65 | 4.4 | 11.8 | 0.3 | 1.4 |
| Lentil & Red Pepper, Sainsbury's* | ½ Pot/300g | 162.0 | 4.0 | 54 | 3.5 | 7.4 | 1.2 | 1.6 |
| Lentil & Smoked Bacon, Fresh, Tesco* | 1 Pack/600g | 420.0 | 11.0 | 70 | 3.9 | 8.5 | 1.9 | 1.6 |
| Lentil & Tomato, New Covent Garden Food Co* | ½ Pack/284g | 162.0 | 3.0 | 57 | 3.6 | 8.1 | 1.1 | 0.7 |
| Lentil & Tomato, Spicy, Chunky, Fresh, Tesco* | ½ Pot/300g | 195.0 | 5.0 | 65 | 2.6 | 9.7 | 1.8 | 1.3 |
| Lentil & Vegetable, Light Choices, Tesco* | 1 Can/400g | 188.0 | 1.0 | 47 | 2.5 | 8.8 | 0.2 | 1.1 |
| Lentil & Vegetable with Bacon, Organic, Baxters* | ½ Can/211g | 93.0 | 1.0 | 44 | 1.9 | 7.6 | 0.7 | 1.0 |
| Lentil,with Red Lentils, Carrots, Potato & Onion, Asda* | 1 Can/400g | 192.0 | 1.0 | 48 | 1.4 | 10.2 | 0.2 | 1.2 |
| Lincolnshire Sausage Hotpot, Taste of Home, Heinz* | 1 Pot/430g | 301.0 | 13.0 | 70 | 2.4 | 7.9 | 3.1 | 1.0 |
| Lobster Bisque, Baxters* | 1 Can/415g | 187.0 | 9.0 | 45 | 3.0 | 3.6 | 2.1 | 0.2 |
| Lobster Bisque, New Covent Garden Food Co* | ½ Carton/300g | 108.0 | 2.0 | 36 | 3.2 | 4.4 | 0.6 | 0.4 |
| Lobster Bisque, Waitrose* | ½ Carton/300g | 201.0 | 14.0 | 67 | 0.9 | 5.5 | 4.6 | 0.6 |
| Londoner's Pea Souper, New Covent Garden Food Co* | ½ Carton/300g | 153.0 | 6.0 | 51 | 4.3 | 4.1 | 2.0 | 1.1 |
| Luxury Game, Baxters* | 1 Can/415g | 187.0 | 3.0 | 45 | 3.7 | 5.9 | 0.7 | 0.5 |
| Malaysian Chicken & Sweetcorn, Dry, Knorr* | 1 Pack/57g | 211.0 | 6.0 | 370 | 10.6 | 56.3 | 11.4 | 1.8 |
| Mediterranean Fish, Waitrose* | ½ Pot/300g | 108.0 | 3.0 | 36 | 3.4 | 3.5 | 0.9 | 0.7 |
| Mediterranean Minestrone, Campbell's* | ½ Carton/250ml | 95.0 | 3.0 | 38 | 0.9 | 6.1 | 1.1 | 0.6 |
| Mediterranean Tomato, Baxters* | 1 Can/415g | 129.0 | 1.0 | 31 | 0.9 | 6.3 | 0.2 | 0.7 |
| Mediterranean Tomato, Campbell's* | 1 Can/295g | 83.0 | 0.0 | 28 | 0.6 | 6.4 | 0.0 | 0.0 |
| Mediterranean Tomato, COU, M & S* | 1 Pack/415g | 104.0 | 2.0 | 25 | 0.7 | 4.8 | 0.5 | 0.6 |
| Mediterranean Tomato, Dry, Slim Fast* | 1 Sachet/62g | 213.0 | 6.0 | 343 | 22.6 | 39.8 | 9.0 | 10.7 |
| Mediterranean Tomato, Fresh, Organic, Sainsbury's* | 1 Serving/250ml | 77.0 | 3.0 | 31 | 1.3 | 3.3 | 1.4 | 1.0 |
| Mediterranean Tomato, in a Cup, Waitrose* | 1 Sachet/18g | 52.0 | 1.0 | 289 | 8.3 | 45.6 | 8.3 | 10.0 |
| Mediterranean Tomato, Instant, Weight Watchers* | 1 Serving/200ml | 50.0 | 0.0 | 25 | 0.7 | 5.2 | 0.1 | 0.1 |
| Mediterranean Tomato, Slim a Soup, Cup, Batchelors* | 1 Serving/208g | 56.0 | 1.0 | 27 | 0.5 | 4.8 | 0.6 | 0.4 |
| Mediterranean Tomato & Vegetable, Fresh, Tesco* | ½ Pot/300g | 105.0 | 2.0 | 35 | 1.0 | 6.2 | 0.7 | 0.7 |
| Mediterranean Tomato & Vegetable, Soupfulls, Batchelors* | 1 Pouch/400g | 180.0 | 1.0 | 45 | 1.5 | 9.1 | 0.3 | 1.1 |
| Mediterranean Vegetable, GFY, Asda* | ½ Pot/250g | 80.0 | 4.0 | 32 | 0.5 | 3.6 | 1.7 | 1.6 |
| Mediterranean Vegetable, Homepride* | 1 Serving/250ml | 82.0 | 3.0 | 33 | 0.9 | 4.3 | 1.3 | 0.0 |
| Melon & Carrot, New Covent Garden Food Co* | 1 Serving/300g | 60.0 | 1.0 | 20 | 0.6 | 3.6 | 0.4 | 0.6 |
| Mexican Beef Chilli, Mighty, Asda* | 1 Can/400g | 192.0 | 3.0 | 48 | 3.3 | 7.0 | 0.7 | 0.9 |

S

## SOUP

| | Measure INFO/WEIGHT | per Measure KCAL | per Measure FAT | Nutrition Values per 100g / 100ml KCAL | PROT | CARB | FAT | FIBRE |
|---|---|---|---|---|---|---|---|---|
| Mexican Black Bean, Extra Special, Asda* | ½ Pot/263g | 194.0 | 11.0 | 74 | 2.3 | 7.0 | 4.1 | 1.7 |
| Mexican Chilli Beef & Bean, Soups of the World, Heinz* | 1 Can/515g | 360.0 | 9.0 | 70 | 4.5 | 9.0 | 1.8 | 1.6 |
| Mexican Mixed Pepper & Chilli, Cup Soup, Ainsley Harriott* | 1 Sachet/223g | 71.0 | 0.0 | 32 | 0.8 | 7.0 | 0.1 | 0.8 |
| Mexican Spicy Bean, Weight Watchers* | 1 Can/400g | 160.0 | 2.0 | 40 | 1.4 | 7.4 | 0.5 | 1.0 |
| Minestrone, Average | 1 Serving/220g | 139.0 | 7.0 | 63 | 1.8 | 7.6 | 3.0 | 0.9 |
| Minestrone, Baxters* | 1 Can/425g | 144.0 | 2.0 | 34 | 1.5 | 5.9 | 0.5 | 0.9 |
| Minestrone, Canned | 1oz/28g | 9.0 | 0.0 | 32 | 1.4 | 5.1 | 0.8 | 0.6 |
| Minestrone, Canned, M & S* | ½ Can/200g | 60.0 | 1.0 | 30 | 1.2 | 5.7 | 0.5 | 1.5 |
| Minestrone, Carton, Tesco* | ½ Carton/300g | 114.0 | 2.0 | 38 | 1.5 | 6.5 | 0.7 | 1.3 |
| Minestrone, Chilled, M & S* | ½ Pot/300g | 135.0 | 4.0 | 45 | 2.0 | 5.8 | 1.3 | 1.9 |
| Minestrone, Chunky, Big Soup, Heinz* | ½ Can/200g | 74.0 | 2.0 | 37 | 1.3 | 6.2 | 0.8 | 1.1 |
| Minestrone, Chunky, Canned, Sainsbury's* | ½ Can/200g | 80.0 | 1.0 | 40 | 1.5 | 7.2 | 0.6 | 1.2 |
| Minestrone, Chunky, Classic, Fresh, Tesco* | ½ Pot/300g | 126.0 | 2.0 | 42 | 1.2 | 7.8 | 0.7 | 1.2 |
| Minestrone, Chunky, Classic, Meal, Canned, Tesco* | ½ Can/200g | 92.0 | 1.0 | 46 | 2.0 | 8.3 | 0.6 | 1.2 |
| Minestrone, Chunky, COU, M & S* | 1 Bowl/400g | 300.0 | 7.0 | 75 | 3.0 | 11.8 | 1.8 | 0.8 |
| Minestrone, Chunky, Fresh, Baxters* | 1 Serving/250g | 95.0 | 2.0 | 38 | 1.5 | 6.5 | 0.7 | 1.1 |
| Minestrone, Chunky, Fresh, Sainsbury's* | ½ Pot/300g | 93.0 | 1.0 | 31 | 1.4 | 6.1 | 0.2 | 2.3 |
| Minestrone, Classic, Heinz* | 1 Can/400g | 128.0 | 1.0 | 32 | 1.1 | 6.5 | 0.2 | 0.9 |
| Minestrone, Fresh, Asda* | ½ Pot/254g | 89.0 | 2.0 | 35 | 0.8 | 6.0 | 0.9 | 1.2 |
| Minestrone, Fresh, Baxters* | 1 Box/568ml | 233.0 | 6.0 | 41 | 1.8 | 6.2 | 1.0 | 0.6 |
| Minestrone, Healthy Choice, Baxters* | ½ Can/208g | 71.0 | 0.0 | 34 | 0.9 | 7.0 | 0.2 | 1.0 |
| Minestrone, Hearty, 99% Fat Free, Campbell's* | 1 Can/295g | 77.0 | 0.0 | 26 | 0.7 | 5.6 | 0.1 | 0.0 |
| Minestrone, Hearty, Chilled, Farmers Market, Heinz* | ½ Carton/300g | 123.0 | 3.0 | 41 | 1.4 | 6.9 | 0.9 | 0.5 |
| Minestrone, in a Cup, BGTY, Sainsbury's* | 1 Serving/200ml | 54.0 | 0.0 | 27 | 0.8 | 6.0 | 0.1 | 0.6 |
| Minestrone, in a Mug, HL, Tesco* | 1 Sachet/21g | 72.0 | 1.0 | 342 | 3.6 | 67.7 | 6.3 | 3.8 |
| Minestrone, Instant, Under 60 Calories, Tesco* | 1 Sachet/19g | 58.0 | 0.0 | 307 | 7.3 | 63.6 | 2.6 | 2.3 |
| Minestrone, Instant, with Croutons, Value, Tesco* | 1 Sachet/21g | 68.0 | 1.0 | 325 | 6.4 | 60.2 | 6.5 | 1.7 |
| Minestrone, Italian, Canned, Sainsbury's* | 1 Can/415g | 212.0 | 7.0 | 51 | 2.0 | 6.6 | 1.8 | 1.1 |
| Minestrone, Mighty, Dry, Asda* | 1 Serving/38g | 131.0 | 0.0 | 343 | 9.0 | 74.0 | 1.2 | 2.4 |
| Minestrone, New Covent Garden Food Co* | ½ Carton/300g | 111.0 | 4.0 | 37 | 1.5 | 4.7 | 1.4 | 0.9 |
| Minestrone, Organic, M & S* | 1 Pack/208g | 83.0 | 1.0 | 40 | 1.4 | 8.9 | 0.5 | 1.1 |
| Minestrone, Organic, Seeds of Change* | 1 Pack/350g | 227.0 | 12.0 | 65 | 1.4 | 7.4 | 3.3 | 0.9 |
| Minestrone, Packet, Dry, Knorr* | 1 Pack/61g | 178.0 | 3.0 | 292 | 9.2 | 53.9 | 4.4 | 6.5 |
| Minestrone, Sainsbury's* | ½ Can/200g | 66.0 | 1.0 | 33 | 1.1 | 6.3 | 0.4 | 0.9 |
| Minestrone, Simmer, Dry, Asda* | 1 Pack/50g | 131.0 | 1.0 | 262 | 6.0 | 57.0 | 1.1 | 15.0 |
| Minestrone, Simmer & Serve, Dried, Sainsbury's* | 1 Pack/600ml | 108.0 | 0.0 | 18 | 0.5 | 3.9 | 0.0 | 0.4 |
| Minestrone, Soup a Slim, Asda* | 1 Serving/17g | 53.0 | 0.0 | 311 | 6.0 | 69.0 | 1.2 | 4.5 |
| Minestrone, Tuscan, Weight Watchers* | ½ Can/200g | 86.0 | 2.0 | 43 | 1.1 | 7.0 | 1.1 | 0.9 |
| Minestrone, with Borlotti Beans, Tuscan Style, Heinz* | ½ Can/200g | 90.0 | 1.0 | 45 | 1.4 | 8.0 | 0.7 | 1.1 |
| Minestrone, with Croutons, in a Cup, Sainsbury's* | 1 Sachet/225ml | 72.0 | 1.0 | 32 | 0.9 | 6.3 | 0.4 | 0.5 |
| Minestrone, with Croutons, in a Mug, Tesco* | 1 Sachet/23g | 83.0 | 2.0 | 360 | 9.0 | 62.6 | 8.1 | 2.7 |
| Minestrone, with Croutons, Slim a Soup, Batchelors* | 1 Serving/203g | 55.0 | 1.0 | 27 | 0.6 | 4.8 | 0.6 | 0.6 |
| Minestrone, with Pasta, Chunky, Co-Op* | 1 Pack/400g | 140.0 | 2.0 | 35 | 1.0 | 6.0 | 0.6 | 0.7 |
| Minestrone with Wholemeal Pasta, Baxters* | 1 Can/400g | 136.0 | 1.0 | 34 | 0.9 | 7.0 | 0.2 | 1.0 |
| Minted Lamb Hot Pot, Big Soup, Heinz* | 1 Can/400g | 220.0 | 5.0 | 55 | 2.6 | 8.5 | 1.2 | 1.0 |
| Miso, Instant, Blue Dragon* | 1 Sachet/18g | 25.0 | 1.0 | 139 | 10.0 | 14.4 | 3.9 | 0.0 |
| Miso, Instant, Dry, Sanchi* | 1 Sachet/8g | 27.0 | 1.0 | 336 | 18.4 | 48.6 | 7.6 | 0.0 |
| Miso, Organic, Instant, Sanchi* | 1 Sachet/10g | 27.0 | 0.0 | 270 | 14.0 | 47.0 | 3.0 | 0.0 |
| Miso, Wakama* | 1 Sachet/8g | 27.0 | 1.0 | 336 | 18.7 | 48.6 | 7.6 | 0.0 |
| Miso, with Tofu, Instant, Wakama* | 1 Serving/8g | 27.0 | 1.0 | 338 | 17.0 | 51.0 | 7.3 | 0.0 |
| Mixed Bean & Pepper, Organic, M & S* | 1 Pack/208g | 94.0 | 1.0 | 45 | 2.3 | 7.7 | 0.3 | 1.8 |
| Moroccan Chicken, Finest, Tesco* | ½ Pot/300g | 180.0 | 5.0 | 60 | 3.6 | 6.8 | 1.7 | 1.2 |
| Moroccan Chicken, New Covent Garden Food Co* | 1 Serving/300g | 108.0 | 6.0 | 36 | 2.1 | 2.7 | 1.9 | 0.4 |

| | Measure INFO/WEIGHT | per Measure | | Nutrition Values per 100g / 100ml | | | | |
|---|---|---|---|---|---|---|---|---|
| | | KCAL | FAT | KCAL | PROT | CARB | FAT | FIBRE |
| **SOUP** | | | | | | | | |
| Moroccan Lentil, Waitrose* | ½ Pot/300g | 153.0 | 1.0 | 51 | 3.5 | 8.2 | 0.5 | 3.4 |
| Moroccan Style, Extra Special, Asda* | ½ Pot/300g | 183.0 | 4.0 | 61 | 2.9 | 9.4 | 1.3 | 1.0 |
| Mulligatawny | 1 Serving/220g | 213.0 | 15.0 | 97 | 1.4 | 8.2 | 6.8 | 0.9 |
| Mulligatawny, Asda* | 1 Can/400g | 172.0 | 4.0 | 43 | 2.2 | 6.0 | 1.1 | 0.3 |
| Mulligatawny, Canned, Tesco* | 1 Can/400g | 188.0 | 4.0 | 47 | 1.3 | 8.1 | 1.0 | 0.3 |
| Mulligatawny, Classic, Heinz* | 1 Can/400g | 208.0 | 7.0 | 52 | 2.0 | 7.1 | 1.8 | 0.6 |
| Mushroom, 98% Fat Free, Baxters* | 1 Can/425g | 170.0 | 7.0 | 40 | 0.9 | 5.6 | 1.6 | 0.3 |
| Mushroom, Canned, HL, Tesco* | 1 Can/400g | 132.0 | 6.0 | 33 | 0.5 | 4.4 | 1.4 | 0.2 |
| Mushroom, Cream Of, Canned | 1 Serving/220g | 101.0 | 7.0 | 46 | 1.1 | 3.9 | 3.0 | 0.1 |
| Mushroom, Cream Of, Canned, Tesco* | ½ Can/200g | 94.0 | 6.0 | 47 | 0.7 | 4.8 | 2.9 | 0.2 |
| Mushroom, Field, Morrisons* | 1 Pack/600g | 192.0 | 10.0 | 32 | 0.8 | 3.3 | 1.7 | 0.0 |
| Mushroom, Fresh, M & S* | ½ Pack/300g | 165.0 | 12.0 | 55 | 1.8 | 3.5 | 3.9 | 0.9 |
| Mushroom, Hi Taste Low Cal, Cup Soup, Ainsley Harriott* | 1 Sachet/22g | 80.0 | 1.0 | 364 | 12.7 | 63.6 | 4.7 | 3.2 |
| Mushroom, in a Cup, Sainsbury's* | 1 Serving/200ml | 96.0 | 4.0 | 48 | 0.5 | 7.0 | 1.9 | 0.2 |
| Mushroom, Low Fat, Fresh, Sainsbury's* | ½ Pot/300g | 132.0 | 9.0 | 44 | 0.7 | 3.7 | 2.9 | 0.6 |
| Mushroom, Morrisons* | 1 Serving/500g | 250.0 | 18.0 | 50 | 1.3 | 3.2 | 3.6 | 0.3 |
| Mushroom, Simmer & Serve, Dried, Sainsbury's* | ½ Pack/600ml | 234.0 | 10.0 | 39 | 0.6 | 5.5 | 1.6 | 0.3 |
| Mushroom, Weight Watchers* | 1 Can/295g | 83.0 | 2.0 | 28 | 1.1 | 4.5 | 0.7 | 0.1 |
| Mushroom, Wild, New Covent Garden Food Co* | 1 Carton/600g | 228.0 | 10.0 | 38 | 1.2 | 4.8 | 1.6 | 0.6 |
| Mushroom, with Croutons, Soup in a Mug, Tesco* | 1 Pack/26g | 113.0 | 5.0 | 435 | 6.1 | 63.3 | 17.5 | 2.9 |
| Mushroom & Chestnut, Fresh, Finest, Tesco* | 1 Serving/250g | 130.0 | 8.0 | 52 | 1.1 | 4.7 | 3.3 | 0.7 |
| Mushroom & Chicken, Co-Op* | 1 Pack/400g | 220.0 | 16.0 | 55 | 0.9 | 5.0 | 4.0 | 0.0 |
| Mushroom & Crouton, Cup Soup, Made Up, Heinz* | 1 Cup/200ml | 80.0 | 4.0 | 40 | 0.7 | 4.5 | 2.1 | 0.0 |
| Mushroom & Garlic, Slimming Cup a Soup, Tesco* | 1 Serving/16g | 58.0 | 2.0 | 360 | 5.8 | 61.1 | 10.3 | 3.2 |
| Mushroom & Madeira Flavour, Soup in a Mug, Safeway* | 1 Sachet/28g | 114.0 | 4.0 | 406 | 3.2 | 67.3 | 13.8 | 1.0 |
| Mushroom & Mascarpone, Fresh, TTD, Sainsbury's* | ½ Carton/300ml | 108.0 | 7.0 | 36 | 0.6 | 2.8 | 2.5 | 0.4 |
| Mushroom & Tarragon, Fresh, TTD, Sainsbury's* | ½ Pot/300ml | 201.0 | 13.0 | 67 | 1.4 | 5.8 | 4.2 | 0.7 |
| Mushroom Creme Fraiche, Waistline, Crosse & Blackwell* | 1 Carton/300g | 69.0 | 2.0 | 23 | 1.2 | 2.8 | 0.8 | 0.3 |
| Mushroom Potage, Baxters* | 1 Can/415g | 320.0 | 22.0 | 77 | 1.5 | 6.1 | 5.2 | 0.3 |
| Oxtail, Baxters* | 1 Can/415g | 187.0 | 5.0 | 45 | 1.9 | 6.4 | 1.3 | 0.5 |
| Oxtail, Canned | 1 Serving/220g | 97.0 | 4.0 | 44 | 2.4 | 5.1 | 1.7 | 0.1 |
| Oxtail, Canned, Sainsbury's* | 1 Can/400g | 132.0 | 2.0 | 33 | 2.3 | 5.1 | 0.4 | 0.2 |
| Oxtail, Canned, Tesco* | 1 Can/400g | 152.0 | 3.0 | 38 | 2.0 | 5.9 | 0.7 | 0.3 |
| Oxtail, Classic, Heinz* | 1 Can/400g | 156.0 | 2.0 | 39 | 1.9 | 6.7 | 0.5 | 0.3 |
| Oxtail, Condensed, Classics, Diluted, Campbell's* | 1 Can/590g | 236.0 | 9.0 | 40 | 1.4 | 5.3 | 1.5 | 0.0 |
| Oxtail, M & S* | 1 Serving/415g | 207.0 | 6.0 | 50 | 2.1 | 6.9 | 1.4 | 0.5 |
| Oxtail, Soup in a Cup, Sainsbury's* | 1 Serving/223ml | 69.0 | 1.0 | 31 | 1.0 | 5.7 | 0.5 | 0.2 |
| Paddestoelen, Cup a Soup, Made Up, Batchelors* | 1 Serving/100ml | 5.0 | 0.0 | 5 | 0.4 | 0.6 | 0.1 | 0.2 |
| Pamplona Picante Chorizo & 3 Bean, TTD, Sainsbury's* | 1 Pack/300g | 162.0 | 2.0 | 54 | 4.0 | 7.6 | 0.8 | 5.8 |
| Parsnip, Fresh, Morrisons* | ½ Pot/250g | 100.0 | 4.0 | 40 | 0.9 | 5.8 | 1.5 | 1.4 |
| Parsnip, Fresh, VLH Kitchens* | 1 Serving/400g | 180.0 | 6.4 | 45 | 0.9 | 5.8 | 1.6 | 1.4 |
| Parsnip, Honey & Ginger, COU, M & S* | 1 Can/415g | 124.0 | 2.0 | 30 | 0.7 | 5.3 | 0.6 | 0.7 |
| Parsnip, Leek & Ginger, New Covent Garden Food Co* | 1 Carton/600g | 162.0 | 2.0 | 27 | 1.2 | 4.9 | 0.3 | 1.3 |
| Parsnip, Spicy, Fresh, Tesco* | 1 Serving/300g | 123.0 | 6.0 | 41 | 0.8 | 4.6 | 2.1 | 1.9 |
| Parsnip & Apple, COU, M & S* | 1 Can/415g | 187.0 | 10.0 | 45 | 0.7 | 5.4 | 2.5 | 1.2 |
| Parsnip & Honey, Fresh, Sainsbury's* | ½ Carton/300g | 192.0 | 13.0 | 64 | 1.1 | 5.4 | 4.2 | 1.5 |
| Pea, Artichoke & Parmesan, The Best, Morrisons* | ½ Pot/300g | 171.0 | 8.0 | 57 | 2.8 | 5.6 | 2.6 | 1.0 |
| Pea, in a Cup, Symingtons* | 1 Sachet/31g | 95.0 | 2.0 | 311 | 7.2 | 54.1 | 7.2 | 6.9 |
| Pea, Organic, Suma* | 1 Can /400g | 272.0 | 9.0 | 68 | 2.7 | 9.4 | 2.2 | 0.7 |
| Pea & Ham | 1oz/28g | 20.0 | 1.0 | 70 | 4.0 | 9.2 | 2.1 | 1.4 |
| Pea & Ham, Baxters* | 1 Can/425g | 212.0 | 2.0 | 50 | 3.0 | 8.3 | 0.5 | 0.9 |
| Pea & Ham, Canned, Tesco* | 1 Can/400g | 240.0 | 4.0 | 60 | 2.6 | 9.0 | 1.1 | 0.8 |
| Pea & Ham, Classic, Heinz* | 1 Can/400g | 216.0 | 3.0 | 54 | 2.7 | 9.0 | 0.7 | 1.0 |

# SOUP

| INFO/WEIGHT | Measure | per Measure KCAL | FAT | Nutrition Values per 100g / 100ml KCAL | PROT | CARB | FAT | FIBRE |
|---|---|---|---|---|---|---|---|---|
| Pea & Ham, Creamy, Chunky, Meal, Weight Watchers* | 1 Pack/340g | 156.0 | 4.0 | 46 | 2.3 | 6.8 | 1.1 | 2.0 |
| Pea & Ham, Extra Thick, In A Cup, Sainsbury's* | 1 Sachet/224ml | 85.0 | 2.0 | 38 | 1.1 | 6.7 | 0.8 | 0.4 |
| Pea & Ham, Fresh, Sainsbury's* | ½ Pack/300ml | 120.0 | 1.0 | 40 | 1.9 | 7.0 | 0.5 | 0.3 |
| Pea & Mint, Baxters* | 1 Serving/300g | 186.0 | 10.0 | 62 | 2.3 | 6.1 | 3.2 | 1.5 |
| Pea & Mint, Fresh, Sainsbury's* | ½ Pot/300g | 141.0 | 7.0 | 47 | 1.8 | 4.8 | 2.3 | 2.3 |
| Pea & Mint, Fresh, Tesco* | 1 Serving/300g | 207.0 | 13.0 | 69 | 2.4 | 5.1 | 4.4 | 0.0 |
| Pea & Mint, New Covent Garden Food Co* | ½ Pack/300g | 168.0 | 6.0 | 56 | 2.5 | 7.1 | 1.9 | 1.7 |
| Pea & Mint, Tinned, Tesco* | 1 Can/400g | 180.0 | 3.0 | 45 | 2.0 | 7.8 | 0.7 | 1.3 |
| Pea & Smoked Ham, Farmers Market, Heinz* | ½ Can/258g | 103.0 | 1.0 | 40 | 3.5 | 5.6 | 0.4 | 0.8 |
| Peking Shiitake Mushroom Noodle, Baxters* | 1 Serving/215g | 90.0 | 2.0 | 42 | 1.3 | 7.5 | 0.8 | 0.2 |
| Pepper & Chorizo, Canned, Sainsbury's* | 1 Can/400ml | 172.0 | 4.0 | 43 | 7.0 | 2.0 | 1.0 | 0.0 |
| Peppered Steak Casserole, Taste of Home, Heinz* | 1 Pot/430g | 219.0 | 4.0 | 51 | 2.8 | 7.7 | 0.9 | 0.7 |
| Plum Tomato & Basil, New Covent Garden Food Co* | ½ Carton/300g | 132.0 | 6.0 | 44 | 1.3 | 5.2 | 2.0 | 1.3 |
| Plum Tomato & Basil Soup, Farmers Market, Heinz* | 1 Can/515g | 247.0 | 14.0 | 48 | 0.7 | 5.3 | 2.7 | 0.7 |
| Pork, Chinese Dumpling, New Cultural Revolution* | 1 Serving/250ml | 156.0 | 4.0 | 62 | 6.4 | 6.0 | 1.6 | 0.4 |
| Pork & Stuffing, Taste of Home, Heinz* | 1 Pot/408g | 241.0 | 6.0 | 59 | 3.0 | 8.6 | 1.4 | 1.0 |
| Potato, Leek & Bacon, Fresh, Baxters* | ½ Pot/300g | 249.0 | 17.0 | 83 | 2.0 | 6.1 | 5.6 | 0.7 |
| Potato, Leek & Chicken, Canned, BGTY, Sainsbury's* | ½ Can/200g | 62.0 | 1.0 | 31 | 1.6 | 5.3 | 0.4 | 0.4 |
| Potato, Leek & Thyme, Farmers Market, Heinz* | 1 Can/515g | 294.0 | 15.0 | 57 | 0.9 | 6.7 | 3.0 | 0.6 |
| Potato & Leek | 1oz/28g | 15.0 | 1.0 | 52 | 1.5 | 6.2 | 2.6 | 0.8 |
| Potato & Leek, Canned, Baxters* | 1 Can/415g | 183.0 | 3.0 | 44 | 1.2 | 8.1 | 0.8 | 0.9 |
| Potato & Leek, Classics, Canned, Heinz* | 1 Can/400g | 184.0 | 7.0 | 46 | 0.8 | 6.7 | 1.8 | 0.6 |
| Potato & Leek with Peppers & Chicken, Stockmeyer* | ½ Can/200g | 118.0 | 5.0 | 59 | 2.6 | 6.7 | 2.4 | 0.8 |
| Proscuitto, Pea, & Potato Soup, Pret a Manger* | 1 Pack/291g | 178.0 | 13.0 | 61 | 2.7 | 6.6 | 4.6 | 0.8 |
| Pumpkin, Creamy, Very Special, Heinz* | 1 Sm Can/290g | 188.0 | 6.0 | 65 | 1.3 | 9.9 | 1.9 | 1.1 |
| Pumpkin, New Covent Garden Food Co* | ½ Pint/284ml | 97.0 | 3.0 | 34 | 0.4 | 5.5 | 1.1 | 0.6 |
| Pumpkin, Spicy, Fresh, Sainsbury's* | ½ Pot/300g | 87.0 | 3.0 | 29 | 0.9 | 4.2 | 1.0 | 1.3 |
| Pumpkin & Bramley Apple, New Covent Garden Food Co* | ½ Carton/300g | 99.0 | 2.0 | 33 | 1.1 | 5.9 | 0.6 | 0.8 |
| Pumpkin & Ginger, in a Cup, Symingtons* | 1 Serving/200ml | 66.0 | 3.0 | 33 | 0.4 | 4.7 | 1.4 | 0.4 |
| Puy Lentil & Tomato, Healthy Choice, Baxters* | ½ Can/207g | 118.0 | 1.0 | 57 | 3.1 | 10.5 | 0.3 | 2.7 |
| Puy Lentil & Vine Ripened Tomato, Finest, Tesco* | 1 Pot/600g | 360.0 | 8.0 | 60 | 2.8 | 9.2 | 1.3 | 1.5 |
| Red Lentil & Ham, Waitrose* | ½ Pot/300g | 147.0 | 3.0 | 49 | 3.9 | 5.8 | 1.1 | 2.0 |
| Red Lentil & Tomato, Canned, Tesco* | ½ Can/300g | 189.0 | 4.0 | 63 | 4.0 | 8.9 | 1.3 | 1.1 |
| Red Lentil & Vegetable, Favourties, Canned, Baxters* | 1 Can/415g | 166.0 | 1.0 | 40 | 2.2 | 7.4 | 0.2 | 1.0 |
| Red Pepper, Tomato & Basil, M & S* | 1 Can/415g | 83.0 | 1.0 | 20 | 1.3 | 2.7 | 0.3 | 0.8 |
| Red Pepper & Tomato, Canned, Sainsbury's* | 1 Can/400g | 120.0 | 4.0 | 30 | 0.9 | 4.1 | 1.1 | 1.6 |
| Red Pepper & Tomato, Canned, Weight Watchers* | 1 Can /295g | 35.0 | 0.0 | 12 | 0.4 | 2.4 | 0.1 | 0.4 |
| Red Pepper & Tomato, Vie, Knorr* | 1 Pack/500ml | 195.0 | 6.0 | 39 | 0.8 | 6.4 | 1.2 | 1.0 |
| Roasted Red Pepper, Fresh, Waitrose* | 1 Pack/600g | 172.0 | 9.0 | 29 | 0.8 | 3.0 | 1.5 | 1.0 |
| Roasted Vegetable, Chunky, M & S* | 1 Can/400g | 140.0 | 2.0 | 35 | 1.3 | 5.8 | 0.6 | 1.1 |
| Roasted Vegetable, Fresh, Sainsbury's* | ½ Pot/300ml | 78.0 | 1.0 | 26 | 0.5 | 4.8 | 0.5 | 1.2 |
| Roasted Winter Vegetable, Fresh, TTD, Sainsbury's* | ½ Pot/300ml | 129.0 | 9.0 | 43 | 0.5 | 3.4 | 3.0 | 1.0 |
| Root Vegetable, & Butternut Squash, Deli Inspired, Baxters* | 1 Can/415g | 187.0 | 1.0 | 45 | 1.9 | 8.7 | 0.3 | 1.4 |
| Root Vegetable & Barley, Broth, Special, Heinz* | 1 Can/400g | 188.0 | 6.0 | 47 | 0.9 | 7.4 | 1.5 | 1.1 |
| San Marzano Tomato & Mascarpone, Finest, Tesco* | ½ Pot/300g | 225.0 | 13.0 | 75 | 1.3 | 6.7 | 4.5 | 0.7 |
| San Marzano Tomato & Mascarpone, M & S* | 1 Serving/150g | 97.0 | 6.0 | 65 | 1.4 | 5.7 | 4.3 | 2.0 |
| Sausage & Bean, Spicy, Meal, Canned, Tesco* | 1 Can/500g | 265.0 | 7.0 | 53 | 2.8 | 6.4 | 1.4 | 1.2 |
| Scotch Broth, Baxters* | 1 Can/415g | 166.0 | 4.0 | 40 | 1.6 | 6.4 | 0.9 | 0.7 |
| Scotch Broth, British, Sainsbury's* | 1 Can/415g | 149.0 | 3.0 | 36 | 1.9 | 5.4 | 0.7 | 0.9 |
| Scotch Broth, Canned, Tesco* | ½ Can/200g | 72.0 | 2.0 | 36 | 1.4 | 6.4 | 0.9 | 0.8 |
| Scotch Broth, Classic, Heinz* | 1 Can/400g | 168.0 | 5.0 | 42 | 1.5 | 6.0 | 1.3 | 0.8 |
| Scotch Broth, Fresh, Baxters* | 1 Serving/300g | 108.0 | 2.0 | 36 | 1.6 | 5.9 | 0.7 | 0.6 |
| Scotch Broth, Fresh, Tesco* | ½ Pack/300g | 129.0 | 5.0 | 43 | 1.7 | 5.0 | 1.8 | 1.4 |

S

| | Measure INFO/WEIGHT | per Measure | | Nutrition Values per 100g / 100ml | | | | |
|---|---|---|---|---|---|---|---|---|
| | | KCAL | FAT | KCAL | PROT | CARB | FAT | FIBRE |

## SOUP

| | Measure INFO/WEIGHT | KCAL | FAT | KCAL | PROT | CARB | FAT | FIBRE |
|---|---|---|---|---|---|---|---|---|
| Scotch Broth, New Covent Garden Food Co* | 1 Carton/600g | 240.0 | 15.0 | 40 | 1.6 | 2.8 | 2.5 | 0.5 |
| Scotch Vegetable, Baxters* | 1 Can/425g | 183.0 | 3.0 | 43 | 1.9 | 7.4 | 0.6 | 1.2 |
| Scottish Vegetable with Lentils & Beef, Heinz* | 1 Can/404g | 210.0 | 3.0 | 52 | 3.4 | 8.2 | 0.7 | 1.2 |
| Seasoned Chicken with Sweetcorn & Croutons, Slim Fast* | 1 Pack/60g | 211.0 | 6.0 | 351 | 23.7 | 36.8 | 10.6 | 9.7 |
| Smoked Haddock Chowder, New Covent Garden Food Co* | ½ Carton/300g | 177.0 | 5.0 | 59 | 2.2 | 8.3 | 1.8 | 0.9 |
| Smoked Salmon & Dill, Fresh, Finest, Tesco* | ½ Carton/300g | 240.0 | 16.0 | 80 | 2.2 | 5.3 | 5.5 | 0.6 |
| Smokey Bacon, Leek & Potato, Big Soup, Canned, Heinz* | 1 Can/515g | 278.0 | 11.0 | 54 | 1.9 | 6.6 | 2.1 | 0.6 |
| Smoky Chicken & Wild Rice, Heinz* | 1 Can/535g | 182.0 | 3.0 | 34 | 2.1 | 5.3 | 0.6 | 0.8 |
| Soup, Leek & Potato, Fresh, Sainsbury's* | ½ Pot/300g | 114.0 | 4.0 | 38 | 0.7 | 6.1 | 1.2 | 1.3 |
| Spiced Chicken & Chickpea, Moroccan, TTD, Sainsbury's* | ½ Pot/300g | 192.0 | 4.0 | 64 | 3.6 | 9.2 | 1.4 | 1.8 |
| Spiced Chickpea & Fresh Red Pepper, M & S* | 1 Serving/300g | 165.0 | 7.0 | 55 | 2.2 | 5.8 | 2.3 | 2.5 |
| Spiced Spinach & Green Lentil, Asda* | ½ Pot/250g | 122.0 | 5.0 | 49 | 2.7 | 5.0 | 2.0 | 0.0 |
| Spicy, Three Bean, Tesco* | ½ Carton/300g | 165.0 | 4.0 | 55 | 2.8 | 7.3 | 1.5 | 2.1 |
| Spicy Lentil, COU, M & S* | 1 Pack/415g | 187.0 | 4.0 | 45 | 2.6 | 6.7 | 0.9 | 1.2 |
| Spicy Lentil, Cup, Made Up, Ainsley Harriott* | 1 Sachet/226ml | 86.0 | 1.0 | 38 | 1.1 | 7.3 | 0.5 | 0.4 |
| Spicy Lentil, Hi Taste Low Cal, Cup Soup, Ainsley Harriott* | 1 Sachet/22g | 67.0 | 0.0 | 305 | 12.3 | 60.4 | 1.4 | 4.1 |
| Spicy Lentil, In A Mug, Light Choices, Tesco* | 1 Sachet/221ml | 62.0 | 0.0 | 28 | 1.1 | 5.9 | 0.0 | 0.0 |
| Spicy Lentil, Seeds of Change* | 1 Pack/422g | 190.0 | 1.0 | 45 | 2.5 | 8.2 | 0.2 | 1.9 |
| Spicy Lentil & Vegetable, Chilled, M & S* | ½ Serving/600g | 300.0 | 5.0 | 50 | 2.7 | 8.0 | 0.8 | 1.1 |
| Spicy Lentil & Vegetable, Micro, Tesco* | 1 Serving/330g | 214.0 | 6.0 | 65 | 2.2 | 9.4 | 1.9 | 0.9 |
| Spicy Mixed Bean, Big Soup, Heinz* | 1 Serving/200g | 78.0 | 1.0 | 39 | 2.3 | 6.7 | 0.3 | 2.0 |
| Spicy Parsnip, New Covent Garden Food Co* | ½ Box/297g | 116.0 | 4.0 | 39 | 0.9 | 5.8 | 1.3 | 1.8 |
| Spicy Parsnip, Vegetarian, Baxters* | 1 Can/425g | 217.0 | 11.0 | 51 | 1.1 | 6.1 | 2.5 | 1.5 |
| Spicy Red Curry, Blue Dragon* | 1 Serving/205g | 97.0 | 5.0 | 47 | 0.4 | 5.8 | 2.5 | 0.3 |
| Spicy Tomato, Cup a Soup, Batchelors* | 1 Sachet/23g | 74.0 | 1.0 | 322 | 7.6 | 65.8 | 3.2 | 3.2 |
| Spinach & Nutmeg, New Covent Garden Food Co* | ½ Carton/300g | 147.0 | 7.0 | 49 | 1.9 | 5.3 | 2.2 | 1.0 |
| Spinach & Watercress, New Covent Garden Food Co* | ½ Carton/298g | 60.0 | 1.0 | 20 | 1.3 | 2.8 | 0.4 | 0.8 |
| Split Pea & Ham, Asda* | 1 Serving/300g | 129.0 | 1.0 | 43 | 3.5 | 6.9 | 0.2 | 0.7 |
| Split Peas, Yellow, Simply Organic* | 1 Pot/600g | 354.0 | 3.0 | 59 | 4.3 | 10.4 | 0.5 | 2.6 |
| Spring Vegetable, Classic, Heinz* | 1 Can/400g | 136.0 | 2.0 | 34 | 0.8 | 6.8 | 0.4 | 0.7 |
| Spring Vegetable, Condensed, Campbell's* | 1 Can/295g | 62.0 | 0.0 | 21 | 0.5 | 4.5 | 0.1 | 0.0 |
| Steak, Potato & Ale, Chunky, Sainsbury's* | 1 Can/400g | 152.0 | 2.0 | 38 | 2.2 | 5.9 | 0.6 | 0.8 |
| Steak & Guiness Casserole, Taste of Home, Heinz* | 1 Pot/430g | 271.0 | 7.0 | 63 | 3.2 | 8.4 | 1.7 | 0.0 |
| Steak & Potato, Big Soup, Heinz* | ½ Can/258g | 129.0 | 2.0 | 50 | 3.0 | 7.7 | 0.8 | 0.8 |
| Stilton, Celery & Watercress, Morrisons* | 1 Serving/250g | 272.0 | 23.0 | 109 | 3.9 | 3.1 | 9.2 | 0.3 |
| Summer Vegetable, with Pasta, Cup a Soup, Batchelors* | 1 Serving/33g | 16.0 | 0.0 | 50 | 1.4 | 8.5 | 1.1 | 1.0 |
| Sun Dried Tomato & Basil, Heinz* | 1 Serving/275ml | 124.0 | 5.0 | 45 | 0.6 | 6.5 | 1.9 | 0.1 |
| Sweet Cherry Tomato, Fresh, TTD, Sainsbury's* | 1 Pack/300g | 120.0 | 4.0 | 40 | 0.7 | 6.0 | 1.5 | 1.0 |
| Sweet Potato, Chickpea & Coriander, BGTY, Sainsbury's* | 1 Can/400g | 188.0 | 2.0 | 47 | 1.4 | 9.3 | 0.5 | 1.3 |
| Sweet Potato & Coconut, COU, M & S* | 1 Can/415g | 166.0 | 5.0 | 40 | 0.7 | 6.7 | 1.3 | 0.8 |
| Sweetcorn & Chicken, Cup, Calorie Counter, Co-Op* | 1 Sachet/11g | 35.0 | 1.0 | 315 | 5.0 | 49.0 | 11.0 | 11.0 |
| Sweetcorn & Chilli, COU, M & S* | ½ Can/275g | 137.0 | 7.0 | 50 | 0.9 | 6.1 | 2.4 | 0.4 |
| Sweetcorn & Chilli Chowder, Simply Organic* | ½ Pot/300g | 126.0 | 3.0 | 42 | 2.2 | 6.1 | 0.9 | 3.8 |
| Tangy Tomato, Extra, Slim a Soup, Batchelors* | 1 Pack/253g | 121.0 | 2.0 | 48 | 1.2 | 9.0 | 0.8 | 0.4 |
| Tangy Tomato, Slim a Soup, Batchelors* | 1 Serving/230ml | 81.0 | 1.0 | 35 | 1.1 | 6.7 | 0.4 | 0.5 |
| Tangy Tomato & Rice, Weight Watchers* | 1 Can/295g | 115.0 | 0.0 | 39 | 1.1 | 8.4 | 0.1 | 0.4 |
| Thai Chicken, New Covent Garden Food Co* | ½ Carton/300g | 174.0 | 10.0 | 58 | 2.6 | 4.1 | 3.5 | 0.8 |
| Thai Green Curry, with Chicken, Soups of the World, Heinz* | ½ Can/258g | 183.0 | 11.0 | 71 | 2.1 | 6.5 | 4.1 | 0.4 |
| Thai Pumpkin Coconut, New Covent Garden Food Co* | 1 Carton/568ml | 182.0 | 7.0 | 32 | 1.3 | 3.5 | 1.3 | 1.1 |
| Three Bean, Chunky, M & S* | 1 Can/415g | 207.0 | 5.0 | 50 | 2.3 | 7.5 | 1.2 | 1.8 |
| Three Bean & Smoked Bacon, Farmers Market, Heinz* | 1 Can/515g | 340.0 | 11.0 | 66 | 4.0 | 7.5 | 2.2 | 1.9 |
| Three Bean & Tomato, Autumn, Farmers Market, Heinz* | ½ Carton/300g | 132.0 | 1.0 | 44 | 2.3 | 7.5 | 0.5 | 0.5 |
| Tomato, & Lentil, Mediterranean, Weight Watchers* | 1 Can/400g | 184.0 | 2.0 | 46 | 2.3 | 7.8 | 0.6 | 1.0 |

S

| | Measure INFO/WEIGHT | KCAL | FAT | KCAL | PROT | CARB | FAT | FIBRE |
|---|---|---|---|---|---|---|---|---|
| **SOUP** | | | | | | | | |
| Tomato, 99% Fat Free, Wattie's* | 1 Serving/105g | 32.0 | 0.0 | 31 | 1.0 | 5.6 | 0.4 | 1.1 |
| Tomato, Basil & Chilli, Microwave, Sainsbury's* | 1 Pot/345g | 100.0 | 2.0 | 29 | 1.0 | 5.0 | 0.6 | 1.2 |
| Tomato, Canned, HL, Tesco* | ½ Can/200g | 110.0 | 4.0 | 55 | 0.7 | 7.4 | 2.0 | 0.5 |
| Tomato, Cannellini & Borlotti Bean, M & S* | ½ Pot/300g | 195.0 | 10.0 | 65 | 2.1 | 6.7 | 3.3 | 2.5 |
| Tomato, Cream Of, Asda* | ½ Can/200g | 122.0 | 6.0 | 61 | 0.7 | 7.3 | 3.2 | 0.7 |
| Tomato, Cream Of, Canned | 1oz/28g | 15.0 | 1.0 | 52 | 0.8 | 5.9 | 3.0 | 0.7 |
| Tomato, Cream Of, Classic, Heinz* | ½ Can/200g | 114.0 | 6.0 | 57 | 0.9 | 6.7 | 3.0 | 0.4 |
| Tomato, Cream Of, Condensed, Batchelors* | 1 Can/295g | 454.0 | 19.0 | 154 | 1.7 | 21.9 | 6.6 | 0.6 |
| Tomato, Cream Of, Dry, Knorr* | 1 Pack/90g | 391.0 | 21.0 | 435 | 4.3 | 51.3 | 23.6 | 3.3 |
| Tomato, Cream Of, Favourites, Baxters* | 1 Can/415g | 257.0 | 11.0 | 62 | 1.0 | 8.4 | 2.7 | 0.3 |
| Tomato, Cream Of, Fresh, Sainsbury's* | ½ Pot/300ml | 126.0 | 4.0 | 42 | 0.9 | 7.0 | 1.2 | 0.6 |
| Tomato, Cream Of, Fresh, Tesco* | ½ Tub/300g | 168.0 | 6.0 | 56 | 1.4 | 8.4 | 1.9 | 0.4 |
| Tomato, Cream Of, Homepride* | ¼ Bottle/250ml | 137.0 | 6.0 | 55 | 0.9 | 7.7 | 2.6 | 0.0 |
| Tomato, Cream Of, In A Cup, Sainsbury's* | 1 Sachet/233ml | 112.0 | 2.0 | 48 | 0.7 | 9.3 | 0.9 | 0.1 |
| Tomato, Cream Of, Microwaveable Cup, Heinz* | 1 Cup/275ml | 169.0 | 9.0 | 61 | 0.8 | 6.9 | 3.4 | 0.4 |
| Tomato, Cream Of, Organic, Heinz* | 1 Can/400g | 220.0 | 10.0 | 55 | 1.0 | 7.0 | 2.6 | 0.4 |
| Tomato, Cream Of, Prepared, Campbell's* | ½ Can/295g | 195.0 | 9.0 | 66 | 0.8 | 8.5 | 3.2 | 0.0 |
| Tomato, Cream Of, Sainsbury's* | 1 Can/400g | 244.0 | 13.0 | 61 | 0.7 | 7.3 | 3.2 | 0.7 |
| Tomato, Cream Of, with a Hint of Basil, Heinz* | ½ Can/200g | 114.0 | 6.0 | 57 | 0.9 | 6.6 | 3.0 | 0.4 |
| Tomato, Cream Of, With Red Pepper, Classic, Heinz* | 1 Can/400g | 232.0 | 12.0 | 58 | 0.9 | 7.0 | 2.9 | 0.6 |
| Tomato, Creamy, Fresh, Asda* | 1 Tub/300g | 135.0 | 6.0 | 45 | 1.2 | 5.5 | 2.0 | 1.4 |
| Tomato, Creme Fraiche & Basil, The Best, Safeway* | 1/3 Pot/200g | 130.0 | 8.0 | 65 | 1.0 | 5.0 | 4.2 | 1.0 |
| Tomato, Cup a Soup, Made Up, Batchelors* | 1 Sachet/256g | 92.0 | 2.0 | 36 | 0.3 | 6.7 | 0.9 | 0.3 |
| Tomato, Hi Taste Low Cal, Cup Soup, Ainsley Harriott* | 1 Sachet/22g | 70.0 | 0.0 | 318 | 8.6 | 65.9 | 2.3 | 3.6 |
| Tomato, in a Cup, Tesco* | 1 Serving/23g | 75.0 | 1.0 | 328 | 6.4 | 68.5 | 3.2 | 0.1 |
| Tomato, Meditarranean, In A Mug, Light Choices, Tesco* | 1 Sachet/220ml | 62.0 | 0.0 | 28 | 0.6 | 6.0 | 0.2 | 0.6 |
| Tomato, Mediterranean, Rich, Fresh, Baxters* | 1 Carton/600g | 318.0 | 10.0 | 53 | 1.8 | 7.7 | 1.7 | 1.1 |
| Tomato, Onion & Basil, GFY, Asda* | 1 Can/400g | 96.0 | 3.0 | 24 | 1.0 | 3.4 | 0.7 | 1.7 |
| Tomato, Red Pepper & Basil, Thick & Creamy, Asda* | 1 Sachet/24g | 89.0 | 2.0 | 370 | 5.6 | 65.7 | 9.4 | 5.5 |
| Tomato, Rice & Sweetcorn, Baxters* | 1 Serving/400ml | 256.0 | 7.0 | 64 | 2.0 | 9.9 | 1.8 | 1.1 |
| Tomato, San Marzano, & Fresh Basil, TTD, Sainsbury's* | ½ Pot/300g | 168.0 | 9.0 | 56 | 1.6 | 5.7 | 3.0 | 1.8 |
| Tomato, Simmer & Serve, Dried, Sainsbury's* | 1 Serving/200ml | 70.0 | 2.0 | 35 | 0.3 | 6.0 | 1.1 | 0.4 |
| Tomato, Sweet Chilli, & Pasta, Classic, Heinz* | ½ Can/200g | 74.0 | 0.0 | 37 | 0.8 | 8.0 | 0.1 | 0.3 |
| Tomato, Three Bean & Bacon, Sainsbury's* | ½ Can/200g | 86.0 | 2.0 | 43 | 3.1 | 5.4 | 1.0 | 3.0 |
| Tomato, Vegetable Garden, Campbell's* | 1 Can/310g | 240.0 | 3.0 | 77 | 1.6 | 16.1 | 0.9 | 0.0 |
| Tomato, Weight Watchers* | 1 Can/295g | 74.0 | 1.0 | 25 | 0.7 | 4.5 | 0.5 | 0.5 |
| Tomato & Basil, Campbell's* | 1 Pack/500ml | 205.0 | 6.0 | 41 | 0.7 | 6.7 | 1.3 | 1.1 |
| Tomato & Basil, Cup a Soup, Made Up, GFY, Asda* | 1 Serving/250ml | 50.0 | 0.0 | 20 | 0.4 | 4.4 | 0.1 | 0.2 |
| Tomato & Basil, Fresh, Finest, Tesco* | ½ Pot/300g | 219.0 | 15.0 | 73 | 1.0 | 6.3 | 4.9 | 0.6 |
| Tomato & Basil, Fresh, Low Fat, Sainsbury's* | ½ Carton/300ml | 75.0 | 2.0 | 25 | 1.1 | 4.1 | 0.6 | 0.7 |
| Tomato & Basil, Fresh, Morrisons* | Pot/600g | 234.0 | 4.0 | 39 | 1.5 | 6.6 | 0.7 | 1.0 |
| Tomato & Basil, Fresh, Sainsbury's* | ½ Pot/300g | 93.0 | 1.0 | 31 | 0.9 | 5.7 | 0.5 | 0.6 |
| Tomato & Basil, Fresh, So Organic, Sainsbury's* | ½ Carton/200g | 100.0 | 4.0 | 50 | 0.5 | 7.5 | 2.0 | 0.2 |
| Tomato & Basil, Fresh, Tesco* | ½ Pack/300g | 138.0 | 5.0 | 46 | 0.9 | 6.9 | 1.6 | 0.6 |
| Tomato & Basil, GFY, Asda* | 1 Serving/250ml | 100.0 | 3.0 | 40 | 0.9 | 6.0 | 1.4 | 1.6 |
| Tomato & Basil, Italian, 99% Fat Free, Baxters* | ½ Can/208g | 119.0 | 2.0 | 57 | 2.6 | 9.3 | 1.0 | 1.1 |
| Tomato & Basil, Loyd Grossman* | ½ Pack/210g | 97.0 | 4.0 | 46 | 0.8 | 6.4 | 1.9 | 0.2 |
| Tomato & Basil, Soup-A-Slim, Asda* | 1 Sachet/16g | 52.0 | 0.0 | 326 | 7.0 | 70.0 | 2.0 | 3.9 |
| Tomato & Basil, Vie, Knorr* | 1 Pack/500ml | 145.0 | 2.0 | 29 | 0.8 | 5.5 | 0.4 | 0.9 |
| Tomato & Basil with Onion, Waistline, Crosse & Blackwell* | 1 Serving/300g | 87.0 | 2.0 | 29 | 0.9 | 5.1 | 0.6 | 0.3 |
| Tomato & Brown Lentil, Healthy Choice, Baxters* | 1 Can/415g | 199.0 | 1.0 | 48 | 2.6 | 9.0 | 0.2 | 2.7 |
| Tomato & Brown Lentil, Healthy Choice, Heinz* | ½ Can/208g | 112.0 | 1.0 | 54 | 3.1 | 9.6 | 0.3 | 1.5 |
| Tomato & Butterbean, Baxters* | 1 Can/415g | 166.0 | 5.0 | 40 | 1.2 | 6.1 | 1.2 | 1.0 |

| | Measure INFO/WEIGHT | per Measure KCAL | FAT | Nutrition Values per 100g / 100ml KCAL | PROT | CARB | FAT | FIBRE |
|---|---|---|---|---|---|---|---|---|
| **SOUP** | | | | | | | | |
| Tomato & Chorizo, Mediterranean, Tesco* | 1 Serving/200g | 130.0 | 7.0 | 65 | 2.0 | 6.1 | 3.4 | 0.3 |
| Tomato & Herb, Campbell's* | 1 Carton/500ml | 180.0 | 6.0 | 36 | 1.0 | 5.0 | 1.3 | 0.0 |
| Tomato & Lentil, M & S* | ½ Can/211g | 95.0 | 0.0 | 45 | 2.3 | 8.4 | 0.2 | 1.5 |
| Tomato & Lentil, Mediteranean, Weight Watchers* | 1 Can/400g | 184.0 | 2.0 | 46 | 2.3 | 7.8 | 0.6 | 1.0 |
| Tomato & Lentil, Spicy, Canned, Tesco* | 1 Can/400g | 180.0 | 1.0 | 45 | 2.1 | 8.7 | 0.2 | 0.8 |
| Tomato & Orange, Baxters* | 1 Can/425g | 178.0 | 2.0 | 42 | 1.0 | 8.3 | 0.5 | 0.4 |
| Tomato & Orange, HE, Tesco* | 1 Pack/400g | 132.0 | 1.0 | 33 | 0.6 | 7.1 | 0.2 | 0.4 |
| Tomato & Puy Lentil, Canned, Tesco* | ½ Can/200g | 64.0 | 1.0 | 32 | 0.7 | 6.5 | 0.3 | 0.6 |
| Tomato & Red Pepper, Campbell's* | 1 Can/590g | 366.0 | 19.0 | 62 | 0.5 | 7.7 | 3.3 | 0.0 |
| Tomato & Red Pepper, to Go, Asda* | 1 Pot/330g | 102.0 | 4.0 | 31 | 0.6 | 4.3 | 1.3 | 0.6 |
| Tomato & Red Pepper with Basil, Farmers Market, Heinz* | ½ Carton/300g | 117.0 | 4.0 | 39 | 1.3 | 5.2 | 1.4 | 0.5 |
| Tomato & Roasted Red Pepper, COU, M & S* | 1 Serving/415g | 145.0 | 0.0 | 35 | 1.0 | 7.6 | 0.1 | 0.9 |
| Tomato & Spinach, Organic, Waitrose* | 1 Serving/300g | 126.0 | 6.0 | 42 | 1.4 | 4.9 | 1.9 | 0.7 |
| Tomato & Three Bean, Canned, BGTY, Sainsbury's* | ½ Can/200g | 118.0 | 2.0 | 59 | 3.7 | 9.1 | 0.9 | 1.7 |
| Tomato & Three Bean, Co-Op* | ½ Can/200g | 130.0 | 2.0 | 65 | 3.7 | 10.2 | 0.9 | 2.0 |
| Tomato & Vegetable, Cup a Soup, Batchelors* | 1 Serving/218g | 107.0 | 3.0 | 49 | 1.1 | 8.5 | 1.2 | 0.6 |
| Tomato & Vegetable, Organic, Baxters* | 1 Can/400g | 200.0 | 3.0 | 50 | 1.6 | 9.2 | 0.8 | 0.8 |
| Tomato & Vegetable, Spicy, Meal in a Mug, Tesco* | 1 Sachet/20g | 74.0 | 2.0 | 370 | 5.5 | 62.3 | 10.5 | 4.3 |
| Tomato with Basil, Italian, Baxters* | 1 Can/415g | 199.0 | 4.0 | 48 | 2.1 | 7.9 | 0.9 | 0.8 |
| Tuscan Bean, Canned, HL, Tesco* | ½ Can/200ml | 130.0 | 4.0 | 65 | 3.5 | 10.3 | 1.8 | 1.3 |
| Tuscan Bean, GFY, Asda* | 1 Carton/400ml | 224.0 | 4.0 | 56 | 2.9 | 9.0 | 0.9 | 0.8 |
| Tuscan Bean, New Covent Garden Food Co* | ½ Carton/300g | 84.0 | 2.0 | 28 | 1.6 | 3.7 | 0.8 | 1.0 |
| Tuscan Bean, Organic, Fresh, Sainsbury's* | 1 Pack/400g | 171.0 | 3.0 | 43 | 2.6 | 6.3 | 0.8 | 2.0 |
| Tuscan Style Bean & Sausage, Chunky, M & S* | 1 Can/415g | 249.0 | 9.0 | 60 | 2.4 | 7.7 | 2.2 | 1.0 |
| Vegetable, & Rosemary, Chunky, Tesco* | ½ Pot/250g | 112.0 | 5.0 | 45 | 1.0 | 5.8 | 2.0 | 1.4 |
| Vegetable, Asda* | 1 Can/400g | 144.0 | 2.0 | 36 | 1.1 | 7.0 | 0.4 | 0.8 |
| Vegetable, Average | 1 Serving/220g | 114.0 | 9.0 | 52 | 0.9 | 3.2 | 4.0 | 0.9 |
| Vegetable, Bean & Pasta, Organic, Baxters* | 1 Can/415g | 212.0 | 3.0 | 51 | 2.2 | 8.7 | 0.8 | 1.4 |
| Vegetable, Canned | 1oz/28g | 13.0 | 0.0 | 48 | 1.4 | 9.9 | 0.6 | 1.5 |
| Vegetable, Canned, Tesco* | ½ Can/200g | 84.0 | 1.0 | 42 | 0.7 | 9.2 | 0.3 | 0.7 |
| Vegetable, Chunky, Big Soup, Heinz* | 1 Can/400g | 208.0 | 4.0 | 52 | 1.7 | 9.2 | 0.9 | 1.6 |
| Vegetable, Chunky, Fresh, Tesco* | 1 Serving/300g | 123.0 | 6.0 | 41 | 0.6 | 5.5 | 1.9 | 1.0 |
| Vegetable, Chunky, Organic, Tesco* | ½ Pot/300g | 150.0 | 4.0 | 50 | 1.7 | 8.0 | 1.2 | 2.1 |
| Vegetable, Chunky, Tesco* | 1 Pot/600g | 288.0 | 17.0 | 48 | 0.8 | 5.0 | 2.9 | 1.3 |
| Vegetable, Classic, Heinz* | 1 Can/400g | 180.0 | 3.0 | 45 | 1.1 | 8.2 | 0.8 | 0.9 |
| Vegetable, Condensed, Classic, Campbell's* | 1 Can/295g | 221.0 | 5.0 | 75 | 1.7 | 13.2 | 1.7 | 1.7 |
| Vegetable, Cream Of, Cup a Soup, Batchelors* | 1 Sachet/33g | 134.0 | 5.0 | 406 | 5.8 | 59.8 | 16.0 | 6.2 |
| Vegetable, Cream Of, Fresh, Sainsbury's* | 1 Pot/600g | 216.0 | 13.0 | 36 | 0.5 | 3.8 | 2.1 | 1.2 |
| Vegetable, Cup Soup, Dry, Heinz* | 1 Sachet/16g | 54.0 | 1.0 | 348 | 5.8 | 64.5 | 7.1 | 3.2 |
| Vegetable, Extra Thick, Canned, Sainsbury's* | 1 Can/400g | 184.0 | 2.0 | 46 | 1.5 | 8.6 | 0.6 | 1.4 |
| Vegetable, From Heinz, Canned, Weight Watchers* | 1 Can/295g | 86.0 | 1.0 | 29 | 0.9 | 5.6 | 0.3 | 0.8 |
| Vegetable, Golden, in a Mug, Tesco* | 1 Sachet/17g | 60.0 | 1.0 | 351 | 8.2 | 62.0 | 7.8 | 3.7 |
| Vegetable, Hi Taste Low Cal, Cup Soup, Ainsley Harriott* | 1 Sachet/22g | 74.0 | 1.0 | 336 | 8.6 | 68.2 | 3.2 | 4.1 |
| Vegetable, in a Cup, BGTY, Sainsbury's* | 1 Sachet/200g | 52.0 | 2.0 | 26 | 0.5 | 4.4 | 0.8 | 0.9 |
| Vegetable, in a Cup, Weight Watchers* | 1 Serving/100g | 57.0 | 1.0 | 57 | 1.2 | 10.4 | 1.2 | 0.5 |
| Vegetable, Mediterranean, Tesco* | ½ Pot/300g | 105.0 | 2.0 | 35 | 1.0 | 6.2 | 0.7 | 0.7 |
| Vegetable, Provencal, M & S* | 1 Serving/300g | 150.0 | 7.0 | 50 | 1.0 | 6.0 | 2.5 | 1.1 |
| Vegetable, Tesco* | ½ Carton/200g | 78.0 | 3.0 | 39 | 0.9 | 5.8 | 1.3 | 1.0 |
| Vegetable, Thick & Creamy, Soup in a Mug, Tesco* | 1 Serving/26g | 104.0 | 4.0 | 399 | 5.2 | 57.4 | 16.5 | 7.5 |
| Vegetable, Vie, Knorr* | 1 Pack/500ml | 160.0 | 3.0 | 32 | 0.9 | 5.5 | 0.7 | 1.2 |
| Vegetable, with Croutons, Soup in a Mug, Tesco* | 1 Pack/23g | 90.0 | 4.0 | 392 | 6.2 | 55.2 | 16.3 | 8.0 |
| Vegetable & Barley Broth, Canned, Organic, Sainsbury's* | ½ Can/200g | 48.0 | 1.0 | 24 | 1.4 | 3.7 | 0.4 | 0.9 |
| Vegetable & Chilli, Chunky, Fresh, Sainsbury's* | ½ Pot/300g | 117.0 | 2.0 | 39 | 1.6 | 6.9 | 0.6 | 2.6 |

**S**

| | Measure INFO/WEIGHT | per Measure KCAL | FAT | Nutrition Values per 100g / 100ml KCAL | PROT | CARB | FAT | FIBRE |
|---|---|---|---|---|---|---|---|---|
| **SOUP** | | | | | | | | |
| Vegetable & Rosemary, Fresh, Sainsbury's* | ½ Pack/300g | 96.0 | 3.0 | 32 | 0.9 | 4.9 | 1.0 | 1.3 |
| Vegetable Broth, Canned, HL, Tesco* | ½ Can/200g | 74.0 | 0.0 | 37 | 1.2 | 7.4 | 0.2 | 1.0 |
| Vegetable Broth, M & S* | 1 Pack/213g | 85.0 | 3.0 | 40 | 1.0 | 6.3 | 1.4 | 0.8 |
| Vegetable Chowder, New Covent Garden Food Co* | ½ Carton/300g | 159.0 | 5.0 | 53 | 2.9 | 6.6 | 1.7 | 1.1 |
| Vegetable Mulligatawny, Tesco* | ½ Pack/300g | 210.0 | 7.0 | 70 | 1.9 | 9.0 | 2.5 | 1.1 |
| Vine Ripened Tomato & Basil, Fresh, Avonmore* | 1 Serving/300g | 141.0 | 8.0 | 47 | 1.0 | 4.7 | 2.7 | 0.3 |
| Vine Tomato, Harissa & Mint, The Best, Morrisons* | 1 Pot/600g | 294.0 | 11.0 | 49 | 1.5 | 6.4 | 1.9 | 1.1 |
| Watercress, M & S* | ½ Pot/300g | 75.0 | 5.0 | 25 | 1.3 | 1.5 | 1.7 | 0.6 |
| Wild Mushroom, Dry, Slim Fast* | 1 Pack/60g | 209.0 | 6.0 | 349 | 23.3 | 37.5 | 10.2 | 10.4 |
| Wild Mushroom, Farmers Market, Heinz* | ½ Carton/300g | 93.0 | 3.0 | 31 | 0.9 | 4.4 | 1.1 | 0.5 |
| Wild Mushroom, in a Cup, BGTY, Sainsbury's* | 1 Serving/200ml | 56.0 | 2.0 | 28 | 0.4 | 4.5 | 0.9 | 0.2 |
| Wild Mushroom & Maderia, Fresh, Finest, Tesco* | ½ Tub/300g | 156.0 | 9.0 | 52 | 1.5 | 4.9 | 2.9 | 0.5 |
| Wild Mushroom & Truffle, The Best, Safeway* | ½ Pot/300g | 180.0 | 13.0 | 60 | 1.1 | 3.5 | 4.5 | 0.9 |
| Winter Vegetable, Broth, Classic, Heinz* | 1 Serving/200g | 68.0 | 1.0 | 34 | 0.8 | 7.3 | 0.1 | 0.8 |
| Winter Vegetable, New Covent Garden Food Co* | ½ Pack/300g | 162.0 | 3.0 | 54 | 2.4 | 8.7 | 1.1 | 1.5 |
| Winter Vegetable, Organic, Sainsbury's* | ½ Can/200g | 100.0 | 2.0 | 50 | 2.3 | 7.9 | 1.0 | 1.3 |
| Wonton, Blue Dragon* | 1 Can/410g | 102.0 | 5.0 | 25 | 1.2 | 2.0 | 1.3 | 0.2 |
| **SOUTHERN COMFORT** | | | | | | | | |
| ***37.5% Volume*** | **1 Shot/35ml** | **72.0** | **0.0** | **207** | **0.0** | **0.0** | **0.0** | **0.0** |
| **SOYA** | | | | | | | | |
| Bolognese Style, Sainsbury's* | ½ Pack/168g | 113.0 | 1.0 | 67 | 3.1 | 13.9 | 0.7 | 2.7 |
| Chunks, Dried, Cooked, Sainsbury's* | 1oz/28g | 27.0 | 0.0 | 98 | 14.0 | 9.8 | 0.3 | 1.1 |
| Chunks, Protein, Natural, Nature's Harvest* | 1 Serving/50g | 172.0 | 0.0 | 345 | 50.0 | 38.0 | 1.0 | 4.0 |
| ***Mince, Granules*** | **1oz/28g** | **74.0** | **2.0** | **263** | **43.2** | **11.0** | **5.4** | **0.0** |
| Mince, with Onion, Cooked, Sainsbury's* | ½ Pack/180g | 122.0 | 3.0 | 68 | 5.4 | 8.0 | 1.6 | 1.8 |
| **SOYA & POTATO SNACK** | | | | | | | | |
| Cheese & Red Onion Flavour, BGTY, Sainsbury's* | 1 Bag/25g | 97.0 | 2.0 | 388 | 17.6 | 59.6 | 8.8 | 6.6 |
| Paprika Flavour, BGTY, Sainsbury's* | 1 Bag/25g | 98.0 | 1.0 | 391 | 18.0 | 59.8 | 5.9 | 6.2 |
| Thai Style Sweet Chilli Flavour, BGTY, Sainsbury's* | 1 Bag/25g | 97.0 | 2.0 | 388 | 17.5 | 59.7 | 8.9 | 6.5 |
| **SOYA MILK** | | | | | | | | |
| Banana Flavour, Provamel* | 1 Serving/250ml | 195.0 | 5.0 | 78 | 3.8 | 10.4 | 2.2 | 0.6 |
| Choco Flavour, Provamel* | 1 Serving/250ml | 207.0 | 6.0 | 83 | 3.8 | 11.1 | 2.4 | 1.1 |
| Chocolate, So Good Beverages* | 1 Serving/250ml | 160.0 | 2.0 | 64 | 3.6 | 10.8 | 1.0 | 0.0 |
| Flavoured, Average | 1 fl oz/30ml | 12.0 | 1.0 | 40 | 2.8 | 3.6 | 1.7 | 0.0 |
| ***No Added Sugar, Unsweetened, Average*** | **1 Serving/250ml** | **85.0** | **5.0** | **34** | **3.3** | **0.9** | **1.9** | **0.4** |
| Omega Original, So Good Beverages* | 1 Serving/250ml | 130.0 | 3.0 | 52 | 3.6 | 6.8 | 1.2 | 0.0 |
| Omega Vanilla, So Good Beverages* | 1 Serving/250ml | 130.0 | 3.0 | 52 | 3.6 | 7.6 | 1.2 | 0.0 |
| Strawberry, So Good Beverages* | 1 Serving/250ml | 160.0 | 2.0 | 64 | 3.6 | 10.4 | 1.0 | 0.0 |
| Strawberry Flavour, Provamel* | 1 Serving/250ml | 160.0 | 5.0 | 64 | 3.6 | 7.7 | 2.1 | 1.2 |
| ***Sweetened, Average*** | **1 Glass/200ml** | **93.0** | **4.0** | **47** | **3.4** | **3.7** | **2.1** | **0.4** |
| Sweetened, Calcium Enriched, Average | 1 Glass/200ml | 91.0 | 4.0 | 46 | 3.4 | 3.7 | 2.0 | 0.3 |
| Uht, Non Dairy, Alternative to Milk, Waitrose* | 1 Serving/250ml | 102.0 | 5.0 | 41 | 3.3 | 2.7 | 1.9 | 0.2 |
| Vanilla, Fat Free, So Good Beverages* | 1 Serving/250ml | 140.0 | 0.0 | 56 | 3.6 | 10.4 | 0.1 | 0.0 |
| Vanilla, Organic, Heinz* | 1 Serving/200ml | 106.0 | 3.0 | 53 | 2.6 | 6.9 | 1.6 | 0.2 |
| Vanilla, So Good Beverages* | 1 Serving/250ml | 180.0 | 5.0 | 72 | 3.6 | 10.4 | 2.0 | 0.0 |
| Vanilla Flavour, Organic, Provamel* | 1 Serving/250ml | 150.0 | 5.0 | 60 | 3.8 | 6.2 | 2.2 | 0.6 |
| **SPAGHETTI** | | | | | | | | |
| ***Cooked, Average*** | **1oz/28g** | **33.0** | **0.0** | **119** | **4.1** | **24.8** | **0.6** | **1.1** |
| ***Dry, Average*** | **1oz/28g** | **98.0** | **0.0** | **350** | **12.1** | **72.1** | **1.5** | **2.4** |
| Dry, Carb Check, Heinz* | 1 Serving/75g | 219.0 | 2.0 | 292 | 52.7 | 15.2 | 2.3 | 20.8 |
| ***Durum Wheat, Dry, Average*** | **1oz/28g** | **97.0** | **0.0** | **347** | **12.3** | **71.7** | **0.3** | **1.4** |
| ***Fresh, Cooked, Average*** | **1 Serving/125g** | **182.0** | **2.0** | **146** | **6.1** | **26.9** | **1.7** | **1.8** |
| ***Fresh, Dry, Average*** | **1 Serving/100g** | **278.0** | **3.0** | **278** | **10.8** | **53.0** | **3.0** | **2.2** |

S

| | Measure INFO/WEIGHT | per Measure KCAL | FAT | Nutrition Values per 100g / 100ml KCAL | PROT | CARB | FAT | FIBRE |
|---|---|---|---|---|---|---|---|---|
| **SPAGHETTI** | | | | | | | | |
| in Tomato & Cheese, Sainsbury's* | 1 Serving/300g | 345.0 | 10.0 | 115 | 4.4 | 16.8 | 3.4 | 1.4 |
| in Tomato Sauce, Canned | 1oz/28g | 18.0 | 0.0 | 64 | 1.9 | 14.1 | 0.4 | 0.7 |
| in Tomato Sauce, Heinz* | ½ Can/200g | 120.0 | 1.0 | 60 | 1.7 | 12.7 | 0.3 | 2.4 |
| in Tomato Sauce, HP* | 1 Can/410g | 247.0 | 1.0 | 60 | 1.5 | 13.1 | 0.2 | 0.4 |
| in Tomato Sauce, Organic, Sainsbury's* | ½ Can/205g | 133.0 | 0.0 | 65 | 1.8 | 13.9 | 0.2 | 1.0 |
| in Tomato Sauce, Sainsbury's* | 1 Sm Can/212g | 123.0 | 1.0 | 58 | 1.7 | 11.8 | 0.4 | 0.5 |
| in Tomato Sauce, Tesco* | 1 Can/410g | 246.0 | 1.0 | 60 | 1.6 | 12.9 | 0.2 | 0.5 |
| In Tomato Sauce, Value, Tesco* | ½ Can/205g | 98.0 | 1.0 | 48 | 1.4 | 10.0 | 0.3 | 0.7 |
| in Tomato Sauce, Whole Wheat, Sainsbury's* | 1 Serving/205g | 125.0 | 1.0 | 61 | 2.0 | 11.9 | 0.6 | 1.1 |
| Wheat Free, Tesco* | 1 Serving/100g | 340.0 | 2.0 | 340 | 8.0 | 72.5 | 2.0 | 2.5 |
| *Whole Wheat, Cooked, Average* | *1oz/28g* | *32.0* | *0.0* | *113* | *4.7* | *23.2* | *0.9* | *3.5* |
| *Whole Wheat, Dry, Average* | *1 Serving/100g* | *326.0* | *3.0* | *326* | *13.5* | *62.2* | *2.6* | *8.0* |
| with Parsley, in Tomato Sauce, Weight Watchers* | 1 Sm Can/200g | 98.0 | 1.0 | 49 | 1.8 | 10.0 | 0.2 | 0.6 |
| with Sausages, in Tomato Sauce, Heinz* | 1 Can/400g | 352.0 | 14.0 | 88 | 3.5 | 10.8 | 3.4 | 0.5 |
| with Tomato & Cheese, Tesco* | ½ Pack/250g | 280.0 | 6.0 | 112 | 4.0 | 18.1 | 2.6 | 1.1 |
| **SPAGHETTI & MEATBALLS** | | | | | | | | |
| American, Superbowl, Asda* | 1 Pack/453g | 594.0 | 18.0 | 131 | 11.0 | 13.0 | 3.9 | 1.1 |
| BGTY, Sainsbury's* | 1 Pack/300g | 249.0 | 3.0 | 83 | 5.9 | 12.7 | 0.9 | 3.1 |
| Chicken, in Tomato Sauce, Heinz* | 1 Can/400g | 332.0 | 9.0 | 83 | 4.2 | 11.3 | 2.3 | 0.5 |
| COU, M & S* | 1 Pack/400g | 360.0 | 8.0 | 90 | 6.0 | 12.3 | 2.0 | 2.6 |
| GFY, Asda* | 1 Pack/400g | 344.0 | 6.0 | 86 | 7.0 | 11.0 | 1.5 | 1.5 |
| HL, Tesco* | 1 Pack/370g | 407.0 | 14.0 | 110 | 4.7 | 13.8 | 3.9 | 1.6 |
| Italian, Sainsbury's* | 1 Pack/450g | 495.0 | 21.0 | 110 | 5.0 | 11.9 | 4.7 | 2.7 |
| Italian Cuisine, Tesco* | 1 Pack/400g | 500.0 | 18.0 | 125 | 5.9 | 14.6 | 4.4 | 1.7 |
| Sainsbury's* | 1 Pack/400g | 497.0 | 18.0 | 124 | 6.5 | 14.2 | 4.6 | 2.8 |
| Tesco* | 1 Serving/475g | 641.0 | 31.0 | 135 | 5.1 | 14.1 | 6.5 | 0.9 |
| Vegetarian, Safeway* | 1 Pack/350g | 381.0 | 13.0 | 109 | 5.0 | 13.7 | 3.8 | 0.5 |
| **SPAGHETTI BOLOGNESE** | | | | | | | | |
| Al Forno, Sainsbury's* | 1 Pack/400g | 460.0 | 20.0 | 115 | 7.8 | 10.0 | 4.9 | 1.1 |
| Average | 1 Serving/450g | 580.0 | 25.0 | 129 | 7.8 | 12.5 | 5.6 | 0.9 |
| BGTY, Sainsbury's* | 1 Pack/450g | 391.0 | 9.0 | 87 | 4.7 | 12.3 | 2.0 | 2.3 |
| Canned, Asda* | ½ Can/205g | 174.0 | 6.0 | 85 | 4.2 | 10.7 | 2.8 | 0.6 |
| Eat Smart, Morrisons* | 1 Pack/399g | 311.0 | 9.0 | 78 | 4.8 | 9.7 | 2.2 | 1.2 |
| Egg Pasta in Rich Beef Sauce, Waitrose* | 1 Pack/400g | 404.0 | 10.0 | 101 | 7.6 | 11.7 | 2.6 | 1.0 |
| Frozen, Tesco* | 1 Pack/450g | 472.0 | 9.0 | 105 | 5.8 | 15.0 | 2.0 | 1.8 |
| GFY, Asda* | 1 Pack/400g | 352.0 | 6.0 | 88 | 4.9 | 13.4 | 1.6 | 2.2 |
| Good Intentions, Somerfield* | 1 Serving/400g | 380.0 | 9.0 | 95 | 6.2 | 12.4 | 2.3 | 1.4 |
| Hidden Veg, Heinz* | 1 Can/400g | 312.0 | 6.0 | 78 | 3.4 | 12.6 | 1.6 | 0.9 |
| HP* | 1 Pack/410g | 312.0 | 8.0 | 76 | 3.8 | 11.3 | 1.9 | 0.7 |
| in Tomato & Beef Sauce, Canned, Carlini* | 1 Can/410g | 324.0 | 11.0 | 79 | 3.7 | 10.2 | 2.6 | 1.2 |
| Italian, Chilled, Tesco* | 1 Pack/400g | 520.0 | 17.0 | 130 | 6.5 | 15.9 | 4.3 | 1.5 |
| Lean Cuisine, Findus* | 1 Pack/320g | 275.0 | 7.0 | 86 | 4.5 | 11.5 | 2.3 | 1.1 |
| M & S* | 1 Pack/400g | 380.0 | 8.0 | 95 | 7.5 | 11.7 | 2.1 | 1.7 |
| Meat Free, Heinz* | 1 Serving/200g | 162.0 | 3.0 | 81 | 3.3 | 13.1 | 1.7 | 0.6 |
| Perfectly Balanced, Waitrose* | 1 Pack/400g | 380.0 | 7.0 | 95 | 6.7 | 13.4 | 1.7 | 1.1 |
| Ross* | 1 Serving/320g | 288.0 | 4.0 | 90 | 4.2 | 15.7 | 1.1 | 0.9 |
| Sainsbury's* | 1 Pack/400g | 525.0 | 19.0 | 131 | 6.1 | 16.0 | 4.7 | 2.2 |
| Vegetarian, Tesco* | 1 Pack/340g | 374.0 | 13.0 | 110 | 5.1 | 13.7 | 3.9 | 1.2 |
| Weight Watchers* | 1 Pack/320g | 307.0 | 7.0 | 96 | 5.7 | 13.1 | 2.2 | 0.7 |
| **SPAGHETTI CARBONARA** | | | | | | | | |
| Cappelletti, Canned, Balanced Lifestyle, Carlini* | 1 Can/400g | 328.0 | 11.0 | 82 | 4.1 | 10.0 | 2.8 | 0.6 |
| Chicken, Mushroom & Ham, Asda* | 1 Pack/700g | 686.0 | 14.0 | 98 | 10.0 | 10.0 | 2.0 | 1.5 |
| Chicken & Asparagus, Sainsbury's* | 1 Pack/450g | 657.0 | 27.0 | 146 | 6.6 | 16.2 | 6.1 | 1.1 |

**S**

| | Measure INFO/WEIGHT | per Measure KCAL | FAT | Nutrition Values per 100g / 100ml KCAL | PROT | CARB | FAT | FIBRE |
|---|---|---|---|---|---|---|---|---|
| **SPAGHETTI CARBONARA** | | | | | | | | |
| COU, M & S* | 1 Pack/330g | 346.0 | 7.0 | 105 | 5.7 | 15.5 | 2.0 | 1.8 |
| Italian, Chilled, Sainsbury's* | 1 Pack/400g | 492.0 | 16.0 | 123 | 5.5 | 16.1 | 3.9 | 1.4 |
| Italian, Fresh, Chilled, Tesco* | 1 Pack/430g | 606.0 | 26.0 | 141 | 7.6 | 13.9 | 6.1 | 1.3 |
| Italian, Tesco* | 1 Pack/450g | 607.0 | 27.0 | 135 | 5.4 | 14.1 | 5.9 | 0.6 |
| M & S* | 1 Pack/360g | 630.0 | 34.0 | 175 | 7.6 | 14.3 | 9.5 | 0.1 |
| **SPAGHETTI HOOPS** | | | | | | | | |
| & Sausages, Tesco* | 1 Serving/205g | 184.0 | 7.0 | 90 | 3.1 | 11.9 | 3.3 | 0.2 |
| Canned, SmartPrice, Asda* | ½ Can/205g | 127.0 | 1.0 | 62 | 1.7 | 13.0 | 0.3 | 0.4 |
| in Tomato Sauce, Heinz* | ½ Can/200g | 106.0 | 0.0 | 53 | 1.7 | 11.1 | 0.2 | 0.5 |
| in Tomato Sauce, Hidden Veg, Heinz* | 1 Can/400g | 244.0 | 2.0 | 61 | 1.7 | 12.4 | 0.5 | 1.1 |
| in Tomato Sauce, Multigrain, Snap Pot, Heinz* | 1 Pot/190g | 112.0 | 1.0 | 59 | 1.6 | 12.7 | 0.3 | 1.5 |
| Tesco* | ½ Can/205g | 123.0 | 0.0 | 60 | 1.6 | 12.9 | 0.2 | 0.5 |
| **SPAGHETTI MARINARA** | | | | | | | | |
| GFY, Asda* | 1 Pack/400g | 520.0 | 17.0 | 130 | 8.0 | 15.0 | 4.2 | 0.9 |
| **SPAGHETTI RINGS** | | | | | | | | |
| in Tomato Sauce, Canned, Sainsbury's* | 1 Serving/213g | 136.0 | 1.0 | 64 | 1.9 | 13.3 | 0.4 | 0.5 |
| **SPAM*** | | | | | | | | |
| Pork & Ham, Chopped, Spam* | 1 Serving/100g | 296.0 | 24.0 | 296 | 14.5 | 3.2 | 24.2 | 0.0 |
| **SPICE BLEND** | | | | | | | | |
| Balti, Sharwood's* | 1oz/28g | 34.0 | 3.0 | 122 | 1.8 | 7.1 | 9.6 | 1.2 |
| Thai, Sharwood's* | 1 Pack 260g | 424.0 | 31.0 | 163 | 1.8 | 12.0 | 11.9 | 1.0 |
| Tikka, Sharwood's* | 1 Pack/260g | 263.0 | 14.0 | 101 | 2.7 | 10.2 | 5.4 | 1.7 |
| **SPICE MIX** | | | | | | | | |
| for Burritos, Old El Paso* | ½ Packet/23g | 68.0 | 1.0 | 304 | 13.0 | 54.0 | 4.0 | 0.0 |
| for Fajitas, Old El Paso* | 1 Pack/35g | 107.0 | 2.0 | 306 | 9.0 | 54.0 | 6.0 | 0.0 |
| for Mexican Fajitas, Discovery* | ½ Pack/15g | 34.0 | 1.0 | 230 | 8.0 | 35.0 | 6.5 | 17.5 |
| From Fajita Dinner Kit, Original Smoky BBQ, Old El Paso* | 1 Pack/35g | 100.0 | 1.0 | 285 | 7.9 | 56.0 | 1.8 | 0.0 |
| Tex Mex Chili Con Carne, Schwartz* | 1 Sachet/100g | 278.0 | 7.0 | 278 | 12.9 | 66.5 | 6.6 | 24.5 |
| **SPICE PASTE** | | | | | | | | |
| Coriander, Honey & Garlic, Simply Stir Fry, Schwartz* | 1 Tbsp/15g | 40.0 | 2.0 | 265 | 2.2 | 37.0 | 12.1 | 0.0 |
| Garlic, Ginger & Spring Onion, Simply Stir Fry, Schwartz* | 1 Tbsp/15g | 27.0 | 2.0 | 177 | 2.5 | 17.8 | 10.8 | 0.0 |
| Lemongrass, Ginger & Coconut, Simply Stir Fry, Schwartz* | 1 Tbsp/15g | 37.0 | 3.0 | 248 | 1.8 | 20.2 | 17.8 | 0.0 |
| **SPINACH** | | | | | | | | |
| *Baby, Average* | *1 Serving/90g* | *22.0* | *1.0* | *25* | *2.8* | *1.6* | *0.8* | *2.1* |
| *Boiled Or Steamed, Average* | *1 Serving/80g* | *17.0* | *1.0* | *21* | *2.6* | *0.9* | *0.8* | *2.1* |
| *Canned, Average* | *1 Serving/80g* | *18.0* | *0.0* | *22* | *3.0* | *1.4* | *0.5* | *2.9* |
| Chopped, Frozen, Fresh, Somerfield* | 1 Serving/90g | 22.0 | 1.0 | 24 | 2.8 | 1.5 | 0.8 | 2.7 |
| Chopped, Frozen, Waitrose* | 1 Serving/80g | 20.0 | 1.0 | 25 | 2.8 | 1.6 | 0.8 | 2.7 |
| *Raw* | *1 Bunch/340g* | *75.0* | *1.0* | *22* | *2.9* | *3.5* | *0.3* | *2.7* |
| *Raw, Average* | *1 Serving/80g* | *19.0* | *1.0* | *24* | *2.9* | *1.3* | *0.8* | *2.1* |
| **SPIRA** | | | | | | | | |
| Cadbury* | 2 Twists/40g | 210.0 | 12.0 | 525 | 7.8 | 56.8 | 29.4 | 0.0 |
| **SPIRALI** | | | | | | | | |
| *Dry, Average* | *1 Serving/50g* | *176.0* | *1.0* | *351* | *12.1* | *72.5* | *1.6* | *2.7* |
| **SPIRITS** | | | | | | | | |
| *37.5% Volume* | *1 Shot/35ml* | *72.0* | *0.0* | *207* | *0.0* | *0.0* | *0.0* | *0.0* |
| *40% Volume* | *1 Shot/35ml* | *78.0* | *0.0* | *222* | *0.0* | *0.0* | *0.0* | *0.0* |
| **SPLENDIPS** | | | | | | | | |
| Cheesecake, Philadelphia, Kraft* | 1 Pack/85g | 200.0 | 7.0 | 235 | 6.1 | 34.0 | 8.3 | 2.9 |
| Chives, Philadelphia, Kraft* | 1 Pack/85g | 159.0 | 4.0 | 187 | 7.5 | 27.0 | 5.2 | 1.7 |
| Nachos, Philadelphia, Kraft* | 1 Pack/85g | 150.0 | 6.0 | 177 | 6.4 | 20.0 | 7.6 | 1.0 |
| Poppadoms & Mango Chutney, Philadelphia, Kraft* | 1 Pack/76g | 131.0 | 4.0 | 172 | 5.1 | 26.5 | 4.7 | 1.9 |

**S**

| | Measure INFO/WEIGHT | per Measure KCAL | FAT | Nutrition Values per 100g / 100ml KCAL | PROT | CARB | FAT | FIBRE |
|---|---|---|---|---|---|---|---|---|
| **SPLIT PEAS** | | | | | | | | |
| *Dried, Average* | *1oz/28g* | *89.0* | *0.0* | *319* | *22.1* | *57.4* | *1.7* | *3.1* |
| *Green, Dried, Boiled, Average* | *1 Tbsp/35g* | *40.0* | *0.0* | *115* | *8.3* | *19.8* | *0.6* | *3.9* |
| **SPONGE FINGERS** | | | | | | | | |
| Boudoir, Sainsbury's* | 1 Finger/5g | 20.0 | 0.0 | 396 | 8.1 | 82.8 | 3.6 | 0.4 |
| Tesco* | 1 Finger/5g | 19.0 | 0.0 | 386 | 7.6 | 80.6 | 3.7 | 1.0 |
| **SPONGE PUDDING** | | | | | | | | |
| Average | 1 Portion/170g | 578.0 | 28.0 | 340 | 5.8 | 45.3 | 16.3 | 1.1 |
| Banoffee, Heinz* | ¼ Can/78g | 239.0 | 10.0 | 307 | 2.8 | 46.6 | 12.2 | 0.6 |
| Blackberry & Apple, HE, Tesco* | 1 Pot/103g | 159.0 | 1.0 | 155 | 3.1 | 32.6 | 1.4 | 0.7 |
| Blackcurrant, BGTY, Sainsbury's* | 1 Serving/110g | 155.0 | 1.0 | 141 | 2.5 | 30.7 | 0.9 | 3.2 |
| Canned, Average | 1 Serving/75g | 214.0 | 9.0 | 285 | 3.1 | 45.4 | 11.4 | 0.8 |
| Cherry & Almond Flavour, Sainsbury's* | ¼ Pudding/110g | 334.0 | 16.0 | 304 | 3.5 | 40.3 | 14.3 | 0.7 |
| Cherry & Chocolate, Eat Smart, Safeway* | 1 Serving/86g | 150.0 | 2.0 | 175 | 2.7 | 35.6 | 2.4 | 0.8 |
| Chocolate, BGTY, Sainsbury's* | 1 Pudding/105g | 137.0 | 3.0 | 131 | 4.4 | 23.1 | 2.4 | 2.7 |
| Chocolate, Cadbury* | 1 Pack/370g | 1276.0 | 73.0 | 345 | 4.9 | 36.7 | 19.8 | 0.0 |
| Chocolate, Free From, Sainsbury's* | 1 Pudding/110g | 388.0 | 10.0 | 353 | 5.2 | 62.0 | 9.3 | 0.3 |
| Chocolate, GFY, Asda* | 1 Pudding/105g | 187.0 | 4.0 | 178 | 3.0 | 32.0 | 4.2 | 2.6 |
| Chocolate, Heinz* | ¼ Pudding/77g | 229.0 | 9.0 | 298 | 4.6 | 44.0 | 11.5 | 1.2 |
| Chocolate, HL, Tesco* | 1 Serving/125g | 239.0 | 5.0 | 191 | 4.4 | 34.7 | 3.8 | 0.9 |
| Chocolate, Less Than 3% Fat, BGTY, Sainsbury's* | 1 Pudding/105g | 180.0 | 2.0 | 171 | 4.5 | 34.0 | 1.9 | 0.9 |
| Chocolate, M & S* | ¼ Pudding/131g | 524.0 | 32.0 | 400 | 6.1 | 38.6 | 24.6 | 1.8 |
| Chocolate, Sainsbury's* | ¼ Pudding/110g | 464.0 | 28.0 | 422 | 5.4 | 42.3 | 25.7 | 0.8 |
| Chocolate, Tesco* | 1 Pudding/110g | 337.0 | 17.0 | 306 | 4.7 | 37.7 | 15.1 | 1.8 |
| Chocolate, Trufree* | 1 Serving/115g | 374.0 | 17.0 | 325 | 2.5 | 44.0 | 15.0 | 2.0 |
| Chocolate, TTD, Sainsbury's* | ¼ Pack/100g | 367.0 | 20.0 | 367 | 4.1 | 43.3 | 19.7 | 2.3 |
| Chocolate, Waitrose* | 1 Pudding/105g | 208.0 | 2.0 | 198 | 4.6 | 40.0 | 2.2 | 1.8 |
| Chocolate, with Cadbury's Caramel Sticky Sauce, Heinz* | 1 Serving/200g | 762.0 | 34.0 | 381 | 3.5 | 52.3 | 16.9 | 0.6 |
| Chocolate & Chocolate Sauce, HE, Tesco* | 1 Pudding/90g | 186.0 | 4.0 | 207 | 3.9 | 38.7 | 4.1 | 2.1 |
| Chocolate & Sauce, Iceland* | 1 Serving/130g | 407.0 | 23.0 | 313 | 3.8 | 35.4 | 17.4 | 1.9 |
| Chocolate Chip, HE, Tesco* | 1 Serving/103g | 197.0 | 4.0 | 191 | 4.4 | 34.7 | 3.8 | 0.9 |
| Circus, & Custard, Weight Watchers* | 1 Serving/140g | 239.0 | 4.0 | 171 | 4.2 | 32.1 | 2.9 | 0.9 |
| Citrus, BGTY, Sainsbury's* | 1 Pudding/110g | 230.0 | 4.0 | 209 | 3.5 | 39.7 | 4.0 | 0.7 |
| Fruit, Co-Op* | 1 Can/300g | 1110.0 | 48.0 | 370 | 3.0 | 53.0 | 16.0 | 2.0 |
| Fruited with Brandy Sauce, Sainsbury's* | 1 Pudding/125g | 261.0 | 8.0 | 209 | 3.6 | 33.6 | 6.7 | 0.8 |
| Fruits of the Forest, Asda* | 1 Pudding/115g | 323.0 | 4.0 | 281 | 2.8 | 59.0 | 3.8 | 1.3 |
| Ginger, with Plum Sauce, Waitrose* | 1 Pudding/120g | 424.0 | 18.0 | 353 | 3.1 | 51.7 | 14.9 | 0.7 |
| Golden Syrup, Co-Op* | 1 Can/300g | 945.0 | 39.0 | 315 | 2.0 | 47.0 | 13.0 | 0.6 |
| Jam, Tesco* | 1 Pudding/110g | 367.0 | 13.0 | 334 | 3.3 | 53.3 | 11.9 | 0.5 |
| Jam & Custard, Co-Op* | 1 Pack/244g | 598.0 | 22.0 | 245 | 3.0 | 37.0 | 9.0 | 0.3 |
| Lemon, COU, M & S* | 1 Pudding/100g | 157.0 | 2.0 | 157 | 2.0 | 32.1 | 2.3 | 1.9 |
| Lemon, M & S* | 1 Pudding/105g | 325.0 | 16.0 | 310 | 4.3 | 39.4 | 15.2 | 2.3 |
| Lemon, with Lemon Sauce, Eat Smart, Safeway* | 1 Pudding/90g | 135.0 | 2.0 | 150 | 2.2 | 29.0 | 2.6 | 1.4 |
| Lemon Curd, Heinz* | ¼ Can/78g | 236.0 | 9.0 | 302 | 2.6 | 46.7 | 11.7 | 0.6 |
| Pear & Ginger, COU, M & S* | 1 Pudding/100g | 175.0 | 1.0 | 175 | 1.9 | 39.8 | 0.7 | 1.1 |
| St Clements, GFY, Asda* | 1 Pudding/116g | 332.0 | 5.0 | 286 | 2.6 | 60.0 | 3.9 | 1.2 |
| Sticky Toffee, COU, M & S* | 1 Pack/150g | 277.0 | 3.0 | 185 | 2.5 | 39.3 | 1.7 | 1.8 |
| Sticky Toffee, Microwavable, Heinz* | 1 Serving/75g | 233.0 | 9.0 | 311 | 3.3 | 47.4 | 12.0 | 0.7 |
| Sticky Toffee, Mini, Somerfield* | 1 Pudding/110g | 384.0 | 14.0 | 349 | 3.0 | 54.0 | 13.0 | 0.0 |
| Strawberry, Co-Op* | 1 Can/300g | 960.0 | 39.0 | 320 | 2.0 | 48.0 | 13.0 | 0.8 |
| Strawberry Jam, Heinz* | ¼ Can/82g | 230.0 | 6.0 | 281 | 2.6 | 50.4 | 7.6 | 0.6 |
| Sultana, with Toffee Sauce, HL, Tesco* | 1 Serving/80g | 280.0 | 2.0 | 350 | 3.2 | 60.2 | 2.7 | 1.0 |
| Summer Fruits, BGTY, Sainsbury's* | 1 Serving/110g | 243.0 | 5.0 | 221 | 2.7 | 42.9 | 4.3 | 1.0 |
| Syrup, & Custard, Iceland* | 1 Pudding/130g | 409.0 | 21.0 | 315 | 3.6 | 38.8 | 16.2 | 0.4 |

| | Measure INFO/WEIGHT | per Measure KCAL | FAT | Nutrition Values per 100g / 100ml KCAL | PROT | CARB | FAT | FIBRE |
|---|---|---|---|---|---|---|---|---|
| **SPONGE PUDDING** | | | | | | | | |
| Syrup, BGTY, Sainsbury's* | 1 Pudding/110g | 338.0 | 5.0 | 307 | 2.8 | 64.6 | 4.1 | 0.4 |
| Syrup, Finest, Tesco* | 1 Pudding/115g | 330.0 | 9.0 | 287 | 3.1 | 51.2 | 7.8 | 0.6 |
| Syrup, GFY, Asda* | 1 Sponge/105g | 207.0 | 4.0 | 197 | 2.0 | 38.0 | 4.1 | 2.6 |
| Syrup, Individual, Tesco* | 1 Pudding/110g | 390.0 | 15.0 | 355 | 3.1 | 55.6 | 13.2 | 0.5 |
| Syrup, Sainsbury's* | ¼ Pudding/110g | 408.0 | 13.0 | 371 | 2.7 | 63.5 | 11.8 | 0.4 |
| Treacle, Heinz* | 1 Serving/160g | 445.0 | 13.0 | 278 | 2.5 | 48.9 | 8.1 | 0.6 |
| Treacle, Super Sticky, Heinz* | 1 Pudding/110g | 318.0 | 12.0 | 289 | 1.9 | 45.3 | 11.1 | 1.6 |
| Treacle, Waitrose* | 1 Pudding/105g | 385.0 | 14.0 | 367 | 2.8 | 59.5 | 13.1 | 0.5 |
| Very Fruity Cherry, M & S* | 1 Pot/110g | 286.0 | 11.0 | 260 | 3.5 | 38.6 | 10.3 | 1.8 |
| with Dried Fruit | 1oz/28g | 93.0 | 4.0 | 331 | 5.4 | 48.1 | 14.3 | 1.2 |
| with Jam or Treacle | 1oz/28g | 93.0 | 4.0 | 333 | 5.1 | 48.7 | 14.4 | 1.0 |
| with Lyles Golden Syrup, Heinz* | ½ Pudding/95g | 368.0 | 14.0 | 386 | 3.1 | 53.3 | 15.1 | 0.5 |
| **SPOTTED DICK** | | | | | | | | |
| Asda* | 1 Serving/105g | 282.0 | 14.0 | 269 | 2.9 | 34.3 | 13.3 | 1.3 |
| Average | 1oz/28g | 92.0 | 5.0 | 327 | 4.2 | 42.7 | 16.7 | 1.0 |
| Individual, Tesco* | 1 Pudding/121g | 417.0 | 15.0 | 345 | 3.2 | 55.2 | 12.0 | 1.2 |
| Pudding, Individual, Sainsbury's* | 1 Serving/110g | 346.0 | 13.0 | 315 | 3.8 | 48.7 | 11.7 | 2.2 |
| Sainsbury's* | ¼ Pudding/82g | 270.0 | 10.0 | 329 | 4.1 | 50.9 | 12.1 | 1.6 |
| **SPRATS** | | | | | | | | |
| *Fried* | *1oz/28g* | *116.0* | *10.0* | *415* | *24.9* | *0.0* | *35.0* | *0.0* |
| *Raw* | *1oz/28g* | *48.0* | *3.0* | *172* | *18.3* | *0.0* | *11.0* | *0.0* |
| **SPREAD** | | | | | | | | |
| Butter Me Up, Light, Tesco* | 1 Thin Spread/7g | 24.0 | 3.0 | 350 | 0.3 | 0.5 | 38.0 | 0.0 |
| Butter Mc Up, Tesco* | 1 Thin Spread/7g | 38.0 | 4.0 | 540 | 0.8 | 1.2 | 59.0 | 0.0 |
| Butterlicious, Vegetable, Sainsbury's* | 1 Thin Spread/7g | 44.0 | 5.0 | 628 | 0.6 | 1.1 | 69.0 | 0.0 |
| Buttersoft, Light, Reduced Fat, Sainsbury's* | 1 Thin Spread/7g | 38.0 | 4.0 | 544 | 0.4 | 0.5 | 60.0 | 0.0 |
| Buttery Taste, Benecol* | 1 Thin Spread/7g | 40.0 | 4.0 | 575 | 0.0 | 0.8 | 63.3 | 0.0 |
| Dairy Free, Organic, Pure Spreads* | 1 Thin Spread/7g | 37.0 | 4.0 | 533 | 0.5 | 0.0 | 59.0 | 0.0 |
| Diet, Delight* | 1 Thin Spread/7g | 16.0 | 2.0 | 228 | 3.6 | 1.6 | 23.0 | 0.0 |
| Enriched Olive, Tesco* | 1 Thin Spread/7g | 38.0 | 4.0 | 540 | 0.2 | 1.2 | 59.0 | 0.0 |
| From Soya, Kallo* | 1 Thin Spread/7g | 27.0 | 3.0 | 380 | 7.0 | 6.0 | 37.0 | 0.0 |
| Gold, Low Fat, Omega 3, St Ivel* | 1 Thin Spread/7g | 25.0 | 3.0 | 360 | 0.5 | 3.1 | 38.0 | 0.0 |
| Gold, Low Fat, St Ivel* | 1 Thin Spread/7g | 23.0 | 2.0 | 330 | 0.5 | 3.1 | 35.0 | 0.0 |
| Gold, Lowest Fat, with Omega 3, St Ivel* | 1 Thin Spread/7g | 13.0 | 1.0 | 192 | 0.8 | 4.3 | 19.0 | 1.3 |
| Heart, Cholesterol Reducing, Dairygold | 1 Thin Spread/7g | 24.0 | 3.0 | 338 | 0.7 | 2.8 | 36.0 | 0.0 |
| Light, Benecol* | 1 Thin Spread/7g | 23.0 | 2.0 | 333 | 2.5 | 0.0 | 35.0 | 0.0 |
| Low Fat, Average | 1 Thin Spread/7g | 27.0 | 3.0 | 390 | 5.8 | 0.5 | 40.5 | 0.0 |
| Low Fat, Better By Far, Morrisons* | 1 Thin Spread/7g | 44.0 | 5.0 | 627 | 0.5 | 1.0 | 69.0 | 0.0 |
| Morning Gold, Low Fat, Morrisons* | 1 Thin Spread/7g | 26.0 | 3.0 | 372 | 7.5 | 0.0 | 38.0 | 0.0 |
| Olive, Gold, Reduced Fat, Sainsbury's* | 1 Thin Spread/7g | 38.0 | 4.0 | 536 | 0.1 | 1.2 | 59.0 | 0.0 |
| Olive, Light, Low Fat, HL, Tesco* | 1 Thin Spread/7g | 24.0 | 3.0 | 348 | 1.5 | 0.0 | 38.0 | 0.0 |
| Olive, Low Fat, Morrisons* | 1 Thin Spread/7g | 24.0 | 3.0 | 346 | 0.9 | 0.0 | 38.0 | 0.0 |
| Olive, Reduced Fat, Asda* | 1 Thin Spread/7g | 38.0 | 4.0 | 536 | 0.2 | 1.1 | 59.0 | 0.0 |
| Olive, Reduced Fat, Morrisons* | 1 Thin Spread/7g | 38.0 | 4.0 | 537 | 0.9 | 0.0 | 59.3 | 0.3 |
| Olive, Reduced Fat, So Organic, Sainsbury's* | 1 Thin Spread/7g | 38.0 | 4.0 | 537 | 0.1 | 0.4 | 59.5 | 0.0 |
| Olive, Waitrose* | 1 Thin Spread/7g | 37.0 | 4.0 | 534 | 0.2 | 0.5 | 59.0 | 0.0 |
| Olive Light, GFY, Asda* | 1 Thin Spread/7g | 24.0 | 3.0 | 345 | 0.8 | 0.0 | 38.0 | 0.0 |
| Olive Light, Low Fat, BGTY, Sainsbury's* | 1 Thin Spread/ 7g | 19.0 | 2.0 | 265 | 0.1 | 0.8 | 29.0 | 0.0 |
| Olive Light, Sainsbury's* | 1 Thin Spread/7g | 24.0 | 3.0 | 348 | 1.5 | 0.0 | 38.0 | 0.0 |
| Olive Oil, 55% Reduced Fat, Benecol* | 1 Thin Spread/7g | 35.0 | 4.0 | 498 | 0.3 | 0.5 | 55.0 | 0.0 |
| Olive Oil, Bertolli* | 1 Thin Spread/7g | 38.0 | 4.0 | 536 | 0.2 | 1.0 | 59.0 | 0.0 |
| Olivite, Low Fat, Weight Watchers* | 1 Thin Spread/7g | 25.0 | 3.0 | 351 | 0.0 | 0.2 | 38.9 | 0.0 |
| Organic, Dairy Free, M & S* | 1 Thin Spread/7g | 37.0 | 4.0 | 531 | 0.0 | 0.0 | 59.0 | 0.0 |

S

| | Measure INFO/WEIGHT | per Measure KCAL | FAT | Nutrition Values per 100g / 100ml KCAL | PROT | CARB | FAT | FIBRE |
|---|---|---|---|---|---|---|---|---|
| **SPREAD** | | | | | | | | |
| Pure Gold, Light, 65% Less Fat, Asda* | 1 Thin Spread/7g | 17.0 | 2.0 | 239 | 2.5 | 1.0 | 25.0 | 0.0 |
| Sandwich, Heinz* | 1 Tbsp/10ml | 22.0 | 1.0 | 220 | 1.0 | 24.0 | 13.0 | 1.0 |
| Sandwich, Light, Heinz* | 1 Tbsp/10g | 16.0 | 1.0 | 161 | 1.1 | 18.2 | 9.2 | 0.9 |
| Soft, Reduced Fat, Basics, Sainsbury's* | 1 Thin Spread/7g | 30.0 | 3.0 | 425 | 0.0 | 0.0 | 48.1 | 0.0 |
| Soft, Sainsbury's* | 1 Thin Spread/7g | 44.0 | 5.0 | 630 | 0.1 | 0.1 | 70.0 | 0.0 |
| Soft, Value, Tesco* | 1 Thin Spread/7g | 30.0 | 3.0 | 435 | 0.0 | 0.0 | 48.0 | 0.0 |
| Sunflower, Asda* | 1 Thin Spread/7g | 44.0 | 5.0 | 635 | 0.2 | 1.0 | 70.0 | 0.0 |
| Sunflower, Enriched, Light, HL, Tesco* | 1 Thin Spread/7g | 24.0 | 3.0 | 350 | 0.3 | 1.0 | 38.0 | 0.0 |
| Sunflower, Enriched, Tesco* | 1 Thin Spread/7g | 37.0 | 4.0 | 535 | 0.1 | 0.2 | 59.0 | 0.0 |
| Sunflower, Light, BFY, Morrisons* | 1 Thin Spread/7g | 24.0 | 3.0 | 342 | 0.0 | 0.0 | 38.0 | 0.0 |
| Sunflower, Light, BGTY, Sainsbury's* | 1 Thin Spread/7g | 19.0 | 2.0 | 265 | 0.1 | 0.8 | 29.0 | 0.0 |
| Sunflower, Light, Reduced Fat, Asda* | 1 Thin Spread/7g | 24.0 | 3.0 | 347 | 0.3 | 1.0 | 38.0 | 0.1 |
| Sunflower, Low Fat, M & S* | 1 Thin Spread/7g | 24.0 | 3.0 | 342 | 0.0 | 0.0 | 38.0 | 1.0 |
| Sunflower, M & S* | 1 Thin Spread/7g | 44.0 | 5.0 | 630 | 0.0 | 0.0 | 70.0 | 3.0 |
| Sunflower, Morrisons* | 1 Thin Spread/7g | 44.0 | 5.0 | 631 | 0.0 | 0.2 | 70.0 | 0.0 |
| Sunflower, Reduced Fat, Suma* | 1 Thin Spread/7g | 38.0 | 4.0 | 537 | 0.0 | 0.4 | 59.5 | 0.0 |
| Sunflower, Sainsbury's* | 1 Thin Spread/7g | 37.0 | 4.0 | 532 | 0.1 | 0.2 | 59.0 | 0.0 |
| Sunflower, Value, Tesco* | 1 Thin Spread/7g | 31.0 | 3.0 | 439 | 0.1 | 0.4 | 48.6 | 0.0 |
| Toast Topper, Bacon & Mushroom, Heinz* | 1 Can/128g | 120.0 | 6.0 | 94 | 6.9 | 6.6 | 4.4 | 0.3 |
| Toast Topper, Chicken & Mushroom, Heinz* | 1 Can/128g | 72.0 | 2.0 | 56 | 5.1 | 5.7 | 1.4 | 0.2 |
| Toast Topper, Ham & Cheese, Heinz* | 1 Can/128g | 122.0 | 5.0 | 95 | 7.3 | 7.3 | 4.1 | 0.1 |
| Toast Topper, Ham & Mushroom, Heinz* | 1 Can/128g | 122.0 | 5.0 | 95 | 7.3 | 7.3 | 4.1 | 0.1 |
| Vegetable, Dairy Free, Free From, Sainsbury's* | 1 Thin Spread/7g | 44.0 | 5.0 | 630 | 0.0 | 0.0 | 70.0 | 3.0 |
| Vegetable, Soft, Tesco* | 1 Thin Spread/7g | 46.0 | 5.0 | 661 | 0.1 | 1.0 | 73.0 | 0.0 |
| Vitalite, St Ivel* | 1 Thin Spread/7g | 35.0 | 4.0 | 503 | 0.0 | 0.0 | 56.0 | 0.8 |
| **SPRING ROLLS** | | | | | | | | |
| Cantonese Selection, Sainsbury's* | 1 Serving/35g | 68.0 | 3.0 | 193 | 4.1 | 26.9 | 7.7 | 1.4 |
| Char Sui Pork & Bacon, M & S* | 1 Pack/220g | 528.0 | 21.0 | 240 | 4.8 | 33.9 | 9.4 | 0.6 |
| Chicken, & Chilli, Cantonese, Sainsbury's* | 1 Roll/51g | 85.0 | 3.0 | 166 | 9.7 | 19.4 | 5.5 | 0.6 |
| Chicken, & Chilli, Sainsbury's* | 1 Roll/50g | 92.0 | 5.0 | 185 | 9.6 | 15.6 | 9.3 | 2.8 |
| Chicken, Asda* | 1 Roll/58g | 115.0 | 5.0 | 199 | 4.6 | 25.0 | 9.0 | 3.4 |
| Chicken, Finest, Tesco* | 1 Roll/60g | 118.0 | 5.0 | 196 | 10.1 | 20.1 | 8.3 | 1.0 |
| Chicken, Oriental, Asda* | 1 Roll/60g | 106.0 | 4.0 | 178 | 3.7 | 25.0 | 7.0 | 0.4 |
| Chicken, Oriental Snack Selection, Sainsbury's* | 1 Roll/15g | 38.0 | 1.0 | 256 | 11.5 | 30.3 | 9.9 | 1.7 |
| Chicken, Tesco* | 1 Roll/50g | 115.0 | 6.0 | 231 | 8.1 | 24.5 | 11.2 | 1.5 |
| Chinese Takeaway, Tesco* | 1 Roll/50g | 100.0 | 4.0 | 201 | 4.4 | 26.4 | 8.6 | 1.5 |
| Dim Sum, Sainsbury's* | 1 Roll/12g | 26.0 | 1.0 | 216 | 4.1 | 28.2 | 9.6 | 2.9 |
| Duck, M & S* | 1 Roll/30g | 75.0 | 3.0 | 250 | 9.8 | 27.7 | 11.2 | 1.5 |
| Duck, Mini, Asda* | 1 Roll/18g | 47.0 | 2.0 | 259 | 8.7 | 32.8 | 10.3 | 1.9 |
| Duck, Morrisons* | 1 Roll/65g | 147.0 | 7.0 | 226 | 6.2 | 27.2 | 10.3 | 1.2 |
| Duck, Party Bites, Sainsbury's* | 1 Roll/20g | 49.0 | 2.0 | 245 | 10.1 | 31.4 | 8.8 | 1.0 |
| Mini, Asda* | 1 Roll/20g | 35.0 | 1.0 | 175 | 3.5 | 33.6 | 3.0 | 1.9 |
| Mini, Sainsbury's* | 1 Roll/12g | 27.0 | 1.0 | 221 | 4.2 | 28.7 | 9.9 | 1.6 |
| Oriental Vegetable, Tesco* | 1 Roll/68g | 152.0 | 8.0 | 225 | 4.0 | 25.9 | 11.3 | 1.6 |
| Prawn, Cantonese, Sainsbury's* | 1 Roll/28g | 46.0 | 2.0 | 162 | 6.8 | 20.3 | 6.0 | 2.5 |
| Prawn, Crispy, M & S* | 1 Roll/34g | 75.0 | 3.0 | 220 | 10.0 | 22.2 | 9.9 | 1.3 |
| Prawn, Tesco* | 1 Roll/33g | 70.0 | 3.0 | 211 | 8.7 | 22.8 | 9.4 | 1.4 |
| Thai, Sainsbury's* | 1 Roll/30g | 69.0 | 3.0 | 229 | 2.9 | 28.8 | 11.3 | 3.5 |
| Thai Prawn, Waitrose* | 1 Roll/50g | 109.0 | 5.0 | 219 | 8.0 | 25.4 | 9.5 | 2.4 |
| Vegetable, Asda* | 1 Roll/62g | 126.0 | 6.0 | 203 | 3.5 | 27.0 | 9.0 | 2.7 |
| Vegetable, Cantonese, Large, Sainsbury's* | 1 Roll/63g | 130.0 | 6.0 | 205 | 3.6 | 25.3 | 9.9 | 1.5 |
| Vegetable, Cantonese, Sainsbury's* | 1 Roll/36g | 84.0 | 4.0 | 233 | 3.6 | 28.1 | 11.7 | 1.4 |
| Vegetable, Chilled, Tesco* | 1 Roll/68g | 149.0 | 8.0 | 221 | 4.0 | 25.9 | 11.3 | 1.6 |

**S**

## SPRING ROLLS

| | Measure INFO/WEIGHT | KCAL | FAT | KCAL | PROT | CARB | FAT | FIBRE |
|---|---|---|---|---|---|---|---|---|
| Vegetable, Chinese, Sainsbury's* | 1 Roll/26g | 50.0 | 2.0 | 193 | 4.1 | 26.9 | 7.7 | 1.4 |
| Vegetable, Chinese Takeaway, Sainsbury's* | 1 Roll/59g | 100.0 | 4.0 | 170 | 4.0 | 24.4 | 6.3 | 2.8 |
| Vegetable, Cocktail, Tiger Tiger* | 1 Roll/15g | 38.0 | 2.0 | 254 | 6.4 | 26.7 | 13.4 | 2.0 |
| Vegetable, Frozen, Tesco* | 1 Roll/60g | 123.0 | 6.0 | 205 | 3.5 | 23.0 | 10.6 | 1.3 |
| Vegetable, M & S* | 1 Roll/29g | 62.0 | 3.0 | 215 | 3.2 | 27.7 | 10.3 | 2.4 |
| Vegetable, Mini, Occasions, Sainsbury's* | 1 Roll/24g | 52.0 | 2.0 | 216 | 4.1 | 28.2 | 9.6 | 2.9 |
| Vegetable, Mini, Oriental Selection, Waitrose* | 1 Roll/18g | 35.0 | 1.0 | 192 | 4.2 | 28.6 | 6.8 | 1.7 |
| Vegetable, Mini, Party Food, M & S* | 1 Roll/17g | 35.0 | 2.0 | 205 | 3.5 | 26.3 | 9.7 | 2.0 |
| Vegetable, Mini, Tesco* | 1 Roll/18g | 36.0 | 2.0 | 205 | 4.4 | 26.4 | 8.6 | 1.5 |
| Vegetable, Oriental Selection, Party, Iceland* | 1 Roll/15g | 36.0 | 1.0 | 241 | 4.3 | 34.1 | 9.7 | 2.1 |
| Vegetable, Tempura, M & S* | 1 Pack/140g | 280.0 | 12.0 | 200 | 2.8 | 27.9 | 8.6 | 1.8 |
| Vegetable & Chicken, Tesco* | 1 Roll/60g | 110.0 | 5.0 | 183 | 6.1 | 22.2 | 7.7 | 2.5 |

## SPRITE*

| | | | | | | | | |
|---|---|---|---|---|---|---|---|---|
| Zero, Sprite* | 1 Can/330ml | 3.0 | 0.0 | 1 | 0.0 | 0.0 | 0.0 | 0.0 |

## SPRITZER

| | | | | | | | | |
|---|---|---|---|---|---|---|---|---|
| Red Grape, Non-Alcoholic, Extra Special, Asda* | 1 Lge Bottle/750ml | 330.0 | 0.0 | 44 | 0.0 | 11.0 | 0.0 | 0.0 |
| Rose & Grape, Non Alchoholic, Extra Special, Asda* | 1 Bottle/750ml | 90.0 | 0.0 | 12 | 0.0 | 3.0 | 0.0 | 0.0 |

## SQUARES

| | | | | | | | | |
|---|---|---|---|---|---|---|---|---|
| Rice Krispies, Chewy, Marshmallow, Kellogg's* | 1 Lge Bar/28g | 116.0 | 3.0 | 415 | 3.0 | 76.0 | 11.0 | 0.9 |
| Rice Krispies, Chocolate & Caramel, Kellogg's* | 1 Bar/36g | 155.0 | 5.0 | 430 | 4.5 | 71.0 | 14.0 | 2.0 |
| Rice Krispies, Crazy Choc, Kellogg's* | 1 Bar/28g | 118.0 | 3.0 | 422 | 3.0 | 76.0 | 12.0 | 1.5 |

## SQUASH

| | | | | | | | | |
|---|---|---|---|---|---|---|---|---|
| Apple, Blackcurrant, Low Sugar, Diluted, Sainsbury's* | 1 Glass/250ml | 5.0 | 0.0 | 2 | 0.1 | 0.2 | 0.1 | 0.1 |
| Apple, No Added Sugar, Morrisons* | 1 Serving/40ml | 8.0 | 0.0 | 21 | 0.1 | 4.1 | 0.0 | 0.0 |
| Apple & Blackcurrant, Fruit, Robinson's* | 100ml | 43.0 | 0.0 | 43 | 0.1 | 9.7 | 0.0 | 0.0 |
| Apple & Blackcurrant, No Added Sugar, Tesco* | 1 Serving/30ml | 4.0 | 0.0 | 15 | 0.2 | 2.0 | 0.0 | 0.0 |
| Apple & Blackcurrant, Special R, Diluted, Robinson's* | 1 fl oz/30ml | 2.0 | 0.0 | 8 | 0.1 | 1.1 | 0.1 | 0.0 |
| Apple & Blackcurrant, Special R, Robinson's* | 1 Serving/30ml | 2.0 | 0.0 | 8 | 0.1 | 1.1 | 0.0 | 0.0 |
| Apple & Cranberry, Fruit Spring, Robinson's* | 100ml | 39.0 | 0.0 | 39 | 0.0 | 9.3 | 0.0 | 0.0 |
| Apple & Strawberry High Juice, Sainsbury's* | 1 Serving/250ml | 82.0 | 0.0 | 33 | 0.1 | 8.2 | 0.1 | 0.1 |
| Blackcurrant, High Juice, M & S* | 1 Glass/250ml | 50.0 | 0.0 | 20 | 0.1 | 5.2 | 0.0 | 0.1 |
| Blackcurrent, No Added Sugar, Tesco* | 1 Serving/25ml | 3.0 | 0.0 | 14 | 0.4 | 1.7 | 0.0 | 0.0 |
| Cherries & Berries, Tesco* | 1 Serving/25ml | 5.0 | 0.0 | 21 | 0.2 | 3.2 | 0.0 | 0.0 |
| Forest Fruits, Fruit & Barley, Diluted, Morrisons* | 1 fl oz/30ml | 4.0 | 0.0 | 12 | 0.1 | 1.7 | 0.0 | 0.0 |
| Fruit & Barley, No Added Sugar, Robinson's* | 1 fl oz/30ml | 4.0 | 0.0 | 14 | 0.3 | 2.0 | 0.0 | 0.0 |
| Fruit & Barley, Tropical, No Added Sugar, Robinson's* | 1 fl oz/30ml | 4.0 | 0.0 | 14 | 0.3 | 2.0 | 0.0 | 0.0 |
| Fruit & Barley Orange, Diluted, Robinson's* | 1 Serving/50ml | 6.0 | 0.0 | 12 | 0.2 | 1.7 | 0.0 | 0.1 |
| Grape & Passion Fruit, High Juice, Diluted, Sainsbury's* | 1 Serving/250ml | 100.0 | 0.0 | 40 | 0.1 | 9.8 | 0.1 | 0.1 |
| Grapefruit, High Juice, No Added Sugar, Sainsbury's* | 1 Serving/25ml | 1.0 | 0.0 | 6 | 0.1 | 1.1 | 0.0 | 0.0 |
| Lemon, Double Concentrate, Value, Tesco* | 1 Serving/25ml | 3.0 | 0.0 | 11 | 0.2 | 0.3 | 0.0 | 0.0 |
| Lemon, High Juice, Diluted, Sainsbury's* | 1 Glass /250ml | 97.0 | 0.0 | 39 | 0.1 | 9.1 | 0.1 | 0.1 |
| Lemon, No Added Sugar, Double Concentrate, Tesco* | 1 Serving/25ml | 4.0 | 0.0 | 16 | 0.3 | 0.7 | 0.0 | 0.0 |
| Lemon, No Sugar, Asda* | 1 Serving/200ml | 5.0 | 0.0 | 2 | 0.1 | 0.3 | 0.1 | 0.1 |
| Lemon, Whole, Low Sugar, Sainsbury's* | 1 Glass/250ml | 5.0 | 0.0 | 2 | 0.1 | 0.2 | 0.1 | 0.1 |
| Mixed Fruit, Low Sugar, Sainsbury's* | 1 Glass/250ml | 5.0 | 0.0 | 2 | 0.1 | 0.2 | 0.1 | 0.1 |
| Mixed Fruit, Tesco* | 1 Serving/75ml | 13.0 | 0.0 | 17 | 0.0 | 3.5 | 0.0 | 0.0 |
| Orange, No Added Sugar, High Juice, Sainsbury's* | 1 Serving/100ml | 6.0 | 0.0 | 6 | 0.1 | 1.1 | 0.1 | 0.1 |
| Orange, No Added Sugar, Undiluted, Pennywise, Crystal* | 1 Serving/40ml | 3.0 | 0.0 | 8 | 0.1 | 1.2 | 0.0 | 0.0 |
| Orange, Sainsbury's* | 1 Glass/250ml | 7.0 | 0.0 | 3 | 0.1 | 0.5 | 0.1 | 0.1 |
| Orange, Special R, Diluted, Robinson's* | 1 fl oz/30ml | 2.0 | 0.0 | 8 | 0.2 | 0.7 | 0.1 | 0.0 |
| Orange, Undiluted, Pennywise, Crystal* | 1 Serving/40ml | 7.0 | 0.0 | 17 | 0.1 | 3.5 | 0.0 | 0.0 |
| Orange & Mandarin, Fruit Spring, Robinson's* | 1 Serving/440ml | 26.0 | 0.0 | 6 | 0.1 | 0.8 | 0.0 | 0.0 |
| Orange & Mango, Low Sugar, Sainsbury's* | 1 Serving/250ml | 5.0 | 0.0 | 2 | 0.1 | 0.2 | 0.1 | 0.1 |

S

| | Measure INFO/WEIGHT | per Measure KCAL | FAT | Nutrition Values per 100g / 100ml KCAL | PROT | CARB | FAT | FIBRE |
|---|---|---|---|---|---|---|---|---|
| **SQUASH** | | | | | | | | |
| Orange & Mango, No Added Sugar, Robinson's* | 1 Serving/25ml | 2.0 | 0.0 | 8 | 0.2 | 0.9 | 0.0 | 0.0 |
| Orange & Mango, Special R, Diluted, Robinson's* | 1 Serving/250ml | 20.0 | 0.0 | 8 | 0.2 | 0.9 | 0.0 | 0.0 |
| Orange & Pineapple, Original, Undiluted, Robinson's* | 1 Serving/250ml | 137.0 | 0.0 | 55 | 1.0 | 13.0 | 0.0 | 0.0 |
| Pink Grapefruit, High Juice, Low Sugar, Tesco* | 1 Serving/75ml | 12.0 | 0.0 | 16 | 0.2 | 3.7 | 0.1 | 0.0 |
| Pink Grapefruit, High Juice, Sainsbury's* | 1 Serving/250ml | 102.0 | 0.0 | 41 | 0.1 | 9.9 | 0.1 | 0.1 |
| *Spaghetti, Baked* | *1oz/28g* | *6.0* | *0.0* | *23* | *0.7* | *4.3* | *0.3* | *2.1* |
| *Spaghetti, Including Pips & Rind, Raw* | *1oz/28g* | *7.0* | *0.0* | *26* | *0.6* | *4.6* | *0.6* | *2.3* |
| Summer Fruits, High Juice, Waitrose* | 1 Serving/250ml | 102.0 | 0.0 | 41 | 0.0 | 10.0 | 0.0 | 0.0 |
| Summer Fruits, No Added Sugar, Double Strength, Asda* | 1 Serving/50ml | 1.0 | 0.0 | 2 | 0.0 | 0.2 | 0.0 | 0.0 |
| Summer Fruits, No Added Sugar, Made Up, Morrisons* | 1 Glass/200ml | 3.0 | 0.0 | 1 | 0.0 | 0.2 | 0.0 | 0.0 |
| Summerfruits. High Juice, Tesco* | 1 Serving/50ml | 11.0 | 0.0 | 23 | 0.2 | 4.5 | 0.0 | 0.0 |
| Tropical, No Added Sugar, Diluted, Tesco* | 1 Glass/200ml | 18.0 | 0.0 | 9 | 0.2 | 0.9 | 0.0 | 0.0 |
| Tropical Fruits, Sainsbury's* | 1 Serving/250ml | 95.0 | 0.0 | 38 | 0.1 | 9.3 | 0.1 | 0.1 |
| Whole Orange, Tesco* | 1 Serving/100ml | 45.0 | 1.0 | 45 | 0.2 | 10.1 | 1.0 | 1.0 |
| *Winter, Acorn, Baked, Average* | *1oz/28g* | *16.0* | *0.0* | *56* | *1.1* | *12.6* | *0.1* | *3.2* |
| *Winter, Acorn, Raw, Average* | *1oz/28g* | *11.0* | *0.0* | *40* | *0.8* | *9.0* | *0.1* | *2.3* |
| *Winter, All Varieties, Flesh Only, Raw* | *1oz/28g* | *10.0* | *0.0* | *34* | *0.9* | *8.6* | *0.1* | *1.5* |
| *Winter, Butternut, Baked, Average* | *1oz/28g* | *9.0* | *0.0* | *32* | *0.9* | *7.4* | *0.1* | *1.4* |
| *Winter, Butternut, Raw, Unprepared, Average* | *1 Serving/80g* | *30.0* | *0.0* | *37* | *1.1* | *8.3* | *0.1* | *1.6* |
| **SQUID** | | | | | | | | |
| Calamari, Battered, with Tartar Sauce Dip, Tesco* | 1 Pack/210g | 573.0 | 41.0 | 273 | 8.9 | 15.4 | 19.5 | 0.6 |
| *Dried, Average* | *1oz/28g* | *88.0* | *1.0* | *313* | *63.3* | *4.8* | *4.6* | *0.0* |
| in Batter, Fried in Blended Oil, Average | 1oz/28g | 55.0 | 3.0 | 195 | 11.5 | 15.7 | 10.0 | 0.5 |
| Pieces in Squid Ink, Palacio De Oriente* | 1 Can/120g | 274.0 | 22.0 | 228 | 13.0 | 3.6 | 18.0 | 0.0 |
| *Raw, Average* | *1oz/28g* | *23.0* | *0.0* | *81* | *15.4* | *1.2* | *1.7* | *0.0* |
| **STAR FRUIT** | | | | | | | | |
| *Average, Tesco* | *1oz/28g* | *9.0* | *0.0* | *32* | *0.5* | *7.3* | *0.3* | *1.3* |
| **STARBAR** | | | | | | | | |
| Cadbury* | 1 Bar/53g | 260.0 | 15.0 | 491 | 10.7 | 49.0 | 27.9 | 0.0 |
| **STARBURST** | | | | | | | | |
| Fruit Chews, Tropical, Mars* | 1 Tube/45g | 168.0 | 3.0 | 373 | 0.0 | 76.9 | 7.3 | 0.0 |
| Joosters, Mars* | 1 Pack/45g | 160.0 | 0.0 | 356 | 0.0 | 88.8 | 0.1 | 0.0 |
| Juicy Gums, Mars* | 1 Pack/45g | 139.0 | 2.0 | 309 | 5.9 | 71.0 | 4.1 | 0.0 |
| Mars* | 1 Pack/45g | 185.0 | 3.0 | 411 | 0.3 | 85.3 | 7.6 | 0.0 |
| **STEAK &** | | | | | | | | |
| Ale, with Vintage Cheddar Mash, Finest, Tesco* | 1 Serving/550g | 594.0 | 25.0 | 108 | 8.0 | 8.6 | 4.6 | 0.6 |
| Vegetable Medley, HE, Tesco* | 1 Pack/400g | 264.0 | 6.0 | 66 | 7.6 | 5.3 | 1.6 | 0.8 |
| **STEAK & KIDNEY PUDDING** | | | | | | | | |
| Fray Bentos* | 1 Tin/213g | 477.0 | 27.0 | 224 | 7.8 | 19.8 | 12.6 | 0.0 |
| M & S* | 1 Pudding/121g | 260.0 | 13.0 | 215 | 9.2 | 19.4 | 11.1 | 3.2 |
| Sainsbury's* | 1 Pudding/435g | 1135.0 | 63.0 | 261 | 10.5 | 22.3 | 14.4 | 0.8 |
| Tesco* | 1 Serving/190g | 437.0 | 23.0 | 230 | 10.0 | 20.7 | 11.9 | 1.2 |
| **STEAK CHASSEUR** | | | | | | | | |
| HE, Tesco* | 1 Pack/450g | 346.0 | 8.0 | 77 | 10.0 | 5.3 | 1.8 | 0.5 |
| **STEAK IN** | | | | | | | | |
| Rich Gravy, Stewed, Extra Lean, Sainsbury's* | 1 Sm Can/220g | 249.0 | 6.0 | 113 | 20.3 | 1.6 | 2.8 | 1.6 |
| **STEAK STEWED** | | | | | | | | |
| & Onions with Gravy, John West* | ½ Can/205g | 269.0 | 14.0 | 131 | 14.0 | 3.0 | 7.0 | 0.0 |
| Tesco* | ½ Can/200g | 230.0 | 6.0 | 115 | 17.5 | 4.5 | 3.0 | 0.0 |
| with Gravy, John West* | 1oz/28g | 30.0 | 1.0 | 107 | 18.0 | 2.0 | 3.0 | 0.2 |
| **STEAK WITH** | | | | | | | | |
| Red Wine & Shallot Sauce, Rump, Waitrose* | 1 Serving/205g | 242.0 | 11.0 | 118 | 16.4 | 0.9 | 5.6 | 0.3 |

**S**

| | Measure INFO/WEIGHT | per Measure KCAL | per Measure FAT | Nutrition Values per 100g / 100ml KCAL | PROT | CARB | FAT | FIBRE |
|---|---|---|---|---|---|---|---|---|
| **STEW** | | | | | | | | |
| Beef, & Dumplings, Frozen, Tesco* | 1 Serving/400g | 380.0 | 13.0 | 95 | 5.7 | 10.5 | 3.2 | 1.5 |
| Beef, Asda* | ½ Can/196g | 178.0 | 5.0 | 91 | 10.0 | 7.0 | 2.5 | 1.5 |
| Beef, Meal for One, M & S* | 1 Pack/440g | 350.0 | 8.0 | 80 | 7.0 | 8.7 | 1.9 | 2.0 |
| Beef, Value, Tesco* | 1 Serving/200g | 170.0 | 10.0 | 85 | 4.0 | 6.2 | 4.9 | 1.0 |
| Beef & Dumplings, Asda* | 1 Pack/400g | 392.0 | 13.0 | 98 | 6.0 | 11.0 | 3.3 | 0.8 |
| Beef & Dumplings, Birds Eye* | 1 Pack/400g | 308.0 | 8.0 | 77 | 4.4 | 10.0 | 2.1 | 0.9 |
| Beef & Dumplings, British Classics, Tesco* | 1 Pack/450g | 563.0 | 30.0 | 125 | 7.9 | 8.6 | 6.6 | 0.5 |
| Beef & Dumplings, Frozen, Asda* | 1 Pack/400g | 392.0 | 13.0 | 98 | 6.0 | 11.0 | 3.3 | 0.8 |
| Beef & Dumplings, Iceland* | 1 Serving/400g | 468.0 | 20.0 | 117 | 4.5 | 13.5 | 5.0 | 0.5 |
| Beef & Dumplings, Weight Watchers* | 1 Pack/327g | 262.0 | 7.0 | 80 | 5.2 | 10.0 | 2.1 | 0.8 |
| Beef with Dumplings, Classic British, Sainsbury's* | 1 Pack/450g | 531.0 | 23.0 | 118 | 7.7 | 10.2 | 5.2 | 0.5 |
| Beef with Dumplings, COU, M & S* | 1 Pack/454g | 431.0 | 12.0 | 95 | 8.9 | 9.1 | 2.6 | 0.8 |
| Beef with Dumplings, Sainsbury's* | 1 Pack/450g | 603.0 | 27.0 | 134 | 9.3 | 10.5 | 6.1 | 0.7 |
| Chicken, Morrisons* | 1 Pack/400g | 492.0 | 8.0 | 123 | 17.6 | 8.9 | 1.9 | 0.5 |
| Chicken & Dumplings, Birds Eye* | 1 Pack/320g | 282.0 | 9.0 | 88 | 7.0 | 8.9 | 2.7 | 0.5 |
| Chicken & Dumplings, Tesco* | 1 Serving/450g | 567.0 | 30.0 | 126 | 7.6 | 9.1 | 6.6 | 0.7 |
| Irish, Asda* | ¼ Can/196g | 172.0 | 8.0 | 88 | 6.0 | 7.0 | 4.0 | 1.0 |
| Irish, Morrisons* | 1 Can/392g | 243.0 | 5.0 | 62 | 3.8 | 8.9 | 1.2 | 0.0 |
| Irish, Sainsbury's* | 1 Pack/450g | 274.0 | 9.0 | 61 | 5.7 | 4.8 | 2.1 | 0.5 |
| Irish, SmartPrice, Asda* | 1 Can/392g | 298.0 | 14.0 | 76 | 3.0 | 8.0 | 3.6 | 0.9 |
| Irish, Tesco* | 1 Can/400g | 308.0 | 11.0 | 77 | 7.0 | 5.9 | 2.8 | 0.8 |
| Lentil & Vegetable, Organic, Simply Organic* | 1 Pack/400g | 284.0 | 6.0 | 71 | 3.5 | 11.0 | 1.5 | 1.3 |
| Lentil & Winter Vegetable, Organic, Pure & Pronto* | 1 Pack/400g | 364.0 | 10.0 | 91 | 3.6 | 14.0 | 2.4 | 4.0 |
| Mixed Vegetable Topped with Herb Dumplings, Tesco* | 1 Pack/420g | 508.0 | 26.0 | 121 | 1.9 | 14.5 | 6.2 | 1.3 |
| **STIR FRY** | | | | | | | | |
| Baby Leaf, Ready Prepared, M & S* | 1 Serving/125g | 25.0 | 0.0 | 20 | 1.7 | 4.9 | 0.1 | 2.5 |
| Baby Vegetable & Pak Choi, Two Step, Tesco* | ½ Pack/95g | 29.0 | 1.0 | 31 | 2.1 | 4.0 | 0.8 | 2.3 |
| Bean Sprout, Chinese, Sainsbury's* | 1 Pack/300g | 144.0 | 8.0 | 48 | 1.9 | 5.1 | 2.8 | 1.5 |
| Bean Sprout, Ready to Eat, Washed, Sainsbury's* | 1 Serving/150g | 82.0 | 6.0 | 55 | 1.5 | 3.3 | 3.9 | 1.8 |
| Bean Sprout & Vegetable, with Red Peppers, Asda* | 1 Pack/350g | 126.0 | 4.0 | 36 | 1.8 | 4.7 | 1.1 | 2.3 |
| Bean Sprouts, Asda* | ½ Pack/175g | 56.0 | 1.0 | 32 | 2.9 | 4.0 | 0.5 | 1.5 |
| Bean Sprouts, Morrisons* | 1 Serving/150g | 46.0 | 1.0 | 31 | 2.0 | 4.8 | 0.4 | 1.8 |
| Bean Sprouts & Vegetables, Asda* | ½ Pack/173g | 107.0 | 7.0 | 62 | 2.0 | 4.5 | 4.0 | 1.8 |
| Beef, BGTY, Sainsbury's* | ½ Pack/125g | 156.0 | 5.0 | 125 | 22.0 | 0.1 | 4.1 | 0.0 |
| Beef, Less Than 10% Fat, Asda* | 1 Pack/227g | 275.0 | 6.0 | 121 | 24.0 | 0.0 | 2.8 | 0.8 |
| Beef, Less Than 3% Fat, BGTY, Sainsbury's* | ½ Pack/125g | 134.0 | 3.0 | 107 | 22.1 | 0.0 | 2.1 | 0.0 |
| Cherry Tomato & Noodle, Waitrose* | 1 Pack/400g | 304.0 | 15.0 | 76 | 2.1 | 8.5 | 3.8 | 1.5 |
| Chicken Chow Mein, Fresh, Heathly Living, Tesco* | 1 Pack/400g | 312.0 | 5.0 | 78 | 5.7 | 11.4 | 1.2 | 1.3 |
| Chicken Chow Mein, Orient Express, Oriental Express* | 1 Pack/400g | 384.0 | 11.0 | 96 | 7.3 | 10.7 | 2.7 | 2.2 |
| Chicken Noodle, GFY, Asda* | 1 Pack/330g | 403.0 | 11.0 | 122 | 7.0 | 16.0 | 3.3 | 2.4 |
| Chinese, Eastern Inspirations* | ½ Pack/170g | 49.0 | 1.0 | 29 | 2.7 | 3.5 | 0.5 | 1.8 |
| Chinese, Family, Sainsbury's* | 1 Serving/150g | 60.0 | 3.0 | 40 | 2.3 | 3.3 | 2.0 | 3.6 |
| Chinese, with Oriental Sauce, Tesco* | 1 Pack/530g | 180.0 | 2.0 | 34 | 2.3 | 5.4 | 0.4 | 1.5 |
| Chinese, With Soy, Garlic & Ginger, Tesco* | 1 Pack/150g | 90.0 | 0.0 | 60 | 1.5 | 12.6 | 0.1 | 0.5 |
| Chinese Bean Sprout, Sainsbury's* | ½ Pack/313g | 150.0 | 9.0 | 48 | 1.9 | 5.1 | 2.8 | 1.5 |
| Chinese Chicken, Iceland* | 1 Pack/298g | 262.0 | 4.0 | 88 | 6.2 | 12.7 | 1.4 | 2.9 |
| Chinese Chicken, Sizzling, Oriental Express* | 1 Pack/400g | 400.0 | 8.0 | 100 | 6.6 | 13.8 | 2.0 | 1.7 |
| Chinese Exotic Vegetable, Sainsbury's* | 1 Pack/350g | 133.0 | 8.0 | 38 | 1.7 | 2.8 | 2.2 | 1.8 |
| Chinese Leaf & Mixed Peppers, Cook Asian, M & S* | 1 Pack/260g | 65.0 | 1.0 | 25 | 1.4 | 3.4 | 0.5 | 1.8 |
| Chinese Mushroom, Sainsbury's* | 1 Serving/175g | 66.0 | 4.0 | 38 | 1.7 | 2.4 | 2.4 | 1.7 |
| Chinese Noodles, Oriental Express* | 1oz/28g | 20.0 | 0.0 | 70 | 2.7 | 14.7 | 0.5 | 1.4 |
| Chinese Prawn, Asda* | 1 Serving/375g | 345.0 | 2.0 | 92 | 3.6 | 18.0 | 0.6 | 1.8 |
| Chinese Prawn, Iceland* | 1 Pack/340g | 235.0 | 4.0 | 69 | 3.1 | 11.1 | 1.3 | 2.1 |

**S**

| | Measure INFO/WEIGHT | per Measure KCAL | FAT | Nutrition Values per 100g / 100ml KCAL | PROT | CARB | FAT | FIBRE |
|---|---|---|---|---|---|---|---|---|

## STIR FRY

| | Measure INFO/WEIGHT | KCAL | FAT | KCAL | PROT | CARB | FAT | FIBRE |
|---|---|---|---|---|---|---|---|---|
| Chinese Style, Tesco* | 1oz/28g | 8.0 | 0.0 | 30 | 2.2 | 4.4 | 0.4 | 2.1 |
| Chinese Style Chicken, GFY, Asda* | 1 Pack/338g | 362.0 | 6.0 | 107 | 6.0 | 17.0 | 1.7 | 1.5 |
| Chinese Style Prawn, GFY, Asda* | 1 Pack/400g | 324.0 | 6.0 | 81 | 3.6 | 13.0 | 1.6 | 1.6 |
| Chinese Style Rice with Vegetables, Tesco* | 1 Serving/550g | 495.0 | 14.0 | 90 | 2.2 | 14.8 | 2.5 | 0.3 |
| Chinese Style Turkey, Asda* | ½ Pack/210g | 321.0 | 6.0 | 153 | 23.8 | 8.1 | 2.9 | 0.8 |
| Chinese Vegetable & Oyster Sauce, Asda* | 1 Serving/150g | 93.0 | 4.0 | 62 | 1.9 | 8.0 | 2.5 | 0.0 |
| Chinese Vegetables, Oriental Express* | ½ Pack/200g | 44.0 | 0.0 | 22 | 1.4 | 3.7 | 0.2 | 2.2 |
| Chinese Vegetables, Tesco* | 1 Serving/175g | 93.0 | 1.0 | 53 | 1.6 | 10.8 | 0.4 | 1.3 |
| Chinese Vegetables, with Chinese Style Sauce, Tesco* | 1 Serving/350g | 133.0 | 3.0 | 38 | 1.4 | 5.6 | 1.0 | 1.2 |
| Chinese Vegetables, with Oyster Sauce, Tesco* | 1 Pack/350g | 98.0 | 1.0 | 28 | 2.0 | 4.6 | 0.2 | 1.1 |
| Classic Medley, Veg Cuisine* | ½ Pack/150g | 45.0 | 1.0 | 30 | 2.5 | 4.1 | 0.4 | 2.1 |
| Creamy Coconut & Lime, The Best, Safeway* | ½ Pack/165g | 231.0 | 12.0 | 140 | 3.4 | 14.4 | 7.2 | 2.1 |
| Edamame Bean & Ginger, Tesco* | 1 Pack/290g | 145.0 | 5.0 | 50 | 4.1 | 4.9 | 1.6 | 2.5 |
| Exotic, Asda* | 1 Serving/250g | 102.0 | 4.0 | 41 | 2.3 | 4.2 | 1.7 | 2.7 |
| Exotic, Tesco* | 1 Pack/191g | 42.0 | 0.0 | 22 | 1.3 | 3.8 | 0.2 | 1.5 |
| Family, Tesco* | 1 Pack/600g | 210.0 | 3.0 | 35 | 2.3 | 5.2 | 0.5 | 2.1 |
| Family Pack, Vegetables & Beansprouts, Fresh, Tesco* | 1 Pack/600g | 108.0 | 1.0 | 18 | 2.0 | 2.2 | 0.1 | 2.1 |
| Green Vegetable, M & S* | 1 Pack/220g | 165.0 | 13.0 | 75 | 3.1 | 2.5 | 5.9 | 2.2 |
| Mediterranean Style, Eastern Inspirations* | ½ Pack/153g | 41.0 | 1.0 | 27 | 1.6 | 4.0 | 0.4 | 2.2 |
| Mediterranean Style, Waitrose* | 1 Pack/305g | 82.0 | 1.0 | 27 | 1.6 | 4.6 | 0.4 | 2.2 |
| Mixed Pepper, Fresh Tastes, Asda* | ½ Pack/160g | 75.0 | 4.0 | 47 | 1.4 | 4.6 | 2.6 | 2.0 |
| Mixed Pepper, HL, Tesco* | 1 Pack/325g | 62.0 | 0.0 | 19 | 1.9 | 2.6 | 0.1 | 1.5 |
| Mixed Pepper, Just Stir Fry, Sainsbury's* | ½ Pack/175g | 66.0 | 3.0 | 38 | 1.7 | 4.4 | 1.5 | 2.5 |
| Mixed Pepper, Tesco* | 1/3 Pack/100g | 23.0 | 0.0 | 23 | 1.9 | 3.7 | 0.1 | 1.9 |
| Mixed Pepper & Sweet Chilli Sauce, Asda* | 1 Pack/300g | 180.0 | 6.0 | 60 | 1.6 | 9.0 | 2.0 | 2.6 |
| Mixed Pepper & Vegetable, Asda* | ½ Pack/150g | 42.0 | 1.0 | 28 | 1.6 | 3.2 | 1.0 | 2.6 |
| Mixed Vegetable, Asda* | 1 Serving/200g | 96.0 | 5.0 | 48 | 1.7 | 4.7 | 2.5 | 3.0 |
| Mixed Vegetable, Safeway* | 1 Serving/150g | 105.0 | 5.0 | 70 | 2.1 | 6.2 | 3.6 | 2.5 |
| Mixed Vegetables, Sainsbury's* | ½ Pack/140g | 70.0 | 4.0 | 50 | 1.7 | 4.7 | 2.7 | 3.0 |
| Mushroom, Just Stir Fry, Sainsbury's* | 1 Pack/350g | 171.0 | 9.0 | 49 | 2.8 | 3.3 | 2.7 | 2.8 |
| Mushroom, Somerfield* | 1 Serving/175g | 89.0 | 6.0 | 51 | 2.2 | 3.0 | 3.4 | 1.0 |
| Mushroom, Tesco* | ½ Pack/180g | 56.0 | 1.0 | 31 | 2.6 | 4.0 | 0.5 | 1.9 |
| Orient Inspired, M & S* | 1 Serving/250g | 50.0 | 1.0 | 20 | 1.6 | 3.4 | 0.3 | 1.6 |
| Oriental, Ready Prepared, M & S* | ½ Pack/260g | 65.0 | 2.0 | 25 | 2.3 | 2.1 | 0.6 | 1.9 |
| Oriental Leaf, M & S* | ½ Pack/125g | 25.0 | 1.0 | 20 | 1.9 | 2.5 | 0.5 | 2.2 |
| Oriental Style Pak Choi, M & S* | 1 Pack/220g | 165.0 | 13.0 | 75 | 2.2 | 3.5 | 5.7 | 2.4 |
| Oriental Vegetable, Frozen, Asda* | 1 Serving/150g | 115.0 | 7.0 | 77 | 2.1 | 7.0 | 4.5 | 1.7 |
| Oriental Vegetable, Szechuan, Spicy, Sainsbury's* | 1 Pack/350g | 224.0 | 15.0 | 64 | 1.3 | 4.9 | 4.4 | 1.7 |
| Oriental Vegetables, Safeway* | 1 Serving/175g | 196.0 | 8.0 | 112 | 2.6 | 15.5 | 4.4 | 0.5 |
| Singaporean Noodle, Sainsbury's* | ½ Pack/160g | 202.0 | 12.0 | 126 | 3.2 | 11.9 | 7.3 | 2.4 |
| SmartPrice, Asda* | 1 Pack/350g | 126.0 | 4.0 | 36 | 1.8 | 4.7 | 1.1 | 2.3 |
| Spicy Thai Style Noodle, Tesco* | 1 Pack/500g | 335.0 | 13.0 | 67 | 2.6 | 8.4 | 2.6 | 1.3 |
| Sweet & Sour, Tesco* | 1 Pack/350g | 161.0 | 1.0 | 46 | 1.8 | 9.1 | 0.3 | 1.3 |
| Sweet & Sour Vegetable, Somerfield* | 1 Pack/350g | 248.0 | 3.0 | 71 | 2.0 | 14.0 | 1.0 | 0.0 |
| Sweet Pepper, M & S* | 1 Pack/400g | 160.0 | 7.0 | 40 | 2.3 | 3.5 | 1.8 | 0.6 |
| Tatsoi & Sugar Snap Pea, M & S* | ½ Pack/125g | 25.0 | 0.0 | 20 | 2.0 | 3.0 | 0.3 | 1.9 |
| Tender Shoot, Sainsbury's* | ½ Pack/126g | 113.0 | 8.0 | 90 | 4.4 | 2.8 | 6.6 | 0.8 |
| Thai Style, Eastern Inspirations* | 1 Pack/330g | 92.0 | 2.0 | 28 | 2.9 | 3.2 | 0.5 | 1.3 |
| Thai Style, M & S* | 1 Serving/150g | 75.0 | 4.0 | 50 | 2.3 | 3.0 | 3.0 | 1.2 |
| Thai Style, Tesco* | 1 Pack/350g | 301.0 | 18.0 | 86 | 3.9 | 6.2 | 5.1 | 1.9 |
| Tomato & Basil, Sundried, Tesco* | 1 Pack/325g | 205.0 | 12.0 | 63 | 1.6 | 6.2 | 3.6 | 2.2 |
| Turkey, Fresh, Good Intentions, Somerfield* | ½ Pack/150g | 246.0 | 7.0 | 164 | 31.0 | 0.0 | 4.5 | 0.0 |
| Vegetable, Asda* | 1 Pack/300g | 132.0 | 7.0 | 44 | 1.6 | 4.2 | 2.3 | 3.1 |

## STIR FRY

| | INFO/WEIGHT | | KCAL | FAT | KCAL | PROT | CARB | FAT | FIBRE |
|---|---|---|---|---|---|---|---|---|---|
| Vegetable, Basics, Sainsbury's* | ½ Bag/325g | | 101.0 | 3.0 | 31 | 2.1 | 3.5 | 0.9 | 2.2 |
| Vegetable, Cantonese, Sainsbury's* | 1 Serving/150g | | 90.0 | 5.0 | 60 | 2.8 | 4.2 | 3.5 | 2.7 |
| Vegetable, Chinese Style, Asda* | 1 Pack/300g | | 81.0 | 2.0 | 27 | 1.6 | 3.6 | 0.7 | 2.8 |
| Vegetable, Chinese Style, Tesco* | 1 Pack/360g | | 79.0 | 1.0 | 22 | 1.9 | 3.2 | 0.2 | 1.4 |
| Vegetable, Crunchy, Sainsbury's* | ½ Pack/150g | | 85.0 | 6.0 | 57 | 1.4 | 4.1 | 3.9 | 2.1 |
| Vegetable, Oriental, Frozen, Freshly, Asda* | 1 Serving/100g | | 25.0 | 0.0 | 25 | 2.2 | 3.4 | 0.3 | 2.0 |
| Vegetable, Oriental, Just Stir Fry, Sainsbury's* | ½ Pack/135g | | 94.0 | 7.0 | 70 | 2.2 | 3.4 | 5.3 | 1.3 |
| Vegetable, Premium, Sainsbury's* | ½ Pack/150g | | 90.0 | 5.0 | 60 | 2.8 | 4.2 | 3.5 | 2.7 |
| Vegetable, Ready Prepared, M & S* | ½ Pack/150g | | 37.0 | 0.0 | 25 | 2.2 | 3.5 | 0.3 | 2.2 |
| Vegetable, Sweet & Crunchy, Waitrose* | 1 Pack/300g | | 69.0 | 0.0 | 23 | 1.8 | 3.6 | 0.1 | 1.4 |
| Vegetable, Thai Style, Tesco* | ½ Pack/135g | | 42.0 | 1.0 | 31 | 2.3 | 4.2 | 0.5 | 2.1 |
| Vegetable & Beansprout, Tesco* | 1 Pack/380g | | 129.0 | 2.0 | 34 | 2.0 | 5.4 | 0.5 | 2.2 |
| Vegetable & Beansprout, Waitrose* | 1 Pack/300g | | 78.0 | 1.0 | 26 | 1.4 | 4.5 | 0.3 | 2.1 |
| Vegetable & Beansprout, with Peanut Sauce, Tesco* | 1 Serving/475g | | 408.0 | 24.0 | 86 | 3.9 | 6.2 | 5.0 | 1.9 |
| Vegetable & Mushroom, Asda* | ½ Pack/160g | | 59.0 | 2.0 | 37 | 2.4 | 3.4 | 1.5 | 3.4 |
| Vegetable Noodles, BGTY, Sainsbury's* | 1 Pack/455g | | 391.0 | 9.0 | 86 | 3.2 | 14.0 | 2.0 | 1.4 |
| Vegetables, Cantonese Style, Tesco* | 1 Serving/125g | | 40.0 | 1.0 | 32 | 2.0 | 4.1 | 0.9 | 1.4 |
| Vegetables, Family, Sainsbury's* | 1 Serving/300g | | 123.0 | 7.0 | 41 | 1.6 | 3.8 | 2.2 | 2.1 |
| Vegetables, Fresh, Asda* | ½ Pack/150g | | 106.0 | 7.0 | 71 | 1.7 | 4.9 | 5.0 | 1.7 |
| Vegetables, Mixed, with Slices of Pepper, Tesco* | 1 Pack/300g | | 57.0 | 0.0 | 19 | 1.9 | 2.6 | 0.1 | 1.5 |
| Vegetables, Sunshine, Tesco* | ½ Pack/150g | | 42.0 | 0.0 | 28 | 1.8 | 4.6 | 0.3 | 2.1 |
| Vegetables & Bean Sprout, M & S* | 1 Pack/350g | | 105.0 | 1.0 | 30 | 1.8 | 4.6 | 0.4 | 2.0 |
| Vegetables with Oyster Sauce, Asda* | 1 Serving/150g | | 93.0 | 4.0 | 62 | 1.9 | 8.0 | 2.5 | 0.0 |
| Water Chestnut & Bamboo Shoot, Asda* | ½ Pack/175g | | 61.0 | 2.0 | 35 | 1.4 | 4.3 | 1.4 | 1.7 |

## STOCK

| | INFO/WEIGHT | | KCAL | FAT | KCAL | PROT | CARB | FAT | FIBRE |
|---|---|---|---|---|---|---|---|---|---|
| Beef, Fresh, Tesco* | 1 Serving/300ml | | 54.0 | 1.0 | 18 | 2.1 | 1.6 | 0.3 | 0.5 |
| Beef, Slowly Prepared, Sainsbury's* | 1 Serving/100g | | 7.0 | 0.0 | 7 | 0.7 | 0.3 | 0.3 | 0.5 |
| Chicken, Asda* | ½ Pot/150g | | 25.0 | 1.0 | 17 | 1.8 | 0.7 | 0.9 | 0.2 |
| Chicken, Fresh, Sainsbury's* | ½ Pot/142ml | | 23.0 | 0.0 | 16 | 3.7 | 0.1 | 0.1 | 0.3 |
| Chicken, Fresh, Tesco* | 1 Serving/300ml | | 27.0 | 0.0 | 9 | 1.6 | 0.5 | 0.1 | 0.5 |
| *Chicken, Home Prepared, Average* | *1 Fl oz/28ml* | | *5.0* | *0.0* | *16* | *3.7* | *0.1* | *0.1* | *0.3* |
| Chicken, Knorr* | 1 Pack/150g | | 348.0 | 6.0 | 232 | 13.1 | 36.5 | 3.7 | 0.4 |
| Chicken, Prepared, Tesco* | 1 Serving/300ml | | 54.0 | 0.0 | 18 | 2.4 | 1.8 | 0.1 | 0.5 |
| Chicken, Simply, Knorr* | 1 Pack/450ml | | 27.0 | 0.0 | 6 | 1.5 | 0.1 | 0.0 | 0.1 |
| Chicken, Slowly Prepared, Sainsbury's* | 1 Pot/300g | | 27.0 | 0.0 | 9 | 0.6 | 1.3 | 0.1 | 0.5 |
| Fish, Fresh, Finest, Tesco* | 1 Serving/100g | | 10.0 | 0.0 | 10 | 0.6 | 1.8 | 0.0 | 0.5 |
| *Fish, Home Prepared, Average* | *1 Serving/250ml* | | *42.0* | *2.0* | *17* | *2.3* | *0.0* | *0.8* | *0.0* |
| Fresh, Finest, Tesco* | 1 Pot/300g | | 33.0 | 0.0 | 11 | 1.9 | 0.8 | 0.0 | 0.2 |
| Vegetable, Campbell's* | 1 Serving/250ml | | 37.0 | 2.0 | 15 | 0.3 | 2.0 | 0.7 | 0.0 |
| Vegetable, Cooks Ingredients, Waitrose* | 1 Pouch/500ml | | 15.0 | 0.0 | 3 | 0.2 | 0.4 | 0.1 | 0.5 |
| Vegetable, Knorr* | 1 Serving/9g | | 18.0 | 0.0 | 199 | 8.5 | 39.9 | 0.6 | 0.9 |
| Vegetable, Tablets, Sainsbury's* | 1 Tablet/11g | | 1.0 | 0.0 | 7 | 0.4 | 0.2 | 0.5 | 0.1 |

## STOCK CUBES

| | INFO/WEIGHT | | KCAL | FAT | KCAL | PROT | CARB | FAT | FIBRE |
|---|---|---|---|---|---|---|---|---|---|
| Basil, Herb Cubes, Knorr* | 1 Cube/10g | | 47.0 | 3.0 | 472 | 6.1 | 35.9 | 33.8 | 0.6 |
| Beef, Dry Weight, Bovril* | 1 Cube/6g | | 12.0 | 0.0 | 197 | 10.8 | 29.3 | 4.1 | 0.0 |
| Beef, Dry Weight, Oxo* | 1 Cube/6g | | 15.0 | 0.0 | 265 | 17.3 | 38.4 | 4.7 | 1.5 |
| Beef, Knorr* | 1 Cube/10g | | 33.0 | 2.0 | 347 | 9.5 | 17.9 | 25.3 | 0.0 |
| Beef, Organic, Kallo* | 1 Cube/12g | | 25.0 | 1.0 | 208 | 16.7 | 16.7 | 8.3 | 0.0 |
| Beef, Tesco* | 1 Cube/7g | | 17.0 | 0.0 | 260 | 9.7 | 48.9 | 2.8 | 1.3 |
| Beef, Value, Tesco* | 1 Cube/10g | | 19.0 | 1.0 | 189 | 11.2 | 17.0 | 8.5 | 0.1 |
| Chicken | 1 Cube/6g | | 14.0 | 1.0 | 237 | 15.4 | 9.9 | 15.4 | 0.0 |
| Chicken, Dry, Oxo* | 1 Cube/6g | | 15.0 | 0.0 | 249 | 11.7 | 42.9 | 3.4 | 1.6 |
| Chicken, Just Bouillon, Kallo* | 1 Cube/12g | | 30.0 | 1.0 | 247 | 11.8 | 26.1 | 10.6 | 1.0 |

**S**

| | Measure INFO/WEIGHT | per Measure KCAL | FAT | Nutrition Values per 100g / 100ml KCAL | PROT | CARB | FAT | FIBRE |
|---|---|---|---|---|---|---|---|---|
| **STOCK CUBES** | | | | | | | | |
| Chicken, Knorr* | 1 Cube/10g | 30.0 | 2.0 | 301 | 10.1 | 23.6 | 18.5 | 0.2 |
| Chicken, Made Up, Sainsbury's* | 1 Cube/200ml | 16.0 | 0.0 | 8 | 0.3 | 1.4 | 0.1 | 0.1 |
| Chicken, Tesco* | 1 Cube/11g | 32.0 | 2.0 | 290 | 10.5 | 11.1 | 22.6 | 0.7 |
| Chinese, Dry Weight, Oxo* | 1 Cube/6g | 16.0 | 0.0 | 274 | 9.5 | 42.9 | 7.2 | 3.6 |
| Fish, Knorr* | 1 Cube/10g | 32.0 | 2.0 | 321 | 18.9 | 15.9 | 20.2 | 0.7 |
| Fish, Sainsbury's* | 1 Cube/11g | 31.0 | 2.0 | 282 | 19.1 | 7.3 | 20.0 | 0.9 |
| Garlic, Dry Weight, Oxo* | 1 Cube/6g | 18.0 | 0.0 | 298 | 13.4 | 48.5 | 5.5 | 3.6 |
| Ham, Knorr* | 1 Cube/10g | 31.0 | 2.0 | 313 | 11.8 | 24.4 | 18.7 | 0.0 |
| Indian, Dry Weight, Oxo* | 1 Cube/6g | 17.0 | 0.0 | 291 | 11.5 | 43.9 | 7.7 | 6.7 |
| Italian, Dry Weight, Oxo* | 1 Cube/6g | 19.0 | 0.0 | 309 | 11.9 | 48.9 | 7.3 | 4.6 |
| Lamb, Made Up, Knorr* | 1 Cube/10g | 30.0 | 2.0 | 301 | 14.7 | 12.9 | 21.2 | 0.2 |
| Mexican, Dry Weight, Oxo* | 1 Cube/6g | 15.0 | 0.0 | 248 | 11.8 | 36.8 | 6.0 | 3.7 |
| Parsley & Garlic, Herb Cubes, Knorr* | 1 Cube/10g | 42.0 | 3.0 | 422 | 8.6 | 35.2 | 27.4 | 1.8 |
| Vegetable, Average | 1 Cube/7g | 18.0 | 1.0 | 253 | 13.5 | 11.6 | 17.3 | 0.0 |
| Vegetable, Dry, Oxo* | 1 Cube/6g | 15.0 | 0.0 | 258 | 9.8 | 45.3 | 4.2 | 1.7 |
| Vegetable, Knorr* | 1 Cube/10g | 33.0 | 2.0 | 330 | 10.0 | 25.0 | 24.0 | 1.0 |
| Vegetable, Low Salt, Organic, Made Up, Kallo* | 1 Serving/500ml | 50.0 | 3.0 | 10 | 0.3 | 0.7 | 0.7 | 0.2 |
| Vegetable, Made Up, Organic, Kallo* | 2 Cubes/100ml | 7.0 | 0.0 | 7 | 0.1 | 0.5 | 0.4 | 0.1 |
| Vegetable Bouillon, Vegetarian, Amoy* | 1 Cube/10g | 30.0 | 2.0 | 300 | 0.0 | 20.0 | 20.0 | 0.0 |
| Vegetable Bouillon, Yeast Free, Made Up, Marigold* | 1 Serving/250ml | 19.0 | 2.0 | 8 | 0.0 | 0.5 | 0.6 | 0.0 |
| **STOCK POT** | | | | | | | | |
| Chicken, Knorr* | 1 Cube/28g | 27.0 | 2.0 | 95 | 2.4 | 4.9 | 7.3 | 0.8 |
| **STORTELLI** | | | | | | | | |
| Microwaveable, Dolmio* | 1 Serving/220g | 299.0 | 2.0 | 136 | 5.3 | 26.3 | 1.0 | 0.0 |
| **STRAWBERRIES** | | | | | | | | |
| & Creme Fraiche, Shapers, Boots* | 1 Pack/100g | 77.0 | 6.0 | 77 | 1.4 | 5.1 | 5.7 | 0.8 |
| Dried, Graze* | 1 Pack/35g | 131.0 | 0.0 | 374 | 1.0 | 91.0 | 0.7 | 0.0 |
| Dried, Urban Fresh Fruit* | 1 Pack/35g | 111.0 | 0.0 | 318 | 1.6 | 77.0 | 0.4 | 5.9 |
| *Fresh, Raw, Average* | *1oz/28g* | *8.0* | *0.0* | *28* | *0.8* | *6.0* | *0.1* | *0.9* |
| *in Fruit Juice, Canned, Average* | *1/3 Can/127g* | *58.0* | *0.0* | *45* | *0.4* | *11.0* | *0.0* | *1.0* |
| in Light Syrup, Canned, Drained, Tesco* | 1 Can/149g | 100.0 | 0.0 | 67 | 0.5 | 16.0 | 0.1 | 0.7 |
| **STROGANOFF** | | | | | | | | |
| Beef, Asda* | 1 Serving/120g | 276.0 | 20.0 | 230 | 16.0 | 3.3 | 17.0 | 0.6 |
| Beef, BGTY, Sainsbury's* | 1 Pack/400g | 416.0 | 10.0 | 104 | 5.6 | 14.6 | 2.6 | 0.6 |
| Beef, Eat Smart, Morrisons* | 1 Pack/400g | 344.0 | 9.0 | 86 | 5.0 | 11.2 | 2.3 | 0.9 |
| Beef, Finest, Tesco* | ½ Pack/200g | 330.0 | 13.0 | 165 | 9.4 | 16.2 | 6.7 | 0.7 |
| Beef, HL, Tesco* | 1 Pack/400g | 400.0 | 9.0 | 100 | 7.0 | 13.0 | 2.2 | 1.3 |
| Beef, Sainsbury's* | 1 Can/200g | 232.0 | 12.0 | 116 | 12.5 | 3.0 | 6.0 | 0.2 |
| Beef, Slow Cooked, With Herby Rice, Sainsbury's* | 1 Pack/450g | 652.0 | 23.0 | 145 | 9.6 | 15.2 | 5.1 | 1.7 |
| Beef, TTD, Sainsbury's* | 1 Pack/400g | 656.0 | 42.0 | 164 | 11.9 | 5.2 | 10.5 | 0.4 |
| Beef, Weight Watchers* | 1 Pack/330g | 297.0 | 8.0 | 90 | 4.3 | 13.0 | 2.3 | 0.1 |
| Beef, with Rice, Naturally Good Food, Tesco* | 1 Pack/400g | 425.0 | 9.0 | 106 | 7.1 | 13.9 | 2.3 | 1.3 |
| Beef, with Rice 'n' Peppers, Tesco* | 1 Pack/450g | 562.0 | 20.0 | 125 | 7.5 | 13.1 | 4.4 | 0.4 |
| Beef, with White & Wild Rice, Classic, Tesco* | 1 Pack/500g | 770.0 | 30.0 | 154 | 9.5 | 15.5 | 5.9 | 2.3 |
| Chicken, with Rice, BGTY, Sainsbury's* | 1 Pack/415g | 448.0 | 5.0 | 108 | 7.0 | 17.1 | 1.3 | 1.1 |
| Chicken & Mushroom, COU, M & S* | 1 Serving/400g | 400.0 | 8.0 | 100 | 3.2 | 16.7 | 2.0 | 0.1 |
| Mushroom, with Rice, BGTY, Sainsbury's* | 1 Serving/450g | 418.0 | 7.0 | 93 | 3.3 | 16.6 | 1.5 | 1.0 |
| Mushroom, with Rice, Vegetarian, HL, Tesco* | 1 Pack/450g | 526.0 | 22.0 | 117 | 3.2 | 15.2 | 4.8 | 1.2 |
| Pork with Rice, HE, Tesco* | 1 Pack/450g | 481.0 | 8.0 | 107 | 7.0 | 15.8 | 1.8 | 0.5 |
| **STRUDEL** | | | | | | | | |
| Apple, Frozen, Sainsbury's* | 1 Serving/100g | 283.0 | 15.0 | 283 | 3.2 | 32.8 | 15.4 | 1.9 |
| Apple, Sainsbury's* | 1/6 Strudel/90g | 255.0 | 14.0 | 283 | 3.2 | 32.8 | 15.4 | 1.9 |
| Apple, Tesco* | 1 Serving/150g | 432.0 | 22.0 | 288 | 3.3 | 36.4 | 14.4 | 2.8 |

| | Measure INFO/WEIGHT | per Measure KCAL | FAT | Nutrition Values per 100g / 100ml KCAL | PROT | CARB | FAT | FIBRE |
|---|---|---|---|---|---|---|---|---|
| **STRUDEL** | | | | | | | | |
| Apple, with Sultanas, Tesco* | 1/6 Strudel/100g | 245.0 | 12.0 | 245 | 2.9 | 30.9 | 12.0 | 0.7 |
| Apple & Mincemeat, Tesco* | 1 Serving/100g | 322.0 | 17.0 | 322 | 3.3 | 39.6 | 16.7 | 2.0 |
| Woodland Fruit, Sainsbury's* | 1/6 Strudel/95g | 276.0 | 15.0 | 290 | 3.7 | 34.0 | 15.5 | 2.0 |
| Woodland Fruit, Tesco* | 1 Serving/100g | 257.0 | 13.0 | 257 | 3.2 | 31.5 | 13.1 | 1.8 |
| **STUFFED PEPPERS** | | | | | | | | |
| Filled with Rice, Average | 1oz/28g | 24.0 | 1.0 | 85 | 1.5 | 15.4 | 2.4 | 1.3 |
| Filled with Vegetables, Cheese Topping, Average | 1oz/28g | 31.0 | 2.0 | 111 | 3.4 | 9.8 | 6.7 | 1.5 |
| Fresh, Asda* | 1 Pepper/150g | 144.0 | 7.0 | 96 | 3.8 | 9.0 | 5.0 | 1.2 |
| Perfectly Balanced, Waitrose* | 1 Pack/300g | 243.0 | 7.0 | 81 | 3.0 | 11.8 | 2.4 | 1.3 |
| Sainsbury's* | 1 Serving/137g | 169.0 | 9.0 | 123 | 3.3 | 11.8 | 6.9 | 1.0 |
| Yellow, Italian, Ready to Roast, Sainsbury's* | 1 Pack/136g | 144.0 | 7.0 | 106 | 5.3 | 9.9 | 5.0 | 1.3 |
| **STUFFING** | | | | | | | | |
| Apricot & Walnut, Made Up, Celebrations, Paxo* | 1 Serving/50g | 80.0 | 2.0 | 161 | 4.3 | 28.0 | 3.5 | 2.8 |
| Chestnut & Pork, M & S* | 1oz/28g | 67.0 | 5.0 | 240 | 6.6 | 16.3 | 16.7 | 2.9 |
| Olde English Chestnut, Sainsbury's* | 1 Serving/110g | 216.0 | 13.0 | 196 | 9.4 | 13.5 | 11.6 | 2.1 |
| Parsley, Thyme & Lemon Stuffing, Paxo* | 1 Serving/45g | 67.0 | 1.0 | 150 | 4.3 | 28.4 | 2.1 | 2.4 |
| Parsley & Thyme, Co-Op* | 1 Serving/28g | 95.0 | 1.0 | 340 | 10.0 | 67.0 | 3.0 | 6.0 |
| Sage & Onion, for Chicken, Paxo* | 1 Serving/50g | 61.0 | 1.0 | 123 | 3.6 | 23.0 | 1.8 | 1.7 |
| Sage & Onion, Made Up, Paxo* | 1 Serving/50g | 71.0 | 1.0 | 143 | 3.2 | 29.9 | 1.2 | 1.9 |
| Sage & Onion, Made Up, Safeway* | 1 Serving/60g | 90.0 | 0.0 | 150 | 4.5 | 30.8 | 0.7 | 3.2 |
| Sage & Onion, with Lemon, Paxo* | 1 Serving/50g | 61.0 | 1.0 | 122 | 3.4 | 24.2 | 1.2 | 1.9 |
| Sausagemeat, Sainsbury's* | 1 Serving/100g | 175.0 | 4.0 | 175 | 7.0 | 27.0 | 4.2 | 2.3 |
| Sausagemeat & Thyme, Made Up, Celebrations, Paxo* | 1 Serving/50g | 80.0 | 2.0 | 160 | 6.3 | 25.8 | 3.5 | 4.0 |
| **STUFFING BALLS** | | | | | | | | |
| Pork, Sausagemeat, Aunt Bessie's* | 1 Ball/26g | 55.0 | 2.0 | 212 | 7.2 | 27.3 | 8.2 | 3.0 |
| Sage & Onion, Aunt Bessie's* | 1 Ball/26g | 63.0 | 2.0 | 243 | 6.4 | 34.4 | 8.9 | 3.1 |
| Sage & Onion, Meat-Free, Aunt Bessie's* | 1 Ball/28g | 54.0 | 2.0 | 193 | 5.4 | 28.0 | 6.7 | 1.7 |
| Sage & Onion, Tesco* | 1 Serving/20g | 64.0 | 4.0 | 322 | 10.0 | 21.1 | 22.0 | 1.9 |
| Tesco* | 1 Ball/21g | 65.0 | 4.0 | 315 | 9.6 | 23.5 | 20.0 | 1.4 |
| **STUFFING MIX** | | | | | | | | |
| Apple, Mustard & Herb, Paxo* | 1 Serving/50g | 83.0 | 1.0 | 166 | 4.2 | 32.8 | 2.0 | 4.0 |
| Apple & Herb, Special Recipe, Sainsbury's* | 1 Serving/41g | 68.0 | 1.0 | 165 | 3.8 | 32.4 | 2.2 | 2.2 |
| Chestnut, Morrisons* | 1 Serving/20g | 33.0 | 1.0 | 165 | 4.6 | 29.1 | 3.4 | 3.7 |
| Chestnut & Cranberry, Celebration, Paxo* | 1 Serving/25g | 35.0 | 0.0 | 141 | 4.0 | 26.7 | 2.0 | 2.4 |
| Date, Walnut & Stilton, Special Recipe, Sainsbury's* | 1 Serving/25g | 49.0 | 2.0 | 196 | 5.2 | 25.0 | 8.4 | 2.0 |
| Date & Walnut, TTD, Sainsbury's* | 1 Serving/50g | 65.0 | 1.0 | 131 | 4.4 | 24.2 | 1.8 | 3.4 |
| Herb & Onion, Gluten Free, Allergycare* | 1 Serving/12g | 43.0 | 0.0 | 360 | 7.9 | 76.8 | 2.4 | 0.0 |
| Parsley, Thyme & Lemon, Sainsbury's* | 1 Pack/170g | 240.0 | 2.0 | 141 | 4.2 | 28.2 | 1.3 | 1.3 |
| Sage, Red Onion & Lemon, TTD, Sainsbury's* | 1 Serving/50g | 53.0 | 1.0 | 106 | 3.8 | 23.9 | 1.3 | 4.2 |
| Sage & Onion, Asda* | 1 Serving/27g | 29.0 | 0.0 | 107 | 3.4 | 22.0 | 0.6 | 1.3 |
| Sage & Onion, Co-Op* | 1 Serving/28g | 94.0 | 1.0 | 335 | 10.0 | 68.0 | 2.0 | 6.0 |
| Sage & Onion, Dry Weight, Tesco* | 1 Std Pack/170g | 578.0 | 4.0 | 340 | 10.3 | 69.3 | 2.4 | 6.3 |
| Sage & Onion, Made Up, Paxo* | 1 Serving/60g | 74.0 | 1.0 | 123 | 3.6 | 23.0 | 1.8 | 1.7 |
| Sage & Onion, Prepared, Tesco* | 1 Serving/100g | 50.0 | 0.0 | 50 | 1.5 | 10.1 | 0.4 | 0.9 |
| Sage & Onion, SmartPrice, Asda* | ¼ Pack/75g | 262.0 | 3.0 | 349 | 11.0 | 68.0 | 3.7 | 4.7 |
| Sausage Meat, Morrisons* | 1 Serving/20g | 35.0 | 1.0 | 174 | 6.8 | 30.8 | 2.6 | 2.9 |
| **SUET** | | | | | | | | |
| Beef, Shredded, Original, Atora* | 1 Pack/250g | 2075.0 | 218.0 | 830 | 0.9 | 10.1 | 87.4 | 0.4 |
| Beef, Tesco* | 1 Serving/100g | 854.0 | 92.0 | 854 | 0.6 | 6.2 | 91.9 | 0.1 |
| *Vegetable, Average* | *1oz/28g* | *234.0* | *25.0* | *836* | *1.2* | *10.1* | *87.9* | *0.0* |
| **SUET PUDDING** | | | | | | | | |
| *Average* | *1oz/28g* | *94.0* | *5.0* | *335* | *4.4* | *40.5* | *18.3* | *0.9* |

S

|  | Measure INFO/WEIGHT | per Measure KCAL | FAT | Nutrition Values per 100g / 100ml KCAL | PROT | CARB | FAT | FIBRE |
|---|---|---|---|---|---|---|---|---|
| **SUGAR** | | | | | | | | |
| *Brown, Soft, Average* | *1 Tsp/4g* | *15.0* | *0.0* | *382* | *0.0* | *96.5* | *0.0* | *0.0* |
| *Caster, Average* | *1 Tbsp/12g* | *48.0* | *0.0* | *399* | *0.0* | *99.8* | *0.0* | *0.0* |
| *Dark Brown, Muscovado, Average* | *1 Tsp/7g* | *27.0* | *0.0* | *380* | *0.2* | *94.7* | *0.0* | *0.0* |
| *Dark Brown, Soft, Average* | *1 Tsp/5g* | *18.0* | *0.0* | *369* | *0.1* | *92.0* | *0.0* | *0.0* |
| *Demerara, Average* | *1 Tsp/5g* | *18.0* | *0.0* | *367* | *0.2* | *99.1* | *0.0* | *0.0* |
| for Making Jam, Silver Spoon* | 1oz/28g | 111.0 | 0.0 | 398 | 0.0 | 99.5 | 0.0 | 0.0 |
| Fructose, Fruit Sugar, Tate & Lyle* | 1 Tsp/4g | 16.0 | 0.0 | 400 | 0.0 | 100.0 | 0.0 | 0.0 |
| *Golden, Unrefined, Average* | *1 Tsp/4g* | *16.0* | *0.0* | *399* | *0.0* | *99.8* | *0.0* | *0.0* |
| *Granulated, Organic, Average* | *1 Tsp/4g* | *16.0* | *0.0* | *398* | *0.2* | *99.7* | *0.0* | *0.0* |
| *Icing, Average* | *1 Tsp/4g* | *16.0* | *0.0* | *394* | *0.0* | *102.1* | *0.0* | *0.0* |
| *Light Or Diet, Average* | *1 Tsp/4g* | *16.0* | *0.0* | *394* | *0.0* | *98.5* | *0.0* | *0.0* |
| *White, Granulated, Average* | *1 Tsp/5g* | *20.0* | *0.0* | *397* | *0.0* | *100.7* | *0.0* | *0.0* |
| **SULTANAS** | | | | | | | | |
| *Average* | *1oz/28g* | *82.0* | *0.0* | *292* | *2.5* | *69.7* | *0.4* | *2.0* |
| **SUNDAE** | | | | | | | | |
| Banoffee, Perfectly Balanced, Waitrose* | 1 Pot/115g | 143.0 | 2.0 | 124 | 3.1 | 23.6 | 1.9 | 0.8 |
| Blackcurrant, M & S* | 1 Sundae/53g | 212.0 | 10.0 | 400 | 3.0 | 54.2 | 19.2 | 1.9 |
| Blackcurrant, Tesco* | 1 Cake/48g | 183.0 | 9.0 | 385 | 3.4 | 52.2 | 18.1 | 5.1 |
| Butter Toffee, Mini, Eat Smart, Safeway* | 1 Pot/63g | 100.0 | 1.0 | 160 | 2.9 | 32.5 | 1.8 | 3.7 |
| Chocolate, HE, Tesco* | 1 Serving/130g | 199.0 | 5.0 | 153 | 4.5 | 24.9 | 3.9 | 0.6 |
| Chocolate, Mini, Asda* | 1 Pot/86g | 199.0 | 13.0 | 231 | 3.1 | 21.0 | 15.0 | 1.7 |
| Chocolate, Sainsbury's* | 1 Pot/140g | 393.0 | 30.0 | 281 | 2.5 | 19.3 | 21.3 | 0.6 |
| Chocolate & Cookie, Weight Watchers* | 1 Pot/82g | 128.0 | 3.0 | 156 | 2.5 | 30.3 | 3.4 | 2.2 |
| Chocolate & Sticky Toffee, Asda* | 1 Sundae/215g | 755.0 | 52.0 | 351 | 2.8 | 31.0 | 24.0 | 0.5 |
| Chocolate & Vanilla, HL, Tesco* | 1 Sundae/120g | 193.0 | 3.0 | 161 | 2.8 | 31.5 | 2.6 | 0.6 |
| Chocolate & Vanilla, Tesco* | 1 Sundae/70g | 140.0 | 6.0 | 199 | 2.8 | 27.5 | 8.6 | 0.5 |
| Chocolate Brownie, Finest, Tesco* | 1 Serving/215g | 778.0 | 57.0 | 362 | 2.7 | 28.7 | 26.3 | 2.3 |
| Chocolate Mint, COU, M & S* | 1 Pot/90g | 108.0 | 2.0 | 120 | 5.4 | 17.8 | 2.6 | 0.5 |
| Chocolate Nut | 1 Serving/70g | 195.0 | 11.0 | 278 | 3.0 | 34.2 | 15.3 | 0.1 |
| Galaxy Caramel, Eden Vale* | 1 Serving/128g | 300.0 | 16.0 | 234 | 4.8 | 26.5 | 12.4 | 0.7 |
| Hot Fudge, Two Scoop, Baskin Robbins* | 1 Serving/203g | 530.0 | 29.0 | 261 | 3.9 | 30.5 | 14.3 | 0.0 |
| Mango & Passionfruit, Tesco* | 1 Pot/78g | 112.0 | 1.0 | 143 | 1.1 | 32.7 | 0.8 | 0.4 |
| Peach & Apricot, Perfectly Balanced, Waitrose* | 1 Pot/175ml | 142.0 | 1.0 | 81 | 1.7 | 17.7 | 0.4 | 0.0 |
| Raspberry, Eat Smart, Safeway* | 1 Serving/97g | 150.0 | 2.0 | 155 | 3.0 | 30.9 | 2.1 | 2.8 |
| Raspberry, Perfectly Balanced, Waitrose* | 1 Pot/175ml | 150.0 | 1.0 | 86 | 1.7 | 18.9 | 0.6 | 0.0 |
| Strawberry, M & S* | 1 Sundae/45g | 173.0 | 8.0 | 385 | 3.4 | 53.3 | 17.8 | 1.0 |
| Strawberry, Tesco* | 1 Sundae/48g | 194.0 | 9.0 | 408 | 3.3 | 57.6 | 18.3 | 1.3 |
| Strawberry & Vanilla, Tesco* | 1 Serving/68g | 120.0 | 4.0 | 177 | 2.0 | 29.5 | 5.7 | 0.1 |
| Strawberry & Vanilla, Weight Watchers* | 1 Pot/105g | 148.0 | 2.0 | 141 | 1.2 | 29.1 | 2.1 | 0.3 |
| Toffee, Asda* | 1 Serving/120g | 322.0 | 19.0 | 268 | 2.1 | 29.0 | 16.0 | 0.0 |
| Toffee & Vanilla, Tesco* | 1 Serving/70g | 133.0 | 5.0 | 189 | 2.1 | 30.7 | 6.4 | 0.1 |
| **SUNNY DELIGHT*** | | | | | | | | |
| Apple & Kiwi Kick, Sunny Delight* | 1 Glass/200ml | 15.0 | 0.0 | 7 | 0.2 | 1.3 | 0.2 | 0.2 |
| Californian Style, No Added Sugar, Sunny Delight* | 1 Serving/200ml | 20.0 | 0.0 | 10 | 0.1 | 1.4 | 0.2 | 0.1 |
| Original, Sunny Delight* | 1 Glass/200ml | 88.0 | 0.0 | 44 | 0.1 | 10.0 | 0.2 | 0.0 |
| **SUSHI** | | | | | | | | |
| Aya Set, Waitrose* | 1 Pack/110g | 200.0 | 4.0 | 182 | 5.4 | 31.7 | 3.9 | 1.5 |
| California Roll Box, M & S* | 1 Pack/230g | 391.0 | 12.0 | 170 | 7.0 | 22.0 | 5.2 | 1.1 |
| California Roll Selection, Classics, M & S* | 1 Pack/225g | 326.0 | 6.0 | 145 | 7.0 | 23.2 | 2.7 | 1.1 |
| California Set, Waitrose* | 1 Pack/120g | 223.0 | 9.0 | 186 | 3.8 | 25.2 | 7.6 | 1.7 |
| Californian, Yakatori, M & S* | 1 Serving/200g | 340.0 | 9.0 | 170 | 6.4 | 25.0 | 4.7 | 1.0 |
| Californian Roll, Nigiri & Maki Selection, M & S* | 1 Pack/210g | 294.0 | 4.0 | 140 | 4.4 | 25.9 | 2.1 | 2.2 |
| Californian Roll & Nigiri, Selection, M & S* | 1 Pack/215g | 355.0 | 6.0 | 165 | 7.1 | 28.0 | 2.7 | 1.1 |

**S**

| | Measure INFO/WEIGHT | per Measure KCAL | per Measure FAT | Nutrition Values per 100g / 100ml KCAL | PROT | CARB | FAT | FIBRE |
|---|---|---|---|---|---|---|---|---|
| **SUSHI** | | | | | | | | |
| Chicken, M & S* | 1 Pack/186g | 260.0 | 4.0 | 140 | 6.0 | 24.4 | 2.2 | 1.0 |
| Chicken, Tesco* | 1 Pack/147g | 243.0 | 4.0 | 165 | 5.2 | 30.0 | 2.4 | 1.0 |
| Classic, Finest, Tesco* | 1 Pack/232g | 330.0 | 1.0 | 142 | 6.6 | 27.6 | 0.4 | 0.6 |
| Deluxe, Shapers, Boots* | 1 Serving/235g | 355.0 | 4.0 | 151 | 5.3 | 29.0 | 1.5 | 2.7 |
| Fish, Snack, Tesco* | 1 Pack/104g | 159.0 | 3.0 | 153 | 4.5 | 28.0 | 2.5 | 1.5 |
| Fish & Veg Selection, Tesco* | 1 Pack/150g | 247.0 | 3.0 | 165 | 6.7 | 29.2 | 2.3 | 0.4 |
| Fish Nigiri, Adventurous, Tesco* | 1 Pack/200g | 270.0 | 4.0 | 135 | 7.1 | 21.7 | 2.2 | 0.5 |
| Fish Roll, Nigiri & Maki Selection, M & S* | 1 Pack/210g | 315.0 | 5.0 | 150 | 6.5 | 25.8 | 2.3 | 1.0 |
| Fish Selection, M & S* | 1 Pack/210g | 346.0 | 7.0 | 165 | 7.4 | 26.3 | 3.1 | 1.4 |
| Hagi Set, Waitrose* | 1 Pack/370g | 688.0 | 10.0 | 186 | 7.1 | 33.6 | 2.6 | 1.1 |
| Hana Set, Waitrose* | 1 Serving/175g | 324.0 | 4.0 | 185 | 5.4 | 35.7 | 2.3 | 1.4 |
| Irodori Set, with Fish, Cucumber, & Avocado, Waitrose* | 1 Pack/281g | 472.0 | 12.0 | 168 | 5.2 | 26.7 | 4.4 | 1.3 |
| Komachi Set, with Salmon, Whiting & Handroll, Waitrose* | 1 Pack/257g | 447.0 | 14.0 | 174 | 5.3 | 25.8 | 5.4 | 1.2 |
| Large, Boots* | 1 Pack/324g | 480.0 | 6.0 | 148 | 5.0 | 28.0 | 1.8 | 0.7 |
| Large Pack, Tesco* | 1 Pack/250g | 357.0 | 5.0 | 143 | 6.1 | 24.8 | 2.2 | 2.7 |
| Maki Rolls Box, Sainsbury's* | 1 Pack/127g | 197.0 | 2.0 | 155 | 4.5 | 30.5 | 1.7 | 0.8 |
| Maki Selection, Shapers, Boots* | 1 Pack/158g | 225.0 | 2.0 | 142 | 3.5 | 29.0 | 1.3 | 1.1 |
| Medium Pack, Tesco* | 1 Pack/139g | 211.0 | 3.0 | 152 | 6.3 | 26.6 | 2.3 | 2.3 |
| Mini, Boots* | 1 Pack/99g | 153.0 | 2.0 | 155 | 5.5 | 29.0 | 1.9 | 0.8 |
| Nigiri, M & S* | 1 Serving/190g | 303.0 | 6.0 | 159 | 7.3 | 25.3 | 3.1 | 0.6 |
| Nigiri, Selection, Tesco* | 1 Pack/152g | 236.0 | 2.0 | 155 | 4.6 | 31.2 | 1.0 | 0.6 |
| Nigiri Set, Waitrose* | 1 Pack/150g | 229.0 | 4.0 | 153 | 6.3 | 26.0 | 2.6 | 0.6 |
| Nigri, Californian Roll, Maki Roll, Sainsbury's* | 1 Pack/195g | 283.0 | 3.0 | 145 | 5.3 | 27.4 | 1.5 | 1.9 |
| Oriental Fish Box, M & S* | 1 Pack/205g | 318.0 | 8.0 | 155 | 6.1 | 23.3 | 4.1 | 0.9 |
| Prawn & Salmon Selection, M & S* | 1 Serving/175g | 255.0 | 3.0 | 146 | 5.5 | 27.4 | 1.7 | 0.6 |
| Prawn Feast, M & S* | 1 Pack/219g | 350.0 | 8.0 | 160 | 5.7 | 25.8 | 3.7 | 1.1 |
| Roll Selection, Sainsbury's* | 1 Pack/217g | 363.0 | 8.0 | 167 | 5.0 | 28.4 | 3.7 | 0.5 |
| Roll Selection, Tesco* | 1 Pack/214g | 327.0 | 5.0 | 153 | 5.0 | 27.6 | 2.5 | 1.2 |
| Rolls, Shapers, Boots* | 1 Pack/168g | 259.0 | 4.0 | 154 | 4.7 | 28.0 | 2.4 | 0.5 |
| Salmon, Nigri Crayfish, Red Pepper, Sainsbury's* | 1 Serving/150g | 232.0 | 4.0 | 155 | 5.5 | 26.4 | 3.0 | 1.0 |
| Salmon & Roll Set, Sainsbury's* | 1 Serving/101g | 167.0 | 3.0 | 165 | 4.9 | 30.4 | 2.6 | 0.8 |
| Salmon Feast Box, M & S* | 1 Pack/200g | 330.0 | 6.0 | 165 | 5.6 | 27.0 | 2.9 | 1.0 |
| Selection, Boots* | 1 Pack/268g | 434.0 | 10.0 | 162 | 5.5 | 27.0 | 3.6 | 1.6 |
| Selection, Shapers, Boots* | 1 Pack/162g | 245.0 | 3.0 | 151 | 5.6 | 29.0 | 1.6 | 1.7 |
| to Share, Tesco* | 1 Pack/385g | 616.0 | 6.0 | 160 | 5.7 | 30.6 | 1.6 | 0.7 |
| Tokyo Set, M & S* | 1 Pack/150g | 240.0 | 5.0 | 160 | 7.3 | 25.3 | 3.1 | 0.6 |
| Tuna, to Snack Selection, Food to Go, M & S* | 1 Serving/150g | 225.0 | 4.0 | 150 | 5.2 | 26.4 | 2.6 | 2.3 |
| Vegetarian, Snack Selection, Tesco* | 1 Pack/85g | 106.0 | 3.0 | 125 | 3.7 | 20.1 | 3.3 | 0.6 |
| Vegetarian, with Pickled Vegetables, Waitrose* | 1 Pack/135g | 244.0 | 5.0 | 181 | 5.0 | 27.8 | 3.6 | 1.7 |
| Yo!, Bento Box, Sainsbury's* | 1 Pack/208g | 530.0 | 6.0 | 255 | 8.4 | 48.7 | 3.0 | 0.9 |
| Yo!, Salmon Lunch Set, Sainsbury's* | 1 Pack/150g | 241.0 | 4.0 | 161 | 5.9 | 28.1 | 2.8 | 0.8 |
| **SWEDE** | | | | | | | | |
| *Boiled, Average* | *1oz/28g* | *3.0* | *0.0* | *11* | *0.3* | *2.3* | *0.1* | *0.7* |
| Mash, COU, M & S* | 1oz/28g | 15.0 | 0.0 | 55 | 1.1 | 9.5 | 1.2 | 2.1 |
| *Raw, Unprepared, Average* | *1oz/28g* | *6.0* | *0.0* | *21* | *0.8* | *4.4* | *0.3* | *1.9* |
| **SWEET & SOUR** | | | | | | | | |
| Beef, Feeling Great, New, Findus* | 1 Pack/350g | 420.0 | 9.0 | 120 | 4.5 | 20.0 | 2.5 | 1.3 |
| Chicken, & Noodles, BGTY, Sainsbury's* | 1 Pack/400g | 356.0 | 2.0 | 89 | 7.5 | 13.3 | 0.6 | 0.7 |
| Chicken, & Noodles, Chinese Takeaway, Tesco* | 1 Pack/350g | 350.0 | 1.0 | 100 | 5.7 | 18.8 | 0.2 | 0.2 |
| Chicken, & Rice, Chilled, Tesco* | 1 Pack/450g | 540.0 | 6.0 | 120 | 4.9 | 21.9 | 1.3 | 0.9 |
| Chicken, & Rice, Mega, Value, Tesco* | 1 Pack/500g | 675.0 | 9.0 | 135 | 4.4 | 25.0 | 1.9 | 1.9 |
| Chicken, & Rice, Morrisons* | 1 Pack/400g | 452.0 | 10.0 | 113 | 3.6 | 18.8 | 2.6 | 0.8 |
| Chicken, Breasts, Tesco* | 1 Serving/185g | 172.0 | 2.0 | 93 | 14.6 | 6.5 | 1.0 | 0.1 |

| | Measure INFO/WEIGHT | per Measure KCAL | per Measure FAT | Nutrition Values per 100g / 100ml KCAL | PROT | CARB | FAT | FIBRE |
|---|---|---|---|---|---|---|---|---|
| **SWEET & SOUR** | | | | | | | | |
| Chicken, Canned, Tesco* | 1 Can/400g | 408.0 | 6.0 | 102 | 9.6 | 12.4 | 1.6 | 1.1 |
| Chicken, Crispy, Fillets, Tesco* | 1 Pack/350g | 507.0 | 20.0 | 145 | 7.2 | 15.3 | 5.6 | 0.9 |
| Chicken, Crispy, Iceland* | 1 Serving/125g | 221.0 | 6.0 | 177 | 18.3 | 14.2 | 5.2 | 1.2 |
| Chicken, Healthy Options, Birds Eye* | 1 Meal/348g | 390.0 | 4.0 | 112 | 4.8 | 20.7 | 1.1 | 0.6 |
| Chicken, in Batter, Cantonese, Chilled, Sainsbury's* | 1 Pack/350g | 560.0 | 21.0 | 160 | 8.9 | 22.4 | 6.0 | 0.9 |
| Chicken, in Crispy Batter, Morrisons* | 1 Pack/350g | 511.0 | 14.0 | 146 | 10.1 | 17.6 | 3.9 | 1.2 |
| Chicken, Low Fat, Iceland* | 1 Pack/400g | 444.0 | 7.0 | 111 | 8.1 | 15.7 | 1.7 | 1.1 |
| Chicken, M & S* | 1 Pack/300g | 465.0 | 11.0 | 155 | 6.6 | 24.4 | 3.6 | 0.8 |
| Chicken, Oriental, Tesco* | 1 Pack/350g | 340.0 | 4.0 | 97 | 9.3 | 12.2 | 1.1 | 0.8 |
| Chicken, Take It Away, M & S* | 1 Pack/200g | 200.0 | 2.0 | 100 | 9.4 | 13.2 | 0.8 | 1.2 |
| Chicken, Waitrose* | 1 Serving/400g | 372.0 | 3.0 | 93 | 9.8 | 11.7 | 0.8 | 1.4 |
| Chicken, Weight Watchers* | 1 Pack/330g | 310.0 | 1.0 | 94 | 5.0 | 17.5 | 0.4 | 0.3 |
| Chicken, with Egg Rice, Chilled, HL, Tesco* | 1 Pack/450g | 499.0 | 3.0 | 111 | 6.8 | 19.2 | 0.7 | 0.6 |
| Chicken, with Noodles, Feeling Great, Findus* | 1 Pack/350g | 385.0 | 9.0 | 110 | 5.0 | 17.0 | 2.5 | 1.5 |
| Chicken, with Noodles, Steamed, HE, Tesco* | 1 Pack/370g | 289.0 | 1.0 | 78 | 8.3 | 10.8 | 0.2 | 0.6 |
| Chicken, with Rice, Big Eat, Heinz* | 1 Pot/350g | 329.0 | 7.0 | 94 | 4.4 | 14.9 | 1.9 | 0.6 |
| Chicken, with Rice, Chilled, BGTY, Sainsbury's* | 1 Pack/400g | 344.0 | 4.0 | 86 | 6.0 | 13.5 | 0.9 | 1.0 |
| Chicken, with Rice, Good Intentions, Somerfield* | 1 Serving/400g | 448.0 | 2.0 | 112 | 6.6 | 20.1 | 0.6 | 0.3 |
| Chicken, with Rice, Oriental Express* | 1 Pack/340g | 350.0 | 2.0 | 103 | 4.4 | 21.3 | 0.6 | 0.7 |
| Chicken, with Rice, Value, Tesco* | 1 Pack/300g | 348.0 | 1.0 | 116 | 5.9 | 22.3 | 0.3 | 0.7 |
| Chicken, with Rice, Weight Watchers* | 1 Pack/400g | 341.0 | 2.0 | 85 | 6.3 | 14.6 | 0.4 | 1.1 |
| Chicken, with Vegetable Rice, COU, M & S* | 1 Pack/400g | 400.0 | 6.0 | 100 | 6.9 | 14.9 | 1.4 | 1.1 |
| Chicken, without Batter, Cantonese, Chilled, Sainsbury's* | 1 Pack/350g | 409.0 | 5.0 | 117 | 8.5 | 17.6 | 1.4 | 1.0 |
| Chicken Balls, Chinese Takeaway, Iceland* | 1 Pack/255g | 311.0 | 3.0 | 122 | 9.9 | 17.5 | 1.3 | 6.0 |
| Pork | 1oz/28g | 48.0 | 2.0 | 172 | 12.7 | 11.3 | 8.8 | 0.6 |
| Pork, Battered, Sainsbury's* | ½ Pack/175g | 306.0 | 9.0 | 175 | 7.3 | 25.1 | 5.0 | 0.6 |
| Roasted Vegetables, Cantonese, Sainsbury's* | 1 Pack/348g | 327.0 | 4.0 | 94 | 1.1 | 19.6 | 1.2 | 0.9 |
| Vegetables, with Rice, Waitrose* | 1 Pack/400g | 384.0 | 4.0 | 96 | 1.9 | 19.5 | 1.1 | 1.1 |
| **SWEET POTATO** | | | | | | | | |
| *Baked, Average* | *1 Med/130g* | *149.0* | *1.0* | *115* | *1.6* | *27.9* | *0.4* | *3.3* |
| *Boiled in Salted Water, Average* | *1 Med/130g* | *109.0* | *0.0* | *84* | *1.1* | *20.5* | *0.3* | *2.3* |
| *Raw, Unprepared, Average* | *1 Med/130g* | *113.0* | *0.0* | *87* | *1.2* | *21.3* | *0.3* | *2.4* |
| *Steamed, Average* | *1 Med/130g* | *109.0* | *0.0* | *84* | *1.1* | *20.4* | *0.3* | *2.3* |
| with Rosemary & Garlic, Frozen, McCain* | 1 Serving/150g | 172.0 | 6.0 | 115 | 2.1 | 18.4 | 3.7 | 2.8 |
| **SWEETBREAD** | | | | | | | | |
| *Lamb, Fried* | *1oz/28g* | *61.0* | *3.0* | *217* | *28.7* | *0.0* | *11.4* | *0.0* |
| *Lamb, Raw* | *1oz/28g* | *37.0* | *2.0* | *131* | *15.3* | *0.0* | *7.8* | *0.0* |
| **SWEETCORN** | | | | | | | | |
| & Petit Pois, M & S* | 1oz/28g | 20.0 | 0.0 | 73 | 4.6 | 10.8 | 1.3 | 3.6 |
| Baby, & Mangetout, Somerfield* | 1 Pack/150g | 42.0 | 0.0 | 28 | 3.2 | 3.0 | 0.3 | 1.9 |
| *Baby, Canned, Drained, Average* | *1oz/28g* | *6.0* | *0.0* | *23* | *2.9* | *2.0* | *0.4* | *1.5* |
| *Baby, Frozen, Average* | *1oz/28g* | *7.0* | *0.0* | *24* | *2.5* | *2.7* | *0.4* | *1.7* |
| *Boiled, Average* | *1oz/28g* | *31.0* | *1.0* | *111* | *4.2* | *19.6* | *2.3* | *2.2* |
| *Canned, in Water, No Sugar & Salt, Average* | *½ Can/125g* | *99.0* | *1.0* | *79* | *2.7* | *14.9* | *1.1* | *1.6* |
| *Canned, with Sugar & Salt, Average* | *½ Can/71g* | *79.0* | *1.0* | *111* | *3.2* | *21.9* | *1.2* | *1.9* |
| *Frozen, Average* | *1 Sachet/115g* | *121.0* | *2.0* | *105* | *3.8* | *17.9* | *2.1* | *1.8* |
| *with Peppers, Canned, Average* | *1 Serving/50g* | *39.0* | *0.0* | *79* | *2.6* | *16.4* | *0.3* | *0.6* |
| **SWEETENER** | | | | | | | | |
| Aspartamo, Artificial Sugar, Zen* | 1 Tbsp/2g | 8.0 | 0.0 | 383 | 1.8 | 94.0 | 0.0 | 0.0 |
| Canderel, Spoonful, Canderel* | 1 Tsp/0.5g | 2.0 | 0.0 | 384 | 2.9 | 93.0 | 0.0 | 0.0 |
| Canderel* | 1 Tbsp/2g | 8.0 | 0.0 | 379 | 24.7 | 7.0 | 0.0 | 5.3 |
| Granulated, Asda* | 1 Tsp/1g | 4.0 | 0.0 | 400 | 0.0 | 100.0 | 0.0 | 0.0 |
| Granulated, Low Calorie, Splenda* | 1 Tsp/0.5g | 2.0 | 0.0 | 391 | 0.0 | 97.7 | 0.0 | 0.0 |

**S**

| | Measure INFO/WEIGHT | per Measure KCAL | FAT | Nutrition Values per 100g / 100ml KCAL | PROT | CARB | FAT | FIBRE |
|---|---|---|---|---|---|---|---|---|
| **SWEETENER** | | | | | | | | |
| Granulated, Safeway* | 1 Tsp/1g | 4.0 | 0.0 | 392 | 3.0 | 95.0 | 0.0 | 0.0 |
| Granulated, Silver Spoon* | 1 Tsp/0.5g | 2.0 | 0.0 | 387 | 1.0 | 96.8 | 0.0 | 0.0 |
| Granulated, Tesco* | 1 Tsp/1g | 4.0 | 0.0 | 383 | 1.8 | 94.0 | 0.0 | 0.0 |
| Low Calorie, Somerfield* | 1 Tsp/1g | 2.0 | 0.0 | 380 | 3.0 | 92.0 | 0.0 | 0.0 |
| Silver Spoon* | 1 Tablet/0.05g | 0.0 | 0.0 | 325 | 10.0 | 71.0 | 0.0 | 0.0 |
| Simply Sweet* | 1 Tbsp/2g | 7.0 | 0.0 | 375 | 1.4 | 92.3 | 0.0 | 0.0 |
| Slendasweet, Sainsbury's* | 1 Tsp/1g | 4.0 | 0.0 | 395 | 1.8 | 97.0 | 0.0 | 0.1 |
| Spoonfull, Low Calorie, SupaSweet* | 1 Tsp/1g | 4.0 | 0.0 | 392 | 3.0 | 95.0 | 0.0 | 0.0 |
| Sweet'N Low* | 1 Sachet/1g | 3.0 | 0.0 | 368 | 0.0 | 92.0 | 0.0 | 0.0 |
| Sweetex* | 1oz/28g | 0.0 | 0.0 | 0 | 0.0 | 0.0 | 0.0 | 0.0 |
| Tablets, Low Calorie, Canderel* | 1 Tablet/0.1g | 0.0 | 0.0 | 342 | 13.0 | 72.4 | 0.0 | 0.0 |
| Tablets, Splenda* | 1 Tablet/0.1g | 0.0 | 0.0 | 345 | 10.0 | 76.2 | 0.0 | 1.6 |
| Tablets, Tesco* | 1 Tablet/1g | 0.0 | 0.0 | 20 | 2.0 | 2.0 | 0.5 | 0.0 |
| Xylosweet, Xylitol* | 1 Serving/4g | 10.0 | 0.0 | 240 | 0.0 | 100.0 | 0.0 | 0.0 |
| **SWEETS** | | | | | | | | |
| Alphabet Candies, Asda* | 1 Pack/80g | 306.0 | 0.0 | 382 | 0.5 | 95.0 | 0.0 | 0.0 |
| Aquadrops, Citrus & Apple, Mars* | 1 Serving/3g | 6.0 | 0.0 | 247 | 0.1 | 94.5 | 1.0 | 0.0 |
| Banana, Baby Foam, M & S* | 1/3 Pack/34g | 131.0 | 0.0 | 385 | 4.1 | 92.7 | 0.0 | 0.0 |
| Black Jacks & Fruit Salad, Bassett's* | 1 Serving/190g | 760.0 | 12.0 | 400 | 0.7 | 84.9 | 6.2 | 0.0 |
| Blackcurrant & Liquorice, M & S* | 1 Sweet/8g | 32.0 | 0.0 | 400 | 0.6 | 89.0 | 4.3 | 0.0 |
| Body Parts, Rowntree's* | 1 Pack/42g | 146.0 | 0.0 | 348 | 4.3 | 82.9 | 0.0 | 0.0 |
| Bursting Bugs, Rowntree's* | 1 Pack/175g | 583.0 | 0.0 | 333 | 4.8 | 78.1 | 0.2 | 0.0 |
| Butter Candies, Original, Werther's* | 1 Sweet/5g | 21.0 | 0.0 | 424 | 0.1 | 85.7 | 8.9 | 0.1 |
| Campino, Oranges & Cream, Bendicks* | 1oz/28g | 116.0 | 2.0 | 416 | 0.1 | 85.8 | 8.1 | 0.0 |
| Campino, Strawberries & Cream, Bendicks* | 1oz/28g | 117.0 | 2.0 | 418 | 0.1 | 86.2 | 8.1 | 0.0 |
| Candy Cane, Average | 1oz/28g | 100.0 | 0.0 | 357 | 3.6 | 85.7 | 0.0 | 0.0 |
| Candy Floss, Asda* | 1 Tub/75g | 292.0 | 0.0 | 390 | 0.0 | 100.0 | 0.0 | 0.0 |
| Candy Foam Shapes, Fun Fruits, Value, Tesco* | 1 Serving/25g | 96.0 | 0.0 | 384 | 3.6 | 94.0 | 0.3 | 0.1 |
| Chewitts, Blackcurrant | 1 Pack/33g | 125.0 | 1.0 | 378 | 0.3 | 86.9 | 2.7 | 0.0 |
| Chews, Calcium, Ellactiva* | 1 Sweet/7g | 24.0 | 1.0 | 350 | 1.4 | 51.4 | 15.7 | 0.0 |
| Chews, Just Fruit, Fruit-tella* | 1 Serving/43g | 170.0 | 3.0 | 400 | 0.9 | 79.5 | 6.5 | 0.0 |
| Chews, Strawberry Mix, Starburst* | 1 Sweet/4g | 15.0 | 0.0 | 401 | 0.0 | 83.9 | 7.3 | 0.0 |
| Choco Toffee, Sula* | 1 Sweet/8g | 21.0 | 1.0 | 267 | 3.3 | 31.7 | 15.8 | 0.0 |
| Chocolate Caramels, Milk, Tesco* | 1 Sweet/3g | 15.0 | 1.0 | 444 | 2.7 | 72.1 | 16.1 | 0.1 |
| Chocolate Eclairs, Cadbury* | 1 Sweet/8g | 36.0 | 1.0 | 455 | 4.5 | 68.9 | 17.9 | 0.0 |
| Chocolate Limes, Pascall* | 1 Sweet/8g | 27.0 | 0.0 | 333 | 0.3 | 77.2 | 2.5 | 0.0 |
| Cola Bottles, Asda* | 1 Serving/100g | 329.0 | 0.0 | 329 | 9.0 | 73.0 | 0.2 | 0.0 |
| Cola Bottles, Fizzy, M & S* | 1 Pack/200g | 650.0 | 0.0 | 325 | 6.4 | 75.0 | 0.0 | 0.0 |
| Cough, Herbs, Swiss, Orginal, Ricola* | 1 Packet/37g | 148.0 | 0.0 | 400 | 0.0 | 98.0 | 0.0 | 0.0 |
| Cream Caramel, Sula* | 1 Sweet/3g | 10.0 | 0.0 | 297 | 0.4 | 86.1 | 0.0 | 0.0 |
| Crunchies, Fruit, Fruit-tella* | 1 Box/23g | 90.0 | 1.0 | 390 | 0.7 | 86.0 | 5.0 | 0.0 |
| Dolly Mix, Bassett's* | 1 Bag/45g | 171.0 | 1.0 | 380 | 3.0 | 85.1 | 3.1 | 0.4 |
| Drops, Lemon & Orange, M & S* | 1 Pack42g | 97.0 | 0.0 | 230 | 0.0 | 61.0 | 0.0 | 0.0 |
| Drumstick, Matlow's* | 1 Pack/40g | 164.0 | 2.0 | 409 | 0.4 | 88.3 | 5.5 | 0.0 |
| Fizzy Lemon Fish, Asda* | 1 Sweet/4g | 14.0 | 0.0 | 325 | 5.0 | 76.0 | 0.1 | 0.0 |
| Fizzy Mix, Tesco* | ½ Bag/50g | 166.0 | 0.0 | 332 | 5.2 | 75.2 | 0.0 | 0.0 |
| Flipsters, Starburst* | 1pack/37g | 145.0 | 0.0 | 392 | 0.0 | 98.1 | 0.0 | 0.0 |
| Flumps, Bassett's* | 1 Serving/5g | 16.0 | 0.0 | 325 | 4.0 | 77.0 | 0.0 | 0.0 |
| Flying Saucers, Morrisons* | 1 Pack/22g | 73.0 | 0.0 | 333 | 0.0 | 84.0 | 0.0 | 0.0 |
| Flying Suacers, Asda* | 1 Serving/23g | 82.0 | 1.0 | 355 | 0.1 | 83.0 | 2.5 | 0.8 |
| Foamy Mushrooms, Chewy, Asda* | 1 Sweet/3g | 9.0 | 0.0 | 347 | 4.2 | 82.0 | 0.2 | 0.0 |
| Fruit Gums & Jellies | 1 Tube/33g | 107.0 | 0.0 | 324 | 6.5 | 79.5 | 0.0 | 0.0 |
| Fruit Tingles, Wonka* | 1 Sweet/8g | 8.0 | 0.0 | 104 | 0.0 | 26.0 | 0.0 | 0.0 |

S

| | Measure INFO/WEIGHT | per Measure KCAL | FAT | Nutrition Values per 100g / 100ml KCAL | PROT | CARB | FAT | FIBRE |
|---|---|---|---|---|---|---|---|---|

## SWEETS

| | Measure INFO/WEIGHT | KCAL | FAT | KCAL | PROT | CARB | FAT | FIBRE |
|---|---|---|---|---|---|---|---|---|
| Fruities, Lemon & Lime, Weight Watchers* | 1 Sweet/2g | 3.0 | 0.0 | 134 | 0.0 | 54.0 | 0.0 | 33.0 |
| Fruity Babies, Bassett's* | 1 Sweet/3g | 10.0 | 0.0 | 310 | 4.6 | 72.7 | 0.2 | 0.0 |
| Fruity Chews, Starburst* | 1 Sweet/8g | 34.0 | 1.0 | 404 | 0.0 | 83.4 | 7.4 | 0.0 |
| Fruity Frogs, Rowntree's* | 1 Serving/40g | 128.0 | 0.0 | 321 | 4.7 | 74.5 | 0.2 | 0.0 |
| Fruity Mallows, Fizzy, Asda* | 1 Pack/400g | 1252.0 | 0.0 | 313 | 4.3 | 74.0 | 0.0 | 0.0 |
| Gummy Bears | 10 Bears/22g | 85.0 | 0.0 | 386 | 0.0 | 98.9 | 0.0 | 98.9 |
| Gummy Mix, Tesco* | 1 Pack/100g | 327.0 | 0.0 | 327 | 5.9 | 75.7 | 0.1 | 0.0 |
| Gummy Worms | 10 Worms/74g | 286.0 | 0.0 | 386 | 0.0 | 98.9 | 0.0 | 98.9 |
| Gummy Zingy Fruits, Bassett's* | 1 Sm Bag/40g | 135.0 | 0.0 | 337 | 5.1 | 79.2 | 0.0 | 0.0 |
| Hazardously Sour, Toxic Waste* | 1 Sweet/3g | 12.0 | 0.0 | 400 | 0.0 | 100.0 | 0.0 | 0.0 |
| Ice Cream Sundae, Asda* | 1 Sweet/2g | 8.0 | 0.0 | 343 | 4.1 | 81.0 | 0.2 | 0.1 |
| Kisses, Hershey* | 1 Sweet/5g | 28.0 | 2.0 | 561 | 7.0 | 59.0 | 32.0 | 0.0 |
| Lances, Fizzy, Strawberry, Somerfield* | 1 Sweet/4g | 13.0 | 0.0 | 362 | 2.8 | 79.8 | 2.7 | 1.5 |
| Lances, Strawberry & Cream Flavour, Tesco* | 1 Bag/75g | 276.0 | 1.0 | 368 | 3.2 | 86.1 | 1.2 | 2.1 |
| Lances, Strawberry Flavour, Fizzy, Tesco* | ½ Pack/50g | 177.0 | 1.0 | 354 | 2.8 | 79.8 | 2.6 | 1.8 |
| Liquorice and Fruit, Fruit-tella* | 1 Sweet/4g | 16.0 | 0.0 | 395 | 0.9 | 83.0 | 6.5 | 0.0 |
| Lovehearts, Giant, Swizzels* | 1 Pack/42g | 165.0 | 0.0 | 393 | 0.0 | 100.0 | 0.0 | 0.0 |
| Lovehearts, Swizzels* | 1oz/28g | 100.0 | 0.0 | 359 | 0.7 | 88.2 | 0.0 | 0.0 |
| Maynards Sours, Bassett's* | 1 Pack/52g | 166.0 | 0.0 | 320 | 3.9 | 74.9 | 0.1 | 0.0 |
| Milk Chocolate Eclairs, Sainsbury's* | 1 Sweet/8g | 33.0 | 1.0 | 442 | 2.1 | 75.7 | 14.5 | 0.5 |
| Milk Duds | 13 Pieces/33g | 170.0 | 6.0 | 510 | 3.0 | 84.0 | 18.0 | 0.0 |
| Milky Babies, Bassett's* | 1 Sweet/3g | 10.0 | 0.0 | 330 | 6.9 | 72.7 | 1.1 | 0.0 |
| Parma Violets, Swizzlers* | 1 Small Tube/10g | 41.0 | 0.0 | 406 | 0.9 | 99.1 | 0.0 | 0.0 |
| Percy Pig & Pals, Soft, M & S* | 1 Sweet/8g | 26.0 | 0.0 | 344 | 5.8 | 80.0 | 0.1 | 0.0 |
| Randoms, Rowntrees* | 1 Pack/50g | 164.0 | 0.0 | 328 | 4.9 | 75.7 | 0.3 | 0.6 |
| Raspberry Vines, Candy Tree* | 1 Pack/75g | 267.0 | 0.0 | 356 | 2.0 | 86.6 | 0.2 | 0.0 |
| Rhubarb & Custard, Sainsbury's* | 1 Sweet/8g | 28.0 | 0.0 | 351 | 0.1 | 87.7 | 0.0 | 0.0 |
| Scary Mix, Tesco* | 1 Bag/100g | 327.0 | 0.0 | 327 | 9.5 | 71.1 | 0.5 | 0.3 |
| Scary Sours, Rowntree's* | 1 Serving/100g | 321.0 | 0.0 | 321 | 3.5 | 74.7 | 0.0 | 0.0 |
| Sherbert Cocktails, Sainsbury's* | 1 Sweet/9g | 36.0 | 1.0 | 400 | 0.0 | 83.1 | 7.5 | 0.0 |
| Sherbert Lemons, M & S* | 1 Serving/20g | 76.0 | 0.0 | 380 | 0.0 | 93.9 | 0.0 | 0.0 |
| Sherbet Lemons, Bassett's* | 1 Sweet/7g | 25.0 | 0.0 | 375 | 0.0 | 93.9 | 0.0 | 0.0 |
| Shrimps & Bananas, Sainsbury's* | ½ Pack/50g | 188.0 | 0.0 | 376 | 2.5 | 91.3 | 0.1 | 0.5 |
| Snakes, Bassett's* | 1 Sweet/9g | 30.0 | 0.0 | 320 | 3.5 | 76.8 | 0.1 | 0.0 |
| Sour Squirms, Bassett's* | 1 Serving/7g | 21.0 | 0.0 | 325 | 3.1 | 78.1 | 0.0 | 0.0 |
| Strawberry & Cream, Sugar Free, Sula* | 1 Serving/10g | 27.0 | 1.0 | 267 | 0.2 | 90.5 | 5.4 | 0.0 |
| Sugar Free, Sula* | 1 Sweet/3g | 7.0 | 0.0 | 231 | 0.0 | 96.1 | 0.0 | 0.0 |
| Sweetshop Favourites, Bassett's* | 1 Sweet/5g | 17.0 | 0.0 | 340 | 0.0 | 84.3 | 0.0 | 0.0 |
| Toffo* | 1 Tube/43g | 194.0 | 9.0 | 451 | 2.2 | 69.8 | 22.0 | 0.0 |
| Tootsie Roll, Small Midgees, Tootsie* | 1 Sweet/3g | 11.0 | 1.0 | 361 | 0.0 | 20.0 | 33.0 | 0.0 |
| Tooty Frooties, Rowntree's* | 1 Bag/28g | 111.0 | 1.0 | 397 | 0.1 | 91.5 | 3.5 | 0.0 |
| Wazzly Wobble Drops, Wonka* | 1 Bag/42g | 186.0 | 7.0 | 443 | 3.0 | 71.6 | 16.1 | 0.2 |
| Wiggly Worms, Sainsbury's* | 1 Serving/10g | 32.0 | 0.0 | 317 | 5.6 | 72.7 | 0.4 | 0.2 |
| Xtra Sour Spiders, Rowntree's* | 1 Pack/35g | 112.0 | 0.0 | 321 | 3.5 | 74.8 | 0.0 | 0.0 |

## SWORDFISH

| | Measure INFO/WEIGHT | KCAL | FAT | KCAL | PROT | CARB | FAT | FIBRE |
|---|---|---|---|---|---|---|---|---|
| *Grilled, Average* | *1oz/28g* | *39.0* | *1.0* | *139* | *22.9* | *0.0* | *5.2* | *0.0* |
| *Raw, Average* | *1oz/28g* | *42.0* | *2.0* | *149* | *21.1* | *0.0* | *7.2* | *0.0* |

## SYRUP

| | Measure INFO/WEIGHT | KCAL | FAT | KCAL | PROT | CARB | FAT | FIBRE |
|---|---|---|---|---|---|---|---|---|
| Caramel, for Coffee, Lyle's* | 2 Tsps/10ml | 33.0 | 0.0 | 329 | 0.0 | 83.0 | 0.0 | 0.0 |
| *Corn, Dark, Average* | *1 Tbsp/20g* | *56.0* | *0.0* | *282* | *0.0* | *76.6* | *0.0* | *0.0* |
| *Golden, Average* | *1 Tbsp/20g* | *61.0* | *0.0* | *304* | *0.4* | *78.2* | *0.0* | *0.0* |
| *Maple, Average* | *1 Tbsp/20g* | *52.0* | *0.0* | *262* | *0.0* | *67.2* | *0.2* | *0.0* |
| Strawberry, Milk Shake Mix, Crusha* | 1 Serving/20ml | 25.0 | 0.0 | 125 | 0.5 | 30.0 | 0.5 | 0.0 |

**S**

| | Measure INFO/WEIGHT | per Measure KCAL | FAT | Nutrition Values per 100g / 100ml KCAL | PROT | CARB | FAT | FIBRE |
|---|---|---|---|---|---|---|---|---|
| **TABOO*** | | | | | | | | |
| Average, Taboo* | 1 Shot/35ml | 80.0 | 0.0 | 230 | 0.0 | 33.0 | 0.0 | 0.0 |
| **TABOULEH** | | | | | | | | |
| *Average* | *1oz/28g* | *33.0* | *1.0* | *119* | *2.6* | *17.2* | *4.6* | *0.0* |
| **TACO SHELLS** | | | | | | | | |
| Corn, Crunchy, Old El Paso* | 1 Taco/10g | 51.0 | 3.0 | 506 | 7.0 | 61.0 | 26.0 | 0.0 |
| Old El Paso* | 1 Taco/12g | 57.0 | 3.0 | 478 | 7.4 | 60.8 | 22.8 | 0.0 |
| Traditional, Discovery* | 1 Taco/11g | 55.0 | 3.0 | 489 | 5.7 | 53.4 | 28.1 | 6.0 |
| **TAGINE** | | | | | | | | |
| Giant Cous Cous, Moroccan, Tasty Veg Pot, Innocent* | 1 Pot/400g | 308.0 | 9.0 | 77 | 3.3 | 11.0 | 2.3 | 4.4 |
| Spicy Chermoula, Tasty Veg Pot, Innocent* | 1 Pot/400g | 356.0 | 10.0 | 89 | 3.4 | 13.8 | 2.4 | 5.0 |
| Vegetable, Filo Topped, M & S* | 1 Serving/282g | 310.0 | 6.0 | 110 | 3.3 | 18.7 | 2.3 | 3.9 |
| **TAGLIATELLE** | | | | | | | | |
| Basil, M & S* | 1 Serving/100g | 365.0 | 3.0 | 365 | 15.1 | 69.0 | 2.8 | 4.0 |
| Bicolore, Asda* | ¼ Pack/125g | 202.0 | 3.0 | 162 | 7.0 | 28.0 | 2.4 | 1.4 |
| Carbonara, Frozen, Tesco* | 1 Pack/450g | 427.0 | 9.0 | 95 | 5.2 | 14.1 | 1.9 | 0.9 |
| Carbonara, Italiano, Tesco* | 1 Serving/325g | 757.0 | 37.0 | 233 | 8.6 | 23.8 | 11.5 | 1.2 |
| Carbonara, Low Fat, Bertorelli* | 1 Pack/350g | 301.0 | 8.0 | 86 | 5.3 | 12.0 | 2.2 | 0.9 |
| Carbonara, Naturally Less 5% Fat, Asda* | 1 Pack/400g | 440.0 | 10.0 | 110 | 4.2 | 18.0 | 2.4 | 0.8 |
| Carbonara, Perfectly Balanced, Waitrose* | 1 Pack/350g | 357.0 | 13.0 | 102 | 5.3 | 12.1 | 3.6 | 0.7 |
| Chargrilled Chicken & Tomato, Asda* | 1 Pack/400g | 392.0 | 12.0 | 98 | 5.8 | 11.7 | 3.1 | 1.4 |
| Chicken, Italia, M & S* | 1 Pack/360g | 342.0 | 6.0 | 95 | 8.1 | 12.1 | 1.8 | 1.2 |
| Chicken, Italian, Sainsbury's* | 1 Pack/450g | 567.0 | 16.0 | 126 | 6.5 | 17.0 | 3.5 | 2.6 |
| Chicken & Mushroom, GFY, Asda* | 1 Pack/400g | 359.0 | 7.0 | 90 | 7.2 | 11.2 | 1.7 | 0.7 |
| Chicken & Tomato, Italiano, Tesco* | 1 Pack/400g | 416.0 | 8.0 | 104 | 6.6 | 14.8 | 2.1 | 0.8 |
| *Dry, Average* | *1 Serving/100g* | *356.0* | *2.0* | *356* | *12.6* | *72.4* | *1.8* | *1.0* |
| *Egg, Dry, Average* | *1 Serving/75g* | *271.0* | *2.0* | *362* | *14.2* | *68.8* | *3.3* | *2.3* |
| *Egg, Fresh, Dry, Average* | *1 Serving/125g* | *345.0* | *3.0* | *276* | *10.6* | *53.0* | *2.8* | *2.1* |
| Egg & Spinach, Safeway* | 1 Serving/83g | 289.0 | 2.0 | 348 | 13.2 | 67.3 | 2.9 | 2.9 |
| *Fresh, Dry, Average* | *1 Serving/75g* | *211.0* | *2.0* | *281* | *11.4* | *53.3* | *2.6* | *2.6* |
| Garlic & Herb, Cooked, Sainsbury's* | 1oz/28g | 41.0 | 1.0 | 147 | 6.5 | 26.3 | 1.8 | 1.9 |
| Garlic & Herb, Fresh, Asda* | ½ Pack/151g | 202.0 | 6.0 | 134 | 3.5 | 21.0 | 4.0 | 2.1 |
| Garlic & Herb, Fresh, Sainsbury's* | 1 Serving/125g | 184.0 | 2.0 | 147 | 6.5 | 26.2 | 1.8 | 1.9 |
| Garlic & Herb, Fresh, Tesco* | 1 Serving/125g | 361.0 | 5.0 | 289 | 12.0 | 51.8 | 3.7 | 1.5 |
| Garlic & Herb, Italiano, Tesco* | 1 Serving/85g | 236.0 | 2.0 | 278 | 11.4 | 52.0 | 2.7 | 2.4 |
| Garlic & Herbs, Cooked, Pasta Reale* | 1 Pack/250g | 390.0 | 3.0 | 156 | 6.2 | 30.4 | 1.1 | 1.0 |
| Garlic Mushroom, BGTY, Sainsbury's* | 1 Pack/400g | 416.0 | 9.0 | 104 | 4.7 | 16.2 | 2.3 | 2.0 |
| Garlic Mushroom, Italiano, Tesco* | 1 Pack/450g | 738.0 | 41.0 | 164 | 5.2 | 15.2 | 9.1 | 0.6 |
| Ham & Mushroom, Asda* | 1 Pack/340g | 469.0 | 13.0 | 138 | 6.0 | 20.0 | 3.8 | 0.2 |
| Ham & Mushroom, BGTY, Sainsbury's* | 1 Pack/450g | 486.0 | 14.0 | 108 | 5.3 | 14.5 | 3.2 | 0.8 |
| Ham & Mushroom, Light Choices, Tesco* | 1 Pack/400g | 400.0 | 9.0 | 100 | 6.0 | 13.8 | 2.2 | 1.8 |
| Ham & Mushroom, Safeway* | 1 Serving/400g | 480.0 | 20.0 | 120 | 5.2 | 12.9 | 5.1 | 1.0 |
| Ham & Roasted Mushroom, Finest, Tesco* | 1 Pack/450g | 562.0 | 24.0 | 125 | 7.3 | 12.0 | 5.3 | 2.4 |
| Multigrain, BGTY, Uncooked, Sainsbury's* | 1 Serving/190g | 294.0 | 5.0 | 155 | 7.0 | 26.0 | 2.5 | 3.0 |
| Mushroom & Bacon, BGTY, Sainsbury's* | 1 Pack/400g | 368.0 | 10.0 | 92 | 4.0 | 13.5 | 2.4 | 1.0 |
| Mushroom & Bacon, Sainsbury's* | 1 Pack/450g | 585.0 | 23.0 | 130 | 7.1 | 13.8 | 5.2 | 0.5 |
| Mushroom & Ham, GFY, Asda* | 1 Pack/399g | 323.0 | 9.0 | 81 | 5.4 | 9.6 | 2.3 | 0.7 |
| Mushroom & Tomato, Asda* | 1 Pack/340g | 211.0 | 4.0 | 62 | 2.5 | 10.0 | 1.3 | 1.2 |
| Nests, Dry Weight, Napolina* | 1oz/28g | 93.0 | 0.0 | 332 | 11.5 | 68.0 | 1.5 | 3.7 |
| Prawn, Eat Smart, Morrisons* | 1 Pack/380g | 296.0 | 7.0 | 78 | 6.1 | 9.4 | 1.8 | 0.9 |
| Red Pepper, Organic, Sainsbury's* | ½ Bag/125g | 182.0 | 2.0 | 146 | 5.4 | 27.8 | 1.5 | 1.4 |
| Salmon, Hot Smoked, HL, Tesco* | 1 Packet/400g | 420.0 | 12.0 | 105 | 6.0 | 12.8 | 2.9 | 1.4 |
| Salmon, Perfectly Balanced, Waitrose* | 1 Pack/400g | 376.0 | 11.0 | 94 | 5.4 | 11.7 | 2.7 | 0.8 |
| Salmon & King Prawn, HL, Tesco* | 1 Pack/400g | 480.0 | 10.0 | 120 | 6.5 | 17.2 | 2.4 | 1.7 |

T

| | Measure INFO/WEIGHT | per Measure KCAL | per Measure FAT | Nutrition Values per 100g / 100ml KCAL | PROT | CARB | FAT | FIBRE |
|---|---|---|---|---|---|---|---|---|
| **TAGLIATELLE** | | | | | | | | |
| Salmon & Prawn, Perfectly Balanced, Waitrose* | 1 Pack/401g | 341.0 | 13.0 | 85 | 6.8 | 7.1 | 3.3 | 1.1 |
| Smoked Salmon, Ready Meals, M & S* | 1 Pack/360g | 612.0 | 40.0 | 170 | 6.2 | 10.6 | 11.2 | 0.9 |
| Sundried Tomato, Fresh, Morrisons* | 1 Pack/250g | 747.0 | 8.0 | 299 | 11.1 | 56.4 | 3.3 | 3.5 |
| Sweet Chilli & Prawn, Tesco* | 1 Pack/400g | 440.0 | 12.0 | 110 | 5.5 | 14.9 | 3.1 | 1.3 |
| Tomato & Basil Chicken, Weight Watchers* | 1 Pack/330g | 322.0 | 4.0 | 98 | 7.5 | 14.1 | 1.2 | 0.3 |
| Tricolore, Waitrose* | ½ Pack/125g | 351.0 | 4.0 | 281 | 12.0 | 51.6 | 2.9 | 1.6 |
| Vegetables, Retail | 1oz/28g | 21.0 | 1.0 | 74 | 1.6 | 11.0 | 3.0 | 0.7 |
| Verdi, Dry, Barilla* | 1 Serving/150g | 555.0 | 5.0 | 370 | 14.0 | 70.5 | 3.5 | 0.0 |
| *Verdi, Fresh, Average* | *1 Serving/125g* | *171.0* | *2.0* | *137* | *5.5* | *25.5* | *1.5* | *1.8* |
| with Chicken, Garlic & Lemon, BGTY, Sainsbury's* | 1 Pack/450g | 409.0 | 1.0 | 91 | 7.8 | 14.2 | 0.3 | 1.7 |
| with Chicken, Garlic & Lemon, New, BGTY, Sainsbury's* | 1 Pack/300g | 324.0 | 4.0 | 108 | 9.2 | 15.1 | 1.2 | 1.7 |
| with Chicken & Pancetta, Sainsbury's* | ½ Pack/351g | 453.0 | 19.0 | 129 | 9.5 | 10.4 | 5.5 | 0.7 |
| with Ham & Mushroom, New, BGTY, Sainsbury's* | 1 Pack/450g | 400.0 | 10.0 | 89 | 5.3 | 11.8 | 2.3 | 1.4 |
| **TAHINI PASTE** | | | | | | | | |
| *Average* | *1 Tsp/6g* | *36.0* | *4.0* | *607* | *18.5* | *0.9* | *58.9* | *8.0* |
| **TAMARILLOS** | | | | | | | | |
| *Fresh, Raw, Average* | *1oz/28g* | *8.0* | *0.0* | *28* | *2.0* | *4.7* | *0.3* | *0.0* |
| **TAMARIND** | | | | | | | | |
| *Leaves, Fresh* | *1oz/28g* | *32.0* | *1.0* | *115* | *5.8* | *18.2* | *2.1* | *0.0* |
| Paste, Barts* | 1 Tbsp/15g | 20.0 | 0.0 | 133 | 0.9 | 32.1 | 0.1 | 0.0 |
| *Pulp* | *1oz/28g* | *76.0* | *0.0* | *273* | *3.2* | *64.5* | *0.3* | *0.0* |
| *Whole, Raw, Weighed with Pod, Average* | *1oz/28g* | *67.0* | *0.0* | *239* | *2.8* | *62.5* | *0.6* | *5.1* |
| **TANGERINES** | | | | | | | | |
| *Fresh, Raw* | *1oz/28g* | *10.0* | *0.0* | *35* | *0.9* | *8.0* | *0.1* | *1.3* |
| *Weighed with Peel & Pips* | *1 Med/70g* | *17.0* | *0.0* | *25* | *0.7* | *5.8* | *0.1* | *0.9* |
| **TANGO*** | | | | | | | | |
| Cherry, Britvic* | 1 Bottle/500ml | 55.0 | 0.0 | 11 | 0.0 | 2.4 | 0.0 | 0.0 |
| Orange, Britvic* | 1 Can/330ml | 63.0 | 0.0 | 19 | 0.1 | 4.4 | 0.0 | 0.0 |
| **TAPENADE** | | | | | | | | |
| Green Olive, The Best, Safeway* | 1 Tsp/15g | 70.0 | 7.0 | 470 | 1.6 | 10.2 | 47.0 | 1.7 |
| Olive with Capers & Anchovy, Safeway* | 1 Tbsp/20g | 103.0 | 11.0 | 513 | 2.1 | 1.0 | 55.6 | 2.2 |
| Sundried Tomato & Jalapeno Pepper, Finest, Tesco* | 1 Jar/90g | 392.0 | 37.0 | 436 | 3.4 | 13.1 | 41.0 | 5.0 |
| **TAPIOCA** | | | | | | | | |
| Creamed, Ambrosia* | ½ Can/213g | 159.0 | 3.0 | 75 | 2.6 | 12.6 | 1.6 | 0.2 |
| *Raw* | *1oz/28g* | *101.0* | *0.0* | *359* | *0.4* | *95.0* | *0.1* | *0.4* |
| **TARAMASALATA** | | | | | | | | |
| Average | 1oz/28g | 141.0 | 15.0 | 504 | 3.2 | 4.1 | 52.9 | 0.0 |
| BGTY, Sainsbury's* | 1oz/28g | 71.0 | 6.0 | 253 | 4.3 | 13.5 | 20.2 | 0.7 |
| M & S* | 1 Serving/100g | 480.0 | 49.0 | 480 | 4.9 | 6.4 | 48.9 | 0.7 |
| Reduced Fat, Tesco* | ½ Pot/85g | 256.0 | 23.0 | 301 | 3.8 | 10.5 | 27.1 | 1.5 |
| Reduced Fat, Waitrose* | 1 Pack/170g | 522.0 | 48.0 | 307 | 4.0 | 8.9 | 28.4 | 1.5 |
| Sainsbury's* | ¼ Tub/50g | 236.0 | 24.0 | 472 | 4.0 | 7.5 | 48.1 | 0.0 |
| Smoked Salmon, Tesco* | 1 Serving/95g | 474.0 | 48.0 | 499 | 3.0 | 7.7 | 50.7 | 0.3 |
| Supreme, Waitrose* | 1 Serving/20g | 84.0 | 8.0 | 421 | 7.4 | 6.3 | 40.7 | 2.9 |
| Tesco* | 1/8 Tub/25g | 115.0 | 11.0 | 460 | 2.9 | 10.5 | 44.8 | 1.0 |
| **TARRAGON** | | | | | | | | |
| *Dried, Ground* | *1 Tsp/2g* | *5.0* | *0.0* | *295* | *22.8* | *42.8* | *7.2* | *0.0* |
| *Fresh, Average* | *1 Tbsp/4g* | *2.0* | *0.0* | *49* | *3.4* | *6.3* | *1.1* | *0.0* |
| **TART** | | | | | | | | |
| Apple & Custard, Asda* | 1 Tart/84g | 227.0 | 11.0 | 270 | 3.1 | 35.0 | 13.1 | 0.1 |
| Apple & Fresh Cream, Asda* | ½ Tart/50g | 133.0 | 8.0 | 267 | 3.4 | 33.0 | 16.0 | 0.8 |
| Apricot Lattice, Sainsbury's* | 1 Slice/125g | 321.0 | 14.0 | 257 | 3.4 | 35.3 | 11.4 | 2.6 |
| Assorted, Oakdale Bakeries* | 1 Serving/27g | 104.0 | 4.0 | 386 | 3.1 | 62.0 | 14.0 | 1.7 |

T

## TART

| INFO/WEIGHT | | per Measure | | Nutrition Values per 100g / 100ml | | | | |
|---|---|---|---|---|---|---|---|---|
| Measure | | KCAL | FAT | KCAL | PROT | CARB | FAT | FIBRE |
| Aubergine & Feta, Roast Marinated, Sainsbury's* | 1 Serving/105g | 227.0 | 15.0 | 216 | 4.8 | 16.6 | 14.5 | 1.7 |
| Bakewell, Average | 1 Tart/50g | 228.0 | 15.0 | 456 | 6.3 | 43.5 | 29.7 | 1.9 |
| Bakewell, Free From, Tesco* | 1 Tart/50g | 170.0 | 5.0 | 340 | 1.6 | 63.0 | 9.2 | 4.8 |
| Bakewell, Lyons* | 1/6 Tart/52g | 205.0 | 9.0 | 397 | 3.8 | 56.7 | 17.2 | 0.9 |
| Bakewell, M & S* | ¼ Tart/75g | 345.0 | 20.0 | 460 | 7.5 | 48.1 | 26.7 | 2.1 |
| Bakewell, Weight Watchers* | 1 Tart/43g | 156.0 | 5.0 | 363 | 3.6 | 65.2 | 11.7 | 3.2 |
| Bannoffi, Finest, Tesco* | 1/6 Tart/87g | 291.0 | 17.0 | 334 | 3.0 | 37.2 | 19.3 | 0.5 |
| Blackcurrant Sundae, Asda* | 1 Tart/55g | 227.0 | 10.0 | 413 | 3.5 | 57.0 | 19.0 | 2.3 |
| Cherry Bakewell, Morrisons* | 1 Tart/46g | 198.0 | 10.0 | 430 | 4.6 | 54.9 | 21.4 | 1.3 |
| Cherry Tomato & Mascarpone, Extra Special, Asda* | 1 Tart/153g | 290.0 | 18.0 | 190 | 4.6 | 16.0 | 12.0 | 1.1 |
| Chocolate, Co-Op* | 1 Tart/22g | 102.0 | 7.0 | 465 | 4.0 | 42.0 | 31.0 | 0.7 |
| Chocolate, TTD, Sainsbury's* | 1 Tart/93g | 389.0 | 26.0 | 418 | 4.8 | 37.6 | 27.6 | 3.0 |
| Coconut, M & S* | 1 Tart/53g | 220.0 | 10.0 | 415 | 5.8 | 57.8 | 18.1 | 3.6 |
| Coconut & Cherry, Asda* | 1 Serving/50g | 215.0 | 10.0 | 430 | 4.4 | 58.0 | 20.0 | 4.0 |
| Coconut & Raspberry, Waitrose* | 1 Tart/48g | 204.0 | 12.0 | 426 | 5.0 | 45.0 | 24.0 | 3.9 |
| Congress, Morrisons* | 1 Tart/38g | 149.0 | 5.0 | 393 | 6.0 | 59.7 | 14.4 | 2.4 |
| Custard, Individual, Average | 1 Tart/94g | 260.0 | 14.0 | 277 | 6.3 | 32.4 | 14.5 | 1.2 |
| Date Pecan & Almond, Sticky, Sainsbury's* | 1/8 Tart/75g | 298.0 | 10.0 | 397 | 5.0 | 63.5 | 13.7 | 1.7 |
| Egg Custard, Tesco* | 1 Tart/82g | 214.0 | 10.0 | 261 | 6.2 | 31.5 | 12.2 | 1.1 |
| Feta Cheese & Spinach, Puff Pastry, Tesco* | 1 Tart/108g | 306.0 | 19.0 | 283 | 7.1 | 23.5 | 17.8 | 0.9 |
| Filo Asparagus Tartlette, M & S* | 1 Serving/15g | 45.0 | 3.0 | 300 | 4.4 | 25.2 | 20.4 | 2.1 |
| Frangipane, Chocolate & William Pear, Waitrose* | 1/6 Pack/80g | 219.0 | 12.0 | 274 | 3.5 | 29.9 | 15.5 | 2.5 |
| Frangipane, Lutowska Cherry Amaretto, Sainsbury's* | 1 Serving/66g | 264.0 | 13.0 | 400 | 6.0 | 50.0 | 19.5 | 1.3 |
| Frangipane, Spiced Winter Fruit, Rustic Bake, Waitrose* | 1 Slice/87g | 315.0 | 14.0 | 363 | 7.2 | 48.3 | 15.7 | 2.1 |
| Gruyere Pancetta & Balsamic Onion, Finest, Tesco* | ¼ Tart/106g | 320.0 | 22.0 | 301 | 7.7 | 21.3 | 20.6 | 3.3 |
| Italian Lemon & Almond, Sainsbury's* | 1 Slice/49g | 182.0 | 12.0 | 371 | 7.4 | 31.9 | 23.7 | 4.1 |
| Jam, Assorted, Tesco* | 1 Tart/35g | 123.0 | 5.0 | 351 | 3.4 | 51.9 | 14.4 | 1.2 |
| Jam, Assorted, VLH Kitchens* | 1 Tart/34g | 44.2 | 4.9 | 130 | 3.4 | 56.0 | 14.4 | 1.3 |
| Jam, Average | 1 Slice/90g | 342.0 | 13.0 | 380 | 3.3 | 62.0 | 14.9 | 1.6 |
| Jam, Real Fruit, Mr Kipling* | 1 Tart/35g | 136.0 | 5.0 | 388 | 3.8 | 67.9 | 14.9 | 1.7 |
| Leek & Stilton, Morrisons* | 1 Serving/125g | 392.0 | 27.0 | 314 | 6.9 | 23.1 | 21.5 | 0.3 |
| Lemon, M & S* | 1/6 Tart/50g | 207.0 | 15.0 | 415 | 5.0 | 32.7 | 29.3 | 0.9 |
| Lemon, Sainsbury's* | 1/8 Tart/56g | 192.0 | 8.0 | 341 | 5.1 | 46.8 | 14.9 | 2.4 |
| Lemon & Raspberry, Finest, Tesco* | 1 Tart/120g | 360.0 | 17.0 | 300 | 5.2 | 38.4 | 14.0 | 2.9 |
| Lemon Bakewell, Easter, Morrisons* | 1 Tart/45g | 186.0 | 7.0 | 413 | 3.1 | 64.8 | 15.7 | 1.8 |
| Lemon Curd, Asda* | 1 Tart/30g | 121.0 | 5.0 | 402 | 2.8 | 64.0 | 15.0 | 2.2 |
| Lemon Curd, Lyons* | 1 Tart/30g | 122.0 | 5.0 | 406 | 3.7 | 59.3 | 17.0 | 0.0 |
| Mixed Fruit, Waitrose* | 1 Tart/146g | 318.0 | 16.0 | 218 | 2.3 | 27.3 | 11.2 | 1.0 |
| Pear & Chocolate with Brandy, TTD, Sainsbury's* | 1/6 Tart/90g | 261.0 | 15.0 | 290 | 3.5 | 32.0 | 16.4 | 1.4 |
| Raspberry, Reduced Sugar, Asda* | 1 Tart/34g | 129.0 | 3.0 | 380 | 4.6 | 67.5 | 10.1 | 1.2 |
| Raspberry & Blueberry, Tesco* | 1 Serving/85g | 168.0 | 7.0 | 198 | 2.7 | 27.0 | 8.8 | 2.8 |
| Raspberry Flavoured, Value, Tesco* | 1 Tart/29g | 113.0 | 5.0 | 389 | 3.8 | 56.6 | 16.4 | 1.6 |
| Roasted Vegetable, Finest, Tesco* | ¼ Tart/113g | 226.0 | 13.0 | 200 | 3.1 | 20.6 | 11.7 | 2.3 |
| Sao Tome Chocolate, TTD, Sainsbury's* | 1 Slice/66g | 314.0 | 19.0 | 476 | 5.6 | 46.1 | 29.1 | 1.8 |
| Strawberry, Fresh, M & S* | 1 Tart/120g | 305.0 | 18.0 | 255 | 3.1 | 26.4 | 15.4 | 2.4 |
| Strawberry, Reduced Sugar, Asda* | 1 Tart/37g | 141.0 | 4.0 | 380 | 4.6 | 67.5 | 10.1 | 1.2 |
| Strawberry, Sainsbury's* | 1 Serving/206g | 521.0 | 26.0 | 253 | 2.6 | 32.0 | 12.7 | 0.7 |
| Strawberry, Waitrose* | 1 Serving/101g | 241.0 | 12.0 | 239 | 3.8 | 29.2 | 11.9 | 1.2 |
| Strawberry & Fresh Cream, Finest, Tesco* | 1 Tart/129g | 350.0 | 19.0 | 271 | 3.3 | 31.1 | 14.8 | 1.2 |
| Strawberry Custard, Asda* | 1 Tart/100g | 335.0 | 15.0 | 335 | 3.1 | 47.0 | 15.0 | 0.0 |
| Strawberry Sundae, Asda* | 1 Tart/46g | 187.0 | 8.0 | 407 | 3.3 | 58.0 | 18.0 | 1.3 |
| Summer Fruit Crumble, Morrisons* | 1 Tart/128g | 379.0 | 15.0 | 296 | 3.6 | 43.8 | 11.8 | 1.3 |
| Toffee Apple, Co-Op* | 1 Tart/20g | 69.0 | 3.0 | 345 | 3.0 | 47.0 | 16.0 | 0.7 |

T

| | Measure INFO/WEIGHT | per Measure KCAL | FAT | Nutrition Values per 100g / 100ml KCAL | PROT | CARB | FAT | FIBRE |
|---|---|---|---|---|---|---|---|---|
| **TART** | | | | | | | | |
| Toffee Bakewell, Sainsbury's* | 1 Tart/45g | 200.0 | 9.0 | 444 | 3.4 | 64.2 | 19.3 | 1.1 |
| Toffee Pecan, M & S* | 1 Tart/91g | 414.0 | 24.0 | 455 | 6.0 | 48.5 | 26.5 | 2.0 |
| Toffee Pecan, Waitrose* | ¼ Tart/133g | 564.0 | 19.0 | 423 | 4.3 | 69.3 | 14.3 | 1.6 |
| Tomato, Mozzarella & Basil Puff, Sainsbury's* | 1/3 Tart/120g | 318.0 | 25.0 | 265 | 9.2 | 10.2 | 20.8 | 0.9 |
| Treacle, Average | 1oz/28g | 103.0 | 4.0 | 368 | 3.7 | 60.4 | 14.1 | 1.1 |
| Treacle, Large, Tesco* | 1/6 Tart/59g | 237.0 | 6.0 | 402 | 3.3 | 74.1 | 10.3 | 1.7 |
| Treacle, Lattice, Lyons* | 1/6 Tart/70g | 255.0 | 8.0 | 364 | 4.4 | 59.3 | 12.0 | 1.1 |
| Treacle & Pecan, Mini, TTD, Sainsbury's* | 1 Tart/27g | 107.0 | 4.0 | 395 | 4.4 | 59.3 | 15.6 | 1.7 |
| Treacle Lattice, Mr Kipling* | 1/6 Tart/70g | 255.0 | 8.0 | 365 | 4.4 | 59.8 | 12.1 | 1.1 |
| **TARTAR** | | | | | | | | |
| *Cream of, Leavening Agent* | *1 Tsp/3g* | *8.0* | *0.0* | *258* | *0.0* | *61.5* | *0.0* | *0.0* |
| **TARTE** | | | | | | | | |
| Au Citron, Frozen, Tesco* | 1/6 Tarte/81g | 255.0 | 12.0 | 315 | 5.4 | 39.4 | 14.6 | 0.7 |
| Au Citron, Waitrose* | 1 Tarte/100g | 325.0 | 18.0 | 325 | 4.9 | 35.7 | 18.1 | 1.0 |
| Aux Cerises, Finest, Tesco* | 1 Serving/98g | 219.0 | 7.0 | 225 | 4.9 | 35.4 | 7.2 | 0.6 |
| Bacon, Leek & Roquefort, Bistro, Waitrose* | ¼ Tarte/100g | 277.0 | 18.0 | 277 | 8.4 | 19.8 | 18.2 | 0.6 |
| Goats Cheese & Spinach Flamme, TTD, Sainsbury's* | 1/3 Tarte/77g | 220.0 | 15.0 | 287 | 7.2 | 19.3 | 20.1 | 1.3 |
| Normande, French Style, M & S* | 1/6 Tarte/85g | 245.0 | 16.0 | 290 | 3.3 | 26.8 | 19.0 | 0.7 |
| Tatin, Sainsbury's* | 1 Serving/120g | 244.0 | 8.0 | 203 | 2.9 | 32.8 | 6.7 | 1.9 |
| **TARTLETS** | | | | | | | | |
| Caramelised Onion & Gruyere, Sainsbury's* | 1 Tartlet/145g | 381.0 | 28.0 | 263 | 5.8 | 17.3 | 19.0 | 1.3 |
| Cheese & Roast Onion, Asda* | 1 Tartlet/50g | 135.0 | 7.0 | 270 | 6.0 | 28.0 | 15.0 | 1.9 |
| Cherry Tomato & Aubergine, M & S* | 1 Tartlet/160g | 320.0 | 20.0 | 200 | 3.1 | 17.8 | 12.6 | 1.7 |
| Mandarin, Mini, M & S* | 1 Tartlet/29g | 80.0 | 5.0 | 280 | 3.4 | 30.4 | 16.3 | 0.6 |
| Mushroom, Bacon & Spinach, Safeway* | 1 Tartlet/120g | 312.0 | 24.0 | 260 | 7.0 | 13.0 | 20.0 | 1.0 |
| Mushroom & Watercress, Waitrose* | 1 Tartlet/120g | 308.0 | 25.0 | 257 | 8.4 | 19.1 | 20.5 | 2.6 |
| Mushroom Medley, BGTY, Sainsbury's* | 1 Serving/80g | 134.0 | 8.0 | 167 | 4.7 | 14.5 | 10.0 | 3.4 |
| Onion, Caramelised, Creamy, Somerfield* | 1 Tartlet/105g | 310.0 | 23.0 | 295 | 4.0 | 21.0 | 22.0 | 0.0 |
| Raspberry, Mini, M & S* | 1 Tartlet/27g | 90.0 | 5.0 | 330 | 4.3 | 34.4 | 19.6 | 0.5 |
| Red Onion & Goats Cheese, Sainsbury's* | 1 Tartlet/113g | 335.0 | 22.0 | 297 | 7.0 | 23.7 | 19.3 | 1.5 |
| Redcurrant & Blackcurrant, Mini, M & S* | 1 Tartlet/29g | 85.0 | 5.0 | 290 | 3.9 | 30.5 | 16.8 | 1.1 |
| Roast Pepper & Mascarpone, Sainsbury's* | 1 Tartlet/100g | 232.0 | 16.0 | 232 | 3.5 | 17.7 | 16.4 | 1.5 |
| Roasted Red Pepper, BGTY, Sainsbury's* | 1 Tartlet/80g | 143.0 | 7.0 | 179 | 3.1 | 21.0 | 9.2 | 3.4 |
| Salmon & Watercress, Hot Smoked, Waitrose* | 1 Serving/130g | 315.0 | 20.0 | 242 | 8.1 | 18.0 | 15.3 | 3.0 |
| Sausage & Tomato, Sainsbury's* | 1 Tartlet/135g | 323.0 | 21.0 | 239 | 4.8 | 19.5 | 15.8 | 1.6 |
| Spinach Ricotta & Sundried Tomato, Filo, Tesco* | 1 Tartlet/135g | 358.0 | 23.0 | 265 | 5.2 | 22.4 | 17.1 | 1.9 |
| Tomato & Goats Cheese, Waitrose* | 1 Tartlet/130g | 295.0 | 19.0 | 227 | 6.6 | 17.4 | 14.6 | 2.0 |
| **TEA** | | | | | | | | |
| Blackcurrant, Fruit Creations, Typhoo* | 1 Sm Cup/100ml | 5.0 | 0.0 | 5 | 0.2 | 0.8 | 0.0 | 0.2 |
| Camomile, Smile, Tetley* | 1oz/28g | 1.0 | 0.0 | 2 | 0.0 | 0.5 | 0.0 | 0.0 |
| Decaf, Tetley* | 1 Cup/100ml | 1.0 | 0.0 | 1 | 0.0 | 0.3 | 0.0 | 0.0 |
| Earl Grey, Infusion with Water, Average | 1 Mug/250ml | 2.0 | 0.0 | 1 | 0.0 | 0.2 | 0.0 | 0.0 |
| Fennel Seeds & Peppermint, Refreshing Infusion, Twinings* | 1 Cup/200ml | 4.0 | 0.0 | 2 | 0.0 | 0.3 | 0.0 | 0.0 |
| Fruit, Twinings* | 1 Mug/227ml | 4.0 | 0.0 | 2 | 0.0 | 0.4 | 0.0 | 0.0 |
| Fruit Or Herbal, Made with Water, Twinings* | 1 Mug/200ml | 8.0 | 0.0 | 4 | 0.0 | 1.0 | 0.0 | 0.0 |
| Fruit Punch, Fruit & Herb Company, The Bombay Brasserie* | 1 Mug/200ml | 4.0 | 0.0 | 2 | 0.0 | 0.5 | 0.0 | 0.0 |
| Green, with Citrus, Twinings* | 1 Serving/200ml | 0.0 | 0.0 | 0 | 1.0 | 0.2 | 0.0 | 0.0 |
| Green, with Jasmine, Twinings* | 1 Serving/100ml | 1.0 | 0.0 | 1 | 0.0 | 0.2 | 0.0 | 0.0 |
| Green, with Jasmine, Wellbeing Selection, Flavia* | 1 Cup/200ml | 14.0 | 0.0 | 7 | 0.5 | 1.2 | 0.1 | 0.0 |
| Green, with Lemon, Jackson's* | 1 Serving/200ml | 2.0 | 0.0 | 1 | 0.0 | 0.2 | 0.0 | 0.0 |
| Green, with Mango, Brewed with Water, Twinings* | 1 Cup/200ml | 2.0 | 0.0 | 1 | 0.0 | 0.2 | 0.0 | 0.0 |
| Green & Lemon, Twinings* | 1 Serving/250ml | 65.0 | 0.0 | 26 | 0.0 | 7.3 | 0.0 | 0.0 |
| Green with Mint, Whittards of Chelsea* | 1 Cup/100ml | 1.0 | 0.0 | 1 | 0.2 | 0.1 | 0.0 | 0.0 |

**T**

| | Measure INFO/WEIGHT | per Measure | | Nutrition Values per 100g / 100ml | | | | |
|---|---|---|---|---|---|---|---|---|
| | | KCAL | FAT | KCAL | PROT | CARB | FAT | FIBRE |
| **TEA** | | | | | | | | |
| Herbal, Wellbeing Blends, Infusions, Twinings* | 1 Serving/200ml | 4.0 | 0.0 | 2 | 0.0 | 0.3 | 0.0 | 0.0 |
| Iced, Green, Orange, Lipton* | 1 Bottle/500ml | 100.0 | 0.0 | 20 | 0.0 | 5.0 | 0.0 | 0.0 |
| Iced, Green & Lemon, Twinings* | 1 Serving/250ml | 75.0 | 0.0 | 30 | 0.1 | 7.3 | 0.1 | 0.0 |
| Iced, Lemon, San Benedetto* | 1 Bottle/500ml | 170.0 | 0.0 | 34 | 0.1 | 8.3 | 0.0 | 0.0 |
| Iced, Mango, Lipton* | 1 fl oz/30ml | 10.0 | 0.0 | 33 | 0.0 | 8.1 | 0.0 | 0.0 |
| Iced, Peach, Twinings* | 1 Serving/200ml | 60.0 | 0.0 | 30 | 0.1 | 7.3 | 0.1 | 0.0 |
| Iced, Pickwick* | 1 Serving/250ml | 32.0 | 0.0 | 13 | 0.0 | 3.3 | 0.0 | 0.0 |
| Iced, with Lemon, Lipton* | 1 Bottle/325ml | 97.0 | 0.0 | 30 | 0.1 | 7.2 | 0.1 | 0.0 |
| Lemon, Instant, Original, Lift* | 1 Serving/15g | 53.0 | 0.0 | 352 | 0.0 | 87.0 | 0.0 | 0.0 |
| Lemon, Instant, Tesco* | 1 Serving/7g | 23.0 | 0.0 | 326 | 1.0 | 80.5 | 0.0 | 0.0 |
| Lemon & Limeflower, Infused, M & S* | 1 Bottle/330ml | 99.0 | 0.0 | 30 | 0.0 | 7.8 | 0.0 | 0.0 |
| Made with Water | 1 Mug/227ml | 0.0 | 0.0 | 0 | 0.1 | 0.0 | 0.0 | 0.0 |
| Made with Water with Semi-Skimmed Milk, Average | 1 Cup/200ml | 14.0 | 0.0 | 7 | 0.5 | 0.7 | 0.2 | 0.0 |
| Made with Water with Skimmed Milk, Average | 1 Mug/227ml | 14.0 | 0.0 | 6 | 0.5 | 0.7 | 0.2 | 0.0 |
| Made with Water with Whole Milk, Average | 1 Cup/200ml | 16.0 | 1.0 | 8 | 0.4 | 0.5 | 0.4 | 0.0 |
| Nettle & Peppermint, Twinings* | 1 Cup/200ml | 2.0 | 0.0 | 1 | 0.0 | 0.1 | 0.0 | 0.0 |
| Orange, Mango and Cinnamon, Twinings* | 1 Cup/200ml | 4.0 | 0.0 | 2 | 0.0 | 0.3 | 0.0 | 0.0 |
| Peach Flavour, Lift* | 1 Cup/15g | 58.0 | 0.0 | 384 | 0.3 | 95.6 | 0.0 | 0.0 |
| Raspberry & Cranberry, T of Life, Tetley* | 1 Serving/100ml | 36.0 | 0.0 | 36 | 0.0 | 9.0 | 0.0 | 0.0 |
| Red Bush, Made with Water, Tetley* | 1 Mug/227g | 2.0 | 0.0 | 1 | 0.0 | 0.1 | 0.0 | 0.0 |
| with Lemon, Lipton* | 1 Bottle/591ml | 150.0 | 0.0 | 25 | 0.0 | 6.8 | 0.0 | 0.0 |
| **TEACAKES** | | | | | | | | |
| Average | 1 Teacake/60g | 178.0 | 4.0 | 296 | 8.0 | 52.5 | 7.5 | 0.0 |
| Caramel, Highlights, Mallows, Cadbury* | 1 Teacake/15g | 61.0 | 2.0 | 408 | 6.2 | 69.1 | 12.4 | 3.6 |
| Coconut Snowballs, Tunnock's* | 1 Cake/30g | 116.0 | 7.0 | 388 | 3.9 | 47.0 | 21.8 | 0.0 |
| Currant, Sainsbury's* | 1 Teacake/72g | 204.0 | 3.0 | 284 | 8.2 | 53.7 | 4.0 | 2.5 |
| Fruited, M & S* | 1 Teacake/60g | 156.0 | 1.0 | 260 | 8.9 | 53.4 | 1.0 | 2.0 |
| Fruity, Warburton's* | 1 Teacake/63g | 160.0 | 2.0 | 256 | 8.7 | 48.0 | 3.5 | 2.7 |
| G H Sheldon* | 1 Teacake/95g | 274.0 | 3.0 | 288 | 8.5 | 57.4 | 2.7 | 0.0 |
| Jam, Castello* | 1 Teacake/13g | 60.0 | 2.0 | 470 | 5.3 | 70.1 | 18.4 | 1.3 |
| Jarn, with Biscuit & Mallow, Chocolate Covered, Burton's* | 1 Teacake/13g | 57.0 | 2.0 | 455 | 3.8 | 66.9 | 19.3 | 1.1 |
| Lees'* | 1 Teacake/19g | 81.0 | 3.0 | 426 | 4.2 | 67.7 | 15.4 | 0.0 |
| Mallow, Tesco* | 1 Teacake/14g | 63.0 | 3.0 | 450 | 4.1 | 65.4 | 19.1 | 1.0 |
| Marshmallow, Milk Chocolate, Tunnock's* | 1 Teacake/24g | 106.0 | 5.0 | 440 | 4.9 | 61.9 | 19.2 | 2.4 |
| Morrisons* | 1 Teacake/64g | 172.0 | 2.0 | 268 | 9.9 | 50.7 | 2.9 | 2.8 |
| Richly Fruited, Waitrose* | 1 Teacake/72g | 205.0 | 3.0 | 285 | 7.8 | 55.0 | 3.7 | 2.2 |
| Sainsbury's* | 1 Teacake/70g | 171.0 | 3.0 | 244 | 8.0 | 45.0 | 3.6 | 2.6 |
| Tesco* | 1 Teacake/61g | 163.0 | 2.0 | 267 | 7.8 | 51.1 | 3.5 | 2.4 |
| Toasted, Average | 1 Teacake/60g | 197.0 | 5.0 | 329 | 8.9 | 58.3 | 8.3 | 0.0 |
| Value, Tesco* | 1 Teacake/68g | 180.0 | 2.0 | 265 | 9.6 | 47.8 | 3.6 | 4.9 |
| with Orange Filling, M & S* | 1 Teacake/20g | 80.0 | 3.0 | 410 | 4.5 | 66.6 | 14.2 | 0.9 |
| **TEMPEH** | | | | | | | | |
| *Average* | *1oz/28g* | *46.0* | *2.0* | *166* | *20.7* | *6.4* | *6.4* | *4.3* |
| **TEQUILA** | | | | | | | | |
| *Average* | *1 Shot/35ml* | *78.0* | *0.0* | *224* | *0.0* | *0.0* | *0.0* | *0.0* |
| **TERRINE** | | | | | | | | |
| Lobster & Prawn, Slices, M & S* | 1 Serving/55g | 107.0 | 7.0 | 195 | 18.2 | 0.7 | 13.4 | 0.7 |
| Prawn, TTD, Sainsbury's* | 1 Serving/60g | 115.0 | 9.0 | 192 | 9.0 | 3.7 | 15.7 | 0.4 |
| Salmon, Poached, Tesco* | 1 Pack/113g | 349.0 | 31.0 | 309 | 15.5 | 0.8 | 27.1 | 0.0 |
| Salmon, Reduced Fat, Tesco* | 1 Serving/56g | 100.0 | 7.0 | 179 | 15.5 | 1.1 | 12.5 | 3.5 |
| Salmon, Three, M & S* | 1 Serving/80g | 168.0 | 12.0 | 210 | 17.6 | 0.8 | 15.3 | 0.9 |
| Salmon, with Prawn & Lobster, M & S* | 1 Serving/55g | 107.0 | 7.0 | 195 | 18.2 | 0.7 | 13.4 | 0.7 |
| Salmon & Crayfish, Slice, Finest, Tesco* | 1 Serving/110g | 148.0 | 6.0 | 135 | 21.9 | 0.1 | 5.2 | 0.1 |

T

| | Measure INFO/WEIGHT | per Measure KCAL | FAT | Nutrition Values per 100g / 100ml KCAL | PROT | CARB | FAT | FIBRE |
|---|---|---|---|---|---|---|---|---|
| **TERRINE** | | | | | | | | |
| Salmon & King Prawn, Waitrose* | 1 Serving/75g | 97.0 | 4.0 | 130 | 19.3 | 1.3 | 5.3 | 0.0 |
| Salmon & Lemon, Luxury, Tesco* | 1 Serving/50g | 98.0 | 8.0 | 196 | 10.6 | 3.2 | 15.7 | 0.8 |
| Trout, TTD, Sainsbury's* | 1 Serving/60g | 138.0 | 11.0 | 230 | 14.7 | 2.6 | 17.9 | 0.2 |
| **THAI BITES** | | | | | | | | |
| Lightly Salted, Jacob's* | 1 Bag/25g | 94.0 | 1.0 | 375 | 6.9 | 79.7 | 3.2 | 0.1 |
| Mild Thai Flavour, Jacob's* | 1 Bag/25g | 93.0 | 1.0 | 373 | 6.9 | 79.0 | 3.3 | 1.0 |
| Red Curry & Coriander, Fusions, Jacob's* | 1 Bag/30g | 110.0 | 2.0 | 367 | 6.0 | 72.3 | 6.0 | 1.0 |
| Roasted Chilli Flavour, Fusions, Jacob's* | 1 Bag/30g | 109.0 | 2.0 | 363 | 5.5 | 72.3 | 5.8 | 1.2 |
| Seaweed Flavour, Jacob's* | 1 Bag/25g | 94.0 | 1.0 | 377 | 7.1 | 80.0 | 3.2 | 0.5 |
| Sesame & Prawn, Fusions, Jacob's* | 1 Bag/25g | 91.0 | 1.0 | 366 | 6.3 | 71.2 | 5.9 | 1.3 |
| Sweet Herb, Jacob's* | 1 Bag/25g | 93.0 | 1.0 | 372 | 7.1 | 78.8 | 3.2 | 0.2 |
| **THYME** | | | | | | | | |
| *Dried, Ground, Average* | *1 Tsp/1g* | *3.0* | *0.0* | *276* | *9.1* | *45.3* | *7.4* | *0.0* |
| *Fresh, Average* | *1 Tsp/1g* | *1.0* | *0.0* | *95* | *3.0* | *15.1* | *2.5* | *0.0* |
| **TIA MARIA** | | | | | | | | |
| *Original* | *1 Shot/35ml* | *105.0* | *0.0* | *300* | *0.0* | *0.0* | *0.0* | *0.0* |
| **TIC TAC** | | | | | | | | |
| Extra Strong Mint, Ferrero* | 2 Tic tacs/1g | 4.0 | 0.0 | 381 | 0.0 | 95.2 | 0.0 | 0.0 |
| Fresh Mint, Ferrero* | 2 Tic Tacs/1g | 4.0 | 0.0 | 390 | 0.0 | 97.5 | 0.0 | 0.0 |
| Lime & Orange, Ferrero* | 2 Tic Tacs/1g | 4.0 | 0.0 | 386 | 0.0 | 95.5 | 0.0 | 0.0 |
| Orange, Ferrero* | 2 Tic Tacs/1g | 4.0 | 0.0 | 385 | 0.0 | 95.5 | 0.0 | 0.0 |
| Spearmint, Ferrero* | 1 Box/16g | 62.0 | 0.0 | 390 | 0.0 | 97.5 | 0.0 | 0.0 |
| **TIDGY PUDS** | | | | | | | | |
| Aunt Bessie's* | 4 Puds/17g | 55.0 | 3.0 | 326 | 9.6 | 38.4 | 14.8 | 2.1 |
| **TIDGY TOADS** | | | | | | | | |
| Aunt Bessie's* | 1 Serving/45g | 125.0 | 6.0 | 278 | 14.7 | 25.3 | 13.2 | 1.1 |
| **TIKKA MASALA** | | | | | | | | |
| Cauliflower & Potato, with Pilau Rice, Safeway* | 1 Serving/414g | 435.0 | 17.0 | 105 | 2.4 | 13.9 | 4.1 | 2.2 |
| Chicken, & Pilau Basmati Rice, Frozen, Patak's* | 1 Pack/400g | 580.0 | 20.0 | 145 | 9.9 | 15.1 | 5.0 | 0.2 |
| Chicken, & Pilau Rice, BGTY, Sainsbury's* | 1 Pack/400g | 380.0 | 5.0 | 95 | 8.1 | 13.0 | 1.2 | 1.1 |
| Chicken, & Pilau Rice, GFY, Asda* | 1 Pack/450g | 495.0 | 9.0 | 110 | 6.0 | 17.0 | 2.0 | 0.8 |
| Chicken, & Pilau Rice, Takeaway, Asda* | 1 Pack/561g | 852.0 | 27.0 | 152 | 7.0 | 20.0 | 4.9 | 1.5 |
| Chicken, & Pilau Rice, Waitrose* | 1 Pack/500g | 797.0 | 34.0 | 159 | 8.2 | 16.1 | 6.9 | 0.8 |
| Chicken, & Rice, Light Choices, Tesco* | 1 Pack/450g | 472.0 | 7.0 | 105 | 7.9 | 14.6 | 1.6 | 1.3 |
| Chicken, & Rice, M & S* | 1 Pack/400g | 700.0 | 35.0 | 175 | 7.4 | 17.0 | 8.8 | 1.0 |
| Chicken, & Vegetable, HL, Tesco* | 1 Pack/450g | 360.0 | 12.0 | 80 | 6.8 | 6.9 | 2.7 | 1.8 |
| Chicken, Asda* | 1 Pack/340g | 388.0 | 20.0 | 114 | 9.0 | 6.0 | 6.0 | 1.5 |
| Chicken, Birds Eye* | 1 Serving/400g | 420.0 | 7.0 | 105 | 5.6 | 16.6 | 1.8 | 0.3 |
| Chicken, Boiled Rice & Nan, Meal for One, GFY, Asda* | 1 Pack/605g | 823.0 | 19.0 | 136 | 6.0 | 21.0 | 3.1 | 0.0 |
| Chicken, Breast, GFY, Asda* | 1 Pack/380g | 486.0 | 14.0 | 128 | 19.0 | 4.5 | 3.8 | 0.2 |
| Chicken, COU, M & S* | 1 Pack/400g | 400.0 | 7.0 | 100 | 7.6 | 14.1 | 1.7 | 1.3 |
| Chicken, Feeling Great, Findus* | 1 Pack/350g | 420.0 | 12.0 | 120 | 5.5 | 17.0 | 3.5 | 2.0 |
| Chicken, Hot, Sainsbury's* | 1 Pack/400g | 604.0 | 37.0 | 151 | 13.2 | 3.6 | 9.3 | 1.5 |
| Chicken, Hot, Tesco* | 1 Pack/400g | 588.0 | 34.0 | 147 | 8.7 | 8.6 | 8.6 | 1.0 |
| Chicken, Indian, Medium, Sainsbury's* | 1 Pack/400g | 848.0 | 61.0 | 212 | 13.2 | 5.3 | 15.3 | 0.1 |
| Chicken, Indian, Tesco* | 1 Pack/350g | 560.0 | 33.0 | 160 | 11.6 | 7.2 | 9.3 | 0.6 |
| Chicken, Indian Meal for One, BGTY, Sainsbury's* | 1 Serving/241g | 200.0 | 2.0 | 83 | 13.9 | 5.1 | 0.8 | 1.0 |
| Chicken, Indian Takeaway, Tesco* | 1 Serving/125g | 100.0 | 3.0 | 80 | 8.9 | 4.9 | 2.6 | 2.1 |
| Chicken, Large, Sainsbury's* | 1 Pack/650g | 1105.0 | 69.0 | 170 | 11.7 | 7.0 | 10.6 | 0.3 |
| Chicken, Low Fat, Iceland* | 1 Pack/400g | 360.0 | 4.0 | 90 | 7.8 | 12.5 | 1.0 | 0.5 |
| Chicken, Microwave Meal, Good Choice, Iceland* | 1 Pack/400g | 488.0 | 6.0 | 122 | 6.6 | 20.4 | 1.5 | 0.6 |
| Chicken, Morrisons* | 1 Pack/340g | 561.0 | 35.0 | 165 | 12.4 | 5.9 | 10.2 | 1.7 |
| Chicken, Sharwood's* | 1 Pack/375g | 562.0 | 25.0 | 150 | 7.2 | 15.1 | 6.7 | 0.8 |

T

| | Measure INFO/WEIGHT | per Measure KCAL | FAT | Nutrition Values per 100g / 100ml KCAL | PROT | CARB | FAT | FIBRE |
|---|---|---|---|---|---|---|---|---|
| **TIKKA MASALA** | | | | | | | | |
| Chicken, SmartPrice, Asda* | 1 Pack/300g | 414.0 | 18.0 | 138 | 13.0 | 8.0 | 6.0 | 1.6 |
| Chicken, Tinned, Asda* | ½ Can/200g | 238.0 | 14.0 | 119 | 8.0 | 6.0 | 7.0 | 0.9 |
| Chicken, Tinned, M & S* | ½ Can/213g | 309.0 | 18.0 | 145 | 14.5 | 2.9 | 8.5 | 2.2 |
| Chicken, with Basmati Rice, Eat Smart, Safeway* | 1 Pack/363g | 290.0 | 5.0 | 80 | 6.4 | 9.6 | 1.4 | 0.7 |
| Chicken, with Fruit & Nut Pilau Rice, Sainsbury's* | 1 Pack/500g | 885.0 | 45.0 | 177 | 7.6 | 16.1 | 9.1 | 2.8 |
| Chicken, with Golden Rice, Iceland* | 1 Pack/500g | 885.0 | 41.0 | 177 | 6.2 | 19.4 | 8.3 | 1.1 |
| Chicken, with Pilau Rice, Frozen, Waitrose* | 1 Pack/400g | 676.0 | 32.0 | 169 | 9.3 | 14.6 | 8.1 | 2.1 |
| Chicken, with Pilau Rice, Perfectly Balanced, Waitrose* | 1 Pack/400g | 476.0 | 10.0 | 119 | 8.2 | 15.8 | 2.5 | 1.8 |
| Chicken, with Rice, Sainsbury's* | 1 Pack/500g | 960.0 | 41.0 | 192 | 8.3 | 21.2 | 8.2 | 0.1 |
| Cooking Sauce, Under 3% Fat, BGTY, Sainsbury's* | ¼ Jar/126g | 83.0 | 2.0 | 66 | 0.8 | 11.7 | 1.8 | 0.6 |
| King Prawn & Rice, Finest, Tesco* | 1 Pack/475g | 617.0 | 27.0 | 130 | 5.1 | 14.5 | 5.7 | 1.9 |
| Prawn, COU, M & S* | 1 Pack/400g | 400.0 | 6.0 | 100 | 6.9 | 14.7 | 1.6 | 1.9 |
| Prawn, King, Perfectly Balanced, Waitrose* | 1 Pack/400g | 372.0 | 4.0 | 93 | 5.2 | 16.0 | 0.9 | 1.7 |
| Vegetable, Asda* | 1 Pack/340g | 316.0 | 21.0 | 93 | 2.0 | 7.4 | 6.1 | 1.1 |
| Vegetable, Canned, Waitrose* | 1 Can/200g | 152.0 | 4.0 | 76 | 3.6 | 10.5 | 2.2 | 0.0 |
| Vegetable, Indian, Tesco* | 1 Pack/225g | 234.0 | 13.0 | 104 | 2.4 | 10.4 | 6.0 | 2.4 |
| Vegetable, with Rice, Patak's* | 1 Pack/298g | 247.0 | 7.0 | 83 | 2.9 | 12.3 | 2.4 | 1.4 |
| Vegetable, with Rice, Tesco* | 1 Pack/450g | 499.0 | 19.0 | 111 | 2.6 | 15.5 | 4.3 | 0.9 |
| Vegetarian, with Pilau Rice, Tesco* | 1 Serving/440g | 519.0 | 17.0 | 118 | 5.0 | 15.6 | 3.9 | 1.5 |
| **TILAPIA** | | | | | | | | |
| *Raw, Average* | *100g* | *95.0* | *1.0* | *95* | *20.0* | *0.0* | *1.0* | *0.0* |
| **TIME OUT** | | | | | | | | |
| Break Pack, Cadbury* | 1 Serving/20g | 108.0 | 6.0 | 530 | 6.2 | 58.3 | 30.7 | 0.0 |
| Chocolate Fingers, Cadbury* | 2 Fingers/35g | 185.0 | 11.0 | 530 | 6.2 | 58.3 | 30.7 | 0.0 |
| Orange, Snack Size, Cadbury* | 1 Finger/11g | 61.0 | 4.0 | 555 | 5.0 | 59.4 | 32.9 | 0.0 |
| **TIRAMISU** | | | | | | | | |
| Asda* | 1 Pot/100g | 252.0 | 11.0 | 252 | 4.3 | 34.0 | 11.0 | 0.5 |
| BGTY, Sainsbury's* | 1 Pot/90g | 140.0 | 2.0 | 156 | 4.5 | 28.3 | 2.7 | 0.3 |
| Choc & Mascarpone, Tiramigu, Gu* | 1 Pud/90g | 316.0 | 23.0 | 351 | 3.3 | 26.1 | 25.9 | 1.0 |
| COU, M & S* | 1 Tub/95g | 138.0 | 3.0 | 145 | 3.7 | 26.9 | 2.7 | 0.6 |
| Family Size, Tesco* | 1 Serving/125g | 356.0 | 18.0 | 285 | 4.3 | 34.5 | 14.5 | 4.3 |
| Italian, Safeway* | 1 Serving/125g | 352.0 | 17.0 | 282 | 4.4 | 34.4 | 14.0 | 1.6 |
| Light Choices, Tesco* | 1 Pot/90g | 162.0 | 4.0 | 180 | 7.7 | 27.6 | 3.9 | 2.4 |
| Morrisons* | 1 Pot/90g | 248.0 | 10.0 | 276 | 4.0 | 38.0 | 11.0 | 0.0 |
| Raspberry, M & S* | 1 Serving/84g | 197.0 | 12.0 | 235 | 3.8 | 22.9 | 14.4 | 0.2 |
| Single Size, Tesco* | 1 Pot/100g | 290.0 | 13.0 | 290 | 3.8 | 35.1 | 12.9 | 4.5 |
| Somerfield* | 1 Pot/100g | 286.0 | 11.0 | 286 | 5.0 | 39.0 | 11.0 | 0.0 |
| Trifle, Sainsbury's* | 1 Serving/100g | 243.0 | 16.0 | 243 | 2.3 | 23.2 | 15.7 | 0.6 |
| Waitrose* | 1 Pot/90g | 221.0 | 11.0 | 246 | 6.4 | 27.2 | 12.4 | 0.0 |
| **TOAD IN THE HOLE** | | | | | | | | |
| Average | 1oz/28g | 78.0 | 5.0 | 277 | 11.9 | 19.5 | 17.4 | 1.1 |
| Large, Great Value, Asda* | ¼ Pack/81g | 238.0 | 14.0 | 293 | 10.0 | 25.0 | 17.0 | 2.3 |
| Tesco* | 1 Serving/188g | 461.0 | 28.0 | 245 | 8.5 | 18.7 | 15.1 | 2.6 |
| Vegetarian, Aunt Bessie's* | 1 Pack/190g | 502.0 | 19.0 | 264 | 15.6 | 27.5 | 10.2 | 2.7 |
| Vegetarian, Linda McCartney* | 1 Pack/190g | 359.0 | 17.0 | 189 | 13.6 | 13.9 | 8.8 | 1.1 |
| Vegetarian, Meat Free, Asda* | 1 Serving/173g | 407.0 | 19.0 | 235 | 9.0 | 25.0 | 11.0 | 3.1 |
| Vegetarian, Tesco* | 1 Pack/190g | 471.0 | 19.0 | 248 | 13.1 | 26.5 | 10.0 | 2.8 |
| with Three Sausages, Asda* | 1 Pack/150g | 435.0 | 27.0 | 290 | 10.0 | 22.0 | 18.0 | 1.0 |
| **TOASTIE** | | | | | | | | |
| All Day Breakfast, M & S* | 1 Serving/174g | 375.0 | 14.0 | 215 | 11.2 | 25.0 | 7.9 | 1.7 |
| Cheese & Ham, Tayto* | 1 Serving/50g | 259.0 | 15.0 | 519 | 6.8 | 58.0 | 29.7 | 0.0 |
| Cheese & Pickle, M & S* | 1 Toastie/136g | 320.0 | 9.0 | 235 | 10.4 | 33.5 | 6.7 | 2.6 |
| Ham & Cheddar, British, M & S* | 1 Pack/128g | 269.0 | 9.0 | 210 | 15.5 | 22.3 | 6.7 | 1.3 |

**T**

| | Measure INFO/WEIGHT | per Measure KCAL | FAT | Nutrition Values per 100g / 100ml KCAL | PROT | CARB | FAT | FIBRE |
|---|---|---|---|---|---|---|---|---|
| **TOASTIE** | | | | | | | | |
| Ham & Cheese, Tesco* | 1 Serving/138g | 388.0 | 18.0 | 281 | 11.5 | 29.1 | 13.2 | 1.0 |
| **TOFFEE CRISP** | | | | | | | | |
| Biscuit, Nestle* | 1 Biscuit/23g | 116.0 | 6.0 | 516 | 3.9 | 62.6 | 27.8 | 1.1 |
| Mini, Nestle* | 1 Bar/18g | 94.0 | 5.0 | 516 | 3.7 | 63.1 | 27.6 | 1.1 |
| Nestle* | 1 Bar/44g | 227.0 | 12.0 | 516 | 3.7 | 63.1 | 27.7 | 0.0 |
| Snack Size, Nestle* | 1 Bar/30g | 155.0 | 8.0 | 516 | 3.7 | 63.1 | 27.6 | 1.1 |
| **TOFFEES** | | | | | | | | |
| Assorted, Bassett's* | 1 Toffee/8g | 35.0 | 1.0 | 434 | 3.8 | 73.1 | 14.0 | 0.0 |
| Assorted, Sainsbury's* | 1 Sweet/8g | 37.0 | 1.0 | 457 | 2.2 | 76.5 | 15.8 | 0.2 |
| Brazil Nut, Diabetic, Thorntons* | 1 Serving/20g | 93.0 | 7.0 | 467 | 3.2 | 49.0 | 35.1 | 0.5 |
| Butter, SmartPrice, Asda* | 1 Toffee/8g | 37.0 | 1.0 | 440 | 1.3 | 75.0 | 15.0 | 0.0 |
| Chewy, Werther's* | 1 Toffee/5g | 22.0 | 1.0 | 436 | 3.5 | 71.3 | 15.2 | 0.1 |
| Chocolate Coated, Thorntons* | 1 Bag/100g | 521.0 | 31.0 | 521 | 3.5 | 57.9 | 30.7 | 0.3 |
| Dairy, Waitrose* | 1 Toffee/14g | 64.0 | 2.0 | 458 | 2.0 | 80.2 | 14.3 | 0.5 |
| Devon Butter, Thorntons* | 1 Sweet/9g | 40.0 | 2.0 | 444 | 1.7 | 72.2 | 16.7 | 0.0 |
| Liquorice, Thorntons* | 1 Bag/100g | 506.0 | 29.0 | 506 | 1.9 | 58.8 | 29.4 | 0.0 |
| Milk Chocolate Smothered, Thorntons* | 1 Pack/125g | 655.0 | 38.0 | 524 | 4.3 | 57.5 | 30.8 | 1.1 |
| Mixed, Average | 1oz/28g | 119.0 | 5.0 | 426 | 2.2 | 66.7 | 18.6 | 0.0 |
| No Added Sugar, Boots* | 1 Serving/7g | 23.0 | 1.0 | 324 | 1.3 | 52.0 | 14.0 | 0.0 |
| Original, Thorntons* | 1 Bag/100g | 514.0 | 30.0 | 514 | 1.8 | 59.3 | 30.1 | 0.0 |
| Strawberries & Cream, Special, Thorntons* | 25g | 126.0 | 7.0 | 505 | 1.9 | 57.3 | 29.8 | 0.2 |
| **TOFU** | | | | | | | | |
| *Average* | *1 Pack/250g* | *297.0* | *16.0* | *119* | *13.4* | *1.4* | *6.6* | *0.1* |
| Beech Smoked, Organic, Cauldron Foods* | ½ Pack/110g | 124.0 | 8.0 | 113 | 10.9 | 1.0 | 7.1 | 0.5 |
| Firm Silken Style, Blue Dragon* | 1 Pack/216g | 134.0 | 6.0 | 62 | 6.9 | 2.4 | 2.7 | 0.0 |
| Fresh, Drained, Kong Nam* | 1 Tub/575g | 397.0 | 21.0 | 69 | 7.7 | 1.3 | 3.7 | 0.5 |
| *Fried, Average* | *1oz/28g* | *75.0* | *4.0* | *268* | *28.6* | *9.3* | *14.1* | *0.0* |
| Original, Organic, Cauldron Foods* | ½ Pack/125g | 131.0 | 7.0 | 105 | 12.1 | 0.6 | 6.0 | 0.5 |
| Sheets, Dried, H.k. Huizenhou Foods* | 10g | 5.0 | 0.0 | 50 | 4.0 | 5.0 | 4.0 | 0.0 |
| Smoked, Organic, Evernat* | 1oz/28g | 36.0 | 2.0 | 127 | 16.3 | 0.8 | 6.6 | 0.0 |
| **TOMATILLOS** | | | | | | | | |
| *Raw* | *1 Med/34g* | *11.0* | *0.0* | *32* | *1.0* | *5.8* | *1.0* | *1.9* |
| **TOMATO PASTE** | | | | | | | | |
| *Average* | *1 Tbsp/20g* | *19.0* | *0.0* | *96* | *4.9* | *19.2* | *0.2* | *1.5* |
| *Sun Dried, Average* | *1 Heaped Tsp/10g* | *38.0* | *4.0* | *385* | *3.2* | *13.8* | *35.1* | *0.0* |
| **TOMATO PUREE** | | | | | | | | |
| *Average* | *1oz/28g* | *21.0* | *0.0* | *76* | *4.5* | *14.1* | *0.2* | *2.3* |
| Sun Dried, & Olive Oil & Herbs, GIA* | 1 Serving/20g | 41.0 | 4.0 | 204 | 2.6 | 0.5 | 21.6 | 0.0 |
| with Garlic, Heinz* | 1 Serving/10g | 6.0 | 0.0 | 57 | 3.6 | 10.2 | 0.2 | 1.2 |
| **TOMATOES** | | | | | | | | |
| *Cherry, Average* | *1 Serving/80g* | *15.0* | *0.0* | *19* | *0.9* | *3.3* | *0.3* | *1.0* |
| *Cherry, on the Vine, Average* | *1 Serving/80g* | *14.0* | *0.0* | *18* | *0.7* | *3.1* | *0.3* | *1.0* |
| *Cherry, Raw* | *1oz/28g* | *5.0* | *0.0* | *18* | *0.8* | *3.0* | *0.4* | *1.0* |
| *Chopped, Canned, Average* | *1 Serving/130g* | *27.0* | *0.0* | *21* | *1.1* | *3.8* | *0.1* | *0.8* |
| *Chopped, Italian, Average* | *½ Can/200g* | *47.0* | *0.0* | *23* | *1.3* | *4.4* | *0.1* | *0.9* |
| Chopped, Italian, with Olive Oil & Garlic, Waitrose* | 1 Serving/100g | 33.0 | 2.0 | 33 | 1.1 | 3.6 | 1.6 | 0.0 |
| Chopped, Italian, with Olives, Waitrose* | 1 Can/400g | 184.0 | 7.0 | 46 | 1.4 | 6.0 | 1.8 | 0.8 |
| Chopped, with Chilli, Sainsbury's* | ½ Can/200g | 44.0 | 1.0 | 22 | 1.0 | 3.5 | 0.5 | 0.9 |
| Chopped, with Chilli & Peppers, Asda* | 1 Pack/400g | 92.0 | 1.0 | 23 | 1.0 | 4.0 | 0.3 | 0.0 |
| *Chopped, with Garlic, Average* | *½ Can/200g* | *43.0* | *0.0* | *21* | *1.2* | *3.8* | *0.1* | *0.8* |
| *Chopped, with Herbs, Average* | *½ Can/200g* | *42.0* | *0.0* | *21* | *1.1* | *3.8* | *0.1* | *0.8* |
| Chopped, with Olive Oil & Roasted Garlic, Sainsbury's* | 1 Pack/390g | 187.0 | 8.0 | 48 | 1.3 | 5.9 | 2.1 | 1.0 |
| Chopped, with Onion & Herbs, Napolina* | 1 Can/400g | 84.0 | 0.0 | 21 | 1.0 | 4.0 | 0.1 | 0.4 |

T

| | Measure INFO/WEIGHT | per Measure KCAL | FAT | Nutrition Values per 100g / 100ml KCAL | PROT | CARB | FAT | FIBRE |
|---|---|---|---|---|---|---|---|---|
| **TOMATOES** | | | | | | | | |
| Chopped, with Onions, Italian, Tesco* | ½ Can/200g | 46.0 | 0.0 | 23 | 1.4 | 4.0 | 0.2 | 0.9 |
| Chopped, with Peppers & Onions, Sainsbury's* | ½ Can/200g | 40.0 | 0.0 | 20 | 1.2 | 3.5 | 0.1 | 0.9 |
| Chopped, with Sliced Green & Black Olives, Sainsbury's* | 1 Pack/390g | 183.0 | 8.0 | 47 | 1.3 | 5.6 | 2.1 | 0.7 |
| Creamed, Sainsbury's* | 1oz/28g | 6.0 | 0.0 | 22 | 1.5 | 5.0 | 0.1 | 1.6 |
| *Fresh, Raw, Average* | *1 Med (2-3in)/123g* | *22.0* | *0.0* | *18* | *0.9* | *3.9* | *0.2* | *1.2* |
| Fried in Blended Oil | 1 Med/85g | 77.0 | 7.0 | 91 | 0.7 | 5.0 | 7.7 | 1.3 |
| Green Tiger, Raw, M & S* | 1 Serving/80g | 16.0 | 0.0 | 20 | 0.7 | 3.1 | 0.3 | 1.0 |
| Grilled, Average | 1oz/28g | 14.0 | 0.0 | 49 | 2.0 | 8.9 | 0.9 | 2.9 |
| Mediterranean, Sunblush, TTD, Sainsbury's* | 1 Sm Pot/240g | 319.0 | 18.0 | 133 | 2.9 | 17.9 | 7.4 | 4.3 |
| *Plum, Baby, Average* | *1 Serving/50g* | *9.0* | *0.0* | *18* | *1.5* | *2.3* | *0.3* | *1.0* |
| *Plum, in Tomato Juice, Average* | *1 Can/400g* | *71.0* | *0.0* | *18* | *0.9* | *3.3* | *0.1* | *0.7* |
| *Plum, in Tomato Juice, Premium, Average* | *1 Can/400g* | *93.0* | *1.0* | *23* | *1.3* | *3.8* | *0.3* | *0.7* |
| Pomodorino, TTD, Sainsbury's* | 1 Serving/80g | 14.0 | 0.0 | 18 | 0.8 | 3.0 | 0.4 | 1.0 |
| *Ripened on the Vine, Average* | *1 Med/123g* | *22.0* | *0.0* | *18* | *0.7* | *3.0* | *0.3* | *0.7* |
| Santini, M & S* | 1 Serving/80g | 16.0 | 0.0 | 20 | 0.7 | 3.1 | 0.3 | 1.0 |
| Semi Dried, in Olive Oil, TTD, Sainsbury's* | 1 Serving/20g | 33.0 | 2.0 | 167 | 4.2 | 19.5 | 8.0 | 0.0 |
| Stuffed with Rice, Average | 1oz/28g | 59.0 | 4.0 | 212 | 2.1 | 22.2 | 13.4 | 1.1 |
| *Sun Dried, Average* | *3 Pieces/20g* | *43.0* | *3.0* | *213* | *4.7* | *12.9* | *15.9* | *3.3* |
| Sun Dried, in Oil, GIA* | 1 Serving/10g | 15.0 | 1.0 | 153 | 1.9 | 7.5 | 13.9 | 0.0 |
| Sun Dried, in Olive Oil, M & S* | 1 Jar/280g | 644.0 | 57.0 | 230 | 3.9 | 7.9 | 20.4 | 6.7 |
| Sun Dried, in Sunflower Oil, Deli Express, Asda* | 1 Serving/50g | 76.0 | 3.0 | 153 | 5.8 | 15.9 | 6.0 | 9.0 |
| Sun Dried, with Herbs & Extra Virgin Olive Oil, Waitrose* | 1 Serving/50g | 72.0 | 5.0 | 145 | 3.4 | 9.1 | 10.5 | 7.1 |
| Sundried, with Chianti, TTD, Sainsbury's* | ½ Pot/150g | 108.0 | 5.0 | 72 | 1.8 | 8.2 | 3.5 | 1.0 |
| **TONGUE** | | | | | | | | |
| *Lunch, Average* | *1oz/28g* | *51.0* | *3.0* | *181* | *20.1* | *1.8* | *10.6* | *0.0* |
| *Slices, Average* | *1oz/28g* | *56.0* | *4.0* | *201* | *18.7* | *0.0* | *14.0* | *0.0* |
| **TONIC WATER** | | | | | | | | |
| Average | 1 Glass/250ml | 82.0 | 0.0 | 33 | 0.0 | 8.8 | 0.0 | 0.0 |
| Diet, Asda* | 1 Glass/200ml | 2.0 | 0.0 | 1 | 0.0 | 0.0 | 0.0 | 0.0 |
| Indian, Diet, Schweppes* | 1 Glass/100ml | 1.0 | 0.0 | 1 | 0.0 | 0.0 | 0.0 | 0.0 |
| Indian, Schweppes* | 1 Serving/500ml | 110.0 | 0.0 | 22 | 0.0 | 5.1 | 0.0 | 0.0 |
| Indian, Slimline, Schweppes* | 1 Serving/188ml | 3.0 | 0.0 | 2 | 0.4 | 0.0 | 0.0 | 0.0 |
| Indian, with a Hint of Lemon, Low Calorie, Asda* | 1 Serving/300ml | 3.0 | 0.0 | 1 | 0.0 | 0.0 | 0.1 | 0.0 |
| Low Calorie, Tesco* | 1 Serving/200ml | 4.0 | 0.0 | 2 | 0.0 | 0.5 | 0.0 | 0.0 |
| Quinine, Schweppes* | 1 Glass/125ml | 46.0 | 0.0 | 37 | 0.0 | 9.0 | 0.0 | 0.0 |
| **TOPIC** | | | | | | | | |
| Mars* | 1 Bar/47g | 234.0 | 12.0 | 498 | 6.2 | 59.6 | 26.2 | 1.7 |
| **TOPPING** | | | | | | | | |
| Bruschetta, Safeway* | 1 Serving/100g | 26.0 | 1.0 | 26 | 1.2 | 3.6 | 0.8 | 0.0 |
| Bruschetta, Sainsbury's* | 1 Sm Can/230g | 60.0 | 2.0 | 26 | 1.2 | 3.6 | 0.8 | 1.1 |
| Bruschetta, Tesco* | 1 Can/230g | 57.0 | 2.0 | 25 | 1.2 | 3.2 | 0.8 | 1.1 |
| Cake Covering, Milk Chocolate Flavoured, Tesco* | 1 Pack/300g | 1761.0 | 116.0 | 587 | 2.1 | 57.3 | 38.8 | 2.6 |
| Creamy, Tip Top, Nestle* | 1 Serving/50g | 53.0 | 3.0 | 107 | 3.5 | 8.6 | 6.4 | 0.1 |
| for Cappuccino, Creamy, Flavia* | 1 Serving/15g | 38.0 | 1.0 | 253 | 14.7 | 33.3 | 6.7 | 0.0 |
| Ice Cream, Monster Crackin, Silver Spoon* | 1 Tbsp/15g | 92.0 | 7.0 | 612 | 0.0 | 50.7 | 45.5 | 0.0 |
| Pizza, Italian Tomato & Herb, Sainsbury's* | 1/5 Jar/50g | 19.0 | 0.0 | 38 | 1.6 | 7.1 | 0.4 | 1.1 |
| Pizza, Tomato with Cheese & Onion, Napolina* | 1 Jar/250g | 195.0 | 10.0 | 78 | 2.9 | 7.0 | 4.0 | 0.8 |
| Pizza, Traditional Tomato with Basil, Napolina* | 1 Jar/250g | 152.0 | 6.0 | 61 | 1.2 | 7.8 | 2.6 | 0.7 |
| Pizza, with Herbs, Napolina* | 1 Serving/100g | 49.0 | 2.0 | 49 | 0.9 | 6.3 | 2.2 | 0.6 |
| **TORTE** | | | | | | | | |
| Chocolate, Half Fat, Waitrose* | 1/6 Torte/70g | 135.0 | 4.0 | 193 | 5.4 | 29.7 | 5.8 | 2.2 |
| Chocolate, Mint, Weight Watchers* | 1 Pot/88g | 174.0 | 4.0 | 198 | 4.7 | 34.3 | 4.7 | 5.2 |
| Chocolate, Safeway* | 1/6 Torte/55g | 122.0 | 6.0 | 221 | 4.1 | 27.6 | 10.5 | 1.5 |

T

| | Measure INFO/WEIGHT | per Measure KCAL | per Measure FAT | Nutrition Values per 100g / 100ml KCAL | PROT | CARB | FAT | FIBRE |
|---|---|---|---|---|---|---|---|---|

## TORTE

| | Measure INFO/WEIGHT | KCAL | FAT | KCAL | PROT | CARB | FAT | FIBRE |
|---|---|---|---|---|---|---|---|---|
| Chocolate, Tesco* | 1 Serving/50g | 125.0 | 6.0 | 251 | 3.6 | 32.3 | 11.9 | 1.0 |
| Chocolate Orange & Almond, Gu* | 1 Serving/65g | 273.0 | 20.0 | 420 | 5.0 | 28.2 | 30.5 | 2.7 |
| Chocolate Truffle, Waitrose* | 1 Serving/116g | 359.0 | 20.0 | 309 | 4.6 | 30.1 | 17.3 | 1.4 |
| Lemon, Somerfield* | 1 Serving/45g | 71.0 | 1.0 | 157 | 0.8 | 32.6 | 2.6 | 0.8 |
| Lemon, Tesco* | 1 Serving/62g | 142.0 | 6.0 | 230 | 2.3 | 32.9 | 9.9 | 0.5 |
| Lemon & Mango, Waitrose* | 1 Serving/80g | 142.0 | 2.0 | 177 | 3.9 | 33.6 | 3.0 | 0.6 |
| Raspberry, Safeway* | 1/6 Torte/54g | 93.0 | 4.0 | 172 | 1.2 | 25.1 | 7.4 | 1.5 |

## TORTELLINI

| | Measure INFO/WEIGHT | KCAL | FAT | KCAL | PROT | CARB | FAT | FIBRE |
|---|---|---|---|---|---|---|---|---|
| 3 Cheese, Sainsbury's* | 1 Serving/50g | 195.0 | 4.0 | 391 | 14.4 | 63.8 | 8.7 | 3.0 |
| Aubergine & Pecorino, Sainsbury's* | ½ Pack/150g | 354.0 | 6.0 | 236 | 8.9 | 40.3 | 4.3 | 3.2 |
| Basil, Mozzarella & Tomato, Weight Watchers* | ½ Pack/125g | 278.0 | 3.0 | 222 | 9.0 | 40.5 | 2.7 | 4.8 |
| Beef & Red Wine, Italian, Asda* | ½ Pack/150g | 242.0 | 4.0 | 161 | 9.0 | 25.0 | 2.8 | 0.0 |
| Beef & Red Wine, Italiano, Tesco* | 1 Serving/150g | 324.0 | 5.0 | 216 | 11.7 | 35.3 | 3.2 | 3.3 |
| Beef Bolognese, Rich, Italian, Giovanni Rana* | ½ Pack/125g | 222.0 | 9.0 | 178 | 7.6 | 20.6 | 7.2 | 4.1 |
| Cheese, Fresh, Sainsbury's* | ½ Pack/180g | 329.0 | 9.0 | 183 | 7.6 | 26.8 | 5.0 | 1.7 |
| Cheese, Heinz* | 1 Can/395g | 233.0 | 7.0 | 59 | 2.1 | 8.6 | 1.8 | 0.5 |
| Cheese, HL, Tesco* | 1 Serving/400g | 368.0 | 11.0 | 92 | 3.2 | 13.4 | 2.8 | 0.6 |
| Cheese, Tomato & Basil, Tesco* | 1 Serving/150g | 387.0 | 8.0 | 258 | 13.0 | 39.5 | 5.4 | 3.3 |
| Cheese, Weight Watchers* | 1 Can/395g | 245.0 | 6.0 | 62 | 2.3 | 9.7 | 1.6 | 0.4 |
| Cheese & Ham, Italiano, Tesco* | ½ Pack/150g | 396.0 | 12.0 | 264 | 12.8 | 34.8 | 8.2 | 3.0 |
| Chicken, Spicy, Big Eat, Heinz* | 1 Pot/350g | 404.0 | 23.0 | 115 | 2.9 | 11.2 | 6.6 | 0.4 |
| Four Cheese, Italian, Asda* | 1 Serving/150g | 295.0 | 7.0 | 197 | 8.0 | 30.0 | 5.0 | 3.4 |
| Four Cheese, Tesco* | ½ Pack/150g | 405.0 | 12.0 | 270 | 12.3 | 37.3 | 7.9 | 3.4 |
| Four Cheese & Tomato, Italian, Asda* | 1 Serving/150g | 249.0 | 6.0 | 166 | 8.0 | 25.0 | 3.8 | 0.0 |
| Four Cheese with Tomato & Basil Sauce, Tesco* | 1 Pack/400g | 500.0 | 15.0 | 125 | 6.1 | 16.9 | 3.7 | 0.6 |
| Garlic, Basil & Ricotta, Asda* | ½ Pack/175g | 318.0 | 10.0 | 182 | 6.0 | 26.0 | 6.0 | 2.6 |
| Garlic & Herb, Fresh, Sainsbury's* | ½ Pack/150g | 364.0 | 12.0 | 243 | 11.1 | 32.2 | 7.8 | 1.8 |
| Ham & Cheese, Fresh, Asda* | ½ Pack/150g | 255.0 | 9.0 | 170 | 6.0 | 23.0 | 6.0 | 1.7 |
| Ham & Cheese, Tesco* | 1 Serving/225g | 578.0 | 13.0 | 257 | 13.5 | 38.1 | 5.6 | 1.8 |
| Meat, Italian, Tesco* | 1 Serving/125g | 332.0 | 9.0 | 266 | 10.6 | 38.9 | 7.6 | 2.3 |
| Mushroom, Asda* | 1 Serving/125g | 217.0 | 5.0 | 174 | 6.0 | 28.0 | 4.2 | 2.3 |
| Mushroom, BGTY, Sainsbury's* | ½ Can/200g | 180.0 | 6.0 | 90 | 2.2 | 13.2 | 3.1 | 0.7 |
| Mushroom, Perfectly Balanced, Waitrose* | 1 Pack/250g | 572.0 | 9.0 | 229 | 9.4 | 39.8 | 3.6 | 2.4 |
| Pepperoni, Italian, Asda* | ½ Pack/150g | 250.0 | 6.0 | 167 | 6.7 | 26.0 | 4.0 | 0.0 |
| Pesto & Goats Cheese, Fresh, Sainsbury's* | ½ Pack/150g | 310.0 | 12.0 | 207 | 8.9 | 24.6 | 8.1 | 2.6 |
| Pork & Beef, BGTY, Sainsbury's* | ½ Can/200g | 148.0 | 3.0 | 74 | 3.7 | 11.2 | 1.5 | 0.6 |
| Ricotta & Spinach, Giovanni Rana* | ½ Pack/125g | 340.0 | 14.0 | 272 | 10.1 | 34.6 | 10.9 | 10.0 |
| Sausage & Ham, Italiano, Tesco* | 1 Pack/300g | 816.0 | 28.0 | 272 | 13.1 | 34.0 | 9.3 | 3.7 |
| Smoked Bacon & Tomato, Asda* | 1 Pack/300g | 591.0 | 15.0 | 197 | 9.0 | 29.0 | 5.0 | 0.0 |
| Spicy Pepperoni, Asda* | ½ Pack/150g | 252.0 | 6.0 | 168 | 7.0 | 26.0 | 4.0 | 0.0 |
| Spicy Pepperoni, Fresh, Asda* | ½ Pack/150g | 249.0 | 6.0 | 166 | 7.0 | 26.0 | 4.0 | 0.0 |
| Spinach & Ricotta, Canned, Somerfield* | 1 Can/250g | 282.0 | 15.0 | 113 | 12.0 | 4.0 | 6.0 | 0.0 |
| Spinach & Ricotta, Italian, Asda* | ½ Pack/150g | 189.0 | 4.0 | 126 | 5.0 | 21.0 | 2.4 | 0.6 |
| Spinach & Ricotta, Pasta Reale* | ½ Pack/125g | 319.0 | 5.0 | 255 | 11.2 | 45.5 | 4.2 | 2.6 |
| Spinach & Ricotta, Verdi, Asda* | 1 Serving/125g | 186.0 | 6.0 | 149 | 6.0 | 21.0 | 4.5 | 2.4 |
| Spinach & Ricotta, Waistline, Crosse & Blackwell* | 1 Serving/300g | 219.0 | 7.0 | 73 | 2.9 | 10.1 | 2.4 | 1.3 |
| Tomato & Mozzarella, Fresh, Asda* | ½ Pack/150g | 235.0 | 4.0 | 157 | 8.0 | 25.0 | 2.8 | 0.0 |
| Tomato & Mozzarella, Fresh, Sainsbury's* | ½ Pack/150g | 291.0 | 12.0 | 194 | 7.5 | 23.0 | 8.0 | 3.4 |
| Trio, Fresh, Tesco* | ½ Pack/125g | 322.0 | 9.0 | 258 | 12.8 | 35.8 | 7.1 | 2.0 |
| with Tomato, Basil, & Paprika, Easy Cook, Napolina* | 1 Pack/120g | 481.0 | 15.0 | 401 | 12.4 | 60.7 | 12.1 | 0.0 |

## TORTELLONI

| | Measure INFO/WEIGHT | KCAL | FAT | KCAL | PROT | CARB | FAT | FIBRE |
|---|---|---|---|---|---|---|---|---|
| Arrabbiata, Sainsbury's* | ½ Pack/210g | 407.0 | 12.0 | 194 | 7.1 | 28.8 | 5.6 | 2.6 |
| Beef & Pancetta, Aberdeen Angus, Grandi, Budgens* | ½ Pack/125g | 314.0 | 5.0 | 251 | 12.4 | 40.5 | 4.3 | 2.9 |

T

| | Measure INFO/WEIGHT | per Measure KCAL | FAT | Nutrition Values per 100g / 100ml KCAL | PROT | CARB | FAT | FIBRE |
|---|---|---|---|---|---|---|---|---|
| **TORTELLONI** | | | | | | | | |
| Bell Pepper & Sundried Tomato, Morrisons* | ½ Pack/150g | 375.0 | 6.0 | 250 | 12.1 | 40.7 | 4.3 | 2.9 |
| Carbonara, Sainsbury's* | 1 Pack/300g | 579.0 | 18.0 | 193 | 8.4 | 26.3 | 6.0 | 2.2 |
| Cheese, Tomato, & Basil, Sainsbury's* | ½ Pack/150g | 271.0 | 10.0 | 181 | 8.0 | 22.7 | 6.5 | 1.7 |
| Cheese & Pesto, Somerfield* | 1 Pack/250g | 787.0 | 30.0 | 315 | 12.0 | 40.0 | 12.0 | 0.0 |
| Cheese & Smoked Ham, Tesco* | ½ Pack/150g | 315.0 | 11.0 | 210 | 8.9 | 26.5 | 7.1 | 1.7 |
| Cheese & Smoked Ham, Waitrose* | 1 Serving/250g | 625.0 | 17.0 | 250 | 11.5 | 35.8 | 6.8 | 1.8 |
| Cheese & Sun Dried Tomato, Fresh, Safeway* | ½ Pack/199g | 364.0 | 12.0 | 183 | 7.7 | 24.2 | 6.2 | 2.7 |
| Cheese Garlic & Herb, Fresh, Budgens* | ½ Pack/125g | 334.0 | 7.0 | 267 | 10.3 | 46.1 | 6.0 | 3.3 |
| Chicken & Bacon, Italiano, Tesco* | 1 Pack/300g | 660.0 | 22.0 | 220 | 7.8 | 29.8 | 7.3 | 2.1 |
| Chicken & Ham, Morrisons* | 1 Serving/150g | 366.0 | 6.0 | 244 | 12.3 | 38.6 | 3.9 | 2.4 |
| Chorizo & Tomato, Morrisons* | 1 Serving/150g | 447.0 | 13.0 | 298 | 12.8 | 45.1 | 8.6 | 2.6 |
| Five Cheese, Safeway* | 1 Serving/150g | 274.0 | 9.0 | 183 | 7.8 | 24.2 | 6.2 | 2.7 |
| Five Cheese, Sainsbury's* | 1 Serving/125g | 285.0 | 12.0 | 228 | 10.8 | 25.2 | 9.3 | 2.9 |
| Four Cheese, Express, Dolmio* | 1 Pack/220g | 411.0 | 17.0 | 187 | 7.6 | 22.1 | 7.6 | 0.0 |
| Four Cheese, Tesco* | 1 Serving/200g | 390.0 | 13.0 | 195 | 8.0 | 25.5 | 6.7 | 1.8 |
| Four Cheese, Waitrose* | ½ Pack/125g | 297.0 | 8.0 | 238 | 10.3 | 34.2 | 6.7 | 1.6 |
| Fresh, Ham & Cheese, Asda* | ½ Pack/150g | 315.0 | 11.0 | 210 | 8.8 | 26.7 | 7.6 | 1.4 |
| Garlic & Herb, Cooked, Pasta Reale* | 1 Pack/300g | 546.0 | 12.0 | 182 | 6.7 | 30.1 | 3.9 | 0.9 |
| Garlic Mushroom & Onion, Eat Smart, Safeway* | 1 Serving/125g | 231.0 | 2.0 | 185 | 9.3 | 31.4 | 2.0 | 1.4 |
| Goats Cheese & Basil, Somerfield* | 1 Serving/250g | 650.0 | 17.0 | 260 | 11.1 | 38.7 | 6.8 | 1.8 |
| Goats Cheese & Red Pepper, Morrisons* | 1 Pack/150g | 450.0 | 17.0 | 300 | 11.5 | 38.4 | 11.1 | 3.8 |
| Italian Style Sausage & Red Wine, Morrisons* | ½ Pack/150g | 420.0 | 11.0 | 280 | 11.1 | 45.5 | 7.2 | 2.7 |
| Meat & Cheese, Fresh, Sainsbury's* | ½ Pack/125g | 304.0 | 10.0 | 243 | 13.5 | 28.3 | 8.4 | 2.6 |
| Mediterranean Vegetable, Perfectly Balanced, Waitrose* | ½ Pack/125g | 286.0 | 4.0 | 229 | 9.1 | 40.1 | 3.6 | 2.5 |
| Mozzarella, Tomato & Basil, Italian, Somerfield* | ½ Pack/125g | 314.0 | 5.0 | 251 | 10.5 | 43.1 | 4.1 | 1.9 |
| Mushroom, Basics, Sainsbury's* | ¼ Pack/125g | 196.0 | 6.0 | 157 | 6.1 | 21.8 | 5.0 | 3.0 |
| Mushroom, Perfectly Balanced, Waitrose* | ½ Pack/125g | 300.0 | 4.0 | 240 | 10.9 | 41.8 | 3.2 | 2.2 |
| Olive & Ricotta, Sainsbury's* | ½ Pack/175g | 403.0 | 18.0 | 230 | 8.8 | 25.1 | 10.5 | 2.3 |
| Parma Ham & Parmesan, Safeway* | 1 Serving/125g | 269.0 | 8.0 | 215 | 9.9 | 27.8 | 6.7 | 1.5 |
| Pasta, Fresh, Cream Cheese, Garlic & Herb, Morrisons* | 1 Serving/150g | 400.0 | 9.0 | 267 | 10.3 | 46.1 | 6.0 | 3.2 |
| Pesto, Italian, Tesco* | 1 Pack/300g | 885.0 | 34.0 | 295 | 10.7 | 36.7 | 11.3 | 3.0 |
| Pesto, Light Choices, Tesco* | ½ Pack/150g | 277.0 | 9.0 | 185 | 6.5 | 26.5 | 5.8 | 2.0 |
| Porcini & Pancetta, TTD, Sainsbury's* | 1 Serving/175g | 294.0 | 11.0 | 168 | 7.1 | 20.8 | 6.3 | 3.4 |
| Potato & Rosemary, Fresh, Sainsbury's* | ½ Pack/175g | 364.0 | 15.0 | 208 | 5.7 | 26.6 | 8.8 | 2.3 |
| Red Pepper & Mozzarella, Cooked, Somerfield* | ½ Pack/124g | 325.0 | 8.0 | 263 | 10.8 | 40.1 | 6.6 | 1.8 |
| Ricotta & Tender Spinach, Cooked, Giovanni Rana* | ½ Pack/190g | 376.0 | 12.0 | 198 | 7.8 | 27.0 | 6.5 | 3.1 |
| Roasted Vegetable, TTD, Sainsbury's* | ½ Pack/125g | 259.0 | 11.0 | 207 | 8.4 | 23.3 | 8.9 | 4.0 |
| Sausage & Ham, Italiano, Tesco* | 1 Serving/150g | 285.0 | 10.0 | 190 | 8.5 | 22.5 | 7.0 | 1.8 |
| Sicilian Style & Tuna, Morrisons* | ½ Pack/150g | 397.0 | 9.0 | 265 | 12.1 | 43.0 | 5.9 | 2.3 |
| Spicy Red Pepper & Tomato, Pasta Reale* | ½ Pack/125g | 310.0 | 5.0 | 248 | 10.0 | 42.0 | 4.4 | 3.3 |
| Spinach & Ricotta, Chilled, Italiano, Tesco* | ½ Pack/150g | 412.0 | 13.0 | 275 | 10.4 | 38.1 | 8.5 | 3.3 |
| Spinach & Ricotta, Fresh, Safeway* | ½ Pack/202g | 341.0 | 10.0 | 169 | 7.4 | 24.0 | 4.8 | 2.4 |
| Spinach & Ricotta, Italian, Somerfield* | 1 Serving/125g | 320.0 | 8.0 | 256 | 10.9 | 38.8 | 6.3 | 2.2 |
| Spinach & Ricotta, Sainsbury's* | ½ Pack/150g | 325.0 | 11.0 | 217 | 7.8 | 30.2 | 7.2 | 2.4 |
| Sun Ripened Tomato & Mozzarella, Giovanni Rana* | ½ Pack/125g | 215.0 | 7.0 | 172 | 6.9 | 23.0 | 5.8 | 3.9 |
| Taleggio & Leek, Fresh, Sainsbury's* | ½ Pack/175g | 450.0 | 12.0 | 257 | 9.7 | 38.8 | 7.1 | 2.6 |
| Tomato & Mozzarella, Sainsbury's* | 1 Serving/175g | 339.0 | 14.0 | 194 | 7.5 | 23.0 | 8.0 | 3.4 |
| Walnut & Gorgonzola, Fresh, Sainsbury's* | ½ Pack/210g | 414.0 | 12.0 | 197 | 8.4 | 27.8 | 5.8 | 2.4 |
| Wild Mushroom, Italian, Sainsbury's* | ½ Pack/150g | 309.0 | 12.0 | 206 | 7.7 | 25.4 | 8.2 | 2.3 |
| Wild Mushroom, Italiano, Tesco* | 1 Pack/300g | 645.0 | 24.0 | 215 | 6.5 | 28.5 | 8.0 | 2.5 |
| **TORTELLONO** | | | | | | | | |
| Cheese & Smoked Ham, Italiano, Tesco* | ½ Pack/150g | 315.0 | 11.0 | 210 | 8.9 | 26.5 | 7.1 | 1.7 |
| Sun Ripened Tomato & Mozarella, Giovanni Rana* | ½ Pack/125g | 215.0 | 7.0 | 172 | 6.9 | 23.0 | 5.8 | 3.9 |

| | Measure INFO/WEIGHT | per Measure KCAL | FAT | Nutrition Values per 100g / 100ml KCAL | PROT | CARB | FAT | FIBRE |
|---|---|---|---|---|---|---|---|---|
| **TORTIGLIONI** | | | | | | | | |
| *Dry, Average* | *1 Serving/75g* | *266.0* | *1.0* | *355* | *12.5* | *72.2* | *1.9* | *2.1* |
| **TORTILLA CHIPS** | | | | | | | | |
| Blazing BBQ, Sainsbury's* | 1 Serving/50g | 237.0 | 12.0 | 474 | 6.8 | 58.9 | 23.5 | 4.6 |
| Blue, Organic, Sainsbury's* | 1 Serving/50g | 252.0 | 12.0 | 504 | 7.7 | 65.8 | 23.4 | 5.6 |
| Chilli Flavour, Somerfield* | 1 Serving/50g | 242.0 | 12.0 | 484 | 6.8 | 60.1 | 24.1 | 5.3 |
| Classic Mexican, Phileas Fogg* | 1 Serving/35g | 162.0 | 7.0 | 464 | 5.9 | 67.2 | 19.1 | 3.8 |
| Cool, Salted, Sainsbury's* | 1 Serving/50g | 253.0 | 14.0 | 506 | 6.5 | 58.6 | 27.3 | 4.3 |
| Cool, Tesco* | 1 Serving/40g | 190.0 | 10.0 | 474 | 6.3 | 56.7 | 24.7 | 7.8 |
| Cool Flavour, Safeway* | 1 Serving/50g | 227.0 | 11.0 | 454 | 6.6 | 58.3 | 21.6 | 7.2 |
| Cool Flavour, Sainsbury's* | 1 Serving/50g | 231.0 | 9.0 | 463 | 5.7 | 68.1 | 18.7 | 3.7 |
| Easy Cheesy!, Sainsbury's* | 1 Serving/50g | 249.0 | 13.0 | 498 | 7.1 | 58.7 | 26.1 | 4.5 |
| Hot Chilli Flavour, Weight Watchers* | 1 Bag/18g | 77.0 | 3.0 | 430 | 5.7 | 66.7 | 15.6 | 5.3 |
| Lightly Salted, M & S* | 1 Serving/20g | 98.0 | 5.0 | 490 | 7.2 | 61.5 | 24.1 | 4.5 |
| Lightly Salted, Tesco* | 1 Serving/50g | 247.0 | 14.0 | 495 | 4.8 | 56.8 | 27.6 | 7.5 |
| Lighty Salted, Basics, Sainsbury's* | ½ Pack/50g | 241.0 | 12.0 | 483 | 6.5 | 60.7 | 23.8 | 5.3 |
| Mexicana Cheddar, Kettle Chips* | 1 Serving/50g | 249.0 | 13.0 | 498 | 7.9 | 56.7 | 26.6 | 5.1 |
| Nacho Cheese Flavour, M & S* | 1 Serving/30g | 144.0 | 7.0 | 480 | 7.5 | 62.0 | 22.4 | 4.2 |
| Nacho Cheese Flavour, Morrisons* | 1 Serving/25g | 126.0 | 7.0 | 504 | 7.2 | 59.4 | 26.4 | 3.6 |
| Nachos Kit, Asda* | 1 Serving/100g | 448.0 | 24.0 | 448 | 7.0 | 51.0 | 24.0 | 0.7 |
| Salsa, Asda* | 1 Serving/25g | 122.0 | 6.0 | 488 | 6.0 | 62.0 | 24.0 | 6.0 |
| Salsa, M & S* | ½ Bag/75g | 364.0 | 19.0 | 485 | 5.7 | 59.1 | 25.1 | 6.1 |
| Slightly Salted, Organic, Sainsbury's* | 1 Serving/50g | 226.0 | 7.0 | 453 | 10.0 | 73.3 | 13.3 | 13.3 |
| Taco, Tesco* | 1 Serving/50g | 247.0 | 13.0 | 495 | 7.4 | 59.3 | 25.4 | 4.4 |
| **TORTILLAS** | | | | | | | | |
| Corn, Gluten Free, Discovery* | 1 Tortilla/22g | 53.0 | 1.0 | 243 | 5.4 | 53.8 | 2.3 | 3.8 |
| Corn, Soft, Old El Paso* | 1 Tortilla/38g | 129.0 | 3.0 | 343 | 10.0 | 60.0 | 7.0 | 0.0 |
| Flour, 10 Pack, Asda* | 1 Tortilla/30g | 94.0 | 2.0 | 315 | 9.0 | 54.0 | 7.0 | 2.5 |
| Flour, American Style, Sainsbury's* | 1 Tortilla/35g | 108.0 | 2.0 | 313 | 8.6 | 53.9 | 7.0 | 2.5 |
| Flour, Bakery, Asda* | 1 Tortilla/43g | 129.0 | 3.0 | 303 | 9.1 | 50.9 | 7.1 | 2.6 |
| Flour, From Dinner Kit, Old El Paso* | 1 Tortilla/42g | 144.0 | 5.0 | 344 | 8.7 | 51.1 | 11.7 | 0.0 |
| Flour, Mexican Style, Morrisons* | 1 Tortilla/33g | 103.0 | 2.0 | 313 | 8.6 | 53.9 | 7.0 | 2.5 |
| Flour, Salsa, Old El Paso* | 1 Tortilla/41g | 132.0 | 4.0 | 323 | 9.0 | 52.0 | 9.0 | 0.0 |
| Flour, Soft, Chilli & Jalapeno, Discovery* | 1 Tortilla/40g | 131.0 | 5.0 | 328 | 7.8 | 44.8 | 13.1 | 2.2 |
| Flour, Soft, Discovery* | 1 Tortilla/40g | 119.0 | 3.0 | 298 | 8.0 | 49.6 | 7.1 | 2.4 |
| Flour, Soft, Garlic & Coriander, Discovery* | 1 Tortilla/40g | 116.0 | 2.0 | 289 | 8.1 | 50.6 | 6.0 | 1.7 |
| Flour, Tex "N" Mex 12, Sainsbury's* | 1 Tortilla/26g | 85.0 | 2.0 | 326 | 8.6 | 53.9 | 9.6 | 2.5 |
| Flour, Wheat, Waitrose* | 1 Tortilla/62g | 203.0 | 6.0 | 327 | 8.5 | 51.5 | 9.8 | 0.0 |
| Made with Wheat Flour | 1oz/28g | 73.0 | 0.0 | 262 | 7.2 | 59.7 | 1.0 | 2.4 |
| Mexican Cheese, Phileas Fogg* | 1 Pack/278g | 1404.0 | 72.0 | 505 | 6.5 | 61.4 | 26.0 | 3.0 |
| Plain, Morrisons* | 1 Serving/35g | 92.0 | 1.0 | 263 | 8.5 | 51.2 | 2.7 | 2.5 |
| Plain, Wheat, Waitrose* | 1 Tortilla/43g | 134.0 | 3.0 | 311 | 8.1 | 51.5 | 8.1 | 3.0 |
| Plain, Wraps, Tesco* | 1 Tortilla/64g | 192.0 | 4.0 | 300 | 8.4 | 52.2 | 5.9 | 2.7 |
| White, Wraps, M & S* | 1 Tortilla/64g | 170.0 | 2.0 | 265 | 7.9 | 49.0 | 3.8 | 1.6 |
| Wholewheat, Asda* | 1 Tortilla/35g | 88.0 | 3.0 | 252 | 9.8 | 35.7 | 7.8 | 7.1 |
| Wrap, 8 Pack, Asda* | 1 Tortilla/50g | 143.0 | 3.0 | 286 | 8.0 | 50.0 | 6.0 | 1.9 |
| Wrap, 8 Pack, Light Choices, Tesco* | 1 Tortilla/68g | 180.0 | 2.0 | 265 | 8.5 | 50.7 | 2.8 | 3.4 |
| Wrap, Flour, Soft, Old El Paso* | 1 Tortilla/41g | 141.0 | 5.0 | 344 | 8.7 | 51.1 | 11.7 | 0.0 |
| Wrap, Garlic & Parsley, Sainsbury's* | 1 Tortilla/60g | 166.0 | 4.0 | 277 | 7.2 | 48.0 | 6.2 | 1.8 |
| Wrap, Low Carb, Tesco* | 1 Tortilla/17g | 77.0 | 2.0 | 453 | 39.4 | 53.5 | 8.8 | 23.5 |
| Wrap, Morrisons* | 1 Serving/60g | 132.0 | 2.0 | 220 | 6.2 | 42.0 | 3.5 | 1.7 |
| Wrap, Organic, Sainsbury's* | 1 Tortilla/56g | 167.0 | 4.0 | 298 | 8.6 | 48.7 | 7.7 | 2.1 |
| Wrap, Organic, Tesco* | 1 Tortilla/57g | 173.0 | 4.0 | 306 | 8.1 | 51.0 | 7.7 | 2.0 |
| Wrap, Plain, Mini, Morrisons* | 1 Tortilla/34g | 91.0 | 1.0 | 267 | 8.1 | 48.9 | 4.0 | 2.8 |

| | Measure INFO/WEIGHT | per Measure | | Nutrition Values per 100g / 100ml | | | | |
|---|---|---|---|---|---|---|---|---|
| | | KCAL | FAT | KCAL | PROT | CARB | FAT | FIBRE |
| **TORTILLAS** | | | | | | | | |
| Wrap, Spicy Tomato, Morrisons* | 1 Tortilla/55g | 158.0 | 3.0 | 288 | 8.6 | 50.5 | 5.7 | 0.7 |
| Wrap, Spicy Tomato, Tesco* | 1 Tortilla/63g | 175.0 | 4.0 | 278 | 7.8 | 49.2 | 5.6 | 2.4 |
| Wrap, Tomato & Herb, Tesco* | 1 Serving/63g | 165.0 | 3.0 | 262 | 7.9 | 45.1 | 5.5 | 2.1 |
| Wrap, Tomato & Herbs, Sainsbury's* | 1 Tortilla/52g | 157.0 | 3.0 | 302 | 7.8 | 54.1 | 6.0 | 2.4 |
| Wrap, Weight Watchers* | 1 Tortilla/42g | 102.0 | 1.0 | 244 | 8.3 | 47.8 | 2.3 | 6.9 |
| Wrap, Whole And White, Mini, Kids, Sainsbury's* | 1 Tortilla/26g | 67.0 | 1.0 | 258 | 9.2 | 42.9 | 5.5 | 6.2 |
| Wraps, Deli, Multigrain, Mission* | 1 Tortilla/61g | 185.0 | 4.0 | 302 | 8.3 | 52.6 | 6.5 | 3.6 |
| Wraps, Healthy 'n' White, Wrap 'n' Roll, Discovery* | 1 Tortilla/56g | 156.0 | 3.0 | 279 | 9.1 | 49.6 | 4.9 | 3.0 |
| Wraps, Less Than 3% Fat, BGTY, Sainsbury's* | 1 Tortilla/51g | 127.0 | 1.0 | 250 | 7.8 | 50.1 | 2.2 | 2.9 |
| Wraps, Mexican, Asda* | 1 Tortilla/34g | 100.0 | 3.0 | 295 | 7.9 | 47.2 | 8.3 | 3.9 |
| Wraps, Multiseed, Discovery* | 1 Tortilla/57g | 160.0 | 3.0 | 280 | 8.7 | 50.1 | 5.0 | 3.6 |
| Wraps, Plain, Sainsbury's* | 1 Tortilla/56g | 167.0 | 4.0 | 299 | 8.1 | 49.2 | 7.8 | 3.6 |
| **TRAIL MIX** | | | | | | | | |
| Average | 1oz/28g | 121.0 | 8.0 | 432 | 9.1 | 37.2 | 28.5 | 4.3 |
| **TREACLE** | | | | | | | | |
| ***Black, Average*** | ***1 Tbsp/20g*** | ***51.0*** | ***0.0*** | ***257*** | ***1.2*** | ***67.2*** | ***0.0*** | ***0.0*** |
| **TRIFLE** | | | | | | | | |
| Average | 1oz/28g | 45.0 | 2.0 | 160 | 3.6 | 22.3 | 6.3 | 0.5 |
| Banana & Mandarin, Co-Op* | ¼ Trifle/125g | 237.0 | 14.0 | 190 | 2.0 | 21.0 | 11.0 | 0.1 |
| Blackforest, BGTY, Sainsbury's* | 1 Pot/125g | 171.0 | 6.0 | 137 | 2.1 | 21.9 | 4.5 | 1.6 |
| Caramel, Galaxy, Mars* | 1 Pot/100g | 255.0 | 13.0 | 255 | 4.5 | 30.0 | 13.0 | 1.0 |
| Cherry, Finest, Tesco* | ¼ Trifle/163g | 340.0 | 19.0 | 209 | 2.6 | 22.9 | 11.9 | 0.3 |
| Cherry & Almond, Somerfield* | 1 Trifle/125g | 230.0 | 11.0 | 184 | 2.0 | 23.0 | 9.0 | 0.0 |
| Chocolate, Asda* | 1 Serving/125g | 272.0 | 16.0 | 217 | 4.1 | 21.0 | 13.0 | 0.5 |
| Chocolate, BGTY, Sainsbury's* | 1 Pot/100g | 137.0 | 3.0 | 137 | 4.8 | 23.4 | 2.7 | 1.6 |
| Chocolate, Cadbury* | 1 Pot/100g | 282.0 | 18.0 | 282 | 5.2 | 24.3 | 18.5 | 0.0 |
| Chocolate, HL, Tesco* | 1 Serving/150g | 189.0 | 4.0 | 126 | 4.0 | 21.4 | 2.7 | 4.6 |
| Chocolate, Light, Cadbury* | 1 Pot/90g | 166.0 | 7.0 | 185 | 5.5 | 23.4 | 7.5 | 0.0 |
| Chocolate, Tesco* | 1 Serving/125g | 312.0 | 19.0 | 250 | 4.3 | 24.0 | 15.2 | 0.7 |
| Cream Mandarin, GFY, Asda* | 1 Serving/113g | 151.0 | 5.0 | 134 | 1.6 | 27.0 | 4.4 | 0.2 |
| Fruit, Sainsbury's* | 1 Serving/125g | 232.0 | 12.0 | 186 | 2.3 | 21.7 | 10.0 | 0.3 |
| Fruit Cocktail, COU, M & S* | 1 Trifle/140g | 175.0 | 3.0 | 125 | 2.8 | 23.1 | 2.3 | 0.5 |
| Fruit Cocktail, Individual, Shape, Danone* | 1 Trifle/115g | 136.0 | 3.0 | 118 | 3.2 | 19.6 | 2.7 | 1.6 |
| Fruit Cocktail, Individual, Tesco* | 1 Pot/113g | 175.0 | 9.0 | 155 | 1.7 | 19.6 | 7.8 | 0.6 |
| Fruit Cocktail, Low Fat, Danone* | 1 Pot/115g | 140.0 | 2.0 | 122 | 2.2 | 24.0 | 1.8 | 0.4 |
| Fruit Cocktail, Luxury Devonshire, St Ivel* | 1 Trifle/125g | 211.0 | 10.0 | 169 | 1.9 | 22.6 | 7.9 | 0.2 |
| Fruit Cocktail, M & S* | 1 Serving/165g | 272.0 | 14.0 | 165 | 2.4 | 19.6 | 8.3 | 0.9 |
| Fruit Cocktail, Sainsbury's* | 1 Trifle/150g | 241.0 | 9.0 | 161 | 1.8 | 24.8 | 6.0 | 0.4 |
| Peach & Zabaglione, COU, M & S* | 1 Glass/130g | 149.0 | 3.0 | 115 | 2.8 | 20.6 | 2.3 | 0.8 |
| Raspberry, Asda* | 1 Serving/100g | 175.0 | 8.0 | 175 | 1.8 | 24.0 | 8.0 | 0.1 |
| Raspberry, Individual, Safeway* | 1 Pot/125g | 259.0 | 13.0 | 207 | 2.7 | 26.2 | 10.2 | 0.0 |
| Raspberry, Sainsbury's* | 1 Pot/125g | 204.0 | 10.0 | 163 | 1.7 | 21.5 | 7.8 | 0.6 |
| Raspberry, Somerfield* | 1 Trifle/125g | 207.0 | 10.0 | 166 | 2.0 | 22.0 | 8.0 | 0.0 |
| Raspberry, Tesco* | 1 Pot/150g | 210.0 | 10.0 | 140 | 1.7 | 18.5 | 6.5 | 1.0 |
| Sherry, BGTY, Sainsbury's* | 1 Pot/135g | 146.0 | 2.0 | 108 | 3.0 | 20.2 | 1.7 | 0.5 |
| Sherry, TTD, Sainsbury's* | 1 Serving/125g | 219.0 | 11.0 | 175 | 1.7 | 21.5 | 9.1 | 0.5 |
| Strawberry, BGTY, Sainsbury's* | 1 Pot/125g | 135.0 | 3.0 | 108 | 2.4 | 19.9 | 2.1 | 0.5 |
| Strawberry, COU, M & S* | 1 Pot/140g | 154.0 | 3.0 | 110 | 2.8 | 20.6 | 2.0 | 1.2 |
| Strawberry, Individual, Safeway* | 1 Pot/125g | 215.0 | 10.0 | 172 | 2.3 | 22.0 | 8.0 | 0.5 |
| Strawberry, Individual, Shape, Danone* | 1 Pot/115g | 137.0 | 3.0 | 119 | 3.3 | 19.8 | 2.7 | 1.6 |
| Strawberry, Individual, Somerfield* | 1 Trifle/125g | 186.0 | 8.0 | 149 | 1.8 | 20.5 | 6.6 | 0.6 |
| Strawberry, Low Fat Goodies, Danone* | 1 Pot/115g | 148.0 | 2.0 | 129 | 2.2 | 26.0 | 1.8 | 0.3 |
| Strawberry, Luxury Devonshire, St Ivel* | 1 Trifle/125g | 207.0 | 10.0 | 166 | 2.0 | 21.7 | 7.9 | 0.2 |

T

| | Measure INFO/WEIGHT | per Measure KCAL | FAT | Nutrition Values per 100g / 100ml KCAL | PROT | CARB | FAT | FIBRE |
|---|---|---|---|---|---|---|---|---|
| **TRIFLE** | | | | | | | | |
| Strawberry, Sainsbury's* | ¼ Tub/150g | 261.0 | 15.0 | 174 | 2.2 | 18.1 | 10.3 | 1.0 |
| Strawberry, St Ivel* | 1 Trifle/113g | 194.0 | 10.0 | 172 | 2.4 | 21.0 | 8.7 | 0.2 |
| Strawberry, Tesco* | 1 Trifle/605g | 998.0 | 56.0 | 165 | 1.5 | 19.1 | 9.2 | 0.8 |
| Summerfruit, BGTY, Sainsbury's* | 1 Trifle/125g | 151.0 | 5.0 | 121 | 1.2 | 19.2 | 4.4 | 0.5 |
| **TRIFLE MIX** | | | | | | | | |
| Strawberry Flavour, Bird's* | 1oz/28g | 119.0 | 3.0 | 425 | 2.7 | 78.0 | 10.5 | 1.2 |
| **TRIFLE SPONGES** | | | | | | | | |
| Sainsbury's* | 1 Sponge/24g | 77.0 | 0.0 | 323 | 5.3 | 71.9 | 1.6 | 1.1 |
| Somerfield* | 1 Sponge/24g | 81.0 | 0.0 | 339 | 5.0 | 76.0 | 2.0 | 0.0 |
| Tesco* | 1 Sponge/24g | 75.0 | 1.0 | 311 | 5.3 | 66.6 | 2.6 | 1.1 |
| **TRIPE &** | | | | | | | | |
| Onions, Stewed | 1oz/28g | 26.0 | 1.0 | 93 | 8.3 | 9.5 | 2.7 | 0.7 |
| **TROMPRETTI** | | | | | | | | |
| Fresh, Waitrose* | 1 Serving/125g | 339.0 | 3.0 | 271 | 11.7 | 50.6 | 2.4 | 2.0 |
| Tricolour, Fresh, Tesco* | 1 Pack/250g | 675.0 | 8.0 | 270 | 11.2 | 48.6 | 3.4 | 4.0 |
| **TROTTOLE** | | | | | | | | |
| Dry, Sainsbury's* | 1 Serving/90g | 337.0 | 2.0 | 375 | 12.3 | 73.1 | 1.7 | 2.5 |
| Tricolore, Sainsbury's* | 1 Serving/90g | 321.0 | 2.0 | 357 | 12.3 | 73.1 | 1.7 | 2.5 |
| **TROUT** | | | | | | | | |
| *Brown, Steamed, Average* | *1 Serving/120g* | *162.0* | *5.0* | *135* | *23.5* | *0.0* | *4.5* | *0.0* |
| Rainbow, Fillets, with Thyme & Lemon Butter, Asda* | 1 Serving/147g | 210.0 | 10.0 | 143 | 20.0 | 0.9 | 7.0 | 0.5 |
| *Rainbow, Grilled, Average* | *1 Serving/120g* | *162.0* | *6.0* | *135* | *21.5* | *0.0* | *5.4* | *0.0* |
| Rainbow, Marinated with Lemon Dill & Pepper, Sainsbury's* | 1 Fish/115g | 202.0 | 13.0 | 176 | 17.8 | 0.0 | 11.4 | 0.5 |
| *Rainbow, Raw, Average* | *1oz/28g* | *36.0* | *1.0* | *127* | *20.5* | *0.0* | *5.1* | *0.0* |
| *Rainbow, Smoked, Average* | *1 Pack/135g* | *190.0* | *8.0* | *140* | *21.7* | *0.7* | *5.6* | *0.0* |
| *Raw, Average* | *1 Serving/120g* | *159.0* | *6.0* | *132* | *20.6* | *0.0* | *5.4* | *0.0* |
| Roasting, Lemon & Rosemary, TTD, Sainsbury's* | 1 Fish/270g | 475.0 | 29.0 | 176 | 20.2 | 0.0 | 10.6 | 0.5 |
| Rosemary Crusted, Finest, Tesco* | 1 Fillet/150g | 352.0 | 26.0 | 235 | 16.1 | 3.1 | 17.5 | 1.0 |
| *Smoked, Average* | *1oz/28g* | *39.0* | *1.0* | *138* | *22.7* | *0.3* | *5.2* | *0.1* |
| **TUACA*** | | | | | | | | |
| Alcoholic Beverage, Average, Tuaca* | 1 Serving/25ml | 67.0 | 0.0 | 267 | 0.0 | 0.0 | 0.0 | 0.0 |
| **TUNA** | | | | | | | | |
| *Bluefin, Cooked, Dry Heat, Average* | *1 Serving/100g* | *184.0* | *6.0* | *184* | *29.9* | *0.0* | *6.3* | *0.0* |
| *Chunks, in Brine, Average, Drained* | *1 Can /130g* | *141.0* | *1.0* | *108* | *25.9* | *0.0* | *0.5* | *0.0* |
| *Chunks, in Spring Water, Average, Drained* | *1 Can /130g* | *140.0* | *1.0* | *108* | *25.4* | *0.0* | *0.6* | *0.1* |
| *Chunks, in Sunflower Oil, Average, Drained* | *1 Can/138g* | *260.0* | *13.0* | *188* | *26.5* | *0.0* | *9.1* | *0.0* |
| *Chunks, Skipjack, in Brine, Average* | *1 Can/138g* | *141.0* | *1.0* | *102* | *24.3* | *0.0* | *0.6* | *0.0* |
| Coronation, BGTY, Sainsbury's* | 1 Can/80g | 90.0 | 2.0 | 112 | 16.5 | 5.7 | 2.6 | 1.0 |
| Coronation Style, By John West, Weight Watchers* | 1 Can/80g | 75.0 | 2.0 | 94 | 9.3 | 8.7 | 2.5 | 0.4 |
| Coronation Style, Canned, Average | 1 Can/80g | 122.0 | 8.0 | 152 | 10.2 | 6.5 | 9.5 | 0.6 |
| Fillets, in Tomato Sauce, Princes* | 1 Can/120g | 131.0 | 3.0 | 109 | 19.0 | 2.5 | 2.5 | 0.0 |
| *Flakes, in Brine, Average* | *1oz/28g* | *29.0* | *0.0* | *104* | *24.7* | *0.0* | *0.5* | *0.0* |
| French Style, Light Lunch, John West* | 1 Pack/240g | 221.0 | 6.0 | 92 | 7.9 | 9.4 | 2.6 | 0.9 |
| in a Light Lemon Mayonnise, Slimming World, Princes* | 1 Can/80g | 99.0 | 4.0 | 124 | 16.8 | 3.5 | 4.8 | 0.0 |
| in a Light Mayonnaise. Slimming World, Princes* | 1 Can/80g | 96.0 | 3.0 | 120 | 17.3 | 3.6 | 4.1 | 0.0 |
| in a Red Chilli & Lime Dressing, Princes* | 1 Sachet/85g | 102.0 | 3.0 | 120 | 21.5 | 1.0 | 3.3 | 0.0 |
| in a Tikka Dressing, Slimming World, Princes* | 1 Can/80g | 108.0 | 5.0 | 135 | 16.8 | 4.0 | 5.7 | 0.0 |
| in Chilli Sauce, Safeway* | 1 Serving/100g | 158.0 | 8.0 | 158 | 16.8 | 4.8 | 7.9 | 0.5 |
| in Sweet & Sour Sauce, Safeway* | 1 Can/185g | 148.0 | 3.0 | 80 | 10.9 | 5.6 | 1.6 | 1.0 |
| in Thousand Island Dressing, John West* | 1 Can/185g | 287.0 | 13.0 | 155 | 18.0 | 5.1 | 7.0 | 0.2 |
| In Thousand Island Dressing, Weight Watchers* | 1 Can/79g | 67.0 | 2.0 | 85 | 8.3 | 7.8 | 2.2 | 0.4 |
| *in Water, Average* | *1 Serving/120g* | *126.0* | *1.0* | *105* | *24.0* | *0.1* | *0.8* | *0.0* |
| Light Lunch, Indian Style, John West* | 1 Pack/240g | 401.0 | 23.0 | 167 | 7.7 | 12.3 | 9.6 | 0.6 |

| | INFO/WEIGHT | KCAL | FAT | KCAL | PROT | CARB | FAT | FIBRE |
|---|---|---|---|---|---|---|---|---|
| **TUNA** | | | | | | | | |
| Light Lunch, Mediterranean Style, John West* | 1 Pack/240g | 218.0 | 6.0 | 91 | 7.9 | 9.3 | 2.5 | 1.7 |
| Light Lunch, Nicoise Style, John West* | 1 Pack/250g | 245.0 | 6.0 | 98 | 10.3 | 9.0 | 2.3 | 2.7 |
| Light Lunch, Tomato Salsa Style, John West* | 1 Pack/250g | 180.0 | 3.0 | 72 | 8.0 | 7.5 | 1.1 | 1.1 |
| Lime & Black Pepper, John West* | 1 Serving/85g | 133.0 | 8.0 | 156 | 15.6 | 2.8 | 9.2 | 0.0 |
| *Steaks, in Brine, Average* | *1 Sm Can/99g* | *106.0* | *1.0* | *107* | *25.6* | *0.0* | *0.5* | *0.0* |
| Steaks, in Cajun Marinade, Sainsbury's* | 1 Steak/100g | 141.0 | 2.0 | 141 | 29.8 | 0.0 | 2.4 | 0.0 |
| *Steaks, in Olive Oil, Average* | *1 Serving/111g* | *211.0* | *11.0* | *190* | *25.8* | *0.0* | *9.6* | *0.0* |
| *Steaks, in Sunflower Oil, Average* | *1 Can/150g* | *276.0* | *13.0* | *184* | *26.7* | *0.0* | *8.6* | *0.0* |
| *Steaks, in Water, Average* | *1 Serving/200g* | *215.0* | *1.0* | *107* | *25.6* | *0.0* | *0.4* | *0.0* |
| Steaks, Lemon & Herb Marinade, Seared, Sainsbury's* | ½ Pack/119g | 191.0 | 9.0 | 161 | 23.4 | 0.1 | 7.4 | 0.0 |
| Steaks, Marinated, Sainsbury's* | 1 Serving/100g | 153.0 | 5.0 | 153 | 25.1 | 1.3 | 5.3 | 0.5 |
| *Steaks, Raw, Average* | *1 Serving/140g* | *185.0* | *3.0* | *132* | *28.5* | *0.1* | *2.0* | *0.2* |
| *Steaks, Skipjack, in Brine, Average* | *½ Can/75g* | *73.0* | *0.0* | *97* | *23.2* | *0.0* | *0.5* | *0.0* |
| Steaks, Thai Style Butter, Tesco* | 1 Serving/110g | 191.0 | 9.0 | 174 | 24.7 | 0.0 | 8.3 | 0.0 |
| Steaks, with Lime & Coriander Dressing, Tesco* | 1 Serving/150g | 156.0 | 1.0 | 104 | 21.6 | 3.6 | 0.4 | 0.6 |
| Steaks, with Sweet Red Pepper Glaze, Sainsbury's* | 1 Steak/100g | 135.0 | 0.0 | 135 | 28.5 | 5.0 | 0.1 | 0.1 |
| with a Twist, French Dressing, John West* | 1 Pack/85g | 135.0 | 8.0 | 159 | 15.2 | 2.8 | 9.7 | 0.1 |
| with a Twist, Oven Dried Tomato & Herb, John West* | 1 Pack/85g | 129.0 | 7.0 | 152 | 16.1 | 3.9 | 8.0 | 0.1 |
| with Basil Butter, Microwave Easy Steam, Sainsbury's* | 1 Pack/170g | 292.0 | 14.0 | 172 | 23.3 | 0.5 | 8.5 | 0.1 |
| with Ginger & Soy, Heinz* | 1 Can/171g | 264.0 | 12.0 | 154 | 22.3 | 0.9 | 7.0 | 0.0 |
| with Salsa Verde, Sainsbury's* | 1 Serving/125g | 310.0 | 20.0 | 248 | 25.5 | 0.6 | 16.0 | 0.0 |
| *Yellowfin, Cooked, Dry Heat, Average* | *1 Serving/100g* | *139.0* | *1.0* | *139* | *30.0* | *0.0* | *1.2* | *0.0* |
| **TUNA MAYONNAISE** | | | | | | | | |
| & Sweetcorn, Canned, BGTY, Sainsbury's* | 1 Can/80g | 78.0 | 2.0 | 97 | 15.2 | 4.0 | 2.3 | 0.7 |
| Garlic & Herb, John West* | ½ Can/92g | 243.0 | 20.0 | 264 | 12.0 | 4.0 | 22.2 | 0.2 |
| Light, Slimming World* | 1 Serving/80g | 96.0 | 3.0 | 120 | 17.3 | 3.6 | 4.1 | 0.0 |
| with Sweetcorn, From Heinz, Weight Watchers* | 1 Can/80g | 114.0 | 6.0 | 142 | 11.5 | 6.2 | 7.9 | 0.1 |
| with Sweetcorn, John West* | ½ Can/92g | 231.0 | 19.0 | 251 | 12.0 | 4.5 | 20.6 | 0.2 |
| with Sweetcorn & Green Peppers, GFY, Asda* | 1 Pack/100g | 103.0 | 3.0 | 103 | 14.0 | 5.0 | 3.0 | 0.8 |
| **TUNA SNACK POT** | | | | | | | | |
| Italian, Weight Watchers* | 1 Pot/240g | 245.0 | 9.0 | 102 | 9.1 | 8.5 | 3.6 | 0.5 |
| Oriental, Weight Watchers* | 1 Pot/240g | 269.0 | 7.0 | 112 | 9.0 | 12.6 | 2.9 | 0.3 |
| Provencale, Weight Watchers* | 1 Pot/240g | 266.0 | 8.0 | 111 | 9.8 | 10.2 | 3.4 | 0.5 |
| **TUNA WITH** | | | | | | | | |
| 3 Bean Salad, Potatoes & Red Peppers, M & S* | 1 Pack/360g | 360.0 | 9.0 | 100 | 8.7 | 10.9 | 2.6 | 5.1 |
| **TURBOT** | | | | | | | | |
| *Grilled* | *1oz/28g* | *34.0* | *1.0* | *122* | *22.7* | *0.0* | *3.5* | *0.0* |
| *Raw* | *1oz/28g* | *27.0* | *1.0* | *95* | *17.7* | *0.0* | *2.7* | *0.0* |
| **TURKEY** | | | | | | | | |
| *Breast, Butter Basted, Average* | *1 Serving/75g* | *110.0* | *4.0* | *146* | *23.7* | *1.9* | *4.9* | *0.4* |
| *Breast, Canned, Average* | *1 Can/200g* | *194.0* | *5.0* | *97* | *18.3* | *0.7* | *2.3* | *0.0* |
| *Breast, Diced, Healthy Range, Average* | *1oz/28g* | *30.0* | *0.0* | *107* | *23.8* | *0.0* | *1.3* | *0.0* |
| *Breast, Honey Roast, Sliced, Average* | *1 Serving/50g* | *57.0* | *1.0* | *114* | *24.0* | *1.6* | *1.3* | *0.2* |
| Breast, Joint, Lemon & Pepper Basted, Tesco* | ¼ Pack/132g | 238.0 | 15.0 | 180 | 19.7 | 0.0 | 11.2 | 0.0 |
| *Breast, Joint, Raw, Average* | *1 Serving/125g* | *134.0* | *3.0* | *107* | *21.3* | *0.7* | *2.1* | *0.6* |
| Breast, Joint, with Sage & Onion Stuffing, Waitrose* | 1 Serving/325g | 377.0 | 13.0 | 116 | 19.2 | 1.4 | 4.1 | 0.1 |
| *Breast, Raw, Average* | *1oz/28g* | *33.0* | *1.0* | *117* | *24.1* | *0.5* | *2.0* | *0.1* |
| *Breast, Roasted, Average* | *1oz/28g* | *37.0* | *1.0* | *131* | *24.6* | *0.7* | *3.3* | *0.1* |
| *Breast, Roll, Cooked, Average* | *1 Slice/10g* | *9.0* | *0.0* | *92* | *17.6* | *3.5* | *0.8* | *0.0* |
| *Breast, Slices, Cooked, Average* | *1 Slice/20g* | *23.0* | *0.0* | *114* | *24.0* | *1.2* | *1.4* | *0.3* |
| *Breast, Smoked, Sliced, Average* | *1 Slice/20g* | *23.0* | *0.0* | *113* | *23.4* | *0.7* | *1.9* | *0.0* |
| Breast, Steaks, in Crumbs, Average | 1 Steak/76g | 217.0 | 14.0 | 286 | 13.7 | 16.4 | 18.5 | 0.2 |
| *Breast, Steaks, Raw, Average* | *1oz/28g* | *30.0* | *0.0* | *107* | *24.3* | *0.0* | *1.1* | *0.0* |

**T**

# TURKEY

| | Measure INFO/WEIGHT | per Measure KCAL | per Measure FAT | Nutrition Values per 100g / 100ml KCAL | PROT | CARB | FAT | FIBRE |
|---|---|---|---|---|---|---|---|---|
| Breast, Steaks, Thai, Bernard Matthews* | 1 Serving/175g | 280.0 | 5.0 | 160 | 29.4 | 4.6 | 2.7 | 0.0 |
| Breast, Strips, Chinese Style, Sainsbury's* | ¼ Pack/163g | 318.0 | 7.0 | 196 | 26.4 | 12.5 | 4.5 | 0.5 |
| *Breast, Strips, for Stir Fry, Average* | *1 Serving/175g* | *205.0* | *3.0* | *117* | *25.6* | *0.1* | *1.6* | *0.0* |
| Breast, Stuffed, Just Roast, Sainsbury's* | 1 Serving/100g | 155.0 | 7.0 | 155 | 21.1 | 2.9 | 6.6 | 0.6 |
| Breast, Wafer Thin, Chinese Style, Bernard Matthews* | 1 Pack/100g | 110.0 | 1.0 | 110 | 18.0 | 6.1 | 1.5 | 0.0 |
| *Dark Meat, Raw, Average* | *1oz/28g* | *29.0* | *1.0* | *104* | *20.4* | *0.0* | *2.5* | *0.0* |
| *Dark Meat, Roasted, Average* | *1oz/28g* | *50.0* | *2.0* | *177* | *29.4* | *0.0* | *6.6* | *0.0* |
| Drummers, Golden, Bernard Matthews* | 1 Drummer/57g | 147.0 | 10.0 | 258 | 13.1 | 11.0 | 18.0 | 1.1 |
| Drummers, Golden, Grilled, Bernard Matthews* | 1 Drummer/50g | 147.0 | 11.0 | 294 | 15.6 | 10.0 | 21.2 | 1.0 |
| Drumsticks, Tesco* | 1 Serving/200g | 272.0 | 13.0 | 136 | 19.9 | 0.0 | 6.3 | 0.0 |
| *Escalope, Average* | *1 Escalope/138g* | *341.0* | *19.0* | *247* | *13.5* | *16.7* | *14.0* | *0.6* |
| Escalope, Creamy Pepper Topped, Tesco* | 1 Escalope/165g | 337.0 | 18.0 | 204 | 11.5 | 15.3 | 10.7 | 1.7 |
| Escalope, Lemon & Pepper, Average | 1 Escalope/143g | 371.0 | 23.0 | 259 | 12.6 | 16.7 | 15.8 | 0.4 |
| Escalope, Spicy Mango, Bernard Matthews* | 1 Escalope/136g | 354.0 | 17.0 | 260 | 11.6 | 24.6 | 12.8 | 0.0 |
| Escalope, Tomato & Herb, Bernard Matthews* | 1 Escalope/143g | 336.0 | 19.0 | 236 | 10.5 | 18.0 | 13.5 | 0.0 |
| Fillets, Chinese Marinated, Bernard Matthews* | 1 Pack/200g | 304.0 | 7.0 | 152 | 23.4 | 7.2 | 3.3 | 0.0 |
| Fillets, Tikka Marinated, 93% Fat Free, Bernard Matthews* | 1 Pack/200g | 310.0 | 10.0 | 155 | 21.8 | 5.2 | 5.2 | 1.5 |
| Goujons, Cooked, Bernard Matthews* | 4 Goujons/128g | 355.0 | 23.0 | 277 | 11.8 | 16.6 | 18.2 | 1.1 |
| Leg, Roast, Uncooked, Bernard Matthews* | 1 Serving/283g | 317.0 | 15.0 | 112 | 15.4 | 0.5 | 5.4 | 0.0 |
| *Light Meat, Raw, Average* | *1oz/28g* | *29.0* | *0.0* | *105* | *24.4* | *0.0* | *0.8* | *0.0* |
| *Light Meat, Roasted* | *1 Cup/140g* | *220.0* | *5.0* | *157* | *29.9* | *0.0* | *3.2* | *0.0* |
| Medallions, Tomato Salsa, Morrisons* | ½ Pack/125g | 184.0 | 3.0 | 147 | 30.4 | 0.8 | 2.5 | 0.9 |
| *Mince, Average* | *1oz/28g* | *45.0* | *2.0* | *161* | *23.9* | *0.0* | *7.2* | *0.0* |
| *Mince, Lean, Healthy Range, Average* | *1oz/28g* | *33.0* | *1.0* | *118* | *20.3* | *0.0* | *4.1* | *0.0* |
| *Rashers, Average* | *1 Rasher/26g* | *26.0* | *0.0* | *101* | *19.1* | *2.3* | *1.6* | *0.0* |
| *Rashers, Smoked, Average* | *1 Serving/75g* | *76.0* | *1.0* | *101* | *19.8* | *1.5* | *1.8* | *0.0* |
| Ready to Roast, with Stuffing & Bacon, M & S* | 1/3 Pack/169g | 245.0 | 10.0 | 145 | 20.2 | 2.1 | 6.2 | 1.1 |
| *Roast, Meat & Skin, Average* | *1oz/28g* | *48.0* | *2.0* | *171* | *28.0* | *0.0* | *6.5* | *0.0* |
| *Roast, Meat Only, Average* | *1 Serving/100g* | *157.0* | *3.0* | *157* | *29.9* | *0.0* | *3.2* | *0.0* |
| Roast, Sugar Marinade, Slices, M & S* | ½ Pack/120g | 156.0 | 2.0 | 130 | 29.0 | 0.2 | 1.6 | 0.5 |
| Roll, Dinosaur, Cooked, Bernard Matthews* | 1 Slice/10g | 17.0 | 1.0 | 170 | 13.6 | 6.0 | 10.2 | 1.1 |
| Steaks, Breaded, Bernard Matthews* | 1 Steak/110g | 319.0 | 20.0 | 290 | 11.0 | 20.5 | 18.2 | 1.5 |
| Sticks, Honey Roast, Mini, Tesco* | 1 Serving/90g | 101.0 | 2.0 | 112 | 20.0 | 3.6 | 1.9 | 0.0 |
| Strips, Stir-Fried, Average | 1oz/28g | 46.0 | 1.0 | 164 | 31.0 | 0.0 | 4.5 | 0.0 |
| *Thigh, Diced, Average* | *1oz/28g* | *33.0* | *1.0* | *117* | *19.6* | *0.0* | *4.3* | *0.0* |
| Wafer Thin, Cooked, Average | 1 Slice/10g | 12.0 | 0.0 | 122 | 19.0 | 3.2 | 3.7 | 0.0 |
| Wafer Thin, Honey Roast, Average | 1 Slice/10g | 11.0 | 0.0 | 109 | 19.2 | 4.2 | 1.7 | 0.2 |
| Wafer Thin, Smoked, Average | 1 Slice/10g | 12.0 | 0.0 | 119 | 18.1 | 3.6 | 3.7 | 0.0 |
| *Whole, Raw, Average* | *½ Joint/254g* | *389.0* | *17.0* | *153* | *22.5* | *0.8* | *6.6* | *0.0* |

# TURKEY DINNER

| | | | | | | | | |
|---|---|---|---|---|---|---|---|---|
| Roast, Asda* | 1 Pack/400g | 344.0 | 6.0 | 86 | 7.0 | 11.0 | 1.6 | 2.0 |
| Roast, Iceland* | 1 Meal/400g | 374.0 | 7.0 | 93 | 8.4 | 10.9 | 1.8 | 1.3 |
| Roast, Meal for One, M & S* | 1 Pack/370g | 462.0 | 16.0 | 125 | 9.1 | 12.4 | 4.4 | 2.7 |
| Roast, Sainsbury's* | 1 Pack/450g | 354.0 | 9.0 | 79 | 6.8 | 8.4 | 2.0 | 1.9 |

# TURKEY HAM

| | | | | | | | | |
|---|---|---|---|---|---|---|---|---|
| *Average* | *1 Serving/75g* | *81.0* | *3.0* | *108* | *15.6* | *2.8* | *3.9* | *0.0* |

# TURKEY IN

| | | | | | | | | |
|---|---|---|---|---|---|---|---|---|
| BBQ Marinade, Steaks, Asda* | 1 Serving/225g | 355.0 | 5.0 | 158 | 30.0 | 4.4 | 2.3 | 0.9 |
| Pepper Sauce, Escalope, Bernard Matthews* | 1 Escalope/143g | 350.0 | 21.0 | 245 | 9.4 | 18.2 | 15.0 | 1.5 |

# TURKEY WITH

| | | | | | | | | |
|---|---|---|---|---|---|---|---|---|
| Cranberry & Orange Glaze, Breast Joint, Sainsbury's* | 1 Serving/180g | 281.0 | 5.0 | 156 | 29.6 | 3.0 | 2.9 | 1.0 |

# TURKEY WITH

| | | | | | | | | |
|---|---|---|---|---|---|---|---|---|
| Nacho Cheese Dip, Sticks, Tesco* | 1 Serving/35g | 161.0 | 17.0 | 459 | 5.5 | 1.5 | 47.9 | 0.0 |

| | Measure INFO/WEIGHT | KCAL | FAT | KCAL | PROT | CARB | FAT | FIBRE |
|---|---|---|---|---|---|---|---|---|
| **TURKEY WITH** | | | | | | | | |
| Sage & Onion, Breast Joint, Glazed, GFY, Asda* | 1 Serving/100g | 101.0 | 2.0 | 101 | 19.0 | 2.5 | 1.7 | 1.0 |
| Sausagemeat, Sage & Onion Stuffing, Breast, Tesco* | 1 Serving/300g | 417.0 | 19.0 | 139 | 17.9 | 2.8 | 6.2 | 0.8 |
| Stuffing, Breast, Cooked, Somerfield* | 1oz/28g | 29.0 | 1.0 | 104 | 17.0 | 6.0 | 2.0 | 0.0 |
| **TURKISH DELIGHT** | | | | | | | | |
| Assorted Flavours, Julian Graves* | 1 Square/30g | 110.0 | 0.0 | 366 | 0.5 | 91.1 | 0.1 | 0.0 |
| Dark Chocolate Covered, Thorntons* | 1 Chocolate/10g | 39.0 | 1.0 | 390 | 2.7 | 69.0 | 11.0 | 2.0 |
| Fry's* | 1 Bar/51g | 186.0 | 4.0 | 365 | 2.0 | 73.3 | 7.2 | 0.0 |
| Milk Chocolate, M & S* | 1 Pack/55g | 220.0 | 5.0 | 400 | 1.6 | 79.0 | 8.5 | 0.0 |
| **TURMERIC** | | | | | | | | |
| *Powder* | *1 Tsp/3g* | *11.0* | *0.0* | *354* | *7.8* | *58.2* | *9.9* | *0.0* |
| **TURNIP** | | | | | | | | |
| *Boiled, Average* | *1oz/28g* | *3.0* | *0.0* | *12* | *0.6* | *2.0* | *0.2* | *1.9* |
| *Raw, Unprepared, Average* | *1oz/28g* | *6.0* | *0.0* | *23* | *0.9* | *4.7* | *0.3* | *2.4* |
| **TURNOVER** | | | | | | | | |
| Apple, Bramley, Tesco* | 1 Turnover/88g | 304.0 | 23.0 | 346 | 2.7 | 25.4 | 25.9 | 0.9 |
| Apple, Dairy Cream, Safeway* | 1 Turnover/92g | 349.0 | 24.0 | 380 | 3.8 | 32.9 | 25.9 | 0.9 |
| Apple, Dutch, Sainsbury's* | 1 Serving/33g | 130.0 | 6.0 | 393 | 3.6 | 56.9 | 16.8 | 1.4 |
| Apple, Fresh Cream, Sainsbury's* | 1 Turnover/84g | 292.0 | 21.0 | 347 | 4.1 | 26.9 | 24.8 | 2.5 |
| Apple, Tesco* | 1 Turnover/88g | 294.0 | 20.0 | 334 | 3.2 | 29.8 | 22.4 | 0.9 |
| Mincemeat, Fresh Cream, Tesco* | 1 Turnover/83g | 334.0 | 22.0 | 405 | 3.1 | 37.5 | 26.9 | 1.1 |
| Raspberry, Fresh Cream, Asda* | 1 Turnover/100g | 411.0 | 23.0 | 411 | 6.0 | 45.0 | 23.0 | 2.1 |
| Raspberry, Tesco* | 1 Turnover/84g | 290.0 | 20.0 | 345 | 4.0 | 27.2 | 24.1 | 2.1 |
| **TWIGLETS** | | | | | | | | |
| Curry, Jacob's* | 1 Bag/30g | 134.0 | 6.0 | 448 | 8.0 | 55.7 | 21.5 | 6.0 |
| Original, Jacob's* | 1 Bag/30g | 117.0 | 3.0 | 390 | 12.0 | 61.3 | 10.8 | 11.8 |
| Tangy, Jacob's* | 1 Bag/30g | 136.0 | 7.0 | 454 | 8.1 | 55.9 | 22.0 | 5.4 |
| **TWIRL** | | | | | | | | |
| Cadbury* | 1 Finger/22g | 115.0 | 7.0 | 525 | 8.1 | 55.9 | 30.1 | 0.0 |
| **TWIRLS** | | | | | | | | |
| Prawn Cocktail, Bobby's* | 1 Pack/26g | 116.0 | 5.0 | 445 | 3.4 | 65.9 | 18.6 | 0.0 |
| Salt & Vinegar, Co-Op* | 1 Bag/40g | 170.0 | 8.0 | 425 | 5.0 | 57.5 | 20.0 | 5.0 |
| Salt & Vinegar, Sainsbury's* | ½ Bag/40g | 167.0 | 6.0 | 418 | 3.0 | 70.1 | 14.0 | 3.0 |
| Salt & Vinegar, Tesco* | 1 Bag/80g | 349.0 | 14.0 | 436 | 3.9 | 65.8 | 17.5 | 2.4 |
| **TWISTS** | | | | | | | | |
| Apple, Sainsbury's* | 1 Serving/10g | 37.0 | 0.0 | 375 | 1.7 | 82.7 | 3.0 | 0.1 |
| Black Olive & Basil, Finest, Tesco* | ¼ Pack/31g | 151.0 | 8.0 | 483 | 11.3 | 53.1 | 25.1 | 3.9 |
| Strawberry, Sainsbury's* | 1 Serving/10g | 37.0 | 0.0 | 375 | 1.7 | 82.7 | 3.0 | 0.1 |
| Tomato & Herb, Shapers, Boots* | 1 Pack/20g | 94.0 | 4.0 | 468 | 3.7 | 66.0 | 21.0 | 3.9 |
| **TWIX** | | | | | | | | |
| Fun Size, Mars* | 1 Bar/21g | 103.0 | 5.0 | 492 | 4.7 | 65.5 | 23.7 | 1.5 |
| Standard, Mars* | 1 Pack/58g | 284.0 | 14.0 | 490 | 4.7 | 65.5 | 23.7 | 1.5 |
| Top, Mars* | 1 Bar/28g | 143.0 | 8.0 | 511 | 5.2 | 60.2 | 27.7 | 0.0 |
| Twixels, Mars* | 1 Finger/6g | 31.0 | 2.0 | 513 | 5.0 | 64.0 | 26.1 | 0.0 |
| Xtra, Mars* | 1 Pack/85g | 416.0 | 20.0 | 490 | 4.7 | 65.5 | 23.7 | 1.5 |
| **TZATZIKI** | | | | | | | | |
| Asda* | 1 Serving/50g | 54.0 | 4.0 | 108 | 3.8 | 4.6 | 8.5 | 1.2 |
| Average | 1oz/28g | 18.0 | 1.0 | 66 | 3.7 | 2.0 | 4.9 | 0.2 |
| Fresh, Sainsbury's* | 1oz/28g | 35.0 | 3.0 | 126 | 4.0 | 3.7 | 10.6 | 0.3 |
| Greek, Authentic, Total, Fage* | 1 Serving/50g | 49.0 | 3.0 | 99 | 4.9 | 4.1 | 7.0 | 1.0 |
| Morrisons* | ½ Pot/85g | 82.0 | 5.0 | 97 | 3.6 | 6.4 | 6.3 | 0.5 |
| Tesco* | ¼ Pack/50g | 72.0 | 6.0 | 145 | 4.0 | 5.1 | 12.0 | 0.2 |
| Waitrose* | 1 Serving/50g | 54.0 | 3.0 | 108 | 6.7 | 8.4 | 5.3 | 0.8 |

**T**

| | Measure INFO/WEIGHT | per Measure KCAL | FAT | Nutrition Values per 100g / 100ml KCAL | PROT | CARB | FAT | FIBRE |
|---|---|---|---|---|---|---|---|---|
| **VANILLA** | | | | | | | | |
| *Bean, Average* | *1oz/28g* | *81.0* | *0.0* | *288* | *0.0* | *13.0* | *0.0* | *0.0* |
| Flavouring, Supercook* | 1 Tsp/4g | 2.0 | 0.0 | 50 | 6.2 | 0.0 | 0.0 | 0.0 |
| Madagascan, Extra Special, Asda* | 1 Pot/150g | 232.0 | 11.0 | 155 | 3.5 | 19.0 | 7.2 | 0.0 |
| **VANILLA EXTRACT** | | | | | | | | |
| *Average* | *1 Tbsp/13g* | *37.0* | *0.0* | *288* | *0.1* | *12.6* | *0.1* | *0.0* |
| Pure, Nielsen Massey Vanillas* | 1 Tsp/5ml | 8.0 | 0.0 | 160 | 0.1 | 39.5 | 0.2 | 0.1 |
| **VEAL** | | | | | | | | |
| Escalope, Fried, Average | 1oz/28g | 55.0 | 2.0 | 196 | 33.7 | 0.0 | 6.8 | 0.0 |
| *Mince, Raw, Average* | *1oz/28g* | *40.0* | *2.0* | *144* | *20.3* | *0.0* | *7.0* | *0.0* |
| *Shoulder, Lean & Fat, Roasted, Average* | *1oz/28g* | *52.0* | *2.0* | *183* | *25.5* | *0.0* | *8.2* | *0.0* |
| *Shoulder, Lean Only, Roasted, Average* | *1oz/28g* | *46.0* | *2.0* | *164* | *26.1* | *0.0* | *5.8* | *0.0* |
| *Sirloin, Lean & Fat, Roasted, Average* | *1oz/28g* | *57.0* | *3.0* | *202* | *25.1* | *0.0* | *10.4* | *0.0* |
| *Sirloin, Lean Only, Roasted, Average* | *1oz/28g* | *48.0* | *2.0* | *168* | *26.3* | *0.0* | *6.2* | *0.0* |
| **VEGEMITE** | | | | | | | | |
| Australian, Kraft* | 1 Tsp/5g | 9.0 | 0.0 | 173 | 23.5 | 19.7 | 0.0 | 0.0 |
| **VEGETABLE ARRABIATA** | | | | | | | | |
| Roast, HE, Tesco* | 1 Pack/450g | 436.0 | 5.0 | 97 | 3.3 | 18.4 | 1.1 | 1.1 |
| **VEGETABLE CHIPS** | | | | | | | | |
| Beetroot, Carrot & Parsnips, Hand Fried, Tyrells* | ½ Pack/25g | 103.0 | 7.0 | 413 | 3.9 | 36.0 | 28.1 | 11.5 |
| Cassava, Average | 1oz/28g | 99.0 | 0.0 | 353 | 1.8 | 91.4 | 0.4 | 4.0 |
| Mixed Root, Tyrells* | 1oz/28g | 133.0 | 8.0 | 476 | 5.7 | 35.4 | 29.8 | 12.8 |
| Parsnip, Golden, Kettle Chips* | ½ Pack/50g | 257.0 | 19.0 | 515 | 4.6 | 39.5 | 37.6 | 8.4 |
| Sweet Potato, Kettle Chips* | ½ Pack/50g | 241.0 | 16.0 | 483 | 2.4 | 44.4 | 32.8 | 9.3 |
| **VEGETABLE ESCALOPE** | | | | | | | | |
| Italian Style, Dalepak* | 1 Escalope/163g | 355.0 | 19.0 | 218 | 4.3 | 26.5 | 11.9 | 1.0 |
| **VEGETABLE FAT** | | | | | | | | |
| Pure, Trex* | 1 Tbsp/12g | 108.0 | 12.0 | 900 | 0.0 | 0.0 | 100.0 | 0.0 |
| **VEGETABLE FINGERS** | | | | | | | | |
| Crispy, Captain Birds Eye, Birds Eye* | 1 Fingers/60g | 115.0 | 5.0 | 191 | 4.8 | 23.8 | 8.5 | 1.8 |
| Crispy Crunchy, Dalepak* | 1 Finger/28g | 62.0 | 3.0 | 223 | 4.2 | 26.7 | 11.0 | 15.0 |
| Sweetcorn, Tesco* | 1 Finger/28g | 66.0 | 4.0 | 236 | 7.7 | 23.0 | 12.6 | 3.0 |
| **VEGETABLE MEDLEY** | | | | | | | | |
| & New Potato, Asda* | ½ Pack/175g | 101.0 | 4.0 | 58 | 2.5 | 7.0 | 2.2 | 5.0 |
| Asda* | 1 Pack/300g | 84.0 | 1.0 | 28 | 2.8 | 3.9 | 0.2 | 2.9 |
| Asparagus Tips, Perfectly Balanced, Waitrose* | 1 Serving/225g | 121.0 | 8.0 | 54 | 1.3 | 4.6 | 3.4 | 1.4 |
| Basil & Oregano Butter, Waitrose* | 1 Serving/113g | 59.0 | 4.0 | 52 | 1.7 | 3.7 | 3.4 | 1.9 |
| Buttered, Sainsbury's* | ½ Pack/175g | 122.0 | 7.0 | 70 | 1.7 | 7.0 | 3.9 | 1.8 |
| Carrot, Courgette, Fine Bean & Baby Corn, Tesco* | 1 Serving/100g | 36.0 | 2.0 | 36 | 1.1 | 2.4 | 2.4 | 3.0 |
| Carrots, Broccoli, Baby Corn, Sugar Snap Peas, Co-Op* | 1/3 Pack/89g | 40.0 | 1.0 | 45 | 3.0 | 7.0 | 0.8 | 3.0 |
| Crunchy, M & S* | 1 Pack/250g | 75.0 | 2.0 | 30 | 3.1 | 2.8 | 0.8 | 2.5 |
| Frozen, M & S* | 1 Pack/500g | 175.0 | 4.0 | 35 | 3.4 | 3.9 | 0.8 | 3.1 |
| Green, HL, Tesco* | 1 Serving/125g | 59.0 | 2.0 | 47 | 3.7 | 4.1 | 1.8 | 4.1 |
| Green, M & S* | 1 Serving/250g | 62.0 | 1.0 | 25 | 3.0 | 1.8 | 0.5 | 1.8 |
| Green, Sainsbury's* | 1 Pack/220g | 178.0 | 14.0 | 81 | 3.0 | 2.5 | 6.5 | 2.9 |
| HL, Tesco* | 1 Serving/100g | 23.0 | 1.0 | 23 | 0.8 | 2.3 | 1.2 | 1.3 |
| Mediterranean Style, Asda* | 1 Pack/410g | 225.0 | 7.0 | 55 | 1.7 | 8.0 | 1.8 | 1.3 |
| with Herby Butter, M & S* | 1 Pack/300g | 225.0 | 15.0 | 75 | 1.5 | 6.2 | 5.0 | 2.6 |
| **VEGETABLE SELECTION** | | | | | | | | |
| Baby, Tesco* | ½ Pack/100g | 25.0 | 0.0 | 25 | 1.6 | 3.7 | 0.4 | 1.0 |
| Chefs, M & S* | 1 Pack/250g | 87.0 | 1.0 | 35 | 2.6 | 4.5 | 0.5 | 2.9 |
| Five, Sainsbury's* | ½ Pack/125g | 42.0 | 1.0 | 34 | 2.6 | 4.3 | 0.8 | 3.1 |
| Fresh, Finest, Tesco* | 1 Pack/250g | 182.0 | 14.0 | 73 | 1.9 | 3.2 | 5.8 | 2.2 |
| Garden, Tesco* | 1 Pack/275g | 124.0 | 9.0 | 45 | 1.2 | 2.7 | 3.3 | 1.2 |

| | Measure INFO/WEIGHT | per Measure KCAL | FAT | Nutrition Values per 100g / 100ml KCAL | PROT | CARB | FAT | FIBRE |
|---|---|---|---|---|---|---|---|---|
| **VEGETABLE SELECTION** | | | | | | | | |
| Lightly Buttered & Seasoned, M & S* | 1 Pack/300g | 195.0 | 11.0 | 65 | 1.6 | 6.3 | 3.6 | 2.8 |
| Ready to Cook, Morrisons* | 1 Serving/150g | 51.0 | 1.0 | 34 | 2.4 | 4.8 | 0.6 | 2.3 |
| Roast, COU, M & S* | 1 Serving/250g | 95.0 | 2.0 | 38 | 1.2 | 6.1 | 0.8 | 0.6 |
| Winter, M & S* | 1 Bag/400g | 80.0 | 0.0 | 20 | 2.2 | 3.2 | 0.0 | 3.1 |
| with Chilli & Garlic Dressing, Finest, Tesco* | 1 Serving/250g | 257.0 | 12.0 | 103 | 2.0 | 12.8 | 4.9 | 1.0 |
| with Herb Butter, Waitrose* | 1 Pack/300g | 270.0 | 17.0 | 90 | 1.9 | 8.1 | 5.6 | 2.1 |
| **VEGETABLES** | | | | | | | | |
| & Feta Cheese, Roasted, BGTY, Sainsbury's* | 1 Pack/200g | 264.0 | 4.0 | 132 | 6.4 | 21.7 | 2.2 | 0.0 |
| Baby, Frozen, Asda* | 1 Serving/100g | 25.0 | 0.0 | 25 | 1.9 | 3.7 | 0.3 | 1.9 |
| Baby Mix, Freshly Frozen, Iceland* | 1 Serving/100g | 26.0 | 0.0 | 26 | 1.8 | 3.9 | 0.3 | 1.9 |
| Broccoli & Cauliflower, Layered, M & S* | ½ Pack/135g | 94.0 | 5.0 | 70 | 1.5 | 7.6 | 3.4 | 1.2 |
| Butternut Squash & Sweet Potato, Fresh Tastes, Asda* | ½ Pack/225g | 128.0 | 0.0 | 57 | 1.0 | 12.9 | 0.2 | 1.8 |
| Carrot, Broccoli & Cauliflower, Organic, Sainsbury's* | 1 Serving/250g | 62.0 | 1.0 | 25 | 1.9 | 3.0 | 0.6 | 2.2 |
| Cauliflower Florets, Peas & Carrots, Freshly Frozen, Asda* | 1 Serving/119g | 44.0 | 1.0 | 37 | 3.0 | 5.0 | 0.6 | 2.8 |
| Chargrilled, With Pasta & Sweet Chilli Sauce, HL, Tesco* | 1 Pack/370g | 499.0 | 12.0 | 135 | 4.7 | 21.8 | 3.3 | 1.7 |
| Chargrilled with Tomato Sauce, GFY, Asda* | 1 Serving/260g | 164.0 | 7.0 | 63 | 1.4 | 8.0 | 2.8 | 0.0 |
| Chinese Glazed, Tesco* | 1 Pack/200g | 110.0 | 4.0 | 55 | 1.3 | 7.7 | 2.2 | 1.2 |
| Chinese Inspired, Crisp, M & S* | 1 Pack/250g | 62.0 | 1.0 | 25 | 1.7 | 4.6 | 0.3 | 1.9 |
| Crisp & Crunchy, Stir Fry, M & S* | ½ Pack/115g | 29.0 | 0.0 | 25 | 1.9 | 3.9 | 0.2 | 1.7 |
| Crispy, Asda* | 1 Serving/50g | 17.0 | 0.0 | 35 | 0.1 | 8.0 | 0.3 | 2.2 |
| Crispy, Ready to Cook, Sainsbury's* | 1 Serving/100g | 24.0 | 0.0 | 24 | 1.8 | 3.6 | 0.3 | 2.2 |
| Crispy, Tesco* | 1 Pack/200g | 54.0 | 1.0 | 27 | 1.9 | 3.9 | 0.4 | 2.3 |
| Diamond Sliced, Ready to Cook, Waitrose* | ½ Pack/125g | 31.0 | 1.0 | 25 | 1.6 | 3.7 | 0.5 | 2.1 |
| Farmhouse Mix, Frozen, Asda* | 1 Serving/100g | 25.0 | 1.0 | 25 | 2.5 | 2.2 | 0.8 | 0.0 |
| Favourite Five Selection, M & S* | ½ Pack/125g | 25.0 | 1.0 | 20 | 1.8 | 2.4 | 0.6 | 2.9 |
| for Roasting, M & S* | ½ Pack/224g | 190.0 | 13.0 | 85 | 1.2 | 7.7 | 5.6 | 2.4 |
| Garden, Washed, Tesco* | 1 Bag/250g | 65.0 | 2.0 | 26 | 3.0 | 1.9 | 0.7 | 2.0 |
| Grilled, Frozen, Sainsbury's* | 1 Serving/80g | 42.0 | 3.0 | 52 | 1.2 | 3.8 | 3.6 | 1.5 |
| Italiano Marinated, Roasted, Tesco* | ½ Tub/100g | 121.0 | 9.0 | 121 | 1.7 | 9.2 | 8.6 | 0.8 |
| Julienne, Tesco* | 1 Serving/100g | 30.0 | 0.0 | 30 | 1.1 | 5.7 | 0.3 | 1.9 |
| Layered, GFY, Asda* | ½ Pack/150g | 81.0 | 4.0 | 54 | 1.2 | 6.0 | 2.8 | 2.0 |
| Layered, Tesco* | 1 Serving/280g | 202.0 | 15.0 | 72 | 1.6 | 4.8 | 5.2 | 1.6 |
| Layered, with Butter, Waitrose* | 1 Pack/280g | 207.0 | 16.0 | 74 | 1.7 | 3.6 | 5.8 | 2.4 |
| Mediterranean, in Tomato Sauce, COU, M & S* | 1 Pack/300g | 105.0 | 2.0 | 35 | 2.5 | 4.3 | 0.7 | 2.2 |
| Mediterranean, Ready to Roast, Waitrose* | 1 Serving/200g | 128.0 | 8.0 | 64 | 1.3 | 5.6 | 4.0 | 1.6 |
| Mediterranean, Sainsbury's* | 1 Pack/400g | 180.0 | 10.0 | 45 | 1.2 | 4.5 | 2.4 | 3.1 |
| Mediterranean Style, Asda* | ½ Pack/205g | 113.0 | 4.0 | 55 | 1.7 | 7.9 | 1.8 | 1.3 |
| Mediterranean Style, COOK!, M & S* | ½ Pack/200g | 60.0 | 2.0 | 30 | 1.2 | 5.5 | 0.9 | 1.0 |
| Mediterranean Style, Finest, Tesco* | ½ Pack/150g | 155.0 | 12.0 | 103 | 1.5 | 5.5 | 8.1 | 3.0 |
| Mediterranean Style, Ready to Roast, Sainsbury's* | ½ Pack/200g | 138.0 | 4.0 | 69 | 2.3 | 9.9 | 2.2 | 2.2 |
| Mediterranean Style, Roasting, Tesco* | 1 Serving/200g | 72.0 | 2.0 | 36 | 1.1 | 5.7 | 1.0 | 1.3 |
| Mixed, Frozen, Sainsbury's* | 1 Serving/100g | 50.0 | 1.0 | 50 | 2.9 | 7.9 | 0.7 | 3.5 |
| Moroccan, COU, M & S* | 1 Pack/300g | 165.0 | 4.0 | 55 | 2.4 | 8.2 | 1.5 | 1.7 |
| Oriental, Waitrose* | 1 Pack/300g | 108.0 | 1.0 | 36 | 0.8 | 7.8 | 0.2 | 1.4 |
| Oriental Inspired, M & S* | 1 Pack/260g | 78.0 | 1.0 | 30 | 1.9 | 4.6 | 0.5 | 2.7 |
| Oriental Stir Fry, Frozen, Sainsbury's* | ½ Pack/225g | 142.0 | 9.0 | 63 | 1.5 | 5.4 | 3.9 | 1.5 |
| Roast, M & S* | 1 Pack/420g | 273.0 | 18.0 | 65 | 1.4 | 4.9 | 4.2 | 0.4 |
| Roasted, & Olive Sauce, TTD, Sainsbury's* | 1 Serving/75g | 42.0 | 2.0 | 56 | 1.7 | 6.9 | 2.4 | 2.0 |
| Roasted, Italian, M & S* | 1 Serving/95g | 218.0 | 20.0 | 230 | 1.8 | 7.1 | 21.0 | 1.7 |
| Roasted, Selection, COU, M & S* | 1 Pack/250g | 87.0 | 2.0 | 35 | 1.2 | 6.1 | 0.8 | 0.6 |
| Roasted Root, Extra Special, Asda* | ½ Pack/205g | 160.0 | 3.0 | 78 | 1.1 | 15.0 | 1.5 | 6.0 |
| Roasted Winter, HL, Tesco* | ½ Pack/200g | 160.0 | 5.0 | 80 | 1.9 | 12.7 | 2.5 | 3.6 |
| Roasting, Tesco* | 1 Serving/350g | 152.0 | 2.0 | 43 | 1.2 | 8.0 | 0.5 | 3.0 |

| | Measure INFO/WEIGHT | per Measure KCAL | FAT | Nutrition Values per 100g / 100ml KCAL | PROT | CARB | FAT | FIBRE |
|---|---|---|---|---|---|---|---|---|
| **VEGETABLES** | | | | | | | | |
| Root, Honey Roast, BGTY, Sainsbury's* | ½ Pack/150g | 174.0 | 2.0 | 116 | 2.5 | 23.1 | 1.5 | 5.5 |
| Root, Honey Roast, Sainsbury's* | 1 Pack/400g | 748.0 | 35.0 | 187 | 0.0 | 25.8 | 8.7 | 5.2 |
| Seasonal, Pack, Sainsbury's* | 1 Serving/261g | 60.0 | 1.0 | 23 | 0.7 | 4.6 | 0.3 | 2.0 |
| Special Mix, Sainsbury's* | 1 Serving/80g | 54.0 | 1.0 | 68 | 3.4 | 9.7 | 1.7 | 3.2 |
| Steam & Serve, Morrisons* | 1 Serving/120g | 66.0 | 1.0 | 55 | 2.4 | 8.8 | 1.1 | 2.6 |
| Stir Fry, Tesco* | 1 Serving/150g | 37.0 | 0.0 | 25 | 0.9 | 5.0 | 0.1 | 1.4 |
| Summer, Layered With Butter, Asda* | ¼ Pack/80g | 50.0 | 2.0 | 62 | 2.6 | 8.2 | 2.1 | 0.0 |
| Summer, Roasting, Tesco* | ½ Pack/175g | 105.0 | 7.0 | 60 | 1.0 | 5.1 | 3.8 | 1.6 |
| Sun Dried Tomato, Selection, Finest, Tesco* | 1 Pack/340g | 303.0 | 17.0 | 89 | 1.8 | 8.9 | 5.1 | 1.1 |
| Sweet & Crunchy, Tesco* | 1 Serving/50g | 21.0 | 0.0 | 43 | 2.3 | 7.0 | 0.6 | 2.4 |
| Szechuan Style, Ready Prepared, Waitrose* | 1 Pack/300g | 132.0 | 4.0 | 44 | 2.3 | 5.7 | 1.3 | 1.9 |
| Tender, Green, Medley, Sainsbury's* | ½ Pack/88g | 35.0 | 1.0 | 40 | 3.6 | 5.1 | 0.6 | 3.3 |
| Vietnamese, Wok, Findus* | 1 Serving/100g | 25.0 | 0.0 | 25 | 1.5 | 4.5 | 0.5 | 0.0 |
| Winter, Fresh, Asda* | 1 Bag/250g | 75.0 | 2.0 | 30 | 3.0 | 2.2 | 1.0 | 2.3 |
| Winter, Ready to Roast, Fresh, Sainsbury's* | 1 Pack/272g | 226.0 | 8.0 | 83 | 1.2 | 13.2 | 2.8 | 0.0 |
| Winter, Sainsbury's* | 1 Serving/125g | 37.0 | 1.0 | 30 | 2.0 | 3.6 | 0.8 | 2.2 |
| Winter Crunchy, M & S* | ½ Pack/125g | 31.0 | 1.0 | 25 | 2.0 | 3.1 | 0.8 | 2.7 |
| with Sun Dried Tomato, Roasted, Finest, Tesco* | ½ Pack/150g | 153.0 | 11.0 | 102 | 1.9 | 7.3 | 7.2 | 1.2 |
| Wok, Chinese, Stir Fry, Classic, Findus* | 1 Pack/500g | 150.0 | 2.0 | 30 | 1.0 | 5.0 | 0.5 | 3.5 |
| Wok, Thai, Findus* | ½ Pack/250g | 87.0 | 1.0 | 35 | 1.5 | 7.0 | 0.3 | 0.0 |
| **VEGETARIAN** | | | | | | | | |
| Chicken Style Pieces, Sainsbury's* | 1 Pack/375g | 754.0 | 26.0 | 201 | 25.5 | 9.0 | 7.0 | 0.6 |
| Fingers, Fish Style, Breaded, Redwood* | 1 Finger/36g | 94.0 | 5.0 | 262 | 16.5 | 16.0 | 14.5 | 0.0 |
| Pepperoni Style Slices, Meat Free, Cheatin', Redwood* | 1 Slice/10g | 28.0 | 2.0 | 282 | 25.3 | 5.2 | 17.7 | 0.2 |
| Slices, Sage & Onion, Vegi Deli, Redwood* | 1 Slice/10g | 23.0 | 1.0 | 233 | 21.4 | 5.0 | 14.1 | 0.0 |
| Slices, Vegetable, Tesco* | 1 Slice/165g | 452.0 | 31.0 | 274 | 5.6 | 21.4 | 18.5 | 3.3 |
| **VEGETARIAN MINCE** | | | | | | | | |
| Easy Cook, Linda McCartney* | 1oz/28g | 35.0 | 0.0 | 126 | 21.4 | 9.3 | 0.4 | 1.7 |
| Frozen, Meatfree, Sainsbury's* | 1oz/28g | 49.0 | 2.0 | 174 | 20.0 | 9.5 | 6.2 | 6.0 |
| Meat Free, Asda* | 1oz/28g | 49.0 | 1.0 | 176 | 27.0 | 7.0 | 4.4 | 4.1 |
| Tesco* | 1 Serving/76g | 116.0 | 4.0 | 153 | 18.0 | 7.2 | 5.8 | 6.0 |
| Vegemince, Realeat* | 1 Serving/125g | 217.0 | 12.0 | 174 | 18.0 | 3.0 | 10.0 | 3.0 |
| **VENISON** | | | | | | | | |
| *Grill Steak, Average* | *1 Grillsteak/150g* | *178.0* | *4.0* | *119* | *19.0* | *5.0* | *2.5* | *0.9* |
| *Minced, Cooked, Average* | *1 Serving/100g* | *187.0* | *8.0* | *187* | *26.4* | *0.0* | *8.2* | *0.0* |
| *Minced, Raw, Average* | *1 Serving/100g* | *157.0* | *7.0* | *157* | *21.8* | *0.0* | *7.1* | *0.0* |
| *Roasted, Average* | *1oz/28g* | *46.0* | *1.0* | *165* | *35.6* | *0.0* | *2.5* | *0.0* |
| *Steak, Raw, Average* | *1oz/28g* | *30.0* | *1.0* | *108* | *22.8* | *0.0* | *1.9* | *0.0* |
| **VENISON IN** | | | | | | | | |
| Red Wine & Port, Average | 1oz/28g | 21.0 | 1.0 | 76 | 9.8 | 3.5 | 2.6 | 0.4 |
| **VERMICELLI** | | | | | | | | |
| *Dry* | *1oz/28g* | *99.0* | *0.0* | *355* | *8.7* | *78.3* | *0.4* | *0.0* |
| *Egg, Cooked, Average* | *1 Serving/185g* | *239.0* | *3.0* | *129* | *5.0* | *24.0* | *1.4* | *1.0* |
| **VERMOUTH** | | | | | | | | |
| *Dry* | *1 Shot/50ml* | *54.0* | *0.0* | *109* | *0.1* | *3.0* | *0.0* | *0.0* |
| *Sweet* | *1 Shot/50ml* | *75.0* | *0.0* | *151* | *0.0* | *15.9* | *0.0* | *0.0* |
| **VICE VERSAS** | | | | | | | | |
| Nestle* | 1 Bag/46g | 221.0 | 10.0 | 485 | 5.0 | 69.3 | 20.9 | 0.0 |
| **VIMTO*** | | | | | | | | |
| Cordial, No Added Sugar, Diluted, Vimto* | 1 Glass/250ml | 6.0 | 0.0 | 2 | 0.1 | 0.4 | 0.1 | 0.0 |
| Cordial, Original, Diluted, Vimto* | 1 Serving/200ml | 60.0 | 0.0 | 30 | 0.0 | 7.4 | 0.0 | 0.0 |
| Grape, Blackcurrant & Raspberry Juice Drink, Fizzy, Vimto* | 1 Can/330ml | 147.0 | 0.0 | 44 | 0.0 | 11.0 | 0.0 | 0.0 |

V

| | Measure INFO/WEIGHT | per Measure KCAL | FAT | Nutrition Values per 100g / 100ml KCAL | PROT | CARB | FAT | FIBRE |
|---|---|---|---|---|---|---|---|---|
| **VINAIGRETTE** | | | | | | | | |
| Balsamic, Hellmann's* | 1 Tbsp/15ml | 12.0 | 0.0 | 82 | 0.1 | 15.3 | 2.7 | 0.6 |
| Balsamic, Newman's Own* | 1 Serving/20g | 67.0 | 7.0 | 333 | 0.5 | 3.9 | 35.0 | 0.0 |
| Balsamic Vinegar & Pistachio, Finest, Tesco* | 1 Tbsp/15ml | 55.0 | 6.0 | 370 | 0.2 | 2.8 | 39.2 | 0.0 |
| Blush Wine, Briannas* | 2 Tbsp/30ml | 100.0 | 6.0 | 333 | 0.0 | 40.0 | 20.0 | 0.0 |
| Fat Free, Hellmann's* | 1 Serving/15ml | 7.0 | 0.0 | 49 | 0.1 | 10.9 | 0.0 | 0.3 |
| French, Real, Briannas* | 2 Tbsp/30ml | 150.0 | 17.0 | 500 | 0.0 | 0.0 | 56.7 | 0.0 |
| French Style, Finest, Tesco* | 1 Tbsp/15ml | 93.0 | 10.0 | 620 | 0.6 | 6.3 | 65.3 | 0.2 |
| Luxury French, Hellmann's* | 1 Tsp/5ml | 15.0 | 1.0 | 305 | 0.8 | 16.0 | 26.1 | 0.4 |
| Olive Oil & Lemon, Amoy* | ½ Sachet/15ml | 37.0 | 4.0 | 250 | 0.3 | 3.0 | 24.0 | 0.0 |
| Perfectly Balanced, Waitrose* | 1 Tsp/5ml | 4.0 | 0.0 | 89 | 0.4 | 20.9 | 0.4 | 0.5 |
| Portuguese, Nando's* | 1 Tbsp/15g | 61.0 | 7.0 | 409 | 1.0 | 2.0 | 44.0 | 0.3 |
| Waistline, 99% Fat Free, Crosse & Blackwell* | 1 Tbsp/15ml | 1.0 | 0.0 | 9 | 1.0 | 0.7 | 0.2 | 0.2 |
| **VINE LEAVES** | | | | | | | | |
| **Preserved in Brine** | **1oz/28g** | **4.0** | **0.0** | **15** | **3.6** | **0.2** | **0.0** | **0.0** |
| Stuffed, Sainsbury's* | 1 Parcel/38g | 46.0 | 2.0 | 124 | 2.9 | 15.3 | 5.7 | 3.1 |
| Stuffed with Rice | 1oz/28g | 73.0 | 5.0 | 262 | 2.8 | 23.8 | 18.0 | 0.0 |
| Stuffed with Rice, Dolmades, M & S* | 1 Leaf/38g | 40.0 | 2.0 | 105 | 2.6 | 14.2 | 4.1 | 1.2 |
| Stuffed with Rice & Mixed Herbs, Sainsbury's* | 1 Leaf/37g | 44.0 | 2.0 | 120 | 2.6 | 16.3 | 4.9 | 1.2 |
| **VINEGAR** | | | | | | | | |
| **Balsamic, Average** | **1 Tsp/5ml** | **4.0** | **0.0** | **88** | **0.5** | **17.0** | **0.0** | **0.0** |
| **Cider** | **1 Tbsp/15ml** | **2.0** | **0.0** | **14** | **0.0** | **5.9** | **0.0** | **0.0** |
| **Malt** | **1 Tbsp/15g** | **1.0** | **0.0** | **4** | **0.4** | **0.6** | **0.0** | **0.0** |
| Red Wine, Average | 1 Tbsp/15ml | 3.0 | 0.0 | 19 | 0.0 | 0.3 | 0.0 | 0.0 |
| Rice, White, Amoy* | 1 Tsp/5ml | 0.0 | 0.0 | 4 | 0.0 | 1.0 | 0.0 | 0.0 |
| **White Wine, Average** | **1 Tsp/5ml** | **1.0** | **0.0** | **19** | **0.4** | **0.3** | **0.0** | **0.0** |
| **VODKA** | | | | | | | | |
| **37.5% Volume** | **1 Shot/35ml** | **72.0** | **0.0** | **207** | **0.0** | **0.0** | **0.0** | **0.0** |
| **40% Volume** | **1 Shot/35ml** | **78.0** | **0.0** | **222** | **0.0** | **0.0** | **0.0** | **0.0** |
| **VOL AU VENTS** | | | | | | | | |
| Garlic Mushroom, Mini, Asda* | 1 Serving/17g | 59.0 | 5.0 | 347 | 5.0 | 21.0 | 27.0 | 0.0 |
| Mushroom, Sainsbury's* | 1 Serving/14g | 49.0 | 3.0 | 350 | 6.9 | 30.8 | 22.1 | 1.4 |
| Mushroom & Roast Garlic, M & S* | 1 Serving/19g | 65.0 | 5.0 | 345 | 6.2 | 25.2 | 24.3 | 1.9 |
| Seafood, Party, Youngs* | 1 Serving/17g | 60.0 | 4.0 | 354 | 8.3 | 26.0 | 24.8 | 1.0 |

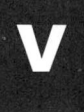

| | Measure INFO/WEIGHT | per Measure KCAL | FAT | Nutrition Values per 100g / 100ml KCAL | PROT | CARB | FAT | FIBRE |
|---|---|---|---|---|---|---|---|---|

## WAFERS

| | Measure INFO/WEIGHT | KCAL | FAT | KCAL | PROT | CARB | FAT | FIBRE |
|---|---|---|---|---|---|---|---|---|
| Apricot & Peach, Highlights, Cadbury* | 1 Wafer/19g | 80.0 | 3.0 | 430 | 5.2 | 70.6 | 14.3 | 1.4 |
| Caramel, Dark Chocolate, Tunnock's* | 1 Wafer/26g | 128.0 | 7.0 | 492 | 5.2 | 60.7 | 25.4 | 0.0 |
| Caramel, Milk Chocolate Coated, Value, Tesco* | 1 Wafer/23g | 110.0 | 5.0 | 475 | 5.6 | 67.6 | 20.2 | 0.6 |
| Caramel, Tunnock's* | 1 Wafer/26g | 116.0 | 5.0 | 448 | 3.6 | 69.2 | 17.4 | 2.5 |
| Caramel Log, Tunnock's* | 1 Wafer/32g | 152.0 | 8.0 | 474 | 4.2 | 64.3 | 24.0 | 0.0 |
| Chocolate, Cadbury* | 1oz/28g | 147.0 | 8.0 | 526 | 7.0 | 61.2 | 29.8 | 0.0 |
| Cream, Tunnock's* | 1 Wafer/20g | 103.0 | 6.0 | 513 | 6.6 | 63.2 | 28.0 | 0.0 |
| Filled, Average | 1oz/28g | 150.0 | 8.0 | 535 | 4.7 | 66.0 | 29.9 | 0.0 |
| Florida Orange, Tunnock's* | 1 Wafer/20g | 104.0 | 6.0 | 519 | 5.1 | 64.0 | 29.0 | 0.0 |
| for Ice Cream, Askeys* | 1 Wafer/1.5g | 6.0 | 0.0 | 388 | 11.4 | 79.0 | 2.9 | 0.0 |
| Milk Chocolate, Sainsbury's* | 1 Wafer/10g | 51.0 | 3.0 | 506 | 6.2 | 60.5 | 26.7 | 1.4 |
| Orange, Highlights, Cadbury* | 1 Wafer/19g | 80.0 | 3.0 | 430 | 5.2 | 70.6 | 14.3 | 1.4 |

## WAFFLES

| | | | | | | | | |
|---|---|---|---|---|---|---|---|---|
| Belgian, TTD, Sainsbury's* | 1 Waffle/25g | 123.0 | 7.0 | 490 | 6.0 | 50.6 | 29.3 | 1.2 |
| Caramel, Asda* | 1 Waffle/8g | 37.0 | 2.0 | 459 | 3.3 | 62.0 | 22.0 | 1.1 |
| Milk Chocolate, Tregroes* | 1 Waffle/49g | 220.0 | 21.0 | 450 | 4.5 | 57.0 | 42.0 | 0.5 |
| Sweet, American Style, Sainsbury's* | 1 Waffle/35g | 160.0 | 9.0 | 457 | 7.2 | 50.6 | 25.3 | 1.1 |
| Toasting, McVitie's* | 1 Waffle/25g | 118.0 | 6.0 | 474 | 6.0 | 52.6 | 25.5 | 0.6 |

## WAGON WHEEL

| | | | | | | | | |
|---|---|---|---|---|---|---|---|---|
| Chocolate, Burton's* | 1 Biscuit/39g | 165.0 | 6.0 | 424 | 5.3 | 67.4 | 14.6 | 1.9 |
| Jammie, Burton's* | 1 Biscuit/40g | 168.0 | 6.0 | 420 | 5.1 | 67.7 | 14.1 | 1.9 |

## WALNUT WHIP

| | | | | | | | | |
|---|---|---|---|---|---|---|---|---|
| Nestle* | 1 Whip/35g | 173.0 | 9.0 | 494 | 5.3 | 61.3 | 25.2 | 0.7 |
| The, Classics, M & S* | 1 Whip/26g | 127.0 | 7.0 | 490 | 7.2 | 54.9 | 27.4 | 1.1 |
| Vanilla, Nestle* | 1 Whip/34g | 165.0 | 8.0 | 486 | 5.7 | 60.5 | 24.6 | 0.0 |

## WALNUTS

| | | | | | | | | |
|---|---|---|---|---|---|---|---|---|
| *Average* | *6 Halves/20g* | *138.0* | *14.0* | *691* | *15.6* | *3.2* | *68.5* | *3.5* |
| *Halves, Average* | *1 Serving/25g* | *167.0* | *16.0* | *669* | *17.4* | *6.3* | *65.0* | *4.7* |

## WASABI

| | | | | | | | | |
|---|---|---|---|---|---|---|---|---|
| Paste, Ready Mixed, Japanese, Yutaka* | 1 Tsp/5g | 14.0 | 0.0 | 286 | 2.7 | 53.0 | 7.0 | 0.0 |

## WATER

| | | | | | | | | |
|---|---|---|---|---|---|---|---|---|
| Berry Blast, Revive, Volvic* | 1 Bottle/500ml | 9.0 | 0.0 | 2 | 0.3 | 0.4 | 0.0 | 0.0 |
| Blackcurrant Flavour, Still, Danone* | 1 Serving/120ml | 25.0 | 0.0 | 21 | 0.0 | 5.0 | 0.0 | 0.0 |
| Cranberries & Raspberries, Juicy, Innocent* | 1 Bottle/380ml | 118.0 | 1.0 | 31 | 0.1 | 6.7 | 0.3 | 0.0 |
| Cranberries & Raspberries, Spring Water, This Water* | 1 Bottle/420ml | 122.0 | 0.0 | 29 | 0.1 | 6.9 | 0.1 | 0.0 |
| Cranberry & Blueberry, Lightly Sparkling, Waitrose* | 1 Glass/250ml | 10.0 | 0.0 | 4 | 0.0 | 0.7 | 0.0 | 0.0 |
| Grapefruit, Slightly Sparkling, Tesco* | 1 Serving/200ml | 4.0 | 0.0 | 2 | 0.0 | 0.2 | 0.0 | 0.0 |
| Lemon, Vittel* | 1 Bottle/500ml | 5.0 | 0.0 | 1 | 0.0 | 0.0 | 0.0 | 0.0 |
| Lemon & Lime, Still, M & S* | 1 Bottle/500ml | 5.0 | 0.0 | 1 | 0.0 | 0.2 | 0.0 | 0.0 |
| Lemon & Lime, Sugar Free, Touch of Fruit, Volvic* | 1 Bottle/150ml | 2.0 | 0.0 | 1 | 0.0 | 0.0 | 0.0 | 0.0 |
| Mandarin & Cranberry, Still, M & S* | 1 Bottle/500ml | 100.0 | 0.0 | 20 | 0.0 | 5.0 | 0.0 | 0.0 |
| *Mineral Or Tap* | *1 Glass/200ml* | *0.0* | *0.0* | *0* | *0.0* | *0.0* | *0.0* | *0.0* |
| Peach & Lemon, Still, M & S* | 1 Bottle/500ml | 100.0 | 0.0 | 20 | 0.0 | 5.0 | 0.0 | 0.0 |
| Peach & Raspberry, Still, M & S* | 1 Bottle/500ml | 10.0 | 0.0 | 2 | 0.0 | 0.0 | 0.0 | 0.0 |
| Pomegranates & Blackcurrants, Spring Water, This Water* | 1 Bottle/420ml | 147.0 | 0.0 | 35 | 0.0 | 8.7 | 0.0 | 0.0 |
| Raspberry & Apple, Still, Shapers, Boots* | 1 Serving/250ml | 10.0 | 0.0 | 4 | 0.0 | 0.8 | 0.0 | 0.0 |
| Sparkling, Fruit, Aqua Libra* | 1 Glass/200ml | 54.0 | 0.0 | 27 | 0.0 | 5.1 | 0.0 | 0.0 |
| Sparkling, Strawberry & Kiwi, Sugar Free, Perfectly Clear* | 1 Glass/250ml | 1.0 | 0.0 | 1 | 0.0 | 0.0 | 0.0 | 0.0 |
| Spring, Apple & Blackcurrant, Hadrian* | 1 Bottle/365ml | 3.0 | 0.0 | 1 | 0.1 | 0.1 | 0.0 | 0.0 |
| Spring, Apple & Cherry Flavoured, Sparkling, Sainsbury's* | 1 Glass/250ml | 5.0 | 0.0 | 2 | 0.1 | 0.2 | 0.1 | 0.1 |
| Spring, Apple & Lemongrass, Food to Go, M & S* | 1 Bottle/500ml | 4.0 | 0.0 | 1 | 0.0 | 0.2 | 0.0 | 0.0 |
| Spring, Apple & Mango, Sparkling, Asda* | 1 Glass/200ml | 2.0 | 0.0 | 1 | 0.0 | 0.2 | 0.0 | 0.0 |
| Spring, Apple & Raspberry, Shapers, Boots* | 1 Bottle/500ml | 10.0 | 0.0 | 2 | 0.0 | 0.2 | 0.0 | 0.0 |

| | Measure INFO/WEIGHT | per Measure KCAL | FAT | Nutrition Values per 100g / 100ml KCAL | PROT | CARB | FAT | FIBRE |
|---|---|---|---|---|---|---|---|---|
| **WATER** | | | | | | | | |
| Spring, Elderflower & Pear, Sainsbury's* | 1 Glass/250g | 5.0 | 0.0 | 2 | 0.1 | 0.2 | 0.1 | 0.1 |
| Spring, Lemon & Lime, Slightly Sparkling, Tesco* | 1 Serving/200ml | 4.0 | 0.0 | 2 | 0.1 | 0.2 | 0.1 | 0.1 |
| Spring, Lemon & Lime Flavour, Sparkling, Superdrug* | 1 Bottle/500ml | 8.0 | 0.0 | 2 | 0.1 | 0.1 | 0.1 | 0.1 |
| Spring, Lemon & Lime Flavoured, Sparkling, Sainsbury's* | 1 Glass/250ml | 4.0 | 0.0 | 2 | 0.1 | 0.1 | 0.1 | 0.1 |
| Spring, Orange & Passionfruit, Drench* | 1 Serving/250ml | 95.0 | 0.0 | 38 | 0.1 | 9.0 | 0.2 | 0.0 |
| Spring, Peach Flavour, Sparkling, Co-Op* | 1 Glass/250ml | 2.0 | 0.0 | 1 | 0.0 | 0.0 | 0.0 | 0.0 |
| Spring, Peach Flavoured, No Added Sugar, Asda* | 1 Glass/200ml | 4.0 | 0.0 | 2 | 0.0 | 0.2 | 0.0 | 0.0 |
| Spring, Peach Flavoured, Sainsbury's* | 1 Glass/250ml | 5.0 | 0.0 | 2 | 0.1 | 0.2 | 0.1 | 0.1 |
| Spring, Raspberry & Cranberry, Shapers, Boots* | 1 Bottle/500ml | 10.0 | 0.0 | 2 | 0.0 | 0.5 | 0.0 | 0.0 |
| Spring, Strawberry & Aloe Vera, Botanical, M & S* | 1 Bottle/500ml | 5.0 | 0.0 | 1 | 0.0 | 0.2 | 0.0 | 0.0 |
| Spring, Strawberry & Kiwi, Still, Shapers, Boots* | 1 Glass/250ml | 2.0 | 0.0 | 1 | 0.0 | 0.1 | 0.0 | 0.9 |
| Spring, Strawberry & Vanilla, Sainsbury's* | 1 Glass/250ml | 5.0 | 0.0 | 2 | 0.1 | 0.2 | 0.1 | 0.1 |
| Spring, White Grape & Blackberry, Tesco* | 1 Glass/200ml | 4.0 | 0.0 | 2 | 0.0 | 0.5 | 0.0 | 0.0 |
| Spring, with Cranberry, Tesco* | 1 Glass/250ml | 2.0 | 0.0 | 1 | 0.0 | 0.2 | 0.0 | 0.0 |
| Spring, with Grapefruit, Tesco* | 1 Serving/200ml | 4.0 | 0.0 | 2 | 0.0 | 0.2 | 0.0 | 0.0 |
| Strawberry, Touch Of Fruit, Volvic* | 1 Bottle/500ml | 7.0 | 0.0 | 1 | 0.0 | 0.1 | 0.0 | 0.0 |
| Strawberry & Guava, Still, M & S* | 1 Glass/250ml | 5.0 | 0.0 | 2 | 0.0 | 0.1 | 0.0 | 0.0 |
| **WATER CHESTNUTS** | | | | | | | | |
| *Raw, Average* | *1oz/28g* | *10.0* | *0.0* | *34* | *1.0* | *7.8* | *0.0* | *0.1* |
| Whole, in Water, Drained, Sainsbury's* | 1 Can/140g | 25.0 | 0.0 | 18 | 0.8 | 3.4 | 0.1 | 0.4 |
| with Bamboo Shoots, Sainsbury's* | 1 Serving/50g | 29.0 | 0.0 | 58 | 2.0 | 12.0 | 0.2 | 1.1 |
| **WATER ICE** | | | | | | | | |
| Orange, Iceland* | 1 Ice/75ml | 73.0 | 0.0 | 98 | 0.2 | 24.4 | 0.0 | 0.2 |
| Pineapple, Iceland* | 1 Ice/75ml | 64.0 | 0.0 | 86 | 0.0 | 21.5 | 0.0 | 0.2 |
| Raspberry, Iceland* | 1 Ice/75ml | 67.0 | 0.0 | 89 | 0.0 | 22.2 | 0.0 | 0.2 |
| **WATERCRESS** | | | | | | | | |
| *Raw, Average* | *1oz/28g* | *3.0* | *0.0* | *11* | *2.3* | *1.3* | *0.1* | *0.5* |
| **WATERMELON** | | | | | | | | |
| *Flesh Only, Average* | *1 Serving/250g* | *75.0* | *1.0* | *30* | *0.4* | *7.0* | *0.3* | *0.4* |
| *Raw* | *1 Wedge/286g* | *92.0* | *1.0* | *32* | *0.6* | *7.2* | *0.4* | *0.5* |
| **WHEAT** | | | | | | | | |
| *Whole Grain, Split, Average* | *1 Serving/60g* | *205.0* | *1.0* | *342* | *11.3* | *75.9* | *1.7* | *12.2* |
| **WHEAT BRAN** | | | | | | | | |
| *Average* | *1 Tbsp/7g* | *14.0* | *0.0* | *206* | *14.1* | *26.8* | *5.5* | *36.4* |
| Coarse, Holland & Barrett* | 1 Tablespoon/4g | 8.0 | 0.0 | 206 | 14.1 | 26.8 | 5.5 | 36.4 |
| Natural, Jordans* | 1 Tbsp/7g | 13.0 | 0.0 | 188 | 16.3 | 17.4 | 5.9 | 44.5 |
| **WHEAT CRUNCHIES** | | | | | | | | |
| Golden Wonder* | 1 Pack/35g | 172.0 | 9.0 | 491 | 11.1 | 55.9 | 24.8 | 0.0 |
| Salt & Vinegar, Golden Wonder* | 1 Bag/34g | 165.0 | 8.0 | 484 | 10.5 | 54.5 | 24.9 | 2.8 |
| Worcester Sauce, Golden Wonder* | 1 Bag/35g | 172.0 | 9.0 | 492 | 9.3 | 56.4 | 25.5 | 3.9 |
| **WHEAT GERM** | | | | | | | | |
| *Average* | *1oz/28g* | *100.0* | *3.0* | *357* | *26.7* | *44.7* | *9.2* | *15.6* |
| Natural, Jordans* | 2 Tbsp/16g | 54.0 | 1.0 | 340 | 28.0 | 36.0 | 9.3 | 13.1 |
| **WHELKS** | | | | | | | | |
| *Boiled* | *1oz/28g* | *25.0* | *0.0* | *89* | *19.5* | *0.0* | *1.2* | *0.0* |
| **WHEY** | | | | | | | | |
| Chocolate, White, Diet, PhD Nutrition* | 1 Serving/50g | 195.0 | 2.0 | 390 | 70.0 | 12.5 | 5.0 | 3.7 |
| Powder, Molkosan Vitality, Vogel* | 1oz/28g | 56.0 | 0.0 | 200 | 1.0 | 20.0 | 0.1 | 61.0 |
| **WHEY PROTEIN** | | | | | | | | |
| Profusion, Reloaded, Boditronics* | 1 Serving/70g | 292.0 | 4.0 | 417 | 62.9 | 28.5 | 5.7 | 5.3 |
| **WHISKEY** | | | | | | | | |
| *37.5% Volume* | *1 Shot/35ml* | *72.0* | *0.0* | *207* | *0.0* | *0.0* | *0.0* | *0.0* |
| *40% Volume* | *1 Shot/35ml* | *78.0* | *0.0* | *222* | *0.0* | *0.0* | *0.0* | *0.0* |

**W**

| | Measure<br>INFO/WEIGHT | per Measure<br>KCAL | <br>FAT | Nutrition Values per 100g / 100ml<br>KCAL | <br>PROT | <br>CARB | <br>FAT | <br>FIBRE |
|---|---|---|---|---|---|---|---|---|
| **WHISKEY** | | | | | | | | |
| *86% Proof* | *1.5 fl oz/42g* | *105.0* | *0.0* | *250* | *0.0* | *0.1* | *0.0* | *0.0* |
| Jack Daniel's* | 1 Shot/35ml | 78.0 | 0.0 | 222 | 0.0 | 0.0 | 0.0 | 0.0 |
| Teacher's* | 1 Shot/35ml | 78.0 | 0.0 | 222 | 0.0 | 0.0 | 0.0 | 0.0 |
| **WHISKY** | | | | | | | | |
| *Scotch, 37.5% Volume* | *1 Shot/35ml* | *72.0* | *0.0* | *207* | *0.0* | *0.0* | *0.0* | *0.0* |
| *Scotch, 40% Volume* | *1 Shot/35ml* | *78.0* | *0.0* | *222* | *0.0* | *0.0* | *0.0* | *0.0* |
| **WHITE PUDDING** | | | | | | | | |
| *Average* | *1oz/28g* | *126.0* | *9.0* | *450* | *7.0* | *36.3* | *31.8* | *0.0* |
| **WHITEBAIT** | | | | | | | | |
| *in Flour, Fried* | *1oz/28g* | *147.0* | *13.0* | *525* | *19.5* | *5.3* | *47.5* | *0.2* |
| **WHITECURRANTS** | | | | | | | | |
| *Raw, Average* | *1oz/28g* | *7.0* | *0.0* | *26* | *1.3* | *5.6* | *0.0* | *3.4* |
| **WHITING** | | | | | | | | |
| in Crumbs, Fried in Blended Oil | 1 Serving/180g | 344.0 | 19.0 | 191 | 18.1 | 7.0 | 10.3 | 0.2 |
| *Raw* | *1oz/28g* | *23.0* | *0.0* | *81* | *18.7* | *0.0* | *0.7* | *0.0* |
| *Steamed* | *1 Serving/85g* | *78.0* | *1.0* | *92* | *20.9* | *0.0* | *0.9* | *0.0* |
| **WIENER SCHNITZEL** | | | | | | | | |
| Average | 1oz/28g | 62.0 | 3.0 | 223 | 20.9 | 13.1 | 10.0 | 0.4 |
| **WINE** | | | | | | | | |
| Cherry, Lambrini* | 1 Sm Glass/125ml | 80.0 | 0.0 | 64 | 0.0 | 0.0 | 0.0 | 0.0 |
| Diet, Lambrini* | 1 Sm Glass/125ml | 43.0 | 0.0 | 35 | 0.0 | 0.0 | 0.0 | 0.0 |
| Elderberry & Lemon, Ame* | 1 Sml Glass/125ml | 46.0 | 0.0 | 37 | 0.0 | 6.4 | 0.0 | 0.0 |
| *Fruit, Average* | *1 Sm Glass/125ml* | *115.0* | *0.0* | *92* | *0.0* | *5.5* | *0.0* | *0.0* |
| Grape & Apricot, Ame* | 1 Sm Glass/125ml | 49.0 | 1.0 | 39 | 1.3 | 6.7 | 1.0 | 0.0 |
| *Mulled, Homemade, Average* | *1 Sm Glass/125ml* | *245.0* | *0.0* | *196* | *0.1* | *25.2* | *0.0* | *0.0* |
| Mulled, Sainsbury's* | 1 Sm Glass/125ml | 112.0 | 0.0 | 90 | 0.0 | 8.6 | 0.0 | 0.0 |
| Original, Lambrini* | 1 Glass/125ml | 88.0 | 0.0 | 70 | 0.0 | 0.0 | 0.0 | 0.0 |
| Red, Amarone, Average* | 1 Sm Glass/125ml | 120.0 | 0.0 | 96 | 0.1 | 3.0 | 0.0 | 0.0 |
| *Red, Average* | *1 Sm Glass/125ml* | *85.0* | *0.0* | *68* | *0.1* | *0.2* | *0.0* | *0.0* |
| Red, Burgundy, 12.9% Abv, Average | 1 Sm Glass/125ml | 110.0 | 0.0 | 88 | 0.1 | 3.7 | 0.0 | 0.0 |
| Red, Cabernet Sauvignon, 13.1% Abv, Average | 1 Sm Glass/125ml | 105.0 | 0.0 | 84 | 0.1 | 2.6 | 0.0 | 0.0 |
| Red, Claret, 12.8% Abv, Average | 1 Sm Glass/120ml | 101.0 | 0.0 | 84 | 0.1 | 3.0 | 0.0 | 0.0 |
| Red, Gamay, 12.3% Abv, Average | 1 Sm Glass/120ml | 95.0 | 0.0 | 79 | 0.1 | 2.4 | 0.0 | 0.0 |
| Red, Low Calorie, Asda* | 1 Glass/125ml | 49.0 | 0.0 | 39 | 0.0 | 0.1 | 0.0 | 0.0 |
| Red, Merlot, 13.3% Abv, Average | 1 Sm Glass/120ml | 101.0 | 0.0 | 84 | 0.1 | 2.5 | 0.0 | 0.0 |
| Red, Petit Sirah, 13.5% Abv, Average | 1 Sm Glass/120ml | 103.0 | 0.0 | 86 | 0.1 | 2.7 | 0.0 | 0.0 |
| Red, Pinot Noir, 13% Abv, Average | 1 Sm Glass/120ml | 100.0 | 0.0 | 83 | 0.1 | 2.3 | 0.0 | 0.0 |
| Red, Sangiovese, 13.6% Abv, Average | 1 Sm Glass/120ml | 104.0 | 0.0 | 87 | 0.1 | 2.6 | 0.0 | 0.0 |
| Red, Syrah, 13.1% Abv, Average | 1 Sm Glass/120ml | 101.0 | 0.0 | 84 | 0.1 | 2.6 | 0.0 | 0.0 |
| Red, Zinfandel, 13.9% Abv, Average | 1 Sm Glass/120ml | 107.0 | 0.0 | 89 | 0.1 | 2.9 | 0.0 | 0.0 |
| *Rose, Medium, Average* | *1 Glass/120ml* | *85.0* | *0.0* | *71* | *0.1* | *2.5* | *0.0* | *0.0* |
| Rose, White Grenache, Blossom Hill* | 1 Glass/250ml | 210.0 | 0.0 | 84 | 0.0 | 3.2 | 0.0 | 0.0 |
| Rose, White Zinfandel, Ernest & Julio Gallo* | 1 Sm Glass/125ml | 89.0 | 0.0 | 71 | 0.0 | 0.0 | 0.0 | 0.0 |
| Sangria, Average | 1 Glass/120ml | 91.0 | 0.0 | 76 | 0.1 | 9.9 | 0.0 | 0.1 |
| Spritzer, White, Echo Falls* | 1 Serving/200ml | 78.0 | 0.0 | 39 | 0.0 | 0.0 | 0.0 | 0.0 |
| White, Chenin Blanc, 12% Abv, Average | 1 Sm Glass/120ml | 97.0 | 0.0 | 81 | 0.1 | 3.3 | 0.0 | 0.0 |
| *White, Dry, Average* | *1 Glass/120ml* | *79.0* | *0.0* | *66* | *0.1* | *0.6* | *0.0* | *0.0* |
| White, Fume Blanc, 13.1% Abv, Average | 1 Sm Glass/120ml | 100.0 | 0.0 | 83 | 0.1 | 2.3 | 0.0 | 0.0 |
| White, Gewurztraminer, 12.6% Abv, Average | 1 Sm Glass/120ml | 98.0 | 0.0 | 82 | 0.1 | 2.6 | 0.0 | 0.0 |
| White, Late Harvest, 10.6% Abv, Average | 1 Sm Glass/120ml | 136.0 | 0.0 | 113 | 0.1 | 13.4 | 0.0 | 0.0 |
| *White, Medium, Average* | *1 Small Glass/120ml* | *89.0* | *0.0* | *74* | *0.1* | *3.0* | *0.0* | *0.0* |
| White, Muller-Thurgau, 11.3% Abv, Average | 1 Sm Glass/120ml | 92.0 | 0.0 | 77 | 0.1 | 3.5 | 0.0 | 0.0 |
| White, Muscat, 11% Abv, Average | 1 Sm Glass/120ml | 100.0 | 0.0 | 83 | 0.1 | 5.2 | 0.0 | 0.0 |

**W**

| | Measure INFO/WEIGHT | per Measure KCAL | per Measure FAT | Nutrition Values per 100g / 100ml KCAL | PROT | CARB | FAT | FIBRE |
|---|---|---|---|---|---|---|---|---|
| **WINE** | | | | | | | | |
| White, Non Alcoholic, Ame* | 1 Glass/120ml | 46.0 | 0.0 | 38 | 0.0 | 9.5 | 0.0 | 0.0 |
| White, Pinot Blanc, 13.3% Abv, Average | 1 Sm Glass/120ml | 98.0 | 0.0 | 82 | 0.1 | 0.0 | 0.0 | 0.0 |
| White, Pinot Grigio, 13.4% Abv, Average | 1 Sm Glass/120ml | 101.0 | 0.0 | 84 | 0.1 | 2.1 | 0.0 | 0.0 |
| White, Riesling, 11.9% Abv, Average | 1 Sm Glass/120ml | 97.0 | 0.0 | 81 | 0.1 | 3.7 | 0.0 | 0.0 |
| White, Sauvignon Blanc, 13.1% Abv, Average | 1 Sm Glass/120ml | 98.0 | 0.0 | 82 | 0.1 | 2.0 | 0.0 | 0.0 |
| White, Semillon, 12.5% Abv, Average | 1 Sm Glass/120ml | 100.0 | 0.0 | 83 | 0.1 | 3.1 | 0.0 | 0.0 |
| *White, Sparkling, Average* | *1 Glass/120ml* | *89.0* | *0.0* | *74* | *0.3* | *5.1* | *0.0* | *0.0* |
| *White, Sweet, Average* | *1 Glass/120ml* | *113.0* | *0.0* | *94* | *0.2* | *5.9* | *0.0* | *0.0* |
| **WINE GUMS** | | | | | | | | |
| Co-Op* | 1 Sweet/6g | 20.0 | 0.0 | 337 | 3.5 | 80.8 | 0.0 | 0.0 |
| Haribo* | 1 Pack/175g | 609.0 | 0.0 | 348 | 0.1 | 86.4 | 0.2 | 0.4 |
| Light, Maynards* | 1 Pack/42g | 90.0 | 0.0 | 215 | 4.6 | 48.0 | 0.2 | 27.9 |
| Maynards* | 1 Sweet/6g | 20.0 | 0.0 | 325 | 5.8 | 74.2 | 0.6 | 0.0 |
| Mini, Co-Op* | 1 Sweet/2g | 7.0 | 0.0 | 330 | 6.0 | 76.0 | 0.1 | 0.0 |
| Mini, Rowntree's* | 1 Sm Bag/36g | 125.0 | 0.0 | 348 | 6.7 | 80.5 | 0.0 | 0.0 |
| Sainsbury's* | 1 Sweet/6g | 19.0 | 0.0 | 314 | 7.7 | 70.3 | 0.2 | 0.0 |
| SmartPrice, Asda* | 1 Sweet/6g | 20.0 | 0.0 | 332 | 4.0 | 79.0 | 0.0 | 0.0 |
| Somerfield* | 1 Sweet/6g | 22.0 | 0.0 | 343 | 6.4 | 76.9 | 0.4 | 0.5 |
| Sour, Bassett's* | ¼ Bag/50g | 159.0 | 0.0 | 319 | 3.7 | 78.0 | 0.0 | 0.0 |
| Tesco* | 1 Serving/100g | 316.0 | 0.0 | 316 | 7.7 | 70.7 | 0.2 | 0.1 |
| **WINKLES** | | | | | | | | |
| *Boiled* | *1oz/28g* | *20.0* | *0.0* | *72* | *15.4* | *0.0* | *1.2* | *0.0* |
| **WISPA** | | | | | | | | |
| Bite, with Biscuit in Caramel, Cadbury* | 1 Bar/47g | 240.0 | 13.0 | 510 | 6.4 | 56.9 | 28.6 | 0.0 |
| Cadbury* | 1 Bar/40g | 210.0 | 13.0 | 525 | 6.7 | 53.0 | 32.2 | 0.7 |
| Gold, Cadbury* | 1 Bar/52g | 263.0 | 15.0 | 505 | 5.7 | 57.0 | 28.0 | 0.0 |
| Mint, Cadbury* | 1 Bar/50g | 275.0 | 17.0 | 550 | 7.0 | 54.7 | 33.6 | 0.0 |
| **WONTON** | | | | | | | | |
| Prawn, Dim Sum Selection, Sainsbury's* | 1 Wonton/10g | 26.0 | 1.0 | 259 | 11.3 | 26.8 | 11.8 | 1.3 |
| Prawn, Oriental Selection, Waitrose* | 1 Wonton/18g | 45.0 | 2.0 | 252 | 9.1 | 29.2 | 11.0 | 1.1 |
| Prawn, Oriental Snack Selection, Sainsbury's* | 1 Wonton/20g | 53.0 | 3.0 | 265 | 10.6 | 25.6 | 13.4 | 2.0 |
| **WOTSITS** | | | | | | | | |
| BBQ, Walkers* | 1 Bag/21g | 108.0 | 6.0 | 515 | 4.5 | 57.0 | 30.0 | 1.3 |
| Flamin' Hot, Walkers* | 1 Bag/19g | 99.0 | 6.0 | 520 | 5.0 | 57.0 | 30.0 | 1.2 |
| Prawn Cocktail, Walkers* | 1 Bag/19g | 101.0 | 6.0 | 530 | 5.5 | 57.0 | 31.0 | 1.1 |
| Really Cheesy, Big Eat, Walkers* | 1 Bag/36g | 196.0 | 12.0 | 545 | 5.5 | 56.0 | 33.0 | 1.1 |
| Really Cheesy, Walkers* | 1 Bag/19g | 104.0 | 6.0 | 545 | 5.5 | 56.0 | 33.0 | 1.1 |
| **WRAP** | | | | | | | | |
| All Day Breakfast, M & S* | 1 Pack/196g | 529.0 | 31.0 | 270 | 10.8 | 21.2 | 16.0 | 1.4 |
| American Deli, Shapers, Boots* | 1 Pack/172g | 249.0 | 4.0 | 145 | 9.5 | 21.0 | 2.6 | 2.0 |
| Beef Fajita, Boots* | 1 Pack/200g | 352.0 | 8.0 | 176 | 9.5 | 25.5 | 4.2 | 3.1 |
| Beef in Black Bean, M & S* | 1 Pack/150g | 337.0 | 17.0 | 225 | 10.2 | 20.5 | 11.4 | 1.6 |
| Brie & Cranberry, M & S* | 1 Pack/225g | 550.0 | 28.0 | 245 | 6.1 | 27.3 | 12.4 | 1.7 |
| Cajun, GFY, Asda* | 1 Pack/176g | 231.0 | 2.0 | 131 | 9.0 | 21.0 | 1.2 | 0.9 |
| Cajun Chicken, Tesco* | 1 Pack/184g | 415.0 | 17.0 | 225 | 9.8 | 25.1 | 9.0 | 1.9 |
| Chargrilled Chicken, Perfectly Balanced, Waitrose* | 1 Pack/230g | 361.0 | 7.0 | 157 | 10.3 | 22.7 | 2.9 | 2.9 |
| Cheese & Bean, Tesco* | 1 Pack/105g | 235.0 | 9.0 | 224 | 7.0 | 28.6 | 9.0 | 1.0 |
| Chicken, Barbecue, GFY, Asda* | 1 Pack/176g | 294.0 | 4.0 | 167 | 9.6 | 26.4 | 2.5 | 1.8 |
| Chicken, Barbecue, Shapers, Boots* | 1 Pack/196g | 271.0 | 4.0 | 138 | 15.0 | 16.0 | 1.8 | 3.5 |
| Chicken, Cheddar & Peppers, Cajun, Sainsbury's* | 1 Pack/242g | 535.0 | 27.0 | 221 | 10.4 | 19.8 | 11.0 | 2.1 |
| Chicken, Chilli, GFY, Asda* | 1 Pack/194g | 277.0 | 4.0 | 143 | 9.1 | 21.6 | 2.2 | 2.3 |
| Chicken, Louisiana Style, GFY, Asda* | 1 Pack/195g | 355.0 | 3.0 | 182 | 11.0 | 31.0 | 1.5 | 2.0 |
| Chicken, M & S* | 1 Pack/247g | 530.0 | 25.0 | 215 | 8.2 | 23.4 | 10.1 | 1.6 |

## WRAP

| INFO/WEIGHT | Measure KCAL | per Measure FAT | KCAL | PROT | CARB | FAT | FIBRE |
|---|---|---|---|---|---|---|---|
| Chicken, Mediterranean Style, Waitrose* | 1 Pack/183g | 296.0 | 11.0 | 162 | 8.3 | 18.6 | 6.0 | 2.3 |
| Chicken, Mexican Style, Co-Op* | 1 Pack/163g | 367.0 | 15.0 | 225 | 11.0 | 26.0 | 9.0 | 3.0 |
| Chicken, Moroccan, BGTY, Sainsbury's* | 1 Pack/207g | 315.0 | 3.0 | 152 | 9.4 | 25.3 | 1.5 | 0.0 |
| Chicken, Nacho, No Mayo, Asda* | 1 Pack/183g | 392.0 | 14.0 | 214 | 12.0 | 24.3 | 7.6 | 3.1 |
| Chicken, Salsa, Light Choices, Tesco* | 1 Pack/219g | 340.0 | 6.0 | 155 | 9.7 | 22.6 | 2.7 | 1.9 |
| Chicken, Southern Fried, Fresh for You, Tesco* | 1 Pack/206g | 485.0 | 24.0 | 235 | 8.6 | 22.7 | 11.8 | 2.0 |
| Chicken, Southern Style, Ginsters* | 1 Wrap/210g | 527.0 | 28.0 | 251 | 7.4 | 24.8 | 13.5 | 2.2 |
| Chicken, Tasties* | 1 Pack/149g | 324.0 | 11.0 | 218 | 11.7 | 26.5 | 7.1 | 0.0 |
| Chicken, Thai, Spiced, Salad, Eat Well, M & S* | 1 Pack/122g | 91.0 | 1.0 | 75 | 5.2 | 9.5 | 1.2 | 1.5 |
| Chicken & Bacon, Simple Solutions, Tesco* | 1 Pack/300g | 474.0 | 23.0 | 158 | 20.7 | 1.2 | 7.8 | 0.5 |
| Chicken & Bacon Caesar, COU, M & S* | 1 Pack/170g | 260.0 | 4.0 | 153 | 10.6 | 22.0 | 2.5 | 2.1 |
| Chicken & Bacon Caesar Salad, Asda* | 1 Pack/160g | 565.0 | 35.0 | 353 | 18.0 | 20.8 | 22.0 | 0.9 |
| Chicken & Cous Cous, BGTY, Sainsbury's* | 1 Pack/230g | 359.0 | 9.0 | 156 | 8.8 | 21.5 | 3.9 | 0.0 |
| Chicken & Cous Cous, Moroccan Style, GFY, Asda* | 1 Pack/164g | 307.0 | 2.0 | 187 | 12.0 | 32.0 | 1.2 | 1.8 |
| Chicken Caesar, HL, Tesco* | 1 Pack/200g | 296.0 | 4.0 | 148 | 10.2 | 22.3 | 2.0 | 2.2 |
| Chicken Caesar, Tesco* | 1 Pack /215g | 516.0 | 24.0 | 240 | 11.6 | 23.0 | 11.3 | 1.2 |
| Chicken Fajita, Asda* | 1 Pack/180g | 369.0 | 17.0 | 205 | 9.4 | 20.6 | 9.4 | 0.4 |
| Chicken Fajita, Daily Bread* | 1 Pack/191g | 392.0 | 11.0 | 205 | 9.4 | 29.4 | 5.5 | 0.0 |
| Chicken Fajita, Finest, Tesco* | 1 Pack/213g | 422.0 | 16.0 | 198 | 9.0 | 24.0 | 7.3 | 1.9 |
| Chicken Fajita, Shapers, Boots* | 1 Pack/216g | 291.0 | 5.0 | 135 | 14.0 | 15.0 | 2.4 | 3.1 |
| Chicken Fajita, Tesco* | 1 Pack/220g | 407.0 | 12.0 | 185 | 10.6 | 23.2 | 5.3 | 1.8 |
| Chicken Fajita, VLH Kitchens | 1 Pack/170g | 311.0 | 8.8 | 183 | 10.6 | 25.0 | 5.2 | 0.0 |
| Chicken Fillet with Cheese & Bacon, Asda* | 1 Pack/164g | 366.0 | 21.0 | 223 | 25.0 | 1.4 | 13.0 | 0.0 |
| Chicken Jalfrezi, Boots* | 1 Pack/215g | 456.0 | 16.0 | 212 | 8.6 | 28.0 | 7.3 | 1.7 |
| Chicken Nacho, HL, Tesco* | 1 Pack/223g | 390.0 | 10.0 | 175 | 12.3 | 21.2 | 4.5 | 2.6 |
| Chicken Salad, Roast, Sainsbury's* | 1 Pack/214g | 443.0 | 20.0 | 207 | 10.0 | 20.9 | 9.3 | 2.5 |
| Chicken Sweet & Sour, Ginsters* | 1 Pack/150g | 378.0 | 6.0 | 252 | 13.4 | 40.8 | 3.9 | 2.4 |
| Chicken Thai Style, Boots* | 1 Pack/156g | 290.0 | 10.0 | 186 | 11.0 | 21.0 | 6.4 | 2.2 |
| Chicken Tikka, Finest, Tesco* | 1 Pack/227g | 402.0 | 14.0 | 177 | 5.1 | 24.9 | 6.3 | 2.0 |
| Chicken Tikka, Ginsters* | 1 Pack/150g | 277.0 | 8.0 | 185 | 8.9 | 25.5 | 5.3 | 1.6 |
| Chicken Tikka, HL, Tesco* | 1 Pack/206g | 317.0 | 5.0 | 154 | 11.3 | 22.1 | 2.3 | 1.3 |
| Chicken Tikka, Shaw & Lisle* | 1 Pack/196g | 311.0 | 6.0 | 159 | 9.4 | 18.2 | 3.1 | 0.0 |
| Chicken Tikka Masala, Patak's* | 1 Pack/150g | 252.0 | 10.0 | 168 | 7.8 | 19.3 | 6.6 | 0.0 |
| Chilli Bean & Cheese, Meat Free, Asda* | 1 Wrap/151g | 263.0 | 7.0 | 174 | 7.9 | 25.1 | 4.7 | 4.9 |
| Chilli Beef, Co-Op* | 1 Pack/163g | 310.0 | 10.0 | 190 | 10.0 | 26.0 | 6.0 | 2.0 |
| Chilli Beef, COU, M & S* | 1 Pack/179g | 268.0 | 3.0 | 150 | 10.1 | 23.4 | 1.6 | 2.6 |
| Chilli Chicken, BGTY, Sainsbury's* | 1 Pack/180g | 313.0 | 4.0 | 174 | 10.2 | 28.0 | 2.4 | 0.0 |
| Chinese Chicken, Asda* | 1 Pack/200g | 404.0 | 12.0 | 202 | 9.0 | 28.0 | 6.0 | 0.0 |
| Chinese Chicken, M & S* | 1 Pack/155g | 239.0 | 2.0 | 154 | 14.0 | 22.3 | 1.0 | 2.0 |
| Coronation Chicken, Waitrose* | 1 Pack/164g | 283.0 | 8.0 | 173 | 10.1 | 21.3 | 5.1 | 2.2 |
| Crayfish, Lemon Dressing & Rocket, COU, M & S* | 1 Pack/183g | 274.0 | 5.0 | 150 | 9.5 | 22.5 | 2.7 | 1.2 |
| Crayfish & Rocket, HL, Tesco* | 1 Pack/164g | 270.0 | 5.0 | 165 | 7.5 | 25.9 | 3.1 | 1.9 |
| Dhansak Prawn, M & S* | 1 Pack/208g | 385.0 | 15.0 | 185 | 7.1 | 23.3 | 7.2 | 2.4 |
| Duck, Food to Go, M & S* | 1 Pack/257g | 475.0 | 14.0 | 185 | 8.5 | 25.5 | 5.4 | 1.0 |
| Duck, Hoi Sin, Delicious, Boots* | 1 Pack/214g | 393.0 | 11.0 | 184 | 10.0 | 25.0 | 5.1 | 1.8 |
| Duck, Hoisin, M & S* | 1 Pack/225g | 405.0 | 8.0 | 180 | 8.4 | 27.7 | 3.7 | 1.5 |
| Duck, Hoisin, No Mayo, Tesco* | 1 Pack/184g | 396.0 | 10.0 | 215 | 12.6 | 28.4 | 5.6 | 3.4 |
| Egg Mayonnaise, Tomato & Cress, Sainsbury's* | 1 Pack/255g | 592.0 | 38.0 | 232 | 7.3 | 17.7 | 15.0 | 0.0 |
| Fajita, Steak, Delicatessen, Waitrose* | 1 Pack/232g | 489.0 | 21.0 | 211 | 10.5 | 22.7 | 9.1 | 2.7 |
| Feta Cheese, GFY, Asda* | 1 Pack/165g | 256.0 | 7.0 | 155 | 7.0 | 22.0 | 4.3 | 2.1 |
| Feta Cheese Flat Bread, COU, M & S* | 1 Pack/180g | 225.0 | 4.0 | 125 | 6.3 | 20.6 | 2.2 | 1.9 |
| Fiery Mexican Cheese, Ginsters* | 1 Pack/150g | 291.0 | 11.0 | 194 | 7.4 | 25.0 | 7.3 | 1.8 |
| Goats Cheese & Tomato, TTD, Sainsbury's* | 1 Pack/204g | 420.0 | 17.0 | 206 | 7.0 | 25.6 | 8.4 | 0.0 |

W

| | Measure INFO/WEIGHT | per Measure KCAL | FAT | Nutrition Values per 100g / 100ml KCAL | PROT | CARB | FAT | FIBRE |
|---|---|---|---|---|---|---|---|---|

## WRAP

| | Measure INFO/WEIGHT | per Measure KCAL | FAT | KCAL | PROT | CARB | FAT | FIBRE |
|---|---|---|---|---|---|---|---|---|
| Greek Feta, Tortilla, Shapers, Boots* | 1 Pack/169g | 271.0 | 5.0 | 160 | 6.7 | 27.0 | 2.7 | 1.6 |
| Greek Feta Salad, Shapers, Boots* | 1 Pack/158g | 241.0 | 6.0 | 153 | 6.4 | 24.0 | 3.6 | 1.2 |
| Greek Salad, COU, M & S* | 1 Pack/180g | 288.0 | 5.0 | 160 | 6.0 | 27.2 | 2.7 | 2.3 |
| Greek Salad, M & S* | 1 Pack/179g | 250.0 | 4.0 | 140 | 8.1 | 21.5 | 2.5 | 1.0 |
| Greek Salad, Sainsbury's* | 1 Pack/167g | 242.0 | 6.0 | 145 | 6.7 | 21.2 | 3.7 | 1.8 |
| Green Thai Prawn, BGTY, Sainsbury's* | 1 Pack/200g | 237.0 | 3.0 | 118 | 7.0 | 19.2 | 1.5 | 1.5 |
| Gressingham Duck & Hoi Sin Sauce, TTD, Sainsbury's* | 1 Pack/199g | 354.0 | 9.0 | 178 | 9.3 | 24.8 | 4.6 | 0.0 |
| Ham, Cheese & Pickle Tortilla, Weight Watchers* | 1 Pack/170g | 296.0 | 5.0 | 174 | 10.9 | 26.4 | 2.8 | 1.2 |
| Houmous, Royal London Hospital* | 1 Pack/200g | 318.0 | 13.0 | 159 | 6.3 | 20.0 | 6.7 | 0.0 |
| Houmous & Chargrilled Vegetables, Shapers, Boots* | 1 Pack/186g | 301.0 | 5.0 | 162 | 5.8 | 29.0 | 2.7 | 3.2 |
| King Prawn, Shapers, Boots* | 1 Pack/154g | 227.0 | 2.0 | 147 | 9.2 | 24.0 | 1.4 | 2.1 |
| Mexican Bean, BGTY, Sainsbury's* | 1 Pack/216g | 341.0 | 5.0 | 158 | 9.2 | 24.9 | 2.5 | 1.5 |
| Mexican Bean, GFY, Asda* | 1 Pack/173g | 303.0 | 6.0 | 175 | 5.0 | 31.0 | 3.4 | 2.3 |
| Mexican Bean & Potato in Spinach Tortilla, Daily Bread* | 1 Pack/196g | 329.0 | 11.0 | 168 | 4.9 | 25.0 | 5.4 | 0.0 |
| Mexican Three Bean, M & S* | 1 Pack/235g | 435.0 | 18.0 | 185 | 6.1 | 21.6 | 7.8 | 2.8 |
| Mexican Tortilla, Ainsley Harriott* | 1 Pack/230g | 421.0 | 17.0 | 183 | 7.1 | 22.4 | 7.5 | 0.0 |
| Mild Chicken Curry, Patak's* | 1 Pack/150g | 238.0 | 9.0 | 159 | 8.1 | 21.3 | 6.0 | 2.8 |
| Monterey Jack & Ham, Tesco* | 1 Pack/200g | 522.0 | 28.0 | 261 | 7.9 | 25.9 | 14.1 | 0.2 |
| Nacho Chicken, COU, M & S* | 1 Pack/175g | 280.0 | 4.0 | 160 | 10.2 | 24.4 | 2.4 | 2.0 |
| Peking Duck, Asda* | 1 Pack/172g | 427.0 | 18.0 | 248 | 9.4 | 28.5 | 10.7 | 1.1 |
| Peking Duck, Bells* | 1 Pack/139g | 266.0 | 9.0 | 192 | 8.9 | 24.0 | 6.8 | 0.0 |
| Peking Duck, Boots* | 1 Pack/229g | 440.0 | 10.0 | 192 | 8.3 | 30.0 | 4.3 | 2.6 |
| Peking Duck, Finest, Tesco* | 1 Pack/200g | 378.0 | 8.0 | 189 | 8.4 | 29.5 | 4.2 | 0.3 |
| Peking Duck, Shapers, Boots* | 1 Pack/162g | 257.0 | 2.0 | 159 | 9.1 | 28.0 | 1.1 | 1.6 |
| Peking Duck, Shell* | 1 Pack/173g | 337.0 | 12.0 | 195 | 8.7 | 24.2 | 7.1 | 0.0 |
| Peking Duck, Waitrose* | 1 Pack/182g | 319.0 | 6.0 | 175 | 10.0 | 25.9 | 3.5 | 1.6 |
| Pepperoni, Tesco* | 1 Pack/153g | 271.0 | 7.0 | 177 | 6.4 | 26.9 | 4.9 | 1.4 |
| Pork Caribbean Spicy, Ginsters* | 1 Pack/150g | 396.0 | 14.0 | 264 | 11.3 | 34.1 | 9.1 | 2.3 |
| Red Thai Chicken, BGTY, Sainsbury's* | 1 Pack/194g | 384.0 | 8.0 | 198 | 11.3 | 29.3 | 3.9 | 1.0 |
| Red Thai Chicken, Shapers, Boots* | 1 Pack/158g | 254.0 | 4.0 | 161 | 12.0 | 22.0 | 2.6 | 1.4 |
| Roasted Vegetable & Feta, BGTY, Sainsbury's* | 1 Serving/200g | 318.0 | 8.0 | 159 | 5.8 | 25.0 | 4.0 | 0.0 |
| Selection, Chicken, BBQ Steak, Hoisin Duck, M & S* | 1 Pack/334g | 685.0 | 24.0 | 205 | 10.9 | 24.3 | 7.1 | 1.7 |
| Sicilian Lemon & Roasted Vegetable, COU, M & S* | 1 Pack/178g | 240.0 | 4.0 | 135 | 4.9 | 23.8 | 2.1 | 1.9 |
| Smoked Salmon, Finest, Tesco* | 1 Pack/58g | 113.0 | 8.0 | 194 | 15.5 | 0.6 | 14.4 | 0.3 |
| Southern Fried Chicken, Tesco* | 1 Pack/214g | 395.0 | 15.0 | 185 | 9.9 | 20.8 | 6.9 | 2.1 |
| Sushi Salmon & Cucumber, Waitrose* | 1 Pack/180g | 299.0 | 6.0 | 166 | 6.3 | 27.2 | 3.6 | 1.6 |
| Sweet Chilli Chicken, Shapers, Boots* | 1 Pack/195g | 290.0 | 4.0 | 149 | 13.0 | 20.0 | 1.8 | 3.7 |
| Sweet Chilli Chicken, Waitrose* | 1 Pack/200g | 390.0 | 15.0 | 195 | 10.2 | 22.0 | 7.3 | 2.4 |
| Sweet Chilli Noodle, Sainsbury's* | 1 Pack/210g | 399.0 | 10.0 | 190 | 10.6 | 26.1 | 4.8 | 2.1 |
| Tandoori Chicken, GFY, Asda* | 1 Pack/167g | 281.0 | 5.0 | 168 | 10.0 | 26.0 | 2.7 | 1.7 |
| Thai Prawn, COU, M & S* | 1 Pack/181g | 235.0 | 3.0 | 130 | 8.3 | 20.4 | 1.6 | 1.9 |
| Tuna, Sweetcorn & Red Pepper, BGTY, Sainsbury's* | 1 Pack/178g | 306.0 | 8.0 | 172 | 11.5 | 21.2 | 4.6 | 2.1 |
| Tuna Nicoise, BGTY, Sainsbury's* | 1 Pack/181g | 273.0 | 7.0 | 151 | 11.0 | 18.0 | 3.9 | 0.0 |
| Tuna Nicoise, HE, Tesco* | 1 Pack/117g | 160.0 | 3.0 | 137 | 8.3 | 20.6 | 2.3 | 0.5 |
| Turkey, Bacon & Cranberry, COU, M & S* | 1 Pack/144g | 230.0 | 2.0 | 160 | 9.6 | 27.1 | 1.5 | 2.3 |
| Yellow Thai Prawn, COU, M & S* | 1 Pack/171g | 266.0 | 5.0 | 155 | 7.6 | 23.4 | 2.9 | 1.7 |

## WRAP KIT

| | Measure INFO/WEIGHT | per Measure KCAL | FAT | KCAL | PROT | CARB | FAT | FIBRE |
|---|---|---|---|---|---|---|---|---|
| Moroccan Style, Sainsbury's* | 1 Wrap/62g | 205.0 | 9.0 | 332 | 8.0 | 41.1 | 15.1 | 3.6 |

| | Measure INFO/WEIGHT | per Measure | | Nutrition Values per 100g / 100ml | | | | |
|---|---|---|---|---|---|---|---|---|
| | | KCAL | FAT | KCAL | PROT | CARB | FAT | FIBRE |
| **YAM** | | | | | | | | |
| *Baked* | *1oz/28g* | *43.0* | *0.0* | *153* | *2.1* | *37.5* | *0.4* | *1.7* |
| *Boiled, Average* | *1oz/28g* | *37.0* | *0.0* | *133* | *1.7* | *33.0* | *0.3* | *1.4* |
| *Raw* | *1oz/28g* | *32.0* | *0.0* | *114* | *1.5* | *28.2* | *0.3* | *1.3* |
| **YEAST** | | | | | | | | |
| *Bakers, Compressed* | *1oz/28g* | *15.0* | *0.0* | *53* | *11.4* | *1.1* | *0.4* | *0.0* |
| *Dried, Average* | *1 Tbsp/6g* | *10.0* | *0.0* | *169* | *35.6* | *3.5* | *1.5* | *0.0* |
| *Extract* | *1 Tsp/9g* | *16.0* | *0.0* | *180* | *40.7* | *3.5* | *0.4* | *0.0* |
| **YOGHURT** | | | | | | | | |
| 0.1% Fat, Lidl* | 1 Pot/150g | 118.0 | 0.0 | 79 | 4.0 | 15.6 | 0.1 | 0.0 |
| Activia, Danone* | 1 Pot/132g | 125.0 | 4.0 | 94 | 3.5 | 12.8 | 3.2 | 2.0 |
| Apple, Light, Muller* | 1 Pot/200g | 108.0 | 0.0 | 54 | 4.4 | 9.0 | 0.1 | 0.0 |
| Apple & Blackberry, Bio, Sainsbury's* | 1 Pot/125g | 134.0 | 3.0 | 107 | 4.1 | 16.6 | 2.7 | 0.2 |
| Apple & Blackberry, Organic, Yeo Valley* | 1 Pot/125g | 121.0 | 4.0 | 97 | 4.3 | 12.5 | 3.3 | 0.1 |
| Apple & Cinnamon, COU, M & S* | 1 Pot/150g | 67.0 | 0.0 | 45 | 4.2 | 6.1 | 0.1 | 0.2 |
| Apple & Cinnamon, Dessert, Low Fat, Sainsbury's* | 1 Pot/125g | 115.0 | 2.0 | 92 | 4.5 | 14.7 | 1.7 | 0.1 |
| Apple & Cranberry, Smooth, Bio, Fat Free, Shape, Danone* | 1 Pot/120g | 86.0 | 0.0 | 72 | 4.2 | 13.5 | 0.1 | 0.0 |
| Apple & Custard, Low Fat, Sainsbury's* | 1 Pot/125g | 116.0 | 2.0 | 93 | 4.3 | 15.5 | 1.5 | 0.2 |
| Apple & Pear, Low Fat, Sainsbury's* | 1 Pot/125g | 115.0 | 2.0 | 92 | 4.3 | 15.2 | 1.5 | 0.2 |
| Apple & Prune, Fat Free, Yeo Valley* | 1 Pot/125g | 97.0 | 0.0 | 78 | 5.1 | 14.1 | 0.1 | 0.2 |
| Apple & Spice Bio, Virtually Fat Free, Shape, Danone* | 1 Pot/120g | 67.0 | 0.0 | 56 | 5.6 | 7.3 | 0.1 | 0.2 |
| Apricot, Bio, Low Fat, Benecol* | 1 Pot/125g | 98.0 | 1.0 | 78 | 3.9 | 14.3 | 0.6 | 0.0 |
| Apricot, Bio Activia, Danone* | 1 Pot/125g | 121.0 | 4.0 | 97 | 3.7 | 13.3 | 3.2 | 1.7 |
| Apricot, French Style Smooth, Tesco* | 1 Pot/125g | 122.0 | 4.0 | 98 | 3.6 | 14.1 | 3.0 | 0.0 |
| Apricot, Fruity, Mullerlight, Muller* | 1 Pot/200g | 100.0 | 0.0 | 50 | 4.1 | 7.5 | 0.1 | 0.1 |
| Apricot, HL, Tesco* | 1 Pot/125g | 67.0 | 0.0 | 54 | 5.1 | 7.9 | 0.3 | 1.1 |
| Apricot, Layered Fruit, Thick & Creamy, Sainsbury's* | 1 Pot/125g | 141.0 | 3.0 | 113 | 4.1 | 18.0 | 2.7 | 0.2 |
| Apricot, Light, HL, Tesco* | 1 Pot/125g | 54.0 | 0.0 | 43 | 4.1 | 6.3 | 0.2 | 0.9 |
| Apricot, Low Fat, Organic, Sainsbury's* | 1 Pot/125g | 102.0 | 1.0 | 82 | 5.3 | 13.0 | 1.0 | 0.1 |
| Apricot, Low Fat, Tesco* | 1 Pot/125g | 112.0 | 2.0 | 90 | 4.3 | 14.1 | 1.8 | 0.0 |
| Apricot, Organic, Low Fat, Tesco* | 1 Pot/125g | 111.0 | 1.0 | 89 | 5.3 | 14.6 | 1.0 | 0.2 |
| Apricot, Smooth Set French, Sainsbury's* | 1 Pot/125g | 100.0 | 1.0 | 80 | 3.5 | 13.6 | 1.2 | 0.0 |
| Apricot & Mango, 25% Extra Fruit, Low Fat, Asda* | 1 Pot/125g | 120.0 | 1.0 | 96 | 4.6 | 17.0 | 1.1 | 0.0 |
| Apricot & Mango, Low Fat, Tesco* | 1 Pot/125g | 126.0 | 2.0 | 101 | 4.9 | 16.3 | 1.8 | 0.0 |
| Apricot & Mango, Thick & Creamy, Sainsbury's* | 1 Pot/150g | 178.0 | 5.0 | 119 | 4.3 | 17.3 | 3.6 | 0.2 |
| Apricot & Nectarine, HE, Tesco* | 1 Pot/175g | 79.0 | 0.0 | 45 | 2.1 | 8.9 | 0.1 | 0.3 |
| Apricot & Nectarine, Sunshine Selection, Sainsbury's* | 1 Pot/125g | 115.0 | 2.0 | 92 | 4.4 | 15.3 | 1.5 | 0.1 |
| Apricot & Passion Fruit, Fat Free, Yeo Valley* | 1 Pot/125g | 94.0 | 0.0 | 75 | 5.3 | 13.2 | 0.1 | 0.1 |
| Banana, Custard Style, Asda* | 1 Pot/150g | 223.0 | 9.0 | 149 | 3.7 | 20.0 | 6.0 | 0.2 |
| Banana, Low Fat, Asda* | 1 Pot/150g | 148.0 | 1.0 | 99 | 4.6 | 18.0 | 1.0 | 0.1 |
| Banana, Low Fat, Sainsbury's* | 1 Pot/125g | 116.0 | 2.0 | 93 | 4.4 | 15.4 | 1.5 | 0.1 |
| Banana, Low Fat, Tesco* | 1 Pot/125g | 127.0 | 2.0 | 102 | 4.9 | 16.8 | 1.7 | 0.1 |
| Banana & Custard, Smooth, Mullerlight, Muller* | 1 Pot/200g | 106.0 | 0.0 | 53 | 4.0 | 8.4 | 0.1 | 0.6 |
| Banana & Orange, Low Fat, 25% Extra Fruit, Asda* | 1 Pot/125g | 125.0 | 1.0 | 100 | 4.6 | 18.0 | 1.1 | 0.0 |
| Banana Choco Flakes, Crunch Corner, Muller* | 1 Pot/150g | 214.0 | 8.0 | 143 | 4.1 | 22.5 | 5.1 | 0.3 |
| Banana Smooth, M & S* | 1 Pot/150g | 165.0 | 3.0 | 110 | 4.8 | 19.3 | 1.7 | 0.2 |
| Banoffee, Dessert, Low Fat, Sainsbury's* | 1 Pot/125g | 122.0 | 2.0 | 98 | 4.5 | 16.1 | 1.7 | 0.2 |
| Banoffee, Low Fat, Asda* | 1 Pot/125g | 126.0 | 1.0 | 101 | 4.6 | 18.2 | 1.2 | 1.0 |
| Bio Activia, Raspberry, Fat Free, Danone* | 1 Pot/125g | 59.0 | 0.0 | 47 | 4.6 | 6.9 | 0.1 | 2.5 |
| Bio Activia, with Raspberry, Danone* | 1 Pot/125g | 112.0 | 3.0 | 90 | 3.5 | 12.8 | 2.8 | 2.0 |
| Bio Fruits with Cherries, 0% Fat, Danone* | 1 Pot/125g | 65.0 | 0.0 | 52 | 3.6 | 9.1 | 0.1 | 0.0 |
| Black Cherry, Extremely Fruity, Bio, M & S* | 1 Pot/150g | 165.0 | 2.0 | 110 | 4.9 | 18.4 | 1.5 | 0.2 |
| Black Cherry, Extremely Fruity, Low Fat Probiotic, M & S* | 1 Pot/170g | 161.0 | 2.0 | 95 | 4.4 | 17.2 | 1.0 | 0.5 |
| Black Cherry, Extremely Fruity, M & S* | 1 Pot/200g | 220.0 | 3.0 | 110 | 4.9 | 18.4 | 1.5 | 0.2 |

## YOGHURT

| | Measure INFO/WEIGHT | per Measure KCAL | FAT | Nutrition Values per 100g / 100ml KCAL | PROT | CARB | FAT | FIBRE |
|---|---|---|---|---|---|---|---|---|
| Black Cherry, Juicy, Shapers, Boots* | 1 Pot/152g | 91.0 | 2.0 | 60 | 4.0 | 8.4 | 1.1 | 0.5 |
| Black Cherry, Live Bio, Perfeclty Balanced, Waitrose* | 1 Pot/125g | 115.0 | 0.0 | 92 | 4.6 | 18.3 | 0.1 | 0.1 |
| Black Cherry, Low Fat, Asda* | 1 Pot/150g | 142.0 | 1.0 | 95 | 4.6 | 17.4 | 1.0 | 0.2 |
| Black Cherry, Low Fat, Value, Tesco* | 1 Pot/125g | 100.0 | 1.0 | 80 | 2.3 | 16.0 | 0.7 | 0.1 |
| Black Cherry, Perfectly Balanced, Waitrose* | 1 Pot/150g | 120.0 | 0.0 | 80 | 4.2 | 15.6 | 0.1 | 0.3 |
| Black Cherry, Thick & Creamy, Waitrose* | 1 Pot/125g | 139.0 | 3.0 | 111 | 3.7 | 18.3 | 2.5 | 0.4 |
| Black Cherry, Very Cherry, Activ8, Ski, Nestle* | 1 Pot/120g | 116.0 | 2.0 | 97 | 4.3 | 16.1 | 1.7 | 0.2 |
| Black Cherry, Virtually Fat Free, Shapers, Boots* | 1 Pot/125g | 71.0 | 0.0 | 57 | 5.3 | 8.8 | 0.1 | 0.1 |
| Black Cherry, VLH Kitchens* | 1 Pot/150g | 188.0 | 5.6 | 125 | 3.7 | 19.6 | 3.7 | 1.0 |
| Blackberry, BGTY, Sainsbury's* | 1 Pot/150g | 106.0 | 1.0 | 71 | 3.4 | 13.5 | 0.4 | 1.6 |
| Blackberry, Boysenberry & William Pear, M & S* | 1 Pot/150g | 187.0 | 10.0 | 125 | 4.0 | 13.6 | 6.5 | 2.4 |
| Blackberry, Farmhouse, BGTY, Sainsbury's* | 1 Pot/150g | 106.0 | 1.0 | 71 | 3.4 | 13.5 | 0.4 | 1.6 |
| Blackberry, Fat Free, BGTY, Sainsbury's* | 1 Pot/150g | 100.0 | 0.0 | 67 | 3.4 | 13.6 | 0.1 | 1.6 |
| Blackberry, Fat Free, Danone, Shape* | 1 Pot/120g | 74.0 | 0.0 | 62 | 6.7 | 8.4 | 0.2 | 2.4 |
| Blackberry, Sveltesse, Nestle* | 1 Pot/125g | 67.0 | 0.0 | 54 | 4.9 | 8.2 | 0.1 | 0.4 |
| Blackberry, Very Berry, Activ8, Ski, Nestle* | 1 Pot/120g | 114.0 | 2.0 | 95 | 4.4 | 15.5 | 1.7 | 0.7 |
| Blackberry & Apple, BGTY, Sainsbury's* | 1 Pot/122g | 61.0 | 0.0 | 50 | 4.7 | 7.2 | 0.2 | 0.3 |
| Blackberry & Apple, HL, Tesco* | 1 Pot/176g | 86.0 | 0.0 | 49 | 2.1 | 10.0 | 0.1 | 1.5 |
| Blackberry & Raspberry, Fruit Corner, Muller* | 1 Pot/175g | 185.0 | 7.0 | 106 | 3.8 | 14.0 | 3.9 | 1.0 |
| Blackberry & Raspberry Flip, Morrisons* | 1 Pot/175g | 206.0 | 8.0 | 118 | 3.4 | 15.8 | 4.6 | 0.5 |
| Blackcurrant, BGTY, Sainsbury's* | 1 Pot/200g | 100.0 | 0.0 | 50 | 4.8 | 7.3 | 0.2 | 0.1 |
| Blackcurrant, Bio Live, Organic, Yeo Valley* | 1 Pot/150g | 151.0 | 6.0 | 101 | 4.1 | 12.4 | 3.9 | 0.2 |
| Blackcurrant, Extra Special, Asda* | 1 Pot/100g | 163.0 | 9.0 | 163 | 2.6 | 18.0 | 9.0 | 0.0 |
| Blackcurrant, Fat Free, BGTY, Sainsbury's* | 1 Pot/125g | 64.0 | 0.0 | 51 | 4.6 | 8.0 | 0.1 | 1.6 |
| Blackcurrant, Fruity, Mullerlight, Muller* | 1 Pot/200g | 102.0 | 0.0 | 51 | 4.1 | 7.9 | 0.1 | 0.8 |
| Blackcurrant, Low Fat, Sainsbury's* | 1 Pot/125g | 116.0 | 2.0 | 93 | 4.2 | 15.9 | 1.4 | 0.6 |
| Blackcurrant, Munch Bunch, Nestle* | 1 Pot/100g | 107.0 | 3.0 | 107 | 4.4 | 15.3 | 3.1 | 0.5 |
| Blackcurrant, Thick & Creamy, Sainsbury's* | 1 Pot/150g | 171.0 | 5.0 | 114 | 4.3 | 15.9 | 3.6 | 0.4 |
| Blackcurrant & Raspberry, Layers, Mullerlight, Muller* | 1 Pot/175g | 94.0 | 0.0 | 54 | 3.1 | 9.7 | 0.1 | 0.7 |
| Blackcurrant & Vanilla, TTD, Sainsbury's* | 1 Pot/143g | 136.0 | 4.0 | 95 | 3.6 | 13.6 | 2.9 | 1.0 |
| Blackcurrant with Liquorice, Tesco* | 1 Pot/150g | 138.0 | 2.0 | 92 | 4.6 | 15.8 | 1.1 | 0.4 |
| Blueberry, Extremely Fruity, Low Fat, Probiotic, M & S* | 1 Pot/150g | 142.0 | 2.0 | 95 | 4.7 | 14.7 | 1.4 | 1.5 |
| Blueberry, Fat Free, Activia, Danone* | 1 Pot/125g | 64.0 | 0.0 | 51 | 4.7 | 7.8 | 0.1 | 2.4 |
| Blueberry, Fruit Corner, Muller* | 1 Pot/175g | 184.0 | 7.0 | 105 | 3.8 | 13.7 | 3.9 | 0.4 |
| Blueberry, Probiotic, Natural Balance, Asda* | 1 Pot/125g | 102.0 | 3.0 | 82 | 2.1 | 13.1 | 2.3 | 2.6 |
| Blueberry, Wholemilk, Organic, Sainsbury's* | 1 Pot/150g | 123.0 | 5.0 | 82 | 3.5 | 9.2 | 3.5 | 0.1 |
| Blueberry Loganberry, Layered, Bio, Sainsbury's* | 1 Pot/125g | 134.0 | 3.0 | 107 | 4.0 | 16.6 | 2.7 | 0.2 |
| Boysenberry, Low Fat, Yoplait* | 1 Pot/100g | 49.0 | 0.0 | 49 | 5.3 | 6.7 | 0.1 | 0.0 |
| Cappuccino, Thick & Creamy, Safeway* | 1 Pot/150g | 228.0 | 8.0 | 152 | 4.5 | 20.8 | 5.6 | 0.0 |
| Caramel & Praline, Indulgent Greek Style, Somerfield* | 1 Pot/125g | 245.0 | 10.0 | 196 | 4.0 | 28.0 | 8.0 | 0.0 |
| Caramelised Orange, COU, M & S* | 1 Pot/145g | 65.0 | 0.0 | 45 | 4.2 | 6.1 | 0.1 | 0.2 |
| Cereals, Fibre, Bio Activia, Danone* | 1 Pot/120g | 119.0 | 4.0 | 99 | 3.7 | 13.5 | 3.4 | 3.0 |
| Champagne Rhubarb & Vanilla, M & S* | 1 Pot/150g | 195.0 | 9.0 | 130 | 3.8 | 15.7 | 5.8 | 0.8 |
| Cherry, 0% Fat, Yoplait* | 1 Pot/125g | 70.0 | 0.0 | 56 | 3.8 | 9.8 | 0.1 | 0.0 |
| Cherry, 0.1% Fat, Shape, Danone* | 1 Pot/120g | 56.0 | 0.0 | 47 | 4.6 | 6.8 | 0.1 | 2.1 |
| Cherry, Bio, Low Fat, Benecol* | 1 Pot/150g | 121.0 | 1.0 | 81 | 3.8 | 15.2 | 0.6 | 0.0 |
| Cherry, Fat Free, Activia, Danone* | 1 Pot/125g | 71.0 | 0.0 | 57 | 4.7 | 9.4 | 0.1 | 0.9 |
| Cherry, Fruit Corner, Muller* | 1 Pot/175g | 187.0 | 7.0 | 107 | 3.9 | 14.0 | 3.9 | 0.4 |
| Cherry, Greek Style, Shape, Danone* | 1 Pot/125g | 143.0 | 3.0 | 114 | 6.0 | 16.4 | 2.7 | 0.0 |
| Cherry, Light, Fat Free, Muller* | 1 Pot/200g | 94.0 | 0.0 | 47 | 4.1 | 6.7 | 0.1 | 0.2 |
| Cherry, Low Fat, Asda* | 1 Pot/125g | 120.0 | 1.0 | 96 | 4.6 | 17.0 | 1.1 | 0.0 |
| Cherry Bakewell Tart Flavour, Muller* | 1 Pot/175g | 119.0 | 0.0 | 68 | 4.8 | 11.8 | 0.2 | 0.2 |
| Cherry Bio, Co-Op* | 1 Pot/125g | 144.0 | 3.0 | 115 | 4.5 | 17.0 | 2.8 | 0.1 |

# YOGHURT

| INFO/WEIGHT | Measure KCAL | FAT | per Measure KCAL | PROT | CARB | FAT | FIBRE |
|---|---|---|---|---|---|---|---|
| | | | Nutrition Values per 100g / 100ml | | | | |

| | Measure INFO/WEIGHT | KCAL | FAT | KCAL | PROT | CARB | FAT | FIBRE |
|---|---|---|---|---|---|---|---|---|
| Cherry Flip, BFY, Morrisons* | 1 Pot/175g | 93.0 | 1.0 | 53 | 3.9 | 8.7 | 0.3 | 0.4 |
| Cherry Morello Bio, Tesco* | 1 Pot/124g | 51.0 | 0.0 | 41 | 4.4 | 5.4 | 0.2 | 0.9 |
| Chocolate, GFY, Asda* | 1 Pot/200g | 110.0 | 1.0 | 55 | 4.7 | 8.0 | 0.5 | 0.1 |
| Chocolate, Seriously Smooth, Waitrose* | 1 Pot/125g | 157.0 | 3.0 | 126 | 6.0 | 20.1 | 2.4 | 0.1 |
| Chocolate, Vitaline* | 1 Pot/125g | 102.0 | 1.0 | 82 | 3.5 | 15.8 | 0.5 | 0.0 |
| Compote, Greek Style, Natural, With Greek Cherry, M & S* | 1 Pack/240g | 312.0 | 16.0 | 130 | 3.7 | 14.1 | 6.5 | 0.3 |
| Cranberry, Fruit Yoghurt, Bio Activia, Danone* | 1 Pot/125g | 115.0 | 4.0 | 92 | 3.6 | 12.3 | 3.2 | 1.7 |
| Cranberry & Blackcurrant, Fat Free, Bio, Shape, Danone* | 1 Pot/120g | 54.0 | 0.0 | 45 | 4.6 | 5.7 | 0.1 | 0.3 |
| Creamy Cranberry & Raspberry, Shapers, Boots* | 1 Pot/150g | 85.0 | 2.0 | 57 | 4.0 | 7.0 | 1.1 | 1.1 |
| Devon Toffee, Low Fat, Sainsbury's* | 1 Pot/126g | 137.0 | 2.0 | 109 | 4.3 | 19.6 | 1.5 | 0.0 |
| English Plum, The Best, Safeway* | 1 Pot/175g | 245.0 | 11.0 | 140 | 3.2 | 17.4 | 6.4 | 0.3 |
| Exotic Fruits French Set Wholemilk, Asda* | 1 Pot/125g | 125.0 | 4.0 | 100 | 3.6 | 14.1 | 3.2 | 0.0 |
| Fig, Fruit Yoghurt, Bio Activia, Danone* | 1 Pot/125g | 121.0 | 4.0 | 97 | 3.7 | 13.3 | 3.2 | 1.6 |
| Forest Fruits, 0.1% Fat, Shape, Danone* | 1 Pot/120g | 55.0 | 0.0 | 46 | 4.6 | 6.7 | 0.1 | 2.1 |
| Forest Fruits, Fat Free, Bio Activia, Danone* | 1 Pot/125g | 66.0 | 0.0 | 53 | 4.5 | 8.5 | 0.1 | 1.1 |
| Forest Fruits, French Set Wholemilk, Asda* | 1 Pot/125g | 125.0 | 4.0 | 100 | 3.6 | 14.1 | 3.2 | 0.0 |
| Forest Fruits, Layered Greek Style, Shapers, Boots* | 1 Pot/150g | 85.0 | 2.0 | 57 | 3.2 | 7.9 | 1.4 | 2.2 |
| Forest Fruits, M & S* | 1 Pot/150g | 148.0 | 2.0 | 99 | 4.7 | 16.8 | 1.6 | 0.5 |
| French Set, Waitrose* | 1 Pot/125g | 120.0 | 4.0 | 96 | 3.5 | 13.4 | 3.1 | 0.0 |
| French Style, Whole Milk, Smooth Set, Tesco* | 1 Pot/125g | 122.0 | 4.0 | 98 | 3.6 | 14.1 | 3.0 | 0.0 |
| Fruit, Low Fat | 1 Pot/120g | 108.0 | 1.0 | 90 | 4.1 | 17.9 | 0.7 | 0.0 |
| Fruit, Luscious, Low Fat, Bio-Live, Rachel's Organic* | 1 Pot/125g | 115.0 | 2.0 | 92 | 4.0 | 15.3 | 1.6 | 0.0 |
| Fruit Bio, Low Fat, Sainsbury's* | 1 Pot/150g | 156.0 | 2.0 | 104 | 4.6 | 18.9 | 1.1 | 0.3 |
| Fruit Whole Milk | 1 Pot/150g | 157.0 | 4.0 | 105 | 5.1 | 15.7 | 2.8 | 0.0 |
| Fruits of the Forest, Nestle* | 1 Pot/125g | 122.0 | 2.0 | 98 | 3.4 | 16.7 | 1.6 | 0.0 |
| Fruits of the Forest, Smooth Set, Co-Op* | 1 Pot/125g | 95.0 | 1.0 | 76 | 3.7 | 12.5 | 0.9 | 0.0 |
| Fruity Favourites, Organic, Yeo Valley* | 1 Pot/125g | 126.0 | 5.0 | 101 | 4.1 | 12.4 | 3.9 | 0.2 |
| Fudge, Devonshire Style, Finest, Tesco* | 1 Pot/150g | 281.0 | 14.0 | 187 | 3.7 | 22.4 | 9.2 | 0.0 |
| Fudge, Thick & Creamy, Co-Op* | 1 Pot/150g | 196.0 | 7.0 | 131 | 3.8 | 17.6 | 5.0 | 0.0 |
| Fudge, Thick & Creamy, M & S* | 1 Pot/150g | 195.0 | 7.0 | 130 | 4.4 | 17.3 | 5.0 | 0.7 |
| Fudge, Thick & Creamy, Waitrose* | 1 Pot/150g | 196.0 | 4.0 | 131 | 4.4 | 21.5 | 3.0 | 0.0 |
| Garden Fruit, Wholemilk, Bio Live, Rachel's Organic* | 1 Pot/125g | 109.0 | 4.0 | 87 | 3.5 | 10.5 | 3.4 | 0.0 |
| **Goats Whole Milk** | **1 Carton/150g** | **94.0** | **6.0** | **63** | **3.5** | **3.9** | **3.8** | **0.0** |
| Gooseberry, Custard Style, Co-Op* | 1 Pot/150g | 216.0 | 8.0 | 144 | 3.7 | 19.3 | 5.3 | 0.3 |
| Gooseberry, Custard Style, Shapers, Boots* | 1 Pot/151g | 106.0 | 1.0 | 70 | 3.9 | 12.0 | 0.7 | 0.2 |
| Gooseberry, Low Fat, Sainsbury's* | 1 Pot/125g | 112.0 | 2.0 | 90 | 4.4 | 14.6 | 1.5 | 0.2 |
| Gooseberry, Low Fat, Tesco* | 1 Pot/125g | 119.0 | 2.0 | 95 | 4.3 | 14.5 | 1.8 | 0.0 |
| Gooseberry & Vanilla, TTD, Sainsbury's* | 1 Pot/150g | 142.0 | 4.0 | 95 | 3.7 | 13.6 | 2.9 | 0.4 |
| Greek, 0% Fat, Strained, Authentic, Total, Fage* | ¼ Pot/125g | 65.0 | 0.0 | 52 | 9.0 | 4.0 | 0.0 | 0.0 |
| Greek, 2% Fat, Strained, Authentic, Total, Fage* | 1 Pot/150g | 100.0 | 3.0 | 67 | 8.4 | 3.8 | 2.0 | 0.0 |
| Greek, Strained, Authentic, Original, Total, Fage* | 1 Pot/200g | 260.0 | 20.0 | 130 | 6.8 | 3.2 | 10.0 | 0.0 |
| Greek, with Honey, Strained, Authentic, Total, Fage* | 1 Pot/150g | 255.0 | 12.0 | 170 | 5.4 | 19.0 | 8.0 | 0.0 |
| Greek, with Strawberry, 2% Fat, Total, Fage* | 1 Pot/150g | 139.0 | 2.0 | 93 | 6.7 | 12.9 | 1.6 | 0.0 |
| Greek Style, & Nectarines, Food to Go, M & S* | 1 Pack/200g | 100.0 | 4.0 | 50 | 2.9 | 6.3 | 2.1 | 1.0 |
| Greek Style, Honey, Selection Pack, Organic, Tesco* | 1 Pot/100g | 156.0 | 9.0 | 156 | 4.1 | 15.3 | 8.7 | 0.0 |
| Greek Style, Honey Topped, Tesco* | 1 Pot/140g | 203.0 | 12.0 | 145 | 3.6 | 13.4 | 8.6 | 0.0 |
| Greek Style, Layered, Honey, Shapers, Boots* | 1 Pot/150g | 136.0 | 3.0 | 91 | 4.2 | 14.0 | 2.0 | 0.0 |
| Greek Style, Natural, Fat Free, Tesco* | ½ Pot/100g | 55.0 | 0.0 | 55 | 7.5 | 4.8 | 0.2 | 0.4 |
| Greek Style with Honey, Asda* | 1 Pot/150g | 225.0 | 13.0 | 150 | 4.0 | 13.9 | 8.7 | 0.0 |
| Greek Style with Strawberries, Asda* | 1 Pot/125g | 159.0 | 8.0 | 127 | 3.2 | 13.6 | 6.6 | 0.2 |
| Greek Style with Strawberry, Morrisons* | 1 Pot/125g | 162.0 | 8.0 | 130 | 3.3 | 14.4 | 6.6 | 0.0 |
| Greek Style with Toffee & Hazelnuts, Asda* | 1 Pot/125g | 230.0 | 11.0 | 184 | 3.7 | 23.1 | 8.6 | 0.1 |
| Greek Style with Tropical Fruits, Asda* | 1 Pot/125g | 164.0 | 8.0 | 131 | 3.3 | 14.5 | 6.6 | 0.3 |

Y

## YOGHURT

| | Measure INFO/WEIGHT | per Measure KCAL | per Measure FAT | KCAL | PROT | CARB | FAT | FIBRE |
|---|---|---|---|---|---|---|---|---|
| | | | | Nutrition Values per 100g / 100ml | | | | |
| Guava & Orange, Fat Free, Organic, Yeo Valley* | 1 Pot/125g | 92.0 | 0.0 | 74 | 5.3 | 13.0 | 0.1 | 0.2 |
| Guava & Passion Fruit, Virtualy Fat Free, Tesco* | 1 Pot/125g | 56.0 | 0.0 | 45 | 4.2 | 6.7 | 0.2 | 1.2 |
| Hazelnut, Low Fat, Asda* | 1 Pot/150g | 150.0 | 3.0 | 100 | 5.1 | 14.7 | 2.3 | 0.2 |
| Hazelnut, Low Fat, Sainsbury's* | 1 Pot/125g | 135.0 | 3.0 | 108 | 4.5 | 16.4 | 2.7 | 0.2 |
| Hazelnut, Low Fat, Tesco* | 1 Pot/150g | 159.0 | 4.0 | 106 | 4.5 | 16.0 | 2.7 | 0.0 |
| Hazelnut, Morrisons* | 1 Pot/150g | 159.0 | 4.0 | 106 | 3.9 | 16.9 | 2.6 | 0.0 |
| Hazelnut Crunchy, Jordans* | 1 Pot/150g | 231.0 | 6.0 | 154 | 5.2 | 22.2 | 4.0 | 1.1 |
| Honey, Greek Style, Co-Op* | 1 Pot/150g | 228.0 | 13.0 | 152 | 4.0 | 13.8 | 8.5 | 0.0 |
| Honey, Greek Style, Organic, Sainsbury's* | 1 Pot/100g | 156.0 | 9.0 | 156 | 4.1 | 15.3 | 8.7 | 0.1 |
| Honey, Low Fat, Asda* | 1 Pot/125g | 130.0 | 1.0 | 104 | 4.6 | 19.0 | 1.1 | 0.0 |
| Honey & Ginger, Enhanced, Low Fat, Asda* | 1 Pot/150g | 150.0 | 2.0 | 100 | 4.6 | 18.0 | 1.1 | 0.0 |
| Honey & Ginger, Tesco* | 1 Pot/150g | 150.0 | 2.0 | 100 | 4.6 | 18.0 | 1.1 | 0.0 |
| Honey & Ginger, Waitrose* | 1 Pot/150g | 226.0 | 11.0 | 151 | 3.7 | 17.0 | 7.6 | 0.1 |
| Honey & Muesli, Breakfast Break, Tesco* | 1 Pot/170g | 207.0 | 5.0 | 122 | 3.9 | 20.5 | 2.7 | 0.6 |
| Honey & Multigrain, Breakfast Selection, Sainsbury's* | 1 Pot/125g | 126.0 | 2.0 | 101 | 4.4 | 17.4 | 1.5 | 0.2 |
| Italian Lemon, Amore Luxury, Muller* | 1 Pot/150g | 219.0 | 12.0 | 146 | 2.8 | 16.2 | 7.8 | 0.1 |
| Jaffa Orange, Low Fat, Co-Op* | 1 Pot/150g | 126.0 | 1.0 | 84 | 3.9 | 15.0 | 0.9 | 0.4 |
| Jaffa Orange, Morrisons* | 1 Pot/150g | 133.0 | 2.0 | 89 | 3.6 | 16.2 | 1.1 | 0.0 |
| Kiwi, BGTY, Sainsbury's* | 1 Pot/125g | 61.0 | 0.0 | 49 | 4.6 | 7.5 | 0.1 | 0.2 |
| Kiwi, Fruit, Activia, Danone* | 1 Pot/125g | 119.0 | 4.0 | 95 | 3.6 | 12.7 | 3.3 | 0.3 |
| Kiwi Cereal, Fibre, Bio Activia, Danone* | 1 Pot/120g | 124.0 | 4.0 | 103 | 3.8 | 14.5 | 3.3 | 3.0 |
| Layered, Eat Smart, Safeway* | 1 Pot/125g | 81.0 | 0.0 | 65 | 4.1 | 11.3 | 0.1 | 0.4 |
| Lemon, COU, M & S* | 1 Pot/200g | 90.0 | 0.0 | 45 | 4.2 | 6.6 | 0.1 | 0.4 |
| Lemon, Greek Style, GFY, Asda* | 1 Pot/150g | 124.0 | 4.0 | 83 | 4.1 | 10.0 | 2.9 | 0.1 |
| Lemon, Greek Style, Shape, Danone* | 1 Pot/125g | 140.0 | 3.0 | 112 | 5.9 | 15.9 | 2.7 | 0.0 |
| Lemon, Low Fat, Asda* | 1 Pot/125g | 130.0 | 1.0 | 104 | 4.6 | 19.0 | 1.1 | 0.0 |
| Lemon, Low Fat, Organic, Sainsbury's* | 1 Pot/125g | 121.0 | 1.0 | 97 | 5.1 | 17.0 | 1.0 | 0.1 |
| Lemon, Low Fat, Safeway* | 1 Pot/150g | 154.0 | 2.0 | 103 | 4.6 | 18.7 | 1.1 | 0.1 |
| Lemon, Smooth Set French, Low Fat, Sainsbury's* | 1 Pot/125g | 100.0 | 1.0 | 80 | 3.5 | 13.6 | 1.2 | 0.0 |
| Lemon, Summer, Biopot, Onken* | 1 Pot/150g | 154.0 | 4.0 | 103 | 3.9 | 15.9 | 2.6 | 0.1 |
| Lemon, Thick & Fruity, Citrus Fruits, Weight Watchers* | 1 Pot/120g | 49.0 | 0.0 | 41 | 4.0 | 5.8 | 0.1 | 0.1 |
| Lemon & Lime, BGTY, Sainsbury's* | 1 Pot/125g | 66.0 | 0.0 | 53 | 4.6 | 8.3 | 0.1 | 1.1 |
| Lemon & Lime, Fat Free, Shape, Danone* | 1 Pot/120g | 61.0 | 0.0 | 51 | 4.5 | 7.3 | 0.1 | 0.1 |
| Lemon Cheesecake, Dessert Style, Mullerlight, Muller* | 1 Pot/175g | 108.0 | 0.0 | 62 | 4.4 | 10.0 | 0.2 | 0.0 |
| Lemon Cheesecake, Probiotic, GFY, Asda* | 1 Pot/125g | 66.0 | 0.0 | 53 | 4.7 | 8.4 | 0.1 | 0.2 |
| Lemon Cheesecake, Sveltesse, Nestle* | 1 Pot/125g | 96.0 | 0.0 | 77 | 4.9 | 14.0 | 0.2 | 0.3 |
| Lemon Curd, Farmhouse, TTD, Sainsbury's* | 1 Pot/150g | 181.0 | 6.0 | 121 | 4.1 | 17.7 | 3.7 | 0.2 |
| Lemon Curd, Indulgent, Dessert, Waitrose* | 1 Pot/150g | 277.0 | 14.0 | 185 | 4.1 | 21.5 | 9.2 | 0.0 |
| Lemon Lime Mousse, Shapers, Boots* | 1 Pot/90g | 89.0 | 4.0 | 99 | 4.2 | 11.0 | 4.2 | 0.1 |
| Lemon Meringue, Eat Smart, Safeway* | 1 Pot/125g | 67.0 | 0.0 | 54 | 4.7 | 8.6 | 0.1 | 0.4 |
| Lemon Meringue, Sveltesse, Nestle* | 1 Pot/125g | 60.0 | 0.0 | 48 | 4.1 | 7.7 | 0.1 | 0.1 |
| Lemon Smooth Set, Co-Op* | 1 Pot/125g | 95.0 | 1.0 | 76 | 3.7 | 12.5 | 0.9 | 0.0 |
| Light, Fat Free, Apricot, Muller* | 1 Pot/200g | 98.0 | 0.0 | 49 | 4.1 | 7.3 | 0.1 | 0.1 |
| Loganberry, Low Fat, Sainsbury's* | 1 Pot/125g | 111.0 | 2.0 | 89 | 4.2 | 14.5 | 1.5 | 0.2 |
| Loganberry, Sainsbury's* | 1 Pot/150g | 193.0 | 9.0 | 129 | 3.9 | 14.2 | 6.2 | 0.6 |
| Low Calorie | 1 Pot/120g | 49.0 | 0.0 | 41 | 4.3 | 6.0 | 0.2 | 0.0 |
| Madagascan Vanilla, Indulgent, Dessert, Waitrose* | 1 Pot/150g | 240.0 | 11.0 | 160 | 3.7 | 19.2 | 7.6 | 0.0 |
| Mandarin, Fat Free, Mullerlight, Muller* | 1 Pot/200g | 104.0 | 0.0 | 52 | 4.0 | 8.2 | 0.1 | 0.0 |
| Mandarin, Longley Farm* | 1 Pot/150g | 160.0 | 6.0 | 107 | 4.9 | 13.3 | 3.8 | 0.0 |
| Mandarin, Low Fat, Asda* | 1 Pot/125g | 101.0 | 1.0 | 81 | 4.6 | 13.0 | 1.2 | 0.0 |
| S | 1 Pot/120g | 74.0 | 0.0 | 62 | 6.6 | 8.6 | 0.1 | 2.2 |
| Mango, Fruit Yoghurt, Bio Activia, Danone* | 1 Pot/125g | 121.0 | 4.0 | 97 | 3.7 | 13.4 | 3.2 | 1.6 |
| Mango, Light, Muller* | 1 Pot/200g | 110.0 | 0.0 | 55 | 4.3 | 9.2 | 0.1 | 0.0 |

# YOGHURT

| | Measure INFO/WEIGHT | per Measure KCAL | FAT | Nutrition Values per 100g / 100ml KCAL | PROT | CARB | FAT | FIBRE |
|---|---|---|---|---|---|---|---|---|
| Mango, Thick & Fruity, Tropical Fruit, Weight Watchers* | 1 Pot/120g | 49.0 | 0.0 | 41 | 3.9 | 6.0 | 0.1 | 1.1 |
| Mango, Virtually Fat Free, Tesco* | 1 Pot/125g | 56.0 | 0.0 | 45 | 4.1 | 6.6 | 0.2 | 0.9 |
| Mango & Guava, Sunshine Selection, Sainsbury's* | 1 Pot/125g | 145.0 | 2.0 | 116 | 5.4 | 19.3 | 1.9 | 0.3 |
| Mango & Passion Fruit, Tropical Fruit, Activ8, Ski, Nestle* | 1 Pot/120g | 114.0 | 2.0 | 95 | 4.3 | 15.6 | 1.7 | 0.2 |
| Mango & Pineapple, BGTY, Sainsbury's* | 1 Pot/124g | 63.0 | 0.0 | 51 | 4.6 | 7.6 | 0.2 | 0.2 |
| Mango Bio, HE, Tesco* | 1 Pot/125g | 59.0 | 0.0 | 47 | 4.7 | 6.8 | 0.1 | 0.2 |
| Maple & Cinnamon Granola, Low Fat, Natural, Asda* | 1 Pot/140g | 196.0 | 5.0 | 140 | 6.1 | 21.5 | 3.3 | 0.8 |
| Mississippi Mud Pie, Crunchable, Brooklea* | 1 Pot/140g | 237.0 | 6.0 | 169 | 4.0 | 28.0 | 4.5 | 0.3 |
| Mixed Berries, Jogood, Imlek* | 1 Pot/200g | 172.0 | 4.0 | 86 | 2.9 | 13.4 | 2.2 | 0.0 |
| Mixed Seeds, Probiotic, Yoplait* | 1 Pot/125g | 139.0 | 6.0 | 111 | 4.5 | 13.2 | 4.5 | 3.1 |
| Morello Cherry, Amore Luxury, Muller* | 1 Pot/150g | 216.0 | 12.0 | 144 | 2.8 | 16.3 | 7.8 | 0.1 |
| Morello Cherry, HE, Tesco* | 1 Pot/125g | 57.0 | 0.0 | 46 | 4.2 | 7.1 | 0.1 | 0.1 |
| Morello Cherry, HL, Tesco* | 1 Pot/125g | 56.0 | 0.0 | 45 | 4.1 | 6.6 | 0.2 | 0.9 |
| Muesli Nut, Low Fat | 1 Pot/120g | 134.0 | 3.0 | 112 | 5.0 | 19.2 | 2.2 | 0.0 |
| Natural, Bio, Fat Free, Waitrose* | 1 Pot/150g | 90.0 | 0.0 | 60 | 6.1 | 8.6 | 0.1 | 0.0 |
| Natural, Bio, Very Low Fat, Somerfield* | 1 Pot/150g | 97.0 | 0.0 | 65 | 7.0 | 9.0 | 0.0 | 0.0 |
| Natural, Bio Activia, Individual Pots, Danone* | 1 Pot/125g | 86.0 | 4.0 | 69 | 4.2 | 5.5 | 3.4 | 0.0 |
| Natural, Bio Life, Easiyo* | 1 Pot/150g | 95.0 | 3.0 | 63 | 5.0 | 6.7 | 1.8 | 0.0 |
| Natural, Bio Live, Fat Free, Organic, Yeo Valley* | 1 Pot/150g | 87.0 | 0.0 | 58 | 5.9 | 8.4 | 0.1 | 0.0 |
| Natural, Bio Live, Low Fat, Organic, Waitrose* | ¼ Pot/125g | 81.0 | 1.0 | 65 | 5.8 | 8.3 | 1.0 | 0.0 |
| Natural, Bio Live, Organic, Yeo Valley* | 1 Pot/150g | 123.0 | 6.0 | 82 | 4.5 | 6.6 | 4.2 | 0.0 |
| Natural, Bio Live, Very Low Fat, Ann Forshaw's* | 1 Pot/125g | 52.0 | 0.0 | 42 | 5.0 | 5.5 | 0.1 | 0.0 |
| Natural, Bio Set, Low Fat, Sainsbury's* | 1 Pot/150g | 78.0 | 2.0 | 52 | 3.9 | 5.7 | 1.5 | 0.0 |
| Natural, Danone* | 1 Pot/125g | 71.0 | 4.0 | 57 | 3.2 | 3.8 | 2.9 | 0.0 |
| Natural, Fat Free, Rachel's Organic* | 1 Pot/500g | 180.0 | 0.0 | 36 | 3.9 | 4.8 | 0.1 | 0.0 |
| Natural, Greek Style, Asda* | 1 Pot/450g | 580.0 | 49.0 | 129 | 4.6 | 4.8 | 10.8 | 0.0 |
| Natural, Greek Style, Bio Live, Rachel's Organic* | 1 Pot/450g | 513.0 | 40.0 | 114 | 3.7 | 4.6 | 9.0 | 0.0 |
| Natural, Greek Style, Less Than 3% Fat, BGTY, Sainsbury's* | ¼ Pot/125g | 99.0 | 3.0 | 79 | 5.6 | 8.1 | 2.7 | 0.0 |
| Natural, Greek Style, Low Fat, Morrisons* | 1 Pot/125g | 96.0 | 3.0 | 77 | 6.4 | 6.7 | 2.7 | 0.0 |
| Natural, Greek Style, Organic, Tesco* | 1 Pot/500g | 665.0 | 50.0 | 133 | 4.5 | 6.2 | 10.0 | 0.0 |
| Natural, Greek Style, with Cow's Milk, Tesco* | 1 Pot/150g | 214.0 | 16.0 | 143 | 4.5 | 6.6 | 10.9 | 0.0 |
| Natural, Greek Style, with Honey Sauce, Sainsbury's* | 1 Pot/140g | 206.0 | 11.0 | 147 | 3.3 | 15.7 | 7.9 | 0.0 |
| Natural, Longley Farm* | 1 Pot/150g | 118.0 | 5.0 | 79 | 4.8 | 7.0 | 3.5 | 0.0 |
| Natural, Low Fat, Asda* | 1 Pot/450g | 279.0 | 4.0 | 62 | 6.1 | 7.1 | 1.0 | 0.0 |
| *Natural, Low Fat, Average* | *1 Pot/ 112g* | *67.0* | *1.0* | *60* | *5.4* | *7.0* | *1.3* | *0.0* |
| Natural, Low Fat, Bio, Co-Op* | 1 Pot/150g | 97.0 | 1.0 | 65 | 6.0 | 8.0 | 1.0 | 0.0 |
| Natural, Low Fat, Bio, Sainsbury's* | 1 Pot/125g | 85.0 | 2.0 | 68 | 5.6 | 7.9 | 1.5 | 0.0 |
| Natural, Low Fat, Live, Waitrose* | 1 Pot/175g | 114.0 | 2.0 | 65 | 5.8 | 8.2 | 1.0 | 0.0 |
| Natural, Low Fat, Morrisons* | 1 Pot/150g | 93.0 | 1.0 | 62 | 6.1 | 7.1 | 1.0 | 0.0 |
| Natural, Low Fat, Somerfield* | 1 Pot/150g | 78.0 | 2.0 | 52 | 4.5 | 5.9 | 1.1 | 0.0 |
| Natural, Low Fat, Tesco* | ¼ Pot/125g | 87.0 | 2.0 | 70 | 5.5 | 7.8 | 1.5 | 0.0 |
| Natural, Low Fat, TTD, Sainsbury's* | 1 Pot/125g | 80.0 | 2.0 | 64 | 6.7 | 4.6 | 1.8 | 0.0 |
| Natural, Luxury, Bio Live, Jersey Dairy* | 1 Pot/150g | 225.0 | 12.0 | 150 | 4.6 | 8.2 | 8.0 | 0.0 |
| Natural, Organic, Yeo Valley* | 1 Pot/150g | 120.0 | 6.0 | 80 | 4.7 | 6.9 | 3.7 | 0.0 |
| Natural, Probiotic, 2% Fat, Sainsbury's* | ¼ Pot/125g | 76.0 | 2.0 | 61 | 4.9 | 7.0 | 1.5 | 0.0 |
| Natural, Probiotic, Eat Smart, Morrisons* | ¼ Pot/125g | 76.0 | 0.0 | 61 | 6.3 | 8.3 | 0.3 | 0.0 |
| Natural, Set, Asda* | 1 Pot/450g | 256.0 | 4.0 | 57 | 5.1 | 6.8 | 1.0 | 0.0 |
| Natural, Set, Low Fat, Waitrose* | 1 Pot/150g | 99.0 | 2.0 | 66 | 5.7 | 8.1 | 1.2 | 0.0 |
| Natural, Whole Milk, Set, Biopot, Onken* | 1 Pot/150g | 108.0 | 6.0 | 72 | 3.9 | 5.7 | 3.7 | 0.0 |
| Natural, Wholemilk, Organic, Sainsbury's* | 1 Pot/125g | 86.0 | 5.0 | 69 | 3.7 | 5.0 | 3.8 | 0.1 |
| Natural, with Cow's Milk, Greek Style, Sainsbury's* | ½ Pot/100g | 143.0 | 11.0 | 143 | 4.5 | 6.6 | 10.9 | 0.0 |
| Nectarine & Orange, Best There Is, Yoplait* | 1 Pot/122g | 131.0 | 2.0 | 107 | 4.7 | 18.0 | 1.6 | 0.0 |
| Nectarine & Orange, Channel Island, M & S* | 1 Pot/150g | 157.0 | 5.0 | 105 | 4.5 | 14.7 | 3.3 | 0.3 |

## YOGHURT

| | Measure INFO/WEIGHT | per Measure KCAL | per Measure FAT | Nutrition Values per 100g / 100ml KCAL | PROT | CARB | FAT | FIBRE |
|---|---|---|---|---|---|---|---|---|
| Nectarine & Orange, M & S* | 1 Pot/150g | 147.0 | 2.0 | 98 | 4.9 | 16.0 | 1.6 | 0.3 |
| Nectarine & Orange, Virtually Fat Free, Shape, Danone* | 1 Pot/120g | 55.0 | 0.0 | 46 | 4.7 | 5.8 | 0.1 | 0.1 |
| Nectarine & Orange, Virtually Fat Free, Tesco* | 1 Pot/125g | 57.0 | 0.0 | 46 | 4.1 | 7.2 | 0.1 | 0.0 |
| Nectarine & Passion Fruit, 0.1% Fat, Shape, Danone* | 1 Pot/120g | 55.0 | 0.0 | 46 | 4.6 | 6.7 | 0.1 | 2.1 |
| Nectarine & Passion Fruit, BGTY, Sainsbury's* | 1 Pot/151g | 122.0 | 1.0 | 81 | 3.2 | 16.3 | 0.4 | 0.6 |
| Orange, Greek Style, Boots* | 1 Pot/140g | 207.0 | 12.0 | 148 | 3.7 | 14.0 | 8.6 | 0.2 |
| Orange, Greek Style, Shape, Danone* | 1 Pot/125g | 140.0 | 3.0 | 112 | 6.0 | 16.0 | 2.7 | 0.1 |
| Orange, Low Fat, Tesco* | 1 Pot/125g | 114.0 | 2.0 | 91 | 4.3 | 14.5 | 1.8 | 0.0 |
| Orange, Sprinkled with Dark Chocolate, Light, Muller* | 1 Pot/165g | 84.0 | 1.0 | 51 | 4.0 | 7.1 | 0.5 | 0.1 |
| Orange & Pineapple, Tropical Fruit, Activ8, Ski, Nestle* | 1 Pot/120g | 112.0 | 2.0 | 93 | 4.4 | 15.1 | 1.7 | 0.2 |
| Orange Blossom Honey, Finest, Tesco* | 1 Pot/150g | 237.0 | 11.0 | 158 | 3.5 | 20.1 | 7.1 | 0.0 |
| Passion Fruit with Elderflower Extract, Tesco* | 1 Pot/150g | 147.0 | 2.0 | 98 | 4.7 | 17.3 | 1.1 | 0.2 |
| Peach, BGTY, Sainsbury's* | 1 Pot/125g | 61.0 | 0.0 | 49 | 4.7 | 7.2 | 0.2 | 0.2 |
| Peach, Custard Style, Low Fat, Sainsbury's* | 1 Pot/125g | 110.0 | 2.0 | 88 | 4.4 | 14.2 | 1.5 | 0.1 |
| Peach, Economy, Sainsbury's* | 1 Pot/125g | 92.0 | 0.0 | 74 | 2.8 | 14.7 | 0.4 | 0.0 |
| Peach, Fat Free, Bio Activia, Danone* | 1 Sm Pot/125g | 71.0 | 0.0 | 57 | 4.7 | 9.3 | 0.1 | 1.0 |
| Peach, Forbidden Fruits, Rachel's Organic* | 1 Pot/125g | 156.0 | 8.0 | 125 | 3.4 | 14.0 | 6.1 | 0.0 |
| Peach, Low Fat, Asda* | 1 Pot/125g | 118.0 | 1.0 | 95 | 4.7 | 16.7 | 1.1 | 0.2 |
| Peach, Low Fat, Basics, Sainsbury's* | 1 Pot/125g | 84.0 | 1.0 | 67 | 4.0 | 10.4 | 1.0 | 0.1 |
| Peach, Low Fat, Probiotic, Tesco* | 1 Pot/125g | 106.0 | 2.0 | 85 | 3.9 | 14.3 | 1.4 | 0.3 |
| Peach, Low Fat, Yeo Valley* | 1 Pot/125g | 112.0 | 1.0 | 90 | 4.6 | 15.3 | 1.1 | 0.1 |
| Peach, Luscious, Low Fat, Rachel's Organic* | 1 Pot/125g | 112.0 | 2.0 | 90 | 4.0 | 14.9 | 1.6 | 0.2 |
| Peach, Smooth Style, Mullerlight, Muller* | 1 Pot/125g | 59.0 | 0.0 | 47 | 4.1 | 6.9 | 0.1 | 0.2 |
| Peach & Apricot, 0.1% Fat, Shape, Danone* | 1 Pot/120g | 55.0 | 0.0 | 46 | 4.6 | 6.7 | 0.1 | 2.1 |
| Peach & Apricot, Fruit Corner, Muller* | 1 Pot/175g | 191.0 | 7.0 | 109 | 3.9 | 14.5 | 3.9 | 0.3 |
| Peach & Apricot, HL, Tesco* | 1 Pot/92g | 42.0 | 0.0 | 46 | 4.0 | 7.4 | 0.1 | 1.0 |
| Peach & Apricot, Light, HL, Tesco* | 1 Pot/200g | 82.0 | 0.0 | 41 | 3.9 | 6.2 | 0.1 | 1.0 |
| Peach & Lemon Balm, Biowild, Onken* | 1 Pot/175g | 157.0 | 3.0 | 90 | 4.3 | 14.9 | 1.5 | 0.1 |
| Peach & Mango, Juicy, Shapers, Boots* | 1 Pot/150g | 88.0 | 2.0 | 59 | 4.0 | 8.3 | 1.1 | 0.5 |
| Peach & Mango, Thick & Creamy, Waitrose* | 1 Pot/125g | 136.0 | 3.0 | 109 | 3.7 | 17.8 | 2.5 | 0.3 |
| Peach & Maracuya, Mullerlight, Muller* | 1 Pot/200g | 102.0 | 0.0 | 51 | 4.5 | 8.1 | 0.1 | 0.0 |
| Peach & Papaya, Fat Free, Yeo Valley* | 1 Pot/125g | 94.0 | 0.0 | 75 | 5.3 | 13.1 | 0.1 | 0.1 |
| Peach & Papaya, Waitrose* | 1 Pot/150g | 129.0 | 0.0 | 86 | 4.2 | 17.1 | 0.1 | 0.2 |
| Peach & Passion Fruit, Fat Free, Shape, Danone* | 1 Pot/120g | 74.0 | 0.0 | 62 | 6.6 | 8.6 | 0.1 | 2.3 |
| Peach & Passion Fruit, Fruit Layered, Bio, GFY, Asda* | 1 Pot/126g | 77.0 | 0.0 | 61 | 4.0 | 11.0 | 0.1 | 0.5 |
| Peach & Passion Fruit, Layers, Mullerlight, Muller* | 1 Pot/175g | 94.0 | 0.0 | 54 | 3.1 | 9.7 | 0.1 | 0.2 |
| Peach & Passion Fruit, Lite Biopot, Onken* | 1/5 Pot/100g | 45.0 | 0.0 | 45 | 4.6 | 6.0 | 0.2 | 0.2 |
| Peach & Passion Fruit, Tropical Fruit, Activ8, Ski, Nestle* | 1 Pot/120g | 112.0 | 2.0 | 93 | 4.4 | 15.1 | 1.7 | 0.2 |
| Peach & Passion Fruit Flip, Morrisons* | 1 Pot/175g | 89.0 | 1.0 | 51 | 3.9 | 8.2 | 0.3 | 0.6 |
| Peach & Passionfruit, BGTY, Sainsbury's* | 1 Pot/125g | 69.0 | 0.0 | 55 | 4.9 | 8.6 | 0.1 | 0.1 |
| Peach & Pear, Seriously Fruity, Low Fat, Waitrose* | 1 Pot/125g | 110.0 | 1.0 | 88 | 4.5 | 15.3 | 1.0 | 0.3 |
| Peach & Vanilla, HL, Tesco* | 1 Pot/125g | 54.0 | 0.0 | 43 | 4.1 | 6.3 | 0.2 | 1.0 |
| Peach & Vanilla, Thick & Creamy, Co-Op* | 1 Pot/150g | 180.0 | 7.0 | 120 | 3.6 | 16.0 | 4.6 | 0.1 |
| Peach & Vanilla Flip, Morrisons* | 1 Pot/175g | 212.0 | 8.0 | 121 | 3.4 | 16.5 | 4.6 | 0.6 |
| Peach Melba, Everyday Low Fat, Co-Op* | 1 Pot/125g | 87.0 | 1.0 | 70 | 3.0 | 13.0 | 0.7 | 0.0 |
| Peach Melba, Low Fat, Tesco* | 1 Pot/125g | 100.0 | 1.0 | 80 | 2.3 | 16.0 | 0.7 | 0.1 |
| Peach Melba, Sveltesse, Nestle* | 1 Pot/126g | 70.0 | 0.0 | 56 | 4.7 | 9.1 | 0.1 | 0.2 |
| Peach Melba, Value, Tesco* | 1 Pot/125g | 100.0 | 1.0 | 80 | 2.3 | 16.0 | 0.7 | 0.1 |
| Peaches, Farmhouse, BGTY, Sainsbury's* | 1 Pot/150g | 133.0 | 1.0 | 89 | 3.2 | 17.8 | 0.4 | 0.3 |
| Pear, Rosehip & Marigold, Biowild, Onken* | 1 Pot/175g | 161.0 | 3.0 | 92 | 4.4 | 15.1 | 1.5 | 0.3 |
| Pear & Butterscotch, Finest, Tesco* | 1 Pot/150g | 412.0 | 21.0 | 275 | 5.0 | 32.3 | 14.0 | 0.5 |
| Pear & Vanilla, Thick & Creamy, Weight Watchers* | 1 Pot/120g | 54.0 | 1.0 | 45 | 4.2 | 5.8 | 0.5 | 0.2 |
| Phish Food, Frozen, Lower Fat, Ben & Jerry's* | ½ Pot/211g | 464.0 | 11.0 | 220 | 4.0 | 40.0 | 5.0 | 1.5 |

| | Measure INFO/WEIGHT | per Measure KCAL | FAT | Nutrition Values per 100g / 100ml KCAL | PROT | CARB | FAT | FIBRE |
|---|---|---|---|---|---|---|---|---|
| **YOGHURT** | | | | | | | | |
| Pineapple, Channel Island, M & S* | 1 Pot/150g | 165.0 | 5.0 | 110 | 4.3 | 15.9 | 3.3 | 0.3 |
| Pineapple, Extremely Fruity, M & S* | 1 Pot/200g | 200.0 | 3.0 | 100 | 4.3 | 17.6 | 1.4 | 0.2 |
| Pineapple, Finest, Tesco* | 1 Pot/200g | 220.0 | 6.0 | 110 | 3.5 | 17.5 | 2.9 | 0.2 |
| Pineapple, HL, Tesco* | 1 Pot/125g | 69.0 | 0.0 | 55 | 5.1 | 8.1 | 0.3 | 1.1 |
| Pineapple, Low Fat, Bio, Asda* | 1 Pot/150g | 144.0 | 2.0 | 96 | 4.6 | 17.0 | 1.1 | 0.1 |
| Pineapple, Low Fat, Tesco* | 1 Pot/125g | 111.0 | 2.0 | 89 | 4.6 | 13.4 | 1.7 | 0.0 |
| Pineapple, Thick & Creamy, Waitrose* | 1 Pot/125g | 136.0 | 3.0 | 109 | 3.6 | 17.9 | 2.5 | 0.2 |
| Pineapple, Thick & Fruity, Tropical Fruit, Weight Watchers* | 1 Pot/120g | 56.0 | 0.0 | 47 | 3.9 | 7.7 | 0.1 | 0.9 |
| Pineapple, Virtually Fat Free, Tesco* | 1 Pot/125g | 55.0 | 0.0 | 44 | 4.1 | 6.5 | 0.2 | 0.9 |
| Pineapple, Vitality, Low Fat, with Omega 3, Muller* | 1 Pot/150g | 138.0 | 3.0 | 92 | 4.2 | 13.8 | 1.9 | 0.7 |
| Pineapple & Grapefruit, BGTY, Sainsbury's* | 1 Pot/125g | 67.0 | 0.0 | 54 | 4.4 | 8.8 | 0.1 | 0.1 |
| Pineapple & Passion Fruit, Soya, Light, Alpro* | 1 Pot/120g | 62.0 | 1.0 | 52 | 2.1 | 7.3 | 1.1 | 0.8 |
| Pineapple & Peach, Fruity, Mullerlight, Muller* | 1 Pot/200g | 100.0 | 0.0 | 50 | 4.1 | 7.6 | 0.1 | 0.2 |
| Pink Grapefruit, Breakfast Selection, Sainsbury's* | 1 Pot/117g | 109.0 | 2.0 | 93 | 4.2 | 15.9 | 1.4 | 0.1 |
| Pink Grapefruit, Low Fat, Sainsbury's* | 1 Pot/125g | 116.0 | 2.0 | 93 | 4.2 | 15.9 | 1.4 | 0.1 |
| Pink Grapefruit, Thick & Fruity, Weight Watchers* | 1 Pot/120g | 49.0 | 0.0 | 41 | 3.9 | 6.2 | 0.1 | 1.0 |
| *Plain, Low Fat, Average* | *1 Serving/100g* | *63.0* | *2.0* | *63* | *5.2* | *7.0* | *1.5* | *0.0* |
| *Plain, Whole Milk, Average* | *1oz/28g* | *22.0* | *1.0* | *79* | *5.7* | *7.8* | *3.0* | *0.0* |
| Plum, BGTY, Sainsbury's* | 1 Pot/125g | 69.0 | 0.0 | 55 | 4.8 | 8.8 | 0.1 | 0.1 |
| Plum, Bio Live, Summer Selection, Yeo Valley* | 1 Pot/125g | 126.0 | 5.0 | 101 | 4.1 | 12.4 | 3.9 | 0.1 |
| Plum, Low Fat, Sainsbury's* | 1 Pot/125g | 117.0 | 2.0 | 94 | 4.5 | 15.2 | 1.7 | 0.1 |
| Plum & Hop, Biowild, Onken* | 1 Pot/175g | 157.0 | 3.0 | 90 | 4.3 | 14.9 | 1.5 | 0.3 |
| Prune, Breakfast Selection, Sainsbury's* | 1 Pot/125g | 119.0 | 2.0 | 95 | 4.2 | 16.3 | 1.4 | 0.2 |
| Prune, Fruit Yoghurt, Bio Activia, Danone* | 1 Pot/125g | 110.0 | 3.0 | 88 | 3.5 | 12.2 | 2.8 | 0.2 |
| Prune, Vitality, Low Fat, with Omega 3, Muller* | 1 Pot/150g | 144.0 | 3.0 | 96 | 4.7 | 15.0 | 1.9 | 1.1 |
| Raspberry, Bio, Low Fat, Benecol* | 1 Pot/125g | 99.0 | 1.0 | 79 | 3.8 | 14.5 | 0.6 | 0.0 |
| Raspberry, Eat Smart, Safeway* | 1 Pot/127g | 70.0 | 0.0 | 55 | 5.2 | 8.5 | 0.1 | 0.7 |
| Raspberry, Economy, Sainsbury's* | 1 Pot/125g | 85.0 | 1.0 | 68 | 3.0 | 11.9 | 1.0 | 0.0 |
| Raspberry, Extremely Fruity, M & S* | 1 Pot/200g | 190.0 | 3.0 | 95 | 5.0 | 15.6 | 1.5 | 0.5 |
| Raspberry, Farmhouse, TTD, Sainsbury's* | 1 Pot/150g | 148.0 | 4.0 | 99 | 3.6 | 15.0 | 2.8 | 1.6 |
| Raspberry, Fat Free, Activ8, Ski, Nestle* | 1 Pot/120g | 91.0 | 0.0 | 76 | 4.6 | 14.1 | 0.1 | 0.7 |
| Raspberry, Fat Free, BGTY, Sainsbury's* | 1 Pot/125g | 64.0 | 0.0 | 51 | 4.8 | 7.7 | 0.1 | 1.7 |
| Raspberry, Fat Free, Bio Live, Organic, Yeo Valley* | 1 Pot/125g | 97.0 | 0.0 | 78 | 5.2 | 14.0 | 0.1 | 0.4 |
| Raspberry, Forbidden Fruit, Rachel's Organic* | 1 Pot/125g | 155.0 | 8.0 | 124 | 3.4 | 13.8 | 6.1 | 0.1 |
| Raspberry, French Set, Waitrose* | 1 Pot/125g | 120.0 | 4.0 | 96 | 3.5 | 13.4 | 3.1 | 2.0 |
| Raspberry, French Set Wholemilk, Asda* | 1 Pot/125g | 125.0 | 4.0 | 100 | 3.6 | 14.1 | 3.2 | 0.0 |
| Raspberry, Incredibly Fruity, Fat Free, Tesco* | 1 Pot/150g | 112.0 | 0.0 | 75 | 4.8 | 13.1 | 0.1 | 1.0 |
| Raspberry, Light, HL, Tesco* | 1 Pot/200g | 88.0 | 0.0 | 44 | 3.9 | 7.0 | 0.1 | 1.7 |
| Raspberry, Low Fat, Bio, Sainsbury's* | 1 Pot/150g | 145.0 | 2.0 | 97 | 4.7 | 17.0 | 1.1 | 0.7 |
| Raspberry, Low Fat, Probiotic, Tesco* | 1 Pot/170g | 144.0 | 2.0 | 85 | 3.9 | 14.3 | 1.4 | 0.3 |
| Raspberry, Low Fat, Tesco* | 1 Pot/125g | 116.0 | 2.0 | 93 | 4.3 | 14.9 | 1.8 | 0.0 |
| Raspberry, Meadow Fresh* | 1 Sm Pot/125g | 130.0 | 1.0 | 104 | 4.5 | 18.9 | 1.0 | 0.0 |
| Raspberry, Orange & Grain, Eat Smart, Safeway* | 1 Pot/200g | 120.0 | 0.0 | 60 | 4.7 | 9.1 | 0.2 | 0.6 |
| Raspberry, Organic, Yeo Valley* | 1 Pot/150g | 151.0 | 6.0 | 101 | 4.2 | 12.3 | 3.9 | 0.4 |
| Raspberry, Probiotic, Live, Yeo Valley* | 1 Pot/125g | 106.0 | 1.0 | 85 | 5.1 | 14.0 | 1.0 | 0.4 |
| Raspberry, Probiotic, Low Fat, Organic, M & S* | 1 Pot/170g | 127.0 | 2.0 | 75 | 4.4 | 11.5 | 1.4 | 0.4 |
| Raspberry, Sveltesse, Nestle* | 1 Pot/125g | 61.0 | 0.0 | 49 | 4.9 | 7.2 | 0.1 | 0.6 |
| Raspberry & Blackberry, Thick & Creamy, Co-Op* | 1 Pot/150g | 187.0 | 7.0 | 125 | 3.6 | 17.3 | 4.6 | 0.1 |
| Raspberry & Cranberry, BGTY, Sainsbury's* | 1 Pot/125g | 65.0 | 0.0 | 52 | 4.4 | 8.4 | 0.1 | 0.5 |
| Raspberry & Cranberry, Fat Free, Mullerlight, Muller* | 1 Pot/200g | 100.0 | 0.0 | 50 | 4.1 | 7.6 | 0.1 | 0.5 |
| Raspberry & Cranberry, Light, HL, Tesco* | 1 Pot/125g | 55.0 | 0.0 | 44 | 4.2 | 6.3 | 0.2 | 1.1 |
| Raspberry & Redcurrant, Low Fat, Morrisons* | 1 Pot/125g | 117.0 | 2.0 | 94 | 4.4 | 15.4 | 1.6 | 0.7 |
| Raspberry & Redcurrant, Low Fat, Sainsbury's* | 1 Pot/125g | 109.0 | 2.0 | 87 | 4.2 | 14.5 | 1.4 | 0.5 |

Y

## YOGHURT

| INFO/WEIGHT | Measure KCAL | per Measure FAT | KCAL | PROT | CARB | FAT | FIBRE |
|---|---|---|---|---|---|---|---|
| Raspberry Tart, Sveltesse, Nestle* | 1 Pot/125g | 64.0 | 0.0 | 51 | 4.5 | 7.1 | 0.1 | 0.1 |
| Red Berry, Healthy Balance, Corner, Muller* | 1 Pot/150g | 178.0 | 4.0 | 119 | 5.0 | 18.0 | 2.7 | 0.5 |
| Red Berry, Vitality, Low Fat, with Omega 3, Muller* | 1 Pot/150g | 138.0 | 3.0 | 92 | 4.3 | 13.8 | 1.9 | 0.7 |
| Red Cherry, Fat Free, Ski, Nestle* | 1 Pot 120g | 97.0 | 0.0 | 81 | 4.5 | 15.6 | 0.1 | 0.1 |
| Red Cherry, Fruit Layered, GFY, Asda* | 1 Pot/125g | 75.0 | 0.0 | 60 | 3.7 | 11.0 | 0.1 | 0.0 |
| Red Fruits, Crumble Style, Sveltesse, Nestle* | 1 Pot/125g | 100.0 | 0.0 | 80 | 4.9 | 14.6 | 0.2 | 0.4 |
| Rhubarb, Custard Style, Co-Op* | 1 Pot/150g | 202.0 | 8.0 | 135 | 3.7 | 17.2 | 5.3 | 0.3 |
| Rhubarb, Eat Smart, Morrisons* | 1 Pot/200g | 112.0 | 1.0 | 56 | 5.7 | 7.9 | 0.3 | 0.2 |
| Rhubarb, Extremely Fruity, Low Fat, Probiotic, M & S* | 1 Pot/170g | 153.0 | 2.0 | 90 | 4.4 | 15.5 | 1.0 | 0.7 |
| Rhubarb, Farmhouse, TTD, Sainsbury's* | 1 Pot/150g | 148.0 | 5.0 | 99 | 4.3 | 13.4 | 3.1 | 0.3 |
| Rhubarb, Fruit Yoghurt, Bio Activia, Danone* | 1 Pot/125g | 112.0 | 4.0 | 90 | 3.5 | 11.8 | 3.2 | 2.2 |
| Rhubarb, Live Bio, Low Fat, Perfectly Balanced, Waitrose* | 1 Pot/150g | 114.0 | 0.0 | 76 | 4.2 | 14.5 | 0.1 | 0.2 |
| Rhubarb, Longley Farm* | 1 Pot/150g | 165.0 | 6.0 | 110 | 4.9 | 14.3 | 3.7 | 0.0 |
| Rhubarb, Low Fat, Organic, M & S* | 1 Pot/170g | 119.0 | 2.0 | 70 | 4.1 | 10.6 | 1.2 | 0.2 |
| Rhubarb, Low Fat, Organic, Sainsbury's* | 1 Pot/125g | 99.0 | 1.0 | 79 | 5.1 | 12.3 | 1.0 | 0.2 |
| Rhubarb, Low Fat, Sainsbury's* | 1 Pot/125g | 114.0 | 2.0 | 91 | 4.5 | 14.5 | 1.7 | 0.2 |
| Rhubarb, Luscious, Low Fat, Bio Live, Rachel's Organic* | 1 Pot/125g | 104.0 | 2.0 | 83 | 4.0 | 13.1 | 1.6 | 0.1 |
| Rhubarb, M & S* | 1 Pot/150g | 148.0 | 2.0 | 99 | 4.4 | 17.4 | 1.4 | 0.3 |
| Rhubarb, Spiced, Thick & Creamy, COU, M & S* | 1 Pot/170g | 68.0 | 0.0 | 40 | 4.3 | 5.8 | 0.1 | 0.5 |
| Rhubarb & Champagne, Truly Irresistible, Co-Op* | 1 Pot/150g | 195.0 | 8.0 | 130 | 3.5 | 16.6 | 5.5 | 0.2 |
| Rhubarb & Orange, Tesco* | 1 Pot/150g | 145.0 | 2.0 | 97 | 4.6 | 17.1 | 1.1 | 0.5 |
| Rhubarb & Vanilla, Summer, Biopot, Onken* | 1/5 Pot/100g | 106.0 | 3.0 | 106 | 3.8 | 16.9 | 2.6 | 0.3 |
| Rhubarb Crumble, Crunch Corner, Muller* | 1 Pot/150g | 238.0 | 8.0 | 159 | 3.6 | 23.5 | 5.6 | 0.5 |
| Rhubarb Crumble, Layered Style, HE, Tesco* | 1 Pot/125g | 92.0 | 1.0 | 74 | 4.1 | 12.9 | 0.7 | 0.2 |
| Sheep's Milk, Total, Fage* | 1 Pot/200g | 180.0 | 12.0 | 90 | 4.8 | 4.3 | 6.0 | 0.0 |
| Smooth Toffee & Apple, Low Fat, Co-Op* | 1 Pot/125g | 150.0 | 1.0 | 120 | 6.0 | 22.0 | 1.0 | 0.1 |
| Smooth Toffee & Orange, Co-Op* | 1 Pot/125g | 181.0 | 1.0 | 145 | 6.0 | 27.0 | 1.0 | 0.0 |
| Smoothie, Apple, Raspberry & Banana, Sveltesse, Nestle* | 1 Pot/125g | 61.0 | 0.0 | 49 | 4.8 | 7.3 | 0.1 | 0.2 |
| Smoothie, Apple, Strawberry & Peach, Sveltesse, Nestle* | 1 Pot/125g | 61.0 | 0.0 | 49 | 4.8 | 7.3 | 0.1 | 0.1 |
| Smoothie, Orange, Pineapple & Banana, Sveltesse, Nestle* | 1 Pot/125g | 61.0 | 0.0 | 49 | 4.8 | 7.3 | 0.1 | 0.1 |
| Somerset with Vanilla, TTD, Sainsbury's* | 1 Pot/150g | 222.0 | 10.0 | 148 | 4.0 | 18.1 | 6.6 | 0.0 |
| **Soya, Plain, Average** | **1oz/28g** | **20.0** | **1.0** | **72** | **5.0** | **3.9** | **4.2** | **0.0** |
| Soya, Plain, Natural, Dairy Free, Organic, Yofu, Provamel* | 1 Pot/125g | 72.0 | 3.0 | 58 | 4.7 | 2.8 | 2.7 | 0.8 |
| Soya, Red Cherry, Dairy Free, Organic, Yofu, Provamel* | 1 Pot/125g | 101.0 | 3.0 | 81 | 3.9 | 10.5 | 2.2 | 0.8 |
| Spanish Orange, Amore Luxury, Muller* | 1 Pot/150g | 226.0 | 12.0 | 151 | 2.9 | 17.2 | 7.8 | 0.1 |
| Spiced Orange, Dessert, Low Fat, Sainsbury's* | 1 Pot/125g | 121.0 | 2.0 | 97 | 4.5 | 16.0 | 1.7 | 0.1 |
| Sticky Toffee Pudding, Dessert Style, Mullerlight, Muller* | 1 Pot/175g | 108.0 | 0.0 | 62 | 4.4 | 9.9 | 0.2 | 0.2 |
| Strawberries & Cream, Finest, Tesco* | 1 Pot/150g | 205.0 | 10.0 | 137 | 3.4 | 15.4 | 6.9 | 0.5 |
| Strawberry, & Muesli, Breakfast, Tesco* | 1 Pot/170g | 192.0 | 5.0 | 113 | 4.1 | 17.9 | 2.8 | 0.5 |
| Strawberry, & Whole Grain, Bio Break, Tesco* | 1 Pot/175g | 175.0 | 2.0 | 100 | 4.7 | 17.8 | 1.1 | 0.2 |
| Strawberry, Amore for Me, Muller* | 1 Pot/150g | 216.0 | 11.0 | 144 | 2.6 | 17.0 | 7.3 | 0.2 |
| Strawberry, Bettabuy, Morrisons* | 1 Pot/115g | 91.0 | 1.0 | 79 | 4.4 | 12.8 | 1.3 | 0.3 |
| Strawberry, BGTY, Sainsbury's* | 1 Pot/125g | 64.0 | 0.0 | 51 | 4.8 | 7.7 | 0.1 | 1.2 |
| Strawberry, Bio, Co-Op* | 1 Pot/125g | 142.0 | 3.0 | 114 | 4.5 | 16.7 | 2.8 | 0.1 |
| Strawberry, Bio, HE, Tesco* | 1 Pot/125g | 61.0 | 0.0 | 49 | 4.7 | 7.0 | 0.2 | 0.2 |
| Strawberry, Bio Live, Organic, Yeo Valley* | 1 Pot/125g | 125.0 | 5.0 | 100 | 4.4 | 11.7 | 4.0 | 0.1 |
| Strawberry, Bio Virtually Fat Free, Tesco* | 1 Pot/125g | 50.0 | 0.0 | 40 | 4.4 | 5.3 | 0.2 | 0.9 |
| Strawberry, Carb Control, Tesco* | 1 Pot/125g | 61.0 | 1.0 | 49 | 3.7 | 6.3 | 1.0 | 0.2 |
| Strawberry, Childrens, Co-Op* | 1 Pot/125g | 121.0 | 3.0 | 97 | 3.5 | 14.9 | 2.7 | 0.2 |
| Strawberry, Custard Style, Shapers, Boots* | 1 Pot/150g | 117.0 | 1.0 | 78 | 3.9 | 14.0 | 0.7 | 0.5 |
| Strawberry, Duo, Co-Op* | 1 Pot/175g | 219.0 | 9.0 | 125 | 3.0 | 17.0 | 5.0 | 0.7 |
| Strawberry, Eat Smart, Morrisons* | 1 Pot/200g | 116.0 | 1.0 | 58 | 5.7 | 8.5 | 0.3 | 0.3 |
| Strawberry, Everyday Low Fat, Co-Op* | 1 Pot/125g | 87.0 | 1.0 | 70 | 3.0 | 13.0 | 0.7 | 0.0 |

## YOGHURT

| INFO/WEIGHT | Measure KCAL | per Measure FAT | KCAL | PROT | CARB | FAT | FIBRE |
|---|---|---|---|---|---|---|---|
| | | | Nutrition Values per 100g / 100ml | | | | |
| Strawberry, Farmhouse, BGTY, Sainsbury's* | 1 Pot/150g | 106.0 | 1.0 | 71 | 3.2 | 13.7 | 0.4 | 0.5 |
| Strawberry, Fat Free, Activ8, Ski, Nestle* | 1 Pot/120g | 89.0 | 0.0 | 74 | 4.5 | 13.7 | 0.2 | 0.3 |
| Strawberry, Fat Free, Bio Activia, Danone* | 1 Pot/125g | 67.0 | 0.0 | 54 | 4.7 | 8.6 | 0.1 | 0.8 |
| Strawberry, Fat Free, Bio Live, Organic, Yeo Valley* | 1 Pot/125g | 107.0 | 1.0 | 86 | 5.1 | 14.1 | 1.0 | 0.1 |
| Strawberry, Fat Free, Shape, Danone* | 1 Pot/120g | 72.0 | 0.0 | 60 | 6.6 | 8.2 | 0.1 | 2.2 |
| Strawberry, Fat Free, Waitrose* | 1 Pot/150g | 135.0 | 0.0 | 90 | 4.6 | 17.8 | 0.1 | 0.1 |
| Strawberry, Fruit Yoghurt, Bio Activia, Danone* | 1 Pot/125g | 117.0 | 4.0 | 94 | 3.5 | 12.8 | 3.2 | 2.0 |
| Strawberry, Fruity, Mullerlight, Muller* | 1 Pot/200g | 102.0 | 0.0 | 51 | 4.1 | 7.9 | 0.1 | 0.0 |
| Strawberry, Healthy Balance, Corner, Muller* | 1 Pot/135g | 161.0 | 4.0 | 119 | 5.4 | 17.9 | 2.6 | 0.8 |
| Strawberry, Incredibly Fruity, Low Fat, Tesco* | 1 Pot/150g | 135.0 | 1.0 | 90 | 4.0 | 15.3 | 1.0 | 0.4 |
| Strawberry, Light, Fat Free, Muller* | 1 Pot/200g | 102.0 | 0.0 | 51 | 4.1 | 7.7 | 0.1 | 0.2 |
| Strawberry, Light, HL, Tesco* | 1 Pot/200g | 80.0 | 0.0 | 40 | 3.5 | 6.4 | 0.1 | 0.8 |
| Strawberry, Light Choices, Tesco* | 1 Pot/200g | 86.0 | 0.0 | 43 | 4.1 | 6.3 | 0.1 | 0.6 |
| Strawberry, Low Fat, Asda* | 1 Pot/125g | 114.0 | 1.0 | 91 | 4.4 | 16.0 | 1.0 | 0.0 |
| Strawberry, Low Fat, Benecol* | 1 Pot/125g | 98.0 | 1.0 | 78 | 3.7 | 14.5 | 0.6 | 0.0 |
| Strawberry, Low Fat, Organic, Sainsbury's* | 1 Pot/125g | 100.0 | 1.0 | 80 | 5.3 | 12.6 | 1.0 | 0.1 |
| Strawberry, Low Fat, Probiotic, Organic, M & S* | 1 Pot/170g | 136.0 | 2.0 | 80 | 4.8 | 11.6 | 1.4 | 0.4 |
| Strawberry, Low Fat, Tesco* | 1 Pot/125g | 112.0 | 2.0 | 90 | 4.2 | 14.4 | 1.7 | 0.0 |
| Strawberry, Low Fat, Value, Tesco* | 1 Pot/125g | 81.0 | 1.0 | 65 | 2.7 | 11.8 | 0.7 | 0.1 |
| Strawberry, Luscious, Low Fat, Bio Live, Rachel's Organic* | 1 Pot/125g | 100.0 | 2.0 | 80 | 3.9 | 12.5 | 1.6 | 0.1 |
| Strawberry, Luscious, Shapers, Boots* | 1 Pot/150g | 82.0 | 2.0 | 55 | 4.0 | 7.3 | 1.1 | 0.6 |
| Strawberry, Organic, Yeo Valley* | 1 Pot/150g | 144.0 | 5.0 | 96 | 4.3 | 12.4 | 3.3 | 0.1 |
| Strawberry, Perfectly Balanced, Waitrose* | 1 Pot/150g | 136.0 | 0.0 | 91 | 4.6 | 17.8 | 0.1 | 0.1 |
| Strawberry, Petit Filou, Yoplait* | 1 Pot/60g | 62.0 | 2.0 | 104 | 6.6 | 12.6 | 2.9 | 0.2 |
| Strawberry, Senga, Low Fat, Sainsbury's* | 1 Pot/125g | 112.0 | 1.0 | 90 | 4.6 | 15.7 | 1.0 | 0.3 |
| Strawberry, Seriously Fruity, Low Fat, Waitrose* | 1 Pot/150g | 130.0 | 1.0 | 87 | 4.5 | 15.0 | 1.0 | 0.3 |
| Strawberry, Smooth, Activ8, Ski, Nestle* | 1 Pot/120g | 113.0 | 2.0 | 94 | 4.6 | 14.8 | 1.7 | 0.7 |
| Strawberry, Smooth Set French, Low Fat, Sainsbury's* | 1 Pot/125g | 112.0 | 4.0 | 90 | 3.7 | 11.8 | 3.2 | 0.0 |
| Strawberry, Soya, Dairy Free, Organic, Yofu, Provamel* | 1 Pot/125g | 101.0 | 3.0 | 81 | 3.9 | 10.6 | 2.2 | 0.8 |
| Strawberry, Thick & Creamy, Co-Op* | 1 Pot/150g | 181.0 | 7.0 | 121 | 3.6 | 16.4 | 4.6 | 0.1 |
| Strawberry, Thick & Creamy, Waitrose* | 1 Pot/125g | 135.0 | 3.0 | 108 | 3.7 | 17.6 | 2.5 | 0.4 |
| Strawberry, Thick & Fruity, Fat Free, Weight Watchers* | 1 Pot/120g | 48.0 | 0.0 | 40 | 4.1 | 5.7 | 0.1 | 0.5 |
| Strawberry, Thick & Fruity, Probiotic, COU, M & S* | 1 Pot/170g | 76.0 | 0.0 | 45 | 4.1 | 7.3 | 0.1 | 0.4 |
| Strawberry, Very Berry, Activ8, Ski, Nestle* | 1 Pot/120g | 110.0 | 2.0 | 92 | 4.3 | 15.0 | 1.7 | 0.3 |
| Strawberry, Virtually Fat Free, Morrisons* | 1 Pot/200g | 114.0 | 0.0 | 57 | 5.4 | 8.4 | 0.2 | 0.0 |
| Strawberry, Virtually Fat Free, Organic, Yeo Valley* | 1 Pot/125g | 97.0 | 0.0 | 78 | 5.1 | 14.3 | 0.1 | 0.1 |
| Strawberry, Virtually Fat Free, Shapers, Boots* | 1 Pot/124g | 67.0 | 0.0 | 54 | 5.2 | 8.1 | 0.1 | 0.1 |
| Strawberry, Virtually Fat Free, Tesco* | 1 Pot/125g | 52.0 | 0.0 | 42 | 4.1 | 6.0 | 0.2 | 1.0 |
| Strawberry, Vitality, Low Fat, with Omega 3, Muller* | 1 Pot/150g | 139.0 | 3.0 | 93 | 4.3 | 14.0 | 1.9 | 0.8 |
| Strawberry, Wholemilk, Organic, Sainsbury's* | 1 Pot/150g | 123.0 | 5.0 | 82 | 3.5 | 9.2 | 3.5 | 0.1 |
| Strawberry, Yoplait* | 1 Pot/125g | 61.0 | 0.0 | 49 | 4.2 | 7.6 | 0.2 | 0.9 |
| Strawberry & Cornish Clotted Cream, M & S* | 1 Pot/150g | 217.0 | 12.0 | 145 | 3.2 | 15.4 | 7.7 | 0.5 |
| Strawberry & French Vanilla, Amore Luxury, Muller* | 1 Pot/150g | 225.0 | 12.0 | 150 | 2.9 | 17.0 | 7.8 | 0.1 |
| Strawberry & Raspberry, Bio Live, Organic, Yeo Valley* | 1 Pot/125g | 125.0 | 5.0 | 100 | 4.2 | 12.0 | 3.9 | 0.1 |
| Strawberry & Raspberry, HL, Tesco* | 1 Pot/125g | 57.0 | 0.0 | 46 | 4.2 | 7.0 | 0.1 | 0.0 |
| Strawberry & Raspberry, Low Fat, Asda* | 1 Pot/150g | 142.0 | 1.0 | 95 | 4.6 | 17.4 | 1.0 | 0.2 |
| Strawberry & Raspberry, Low Fat, Sainsbury's* | 1 Pot/125g | 109.0 | 2.0 | 87 | 4.2 | 14.3 | 1.4 | 0.2 |
| Strawberry & Rhubarb, Channel Island, M & S* | 1 Pot/150g | 157.0 | 4.0 | 105 | 3.9 | 15.4 | 3.0 | 0.0 |
| Strawberry & Rhubarb, Low Fat, Sainsbury's* | 1 Pot/125g | 107.0 | 2.0 | 86 | 4.2 | 14.1 | 1.4 | 0.2 |
| Strawberry Cheesecake, Eat Smart, Safeway* | 1 Pot/125g | 64.0 | 0.0 | 51 | 4.7 | 7.7 | 0.1 | 0.3 |
| Strawberry Crumble, Crunch Corner, Muller* | 1 Pot/150g | 234.0 | 8.0 | 156 | 3.6 | 22.9 | 5.6 | 0.5 |
| Strawberry Orange Balls. Crunch Corner, Muller* | 1 Pot/150g | 222.0 | 8.0 | 148 | 4.0 | 20.8 | 5.4 | 0.2 |
| Strawberry Shortcake, Crunch Corner, Muller* | 1 Pot/150g | 231.0 | 9.0 | 154 | 3.9 | 21.0 | 5.7 | 0.1 |

**Y**

## YOGHURT

| | Measure INFO/WEIGHT | per Measure KCAL | FAT | Nutrition Values per 100g / 100ml KCAL | PROT | CARB | FAT | FIBRE |
|---|---|---|---|---|---|---|---|---|
| Summer Selection, Fat Free, Organic, Yeo Valley* | 1 Pot/125g | 89.0 | 0.0 | 71 | 5.2 | 12.3 | 0.1 | 0.2 |
| Summer Selection, Thick & Fruity, COU, M & S* | 1 Pot/145g | 75.0 | 0.0 | 52 | 4.2 | 7.8 | 0.1 | 0.5 |
| Summerfruits, Fat Free, Bio Live, Rachel's Organic* | 1 Pot/125g | 120.0 | 2.0 | 96 | 4.7 | 15.3 | 1.8 | 0.0 |
| Summerfruits Bio, Boots* | 1 Pot/150g | 139.0 | 4.0 | 93 | 4.1 | 13.0 | 2.7 | 0.4 |
| Timperley Rhubarb, Seriously Fruity, Waitrose* | 1 Pot/150g | 127.0 | 1.0 | 85 | 4.6 | 14.4 | 1.0 | 0.0 |
| Toffee, Benecol* | 1 Pot/125g | 124.0 | 1.0 | 99 | 3.8 | 19.3 | 0.7 | 0.0 |
| Toffee, Childrens, Co-Op* | 1 Pot/125g | 142.0 | 3.0 | 114 | 3.6 | 18.6 | 2.8 | 0.0 |
| Toffee, COU, M & S* | 1 Pot/145g | 65.0 | 0.0 | 45 | 4.2 | 7.7 | 0.2 | 0.0 |
| Toffee, Economy, Sainsbury's* | 1 Pot/126g | 91.0 | 1.0 | 72 | 3.0 | 12.8 | 1.0 | 0.0 |
| Toffee, Light, HL, Tesco* | 1 Pot/200g | 80.0 | 0.0 | 40 | 3.9 | 5.9 | 0.1 | 1.0 |
| Toffee, Live Bio, Perfectly Balanced, Waitrose* | 1 Pot/150g | 156.0 | 0.0 | 104 | 4.2 | 21.1 | 0.3 | 0.0 |
| Toffee, Low Fat, Co-Op* | 1 Pot/150g | 124.0 | 1.0 | 83 | 3.8 | 15.0 | 0.9 | 0.2 |
| Toffee, Low Fat, M & S* | 1 Pot/150g | 180.0 | 3.0 | 120 | 4.9 | 21.6 | 1.7 | 0.0 |
| Toffee, Seriously Smooth, Low Fat, Waitrose* | 1 Pot/150g | 156.0 | 3.0 | 104 | 4.7 | 16.5 | 2.1 | 0.1 |
| Toffee, Smooth, Mullerlight, Fat Free, Muller* | 1 Pot/200g | 100.0 | 0.0 | 50 | 4.0 | 7.7 | 0.1 | 0.0 |
| Toffee, Smooth & Creamy, Fat Free, Weight Watchers* | 1 Pot/120g | 48.0 | 0.0 | 40 | 3.9 | 5.9 | 0.1 | 0.8 |
| Toffee, Virtually Fat Free, Boots* | 1 Pot/125g | 69.0 | 0.0 | 55 | 5.1 | 8.3 | 0.1 | 0.0 |
| Toffee Apple, COU, M & S* | 1 Pot/200g | 90.0 | 0.0 | 45 | 4.2 | 6.3 | 0.2 | 0.2 |
| Toffee Fudge, Low Fat, Sainsbury's* | 1 Pot/125g | 146.0 | 2.0 | 117 | 4.3 | 20.4 | 2.0 | 0.0 |
| Toffee Hoops, Crunch Corner, Muller* | 1 Pot/150g | 232.0 | 8.0 | 155 | 4.0 | 22.6 | 5.5 | 0.2 |
| Totally Vanilla, Low Fat, Asda* | 1 Pot/150g | 133.0 | 2.0 | 89 | 4.7 | 15.1 | 1.1 | 0.0 |
| Treacle Toffee, Dessert, Low Fat, Sainsbury's* | 1 Pot/125g | 149.0 | 2.0 | 119 | 4.3 | 21.2 | 1.9 | 0.0 |
| Tropical, Luscious, Low Fat, Rachel's Organic* | 1 Pot/125g | 115.0 | 2.0 | 92 | 4.0 | 15.3 | 1.6 | 0.0 |
| Tropical Crunch, Healthy Balance, Fruit Corner, Muller* | 1 Pot/150g | 169.0 | 3.0 | 113 | 4.7 | 18.2 | 2.1 | 0.5 |
| Tropical Fruit, Greek Style, Asda* | 1 Pot/125g | 170.0 | 9.0 | 136 | 3.3 | 15.0 | 7.0 | 0.0 |
| Tropical Fruit, Greek Style, Shapers, Boots* | 1 Pot/150g | 100.0 | 2.0 | 67 | 3.6 | 9.8 | 1.5 | 0.8 |
| Valencia Orange, Layered, Bio, GFY, Asda* | 1 Pot/125g | 80.0 | 0.0 | 64 | 3.7 | 12.0 | 0.1 | 0.0 |
| Valencia Orange, Seriously Fruity, Low Fat, Waitrose* | 1 Pot/150g | 147.0 | 1.0 | 98 | 4.3 | 18.0 | 1.0 | 0.3 |
| Vanilla, BGTY, Sainsbury's* | 1 Pot/200g | 98.0 | 0.0 | 49 | 4.5 | 7.5 | 0.1 | 0.0 |
| Vanilla, Bio, BFY, Morrisons* | 1 Pot/150g | 82.0 | 0.0 | 55 | 5.7 | 8.4 | 0.3 | 0.0 |
| Vanilla, Breakfast, Tesco* | 1 Pot/150g | 108.0 | 1.0 | 72 | 2.9 | 13.9 | 0.5 | 0.0 |
| Vanilla, Creamy, Smarties, Nestle* | 1 Pot/120g | 200.0 | 7.0 | 167 | 4.1 | 23.7 | 6.2 | 0.0 |
| Vanilla, Eat Smart, Morrisons* | 1 Pot/200g | 116.0 | 1.0 | 58 | 5.6 | 8.4 | 0.3 | 0.1 |
| Vanilla, French Set Wholemilk, Asda* | 1 Pot/125g | 125.0 | 4.0 | 100 | 3.6 | 14.1 | 3.2 | 0.0 |
| Vanilla, Lifestyle, Co-Op* | 1 Pot/180g | 81.0 | 0.0 | 45 | 5.0 | 6.0 | 0.1 | 0.0 |
| Vanilla, Live Bio, Low Fat, Perfectly Balanced, Waitrose* | 1 Pot/150g | 114.0 | 0.0 | 76 | 4.1 | 14.7 | 0.1 | 0.0 |
| Vanilla, Low Fat, Bio, Sainsbury's* | 1 Pot/150g | 147.0 | 2.0 | 98 | 4.8 | 17.2 | 1.1 | 0.0 |
| Vanilla, Low Fat, Tesco* | 1 Pot/125g | 125.0 | 2.0 | 100 | 4.9 | 16.3 | 1.7 | 0.0 |
| Vanilla, Organic, Low Fat, Sainsbury's* | 1 Pot/125g | 114.0 | 1.0 | 91 | 5.3 | 15.3 | 1.0 | 0.0 |
| Vanilla, Organic, Probiotic, Fat Free, Yeo Valley* | 1 Pot/500g | 400.0 | 0.0 | 80 | 5.4 | 14.2 | 0.1 | 0.0 |
| Vanilla, Smooth, Light, Fat Free, Muller* | 1 Pot/200g | 100.0 | 0.0 | 50 | 4.3 | 7.2 | 0.1 | 0.0 |
| Vanilla, Smooth & Creamy, Fat Free, Weight Watchers* | 1 Pot/120g | 50.0 | 0.0 | 42 | 3.9 | 6.5 | 0.1 | 0.1 |
| Vanilla, Smooth Set, Co-Op* | 1 Pot/125g | 95.0 | 1.0 | 76 | 3.7 | 12.5 | 0.9 | 0.0 |
| Vanilla, Thick & Creamy, Channel Island, M & S* | 1 Pot/150g | 187.0 | 7.0 | 125 | 4.5 | 17.5 | 4.4 | 1.0 |
| Vanilla, Thick & Creamy, Probiotic, COU, M & S* | 1 Pot/170g | 76.0 | 0.0 | 45 | 4.5 | 6.3 | 0.1 | 0.5 |
| Vanilla, Virtually Fat Free, Shapers, Boots* | 1 Pot/125g | 66.0 | 0.0 | 53 | 5.0 | 7.9 | 0.1 | 0.0 |
| Vanilla, Virtually Fat Free, Yeo Valley* | 1 Pot/150g | 121.0 | 0.0 | 81 | 5.1 | 15.0 | 0.1 | 0.0 |
| Vanilla & Pineapple, Nestle* | 1 Pot/125g | 120.0 | 2.0 | 96 | 4.2 | 16.7 | 1.5 | 0.0 |
| Vanilla Choco Balls, Crunch Corner, Muller* | 1 Pot/150g | 228.0 | 7.0 | 152 | 4.0 | 22.0 | 5.0 | 0.2 |
| Vanilla Flavour, Healthy Living, Light, Tesco* | 1 Pot/200g | 90.0 | 0.0 | 45 | 4.1 | 7.0 | 0.1 | 0.0 |
| Vanilla Flavour, Organic, Low Fat, Tesco* | 1 Pot/125g | 114.0 | 1.0 | 91 | 5.3 | 15.3 | 1.0 | 0.0 |
| Vanilla Toffee, Low Fat, Sainsbury's* | 1 Pot/125g | 145.0 | 2.0 | 116 | 4.3 | 20.6 | 1.8 | 0.0 |
| Walnut & Greek Honey, Amore Luxury, Muller* | 1 Pot/150g | 241.0 | 13.0 | 161 | 3.0 | 17.6 | 8.7 | 0.1 |

| | Measure INFO/WEIGHT | per Measure KCAL | FAT | Nutrition Values per 100g / 100ml KCAL | PROT | CARB | FAT | FIBRE |
|---|---|---|---|---|---|---|---|---|
| **YOGHURT** | | | | | | | | |
| White Peach, Seriously Fruity, Waitrose* | 1 Pot/150g | 151.0 | 3.0 | 101 | 4.8 | 16.5 | 1.7 | 0.2 |
| Wholegrain, Lite, Fig, Date & Grape, Biopot, Onken* | ¼ Pot/120g | 102.0 | 0.0 | 85 | 4.8 | 16.0 | 0.2 | 1.0 |
| Wholegrain, Lite, Summer Berries, Biopot, Onken* | ¼ Pot/120g | 100.0 | 0.0 | 83 | 4.6 | 15.8 | 0.2 | 1.4 |
| Wholemilk, Organic, M & S* | 1 Pot/454ml | 409.0 | 16.0 | 90 | 6.1 | 7.4 | 3.6 | 0.0 |
| Wholemilk, with Maple Syrup, Bio Live, Rachel's Organic* | 1 Pot/142g | 139.0 | 5.0 | 98 | 3.5 | 13.0 | 3.5 | 0.0 |
| Wicked Wholemilk Vanilla, Bio Live, Rachel's Organic* | 1 Pot/125g | 125.0 | 4.0 | 100 | 5.2 | 12.1 | 3.5 | 0.0 |
| Wild Blackberry, Seriously Fruity, Waitrose* | 1 Pot/125g | 120.0 | 1.0 | 96 | 4.4 | 17.2 | 1.0 | 0.4 |
| Wild Blueberry, Finest, Tesco* | 1 Pot/150g | 211.0 | 10.0 | 141 | 3.4 | 16.6 | 6.8 | 0.5 |
| Wild Blueberry, Light, Fat Free, Muller* | 1 Pot/200g | 94.0 | 0.0 | 47 | 4.1 | 6.9 | 0.1 | 0.7 |
| Winter Medley, COU, M & S* | 1 Pot/150g | 67.0 | 0.0 | 45 | 4.2 | 6.2 | 0.1 | 0.1 |
| Yellow Fruit, Yoplait* | 1 Pot/125g | 139.0 | 4.0 | 111 | 3.3 | 18.0 | 2.9 | 0.0 |
| Zesty Lemon, Intensley Creamy, Activia, Danone* | 1 Pot/120g | 119.0 | 4.0 | 99 | 4.8 | 13.3 | 3.0 | 0.1 |
| **YOGHURT BREAK** | | | | | | | | |
| Forest Fruit, Go Ahead, McVitie's* | 1 Slice/18g | 73.0 | 2.0 | 404 | 5.6 | 71.4 | 10.7 | 2.2 |
| Plain, Go Ahead, McVitie's* | 1 Bar/18g | 72.0 | 2.0 | 394 | 6.5 | 66.0 | 11.5 | 3.3 |
| Strawberry, Go Ahead, McVitie's* | 1 Slice/18g | 72.0 | 2.0 | 397 | 5.9 | 68.0 | 11.1 | 2.1 |
| Tropical, Go Ahead, McVitie's* | 1 Slice/18g | 77.0 | 2.0 | 430 | 5.9 | 76.3 | 11.0 | 2.3 |
| **YOGHURT DRINK** | | | | | | | | |
| Actimel, Multi Fruit, Danone* | 1 Bottle/100g | 85.0 | 1.0 | 85 | 2.7 | 14.4 | 1.5 | 0.1 |
| Actimel, Orange, Danone* | 1 Bottle/100g | 74.0 | 1.0 | 74 | 2.9 | 11.5 | 1.5 | 0.0 |
| Actimel, Original, 0.1% Fat, Danone* | 1 Bottle/100g | 28.0 | 0.0 | 28 | 2.8 | 3.3 | 0.1 | 1.9 |
| Actimel, Original, Danone* | 1 Bottle/100g | 80.0 | 2.0 | 80 | 2.8 | 12.8 | 1.6 | 0.0 |
| Actimel, Pineapple, 0.1% Fat, Danone* | 1 Bottle/100g | 33.0 | 0.0 | 33 | 2.7 | 5.5 | 0.0 | 1.8 |
| Actimel, Strawberry, Danone* | 1 Bottle/100g | 74.0 | 1.0 | 74 | 2.9 | 11.5 | 1.5 | 0.0 |
| Average | 1floz/30ml | 19.0 | 0.0 | 62 | 3.1 | 13.1 | 0.0 | 0.0 |
| Banana & Honey, Ski Up & Go, Nestle* | 1 Bottle/250g | 215.0 | 2.0 | 86 | 0.0 | 16.0 | 0.9 | 0.0 |
| Bioactive, Yagua* | 1 Bottle/200ml | 84.0 | 0.0 | 42 | 0.4 | 9.9 | 0.0 | 0.0 |
| Blueberry, Low Fat, Prebiotic and Probiotic, Muller* | 1 Pot/100g | 66.0 | 1.0 | 66 | 2.6 | 10.3 | 1.4 | 2.2 |
| Blueberry & Blackcurrant, Orchard Maid* | 1 Carton/250ml | 147.0 | 0.0 | 59 | 1.6 | 13.6 | 0.0 | 0.0 |
| Cholesterol Lowering, Asda* | 1 Bottle/100g | 76.0 | 1.0 | 76 | 2.9 | 13.0 | 1.4 | 1.0 |
| Danacol, Original, Danone* | 1 Bottle/100ml | 64.0 | 1.0 | 64 | 3.2 | 10.0 | 1.0 | 0.0 |
| Danacol, Strawberry, Danone* | 1 Bottle/100g | 68.0 | 1.0 | 68 | 3.2 | 11.2 | 1.2 | 0.0 |
| Fristi* | 1 Carton/330g | 191.0 | 0.0 | 58 | 2.6 | 13.6 | 0.1 | 0.0 |
| Light, Benecol* | 1 Bottle/68g | 40.0 | 1.0 | 60 | 2.8 | 7.3 | 2.1 | 0.1 |
| Light, Yakult* | 1 Bottle/65ml | 27.0 | 0.0 | 42 | 1.4 | 10.2 | 0.0 | 1.8 |
| Mixed Berry, Up & Go, Ski, Nestle* | 1 Bottle/250g | 217.0 | 2.0 | 87 | 3.1 | 16.0 | 0.9 | 0.2 |
| Omega 3 Plus, Raspberry, Pro Biotic, Flora* | 1 Bottle/100g | 58.0 | 2.0 | 58 | 2.6 | 8.5 | 1.6 | 0.0 |
| Orange, Banana & Passion Fruit, One a Day, Muller* | 1 Bottle/310ml | 208.0 | 0.0 | 67 | 2.1 | 14.1 | 0.1 | 0.0 |
| Peach & Apricot, Benecol* | 1 Bottle/68g | 38.0 | 1.0 | 56 | 2.8 | 6.2 | 2.2 | 0.0 |
| Peach & Mango, Fristi* | 1 Carton/330g | 191.0 | 0.0 | 58 | 2.6 | 13.6 | 0.1 | 0.0 |
| Pro Activ, Orange, Cholesterol, Flora* | 1 Bottle/100g | 87.0 | 3.0 | 87 | 2.6 | 12.5 | 2.9 | 0.0 |
| Pro Activ, Original, Blood Pressure, Flora* | 1 Bottle/100g | 80.0 | 1.0 | 80 | 3.9 | 12.7 | 1.5 | 0.3 |
| Pro Activ, Original, Cholesterol, Flora* | 1 Bottle/100g | 87.0 | 3.0 | 87 | 2.6 | 12.5 | 2.9 | 0.0 |
| Pro Activ, Strawberry, Blood Pressure, Flora* | 1 Bottle/100g | 80.0 | 1.0 | 80 | 3.9 | 12.7 | 1.5 | 0.3 |
| Pro Activ, Strawberry, Cholesterol, Flora* | 1 Bottle/100g | 87.0 | 3.0 | 87 | 2.6 | 12.5 | 2.9 | 0.0 |
| Raspberry, Apple, & Cranberry, Smooth, One a Day, Muller* | 1 Bottle/330ml | 155.0 | 0.0 | 47 | 2.0 | 9.0 | 0.1 | 0.5 |
| Raspberry & Passion Fruit, Everybody, Yoplait* | 1 Bottle/90g | 60.0 | 1.0 | 67 | 2.6 | 12.2 | 0.9 | 0.0 |
| Strawberry, Benecol* | 1 Bottle/68g | 38.0 | 1.0 | 56 | 2.9 | 6.2 | 2.2 | 0.0 |
| Strawberry, Fristi* | 1 Carton/250g | 165.0 | 0.0 | 66 | 2.6 | 13.6 | 0.1 | 0.0 |
| Strawberry, Yop, Yoplait* | 1 Bottle/330g | 261.0 | 4.0 | 79 | 2.8 | 14.0 | 1.3 | 0.0 |
| Sveltesse, 0%, Nestle* | 1 Pot/125g | 61.0 | 0.0 | 49 | 4.8 | 7.3 | 0.1 | 0.1 |
| Yakult* | 1 Pot/65ml | 51.0 | 0.0 | 78 | 1.4 | 17.8 | 0.1 | 0.0 |

**Y**

| | Measure INFO/WEIGHT | per Measure | | Nutrition Values per 100g / 100ml | | | | |
|---|---|---|---|---|---|---|---|---|
| | | KCAL | FAT | KCAL | PROT | CARB | FAT | FIBRE |
| **YORK FRUITS** | | | | | | | | |
| Terry's* | 1 Sweet/9g | 30.0 | 0.0 | 328 | 0.0 | 81.4 | 0.0 | 1.0 |
| **YORKIE** | | | | | | | | |
| Honeycomb, Nestle* | 1 Bar/65g | 331.0 | 17.0 | 509 | 5.7 | 63.6 | 25.8 | 0.0 |
| King Size, Nestle* | 1 Bar/83g | 445.0 | 26.0 | 537 | 6.1 | 57.3 | 31.5 | 0.0 |
| Original, Nestle* | 1 Bar/68g | 365.0 | 21.0 | 537 | 6.1 | 57.3 | 31.5 | 0.7 |
| Raisin & Biscuit, Nestle* | 1 Bar/67g | 331.0 | 17.0 | 497 | 5.5 | 59.7 | 26.2 | 0.9 |
| **YORKSHIRE PUDDING** | | | | | | | | |
| & Beef Dripping, M & S* | 4 Puddings/100g | 410.0 | 30.0 | 410 | 9.4 | 25.2 | 30.4 | 3.2 |
| 3", Baked, Aunt Bessie's* | 1 Pudding/36g | 91.0 | 3.0 | 252 | 9.0 | 36.4 | 7.9 | 1.7 |
| 4 Minute, Aunt Bessie's* | 1 Pudding/18g | 52.0 | 2.0 | 291 | 10.5 | 36.6 | 11.3 | 2.2 |
| 7", Baked, Aunt Bessie's* | 1 Pudding/110g | 290.0 | 10.0 | 264 | 8.5 | 37.4 | 9.0 | 2.0 |
| Average | 1 Pudding/30g | 62.0 | 3.0 | 208 | 6.6 | 24.7 | 9.9 | 0.9 |
| Batters, in Foils, Ready to Bake, Frozen, Aunt Bessie's* | 1 Pudding/17g | 47.0 | 2.0 | 276 | 9.1 | 32.6 | 10.8 | 1.4 |
| Chicken & Vegetable, COU, M & S* | 1 Pudding/150g | 195.0 | 3.0 | 130 | 12.2 | 14.3 | 2.2 | 1.3 |
| Filled, with Sausage, Sainsbury's* | 1 Pack/300g | 576.0 | 31.0 | 192 | 6.9 | 17.5 | 10.4 | 0.9 |
| Filled with Beef, Tesco* | 1 Pudding/300g | 408.0 | 16.0 | 136 | 6.1 | 16.2 | 5.2 | 1.1 |
| Filled with Chicken, GFY, Asda* | 1 Pack/381g | 438.0 | 10.0 | 115 | 9.0 | 14.0 | 2.6 | 1.5 |
| Filled with Chicken, Tesco* | 1 Pack/300g | 366.0 | 9.0 | 122 | 6.5 | 17.4 | 2.9 | 1.3 |
| Filled with Chicken & Vegetable, GFY, Asda* | 1 Pack/380g | 376.0 | 10.0 | 99 | 6.0 | 13.0 | 2.6 | 1.1 |
| Frozen, Ovenbaked, Iceland* | 1 Pudding/12g | 36.0 | 1.0 | 290 | 9.7 | 45.1 | 7.9 | 4.1 |
| Fully Prepared, M & S* | 1 Pudding/22g | 63.0 | 3.0 | 285 | 9.4 | 31.6 | 13.2 | 1.2 |
| Giant, Aunt Bessie's* | 1 Pudding/110g | 290.0 | 10.0 | 264 | 8.5 | 37.4 | 9.0 | 2.0 |
| Giant, VLH Kitchens* | 1 Pudding/110g | 284.0 | 11.0 | 259 | 8.5 | 33.6 | 10.0 | 2.3 |
| Large, Aunt Bessie's* | 1 Pudding/40g | 111.0 | 5.0 | 277 | 8.5 | 35.3 | 11.4 | 1.5 |
| Large, Frozen, Co-Op* | 1 Pudding/34g | 84.0 | 2.0 | 250 | 10.0 | 36.0 | 7.0 | 2.0 |
| Large, Iceland* | 1 Pudding/30g | 96.0 | 4.0 | 321 | 10.5 | 38.8 | 13.8 | 1.7 |
| Large, The Real Yorkshire Pudding Co* | 1 Pudding/34g | 103.0 | 4.0 | 304 | 11.5 | 37.3 | 12.1 | 2.5 |
| Made From Batter Mix, Sainsbury's* | 1 Pudding/100g | 248.0 | 5.0 | 248 | 9.9 | 40.1 | 5.3 | 4.0 |
| Mini, Farmfoods* | 1 Pudding/3g | 8.0 | 0.0 | 281 | 9.6 | 43.2 | 7.7 | 1.9 |
| Premium, Bisto* | 1 Pudding/30g | 74.0 | 3.0 | 248 | 7.3 | 30.3 | 10.9 | 2.1 |
| Ready Baked, SmartPrice, Asda* | 1 Pudding/12g | 36.0 | 1.0 | 297 | 10.0 | 44.0 | 9.0 | 2.8 |
| Ready to Bake, Aunt Bessie's* | 1 Pudding/17g | 42.0 | 1.0 | 246 | 8.5 | 35.1 | 8.0 | 1.7 |
| Ready to Bake, Sainsbury's* | 1 Pudding/18g | 48.0 | 2.0 | 263 | 9.9 | 35.9 | 8.9 | 1.3 |
| Riding Lodge* | 1 Pudding/16g | 44.0 | 1.0 | 276 | 10.0 | 41.5 | 7.8 | 0.0 |
| Roast Chicken Filled, COU, M & S* | 1 Pudding/150g | 210.0 | 4.0 | 140 | 12.6 | 15.7 | 2.7 | 0.9 |
| Sage & Onion, Tesco* | 1 Pudding/19g | 53.0 | 2.0 | 280 | 8.0 | 35.0 | 12.0 | 2.6 |
| Sainsbury's* | 1 Pudding/14g | 43.0 | 2.0 | 309 | 7.9 | 37.5 | 14.1 | 2.9 |
| Sausage Filled, Frozen, Tesco* | 1 Pack/340g | 510.0 | 20.0 | 150 | 6.6 | 17.8 | 5.8 | 1.8 |
| The Best, Morrisons* | 1 Pudding/22g | 60.0 | 3.0 | 271 | 8.3 | 43.0 | 8.0 | 1.6 |
| Traditional, Giant, Asda* | 1 Pudding/110g | 310.0 | 11.0 | 282 | 10.0 | 38.0 | 10.0 | 2.3 |
| Traditional Style, Medium, Asda* | 1 Pudding/36g | 86.0 | 3.0 | 241 | 9.0 | 31.0 | 9.0 | 2.4 |
| Traditional Style, Small, Asda* | 1 Pudding/20g | 52.0 | 2.0 | 262 | 8.0 | 35.0 | 10.0 | 2.9 |
| Value, Tesco* | 1 Pudding/16g | 45.0 | 2.0 | 282 | 9.7 | 34.3 | 11.8 | 1.6 |
| **YULE LOG** | | | | | | | | |
| Chocolate, Sainsbury's* | 1/8 Log/49g | 186.0 | 10.0 | 382 | 5.1 | 46.5 | 19.6 | 0.7 |
| Mini, M & S* | 1 Cake/36g | 165.0 | 8.0 | 460 | 5.7 | 56.9 | 23.3 | 1.1 |

| | Measure INFO/WEIGHT | per Measure KCAL | FAT | Nutrition Values per 100g / 100ml KCAL | PROT | CARB | FAT | FIBRE |
|---|---|---|---|---|---|---|---|---|

## BAGEL FACTORY

### BAGEL

| | Measure INFO/WEIGHT | KCAL | FAT | KCAL | PROT | CARB | FAT | FIBRE |
|---|---|---|---|---|---|---|---|---|
| Bacon, Bagel Factory* | 1 Bagel/100g | 613 | 26.0 | 613 | 32.2 | 62.1 | 25.9 | 3.8 |
| Chicken, Tomato & Spinach, Wholemeal, Bagel Factory* | 1 Bagel/100g | 306 | 2.0 | 306 | 23.0 | 49.2 | 1.9 | 9.1 |
| Cream Cheese, Ham & Tomato, Bagel Factory* | 1 Bagel/100g | 421 | 11.0 | 421 | 31.2 | 48.6 | 11.2 | 9.0 |
| Marmite, Wholemeal, Bagel Factory* | 1 Bagel/85g | 312 | 2.0 | 367 | 24.4 | 63.4 | 1.9 | 11.6 |
| Salmon & Cream Cheese, Bagel Factory* | 1 Serving/300g | 515 | 18.0 | 172 | 9.9 | 19.1 | 6.1 | 0.7 |

## BURGER KING

### APPLE

| | | | | | | | | |
|---|---|---|---|---|---|---|---|---|
| Fries, Burger King* | 1 Serving/60g | 28 | 0.0 | 47 | 0.1 | 12.0 | 0.1 | 2.0 |

### BITES

| | | | | | | | | |
|---|---|---|---|---|---|---|---|---|
| Chicken, Kids, Burger King* | 1 Serving/56g | 158 | 7.0 | 282 | 16.0 | 25.0 | 13.0 | 2.0 |

### BURGERS

| | | | | | | | | |
|---|---|---|---|---|---|---|---|---|
| Angus, Burger King* | 1 Burger/239g | 554 | 29.0 | 232 | 12.0 | 18.0 | 12.0 | 1.0 |
| Angus, Double, Burger King* | 1 Burger/323g | 795 | 45.0 | 246 | 16.0 | 14.0 | 14.0 | 1.0 |
| Angus, Mini, Burger King* | 1 Burger/97g | 272 | 11.0 | 280 | 14.0 | 31.0 | 11.0 | 1.0 |
| Angus, Mini with Cheese, Burger King* | 1 Burger/110g | 321 | 15.0 | 292 | 15.0 | 27.0 | 14.0 | 1.0 |
| Angus, Smoked Bacon & Cheddar, Burger King* | 1 Burger/270g | 678 | 38.0 | 251 | 14.0 | 17.0 | 14.0 | 1.0 |
| Angus, Smoked Bacon & Cheddar, Double, Burger King* | 1 Burger/354g | 920 | 53.0 | 260 | 17.0 | 13.0 | 15.0 | 1.0 |
| Bean, Veggie, Kids, Burger King* | 1 Burger/116g | 278 | 7.0 | 240 | 6.0 | 42.0 | 6.0 | 3.0 |
| Big King, Burger King* | 1 Burger/190g | 503 | 27.0 | 265 | 15.0 | 17.0 | 14.0 | 1.0 |
| Big King, XL, Burger King* | 1 Burger/338g | 902 | 54.0 | 267 | 16.0 | 14.0 | 16.0 | 1.0 |
| BK, Veggie Bean Burger, Burger King* | 1 Burger/280g | 588 | 20.0 | 210 | 6.0 | 30.0 | 7.0 | 3.0 |
| Cheeseburger, Bacon Double, Burger King* | 1 Burger/160g | 478 | 26.0 | 299 | 19.0 | 19.0 | 16.0 | 1.0 |
| Cheeseburger, Bacon Double, Extra Large, Burger King* | 1 Burger/302g | 927 | 54.0 | 307 | 21.0 | 15.0 | 18.0 | 1.0 |
| Cheeseburger, Burger King* | 1 Burger/123g | 320 | 14.0 | 260 | 13.0 | 25.0 | 11.0 | 1.0 |
| Cheeseburger, Double, Burger King* | 1 Burger/173g | 465 | 22.0 | 269 | 17.0 | 18.0 | 13.0 | 1.0 |
| Cheeseburger, Kids, Burger King* | 1 Burger/113g | 318 | 14.0 | 281 | 14.0 | 27.0 | 12.0 | 1.0 |
| Chicken, Piri Piri, Sandwich, Burger King* | 1 Burger/196g | 335 | 6.0 | 171 | 13.0 | 21.0 | 3.0 | 1.0 |
| Chicken Royale, Angry, Burger King* | 1 Burger/269g | 764 | 43.0 | 284 | 10.0 | 22.0 | 16.0 | 1.0 |
| Chicken Royale, Burger King* | 1 Burger/210g | 607 | 31.0 | 289 | 11.0 | 25.0 | 15.0 | 1.0 |
| Chicken Royale, Sweet Chilli, Burger King* | 1 Burger/210g | 542 | 23.0 | 258 | 11.0 | 28.0 | 11.0 | 1.0 |
| Chicken Royale, with Cheese, Burger King* | 1 Burger/263g | 697 | 39.0 | 265 | 11.0 | 21.0 | 15.0 | 1.0 |
| Hamburger, Burger King* | 1 Burger/110g | 275 | 9.0 | 250 | 13.0 | 28.0 | 8.0 | 1.0 |
| Hamburger, Kids, Burger King* | 1 Burger/100g | 272 | 9.0 | 272 | 14.0 | 31.0 | 9.0 | 1.0 |
| Ocean Catch, Burger King* | 1 Burger/188g | 494 | 26.0 | 263 | 9.0 | 23.0 | 14.0 | 1.0 |
| Spicy Royale, Burger King* | 1 Burger/210g | 545 | 30.0 | 260 | 12.4 | 20.9 | 14.3 | 2.4 |
| Whopper, Angry, Burger King* | 1 Burger/313g | 808 | 50.0 | 258 | 11.0 | 18.0 | 16.0 | 1.0 |
| Whopper, Angry, Double, Burger King* | 1 Burger/394g | 1052 | 67.0 | 267 | 14.0 | 14.0 | 17.0 | 1.0 |
| Whopper, Burger King* | 1 Burger/274g | 633 | 36.0 | 231 | 11.0 | 18.0 | 13.0 | 1.0 |
| Whopper, Double, Burger King* | 1 Burger/355g | 877 | 53.0 | 247 | 14.0 | 14.0 | 15.0 | 1.0 |
| Whopper, Double, with Cheese, Burger King* | 1 Burger/380g | 961 | 61.0 | 253 | 14.0 | 13.0 | 16.0 | 1.0 |
| Whopper, Junior, Burger King* | 1 Burger/148g | 343 | 16.0 | 232 | 9.0 | 21.0 | 11.0 | 1.0 |
| Whopper, with Cheese, Burger King* | 1 Burger/299g | 721 | 42.0 | 241 | 11.0 | 16.0 | 14.0 | 1.0 |
| Whopper, with Cheese, Junior, Burger King* | 1 Burger/161g | 388 | 19.0 | 241 | 10.0 | 19.0 | 12.0 | 1.0 |

### BUTTY

| | | | | | | | | |
|---|---|---|---|---|---|---|---|---|
| Bacon, with Heinz Ketchup, Burger King* | 1 Butty/126g | 391 | 16.0 | 310 | 15.0 | 33.0 | 13.0 | 2.0 |
| Bacon, with HP Sauce, Burger King* | 1 Butty/126g | 392 | 16.0 | 311 | 15.0 | 33.0 | 13.0 | 2.0 |
| Bacon & Egg, with Heinz Ketchup, Burger King* | 1 Butty/176g | 475 | 23.0 | 270 | 14.0 | 24.0 | 13.0 | 1.0 |
| Bacon & Egg, with HP Sauce, Burger King* | 1 Butty/176g | 475 | 23.0 | 270 | 14.0 | 24.0 | 13.0 | 1.0 |
| Big Breakfast, with Heinz Ketchup, Burger King* | 1 Butty/297g | 849 | 50.0 | 286 | 14.0 | 18.0 | 17.0 | 1.0 |
| Big Breakfast, with HP Sauce, Burger King* | 1 Butty/297g | 852 | 50.0 | 287 | 14.0 | 18.0 | 17.0 | 1.0 |
| Egg & Cheese, with Heinz Ketchup, Burger King* | 1 Butty/164g | 454 | 23.0 | 277 | 11.0 | 26.0 | 14.0 | 1.0 |
| Egg & Cheese, with HP Sauce, Burger King* | 1 Butty/164g | 454 | 23.0 | 277 | 11.0 | 26.0 | 14.0 | 1.0 |

| | Measure INFO/WEIGHT | per Measure KCAL | FAT | Nutrition Values per 100g / 100ml KCAL | PROT | CARB | FAT | FIBRE |
|---|---|---|---|---|---|---|---|---|

## BURGER KING

### BUTTY

| | Measure INFO/WEIGHT | KCAL | FAT | KCAL | PROT | CARB | FAT | FIBRE |
|---|---|---|---|---|---|---|---|---|
| Sausage, Cumberland, with Heinz Ketchup, Burger King* | 1 Butty/193g | 585 | 33.0 | 303 | 11.0 | 25.0 | 17.0 | 2.0 |
| Sausage, Cumberland, with HP Sauce, Burger King* | 1 Butty/193g | 587 | 33.0 | 304 | 11.0 | 25.0 | 17.0 | 2.0 |
| Sausage, Cumberland & Egg, with HP Sauce, Burger King* | 1 Butty/243g | 671 | 39.0 | 276 | 11.0 | 21.0 | 16.0 | 1.0 |

### CAKE

| | | | | | | | | |
|---|---|---|---|---|---|---|---|---|
| Chocolate Fudge, Double, Fusions, Burger King* | 1 Serving/155g | 244 | 7.0 | 157 | 3.9 | 25.2 | 4.5 | 0.6 |

### CHEESE & ONION

| | | | | | | | | |
|---|---|---|---|---|---|---|---|---|
| Fingers, Burger King* | 4 Fingers/88g | 301 | 19.0 | 342 | 14.0 | 24.0 | 22.0 | 2.0 |

### CHEESECAKE

| | | | | | | | | |
|---|---|---|---|---|---|---|---|---|
| Strawberry, Burger King* | 1 Serving/100g | 346 | 24.0 | 346 | 6.0 | 27.0 | 24.0 | 0.1 |

### CHICKEN

| | | | | | | | | |
|---|---|---|---|---|---|---|---|---|
| Bites, Burger King* | 14 Bites/112g | 317 | 15.0 | 283 | 16.0 | 25.0 | 13.0 | 1.0 |
| Fillet, Strips, Chargrilled, Burger King* | 3 Strips/75g | 95 | 2.0 | 127 | 25.0 | 0.1 | 3.0 | 0.1 |

### COFFEE

| | | | | | | | | |
|---|---|---|---|---|---|---|---|---|
| Black, Large, Burger King* | 1 Serving/284ml | 6 | 0.0 | 2 | 0.0 | 0.0 | 0.0 | 0.0 |
| Black, Regular, Burger King* | 1 Reg/200ml | 4 | 0.0 | 2 | 0.0 | 0.0 | 0.0 | 0.0 |
| Cappuccino, Large, Burger King* | 1 Lge Serving/59g | 81 | 3.0 | 137 | 10.0 | 15.0 | 5.0 | 0.0 |
| Cappuccino, Regular, Burger King* | 1 Reg Serving/46g | 64 | 2.0 | 139 | 9.0 | 15.0 | 4.0 | 0.0 |
| Latte, Large, Burger King* | 1 Reg Serving/45g | 60 | 2.0 | 133 | 11.0 | 13.0 | 4.0 | 0.0 |
| Latte, Regular, Burger King* | 1 Lge Serving/62g | 82 | 3.0 | 132 | 10.0 | 15.0 | 5.0 | 0.0 |

### COLA

| | | | | | | | | |
|---|---|---|---|---|---|---|---|---|
| Coca-Cola, Burger King* | 1 Reg/400g | 168 | 0.0 | 42 | 0.0 | 11.0 | 0.0 | 0.0 |
| Coca-Cola, Small, Burger King* | 1 Sm/300g | 126 | 0.0 | 42 | 0.0 | 11.0 | 0.0 | 0.0 |
| Coke, Diet, Burger King* | 1 Reg/400g | 4 | 0.0 | 1 | 0.0 | 0.0 | 0.0 | 0.0 |
| Coke, Diet, Small, Burger King* | 1 Sm/300g | 3 | 0.0 | 1 | 0.0 | 0.0 | 0.0 | 0.0 |

### DIP POT

| | | | | | | | | |
|---|---|---|---|---|---|---|---|---|
| Barbeque Sauce, Heinz, Burger King* | 1 Serving/40g | 48 | 0.0 | 120 | 0.1 | 28.0 | 0.1 | 0.1 |
| Mexican Salsa, Heinz, Burger King* | 1 Pot/25g | 22 | 0.0 | 88 | 0.1 | 20.0 | 0.1 | 0.1 |
| Sweet Chilli, Heinz, Burger King* | 1 Pot/40g | 96 | 0.0 | 240 | 0.0 | 60.0 | 0.0 | 0.0 |

### DOUGHNUTS

| | | | | | | | | |
|---|---|---|---|---|---|---|---|---|
| Diddy, Burger King* | 1 Serving/84g | 256 | 8.0 | 305 | 5.9 | 48.8 | 9.5 | 1.2 |

### DRESSING

| | | | | | | | | |
|---|---|---|---|---|---|---|---|---|
| French, Burger King* | 1 Sachet/40g | 8 | 0.0 | 20 | 90.0 | 2.5 | 0.0 | 0.0 |
| Honey & Mustard, Burger King* | 1 Sachet/40g | 32 | 1.0 | 80 | 2.5 | 15.0 | 2.5 | 0.0 |
| Thousand Island, Burger King* | 1 Sachet/40g | 65 | 6.0 | 162 | 0.0 | 7.5 | 15.0 | 0.0 |
| Tomato & Basil, Burger King* | 1 Sachet/40g | 19 | 1.0 | 47 | 2.5 | 7.5 | 2.5 | 0.0 |

### FANTA

| | | | | | | | | |
|---|---|---|---|---|---|---|---|---|
| Orange, Small, Burger King* | 1 Cup/300g | 117 | 0.0 | 39 | 0.1 | 10.0 | 0.1 | 0.0 |

### FRIES

| | | | | | | | | |
|---|---|---|---|---|---|---|---|---|
| Large, Burger King* | 1 Serving/141g | 381 | 18.0 | 270 | 3.0 | 38.0 | 13.0 | 4.0 |
| Regular, Burger King* | 1 Serving/111g | 300 | 16.0 | 270 | 3.0 | 39.0 | 14.0 | 4.0 |
| Small, Burger King* | 1 Serving/74g | 200 | 10.0 | 270 | 3.0 | 38.0 | 14.0 | 4.0 |
| Super, Burger King* | 1 Serving/174g | 470 | 23.0 | 270 | 3.0 | 39.0 | 13.0 | 4.0 |

### HASH BROWNS

| | | | | | | | | |
|---|---|---|---|---|---|---|---|---|
| Large, Burger King* | 1 Serving/130g | 403 | 27.0 | 310 | 3.0 | 27.0 | 21.0 | 4.0 |
| Regular, Burger King* | 1 Serving/102g | 316 | 22.0 | 310 | 3.0 | 27.0 | 22.0 | 4.0 |

### HOT CHOCOLATE

| | | | | | | | | |
|---|---|---|---|---|---|---|---|---|
| Burger King* | 1 Serving/200ml | 78 | 2.0 | 39 | 0.5 | 7.5 | 1.0 | 0.5 |

### ICE CREAM

| | | | | | | | | |
|---|---|---|---|---|---|---|---|---|
| Apple Crumble, Bramley, Burger King* | 1 Serving/190g | 313 | 11.0 | 165 | 3.2 | 24.2 | 5.8 | 0.0 |
| Cookies & Cream, Burger King* | 1 Serving/170g | 315 | 11.0 | 185 | 3.5 | 27.6 | 6.5 | 0.0 |
| Millionaires Shortbread, Fusions, Burger King* | 1 Serving/175g | 374 | 14.0 | 214 | 3.0 | 32.0 | 8.0 | 0.0 |
| Mint Choc Swirl, Fusions, Burger King* | 1 Serving/145g | 270 | 12.0 | 186 | 4.0 | 26.0 | 8.0 | 1.0 |

| | Measure INFO/WEIGHT | per Measure KCAL | FAT | Nutrition Values per 100g / 100ml KCAL | PROT | CARB | FAT | FIBRE |
|---|---|---|---|---|---|---|---|---|
| **BURGER KING** | | | | | | | | |
| **ICE CREAM** | | | | | | | | |
| Strawberry Shortcake, Fusions, Burger King* | 1 Serving/170g | 345 | 12.0 | 203 | 4.0 | 32.0 | 7.0 | 0.1 |
| Summer Berry Burst, Fusions, Burger King* | 1 Serving/148g | 180 | 3.0 | 122 | 2.7 | 23.0 | 2.0 | 0.0 |
| Vanilla & Chocolate, Burger King* | 1 Cone/102g | 287 | 14.0 | 281 | 2.9 | 36.3 | 13.7 | 2.9 |
| Vanilla & Strawberry, Burger King* | 1 Cone/102g | 269 | 12.0 | 264 | 2.9 | 39.2 | 11.8 | 1.0 |
| **ICE CREAM CONE** | | | | | | | | |
| Vanilla & Chocolate, Burger King* | 1 Serving/102g | 287 | 14.0 | 281 | 2.9 | 36.3 | 13.7 | 2.9 |
| Vanilla & Strawberry, Burger King* | 1 Cone/102g | 269 | 12.0 | 264 | 2.9 | 39.2 | 11.8 | 1.0 |
| **KETCHUP** | | | | | | | | |
| Heinz, Sachet, Burger King* | 1 Sachet/10g | 10 | 0.0 | 100 | 0.1 | 20.0 | 0.1 | 0.1 |
| **MAYONNAISE** | | | | | | | | |
| Heinz, Sachet, Burger King* | 1 Sachet/12g | 80 | 9.0 | 667 | 0.0 | 0.0 | 75.0 | 0.0 |
| **MILK** | | | | | | | | |
| Semi Skimmed, Kids, Burger King* | 1 Carton/250g | 117 | 5.0 | 47 | 4.0 | 5.0 | 2.0 | 0.0 |
| **MILK SHAKE** | | | | | | | | |
| Chocolate, Large, Burger King* | 1 Serving/519g | 612 | 10.0 | 118 | 3.0 | 22.0 | 2.0 | 0.0 |
| Chocolate, Regular, Burger King* | 1 Serving/401g | 449 | 8.0 | 112 | 3.0 | 20.0 | 2.0 | 0.1 |
| Chocolate, Small, Burger King* | 1 Serving/276g | 301 | 8.0 | 109 | 3.0 | 19.0 | 3.0 | 0.1 |
| Strawberry, Large, Burger King* | 1 Serving/519g | 581 | 10.0 | 112 | 3.0 | 20.0 | 2.0 | 0.0 |
| Strawberry, Regular, Burger King* | 1 Serving/401g | 433 | 8.0 | 108 | 3.0 | 19.0 | 2.0 | 0.0 |
| Strawberry, Small, Burger King* | 1 Serving/276g | 293 | 8.0 | 106 | 3.0 | 18.0 | 3.0 | 0.0 |
| Vanilla, Burger King* | 1 Serving/124g | 124 | 4.0 | 100 | 3.0 | 16.0 | 3.0 | 0.0 |
| **ONION RINGS** | | | | | | | | |
| Large, Burger King* | 1 Large/190g | 559 | 28.0 | 294 | 5.0 | 35.0 | 15.0 | 4.0 |
| Regular, Burger King* | 1 Reg/126g | 370 | 19.0 | 294 | 5.0 | 36.0 | 15.0 | 4.0 |
| Super, Burger King* | 1 Super/253g | 744 | 38.0 | 294 | 5.0 | 36.0 | 15.0 | 4.0 |
| **PIE** | | | | | | | | |
| Apple, Burger King* | 1 Pie/150g | 330 | 13.0 | 220 | 2.0 | 33.0 | 9.0 | 1.0 |
| Apple, with Ice Cream, Burger King* | 1 Pie/220g | 431 | 18.0 | 196 | 3.0 | 29.0 | 8.0 | 1.0 |
| Dutch Apple, Burger King* | 1 Pie/113g | 339 | 14.0 | 300 | 1.7 | 46.0 | 12.3 | 0.8 |
| **POTATO WEDGES** | | | | | | | | |
| Burger King* | 1 Portion/100g | 147 | 3.0 | 147 | 2.0 | 21.0 | 3.0 | 3.0 |
| **SALAD** | | | | | | | | |
| Chicken, Flame Grilled, Burger King* | 1 Salad/240g | 127 | 2.0 | 53 | 8.0 | 3.0 | 1.0 | 1.0 |
| Chicken, Flame Grilled, with French Dressing, Burger King* | 1 Serving/280g | 134 | 3.0 | 48 | 7.0 | 3.0 | 1.0 | 1.0 |
| Garden, Burger King* | 1 Serving/165g | 33 | 2.0 | 20 | 1.0 | 4.0 | 1.0 | 1.0 |
| **SPRITE** | | | | | | | | |
| Burger King* | 1 Reg/400g | 148 | 0.0 | 37 | 0.0 | 9.0 | 0.0 | 0.0 |
| **TEA** | | | | | | | | |
| Regular, White, No Sugar, Burger King* | 1 Reg/200ml | 22 | 4.0 | 11 | 1.0 | 1.0 | 2.0 | 0.0 |
| **CAFFE NERO** | | | | | | | | |
| **BARS** | | | | | | | | |
| Chocolate, Milk, Caffe Nero* | 1 Bar/40g | 223 | 14.0 | 558 | 8.0 | 55.0 | 34.0 | 1.0 |
| Chocolate & Hazelnut, Caffe Nero* | 1 Bar/40g | 229 | 15.0 | 572 | 8.0 | 49.5 | 38.0 | 1.8 |
| Exotic Fruit, Organic, Caffe Nero* | 1 Bar/64g | 239 | 11.0 | 374 | 5.6 | 50.3 | 16.8 | 10.0 |
| Granola, Caffe Nero* | 1 Bar/64g | 259 | 14.0 | 404 | 5.9 | 55.3 | 21.7 | 0.0 |
| Granola, Organic, Caffe Nero* | 1 Bar/64g | 269 | 13.0 | 420 | 7.4 | 51.0 | 20.7 | 6.0 |
| Shortbread, Caffe Nero* | 1 Pack/50g | 243 | 14.0 | 485 | 4.8 | 54.6 | 27.6 | 0.0 |
| **BISCOTTI** | | | | | | | | |
| Almond, Caffe Nero* | 1 Pack/52g | 202 | 8.0 | 388 | 9.2 | 53.1 | 15.3 | 2.8 |
| Doppio, Almond & Chocolate, Caffe Nero* | 1 Pack/29g | 228 | 9.0 | 786 | 15.0 | 110.0 | 32.0 | 0.0 |
| **BROWNIE** | | | | | | | | |
| Chocolate, Brownie, Caffe Nero* | 1 Brownie/74g | 321 | 18.0 | 429 | 6.0 | 48.6 | 23.7 | 3.6 |

| | Measure INFO/WEIGHT | per Measure KCAL | FAT | Nutrition Values per 100g / 100ml KCAL | PROT | CARB | FAT | FIBRE |
|---|---|---|---|---|---|---|---|---|
| **CAFFE NERO** | | | | | | | | |
| **BROWNIE** | | | | | | | | |
| Chocolate, Double, Organic, Gluten Free, Caffe Nero* | 1 Brownie/78g | 331 | 16.0 | 425 | 4.3 | 55.4 | 20.7 | 2.0 |
| **BRUSCHETTA** | | | | | | | | |
| Parmesan & Roast Onion, Caffe Nero* | 1 Pack/50g | 239 | 11.0 | 479 | 16.0 | 53.7 | 22.2 | 1.5 |
| Sun Dried Tomato & Basil, Caffe Nero* | 1 Pack/50g | 224 | 9.0 | 448 | 12.1 | 58.4 | 18.3 | 1.7 |
| **CAKE** | | | | | | | | |
| Banana & Caramel, Slice, Caffe Nero* | 1 Serving/82g | 342 | 20.0 | 417 | 4.6 | 45.5 | 24.1 | 0.0 |
| Banana & Sultana, Slice, Caffe Nero* | 1 Serving/80g | 221 | 4.0 | 276 | 4.7 | 53.6 | 4.8 | 0.0 |
| Carrot & Raisin, Slice, Organic, Caffe Nero* | 1 Slice/70g | 283 | 17.0 | 404 | 4.1 | 41.5 | 24.7 | 4.4 |
| Chocolate & Orange, Slice, Caffe Nero* | 1 Serving/70g | 233 | 10.0 | 333 | 4.7 | 46.7 | 14.2 | 1.4 |
| Chocolate & Pecan Fudge Brownie, Caffe Nero* | 1 Serving/113g | 426 | 22.0 | 377 | 3.6 | 47.7 | 19.1 | 0.0 |
| Chocolate Fudge, Caffe Nero* | 1 Serving/143g | 615 | 32.0 | 430 | 5.3 | 51.8 | 22.4 | 1.3 |
| Chocolate Zabaglione, Caffe Nero* | 1 Serving/112g | 420 | 28.0 | 375 | 5.1 | 32.5 | 25.0 | 3.9 |
| Coffee & Pecan, Slice, Caffe Nero* | 1 Serving/87g | 389 | 23.0 | 447 | 5.1 | 46.2 | 26.9 | 0.0 |
| Cranberry & Orange, Slice, Caffe Nero* | 1 Serving/60g | 196 | 7.0 | 326 | 5.1 | 49.8 | 11.9 | 0.0 |
| Fruit, Slice, Organic, Caffe Nero* | 1 Slice/70g | 223 | 8.0 | 319 | 4.7 | 48.0 | 12.0 | 0.0 |
| Ginger, Spicy, Organic, Caffe Nero* | 1 Serving/70g | 236 | 11.0 | 338 | 3.9 | 46.4 | 15.2 | 4.1 |
| Lemon Drizzle, Slice, Organic, Caffe Nero* | 1 Slice/76g | 252 | 10.0 | 331 | 4.3 | 49.2 | 13.0 | 0.7 |
| Mocha, Slice, Caffe Nero* | 1 Serving/89g | 333 | 18.0 | 375 | 4.8 | 43.4 | 20.2 | 0.0 |
| Panettone, Chocolate, Mini, Caffe Nero* | 1 Serving/100g | 420 | 22.0 | 420 | 9.0 | 46.0 | 22.3 | 1.0 |
| Panettone, Classic, Mini, Caffe Nero* | 1 Serving/100g | 385 | 14.0 | 385 | 9.0 | 51.0 | 13.6 | 2.0 |
| Passion, Caffe Nero* | 1 Serving/125g | 518 | 40.0 | 414 | 5.5 | 52.8 | 31.6 | 0.9 |
| Sponge, Victoria, Caffe Nero* | 1 Serving/144g | 474 | 22.0 | 329 | 4.5 | 43.5 | 15.1 | 0.4 |
| Toffee & Banana, Organic, Caffe Nero* | 1 Serving/70g | 188 | 9.0 | 268 | 3.8 | 33.8 | 13.1 | 0.7 |
| White Chocolate & Orange Ganache, Caffe Nero* | 1 Serving/135g | 558 | 42.0 | 413 | 4.0 | 29.0 | 31.3 | 0.0 |
| **CALZONE** | | | | | | | | |
| Mozzarella & Tomato, Caffe Nero* | 1 Serving/155g | 320 | 11.0 | 206 | 9.3 | 25.5 | 7.2 | 1.2 |
| Pepperoni, Spicy, Caffe Nero* | 1 Pack/154g | 298 | 10.0 | 194 | 8.2 | 25.9 | 6.5 | 1.3 |
| **CHEESE TWISTS** | | | | | | | | |
| Caffe Nero* | 1 Serving/90g | 387 | 23.0 | 431 | 14.3 | 36.4 | 25.3 | 1.5 |
| **CHEESECAKE** | | | | | | | | |
| Apple & Blackberry, Reduced Fat, Caffe Nero* | 1 Serving/165g | 277 | 12.0 | 168 | 4.2 | 23.3 | 7.1 | 1.3 |
| Apple & Cinnamon, Baked, Caffe Nero* | 1 Serving/138g | 406 | 25.0 | 294 | 4.1 | 30.6 | 17.9 | 0.0 |
| Blackcurrant, Reduced Fat, Caffe Nero* | 1 Serving/119g | 248 | 11.0 | 209 | 5.4 | 25.7 | 9.4 | 0.5 |
| Chocolate, Simply, Caffe Nero* | 1 Serving/125g | 475 | 25.0 | 380 | 4.4 | 45.6 | 20.0 | 0.0 |
| Chocolate, White & Dark, Caffe Nero* | 1 Serving/171g | 711 | 53.0 | 416 | 5.7 | 30.8 | 30.8 | 0.0 |
| Chocolate, Zucotto, Caffe Nero* | 1 Serving/137g | 512 | 36.0 | 374 | 4.8 | 29.6 | 26.3 | 0.5 |
| Lemon, Dessert Pot, Caffe Nero* | 1 Pot/105g | 390 | 27.0 | 370 | 2.6 | 32.0 | 25.8 | 0.9 |
| Lemon & Mascarpone, Caffe Nero* | 1 Serving/135g | 466 | 30.0 | 345 | 5.2 | 30.2 | 22.5 | 1.0 |
| Rhubarb & Vanilla, Caffe Nero* | 1 Serving/135g | 424 | 30.0 | 314 | 5.4 | 26.9 | 22.0 | 0.0 |
| Summer Fruit, Caffe Nero* | 1 Serving/157g | 388 | 21.0 | 247 | 3.4 | 29.5 | 13.2 | 0.0 |
| Toffee Crunch, Caffe Nero* | 1 Serving/155g | 577 | 35.0 | 372 | 5.8 | 36.8 | 22.5 | 1.0 |
| Toffee Swirl, Caffe Nero* | 1 Serving/133g | 410 | 24.0 | 308 | 6.3 | 30.0 | 18.1 | 0.0 |
| White Chocolate & Orange, Reduced Fat, Caffe Nero* | 1 Serving/120g | 310 | 19.0 | 258 | 6.5 | 23.0 | 15.6 | 0.7 |
| **CHOCOLATE** | | | | | | | | |
| Coin, Caffe Nero* | 1 Serving/25g | 129 | 7.0 | 516 | 6.3 | 59.7 | 27.8 | 2.1 |
| **COFFEE** | | | | | | | | |
| Cappuccino, Semi Skimmed Milk, Regular, Caffe Nero* | 1 Cup/80g | 37 | 1.0 | 46 | 3.5 | 4.7 | 1.7 | 0.0 |
| Cappuccino, Skimmed Milk, Regular, Caffe Nero* | 1 Regular/80g | 27 | 0.0 | 34 | 3.5 | 4.8 | 0.3 | 0.0 |
| Cappuccino, Soya Milk, Regular, Caffe Nero* | 1 Serving/80g | 36 | 2.0 | 45 | 3.7 | 2.5 | 2.2 | 0.6 |
| Latte, Caramel, Semi Skimmed Milk, Caffe Nero* | 1 Latte/421ml | 484 | 25.0 | 115 | 2.3 | 12.3 | 6.0 | 0.0 |
| Latte, Chai, Semi Skimmed Milk, Caffe Nero* | 1 Serving/405ml | 283 | 11.0 | 70 | 3.8 | 8.3 | 2.6 | 0.0 |
| Latte, Chai, Skimmed Milk, Caffe Nero* | 1 Serving/405ml | 239 | 5.0 | 59 | 3.8 | 8.4 | 1.3 | 0.0 |

| | Measure INFO/WEIGHT | KCAL | FAT | KCAL | PROT | CARB | FAT | FIBRE |
|---|---|---|---|---|---|---|---|---|
| **CAFFE NERO** | | | | | | | | |
| **COFFEE** | | | | | | | | |
| Latte, Frappe, Semi Skimmed, Caffe Nero* | 1 Serving/538ml | 307 | 4.0 | 57 | 2.6 | 10.2 | 0.8 | 0.0 |
| Latte, Frappe, Skimmed Milk, Caffe Nero* | 1 Serving/533g | 277 | 1.0 | 52 | 2.6 | 10.3 | 0.2 | 0.0 |
| Latte, Iced, Caffe Nero* | 1 Latte/488g | 117 | 4.0 | 24 | 1.8 | 2.5 | 0.9 | 0.0 |
| Latte, Semi Skimmed Milk, Caffe Nero* | 1 Regular/150g | 69 | 3.0 | 46 | 3.5 | 4.7 | 1.7 | 0.0 |
| Latte, Skimmed Milk, Regular, Caffe Nero* | 1 Regular/150g | 51 | 0.0 | 34 | 3.5 | 4.8 | 0.3 | 0.0 |
| Latte, Soya Milk, Regular, Caffe Nero* | 1 Cup/151g | 68 | 3.0 | 45 | 3.7 | 2.5 | 2.2 | 0.6 |
| Mocha, Whipped Cream, Semi Skimmed Milk, Caffe Nero* | 1 Cup/180ml | 326 | 19.0 | 181 | 4.3 | 17.2 | 10.8 | 0.8 |
| Mocha, White Chocolate, Semi Skimmed Milk, Caffe Nero* | 1 Serving/400ml | 412 | 25.0 | 103 | 2.4 | 6.1 | 6.3 | 0.0 |
| Mocha Latte, Semi Skimmed Milk, Regular, Caffe Nero* | 1 Serving/582g | 483 | 6.0 | 83 | 2.8 | 16.3 | 1.0 | 0.4 |
| Mocha Latte, Skimmed Milk, Caffe Nero* | 1 Serving/587ml | 511 | 4.0 | 87 | 3.8 | 16.6 | 0.7 | 0.8 |
| **COFFEE BEANS** | | | | | | | | |
| Chocolate Coated, Caffe Nero* | 1 Serving/25g | 117 | 7.0 | 469 | 8.5 | 50.0 | 26.2 | 11.9 |
| Cioccafe, Caffe Nero* | 1 Serving/25g | 117 | 6.0 | 468 | 8.5 | 50.0 | 26.0 | 0.0 |
| **COOKIES** | | | | | | | | |
| Belgian Chocolate, Organic, Caffe Nero* | 1 Cookie/50g | 244 | 11.0 | 488 | 6.4 | 64.8 | 22.6 | 0.0 |
| Chocolate Chip, Organic, Caffe Nero* | 1 Cookie/60g | 263 | 12.0 | 438 | 4.5 | 56.6 | 20.1 | 1.5 |
| Milk Chocolate Chunk, Caffe Nero* | 1 Cookie/71g | 338 | 18.0 | 470 | 5.8 | 55.8 | 24.9 | 1.7 |
| Raisin & Oat, Organic, Caffe Nero* | 1 Cookie/60g | 253 | 12.0 | 422 | 5.1 | 56.8 | 19.3 | 2.4 |
| Triple Chocolate, Caffe Nero* | 1 Cookie/72g | 333 | 17.0 | 463 | 5.6 | 55.6 | 24.3 | 3.3 |
| White Chocolate & Cranberry, Caffe Nero* | 1 Cookie/71g | 301 | 11.0 | 419 | 4.4 | 66.3 | 15.2 | 1.5 |
| **COUS COUS** | | | | | | | | |
| Mediterranean, Caffe Nero* | 1 Serving/315g | 403 | 21.0 | 128 | 2.8 | 14.0 | 6.8 | 2.1 |
| **CRISPS** | | | | | | | | |
| Mature Cheddar & Spring Onion, Handcooked, Caffe Nero* | 1 Pack/50g | 240 | 14.0 | 481 | 6.1 | 54.0 | 28.6 | 4.4 |
| Sea Salt, Caffe Nero* | 1 Pack/50g | 247 | 14.0 | 493 | 8.0 | 54.0 | 27.1 | 4.5 |
| Sea Salt & Balsamic Vinegar, Caffe Nero* | 1 Pack/50g | 241 | 13.0 | 482 | 7.0 | 54.1 | 26.4 | 4.0 |
| **CROISSANT** | | | | | | | | |
| Almond, Caffe Nero* | 1 Croissant/90g | 365 | 19.0 | 406 | 7.5 | 46.4 | 21.1 | 1.7 |
| Apricot, Caffe Nero* | 1 Croissant/104g | 286 | 12.0 | 273 | 5.4 | 37.3 | 11.3 | 1.2 |
| Butter, Caffe Nero* | 1 Croissant/53g | 244 | 15.0 | 460 | 9.1 | 44.1 | 27.5 | 1.7 |
| **CUPCAKE** | | | | | | | | |
| Chocolate, Caffe Nero* | 1 Cupcake/68g | 311 | 19.0 | 457 | 3.1 | 48.7 | 28.1 | 0.5 |
| **DANISH PASTRY** | | | | | | | | |
| Apple, Caffe Nero* | 1 Pastry/75g | 255 | 12.0 | 340 | 5.7 | 42.5 | 16.3 | 2.3 |
| Pear & Chocolate, Caffe Nero* | 1 Pastry/90g | 238 | 12.0 | 264 | 4.7 | 36.9 | 12.8 | 0.0 |
| **DRIED FRUIT MIX** | | | | | | | | |
| Caffe Nero* | 1 Bag/75g | 248 | 4.0 | 331 | 1.6 | 69.1 | 5.4 | 5.0 |
| **FARFALLE** | | | | | | | | |
| with Roasted Vegetable Sauce, Caffe Nero* | 1 Serving/324g | 275 | 8.0 | 85 | 2.6 | 13.4 | 2.6 | 1.6 |
| **FRUIT & NUT MIX** | | | | | | | | |
| Caffe Nero* | 1 Serving/75g | 322 | 18.0 | 430 | 9.8 | 44.8 | 23.4 | 3.5 |
| **FRUIT SALAD** | | | | | | | | |
| Classic, Caffe Nero* | 1 Serving/170g | 75 | 0.0 | 44 | 0.5 | 10.9 | 0.1 | 1.5 |
| Spring, Caffe Nero* | 1 Salad/174g | 47 | 0.0 | 27 | 0.6 | 6.2 | 0.1 | 0.0 |
| Tropical, Caffe Nero* | 1 Serving/170g | 70 | 0.0 | 41 | 0.6 | 11.1 | 0.1 | 1.4 |
| **GINGERBREAD** | | | | | | | | |
| Man, Caffe Nero* | 1 Man/54g | 235 | 8.0 | 435 | 6.7 | 70.2 | 14.2 | 1.6 |
| **HOT CHOCOLATE** | | | | | | | | |
| Milano, Caffe Nero* | 1 Cup/240g | 446 | 24.0 | 186 | 3.8 | 19.4 | 10.2 | 2.0 |
| Semi Skimmed Milk, Regular, Caffe Nero* | 1 Cup/211g | 280 | 4.0 | 133 | 4.0 | 25.1 | 2.0 | 1.3 |
| Skimmed Milk, No Cream, Regular, Caffe Nero* | 1 Cup/210ml | 262 | 2.0 | 125 | 4.0 | 25.5 | 1.0 | 1.3 |
| Whipped Cream, Semi Skimmed Milk, Regular, Caffe Nero* | 1 Cup/250ml | 432 | 20.0 | 173 | 3.7 | 21.6 | 8.2 | 1.1 |

## CAFFE NERO

| | Measure INFO/WEIGHT | KCAL | FAT | KCAL | PROT | CARB | FAT | FIBRE |
|---|---|---|---|---|---|---|---|---|
| **JUICE** | | | | | | | | |
| Apple, Organic, Caffe Nero* | 1 Serving/200ml | 94 | 0.0 | 47 | 0.5 | 11.2 | 0.0 | 0.0 |
| Apple, Pressed, 100% Premium Juice, Caffe Nero* | 1 Serving/250ml | 128 | 0.0 | 51 | 0.1 | 11.9 | 0.0 | 0.0 |
| Orange, 100% Squeezed, Caffe Nero* | 1 Bottle/250ml | 95 | 0.0 | 38 | 0.5 | 8.8 | 0.1 | 0.0 |
| Orange, Organic, Caffe Nero* | 1 Serving/200ml | 94 | 0.0 | 47 | 0.5 | 10.4 | 0.0 | 0.0 |
| **JUICE DRINK** | | | | | | | | |
| Fruit Booster, Mango, Caffe Nero* | 1 Drink/644ml | 219 | 1.0 | 34 | 0.5 | 8.2 | 0.1 | 0.6 |
| Pineapple, Orange & Banana, Fruit Booster, Caffe Nero* | 1 Drink/652ml | 202 | 1.0 | 31 | 0.2 | 7.9 | 0.1 | 0.1 |
| Strawberry & Raspberry, Fruit Booster, Caffe Nero* | 1 Drink/638ml | 166 | 1.0 | 26 | 0.3 | 6.4 | 0.1 | 0.5 |
| Summer Fruits, Fruit Booster, Caffe Nero* | 1 Drink/642ml | 244 | 0.0 | 38 | 0.3 | 9.4 | 0.0 | 0.4 |
| **LASAGNE** | | | | | | | | |
| Beef, Al Forno, Caffe Nero* | 1 Serving/350g | 595 | 36.0 | 170 | 10.2 | 8.3 | 10.3 | 0.5 |
| Spinach & Ricotta, Caffe Nero* | 1 Serving/375g | 633 | 36.0 | 169 | 8.4 | 13.3 | 9.5 | 0.9 |
| Vegetable, Caffe Nero* | 1 Serving/371g | 482 | 24.0 | 130 | 5.1 | 13.9 | 6.5 | 0.0 |
| **LEMONADE** | | | | | | | | |
| Sicilian, Still, Caffe Nero* | 1 Serving/250ml | 115 | 0.0 | 46 | 0.0 | 11.2 | 0.0 | 0.0 |
| **MILKSHAKE** | | | | | | | | |
| Banana Frappe, Caffe Nero* | 1 Frappe/549ml | 472 | 7.0 | 86 | 3.1 | 16.1 | 1.2 | 0.0 |
| Double Chocolate, Semi Skimmed, Frappe, Caffe Nero* | 1 Frappe/582ml | 483 | 6.0 | 83 | 2.8 | 16.3 | 1.0 | 0.4 |
| Double Chocolate, Skimmed Milk, Frappe, Caffe Nero* | 1 Frappe/587g | 452 | 2.0 | 77 | 2.8 | 16.3 | 0.4 | 0.4 |
| Mint, Frappe, Caffe Nero* | 1 Frappe/543ml | 462 | 7.0 | 85 | 3.2 | 15.6 | 1.2 | 0.0 |
| Strawberry, Frappe, Caffe Nero* | 1 Frappe/546ml | 475 | 7.0 | 87 | 3.2 | 16.2 | 1.2 | 0.0 |
| Vanilla, Frappe, Caffe Nero* | 1 Frappe/543g | 473 | 7.0 | 87 | 3.1 | 16.2 | 1.2 | 0.0 |
| **MOUSSE** | | | | | | | | |
| Chocolate Brownie, Dessert Pot, Caffe Nero* | 1 Pot/89g | 335 | 19.0 | 375 | 4.3 | 42.8 | 21.0 | 1.5 |
| Sicilian Lemon, Dessert Pot, Caffe Nero* | 1 Pot/125g | 423 | 35.0 | 338 | 1.7 | 20.5 | 27.7 | 0.1 |
| **MUFFIN** | | | | | | | | |
| Apple & Ginger, Caffe Nero* | 1 Muffin/120g | 402 | 22.0 | 335 | 4.4 | 37.8 | 18.4 | 0.7 |
| Blueberry, Caffe Nero* | 1 Muffin/120g | 430 | 23.0 | 358 | 4.5 | 42.7 | 18.8 | 1.1 |
| Blueberry, Reduced Fat, Caffe Nero* | 1 Muffin/120g | 287 | 6.0 | 239 | 4.7 | 44.8 | 4.6 | 2.9 |
| Carrot & Sultana, Low Fat, Caffe Nero* | 1 Muffin/119g | 271 | 4.0 | 227 | 5.0 | 44.8 | 3.0 | 0.0 |
| Chocolate, White & Dark, Caffe Nero* | 1 Muffin/100g | 393 | 21.0 | 393 | 5.7 | 45.0 | 21.2 | 1.7 |
| Lemon & Raspberry, Reduced Fat, Caffe Nero* | 1 Muffin/120g | 365 | 16.0 | 305 | 4.6 | 41.7 | 13.2 | 1.5 |
| Lemon Poppy Seed, Caffe Nero* | 1 Muffin/120g | 449 | 22.0 | 374 | 5.7 | 45.9 | 18.6 | 0.9 |
| Raspberry & White Chocolate, Caffe Nero* | 1 Muffin/120g | 461 | 24.0 | 384 | 5.0 | 46.0 | 20.0 | 0.9 |
| Summer Fruit, Caffe Nero* | 1 Muffin/120g | 410 | 21.0 | 342 | 4.2 | 41.8 | 17.5 | 1.0 |
| Super Seed, Caffe Nero* | 1 Muffin/119g | 398 | 20.0 | 332 | 5.9 | 40.4 | 16.3 | 2.1 |
| Triple Belgian Chocolate, Caffe Nero* | 1 Muffin/124g | 488 | 26.0 | 393 | 5.7 | 45.0 | 21.2 | 1.7 |
| White & Dark Chocolate, Caffe Nero* | 1 Muffin/120g | 472 | 25.0 | 393 | 5.7 | 45.0 | 21.2 | 1.7 |
| White Chocolate & Raspberry, Caffe Nero* | 1 Muffin/120g | 453 | 25.0 | 378 | 6.0 | 41.0 | 21.1 | 0.0 |
| **NUTS** | | | | | | | | |
| Cashew, Roasted & Salted, Caffe Nero* | 1 Serving/40g | 244 | 20.0 | 611 | 20.5 | 18.8 | 50.9 | 3.2 |
| **OLIVES** | | | | | | | | |
| Green, Marinated, Caffe Nero* | 1 Pack/110g | 212 | 23.0 | 193 | 1.0 | 5.0 | 20.6 | 4.1 |
| **PAIN AU CHOCOLAT** | | | | | | | | |
| Almond, Caffe Nero* | 1 Pain/100g | 406 | 22.0 | 406 | 7.9 | 45.9 | 22.3 | 2.5 |
| Caffe Nero* | 1 Pain/62g | 277 | 16.0 | 446 | 8.5 | 46.2 | 25.2 | 1.3 |
| **PAIN AU RAISIN** | | | | | | | | |
| Caffe Nero* | 1 Pain/95g | 325 | 15.0 | 342 | 5.4 | 45.0 | 15.6 | 1.4 |
| **PANINI** | | | | | | | | |
| All Day Breakfast, Caffe Nero* | 1 Panini/250g | 343 | 12.0 | 137 | 9.0 | 14.8 | 4.6 | 2.0 |
| Bacon, Breakfast, Caffe Nero* | 1 Panini/110g | 299 | 11.0 | 272 | 10.0 | 35.2 | 10.1 | 1.7 |
| Butternut Squash & Soft Cheese, Caffe Nero* | 1 Panini/150g | 208 | 6.0 | 139 | 8.2 | 20.2 | 4.1 | 1.4 |

|  | Measure | per Measure | | Nutrition Values per 100g / 100ml | | | | |
|---|---|---|---|---|---|---|---|---|
|  | INFO/WEIGHT | KCAL | FAT | KCAL | PROT | CARB | FAT | FIBRE |

## CAFFE NERO

### PANINI

| Item | Measure | KCAL | FAT | KCAL | PROT | CARB | FAT | FIBRE |
|---|---|---|---|---|---|---|---|---|
| Chicken, & Creme Fraiche, Spicy, Caffe Nero* | 1 Panini/200g | 294 | 7.0 | 147 | 9.5 | 19.4 | 3.4 | 1.0 |
| Chicken, Bacon & Arrabbiata Sauce, Caffe Nero* | 1 Panini/244g | 354 | 9.0 | 145 | 10.1 | 17.6 | 3.8 | 0.9 |
| Chicken, with Herb Creme Fraiche, Caffe Nero* | 1 Panini/190g | 299 | 9.0 | 157 | 9.2 | 20.1 | 4.5 | 1.2 |
| Chicken BLT, Caffe Nero* | 1 Panini/249g | 513 | 29.0 | 206 | 8.7 | 16.4 | 11.8 | 1.3 |
| Chicken Caesar, Caffe Nero* | 1 Panini/237g | 473 | 26.0 | 200 | 8.9 | 16.3 | 11.0 | 0.9 |
| Club, Italian, Caffe Nero* | 1 Panini/212g | 454 | 21.0 | 214 | 12.8 | 17.9 | 10.1 | 1.3 |
| Egg, Mushroom, & Tomato, Breakfast, Caffe Nero* | 1 Panini/145g | 297 | 10.0 | 205 | 8.6 | 27.4 | 6.8 | 1.7 |
| Egg Florentine, Breakfast, Caffe Nero* | 1 Panini/136g | 288 | 10.0 | 212 | 8.6 | 27.0 | 7.7 | 1.7 |
| Ham, & Brie, Caffe Nero* | 1 Panini/229g | 399 | 18.0 | 174 | 9.9 | 16.4 | 7.7 | 0.9 |
| Ham, & Smoked Mozzarella, Caffe Nero* | 1 Panini/229g | 460 | 21.0 | 201 | 13.1 | 17.0 | 9.0 | 0.8 |
| Ham & Egg, Breakfast, Caffe Nero* | 1 Panini/141g | 362 | 17.0 | 257 | 11.3 | 26.2 | 11.9 | 1.4 |
| Ham & Mozzarella, Caffe Nero* | 1 Panini/214g | 417 | 17.0 | 195 | 12.2 | 18.2 | 8.1 | 0.9 |
| Lemon Chicken, Caffe Nero* | 1 Panini/212g | 478 | 17.0 | 225 | 9.1 | 28.8 | 8.2 | 0.0 |
| Meatball, with Tomato Sauce, Italian, Caffe Nero* | 1 Panini/245g | 449 | 20.0 | 183 | 8.9 | 18.5 | 8.2 | 0.9 |
| Mozzarella, & Plum Tomato, Caffe Nero* | 1 Panini/216g | 415 | 21.0 | 192 | 7.9 | 17.9 | 9.8 | 1.1 |
| Mozzarella, & Roasted Mushroom, Caffe Nero* | 1 Panini/214g | 351 | 12.0 | 164 | 8.1 | 20.1 | 5.6 | 1.2 |
| Mozzarella & Meatball, Caffe Nero* | 1 Panini/239g | 481 | 22.0 | 201 | 9.5 | 19.9 | 9.2 | 1.0 |
| Parma Ham, & Mascarpone, Caffe Nero* | 1 Panini/195g | 536 | 23.0 | 275 | 11.3 | 30.6 | 11.9 | 0.0 |
| Pepperoni, Mozzarella & Tomato, Caffe Nero* | 1 Panini/241g | 446 | 22.0 | 185 | 8.3 | 17.1 | 9.3 | 0.9 |
| Prosciutto Ham, & Mascarpone, Caffe Nero* | 1 Panini/195g | 430 | 22.0 | 221 | 10.0 | 19.2 | 11.5 | 0.9 |
| Roasted Mediterranean Vegetable, Caffe Nero* | 1 Panini/204g | 255 | 5.0 | 125 | 5.2 | 20.2 | 2.5 | 3.6 |
| Salami Tomato & Mozzarella, Caffe Nero* | 1 Panini/215g | 417 | 18.0 | 194 | 8.9 | 20.5 | 8.6 | 0.0 |
| Soft Cheese & Sweet Chilli Vegetable, Caffe Nero* | 1 Panini/223g | 308 | 7.0 | 138 | 5.1 | 22.5 | 3.1 | 1.5 |
| Tricolore, Caffe Nero* | 1 Panini/239g | 435 | 23.0 | 182 | 7.2 | 16.4 | 9.7 | 1.3 |
| Tuna, Melt, Caffe Nero* | 1 Panini/224g | 405 | 16.0 | 181 | 11.5 | 17.4 | 7.2 | 1.0 |
| Turkey & Cranberry, Caffe Nero* | 1 Panini/225g | 443 | 15.0 | 197 | 9.9 | 24.4 | 6.6 | 1.2 |

### PANNA COTTA

| Item | Measure | KCAL | FAT | KCAL | PROT | CARB | FAT | FIBRE |
|---|---|---|---|---|---|---|---|---|
| Raspberry, Caffe Nero* | 1 Pot/130g | 384 | 32.0 | 295 | 1.2 | 17.2 | 24.6 | 0.0 |

### PASTA

| Item | Measure | KCAL | FAT | KCAL | PROT | CARB | FAT | FIBRE |
|---|---|---|---|---|---|---|---|---|
| Penne, with Roasted Red Pepper, Caffe Nero* | 1 Serving/341g | 317 | 8.0 | 93 | 3.0 | 14.7 | 2.4 | 0.6 |

### PASTA SALAD

| Item | Measure | KCAL | FAT | KCAL | PROT | CARB | FAT | FIBRE |
|---|---|---|---|---|---|---|---|---|
| Basil Pesto, Caffe Nero* | 1 Serving/200g | 510 | 30.0 | 255 | 5.9 | 24.1 | 15.1 | 0.4 |
| Red Pepper & Pine Nuts, Caffe Nero* | 1 Salad/271g | 506 | 25.0 | 187 | 5.7 | 19.7 | 9.4 | 1.9 |
| Sunkissed Tomato, Caffe Nero* | 1 Salad/285g | 755 | 44.0 | 265 | 6.7 | 24.6 | 15.5 | 0.0 |
| Tomato & Mozzarella, Caffe Nero* | 1 Pack/298g | 391 | 26.0 | 131 | 2.9 | 10.3 | 8.7 | 1.1 |

### PENNE

| Item | Measure | KCAL | FAT | KCAL | PROT | CARB | FAT | FIBRE |
|---|---|---|---|---|---|---|---|---|
| with Roasted Red Pepper Sauce, Caffe Nero* | 1 Serving/341g | 317 | 8.0 | 93 | 3.0 | 14.7 | 2.4 | 0.6 |

### PIZZA

| Item | Measure | KCAL | FAT | KCAL | PROT | CARB | FAT | FIBRE |
|---|---|---|---|---|---|---|---|---|
| Cheese & Tomato, Caffe Nero* | 1 Serving/194g | 444 | 13.0 | 229 | 10.4 | 37.9 | 6.9 | 3.3 |
| Milano Salami & Peppers, Caffe Nero* | 1 Serving/357g | 768 | 24.0 | 215 | 9.7 | 33.7 | 6.7 | 2.9 |

### RAVIOLI

| Item | Measure | KCAL | FAT | KCAL | PROT | CARB | FAT | FIBRE |
|---|---|---|---|---|---|---|---|---|
| Mushroom, with Chestnut Mushroom Sauce, Caffe Nero* | 1 Serving/310g | 565 | 32.0 | 182 | 6.9 | 15.3 | 10.3 | 0.0 |

### SALAD

| Item | Measure | KCAL | FAT | KCAL | PROT | CARB | FAT | FIBRE |
|---|---|---|---|---|---|---|---|---|
| Cous Cous, Mediterranean Style, Caffe Nero* | 1 Pack/275g | 352 | 19.0 | 128 | 2.8 | 14.0 | 6.8 | 2.1 |
| Cous Cous & Roasted Vegetable, Caffe Nero* | 1 Salad/250g | 452 | 14.0 | 181 | 4.3 | 27.5 | 5.8 | 1.4 |
| Crayfish, Caffe Nero* | 1 Salad/205g | 279 | 11.0 | 136 | 5.2 | 17.0 | 5.4 | 0.0 |
| Prosciutto & Pecorino, Caffe Nero* | 1 Salad/217g | 369 | 28.0 | 170 | 3.5 | 10.1 | 12.7 | 0.3 |
| Roast Summer Vegetables, & Feta Cheese, Caffe Nero* | 1 Serving/263g | 460 | 40.0 | 175 | 3.6 | 4.1 | 15.3 | 0.5 |
| Sun Kissed Tomato & Mozzarella, Caffe Nero* | 1 Salad/265g | 446 | 17.0 | 168 | 6.3 | 21.4 | 6.4 | 1.5 |
| Tuna, With Herbed Potatos, Caffe Nero* | 1 Pack/247g | 254 | 14.0 | 103 | 3.4 | 9.6 | 5.8 | 1.7 |
| Tuna Nicoise, Caffe Nero* | 1 Pack/278g | 236 | 12.0 | 85 | 6.0 | 5.9 | 4.2 | 0.8 |

## CAFFE NERO

| | Measure INFO/WEIGHT | per Measure KCAL | per Measure FAT | Nutrition Values per 100g / 100ml KCAL | PROT | CARB | FAT | FIBRE |
|---|---|---|---|---|---|---|---|---|
| **SANDWICH** | | | | | | | | |
| BLT, Caffe Nero* | 1 Sandwich/163g | 322 | 14.0 | 198 | 7.3 | 24.9 | 8.4 | 1.8 |
| Cheese, Simply, Caffe Nero* | 1 Serving/161g | 506 | 26.0 | 314 | 16.1 | 26.4 | 16.0 | 3.1 |
| Chicken, Italian, Caffe Nero* | 1 Serving/174g | 361 | 16.0 | 207 | 9.6 | 21.0 | 9.4 | 0.0 |
| Chicken, Oven Roasted Tomatoes, & Spinach, Caffe Nero* | 1 Sandwich/169g | 289 | 8.0 | 171 | 10.7 | 22.0 | 4.5 | 2.0 |
| Chicken Salad, Caffe Nero* | 1 Pack/177g | 358 | 14.0 | 202 | 11.8 | 22.2 | 8.0 | 1.8 |
| Crayfish, with Lemon Mayonnaise, Caffe Nero* | 1 Serving/156g | 370 | 20.0 | 237 | 8.3 | 22.4 | 12.7 | 0.0 |
| Egg Mayonnaise, & Cress, Caffe Nero* | 1 Serving/168g | 347 | 13.0 | 206 | 10.1 | 26.1 | 7.6 | 2.0 |
| Goats Cheese & Roasted Red Pepper, Caffe Nero* | 1 Focaccia/182g | 344 | 10.0 | 189 | 8.5 | 26.6 | 5.4 | 1.6 |
| Ham, & Cheddar, Caffe Nero* | 1 Pack/179g | 433 | 18.0 | 242 | 15.4 | 22.5 | 10.0 | 1.5 |
| Ham, & Egg, Caffe Nero* | 1 Sandwich/204g | 371 | 16.0 | 181 | 12.3 | 15.6 | 7.7 | 1.1 |
| Ham, Roasted Mushroom & Mozzarella, Caffe Nero* | 1 Pack/206g | 428 | 12.0 | 208 | 12.4 | 27.1 | 5.6 | 1.4 |
| Herbed Ham, Mozzarella & Mushroom, Caffe Nero* | 1 Focaccia/217g | 421 | 10.0 | 194 | 10.7 | 27.3 | 4.7 | 1.3 |
| Mature Cheddar & Pickle, Caffe Nero* | 1 Seving/188g | 426 | 20.0 | 226 | 9.9 | 24.1 | 10.6 | 1.7 |
| Mozzarella, & Tomato, Caffe Nero* | 1 Sandwich/204g | 456 | 25.0 | 223 | 10.2 | 18.2 | 12.1 | 1.2 |
| Prawn, Lemon Dressing & Rocket, Caffe Nero* | 1 Pack/169g | 342 | 13.0 | 202 | 12.4 | 20.9 | 7.7 | 3.2 |
| Salmon, Smoked, & Lemon Mayonnaise, Caffe Nero* | 1 Serving/159g | 497 | 32.0 | 313 | 10.6 | 21.8 | 20.3 | 0.0 |
| Tuna & Salad, Caffe Nero* | 1 Pack/138g | 254 | 5.0 | 183 | 11.6 | 28.5 | 3.3 | 2.1 |
| Tuna Mayonnaise, & Salad, Caffe Nero* | 1 Sandwich/183g | 353 | 15.0 | 192 | 8.8 | 20.4 | 8.4 | 1.3 |
| **SCONE** | | | | | | | | |
| Luxury Fruit, Caffe Nero* | 1 Scone/100g | 330 | 10.0 | 330 | 5.9 | 52.6 | 10.2 | 2.0 |
| **SHORTBREAD** | | | | | | | | |
| Chocolate Chip, Organic, Sharing, Caffe Nero* | 1 Serving/105g | 502 | 29.0 | 478 | 5.3 | 51.8 | 27.7 | 1.7 |
| Organic, Caffe Nero* | 1 Serving/50g | 238 | 14.0 | 477 | 5.4 | 51.3 | 27.7 | 1.5 |
| **SLICES** | | | | | | | | |
| Almond Torta, Pastry, Caffe Nero* | 1 Pastry/126g | 439 | 18.0 | 346 | 2.7 | 51.6 | 14.4 | 0.5 |
| Caramel, Caffe Nero* | 1 Slice/50g | 252 | 15.0 | 505 | 4.6 | 55.5 | 29.4 | 2.1 |
| Caramel, Digestive Biscuit, Caffe Nero* | 1 Serving/80g | 418 | 24.0 | 523 | 4.1 | 59.2 | 29.5 | 1.1 |
| Caramel, Shortcake, Caffe Nero* | 1 Slice/98g | 514 | 31.0 | 524 | 2.7 | 49.6 | 31.1 | 0.0 |
| Creamed Spinach, Savoury, Pastry, Caffe Nero* | 1 Pastry/120g | 372 | 23.0 | 310 | 5.7 | 27.8 | 19.5 | 0.0 |
| Frutt Di Bosco, Torta, Pastry, Caffe Nero* | 1 Torta/97g | 227 | 8.0 | 234 | 2.9 | 37.1 | 8.2 | 1.5 |
| Ham & Cheese, Savoury, Puff Pastry, Caffe Nero* | 1 Pastry/110g | 394 | 25.0 | 358 | 11.5 | 26.9 | 22.7 | 0.0 |
| **SMOOTHIE** | | | | | | | | |
| Mango & Passionfruit, Caffe Nero* | 1 Smoothie/250ml | 155 | 0.0 | 62 | 0.6 | 14.3 | 0.1 | 0.3 |
| Peach & Apricot, Caffe Nero* | 1 Smoothie/250ml | 132 | 0.0 | 53 | 0.6 | 12.1 | 0.0 | 0.5 |
| Peach & Raspberry, Organic, Bio, Caffe Nero* | 1 Smoothie/250ml | 188 | 5.0 | 75 | 3.2 | 11.4 | 1.8 | 0.0 |
| Red Berry, Caffe Nero* | 1 Smoothie/250ml | 130 | 0.0 | 52 | 0.7 | 11.9 | 0.2 | 1.9 |
| Strawberry, Organic, Bio, Caffe Nero* | 1 Smoothie/250ml | 188 | 4.0 | 75 | 2.9 | 11.9 | 1.7 | 0.0 |
| Strawberry & Banana, Caffe Nero* | 1 Smoothie/250ml | 115 | 1.0 | 46 | 0.8 | 10.4 | 0.3 | 5.0 |
| **SNACK** | | | | | | | | |
| Chocolate Coated Coffee Beans, Caffe Nero* | 1 Serving/25g | 117 | 7.0 | 469 | 8.5 | 50.0 | 26.2 | 11.9 |
| Chocolate Crunch, Caffe Nero* | 1 Serving/80g | 434 | 34.0 | 543 | 4.1 | 39.4 | 42.2 | 4.4 |
| **SOUP** | | | | | | | | |
| Broccoli & Blue Cheese, Less Than 5% Fat, Caffe Nero* | 1 Serving/331g | 205 | 16.0 | 62 | 1.8 | 3.0 | 4.8 | 0.0 |
| Butternut Squash & Roasted Garlic, Caffe Nero* | 1 Serving/300g | 114 | 6.0 | 38 | 0.7 | 4.2 | 2.1 | 0.9 |
| Carrot & Coriander, Caffe Nero* | 1 Serving/300g | 186 | 10.0 | 62 | 1.5 | 6.5 | 3.3 | 1.4 |
| Cream of Tomato & Basil, Caffe Nero* | 1 Serving/330g | 234 | 17.0 | 71 | 1.0 | 5.8 | 5.1 | 0.0 |
| Creamy Mushroom, Caffe Nero* | 1 Serving/331g | 185 | 14.0 | 56 | 1.0 | 4.1 | 4.1 | 0.0 |
| Mediterranean Vegetable, Caffe Nero* | 1 Serving/300g | 93 | 6.0 | 31 | 0.7 | 2.8 | 1.9 | 1.0 |
| Potato & Leek, Caffe Nero* | 1 Serving/300g | 195 | 14.0 | 65 | 1.1 | 4.3 | 4.8 | 0.7 |
| Roast Vegetable, Caffe Nero* | 1 Serving/332g | 73 | 4.0 | 22 | 0.6 | 2.2 | 1.3 | 0.0 |
| Roasted Tomato, Caffe Nero* | 1 Serving/329g | 112 | 4.0 | 34 | 0.8 | 5.1 | 1.1 | 0.0 |
| Sun Dried Tomato & Basil, Caffe Nero* | 1 Serving/300g | 144 | 7.0 | 48 | 2.2 | 4.7 | 2.3 | 0.5 |

| | Measure INFO/WEIGHT | per Measure KCAL | FAT | Nutrition Values per 100g / 100ml KCAL | PROT | CARB | FAT | FIBRE |
|---|---|---|---|---|---|---|---|---|

## CAFFE NERO

### TAGLIATELLE

| | Measure INFO/WEIGHT | KCAL | FAT | KCAL | PROT | CARB | FAT | FIBRE |
|---|---|---|---|---|---|---|---|---|
| Carbonara, Caffe Nero* | 1 Serving/349g | 856 | 61.0 | 245 | 6.3 | 15.6 | 17.4 | 0.6 |

### TART

| | | | | | | | | |
|---|---|---|---|---|---|---|---|---|
| Blueberry, Caffe Nero* | 1 Serving/111g | 311 | 18.0 | 280 | 3.2 | 30.3 | 16.2 | 1.2 |
| Lemon & Lime, Caffe Nero* | 1 Serving/109g | 375 | 24.0 | 344 | 4.9 | 12.7 | 22.1 | 0.0 |
| Winter Fruit, Caffe Nero* | 1 Serving/145g | 434 | 16.0 | 299 | 2.9 | 46.6 | 11.2 | 0.0 |

### TEA

| | | | | | | | | |
|---|---|---|---|---|---|---|---|---|
| Chai Latte, Semi Skimmed Milk, Caffe Nero* | 1 Grande/405g | 284 | 11.0 | 70 | 3.8 | 8.3 | 2.6 | 0.0 |
| Chai Latte, Skimmed Milk, Caffe Nero* | 1 Grande/405g | 239 | 5.0 | 59 | 3.8 | 8.4 | 1.3 | 0.0 |
| Chia Latte, Iced, Caffe Nero* | 1 Latte/548g | 466 | 11.0 | 85 | 3.6 | 13.7 | 2.0 | 0.0 |

### TIRAMISU

| | | | | | | | | |
|---|---|---|---|---|---|---|---|---|
| Caffe Nero* | 1 Serving/113g | 386 | 24.0 | 342 | 4.0 | 33.5 | 21.3 | 0.9 |

### WATER

| | | | | | | | | |
|---|---|---|---|---|---|---|---|---|
| Spring, Orange & Passion Fruit, Fruity, Caffe Nero* | 1 Bottle/500ml | 190 | 0.0 | 38 | 0.0 | 9.3 | 0.0 | 0.0 |

### WRAP

| | | | | | | | | |
|---|---|---|---|---|---|---|---|---|
| Chicken, Caesar, Caffe Nero* | 1 Serving/209g | 356 | 12.0 | 170 | 11.1 | 18.8 | 5.6 | 0.9 |
| Chicken, Spicy, Caffe Nero* | 1 Serving/176g | 300 | 6.0 | 170 | 11.4 | 23.7 | 3.4 | 1.2 |
| Chicken, with Yoghurt & Mint, Caffe Nero* | 1 Sandwich/180g | 418 | 20.0 | 232 | 11.8 | 21.3 | 11.1 | 1.0 |
| Cream Cheese, Grilled Vegetable, & Tomato, Caffe Nero* | 1 Serving/216g | 344 | 11.0 | 159 | 4.8 | 22.9 | 5.3 | 0.0 |
| Falafel, Caffe Nero* | 1 Pack/157g | 424 | 22.0 | 270 | 8.7 | 29.4 | 13.9 | 1.8 |
| Ham, Leek, & Cheese, Hot, Caffe Nero* | 1 Pack/165g | 357 | 14.0 | 216 | 11.9 | 23.3 | 8.4 | 1.1 |
| Ham, Mushroom, & Mozzarella, Caffe Nero* | 1 Serving/166g | 345 | 13.0 | 208 | 12.2 | 21.4 | 8.1 | 1.0 |
| Houmous, & Red Pepper, Caffe Nero* | 1 Serving/202g | 303 | 9.0 | 150 | 4.6 | 23.0 | 4.4 | 2.0 |
| Roast Vegetable, Bean & Tomato, Caffe Nero* | 1 Serving/200g | 332 | 8.0 | 166 | 5.0 | 27.9 | 4.1 | 0.0 |
| Three Bean, Caffe Nero* | 1 Wrap/178g | 416 | 20.0 | 233 | 9.3 | 23.7 | 11.2 | 1.8 |
| Tuna Nicoise, Caffe Nero* | 1 Serving/236g | 331 | 12.0 | 140 | 8.1 | 15.9 | 4.9 | 0.8 |

### YOGHURT

| | | | | | | | | |
|---|---|---|---|---|---|---|---|---|
| Bio, Caffe Nero* | 1 Pot/150g | 230 | 15.0 | 153 | 6.1 | 10.4 | 9.8 | 0.0 |
| Blackcurrant, Bio, Caffe Nero* | 1 Pot/150g | 235 | 13.0 | 157 | 5.3 | 14.2 | 8.6 | 0.2 |
| Blueberry, Brunch Pot, Caffe Nero* | 1 Pot/127g | 165 | 6.0 | 130 | 1.3 | 19.8 | 4.8 | 1.0 |
| Fig & Honey, Brunch Pot, Caffe Nero* | 1 Pot/135g | 203 | 7.0 | 150 | 6.2 | 19.2 | 4.9 | 1.0 |
| Forest Fruits, Muesli Topped, Brunch Pot, Caffe Nero* | 1 Pot/150g | 228 | 11.0 | 152 | 5.1 | 13.3 | 7.3 | 0.0 |
| Mango & Passion Fruit, Brunch Pot, Caffe Nero* | 1 Pot/135g | 183 | 6.0 | 136 | 5.6 | 20.7 | 4.7 | 1.0 |
| Strawberry, Brunch Pot, Caffe Nero* | 1 Pot/125g | 150 | 6.0 | 120 | 1.3 | 17.6 | 4.8 | 1.1 |
| Strawberry, Muesli Topped, Brunch Pot, Caffe Nero* | 1 Pot/150g | 300 | 12.0 | 200 | 5.1 | 11.5 | 8.1 | 0.0 |

### YOGHURT DRINK

| | | | | | | | | |
|---|---|---|---|---|---|---|---|---|
| Strawberry, Probiotic, Organic, Caffe Nero* | 1 Bottle/250ml | 187 | 4.0 | 75 | 2.9 | 11.9 | 1.7 | 0.0 |

## COFFEE REPUBLIC

### FLAPJACK

| | | | | | | | | |
|---|---|---|---|---|---|---|---|---|
| Chewy Nutty, Coffee Republic* | 1 Flapjack/33g | 145 | 8.0 | 440 | 7.1 | 50.9 | 23.2 | 2.0 |

### PANINI

| | | | | | | | | |
|---|---|---|---|---|---|---|---|---|
| Ham & Swiss Cheese, Coffee Republic* | 1 Panini/223g | 557 | 26.0 | 250 | 15.7 | 20.5 | 11.7 | 0.0 |
| Mozzarella & Tomato, Coffee Republic* | 1 Panini/255g | 566 | 25.0 | 222 | 11.1 | 23.6 | 10.0 | 0.0 |

### SALAD

| | | | | | | | | |
|---|---|---|---|---|---|---|---|---|
| Chicken Caesar, Bacon, Grana Padano, Coffee Republic* | 1 Pack/139g | 201 | 15.0 | 145 | 10.3 | 1.0 | 11.1 | 0.0 |

### SANDWICH

| | | | | | | | | |
|---|---|---|---|---|---|---|---|---|
| Cheese, & Ham, Toasted, Coffee Republic* | 1 Pack/160g | 429 | 20.0 | 268 | 15.7 | 24.4 | 12.7 | 0.0 |
| Ham, & Salad, Coffee Republic* | 1 Pack/224g | 309 | 6.0 | 138 | 8.6 | 19.9 | 2.7 | 0.0 |
| Mozzarella, & Salad, Coffee Republic* | 1 Pack/242g | 477 | 29.0 | 197 | 8.6 | 14.4 | 11.8 | 0.0 |
| Salmon, Poached, Coffee Republic* | 1 Pack/191g | 350 | 15.0 | 183 | 10.3 | 18.4 | 7.6 | 0.0 |
| Turkey, & Sun Dried Tomato, Coffee Republic* | 1 Pack/215g | 445 | 14.0 | 207 | 11.8 | 25.3 | 6.5 | 0.0 |

### TOASTIE

| | | | | | | | | |
|---|---|---|---|---|---|---|---|---|
| Cheese & Ham, Coffee Republic* | 1 Serving/164g | 436 | 17.0 | 266 | 13.7 | 30.1 | 10.1 | 0.0 |

| | Measure INFO/WEIGHT | per Measure KCAL | FAT | Nutrition Values per 100g / 100ml KCAL | PROT | CARB | FAT | FIBRE |
|---|---|---|---|---|---|---|---|---|
| **COSTA** | | | | | | | | |
| **BISCUIT** | | | | | | | | |
| Linzer, Raspberry, Costa* | 1 Av Serving/65g | 308 | 15.0 | 474 | 4.1 | 63.1 | 22.8 | 0.0 |
| Linzer, with Lemon Curd, Costa* | 1 Av Serving/65g | 308 | 15.0 | 474 | 4.1 | 63.1 | 22.8 | 0.0 |
| **BISCUITS** | | | | | | | | |
| Almond, Mini, Bag, Costa* | 1 Av Bag/78g | 383 | 24.0 | 491 | 14.3 | 40.0 | 30.5 | 0.0 |
| Garibaldi, Costa* | 2 Biscuits/68g | 316 | 16.0 | 464 | 5.3 | 57.3 | 23.8 | 2.9 |
| Raisin, Cranberry & Hazelnut, Costa* | 1 Serving/23g | 84 | 4.0 | 364 | 2.7 | 47.5 | 18.2 | 0.0 |
| Stem Ginger, Costa* | 1 Pack/60g | 286 | 13.0 | 476 | 4.8 | 65.6 | 21.6 | 0.0 |
| **CAKE** | | | | | | | | |
| Carrot, Costa* | 1 Av Slice/138g | 491 | 25.0 | 357 | 5.1 | 43.4 | 18.1 | 0.0 |
| Chocolate, Costa* | 1 Av Slice/172g | 667 | 25.0 | 388 | 4.8 | 58.9 | 14.8 | 0.0 |
| Coffee & Walnut, Costa* | 1 Av Slice/135g | 637 | 38.0 | 472 | 4.9 | 50.3 | 27.9 | 0.0 |
| Lemon, Costa* | 1 Av Slice/135g | 545 | 25.0 | 404 | 4.3 | 55.0 | 18.5 | 0.0 |
| Victoria Sandwich, Costa* | 1 Av Slice/128g | 501 | 25.0 | 390 | 3.2 | 49.8 | 19.5 | 0.0 |
| **CIABATTA** | | | | | | | | |
| Ham, with Plum Tomato & Rocket, Italian, Costa* | 1 Serving/50g | 115 | 2.0 | 230 | 23.1 | 24.9 | 4.4 | 0.0 |
| **COFFEE** | | | | | | | | |
| Caffe Latte, Caramel, Full Fat, Massimo, Costa* | 1 Massimo/409ml | 282 | 10.0 | 69 | 2.4 | 9.4 | 2.4 | 0.0 |
| Caffe Latte, Caramel, Full Fat, Medio, Costa* | 1 Medio/295ml | 221 | 7.0 | 75 | 2.3 | 11.2 | 2.4 | 0.0 |
| Caffe Latte, Caramel, Full Fat, Primo, Costa* | 1 Primo/220ml | 187 | 5.0 | 85 | 1.2 | 14.7 | 2.4 | 0.0 |
| Caffe Latte, Caramel, Skimmed, Massimo, Costa* | 1 Massimo/404ml | 194 | 0.0 | 48 | 2.3 | 9.3 | 0.1 | 0.0 |
| Caffe Latte, Caramel, Skimmed, Medio, Costa* | 1 Medio/291ml | 163 | 0.0 | 56 | 2.3 | 11.3 | 0.1 | 0.0 |
| Caffe Latte, Caramel, Skimmed, Primo, Costa* | 1 Primo/220ml | 143 | 0.0 | 65 | 1.9 | 14.1 | 0.1 | 0.0 |
| Caffe Latte, Full Fat, Massimo, Costa* | 1 Massimo/380ml | 190 | 10.0 | 50 | 2.6 | 4.1 | 2.6 | 0.0 |
| Caffe Latte, Full Fat, Medio, Costa* | 1 Latte/264g | 129 | 7.0 | 49 | 2.5 | 3.8 | 2.6 | 0.0 |
| Caffe Latte, Full Fat, Primo, Costa* | 1 Cup/190ml | 95 | 5.0 | 50 | 1.4 | 5.0 | 2.7 | 0.0 |
| Caffe Latte, Skimmed, Massimo, Costa* | 1 Massimo/378ml | 102 | 0.0 | 27 | 2.5 | 4.0 | 0.1 | 0.0 |
| Caffe Latte, Skimmed, Medio, Costa* | 1 Latte/264ml | 71 | 0.0 | 27 | 2.6 | 3.9 | 0.1 | 0.0 |
| Caffe Latte, Skimmed, Primo, Costa* | 1 Primo/189g | 51 | 0.0 | 27 | 2.2 | 4.3 | 0.1 | 0.0 |
| Caffe Latte, Soya, Massimo, Costa* | 1 Massimo/378ml | 185 | 10.0 | 49 | 2.3 | 4.1 | 2.6 | 0.0 |
| Caffe Latte, Soya, Medio, Costa* | 1 Medio/261ml | 86 | 4.0 | 33 | 2.4 | 2.4 | 1.5 | 0.0 |
| Caffe Latte, Soya, Primo, Costa* | 1 Primo/188ml | 62 | 3.0 | 33 | 2.5 | 2.5 | 1.4 | 0.0 |
| Caffe Latte, Vanilla, Full Fat, Massimo, Costa* | 1 Massimo/408ml | 290 | 10.0 | 71 | 2.4 | 9.9 | 2.4 | 0.0 |
| Caffe Latte, Vanilla, Full Fat, Medio, Costa* | 1 Latte/294g | 229 | 7.0 | 78 | 2.3 | 11.9 | 2.4 | 0.0 |
| Catte Latte, Vanilla, Full Fat, Primo, Costa* | 1 Primo/219ml | 195 | 5.0 | 89 | 1.2 | 15.6 | 2.4 | 0.0 |
| Caffe Latte, Vanilla, Skimmed, Massimo, Costa* | 1 Massimo/404ml | 202 | 0.0 | 50 | 2.3 | 9.8 | 0.1 | 0.0 |
| Caffe Latte, Vanilla, Skimmed, Medio, Costa* | 1 Medio/295ml | 171 | 0.0 | 58 | 2.3 | 11.9 | 0.1 | 0.0 |
| Caffe Latte, Vanilla, Skimmed, Primo, Costa* | 1 Latte/220ml | 151 | 0.0 | 69 | 1.9 | 15.0 | 0.1 | 0.0 |
| Cappucino, Full Fat, Massimo, Costa* | 1 Massimo/279g | 123 | 7.0 | 44 | 2.3 | 3.3 | 2.4 | 0.0 |
| Cappucino, Full Fat, Medio, Costa* | 1 Medio/246g | 101 | 5.0 | 41 | 2.2 | 3.8 | 1.9 | 0.0 |
| Cappucino, Full Fat, Primo, Costa* | 1 Cup/183ml | 71 | 3.0 | 39 | 2.0 | 3.4 | 1.9 | 0.0 |
| Cappucino, Skimmed, Massimo, Costa* | 1 Mug/280ml | 73 | 1.0 | 26 | 2.3 | 3.5 | 0.3 | 0.0 |
| Cappucino, Skimmed, Medio, Costa* | 1 Medio/242g | 58 | 0.0 | 24 | 2.2 | 3.5 | 0.1 | 0.0 |
| Cappucino, Skimmed, Primo, Costa* | 1 Primo Cup/183ml | 40 | 0.0 | 22 | 1.9 | 3.1 | 0.2 | 0.0 |
| Cappucino, Soya, Massimo, Costa* | 1 Massimo/275g | 88 | 4.0 | 32 | 2.3 | 2.2 | 1.5 | 0.0 |
| Cappucino, Soya, Medio, Costa* | 1 Medio/248g | 77 | 3.0 | 31 | 2.3 | 2.6 | 1.3 | 0.0 |
| Cappucino, Soya, Primo, Costa* | 1 Primo/181g | 47 | 2.0 | 26 | 2.0 | 1.9 | 1.1 | 0.0 |
| Frescato, Expresso, Costa* | 1 Primo/360ml | 148 | 0.0 | 41 | 56.1 | 9.4 | 0.0 | 0.0 |
| Latte, Cinnamon, Full Fat, Medio, Costa, Costa* | 1 Medio/291g | 527 | 20.0 | 181 | 6.6 | 23.8 | 6.9 | 0.0 |
| Latte, Cinnamon, Full Fat Milk, Massimo, Costa* | 1 Massimo/400ml | 255 | 10.0 | 64 | 2.4 | 7.9 | 2.4 | 0.0 |
| Latte, Cinnamon, Skimmed Milk, Massimo, Costa* | 1 Massimo/400ml | 167 | 0.0 | 42 | 2.4 | 7.7 | 0.1 | 0.0 |
| Latte, Cinnamon, Soya Milk, Massimo, Costa* | 1 Massimo/400ml | 251 | 10.0 | 63 | 2.2 | 7.9 | 2.4 | 0.0 |
| Mocha, Full Fat, Massimo, Costa* | 1 Massimo/288ml | 170 | 8.0 | 59 | 2.6 | 5.8 | 2.8 | 0.0 |

| | Measure | | | Nutrition Values per 100g / 100ml | | | | |
|---|---|---|---|---|---|---|---|---|
| | INFO/WEIGHT | KCAL | FAT | KCAL | PROT | CARB | FAT | FIBRE |

## COSTA

### COFFEE
| | | | | | | | | |
|---|---|---|---|---|---|---|---|---|
| Mocha, Full Fat, Medio, Costa* | 1 Mocha/253ml | 153 | 7.0 | 60 | 2.6 | 6.7 | 2.6 | 0.0 |
| Mocha, Full Fat, Primo, Costa* | 1 Primo/188ml | 113 | 5.0 | 60 | 2.6 | 6.7 | 2.5 | 0.0 |
| Mocha, Skimmed, Massimo, Costa* | 1 Massimo/288ml | 138 | 2.0 | 48 | 2.8 | 7.6 | 0.7 | 0.0 |
| Mocha, Skimmed, Medio, Costa* | 1 Mocha/253ml | 119 | 2.0 | 47 | 2.5 | 7.8 | 0.6 | 0.0 |
| Mocha, Skimmed, Primo, Costa* | 1 Primo/191ml | 84 | 1.0 | 44 | 2.7 | 7.0 | 0.6 | 0.0 |
| Mocha Flake, Full Fat, Massimo, Costa* | 1 Massimo/332ml | 369 | 24.0 | 111 | 2.9 | 8.7 | 7.1 | 0.0 |
| Mocha Flake, Full Fat, Medio, Costa* | 1 Medio/288ml | 297 | 19.0 | 103 | 2.7 | 8.1 | 6.7 | 0.0 |
| Mocha Flake, Full Fat, Primo, Costa* | 1 Primo/234ml | 257 | 17.0 | 110 | 2.6 | 8.1 | 7.4 | 0.0 |
| Mocha Flake, Skimmed, Massimo, Costa* | 1 Massimo/334ml | 338 | 18.0 | 101 | 3.0 | 10.3 | 5.3 | 0.0 |
| Mocha Flake, Skimmed, Medio, Costa* | 1 Medio/288ml | 262 | 14.0 | 91 | 2.6 | 9.0 | 4.9 | 0.0 |
| Mocha Flake, Skimmed, Primo, Costa* | 1 Primo/234ml | 227 | 14.0 | 97 | 2.7 | 8.3 | 5.9 | 0.0 |

### COOKIES
| | | | | | | | | |
|---|---|---|---|---|---|---|---|---|
| Choc Chunk, Double, Costa* | 1 Av Packet/60g | 296 | 15.0 | 493 | 5.2 | 61.1 | 25.3 | 3.7 |
| Fruit & Oat, Costa* | 1 Av Pack/60g | 283 | 13.0 | 472 | 5.1 | 65.2 | 21.2 | 2.0 |

### CRISPS
| | | | | | | | | |
|---|---|---|---|---|---|---|---|---|
| Sea Salt Flavour, Costa* | 1 Pack/50g | 251 | 14.0 | 503 | 7.1 | 55.9 | 27.9 | 4.2 |

### CROISSANT
| | | | | | | | | |
|---|---|---|---|---|---|---|---|---|
| Almond, Costa* | 1 Croissant/88g | 336 | 17.0 | 382 | 9.3 | 43.0 | 19.2 | 0.0 |
| Butter, Costa* | 1 Croissant/64g | 276 | 17.0 | 431 | 8.3 | 40.6 | 26.1 | 0.0 |

### CRUMBLE
| | | | | | | | | |
|---|---|---|---|---|---|---|---|---|
| Apple, Costa* | 1 Slice/100g | 469 | 30.0 | 469 | 5.6 | 46.7 | 30.1 | 0.0 |

### FLAPJACK
| | | | | | | | | |
|---|---|---|---|---|---|---|---|---|
| Fruity, Costa* | 1 Av Serving/85g | 353 | 12.0 | 415 | 4.9 | 67.0 | 14.2 | 12.5 |
| Nutty, Costa* | 1 Av Serving/85g | 391 | 20.0 | 460 | 7.4 | 54.8 | 23.5 | 5.0 |

### FLATBREAD
| | | | | | | | | |
|---|---|---|---|---|---|---|---|---|
| Cajun Chicken, Costa* | 1 Pack/168g | 310 | 5.0 | 184 | 12.7 | 26.6 | 3.0 | 0.0 |
| Cheddar & Caramelised Onion Chutney, Costa* | 1 Pack/118g | 340 | 13.0 | 288 | 11.9 | 34.8 | 11.3 | 0.0 |
| Chicken, Green Thai, Costa* | 1 Av Pack/173g | 325 | 6.0 | 188 | 12.2 | 26.6 | 3.7 | 0.0 |

### FRUIT SALAD
| | | | | | | | | |
|---|---|---|---|---|---|---|---|---|
| Classic, Costa* | 1 Av Serving/161g | 312 | 0.0 | 194 | 0.6 | 10.5 | 0.1 | 0.0 |

### GRAPES
| | | | | | | | | |
|---|---|---|---|---|---|---|---|---|
| Red, Costa* | 1 Av Serving/91g | 58 | 0.0 | 64 | 0.4 | 15.4 | 0.1 | 0.0 |

### HOT CHOCOLATE
| | | | | | | | | |
|---|---|---|---|---|---|---|---|---|
| Frothed Milk, Full Fat, Massimo, Costa* | 1 Massimo/376ml | 259 | 11.0 | 69 | 3.1 | 7.6 | 2.9 | 0.0 |
| Frothed Milk, Full Fat, Medio, Costa* | 1 Medio/266ml | 157 | 6.0 | 59 | 3.0 | 6.9 | 2.2 | 0.0 |
| Frothed Milk, Full Fat, Primo, Costa* | 1 Primo/192ml | 121 | 5.0 | 63 | 3.1 | 6.9 | 2.5 | 0.0 |
| Frothed Milk, Skimmed, Medio, Costa* | 1 Medio/265ml | 130 | 1.0 | 49 | 3.4 | 7.7 | 0.5 | 0.0 |
| Frothed Milk, Skimmed, Primo, Costa* | 1 Primo/192ml | 98 | 1.0 | 51 | 3.4 | 7.9 | 0.6 | 0.0 |
| Frothed Milk, Skimmmed, Massimo, Costa* | 1 Massimo/380ml | 175 | 2.0 | 46 | 3.1 | 7.6 | 0.4 | 0.0 |
| Marshmallows & Whipped Cream, Full Fat, Costa* | 1 Massimo/419ml | 423 | 21.0 | 101 | 3.1 | 11.2 | 4.9 | 0.0 |
| Marshmallows & Whipped Cream, Full Fat, Costa* | 1 Medio/308ml | 321 | 15.0 | 104 | 3.0 | 11.7 | 5.0 | 0.0 |
| Marshmallows & Whipped Cream, Full Fat, Costa* | 1 Primo/238ml | 285 | 14.0 | 120 | 3.0 | 13.2 | 6.1 | 0.0 |
| Marshmallows & Whipped Cream, Skimmed, Costa* | 1 Massimo/418ml | 339 | 11.0 | 81 | 3.1 | 11.2 | 2.7 | 0.0 |
| Marshmallows & Whipped Cream, Skimmed, Costa* | 1 Medio/309ml | 294 | 11.0 | 95 | 3.3 | 12.4 | 3.5 | 0.0 |
| Marshmallows & Whipped Cream, Skimmed, Costa* | 1 Primo/238ml | 262 | 11.0 | 110 | 3.3 | 14.0 | 4.5 | 0.0 |

### MUFFIN
| | | | | | | | | |
|---|---|---|---|---|---|---|---|---|
| Banana & Toffee, Costa* | 1 Muffin/117g | 462 | 24.0 | 395 | 4.4 | 49.1 | 20.3 | 0.0 |
| Blackcurrant & White Chocolate, Costa* | 1 Muffin/124g | 474 | 21.0 | 382 | 4.3 | 53.0 | 17.0 | 0.0 |
| Blueberry, Costa* | 1 Muffin/136g | 516 | 25.0 | 379 | 4.6 | 48.5 | 18.5 | 0.0 |
| Chocolate, Mini, Costa* | 1 Muffin/19g | 73 | 4.0 | 383 | 4.3 | 44.5 | 20.5 | 0.0 |
| Lemon & Orange, Low Fat, Costa* | 1 Muffin/135g | 319 | 3.0 | 236 | 4.6 | 49.4 | 2.3 | 1.1 |
| Lemon & White Chocolate, Costa* | 1 Muffin/129g | 472 | 20.0 | 366 | 5.4 | 52.3 | 15.8 | 0.0 |

| | Measure INFO/WEIGHT | per Measure KCAL | FAT | Nutrition Values per 100g / 100ml KCAL | PROT | CARB | FAT | FIBRE |
|---|---|---|---|---|---|---|---|---|

## COSTA
### MUFFIN

| | Measure INFO/WEIGHT | KCAL | FAT | KCAL | PROT | CARB | FAT | FIBRE |
|---|---|---|---|---|---|---|---|---|
| Raspberry & White Chocolate, Costa* | 1 Muffin/135g | 511 | 26.0 | 376 | 4.8 | 46.4 | 19.1 | 0.0 |
| Raspberry & White Chocolate, Mini, Costa* | 1 Muffin/19g | 72 | 4.0 | 379 | 4.1 | 45.9 | 19.4 | 0.0 |
| Red Berry, Low Fat, Costa* | 1 Muffin/124g | 381 | 4.0 | 307 | 6.2 | 63.0 | 3.4 | 0.0 |
| Triple Chocolate, Costa* | 1 Muffin/134g | 537 | 27.0 | 401 | 4.4 | 50.1 | 20.3 | 0.0 |
| Very Berry, Costa* | 1 Muffin/140g | 354 | 6.0 | 253 | 4.4 | 48.6 | 4.6 | 0.0 |

### PAIN AU RAISIN

| | | | | | | | | |
|---|---|---|---|---|---|---|---|---|
| Costa* | 1 Pastry/119g | 356 | 14.0 | 299 | 5.1 | 43.7 | 11.5 | 0.0 |

### PANETTINO

| | | | | | | | | |
|---|---|---|---|---|---|---|---|---|
| Chocolate, Costa* | 1 Av Cake/100g | 407 | 20.0 | 407 | 8.3 | 48.4 | 20.0 | 0.0 |

### PANINI

| | | | | | | | | |
|---|---|---|---|---|---|---|---|---|
| Chicken, Red Chilli, Costa* | 1 Av Panini/207g | 370 | 6.0 | 179 | 13.5 | 25.1 | 2.7 | 0.0 |
| Chicken & Baby Spinach, Costa* | 1 Panini/440g | 832 | 11.0 | 189 | 9.8 | 32.5 | 2.5 | 0.0 |
| Chicken Arrabiata, Costa* | 1 Pack/205g | 377 | 6.0 | 184 | 13.7 | 26.1 | 2.7 | 0.0 |
| Ham & Cheese, Costa* | 1 Av Panini/175g | 461 | 21.0 | 263 | 12.5 | 26.2 | 12.1 | 0.0 |
| Mozzarella, Tomato & Basil, Costa* | 1 Av Panini/190g | 512 | 23.0 | 270 | 11.0 | 30.6 | 12.0 | 0.0 |
| Mozzarella, Tomato & Pesto, Costa* | 1 Panini/209g | 487 | 15.0 | 233 | 9.0 | 35.0 | 7.0 | 5.0 |
| Mushroom & Emmental, Costa* | 1 Panini/187g | 456 | 18.0 | 244 | 10.9 | 28.0 | 9.8 | 0.0 |
| Spicy Meatball, Costa* | 1 Av Panini/177g | 506 | 18.0 | 286 | 11.9 | 37.1 | 9.9 | 0.0 |
| Tuna Melt, Costa* | 1 Av Panini/190g | 553 | 25.0 | 291 | 14.8 | 29.4 | 13.3 | 0.0 |

### SALAD

| | | | | | | | | |
|---|---|---|---|---|---|---|---|---|
| Cous Cous, Moroccan Styles, Costa * | 1 Pack/290g | 392 | 7.0 | 135 | 3.6 | 24.6 | 2.5 | 2.2 |

### SANDWICH

| | | | | | | | | |
|---|---|---|---|---|---|---|---|---|
| Bacon & Tomato Sauce, Tostato, Costa* | 1 Tostato/132g | 316 | 7.0 | 239 | 8.5 | 40.2 | 5.0 | 0.0 |
| BLT, Costa* | 1 Av Pack/179g | 442 | 22.0 | 247 | 10.4 | 23.6 | 12.3 | 0.0 |
| Brie, Apple & Grape, Costa* | 1 Serving/225g | 535 | 25.0 | 238 | 8.3 | 28.7 | 10.9 | 0.0 |
| Chicken, Coronation, Costa* | 1 Av Pack/178g | 319 | 6.0 | 179 | 13.1 | 24.9 | 3.1 | 0.0 |
| Chicken, Roast, Costa* | 1 Pack/177g | 325 | 7.0 | 184 | 13.0 | 23.8 | 4.0 | 0.0 |
| Club, All Day Breakfast, Costa* | 1 Av Pack/248g | 587 | 23.0 | 236 | 10.2 | 27.8 | 9.4 | 0.0 |
| Club, Chicken & Bacon, Costa* | 1 Av Pack/230g | 529 | 15.0 | 230 | 14.5 | 30.1 | 6.6 | 0.0 |
| Egg, Free Range, Costa* | 1 Av Pack/172g | 329 | 11.0 | 191 | 7.8 | 25.3 | 6.5 | 0.0 |
| Egg Mayonnaise & Tomato, Free Range, Costa* | 1 Pack/174g | 389 | 24.0 | 223 | 8.6 | 18.3 | 13.8 | 0.0 |
| Houmous, Costa* | 1 Pack/165g | 263 | 5.0 | 160 | 6.4 | 25.9 | 2.8 | 0.0 |
| Ploughmans, Cheese, Costa* | 1 Av Pack/202g | 1795 | 19.0 | 889 | 9.2 | 23.0 | 9.3 | 0.0 |
| Prawn, Tiger, with Lime & Chilli Dressing, Costa* | 1 Pack/185g | 367 | 19.0 | 198 | 8.2 | 21.2 | 10.2 | 0.0 |
| Salmon, & Salad, Poached, Oatmeal, Costa* | 1 Pack/151g | 224 | 4.0 | 148 | 7.7 | 22.9 | 2.8 | 0.0 |
| Sausage, Chorizo, & Vine Ripened Tomato, Costa* | 1 Pack/181g | 315 | 4.0 | 174 | 15.5 | 26.1 | 2.1 | 0.0 |
| Tuna, & Salad, Costa* | 1 Av Pack/177g | 289 | 4.0 | 163 | 11.9 | 25.7 | 2.3 | 0.0 |

### SCONE

| | | | | | | | | |
|---|---|---|---|---|---|---|---|---|
| Fruit, Costa* | 1 Av Serving/110g | 370 | 12.0 | 336 | 5.6 | 55.1 | 10.7 | 0.0 |

### SHORTCAKE

| | | | | | | | | |
|---|---|---|---|---|---|---|---|---|
| Raspberry, Costa* | 1 Shortcake/45g | 215 | 11.0 | 477 | 2.4 | 63.5 | 23.7 | 0.0 |

### SLICES

| | | | | | | | | |
|---|---|---|---|---|---|---|---|---|
| Cheese, Twist, Pastry, Costa* | 1 Av Pastry/103g | 346 | 20.0 | 336 | 11.1 | 29.5 | 19.8 | 0.0 |
| Pecan, Pastry, Costa* | 1 Pastry/105g | 465 | 30.0 | 443 | 5.6 | 42.1 | 28.5 | 3.0 |

### SOUP

| | | | | | | | | |
|---|---|---|---|---|---|---|---|---|
| Fish, Bouillabaisse, Costa* | 1 Serving/400g | 180 | 6.0 | 45 | 5.8 | 2.2 | 1.4 | 0.0 |

### TEA

| | | | | | | | | |
|---|---|---|---|---|---|---|---|---|
| Iced, Lemon, Costa* | 1 Bottle/275ml | 91 | 0.0 | 33 | 0.0 | 8.0 | 0.0 | 0.0 |

### TOASTIE

| | | | | | | | | |
|---|---|---|---|---|---|---|---|---|
| Bacon, Costa* | 1 Av Toastie/142g | 355 | 11.0 | 250 | 11.3 | 33.8 | 7.7 | 5.3 |
| Ham & Cheese, Costa* | 1 Av Pack/160g | 406 | 17.0 | 254 | 9.8 | 29.5 | 10.7 | 0.0 |

| | INFO/WEIGHT | KCAL | FAT | KCAL | PROT | CARB | FAT | FIBRE |
|---|---|---|---|---|---|---|---|---|
| **COSTA** | | | | | | | | |
| **TRAYBAKE** | | | | | | | | |
| Fruit, Seed, Nut & Honey Bar, Costa Coffee* | 1 Av Serving/75g | 317 | 15.0 | 423 | 7.5 | 52.5 | 20.3 | 0.0 |
| Lemon & Coconut Slice, Costa* | 1 Av Serving/85g | 381 | 22.0 | 448 | 5.8 | 48.0 | 25.9 | 0.0 |
| Raspberry & Almond, Costa* | 1 Av Serving/100g | 451 | 28.0 | 451 | 8.5 | 40.8 | 28.2 | 1.0 |
| Shortbread, Caramel, Costa* | 1 Av Serving/77g | 426 | 26.0 | 553 | 4.7 | 55.9 | 34.4 | 0.0 |
| Tiffin Triangle, Chocolate, Costa Coffee* | 1 Av Serving/85g | 433 | 26.0 | 509 | 4.9 | 54.6 | 30.2 | 0.0 |
| **WRAP** | | | | | | | | |
| Sweet Chilli Chicken, Costa* | 1 Wrap/192g | 365 | 8.0 | 190 | 10.7 | 27.1 | 4.3 | 0.0 |
| **CRUSSH JUICE BARS** | | | | | | | | |
| **BREAKFAST CEREAL** | | | | | | | | |
| Museli, Berry, Crussh Juice Bars* | 1 Serving/225g | 295 | 14.0 | 131 | 5.1 | 13.9 | 6.1 | 1.3 |
| Porridge, Cinnamon, Crussh Juice Bars* | 1 Serving/300g | 285 | 6.0 | 95 | 3.1 | 15.7 | 2.1 | 1.8 |
| Porridge, Summer, Crussh Juice Bars* | 1 Serving/330g | 495 | 13.0 | 150 | 1.5 | 27.0 | 4.0 | 0.0 |
| Porridge, Traditional, Organic, Crussh Juice Bars* | 1 Serving/331g | 314 | 7.0 | 95 | 3.1 | 15.7 | 2.1 | 1.8 |
| Porridge, with Soy Milk, Organic, Crussh Juice Bars* | 1 Serving/331g | 330 | 12.0 | 100 | 3.5 | 16.5 | 3.5 | 1.9 |
| **CHOCOLATE** | | | | | | | | |
| Shot, Fairtrade, Crussh Juice Bars* | 1 Shot/100g | 210 | 17.0 | 210 | 2.3 | 12.0 | 17.2 | 0.6 |
| **COOKIE** | | | | | | | | |
| Chocolate Chip & Hazelnut, Organic, Crussh Juice Bars* | 1 Cookie/50g | 228 | 13.0 | 457 | 5.8 | 50.3 | 25.8 | 2.3 |
| Double Chocolate, Crussh Juice Bars* | 1 Cookie/50g | 210 | 9.0 | 421 | 5.0 | 60.8 | 17.6 | 2.7 |
| Oat & Raisin, Organic, Crussh Juice Bars* | 1 Cookie/50g | 203 | 9.0 | 406 | 4.8 | 55.8 | 18.2 | 2.7 |
| **JUICE** | | | | | | | | |
| Apple, Crussh Juice Bars* | 1 Glass/340ml | 119 | 0.0 | 35 | 0.3 | 8.1 | 0.1 | 1.4 |
| Carrot, Crussh Juice Bars* | 1 Glass/339ml | 122 | 1.0 | 36 | 0.6 | 7.7 | 0.3 | 3.0 |
| Clean & Lean, Crussh Juice Bars* | 1 Glass/340ml | 146 | 0.0 | 43 | 0.4 | 10.0 | 0.1 | 2.4 |
| Combo, Superjuice, Crussh Juice Bars* | 1 Glass/330ml | 87 | 1.0 | 26 | 1.3 | 4.5 | 0.4 | 2.0 |
| Energiser, Crussh Juice Bars* | 1 Glass/339ml | 139 | 1.0 | 41 | 0.5 | 9.2 | 0.2 | 2.9 |
| Green Goddess, Crussh Juice Bars* | 1 Glass/341ml | 133 | 1.0 | 39 | 0.7 | 8.5 | 0.2 | 2.4 |
| Liquid Lunch, Crussh Juice Bars* | 1 Glass/340ml | 153 | 1.0 | 45 | 0.4 | 10.5 | 0.2 | 2.1 |
| Love Juice, Crussh Juice Bars* | 1 Glass/340ml | 143 | 0.0 | 42 | 0.7 | 9.6 | 0.1 | 0.6 |
| Orange, Crussh Juice Bars* | 1 Glass/340ml | 92 | 0.0 | 27 | 0.8 | 5.6 | 0.1 | 1.7 |
| Purifier, Crussh Juice Bars* | 1 Glass/339ml | 122 | 1.0 | 36 | 0.6 | 7.9 | 0.2 | 2.7 |
| Super Juice, Crussh Juice Bars* | 1 Glass/342ml | 113 | 1.0 | 33 | 1.0 | 6.5 | 0.3 | 2.7 |
| Zinger, Crussh Juice Bars* | 1 Glass/341ml | 133 | 0.0 | 39 | 0.5 | 9.0 | 0.1 | 1.4 |
| **SALAD** | | | | | | | | |
| Chicken, Bang Bang, Crussh Juice Bars* | 1 Salad/461g | 341 | 26.0 | 74 | 3.8 | 4.0 | 5.7 | 2.2 |
| Chicken Caesar, Free Range, Crussh Juice Bars* | 1 Salad/280g | 333 | 16.0 | 119 | 8.8 | 8.8 | 5.7 | 1.4 |
| Crayfish & Sweet Chilli Noodle, Crussh Juice Bars* | 1 Serving/111g | 169 | 3.0 | 153 | 6.5 | 24.5 | 3.1 | 0.0 |
| Falafel, Crussh Juice Bars* | 1 Salad/300g | 321 | 23.0 | 107 | 3.8 | 5.3 | 7.8 | 1.4 |
| Greek, Crussh Juice Bars* | 1 Salad/196g | 137 | 9.0 | 70 | 2.9 | 4.6 | 4.4 | 0.0 |
| Health Pot, Full O'Beans, Crussh Juice Bars* | 1 Salad/159g | 243 | 11.0 | 152 | 5.3 | 17.4 | 6.8 | 0.1 |
| Health Pot, O-Me-Good, Crussh Juice Bars* | 1 Pack/290g | 705 | 31.0 | 243 | 9.7 | 28.6 | 10.6 | 0.9 |
| Health Pot, Puy Lentil, Crussh Juice Bars* | 1 Salad/100g | 274 | 13.0 | 274 | 12.5 | 26.4 | 13.2 | 6.8 |
| Health Pot, Superfoods, Crussh Juice Bars* | 1 Salad/160g | 440 | 24.0 | 275 | 10.7 | 23.9 | 15.1 | 4.3 |
| Health Pot, Tuna Lean Bean, Crussh Juice Bars* | 1 Pot/159g | 213 | 10.0 | 134 | 8.0 | 11.6 | 6.1 | 2.0 |
| Health Pot, Tuscan Chicken & Barley, Crussh Juice Bars* | 1 Salad/160g | 442 | 7.0 | 276 | 12.2 | 48.3 | 4.1 | 14.3 |
| Super 7, Crussh Juice Bars* | 1 Pack/330g | 297 | 13.0 | 90 | 7.3 | 6.7 | 3.8 | 2.0 |
| Tuna Nicoise, Crussh Juice Bars* | 1 Salad/300g | 207 | 7.0 | 69 | 4.5 | 6.9 | 2.5 | 1.3 |
| **SANDWICH** | | | | | | | | |
| 5-A-Day, Wheat Free, Crussh Juice Bars* | 1 Sandwich/230g | 391 | 19.0 | 170 | 4.2 | 22.1 | 8.2 | 1.3 |
| Chicken, & Salad, Crussh Juice Bars* | 1 Pack/172g | 330 | 11.0 | 192 | 13.6 | 20.0 | 6.3 | 3.0 |
| Egg Mayo & Mustard Cress, Crussh Juice Bars* | 1 Pack/422g | 489 | 5.0 | 116 | 5.6 | 20.6 | 1.3 | 3.7 |
| Ham, Smokey, Swiss, Crussh Juice Bars* | 1 Pack/244g | 490 | 19.0 | 201 | 12.1 | 20.2 | 7.9 | 3.0 |

| | Measure INFO/WEIGHT | per Measure KCAL | per Measure FAT | KCAL | PROT | CARB | FAT | FIBRE |
|---|---|---|---|---|---|---|---|---|
| **CRUSSH JUICE BARS** | | | | | | | | |
| **SANDWICH** | | | | | | | | |
| Mature Cheddar & Friars Chutney, Crussh Juice Bars* | 1 Pack/152g | 390 | 16.0 | 255 | 12.1 | 28.8 | 10.3 | 3.9 |
| Tuna, Cucumber & Mayo, Crussh Juice Bars* | 1 Pack/227g | 340 | 7.0 | 150 | 12.5 | 18.1 | 3.1 | 2.8 |
| **SMOOTHIE** | | | | | | | | |
| Bananarama, Crussh Juice Bars* | 1 Med/339ml | 326 | 1.0 | 96 | 3.0 | 20.1 | 0.4 | 1.0 |
| Berry Blast, Crussh Juice Bars* | 1 Med/339ml | 241 | 1.0 | 71 | 2.0 | 10.5 | 0.2 | 0.6 |
| Berry Breakfast, Crussh Juice Bars* | 1 Med/330ml | 396 | 9.0 | 120 | 4.5 | 19.5 | 2.7 | 1.5 |
| Bliss Blend, Crussh Juice Bars* | 1 Med/339ml | 950 | 1.0 | 280 | 1.6 | 13.9 | 0.2 | 0.8 |
| Brainstorm, Crussh Juice Bars* | 1 Med/340ml | 235 | 1.0 | 69 | 1.8 | 10.6 | 0.2 | 0.9 |
| Brazillian, Crussh Juice Bars* | 1 Med/339ml | 224 | 2.0 | 66 | 1.8 | 10.1 | 0.6 | 0.9 |
| Breakfast, Crussh Juice Bars* | 1 Med/340ml | 507 | 13.0 | 149 | 5.0 | 23.8 | 3.7 | 1.8 |
| Energy Explosion, Crussh Juice Bars* | 1 Med/344ml | 241 | 1.0 | 70 | 1.8 | 11.5 | 0.2 | 0.7 |
| Fat Burner, Crussh Juice Bars* | 1 Med/340ml | 231 | 1.0 | 68 | 1.9 | 10.3 | 0.2 | 0.7 |
| Mango Madness, Crussh Juice Bars* | 1 Med/339ml | 248 | 1.0 | 73 | 1.7 | 15.5 | 0.3 | 0.7 |
| Peach Passion, Crussh Juice Bars* | 1 Med/340ml | 228 | 1.0 | 67 | 1.8 | 13.9 | 0.2 | 0.7 |
| Pineapple Pleasure, Crussh Juice Bars* | 1 Med/339g | 241 | 1.0 | 71 | 1.8 | 15.3 | 0.2 | 0.5 |
| Strawberry Cool, Crussh Juice Bars* | 1 Med/342ml | 229 | 1.0 | 67 | 1.7 | 13.9 | 0.2 | 0.7 |
| Super, Protein Power, Crussh Juice Bars* | 1 Lge/450g | 306 | 5.0 | 68 | 9.9 | 14.0 | 1.2 | 0.8 |
| **SOUP** | | | | | | | | |
| Beef Chilli, Crussh Juice Bars* | 1 Med/300g | 135 | 4.0 | 45 | 4.8 | 3.4 | 1.3 | 0.0 |
| Bengali Tomato, Crussh Juice Bars* | 1 Lrg/400g | 156 | 8.0 | 39 | 1.2 | 4.1 | 1.9 | 0.0 |
| Boston Clam Chowder, Crussh Juice Bars* | 1 Med/331g | 212 | 9.0 | 64 | 2.7 | 7.0 | 2.8 | 0.8 |
| Cauliflower & Brie, Gourmet, Crussh Juice Bars* | 1 Lrg/400g | 264 | 16.0 | 66 | 3.4 | 4.3 | 3.9 | 1.0 |
| Chicken Chowder, Boston, Gourmet, Crussh Juice Bars* | 1 Lrg/400g | 312 | 14.0 | 78 | 4.4 | 7.2 | 3.5 | 0.0 |
| Chicken Provencale, Gourmet, Crussh Juice Bars* | 1 Med/330g | 90 | 3.0 | 27 | 2.6 | 1.9 | 1.0 | 0.0 |
| Chicken Tikka, Organic, Crussh Juice Bars* | 1 Med/330ml | 330 | 17.0 | 100 | 4.6 | 8.7 | 5.2 | 0.0 |
| Farmhouse Chicken, Crussh Juice Bars* | 1 Med/330g | 191 | 9.0 | 58 | 3.4 | 5.2 | 2.6 | 0.0 |
| Hong Kong, Borscht, Crussh Juice Bars* | 1 Med/329g | 138 | 5.0 | 42 | 2.8 | 4.5 | 1.4 | 0.0 |
| Lamb Stew, Irish, Crussh Juice Bars* | 1 Med/340g | 122 | 5.0 | 36 | 2.0 | 4.2 | 1.4 | 1.0 |
| Lentil & Herbs, Crussh Juice Bars* | 1 Med/300g | 162 | 1.0 | 54 | 4.0 | 8.6 | 0.4 | 10.0 |
| Lentil & Tomato, Crussh Juice Bars* | 1 Med/300g | 330 | 3.0 | 110 | 4.8 | 21.4 | 1.0 | 0.0 |
| Mediterranean Vegetable, Crussh Juice Bars* | 1 Lge/400g | 140 | 4.0 | 35 | 2.0 | 4.4 | 1.1 | 1.7 |
| Minestrone, Classic, Italian, Crussh Juice Bars* | 1 Med/300g | 135 | 2.0 | 45 | 2.3 | 7.1 | 0.8 | 2.1 |
| Mixed Vegetable, Organic, Crussh Juice Bars* | 1 Lge/400g | 112 | 2.0 | 28 | 2.1 | 4.0 | 0.5 | 0.0 |
| Mulligatawny, Organic, Crussh Juice Bars* | 1 Lge/400g | 328 | 19.0 | 82 | 3.0 | 6.9 | 4.7 | 0.0 |
| Potato & Leek, Organic, Crussh Juice Bars* | 1 Med/330ml | 162 | 8.0 | 49 | 1.5 | 6.0 | 2.4 | 0.6 |
| Roasted Tomato & Thyme, Organic, Crussh Juice Bars* | 1 Med/330g | 99 | 4.0 | 30 | 0.9 | 4.0 | 1.1 | 0.9 |
| Sun Ripened Tomato & Basil, Crussh Juice Bars* | 1 Med/330g | 132 | 7.0 | 40 | 0.7 | 4.8 | 2.0 | 1.0 |
| Thai Chicken & Sweet Potato, Crussh Juice Bars* | 1 Lge/400g | 280 | 9.0 | 70 | 4.8 | 7.7 | 2.2 | 2.0 |
| Thai Tomato, Crussh Juice Bars* | 1 Med/329g | 313 | 11.0 | 95 | 2.5 | 15.3 | 3.2 | 0.0 |
| Tomato & Basil, Crussh Juice Bars* | 1 Lge/400g | 68 | 2.0 | 17 | 0.6 | 2.4 | 0.5 | 0.8 |
| Tuscan Vegetable, Organic, Crussh Juice Bars* | 1 Med/331ml | 215 | 9.0 | 65 | 2.4 | 8.1 | 2.6 | 0.0 |
| **SUSHI** | | | | | | | | |
| Salmon, Crussh Juice Bars* | 1 Box/280g | 344 | 6.0 | 123 | 4.3 | 21.9 | 2.0 | 0.0 |
| Veggie, Crussh Juice Bars* | 1 Box/380g | 490 | 19.0 | 129 | 2.8 | 18.3 | 4.9 | 0.0 |
| **TOASTIE** | | | | | | | | |
| Cheddar Cheese, Tasty, Crussh Juice Bars* | 1 Toastie/106g | 310 | 10.0 | 295 | 14.5 | 37.9 | 9.5 | 0.0 |
| Edam & Ham, Skinny, Crussh Juice Bars* | 1 Pack/130g | 329 | 9.0 | 253 | 15.4 | 32.9 | 6.7 | 0.0 |
| Jalapeno & Spinach, Crussh Juice Bars* | 1 Toastie/150g | 403 | 16.0 | 269 | 13.9 | 29.3 | 10.7 | 0.3 |
| Spinach & Chorizo, Crussh Juice Bars* | 1 Toastie/150g | 333 | 11.0 | 222 | 11.3 | 28.3 | 7.3 | 0.4 |
| Tuna, Swiss, Crussh Juice Bars* | 1 Toastie/170g | 379 | 12.0 | 223 | 16.3 | 24.0 | 6.8 | 0.1 |
| **VEGETABLES** | | | | | | | | |
| Great Greens, Crussh Juice Bars* | 1 Pot/150g | 91 | 4.0 | 61 | 6.2 | 3.4 | 2.5 | 4.1 |

| | Measure INFO/WEIGHT | per Measure KCAL | FAT | Nutrition Values per 100g / 100ml KCAL | PROT | CARB | FAT | FIBRE |
|---|---|---|---|---|---|---|---|---|

## CRUSSH JUICE BARS
### WRAP
| | | | | | | | | |
|---|---|---|---|---|---|---|---|---|
| Caesar, Simply, Crussh Juice Bars* | 1 Wrap/190g | 538 | 17.0 | 283 | 10.3 | 40.4 | 8.8 | 1.5 |
| Houmous & Falafel, Crussh Juice Bars* | 1 Wrap/150g | 318 | 14.0 | 212 | 7.5 | 23.9 | 9.6 | 1.0 |
| Mushroom & Sushi, with Soy Vinegar, Crussh Juice Bars* | 1 Wrap/298g | 310 | 2.0 | 104 | 1.8 | 22.7 | 0.6 | 0.0 |
| Tuna & Salad, Crussh Juice Bars* | 1 Wrap/210g | 365 | 10.0 | 174 | 12.0 | 20.4 | 4.9 | 0.4 |

### YOGHURT
| | | | | | | | | |
|---|---|---|---|---|---|---|---|---|
| with Honey, Low Fat, Greek, Crussh Juice Bars* | 1 Pot/140g | 209 | 13.0 | 150 | 5.1 | 12.5 | 9.1 | 0.0 |

## DOMINO'S PIZZA
### BROWNIES
| | | | | | | | | |
|---|---|---|---|---|---|---|---|---|
| Chocolate, Squares, Domino's Pizza* | 1 Brownie/22g | 104 | 6.0 | 474 | 5.9 | 54.2 | 25.9 | 1.8 |

### CHICKEN
| | | | | | | | | |
|---|---|---|---|---|---|---|---|---|
| Kickers, Domino's Pizza* | 7 Kickers/168g | 366 | 15.0 | 218 | 18.0 | 17.0 | 8.7 | 0.9 |
| Strippers, Domino's Pizza* | 7 Strippers/189g | 442 | 23.0 | 234 | 17.0 | 13.5 | 12.4 | 1.1 |

### COLESLAW
| | | | | | | | | |
|---|---|---|---|---|---|---|---|---|
| Domino's Pizza* | 1 Tub/200g | 328 | 30.0 | 164 | 1.3 | 6.6 | 14.8 | 1.7 |

### COOKIES
| | | | | | | | | |
|---|---|---|---|---|---|---|---|---|
| Domino's Pizza* | 1 Cookie/40g | 175 | 7.0 | 438 | 5.6 | 66.6 | 18.0 | 3.1 |

### DIP
| | | | | | | | | |
|---|---|---|---|---|---|---|---|---|
| BBQ, Domino's Pizza* | 1 Pot/28g | 46 | 0.0 | 163 | 0.0 | 39.5 | 0.5 | 0.0 |
| Chocolate Sauce, Domino's Pizza* | 1 Pot/28g | 88 | 0.0 | 313 | 0.5 | 76.6 | 0.4 | 0.8 |
| Garlic & Herb, Domino's Pizza* | 1 Pot/28g | 194 | 21.0 | 693 | 1.1 | 1.9 | 75.4 | 0.1 |
| Honey & Mustard, Domino's Pizza* | 1 Pot/28g | 129 | 13.0 | 459 | 1.8 | 7.5 | 46.5 | 0.2 |
| Mango, Domino's Pizza* | 1 Pot/28g | 52 | 0.0 | 185 | 0.2 | 42.5 | 1.1 | 0.6 |
| Sweet Chilli, Domino's Pizza* | 1 Pot/28g | 61 | 0.0 | 217 | 4.0 | 51.0 | 0.9 | 0.6 |
| Toffee, Domino's Pizza* | 1 Pot/28g | 94 | 1.0 | 335 | 1.5 | 75.1 | 3.2 | 0.1 |

### PIZZA
| | | | | | | | | |
|---|---|---|---|---|---|---|---|---|
| American Hot, Dominator, Lg, Domino's Pizza* | 1 Slice/110g | 306 | 12.0 | 279 | 13.2 | 31.7 | 11.0 | 1.9 |
| American Hot, Regular, Lg, Domino's Pizza* | 1 Slice/87g | 217 | 8.0 | 250 | 13.6 | 29.0 | 8.8 | 2.2 |
| American Hot, Regular, Med, Domino's Pizza* | 1 Slice/79g | 194 | 7.0 | 245 | 13.3 | 28.0 | 8.9 | 2.2 |
| American Hot, Regular, Sm, Domino's Pizza* | 1 Slice/72g | 181 | 7.0 | 253 | 14.0 | 28.5 | 9.2 | 2.2 |
| American Hot, Thin, Lg, Domino's Pizza* | 1 Slice/67g | 202 | 10.0 | 303 | 14.7 | 28.4 | 14.5 | 2.2 |
| American Hot, Thin, Med, Domino's Pizza* | 1 Slice/62g | 191 | 9.0 | 308 | 15.0 | 28.4 | 15.0 | 2.5 |
| Americano, Lg, Domino's Pizza* | 1 Slice/114g | 334 | 11.0 | 293 | 14.1 | 37.0 | 10.0 | 1.8 |
| Americano, Med, Domino's Pizza* | 1 Slice/103g | 346 | 15.0 | 336 | 14.8 | 36.1 | 14.7 | 1.8 |
| Americano, Regular, Lg, Domino's Pizza* | 1 Slice/91g | 268 | 8.0 | 295 | 15.7 | 37.2 | 9.3 | 1.9 |
| Americano, Regular, Med, Domino's Pizza* | 1 Slice/84g | 248 | 8.0 | 295 | 15.7 | 37.2 | 9.3 | 1.9 |
| Americano, Regular, Sm, Domino's Pizza* | 1 Slice/76g | 224 | 7.0 | 295 | 15.7 | 37.2 | 9.3 | 1.9 |
| Americano, Thin, Lg, Domino's Pizza* | 1 Slice/71g | 257 | 11.0 | 362 | 17.4 | 39.3 | 15.0 | 2.1 |
| Americano, Thin, Med, Domino's Pizza* | 1 Slice/67g | 243 | 10.0 | 362 | 17.4 | 39.3 | 15.0 | 2.1 |
| Bacon Double Cheese, Decadence, Med, Domino's Pizza* | 1 Slice/108g | 318 | 17.0 | 294 | 13.8 | 24.8 | 15.6 | 2.1 |
| Bacon Double Cheese, Dominator, Lg, Domino's Pizza* | 1 Slice/120g | 328 | 13.0 | 273 | 14.1 | 29.3 | 11.0 | 1.9 |
| Bacon Double Cheese, Regular, Lg, Domino's Pizza* | 1 Slice/97g | 240 | 10.0 | 247 | 14.7 | 24.6 | 10.0 | 1.9 |
| Bacon Double Cheese, Regular, Med, Domino's Pizza* | 1 Slice/88g | 217 | 9.0 | 247 | 14.7 | 24.6 | 10.0 | 1.9 |
| Bacon Double Cheese, Regular, Sm, Domino's Pizza* | 1 Slice/80g | 198 | 8.0 | 247 | 14.7 | 24.6 | 10.0 | 1.9 |
| Bacon Double Cheese, Thin, Lg, Domino's Pizza* | 1 Slice/77g | 224 | 12.0 | 291 | 16.3 | 21.8 | 15.4 | 2.2 |
| Bacon Double Cheese, Thin, Med, Domino's Pizza* | 1 Slice/71g | 215 | 11.0 | 303 | 16.4 | 24.1 | 15.6 | 2.1 |
| Beef & Onion Pie, Decadence, Med, Domino's Pizza* | 1 Slice/98g | 282 | 14.0 | 288 | 12.1 | 27.3 | 14.5 | 2.3 |
| Beef & Onion Pie, Dominator, Lg, Domino's Pizza* | 1 Slice/110g | 290 | 10.0 | 264 | 12.5 | 32.2 | 9.5 | 2.1 |
| Beef & Onion Pie, Regular, Lg, Domino's Pizza* | 1 Slice/87g | 204 | 7.0 | 234 | 12.7 | 27.8 | 8.0 | 2.2 |
| Beef & Onion Pie, Regular, Med, Domino's Pizza* | 1 Slice/79g | 185 | 6.0 | 234 | 12.7 | 27.8 | 8.0 | 2.2 |
| Beef & Onion Pie, Regular, Sm, Domino's Pizza* | 1 Slice/71g | 166 | 6.0 | 234 | 12.7 | 27.8 | 8.0 | 2.2 |
| Beef & Onion Pie, Thin, Lg, Domino's Pizza* | 1 Slice/67g | 188 | 9.0 | 280 | 14.0 | 25.4 | 13.6 | 2.6 |
| Beef & Onion Pie, Thin, Med, Domino's Pizza* | 1 Slice/62g | 182 | 9.0 | 294 | 14.2 | 28.1 | 13.9 | 2.5 |

| | Measure INFO/WEIGHT | per Measure KCAL | FAT | Nutrition Values per 100g / 100ml KCAL | PROT | CARB | FAT | FIBRE |
|---|---|---|---|---|---|---|---|---|

## DOMINO'S PIZZA
### PIZZA

| | Measure INFO/WEIGHT | KCAL | FAT | KCAL | PROT | CARB | FAT | FIBRE |
|---|---|---|---|---|---|---|---|---|
| Calypso, Decadence, Med, Domino's Pizza* | 1 Slice/95g | 273 | 13.0 | 287 | 12.1 | 28.8 | 13.8 | 2.4 |
| Calypso, Dominator, Lg, Domino's Pizza* | 1 Slice/106g | 279 | 9.0 | 263 | 12.5 | 33.9 | 8.7 | 2.2 |
| Calypso, Regular, Lg, Domino's Pizza* | 1 Slice/80g | 185 | 6.0 | 231 | 12.7 | 29.6 | 6.9 | 2.3 |
| Calypso, Regular, Med, Domino's Pizza* | 1 Slice/72g | 166 | 5.0 | 231 | 12.7 | 29.6 | 6.9 | 2.3 |
| Calypso, Regular, Sm, Domino's Pizza* | 1 Slice/65g | 150 | 4.0 | 231 | 12.7 | 29.6 | 6.9 | 2.3 |
| Calypso, Thin, Lg, Domino's Pizza* | 1 Slice/63g | 176 | 8.0 | 279 | 14.1 | 27.8 | 12.5 | 2.7 |
| Calypso, Thin, Med, Domino's Pizza* | 1 Slice/59g | 132 | 4.0 | 223 | 12.5 | 28.5 | 6.6 | 2.2 |
| Cheese & Tomato, Decadence, Med, Domino's Pizza* | 1 Slice/82g | 259 | 13.0 | 316 | 12.6 | 31.7 | 15.5 | 2.5 |
| Cheese & Tomato, Delight, Regular, Sm, Domino's Pizza* | 1 Slice/56g | 145 | 3.0 | 259 | 16.0 | 35.1 | 6.0 | 2.7 |
| Cheese & Tomato, Dominator, Lg, Domino's Pizza* | 1 Slice/92g | 265 | 9.0 | 288 | 13.0 | 37.6 | 9.5 | 2.3 |
| Cheese & Tomato, Regular, Lg, Domino's Pizza* | 1 Slice/69g | 183 | 5.0 | 265 | 14.0 | 34.7 | 7.8 | 2.4 |
| Cheese & Tomato, Regular, Med, Domino's Pizza* | 1 Slice/63g | 162 | 5.0 | 257 | 13.4 | 33.6 | 7.6 | 2.4 |
| Cheese & Tomato, Regular, Sm, Domino's Pizza* | 1 Slice/56g | 148 | 4.0 | 264 | 14.1 | 34.5 | 7.8 | 2.5 |
| Cheese & Tomato, Thin, Lg, Domino's Pizza* | 1 Slice/49g | 162 | 7.0 | 330 | 15.6 | 32.9 | 15.2 | 3.1 |
| Cheese & Tomato, Thin, Med, Domino's Pizza* | 1 Slice/46g | 160 | 7.0 | 347 | 15.7 | 36.2 | 15.5 | 2.9 |
| Chicken Feast, Decadence, Med, Domino's Pizza* | 1 Slice/100g | 232 | 7.0 | 232 | 14.3 | 28.9 | 6.6 | 2.1 |
| Chicken Feast, Delight, Regular, Sm, Domino's Pizza* | 1 Slice/72g | 165 | 4.0 | 228 | 16.5 | 29.0 | 5.1 | 2.3 |
| Chicken Feast, Dominator, Lg, Domino's Pizza* | 1 Slice/112g | 289 | 9.0 | 258 | 13.9 | 32.3 | 8.2 | 2.0 |
| Chicken Feast, Regular, Lg, Domino's Pizza* | 1 Slice/89g | 201 | 6.0 | 226 | 14.6 | 27.8 | 6.3 | 2.1 |
| Chicken Feast, Regular, Med, Domino's Pizza* | 1 Slice/81g | 183 | 5.0 | 226 | 14.6 | 27.8 | 6.3 | 2.1 |
| Chicken Feast, Regular, Sm, Domino's Pizza* | 1 Slice/72g | 163 | 5.0 | 226 | 14.6 | 27.8 | 6.3 | 2.1 |
| Chicken Feast, Thin, Lg, Domino's Pizza* | 1 Slice/69g | 195 | 8.0 | 283 | 16.5 | 28.1 | 11.6 | 2.4 |
| Chicken Feast, Thin, Med, Domino's Pizza* | 1 Slice/64g | 181 | 7.0 | 283 | 16.5 | 28.1 | 11.6 | 2.4 |
| Chicken Tikka Pizza, Regular, Lg, Domino's Pizza* | 1 Slice/85g | 194 | 6.0 | 229 | 13.1 | 27.8 | 7.3 | 2.3 |
| Chicken Tikka Pizza, Regular, Med, Domino's Pizza* | 1 Slice/77g | 177 | 6.0 | 229 | 13.1 | 27.8 | 7.3 | 2.3 |
| Chicken Tikka Pizza, Regular, Sm, Domino's Pizza* | 1 Slice/69g | 158 | 5.0 | 229 | 13.1 | 27.8 | 7.3 | 2.3 |
| Chicken Tikka Pizza, Thin, Lg, Domino's Pizza* | 1 Slice/62g | 146 | 5.0 | 235 | 13.6 | 27.3 | 7.9 | 2.4 |
| Chicken Tikka Pizza, Thin, Med, Domino's Pizza* | 1 Slice/58g | 136 | 5.0 | 235 | 13.6 | 27.3 | 7.9 | 2.4 |
| Domino's Deluxe, Decadence, Med, Domino's Pizza* | 1 Slice/100g | 296 | 15.0 | 296 | 12.5 | 26.6 | 15.5 | 2.3 |
| Domino's Deluxe, Dominator, Lg, Domino's Pizza* | 1 Slice/111g | 1270 | 12.0 | 1144 | 12.8 | 31.7 | 10.4 | 2.1 |
| Domino's Deluxe, Regular, Lg, Domino's Pizza* | 1 Slice/88g | 216 | 8.0 | 245 | 13.2 | 26.9 | 9.4 | 2.1 |
| Domino's Deluxe, Regular, Med, Domino's Pizza* | 1 Slice/81g | 198 | 8.0 | 245 | 13.2 | 26.9 | 9.4 | 2.1 |
| Domino's Deluxe, Regular, Sm, Domino's Pizza* | 1 Slice/74g | 181 | 7.0 | 245 | 13.2 | 26.9 | 9.4 | 2.1 |
| Domino's Deluxe, Thin, Lg, Domino's Pizza* | 1 Slice/68g | 199 | 10.0 | 292 | 14.5 | 24.7 | 15.1 | 2.5 |
| Domino's Deluxe, Thin, Med, Domino's Pizza* | 1 Slice/64g | 196 | 10.0 | 307 | 14.7 | 27.0 | 15.5 | 2.4 |
| Domino's Meateor, Decadence, Med, Domino's Pizza* | 1 Slice/103g | 368 | 18.0 | 356 | 13.9 | 35.7 | 17.5 | 1.8 |
| Domino's Meateor, Dominator, Lg, Domino's Pizza* | 1 Slice/114g | 357 | 14.0 | 313 | 13.3 | 36.6 | 12.7 | 1.8 |
| Domino's Meateor, Regular, Lg, Domino's Pizza* | 1 Slice/88g | 280 | 11.0 | 319 | 14.5 | 36.7 | 12.7 | 1.8 |
| Domino's Meateor, Regular, Med, Domino's Pizza* | 1 Slice/81g | 258 | 10.0 | 319 | 14.5 | 36.7 | 12.7 | 1.8 |
| Domino's Meateor, Regular, Sm, Domino's Pizza* | 1 Slice/74g | 236 | 9.0 | 319 | 14.5 | 36.7 | 12.7 | 1.8 |
| Domino's Meateor, Thin, Lg, Domino's Pizza* | 1 Slice/68g | 239 | 12.0 | 352 | 15.3 | 32.8 | 17.7 | 1.7 |
| Domino's Meateor, Thin, Med, Domino's Pizza* | 1 Slice/64g | 250 | 12.0 | 392 | 16.0 | 38.6 | 19.3 | 2.0 |
| Domino's Scrummy, Decadence, Med, Domino's Pizza* | 1 Slice/119g | 369 | 20.0 | 310 | 15.9 | 23.2 | 17.1 | 1.9 |
| Domino's Scrummy, Dominator, Lg, Domino's Pizza* | 1 Slice/130g | 1585 | 17.0 | 1219 | 16.0 | 27.8 | 12.8 | 1.8 |
| Domino's Scrummy, Regular, Lg, Domino's Pizza* | 1 Slice/107g | 290 | 13.0 | 271 | 17.0 | 22.8 | 12.4 | 1.7 |
| Domino's Scrummy, Regular, Med, Domino's Pizza* | 1 Slice/99g | 268 | 12.0 | 271 | 17.0 | 22.8 | 12.4 | 1.7 |
| Domino's Scrummy, Regular, Sm, Domino's Pizza* | 1 Slice/92g | 249 | 11.0 | 271 | 17.0 | 22.8 | 12.4 | 1.7 |
| Domino's Scrummy, Thin, Lg, Domino's Pizza* | 1 Slice/87g | 283 | 15.0 | 325 | 19.0 | 22.2 | 17.8 | 1.9 |
| Domino's Scrummy, Thin, Med, Domino's Pizza* | 1 Slice/82g | 266 | 15.0 | 324 | 19.1 | 21.9 | 17.8 | 1.9 |
| Extravaganza, Decadence, Med, Domino's Pizza* | 1 Slice/114g | 327 | 18.0 | 287 | 13.1 | 23.7 | 15.5 | 2.1 |
| Extravaganza, Dominator, Lg, Domino's Pizza* | 1 Slice/127g | 338 | 14.0 | 266 | 13.3 | 28.2 | 11.1 | 1.9 |
| Extravaganza, Regular, Lg, Domino's Pizza* | 1 Slice/104g | 252 | 11.0 | 242 | 13.7 | 23.4 | 10.3 | 1.9 |

| | Measure INFO/WEIGHT | per Measure KCAL | FAT | Nutrition Values per 100g / 100ml KCAL | PROT | CARB | FAT | FIBRE |
|---|---|---|---|---|---|---|---|---|

## DOMINO'S PIZZA
### PIZZA

| | Measure INFO/WEIGHT | KCAL | FAT | KCAL | PROT | CARB | FAT | FIBRE |
|---|---|---|---|---|---|---|---|---|
| Extravaganza, Regular, Med, Domino's Pizza* | 1 Slice/95g | 230 | 10.0 | 242 | 13.7 | 23.4 | 10.3 | 1.9 |
| Extravaganza, Regular, Sm, Domino's Pizza* | 1 Slice/86g | 208 | 9.0 | 242 | 13.7 | 23.4 | 10.3 | 1.9 |
| Extravaganza, Thin, Lg, Domino's Pizza* | 1 Slice/84g | 235 | 13.0 | 280 | 15.0 | 20.7 | 15.2 | 2.2 |
| Extravaganza, Thin, Med, Domino's Pizza* | 1 Slice/78g | 227 | 12.0 | 291 | 15.1 | 22.6 | 15.5 | 2.1 |
| Farmhouse, Decadence, Med, Domino's Pizza* | 1 Slice/100g | 277 | 13.0 | 277 | 12.7 | 26.5 | 13.4 | 2.3 |
| Farmhouse, Dominator, Lg, Domino's Pizza* | 1 Slice/111g | 283 | 9.0 | 255 | 13.0 | 31.7 | 8.5 | 2.0 |
| Farmhouse, Regular, Lg, Domino's Pizza* | 1 Slice/88g | 195 | 6.0 | 222 | 13.4 | 26.8 | 6.8 | 2.1 |
| Farmhouse, Regular, Med, Domino's Pizza* | 1 Slice/81g | 180 | 6.0 | 222 | 13.4 | 26.8 | 6.8 | 2.1 |
| Farmhouse, Regular, Sm, Domino's Pizza* | 1 Slice/73g | 162 | 5.0 | 222 | 13.4 | 26.8 | 6.8 | 2.1 |
| Farmhouse, Thin, Lg, Domino's Pizza* | 1 Slice/68g | 180 | 8.0 | 265 | 14.8 | 24.6 | 11.9 | 2.5 |
| Farmhouse, Thin, Med, Domino's Pizza* | 1 Slice/63g | 175 | 8.0 | 277 | 15.1 | 26.9 | 12.2 | 2.4 |
| Full House, , Delight, Regular, Sm, Domino's Pizza* | 1 Slice/80g | 190 | 6.0 | 238 | 14.8 | 27.1 | 7.8 | 2.3 |
| Full House, Decadence, Med, Domino's Pizza* | 1 Slice/107g | 306 | 16.0 | 286 | 12.4 | 25.9 | 14.7 | 2.2 |
| Full House, Dominator, Lg, Domino's Pizza* | 1 Slice/119g | 312 | 12.0 | 262 | 12.6 | 31.0 | 9.7 | 2.0 |
| Full House, Regular, Lg, Domino's Pizza* | 1 Slice/96g | 231 | 9.0 | 241 | 13.2 | 27.0 | 8.9 | 2.1 |
| Full House, Regular, Med, Domino's Pizza* | 1 Slice/88g | 208 | 8.0 | 236 | 13.0 | 26.0 | 8.9 | 2.0 |
| Full House, Regular, Sm, Domino's Pizza* | 1 Slice/80g | 194 | 7.0 | 242 | 13.5 | 26.3 | 9.2 | 2.1 |
| Full House, Thin, Lg, Domino's Pizza* | 1 Slice/76g | 210 | 11.0 | 276 | 14.0 | 23.7 | 13.9 | 2.4 |
| Full House, Thin, Med, Domino's Pizza* | 1 Slice/71g | 206 | 10.0 | 290 | 14.3 | 25.9 | 14.3 | 2.3 |
| Ham & Pineapple, Decadence, Med, Domino's Pizza* | 1 Slice/97g | 278 | 13.0 | 287 | 12.9 | 27.8 | 13.8 | 2.2 |
| Ham & Pineapple, Delight, Regular, Sm, Domino's Pizza* | 1 Slice/70g | 163 | 4.0 | 233 | 15.7 | 29.7 | 5.7 | 2.3 |
| Ham & Pineapple, Dominator, Lg, Domino's Pizza* | 1 Slice/106g | 281 | 9.0 | 265 | 13.2 | 33.3 | 8.8 | 2.0 |
| Ham & Pineapple, Regular, Lg, Domino's Pizza* | 1 Slice/84g | 194 | 6.0 | 231 | 13.7 | 28.5 | 7.0 | 2.0 |
| Ham & Pineapple, Regular, Med, Domino's Pizza* | 1 Slice/77g | 178 | 5.0 | 231 | 13.7 | 28.5 | 7.0 | 2.0 |
| Ham & Pineapple, Regular, Sm, Domino's Pizza* | 1 Slice/70g | 162 | 5.0 | 231 | 13.7 | 28.5 | 7.0 | 2.0 |
| Ham & Pineapple, Thin, Lg, Domino's Pizza* | 1 Slice/64g | 181 | 8.0 | 283 | 15.4 | 26.8 | 12.7 | 2.5 |
| Ham & Pineapple, Thin, Med, Domino's Pizza* | 1 Slice/60g | 175 | 8.0 | 292 | 15.4 | 29.0 | 12.7 | 2.3 |
| Hawaiian, Decadence, Med, Domino's Pizza* | 1 Slice/106g | 290 | 14.0 | 275 | 13.0 | 25.5 | 13.4 | 2.1 |
| Hawaiian, Delight, Regular, Sm, Domino's Pizza* | 1 Slice/79g | 176 | 5.0 | 224 | 15.6 | 26.7 | 6.1 | 2.2 |
| Hawaiian, Dominator, Lg, Domino's Pizza* | 1 Slice/117g | 298 | 10.0 | 254 | 13.3 | 30.4 | 8.8 | 1.9 |
| Hawaiian, Regular, Lg, Domino's Pizza* | 1 Slice/94g | 216 | 7.0 | 229 | 14.1 | 26.5 | 7.4 | 1.9 |
| Hawaiian, Regular, Med, Domino's Pizza* | 1 Slice/86g | 192 | 6.0 | 223 | 13.8 | 25.6 | 7.3 | 1.9 |
| Hawaiian, Regular, Sm, Domino's Pizza* | 1 Slice/79g | 178 | 6.0 | 227 | 14.3 | 25.9 | 7.4 | 2.0 |
| Hawaiian, Thin, Lg, Domino's Pizza* | 1 Slice/75g | 195 | 9.0 | 262 | 15.1 | 23.1 | 12.1 | 2.2 |
| Hawaiian, Thin, Med, Domino's Pizza* | 1 Slice/69g | 190 | 9.0 | 274 | 15.3 | 25.3 | 12.4 | 2.1 |
| Hot & Spicy, Decadence, Med, Domino's Pizza* | 1 Slice/96g | 276 | 14.0 | 288 | 11.8 | 28.0 | 14.3 | 2.4 |
| Hot & Spicy, Dominator, Lg, Domino's Pizza* | 1 Slice/107g | 284 | 10.0 | 264 | 12.2 | 33.0 | 9.2 | 2.2 |
| Hot & Spicy, Regular, Lg, Domino's Pizza* | 1 Slice/85g | 201 | 7.0 | 238 | 12.7 | 29.5 | 7.7 | 2.3 |
| Hot & Spicy, Regular, Med, Domino's Pizza* | 1 Slice/77g | 178 | 6.0 | 232 | 12.3 | 28.7 | 7.6 | 2.3 |
| Hot & Spicy, Regular, Sm, Domino's Pizza* | 1 Slice/69g | 163 | 5.0 | 237 | 12.8 | 29.3 | 7.7 | 2.3 |
| Hot & Spicy, Thin, Lg, Domino's Pizza* | 1 Slice/65g | 181 | 9.0 | 280 | 9.3 | 26.5 | 13.3 | 2.7 |
| Hot & Spicy, Thin, Med, Domino's Pizza* | 1 Slice/60g | 175 | 8.0 | 294 | 13.7 | 29.2 | 13.6 | 2.6 |
| Hot Dog, Decadence, Med, Domino's Pizza* | 1 Slice/117g | 358 | 21.0 | 306 | 13.7 | 23.1 | 17.6 | 2.1 |
| Hot Dog, Dominator, Lg, Domino's Pizza* | 1 Slice/129g | 368 | 17.0 | 285 | 14.0 | 27.7 | 13.1 | 1.9 |
| Hot Dog, Regular, Lg, Domino's Pizza* | 1 Slice/106g | 323 | 14.0 | 305 | 14.1 | 31.6 | 13.5 | 1.8 |
| Hot Dog, Regular, Med, Domino's Pizza* | 1 Slice/98g | 299 | 13.0 | 305 | 14.1 | 31.6 | 13.5 | 1.8 |
| Hot Dog, Regular, Sm, Domino's Pizza* | 1 Slice/90g | 274 | 12.0 | 305 | 14.1 | 31.6 | 13.5 | 1.8 |
| Hot Dog, Thin, Lg, Domino's Pizza* | 1 Slice/86g | 265 | 16.0 | 308 | 15.9 | 20.1 | 18.1 | 2.2 |
| Hot Dog, Thin, Med, Domino's Pizza* | 1 Slice/81g | 258 | 15.0 | 319 | 16.0 | 21.8 | 18.5 | 2.1 |
| House Special, Decadence, Med, Domino's Pizza* | 1 Slice/110g | 319 | 16.0 | 290 | 14.8 | 24.1 | 14.9 | 2.1 |
| House Special, Dominator, Lg, Domino's Pizza* | 1 Slice/122g | 328 | 13.0 | 269 | 15.0 | 28.7 | 10.4 | 1.9 |
| House Special, Regular, Lg, Domino's Pizza* | 1 Slice/100g | 243 | 9.0 | 243 | 15.8 | 23.8 | 9.4 | 1.9 |

| | Measure INFO/WEIGHT | per Measure KCAL | FAT | Nutrition Values per 100g / 100ml KCAL | PROT | CARB | FAT | FIBRE |
|---|---|---|---|---|---|---|---|---|

## DOMINO'S PIZZA

### PIZZA

| | Measure INFO/WEIGHT | KCAL | FAT | KCAL | PROT | CARB | FAT | FIBRE |
|---|---|---|---|---|---|---|---|---|
| House Special, Regular, Med, Domino's Pizza* | 1 Slice/91g | 221 | 9.0 | 243 | 15.8 | 23.8 | 9.4 | 1.9 |
| House Special, Regular, Sm, Domino's Pizza* | 1 Slice/82g | 199 | 8.0 | 243 | 15.8 | 23.8 | 9.4 | 1.9 |
| House Special, Thin, Lg, Domino's Pizza* | 1 Slice/80g | 227 | 12.0 | 284 | 17.6 | 21.0 | 14.4 | 2.2 |
| House Special, Thin, Med, Domino's Pizza* | 1 Slice/74g | 219 | 11.0 | 296 | 17.8 | 23.1 | 14.6 | 2.1 |
| Jamaican Bombastic, Decadence, Med, Domino's Pizza* | 1 Slice/102g | 280 | 13.0 | 275 | 12.2 | 28.0 | 12.7 | 2.4 |
| Jamaican Bombastic, Dominator, Lg, Domino's Pizza* | 1 Slice/114g | 288 | 9.0 | 253 | 12.5 | 32.8 | 7.9 | 2.2 |
| Jamaican Bombastic, Regular, Lg, Domino's Pizza* | 1 Slice/91g | 201 | 6.0 | 221 | 12.8 | 28.7 | 6.1 | 2.3 |
| Jamaican Bombastic, Regular, Med, Domino's Pizza* | 1 Slice/83g | 183 | 5.0 | 221 | 12.8 | 28.7 | 6.1 | 2.3 |
| Jamaican Bombastic, Regular, Sm, Domino's Pizza* | 1 Slice/75g | 166 | 5.0 | 221 | 12.8 | 28.7 | 6.1 | 2.3 |
| Jamaican Bombastic, Thin, Lg, Domino's Pizza* | 1 Slice/71g | 185 | 8.0 | 260 | 14.0 | 26.7 | 10.8 | 2.7 |
| Jamaican Bombastic, Thin, Med, Domino's Pizza* | 1 Slice/66g | 181 | 7.0 | 274 | 14.2 | 29.2 | 11.1 | 2.6 |
| Meat Lovers, Decadence, Med, Domino's Pizza* | 1 Slice/101g | 314 | 16.0 | 311 | 14.9 | 26.3 | 16.3 | 2.1 |
| Meat Lovers, Dominator, Lg, Domino's Pizza* | 1 Slice/111g | 320 | 13.0 | 288 | 15.1 | 31.4 | 11.3 | 1.9 |
| Meat Lovers, Regular, Lg, Domino's Pizza* | 1 Slice/89g | 235 | 9.0 | 264 | 16.1 | 26.5 | 10.4 | 1.9 |
| Meat Lovers, Regular, Med, Domino's Pizza* | 1 Slice/81g | 214 | 8.0 | 264 | 16.1 | 26.5 | 10.4 | 1.9 |
| Meat Lovers, Regular, Sm, Domino's Pizza* | 1 Slice/74g | 195 | 8.0 | 264 | 16.1 | 26.5 | 10.4 | 1.9 |
| Meat Lovers, Thin, Lg, Domino's Pizza* | 1 Slice/69g | 219 | 11.0 | 318 | 18.3 | 24.2 | 16.5 | 2.3 |
| Meat Lovers, Thin, Med, Domino's Pizza* | 1 Slice/64g | 211 | 11.0 | 330 | 18.5 | 26.5 | 16.7 | 2.2 |
| Meat Packer, Decadence, Med, Domino's Pizza* | 1 Slice/106g | 329 | 17.0 | 310 | 15.5 | 25.1 | 16.4 | 2.0 |
| Meat Packer, Dominator, Lg, Domino's Pizza* | 1 Slice/116g | 334 | 13.0 | 288 | 15.6 | 30.1 | 11.6 | 1.8 |
| Meat Packer, Regular, Lg, Domino's Pizza* | 1 Slice/94g | 249 | 10.0 | 265 | 16.8 | 25.1 | 10.9 | 1.8 |
| Meat Packer, Regular, Med, Domino's Pizza* | 1 Slice/86g | 228 | 9.0 | 265 | 16.8 | 25.1 | 10.9 | 1.8 |
| Meat Packer, Regular, Sm, Domino's Pizza* | 1 Slice/79g | 209 | 9.0 | 265 | 16.8 | 25.1 | 10.9 | 1.8 |
| Meat Packer, Thin, Lg, Domino's Pizza* | 1 Slice/74g | 234 | 12.0 | 316 | 18.9 | 22.7 | 16.6 | 2.1 |
| Meat Packer, Thin, Med, Domino's Pizza* | 1 Slice/69g | 226 | 12.0 | 327 | 19.1 | 24.7 | 16.8 | 2.0 |
| Meatball Mayham, Decadence, Med, Domino's Pizza* | 1 Slice/111g | 362 | 17.0 | 327 | 11.8 | 35.2 | 15.5 | 1.9 |
| Meatball Mayham, Dominator, Lg, Domino's Pizza* | 1 Slice/122g | 350 | 13.0 | 288 | 11.2 | 36.1 | 11.0 | 1.9 |
| Meatball Mayham, Regular, Lg, Domino's Pizza* | 1 Slice/99g | 285 | 11.0 | 288 | 12.0 | 36.0 | 10.7 | 2.0 |
| Meatball Mayham, Regular, Med, Domino's Pizza* | 1 Slice/91g | 263 | 10.0 | 288 | 12.0 | 36.0 | 10.7 | 2.0 |
| Meatball Mayham, Regular, Sm, Domino's Pizza* | 1 Slice/84g | 241 | 9.0 | 288 | 12.0 | 36.0 | 10.7 | 2.0 |
| Meatball Mayham, Thin, Lg, Domino's Pizza* | 1 Slice/79g | 244 | 12.0 | 309 | 12.0 | 32.5 | 14.6 | 2.0 |
| Meatball Mayham, Thin, Med, Domino's Pizza* | 1 Slice/74g | 257 | 12.0 | 346 | 12.7 | 37.5 | 16.1 | 2.2 |
| Meatzza Pizza, Decadence, Med, Domino's Pizza* | 1 Slice/105g | 333 | 18.0 | 317 | 14.6 | 25.5 | 17.4 | 2.1 |
| Meatzza Pizza, Dominator, Lg, Domino's Pizza* | 1 Slice/115g | 338 | 14.0 | 294 | 14.8 | 30.6 | 12.5 | 1.9 |
| Meatzza Pizza, Regular, Lg, Domino's Pizza* | 1 Slice/89g | 235 | 9.0 | 264 | 16.1 | 26.5 | 10.4 | 1.9 |
| Meatzza Pizza, Regular, Med, Domino's Pizza* | 1 Slice/81g | 214 | 8.0 | 264 | 16.1 | 26.5 | 10.4 | 1.9 |
| Meatzza Pizza, Regular, Sm, Domino's Pizza* | 1 Slice/74g | 195 | 8.0 | 264 | 16.1 | 26.5 | 10.4 | 1.9 |
| Meatzza Pizza, Thin, Lg, Domino's Pizza* | 1 Slice/69g | 228 | 12.0 | 330 | 18.5 | 26.5 | 16.7 | 2.2 |
| Meatzza Pizza, Thin, Med, Domino's Pizza* | 1 Slice/64g | 211 | 11.0 | 330 | 18.5 | 26.5 | 16.7 | 2.2 |
| Mediterranean Spice, Decadence, Med, Domino's Pizza* | 1 Slice/117g | 300 | 15.0 | 256 | 12.8 | 23.2 | 12.4 | 2.0 |
| Mediterranean Spice, Dominator, Lg, Domino's Pizza* | 1 Slice/129g | 306 | 11.0 | 237 | 12.9 | 27.8 | 8.3 | 1.9 |
| Mediterranean Spice, Regular, Lg, Domino's Pizza* | 1 Slice/106g | 218 | 7.0 | 206 | 13.4 | 22.8 | 6.8 | 1.9 |
| Mediterranean Spice, Regular, Med, Domino's Pizza* | 1 Slice/97g | 200 | 7.0 | 206 | 13.4 | 22.8 | 6.8 | 1.9 |
| Mediterranean Spice, Regular, Sm, Domino's Pizza* | 1 Slice/89g | 183 | 6.0 | 206 | 13.4 | 22.8 | 6.8 | 1.9 |
| Mediterranean Spice, Thin, Lg, Domino's Pizza* | 1 Slice/86g | 202 | 9.0 | 235 | 14.3 | 20.2 | 10.8 | 2.1 |
| Mediterranean Spice, Thin, Med, Domino's Pizza* | 1 Slice/80g | 197 | 9.0 | 246 | 14.7 | 22.0 | 11.0 | 2.0 |
| Mexican Hot, Decadence, Med, Domino's Pizza* | 1 Slice/103g | 302 | 16.0 | 293 | 12.9 | 26.2 | 15.1 | 2.3 |
| Mexican Hot, Dominator, Lg, Domino's Pizza* | 1 Slice/114g | 308 | 12.0 | 270 | 13.2 | 31.1 | 10.2 | 2.1 |
| Mexican Hot, Regular, Lg, Domino's Pizza* | 1 Slice/98g | 238 | 9.0 | 243 | 13.7 | 26.4 | 9.1 | 2.1 |
| Mexican Hot, Regular, Med, Domino's Pizza* | 1 Slice/90g | 219 | 8.0 | 243 | 13.7 | 26.4 | 9.1 | 2.1 |
| Mexican Hot, Regular, Sm, Domino's Pizza* | 1 Slice/81g | 197 | 7.0 | 243 | 13.7 | 26.4 | 9.1 | 2.1 |
| Mexican Hot, Thin, Lg, Domino's Pizza* | 1 Slice/71g | 204 | 10.0 | 287 | 15.1 | 24.0 | 14.5 | 2.5 |

## DOMINO'S PIZZA

### PIZZA

| | INFO/WEIGHT | KCAL | FAT | KCAL | PROT | CARB | FAT | FIBRE |
|---|---|---|---|---|---|---|---|---|
| Mexican Hot, Thin, Med, Domino's Pizza* | 1 Slice/66g | 199 | 10.0 | 301 | 15.3 | 26.4 | 14.9 | 2.4 |
| Mighty Meaty, Decadence, Med, Domino's Pizza* | 1 Slice/107g | 319 | 17.0 | 298 | 13.8 | 25.1 | 15.8 | 2.1 |
| Mighty Meaty, Delight, Regular, Sm, Domino's Pizza* | 1 Slice/80g | 202 | 7.0 | 253 | 16.5 | 26.1 | 9.1 | 2.2 |
| Mighty Meaty, Dominator, Lg, Domino's Pizza* | 1 Slice/118g | 326 | 13.0 | 276 | 14.0 | 30.0 | 11.1 | 1.9 |
| Mighty Meaty, Regular, Lg, Domino's Pizza* | 1 Slice/95g | 243 | 10.0 | 256 | 15.0 | 26.1 | 10.2 | 2.0 |
| Mighty Meaty, Regular, Med, Domino's Pizza* | 1 Slice/87g | 218 | 9.0 | 251 | 14.7 | 25.0 | 10.3 | 1.9 |
| Mighty Meaty, Regular, Sm, Domino's Pizza* | 1 Slice/80g | 206 | 8.0 | 257 | 15.3 | 25.2 | 10.6 | 2.0 |
| Mighty Meaty, Thin, Lg, Domino's Pizza* | 1 Slice/75g | 222 | 12.0 | 296 | 16.2 | 22.6 | 15.7 | 2.3 |
| Mighty Meaty, Thin, Med, Domino's Pizza* | 1 Slice/70g | 216 | 11.0 | 309 | 16.5 | 24.6 | 16.0 | 2.1 |
| Mixed Grill, Decadence, Med, Domino's Pizza* | 1 Slice/106g | 319 | 18.0 | 301 | 12.8 | 25.1 | 16.7 | 2.2 |
| Mixed Grill, Dominator, Lg, Domino's Pizza* | 1 Slice/117g | 325 | 14.0 | 278 | 13.1 | 30.0 | 11.8 | 1.9 |
| Mixed Grill, Regular, Lg, Domino's Pizza* | 1 Slice/94g | 240 | 11.0 | 255 | 13.5 | 25.0 | 11.2 | 2.0 |
| Mixed Grill, Regular, Med, Domino's Pizza* | 1 Slice/87g | 222 | 10.0 | 255 | 13.5 | 25.0 | 11.2 | 2.0 |
| Mixed Grill, Regular, Sm, Domino's Pizza* | 1 Slice/79g | 201 | 9.0 | 255 | 13.5 | 25.0 | 11.2 | 2.0 |
| Mixed Grill, Thin, Lg, Domino's Pizza* | 1 Slice/74g | 223 | 12.0 | 301 | 14.9 | 22.5 | 16.8 | 2.3 |
| Mixed Grill, Thin, Med, Domino's Pizza* | 1 Slice/70g | 220 | 12.0 | 314 | 15.0 | 24.6 | 17.3 | 2.2 |
| New Yorker, Decadence, Med, Domino's Pizza* | 1 Slice/100g | 254 | 9.0 | 254 | 15.1 | 28.0 | 9.0 | 2.0 |
| New Yorker, Dominator, Lg, Domino's Pizza* | 1 Slice/110g | 307 | 12.0 | 279 | 14.6 | 31.6 | 10.5 | 1.9 |
| New Yorker, Regular, Lg, Domino's Pizza* | 1 Slice/87g | 220 | 8.0 | 253 | 15.5 | 26.7 | 9.4 | 2.0 |
| New Yorker, Regular, Med, Domino's Pizza* | 1 Slice/80g | 202 | 8.0 | 253 | 15.5 | 26.7 | 9.4 | 2.0 |
| New Yorker, Regular, Sm, Domino's Pizza* | 1 Slice/73g | 185 | 7.0 | 253 | 15.5 | 26.7 | 9.4 | 2.0 |
| New Yorker, Thin, Lg, Domino's Pizza* | 1 Slice/67g | 212 | 10.0 | 317 | 17.6 | 26.7 | 15.5 | 2.2 |
| New Yorker, Thin, Med, Domino's Pizza* | 1 Slice/63g | 200 | 10.0 | 317 | 17.6 | 26.7 | 15.5 | 2.2 |
| Pepperoni Passion, Decadence, Med, Domino's Pizza* | 1 Slice/104g | 341 | 19.0 | 328 | 15.9 | 25.4 | 17.9 | 2.0 |
| Pepperoni Passion, Dominator, Lg, Domino's Pizza* | 1 Slice/115g | 351 | 15.0 | 305 | 16.1 | 30.4 | 13.0 | 1.8 |
| Pepperoni Passion, Regular, Lg, Domino's Pizza* | 1 Slice/92g | 269 | 11.0 | 292 | 17.6 | 26.5 | 12.5 | 1.8 |
| Pepperoni Passion, Regular, Med, Domino's Pizza* | 1 Slice/85g | 244 | 11.0 | 287 | 17.3 | 25.4 | 12.6 | 1.8 |
| Pepperoni Passion, Regular, Sm, Domino's Pizza* | 1 Slice/77g | 226 | 10.0 | 294 | 17.9 | 25.8 | 12.9 | 1.9 |
| Pepperoni Passion, Thin, Lg, Domino's Pizza* | 1 Slice/72g | 248 | 14.0 | 344 | 19.6 | 22.9 | 18.8 | 2.1 |
| Pepperoni Passion, Thin, Med, Domino's Pizza* | 1 Slice/68g | 242 | 13.0 | 356 | 19.8 | 25.1 | 19.1 | 2.0 |
| Piri Piri Pizza, Regular, Lg, Domino's Pizza* | 1 Slice/61g | 155 | 5.0 | 256 | 14.7 | 30.8 | 8.2 | 1.6 |
| Piri Piri Pizza, Regular, Med, Domino's Pizza* | 1 Slice/55g | 142 | 5.0 | 256 | 14.7 | 30.8 | 8.2 | 1.6 |
| Piri Piri Pizza, Regular, Sm, Domino's Pizza* | 1 Slice/49g | 126 | 4.0 | 256 | 14.7 | 30.8 | 8.2 | 1.6 |
| Piri Piri Pizza, Thin, Lg, Domino's Pizza* | 1 Slice/41g | 126 | 6.0 | 310 | 17.7 | 26.9 | 14.7 | 1.9 |
| Piri Piri Pizza, Thin, Med, Domino's Pizza* | 1 Slice/38g | 119 | 6.0 | 310 | 17.7 | 26.9 | 14.7 | 1.9 |
| Premiere, Regular, Lg, Domino's Pizza* | 1 Slice/83g | 213 | 7.0 | 257 | 15.4 | 30.0 | 8.3 | 2.2 |
| Premiere, Regular, Med, Domino's Pizza* | 1 Slice/77g | 198 | 6.0 | 257 | 15.4 | 30.0 | 8.3 | 2.2 |
| Premiere, Regular, Sm, Domino's Pizza* | 1 Slice/69g | 177 | 6.0 | 257 | 15.4 | 30.0 | 8.3 | 2.2 |
| Tandoori Hot, Decadence, Med, Domino's Pizza* | 1 Slice/101g | 275 | 13.0 | 273 | 12.4 | 26.9 | 12.9 | 2.3 |
| Tandoori Hot, Delight, Regular, Sm, Domino's Pizza* | 1 Slice/73g | 159 | 4.0 | 218 | 15.0 | 28.4 | 4.9 | 2.4 |
| Tandoori Hot, Dominator, Lg, Domino's Pizza* | 1 Slice/112g | 280 | 9.0 | 250 | 12.7 | 31.8 | 8.0 | 2.1 |
| Tandoori Hot, Regular, Lg, Domino's Pizza* | 1 Slice/89g | 199 | 6.0 | 223 | 13.4 | 28.1 | 6.3 | 2.2 |
| Tandoori Hot, Regular, Med, Domino's Pizza* | 1 Slice/81g | 176 | 5.0 | 217 | 13.0 | 27.2 | 6.2 | 2.2 |
| Tandoori Hot, Regular, Sm, Domino's Pizza* | 1 Slice/73g | 162 | 5.0 | 222 | 13.5 | 27.9 | 6.3 | 2.3 |
| Tandoori Hot, Thin, Lg, Domino's Pizza* | 1 Slice/69g | 178 | 8.0 | 257 | 14.3 | 24.9 | 11.1 | 2.6 |
| Tandoori Hot, Thin, Med, Domino's Pizza* | 1 Slice/64g | 173 | 7.0 | 270 | 14.5 | 27.4 | 11.4 | 2.5 |
| Texas BBQ, Decadence, Med, Domino's Pizza* | 1 Slice/98g | 321 | 14.0 | 328 | 13.5 | 37.0 | 14.0 | 1.8 |
| Texas BBQ, Delight, Regular, Sm, Domino's Pizza* | 1 Slice/71g | 167 | 4.0 | 235 | 13.0 | 33.4 | 5.5 | 2.2 |
| Texas BBQ, Dominator, Lg, Domino's Pizza* | 1 Slice/110g | 312 | 10.0 | 284 | 12.8 | 37.6 | 9.2 | 1.8 |
| Texas BBQ, Regular, Lg, Domino's Pizza* | 1 Slice/87g | 245 | 7.0 | 282 | 14.1 | 38.4 | 8.0 | 1.9 |
| Texas BBQ, Regular, Med, Domino's Pizza* | 1 Slice/79g | 223 | 6.0 | 282 | 14.1 | 38.4 | 8.0 | 1.9 |
| Texas BBQ, Regular, Sm, Domino's Pizza* | 1 Slice/71g | 200 | 6.0 | 282 | 14.1 | 38.4 | 8.0 | 1.9 |

## DOMINO'S PIZZA

| | Measure INFO/WEIGHT | per Measure | | Nutrition Values per 100g / 100ml | | | | |
|---|---|---|---|---|---|---|---|---|
| | | KCAL | FAT | KCAL | PROT | CARB | FAT | FIBRE |

### PIZZA

| | Measure INFO/WEIGHT | KCAL | FAT | KCAL | PROT | CARB | FAT | FIBRE |
|---|---|---|---|---|---|---|---|---|
| Texas BBQ, Thin, Lg, Domino's Pizza* | 1 Slice/67g | 206 | 8.0 | 307 | 14.8 | 34.3 | 12.2 | 1.8 |
| Texas BBQ, Thin, Med, Domino's Pizza* | 1 Slice/62g | 217 | 9.0 | 350 | 15.5 | 40.9 | 13.8 | 2.1 |
| The Sizzler, Decadence, Med, Domino's Pizza* | 1 Slice/106g | 334 | 17.0 | 315 | 13.5 | 29.3 | 16.0 | 2.3 |
| The Sizzler, Dominator, Lg, Domino's Pizza* | 1 Slice/118g | 344 | 13.0 | 293 | 13.7 | 34.1 | 11.4 | 2.1 |
| The Sizzler, Regular, Lg, Domino's Pizza* | 1 Slice/95g | 270 | 11.0 | 285 | 14.7 | 31.5 | 11.2 | 2.2 |
| The Sizzler, Regular, Med, Domino's Pizza* | 1 Slice/87g | 247 | 10.0 | 285 | 14.7 | 31.5 | 11.2 | 2.2 |
| The Sizzler, Regular, Sm, Domino's Pizza* | 1 Slice/78g | 223 | 9.0 | 285 | 14.7 | 31.5 | 11.2 | 2.2 |
| The Sizzler, Thin, Lg, Domino's Pizza* | 1 Slice/75g | 227 | 11.0 | 303 | 14.7 | 28.4 | 14.5 | 2.2 |
| The Sizzler, Thin, Med, Domino's Pizza* | 1 Slice/70g | 242 | 12.0 | 347 | 16.1 | 32.1 | 17.1 | 2.4 |
| Tuna Delight, Decadence, Med, Domino's Pizza* | 1 Slice/97g | 279 | 13.0 | 288 | 12.4 | 28.8 | 13.8 | 2.4 |
| Tuna Delight, Dominator, Lg, Domino's Pizza* | 1 Slice/108g | 286 | 9.0 | 265 | 12.8 | 33.8 | 8.7 | 2.1 |
| Tuna Delight, Regular, Lg, Domino's Pizza* | 1 Slice/80g | 186 | 6.0 | 233 | 13.1 | 29.6 | 6.9 | 2.2 |
| Tuna Delight, Regular, Med, Domino's Pizza* | 1 Slice/72g | 168 | 5.0 | 233 | 13.1 | 29.6 | 6.9 | 2.2 |
| Tuna Delight, Regular, Sm, Domino's Pizza* | 1 Slice/65g | 151 | 4.0 | 233 | 13.1 | 29.6 | 6.9 | 2.2 |
| Tuna Delight, Thin, Lg, Domino's Pizza* | 1 Slice/65g | 183 | 8.0 | 281 | 14.6 | 27.8 | 12.4 | 2.6 |
| Tuna Delight, Thin, Med, Domino's Pizza* | 1 Slice/60g | 177 | 8.0 | 295 | 14.7 | 30.5 | 12.7 | 2.6 |
| Veg-A-Roma, Delight, Regular, Sm, Domino's Pizza* | 1 Slice/70g | 153 | 5.0 | 219 | 10.4 | 29.3 | 6.7 | 2.4 |
| Veg-A-Roma, Regular, Lg, Domino's Pizza* | 1 Slice/86g | 240 | 9.0 | 279 | 12.3 | 34.3 | 10.4 | 2.4 |
| Veg-A-Roma, Regular, Med, Domino's Pizza* | 1 Slice/78g | 218 | 8.0 | 279 | 12.3 | 34.3 | 10.4 | 2.4 |
| Veg-A-Roma, Regular, Sm, Domino's Pizza* | 1 Slice/70g | 195 | 7.0 | 279 | 12.3 | 34.3 | 10.4 | 2.4 |
| Veg-A-Roma, Thin, Lg, Domino's Pizza* | 1 Slice/66g | 180 | 8.0 | 273 | 12.5 | 29.2 | 11.8 | 2.8 |
| Veg-A-Roma, Thin, Med, Domino's Pizza* | 1 Slice/61g | 167 | 7.0 | 273 | 12.5 | 29.2 | 11.8 | 2.8 |
| Vegetarian Supreme, Decadence, Med, Domino's Pizza* | 1 Slice/99g | 267 | 13.0 | 270 | 10.8 | 27.7 | 13.0 | 2.4 |
| Vegetarian Supreme, Delight, Regular, Sm, Domino's Pizza* | 1 Slice/72g | 154 | 4.0 | 214 | 13.1 | 29.5 | 4.9 | 2.5 |
| Vegetarian Supreme, Dominator, Lg, Domino's Pizza* | 1 Slice/111g | 274 | 9.0 | 247 | 11.2 | 32.6 | 8.0 | 2.2 |
| Vegetarian Supreme, Regular, Lg, Domino's Pizza* | 1 Slice/88g | 192 | 6.0 | 218 | 11.5 | 29.1 | 6.3 | 2.3 |
| Vegetarian Supreme, Regular, Med, Domino's Pizza* | 1 Slice/80g | 170 | 5.0 | 213 | 11.0 | 28.3 | 6.1 | 2.3 |
| Vegetarian Supreme, Regular, Sm, Domino's Pizza* | 1 Slice/72g | 156 | 4.0 | 217 | 11.5 | 28.9 | 6.2 | 2.3 |
| Vegetarian Supreme, Thin, Lg, Domino's Pizza* | 1 Slice/68g | 171 | 8.0 | 252 | 11.8 | 26.1 | 11.1 | 2.7 |
| Vegetarian Supreme, Thin, Med, Domino's Pizza* | 1 Slice/63g | 168 | 7.0 | 266 | 12.0 | 28.7 | 11.5 | 2.6 |
| Vegi Lite, Decadence, Med, Domino's Pizza* | 1 Slice/97g | 266 | 13.0 | 274 | 11.0 | 27.6 | 13.3 | 2.4 |
| Vegi Lite, Dominator, Lg, Domino's Pizza* | 1 Slice/108g | 270 | 9.0 | 250 | 11.4 | 32.6 | 8.2 | 2.2 |
| Vegi Lite, Regular, Lg, Domino's Pizza* | 1 Slice/85g | 183 | 5.0 | 215 | 11.4 | 28.2 | 6.3 | 2.3 |
| Vegi Lite, Regular, Med, Domino's Pizza* | 1 Slice/77g | 166 | 5.0 | 215 | 11.4 | 28.2 | 6.3 | 2.3 |
| Vegi Lite, Regular, Sm, Domino's Pizza* | 1 Slice/69g | 148 | 4.0 | 215 | 11.4 | 28.2 | 6.3 | 2.3 |
| Vegi Lite, Thin, Lg, Domino's Pizza* | 1 Slice/60g | 163 | 7.0 | 272 | 12.5 | 28.6 | 11.9 | 2.7 |
| Vegi Lite, Thin, Med, Domino's Pizza* | 1 Slice/65g | 166 | 7.0 | 256 | 12.3 | 25.8 | 11.5 | 2.8 |
| Vegi-Delight, Decadence, Med, Domino's Pizza* | 1 Slice/103g | 288 | 15.0 | 280 | 11.8 | 26.4 | 14.1 | 2.4 |
| Vegi-Delight, Dominator, Lg, Domino's Pizza* | 1 Slice/115g | 297 | 11.0 | 258 | 12.2 | 31.1 | 9.4 | 2.1 |
| Vegi-Delight, Regular, Lg, Domino's Pizza* | 1 Slice/92g | 209 | 7.0 | 227 | 12.3 | 26.6 | 7.9 | 2.2 |
| Vegi-Delight, Regular, Med, Domino's Pizza* | 1 Slice/84g | 191 | 7.0 | 227 | 12.3 | 26.6 | 7.9 | 2.2 |
| Vegi-Delight, Regular, Sm, Domino's Pizza* | 1 Slice/75g | 170 | 6.0 | 227 | 12.3 | 26.6 | 7.9 | 2.2 |
| Vegi-Delight, Thin, Lg, Domino's Pizza* | 1 Slice/72g | 193 | 9.0 | 268 | 13.4 | 24.1 | 13.1 | 2.6 |
| Vegi-Delight, Thin, Med, Domino's Pizza* | 1 Slice/67g | 189 | 9.0 | 282 | 13.6 | 26.6 | 13.4 | 2.5 |
| Vegi-Volcano, Decadence, Med, Domino's Pizza* | 1 Slice/102g | 282 | 14.0 | 276 | 11.7 | 26.3 | 13.7 | 2.3 |
| Vegi-Volcano, Delight, Regular, Sm, Domino's Pizza* | 1 Slice/75g | 167 | 5.0 | 223 | 14.2 | 27.7 | 6.2 | 2.4 |
| Vegi-Volcano, Dominator, Lg, Domino's Pizza* | 1 Slice/114g | 1215 | 10.0 | 1066 | 12.1 | 31.1 | 9.0 | 2.1 |
| Vegi-Volcano, Regular, Lg, Domino's Pizza* | 1 Slice/91g | 202 | 7.0 | 222 | 12.2 | 26.5 | 7.4 | 2.2 |
| Vegi-Volcano, Regular, Med, Domino's Pizza* | 1 Slice/83g | 184 | 6.0 | 222 | 12.2 | 26.5 | 7.4 | 2.2 |
| Vegi-Volcano, Regular, Sm, Domino's Pizza* | 1 Slice/75g | 166 | 6.0 | 222 | 12.2 | 26.5 | 7.4 | 2.2 |
| Vegi-Volcano, Thin, Lg, Domino's Pizza* | 1 Slice/72g | 189 | 9.0 | 262 | 13.3 | 23.9 | 12.5 | 2.6 |
| Vegi-Volcano, Thin, Med, Domino's Pizza* | 1 Slice/66g | 181 | 8.0 | 275 | 13.5 | 26.5 | 12.8 | 2.5 |

| | Measure INFO/WEIGHT | per Measure | | Nutrition Values per 100g / 100ml | | | | |
|---|---|---|---|---|---|---|---|---|
| | | KCAL | FAT | KCAL | PROT | CARB | FAT | FIBRE |
| **DOMINO'S PIZZA** | | | | | | | | |
| **POTATO** | | | | | | | | |
| Wedges, Domino's Pizza* | 1 Serving/190g | 298 | 12.0 | 157 | 2.5 | 21.9 | 6.5 | 2.2 |
| **POTATO SKINS** | | | | | | | | |
| Cheese & Bacon, Loaded, Domino's Pizza* | 1 Skin/56g | 99 | 5.0 | 176 | 5.3 | 19.0 | 8.8 | 3.9 |
| Cheese & Onion, Loaded, Domino's Pizza* | 1 Skin/56g | 96 | 4.0 | 172 | 3.8 | 23.8 | 6.8 | 4.1 |
| **SAUCE** | | | | | | | | |
| Hot, Domino's Pizza* | 1 Pot/28g | 7 | 0.0 | 25 | 0.8 | 1.8 | 1.1 | 1.1 |
| **WAFFLES** | | | | | | | | |
| Domino's Pizza* | 1 Serving/104g | 491 | 25.0 | 472 | 5.0 | 58.2 | 24.4 | 1.2 |
| **EAT** | | | | | | | | |
| **ANTIPASTO** | | | | | | | | |
| Italian, EAT* | 1 Serving/100g | 353 | 29.0 | 353 | 19.9 | 2.4 | 29.3 | 1.5 |
| **BAGUETTE** | | | | | | | | |
| Brie, Tomato & Basil, EAT* | 1 Baguette/231g | 554 | 24.0 | 240 | 9.8 | 27.0 | 10.3 | 1.7 |
| Cheddar, Simple, Kids, EAT* | 1 Baguette/95g | 311 | 15.0 | 327 | 13.4 | 32.3 | 16.0 | 1.8 |
| Cheddar,& Branston, Farmhouse, Mature, EAT* | 1 Baguette/240g | 704 | 34.0 | 293 | 10.8 | 30.7 | 14.1 | 1.8 |
| Chicken, Thai, EAT* | 1 Baguette/233g | 645 | 30.0 | 277 | 13.6 | 26.6 | 12.9 | 1.6 |
| Chorizo & Peppers, EAT* | 1 Baguette/220g | 607 | 28.0 | 276 | 10.8 | 29.6 | 12.7 | 2.0 |
| Ham, Brie, & Cranberry, EAT* | 1 Baguette/306g | 792 | 41.0 | 259 | 10.5 | 24.0 | 13.4 | 1.4 |
| Ham, Simple, Kids, EAT* | 1 Baguette/102g | 240 | 7.0 | 234 | 12.6 | 29.9 | 7.0 | 1.7 |
| Ham & Jarlsberg, EAT* | 1 Baguette/245g | 622 | 25.0 | 254 | 14.9 | 22.0 | 10.4 | 1.5 |
| Roast Beef & Rocket, EAT* | 1 Baguette/233g | 657 | 30.0 | 282 | 14.8 | 26.5 | 12.9 | 1.5 |
| Tuna & Cucumber, EAT* | 1 Baguette/260g | 637 | 31.0 | 245 | 10.0 | 24.0 | 12.1 | 1.5 |
| Tuna & Cucumber, Kids, EAT* | 1 Baguette/130g | 318 | 16.0 | 245 | 10.0 | 24.0 | 12.1 | 1.5 |
| **BARS** | | | | | | | | |
| Cereal, Zesty Citrus, EAT* | 1 Bar/25g | 84 | 1.0 | 336 | 5.6 | 66.4 | 5.2 | 3.6 |
| Oat, Fruit & Nut, EAT* | 1 Bar/65g | 396 | 22.0 | 609 | 8.6 | 66.9 | 34.2 | 5.2 |
| **BREAD** | | | | | | | | |
| Wholemeal, Chunk, EAT* | 1 Serving/67g | 138 | 2.0 | 206 | 9.0 | 37.2 | 2.4 | 7.9 |
| **BREAKFAST CEREAL** | | | | | | | | |
| Muesli, Mango & Banana, Bircher, EAT* | 1 Pot/254g | 345 | 7.0 | 136 | 4.5 | 23.2 | 2.9 | 2.2 |
| Muesli, Swiss Bircher, EAT* | 1 Pot/255g | 342 | 5.0 | 134 | 5.0 | 23.7 | 2.1 | 1.4 |
| Museli, Mango & Coconut, EAT* | 1 Pot/220g | 485 | 27.0 | 220 | 4.9 | 23.2 | 12.0 | 2.9 |
| Porridge, Plain, EAT* | 1 Serving/12oz | 227 | 4.0 | 81 | 4.5 | 12.6 | 1.4 | 1.0 |
| Porridge, with Apple, Cinnamon & Sultana Compote, EAT* | 1 Serving/12oz | 291 | 4.0 | 88 | 3.9 | 15.7 | 1.2 | 1.2 |
| Porridge, with Apple & Blackberry Compote, EAT* | 1 Serving/12oz | 291 | 4.0 | 88 | 4.0 | 15.4 | 1.2 | 1.3 |
| Porridge, with Banana, EAT* | 1 Serving/12oz | 257 | 4.0 | 83 | 4.2 | 13.6 | 1.3 | 1.1 |
| Porridge, with Banana & Maple Syrup, EAT* | 1 Serving/12oz | 296 | 4.0 | 91 | 4.0 | 15.9 | 1.2 | 1.1 |
| Porridge, with Maple Syrup, EAT* | 1 Serving/12oz | 266 | 4.0 | 90 | 4.3 | 15.2 | 1.3 | 0.9 |
| **BROWNIE** | | | | | | | | |
| Chocolate, EAT* | 1 Brownie/50g | 341 | 18.0 | 682 | 8.4 | 80.0 | 36.4 | 2.6 |
| EAT* | 1 Slice/70g | 345 | 18.0 | 493 | 5.9 | 61.3 | 25.4 | 2.9 |
| **CAKE** | | | | | | | | |
| Banana & Walnut, EAT* | 1 Av Pack/86g | 292 | 14.0 | 340 | 3.8 | 43.9 | 16.7 | 1.7 |
| Carrot, EAT* | 1 Av Slice/90g | 329 | 16.0 | 365 | 3.5 | 46.6 | 18.1 | 1.3 |
| Chocolate, EAT* | 1 Av Slice/86g | 334 | 18.0 | 388 | 5.4 | 44.6 | 20.9 | 1.5 |
| Lemon, EAT* | 1 Av Slice/84g | 326 | 15.0 | 388 | 4.5 | 51.0 | 18.3 | 0.9 |
| **CHEESECAKE** | | | | | | | | |
| Lemon, EAT* | 1 Serving/115g | 454 | 35.0 | 395 | 3.2 | 26.5 | 30.3 | 0.7 |
| **COFFEE** | | | | | | | | |
| Cappuccino, Skimmed Milk, EAT* | 1 Tall/12oz | 118 | 4.0 | 33 | 2.4 | 3.4 | 1.1 | 0.0 |
| Cappuccino, Soya Milk, EAT* | 1 Tall/12oz | 131 | 5.0 | 37 | 3.2 | 3.5 | 1.4 | 0.9 |
| Cappuccino, Whole Milk, EAT* | 1 Tall/12oz | 168 | 9.0 | 47 | 2.4 | 3.4 | 2.6 | 0.0 |

| | Measure INFO/WEIGHT | per Measure KCAL | per Measure FAT | Nutrition Values per 100g / 100ml KCAL | PROT | CARB | FAT | FIBRE |
|---|---|---|---|---|---|---|---|---|
| **EAT** | | | | | | | | |
| **COFFEE** | | | | | | | | |
| Espresso, Macchiato, Skimmed Milk, EAT* | 1 Espresso/4oz | 8 | 0.0 | 7 | 0.5 | 0.6 | 0.3 | 0.0 |
| Espresso, Macchiato, Soya Milk, EAT* | 1 Espresso/4oz | 9 | 0.0 | 8 | 0.6 | 0.7 | 0.3 | 0.2 |
| Espresso, Macchiato, Whole Milk, EAT* | 1 Espresso/4oz | 11 | 1.0 | 9 | 0.5 | 0.6 | 0.5 | 0.0 |
| Latte, Chai, Skimmed Milk, EAT* | 1 Tall/12oz | 305 | 1.0 | 86 | 3.2 | 17.7 | 0.3 | 0.0 |
| Latte, Chai, Soya Milk, EAT* | 1 Tall/12oz | 279 | 5.0 | 79 | 2.4 | 13.9 | 1.5 | 0.5 |
| Latte, Chai, Whole Milk, EAT* | 1 Tall/12oz | 408 | 13.0 | 115 | 3.1 | 17.5 | 3.6 | 0.0 |
| Latte, Chiller, Skimmed Milk, EAT* | 1 Tall/12oz | 241 | 3.0 | 68 | 3.1 | 11.9 | 0.9 | 0.0 |
| Latte, Chiller, Soya Milk, EAT* | 1 Tall/12oz | 251 | 4.0 | 71 | 3.7 | 12.0 | 1.1 | 0.7 |
| Latte, Chiller, Whole Milk, EAT* | 1 Tall/12oz | 412 | 15.0 | 116 | 1.8 | 17.7 | 4.2 | 0.2 |
| Latte, Iced, Skimmed Milk, EAT* | 1 Tall/12oz | 95 | 3.0 | 27 | 1.9 | 2.7 | 0.9 | 0.0 |
| Latte, Iced, Soya Milk, EAT* | 1 Tall/12oz | 105 | 4.0 | 30 | 2.5 | 2.8 | 1.1 | 0.7 |
| Latte, Iced, Whole Milk, EAT* | 1 Tall/12oz | 135 | 7.0 | 38 | 1.9 | 2.7 | 2.0 | 0.0 |
| Latte, Matcha, Skimmed Milk, EAT* | 1 Tall/12oz | 204 | 1.0 | 57 | 3.0 | 10.6 | 0.3 | 0.3 |
| Latte, Matcha, Soya Milk, EAT* | 1 Tall/12oz | 201 | 6.0 | 57 | 3.0 | 7.4 | 1.6 | 0.3 |
| Latte, Matcha, Whole Milk, EAT* | 1 Tall/12oz | 297 | 12.0 | 84 | 3.0 | 10.4 | 3.3 | 0.3 |
| Latte, Skimmed Milk, EAT* | 1 Tall/12oz | 142 | 5.0 | 40 | 2.9 | 4.1 | 1.4 | 0.0 |
| Latte, Soya Milk, EAT* | 1 Tall/12oz | 157 | 6.0 | 44 | 3.8 | 4.2 | 1.6 | 1.1 |
| Latte, Whole Milk, EAT* | 1 Tall/12oz | 202 | 11.0 | 57 | 2.9 | 4.1 | 3.1 | 0.0 |
| Mocha, Chiller, Skimmed Milk, EAT* | 1 Tall/12oz | 243 | 3.0 | 68 | 2.5 | 12.6 | 0.9 | 0.0 |
| Mocha, Chiller, Soya Milk, EAT* | 1 Tall/12oz | 253 | 4.0 | 71 | 3.1 | 12.7 | 1.1 | 0.7 |
| Mocha, Chiller, Whole Milk, EAT* | 1 Tall/12oz | 283 | 7.0 | 80 | 2.5 | 12.6 | 2.1 | 0.0 |
| Mocha, Skimmed Milk, EAT* | 1 Tall/12oz | 157 | 5.0 | 44 | 3.0 | 4.8 | 1.4 | 0.0 |
| Mocha, Soya Milk, EAT* | 1 Tall/12oz | 173 | 6.0 | 49 | 4.0 | 5.0 | 1.7 | 1.2 |
| Mocha, Whole Milk, EAT* | 1 Tall/12oz | 219 | 11.0 | 62 | 3.0 | 4.8 | 3.2 | 0.0 |
| **COOKIES** | | | | | | | | |
| Chocolate, EAT* | 1 Pack/150g | 455 | 23.0 | 303 | 3.6 | 37.9 | 15.3 | 0.4 |
| Muesli, EAT* | 1 Av Pack/100g | 376 | 13.0 | 376 | 4.5 | 60.8 | 12.8 | 1.8 |
| **CROISSANT** | | | | | | | | |
| Almond, EAT* | 1 Croissant/200g | 467 | 26.0 | 233 | 4.8 | 23.8 | 13.2 | 1.5 |
| Chocolate, EAT* | 1 Croissant/100g | 407 | 23.0 | 407 | 6.7 | 45.9 | 23.1 | 3.0 |
| Ham & Jarlsberg, EAT* | 1 Pack/115g | 304 | 19.0 | 265 | 16.3 | 18.4 | 16.8 | 0.0 |
| Plain, EAT* | 1 Croissant/100g | 274 | 14.0 | 274 | 5.5 | 32.6 | 14.2 | 1.6 |
| **CUPCAKES** | | | | | | | | |
| Vanilla, EAT* | 1 Av Pack/75g | 352 | 18.0 | 469 | 3.2 | 58.7 | 24.5 | 0.4 |
| **DESSERT** | | | | | | | | |
| Chunky Chocolate Fudge, EAT* | 1 Serving/116g | 447 | 26.0 | 385 | 3.3 | 43.7 | 22.0 | 1.5 |
| Dark Chocolate, Pot, EAT* | 1 Pot/50g | 211 | 17.0 | 422 | 2.2 | 27.0 | 35.0 | 2.0 |
| **DRIED FRUIT & SEED MIX** | | | | | | | | |
| EAT* | 1 Pack/50g | 224 | 9.0 | 448 | 10.0 | 61.3 | 17.8 | 0.0 |
| **FRUIT** | | | | | | | | |
| Salad, Seasonal, Winter, EAT* | 1 Av Pack/137g | 74 | 0.0 | 54 | 0.9 | 12.0 | 0.3 | 2.4 |
| **FRUIT & NUT MIX** | | | | | | | | |
| EAT* | 1 Pack/70g | 253 | 17.0 | 361 | 7.1 | 27.7 | 24.9 | 0.0 |
| **FRUIT SALAD** | | | | | | | | |
| Seasonal, EAT* | 1 Pack/100g | 59 | 0.0 | 59 | 0.7 | 13.8 | 0.1 | 3.5 |
| Tropical, EAT* | 1 Pack/150g | 64 | 0.0 | 43 | 0.5 | 10.5 | 0.2 | 1.6 |
| **FUDGE** | | | | | | | | |
| Vanilla, EAT* | 1 Pack/100g | 405 | 12.0 | 405 | 1.2 | 73.0 | 12.0 | 0.0 |
| **HOT CHOCOLATE** | | | | | | | | |
| Chiller, EAT* | 1 Tall/335ml | 533 | 22.0 | 159 | 2.3 | 24.6 | 6.7 | 0.6 |
| Chiller, Whole Milk, EAT* | 1 Tall/12oz | 19 | 1.0 | 158 | 2.3 | 23.2 | 6.3 | 0.5 |
| Skimmed Milk, EAT* | 1 Tall/12oz | 171 | 5.0 | 48 | 3.3 | 5.2 | 1.5 | 0.0 |

| | Measure INFO/WEIGHT | per Measure KCAL | FAT | Nutrition Values per 100g / 100ml KCAL | PROT | CARB | FAT | FIBRE |
|---|---|---|---|---|---|---|---|---|

## EAT

### HOT CHOCOLATE
| | | | | | | | | |
|---|---|---|---|---|---|---|---|---|
| Soya Milk, EAT* | 1 Tall/12oz | 188 | 7.0 | 53 | 4.3 | 5.4 | 1.9 | 1.3 |
| Whole Milk, EAT* | 1 Tall/12oz | 239 | 12.0 | 67 | 3.3 | 5.2 | 3.5 | 0.0 |

### ICE CREAM
| | | | | | | | | |
|---|---|---|---|---|---|---|---|---|
| Belgian Chocolate, Haagen Das, EAT* | 1 Serving/100g | 227 | 18.0 | 227 | 3.9 | 23.8 | 18.4 | 1.7 |
| Cookies & Cream, Haagen Das, EAT* | 1 Serving/100g | 225 | 14.0 | 225 | 3.7 | 20.0 | 14.4 | 0.7 |
| Strawberry, Haagen Das, EAT* | 1 Serving/100g | 221 | 14.0 | 221 | 3.5 | 20.0 | 14.1 | 0.3 |
| Vanilla, Haagen Das, EAT* | 1 Serving/100g | 225 | 15.0 | 225 | 3.8 | 18.1 | 15.2 | 0.0 |

### JELLY
| | | | | | | | | |
|---|---|---|---|---|---|---|---|---|
| Summer Berry & Elderflower, EAT* | 1 Pack/240g | 281 | 0.0 | 117 | 2.6 | 26.4 | 0.1 | 0.0 |

### JUICE DRINK
| | | | | | | | | |
|---|---|---|---|---|---|---|---|---|
| Mango & Lime, Blast, EAT* | 1 Tall/12oz | 253 | 0.0 | 71 | 0.3 | 17.7 | 0.1 | 0.1 |
| Peach & Mint, Blast, EAT* | 1 Tall/12oz | 216 | 0.0 | 61 | 0.2 | 15.1 | 0.1 | 0.0 |
| Wild Berry, Blast, EAT* | 1 Tall/12oz | 350 | 0.0 | 99 | 0.2 | 23.5 | 0.1 | 0.5 |

### MILK
| | | | | | | | | |
|---|---|---|---|---|---|---|---|---|
| Skimmed, Steamed, EAT* | 1 Tall/12oz | 169 | 6.0 | 48 | 3.5 | 4.9 | 1.6 | 0.0 |
| Soya, Steamed, EAT* | 1 Tall/12oz | 187 | 7.0 | 53 | 4.5 | 5.0 | 1.9 | 1.3 |
| Whole, Steamed, EAT* | 1 Tall/12oz | 241 | 13.0 | 68 | 3.4 | 4.9 | 3.7 | 0.0 |

### MUFFIN
| | | | | | | | | |
|---|---|---|---|---|---|---|---|---|
| Bacon Butty, EAT* | 1 Serving/90g | 279 | 11.0 | 310 | 15.8 | 34.5 | 11.9 | 2.3 |
| Bacon Butty, Large, EAT* | 1 Muffin/190g | 432 | 11.0 | 228 | 10.4 | 33.0 | 6.0 | 2.0 |
| Blueberry, Low Fat, EAT* | 1 Muffin/100g | 280 | 3.0 | 280 | 5.7 | 58.1 | 2.7 | 2.3 |
| Breakfast, Full English, EAT* | 1 Av Pack/293g | 714 | 29.0 | 244 | 10.5 | 26.1 | 10.0 | 2.4 |
| Breakfast, Full Scottish, EAT* | 1 Av Pack/297g | 711 | 28.0 | 239 | 10.5 | 27.3 | 9.3 | 2.3 |
| Cumberland Sausage, EAT* | 1 Sandwich/110g | 323 | 15.0 | 293 | 10.9 | 27.3 | 13.2 | 2.0 |
| Egg, Mushroom & Cheddar, EAT* | 1 Pack/135g | 289 | 11.0 | 214 | 8.9 | 26.8 | 7.8 | 2.0 |
| Eggs Benedict, EAT* | 1 Muffin/120g | 290 | 12.0 | 241 | 10.2 | 26.5 | 10.3 | 1.6 |

### NOUGAT
| | | | | | | | | |
|---|---|---|---|---|---|---|---|---|
| EAT* | 1 Pack/30g | 132 | 3.0 | 440 | 3.7 | 86.3 | 9.0 | 0.7 |

### NUT
| | | | | | | | | |
|---|---|---|---|---|---|---|---|---|
| & Fruit, Honey Toasted, EAT* | 1 Av Pack/50g | 226 | 13.0 | 453 | 11.5 | 44.5 | 25.5 | 5.6 |

### NUTS
| | | | | | | | | |
|---|---|---|---|---|---|---|---|---|
| Honey & Chilli, EAT* | 1 Av Pack/85g | 422 | 27.0 | 496 | 15.9 | 44.4 | 31.7 | 5.6 |

### PAIN AU CHOCOLAT
| | | | | | | | | |
|---|---|---|---|---|---|---|---|---|
| EAT* | 1 Pain/120g | 460 | 19.0 | 383 | 6.6 | 28.6 | 15.8 | 2.4 |

### PEAS
| | | | | | | | | |
|---|---|---|---|---|---|---|---|---|
| Wasabi, EAT* | 1 Pack/92g | 136 | 5.0 | 148 | 1.3 | 22.4 | 5.9 | 7.9 |

### PIE
| | | | | | | | | |
|---|---|---|---|---|---|---|---|---|
| Banoffee, EAT* | 1 Av Pie/114g | 409 | 26.0 | 359 | 3.7 | 34.4 | 23.0 | 1.6 |
| Beef & Stilton, EAT* | 1 Av Pie/270g | 670 | 37.0 | 248 | 11.2 | 20.1 | 13.8 | 0.0 |
| Cheddar Cheese, Potato & Onion, EAT* | 1 Av Pie/270g | 672 | 35.0 | 249 | 6.2 | 26.9 | 12.9 | 0.0 |
| Chicken, Ham & Leek, EAT* | 1 Av Pie/290g | 751 | 47.0 | 259 | 11.9 | 16.4 | 16.1 | 1.3 |
| Chicken & Mushroom, EAT* | 1 Av Pie/280g | 667 | 37.0 | 238 | 9.9 | 19.3 | 13.2 | 1.1 |
| Goats Cheese & Sweet Potato, EAT* | 1 Av Pie/265g | 596 | 28.0 | 225 | 5.1 | 29.9 | 10.7 | 2.9 |
| Steak & Ale, EAT* | 1 Av Pie/270g | 613 | 30.0 | 227 | 8.0 | 27.0 | 11.0 | 0.0 |

### SALAD
| | | | | | | | | |
|---|---|---|---|---|---|---|---|---|
| Baby Plum Tomato & Mozzarella, Side, EAT* | 1 Pack/250g | 221 | 19.0 | 88 | 3.8 | 1.3 | 7.6 | 0.4 |
| Chef's, EAT* | 1 Serving/200g | 414 | 37.0 | 207 | 8.5 | 1.8 | 18.4 | 0.9 |
| Chicken, & Oriental Vegetable, EAT* | 1 Portion/150g | 222 | 10.0 | 148 | 11.7 | 10.1 | 6.6 | 2.2 |
| Chicken, Morrocan & Cous Cous, EAT* | 1 Pack/100g | 688 | 30.0 | 688 | 26.9 | 75.4 | 30.5 | 5.7 |
| Chicken Noodles, Spicy, EAT* | 1 Av Pack/285g | 393 | 10.0 | 138 | 9.5 | 17.3 | 3.4 | 0.9 |
| Courgette, Feta & Lemon, Side, EAT* | 1 Pack/200g | 266 | 13.0 | 133 | 4.9 | 13.8 | 6.4 | 1.3 |
| Crayfish Noodles, Spicy, EAT* | 1 Av Pack/288g | 371 | 10.0 | 129 | 5.9 | 18.6 | 3.4 | 0.7 |

| | Measure INFO/WEIGHT | per Measure KCAL | FAT | Nutrition Values per 100g / 100ml KCAL | PROT | CARB | FAT | FIBRE |
|---|---|---|---|---|---|---|---|---|
| **EAT** | | | | | | | | |
| **SALAD** | | | | | | | | |
| Duck & Mango, EAT* | 1 Pack/300g | 369 | 19.0 | 123 | 5.4 | 11.3 | 6.3 | 1.6 |
| Duck & Mango, without Dressing, EAT* | 1 Pack/299g | 323 | 19.0 | 108 | 6.0 | 6.9 | 6.3 | 1.8 |
| Feta, Lentil & Rice, Side, EAT* | 1 Pack | 525 | 21.0 | 525 | 21.1 | 64.0 | 20.5 | 8.1 |
| Goats Cheese & Pine Nuts, Superfood, EAT* | 1 Pack/250g | 347 | 27.0 | 139 | 5.5 | 5.0 | 10.7 | 2.1 |
| Horiatiki Greek, Side, EAT* | 1 Pack/250g | 298 | 28.0 | 119 | 3.3 | 1.3 | 11.2 | 0.4 |
| Mackerel, Smoked, Super, EAT* | 1 Pack/175g | 683 | 53.0 | 390 | 15.1 | 13.7 | 30.6 | 2.5 |
| Mediterranean Chicken, with Dressing, EAT* | 1 Pack/255g | 354 | 23.0 | 139 | 10.2 | 4.2 | 9.1 | 1.1 |
| Mezze, Side, EAT* | 1 Serving/300g | 420 | 27.0 | 140 | 3.0 | 11.8 | 9.0 | 1.7 |
| Moroccan Chicken Couscous, EAT* | 1 Pack/100g | 688 | 30.0 | 688 | 26.0 | 75.0 | 30.0 | 6.0 |
| Nicoise, EAT* | 1 Pack/200g | 260 | 16.0 | 130 | 8.0 | 6.5 | 8.0 | 0.7 |
| Noodle, Thai, EAT* | 1 Av Pack/287g | 533 | 26.0 | 186 | 4.7 | 21.3 | 9.2 | 2.1 |
| Potato, Spring, EAT* | 1 Pack/250g | 220 | 11.0 | 88 | 1.2 | 10.7 | 4.5 | 1.0 |
| Prawn Cocktail, Side, EAT* | 1 Av Pack/192g | 324 | 31.0 | 169 | 4.4 | 1.9 | 15.9 | 1.1 |
| Rainbow Sprouted, Side Salad, with Dressing, EAT* | 1 Av Pack/186g | 323 | 28.0 | 174 | 7.5 | 17.9 | 15.3 | 5.1 |
| Rainbow Sprouted, Side Salad, without Dressing, EAT* | 1 Av Pack/161g | 217 | 6.0 | 135 | 8.6 | 17.2 | 3.8 | 3.1 |
| Satsuma, Carrot & Watercress, Side, EAT* | 1 Pack/100g | 147 | 10.0 | 147 | 3.2 | 10.3 | 10.3 | 2.9 |
| Smoked Mackerel, Superfood, EAT* | 1 Pack/300g | 683 | 53.0 | 228 | 8.8 | 8.0 | 17.8 | 1.5 |
| Smoked Salmon, Potato & Horseradish, Side, EAT* | 1 Pack/400g | 400 | 29.0 | 100 | 3.6 | 4.9 | 7.3 | 0.6 |
| Superfood, with Dressing, EAT* | 1 Av Pack/325g | 491 | 28.0 | 151 | 7.6 | 10.9 | 8.7 | 3.9 |
| Superfood, without Dressing, EAT* | 1 Av Pack/300g | 396 | 21.0 | 132 | 8.2 | 9.7 | 6.9 | 4.3 |
| Supergreens, Side Salad, with Dressing, EAT* | 1 Av Pack/174g | 148 | 4.0 | 85 | 5.4 | 11.3 | 2.3 | 1.6 |
| Tuna, & Bean, Side, EAT* | 1 Pack/200g | 212 | 9.0 | 106 | 7.4 | 8.3 | 4.7 | 3.3 |
| Tuna, Olive & Bean, Side Salad, with Dressing, EAT* | 1 Av Pack/200g | 236 | 10.0 | 118 | 7.8 | 10.7 | 4.9 | 4.0 |
| Tuna Nicoise, with Dressing, EAT* | 1 Av Pack/303g | 400 | 85.0 | 132 | 7.8 | 4.5 | 27.9 | 3.1 |
| Tuna Nicoise, without Dressing, EAT* | 1 Av Pack/264g | 214 | 9.0 | 81 | 8.7 | 4.0 | 3.3 | 1.0 |
| Tuna Olive & Bean, Side Salad, without Dressing, EAT* | 1 Pack/175g | 170 | 3.0 | 97 | 8.8 | 11.4 | 1.8 | 4.4 |
| **SANDWICH** | | | | | | | | |
| Avocado, Houmous, & Red Pepper, EAT* | 1 Pack/250g | 485 | 25.0 | 194 | 5.8 | 20.6 | 9.9 | 3.2 |
| Bacon Butty, EAT* | 1 Butty/120g | 220 | 8.0 | 183 | 11.8 | 19.4 | 6.5 | 1.0 |
| Beef, & Horseradish, Rare Roast, EAT* | 1 Pack/245g | 475 | 18.0 | 194 | 13.8 | 17.9 | 7.4 | 1.4 |
| BLT, EAT* | 1 Pack/197g | 510 | 30.0 | 259 | 10.7 | 19.9 | 15.3 | 1.8 |
| Bombay Bhaji, EAT* | 1 Pack/237g | 543 | 8.0 | 229 | 5.2 | 25.6 | 3.5 | 1.0 |
| Carrot, & Houmous, EAT* | 1 Pack/250g | 436 | 17.0 | 174 | 6.2 | 21.8 | 7.0 | 2.0 |
| Cheddar, & Branston Pickle, EAT* | 1 Pack/235g | 562 | 28.0 | 239 | 10.9 | 22.5 | 11.7 | 1.8 |
| Cheese, Spring Onion, & Salad, EAT* | 1 Pack/217g | 523 | 29.0 | 241 | 10.7 | 19.2 | 13.5 | 1.5 |
| Chicken, & Bacon, EAT* | 1 Pack/238g | 518 | 26.0 | 218 | 13.9 | 16.3 | 10.9 | 1.5 |
| Chicken, & Mediterranean Vegetables, EAT* | 1 Pack/350g | 434 | 15.0 | 124 | 7.6 | 13.9 | 4.2 | 1.5 |
| Chicken, & Salad, EAT* | 1 Pack/250g | 436 | 17.0 | 174 | 9.3 | 19.3 | 6.6 | 2.1 |
| Chicken, & Salad, Less Than 5% Fat, EAT* | 1 Pack/242g | 337 | 7.0 | 139 | 11.9 | 16.3 | 2.9 | 1.6 |
| Chicken, Aioli, EAT* | 1 Pack/250g | 424 | 17.0 | 170 | 12.8 | 14.0 | 6.9 | 2.6 |
| Chicken, Avocado, Basil, EAT* | 1 Pack/232g | 601 | 38.0 | 259 | 11.5 | 16.4 | 16.4 | 2.4 |
| Chicken, Basil Pesto, & Pine Nuts, EAT* | 1 Pack/228g | 577 | 27.0 | 253 | 11.0 | 25.5 | 11.7 | 4.2 |
| Chicken, Caesar, EAT* | 1 Pack/250g | 605 | 33.0 | 242 | 16.0 | 15.1 | 13.1 | 1.3 |
| Chicken, Lemon, & Black Pepper, EAT* | 1 Pack/237g | 521 | 19.0 | 220 | 12.0 | 24.7 | 8.2 | 3.9 |
| Chicken, Thai Citrus, EAT* | 1 Pack/213g | 420 | 14.0 | 197 | 12.9 | 21.1 | 6.8 | 1.6 |
| Chicken Salad, EAT* | 1 Pack/222g | 340 | 10.0 | 153 | 11.2 | 17.4 | 4.3 | 1.5 |
| Club, EAT* | 1 Pack/267g | 721 | 43.0 | 270 | 15.1 | 16.0 | 16.1 | 1.2 |
| Club, New York, EAT* | 1 Pack/257g | 491 | 22.0 | 191 | 12.7 | 15.5 | 8.7 | 1.7 |
| Corainder, & Lemon Houmous, EAT* | 1 Pack/244g | 486 | 23.0 | 199 | 5.6 | 26.2 | 9.6 | 5.8 |
| Crayfish, Rocket, & Lemon, EAT* | 1 Pack/198g | 341 | 14.0 | 172 | 7.3 | 19.5 | 7.1 | 1.4 |
| Egg, Spinach & Chargrilled Peppers, EAT* | 1 Pack/243g | 558 | 33.0 | 229 | 9.0 | 17.0 | 13.6 | 1.8 |
| Egg Mayonnaise, Free Range, Chunky, EAT* | 1 Pack/203g | 463 | 26.0 | 228 | 8.8 | 19.4 | 12.8 | 1.6 |

| | Measure INFO/WEIGHT | per Measure KCAL FAT | Nutrition Values per 100g / 100ml KCAL PROT CARB FAT FIBRE |
|---|---|---|---|

# EAT

## SANDWICH

| | Measure INFO/WEIGHT | per Measure KCAL | FAT | KCAL | PROT | CARB | FAT | FIBRE |
|---|---|---|---|---|---|---|---|---|
| Ham, & Brie, with Honey Mustard, EAT* | 1 Pack/250g | 618 | 32.0 | 247 | 12.7 | 20.1 | 12.9 | 1.4 |
| Ham, & Mustard Salad, EAT* | 1 Pack/85g | 363 | 10.0 | 427 | 26.8 | 54.9 | 11.2 | 6.1 |
| Ham, Cheddar, & Real Ale Pickle, EAT* | 1 Pack/267g | 587 | 30.0 | 220 | 11.0 | 18.4 | 11.4 | 1.4 |
| Ham, Smoked, & Mature Cheddar, EAT* | 1 Pack/246g | 607 | 30.0 | 247 | 11.2 | 23.6 | 12.0 | 3.7 |
| Ham & Mustard, EAT* | 1 Pack/178g | 381 | 15.0 | 214 | 12.0 | 22.4 | 8.7 | 1.5 |
| Houmous, & Red Pepper, EAT* | 1 Pack/250g | 402 | 12.0 | 161 | 6.0 | 23.8 | 4.7 | 2.5 |
| Houmous, & Roast Vegetables, EAT* | 1 Pack/176g | 243 | 6.0 | 138 | 4.9 | 22.2 | 3.2 | 6.0 |
| New York, EAT* | 1 Pack/249g | 565 | 27.0 | 227 | 9.1 | 23.5 | 10.7 | 3.9 |
| Prawn Cocktail, EAT* | 1 Pack/231g | 550 | 26.0 | 238 | 9.6 | 24.8 | 11.1 | 4.0 |
| Salmon, Smoked, EAT* | 1 Pack/250g | 431 | 17.0 | 172 | 11.3 | 16.9 | 6.6 | 1.3 |
| Steak, Onion, & Cheese, EAT* | 1 Pack/300g | 789 | 32.0 | 263 | 15.5 | 26.5 | 10.6 | 1.8 |
| Superfood, EAT* | 1 Pack/221g | 502 | 24.0 | 227 | 10.1 | 22.6 | 10.7 | 2.3 |
| Toastie, Chicken, & Basil, Smoked, EAT* | 1 Pack/255g | 777 | 43.0 | 305 | 13.9 | 24.1 | 16.9 | 1.6 |
| Toastie, Ham & Cheese, Simply, EAT* | 1 Pack/250g | 760 | 42.0 | 304 | 13.9 | 24.2 | 16.8 | 1.5 |
| Toastie, Steak & Cheese Melt, EAT* | 1 Pack/290g | 853 | 48.0 | 294 | 13.0 | 23.7 | 16.4 | 1.7 |
| Tuna, & Red Onion, EAT* | 1 Pack/195g | 322 | 9.0 | 165 | 11.9 | 19.7 | 4.4 | 1.5 |
| Tuna, Crunch, EAT* | 1 Pack/200g | 377 | 11.0 | 188 | 12.2 | 23.1 | 5.3 | 2.3 |
| Tuna, Ginger, & Wasabi, EAT* | 1 Pack/224g | 519 | 29.0 | 232 | 10.3 | 19.0 | 12.8 | 2.1 |
| Tuna, Mediterranean, EAT* | 1 Pack/234g | 473 | 17.0 | 202 | 8.7 | 26.3 | 7.1 | 4.7 |
| Tuna, Tuscan, EAT* | 1 Pack/250g | 515 | 29.0 | 206 | 8.8 | 16.2 | 11.5 | 2.0 |
| Turkey, & Cranberry, EAT* | 1 Pack/218g | 388 | 10.0 | 178 | 9.9 | 24.8 | 4.4 | 1.3 |

## SEED MIXTURE

| | | | | | | | | |
|---|---|---|---|---|---|---|---|---|
| Goji, Seed & Berry, EAT* | 1 Av Pack/80g | 364 | 19.0 | 455 | 13.0 | 45.0 | 24.0 | 5.0 |

## SLICE

| | | | | | | | | |
|---|---|---|---|---|---|---|---|---|
| Coconut, EAT* | 1 Av Pack/150g | 688 | 42.0 | 459 | 6.1 | 45.2 | 28.1 | 4.4 |

## SOUP

| | | | | | | | | |
|---|---|---|---|---|---|---|---|---|
| Asparagus, Cream & Thyme, EAT* | 1 Small/350ml | 90 | 2.0 | 26 | 1.2 | 3.9 | 0.7 | 0.6 |
| Bean, Mexican, Big, EAT* | 1 Big/400g | 196 | 7.0 | 49 | 2.7 | 5.6 | 1.8 | 1.9 |
| Bean, Mexican, Small, EAT* | 1 Small/300g | 159 | 7.0 | 53 | 2.9 | 5.6 | 2.2 | 1.9 |
| Bean, Mexican, Very Big, EAT* | 1 Very Big/800g | 368 | 12.0 | 46 | 2.6 | 5.5 | 1.5 | 1.9 |
| Beef, Chilli & Ginger Pho, EAT* | 1 Small/300g | 105 | 3.0 | 35 | 2.9 | 3.3 | 1.1 | 0.4 |
| Beetroot Borscht, EAT* | 1 Small/340ml | 98 | 5.0 | 29 | 0.7 | 3.3 | 1.5 | 0.4 |
| Broccoli & Stilton, EAT* | 1 Small/300g | 207 | 12.0 | 69 | 2.5 | 5.6 | 4.1 | 1.2 |
| Carrot, Honey & Ginger, EAT* | 1 Small/350ml | 132 | 6.0 | 38 | 0.7 | 5.0 | 1.8 | 1.0 |
| Carrot & Coriander, EAT* | 1 Small/300g | 111 | 7.0 | 37 | 0.6 | 3.1 | 2.5 | 1.4 |
| Celeriac & Leek, EAT* | 1 Small/350ml | 176 | 15.0 | 50 | 0.9 | 2.3 | 4.1 | 1.5 |
| Chicken, Creamy, EAT* | 1 Small/300g | 213 | 12.0 | 71 | 5.1 | 3.7 | 3.9 | 0.6 |
| Chicken, Thai Green Curry, Big, EAT* | 1 Big/443g | 341 | 20.0 | 77 | 3.3 | 5.6 | 4.6 | 1.1 |
| Chicken, Thai Green Curry, Small, EAT* | 1 Small/340g | 269 | 15.0 | 79 | 3.3 | 6.3 | 4.5 | 1.0 |
| Chicken, Thai Green Curry, Very Big, EAT* | 1 Very Big/862g | 646 | 41.0 | 75 | 3.3 | 5.0 | 4.7 | 1.1 |
| Chicken, Tom Kha Gai, EAT* | 1 Small/12oz | 295 | 20.0 | 87 | 5.0 | 3.3 | 6.0 | 0.9 |
| Chicken & Egg Noodles, Old Fashioned, Big, EAT* | 1 Big/400g | 124 | 2.0 | 31 | 4.8 | 2.1 | 0.4 | 0.6 |
| Chicken & Egg Noodles, Old Fashioned, Small, EAT* | 1 Small/300g | 93 | 1.0 | 31 | 4.8 | 2.1 | 0.4 | 0.6 |
| Chicken & Garden Vegetable, Broth, EAT* | 1 Small/300g | 150 | 2.0 | 50 | 6.1 | 5.0 | 0.7 | 1.3 |
| Chicken Laksa, EAT* | 1 Small/300g | 276 | 15.0 | 92 | 5.8 | 6.1 | 5.0 | 0.8 |
| Chicken Pho, Eat* | 1 Small/300g | 105 | 2.0 | 35 | 3.8 | 3.1 | 0.8 | 0.4 |
| Chicken Pot Pie, Big, EAT* | 1 Big/400g | 352 | 16.0 | 88 | 5.8 | 7.4 | 4.0 | 1.2 |
| Chicken Pot Pie, Small, EAT* | 1 Small/300g | 282 | 13.0 | 94 | 5.8 | 7.8 | 4.4 | 1.2 |
| Chicken Pot Pie, Very Big, EAT* | 1 Very Big/800g | 640 | 26.0 | 80 | 5.8 | 6.8 | 3.3 | 1.2 |
| Chilli Con Carne, Texan, Big, EAT* | 1 Big/400g | 376 | 18.0 | 94 | 6.6 | 7.5 | 4.4 | 2.0 |
| Chilli Con Carne, Texan, Small, EAT* | 1 Small/300g | 297 | 15.0 | 99 | 6.6 | 6.9 | 4.9 | 2.0 |
| Chilli Con Carne, Texan, Very Big, EAT* | 1 Very Big/800g | 720 | 32.0 | 90 | 6.5 | 6.9 | 4.0 | 2.0 |

| | Measure INFO/WEIGHT | per Measure KCAL | per Measure FAT | Nutrition Values per 100g / 100ml KCAL | PROT | CARB | FAT | FIBRE |
|---|---|---|---|---|---|---|---|---|

# EAT
## SOUP

| | Measure INFO/WEIGHT | KCAL | FAT | KCAL | PROT | CARB | FAT | FIBRE |
|---|---|---|---|---|---|---|---|---|
| Chowder, Clam, New England, EAT* | 1 Small/300g | 321 | 19.0 | 107 | 4.6 | 7.8 | 6.4 | 1.0 |
| Chowder, Corn, EAT* | 1 Serving/340g | 383 | 26.0 | 113 | 3.4 | 7.6 | 7.6 | 0.7 |
| Courgette & Coriander, EAT* | 1 Big/454g | 164 | 5.0 | 36 | 1.6 | 4.6 | 1.1 | 0.9 |
| Cream of Corn, EAT* | 1 Small/300g | 288 | 23.0 | 96 | 1.5 | 5.6 | 7.6 | 1.1 |
| Dal, Red, Gugarati, with Raita, Very Big, EAT* | 1 Very Big/800g | 272 | 9.0 | 34 | 1.9 | 4.2 | 1.1 | 0.7 |
| Dal, Red, Gujarati, with Raita, Big, EAT* | 1 Big/400g | 144 | 5.0 | 36 | 2.0 | 4.4 | 1.2 | 0.7 |
| Dal, Red, Gujarati, with Raita, Small, EAT* | 1 Small/300g | 111 | 4.0 | 37 | 2.0 | 4.4 | 1.3 | 0.7 |
| Fish Bouillabaisse with Rouille, Small, EAT* | 1 Small/350g | 243 | 9.0 | 69 | 5.8 | 3.2 | 2.6 | 1.5 |
| French Onion, Big, EAT* | 1 Big/400g | 204 | 7.0 | 51 | 1.6 | 6.8 | 1.7 | 0.6 |
| French Onion, Small, EAT* | 1 Small/300g | 174 | 7.0 | 58 | 1.9 | 7.2 | 2.2 | 0.6 |
| French Onion, Very Big, EAT* | 1 Very Big/800g | 328 | 10.0 | 41 | 1.3 | 6.0 | 1.2 | 0.6 |
| Garden Vegetable, EAT* | 1 Small/300ml | 153 | 9.0 | 51 | 0.8 | 5.4 | 2.9 | 1.2 |
| Gazpacho, EAT* | 1 Small/350ml | 78 | 2.0 | 22 | 0.6 | 3.6 | 0.6 | 0.9 |
| Goulash, Hungarian, EAT* | 1 Small/300g | 210 | 6.0 | 70 | 7.1 | 6.0 | 1.9 | 1.0 |
| Italian Ragu & Pasta, Big, Eat* | 1 Big/400g | 228 | 5.0 | 57 | 2.0 | 9.3 | 1.3 | 0.9 |
| Italian Ragu & Pasta, Small, EAT* | 1 Small/300g | 180 | 4.0 | 60 | 2.2 | 9.3 | 1.5 | 0.9 |
| Italian Ragu & Pasta, Very Big, EAT* | 1 Very Big/800g | 392 | 6.0 | 49 | 1.2 | 9.4 | 0.7 | 0.9 |
| Leek, Potato & Chive, EAT* | 1 Small/300g | 159 | 9.0 | 53 | 1.2 | 5.7 | 2.9 | 1.0 |
| Leek & Potato, EAT* | 1 Small/350ml | 154 | 9.0 | 44 | 0.8 | 4.4 | 2.6 | 0.6 |
| Mexican Chicken Tortilla, Big, EAT* | 1 Big/400g | 252 | 8.0 | 63 | 6.0 | 5.0 | 2.1 | 1.1 |
| Mexican Chicken Tortilla, Small, EAT* | 1 Small/300g | 210 | 8.0 | 70 | 6.3 | 5.5 | 2.6 | 1.1 |
| Minestrone, with Pesto, Chunky, Small, EAT* | 1 Small/300g | 159 | 8.0 | 53 | 1.9 | 4.6 | 2.8 | 1.5 |
| Minestrone, with Pesto, Chunky, Very Big, EAT* | 1 Very Big/800g | 344 | 14.0 | 43 | 1.7 | 4.6 | 1.8 | 1.5 |
| Minestrone with Pesto, Chunky, Big, EAT* | 1 Big/400g | 188 | 9.0 | 47 | 1.8 | 4.7 | 2.3 | 1.5 |
| Moroccan Chicken & Root Vegetable, EAT* | 1 Small/12oz | 220 | 8.0 | 65 | 3.9 | 7.0 | 2.3 | 2.2 |
| Mushroom, Wild, Forest, EAT* | 1 Small/300g | 144 | 9.0 | 48 | 2.0 | 3.6 | 2.9 | 0.9 |
| Parsnip, Spiced, EAT* | 1 Small/300g | 141 | 8.0 | 47 | 1.0 | 5.2 | 2.6 | 1.9 |
| Pea & Mint, EAT* | 1 Big/480ml | 236 | 7.0 | 49 | 1.9 | 7.3 | 1.5 | 1.5 |
| Prawn, Tom Yum, EAT* | 1 Small/300g | 93 | 3.0 | 31 | 1.5 | 3.7 | 1.1 | 0.6 |
| Pumpkin, Roast, EAT* | 1 Small/300g | 156 | 9.0 | 52 | 0.8 | 5.8 | 2.9 | 1.1 |
| Pumpkin, Thai, EAT* | 1 Small/340g | 81 | 2.0 | 24 | 0.7 | 3.8 | 0.6 | 1.0 |
| Red Pepper, Roasted, & Tomato, EAT* | 1 Small/300g | 75 | 2.0 | 25 | 0.9 | 4.1 | 0.6 | 1.0 |
| Roast Tomato & Basil, EAT* | 1 Small/340g | 110 | 4.0 | 32 | 1.3 | 4.4 | 1.1 | 1.0 |
| Sausage, Toulouse, Butter Bean & Lentil, Very Big, EAT* | 1 Very Big/800g | 520 | 26.0 | 65 | 3.6 | 5.5 | 3.2 | 1.7 |
| Smoked Haddock, EAT* | 1 Small/343g | 184 | 7.0 | 54 | 3.1 | 5.8 | 2.0 | 0.5 |
| Smokey Bacon & Lentils, EAT* | 1 Small/300g | 111 | 3.0 | 37 | 2.6 | 4.3 | 1.1 | 0.6 |
| Spicy Carrot & Coconut, EAT* | 1 Small/350ml | 198 | 15.0 | 57 | 0.7 | 4.0 | 4.3 | 1.0 |
| Spicy Cauliflower & Potato, EAT* | 1 Small/12oz | 69 | 1.0 | 20 | 0.8 | 3.3 | 0.4 | 0.7 |
| Spicy Tomato, EAT* | 1 Small/350ml | 113 | 5.0 | 32 | 0.7 | 3.5 | 1.6 | 0.8 |
| Spinach & Ricotta, EAT* | 1 Small/350ml | 196 | 14.0 | 56 | 2.1 | 3.0 | 4.0 | 0.6 |
| Sweet Pepper & Tomato, EAT* | 1 Small/350ml | 79 | 1.0 | 23 | 0.7 | 4.3 | 0.3 | 0.7 |
| Sweet Potato, Curried, EAT* | 1 Small/350ml | 159 | 2.0 | 45 | 0.7 | 9.2 | 0.5 | 1.6 |
| Sweet Red Pepper, EAT* | 1 Small/340g | 75 | 1.0 | 22 | 0.8 | 4.0 | 0.3 | 0.7 |
| Thai Butternut Squash, EAT* | 1 Small/300g | 144 | 7.0 | 48 | 0.8 | 6.2 | 2.2 | 1.6 |
| Tomato, Pancetta, & Mascarpone, EAT* | 1 Small/300g | 153 | 9.0 | 51 | 2.0 | 3.6 | 3.1 | 1.0 |
| Tomato, Spicy, & Basil, EAT* | 1 Small/300g | 63 | 1.0 | 21 | 0.9 | 3.8 | 0.3 | 1.0 |
| Tomato & Creme Fraiche, EAT* | 1 Small/350g | 188 | 14.0 | 54 | 0.9 | 3.4 | 4.0 | 0.8 |
| Tomato & Lentil Rasam, EAT* | 1 Large/454g | 114 | 2.0 | 25 | 1.5 | 3.9 | 0.4 | 0.5 |
| Tomato Rasam, EAT* | 1 Small/12oz | 66 | 2.0 | 19 | 1.1 | 2.7 | 0.5 | 0.7 |
| Toulouse Sausage, Butter Bean & Lentil, Big, Eat* | 1 Big/400g | 260 | 13.0 | 65 | 3.6 | 5.5 | 3.2 | 1.7 |
| Winter Vegetable, EAT* | 1 Small/340g | 164 | 9.0 | 48 | 0.9 | 5.8 | 2.6 | 1.1 |

| | Measure INFO/WEIGHT | per Measure KCAL | FAT | Nutrition Values per 100g / 100ml KCAL | PROT | CARB | FAT | FIBRE |
|---|---|---|---|---|---|---|---|---|

## EAT

### SUSHI

| | | | | | | | | |
|---|---|---|---|---|---|---|---|---|
| Vegetarian, EAT* | 1 Pack/150g | 240 | 2.0 | 160 | 3.9 | 33.5 | 1.1 | 1.3 |

### TEA

| | | | | | | | | |
|---|---|---|---|---|---|---|---|---|
| Chai Latte, Soya, EAT* | 1 Cup/355ml | 208 | 6.0 | 59 | 4.2 | 7.1 | 1.8 | 0.0 |

### TIFFIN

| | | | | | | | | |
|---|---|---|---|---|---|---|---|---|
| Milk Chocolate, EAT* | 1 Av Pack/65g | 331 | 20.0 | 510 | 7.1 | 51.0 | 30.8 | 2.9 |

### TOASTIE

| | | | | | | | | |
|---|---|---|---|---|---|---|---|---|
| Cheese, Mushroom & Roast Tomato, EAT* | 1 Pack/300g | 519 | 22.0 | 173 | 7.5 | 19.5 | 7.3 | 2.4 |
| Ham, Cheese & Mustard, EAT* | 1 Pack/250g | 593 | 28.0 | 237 | 12.5 | 21.9 | 11.1 | 1.9 |
| Three Cheese, & Caramelised Balsamic Onion, EAT* | 1 Pack/100g | 477 | 27.0 | 477 | 18.6 | 40.5 | 26.7 | 2.5 |

### VANILLA

| | | | | | | | | |
|---|---|---|---|---|---|---|---|---|
| Chiller, EAT* | 1 Tall/12oz | 482 | 21.0 | 136 | 1.8 | 19.0 | 5.9 | 0.1 |

### WATER

| | | | | | | | | |
|---|---|---|---|---|---|---|---|---|
| Lemon & Lime, V, EAT* | 1 Bottle/500ml | 50 | 0.0 | 10 | 0.0 | 2.5 | 0.0 | 0.0 |
| Pomegranate & Blueberry, V, EAT* | 1 Bottle/500ml | 50 | 0.0 | 10 | 0.0 | 2.5 | 0.0 | 0.0 |

### WRAP

| | | | | | | | | |
|---|---|---|---|---|---|---|---|---|
| Falafel, Moroccan, EAT* | 1 Av Pack/204g | 367 | 12.0 | 180 | 5.3 | 26.6 | 5.9 | 2.7 |
| Mexican Chicken, EAT* | 1 Av Pack/224g | 410 | 15.0 | 183 | 10.7 | 20.9 | 6.5 | 1.4 |
| Peking Duck, EAT* | 1 Av Pack/208g | 426 | 17.0 | 205 | 10.6 | 22.3 | 8.1 | 1.9 |

### YOGHURT

| | | | | | | | | |
|---|---|---|---|---|---|---|---|---|
| & Granola, EAT* | 1 Av Serving/210g | 349 | 12.0 | 166 | 6.4 | 22.0 | 5.9 | 2.3 |
| Banana Honey & Grapenut, EAT* | 1 Av Pot/249g | 378 | 6.0 | 152 | 4.7 | 28.1 | 2.4 | 1.0 |
| Greek, Fruits of the Forest, EAT* | 1 Pot/125g | 94 | 1.0 | 75 | 5.0 | 12.3 | 0.8 | 0.2 |
| Greek, with Mango, EAT* | 1 Tub/100g | 100 | 1.0 | 100 | 6.6 | 16.6 | 1.0 | 0.1 |
| Rhubarb & Muesli, EAT* | 1 Av Pack/180g | 225 | 6.0 | 125 | 5.1 | 20.3 | 3.1 | 1.5 |
| with Apple & Blackberry (Small), EAT* | 1 Small Pot/135g | 139 | 4.0 | 103 | 4.4 | 15.1 | 2.9 | 1.0 |
| with Apple & Blackberry Compote, EAT* | 1 Av Pack/210g | 365 | 10.0 | 174 | 5.2 | 27.4 | 5.0 | 3.1 |
| with Blueberry & Pomegranate Compote, EAT* | 1 Av Pot/135g | 150 | 4.0 | 111 | 4.5 | 17.0 | 2.9 | 0.9 |
| with Muesli & Mixed Berries, EAT* | 1 Av Pack/210g | 290 | 6.0 | 138 | 4.7 | 24.1 | 2.7 | 2.1 |
| with Raspberries, Honey & Grape Nuts, EAT* | 1 Tub/140g | 184 | 4.0 | 131 | 4.9 | 22.2 | 2.7 | 1.4 |

## ITSU

### BEANS

| | | | | | | | | |
|---|---|---|---|---|---|---|---|---|
| Edamame, Raw, Cold, Itsu* | 1 Pack/80g | 100 | 3.0 | 125 | 10.7 | 12.0 | 4.0 | 5.3 |

### DESSERT

| | | | | | | | | |
|---|---|---|---|---|---|---|---|---|
| If Bounty Went to Heaven, Itsu* | 1 Pot/80g | 347 | 23.0 | 434 | 5.9 | 24.2 | 28.2 | 3.7 |
| Valrhona Chocolate Shot, Itsu* | 1 Serving/44g | 134 | 2.0 | 305 | 7.7 | 21.1 | 3.9 | 0.0 |

### FROZEN YOGHURT

| | | | | | | | | |
|---|---|---|---|---|---|---|---|---|
| Skinny, Original, Itsu* | 1 Pot/166g | 180 | 0.0 | 108 | 3.6 | 24.1 | 0.0 | 0.0 |
| Yo Cream, Itsu* | 1 Pot/166g | 166 | 0.0 | 100 | 3.0 | 20.0 | 0.0 | 0.0 |

### NUTS

| | | | | | | | | |
|---|---|---|---|---|---|---|---|---|
| Squirrel's Dream, Itsu* | 1 Pack/70g | 210 | 24.0 | 300 | 9.1 | 40.3 | 34.0 | 0.0 |

### PEAS

| | | | | | | | | |
|---|---|---|---|---|---|---|---|---|
| Wasabi, Itsu* | 1 Pack/70g | 301 | 21.0 | 430 | 13.9 | 15.4 | 30.7 | 0.0 |

### RICE CRACKERS

| | | | | | | | | |
|---|---|---|---|---|---|---|---|---|
| Peanut, Itsu* | 1 Pack/70g | 232 | 10.0 | 331 | 12.6 | 39.6 | 13.7 | 0.0 |

### SALAD

| | | | | | | | | |
|---|---|---|---|---|---|---|---|---|
| Chicken, Chilli, with Greens, Itsu* | 1 Pack/210g | 270 | 8.0 | 129 | 10.2 | 13.0 | 3.9 | 2.6 |
| Chicken, Sesame, Itsu* | 1 Box/297g | 482 | 25.0 | 162 | 9.7 | 12.1 | 8.3 | 2.5 |
| Graze & Dazzle, Itsu* | 1 Pack/125g | 264 | 11.0 | 211 | 5.9 | 26.6 | 8.8 | 2.2 |
| Gulfstream, Itsu* | 1 Pack/356g | 402 | 6.0 | 113 | 14.8 | 9.5 | 1.8 | 1.1 |
| Hip, Humble & Healthy, Itsu* | 1 Box/314g | 336 | 16.0 | 107 | 4.3 | 11.2 | 5.2 | 5.6 |
| Salmon, Skinny, Itsu* | 1 Salad/182g | 272 | 13.0 | 149 | 11.4 | 9.7 | 7.2 | 1.5 |
| Salmon, Special, Itsu* | 1 Box/473g | 514 | 17.0 | 109 | 5.7 | 13.4 | 3.5 | 1.5 |

| | Measure INFO/WEIGHT | per Measure KCAL | FAT | Nutrition Values per 100g / 100ml KCAL | PROT | CARB | FAT | FIBRE |
|---|---|---|---|---|---|---|---|---|
| **ITSU** | | | | | | | | |
| **SALAD** | | | | | | | | |
| Sirloin Steak & Noodles, Itsu* | 1 Box/397g | 367 | 15.0 | 92 | 7.4 | 8.8 | 3.7 | 1.6 |
| Superfood, Itsu* | 1 Box/314g | 336 | 16.0 | 107 | 4.2 | 11.1 | 5.2 | 5.6 |
| Tuna, Asian Seared, Itsu* | 1 Box/100g | 212 | 0.0 | 212 | 34.0 | 18.0 | 0.5 | 1.0 |
| Tuna, Yellow Fin, Line Caught, Itsu* | 1 Box/328g | 401 | 16.0 | 122 | 9.0 | 10.6 | 4.8 | 1.9 |
| **SOUP** | | | | | | | | |
| Chicken Teriyaki Noodles, Itsu* | 1 Serving/805g | 453 | 3.0 | 56 | 3.8 | 9.2 | 0.4 | 1.2 |
| Dynamite, Detox, Itsu* | 1 Pot/425g | 153 | 1.0 | 36 | 0.6 | 8.1 | 0.1 | 0.6 |
| Dynamite, Duck, Itsu* | 1 Pot/474g | 263 | 4.0 | 55 | 2.1 | 7.7 | 0.8 | 0.6 |
| Dynamite, Itsu* | 1 Serving/425g | 133 | 0.0 | 31 | 0.3 | 7.4 | 0.1 | 0.4 |
| Dynamite, Salmon, Sense, Itsu* | 1 Pot/482g | 179 | 6.0 | 37 | 2.6 | 3.8 | 1.3 | 0.7 |
| Miso, Forever Young, Itsu* | 1 Serving/395g | 86 | 3.0 | 22 | 2.5 | 1.1 | 0.8 | 1.5 |
| Miso, Skinny, Itsu* | 1 Serving/500ml | 19 | 0.0 | 4 | 0.0 | 0.0 | 0.1 | 0.0 |
| Spicy Dumpling Noodles, Itsu* | 1 Serving/782g | 589 | 18.0 | 75 | 2.8 | 10.7 | 2.3 | 1.4 |
| **SUSHI** | | | | | | | | |
| Caviar, Sashimi & Salmon, Itsu* | 1 Pack/362g | 398 | 18.0 | 110 | 15.1 | 0.8 | 5.0 | 7.5 |
| Health & Happiness, Itsu* | 1 Pack/384g | 453 | 21.0 | 118 | 8.1 | 8.9 | 5.5 | 3.7 |
| Maki Roll, Chicken, Free Range, Itsu* | 1 Pack/221g | 241 | 10.0 | 109 | 6.0 | 11.2 | 4.6 | 1.2 |
| Maki Roll, Duck Hoi Sin, Itsu* | 1 Box/162g | 171 | 4.0 | 106 | 5.4 | 14.4 | 2.5 | 0.8 |
| Maki Roll, Salmon & Avocado, Itsu* | 1 Box/211g | 239 | 13.0 | 113 | 4.6 | 9.3 | 6.3 | 1.5 |
| Maki Roll, Spicy Crab, Itsu* | 1 Box/202g | 238 | 13.0 | 118 | 4.3 | 9.8 | 6.7 | 0.8 |
| Maki Roll, Tuna, Itsu* | 1 Serving/98g | 152 | 3.0 | 155 | 5.1 | 24.0 | 3.6 | 0.0 |
| Maki Roll, Vegetarian Sunrise, Itsu* | 1 Box/222g | 213 | 11.0 | 96 | 1.8 | 10.9 | 4.9 | 1.9 |
| Prawn, Itsu* | 1 Portion/98g | 151 | 2.0 | 154 | 6.0 | 28.5 | 1.8 | 0.0 |
| Salmon, Itsu* | 1 Portion/64g | 129 | 4.0 | 202 | 8.3 | 26.4 | 6.9 | 0.0 |
| Salmon, Super, 3 Ways, Itsu* | 1 Pack/391g | 451 | 21.0 | 115 | 7.9 | 8.7 | 5.4 | 4.4 |
| Salmon Rushdie, Itsu* | 1 Box/400g | 488 | 16.0 | 122 | 5.2 | 16.5 | 3.9 | 0.0 |
| Salmon Sashimi, Itsu* | 1 Portion/48g | 53 | 2.0 | 110 | 15.5 | 0.8 | 5.0 | 0.0 |
| Salmon Supreme, Omega 3, Itsu* | 1 Pack/340g | 509 | 25.0 | 150 | 7.4 | 13.6 | 7.2 | 1.1 |
| Tuna, Avocado & Chives, Itsu* | 1 Pack/210g | 234 | 10.0 | 111 | 6.4 | 11.5 | 4.8 | 1.5 |
| Tuna & Salmon, Itsu* | 1 Pack/282g | 315 | 7.0 | 112 | 7.5 | 14.2 | 2.6 | 0.3 |
| Tuna & Salmon, Junior, Itsu* | 1 Pack/175g | 181 | 6.0 | 103 | 9.5 | 9.0 | 3.2 | 8.1 |
| **TEA** | | | | | | | | |
| Green, Beautiful Detox, Itsu* | 1 Bottle/500ml | 58 | 0.0 | 12 | 0.0 | 2.7 | 0.0 | 0.0 |
| **YOGHURT** | | | | | | | | |
| Fruit & Goji Berries, Itsu* | 1 Pack/70g | 320 | 11.0 | 457 | 44.0 | 0.0 | 16.0 | 0.0 |
| **IXXY'S** | | | | | | | | |
| **BAGEL** | | | | | | | | |
| Chicken, Caesar, Ixxy's* | 1 Pack/200g | 530 | 25.0 | 265 | 12.9 | 24.7 | 12.7 | 1.7 |
| Chicken & Bacon, Ixxy's* | 1 Serving/215g | 589 | 27.0 | 274 | 12.8 | 29.3 | 12.5 | 0.0 |
| Cranberry & Honey, Multigrain, Mini, Ixxy's* | 1 Bagel/34g | 95 | 1.0 | 278 | 9.2 | 49.7 | 3.8 | 5.3 |
| Ham & Rosemary Ricotta Cheese, Ixxy's* | 1 Pack/215g | 372 | 7.0 | 173 | 11.1 | 25.0 | 3.2 | 0.3 |
| Plain, Mini, Ixxy's* | 1 Bagel/45g | 120 | 1.0 | 266 | 9.6 | 53.6 | 1.5 | 3.0 |
| Salt Beef & Dill Pickle, Ixxy's* | 1 Bagel/213g | 403 | 10.0 | 189 | 11.1 | 25.5 | 4.7 | 1.8 |
| Sesame, Mini, Ixxy's* | 1 Bagel/49g | 133 | 2.0 | 271 | 9.6 | 51.0 | 3.2 | 3.6 |
| Smoked Salmon & Soft Cheese, Ixxy's* | 1 Pack/192g | 474 | 18.0 | 247 | 11.3 | 28.8 | 9.6 | 1.6 |
| Soft Cheese & Tomato, Low Fat, Ixxy's* | 1 Serving/191g | 332 | 3.0 | 174 | 7.2 | 33.1 | 1.4 | 0.0 |
| Tuna & Cucumber, Ixxy's* | 1 Bagel/260g | 390 | 4.0 | 150 | 11.3 | 23.1 | 1.4 | 0.0 |
| Tuna Mayonnaise, Ixxy's* | 1 Serving/220g | 462 | 15.0 | 210 | 11.1 | 26.1 | 6.8 | 1.4 |
| **JD WETHERSPOON** | | | | | | | | |
| **BAGUETTE** | | | | | | | | |
| BLT, Malted Grain, JD Wetherspoon* | 1 Baguette/399g | 823 | 46.0 | 206 | 8.3 | 17.8 | 11.4 | 1.3 |
| Cheddar Cheese & Pickle, Malted Grain, JD Wetherspoon* | 1 Baguette/361g | 696 | 30.0 | 193 | 7.9 | 21.9 | 8.3 | 1.6 |

| | Measure INFO/WEIGHT | per Measure KCAL | per Measure FAT | Nutrition Values per 100g / 100ml KCAL | PROT | CARB | FAT | FIBRE |
|---|---|---|---|---|---|---|---|---|
| **JD WETHERSPOON** | | | | | | | | |
| **BAGUETTE** | | | | | | | | |
| Chicken, BBQ & Bacon, Malted Grain, JD Wetherspoon* | 1 Baguette/342g | 1271 | 49.0 | 371 | 20.6 | 37.4 | 14.4 | 2.9 |
| Chicken, Southern Fried, Creole Mayo, JD Wetherspoon* | 1 Meal/250g | 817 | 36.0 | 327 | 12.6 | 37.7 | 14.3 | 2.0 |
| Club, Malted Grain, JD Wetherspoon* | 1 Baguette/388g | 768 | 37.0 | 198 | 9.8 | 18.5 | 9.5 | 1.4 |
| Crayfish, Malted Grain, JD Wetherspoon* | 1 Baguette/314g | 594 | 25.0 | 189 | 6.1 | 23.2 | 8.1 | 1.7 |
| Hot Sausage & Tomato Chutney, JD Wetherspoon* | 1 Meal/250g | 839 | 33.0 | 336 | 14.1 | 40.7 | 13.4 | 3.8 |
| Ploughmans, Lloyds, JD Wetherspoon* | 1 Baguette/346g | 778 | 34.0 | 225 | 8.6 | 25.5 | 9.9 | 2.2 |
| Tuna Mayonnaise, Malted Grain, JD Wetherspoon* | 1 Baguette/401g | 710 | 31.0 | 177 | 8.9 | 18.1 | 7.8 | 1.3 |
| Wiltshire Ham, JD Wetherspoon* | 1 Baguette/346g | 536 | 13.0 | 155 | 9.9 | 20.4 | 3.8 | 1.5 |
| **BEEF DINNER** | | | | | | | | |
| Roast Potatoes, Yorkshire Pudding, Veg, JD Wetherspoon* | 1 Portion/837g | 1305 | 63.0 | 156 | 6.1 | 17.7 | 7.5 | 2.3 |
| **BHAJI** | | | | | | | | |
| Onion, JD Wetherspoon* | 1 Bhaji/30g | 43 | 2.0 | 143 | 5.3 | 18.7 | 7.3 | 5.7 |
| **BIRYANI** | | | | | | | | |
| Chicken, Naan, Curry Club Dinner, JD Wetherspoon* | 1 Meal/706g | 897 | 27.0 | 127 | 5.1 | 18.1 | 3.8 | 1.3 |
| Chicken, without Naan, JD Wetherspoon* | 1 Meal/614g | 700 | 25.0 | 114 | 4.7 | 14.8 | 4.0 | 1.3 |
| **BREAD** | | | | | | | | |
| Garlic, Ciabatta, JD Wetherspoon* | 1 Serving/142g | 406 | 18.0 | 286 | 8.0 | 1.0 | 12.6 | 1.5 |
| **BREAKFAST** | | | | | | | | |
| Baguette, Quorn Sausage, JD Wetherspoon* | 1 Baguette/285g | 622 | 18.0 | 218 | 10.5 | 29.4 | 6.4 | 3.4 |
| Blueberry Muffin, JD Wetherspoon* | 1 Muffin/124g | 467 | 26.0 | 374 | 4.7 | 43.2 | 20.7 | 0.4 |
| Bran, Fruit & Nut Muffin, JD Wetherspoon* | 1 Serving/145g | 571 | 32.0 | 394 | 7.2 | 43.0 | 21.9 | 1.1 |
| Children's, JD Wetherspoon* | 1 Serving/341g | 613 | 37.0 | 180 | 10.4 | 10.8 | 10.9 | 2.3 |
| Chocolate Muffin, JD Wetherspoon* | 1 Muffin/125g | 490 | 28.0 | 392 | 5.0 | 43.6 | 22.7 | 4.8 |
| Farmhouse, with Toast, JD Wetherspoon* | 1 Serving/796g | 1647 | 102.0 | 207 | 9.4 | 14.0 | 12.8 | 1.9 |
| Morning Roll, with Bacon, JD Wetherspoon* | 1 Roll/183g | 546 | 35.0 | 298 | 11.1 | 21.7 | 18.9 | 1.1 |
| Morning Roll, with Fried Egg, JD Wetherspoon* | 1 Roll/143g | 400 | 21.0 | 280 | 9.7 | 27.8 | 14.9 | 1.4 |
| Morning Roll, with Sausage, JD Wetherspoon* | 1 Roll/158g | 517 | 28.0 | 327 | 13.8 | 30.1 | 17.7 | 2.3 |
| Sandwich, Sausage, Bacon & Egg, JD Wetherspoon* | 1 Sandwich/357g | 840 | 56.0 | 235 | 12.6 | 11.3 | 15.6 | 1.5 |
| Scrambled Egg, on Toast, JD Wetherspoon* | 1 Serving/265g | 503 | 25.0 | 190 | 8.4 | 17.4 | 9.4 | 1.1 |
| Toast & Preserves, JD Wetherspoon* | 1 Serving/148g | 420 | 15.0 | 284 | 5.7 | 41.8 | 10.3 | 3.2 |
| Traditional, JD Wetherspoon* | 1 Breakfast/523g | 904 | 60.0 | 173 | 8.4 | 9.4 | 11.5 | 1.8 |
| Vegetarian, JD Wetherspoon* | 1 Breakfast/562g | 804 | 47.0 | 143 | 6.7 | 10.2 | 8.4 | 2.1 |
| **BROWNIES** | | | | | | | | |
| Chocolate, Fudge, Vanilla Ice Cream, JD Wetherspoon* | 1 Portion/108g | 334 | 18.0 | 309 | 4.5 | 35.6 | 16.2 | 1.5 |
| **BURGERS** | | | | | | | | |
| Beef, Double, & Chips, JD Wetherspoon* | 1 Serving/598g | 1382 | 82.0 | 231 | 16.8 | 11.4 | 13.6 | 0.5 |
| Beef, Double, Bacon, Cheese, & Chips, JD Wetherspoon* | 1 Serving/729g | 1891 | 119.0 | 259 | 18.1 | 9.4 | 16.4 | 0.4 |
| Beef, Double, Cheese, & Chips, JD Wetherspoon* | 1 Serving/654g | 1565 | 91.0 | 239 | 17.2 | 10.7 | 14.0 | 0.5 |
| Beef, with Bacon, Cheese & Chips, JD Wetherspoon* | 1 Serving/531g | 1295 | 79.0 | 244 | 15.2 | 12.6 | 14.8 | 0.5 |
| Beef, with Cheese, & Chips, JD Wetherspoon* | 1 Serving/456g | 966 | 54.0 | 212 | 13.7 | 13.8 | 11.8 | 0.5 |
| Beef, with Chips, JD Wetherspoon* | 1 Serving/428g | 881 | 46.0 | 206 | 12.8 | 15.7 | 10.8 | 0.6 |
| Chicken, Fillet, with Chips, JD Wetherspoon* | 1 Serving/465g | 727 | 17.0 | 156 | 10.9 | 16.7 | 3.7 | 0.8 |
| Lamb, Double, Minted, with Chips, JD Wetherspoon* | 1 Serving/598g | 1077 | 47.0 | 180 | 14.6 | 14.1 | 7.9 | 0.9 |
| Lamb, Minted, with Chips, JD Wetherspoon* | 1 Serving/428g | 712 | 28.0 | 166 | 11.3 | 17.2 | 6.5 | 0.9 |
| Vegetable, with Chips, JD Wetherspoon* | 1 Meal/488g | 839 | 26.0 | 172 | 4.7 | 27.2 | 5.3 | 2.0 |
| **BUTTY** | | | | | | | | |
| Bacon, Brown Bloomer, JD Wetherspoon* | 1 Serving/309g | 869 | 40.0 | 281 | 23.3 | 18.3 | 12.8 | 1.2 |
| Bacon & Egg, Brown Bloomer, JD Wetherspoon* | 1 Serving/269g | 702 | 31.0 | 261 | 18.2 | 21.0 | 11.6 | 1.4 |
| Bacon & Egg, White Bloomer, JD Wetherspoon* | 1 Serving/269g | 689 | 33.0 | 256 | 16.7 | 20.9 | 12.2 | 1.2 |
| Sausage & Egg, Brown Bloomer, JD Wetherspoon* | 1 Serving/331g | 885 | 49.0 | 267 | 16.8 | 20.8 | 14.8 | 1.3 |
| Sausage & Egg, White Bloomer, JD Wetherspoon* | 1 Serving/331g | 872 | 51.0 | 263 | 11.4 | 20.7 | 15.3 | 1.1 |

| | Measure INFO/WEIGHT | per Measure | | Nutrition Values per 100g / 100ml | | | | |
|---|---|---|---|---|---|---|---|---|
| | | KCAL | FAT | KCAL | PROT | CARB | FAT | FIBRE |

**JD WETHERSPOON**

**CAULIFLOWER CHEESE**

| | | | | | | | | |
|---|---|---|---|---|---|---|---|---|
| JD Wetherspoon* | 1 Portion/220g | 275 | 15.0 | 125 | 4.1 | 3.6 | 6.9 | 0.8 |

**CHEESECAKE**

| | | | | | | | | |
|---|---|---|---|---|---|---|---|---|
| Chocolate Chip, JD Wetherspoon* | 1 Serving/100g | 270 | 11.0 | 270 | 4.9 | 36.8 | 11.5 | 0.5 |
| White Chocolate & Raspberry, JD Wetherspoon* | 1 Serving/175g | 656 | 37.0 | 375 | 5.6 | 40.8 | 21.1 | 0.9 |

**CHICKEN**

| | | | | | | | | |
|---|---|---|---|---|---|---|---|---|
| Wings, Buffalo, JD Wetherspoon* | 1 Portion/328g | 636 | 43.0 | 194 | 15.2 | 4.0 | 13.1 | 0.5 |

**CHICKEN ALFREDO**

| | | | | | | | | |
|---|---|---|---|---|---|---|---|---|
| Pasta, with Dressed Side Salad, JD Wetherspoon* | 1 Meal/576g | 950 | 52.0 | 165 | 8.7 | 12.0 | 9.1 | 0.3 |
| Pasta, with Garlic Bread, JD Wetherspoon* | 1 Meal/501g | 1007 | 48.0 | 201 | 10.8 | 13.0 | 9.5 | 0.3 |
| Pasta, without Garlic Bread, JD Wetherspoon* | 1 Meal/430g | 804 | 39.0 | 187 | 11.3 | 15.0 | 9.0 | 0.1 |

**CHICKEN ROAST**

| | | | | | | | | |
|---|---|---|---|---|---|---|---|---|
| & Chips, Peas, Tomatoes, Mushrooms, JD Wetherspoon* | 1 Meal/742g | 904 | 39.0 | 122 | 13.0 | 5.6 | 5.2 | 1.2 |
| with BBQ Sauce, JD Wetherspoon* | 1 Meal/742g | 948 | 37.0 | 128 | 11.3 | 9.2 | 5.0 | 0.6 |
| with Chips & BBQ Sauce, JD Wetherspoon* | 1 Meal/768g | 1183 | 53.0 | 154 | 11.5 | 12.2 | 6.9 | 0.9 |
| with Chips & Salad, JD Wetherspoon* | 1 Meal/695g | 983 | 52.0 | 141 | 13.1 | 5.9 | 7.5 | 0.6 |
| with Dressed Side Salad & BBQ Sauce, JD Wetherspoon* | 1 Meal/666g | 913 | 46.0 | 137 | 12.2 | 6.0 | 6.9 | 0.9 |
| with Jacket Potato, Salad, & Salsa, JD Wetherspoon* | 1 Meal/785g | 1193 | 57.0 | 152 | 12.2 | 10.2 | 7.3 | 1.3 |

**CHICKEN VINDALOO**

| | | | | | | | | |
|---|---|---|---|---|---|---|---|---|
| JD Wetherspoon* | 1 Meal/500g | 704 | 19.0 | 141 | 6.4 | 21.0 | 3.8 | 1.3 |

**CHILLI**

| | | | | | | | | |
|---|---|---|---|---|---|---|---|---|
| Con Carne, Rice, Tortilla Chips, JD Wetherspoon* | 1 Serving/585g | 744 | 20.0 | 127 | 6.5 | 17.8 | 3.4 | 1.6 |
| Five Bean, Basmati Rice, Tortilla Chips, JD Wetherspoon* | 1 Portion/390g | 511 | 9.0 | 131 | 3.6 | 24.0 | 2.3 | 1.7 |

**CHIPS**

| | | | | | | | | |
|---|---|---|---|---|---|---|---|---|
| with Cheese, JD Wetherspoon* | 1 Serving/501g | 1002 | 52.0 | 200 | 5.2 | 21.9 | 10.3 | 1.8 |
| with Roast Gravy, JD Wetherspoon* | 1 Serving/400g | 392 | 12.0 | 98 | 2.5 | 17.6 | 3.1 | 0.0 |

**CHUTNEY**

| | | | | | | | | |
|---|---|---|---|---|---|---|---|---|
| Mango, JD Wetherspoon* | 1 Serving/25g | 47 | 0.0 | 188 | 0.4 | 44.8 | 0.8 | 0.4 |

**CIABATTA**

| | | | | | | | | |
|---|---|---|---|---|---|---|---|---|
| BBQ Chicken & Bacon Melt, JD Wetherspoon* | 1 Ciabatta/333g | 716 | 34.0 | 215 | 11.3 | 20.4 | 10.1 | 1.8 |
| BLT, JD Wetherspoon* | 1 Ciabatta/390g | 789 | 47.0 | 202 | 8.2 | 15.4 | 12.1 | 1.5 |
| Club, JD Wetherspoon* | 1 Ciabatta/378g | 734 | 39.0 | 194 | 9.7 | 16.1 | 10.2 | 1.6 |
| Crayfish, JD Wetherspoon* | 1 Ciabatta/305g | 561 | 27.0 | 184 | 5.8 | 20.3 | 9.0 | 1.9 |
| Mature Cheddar Cheese & Pickle, JD Wetherspoon* | 1 Ciabatta/350g | 662 | 32.0 | 189 | 7.8 | 19.4 | 9.0 | 1.7 |
| Tuna Mayonnaise, JD Wetherspoon* | 1 Ciabatta/391g | 676 | 33.0 | 173 | 8.8 | 15.8 | 8.4 | 1.5 |
| Wiltshire Ham, JD Wetherspoon* | 1 Ciabatta/335g | 503 | 15.0 | 150 | 9.8 | 17.7 | 4.4 | 1.7 |

**CURRY**

| | | | | | | | | |
|---|---|---|---|---|---|---|---|---|
| Beef, Malaysian, Rendang, with Naan, JD Wetherspoon* | 1 Meal/706g | 1144 | 41.0 | 162 | 6.8 | 20.1 | 5.8 | 1.1 |
| Beef, Malaysian, Rendang, without Naan, JD Wetherspoon* | 1 Meal/615g | 947 | 38.0 | 154 | 6.7 | 17.0 | 6.2 | 1.0 |
| Kashmiri, Lamb, with Naan, JD Wetherspoon* | 1 Meal/704g | 1021 | 33.0 | 145 | 7.2 | 19.5 | 4.7 | 1.2 |
| Kerala, Fish, with Naan, JD Wetherspoon* | 1 Meal/706g | 1066 | 36.0 | 151 | 7.0 | 20.0 | 5.1 | 1.0 |
| Mushroom Dopiaza, with Naan Bread, JD Wetherspoon* | 1 Serving/719g | 899 | 24.0 | 125 | 3.5 | 21.5 | 3.4 | 1.5 |
| Royal Thali, with Naan, JD Wetherspoon* | 1 Meal/948g | 1336 | 48.0 | 141 | 7.1 | 16.8 | 5.1 | 1.3 |
| Thai, Green Chicken, without Naan, JD Wetherspoon* | 1 Meal/617g | 1037 | 47.0 | 168 | 7.5 | 17.6 | 7.6 | 0.5 |
| Vegetarian, Thali, with Naan, JD Wetherspoon* | 1 Meal/950g | 1320 | 43.0 | 139 | 5.3 | 20.3 | 4.5 | 2.4 |

**DHANSAK**

| | | | | | | | | |
|---|---|---|---|---|---|---|---|---|
| Lamb, Meal, JD Wetherspoon* | 1 Serving/720g | 983 | 26.0 | 137 | 7.2 | 19.6 | 3.6 | 0.8 |

**FISH & CHIPS**

| | | | | | | | | |
|---|---|---|---|---|---|---|---|---|
| Haddock, JD Wetherspoon* | 1 Meal/496g | 806 | 41.0 | 162 | 7.2 | 14.4 | 8.2 | 2.4 |
| Plaice, Breaded, & Peas, JD Wetherspoon* | 1 Serving/460g | 550 | 16.0 | 120 | 6.8 | 15.0 | 3.4 | 1.7 |

**FISH CAKES**

| | | | | | | | | |
|---|---|---|---|---|---|---|---|---|
| Salmon & Lime, with Tartare Sauce, JD Wetherspoon* | 1 Serving/355g | 569 | 31.0 | 160 | 5.8 | 14.5 | 8.8 | 1.0 |

| | Measure INFO/WEIGHT | per Measure KCAL | FAT | Nutrition Values per 100g / 100ml KCAL | PROT | CARB | FAT | FIBRE |
|---|---|---|---|---|---|---|---|---|
| **JD WETHERSPOON** | | | | | | | | |
| **GAMMON &** | | | | | | | | |
| Chips, Peas, Tomato, & Egg, JD Wetherspoon* | 1 Meal/564g | 844 | 41.0 | 150 | 15.0 | 6.7 | 7.3 | 1.3 |
| Chips, Peas, Tomato, & Pineapple, JD Wetherspoon* | 1 Meal/575g | 799 | 36.0 | 139 | 13.6 | 7.8 | 6.3 | 1.4 |
| Egg, Chips & Side Salad, JD Wetherspoon* | 1 Meal/593g | 801 | 42.0 | 135 | 10.2 | 9.0 | 7.0 | 0.3 |
| Egg, Jacket Potato & Side Salad, JD Wetherspoon* | 1 Meal/707g | 1040 | 45.0 | 147 | 10.1 | 13.1 | 6.4 | 1.3 |
| Pineapple, Potato, Tomato, Mushroom, JD Wetherspoon* | 1 Meal/763g | 931 | 34.0 | 122 | 8.7 | 12.8 | 4.4 | 1.3 |
| **HAGGIS** | | | | | | | | |
| with Neeps & Tatties, JD Wetherspoon* | 1 Meal/682g | 982 | 53.0 | 144 | 4.6 | 15.0 | 7.7 | 1.9 |
| **HAM** | | | | | | | | |
| & Eggs, JD Wetherspoon* | 1 Serving/396g | 253 | 13.0 | 64 | 4.9 | 3.5 | 3.2 | 0.0 |
| **ICE CREAM** | | | | | | | | |
| Bombe, Mint Chocolate, JD Wetherspoon* | 1 Portion/135g | 300 | 13.0 | 222 | 2.6 | 30.6 | 9.9 | 0.8 |
| Chocolate, Bomb, JD Wetherspoon* | 1 Portion/100g | 259 | 13.0 | 259 | 5.9 | 34.3 | 13.4 | 5.4 |
| Neopolitan, Movenpick, JD Wetherspoon* | 1 Bowl/100g | 181 | 10.0 | 181 | 3.0 | 20.0 | 9.6 | 0.0 |
| **JALFREZI** | | | | | | | | |
| Chicken, Meal, with Naan Bread, JD Wetherspoon* | 1 Meal/705g | 916 | 20.0 | 130 | 6.8 | 19.9 | 2.8 | 1.3 |
| Chicken, without Naan Bread, JD Wetherspoon* | 1 Meal/615g | 719 | 17.0 | 117 | 6.7 | 16.9 | 2.8 | 1.3 |
| **KORMA** | | | | | | | | |
| Chicken, Meal, without Naan, JD Wetherspoon* | 1 Meal/617g | 944 | 38.0 | 153 | 6.4 | 17.0 | 6.2 | 0.8 |
| Chicken, with Naan, JD Wetherspoon* | 1 Meal/704g | 1141 | 41.0 | 162 | 6.6 | 20.1 | 5.8 | 0.9 |
| **LAMB** | | | | | | | | |
| Shoulder, Mashed Potato & Vegetables, JD Wetherspoon* | 1 Meal/844g | 1114 | 67.0 | 132 | 8.9 | 6.8 | 7.9 | 1.0 |
| **LASAGNE** | | | | | | | | |
| Al Forno, Wth Dressed Side Salad, JD Wetherspoon* | 1 Meal/658g | 823 | 41.0 | 125 | 5.5 | 11.4 | 6.2 | 0.8 |
| **MASALA** | | | | | | | | |
| Chicken, Hot, with Naan, JD Wetherspoon* | 1 Meal/707g | 1033 | 31.0 | 146 | 6.9 | 20.1 | 4.4 | 1.2 |
| Chicken, Hot, without Naan, JD Wetherspoon* | 1 Meal/614g | 835 | 28.0 | 136 | 6.8 | 17.1 | 4.6 | 1.1 |
| Prawn, Sri Lankan, with Naan, JD Wetherspoon* | 1 Meal/708g | 1027 | 36.0 | 145 | 5.7 | 19.7 | 5.1 | 0.8 |
| Prawn, Sri Lankan, without Naan, JD Wetherspoon* | 1 Meal/617g | 827 | 33.0 | 134 | 5.4 | 16.6 | 5.4 | 1.0 |
| Vegetable, Tandoori, Meal, JD Wetherspoon* | 1 Serving/720g | 1020 | 36.0 | 142 | 3.4 | 20.7 | 5.0 | 2.3 |
| **MEATBALLS** | | | | | | | | |
| with Linguine Pasta, JD Wetherspoon* | 1 Serving/512g | 614 | 24.0 | 120 | 6.3 | 13.1 | 4.7 | 1.9 |
| **MELT** | | | | | | | | |
| BBQ Chicken, & Chips, & Salad, JD Wetherspoon* | 1 Serving/643g | 849 | 42.0 | 132 | 10.4 | 8.2 | 6.6 | 0.4 |
| **MIXED GRILL** | | | | | | | | |
| with Chips, & Dressed Side Salad, JD Wetherspoon* | 1 Serving/784g | 1324 | 87.0 | 169 | 12.0 | 5.6 | 11.1 | 0.3 |
| **MOUSSAKA** | | | | | | | | |
| Vegetarian, JD Wetherspoon* | 1 Serving/555g | 582 | 39.0 | 105 | 2.7 | 7.6 | 7.0 | 2.7 |
| **NACHOS** | | | | | | | | |
| with Chilli Con Carne, JD Wetherspoon* | 1 Meal/570g | 1505 | 89.0 | 264 | 8.6 | 22.2 | 15.6 | 1.8 |
| with Fajita Chicken, JD Wetherspoon* | 1 Serving/486g | 1225 | 70.0 | 252 | 5.7 | 24.7 | 14.5 | 2.9 |
| with Five Bean Chilli, JD Wetherspoon* | 1 Serving/571g | 1399 | 81.0 | 245 | 7.3 | 21.8 | 14.2 | 2.7 |
| **PANINI** | | | | | | | | |
| BBQ Chicken & Bacon, Melt, JD Wetherspoon* | 1 Panini/337g | 650 | 28.0 | 193 | 9.9 | 19.9 | 8.2 | 1.7 |
| Cheese, Tomato, & Bacon, JD Wetherspoon* | 1 Panini/261g | 630 | 29.0 | 241 | 14.3 | 21.6 | 11.1 | 0.8 |
| Cheese & Tuna, JD Wetherspoon* | 1 Panini/221g | 551 | 22.0 | 249 | 15.5 | 24.9 | 10.1 | 0.7 |
| Club, JD Wetherspoon* | 1 Panini/378g | 734 | 39.0 | 194 | 9.7 | 16.1 | 10.2 | 1.6 |
| Fajita Chicken, JD Wetherspoon* | 1 Panini/235g | 359 | 6.0 | 153 | 4.4 | 28.8 | 2.6 | 1.7 |
| Ham & Mature, Cheddar Cheese, JD Wetherspoon* | 1 Panini/354g | 868 | 50.0 | 245 | 12.7 | 16.7 | 14.1 | 1.5 |
| Mature, Cheddar Cheese & Tomato, JD Wetherspoon* | 1 Panini/330g | 750 | 27.0 | 227 | 10.4 | 18.0 | 8.2 | 1.7 |
| Pepperoni & Mozzarella, JD Wetherspoon* | 1 Panini/205g | 617 | 33.0 | 301 | 11.6 | 27.5 | 16.3 | 1.0 |
| Tomato, Mozzarella & Green Pesto, JD Wetherspoon* | 1 Panini/245g | 502 | 23.0 | 205 | 7.3 | 23.0 | 9.3 | 1.4 |

## JD WETHERSPOON

### PASTA
| | | | | | | | | |
|---|---|---|---|---|---|---|---|---|
| Five Cheese & Bacon, & Garlic Ciabatta, JD Wetherspoon* | 1 Meal/469g | 563 | 23.0 | 120 | 3.6 | 9.7 | 5.0 | 1.5 |

### PASTA BAKE
| | | | | | | | | |
|---|---|---|---|---|---|---|---|---|
| Mediterranean, JD Wetherspoon* | 1 Serving/450g | 577 | 22.0 | 128 | 4.3 | 16.4 | 4.9 | 0.9 |

### PIE
| | | | | | | | | |
|---|---|---|---|---|---|---|---|---|
| Aberdeen Angus, Chips, & Vegetables, JD Wetherspoon* | 1 Serving/780g | 1356 | 87.0 | 174 | 5.5 | 15.7 | 11.1 | 0.9 |
| Beef & Abbot Ale, Chips, Veg & Gravy, JD Wetherspoon* | 1 Meal/850g | 1258 | 68.0 | 148 | 4.0 | 14.9 | 8.0 | 1.0 |
| Cottage, with Chips & Peas, JD Wetherspoon* | 1 Meal/682g | 846 | 33.0 | 124 | 3.7 | 15.6 | 4.9 | 1.9 |
| Fish, Carrot & Broccoli, in Herb Butter, JD Wetherspoon* | 1 Serving/550g | 612 | 38.0 | 111 | 4.6 | 9.7 | 6.9 | 2.4 |
| Scotch, with Chips & Beans, JD Wetherspoon* | 1 Serving/435g | 603 | 22.0 | 139 | 6.8 | 14.9 | 5.1 | 1.5 |

### PLATTER
| | | | | | | | | |
|---|---|---|---|---|---|---|---|---|
| Italian Style, JD Wetherspoon* | 1 Platter/1020g | 1985 | 75.0 | 195 | 10.4 | 22.9 | 7.4 | 0.6 |
| Mexican, Chilli, Sour Cream, JD Wetherspoon* | 1 Platter/1062g | 2560 | 141.0 | 241 | 7.5 | 22.6 | 13.3 | 2.8 |
| Mexican, with Five Bean Chilli, JD Wetherspoon* | 1 Platter/1002g | 2358 | 123.0 | 235 | 6.2 | 25.6 | 12.3 | 3.6 |
| Western, JD Wetherspoon* | 1 Platter/1454g | 2973 | 169.0 | 204 | 16.9 | 9.1 | 11.6 | 0.4 |

### POPPADOMS
| | | | | | | | | |
|---|---|---|---|---|---|---|---|---|
| & Dips, JD Wetherspoon* | 1 Serving/134g | 425 | 11.0 | 317 | 4.6 | 28.4 | 8.1 | 2.5 |

### PORK DINNER
| | | | | | | | | |
|---|---|---|---|---|---|---|---|---|
| Potatoes, Yorkshire Pudding & Veg, JD Wetherspoon* | 1 Meal/1022g | 1543 | 63.0 | 151 | 10.4 | 14.6 | 6.2 | 2.1 |

### POTATO BOMBAY
| | | | | | | | | |
|---|---|---|---|---|---|---|---|---|
| JD Wetherspoon* | 1 Serving/300g | 285 | 15.0 | 95 | 1.8 | 10.8 | 4.9 | 2.5 |

### POTATO SKINS
| | | | | | | | | |
|---|---|---|---|---|---|---|---|---|
| Cheese & Bacon, Loaded, JD Wetherspoon* | 1 Serving/439g | 949 | 58.0 | 216 | 8.9 | 15.2 | 13.3 | 1.5 |
| Cheese & Red Onion, Loaded, JD Wetherspoon* | 1 Serving/414g | 835 | 51.0 | 202 | 6.0 | 16.5 | 12.4 | 1.6 |
| Chilli Con Carne, Loaded, JD Wetherspoon* | 1 Serving/503g | 735 | 36.0 | 146 | 5.0 | 15.7 | 7.1 | 1.9 |

### POTATO WEDGES
| | | | | | | | | |
|---|---|---|---|---|---|---|---|---|
| Spicy, JD Wetherspoon* | 1 Serving/270g | 434 | 16.0 | 161 | 2.2 | 27.7 | 5.8 | 1.8 |
| Spicy, with Sour Cream, JD Wetherspoon* | 1 Serving/330g | 558 | 27.0 | 169 | 2.3 | 23.4 | 8.3 | 1.5 |

### POTATOES
| | | | | | | | | |
|---|---|---|---|---|---|---|---|---|
| Jacket, Coleslaw, JD Wetherspoon* | 1 Meal/596g | 918 | 49.0 | 154 | 2.3 | 17.1 | 8.2 | 1.8 |
| Jacket, Crayfish, Marie Rose Dressing, JD Wetherspoon* | 1 Meal/524g | 796 | 41.0 | 152 | 3.5 | 18.2 | 7.8 | 1.7 |
| Jacket, Mature, Cheddar Cheese, JD Wetherspoon* | 1 Meal/496g | 858 | 45.0 | 173 | 5.6 | 18.7 | 9.0 | 1.8 |
| Jacket, with Baked Beans, Salad, JD Wetherspoon* | 1 Meal/575g | 725 | 25.0 | 126 | 3.3 | 19.6 | 4.3 | 2.4 |
| Jacket, with Five Bean Chilli, Side Salad, JD Wetherspoon* | 1 Meal/597g | 705 | 26.0 | 118 | 3.0 | 17.9 | 4.3 | 2.4 |
| Mashed, Creamy, JD Wetherspoon* | 1 Portion/279g | 349 | 21.0 | 125 | 1.5 | 15.0 | 7.6 | 1.1 |
| Roast, JD Wetherspoon* | 1 Portion/200g | 290 | 9.0 | 145 | 2.5 | 23.0 | 4.7 | 2.3 |

### RIBS
| | | | | | | | | |
|---|---|---|---|---|---|---|---|---|
| Double, with Chips, JD Wetherspoon* | 1 Serving/500g | 949 | 46.0 | 190 | 12.5 | 14.9 | 9.3 | 0.3 |
| Double, with Jacket Potato, JD Wetherspoon* | 1 Serving/590g | 1159 | 51.0 | 196 | 11.4 | 19.2 | 8.6 | 1.3 |

### RICE
| | | | | | | | | |
|---|---|---|---|---|---|---|---|---|
| Basmati, Yellow, JD Wetherspoon* | 1 Portion/200g | 286 | 1.0 | 143 | 3.4 | 31.1 | 0.6 | 0.2 |

### ROGAN JOSH
| | | | | | | | | |
|---|---|---|---|---|---|---|---|---|
| Lamb, Meal, without Naan, JD Wetherspoon* | 1 Meal/617g | 820 | 28.0 | 133 | 7.1 | 17.0 | 4.5 | 1.0 |
| Lamb, with Naan, JD Wetherspoon* | 1 Meal/706g | 1017 | 30.0 | 144 | 7.2 | 20.1 | 4.3 | 1.1 |

### SALAD
| | | | | | | | | |
|---|---|---|---|---|---|---|---|---|
| Caesar, Chicken, JD Wetherspoon* | 1 Meal/230g | 507 | 36.0 | 220 | 14.3 | 5.1 | 15.8 | 0.8 |
| Chicken, BBQ, Croutons & Dressing, JD Wetherspoon* | 1 Portion/350g | 315 | 8.0 | 90 | 9.4 | 7.5 | 2.4 | 0.8 |
| Chicken & Bacon, Warm, JD Wetherspoon* | 1 Meal/426g | 600 | 41.0 | 141 | 9.8 | 3.8 | 9.7 | 0.6 |
| Crayfish, JD Wetherspoon* | 1 Meal/317g | 247 | 18.0 | 78 | 4.4 | 2.7 | 5.7 | 0.6 |
| Side, with Dressing, JD Wetherspoon* | 1 Salad/215g | 263 | 20.0 | 122 | 2.2 | 8.1 | 9.1 | 1.0 |
| Side, with Dressing & Croutons, JD Wetherspoon* | 1 Portion/140g | 221 | 18.0 | 158 | 2.1 | 8.6 | 13.1 | 1.1 |
| Side, with Dressing & No Croutons, JD Wetherspoon* | 1 Portion/129g | 145 | 14.0 | 112 | 1.0 | 3.2 | 10.8 | 0.9 |
| Thai Noodle, JD Wetherspoon* | 1 Portion/394g | 433 | 21.0 | 110 | 2.7 | 12.7 | 5.4 | 1.4 |

## JD WETHERSPOON

| INFO/WEIGHT | Measure | per Measure KCAL | FAT | Nutrition Values per 100g / 100ml KCAL | PROT | CARB | FAT | FIBRE |
|---|---|---|---|---|---|---|---|---|
| **SALAD** | | | | | | | | |
| Thai Noodle, with Chicken, JD Wetherspoon* | 1 Meal/554g | 637 | 28.0 | 115 | 9.2 | 9.6 | 5.0 | 1.4 |
| Tiger Prawn, Dressing, & Chilli Jam, JD Wetherspoon* | 1 Portion/340g | 500 | 33.0 | 147 | 4.7 | 10.1 | 9.7 | 0.9 |
| Tuna, with Eggs, Olives, & Croutons, JD Wetherspoon* | 1 Portion/395g | 679 | 52.0 | 172 | 10.3 | 3.2 | 13.1 | 0.7 |
| **SAMOSAS** | | | | | | | | |
| Lamb, JD Wetherspoon* | 1 Samosa/90g | 160 | 4.0 | 178 | 7.9 | 29.9 | 4.2 | 3.9 |
| Vegetable, JD Wetherspoon* | 1 Samosa/50g | 92 | 3.0 | 184 | 5.4 | 28.4 | 6.2 | 2.2 |
| **SANDWICH** | | | | | | | | |
| Beef, Hot, Brown Bloomer, JD Wetherspoon* | 1 Sandwich/299g | 618 | 27.0 | 207 | 11.4 | 19.9 | 9.1 | 1.3 |
| Beef, Hot, White Poppy Seed Bloomer, JD Wetherspoon* | 1 Sandwich/299g | 605 | 29.0 | 202 | 10.0 | 19.8 | 9.6 | 1.1 |
| BLT, Brown Bloomer, JD Wetherspoon* | 1 Sandwich/404g | 885 | 40.0 | 219 | 18.0 | 14.6 | 9.8 | 1.2 |
| BLT, White Bloomer, JD Wetherspoon* | 1 Sandwich/404g | 872 | 33.0 | 216 | 17.0 | 14.6 | 8.1 | 1.0 |
| Cheddar, & Pickle, Brown Bloomer, JD Wetherspoon* | 1 Sandwich/260g | 665 | 32.0 | 256 | 11.0 | 25.4 | 12.3 | 1.9 |
| Cheddar, & Pickle, White Bloomer, JD Wetherspoon* | 1 Sandwich/260g | 638 | 33.0 | 245 | 9.2 | 0.0 | 12.6 | 1.5 |
| Chicken, Cheese, Bacon, Mayo, White, JD Wetherspoon* | 1 Sandwich/312g | 710 | 40.0 | 228 | 13.5 | 18.8 | 12.7 | 1.2 |
| Chicken, Half Fat Mayo, Brown, Hot, JD Wetherspoon* | 1 Sandwich/289g | 628 | 28.0 | 217 | 11.8 | 20.7 | 9.8 | 1.7 |
| Chicken, Half Fat Mayo, White, Hot, JD Wetherspoon* | 1 Sandwich/289g | 615 | 30.0 | 213 | 11.3 | 20.6 | 10.3 | 1.5 |
| Egg Mayonnaise, Brown Bloomer, JD Wetherspoon* | 1 Sandwich/295g | 704 | 40.0 | 239 | 10.1 | 19.7 | 13.4 | 1.3 |
| Egg Mayonnaise, White Bloomer, JD Wetherspoon* | 1 Sandwich/295g | 692 | 41.0 | 235 | 8.7 | 19.6 | 13.9 | 1.1 |
| Ham, & Tomato, Brown Bloomer, JD Wetherspoon* | 1 Sandwich/239g | 514 | 17.0 | 215 | 11.4 | 24.4 | 7.2 | 1.8 |
| Ham, & Tomato, White Bloomer, JD Wetherspoon* | 1 Sandwich/239g | 501 | 19.0 | 210 | 9.7 | 24.4 | 7.8 | 1.5 |
| Prawn Mayonnaise, Brown Bloomer, JD Wetherspoon* | 1 Sandwich/244g | 579 | 27.0 | 237 | 11.0 | 23.8 | 10.9 | 1.6 |
| Prawn Mayonnaise, White Bloomer, JD Wetherspoon* | 1 Sandwich/244g | 567 | 28.0 | 232 | 9.3 | 23.7 | 11.6 | 1.4 |
| Salmon, Lemon Mayo, Brown Bloomer, JD Wetherspoon* | 1 Sandwich/229g | 637 | 34.0 | 278 | 11.4 | 25.4 | 14.7 | 1.7 |
| Salmon, Lemon Mayo, White Bloomer, JD Wetherspoon* | 1 Sandwich/229g | 625 | 35.0 | 273 | 9.6 | 25.2 | 15.4 | 1.4 |
| Tuna Mayonnaise, Half Fat Mayo, White, JD Wetherspoon* | 1 Sandwich/389g | 828 | 47.0 | 213 | 11.2 | 15.6 | 12.1 | 1.0 |
| **SAUSAGE & MASH** | | | | | | | | |
| with Red Wine Gravy, JD Wetherspoon* | 1 Portion/677g | 887 | 51.0 | 131 | 6.0 | 10.2 | 7.5 | 1.8 |
| **SAUSAGES WITH** | | | | | | | | |
| Bacon & Egg, JD Wetherspoon* | 1 Serving/582g | 1040 | 58.0 | 179 | 11.7 | 11.3 | 9.9 | 1.0 |
| Chips & Beans, JD Wetherspoon* | 1 Meal/554g | 897 | 43.0 | 162 | 7.3 | 16.4 | 7.7 | 2.3 |
| **SCAMPI** | | | | | | | | |
| Breaded, Chips, Peas, Tartare Sauce, JD Wetherspoon* | 1 Serving/561g | 987 | 44.0 | 176 | 5.2 | 19.9 | 7.8 | 2.3 |
| **SORBET** | | | | | | | | |
| Mango & Passionfruit, JD Wetherspoon* | 1 Serving/135g | 115 | 0.0 | 85 | 0.2 | 20.0 | 0.1 | 0.2 |
| **SOUP** | | | | | | | | |
| Leek & Potato, without Bread & Butter, JD Wetherspoon* | 1 Bowl/420 | 105 | 1.0 | 25 | 0.9 | 5.1 | 0.2 | 1.0 |
| Mushroom, No Bread, JD Wetherspoon* | 1 Serving/305g | 252 | 16.0 | 83 | 2.8 | 5.5 | 5.4 | 0.4 |
| Mushroom, with Brown Bloomer, JD Wetherspoon* | 1 Serving/429g | 561 | 24.0 | 131 | 3.4 | 16.0 | 5.5 | 1.2 |
| Mushroom, with White Bloomer, JD Wetherspoon* | 1 Serving/429g | 549 | 25.0 | 128 | 3.4 | 15.9 | 5.9 | 1.1 |
| Tomato, No Bread, JD Wetherspoon* | 1 Serving/305g | 198 | 14.0 | 65 | 0.9 | 3.9 | 4.6 | 0.6 |
| Tomato, with Brown Bloomer, JD Wetherspoon* | 1 Serving/429g | 576 | 26.0 | 134 | 3.7 | 15.7 | 6.0 | 1.3 |
| Tomato, with White Bloomer, JD Wetherspoon* | 1 Serving/429g | 563 | 27.0 | 131 | 2.8 | 15.6 | 6.4 | 1.2 |
| Tomato & Basil, Organic, JD Wetherspoon* | 1 Serving/491g | 584 | 23.0 | 119 | 2.9 | 15.8 | 4.7 | 1.2 |
| Tomato & Basil, Organic, with Bread, JD Wetherspoon* | 1 Bowl/450g | 396 | 9.0 | 88 | 1.0 | 6.0 | 1.9 | 1.1 |
| Tomato & Basil, Organic, without Bread, JD Wetherspoon* | 1 Bowl/350g | 199 | 15.0 | 57 | 0.7 | 3.0 | 4.3 | 0.6 |
| **SPONGE PUDDING** | | | | | | | | |
| Treacle, with Hot Custard, JD Wetherspoon* | 1 Serving/515g | 1267 | 71.0 | 246 | 2.3 | 41.8 | 13.8 | 0.2 |
| **STEAK** | | | | | | | | |
| Ribeye, Chips, Tomato, Mushroom, JD Wetherspoon* | 1 Portion/531g | 945 | 64.0 | 178 | 9.3 | 9.3 | 12.0 | 0.3 |
| Ribeye, Chips & Side Salad, JD Wetherspoon* | 1 Meal/562g | 1006 | 72.0 | 179 | 8.0 | 8.9 | 12.8 | 0.3 |
| Ribeye, Potato, Tomato, Mushroom, JD Wetherspoon* | 1 Meal/674g | 1253 | 154.0 | 186 | 7.8 | 11.5 | 22.8 | 1.9 |
| Ribeye, Potato & Dressed Side Salad, JD Wetherspoon* | 1 Meal/620g | 850 | 43.0 | 137 | 8.2 | 10.1 | 7.0 | 1.1 |

| | Measure INFO/WEIGHT | per Measure KCAL | per Measure FAT | Nutrition Values per 100g / 100ml KCAL | PROT | CARB | FAT | FIBRE |
|---|---|---|---|---|---|---|---|---|
| **JD WETHERSPOON** | | | | | | | | |
| **STEAK** | | | | | | | | |
| Ribeye, Prawns, Chips, & Side Salad, JD Wetherspoon* | 1 Meal/714g | 1093 | 56.0 | 153 | 11.0 | 7.7 | 7.9 | 0.3 |
| Ribeye, Prawns, Chips, Mushroom, JD Wetherspoon* | 1 Meal/768g | 1083 | 51.0 | 141 | 11.0 | 7.0 | 6.6 | 0.9 |
| Ribeye, Prawns, Jacket Potato, Salad, JD Wetherspoon* | 1 Meal/727g | 1178 | 57.0 | 162 | 10.8 | 7.7 | 7.9 | 0.3 |
| Rump, Chips, Dressed Side Salad, JD Wetherspoon* | 1 Meal/787g | 1283 | 72.0 | 163 | 14.3 | 6.3 | 9.1 | 0.2 |
| Rump, Chips, Peas, Tomato, Mushroom, JD Wetherspoon* | 1 Meal/759g | 1268 | 71.0 | 167 | 14.9 | 6.5 | 9.3 | 0.2 |
| Rump, Potato, Dressed Side Salad, JD Wetherspoon* | 1 Meal/867g | 1466 | 71.0 | 169 | 13.6 | 10.7 | 8.2 | 1.0 |
| Rump, Potato, Peas, Tomato, Mushroom, JD Wetherspoon* | 1 Meal/839g | 1451 | 70.0 | 173 | 14.1 | 11.0 | 8.3 | 1.1 |
| T-Bone, Chips, Dressed Side Salad, JD Wetherspoon* | 1 Meal/673g | 1313 | 98.0 | 195 | 9.4 | 7.4 | 14.5 | 0.2 |
| T-Bone, Potato, Dresed Side Salad, JD Wetherspoon* | 1 Meal/756g | 1496 | 97.0 | 198 | 9.1 | 12.3 | 12.8 | 1.2 |
| T-Bone, Potato, Tomato, Mushroom, JD Wetherspoon* | 1 Meal/722g | 1481 | 95.0 | 205 | 9.5 | 12.7 | 13.2 | 1.2 |
| **STEW** | | | | | | | | |
| Irish, JD Wetherspoon* | 1 Serving/600g | 516 | 23.0 | 86 | 7.3 | 5.6 | 3.9 | 0.9 |
| **TART** | | | | | | | | |
| Apple, with Ice Cream, JD Wetherspoon* | 1 Serving/235g | 464 | 20.0 | 197 | 1.6 | 29.8 | 8.5 | 0.4 |
| **TIKKA MASALA** | | | | | | | | |
| Chicken, with Rice & No Naan Bread, JD Wetherspoon* | 1 Meal/614g | 872 | 33.0 | 142 | 6.9 | 16.9 | 5.4 | 1.2 |
| **WAFFLES** | | | | | | | | |
| Belgian, Ice Cream & Maple Syrup, JD Wetherspoon* | 1 Serving/395g | 934 | 34.0 | 236 | 13.8 | 28.4 | 8.5 | 0.8 |
| **WRAP** | | | | | | | | |
| Caesar Wetherwrap, JD Wetherspoon* | 1 Wrap/159g | 478 | 33.0 | 301 | 7.0 | 23.1 | 20.5 | 1.5 |
| Caesar Wetherwrap, Tortillas & Salsa, JD Wetherspoon* | 1 Serving/244g | 624 | 39.0 | 256 | 5.7 | 23.4 | 15.9 | 1.6 |
| Caesar Wetherwrap & Potato Wedges, JD Wetherspoon* | 1 Serving/289g | 687 | 40.0 | 238 | 5.0 | 25.2 | 13.9 | 1.6 |
| Chicken, Cheese, & Potato Wedges, JD Wetherspoon* | 1 Serving/401g | 762 | 34.0 | 190 | 8.0 | 22.2 | 8.5 | 1.5 |
| Chicken, Cheese, Tortilla Chips, Salsa, JD Wetherspoon* | 1 Serving/356g | 699 | 32.0 | 196 | 8.8 | 20.6 | 9.1 | 1.5 |
| Chicken, Guacamole, Potato Wedges, JD Wetherspoon* | 1 Serving/318g | 537 | 18.0 | 169 | 7.2 | 23.7 | 5.8 | 2.0 |
| Chicken, Guacamole, Tortillas, Salsa, JD Wetherspoon* | 1 Serving/273g | 474 | 17.0 | 174 | 8.2 | 21.9 | 6.2 | 2.0 |
| Chicken, Southern Fried, Creole Mayo, JD Wetherspoon* | 1 Wrap/320g | 553 | 30.0 | 173 | 7.1 | 16.3 | 9.4 | 1.4 |
| Chicken, with Chicken Breast, JD Wetherspoon* | 1 Wrap/292g | 450 | 22.0 | 154 | 9.4 | 14.5 | 7.4 | 1.5 |
| Chicken, with Potato Wedges, JD Wetherspoon* | 1 Serving/373g | 647 | 24.0 | 173 | 6.7 | 23.9 | 6.5 | 1.7 |
| Chicken, with Tortilla Chips & Salsa, JD Wetherspoon* | 1 Serving/328g | 584 | 23.0 | 178 | 7.5 | 22.3 | 7.0 | 1.6 |
| Chicken & Cheese, JD Wetherspoon* | 1 Wrap/271g | 553 | 26.0 | 204 | 10.7 | 19.6 | 9.7 | 1.4 |
| Club Wetherwrap, Tortilla Chips, Salsa, JD Wetherspoon* | 1 Serving/336g | 759 | 42.0 | 226 | 12.2 | 17.1 | 12.5 | 1.1 |
| Club Wetherwrap, with Potato Wedges, JD Wetherspoon* | 1 Serving/381g | 822 | 43.0 | 216 | 10.9 | 19.2 | 11.3 | 1.2 |
| Fajita Chicken, JD Wetherspoon* | 1 Wrap/228g | 345 | 14.0 | 151 | 3.8 | 21.2 | 6.2 | 1.9 |
| Fajita Chicken, Tortilla Chips, Salsa, JD Wetherspoon* | 1 Serving/313g | 491 | 20.0 | 157 | 3.5 | 21.9 | 6.5 | 1.9 |
| Fajita Chicken, with Potato Wedges, JD Wetherspoon* | 1 Serving/358g | 554 | 22.0 | 155 | 3.2 | 23.5 | 6.1 | 1.9 |
| Poached Salmon, Tortilla Chips, Salsa, JD Wetherspoon* | 1 Serving/203g | 573 | 33.0 | 282 | 9.9 | 25.8 | 16.2 | 1.6 |
| Poached Salmon, with Potato Wedges, JD Wetherspoon* | 1 Serving/298g | 656 | 34.0 | 220 | 7.1 | 24.2 | 11.5 | 1.5 |
| Poached Salmon & Prawn Salad, JD Wetherspoon* | 1 Wrap/355g | 512 | 34.0 | 144 | 9.8 | 4.5 | 9.6 | 0.5 |
| **YORKSHIRE PUDDING** | | | | | | | | |
| JD Wetherspoon* | 2 Yorkshires/56g | 132 | 5.0 | 236 | 8.2 | 32.9 | 8.2 | 1.1 |
| **KFC** | | | | | | | | |
| **BEANS** | | | | | | | | |
| BBQ, Large, KFC* | 1 Serving/188g | 158 | 1.0 | 84 | 5.3 | 15.1 | 0.7 | 0.0 |
| BBQ, Regular, KFC* | 1 Serving/94g | 79 | 1.0 | 84 | 5.3 | 15.1 | 0.7 | 0.0 |
| **BURGERS** | | | | | | | | |
| Fillet, KFC* | 1 Burger/245g | 441 | 16.0 | 180 | 12.2 | 18.6 | 6.4 | 0.0 |
| Fillet, Mini, KFC* | 1 Burger/114g | 275 | 11.0 | 241 | 14.8 | 23.9 | 9.8 | 0.0 |
| Fillet Tower Burger, KFC* | 1 Burger/163g | 617 | 21.0 | 378 | 24.3 | 41.4 | 12.9 | 0.0 |
| Mini Fillet, Kids, KFC* | 1 Burger/114g | 253 | 6.0 | 222 | 15.8 | 27.0 | 5.6 | 0.0 |
| Tower, KFC* | 1 Burger/210g | 628 | 21.0 | 299 | 15.9 | 30.0 | 9.9 | 0.0 |
| Tower, Zinger, KFC* | 1 Burger/264g | 655 | 33.0 | 248 | 11.2 | 24.3 | 12.4 | 0.0 |

| INFO/WEIGHT | Measure | per Measure | | Nutrition Values per 100g / 100ml | | | | |
|---|---|---|---|---|---|---|---|---|
| | | KCAL | FAT | KCAL | PROT | CARB | FAT | FIBRE |

# KFC
## BURGERS
| | | | | | | | | |
|---|---|---|---|---|---|---|---|---|
| Zinger, Fillet, KFC* | 1 Serving/185g | 445 | 20.0 | 241 | 13.9 | 22.4 | 10.6 | 1.4 |
| Zinger, KFC* | 1 Burger/219g | 481 | 21.0 | 220 | 12.2 | 22.0 | 9.5 | 0.0 |

## CHEESECAKE
| | | | | | | | | |
|---|---|---|---|---|---|---|---|---|
| Boysenberry, Chateau, KFC* | 1 Serving/85g | 196 | 9.0 | 230 | 4.0 | 30.0 | 11.0 | 0.0 |
| Cookies & Cream, KFC* | 1 Serving/80g | 261 | 17.0 | 326 | 4.3 | 29.1 | 21.4 | 0.0 |

## CHICKEN
| | | | | | | | | |
|---|---|---|---|---|---|---|---|---|
| Breast, Original Recipe, KFC* | 1 Breast/137g | 285 | 13.0 | 207 | 24.9 | 5.6 | 9.7 | 0.0 |
| Drumsticks, Original Recipe, KFC* | 1 Drumstick/95g | 161 | 9.0 | 170 | 11.9 | 9.1 | 10.0 | 0.0 |
| Popcorn, Kids, KFC* | 1 Portion/66g | 144 | 8.0 | 219 | 14.1 | 13.2 | 12.7 | 0.0 |
| Popcorn, Large, KFC* | 1 Serving/186g | 494 | 30.0 | 262 | 17.5 | 13.5 | 15.8 | 0.0 |
| Popcorn, Regular, KFC* | 1 Serving/122g | 307 | 19.0 | 251 | 16.8 | 12.9 | 15.2 | 0.0 |
| Ribs, Original Recipe, KFC* | 1 Rib/126g | 238 | 13.0 | 188 | 19.8 | 4.1 | 10.6 | 0.0 |
| Strips, Crispy, KFC* | 1 Strip/46g | 112 | 5.0 | 243 | 15.4 | 20.4 | 11.7 | 0.0 |
| Thighs, Original Recipe, KFC* | 1 Thigh/134g | 218 | 14.0 | 162 | 12.6 | 4.4 | 10.6 | 0.0 |
| Wings, Hot, KFC* | 1 Wing/58g | 102 | 7.0 | 175 | 9.4 | 7.5 | 12.1 | 0.0 |
| Wings, Original Recipe, KFC* | 1 Wing/17g | 150 | 8.0 | 862 | 78.5 | 39.2 | 45.4 | 0.0 |

## COLESLAW
| | | | | | | | | |
|---|---|---|---|---|---|---|---|---|
| Large, KFC* | 1 Serving/200g | 268 | 22.0 | 134 | 0.8 | 9.5 | 11.2 | 0.0 |
| Regular, KFC* | 1 Serving/100g | 134 | 11.0 | 134 | 0.8 | 9.5 | 11.2 | 0.0 |

## CORN
| | | | | | | | | |
|---|---|---|---|---|---|---|---|---|
| Cobs, Cobette, KFC* | 1 Serving/70g | 141 | 8.0 | 201 | 4.3 | 20.1 | 12.1 | 0.0 |

## DRESSING
| | | | | | | | | |
|---|---|---|---|---|---|---|---|---|
| Caesar, KFC* | 1 Sachet/35g | 103 | 11.0 | 295 | 19.2 | 2.7 | 31.1 | 0.0 |
| French, KFC* | 1 Sachet/45g | 30 | 1.0 | 66 | 0.2 | 2.9 | 2.9 | 0.0 |
| Vinaigrette, Low Fat, KFC* | 1 Sachet/35g | 21 | 1.0 | 59 | 0.5 | 8.9 | 2.2 | 0.0 |
| Yoghurt, Coriander & Chilli, KFC* | 1 Sachet/45g | 166 | 16.0 | 369 | 2.2 | 9.3 | 36.0 | 0.0 |

## FRIES
| | | | | | | | | |
|---|---|---|---|---|---|---|---|---|
| Large, KFC* | 1 Serving/162g | 375 | 19.0 | 231 | 3.1 | 32.4 | 11.9 | 0.0 |
| Regular, KFC* | 1 Serving/111g | 257 | 13.0 | 232 | 3.1 | 32.4 | 11.9 | 0.0 |

## GRAVY
| | | | | | | | | |
|---|---|---|---|---|---|---|---|---|
| Large, KFC* | 1 Serving/204g | 144 | 8.0 | 71 | 2.3 | 7.3 | 3.9 | 0.0 |
| Regular, KFC* | 1 Serving/102g | 72 | 4.0 | 71 | 2.3 | 7.3 | 3.9 | 0.0 |

## ICE CREAM
| | | | | | | | | |
|---|---|---|---|---|---|---|---|---|
| Avalanche, KFC* | 1 Pot/28g | 114 | 5.0 | 407 | 10.4 | 51.4 | 18.2 | 0.0 |
| Soft, KFC* | 1 Serving/110g | 171 | 7.0 | 155 | 3.7 | 20.6 | 6.4 | 0.0 |

## PIE
| | | | | | | | | |
|---|---|---|---|---|---|---|---|---|
| Apple Slice, Colonel's Pies, KFC* | 1 Slice/113g | 310 | 14.0 | 274 | 1.7 | 38.9 | 12.3 | 0.0 |
| Strawberry Creme, Slice, KFC* | 1 Slice/78g | 279 | 15.0 | 358 | 5.4 | 41.0 | 19.2 | 2.5 |

## SALAD
| | | | | | | | | |
|---|---|---|---|---|---|---|---|---|
| Chicken, Original Recipe, No Dressing, KFC* | 1 Av Salad/292g | 270 | 10.0 | 92 | 9.0 | 7.0 | 3.3 | 0.0 |
| Chicken, Zinger, No Dressing, KFC* | 1 Av Salad/285g | 307 | 15.0 | 108 | 7.8 | 8.0 | 5.2 | 0.0 |
| Potato, KFC* | 1 Portion/160g | 229 | 14.0 | 143 | 2.5 | 14.3 | 8.7 | 1.8 |

## WRAP
| | | | | | | | | |
|---|---|---|---|---|---|---|---|---|
| Twister, Salsa, Toasted, KFC* | 1 Av Wrap/222g | 516 | 25.0 | 232 | 8.7 | 24.6 | 11.2 | 0.0 |
| Twister, Toasted, KFC* | 1 Av Wrap/217g | 509 | 25.0 | 235 | 8.9 | 24.6 | 11.5 | 0.0 |
| Wrapstar, KFC* | 1 Wrapstar/239g | 642 | 37.0 | 269 | 11.4 | 25.9 | 15.3 | 0.0 |

# KRISPY KREME
## CAKE
| | | | | | | | | |
|---|---|---|---|---|---|---|---|---|
| Chocolate, Glazed, Krispy Kreme* | 1 Doughnut/80g | 309 | 14.0 | 387 | 4.0 | 55.0 | 17.0 | 3.0 |
| Vanilla, Krispy Kreme* | 1 Doughnut/80g | 315 | 14.0 | 391 | 4.0 | 57.0 | 17.0 | 2.0 |

## DOUGHNUTS
| | | | | | | | | |
|---|---|---|---|---|---|---|---|---|
| Blueberry, Powdered, Filled, Krispy Kreme* | 1 Doughnut/86g | 307 | 17.0 | 357 | 7.0 | 36.0 | 20.0 | 5.0 |

| | Measure INFO/WEIGHT | per Measure KCAL | FAT | Nutrition Values per 100g / 100ml KCAL | PROT | CARB | FAT | FIBRE |
|---|---|---|---|---|---|---|---|---|
| **KRISPY KREME** | | | | | | | | |
| **DOUGHNUTS** | | | | | | | | |
| Chocolate Iced, Creme Filled, Krispy Kreme* | 1 Doughnut/87g | 339 | 17.0 | 390 | 6.0 | 47.0 | 20.0 | 4.0 |
| Chocolate Iced, Custard Filled, Krispy Kreme* | 1 Doughnut/87g | 307 | 15.0 | 353 | 6.0 | 43.0 | 17.0 | 2.0 |
| Chocolate Iced, Glazed, Krispy Kreme* | 1 Doughnut/66g | 270 | 13.0 | 410 | 5.0 | 51.0 | 20.0 | 3.0 |
| Chocolate Iced, with Creme Filling, Krispy Kreme* | 1 Doughnut/87g | 350 | 21.0 | 402 | 3.0 | 42.0 | 24.0 | 1.0 |
| Chocolate Iced, with Sprinkles, Krispy Kreme* | 1 Doughnut/71g | 293 | 13.0 | 413 | 5.0 | 56.0 | 19.0 | 3.0 |
| Cinnamon Apple, Filled, Krispy Kreme* | 1 Doughnut/81g | 269 | 15.0 | 332 | 7.0 | 37.0 | 18.0 | 5.0 |
| Cruller, Glazed, Krispy Kreme* | 1 Doughnut/54g | 254 | 16.0 | 471 | 4.0 | 49.0 | 29.0 | 3.0 |
| Glazed, with a Creme Filling, Krispy Kreme* | 1 Doughnut/86g | 309 | 15.0 | 359 | 5.0 | 44.0 | 18.0 | 4.0 |
| Lemon Filled, Glazed, Krispy Kreme* | 1 Doughnut/66g | 218 | 11.0 | 331 | 5.0 | 41.0 | 16.0 | 4.0 |
| Maple Iced, Krispy Kreme* | 1 Doughnut/66g | 279 | 15.0 | 422 | 5.0 | 49.0 | 23.0 | 3.0 |
| Original, Glazed, Krispy Kreme* | 1 Doughnut/52g | 217 | 13.0 | 417 | 6.0 | 43.0 | 25.0 | 4.0 |
| Raspberry, Glazed, Krispy Kreme* | 1 Doughnut/86g | 307 | 14.0 | 357 | 6.0 | 47.0 | 16.0 | 4.0 |
| Sour Cream, Krispy Kreme* | 1 Doughnut/80g | 340 | 18.0 | 425 | 4.0 | 53.0 | 23.0 | 1.0 |
| Strawberry Filled, Powdered, Krispy Kreme* | 1 Doughnut/74g | 248 | 13.0 | 335 | 7.0 | 36.0 | 18.0 | 5.0 |
| **MCDONALD'S** | | | | | | | | |
| **APPLES** | | | | | | | | |
| McDonald's* | 1 Apple/140g | 59 | 0.0 | 42 | 0.3 | 10.0 | 0.0 | 2.2 |
| **BAGEL** | | | | | | | | |
| Plain, Toasted, McDonald's* | 1 Bagel/85g | 210 | 1.0 | 248 | 9.0 | 50.0 | 1.0 | 4.0 |
| Toasted, with Strawberry Jam, McDonald's* | 1 Bagel/105g | 260 | 1.0 | 248 | 8.0 | 52.0 | 1.0 | 3.0 |
| with Bacon, Egg & Cheese, McDonald's* | 1 Bagel/190g | 500 | 23.0 | 263 | 13.0 | 26.0 | 12.0 | 2.0 |
| with Butter & Jam, McDonald's* | 1 Bagel/122g | 399 | 10.0 | 326 | 5.9 | 58.8 | 8.3 | 2.2 |
| with Flora & Jam, McDonald's* | 1 Bagel/120g | 369 | 7.0 | 305 | 6.0 | 59.4 | 5.7 | 2.2 |
| with Philadelphia, McDonald's* | 1 Bagel/125g | 317 | 6.0 | 254 | 7.7 | 47.5 | 4.7 | 2.1 |
| with Sausage, Egg & Cheese, McDonald's* | 1 Bagel/205g | 545 | 27.0 | 266 | 14.0 | 22.0 | 13.0 | 2.0 |
| with Sausage & Egg, McDonald's* | 1 Bagel/207g | 551 | 27.0 | 266 | 13.3 | 23.3 | 12.8 | 1.6 |
| **BREAKFAST** | | | | | | | | |
| Big Breakfast, McDonald's* | 1 Breakfast/264g | 595 | 34.0 | 225 | 11.0 | 15.0 | 13.0 | 1.0 |
| Big Breakfast Bun, McDonald's* | 1 Bun/242g | 571 | 32.0 | 236 | 13.0 | 15.1 | 13.3 | 0.9 |
| **BREAKFAST CEREAL** | | | | | | | | |
| Porridge, Oatso Simple, & Jam, McDonald's* | 1 Serving/232g | 246 | 5.0 | 106 | 4.0 | 17.0 | 2.3 | 0.9 |
| Porridge, Oatso Simple, & Sugar, McDonald's* | 1 Serving/215g | 205 | 5.0 | 95 | 4.3 | 13.7 | 2.5 | 0.9 |
| Porridge, Oatso Simple, Plain, McDonald's* | 1 Serving/233g | 214 | 5.0 | 92 | 5.0 | 13.0 | 2.0 | 1.0 |
| **BROWNIE** | | | | | | | | |
| Belgian Bliss, McDonald's* | 1 Serving/85g | 390 | 22.0 | 459 | 8.0 | 51.0 | 26.0 | 2.0 |
| Chocolate Chip, McMini, McDonald's* | 1 Brownie/19g | 68 | 2.0 | 360 | 4.9 | 58.8 | 12.7 | 1.9 |
| **BURGERS** | | | | | | | | |
| Arizona, Grande, McDonald's* | 1 Burger/251g | 655 | 40.0 | 261 | 16.0 | 15.0 | 16.0 | 2.0 |
| Bacon Cheeseburger, McDonald's* | 1 Burger/136g | 368 | 17.0 | 270 | 16.0 | 23.6 | 12.2 | 2.3 |
| Bacon McDouble, with Cheese, McDonald's* | 1 Burger/141g | 372 | 19.0 | 264 | 16.1 | 19.6 | 13.5 | 2.2 |
| Beef, Deluxe, McDonald's* | 1 Burger/265g | 650 | 34.0 | 245 | 14.0 | 18.0 | 13.0 | 2.0 |
| Beef, Deluxe, with Bacon, McDonald's* | 1 Burger/274g | 689 | 38.0 | 252 | 15.0 | 18.0 | 14.0 | 2.0 |
| Big Mac, McDonald's* | 1 Burger/216g | 496 | 24.0 | 229 | 13.0 | 19.0 | 11.0 | 2.0 |
| Big Mac, No Sauce, No Cheese, McDonald's* | 1 Sandwich/181g | 400 | 16.0 | 221 | 12.1 | 23.8 | 8.8 | 1.1 |
| Big Tasty, McDonald's* | 1 Burger/348g | 804 | 50.0 | 231 | 11.7 | 14.6 | 14.5 | 1.6 |
| Big Tasty, with Bacon, McDonald's* | 1 Burger/360g | 886 | 58.0 | 246 | 13.0 | 14.0 | 16.0 | 2.0 |
| Bigger Big Mac, McDonald's* | 1 Burger/325g | 714 | 34.0 | 220 | 12.9 | 18.5 | 10.5 | 1.6 |
| Cheeseburger, Bacon, McDonald's* | 1 Burger/127g | 336 | 15.0 | 264 | 16.0 | 24.0 | 12.0 | 2.0 |
| Cheeseburger, Double, McDonald's* | 1 Burger/169g | 446 | 22.0 | 263 | 17.0 | 19.0 | 13.0 | 1.0 |
| Cheeseburger, McDonald's* | 1 Burger/119g | 300 | 12.0 | 253 | 14.3 | 26.2 | 10.1 | 2.5 |
| Chicken Deluxe, with Bacon, McDonald's* | 1 Burger/256g | 570 | 23.0 | 223 | 13.0 | 24.0 | 9.0 | 2.0 |
| Chicken Legend, with Cool Mayo, McDonald's* | 1 Burger/218g | 550 | 22.0 | 252 | 14.0 | 28.0 | 10.0 | 2.0 |

| | INFO/WEIGHT | KCAL | FAT | KCAL | PROT | CARB | FAT | FIBRE |
|---|---|---|---|---|---|---|---|---|
| **MCDONALD'S** | | | | | | | | |
| **BURGERS** | | | | | | | | |
| Chicken Legend, with Spicy Tomato Salsa, McDonald's* | 1 Burger/224g | 516 | 13.0 | 230 | 13.0 | 30.0 | 6.0 | 2.0 |
| Filet-O-Fish, McDonald's* | 1 Burger/147g | 341 | 16.0 | 232 | 10.0 | 24.0 | 11.0 | 1.0 |
| Filet-O-Fish, No Tartar Sauce, McDonald's* | 1 Burger/124g | 290 | 9.0 | 234 | 12.1 | 30.6 | 7.3 | 0.8 |
| Grilled Chicken Caprese, McDonald's* | 1 Burger/275g | 470 | 21.0 | 171 | 12.5 | 15.0 | 7.7 | 2.1 |
| Hamburger, McDonald's* | 1 Burger/104g | 249 | 8.0 | 240 | 13.0 | 29.0 | 8.0 | 3.0 |
| Little Chorizo Melt, McDonald's* | 1 Burger/128g | 330 | 17.0 | 258 | 14.0 | 23.0 | 13.0 | 2.0 |
| McChicken Grill with BBQ Sauce, McDonald's* | 1 Sandwich/215g | 309 | 5.0 | 144 | 12.1 | 18.1 | 2.5 | 2.2 |
| McChicken Premiere, McDonald's* | 1 Burger/221g | 464 | 17.0 | 210 | 10.4 | 24.4 | 7.7 | 1.4 |
| McChicken Sandwich, McDonald's* | 1 Sandwich/170g | 380 | 16.0 | 223 | 9.4 | 25.3 | 9.4 | 2.3 |
| Quarter Pounder, Bacon with Cheese, McDonald's* | 1 Burger/230g | 592 | 33.0 | 259 | 16.5 | 15.4 | 14.5 | 1.3 |
| Quarter Pounder, Deluxe, Bacon & Cheese, McDonald's* | 1 Burger/229g | 592 | 33.0 | 259 | 16.5 | 15.4 | 14.5 | 1.3 |
| Quarter Pounder, Deluxe, McDonald's* | 1 Burger/253g | 521 | 27.0 | 206 | 11.4 | 16.1 | 10.6 | 1.7 |
| Quarter Pounder, Double, with Cheese, McDonald's* | 1 Burger/275g | 710 | 40.0 | 259 | 19.5 | 12.2 | 14.7 | 1.1 |
| Quarter Pounder, McDonald's* | 1 Burger/178g | 424 | 19.0 | 238 | 14.5 | 20.9 | 10.7 | 2.1 |
| Quarter Pounder, with Cheese, McDonald's* | 1 Burger/194g | 500 | 25.0 | 257 | 17.0 | 19.0 | 13.0 | 2.0 |
| Steak Premiere, McDonald's* | 1 Burger/229g | 453 | 14.0 | 198 | 14.9 | 19.4 | 6.2 | 1.6 |
| **BURGERS VEGETARIAN** | | | | | | | | |
| Vegetable, Deluxe, McDonald's* | 1 Burger/181g | 411 | 16.0 | 227 | 6.0 | 30.0 | 9.0 | 6.0 |
| **BUTTER** | | | | | | | | |
| McDonald's* | 1 Pack/11g | 85 | 9.0 | 752 | 0.0 | 0.0 | 80.0 | 0.0 |
| **CADBURY BYTE** | | | | | | | | |
| McMini, McDonald's* | 1 Byte/14g | 67 | 3.0 | 478 | 6.5 | 64.7 | 20.7 | 1.7 |
| **CAKE** | | | | | | | | |
| Birthday, McDonald's* | 1 Portion/158g | 640 | 23.0 | 405 | 2.7 | 65.4 | 14.3 | 1.0 |
| **CARROTS** | | | | | | | | |
| Sticks, McDonald's* | 1 Bag/80g | 24 | 0.0 | 30 | 0.0 | 8.0 | 0.0 | 2.0 |
| **CHEESE** | | | | | | | | |
| Soft, Philadelphia, Light, McDonald's* | 1 Serving/35g | 55 | 4.0 | 157 | 9.0 | 3.0 | 11.0 | 0.0 |
| **CHICKEN** | | | | | | | | |
| McNuggets, McDonald's* | 4 Pieces/71g | 175 | 9.0 | 245 | 14.0 | 18.0 | 13.0 | 1.0 |
| McNuggets, McDonald's* | 6 Pieces/106g | 260 | 14.0 | 245 | 14.0 | 18.0 | 13.0 | 1.0 |
| McNuggets, McDonald's* | 9 Pieces/159g | 390 | 21.0 | 245 | 14.0 | 18.0 | 13.0 | 1.0 |
| Selects, 3 Pieces, McDonald's* | 3 Pieces/131g | 366 | 20.0 | 280 | 16.0 | 20.0 | 15.0 | 1.0 |
| Selects, 5 Pieces, McDonald's* | 5 Pieces/219g | 612 | 33.0 | 280 | 16.0 | 20.0 | 15.0 | 1.0 |
| **COFFEE** | | | | | | | | |
| Black, Large, McDonald's* | 1 Serving/428ml | 0 | 0.0 | 0 | 0.0 | 0.0 | 0.0 | 0.0 |
| Black, Regular, McDonald's* | 1 Serving/312ml | 0 | 0.0 | 0 | 0.0 | 0.0 | 0.0 | 0.0 |
| Cappuccino, Large, McDonald's* | 1 Serving/307ml | 120 | 3.0 | 39 | 3.0 | 4.0 | 1.0 | 0.0 |
| Cappuccino, Regular, McDonald's* | 1 Serving/231ml | 90 | 2.0 | 39 | 3.0 | 4.0 | 1.0 | 0.0 |
| Latte, Large, McDonald's* | 1 Serving/451ml | 185 | 5.0 | 41 | 3.0 | 4.0 | 1.0 | 0.0 |
| Latte, Regular, McDonald's* | 1 Serving/337ml | 135 | 3.0 | 40 | 3.0 | 4.0 | 1.0 | 0.0 |
| White, Large, McDonald's* | 1 Serving/428ml | 30 | 0.0 | 7 | 0.0 | 1.0 | 0.0 | 0.0 |
| White, Regular, McDonald's* | 1 Serving/313ml | 25 | 0.0 | 8 | 1.0 | 1.0 | 0.0 | 0.0 |
| **COLA** | | | | | | | | |
| Coca-Cola, Diet, McDonald's* | 1 Super/750ml | 7 | 0.0 | 1 | 0.0 | 0.0 | 0.0 | 0.0 |
| Coca-Cola, McDonald's* | 1 Super/750ml | 322 | 0.0 | 43 | 0.0 | 11.0 | 0.0 | 0.0 |
| Coke, Zero, McDonald's* | 1 Large/300ml | 3 | 0.0 | 1 | 0.0 | 0.0 | 0.0 | 0.0 |
| **CREAMER** | | | | | | | | |
| Uht, McDonald's* | 1 Cup/14ml | 17 | 1.0 | 123 | 4.2 | 4.2 | 10.0 | 0.0 |
| **CROUTONS** | | | | | | | | |
| McDonald's* | 1 Sachet/14g | 60 | 2.0 | 426 | 11.8 | 63.4 | 14.0 | 2.7 |

## MCDONALD'S

| | Measure INFO/WEIGHT | per Measure KCAL | FAT | Nutrition Values per 100g / 100ml KCAL | PROT | CARB | FAT | FIBRE |
|---|---|---|---|---|---|---|---|---|
| **DIP** | | | | | | | | |
| BBQ, McDonald's* | 1 Pot/50g | 83 | 0.0 | 166 | 0.0 | 37.0 | 0.0 | 0.0 |
| Caramelised Onion, McDonald's* | 1 Dip/31g | 45 | 2.0 | 144 | 3.0 | 19.0 | 6.0 | 3.0 |
| Sour Cream & Chive, McDonald's* | 1 Pot/50g | 150 | 16.0 | 300 | 2.0 | 2.0 | 32.0 | 4.0 |
| Sweet Chilli, McDonald's* | 1 Pot/31g | 80 | 1.0 | 256 | 0.0 | 58.0 | 3.0 | 0.0 |
| **DOUGHNUTS** | | | | | | | | |
| Chocolate Donut, McDonald's* | 1 Donut/79g | 345 | 16.0 | 437 | 5.7 | 43.8 | 20.5 | 1.0 |
| Chocolate Donut, McMini, McDonald's* | 1 Donut/17g | 64 | 3.0 | 375 | 6.8 | 46.9 | 17.8 | 1.6 |
| Cinnamon Donut, McDonald's* | 1 Donut/72g | 302 | 18.0 | 419 | 5.1 | 43.1 | 25.1 | 3.8 |
| Sugared Donut, McDonald's* | 1 Donut/49g | 175 | 9.0 | 357 | 6.0 | 45.0 | 18.0 | 2.0 |
| **DRESSING** | | | | | | | | |
| Balsamic, Low Fat, McDonald's* | 1 Sachet/33g | 20 | 1.0 | 60 | 0.0 | 9.0 | 3.0 | 0.0 |
| Caesar, Low Fat, McDonald's* | 1 Sachet/80g | 55 | 2.0 | 68 | 2.0 | 10.0 | 2.0 | 0.0 |
| French, Low Fat, McDonald's* | 1 Serving/22g | 13 | 1.0 | 58 | 0.5 | 7.1 | 2.6 | 1.0 |
| Ranch, Salad, McDonald's* | 1 Sachet/79ml | 107 | 7.0 | 136 | 3.1 | 12.3 | 8.3 | 0.8 |
| **FANTA** | | | | | | | | |
| Orange, McDonald's* | 1 Super/750ml | 315 | 0.0 | 42 | 0.0 | 10.0 | 0.0 | 0.0 |
| **FISH FINGERS** | | | | | | | | |
| McDonald's* | 3 Fingers/74g | 172 | 8.0 | 232 | 15.0 | 19.0 | 11.0 | 1.0 |
| **FLATBREAD** | | | | | | | | |
| Chicken Salsa, McDonald's* | 1 Serving/100g | 480 | 15.0 | 480 | 27.3 | 57.6 | 15.5 | 0.0 |
| Greek, McDonald's* | 1 Flatbread/100g | 433 | 21.0 | 433 | 21.2 | 47.3 | 20.7 | 3.8 |
| **FRIES** | | | | | | | | |
| French, Large, McDonald's* | 1 Serving/160g | 460 | 22.0 | 288 | 3.0 | 38.0 | 14.0 | 4.0 |
| French, Medium, McDonald's* | 1 Serving/114g | 330 | 16.0 | 289 | 3.0 | 37.0 | 14.0 | 4.0 |
| French, Small, McDonald's* | 1 Serving/79g | 228 | 11.0 | 288 | 2.0 | 38.0 | 14.0 | 4.0 |
| **FRUIT** | | | | | | | | |
| & Yoghurt, McDonald's* | 1 Serving/144g | 138 | 3.0 | 96 | 2.8 | 15.9 | 1.9 | 1.1 |
| Bag, Apple & Grape, McDonald's* | 1 Bag/80g | 43 | 0.0 | 54 | 0.3 | 13.0 | 0.1 | 2.3 |
| Bag, McDonald's* | 1 Pack/80g | 40 | 0.0 | 50 | 0.0 | 13.0 | 0.0 | 3.0 |
| Bag, Pineapple & Grape, McDonald's* | 1 Pack/80g | 38 | 0.0 | 47 | 0.4 | 11.1 | 0.2 | 1.2 |
| **HASH BROWNS** | | | | | | | | |
| McDonald's* | 1 Hash Brown/57g | 140 | 8.0 | 246 | 2.0 | 28.0 | 14.0 | 4.0 |
| **HOT CHOCOLATE** | | | | | | | | |
| McDonald's* | 1 Serving/330ml | 164 | 4.0 | 50 | 0.7 | 8.8 | 1.1 | 0.0 |
| **HOT DOG** | | | | | | | | |
| & Ketchup, McDonald's* | 1 Serving/116g | 296 | 15.0 | 255 | 9.6 | 25.8 | 12.6 | 1.3 |
| **ICE CREAM** | | | | | | | | |
| Smartie, McDonald's* | 1 Pot/120g | 260 | 10.0 | 216 | 3.4 | 33.3 | 7.9 | 1.0 |
| **ICE CREAM CONE** | | | | | | | | |
| McDonald's* | 1 Cone/90g | 141 | 5.0 | 156 | 4.5 | 24.4 | 5.0 | 0.0 |
| with Flake, McDonald's* | 1 Cone/107g | 204 | 8.0 | 191 | 4.8 | 27.0 | 7.2 | 0.0 |
| **JAM** | | | | | | | | |
| Strawberry, McDonald's* | 1 Pack/20g | 50 | 0.0 | 250 | 0.0 | 60.0 | 0.0 | 0.0 |
| **JUICE** | | | | | | | | |
| Fruit Shoot, Robinsons, McDonald's* | 1 Bottle200ml | 10 | 0.0 | 5 | 0.0 | 1.0 | 0.0 | 0.0 |
| Tropicana, McDonald's* | 1 Bottle/250ml | 107 | 0.0 | 43 | 1.0 | 9.0 | 0.0 | 0.0 |
| **KETCHUP** | | | | | | | | |
| Tomato, McDonald's* | 1 Portion/23g | 25 | 0.0 | 109 | 0.0 | 26.0 | 0.0 | 0.0 |
| **LEMONADE** | | | | | | | | |
| Sprite, Z, McDonald's* | 1 Lge/500ml | 5 | 0.0 | 1 | 0.0 | 0.0 | 0.0 | 0.0 |
| **MARGARINE** | | | | | | | | |
| Flora, Original, McDonald's* | 1 Portion/10g | 55 | 6.0 | 550 | 0.0 | 0.0 | 60.0 | 0.0 |

## MCDONALD'S

| | Measure INFO/WEIGHT | per Measure KCAL | FAT | Nutrition Values per 100g / 100ml KCAL | PROT | CARB | FAT | FIBRE |
|---|---|---|---|---|---|---|---|---|
| **MCFLURRY** | | | | | | | | |
| After Eight, McDonald's* | 1 McFlurry/204g | 381 | 11.0 | 187 | 2.8 | 31.4 | 5.4 | 0.5 |
| Cadbury, Shortcake, Limited Edition, McDonald's* | 1 McFlurry/206g | 385 | 14.0 | 187 | 3.0 | 28.0 | 7.0 | 1.0 |
| Chocolate, Cornetto, McDonald's* | 1 McFlurry/207g | 400 | 17.0 | 193 | 3.0 | 29.0 | 8.0 | 1.0 |
| Cornetto, Mint Choc, McDonald's* | 1 McFlurry/207g | 400 | 17.0 | 193 | 3.0 | 29.0 | 8.0 | 1.0 |
| Creme Egg, Cadbury's, McDonald's* | 1 McFlurry/203g | 381 | 13.0 | 188 | 2.9 | 29.8 | 6.3 | 0.5 |
| Crunchie, McDonald's* | 1 McFlurry/185g | 330 | 11.0 | 178 | 3.0 | 28.0 | 6.0 | 1.0 |
| Dairy Milk, McDonald's* | 1 McFlurry/184g | 340 | 13.0 | 184 | 3.0 | 28.0 | 7.0 | 1.0 |
| Dairy Milk, with Caramel, McDonald's* | 1 McFlurry/206g | 385 | 13.0 | 187 | 2.9 | 29.1 | 6.3 | 0.0 |
| Jammie Dodger, McDonald's* | 1 McFlurry/128g | 256 | 8.0 | 200 | 3.9 | 33.6 | 6.4 | 0.3 |
| Rolo, McDonald's* | 1 McFlurry/205g | 390 | 13.0 | 190 | 4.0 | 29.2 | 6.5 | 0.1 |
| Smarties, McDonald's* | 1 McFlurry/185g | 330 | 11.0 | 178 | 3.0 | 28.0 | 6.0 | 1.0 |
| Strawberry, Cornetto, McDonald's* | 1 McFlurry/207g | 375 | 12.0 | 181 | 3.0 | 29.0 | 6.0 | 0.0 |
| Toffee Swirl, Oreo Cookie, McDonald's* | 1 McFlurry/206g | 400 | 12.0 | 194 | 3.0 | 31.0 | 6.0 | 1.0 |
| Yorkie, McDonald's* | 1 McFlurry/204g | 379 | 15.0 | 186 | 3.4 | 27.0 | 7.3 | 0.8 |
| **MCMUFFIN** | | | | | | | | |
| Bacon & Egg, Double, McDonald's* | 1 McMuffin/226g | 553 | 29.0 | 244 | 15.0 | 16.0 | 13.0 | 1.0 |
| Bacon & Egg, McDonald's* | 1 McMuffin/143g | 340 | 17.0 | 237 | 14.0 | 18.0 | 12.0 | 1.0 |
| Egg, McDonald's* | 1 McMuffin/127g | 281 | 13.0 | 221 | 12.2 | 20.4 | 10.1 | 3.2 |
| Sausage & Egg, Double, McDonald's* | 1 McMuffin/222g | 560 | 33.0 | 252 | 16.0 | 12.0 | 15.0 | 1.0 |
| Sausage & Egg, McDonald's* | 1 McMuffin/174g | 420 | 23.0 | 242 | 14.0 | 16.0 | 13.0 | 1.0 |
| Scrambled Egg, McDonald's* | 1 McMuffin/147g | 294 | 14.0 | 200 | 10.9 | 17.5 | 9.6 | 1.3 |
| **MELT** | | | | | | | | |
| Toasted Ham & Cheese, McDonald's* | 1 Serving/100g | 239 | 8.0 | 239 | 11.2 | 30.6 | 8.0 | 1.8 |
| **MILK** | | | | | | | | |
| Fresh, Portion, McDonald's* | 1 Portion/14ml | 10 | 0.0 | 69 | 0.0 | 7.0 | 0.0 | 0.0 |
| Organic, McDonald's* | 1 Bottle/250ml | 125 | 10.0 | 50 | 4.0 | 5.0 | 4.0 | 0.0 |
| **MILKSHAKE** | | | | | | | | |
| Banana, Large, McDonald's* | 1 Serving/432ml | 545 | 13.0 | 126 | 3.0 | 21.0 | 3.0 | 0.0 |
| Banana, Medium, McDonald's* | 1 Serving/338ml | 425 | 10.0 | 126 | 3.0 | 21.0 | 3.0 | 0.0 |
| Banana, Small, McDonald's* | 1 Serving/178ml | 226 | 5.0 | 127 | 3.0 | 21.0 | 3.0 | 0.0 |
| Cadbury Dairy Milk, Caramel Flavour, Small, McDonald's* | 1 Serving/177ml | 220 | 5.0 | 124 | 3.0 | 20.0 | 3.0 | 1.0 |
| Cadburys Dairy Milk, Caramel, Large, McDonald's* | 1 Serving/417ml | 505 | 17.0 | 121 | 3.0 | 19.0 | 4.0 | 1.0 |
| Cadburys Dairy Milk, Caramel, Medium, McDonald's* | 1 Serving/394ml | 480 | 16.0 | 122 | 3.0 | 19.0 | 4.0 | 1.0 |
| Chocolate, Large, McDonald's* | 1 Serving/431ml | 530 | 13.0 | 123 | 3.0 | 20.0 | 3.0 | 0.0 |
| Chocolate, Medium, McDonald's* | 1 Serving/337ml | 425 | 10.0 | 126 | 3.0 | 21.0 | 3.0 | 0.0 |
| Chocolate, Small, McDonald's* | 1 Serving/177ml | 225 | 5.0 | 127 | 3.0 | 21.0 | 3.0 | 0.0 |
| Strawberry, Large, McDonald's* | 1 Serving/432ml | 540 | 13.0 | 125 | 3.0 | 21.0 | 3.0 | 0.0 |
| Strawberry, Medium, McDonald's* | 1 Serving/336ml | 420 | 10.0 | 125 | 3.0 | 21.0 | 3.0 | 0.0 |
| Strawberry, Small, McDonald's* | 1 Serving/177ml | 220 | 5.0 | 124 | 3.0 | 21.0 | 3.0 | 0.0 |
| Vanilla, Large, McDonald's* | 1 Serving/431ml | 535 | 13.0 | 124 | 3.0 | 21.0 | 3.0 | 0.0 |
| Vanilla, Medium, McDonald's* | 1 Serving/336ml | 420 | 10.0 | 125 | 3.0 | 21.0 | 3.0 | 0.0 |
| Vanilla, Small, McDonald's* | 1 Serving/177ml | 220 | 5.0 | 124 | 3.0 | 21.0 | 3.0 | 0.0 |
| **MOZZARELLA** | | | | | | | | |
| Dippers, McDonald's* | 3 Dippers/85g | 265 | 14.0 | 312 | 13.0 | 27.0 | 16.0 | 1.0 |
| **MUFFIN** | | | | | | | | |
| Blueberry, Low Fat, McDonald's* | 1 Muffin/126g | 300 | 3.0 | 238 | 5.0 | 50.0 | 2.0 | 2.0 |
| Buttered, McDonald's* | 1 Muffin/63g | 157 | 4.0 | 250 | 8.6 | 40.7 | 5.9 | 2.9 |
| Buttered, with Preserve, McDonald's* | 1 Muffin/93g | 234 | 4.0 | 252 | 5.9 | 48.1 | 4.0 | 2.0 |
| Carrot, McDonald's* | 1 Muffin/135g | 360 | 4.0 | 267 | 4.8 | 55.4 | 2.9 | 1.6 |
| Double Chocolate, McDonald's* | 1 Muffin/123g | 425 | 18.0 | 346 | 6.0 | 48.0 | 15.0 | 2.0 |
| Triple Chocolate, McDonald's* | 1 Muffin/138g | 581 | 34.0 | 420 | 4.7 | 45.7 | 24.3 | 0.9 |

# MCDONALD'S

| | Measure INFO/WEIGHT | per Measure KCAL | FAT | Nutrition Values per 100g / 100ml KCAL | PROT | CARB | FAT | FIBRE |
|---|---|---|---|---|---|---|---|---|
| **ONION RINGS** | | | | | | | | |
| McDonald's* | 1 Serving/80g | 180 | 10.0 | 225 | 4.0 | 26.0 | 13.0 | 1.0 |
| **PANCAKE** | | | | | | | | |
| & Sausage, McDonald's* | 1 Portion/262g | 665 | 29.0 | 254 | 11.0 | 28.0 | 11.0 | 2.0 |
| & Syrup, McDonald's* | 1 Pack/209g | 616 | 15.0 | 294 | 4.0 | 52.0 | 7.0 | 2.0 |
| **PIE** | | | | | | | | |
| Apple, McDonald's* | 1 Pie/80g | 231 | 13.0 | 289 | 2.0 | 35.0 | 16.0 | 0.0 |
| **POTATO WEDGES** | | | | | | | | |
| McDonald's* | 1 Portion/177g | 349 | 18.0 | 197 | 3.3 | 23.3 | 10.0 | 2.8 |
| **QUORN*** | | | | | | | | |
| Burger, Premiere, McDonald's* | 1 Burger/210g | 311 | 6.0 | 148 | 9.1 | 24.2 | 2.9 | 2.7 |
| **ROLL** | | | | | | | | |
| Bacon, McBacon, McDonald's* | 1 Roll/122g | 349 | 14.0 | 286 | 13.5 | 30.5 | 11.5 | 1.7 |
| Bacon, with Brown Sauce, McDonald's* | 1 Roll/118g | 328 | 8.0 | 278 | 15.0 | 37.0 | 7.0 | 2.0 |
| Bacon, with Tomato Ketchup, McDonald's* | 1 Roll/126g | 345 | 9.0 | 273 | 15.0 | 36.0 | 7.0 | 2.0 |
| **SALAD** | | | | | | | | |
| Chicken, No Bacon, Grilled, McDonald's* | 1 Salad/261g | 117 | 3.0 | 45 | 7.0 | 2.0 | 1.0 | 1.0 |
| Chicken, with Bacon, Grilled, McDonald's* | 1 Salad/270g | 167 | 5.0 | 62 | 9.0 | 2.0 | 2.0 | 1.0 |
| Crispy Chicken, No Bacon, McDonald's* | 1 Salad/281g | 271 | 11.0 | 96 | 8.0 | 6.0 | 4.0 | 1.0 |
| Crispy Chicken, with Bacon, McDonald's* | 1 Salad/292g | 326 | 15.0 | 111 | 10.0 | 7.0 | 5.0 | 1.0 |
| Garden, Side, No Dressing, McDonald's* | 1 Salad/93g | 10 | 0.0 | 11 | 1.0 | 2.0 | 0.0 | 1.0 |
| Garden, Side, with Balsamic Dressing, McDonald's* | 1 Salad/128g | 91 | 4.0 | 71 | 1.0 | 11.0 | 3.0 | 1.0 |
| Ranch, Grilled Chicken, No Dressing, McDonald's* | 1 Salad/298g | 268 | 13.0 | 90 | 11.4 | 1.4 | 4.2 | 1.0 |
| **SANDWICH** | | | | | | | | |
| Arizona Grande, McDonald's* | 1 Sandwich/252g | 657 | 40.0 | 261 | 16.0 | 15.0 | 16.0 | 2.0 |
| California Classic, McDonald's* | 1 Sandwich/253g | 617 | 33.0 | 244 | 16.0 | 15.0 | 13.0 | 2.0 |
| Chicken, Grilled, McDonald's* | 1 Serving/211g | 367 | 14.0 | 174 | 11.9 | 16.9 | 6.6 | 0.0 |
| Deli, Chicken, Salad, McDonald's* | 1 Sandwich/216g | 408 | 9.0 | 189 | 7.0 | 25.0 | 4.0 | 2.0 |
| Deli, Chicken, Sweet Chilli, McDonald's* | 1 Sandwich/250g | 585 | 20.0 | 234 | 12.0 | 29.0 | 8.0 | 2.0 |
| Deli, Chicken & Bacon, McDonald's* | 1 Sandwich/193g | 420 | 13.0 | 218 | 10.0 | 28.0 | 7.0 | 2.0 |
| Deli, Spicy Veggie, McDonald's* | 1 Sandwich/216g | 545 | 19.0 | 252 | 8.0 | 37.0 | 9.0 | 4.0 |
| The Miami Melt, McDonald's* | 1 Sandwich/252g | 677 | 40.0 | 268 | 16.0 | 15.0 | 16.0 | 2.0 |
| The New York Supreme, McDonald's* | 1 Sandwich/253g | 657 | 40.0 | 260 | 16.0 | 14.0 | 16.0 | 2.0 |
| **SAUCE** | | | | | | | | |
| Barbeque, McDonald's* | 1 Portion/50g | 85 | 1.0 | 170 | 0.0 | 38.0 | 2.0 | 0.0 |
| Curry, Sweet, McDonald's* | 1 Portion/29g | 50 | 1.0 | 171 | 0.0 | 38.0 | 3.0 | 3.0 |
| Mustard, Mild, McDonald's* | 1 Portion/30g | 64 | 4.0 | 212 | 1.0 | 24.8 | 12.1 | 0.0 |
| Sweet & Sour, McDonald's* | 1 Portion/29g | 50 | 0.0 | 172 | 0.0 | 38.0 | 0.0 | 0.0 |
| **SUNDAE** | | | | | | | | |
| Hot Caramel, McDonald's* | 1 Sundae/189g | 357 | 8.0 | 189 | 3.8 | 33.9 | 4.4 | 0.0 |
| Hot Fudge, McDonald's* | 1 Sundae/187g | 352 | 11.0 | 188 | 4.5 | 30.0 | 5.7 | 0.0 |
| No Topping, McDonald's* | 1 Sundae/149g | 219 | 8.0 | 147 | 4.2 | 21.6 | 5.1 | 0.0 |
| Strawberry, McDonald's* | 1 Sundae/214g | 360 | 6.0 | 168 | 2.0 | 33.0 | 3.0 | 0.0 |
| Toffee, McDonald's* | 1 Sunday/180g | 346 | 9.0 | 192 | 3.0 | 34.0 | 5.0 | 1.0 |
| **SYRUP** | | | | | | | | |
| Pancake, McDonald's* | 1 Pot/55g | 190 | 0.0 | 345 | 0.0 | 84.0 | 0.0 | 0.0 |
| **TEA** | | | | | | | | |
| with Milk, McDonald's* | 1 Serving/333ml | 10 | 0.0 | 3 | 0.0 | 1.0 | 0.0 | 0.0 |
| **TOASTIE** | | | | | | | | |
| Ham & Cheese, McDonald's* | 1 Serving/92g | 214 | 8.0 | 233 | 11.5 | 28.0 | 8.4 | 2.2 |
| **WRAP** | | | | | | | | |
| Chicken, Cajun, McDonald's* | 1 Wrap/222g | 585 | 33.0 | 263 | 9.0 | 22.0 | 15.0 | 2.0 |
| Chicken, Snack, McDonald's* | 1 Wrap/112g | 266 | 11.0 | 237 | 10.0 | 29.0 | 10.0 | 2.0 |

|  | Measure INFO/WEIGHT | per Measure KCAL | per Measure FAT | Nutrition Values per 100g / 100ml KCAL | PROT | CARB | FAT | FIBRE |
|---|---|---|---|---|---|---|---|---|
| **MCDONALD'S** | | | | | | | | |
| **WRAP** | | | | | | | | |
| Chicken Fajita, McDonald's* | 1 Wrap/259g | 647 | 31.0 | 250 | 8.9 | 26.7 | 12.0 | 1.2 |
| Oriental, Snack, McDonald's* | 1 Wrap/125g | 260 | 9.0 | 208 | 10.0 | 25.0 | 7.0 | 2.0 |
| **YOGHURT** | | | | | | | | |
| Berry Crunch, McDonald's* | 1 Serving/195g | 224 | 5.0 | 115 | 3.5 | 18.9 | 2.6 | 1.2 |
| Burst, Strawberry, McDonald's* | 1 Yoghurt/40g | 21 | 0.0 | 52 | 2.9 | 11.0 | 0.0 | 0.9 |
| **PIZZA HUT** | | | | | | | | |
| **BACON BITS** | | | | | | | | |
| Pizza Hut* | 1 Serving/12g | 60 | 4.0 | 496 | 8.3 | 48.7 | 29.8 | 0.0 |
| **BEANS** | | | | | | | | |
| Chocolate Coated, Ice Cream Factory, Pizza Hut* | 1 Serving/30g | 142 | 5.0 | 475 | 5.5 | 72.2 | 18.1 | 0.0 |
| **BEETROOT** | | | | | | | | |
| Pizza Hut* | 1 Portion/25g | 14 | 0.0 | 55 | 0.9 | 12.0 | 0.1 | 0.0 |
| **BISCUIT** | | | | | | | | |
| Cafe Curls, Dessert, Pizza Hut* | 1 Biscuit/9g | 38 | 1.0 | 422 | 5.8 | 80.3 | 8.6 | 0.0 |
| **BREAD** | | | | | | | | |
| Ciabatta, Garlic, Pizza Hut* | 2 Pieces/253g | 820 | 32.0 | 324 | 9.1 | 43.4 | 12.7 | 0.0 |
| Garlic, Ciabatta, Pizza Hut* | 2 Ciabattas/253g | 820 | 32.0 | 324 | 9.1 | 43.4 | 12.7 | 1.0 |
| Garlic, Dipsters, Pizza Hut* | 1 Piece/90g | 308 | 14.0 | 342 | 6.8 | 43.1 | 15.8 | 0.0 |
| Garlic, Pizza Hut* | 4 Pieces/120g | 382 | 18.0 | 318 | 6.8 | 38.1 | 15.4 | 0.0 |
| Garlic, with Cheese, Pizza Hut* | 4 Pieces/187g | 569 | 34.0 | 304 | 16.0 | 19.1 | 18.2 | 0.0 |
| **BREADSTICKS** | | | | | | | | |
| Garlic, Pizza Hut* | 1 Stick/50g | 173 | 7.0 | 347 | 9.8 | 46.9 | 13.4 | 1.0 |
| **BRUSCHETTA** | | | | | | | | |
| Light Lunch, Pizza Hut* | 3 Pieces/211g | 369 | 16.0 | 175 | 4.1 | 22.4 | 7.6 | 0.0 |
| **CAKE** | | | | | | | | |
| Chocolate Fudge, Pizza Hut* | 1 Serving/179g | 686 | 32.0 | 384 | 4.2 | 51.4 | 17.9 | 0.0 |
| **CARBONARA** | | | | | | | | |
| Ham, Buffet, Pizza Hut* | 1 Portion/200g | 180 | 5.0 | 90 | 3.4 | 14.4 | 2.3 | 0.0 |
| **CHEESE** | | | | | | | | |
| 4 & Vegetable, Buffet, Pizza Hut* | 1 Portion/200g | 210 | 9.0 | 105 | 4.0 | 12.6 | 4.3 | 0.0 |
| Hard, Grated, Pizza Hut* | 1 Serving/30g | 121 | 9.0 | 404 | 33.0 | 0.1 | 30.0 | 0.0 |
| **CHEESECAKE** | | | | | | | | |
| Chocolate, Pizza Hut* | 1 Serving/63g | 228 | 11.0 | 360 | 5.6 | 44.9 | 17.5 | 0.0 |
| Clotted Cream, Pizza Hut* | 1 Serving/64g | 205 | 10.0 | 323 | 4.6 | 39.3 | 16.4 | 0.0 |
| Lemon & Ginger, Pizza Hut* | 1 Serving/64g | 205 | 10.0 | 323 | 4.2 | 42.4 | 15.2 | 0.0 |
| New York Style, Baked, Pizza Hut* | 1 Slice/113g | 442 | 16.0 | 391 | 6.6 | 62.3 | 14.3 | 0.0 |
| Vanilla, Madagascan, Dessert, Pizza Hut* | 1 Serving/133g | 397 | 18.0 | 298 | 4.8 | 39.2 | 13.6 | 0.0 |
| **CHICKEN** | | | | | | | | |
| Cheesy Jalapeno Poppers, Pizza Hut* | 6 Pieces/150g | 408 | 20.0 | 272 | 5.2 | 32.8 | 13.3 | 0.0 |
| Dippin, Pizza Hut* | 1 Serving/155g | 332 | 14.0 | 214 | 15.7 | 17.1 | 9.3 | 0.0 |
| Goujons, Pizza Hut* | 5 Pieces/169g | 311 | 14.0 | 184 | 17.0 | 11.0 | 8.0 | 1.5 |
| Strips, Breaded, Pizza Hut* | 5 Pieces/200g | 368 | 16.0 | 184 | 17.0 | 11.0 | 8.0 | 0.0 |
| Strips, Hot n Kicking, Pizza Hut* | 7 Pieces/140g | 276 | 13.0 | 197 | 17.0 | 12.0 | 9.0 | 0.0 |
| Wings, BBQ, Pizza Hut* | 6 Pieces/184g | 287 | 18.0 | 156 | 14.9 | 2.3 | 9.8 | 0.0 |
| Wings, BBQ, Saucy, Pizza Hut* | 6 Wings/159g | 355 | 22.0 | 223 | 21.4 | 3.6 | 13.7 | 0.0 |
| Wings, Buffalo, Saucy, Pizza Hut* | 6 Wings/181g | 380 | 22.0 | 209 | 21.0 | 3.7 | 12.2 | 0.0 |
| Wings, Spicy, Crunch, Pizza Hut* | 1 Portion/218g | 510 | 31.0 | 234 | 17.0 | 10.0 | 14.0 | 0.0 |
| Wings, Texan BBQ Chicken, Pizza Hut* | 6 Pieces/159g | 355 | 22.0 | 223 | 21.4 | 3.6 | 13.7 | 0.0 |
| Wings, with Sour Cream & Chive Dip, Pizza Hut* | 1 Pack/178g | 680 | 56.0 | 382 | 22.8 | 1.9 | 31.5 | 1.3 |
| **CHICKEN STRIPS** | | | | | | | | |
| Breaded, & Wedges, 2, Kids, Pizza Hut* | 1 Serving/231g | 386 | 12.0 | 167 | 6.7 | 23.9 | 5.0 | 0.0 |
| Breaded, & Wedges, 3, Kids, Pizza Hut* | 1 Serving/265g | 451 | 14.0 | 170 | 8.1 | 22.2 | 5.4 | 0.0 |

# PIZZA HUT

| | Measure INFO/WEIGHT | per Measure KCAL | FAT | Nutrition Values per 100g / 100ml KCAL | PROT | CARB | FAT | FIBRE |
|---|---|---|---|---|---|---|---|---|
| **CHICKEN STRIPS** | | | | | | | | |
| Breaded, Wrap Factory, 2, Kids, Pizza Hut* | 1 Serving/247g | 434 | 12.0 | 176 | 8.3 | 24.8 | 4.9 | 0.0 |
| Breaded, Wrap Factory, 3, Kids, Pizza Hut* | 1 Serving/325g | 617 | 18.0 | 190 | 9.2 | 25.9 | 5.5 | 0.0 |
| **COLESLAW** | | | | | | | | |
| Pot, Pizza Hut* | 1 Serving/200g | 268 | 22.0 | 134 | 0.8 | 7.4 | 11.2 | 0.0 |
| **COOKIE** | | | | | | | | |
| Dough, Ice Cream Factory, (Delivery Only), Pizza Hut* | 1 Portion/145g | 650 | 30.0 | 448 | 5.9 | 59.4 | 20.7 | 0.0 |
| **CREAM** | | | | | | | | |
| Single, Dessert, Pizza Hut* | 1 Serving/40g | 75 | 7.0 | 188 | 2.6 | 3.9 | 18.0 | 0.0 |
| UHT, Dessert, Pizza Hut* | 1 Serving/13g | 46 | 4.0 | 367 | 2.3 | 3.4 | 28.4 | 0.0 |
| UHT, Pizza Hut* | 1 Serving/12g | 22 | 2.0 | 188 | 2.7 | 3.9 | 18.0 | 0.0 |
| UHT, Portion, Pizza Hut* | 1 Portion/12g | 23 | 2.0 | 188 | 2.7 | 3.9 | 18.0 | 0.0 |
| **CROUTONS** | | | | | | | | |
| Pizza Flavoured, Pizza Hut* | 1 Serving/12g | 23 | 3.0 | 196 | 10.1 | 55.2 | 26.1 | 0.0 |
| Salad, Large, Pizza Hut* | 1 Portion/20g | 94 | 4.0 | 470 | 11.0 | 59.1 | 21.1 | 0.0 |
| **DESSERT** | | | | | | | | |
| Cherries in Sauce, Pizza Hut* | 1 Serving/20g | 28 | 0.0 | 142 | 0.5 | 34.9 | 0.1 | 0.0 |
| Chocolate Obsession, Pizza Hut* | 1 Serving/100g | 157 | 7.0 | 157 | 2.0 | 22.1 | 6.8 | 0.0 |
| Cookie Dough, Pizza Hut* | 1 Serving/145g | 650 | 30.0 | 448 | 5.9 | 59.4 | 20.7 | 0.0 |
| Toffee Apple Meltdown, Pizza Hut* | 1 Serving/120g | 325 | 11.0 | 271 | 3.3 | 43.7 | 9.2 | 0.0 |
| Vanilla Ice Cream Pots, Pizza Hut* | 1 Serving/55g | 110 | 6.0 | 200 | 2.8 | 19.9 | 11.6 | 0.0 |
| **DIP** | | | | | | | | |
| BBQ Sauce, Pizza Hut* | 1 Pot/28g | 35 | 0.0 | 123 | 1.3 | 29.3 | 0.1 | 0.0 |
| BBQ Tabasco, Pizza Hut* | 1 Serving/25g | 36 | 0.0 | 142 | 1.2 | 33.6 | 0.2 | 0.0 |
| Garlic & Herb, Pizza Hut* | 1 Serving/28g | 93 | 9.0 | 331 | 1.4 | 7.6 | 32.6 | 0.0 |
| Sour Cream & Chive, Pizza Hut* | 1 Pot/28g | 82 | 1.0 | 294 | 0.9 | 4.1 | 4.0 | 0.0 |
| Sweet Chilli Sauce, Pizza Hut* | 1 Pot/28g | 48 | 0.0 | 172 | 0.3 | 32.9 | 0.8 | 0.0 |
| Tomato Ketchup, Pizza Hut* | 1 Pot/28g | 39 | 0.0 | 141 | 1.4 | 34.1 | 0.1 | 0.0 |
| **DRESSING** | | | | | | | | |
| 1000 Island, Pizza Hut* | 1 Serving/38g | 107 | 10.0 | 280 | 0.7 | 11.5 | 25.5 | 0.0 |
| Blue Cheese, Pizza Hut* | 1 Serving/35g | 91 | 8.0 | 258 | 1.7 | 11.5 | 22.7 | 0.0 |
| Caesar, Pizza Hut* | 1 Serving/40g | 27 | 1.0 | 68 | 1.5 | 8.9 | 2.8 | 0.0 |
| Ranch, Pizza Hut* | 1 Serving/32g | 163 | 18.0 | 510 | 1.2 | 1.5 | 56.4 | 0.0 |
| Vinaigrette, Low Fat, Pizza Hut* | 1 Serving/30ml | 23 | 0.0 | 77 | 0.3 | 17.2 | 0.5 | 0.0 |
| **FRIES** | | | | | | | | |
| Seasoned, Savoury, Pizza Hut* | 1 Portion/145g | 247 | 11.0 | 171 | 2.3 | 23.0 | 7.7 | 0.0 |
| **FRUIT** | | | | | | | | |
| Frozen, Dessert, Pizza Hut* | 1 Serving/20g | 7 | 0.0 | 34 | 1.0 | 12.1 | 0.3 | 0.0 |
| **FUDGE BROWNIE** | | | | | | | | |
| Pizza Hut* | 1 Serving/105g | 418 | 16.0 | 398 | 4.3 | 60.1 | 15.6 | 0.0 |
| **ICE CREAM** | | | | | | | | |
| Coco Mango, Pizza Hut* | 1 Serving/100g | 88 | 2.0 | 88 | 0.6 | 17.3 | 1.8 | 0.0 |
| Cookie Craving, Pizza Hut* | 1 Serving/100g | 149 | 7.0 | 149 | 1.6 | 20.1 | 6.9 | 0.0 |
| Dairy, Dessert, Pizza Hut* | 1 Portion/142g | 272 | 13.0 | 192 | 4.6 | 23.3 | 8.9 | 0.2 |
| Mix, Ice Cream Factory, Pizza Hut* | 1 Serving/100g | 147 | 6.0 | 147 | 4.0 | 18.8 | 6.2 | 0.0 |
| Mix, Pizza Hut* | 1 Serving/100g | 147 | 6.0 | 147 | 4.0 | 18.8 | 6.2 | 0.0 |
| Traditional, Dessert, Pizza Hut* | 1 Serving/130g | 251 | 14.0 | 193 | 2.6 | 22.4 | 10.4 | 0.0 |
| Traditional, Kids, Pizza Hut* | 1 Serving/89g | 171 | 9.0 | 193 | 2.6 | 22.4 | 10.4 | 0.0 |
| Vanilla, Pots, Ice Cream Factory, Pizza Hut* | 1 Portion/55g | 110 | 6.0 | 200 | 2.8 | 19.9 | 11.6 | 0.0 |
| **KETCHUP** | | | | | | | | |
| Heinz, Pizza Hut* | 1 Serving/12g | 14 | 0.0 | 119 | 0.5 | 28.4 | 0.1 | 0.0 |
| Tomato, Sachet, Heinz, Pizza Hut* | 1 Sachet/12g | 14 | 0.0 | 119 | 0.0 | 28.4 | 0.1 | 0.0 |

| | INFO/WEIGHT | KCAL | FAT | KCAL | PROT | CARB | FAT | FIBRE |
|---|---|---|---|---|---|---|---|---|
| **PIZZA HUT** | | | | | | | | |
| **MACARONI CHEESE** | | | | | | | | |
| Pizza Hut* | 1 Serving/41g | 57 | 2.0 | 140 | 4.9 | 16.6 | 6.0 | 0.0 |
| **MARSHMALLOWS** | | | | | | | | |
| Mini, Ice Cream Factory, Pizza Hut* | 1 Serving/30g | 96 | 0.0 | 320 | 5.4 | 74.3 | 0.0 | 0.0 |
| **MAYONNAISE** | | | | | | | | |
| Heinz, Pizza Hut* | 1 Serving/12g | 88 | 10.0 | 731 | 1.3 | 1.8 | 81.2 | 0.0 |
| **MEATBALLS** | | | | | | | | |
| in Pomodoro Sauce, Light Lunch, Pizza Hut* | 1 Portion/253g | 342 | 18.0 | 135 | 6.6 | 11.0 | 7.2 | 0.0 |
| **MILK** | | | | | | | | |
| Half Fat, Portions, Millac Maid, Pizza Hut* | 1 Portion/14g | 6 | 0.0 | 45 | 6.0 | 5.1 | 1.6 | 0.0 |
| **MILKSHAKE** | | | | | | | | |
| Strawberry Cheesecake, Pizza Hut* | 1 Serving/236g | 371 | 14.0 | 157 | 3.4 | 22.3 | 5.9 | 0.0 |
| The Chocoholic, Pizza Hut* | 1 Serving/248g | 442 | 20.0 | 178 | 3.6 | 22.8 | 8.2 | 0.0 |
| Toffee Banoffee Shake, Pizza Hut* | 1 Serving/404g | 763 | 23.0 | 189 | 2.4 | 32.3 | 5.6 | 0.0 |
| **MUFFIN** | | | | | | | | |
| Cheesecake, Sicillian Lemon, Pizza Hut* | 1 Portion/130g | 508 | 24.0 | 391 | 5.1 | 50.9 | 18.6 | 0.0 |
| Double Choc Chip, Pizza Hut* | 1 Muffin/108g | 442 | 23.0 | 409 | 6.4 | 48.7 | 21.0 | 0.0 |
| Fruity, Pizza Hut* | 1 Serving/115g | 366 | 14.0 | 318 | 4.1 | 48.4 | 11.9 | 0.0 |
| Mixed Berry, Pizza Hut* | 1 Muffin/108g | 402 | 23.0 | 372 | 4.4 | 41.6 | 20.9 | 0.0 |
| Sicilian Lemon Cheesecake, Pizza Hut* | 1 Serving/130g | 508 | 24.0 | 391 | 5.1 | 50.9 | 18.6 | 0.0 |
| Strawberry & White Chocolate, Pizza Hut* | 1 Muffin/108g | 402 | 23.0 | 372 | 4.4 | 41.6 | 20.9 | 0.0 |
| Triple Choc, Pizza Hut* | 1 Portion/130g | 497 | 29.0 | 382 | 5.0 | 52.5 | 22.0 | 0.0 |
| **MUSHROOMS** | | | | | | | | |
| Breaded, Pizza Hut* | 1 Portion/180g | 410 | 14.0 | 228 | 4.5 | 26.1 | 8.0 | 0.0 |
| Garlic, Crispy Coated, Pizza Hut* | 1 Portion/135g | 240 | 10.0 | 178 | 4.1 | 23.4 | 7.5 | 0.0 |
| Garlic, Pizza Hut* | 1 Serving/230g | 570 | 43.0 | 248 | 7.9 | 6.9 | 18.9 | 0.0 |
| Garlic, with BBQ Dip, Pizza Hut* | 1 Portion/112g | 263 | 11.0 | 234 | 6.2 | 30.5 | 10.0 | 3.4 |
| Garlic, with Sour Cream & Chive Dip, Pizza Hut* | 1 Portion/112g | 426 | 35.0 | 380 | 6.4 | 20.0 | 30.8 | 3.4 |
| **NACHOS** | | | | | | | | |
| Chilli, Pizza Hut* | 1 Serving/190g | 550 | 33.0 | 289 | 8.8 | 27.2 | 17.4 | 0.0 |
| Sharing Starters, Pizza Hut* | 1 Serving/222g | 669 | 40.0 | 301 | 7.7 | 30.2 | 18.1 | 0.0 |
| **OLIVES** | | | | | | | | |
| Mixed, Pizza Hut* | 1 Serving/70g | 140 | 9.0 | 200 | 1.5 | 19.6 | 12.8 | 0.0 |
| **ONION RINGS** | | | | | | | | |
| Chilli, Pizza Hut* | 8 Rings/100g | 212 | 10.0 | 212 | 3.2 | 28.2 | 9.6 | 0.0 |
| **ONIONS** | | | | | | | | |
| White, Pizza Hut* | 1 Serving/24g | 10 | 0.0 | 42 | 1.0 | 10.0 | 0.0 | 0.0 |
| **PANCAKE** | | | | | | | | |
| Fruity, Kids, Pizza Hut* | 1 Serving/156g | 227 | 3.0 | 146 | 1.9 | 30.6 | 2.1 | 0.0 |
| **PASTA** | | | | | | | | |
| 3 Cheese & Vegetable, Pizza Hut* | 1 Serving/300g | 315 | 13.0 | 105 | 4.0 | 12.6 | 4.3 | 0.0 |
| 4 Cheese, Sharing, Pizza Hut* | 1 Serving/1200g | 1860 | 102.0 | 155 | 6.1 | 13.5 | 8.5 | 0.0 |
| Alfredo, Chicken, Sharing, (Delivery Only), Pizza Hut* | 1 Pack/1200g | 1680 | 41.0 | 140 | 8.1 | 19.1 | 3.4 | 0.0 |
| Alfredo, Light Lunch, Pizza Hut* | 1 Portion/226g | 294 | 5.0 | 130 | 4.1 | 23.3 | 2.2 | 0.0 |
| Alfredo, Pizza Hut* | 1 Portion/400g | 520 | 9.0 | 130 | 4.1 | 23.3 | 2.2 | 0.0 |
| Arrabiata, Pizza Hut* | 1 Serving/450g | 441 | 13.0 | 98 | 2.9 | 15.0 | 2.9 | 0.0 |
| Arrabiatta, Light Lunch, Pizza Hut* | 1 Portion/226g | 221 | 7.0 | 98 | 2.9 | 15.0 | 2.9 | 0.0 |
| Bolognese, Sharing, Pizza Hut* | 1 Serving/1200g | 1500 | 65.0 | 125 | 7.2 | 11.9 | 5.4 | 0.0 |
| Cannelloni, Spinach & Ricotta, Pizza Hut* | 1 Portion/404g | 566 | 27.0 | 140 | 6.2 | 13.1 | 6.8 | 0.0 |
| Chicken Alfredo, Sharing, Pizza Hut* | 1 Serving/1200g | 1680 | 41.0 | 140 | 8.1 | 19.1 | 3.4 | 0.0 |
| Ham & Mushroom, Pizza Hut* | 1 Serving/450g | 473 | 10.0 | 105 | 4.2 | 17.0 | 2.3 | 0.0 |
| Lasagne, Traditional, Pizza Hut* | 1 Portion/460g | 589 | 27.0 | 128 | 5.9 | 13.0 | 5.8 | 0.0 |
| Macaroni Cheese, Kids, Pizza Hut* | 1 Portion/250g | 332 | 16.0 | 133 | 4.0 | 14.8 | 6.5 | 0.0 |

| | Measure INFO/WEIGHT | per Measure KCAL | per Measure FAT | Nutrition Values per 100g / 100ml KCAL | PROT | CARB | FAT | FIBRE |
|---|---|---|---|---|---|---|---|---|

## PIZZA HUT

### PASTA

| | Measure INFO/WEIGHT | KCAL | FAT | KCAL | PROT | CARB | FAT | FIBRE |
|---|---|---|---|---|---|---|---|---|
| Mezzaluna, Tomato & Mozzarella, Pizza Hut* | 1 Portion/350g | 339 | 10.0 | 97 | 3.1 | 14.7 | 2.9 | 0.0 |
| Spaghetti Bolognese, New Kids, Pizza Hut* | 1 Portion/235g | 211 | 4.0 | 90 | 7.6 | 11.4 | 1.5 | 0.0 |
| Tagliatelle, Alla Carbonara, Pizza Hut* | 1 Serving/400g | 548 | 32.0 | 137 | 5.6 | 10.4 | 8.1 | 0.0 |
| Tagliatelle, Carbonara, Pizza Hut* | 1 Potion/400g | 548 | 32.0 | 137 | 5.6 | 10.4 | 8.1 | 0.0 |
| Tagliatelle, Meatball, Italian Recipe, Pizza Hut* | 1 Portion/240g | 324 | 11.0 | 135 | 6.9 | 16.6 | 4.4 | 0.0 |
| Tomato & Pepperoni, Pizza Hut* | 1 Serving/300g | 312 | 8.0 | 104 | 3.6 | 16.3 | 2.7 | 0.0 |

### PASTA BAKE

| | | | | | | | | |
|---|---|---|---|---|---|---|---|---|
| Salmon, Light Lunch, Pizza Hut* | 1 Portion/200g | 344 | 20.0 | 172 | 7.5 | 13.0 | 10.0 | 0.0 |
| Salmon, Pizza Hut* | 1 Portion/400g | 692 | 43.0 | 173 | 7.9 | 11.3 | 10.7 | 0.0 |

### PASTA SALAD

| | | | | | | | | |
|---|---|---|---|---|---|---|---|---|
| Sweetcorn & Pepper, Pizza Hut* | 1 Serving/47g | 75 | 3.0 | 159 | 4.6 | 23.1 | 5.3 | 0.0 |
| Tomato & Basil, Pizza Hut* | 1 Serving/50g | 50 | 1.0 | 100 | 3.7 | 17.8 | 1.5 | 0.0 |

### PENNE

| | | | | | | | | |
|---|---|---|---|---|---|---|---|---|
| Mediterranean Vegetable, Pizza Hut* | 1 Portion/448g | 592 | 20.0 | 132 | 3.7 | 18.3 | 4.4 | 0.0 |

### PEPPERS

| | | | | | | | | |
|---|---|---|---|---|---|---|---|---|
| Red & Green Wedges, Pizza Hut* | 1 Serving/40g | 6 | 0.0 | 15 | 0.8 | 2.6 | 0.3 | 0.0 |

### PIE

| | | | | | | | | |
|---|---|---|---|---|---|---|---|---|
| Banoffee, Dessert, Pizza Hut* | 1 Scrving/125g | 428 | 25.0 | 340 | 2.5 | 37.3 | 20.1 | 0.0 |
| Banoffee, Pizza Hut* | 1 Serving/100g | 350 | 21.0 | 350 | 4.2 | 34.9 | 21.5 | 0.0 |

### PIZZA

| | | | | | | | | |
|---|---|---|---|---|---|---|---|---|
| BBQ Deluxe, Cheesy Bites, Pizza Hut* | 1 Av Slice/143g | 358 | 12.0 | 251 | 11.7 | 34.4 | 8.1 | 0.0 |
| BBQ Deluxe, Italian, Individual, Pizza Hut* | 1 Av Slice/78g | 185 | 6.0 | 238 | 10.9 | 34.3 | 7.9 | 0.0 |
| BBQ Deluxe, Italian, Large, Pizza Hut* | 1 Av Slice/95g | 239 | 8.0 | 252 | 14.3 | 29.7 | 8.4 | 0.0 |
| BBQ Deluxe, Italian, Medium, Pizza Hut* | 1 Av Slice/105g | 253 | 8.0 | 241 | 12.0 | 31.1 | 7.6 | 0.0 |
| BBQ Deluxe, Pan, Individual, Pizza Hut* | 1 Av Slice/79g | 200 | 8.0 | 253 | 12.7 | 28.0 | 10.0 | 0.0 |
| BBQ Deluxe, Pan, Large, Pizza Hut* | 1 Av Slice/122g | 306 | 12.0 | 251 | 11.8 | 28.6 | 9.9 | 0.0 |
| BBQ Deluxe, Pan, Medium, Pizza Hut* | 1 Av Slice/107g | 276 | 11.0 | 257 | 11.7 | 28.8 | 10.5 | 0.0 |
| BBQ Deluxe, Stuffed Crust, Pizza Hut* | 1 Av Slice/155g | 337 | 10.0 | 217 | 11.6 | 31.9 | 6.7 | 0.0 |
| Cajun Chicken, Hot One, Italian, Medium, Pizza Hut* | 1 Slice/100g | 250 | 9.0 | 250 | 12.5 | 29.1 | 9.3 | 0.0 |
| Cajun Chicken, Hot One, Pan, Large, Pizza Hut* | 1 Slice/125g | 321 | 15.0 | 257 | 12.9 | 24.7 | 11.8 | 0.0 |
| Cajun Chicken, Hot One, Pan, Medium, Pizza Hut* | 1 Slice/105g | 273 | 12.0 | 259 | 12.7 | 25.6 | 11.7 | 0.0 |
| Cajun Chicken, Hot One, Stuffed Crust, Pizza Hut* | 1 Slice/135g | 331 | 11.0 | 245 | 13.3 | 30.0 | 8.0 | 0.0 |
| Cheese Feast, Italian, Medium, Pizza Hut* | 1 Slice/96g | 260 | 11.0 | 272 | 12.3 | 29.1 | 11.8 | 0.0 |
| Cheese Feast, Pan, Medium, Pizza Hut* | 1 Slice/106g | 299 | 15.0 | 283 | 14.6 | 24.2 | 14.2 | 0.0 |
| Cheese Feast, Stuffed Crust, Pizza Hut* | 1 Slice/132g | 361 | 14.0 | 273 | 14.3 | 30.5 | 10.4 | 0.0 |
| Chicken, Hi Light, Medium, Pizza Hut* | 1 Slice/83g | 189 | 6.0 | 230 | 13.2 | 29.2 | 6.7 | 0.0 |
| Chicken Supreme, Cheesy Bites, Pizza Hut* | 1 Serving/142g | 309 | 10.0 | 218 | 11.8 | 29.5 | 6.8 | 0.0 |
| Chicken Supreme, Italian, Individual, Pizza Hut* | 1 Av Slice/74g | 169 | 4.0 | 229 | 10.7 | 35.4 | 5.9 | 0.0 |
| Chicken Supreme, Italian, Large, Pizza Hut* | 1 Av Slice/111g | 217 | 6.0 | 196 | 9.8 | 29.3 | 5.8 | 0.0 |
| Chicken Supreme, Italian, Medium, Pizza Hut* | 1 Av Slice/102g | 220 | 6.0 | 215 | 10.3 | 31.9 | 6.2 | 0.0 |
| Chicken Supreme, Pan, Individual, Pizza Hut* | 1 Av Slice/81g | 186 | 8.0 | 231 | 11.6 | 26.9 | 9.9 | 0.0 |
| Chicken Supreme, Pan, Large, Pizza Hut* | 1 Av Slice/124g | 271 | 12.0 | 219 | 10.9 | 26.1 | 9.4 | 0.0 |
| Chicken Supreme, Pan, Medium, Pizza Hut* | 1 Av Slice/115g | 251 | 10.0 | 219 | 11.2 | 26.6 | 8.6 | 0.0 |
| Chicken Supreme, Stuffed Crust, Pizza Hut* | 1 Serving/153g | 367 | 11.0 | 240 | 11.6 | 34.8 | 7.2 | 0.0 |
| Country Feast, Italian, Medium, Pizza Hut* | 1 Slice/109g | 252 | 10.0 | 232 | 9.7 | 28.6 | 8.8 | 0.0 |
| Country Feast, Pan, Medium, Pizza Hut* | 1 Slice/115g | 279 | 12.0 | 243 | 11.4 | 25.8 | 10.5 | 0.0 |
| Country Feast, Stuffed Crust, Pizza Hut* | 1 Slice/144g | 326 | 11.0 | 227 | 11.5 | 28.4 | 7.5 | 0.0 |
| Express, Chicken Supreme, Pizza Hut* | 1 Serving/65g | 143 | 6.0 | 221 | 10.1 | 28.1 | 9.0 | 0.0 |
| Express, Hawaiian, Pizza Hut* | 1 Serving/60g | 147 | 6.0 | 245 | 10.5 | 29.9 | 10.6 | 0.0 |
| Express, Margherita, Pizza Hut* | 1 Serving/57g | 153 | 7.0 | 267 | 11.1 | 30.3 | 12.6 | 0.0 |
| Express, Supreme, Pizza Hut* | 1 Serving/68g | 165 | 8.0 | 242 | 10.7 | 27.8 | 11.2 | 0.0 |
| Farmhouse, Cheesy Bites, Pizza Hut* | 1 Slice/133g | 332 | 13.0 | 250 | 13.2 | 30.7 | 9.5 | 0.0 |

## PIZZA HUT
### PIZZA

| | Measure INFO/WEIGHT | KCAL | FAT | KCAL | PROT | CARB | FAT | FIBRE |
|---|---|---|---|---|---|---|---|---|
| Farmhouse, Hi Light, Medium, Pizza Hut* | 1 Slice/82g | 184 | 5.0 | 225 | 12.1 | 29.1 | 6.7 | 0.0 |
| Farmhouse, Italian, Individual, Pizza Hut* | 1 Slice/74g | 188 | 6.0 | 253 | 11.8 | 33.1 | 8.1 | 0.0 |
| Farmhouse, Italian, Large, Pizza Hut* | 1 Slice/92g | 206 | 7.0 | 224 | 10.2 | 34.0 | 7.3 | 0.0 |
| Farmhouse, Italian, Medium, Pizza Hut* | 1 Slice/84g | 192 | 5.0 | 229 | 10.2 | 35.7 | 6.4 | 0.0 |
| Farmhouse, Pan, Individual, Pizza Hut* | 1 Slice/70g | 179 | 7.0 | 256 | 11.3 | 31.6 | 10.6 | 0.0 |
| Farmhouse, Pan, Large, Pizza Hut* | 1 Slice/106g | 257 | 11.0 | 242 | 11.4 | 29.7 | 10.4 | 0.0 |
| Farmhouse, Pan, Medium, Pizza Hut* | 1 Slice/100g | 242 | 10.0 | 242 | 11.3 | 28.6 | 10.4 | 0.0 |
| Farmhouse, Stuffed Crust, Pizza Hut* | 1 Slice/132g | 387 | 10.0 | 293 | 11.8 | 30.0 | 7.6 | 0.0 |
| Ham, Hi Light, Medium, Pizza Hut* | 1 Slice/82g | 184 | 5.0 | 225 | 12.1 | 29.1 | 6.7 | 0.0 |
| Happy Hour, Chicken & Mushroom, Pizza Hut* | 1 Serving/80g | 165 | 5.0 | 207 | 9.6 | 27.6 | 6.8 | 0.0 |
| Happy Hour, Ham & Sweetcorn, Pizza Hut* | 1 Serving/86g | 174 | 6.0 | 202 | 9.4 | 27.0 | 6.5 | 0.0 |
| Happy Hour, Margherita, Pizza Hut* | 1 Serving/78g | 183 | 7.0 | 234 | 10.5 | 28.6 | 8.8 | 0.0 |
| Happy Hour, Pepper & Tomato, Pizza Hut* | 1 Serving/86g | 163 | 5.0 | 189 | 8.0 | 26.1 | 6.3 | 0.0 |
| Happy Hour, Pepperoni & Onion, Pizza Hut* | 1 Serving/80g | 179 | 7.0 | 224 | 9.4 | 28.2 | 8.6 | 0.0 |
| Hawaiian, Cheesy Bites, Pizza Hut* | 1 Serving/136g | 316 | 11.0 | 232 | 11.6 | 31.2 | 7.8 | 0.0 |
| Hawaiian, Italian, Individual, Pizza Hut* | 1 Slice/71g | 164 | 4.0 | 229 | 9.8 | 37.9 | 5.8 | 0.0 |
| Hawaiian, Italian, Large, Pizza Hut* | 1 Slice/99g | 221 | 7.0 | 223 | 10.0 | 33.2 | 7.1 | 0.0 |
| Hawaiian, Italian, Medium, Pizza Hut* | 1 Slice/92g | 201 | 6.0 | 219 | 9.8 | 33.3 | 6.1 | 0.0 |
| Hawaiian, Pan, Individual, Pizza Hut* | 1 Slice/72g | 175 | 6.0 | 240 | 10.9 | 32.2 | 8.9 | 0.0 |
| Hawaiian, Pan, Large, Pizza Hut* | 1 Slice/112g | 293 | 13.0 | 262 | 10.6 | 32.6 | 11.4 | 0.0 |
| Hawaiian, Pan, Medium, Pizza Hut* | 1 Slice/109g | 245 | 10.0 | 224 | 10.1 | 28.5 | 8.9 | 0.0 |
| Hawaiian, Stuffed Crust, Pizza Hut* | 1 Serving/141g | 306 | 10.0 | 217 | 11.0 | 30.7 | 7.3 | 0.0 |
| Hot 'n' Spicy, Cheesy Bites, Pizza Hut* | 1 Av Slice/127g | 331 | 13.0 | 261 | 12.6 | 33.7 | 9.9 | 0.0 |
| Hot 'n' Spicy, Italian, Individual, Pizza Hut* | 1 Av Slice/66g | 180 | 7.0 | 272 | 11.0 | 36.5 | 10.4 | 0.0 |
| Hot 'n' Spicy, Italian, Large, Pizza Hut* | 1 Av Slice/93g | 236 | 9.0 | 254 | 11.2 | 32.7 | 10.1 | 0.0 |
| Hot 'n' Spicy, Italian, Medium, Pizza Hut* | 1 Av Slice/86g | 222 | 8.0 | 259 | 11.0 | 34.5 | 9.8 | 0.0 |
| Hot 'n' Spicy, Pan, Individual, Pizza Hut* | 1 Av Slice/71g | 183 | 8.0 | 259 | 10.9 | 30.4 | 11.2 | 0.0 |
| Hot 'n' Spicy, Pan, Large, Pizza Hut* | 1 Av Slice/105g | 266 | 11.0 | 254 | 12.0 | 30.2 | 10.9 | 0.0 |
| Hot 'n' Spicy, Pan, Medium, Pizza Hut* | 1 Av Slice/93g | 237 | 11.0 | 254 | 11.5 | 29.2 | 11.4 | 0.0 |
| Hot 'n' Spicy, Stuffed Crust, Pizza Hut* | 1 Av Slice/139g | 329 | 11.0 | 236 | 11.8 | 33.1 | 7.9 | 0.0 |
| Margherita, Cheesy Bites, Pizza Hut* | 1 Slice/128g | 337 | 13.0 | 263 | 12.8 | 33.1 | 10.1 | 0.0 |
| Margherita, Fingers, Kids, Pizza Hut* | 1 Serving/95g | 258 | 12.0 | 273 | 11.0 | 28.4 | 12.8 | 0.0 |
| Margherita, Italian, Individual, Pizza Hut* | 1 Slice/67g | 177 | 5.0 | 264 | 11.9 | 39.2 | 8.0 | 0.0 |
| Margherita, Italian, Large, Pizza Hut* | 1 Slice/91g | 229 | 9.0 | 252 | 10.4 | 34.2 | 9.5 | 0.0 |
| Margherita, Italian, Medium, Pizza Hut* | 1 Slice/80g | 205 | 7.0 | 256 | 11.0 | 35.7 | 8.8 | 0.0 |
| Margherita, Pan, Individual, Pizza Hut* | 1 Slice/71g | 189 | 8.0 | 268 | 11.6 | 32.4 | 11.5 | 0.0 |
| Margherita, Pan, Large, Pizza Hut* | 1 Slice/105g | 273 | 12.0 | 261 | 11.6 | 29.8 | 11.9 | 0.0 |
| Margherita, Pan, Medium, Pizza Hut* | 1 Slice/97g | 248 | 11.0 | 256 | 11.6 | 30.6 | 11.8 | 0.0 |
| Margherita, Stuffed Crust, Pizza Hut* | 1 Slice/140g | 349 | 12.0 | 248 | 14.0 | 31.6 | 8.8 | 0.0 |
| Margherita, Thick, Kids, Pizza Hut* | 1 Serving/202g | 506 | 18.0 | 251 | 9.0 | 33.0 | 8.9 | 0.0 |
| Meat Feast, Cheesy Bites, Pizza Hut* | 1 Av Slice/142g | 387 | 16.0 | 272 | 13.9 | 30.3 | 11.4 | 0.0 |
| Meat Feast, Italian, Individual, Pizza Hut* | 1 Av Slice/81g | 220 | 9.0 | 270 | 13.9 | 32.3 | 10.8 | 0.0 |
| Meat Feast, Italian, Large, Pizza Hut* | 1 Av Slice/111g | 279 | 13.0 | 251 | 12.9 | 27.3 | 11.4 | 0.0 |
| Meat Feast, Italian, Medium, Pizza Hut* | 1 Av Slice/100g | 257 | 11.0 | 258 | 13.0 | 30.0 | 11.0 | 0.0 |
| Meat Feast, Pan, Individual, Pizza Hut* | 1 Av Slice/84g | 220 | 10.0 | 262 | 13.3 | 27.6 | 11.8 | 0.0 |
| Meat Feast, Pan, Large, Pizza Hut* | 1 Av Slice/124g | 344 | 16.0 | 277 | 12.6 | 29.1 | 13.2 | 0.0 |
| Meat Feast, Pan, Medium, Pizza Hut* | 1 Av Slice/112g | 294 | 14.0 | 262 | 12.2 | 28.0 | 12.4 | 0.0 |
| Meat Feast, Stuffed Crust, Pizza Hut* | 1 Av Slice/152g | 376 | 16.0 | 247 | 13.5 | 28.0 | 10.4 | 0.0 |
| Meaty, The Edge, Medium, Pizza Hut* | 1 Slice/36g | 110 | 6.0 | 308 | 17.0 | 20.4 | 16.1 | 0.0 |
| Meaty BBQ, Cheesy Bites, Delivery, Pizza Hut* | 1 Serving/115g | 282 | 11.0 | 245 | 11.3 | 31.1 | 9.4 | 0.0 |
| Meaty BBQ, Large Italian, Delivery, Pizza Hut* | 1 Serving/81g | 176 | 6.0 | 217 | 11.1 | 29.4 | 7.4 | 0.0 |
| Meaty BBQ, Large Pan, Delivery, Pizza Hut* | 1 Serving/111g | 313 | 9.0 | 282 | 10.7 | 26.4 | 8.3 | 0.0 |

# PIZZA HUT

## PIZZA

| Measure INFO/WEIGHT | | per Measure | | Nutrition Values per 100g / 100ml | | | | |
|---|---|---|---|---|---|---|---|---|
| | | KCAL | FAT | KCAL | PROT | CARB | FAT | FIBRE |
| Meaty BBQ, Medium Italian, Delivery, Pizza Hut* | 1 Serving/70g | 154 | 5.0 | 220 | 10.9 | 30.0 | 7.2 | 0.0 |
| Meaty BBQ, Medium Pan, Delivery, Pizza Hut* | 1 Serving/92g | 215 | 9.0 | 234 | 11.1 | 25.9 | 9.5 | 0.0 |
| Meaty BBQ, Stuffed Crust, Delivery, Pizza Hut* | 1 Serving/122g | 259 | 9.0 | 213 | 12.0 | 28.3 | 7.4 | 0.0 |
| Mediterranean Meat Deluxe, Cheesy Bites, Pizza Hut* | 1 Slice/201g | 547 | 22.0 | 272 | 13.5 | 33.0 | 10.7 | 0.0 |
| Mediterranean Meat Deluxe, Italian, Individual, Pizza Hut* | 1 Slice/72g | 206 | 9.0 | 288 | 12.6 | 34.7 | 12.3 | 0.0 |
| Mediterranean Meat Deluxe, Italian, Large, Pizza Hut* | 1 Slice/95g | 267 | 11.0 | 280 | 12.4 | 33.0 | 12.0 | 0.0 |
| Mediterranean Meat Deluxe, Italian, Medium, Pizza Hut* | 1 Slice/91g | 245 | 9.0 | 270 | 12.8 | 33.5 | 10.4 | 0.0 |
| Mediterranean Meat Deluxe, Pan, Individual, Pizza Hut* | 1 Slice/75g | 212 | 10.0 | 284 | 13.5 | 29.5 | 13.9 | 0.0 |
| Mediterranean Meat Deluxe, Pan, Large, Pizza Hut* | 1 Av Slice/108g | 285 | 13.0 | 262 | 11.6 | 29.2 | 11.9 | 0.0 |
| Mediterranean Meat Deluxe, Pan, Medium, Pizza Hut* | 1 Slice/98g | 245 | 11.0 | 249 | 11.7 | 28.1 | 11.4 | 0.0 |
| Mediterranean Meat Deluxe, Stuffed Crust, Pizza Hut* | 1 Av Slice/143g | 382 | 16.0 | 268 | 13.4 | 31.9 | 11.1 | 0.0 |
| Mountain Fantastico, Cheesy Bites, Pizza Hut* | 1 Av Slice/141g | 340 | 11.0 | 242 | 10.9 | 33.5 | 8.0 | 0.0 |
| Mountain Fantastico, Italian, Individual, Pizza Hut* | 1 Av Slice/75g | 183 | 6.0 | 245 | 9.3 | 36.4 | 8.5 | 0.0 |
| Mountain Fantastico, Italian, Large, Pizza Hut* | 1 Slice/94g | 222 | 9.0 | 235 | 10.0 | 32.6 | 9.0 | 0.0 |
| Mountain Fantastico, Italian, Medium, Pizza Hut* | 1 Slice/102g | 247 | 9.0 | 242 | 9.6 | 33.1 | 9.1 | 0.0 |
| Mountain Fantastico, Pan, Individual, Pizza Hut* | 1 Slice/74g | 181 | 7.0 | 244 | 10.7 | 31.4 | 9.9 | 0.0 |
| Mountain Fantastico, Pan, Large, Pizza Hut* | 1 Slice/113g | 295 | 14.0 | 261 | 10.6 | 29.1 | 12.5 | 0.0 |
| Mountain Fantastico, Pan, Medium, Pizza Hut* | 1 Slice/106g | 273 | 14.0 | 258 | 9.6 | 28.9 | 12.8 | 0.0 |
| Mountain Fantastico, Stuffed Crust, Pizza Hut* | 1 Slice/151g | 327 | 11.0 | 217 | 10.5 | 30.8 | 7.5 | 0.0 |
| Pepperoni Feast, Cheesy Bites, Pizza Hut* | 1 Slice/135g | 382 | 17.0 | 284 | 15.8 | 29.6 | 12.4 | 0.0 |
| Pepperoni Feast, Italian, Individual, Pizza Hut* | 1 Slice/73g | 205 | 8.0 | 282 | 11.4 | 36.3 | 11.6 | 0.0 |
| Pepperoni Feast, Italian, Large, Pizza Hut* | 1 Av Slice/103g | 286 | 13.0 | 278 | 12.2 | 30.9 | 12.9 | 0.0 |
| Pepperoni Feast, Italian, Medium, Pizza Hut* | 1 Slice/93g | 254 | 10.0 | 273 | 12.3 | 35.0 | 10.5 | 0.0 |
| Pepperoni Feast, Pan, Individual, Pizza Hut* | 1 Av Slice/79g | 227 | 11.0 | 286 | 12.3 | 30.3 | 13.6 | 0.0 |
| Pepperoni Feast, Pan, Large, Pizza Hut* | 1 Slice/115g | 347 | 20.0 | 302 | 12.0 | 26.4 | 17.6 | 0.0 |
| Pepperoni Feast, Pan, Medium, Pizza Hut* | 1 Av Slice/106g | 297 | 16.0 | 279 | 12.6 | 26.2 | 14.9 | 0.0 |
| Pepperoni Feast, Stuffed Crust, Pizza Hut* | 1 Slice/143g | 375 | 16.0 | 261 | 13.1 | 30.4 | 11.3 | 0.0 |
| Seafood Fantastico, Italian, Individual, Pizza Hut* | 1 Slice/81g | 173 | 5.0 | 213 | 15.3 | 25.1 | 5.7 | 0.0 |
| Seafood Fantastico, Italian, Large, Pizza Hut* | 1 Slice/106g | 228 | 7.0 | 215 | 15.1 | 24.6 | 6.2 | 0.0 |
| Seafood Lovers, Cheesy Bites, Pizza Hut* | 1 Av Slice/128g | 328 | 12.0 | 257 | 11.6 | 33.7 | 9.1 | 0.0 |
| Seafood Lovers, Italian, Individual, Pizza Hut* | 1 Av Slice/66g | 170 | 5.0 | 258 | 9.8 | 38.4 | 8.2 | 0.0 |
| Seafood Lovers, Italian, Large, Pizza Hut* | 1 Slice/90g | 215 | 7.0 | 239 | 10.2 | 35.3 | 7.6 | 0.0 |
| Seafood Lovers, Italian, Medium, Pizza Hut* | 1 Av Slice/82g | 202 | 7.0 | 245 | 10.1 | 35.3 | 8.0 | 0.0 |
| Seafood Lovers, Pan, Individual, Pizza Hut* | 1 Av Slice/69g | 160 | 6.0 | 232 | 10.7 | 31.3 | 8.7 | 0.0 |
| Seafood Lovers, Pan, Large, Pizza Hut* | 1 Av Slice/109g | 266 | 12.0 | 245 | 10.4 | 28.2 | 11.3 | 0.0 |
| Seafood Lovers, Pan, Medium, Pizza Hut* | 1 Av Slice/98g | 233 | 10.0 | 237 | 9.7 | 28.3 | 10.6 | 0.0 |
| Seafood Lovers, Stuffed Crust, Pizza Hut* | 1 Av Slice/131g | 314 | 11.0 | 239 | 12.3 | 31.8 | 8.3 | 0.0 |
| Spicy, Hot One, Pan, Medium, Pizza Hut* | 1 Slice/115g | 274 | 13.0 | 239 | 11.2 | 23.1 | 11.3 | 0.0 |
| Spicy, Hot One, Stuffed Crust, Pizza Hut* | 1 Slice/141g | 352 | 14.0 | 249 | 13.0 | 27.6 | 9.6 | 0.0 |
| Stuffed Crust, Cheesy Bites, Delivery, Pizza Hut* | 1 Serving/130g | 312 | 13.0 | 241 | 11.9 | 29.0 | 9.8 | 0.0 |
| Stuffed Crust, Large Italian, Delivery, Pizza Hut* | 1 Serving/85g | 198 | 9.0 | 234 | 11.7 | 26.9 | 10.2 | 0.0 |
| Stuffed Crust, Large Pan, Delivery, Pizza Hut* | 1 Serving/120g | 289 | 15.0 | 241 | 10.9 | 25.0 | 12.1 | 0.0 |
| Stuffed Crust, Medium Italian, Delivery, Pizza Hut* | 1 Serving/76g | 170 | 8.0 | 225 | 11.0 | 25.3 | 10.3 | 0.0 |
| Stuffed Crust, Medium Pan, Delivery, Pizza Hut* | 1 Serving/100g | 234 | 12.0 | 234 | 11.6 | 22.9 | 12.0 | 0.0 |
| Stuffed Crust, Stuffed Crust, Delivery, Pizza Hut* | 1 Serving/136g | 305 | 13.0 | 225 | 11.5 | 27.2 | 9.3 | 0.0 |
| Super Supreme, Cheesy Bites, Pizza Hut* | 1 Serving/162g | 393 | 16.0 | 242 | 12.4 | 26.9 | 10.0 | 0.0 |
| Super Supreme, Italian, Individual, Pizza Hut* | 1 Av Slice/97g | 260 | 11.0 | 267 | 13.9 | 27.3 | 11.3 | 0.0 |
| Super Supreme, Italian, Large, Pizza Hut* | 1 Av Slice/128g | 281 | 13.0 | 219 | 10.6 | 24.4 | 10.3 | 0.0 |
| Super Supreme, Italian, Medium, Pizza Hut* | 1 Slice/119g | 267 | 12.0 | 225 | 11.1 | 26.3 | 9.7 | 0.0 |
| Super Supreme, Pan, Individual, Pizza Hut* | 1 Av Slice/96g | 228 | 11.0 | 237 | 11.9 | 24.8 | 11.3 | 0.0 |
| Super Supreme, Pan, Large, Pizza Hut* | 1 Av Slice/148g | 346 | 18.0 | 234 | 11.4 | 22.5 | 12.0 | 0.0 |
| Super Supreme, Pan, Medium, Pizza Hut* | 1 Av Slice/127g | 323 | 18.0 | 255 | 11.4 | 22.8 | 14.6 | 0.0 |

## PIZZA HUT

### PIZZA

| INFO/WEIGHT | KCAL | FAT | KCAL | PROT | CARB | FAT | FIBRE |
|---|---|---|---|---|---|---|---|
| Super Supreme, Stuffed Crust, Pizza Hut* | 1 Serving/165g | 366 | 16.0 | 222 | 11.9 | 25.2 | 10.0 | 0.0 |
| Supreme, Cheesy Bites, Pizza Hut* | 1 Av Slice/147g | 369 | 14.0 | 251 | 12.6 | 29.9 | 9.8 | 0.0 |
| Supreme, Italian, Individual, Pizza Hut* | 1 Av Slice/81g | 204 | 7.0 | 251 | 10.9 | 33.5 | 9.2 | 0.0 |
| Supreme, Italian, Large, Pizza Hut* | 1 Av Slice/113g | 264 | 11.0 | 233 | 9.7 | 29.6 | 9.7 | 0.0 |
| Supreme, Italian, Medium, Pizza Hut* | 1 Slice/110g | 286 | 12.0 | 261 | 12.2 | 28.9 | 10.7 | 0.0 |
| Supreme, Pan, Individual, Pizza Hut* | 1 Av Slice/84g | 209 | 10.0 | 248 | 11.0 | 28.0 | 11.4 | 0.0 |
| Supreme, Pan, Large, Pizza Hut* | 1 Av Slice/132g | 302 | 15.0 | 228 | 10.4 | 24.0 | 11.6 | 0.0 |
| Supreme, Pan, Medium, Pizza Hut* | 1 Av Slice/120g | 310 | 16.0 | 259 | 10.5 | 27.0 | 13.1 | 0.0 |
| Supreme, Stuffed Crust, Pizza Hut* | 1 Serving/160g | 371 | 14.0 | 232 | 11.9 | 29.7 | 8.6 | 0.0 |
| The Sizzler, Cajun Chicken, Cheesy Bites, Pizza Hut* | 1 Serving/114g | 265 | 9.0 | 232 | 11.4 | 33.1 | 7.7 | 0.0 |
| The Sizzler, Cajun Chicken, Large Italian, Pizza Hut* | 1 Serving/83g | 177 | 6.0 | 213 | 11.2 | 28.1 | 7.4 | 0.0 |
| The Sizzler, Cajun Chicken, Large Pan, Pizza Hut* | 1 Serving/90g | 215 | 8.0 | 238 | 10.8 | 27.2 | 8.8 | 0.0 |
| The Sizzler, Cajun Chicken, Medium Italian, Pizza Hut* | 1 Serving/67g | 147 | 5.0 | 220 | 11.8 | 30.2 | 7.2 | 0.0 |
| The Sizzler, Cajun Chicken, Medium Pan, Pizza Hut* | 1 Serving/75g | 166 | 7.0 | 221 | 10.3 | 27.3 | 9.3 | 0.0 |
| The Sizzler, Cajun Chicken, Stuffed Crust, Pizza Hut* | 1 Serving/114g | 270 | 10.0 | 236 | 11.7 | 31.7 | 8.6 | 0.0 |
| The Sizzler, Spicy Beef, Cheesy Bites, Pizza Hut* | 1 Serving/112g | 266 | 10.0 | 238 | 12.1 | 30.4 | 9.2 | 0.0 |
| The Sizzler, Spicy Beef, Large Italian, Pizza Hut* | 1 Serving/80g | 179 | 6.0 | 223 | 9.6 | 33.1 | 7.4 | 0.0 |
| The Sizzler, Spicy Beef, Large Pan, Pizza Hut* | 1 Serving/96g | 240 | 11.0 | 250 | 10.5 | 29.1 | 11.5 | 0.0 |
| The Sizzler, Spicy Beef, Medium Italian, Pizza Hut* | 1 Serving/68g | 163 | 6.0 | 240 | 10.9 | 31.6 | 9.0 | 0.0 |
| The Sizzler, Spicy Beef, Medium Pan, Pizza Hut* | 1 Serving/76g | 173 | 8.0 | 228 | 10.3 | 32.0 | 10.1 | 0.0 |
| The Sizzler, Spicy Beef, Stuffed Crust, Pizza Hut* | 1 Serving/118g | 275 | 9.0 | 234 | 11.1 | 32.5 | 8.0 | 0.0 |
| The Sizzler, Spicy Mushroom, Cheesy Bites, Pizza Hut* | 1 Serving/112g | 257 | 9.0 | 229 | 10.4 | 32.0 | 7.9 | 0.0 |
| The Sizzler, Spicy Mushroom, Large Italian, Pizza Hut* | 1 Serving/79g | 165 | 6.0 | 209 | 9.3 | 31.2 | 7.0 | 0.0 |
| The Sizzler, Spicy Mushroom, Large Pan, Pizza Hut* | 1 Serving/92g | 207 | 9.0 | 225 | 9.1 | 28.9 | 9.7 | 0.0 |
| The Sizzler, Spicy Mushroom, Medium Italian, Pizza Hut* | 1 Serving/66g | 146 | 5.0 | 223 | 10.5 | 30.1 | 8.2 | 0.0 |
| The Sizzler, Spicy Mushroom, Medium Pan, Pizza Hut* | 1 Serving/78g | 174 | 7.0 | 224 | 9.3 | 27.9 | 9.6 | 0.0 |
| The Sizzler, Spicy Mushroom, Stuffed Crust, Pizza Hut* | 1 Serving/116g | 244 | 8.0 | 210 | 9.7 | 31.7 | 6.8 | 0.0 |
| The Works, The Edge, Medium, Pizza Hut* | 1 Slice/64g | 150 | 7.0 | 235 | 12.7 | 19.5 | 10.4 | 0.0 |
| Tortilla, Thin, Kids, Pizza Hut* | 1 Serving/108g | 264 | 14.0 | 245 | 9.1 | 20.9 | 13.4 | 0.0 |
| Tuscani, Chicken & Mushroom, Pizza Hut* | 1 Pizza/491g | 1032 | 55.0 | 210 | 10.5 | 16.9 | 11.2 | 0.0 |
| Tuscani, Mediterranean Meats, Pizza Hut* | 1 Serving/379g | 1065 | 57.0 | 281 | 13.6 | 21.8 | 15.0 | 0.0 |
| Tuscani, Rocket & Proscuitto, Pizza Hut* | 1 Serving/434g | 829 | 37.0 | 191 | 9.2 | 19.2 | 8.5 | 0.0 |
| Tuscani, Verde, Pizza Hut* | 1 Serving/460g | 878 | 42.0 | 191 | 8.0 | 18.6 | 9.2 | 0.0 |
| Tuscani Caprina, Pizza Hut* | 1 Pizza/474g | 990 | 45.0 | 209 | 9.0 | 20.6 | 9.6 | 0.0 |
| Vegetable Supreme, Cheesy Bites, Pizza Hut* | 1 Av Slice/145g | 312 | 10.0 | 215 | 10.0 | 30.7 | 6.9 | 0.0 |
| Vegetable Supreme, Italian, Individual, Pizza Hut* | 1 Av Slice/77g | 160 | 5.0 | 207 | 8.7 | 32.4 | 6.1 | 0.0 |
| Vegetable Supreme, Italian, Large, Pizza Hut* | 1 Av Slice/111g | 222 | 6.0 | 200 | 7.4 | 32.5 | 5.7 | 0.0 |
| Vegetable Supreme, Italian, Medium, Pizza Hut* | 1 Av Slice/99g | 196 | 6.0 | 198 | 8.3 | 30.7 | 6.1 | 0.0 |
| Vegetable Supreme, Pan, Individual, Pizza Hut* | 1 Av Slice/84g | 180 | 8.0 | 214 | 8.6 | 27.7 | 9.0 | 0.0 |
| Vegetable Supreme, Pan, Large, Pizza Hut* | 1 Av Slice/126g | 258 | 12.0 | 204 | 8.1 | 25.7 | 9.2 | 0.0 |
| Vegetable Supreme, Pan, Medium, Pizza Hut* | 1 Av Slice/109g | 263 | 11.0 | 241 | 9.9 | 30.0 | 10.3 | 0.0 |
| Vegetable Supreme, Stuffed Crust, Pizza Hut* | 1 Av Slice/156g | 307 | 11.0 | 197 | 9.3 | 27.8 | 6.9 | 0.0 |
| Vegetarian, Hi Light, Medium, Pizza Hut* | 1 Slice/77g | 170 | 5.0 | 221 | 10.3 | 30.0 | 6.6 | 0.0 |
| Vegetarian Hot One, Cheesy Bites, Pizza Hut* | 1 Serving/143g | 302 | 10.0 | 212 | 9.8 | 30.3 | 7.1 | 0.0 |
| Vegetarian Hot One, Italian, Individual, Pizza Hut* | 1 Av Slice/78g | 164 | 5.0 | 211 | 8.1 | 34.6 | 5.8 | 0.0 |
| Vegetarian Hot One, Italian, Large, Pizza Hut* | 1 Av Slice/114g | 165 | 7.0 | 145 | 7.5 | 19.1 | 5.9 | 0.0 |
| Vegetarian Hot One, Italian, Medium, Pizza Hut* | 1 Av Slice/98g | 188 | 5.0 | 192 | 9.3 | 29.5 | 5.5 | 0.0 |
| Vegetarian Hot One, Pan, Individual, Pizza Hut* | 1 Av Slice/82g | 174 | 6.0 | 211 | 8.8 | 29.6 | 7.3 | 0.0 |
| Vegetarian Hot One, Pan, Large, Pizza Hut* | 1 Av Slice/126g | 290 | 12.0 | 231 | 9.4 | 29.7 | 9.6 | 0.0 |
| Vegetarian Hot One, Pan, Medium, Pizza Hut* | 1 Av Slice/115g | 234 | 10.0 | 204 | 8.4 | 26.6 | 8.6 | 0.0 |
| Vegetarian Hot One, Stuffed Crust, Pizza Hut* | 1 Serving/161g | 334 | 11.0 | 208 | 10.1 | 30.2 | 6.9 | 0.0 |
| Veggie, The Edge, Medium, Pizza Hut* | 1 Slice/60g | 136 | 5.0 | 227 | 11.2 | 22.2 | 9.0 | 0.0 |

# PIZZA HUT

| | Measure INFO/WEIGHT | per Measure KCAL | FAT | Nutrition Values per 100g / 100ml KCAL | PROT | CARB | FAT | FIBRE |
|---|---|---|---|---|---|---|---|---|
| **POTATO SKINS** | | | | | | | | |
| Jacket, Loaded, with Cheese, Pizza Hut* | 1 Portion/267g | 571 | 34.0 | 214 | 13.6 | 11.2 | 12.8 | 0.0 |
| Jacket, Pizza Hut* | 1 Portion/224g | 571 | 37.0 | 255 | 3.4 | 23.0 | 16.6 | 2.1 |
| Jacket, with Sour Cream & Chive Dip, Pizza Hut* | 1 Portion/224g | 311 | 24.0 | 139 | 1.4 | 9.3 | 10.8 | 0.8 |
| **POTATO WEDGES** | | | | | | | | |
| Pizza Hut* | 1 Portion/224g | 329 | 14.0 | 147 | 2.1 | 20.8 | 6.2 | 0.0 |
| **POTATOES** | | | | | | | | |
| Savoury Seasoned Fries, Pizza Hut* | 1 Serving/144g | 238 | 12.0 | 165 | 2.4 | 20.8 | 8.0 | 0.0 |
| **PROFITEROLES** | | | | | | | | |
| Dessert, Pizza Hut* | 1 Serving/100g | 381 | 31.0 | 381 | 4.6 | 20.1 | 31.3 | 0.0 |
| Pizza Hut* | 1 Serving/100g | 381 | 31.0 | 381 | 4.6 | 20.1 | 31.3 | 0.0 |
| **PUDDING** | | | | | | | | |
| Sticky Toffee, Pizza Hut* | 1 Serving/105g | 400 | 18.0 | 380 | 5.5 | 50.6 | 17.3 | 0.0 |
| **RAISINS** | | | | | | | | |
| Chocolate, Ice Cream Factory, Pizza Hut* | 1 Serving/30g | 121 | 4.0 | 405 | 5.4 | 63.3 | 14.2 | 0.0 |
| **SALAD** | | | | | | | | |
| 4 Leaf Mix, Pizza Hut* | 1 Serving/100g | 14 | 0.0 | 14 | 0.8 | 1.7 | 0.5 | 0.0 |
| Caesar, Chicken, Small, Light Lunch, Pizza Hut* | 1 Portion/172g | 263 | 13.0 | 153 | 14.1 | 7.4 | 7.4 | 0.0 |
| Caesar, Classic, Pizza Hut* | 1 Portion/194g | 367 | 23.0 | 189 | 7.2 | 13.0 | 11.9 | 0.0 |
| Caesar, Classic, Small, Light Lunch, Pizza Hut* | 1 Portion/97g | 183 | 12.0 | 189 | 7.2 | 13.0 | 11.9 | 0.0 |
| Caesar, Pizza Hut* | 1 Salad/195g | 344 | 20.0 | 177 | 6.0 | 14.8 | 10.4 | 0.0 |
| Caesar, Prawn, Small, Light Lunch, Pizza Hut* | 1 Portion/172g | 229 | 12.0 | 133 | 9.6 | 7.6 | 7.0 | 0.0 |
| Chicken & Bacon, Pizza Hut* | 1 Serving/323g | 514 | 32.0 | 159 | 10.3 | 6.9 | 9.9 | 0.0 |
| Chicken Caesar, Pizza Hut* | 1 Serving/344g | 527 | 25.0 | 153 | 14.1 | 7.4 | 7.4 | 0.0 |
| Chicken Caesar, Small, Happy Hour, Pizza Hut* | 1 Serving/172g | 263 | 13.0 | 153 | 14.1 | 7.4 | 7.4 | 0.0 |
| Chicken Caesar, With Bacon, Pizza Hut* | 1 Serving/375g | 588 | 30.0 | 157 | 14.4 | 6.8 | 7.9 | 0.0 |
| Classic Caesar, Pizza Hut* | 1 Serving/194g | 366 | 23.0 | 189 | 7.2 | 13.0 | 11.9 | 0.0 |
| Dressed, Pasta, Tomato, Med, Pizza Hut* | 1 Serving/100g | 112 | 1.0 | 112 | 3.5 | 21.2 | 1.5 | 0.0 |
| Dressed, Tabbouleh, Pizza Hut* | 1 Serving/100g | 189 | 8.0 | 189 | 4.2 | 24.9 | 8.1 | 0.0 |
| Fresh, Apple & Grape, Mix, Pizza Hut* | 1 Portion/80g | 39 | 1.0 | 49 | 0.4 | 12.0 | 1.0 | 0.0 |
| Fresh, Carrot, Grated, Pizza Hut* | 1 Serving/17g | 5 | 0.0 | 30 | 0.7 | 6.0 | 0.5 | 0.0 |
| Fresh, Cucumber, Slices, Pizza Hut* | 1 Serving/80g | 8 | 0.0 | 10 | 0.7 | 1.5 | 0.1 | 0.0 |
| Fresh, Onion, Red, Slices, Pizza Hut* | 1 Portion/80g | 29 | 0.0 | 36 | 1.2 | 7.9 | 0.2 | 0.0 |
| Fresh, Seasonal, Pizza Hut* | 1 Serving/80g | 12 | 0.0 | 15 | 0.7 | 1.8 | 0.6 | 0.0 |
| Fresh, Tomatoes, Cherry, Pizza Hut* | 1 Serving/80g | 15 | 0.0 | 19 | 0.8 | 3.0 | 0.4 | 0.0 |
| Goats Cheese, Pizza Hut* | 1 Portion/340g | 524 | 40.0 | 154 | 7.5 | 4.4 | 11.8 | 0.0 |
| Grated Hard Cheese, Pizza Hut* | 1 Serving/50g | 202 | 15.0 | 404 | 33.0 | 0.0 | 30.0 | 0.0 |
| Leaf Mix, Pizza Hut* | 1 Serving/41g | 7 | 0.0 | 17 | 2.9 | 6.3 | 1.1 | 0.0 |
| Mozzarella & Tomato, Light Lunch, Pizza Hut* | 1 Serving/188g | 387 | 31.0 | 206 | 12.3 | 2.4 | 16.3 | 0.0 |
| Mozzarella & Tomato, Pizza Hut* | 1 Serving/188g | 387 | 31.0 | 206 | 12.3 | 2.4 | 16.3 | 0.0 |
| Olive & Feta, Pizza Hut* | 1 Portion/406g | 345 | 26.0 | 85 | 3.8 | 3.6 | 6.4 | 0.0 |
| Potato, Whole, Pizza Hut* | 1 Serving/100g | 154 | 10.0 | 154 | 1.6 | 13.5 | 10.1 | 0.0 |
| Prawn, Caesar, Pizza Hut* | 1 Portion/345g | 459 | 24.0 | 133 | 9.6 | 7.6 | 7.0 | 0.0 |
| Seasonal, Pizza Hut* | 1 Serving/80g | 12 | 0.0 | 15 | 0.7 | 1.8 | 0.6 | 0.0 |
| Small Chicken Caesar, Pizza Hut* | 1 Serving/172g | 263 | 13.0 | 153 | 14.1 | 7.4 | 7.4 | 0.0 |
| Small Prawn Caesar, Pizza Hut* | 1 Serving/172g | 229 | 12.0 | 133 | 9.6 | 7.6 | 7.0 | 0.0 |
| Tuna, Pizza Hut* | 1 Portion/461g | 378 | 9.0 | 82 | 10.4 | 5.9 | 1.9 | 2.0 |
| Warm Chicken, Pizza Hut* | 1 Salad/342g | 403 | 17.0 | 118 | 11.0 | 6.8 | 5.1 | 0.0 |
| **SALAD BAR** | | | | | | | | |
| Apple & Grape Mix, Fresh, Pizza Hut* | 1 Serving/80g | 39 | 0.0 | 49 | 0.4 | 12.0 | 0.1 | 0.0 |
| Baby Potatoes, Pizza Hut* | 1 Serving/80g | 63 | 1.0 | 79 | 1.2 | 14.6 | 1.8 | 0.0 |
| Beetroot & Carrot, with Balsamic Vinaigrette, Pizza Hut* | 1 Serving/80g | 24 | 0.0 | 30 | 1.1 | 5.7 | 0.3 | 0.0 |
| Carrot Batons, Fresh, Pizza Hut* | 1 Serving/80g | 28 | 0.0 | 35 | 0.6 | 7.9 | 0.3 | 0.0 |

| | Measure<br>INFO/WEIGHT | per Measure<br>KCAL | FAT | Nutrition Values per 100g / 100ml<br>KCAL | PROT | CARB | FAT | FIBRE |
|---|---|---|---|---|---|---|---|---|

## PIZZA HUT

### SALAD BAR

| | Measure INFO/WEIGHT | KCAL | FAT | KCAL | PROT | CARB | FAT | FIBRE |
|---|---|---|---|---|---|---|---|---|
| Cherry Tomatoes, Fresh, Pizza Hut* | 1 Serving/80g | 15 | 0.0 | 19 | 0.8 | 3.0 | 0.4 | 0.0 |
| Coleslaw, Pizza Hut* | 1 Serving/80g | 149 | 15.0 | 186 | 1.1 | 4.5 | 18.2 | 0.0 |
| Cos Lettuce, Fresh, Pizza Hut* | 1 Serving/80g | 10 | 0.0 | 13 | 0.7 | 1.9 | 0.3 | 0.0 |
| Cous Cous, Pizza Hut* | 1 Serving/100g | 219 | 9.0 | 219 | 5.0 | 30.0 | 9.0 | 0.0 |
| Cucumber, Fresh, Pizza Hut* | 1 Serving/80g | 8 | 0.0 | 10 | 0.7 | 1.5 | 0.1 | 0.0 |
| Gemelli Pasta, Pizza Hut* | 1 Serving/100g | 155 | 4.0 | 155 | 4.3 | 26.0 | 4.4 | 0.0 |
| Kids Pasta, Pizza Hut* | 1 Serving/100g | 180 | 9.0 | 180 | 6.9 | 16.5 | 9.4 | 0.0 |
| Melon Pieces, Fresh, Pizza Hut* | 1 Serving/80g | 27 | 0.0 | 34 | 0.8 | 8.2 | 0.0 | 0.0 |
| Mixed Peppers, Fresh, Pizza Hut* | 1 Serving/80g | 12 | 0.0 | 15 | 0.8 | 2.6 | 0.3 | 0.0 |
| Potato Salad, Pizza Hut* | 1 Serving/80g | 123 | 10.0 | 154 | 1.7 | 10.0 | 11.9 | 0.0 |
| Red Onion, Fresh, Pizza Hut* | 1 Serving/80g | 29 | 0.0 | 36 | 1.2 | 7.9 | 0.2 | 0.0 |
| Seasonal Salad, Fresh, Pizza Hut* | 1 Serving/80g | 12 | 0.0 | 15 | 0.7 | 1.8 | 0.6 | 0.0 |
| Sweetcorn, Fresh, Pizza Hut* | 1 Serving/80g | 63 | 1.0 | 79 | 1.8 | 16.8 | 0.8 | 0.0 |
| Tomato Pasta, Pizza Hut* | 1 Serving/80g | 149 | 7.0 | 186 | 3.7 | 21.8 | 9.3 | 0.0 |
| Tomato Slices, Fresh, Pizza Hut* | 1 Serving/80g | 14 | 0.0 | 17 | 0.7 | 3.1 | 0.3 | 0.0 |

### SAUCE

| | | | | | | | | |
|---|---|---|---|---|---|---|---|---|
| Caramel, Ice Cream Factory, Pizza Hut* | 1 Serving/25g | 77 | 1.0 | 307 | 0.7 | 67.2 | 3.9 | 0.0 |
| Chocolate, Ice Cream Factory, Pizza Hut* | 1 Serving/25g | 74 | 1.0 | 298 | 2.0 | 66.8 | 2.5 | 0.0 |
| Lemon, Ice Cream Factory, Pizza Hut* | 1 Serving/25g | 70 | 0.0 | 280 | 0.1 | 69.0 | 0.0 | 0.0 |
| Strawberry, Ice Cream Factory, Pizza Hut* | 1 Serving/25g | 70 | 0.0 | 280 | 0.0 | 69.5 | 0.0 | 0.0 |

### SMOOTHIE

| | | | | | | | | |
|---|---|---|---|---|---|---|---|---|
| BananaBerry Split, Pizza Hut* | 1 Serving/171g | 258 | 0.0 | 151 | 1.5 | 33.6 | 0.2 | 0.0 |
| Truly Tropical, Pizza Hut* | 1 Serving/239g | 234 | 0.0 | 98 | 0.6 | 24.0 | 0.1 | 0.0 |
| Very Berry, Pizza Hut* | 1 Serving/220g | 189 | 0.0 | 86 | 0.6 | 20.4 | 0.1 | 0.0 |

### SPAGHETTI BOLOGNAISE

| | | | | | | | | |
|---|---|---|---|---|---|---|---|---|
| Pizza Hut* | 1 Portion/475g | 745 | 31.0 | 157 | 6.2 | 17.8 | 6.6 | 0.0 |

### SUNDAE

| | | | | | | | | |
|---|---|---|---|---|---|---|---|---|
| Double Chocolate, Pizza Hut* | 1 Sundae/145g | 307 | 16.0 | 212 | 3.1 | 27.0 | 11.2 | 0.0 |

### SWEETCORN

| | | | | | | | | |
|---|---|---|---|---|---|---|---|---|
| Pizza Hut* | 1 Serving/30g | 24 | 0.0 | 79 | 1.8 | 16.8 | 0.8 | 0.0 |

### TIRAMISU

| | | | | | | | | |
|---|---|---|---|---|---|---|---|---|
| Pizza Hut* | 1 Serving/84g | 248 | 11.0 | 297 | 3.9 | 39.5 | 13.7 | 0.0 |

### TOPPINGS

| | | | | | | | | |
|---|---|---|---|---|---|---|---|---|
| Caramel Sauce, Pizza Hut* | 1 Serving/100g | 307 | 4.0 | 307 | 0.7 | 67.2 | 3.9 | 0.0 |
| Chocolate Raisins, Pizza Hut* | 1 Serving/100g | 405 | 14.0 | 405 | 5.4 | 63.3 | 14.2 | 0.0 |
| Chocolate Sauce, Pizza Hut* | 1 Serving/100g | 298 | 2.0 | 298 | 2.0 | 66.8 | 2.5 | 0.0 |
| Coated Chocolate Beans, Pizza Hut* | 1 Serving/100g | 475 | 18.0 | 475 | 5.5 | 72.2 | 18.1 | 0.0 |
| Frozen Fruits, Pizza Hut* | 1 Serving/21g | 7 | 0.0 | 34 | 1.0 | 12.1 | 0.3 | 0.0 |
| Lemon Sauce, Pizza Hut* | 1 Serving/100g | 280 | 0.0 | 280 | 0.1 | 69.0 | 0.0 | 0.0 |
| Mini Marshmallows, Pizza Hut* | 1 Serving/100g | 320 | 0.0 | 320 | 5.4 | 74.3 | 0.0 | 0.0 |
| Single Cream, Pizza Hut* | 1 Serving/40g | 75 | 7.0 | 188 | 2.6 | 3.9 | 18.0 | 0.0 |
| Strawberry Sauce, Pizza Hut* | 1 Serving/100g | 280 | 0.0 | 280 | 0.0 | 69.5 | 0.0 | 0.0 |
| UHT Cream, Pizza Hut* | 1 Serving/13g | 46 | 4.0 | 367 | 2.3 | 3.4 | 28.4 | 0.0 |

### TORTIZZA

| | | | | | | | | |
|---|---|---|---|---|---|---|---|---|
| Margherita, Light Lunch, Pizza Hut* | 1 Portion/209g | 573 | 28.0 | 274 | 13.7 | 25.1 | 13.2 | 0.0 |

### TUSCANI PLATTER

| | | | | | | | | |
|---|---|---|---|---|---|---|---|---|
| Pizza Hut* | 1 Serving/462g | 1223 | 90.0 | 265 | 8.8 | 13.2 | 19.4 | 0.0 |

## PRET A MANGER

### BAGUETTE

| | | | | | | | | |
|---|---|---|---|---|---|---|---|---|
| Bacon, Posh, Pret a Manger* | 1 Serving/318g | 579 | 20.0 | 182 | 9.9 | 21.4 | 6.3 | 2.0 |
| Beef & Rocket, Artisan, Pret a Manger* | 1 Roll/248g | 619 | 22.0 | 250 | 14.8 | 27.6 | 8.9 | 2.1 |
| Brie, Tomato & Basil, Pret a Manger* | 1 Pack/200g | 407 | 16.0 | 203 | 9.3 | 23.9 | 7.8 | 0.3 |

| | Measure INFO/WEIGHT | per Measure KCAL | FAT | Nutrition Values per 100g / 100ml KCAL | PROT | CARB | FAT | FIBRE |
|---|---|---|---|---|---|---|---|---|

## PRET A MANGER

### BAGUETTE

| | Measure INFO/WEIGHT | KCAL | FAT | KCAL | PROT | CARB | FAT | FIBRE |
|---|---|---|---|---|---|---|---|---|
| Brie, Tomato & Whole Leaf Basil, Pret a Manger* | 1 Serving/232g | 432 | 18.0 | 186 | 7.7 | 21.1 | 7.9 | 2.6 |
| Cheddar, & Baby Plum Tomato, Pret a Manger* | 1 Pack/300g | 625 | 36.0 | 208 | 6.7 | 18.5 | 11.9 | 1.0 |
| Cheddar, & Pickle, Artisan, Posh, Pret a Manger* | 1 Baguette/296g | 779 | 39.0 | 264 | 10.1 | 25.9 | 13.2 | 1.8 |
| Cheddar, & Pickle, Posh, Slim, Pret a Manger* | 1 Pack/147g | 390 | 19.0 | 264 | 10.1 | 25.9 | 13.2 | 1.8 |
| Cheese, Kids, Pret a Manger* | 1 Pack/105g | 329 | 16.0 | 313 | 11.0 | 29.9 | 15.1 | 0.5 |
| Chicken Caesar, Pret a Manger* | 1 Baguette/275g | 517 | 24.0 | 188 | 9.2 | 18.0 | 8.7 | 1.3 |
| Egg, & Salmon, Pret a Manger* | 1 Pack/230g | 527 | 24.0 | 229 | 10.9 | 23.0 | 10.4 | 2.2 |
| Egg, & Tomato, Pret a Manger* | 1 Pack/157g | 291 | 11.0 | 185 | 8.1 | 22.8 | 6.8 | 0.7 |
| Egg Mayo & Bacon, Breakfast, Pret a Manger* | 1 Baguette/138g | 372 | 20.0 | 270 | 11.9 | 22.8 | 14.5 | 0.1 |
| Egg Mayo & Roasted Tomato, Breakfast, Pret a Manger* | 1 Pack/152g | 352 | 18.0 | 232 | 8.1 | 23.1 | 11.9 | 0.1 |
| Egg Mayo & Roasted Tomato, Breakfast, Pret a Manger* | 1 Pack/152g | 352 | 18.0 | 232 | 8.1 | 23.1 | 11.9 | 0.1 |
| Goat's Cheese, Asparagus & Peppers, Pret a Manger* | 1 Bagutte/249g | 441 | 12.0 | 177 | 7.1 | 26.0 | 4.9 | 2.5 |
| Ham, Dry Cured & Greve, Pret a Manger* | 1 Baguette/225g | 543 | 24.0 | 241 | 12.3 | 21.9 | 10.9 | 0.3 |
| Ham, Kids, Pret a Manger* | 1 Pack/118g | 308 | 14.0 | 261 | 12.4 | 26.8 | 11.6 | 0.0 |
| Italian Prosciutti Artisan, Pret a Manger* | 1 Baguette/288g | 636 | 29.0 | 221 | 9.3 | 23.5 | 9.9 | 2.0 |
| Mozzarella & Pesto, Pret a Manger* | 1 Pack/277g | 606 | 26.0 | 219 | 9.2 | 24.4 | 9.3 | 1.9 |
| New York Deli, Pret a Manger* | 1 Baguette/260g | 572 | 23.0 | 220 | 10.6 | 25.6 | 8.8 | 2.1 |
| Prosciutto Capreze, Pret a Manger* | 1 Pack/255g | 699 | 33.0 | 274 | 12.6 | 27.0 | 12.9 | 1.9 |
| Proscuitto, Artisan, Italian, Slim, Pret a Manger* | 1 Baguette/144g | 318 | 14.0 | 221 | 9.3 | 23.5 | 9.9 | 1.9 |
| Salmon, Egg Mayo & Cress, Breakfast, Pret a Manger* | 1 Baguette/152g | 349 | 18.0 | 229 | 10.6 | 20.5 | 11.6 | 1.2 |
| Salmon, Smoked & Capers, Artisan, Pret a Manger* | 1 Baguette/239g | 525 | 18.0 | 220 | 11.0 | 26.6 | 7.7 | 2.1 |
| Salmon, Smoked & Capers, Artisan, Slim, Pret a Manger* | 1 Baguette/120g | 263 | 9.0 | 219 | 10.9 | 26.5 | 7.7 | 2.1 |
| Skipjack Tuna, Pret a Manger* | 1 Pack/232g | 484 | 23.0 | 209 | 9.1 | 20.7 | 9.9 | 1.2 |
| Smoked Salmon, Egg Mayo & Cress, Pret a Manger* | 1 Pack/153g | 349 | 18.0 | 229 | 10.6 | 20.5 | 11.6 | 1.2 |
| Tuna, & Salad, Pret a Manger* | 1 Pack/227g | 506 | 24.0 | 223 | 10.0 | 21.7 | 10.7 | 0.9 |
| Tuna, Dolphin Friendly, Pret a Manger* | 1 Baguette/210g | 474 | 22.0 | 226 | 9.7 | 22.7 | 10.3 | 1.3 |
| Tuna Mayonnaise, Pret a Manger* | 1 Pack/230g | 535 | 23.0 | 233 | 10.8 | 25.0 | 10.0 | 1.7 |
| Wiltshire Cured Ham & Greve, Slim, Pret a Manger* | 1 Pack/113g | 271 | 12.0 | 240 | 14.0 | 21.3 | 11.0 | 1.5 |

### BARS

| | | | | | | | | |
|---|---|---|---|---|---|---|---|---|
| Bird, Pret a Manger* | 1 Bar/60g | 245 | 13.0 | 408 | 13.0 | 39.3 | 22.5 | 2.3 |
| Choc, Pret a Manger* | 1 Bar/105g | 555 | 39.0 | 529 | 4.9 | 44.3 | 36.8 | 2.6 |
| Fruit Goodness, Pret a Manger* | 1 Bar/70g | 286 | 17.0 | 408 | 6.8 | 41.3 | 24.0 | 0.0 |
| Love, Pret a Manger* | 1 Bar/72g | 324 | 18.0 | 450 | 5.9 | 49.2 | 25.4 | 0.0 |
| Power, Pret a Manger* | 1 Bar/65g | 265 | 16.0 | 408 | 6.8 | 41.4 | 24.0 | 6.2 |

### BREAKFAST

| | | | | | | | | |
|---|---|---|---|---|---|---|---|---|
| Bowl, All Day Breakfast, Pret a Manger* | 1 Bowl/220g | 363 | 15.0 | 165 | 5.2 | 19.4 | 6.9 | 1.2 |
| Bowl, Gooseberry, Pret a Manger* | 1 Bowl/217g | 386 | 12.0 | 178 | 6.6 | 25.2 | 5.6 | 1.7 |
| Bowl, Scottish Raspberry, Pret a Manger* | 1 Pack/214g | 372 | 12.0 | 174 | 6.7 | 24.1 | 5.7 | 1.7 |
| Bowl, Strawberry, Wild, Pret a Manger* | 1 Bowl/214g | 364 | 12.0 | 170 | 6.6 | 23.1 | 5.7 | 1.6 |
| Bowl, Very Berry, Pret a Manger* | 1 Bowl/218g | 368 | 15.0 | 169 | 5.2 | 20.3 | 6.9 | 1.4 |

### BREAKFAST CEREAL

| | | | | | | | | |
|---|---|---|---|---|---|---|---|---|
| Granola, Hot & Warming, Pret a Manger* | 1 Pack/226g | 579 | 20.0 | 256 | 6.4 | 38.4 | 8.8 | 3.5 |
| Oats & Granola, Pret a Manger* | 1 Serving/211g | 519 | 17.0 | 246 | 7.9 | 35.7 | 8.0 | 3.5 |

### BROWNIE

| | | | | | | | | |
|---|---|---|---|---|---|---|---|---|
| Chocolate, Pret a Manger* | 1 Brownie/60g | 267 | 16.0 | 445 | 4.7 | 47.7 | 26.2 | 1.5 |

### CAKE

| | | | | | | | | |
|---|---|---|---|---|---|---|---|---|
| Apple, Card Box, Pret a Manger* | 1 Pack/116g | 356 | 17.0 | 307 | 3.9 | 39.6 | 14.7 | 1.8 |
| Apple, Pret a Manger* | 1 Pack/120g | 432 | 26.0 | 360 | 5.2 | 38.7 | 21.9 | 2.1 |
| Bakewell, Pret a Manger* | 1 Cake/68g | 315 | 18.0 | 463 | 7.2 | 50.0 | 26.0 | 2.2 |
| Banana, Card Box, Pret a Manger* | 1 Pack/103g | 345 | 18.0 | 335 | 4.6 | 39.0 | 17.8 | 1.9 |
| Carrot, Card Box, Pret a Manger* | 1 Pack/112g | 402 | 22.0 | 359 | 4.0 | 41.0 | 19.9 | 2.3 |
| Carrot, Pret a Manger* | 1 Av Pack/120g | 288 | 8.0 | 240 | 2.9 | 41.6 | 6.9 | 0.2 |

## PRET A MANGER

### CAKE

| | | | | | | | | |
|---|---|---|---|---|---|---|---|---|
| Chocolate, Card Box, Pret a Manger* | 1 Cake/88g | 354 | 21.0 | 402 | 5.3 | 41.7 | 23.7 | 1.4 |
| Fudge, Pret a Manger* | 1 Pack/140g | 537 | 28.0 | 384 | 4.1 | 46.1 | 20.3 | 1.3 |
| Lemon, Card Box, Pret a Manger* | 1 Cake/97g | 318 | 15.0 | 328 | 4.9 | 42.8 | 15.1 | 0.9 |
| Nut Munch, Pret a Manger* | 1 Pack/100g | 497 | 35.0 | 497 | 8.0 | 38.5 | 34.6 | 7.9 |
| Orange, The Amazing Wheatfree, Pret a Manger* | 1 Pack/90g | 326 | 16.0 | 362 | 10.2 | 40.9 | 17.8 | 3.8 |

### CHEESECAKE

| | | | | | | | | |
|---|---|---|---|---|---|---|---|---|
| Caramel Crunch, Pret a Manger* | 1 Serving/105g | 395 | 32.0 | 376 | 5.3 | 21.0 | 30.1 | 1.2 |
| Lemon, Pret a Manger* | 1 Serving/95g | 376 | 29.0 | 396 | 4.3 | 26.4 | 30.3 | 0.6 |

### CHERRIES

| | | | | | | | | |
|---|---|---|---|---|---|---|---|---|
| Summer, Pret a Manger* | 1 Pot/150g | 60 | 0.0 | 40 | 0.8 | 9.0 | 0.1 | 1.8 |

### CHOCOLATE

| | | | | | | | | |
|---|---|---|---|---|---|---|---|---|
| Milk, Organic, Pret a Manger* | 1 Bar/40g | 216 | 13.0 | 540 | 9.5 | 54.0 | 32.0 | 0.0 |
| Plain, Organic, Pret a Manger* | 1 Bar/40g | 230 | 16.0 | 575 | 7.5 | 45.5 | 40.5 | 0.0 |
| White, Organic, Pret a Manger* | 1 Bar/40g | 230 | 15.0 | 575 | 7.5 | 52.5 | 37.5 | 0.0 |

### COFFEE

| | | | | | | | | |
|---|---|---|---|---|---|---|---|---|
| Cappuccino, Chocolate, Pret a Manger* | 1 Serving/340g | 106 | 6.0 | 31 | 1.7 | 2.2 | 1.7 | 0.0 |
| Cappuccino, Chocolate, Skinny, Pret a Manger* | 1 Serving/355ml | 58 | 0.0 | 16 | 1.7 | 2.1 | 0.1 | 0.0 |
| Cappuccino, Chocolate, Tall, Pret a Manger* | 1 Serving/355ml | 106 | 6.0 | 30 | 1.7 | 2.1 | 1.6 | 0.0 |
| Cappuccino, Full-Fat Milk, No Chocolate, Pret a Manger* | 1 Serving/355ml | 102 | 6.0 | 29 | 1.7 | 1.9 | 1.6 | 0.0 |
| Cappuccino, Toffee, Pret a Manger* | 1 Serving/355ml | 187 | 7.0 | 53 | 1.6 | 7.1 | 1.9 | 0.0 |
| Latte, Pret a Manger* | 1 Serving/340ml | 194 | 11.0 | 57 | 3.1 | 3.9 | 3.3 | 0.0 |
| Latte, Toffee, Pret a Manger* | 1 Latte/247ml | 205 | 8.0 | 83 | 2.6 | 10.9 | 3.3 | 0.0 |
| Mocha, Pret a Manger* | 1 Serving/340ml | 233 | 11.0 | 68 | 2.7 | 7.3 | 3.2 | 0.0 |
| Mocha, Skimmed Milk, Pret a Manger* | 1 Serving/340ml | 91 | 1.0 | 27 | 2.6 | 3.6 | 0.2 | 0.0 |

### CRISPS

| | | | | | | | | |
|---|---|---|---|---|---|---|---|---|
| Cheddar & Chive, Pret a Manger* | 1 Bag/40g | 187 | 10.0 | 467 | 7.0 | 53.7 | 24.7 | 6.0 |
| Cheddar & Red Onion, Croxton Manor, Pret a Manger* | 1 Bag/40g | 181 | 10.0 | 452 | 6.5 | 50.5 | 24.7 | 7.0 |
| Cider Vinegar & Sea Salt, Organic, Pret a Manger* | 1 Bag/40g | 178 | 10.0 | 445 | 5.3 | 51.9 | 24.1 | 0.0 |
| Crispy Seaweed & Miso, Pret a Manger* | 1 Bag/40g | 179 | 10.0 | 447 | 6.5 | 50.5 | 24.5 | 5.7 |
| Lightly Salted, Pret a Manger* | 1 Bag/40g | 198 | 11.0 | 495 | 5.7 | 58.0 | 28.5 | 4.2 |
| Maldon Sea Salt, Pret a Manger* | 1 Pack/40g | 184 | 10.0 | 460 | 5.5 | 51.1 | 25.4 | 0.0 |
| Mature Cheddar, & Red Onion, Pret a Manger* | 1 Bag/40g | 196 | 10.0 | 490 | 6.0 | 60.0 | 25.0 | 5.0 |
| Mediterranean Sea Salt, Pret a Manger* | 1 Bag/40g | 198 | 11.0 | 495 | 5.7 | 58.0 | 28.5 | 4.2 |
| Parsnip, Pret a Manger* | 1 Pack/50g | 238 | 15.0 | 476 | 5.8 | 35.4 | 29.8 | 12.8 |
| Pickled Onion, Pret a Manger* | 1 Bag/40g | 177 | 9.0 | 442 | 7.5 | 52.0 | 22.7 | 7.2 |
| Sea Salt & Balsamic Vinegar, Pret a Manger* | 1 Bag/40g | 186 | 10.0 | 465 | 6.7 | 55.0 | 25.0 | 6.0 |
| Sea Salt & Black Pepper, Pret a Manger* | 1 Bag/40g | 186 | 10.0 | 465 | 6.7 | 55.0 | 25.0 | 6.0 |
| Sea Salt & Mixed Peppercorns, Pret a Manger* | 1 Pack/40g | 178 | 10.0 | 445 | 5.5 | 51.0 | 24.3 | 4.1 |
| Spicy Piri Chilli, Pret a Manger* | 1 Pack/40g | 190 | 10.0 | 475 | 5.2 | 56.7 | 25.2 | 5.2 |
| Sweet Chilli, Pret a Manger* | 1 Pack/40g | 190 | 9.0 | 475 | 5.5 | 60.5 | 23.5 | 6.2 |
| Sweet Potato, With Chipotle Chilli, Pret a Manger* | 1 Pack/25g | 123 | 8.0 | 493 | 5.1 | 44.8 | 32.6 | 0.0 |
| Vegetable, Pret a Manger* | 1 Bag/25g | 123 | 9.0 | 493 | 5.5 | 51.2 | 34.6 | 11.4 |

### CROISSANT

| | | | | | | | | |
|---|---|---|---|---|---|---|---|---|
| All Butter, Pret a Manger* | 1 Croissant/80g | 340 | 20.0 | 425 | 7.6 | 42.5 | 24.9 | 2.4 |
| Almond, Pret a Manger* | 1 Croissant/100g | 365 | 21.0 | 365 | 8.8 | 34.9 | 21.1 | 1.1 |
| Cheese & Tomato, Pret a Manger* | 1 Croissant/111g | 376 | 25.0 | 339 | 11.4 | 22.5 | 22.6 | 0.0 |
| Chocolate, Pret a Manger* | 1 Croissant/95g | 364 | 20.0 | 383 | 5.4 | 42.3 | 21.5 | 0.8 |
| Egg & Bacon, Pret a Manger* | 1 Croissant/167g | 483 | 20.0 | 289 | 11.3 | 20.6 | 12.0 | 1.8 |
| Ham, Cheese & Smoked Bacon, Pret a Manger* | 1 Croissant/100g | 359 | 24.0 | 359 | 12.1 | 22.9 | 24.3 | 1.8 |
| Ham, Cheese & Tomato, Pret a Manger* | 1 Croissant/115g | 337 | 21.0 | 293 | 11.6 | 19.6 | 18.3 | 0.0 |
| Ham & Cheese, Pret a Manger* | 1 Croissant/134g | 441 | 27.0 | 329 | 13.3 | 21.4 | 20.0 | 2.2 |
| Mozzarella & Tomato, Pret a Manger* | 1 Croissant/110g | 371 | 24.0 | 337 | 12.7 | 22.7 | 21.8 | 1.8 |

## PRET A MANGER

| | Measure INFO/WEIGHT | per Measure KCAL | FAT | Nutrition Values per 100g / 100ml KCAL | PROT | CARB | FAT | FIBRE |
|---|---|---|---|---|---|---|---|---|
| **CROISSANT** | | | | | | | | |
| Plain, Pret a Manger* | 1 Pack/80g | 324 | 19.0 | 405 | 8.2 | 39.5 | 23.6 | 2.4 |
| **CRUMBLE** | | | | | | | | |
| Mincemeat, Pret a Manger* | 1 Serving/70g | 275 | 13.0 | 393 | 3.9 | 53.0 | 17.9 | 2.1 |
| **DANDELION & BURDOCK** | | | | | | | | |
| Pret a Manger* | 1 Serving/100ml | 27 | 0.0 | 27 | 0.0 | 7.1 | 0.0 | 0.0 |
| **DANISH PASTRY** | | | | | | | | |
| Cinnamon & Raisin, Pret a Manger* | 1 Danish/85g | 408 | 28.0 | 480 | 6.5 | 40.3 | 32.5 | 1.4 |
| **DESSERT** | | | | | | | | |
| Brownie, Pret Pot, Pret a Manger* | 1 Pot/121g | 201 | 10.0 | 166 | 5.7 | 17.7 | 8.3 | 0.7 |
| **DRESSING** | | | | | | | | |
| French, Dijon, Pret a Manger* | 1 Pot/48g | 202 | 20.0 | 421 | 2.3 | 9.2 | 42.1 | 1.0 |
| Sweet Chilli, Pret a Manger* | 1 Pot/48g | 87 | 6.0 | 182 | 3.7 | 16.9 | 11.5 | 0.2 |
| **DRIED FRUIT** | | | | | | | | |
| Nuts & Bolts, Pret a Manger* | 1 Pack/120g | 571 | 39.0 | 476 | 15.5 | 35.7 | 32.5 | 4.4 |
| **FALAFEL** | | | | | | | | |
| No Bread, Pret a Manger* | 1 Pack/256g | 369 | 28.0 | 144 | 3.8 | 7.3 | 11.1 | 1.5 |
| **FOOL** | | | | | | | | |
| Raspberry, Pret a Manger* | 1 Pot/140g | 188 | 12.0 | 134 | 1.7 | 12.4 | 8.9 | 0.4 |
| **FRUIT** | | | | | | | | |
| Berries & Cherries, Bag, Pret a Manger* | 1 Bag/120g | 334 | 1.0 | 278 | 2.2 | 70.4 | 0.7 | 3.8 |
| Melon & Mango, Pret A Manger* | 1 Pot/200g | 72 | 0.0 | 36 | 0.5 | 8.6 | 0.2 | 0.9 |
| Pot, British Berries, Pret a Manger* | 1 Pot/130g | 146 | 0.0 | 112 | 0.9 | 5.4 | 0.1 | 1.6 |
| **FRUIT BOWL** | | | | | | | | |
| British Berries, Pret a Manger* | 1 Pack/130g | 34 | 0.0 | 26 | 0.9 | 5.4 | 0.1 | 1.6 |
| **FRUIT SALAD** | | | | | | | | |
| Fresh, Pret a Manger* | 1 Pack/250g | 98 | 0.0 | 39 | 0.6 | 8.8 | 0.2 | 0.0 |
| **GINGER BEER** | | | | | | | | |
| Pure Pret, Pret a Manger* | 1 Can/330ml | 152 | 0.0 | 46 | 0.0 | 11.4 | 0.0 | 0.0 |
| **GOULASH** | | | | | | | | |
| Hungarian, Pret a Manger* | 1 Serving/455g | 240 | 8.0 | 53 | 3.2 | 6.7 | 1.7 | 1.2 |
| **GRAPES** | | | | | | | | |
| Pret a Manger* | 1 Pack/130g | 78 | 0.0 | 60 | 0.4 | 15.4 | 0.1 | 0.7 |
| **ICE CREAM** | | | | | | | | |
| Chocolate, Organic, Pret a Manger* | 1 Serving/100ml | 192 | 11.0 | 192 | 3.9 | 19.5 | 10.8 | 0.9 |
| Vanilla, Organic, Pret a Manger* | 1 Serving/100ml | 156 | 9.0 | 156 | 3.3 | 14.3 | 9.5 | 0.1 |
| White Chocolate & Caramel, Organic, Pret a Manger* | 1 Serving/100ml | 100 | 6.0 | 100 | 1.4 | 10.0 | 6.0 | 0.0 |
| **JUICE** | | | | | | | | |
| Apple, 100% Premium, Pret a Manger* | 1 Serving/250ml | 128 | 0.0 | 51 | 0.1 | 11.9 | 0.0 | 0.0 |
| Blue Bionic, Pret a Manger* | 1 Serving/250g | 170 | 3.0 | 68 | 2.9 | 11.3 | 1.4 | 1.8 |
| Carrot, Freshly Pressed, Pret a Manger* | 1 Serving/250ml | 60 | 0.0 | 24 | 0.5 | 5.7 | 0.1 | 0.0 |
| Orange, & Raspberry, Pret a Manger* | 1 Serving/250g | 110 | 0.0 | 44 | 0.7 | 10.0 | 0.0 | 0.0 |
| Orange, Pret a Manger* | 1 Serving/260ml | 119 | 0.0 | 46 | 0.6 | 11.4 | 0.0 | 0.1 |
| **JUICE DRINK** | | | | | | | | |
| Hippie, Pret A Manger* | 1 Bottle/500ml | 80 | 0.0 | 16 | 0.0 | 3.9 | 0.0 | 0.0 |
| Mandarin & Lychee, Pret a Manger* | 1 Bottle/250ml | 103 | 0.0 | 41 | 0.7 | 9.5 | 0.0 | 0.1 |
| Red Defence, Pure Pret, Pret a Manger* | 1 Can/330ml | 140 | 0.0 | 42 | 0.0 | 10.3 | 0.0 | 0.0 |
| **MANGO** | | | | | | | | |
| Dried, Pret a Manger* | 1 Pack/60g | 200 | 0.0 | 333 | 1.5 | 84.5 | 0.4 | 4.5 |
| **MELON** | | | | | | | | |
| Fruit Sticks, Pret a Manger* | 1 Pack/200g | 52 | 0.0 | 26 | 0.5 | 5.6 | 0.2 | 0.0 |
| **MOUSSE** | | | | | | | | |
| Chocolate, Pret a Manger* | 1 Pot/90g | 338 | 26.0 | 376 | 3.3 | 24.6 | 29.2 | 1.2 |

| | Measure INFO/WEIGHT | per Measure | | Nutrition Values per 100g / 100ml | | | | |
|---|---|---|---|---|---|---|---|---|
| | | KCAL | FAT | KCAL | PROT | CARB | FAT | FIBRE |

## PRET A MANGER

### MUFFIN

| | Measure INFO/WEIGHT | KCAL | FAT | KCAL | PROT | CARB | FAT | FIBRE |
|---|---|---|---|---|---|---|---|---|
| Double Berry, Pret a Manger* | 1 Muffin/140g | 470 | 24.0 | 336 | 4.5 | 41.4 | 17.0 | 1.3 |
| Morning Glory, Pret a Manger* | 1 Muffin/140g | 521 | 32.0 | 372 | 7.4 | 35.2 | 22.6 | 3.2 |
| Orange, & Lemon, Pret a Manger* | 1 Muffin/160g | 603 | 28.0 | 377 | 4.9 | 38.1 | 17.6 | 1.1 |
| Yoghurt & Pecan, Pret a Manger* | 1 Muffin/140g | 521 | 32.0 | 372 | 7.4 | 35.2 | 22.6 | 3.2 |

### PANNACOTTA

| | | | | | | | | |
|---|---|---|---|---|---|---|---|---|
| Mango & Passion Fruit, Pret a Manger* | 1 Pot/110g | 330 | 26.0 | 300 | 2.1 | 18.8 | 24.0 | 0.4 |

### PIE

| | | | | | | | | |
|---|---|---|---|---|---|---|---|---|
| Pecan, Pret a Manger* | 1 Pie/80g | 376 | 26.0 | 470 | 5.9 | 39.1 | 32.2 | 0.2 |

### POPCORN

| | | | | | | | | |
|---|---|---|---|---|---|---|---|---|
| Honey, Organic, Pret a Manger* | 1 Bag/35g | 157 | 6.0 | 449 | 4.0 | 75.7 | 17.4 | 6.3 |

### PRET POT

| | | | | | | | | |
|---|---|---|---|---|---|---|---|---|
| Caramel, Pret a Manger* | 1 Pot/120g | 391 | 31.0 | 326 | 1.7 | 20.5 | 26.2 | 0.7 |

### PRETZELS

| | | | | | | | | |
|---|---|---|---|---|---|---|---|---|
| Plain, Sesame Or Poppy, Pret a Manger* | 1 Pretzel/120g | 371 | 8.0 | 309 | 10.9 | 51.6 | 6.5 | 2.5 |

### SALAD

| | | | | | | | | |
|---|---|---|---|---|---|---|---|---|
| Chicken, Al Fresco, Pret a Manger* | 1 Pack/287g | 439 | 34.0 | 153 | 6.9 | 4.8 | 12.0 | 1.6 |
| Chicken & Fresh Pesto, Pret a Manger* | 1 Serving/328g | 456 | 32.0 | 139 | 10.6 | 1.3 | 9.7 | 0.7 |
| Chicken Avocado, Pret a Manger* | 1 Salad/311g | 342 | 24.0 | 110 | 7.8 | 2.6 | 7.7 | 2.6 |
| Chicken Caesar, Pret a Manger* | 1 Serving/273g | 319 | 22.0 | 117 | 9.2 | 1.4 | 8.2 | 0.7 |
| Chicken Provencal, No Bread, Pret a Manger* | 1 Pack/288g | 234 | 14.0 | 81 | 6.5 | 3.1 | 4.8 | 1.0 |
| Chicken Tabbouleh & Yoghurt Dressing, Pret a Manger* | 1 Pack/289g | 183 | 5.0 | 63 | 7.5 | 4.5 | 1.8 | 2.3 |
| Crayfish, & Smoked Salmon, Pret a Manger* | 1 Pack/230g | 134 | 4.0 | 58 | 9.4 | 1.4 | 1.7 | 0.9 |
| Crayfish, Pret a Manger* | 1 Pack/320g | 200 | 17.0 | 62 | 3.0 | 0.8 | 5.2 | 0.2 |
| Houmous & Pitta Bread, Pot, Pret a Manger* | 1 Pot/200g | 393 | 29.0 | 196 | 4.7 | 11.9 | 14.4 | 3.3 |
| Humous, Chunky, Pret a Manger* | 1 Salad/268g | 539 | 31.0 | 201 | 6.0 | 18.5 | 11.6 | 2.8 |
| Mezze, Pret a Manger* | 1 Serving/330g | 241 | 11.0 | 73 | 3.0 | 7.4 | 3.5 | 1.6 |
| Pesto Pasta, Pret a Manger* | 1 Pot/320g | 425 | 34.0 | 133 | 2.7 | 6.9 | 10.7 | 0.9 |
| Skipjack Tuna Nicoise, Pret a Manger* | 1 Salad/332g | 238 | 12.0 | 72 | 8.1 | 2.3 | 3.5 | 0.8 |
| Super Club, Pret a Manger* | 1 Pack/200g | 213 | 13.0 | 106 | 10.7 | 1.6 | 6.3 | 0.6 |
| Super Duper Health & Humous, Pret a Manger* | 1 Serving/389g | 342 | 19.0 | 88 | 4.0 | 7.1 | 4.9 | 1.6 |
| Tomato & Mozzarella, No Bread, Pret a Manger* | 1 Pack/180g | 216 | 17.0 | 120 | 6.9 | 1.9 | 9.4 | 0.0 |
| Tuna, Tricolore, Pret a Manger* | 1 Serving/321g | 240 | 12.0 | 75 | 9.2 | 1.5 | 3.6 | 1.3 |
| Tuna Nicoise, Pret a Manger* | 1 Pack/300g | 381 | 27.0 | 127 | 7.9 | 3.7 | 9.1 | 1.2 |

### SALAD BOWL

| | | | | | | | | |
|---|---|---|---|---|---|---|---|---|
| Crayfish, with Sweet Chilli Dressing, Pret a Manger* | 1 Bowl/244g | 149 | 6.0 | 61 | 4.8 | 4.6 | 2.6 | 0.5 |
| Houmous & Feta, Pret a Manger* | 1 Bowl/200g | 422 | 34.0 | 211 | 5.8 | 9.1 | 17.0 | 1.5 |
| Houmous & Feta Salad, Pret a Manger* | 1 Bowl/252g | 399 | 26.0 | 158 | 6.1 | 10.2 | 10.4 | 1.6 |
| Pasta, Basil, Pret a Manger* | 1 Bowl/334g | 629 | 37.0 | 188 | 4.4 | 17.7 | 11.0 | 0.8 |
| Tuna, No Dressing, Dolphin Friendly, Pret a Manger* | 1 Bowl/261g | 178 | 7.0 | 68 | 9.2 | 2.3 | 2.6 | 1.4 |

### SANDWICH

| | | | | | | | | |
|---|---|---|---|---|---|---|---|---|
| All Day Breakfast, Pret a Manger* | 1 Sandwich/306g | 560 | 27.0 | 183 | 9.6 | 16.0 | 9.0 | 1.5 |
| All Day Breakfast, Slim Pret, Pret a Manger* | 1 Pack/149g | 306 | 18.0 | 206 | 8.6 | 15.7 | 12.0 | 1.5 |
| Avocado, & Alfalfa Sprout, Pret a Manger* | 1 Pack/250g | 329 | 20.0 | 132 | 3.4 | 11.6 | 8.0 | 2.4 |
| Avocado, & Bacon, Pret a Manger* | 1 Pack/286g | 543 | 35.0 | 190 | 5.8 | 13.4 | 12.4 | 2.6 |
| Avocado, & Black Olive, Pret a Manger* | 1 Pack/267g | 412 | 21.0 | 154 | 4.7 | 16.6 | 7.7 | 3.5 |
| Avocado, & Italian Cheese Salad, Pret a Manger* | 1 Pack/290g | 552 | 37.0 | 190 | 5.7 | 13.4 | 12.6 | 2.7 |
| Avocado, & Roasted Tomatoes, Pret a Manger* | 1 Pack/300g | 560 | 34.0 | 187 | 5.2 | 14.4 | 11.4 | 2.6 |
| Big Prawn, Pret a Manger* | 1 Pack/209g | 445 | 25.0 | 213 | 10.6 | 16.5 | 11.9 | 1.5 |
| BLT, Beech Smoked, Slim Pret, Pret a Manger* | 1 Sandwich/123g | 248 | 14.0 | 200 | 8.5 | 15.4 | 11.6 | 1.7 |
| BLT, Big, Pret a Manger* | 1 Pack/200g | 398 | 23.0 | 199 | 8.5 | 15.4 | 11.6 | 1.6 |
| BLT, Slim, Pret a Manger* | 1 Pack/124g | 248 | 14.0 | 200 | 8.5 | 15.4 | 11.6 | 1.7 |
| BMT, Italian, Pret a Manger* | 1 Sandwich/218g | 625 | 36.0 | 286 | 13.9 | 18.7 | 16.3 | 0.0 |

## PRET A MANGER

| | Measure INFO/WEIGHT | per Measure KCAL | FAT | Nutrition Values per 100g / 100ml KCAL | PROT | CARB | FAT | FIBRE |
|---|---|---|---|---|---|---|---|---|
| **SANDWICH** | | | | | | | | |
| Brie & Roasted Tomato, Pret a Manger* | 1 Pack/235g | 530 | 30.0 | 226 | 8.3 | 17.2 | 12.8 | 1.5 |
| Cheddar, Christmas, Pret a Manger* | 1 Pack/270g | 671 | 42.0 | 249 | 8.8 | 18.3 | 15.5 | 2.0 |
| Cheddar, Roasted Tomatoes & Pickle, Pret a Manger* | 1 Pack/301g | 648 | 24.0 | 215 | 9.0 | 20.0 | 8.0 | 1.8 |
| Cheese, Three, & Roasted Tomato, Pret a Manger* | 1 Pack/350g | 417 | 22.0 | 119 | 3.8 | 11.5 | 6.2 | 1.5 |
| Chicken, & Basil Salad, Pret a Manger* | 1 Pack/284g | 577 | 35.0 | 203 | 9.7 | 13.6 | 12.3 | 1.8 |
| Chicken, & Coriander, on Rye, Pret a Manger* | 1 Pack/200g | 500 | 28.0 | 250 | 10.8 | 22.0 | 13.9 | 1.9 |
| Chicken, & Mango, Summer, Pret a Manger* | 1 Pack/242g | 486 | 20.0 | 201 | 10.7 | 20.9 | 8.3 | 2.1 |
| Chicken, Black Pepper, Bloomer, Pret a Manger* | 1 Pack/250g | 642 | 24.0 | 257 | 13.0 | 29.5 | 9.7 | 1.8 |
| Chicken, Caesar, Pret a Manger* | 1 Pack/261g | 429 | 20.0 | 164 | 8.5 | 14.5 | 7.8 | 1.7 |
| Chicken, Coronation, Pret a Manger* | 1 Pack/250g | 415 | 14.0 | 166 | 7.9 | 21.2 | 5.4 | 0.2 |
| Chicken, Devonshire Red, Rocket, Pret a Manger* | 1 Sandwich/192g | 504 | 27.0 | 262 | 14.2 | 19.2 | 14.3 | 1.5 |
| Chicken & Pepper Sauce, Special, Pret a Manger* | 1 Pack/215g | 397 | 18.0 | 184 | 10.1 | 17.5 | 8.3 | 1.9 |
| Chicken & Pesto, Pret a Manger* | 1 Sandwich/207g | 408 | 16.0 | 197 | 11.2 | 19.5 | 7.5 | 1.6 |
| Chicken & Whole-Leaf Basil, with Salad, Pret a Manger* | 1 Pack/276g | 480 | 23.0 | 174 | 10.1 | 15.1 | 8.2 | 1.8 |
| Chicken Avocado, Pret a Manger* | 1 Pack/251g | 456 | 24.0 | 182 | 8.7 | 15.8 | 9.4 | 2.9 |
| Chicken Caesar, Slim Pret, Pret a Manger* | 1 Pack/135g | 239 | 13.0 | 177 | 8.3 | 14.2 | 9.3 | 1.7 |
| Chicken Ceaser, No Bread, Pret a Manger* | 1 Pack/226g | 360 | 27.0 | 159 | 8.6 | 2.6 | 12.0 | 1.0 |
| Chicken Valentino, Pret a Manger* | 1 Pack/271g | 516 | 25.0 | 190 | 9.8 | 14.8 | 9.3 | 1.7 |
| Club, Caesar's, Pret a Manger* | 1 Pack/285g | 558 | 28.0 | 196 | 11.3 | 13.9 | 9.8 | 1.5 |
| Club, Cheddar, Pret a Manger* | 1 Pack/298g | 641 | 41.0 | 215 | 8.9 | 13.7 | 13.9 | 1.6 |
| Club, Pret a Manger* | 1 Pack/250g | 542 | 25.0 | 217 | 12.8 | 18.7 | 10.1 | 2.3 |
| Club, Super, Pret a Manger* | 1 Sandwich/227g | 445 | 26.0 | 196 | 10.4 | 13.6 | 11.3 | 1.5 |
| Club, Super, Slim Pret, Pret a Manger* | 1 Pack/143g | 290 | 17.0 | 202 | 10.3 | 13.6 | 12.1 | 1.6 |
| Crayfish, & Avocado, No Bread, Pret a Manger* | 1 Pack/241g | 258 | 22.0 | 107 | 4.2 | 1.8 | 9.2 | 2.0 |
| Crayfish, & White Crab, Pret a Manger* | 1 Pack/250g | 391 | 19.0 | 156 | 5.0 | 16.8 | 7.7 | 2.2 |
| Crayfish & Avocado, Pret a Manger* | 1 Sandwich/279g | 436 | 23.0 | 156 | 5.7 | 14.3 | 8.4 | 2.5 |
| Crayfish & Roacket, Wild, Slim Pret, Pret a Manger* | 1 Sandwich/98g | 185 | 9.0 | 190 | 8.3 | 19.4 | 8.8 | 1.6 |
| Crayfish & Rocket, Pret a Manger* | 1 Pack/195g | 370 | 17.0 | 190 | 8.3 | 19.4 | 8.8 | 1.6 |
| Crayfish & Rocket, Wild, Pret a Manger* | 1 Sandwich/195g | 370 | 17.0 | 190 | 8.3 | 19.4 | 8.8 | 1.6 |
| Duck & Mango, Special, Pret a Manger* | 1 Pack/249g | 376 | 20.0 | 151 | 7.8 | 15.8 | 8.1 | 1.7 |
| Egg, Bacon & Tomato, Free Range, Pret a Manger* | 1 Sandwich/219g | 522 | 29.0 | 238 | 11.8 | 18.1 | 13.1 | 1.5 |
| Egg, Florentine, No Bread, Pret a Manger* | 1 Pack/232g | 263 | 18.0 | 113 | 5.7 | 4.9 | 7.9 | 0.7 |
| Egg, Sunny, & Salad, Pret a Manger* | 1 Sandwich/289g | 488 | 27.0 | 169 | 7.0 | 14.1 | 9.4 | 1.4 |
| Egg Florentine, Pret a Manger* | 1 Sandwich/284g | 504 | 28.0 | 177 | 8.1 | 14.1 | 9.7 | 1.5 |
| Egg Mayonnaise, Pret a Manger* | 1 Pack/250g | 360 | 16.0 | 144 | 6.8 | 14.9 | 6.3 | 1.4 |
| Falafel, Spinach & Tomato, Pret a Manger* | 1 Pack/271g | 360 | 9.0 | 133 | 5.2 | 20.5 | 3.4 | 1.6 |
| Feta & Olive, Pret a Manger* | 1 Pack/181g | 123 | 9.0 | 68 | 4.0 | 2.1 | 4.9 | 1.9 |
| Gourmet Egg, Tomato & Rocket, Pret a Manger* | 1 Sandwich/280g | 436 | 23.0 | 156 | 6.2 | 14.4 | 8.3 | 1.5 |
| Grilled Peppers & Salad, Pret a Manger* | 1 Pack/275g | 421 | 22.0 | 153 | 5.1 | 15.5 | 7.9 | 2.3 |
| Ham, & Egg, Bloomer, Pret a Manger* | 1 Pack/290g | 476 | 26.0 | 164 | 6.0 | 19.0 | 9.0 | 0.0 |
| Ham, & Egg Salad, Pret a Manger* | 1 Pack/287g | 426 | 16.0 | 148 | 9.2 | 15.6 | 5.5 | 1.3 |
| Ham, & Salad, Summer, Pret a Manger* | 1 Pack/286g | 454 | 19.0 | 159 | 10.5 | 14.1 | 6.8 | 1.5 |
| Ham, Cheese, & Pickle, Pret a Manger* | 1 Pack/250g | 592 | 28.0 | 237 | 11.9 | 25.0 | 11.0 | 2.4 |
| Ham, Egg & Greve, Pret a Manger* | 1 Pack/325g | 552 | 27.0 | 170 | 11.5 | 12.7 | 8.2 | 1.4 |
| Herb Chicken & Rocket, Pret a Manger* | 1 Pack/195g | 456 | 23.0 | 234 | 12.8 | 19.1 | 11.8 | 2.4 |
| Houmous, & Oven Roasted Tomato, Pret a Manger* | 1 Pack/350g | 404 | 18.0 | 115 | 3.5 | 13.6 | 5.2 | 3.1 |
| Houmous, & Roasted Peppers, Pret a Manger* | 1 Pack/268g | 477 | 25.0 | 178 | 5.5 | 18.4 | 9.3 | 3.1 |
| Houmous Salad, Slim Pret, Pret a Manger* | 1 Pack/128g | 201 | 9.0 | 157 | 5.1 | 18.4 | 7.1 | 2.6 |
| Lamb, Pea & Mint Relish, Roast, Pret a Manger* | 1 Pack/250g | 937 | 32.0 | 375 | 21.8 | 44.1 | 12.7 | 7.4 |
| Mature Cheddar & Pret Pickle, Slim Pret, Pret a Manger* | 1 Pack/246g | 294 | 17.0 | 119 | 5.2 | 9.3 | 6.9 | 0.9 |
| More Than Mozzarella, Pret a Manger* | 1 Sandwich/250g | 508 | 30.0 | 203 | 9.3 | 15.0 | 11.8 | 1.6 |
| Mozzeralla & Pesto, Bloomer, Pret a Manger* | 1 Pack/270g | 564 | 28.0 | 209 | 8.7 | 18.8 | 10.4 | 0.0 |

| | Measure INFO/WEIGHT | per Measure KCAL | FAT | Nutrition Values per 100g / 100ml KCAL | PROT | CARB | FAT | FIBRE |
|---|---|---|---|---|---|---|---|---|
| **PRET A MANGER** | | | | | | | | |
| **SANDWICH** | | | | | | | | |
| New Tuna Salad, Slim Pret, Pret a Manger* | 1 Pack/116g | 234 | 13.0 | 202 | 1.0 | 16.2 | 11.0 | 2.3 |
| New York Deli, Bloomer, Pret a Manger* | 1 Pack/227g | 513 | 24.0 | 226 | 12.3 | 22.7 | 10.4 | 2.4 |
| New York Deli, Pret a Manger* | 1 Serving/242g | 479 | 23.0 | 198 | 11.9 | 17.3 | 9.4 | 0.0 |
| Pastrami, Bloomer, Pret a Manger* | 1 Pack/301g | 434 | 15.0 | 144 | 7.1 | 18.1 | 4.9 | 2.5 |
| Pastrami, on Rye, Pret a Manger* | 1 Pack/200g | 391 | 15.0 | 195 | 10.2 | 22.6 | 7.6 | 1.9 |
| Prawn, & Rocket, Pret a Manger* | 1 Pack/280g | 435 | 19.0 | 155 | 8.4 | 14.9 | 6.9 | 1.3 |
| Prawn, Gourmet, Pret a Manger* | 1 Pack/250g | 454 | 25.0 | 182 | 7.8 | 15.2 | 10.2 | 1.8 |
| Prawn, with Yummy Yoghurt, Pret a Manger* | 1 Pack/277g | 282 | 6.0 | 102 | 7.5 | 13.6 | 2.1 | 1.4 |
| Roasted Red Peppers & Swiss, Pret a Manger* | 1 Sandwich/252g | 474 | 27.0 | 188 | 6.8 | 16.1 | 10.7 | 2.1 |
| Salmon, & Horseradish, Pret a Manger* | 1 Pack/300g | 462 | 20.0 | 154 | 9.0 | 14.2 | 6.7 | 1.8 |
| Salmon, Really Wild, Pret a Manger* | 1 Sandwich/266g | 440 | 16.0 | 166 | 11.8 | 16.0 | 6.1 | 1.6 |
| Salmon, Really Wild, Summer, Pret a Manger* | 1 Sandwich/221g | 473 | 24.0 | 214 | 12.0 | 17.0 | 11.0 | 1.6 |
| Salmon, Scottish, Smoked, Pret a Manger* | 1 Serving/158g | 348 | 11.0 | 220 | 16.5 | 21.8 | 7.3 | 0.0 |
| Salmon, Smoked & Free Range Egg, Pret a Manger* | 1 Pack/232g | 438 | 18.0 | 189 | 13.0 | 16.3 | 7.9 | 1.6 |
| Salmon, Wild Alaskan & Cucumber, Pret a Manger* | 1 Pack/247g | 479 | 22.0 | 194 | 12.1 | 16.3 | 8.9 | 0.0 |
| Salt Beef Deli, Pret a Manger* | 1 Sandwich/223g | 415 | 19.0 | 186 | 9.7 | 18.5 | 8.6 | 1.8 |
| Sausage & Bacon, Bloomer, Pret a Manger* | 1 Pack/281g | 641 | 32.0 | 228 | 10.7 | 21.0 | 11.2 | 0.0 |
| Simply Ham & Mustard Mayonnaise, Pret a Manger* | 1 Pack/186g | 467 | 23.0 | 251 | 14.5 | 20.3 | 12.4 | 1.6 |
| Smoked Salmon, Pret a Manger* | 1 Pack/158g | 348 | 11.0 | 220 | 16.5 | 21.8 | 7.3 | 1.7 |
| Smoked Turkey & Leaf Spinach, Pret a Manger* | 1 Pack/280g | 537 | 27.0 | 192 | 12.1 | 14.3 | 9.6 | 1.7 |
| Soft Cheese, & Spicy Aubergine, Pret a Manger* | 1 Pack/250g | 319 | 7.0 | 128 | 4.6 | 21.2 | 2.7 | 2.8 |
| Tabbouleh, No Bread, Pret a Manger* | 1 Pack/342g | 250 | 17.0 | 73 | 2.1 | 4.8 | 5.1 | 2.2 |
| Tuna, Dolphin Friendly, Pret a Manger* | 1 Sandwich/227g | 442 | 23.0 | 195 | 8.8 | 16.8 | 10.0 | 1.5 |
| Tuna, Dolphin Friendly, Slim Pret, Pret a Manger* | 1 Pack/116g | 234 | 13.0 | 202 | 9.7 | 16.2 | 11.0 | 2.3 |
| Tuna, Nicoise, Pret a Manger* | 1 Sandwich/305g | 467 | 24.0 | 153 | 8.1 | 12.4 | 7.8 | 2.0 |
| Tuna, St Tropez, Pret a Manger* | 1 Pack/250g | 387 | 19.0 | 155 | 7.4 | 14.7 | 7.6 | 2.0 |
| Tuna Mayonnaise, No Bread, Pret a Manger* | 1 Pack/233g | 193 | 9.0 | 83 | 10.8 | 1.9 | 3.8 | 0.5 |
| Tuna Nicoise, on Whole Grain, Pret a Manger* | 1 Pack/295g | 486 | 27.0 | 165 | 7.9 | 13.4 | 9.0 | 1.9 |
| Turkey Club, Pret a Manger* | 1 Pack/296g | 592 | 31.0 | 200 | 10.0 | 15.1 | 10.6 | 1.8 |
| Veggie Weekly Special, Summer Brie-Ze, Pret a Manger* | 1 Pack/280g | 572 | 37.0 | 204 | 6.7 | 14.7 | 13.0 | 1.8 |
| **SAUSAGE ROLL** | | | | | | | | |
| Pret a Manger* | 1 Serving/150g | 482 | 32.0 | 321 | 12.8 | 19.0 | 21.1 | 2.0 |
| **SHORTBREAD** | | | | | | | | |
| Fingers, Pret a Manger* | 1 Pack/28g | 148 | 10.0 | 521 | 5.6 | 58.4 | 35.2 | 2.8 |
| **SLICES** | | | | | | | | |
| Oat & Fruit, Pret a Manger* | 1 Slice/80g | 342 | 16.0 | 427 | 5.2 | 56.0 | 20.2 | 5.1 |
| **SMOOTHIE** | | | | | | | | |
| Mango, Pret a Manger* | 1 Serving/250g | 130 | 0.0 | 52 | 0.6 | 12.4 | 0.2 | 1.2 |
| Strawberry, With Banana, Pret a Manger* | 1 Bottle/250ml | 127 | 1.0 | 51 | 0.9 | 11.2 | 0.3 | 0.0 |
| Vitamin Volcano, Pret a Manger* | 1 Serving/250ml | 103 | 0.0 | 41 | 0.4 | 10.1 | 0.1 | 0.9 |
| **SNACK POT** | | | | | | | | |
| Banoffee, Pret a Manger* | 1 Pot/198g | 273 | 7.0 | 138 | 5.9 | 21.5 | 3.4 | 0.4 |
| **SOUP** | | | | | | | | |
| Bacon, Tomato & Creme Fraiche, Pret a Manger* | 1 Pack/334g | 220 | 15.0 | 66 | 1.7 | 4.7 | 4.5 | 0.8 |
| Bean & Herb, Summer, Pret a Manger* | 1 Serving/335g | 191 | 13.0 | 57 | 1.8 | 3.8 | 3.8 | 1.3 |
| Carrot, Arabian Spiced, Pret a Manger* | 1 Serving/334g | 194 | 9.0 | 58 | 2.5 | 5.8 | 2.7 | 0.7 |
| Carrot & Roast Cumin, Pret a Manger* | 1 Serving/282g | 167 | 9.0 | 59 | 1.4 | 5.6 | 3.4 | 1.3 |
| Celeriac & Mash, Pret a Manger* | 1 Serving/297g | 125 | 10.0 | 42 | 0.8 | 2.2 | 3.4 | 1.0 |
| Chicken, Malaysian, Pret a Manger* | 1 Serving/347g | 243 | 12.0 | 70 | 5.1 | 4.8 | 3.4 | 0.9 |
| Chicken Salsa, Verde, Pret a Manger* | 1 Serving/345g | 197 | 9.0 | 57 | 4.5 | 3.6 | 2.7 | 4.6 |
| Chilli & Rice, Pret a Manger* | 1 Serving/334g | 244 | 8.0 | 73 | 5.4 | 7.3 | 2.5 | 2.8 |
| Classic Tomato, Pret a Manger* | 1 Serving/336g | 179 | 7.0 | 53 | 0.9 | 7.5 | 2.1 | 0.7 |

| | Measure INFO/WEIGHT | per Measure KCAL | FAT | Nutrition Values per 100g / 100ml KCAL | PROT | CARB | FAT | FIBRE |
|---|---|---|---|---|---|---|---|---|

## PRET A MANGER

### SOUP

| | Measure INFO/WEIGHT | KCAL | FAT | KCAL | PROT | CARB | FAT | FIBRE |
|---|---|---|---|---|---|---|---|---|
| Five Bean Cassoulet, Pret a Manger* | 1 Serving/294g | 174 | 6.0 | 59 | 3.6 | 6.6 | 2.0 | 4.9 |
| Fresh Tomato, & Herb, Pret a Manger* | 1 Serving/307g | 123 | 7.0 | 40 | 0.6 | 3.3 | 2.2 | 0.9 |
| Italian Meatball, Pret a Manger* | 1 Serving/340g | 221 | 14.0 | 65 | 1.8 | 5.1 | 4.1 | 1.2 |
| Kedgeree, Chowder, Pret a Manger* | 1 Serving/334g | 197 | 12.0 | 59 | 1.9 | 4.8 | 3.6 | 1.2 |
| Lentil, Tomato & Tumeric, Pret a Manger* | 1 Pack/345g | 248 | 7.0 | 72 | 4.5 | 8.7 | 2.1 | 5.0 |
| Lentil & Bacon, Hotpot, Pret a Manger* | 1 Serving/296g | 219 | 9.0 | 74 | 5.9 | 6.3 | 3.1 | 1.2 |
| Minestrone, Pret a Manger* | 1 Serving/455g | 187 | 6.0 | 41 | 1.7 | 5.6 | 1.4 | 1.5 |
| Miso, Pork & Rice, Slow Cooked, Pret a Manger* | 1 Pack/370g | 164 | 4.0 | 44 | 2.6 | 5.8 | 1.2 | 0.8 |
| Mushroom Risotto, Pret a Manger* | 1 Serving/347g | 202 | 9.0 | 58 | 1.5 | 7.0 | 2.7 | 1.2 |
| Pea & Mint, Pret a Manger* | 1 Pack/335g | 218 | 14.0 | 65 | 2.4 | 3.9 | 4.3 | 3.6 |
| Pea & Pancetta Risotta, Pret a Manger* | 1 Pot/335g | 214 | 14.0 | 64 | 2.4 | 3.9 | 4.3 | 3.6 |
| Porcini Musroom, Pret a Manger* | 1 Serving/455g | 210 | 8.0 | 46 | 1.4 | 5.6 | 1.8 | 0.9 |
| Red Pepper & Goats Cheese, Pret a Manger* | 1 Pack/367g | 192 | 10.0 | 52 | 2.6 | 4.8 | 2.7 | 0.5 |
| Spinach, Nutmeg & Sage, Pret a Manger* | 1 Serving/334g | 248 | 19.0 | 74 | 1.2 | 4.4 | 5.7 | 1.0 |
| Thai Chicken Curry, Pret a Manger* | 1 Serving/365g | 277 | 14.0 | 76 | 3.1 | 7.6 | 3.7 | 0.2 |
| Thai Corn, On the Hob, Pret a Manger* | 1 Serving/334g | 230 | 7.0 | 69 | 1.6 | 10.9 | 2.1 | 0.9 |
| Tomato & Basil, Pret a Manger* | 1 Serving/454g | 147 | 6.0 | 32 | 0.6 | 4.7 | 1.4 | 0.7 |
| Tomato & Mountain Wheat, Pret a Manger* | 1 Serving/455g | 220 | 6.0 | 48 | 1.3 | 8.1 | 1.3 | 0.7 |
| Tuscan Bean & Sausage, Pret a Manger* | 1 Serving/340g | 267 | 11.0 | 79 | 4.8 | 8.1 | 3.3 | 3.8 |
| Yoghurt, Cumin & Carrot, Spicy, Pret a Manger* | 1 Serving/100g | 191 | 9.0 | 191 | 8.3 | 19.1 | 8.9 | 2.3 |

### STRUDEL

| | Measure INFO/WEIGHT | KCAL | FAT | KCAL | PROT | CARB | FAT | FIBRE |
|---|---|---|---|---|---|---|---|---|
| Cinnamon, Pret a Manger* | 1 Serving/93g | 363 | 18.0 | 392 | 6.0 | 49.0 | 19.1 | 4.6 |

### SUSHI

| | Measure INFO/WEIGHT | KCAL | FAT | KCAL | PROT | CARB | FAT | FIBRE |
|---|---|---|---|---|---|---|---|---|
| Bento, Deluxe, Pret a Manger* | 1 Serving/289g | 432 | 10.0 | 149 | 5.3 | 23.1 | 3.6 | 2.9 |
| Bento, Veggie, Pret a Manger* | 1 Serving/283g | 399 | 7.0 | 141 | 4.3 | 25.3 | 2.4 | 5.4 |
| Maki & Nigiri, Pret a Manger* | 1 Pack/200g | 314 | 8.0 | 157 | 5.4 | 23.4 | 4.2 | 1.0 |
| Salmon, Nigiri, Pret a Manger* | 1 Pack/200g | 314 | 8.0 | 157 | 5.4 | 23.4 | 4.2 | 0.0 |
| Vegetarian, Pret a Manger* | 1 Serving/193g | 277 | 5.0 | 144 | 3.4 | 25.8 | 2.8 | 5.6 |

### VEGETABLE CHIPS

| | Measure INFO/WEIGHT | KCAL | FAT | KCAL | PROT | CARB | FAT | FIBRE |
|---|---|---|---|---|---|---|---|---|
| Parsnip, Beetroot & Carrot, Pret a Manger* | 1 Bag/25g | 126 | 9.0 | 504 | 5.6 | 37.2 | 36.8 | 10.0 |

### WATER

| | Measure INFO/WEIGHT | KCAL | FAT | KCAL | PROT | CARB | FAT | FIBRE |
|---|---|---|---|---|---|---|---|---|
| Blackcurrant, Pure Still, Pret a Manger* | 1 Serving/500ml | 80 | 0.0 | 16 | 0.0 | 3.6 | 0.0 | 0.0 |
| Cranberry, Pure Pret, Pret a Manger* | 1 Serving/330ml | 119 | 0.0 | 36 | 0.0 | 8.6 | 0.0 | 0.0 |
| Grape & Elderflower, Pure Pret, Pret a Manger* | 1 Serving/330ml | 146 | 0.0 | 44 | 0.0 | 10.6 | 0.0 | 0.0 |
| Lemon, Pure Pret, Pret a Manger* | 1 Can/330ml | 175 | 0.0 | 53 | 0.0 | 12.6 | 0.0 | 0.0 |
| Lemon Aid, Pret a Manger* | 1 Bottle/500ml | 75 | 0.0 | 15 | 0.0 | 4.0 | 0.0 | 0.0 |
| Lemon Barley, Pure Pret, Pret a Manger* | 1 Serving/500ml | 80 | 0.0 | 16 | 0.0 | 3.7 | 0.0 | 0.0 |
| Mango & Mandarin, Pret a Manger* | 1 Serving/500ml | 200 | 0.0 | 40 | 0.2 | 9.6 | 0.0 | 0.0 |
| Orange, Pure Pret, Pret a Manger* | 1 Can/330ml | 158 | 0.0 | 48 | 0.0 | 11.3 | 0.0 | 0.0 |
| Orange, Still, Pure Pret, Pret a Manger* | 1 Serving/500ml | 85 | 0.0 | 17 | 0.0 | 3.8 | 0.0 | 0.0 |
| Pomegranate Power, Pret a Manger* | 1 Bottle/500ml | 90 | 0.0 | 18 | 0.0 | 4.4 | 0.0 | 0.0 |
| Yoga Bunny, Pret a Manger* | 1 Can/330ml | 132 | 0.0 | 40 | 0.0 | 9.7 | 0.0 | 0.0 |

### WRAP

| | Measure INFO/WEIGHT | KCAL | FAT | KCAL | PROT | CARB | FAT | FIBRE |
|---|---|---|---|---|---|---|---|---|
| All Day Breakfast, Hot, Pret a Manger* | 1 Pack/255g | 512 | 24.0 | 201 | 10.0 | 18.9 | 9.5 | 1.9 |
| Avocado & Herb Salad, Pret a Manger* | 1 Pack/252g | 461 | 30.0 | 183 | 4.8 | 14.1 | 12.0 | 2.7 |
| Beef, with Salt, Hot, Pret a Manger* | 1 Pack/204g | 392 | 18.0 | 192 | 13.0 | 16.5 | 8.8 | 0.0 |
| Chicken, Jalapeno, Hot, Pret a Manger* | 1 Pack/261g | 433 | 15.0 | 166 | 12.7 | 16.4 | 5.6 | 1.8 |
| Chicken Salad, Pret a Manger* | 1 Pack/230g | 378 | 18.0 | 164 | 8.3 | 15.6 | 7.7 | 1.3 |
| Falafel, Spicy, Melt, Hot, Pret a Manger* | 1 Pack/218g | 380 | 13.0 | 174 | 6.4 | 23.7 | 6.1 | 0.0 |
| Hoisin Duck, Pret a Manger* | 1 Wrap/211g | 433 | 20.0 | 205 | 9.5 | 20.7 | 9.5 | 1.4 |
| Houmous Salad, Pret a Manger* | 1 Pack/230g | 351 | 16.0 | 153 | 5.0 | 17.9 | 6.8 | 3.4 |
| Lamb, Pret a Manger* | 1 Pack/271g | 421 | 21.0 | 155 | 7.9 | 13.7 | 7.7 | 1.7 |

|  | Measure INFO/WEIGHT | per Measure | | Nutrition Values per 100g / 100ml | | | | |
|---|---|---|---|---|---|---|---|---|
|  |  | KCAL | FAT | KCAL | PROT | CARB | FAT | FIBRE |

## PRET A MANGER
### WRAP
| | | | | | | | | |
|---|---|---|---|---|---|---|---|---|
| Meatball Ragu, Swedish, Hot, Pret a Manger* | 1 Pack/219g | 566 | 26.0 | 259 | 13.3 | 24.9 | 11.9 | 2.2 |
| Salmon Fish Cake, Hot, Pret a Manger* | 1 Pack/250g | 460 | 25.0 | 184 | 10.9 | 12.7 | 10.0 | 0.7 |
| Sausage & Mash, Pret a Manger* | 1 Pack/239g | 599 | 36.0 | 251 | 7.7 | 20.8 | 14.9 | 1.5 |
| Tuna Nicoise, Pret a Manger* | 1 Pack/200g | 338 | 18.0 | 169 | 7.0 | 15.1 | 9.1 | 2.1 |
| Tuna Nicoise & Salad, Pret a Manger* | 1 Pack/287g | 430 | 21.0 | 150 | 7.7 | 13.9 | 7.2 | 1.6 |

### YOGHURT
| | | | | | | | | |
|---|---|---|---|---|---|---|---|---|
| Goosberry, Pret Pot, Pret a Manger* | 1 Pot/151g | 161 | 5.0 | 107 | 5.9 | 13.7 | 3.1 | 0.3 |
| Honey & Granola, Pret Pot, Pret a Manger* | 1 Pot/135g | 255 | 8.0 | 189 | 7.6 | 25.8 | 6.2 | 1.7 |
| Red Berry, Blender, Pret a Manger* | 1 Pot/125g | 175 | 4.0 | 140 | 5.6 | 23.0 | 3.0 | 2.4 |
| Vanilla, Blender, Pret a Manger* | 1 Pot/250g | 230 | 7.0 | 92 | 4.5 | 12.8 | 2.7 | 0.0 |
| Vanilla Bean & Honey, Pret a Manger* | 1 Serving/250g | 226 | 5.0 | 90 | 4.0 | 14.5 | 2.1 | 0.0 |
| Very Berry, Pret Pot, Pret a Manger* | 1 Pot/148g | 151 | 5.0 | 102 | 6.0 | 12.5 | 3.2 | 0.3 |

### YOGHURT DRINK
| | | | | | | | | |
|---|---|---|---|---|---|---|---|---|
| Blueberry Blender, Pret a Manger* | 1 Drink/250g | 170 | 3.0 | 68 | 2.9 | 11.3 | 1.4 | 1.8 |
| Mango's & Minerals, Pret a Manger* | 1 Drink/250g | 203 | 3.0 | 81 | 2.6 | 14.4 | 1.4 | 0.1 |
| Vanilla, Pret a Manger* | 1 Drink/250g | 230 | 7.0 | 92 | 4.5 | 12.8 | 2.7 | 0.0 |

## STARBUCKS
### BAGEL
| | | | | | | | | |
|---|---|---|---|---|---|---|---|---|
| Cheese, & Jalapeno, Starbucks* | 1 Bagel/115g | 292 | 4.0 | 254 | 10.8 | 45.8 | 3.1 | 1.5 |
| Cheesy, Starbucks* | 1 Bagel/90g | 253 | 7.0 | 281 | 11.9 | 41.7 | 7.3 | 2.2 |
| Cinamon & Raisin, Starbucks* | 1 Bagel/83g | 190 | 1.0 | 229 | 44.8 | 9.4 | 1.4 | 1.3 |
| Fruity, Starbucks* | 1 Bagel/90g | 338 | 16.0 | 376 | 9.7 | 44.5 | 17.9 | 3.4 |

### BARS
| | | | | | | | | |
|---|---|---|---|---|---|---|---|---|
| Almond, Cranberry & Yoghurt, Starbucks* | 1 Bar/50g | 220 | 13.0 | 440 | 6.6 | 46.0 | 25.5 | 10.2 |
| Chocolate, Milk, Starbucks* | 1 Bar/45g | 252 | 17.0 | 559 | 8.4 | 48.8 | 36.7 | 0.0 |
| Granola, Starbucks* | 1 Bar/80g | 348 | 20.0 | 435 | 7.3 | 46.4 | 24.6 | 4.4 |
| Mango, Pistachio & Cashew, Fruit & Nut, Starbucks* | 1 Bar/50g | 200 | 11.0 | 401 | 7.7 | 45.0 | 21.1 | 16.9 |
| Rocky Road, Starbucks* | 1 Bar/65g | 366 | 27.0 | 563 | 4.2 | 46.6 | 41.1 | 2.2 |

### BISCOTTI
| | | | | | | | | |
|---|---|---|---|---|---|---|---|---|
| Almond, Starbucks* | 1 Biscuit/55g | 219 | 9.0 | 399 | 8.0 | 54.4 | 16.6 | 2.5 |
| Starbucks* | 1 Biscuit/27g | 100 | 4.0 | 370 | 7.4 | 55.6 | 14.8 | 0.0 |

### BISCUITS
| | | | | | | | | |
|---|---|---|---|---|---|---|---|---|
| Ginger Snaps, Organic, Starbucks* | 3 Biscuits/60g | 267 | 9.0 | 445 | 4.8 | 71.9 | 15.4 | 1.5 |
| Golden Crunch, Starbucks* | 1 Biscuit/30g | 144 | 7.0 | 481 | 5.1 | 65.4 | 22.1 | 2.0 |
| Oat & Fruit, Starbucks* | 1 Biscuit/60g | 258 | 10.0 | 430 | 4.2 | 64.0 | 17.5 | 2.2 |

### BREAD
| | | | | | | | | |
|---|---|---|---|---|---|---|---|---|
| Fruit, Luxury, Starbucks* | 1 Serving/145g | 486 | 12.0 | 335 | 7.0 | 58.0 | 8.3 | 2.3 |

### BREAKFAST CEREAL
| | | | | | | | | |
|---|---|---|---|---|---|---|---|---|
| Porridge, Dried Fruit, Made with Full Fat Milk, Starbucks* | 1 Serving/244g | 344 | 10.0 | 141 | 4.3 | 23.1 | 3.9 | 1.6 |
| Porridge, Dried Fruit, Made with Skimmed Milk, Starbucks* | 1 Serving/243g | 292 | 3.0 | 120 | 4.4 | 23.3 | 1.4 | 1.6 |

### CAKE
| | | | | | | | | |
|---|---|---|---|---|---|---|---|---|
| Banana & Date, Skinny, Starbucks* | 1 Slice/120g | 300 | 3.0 | 250 | 3.9 | 52.1 | 2.9 | 2.5 |
| Banana Date & Raisin, Wholemeal, Low Fat, Starbucks* | 1 Slice/70g | 169 | 2.0 | 242 | 5.0 | 49.1 | 2.9 | 3.4 |
| Butterfly, Starbucks* | 1 Slice/80g | 361 | 18.0 | 451 | 3.4 | 58.2 | 22.7 | 0.5 |
| Carrot, Skinny, Starbucks* | 1 Slice/75g | 192 | 2.0 | 256 | 4.0 | 54.1 | 3.3 | 2.1 |
| Carrot & Valencia Orange, Low Fat, Starbucks* | 1 Slice/80g | 200 | 2.0 | 250 | 3.3 | 53.0 | 3.0 | 3.0 |
| Carrot Loaf, Starbucks* | 1 Slice/100g | 352 | 20.0 | 352 | 4.7 | 38.4 | 19.9 | 2.3 |
| Chocolate, Fairtrade, Starbucks* | 1 Serving/70g | 330 | 20.0 | 471 | 10.9 | 40.7 | 28.3 | 4.6 |
| Chocolate Decadence, Starbucks* | 1 Slice/170g | 717 | 41.0 | 422 | 4.4 | 46.9 | 24.1 | 1.4 |
| Chocolate Orange, Starbucks* | 1 Slice/70g | 276 | 15.0 | 395 | 5.7 | 45.4 | 21.2 | 1.9 |
| Coconut & Raspberry, Starbucks* | 1 Cake/62g | 267 | 15.0 | 430 | 4.0 | 49.9 | 23.6 | 1.6 |
| Fruit, Starbucks* | 1 Slice/80g | 236 | 7.0 | 295 | 3.6 | 50.1 | 8.7 | 2.8 |

| | Measure INFO/WEIGHT | per Measure KCAL | FAT | Nutrition Values per 100g / 100ml KCAL | PROT | CARB | FAT | FIBRE |
|---|---|---|---|---|---|---|---|---|

## STARBUCKS

### CAKE

| | Measure INFO/WEIGHT | KCAL | FAT | KCAL | PROT | CARB | FAT | FIBRE |
|---|---|---|---|---|---|---|---|---|
| Ginger, Square, Starbucks* | 1 Square/45g | 202 | 13.0 | 450 | 4.3 | 45.0 | 28.2 | 0.9 |
| Iced Fancies, Starbucks* | 1 Cake/81g | 307 | 11.0 | 379 | 2.3 | 63.7 | 13.0 | 0.6 |
| Marshmallow, Chocolate, Twizzle, Starbucks* | 1 Cake/35g | 143 | 3.0 | 410 | 4.2 | 78.6 | 8.3 | 2.2 |
| Orange, Summer Valencia, Wheat & Dairy Free, Starbucks* | 1 Slice/70g | 190 | 10.0 | 271 | 7.6 | 28.9 | 14.0 | 2.9 |
| Orange, Wheat & Gluten Free, Starbucks* | 1 Serving/55g | 138 | 7.0 | 251 | 7.4 | 25.8 | 13.2 | 3.3 |
| Passion, Starbucks* | 1 Slice/145g | 528 | 32.0 | 364 | 4.3 | 37.2 | 22.0 | 1.8 |
| Victoria Sponge, Classic, Starbucks* | 1 Slice/127g | 490 | 25.0 | 385 | 3.2 | 48.4 | 19.7 | 0.8 |
| Victoria Sponge, Mini, Starbucks* | 1 Cake/65g | 243 | 12.0 | 375 | 3.7 | 47.5 | 18.8 | 0.9 |
| Yoghurt & Berry Loaf, Low Fat, Starbucks* | 1 Slice/94g | 254 | 5.0 | 270 | 5.3 | 50.8 | 5.1 | 1.7 |

### CHEESECAKE

| | Measure INFO/WEIGHT | KCAL | FAT | KCAL | PROT | CARB | FAT | FIBRE |
|---|---|---|---|---|---|---|---|---|
| Blueberry Swirl, Starbucks* | 1 Slice/155g | 463 | 30.0 | 299 | 5.6 | 24.1 | 19.7 | 0.9 |
| Chocolate, Starbucks* | 1 Serving/185g | 723 | 50.0 | 391 | 6.9 | 30.5 | 26.8 | 0.8 |

### COFFEE

| | Measure INFO/WEIGHT | KCAL | FAT | KCAL | PROT | CARB | FAT | FIBRE |
|---|---|---|---|---|---|---|---|---|
| Brewed, Grande, Starbucks* | 1 Cup/473ml | 5 | 0.0 | 1 | 0.1 | 0.0 | 0.0 | 0.0 |
| Brewed, Short, Starbucks* | 1 Cup/236ml | 2 | 0.0 | 1 | 0.1 | 0.0 | 0.0 | 0.0 |
| Brewed, Tall, Starbucks* | 1 Cup/335ml | 4 | 0.0 | 1 | 0.1 | 0.0 | 0.0 | 0.0 |
| Brewed, Venti, Starbucks* | 1 Cup/591ml | 6 | 0.0 | 1 | 0.1 | 0.0 | 0.0 | 0.0 |
| Caffe Americano, Grande, Starbucks* | 1 Cup/473ml | 17 | 0.0 | 4 | 0.2 | 0.6 | 0.0 | 0.0 |
| Caffe Americano, Short, Starbucks* | 1 Cup/236ml | 6 | 0.0 | 3 | 0.2 | 0.4 | 0.0 | 0.0 |
| Caffe Americano, Tall, Starbucks* | 1 Cup/335ml | 11 | 0.0 | 3 | 0.1 | 0.3 | 0.0 | 0.0 |
| Caffe Americano, Venti, Starbucks* | 1 Cup/591ml | 23 | 0.0 | 4 | 0.2 | 0.7 | 0.0 | 0.0 |
| Caffe Latte, Grande, Semi Skimmed Milk, Starbucks* | 1 Cup/473ml | 188 | 7.0 | 40 | 2.6 | 4.0 | 1.5 | 0.0 |
| Caffe Latte, Grande, Skimmed Milk, Starbucks* | 1 Cup/473ml | 131 | 0.0 | 28 | 2.7 | 4.0 | 0.1 | 0.0 |
| Caffe Latte, Grande, Soy, Starbucks* | 1 Cup/473ml | 148 | 5.0 | 31 | 2.2 | 2.7 | 1.1 | 0.3 |
| Caffe Latte, Grande, Whole Milk, Starbucks* | 1 Cup/473ml | 223 | 11.0 | 47 | 2.6 | 3.8 | 2.4 | 0.0 |
| Caffe Latte, Short, Semi Skimmed Milk, Starbucks* | 1 Cup/236ml | 95 | 3.0 | 40 | 2.7 | 3.8 | 1.5 | 0.0 |
| Caffe Latte, Short, Skimmed Milk, Starbucks* | 1 Cup/236ml | 67 | 0.0 | 28 | 2.7 | 4.2 | 0.0 | 0.0 |
| Caffe Latte, Short, Soy, Starbucks* | 1 Cup/236ml | 75 | 3.0 | 32 | 2.2 | 3.0 | 1.1 | 0.3 |
| Caffe Latte, Short, Whole Milk, Starbucks* | 1 Cup/236ml | 113 | 6.0 | 48 | 2.6 | 3.8 | 2.5 | 0.0 |
| Caffe Latte, Tall, Semi Skimmed Milk, Starbucks* | 1 Cup/335ml | 148 | 6.0 | 44 | 2.9 | 4.2 | 1.7 | 0.0 |
| Caffe Latte, Tall, Skimmed Milk, Starbucks* | 1 Cup/335ml | 102 | 0.0 | 30 | 3.0 | 4.5 | 0.1 | 0.0 |
| Caffe Latte, Tall, Soy, Starbucks* | 1 Cup/335ml | 116 | 4.0 | 35 | 2.4 | 3.0 | 1.3 | 0.3 |
| Caffe Latte, Tall, Whole Milk, Starbucks* | 1 Cup/335ml | 176 | 9.0 | 53 | 2.8 | 4.2 | 2.7 | 0.0 |
| Caffe Latte, Venti, Semi Skimmed Milk, Starbucks* | 1 Cup/591ml | 242 | 9.0 | 41 | 2.7 | 4.1 | 1.5 | 0.0 |
| Caffe Latte, Venti, Skimmed Milk, Starbucks* | 1 Cup/591ml | 210 | 0.0 | 36 | 3.4 | 5.3 | 0.1 | 0.0 |
| Caffe Latte, Venti, Soy, Starbucks* | 1 Cup/591ml | 190 | 7.0 | 32 | 2.3 | 2.7 | 1.2 | 0.3 |
| Caffe Latte, Venti, Whole Milk, Starbucks* | 1 Cup/591ml | 289 | 15.0 | 49 | 2.6 | 3.9 | 2.5 | 0.0 |
| Caffe Misto, Cafe Au Lait, Grande, Soy, Starbucks* | 1 Cup/473ml | 82 | 3.0 | 17 | 1.2 | 1.3 | 0.7 | 0.2 |
| Caffe Misto, Cafe Au Lait, Grande, SS Milk, Starbucks* | 1 Cup/473ml | 106 | 4.0 | 22 | 1.5 | 2.1 | 0.9 | 0.0 |
| Caffe Misto, Cafe Au Lait, Grande, Whole Milk, Starbucks* | 1 Cup/473ml | 126 | 7.0 | 27 | 1.5 | 1.9 | 1.4 | 0.0 |
| Caffe Misto, Cafe Au Lait, Short, Skimmed Milk, Starbucks* | 1 Cup/236ml | 37 | 0.0 | 16 | 1.6 | 2.1 | 0.0 | 0.0 |
| Caffe Misto, Cafe Au Lait, Short, Soy, Starbucks* | 1 Cup/236ml | 42 | 2.0 | 18 | 1.3 | 1.3 | 0.7 | 0.2 |
| Caffe Misto, Cafe Au Lait, Short, SS Milk, Starbucks* | 1 Cup/236ml | 54 | 2.0 | 23 | 1.5 | 2.1 | 0.9 | 0.0 |
| Caffe Misto, Cafe Au Lait, Short, Whole Milk, Starbucks* | 1 Cup/236ml | 65 | 3.0 | 28 | 1.5 | 2.1 | 1.5 | 0.0 |
| Caffe Misto, Cafe Au Lait, Tall, Skimmed Milk, Starbucks* | 1 Cup/335ml | 56 | 0.0 | 17 | 1.7 | 2.4 | 0.1 | 0.0 |
| Caffe Misto, Cafe Au Lait, Tall, Soy, Starbucks* | 1 Cup/335ml | 63 | 2.0 | 19 | 1.3 | 1.5 | 0.7 | 0.2 |
| Caffe Misto, Cafe Au Lait, Tall, SS Milk, Starbucks* | 1 Cup/335ml | 81 | 3.0 | 24 | 1.6 | 2.1 | 1.0 | 0.0 |
| Caffe Misto, Cafe Au Lait, Tall, Whole Milk, Starbucks* | 1 Cup/335ml | 97 | 5.0 | 29 | 1.6 | 2.1 | 1.5 | 0.0 |
| Caffe Misto, Cafe Au Lait, Venti, Skimmed Milk, Starbucks* | 1 Cup/591ml | 92 | 0.0 | 16 | 1.6 | 2.2 | 0.0 | 0.0 |
| Caffe Misto, Cafe Au Lait, Venti, Soy, Starbucks* | 1 Cup/591ml | 104 | 4.0 | 18 | 1.3 | 1.3 | 0.7 | 0.2 |
| Caffe Misto, Cafe Au Lait, Venti, SS Milk, Starbucks* | 1 Cup/591ml | 134 | 5.0 | 23 | 1.5 | 2.0 | 0.9 | 0.0 |
| Caffe Misto, Cafe Au Lait, Venti, Whole Milk, Starbucks* | 1 Cup/591ml | 160 | 9.0 | 27 | 1.5 | 2.0 | 1.5 | 0.0 |

| | Measure INFO/WEIGHT | per Measure KCAL | FAT | Nutrition Values per 100g / 100ml KCAL | PROT | CARB | FAT | FIBRE |
|---|---|---|---|---|---|---|---|---|

## STARBUCKS
### COFFEE

| | Measure INFO/WEIGHT | per Measure KCAL | FAT | KCAL | PROT | CARB | FAT | FIBRE |
|---|---|---|---|---|---|---|---|---|
| Caffe Misto, Grande, Whole Milk, Starbucks* | 1 Cup/442ml | 134 | 7.0 | 30 | 1.6 | 2.3 | 1.6 | 0.0 |
| Caffe Misto, Tall, Skimmed Milk, Starbucks* | 1 Cup/354ml | 64 | 0.0 | 18 | 1.8 | 2.5 | 0.0 | 0.0 |
| Caffe Mocha, Tall, Skimmed Milk, Starbucks* | 1 Cup/354ml | 175 | 1.0 | 49 | 0.3 | 9.3 | 0.4 | 0.4 |
| Caffe Mocha, Tall, Whole Milk, Starbucks* | 1 Cup/354ml | 233 | 9.0 | 66 | 2.8 | 8.8 | 2.6 | 0.4 |
| Caffe Mocha, with Whip, Grande, Skim Milk, Starbucks* | 1 Cup/473ml | 324 | 12.0 | 68 | 3.0 | 9.3 | 2.4 | 0.4 |
| Caffe Mocha, with Whip, Grande, Skim Milk, Starbucks* | 1 Cup/473ml | 288 | 10.0 | 61 | 2.8 | 9.3 | 2.0 | 0.4 |
| Caffe Mocha, with Whip, Grande, Soy, Starbucks* | 1 Cup/473ml | 302 | 14.0 | 64 | 2.4 | 8.0 | 2.9 | 0.6 |
| Caffe Mocha, with Whip, Grande, SS Milk, Starbucks* | 1 Cup/473ml | 335 | 15.0 | 71 | 2.8 | 9.1 | 3.2 | 0.4 |
| Caffe Mocha, with Whip, Grande, Whole Milk, Starbucks* | 1 Cup/473ml | 364 | 19.0 | 77 | 2.7 | 8.9 | 3.9 | 0.4 |
| Caffe Mocha, with Whip, Short, Skimmed Milk, Starbucks* | 1 Cup/236ml | 160 | 6.0 | 68 | 2.9 | 9.3 | 2.7 | 0.4 |
| Caffe Mocha, with Whip, Short, Soy, Starbucks* | 1 Cup/236ml | 167 | 8.0 | 71 | 2.5 | 8.5 | 3.6 | 0.6 |
| Caffe Mocha, with Whip, Short, SS Milk, Starbucks* | 1 Cup/236ml | 184 | 9.0 | 78 | 2.8 | 9.3 | 3.9 | 0.4 |
| Caffe Mocha, with Whip, Short, Whole Milk, Starbucks* | 1 Cup/236ml | 198 | 11.0 | 84 | 2.8 | 9.3 | 4.7 | 0.4 |
| Caffe Mocha, with Whip, Tall, Semi Skimmed, Starbucks* | 1 Cup/236ml | 228 | 8.0 | 97 | 4.5 | 14.4 | 3.4 | 0.6 |
| Caffe Mocha, with Whip, Tall, Skimmed Milk, Starbucks* | 1 Cup/335ml | 228 | 8.0 | 68 | 3.2 | 10.1 | 2.4 | 0.4 |
| Caffe Mocha, with Whip, Tall, Soy, Starbucks* | 1 Cup/335ml | 24 | 1.0 | 7 | 0.3 | 0.9 | 0.3 | 0.1 |
| Caffe Mocha, with Whip, Tall, Whole Milk, Starbucks* | 1 Cup/335ml | 290 | 16.0 | 87 | 3.0 | 9.8 | 4.6 | 0.4 |
| Caffe Mocha, with Whip, Tall, Whole Milk, Starbucks* | 1 Cup/354ml | 313 | 17.0 | 88 | 2.8 | 9.0 | 4.9 | 0.4 |
| Caffe Mocha, with Whip, Venti, Skimmed Milk, Starbucks* | 1 Cup/591ml | 347 | 10.0 | 59 | 2.9 | 9.3 | 1.7 | 0.4 |
| Caffe Mocha, with Whip, Venti, Soy, Starbucks* | 1 Cup/591ml | 366 | 16.0 | 62 | 2.5 | 8.1 | 2.7 | 0.6 |
| Caffe Mocha, with Whip, Venti, SS Milk, Starbucks* | 1 Cup/591ml | 409 | 17.0 | 69 | 2.9 | 9.1 | 3.0 | 0.4 |
| Caffe Mocha, with Whip, Venti, Whole Milk, Starbucks* | 1 Cup/591ml | 448 | 23.0 | 76 | 2.8 | 9.0 | 3.8 | 0.4 |
| Cappuccino, Grande, Semi Skimmed Milk, Starbucks* | 1 Cup/473ml | 115 | 4.0 | 24 | 1.6 | 2.5 | 0.9 | 0.0 |
| Cappuccino, Grande, Soy, Starbucks* | 1 Cup/473ml | 92 | 3.0 | 19 | 1.3 | 1.7 | 0.7 | 0.2 |
| Cappuccino, Grande, Whole Milk, Starbucks* | 1 Cup/473ml | 136 | 7.0 | 29 | 1.6 | 2.3 | 1.4 | 0.0 |
| Cappuccino, Short, Semi Skimmed Milk, Starbucks* | 1 Cup/236ml | 78 | 3.0 | 33 | 2.2 | 3.4 | 1.2 | 0.0 |
| Cappuccino, Short, Skimmed Milk, Starbucks* | 1 Cup/236ml | 55 | 0.0 | 23 | 2.2 | 3.4 | 0.0 | 0.0 |
| Cappuccino, Short, Soy, Starbucks* | 1 Cup/236ml | 62 | 2.0 | 26 | 1.8 | 2.5 | 0.9 | 0.2 |
| Cappuccino, Short, Whole Milk, Starbucks* | 1 Cup/236ml | 92 | 5.0 | 39 | 2.1 | 3.4 | 2.0 | 0.0 |
| Cappuccino, Tall, Semi Skimmed Milk, Starbucks* | 1 Cup/335ml | 91 | 3.0 | 27 | 1.8 | 2.7 | 1.0 | 0.0 |
| Cappuccino, Tall, Skimmed Milk, Starbucks* | 1 Cup/335ml | 64 | 0.0 | 19 | 1.8 | 2.7 | 0.0 | 0.0 |
| Cappuccino, Tall, Soy, Starbucks* | 1 Cup/335ml | 72 | 3.0 | 21 | 1.5 | 1.8 | 0.8 | 0.2 |
| Cappuccino, Tall, Whole Milk, Starbucks* | 1 Cup/335ml | 108 | 6.0 | 32 | 1.8 | 2.7 | 1.7 | 0.0 |
| Cappuccino, Venti, Semi Skimmed Milk, Starbucks* | 1 Cup/591ml | 155 | 6.0 | 26 | 1.7 | 2.5 | 1.0 | 0.0 |
| Cappuccino, Venti, Skimmed Milk, Starbucks* | 1 Cup/591ml | 109 | 0.0 | 18 | 1.8 | 2.7 | 0.0 | 0.0 |
| Cappuccino, Venti, Soy, Starbucks* | 1 Cup/591ml | 123 | 4.0 | 21 | 1.5 | 1.9 | 0.7 | 0.2 |
| Cappuccino, Venti, Whole Milk, Starbucks* | 1 Cup/591ml | 184 | 9.0 | 31 | 1.7 | 2.5 | 1.6 | 0.0 |
| Caramel Macchiato, Grande, Skimmed Milk, Starbucks* | 1 Cup/473ml | 193 | 1.0 | 41 | 2.3 | 7.4 | 0.2 | 0.0 |
| Caramel Macchiato, Grande, Soy, Starbucks* | 1 Cup/473ml | 207 | 5.0 | 44 | 1.9 | 6.1 | 1.1 | 0.2 |
| Caramel Macchiato, Grande, SS Milk, Starbucks* | 1 Cup/473ml | 240 | 7.0 | 51 | 2.2 | 7.2 | 1.4 | 0.0 |
| Caramel Macchiato, Grande, Whole Milk, Starbucks* | 1 Cup/473ml | 269 | 11.0 | 57 | 2.2 | 7.2 | 2.2 | 0.0 |
| Caramel Macchiato, Short, Semi Skimmed Milk, Starbucks* | 1 Cup/236ml | 122 | 4.0 | 52 | 2.3 | 6.8 | 1.6 | 0.0 |
| Caramel Macchiato, Short, Skimmed Milk, Starbucks* | 1 Cup/236ml | 97 | 1.0 | 41 | 2.4 | 7.2 | 0.4 | 0.0 |
| Caramel Macchiato, Short, Soy, Starbucks* | 1 Cup/236ml | 104 | 3.0 | 44 | 1.9 | 5.9 | 1.3 | 0.2 |
| Caramel Macchiato, Short, Whole Milk, Starbucks* | 1 Cup/236ml | 137 | 6.0 | 58 | 2.2 | 6.8 | 2.4 | 0.0 |
| Caramel Macchiato, Tall, Semi Skimmed Milk, Starbucks* | 1 Cup/335ml | 178 | 5.0 | 53 | 2.4 | 7.5 | 1.6 | 0.0 |
| Caramel Macchiato, Tall, Skimmed Milk, Starbucks* | 1 Cup/335ml | 142 | 1.0 | 42 | 2.4 | 7.5 | 0.3 | 0.0 |
| Caramel Macchiato, Tall, Skimmed Milk, Starbucks* | 1 Cup/354ml | 173 | 1.0 | 49 | 3.1 | 8.5 | 0.2 | 0.0 |
| Caramel Macchiato, Tall, Soy, Starbucks* | 1 Cup/335ml | 153 | 4.0 | 46 | 2.0 | 6.3 | 1.2 | 0.3 |
| Caramel Macchiato, Tall, Whole Milk, Starbucks* | 1 Cup/335ml | 201 | 8.0 | 60 | 2.3 | 7.2 | 2.4 | 0.0 |
| Caramel Macchiato, Tall, Whole Milk, Starbucks* | 1 Cup/354ml | 244 | 10.0 | 69 | 2.8 | 7.9 | 2.9 | 0.0 |
| Caramel Macchiato, Venti, Skimmed Milk, Starbucks* | 1 Cup/591ml | 239 | 1.0 | 40 | 2.3 | 7.4 | 0.2 | 0.0 |

| | Measure INFO/WEIGHT | per Measure KCAL | FAT | Nutrition Values per 100g / 100ml KCAL | PROT | CARB | FAT | FIBRE |
|---|---|---|---|---|---|---|---|---|

## STARBUCKS

### COFFEE

| | Measure INFO/WEIGHT | KCAL | FAT | KCAL | PROT | CARB | FAT | FIBRE |
|---|---|---|---|---|---|---|---|---|
| Caramel Macchiato, Venti, Whole Milk, Starbucks* | 1 Cup/591ml | 337 | 13.0 | 57 | 2.2 | 7.1 | 2.2 | 0.0 |
| Espresso, Con Panna, Doppio, Starbucks* | 1 Cup/60ml | 111 | 9.0 | 185 | 1.2 | 6.7 | 15.5 | 0.0 |
| Espresso, Con Panna, Solo, Starbucks* | 1 Cup/30ml | 105 | 9.0 | 350 | 1.3 | 10.0 | 31.0 | 0.0 |
| Espresso, Doppio, Starbucks* | 1 Cup/60ml | 11 | 0.0 | 18 | 1.2 | 3.3 | 0.0 | 0.0 |
| Espresso, Solo, Starbucks* | 1 Cup/30ml | 6 | 0.0 | 20 | 1.3 | 3.3 | 0.0 | 0.0 |
| Espresso Con Panna, Doppio, Starbucks* | 1 Cup/60ml | 36 | 3.0 | 60 | 1.5 | 5.0 | 4.2 | 0.0 |
| Espresso Con Panna, Solo, Starbucks* | 1 Cup/30ml | 31 | 2.0 | 103 | 1.7 | 6.7 | 8.3 | 0.0 |
| Espresso Macchiato, Doppio, Skimmed Milk, Starbucks* | 1 Cup/60ml | 13 | 0.0 | 22 | 1.7 | 3.3 | 0.0 | 0.0 |
| Espresso Macchiato, Doppio, Soy, Starbucks* | 1 Cup/60ml | 13 | 0.0 | 22 | 1.5 | 3.3 | 0.2 | 0.0 |
| Espresso Macchiato, Doppio, SS Milk, Starbucks* | 1 Cup/60ml | 14 | 0.0 | 23 | 1.5 | 3.3 | 0.2 | 0.0 |
| Espresso Macchiato, Doppio, Whole Milk, Starbucks* | 1 Cup/60ml | 15 | 0.0 | 25 | 1.5 | 3.3 | 0.3 | 0.0 |
| Espresso Macchiato, Solo, Semi Skimmed Milk, Starbucks* | 1 Cup/30ml | 8 | 0.0 | 27 | 1.7 | 3.3 | 0.3 | 0.0 |
| Espresso Macchiato, Solo, Skimmed Milk, Starbucks* | 1 Cup/30ml | 7 | 0.0 | 23 | 1.7 | 3.3 | 0.0 | 0.0 |
| Espresso Macchiato, Solo, Soy, Starbucks* | 1 Cup/30ml | 7 | 0.0 | 23 | 1.7 | 3.3 | 0.3 | 0.0 |
| Espresso Macchiato, Solo, Whole Milk, Starbucks* | 1 Cup/30ml | 8 | 0.0 | 27 | 1.7 | 3.3 | 0.7 | 0.0 |
| Hazelnut Mocha, with Whip, Grande, Skim Milk, Starbucks* | 1 Cup/335ml | 252 | 7.0 | 75 | 2.7 | 13.1 | 2.0 | 0.4 |
| Hazelnut Mocha, with Whip, Grande, Soy, Starbucks* | 1 Cup/473ml | 369 | 13.0 | 78 | 2.3 | 12.0 | 2.8 | 0.6 |
| Hazelnut Mocha, with Whip, Grande, SS Milk, Starbucks* | 1 Cup/473ml | 399 | 15.0 | 84 | 2.6 | 12.9 | 3.1 | 0.4 |
| Hazelnut Mocha, with Whip, Grande, Wh. Milk, Starbucks* | 1 Cup/473ml | 425 | 18.0 | 90 | 2.6 | 12.7 | 3.8 | 0.4 |
| Hazelnut Mocha, with Whip, Short, Skim Milk, Starbucks* | 1 Cup/236ml | 197 | 6.0 | 83 | 2.8 | 13.6 | 2.6 | 0.4 |
| Hazelnut Mocha, with Whip, Short, Soy, Starbucks* | 1 Cup/236ml | 201 | 8.0 | 85 | 2.3 | 12.3 | 3.5 | 0.6 |
| Hazelnut Mocha, with Whip, Short, SS Milk, Starbucks* | 1 Cup/236ml | 216 | 9.0 | 92 | 2.7 | 13.1 | 3.8 | 0.4 |
| Hazelnut Mocha, with Whip, Short, Whole Milk, Starbucks* | 1 Cup/236ml | 229 | 11.0 | 97 | 2.6 | 13.1 | 4.5 | 0.4 |
| Hazelnut Mocha, with Whip, Tall, Skimmed Milk, Starbucks* | 1 Cup/335ml | 277 | 8.0 | 83 | 3.0 | 13.7 | 2.4 | 0.4 |
| Hazelnut Mocha, with Whip, Tall, Soy, Starbucks* | 1 Cup/335ml | 288 | 11.0 | 86 | 2.6 | 12.5 | 3.3 | 0.7 |
| Hazelnut Mocha, with Whip, Tall, SS Milk, Starbucks* | 1 Cup/335ml | 312 | 12.0 | 93 | 2.9 | 13.7 | 3.6 | 0.4 |
| Hazelnut Mocha, with Whip, Tall, Whole Milk, Starbucks* | 1 Cup/335ml | 334 | 15.0 | 100 | 2.9 | 13.4 | 4.4 | 0.4 |
| Hazelnut Mocha, with Whip, Venti, Skim Milk, Starbucks* | 1 Cup/591ml | 430 | 10.0 | 73 | 2.7 | 13.0 | 1.7 | 0.4 |
| Hazelnut Mocha, with Whip, Venti, Soy, Starbucks* | 1 Cup/591ml | 448 | 15.0 | 76 | 2.4 | 11.8 | 2.6 | 0.6 |
| Hazelnut Mocha, with Whip, Venti, SS Milk, Starbucks* | 1 Cup/591ml | 487 | 17.0 | 82 | 2.7 | 12.9 | 2.8 | 0.4 |
| Hazelnut Mocha, with Whip, Venti, Whole Milk, Starbucks* | 1 Cup/591ml | 523 | 21.0 | 88 | 2.6 | 12.7 | 3.6 | 0.4 |
| Iced, Caffe Americano, Grande, Starbucks* | 1 Cup/473ml | 17 | 0.0 | 4 | 0.2 | 0.6 | 0.0 | 0.0 |
| Iced, Caffe Americano, Tall, Starbucks* | 1 Cup/335ml | 11 | 0.0 | 3 | 0.2 | 0.6 | 0.0 | 0.0 |
| Iced, Caffe Americano, Venti, Starbucks* | 1 Cup/591ml | 23 | 0.0 | 4 | 0.2 | 0.7 | 0.0 | 0.0 |
| Iced, Caffe Latte, Grande, Semi Skimmed Milk, Starbucks* | 1 Cup/473ml | 126 | 4.0 | 27 | 1.8 | 2.7 | 0.9 | 0.0 |
| Iced, Caffe Latte, Grande, Skimmed Milk, Starbucks* | 1 Cup/473ml | 90 | 0.0 | 19 | 1.8 | 2.7 | 0.0 | 0.0 |
| Iced, Caffe Latte, Grande, Soy, Starbucks* | 1 Cup/473ml | 104 | 4.0 | 22 | 1.5 | 1.9 | 0.8 | 0.2 |
| Iced, Caffe Latte, Grande, Whole Milk, Starbucks* | 1 Cup/473ml | 149 | 8.0 | 31 | 1.7 | 2.5 | 1.6 | 0.0 |
| Iced, Caffe Latte, Tall, Semi Skimmed Milk, Starbucks* | 1 Cup/335ml | 97 | 4.0 | 29 | 1.9 | 3.0 | 1.1 | 0.0 |
| Iced, Caffe Latte, Tall, Skimmed Milk, Starbucks* | 1 Cup/335ml | 68 | 0.0 | 20 | 1.9 | 3.0 | 0.1 | 0.0 |
| Iced, Caffe Latte, Tall, Soy, Starbucks* | 1 Cup/335ml | 80 | 3.0 | 24 | 1.7 | 2.1 | 0.9 | 0.2 |
| Iced, Caffe Latte, Tall, Whole Milk, Starbucks* | 1 Cup/335ml | 115 | 6.0 | 34 | 1.8 | 2.7 | 1.8 | 0.0 |
| Iced, Caffe Latte, Venti, Semi Skimmed Milk, Starbucks* | 1 Cup/591ml | 142 | 5.0 | 24 | 1.6 | 2.4 | 0.9 | 0.0 |
| Iced, Caffe Latte, Venti, Skimmed Milk, Starbucks* | 1 Cup/591ml | 100 | 0.0 | 17 | 1.6 | 2.5 | 0.0 | 0.0 |
| Iced, Caffe Latte, Venti, Soy, Starbucks* | 1 Cup/591ml | 118 | 4.0 | 20 | 1.4 | 1.9 | 0.7 | 0.2 |
| Iced, Caffe Latte, Venti, Whole Milk, Starbucks* | 1 Cup/591ml | 168 | 9.0 | 28 | 1.5 | 2.4 | 1.4 | 0.0 |
| Iced, Caffe Mocha, with Whip, Grande, Skim, Starbucks* | 1 Cup/473ml | 289 | 14.0 | 61 | 2.0 | 8.2 | 2.9 | 0.4 |
| Iced, Caffe Mocha, with Whip, Grande, Soy, Starbucks* | 1 Cup/473ml | 300 | 16.0 | 63 | 1.8 | 7.6 | 3.4 | 0.5 |
| Iced, Caffe Mocha, with Whip, Grande, SS Milk, Starbucks* | 1 Cup/473ml | 316 | 17.0 | 67 | 2.0 | 8.0 | 3.5 | 0.4 |
| Iced, Caffe Mocha, with Whip, Tall, Skim Milk, Starbucks* | 1 Cup/335ml | 212 | 10.0 | 63 | 2.1 | 8.7 | 2.9 | 0.4 |
| Iced, Caffe Mocha, with Whip, Tall, Soy, Starbucks* | 1 Cup/335ml | 221 | 12.0 | 66 | 2.0 | 8.1 | 3.5 | 0.6 |
| Iced, Caffe Mocha, with Whip, Tall, SS Milk, Starbucks* | 1 Cup/335ml | 234 | 12.0 | 70 | 2.1 | 8.7 | 3.7 | 0.4 |

| | Measure INFO/WEIGHT | per Measure KCAL | per Measure FAT | Nutrition Values per 100g / 100ml KCAL | PROT | CARB | FAT | FIBRE |
|---|---|---|---|---|---|---|---|---|

## STARBUCKS

### COFFEE

| | Measure INFO/WEIGHT | KCAL | FAT | KCAL | PROT | CARB | FAT | FIBRE |
|---|---|---|---|---|---|---|---|---|
| Iced, Caffe Mocha, with Whip, Tall, Whole Milk, Starbucks* | 1 Cup/335ml | 248 | 14.0 | 74 | 2.1 | 8.4 | 4.2 | 0.4 |
| Iced, Caffe Mocha, with Whip, Venti, Skim Milk, Starbucks* | 1 Cup/591ml | 310 | 13.0 | 52 | 1.8 | 7.8 | 2.2 | 0.4 |
| Iced, Caffe Mocha, with Whip, Venti, Soy, Starbucks* | 1 Cup/591ml | 322 | 16.0 | 54 | 1.6 | 7.1 | 2.7 | 0.5 |
| Iced, Caffe Mocha, with Whip, Venti, SS Milk, Starbucks* | 1 Cup/591ml | 340 | 17.0 | 58 | 1.8 | 7.6 | 2.8 | 0.4 |
| Iced, Caffe Mocha, with Whip, Venti, Whole Milk, Starbucks* | 1 Cup/591ml | 358 | 19.0 | 61 | 1.7 | 7.6 | 3.2 | 0.4 |
| Iced, Caramel Macchiato, Grande, Skim Milk, Starbucks* | 1 Cup/473ml | 188 | 1.0 | 40 | 2.1 | 7.2 | 0.3 | 0.0 |
| Iced, Caramel Macchiato, Grande, Soy, Starbucks* | 1 Cup/473ml | 206 | 5.0 | 44 | 1.8 | 6.3 | 1.1 | 0.2 |
| Iced, Caramel Macchiato, Grande, SS Milk, Starbucks* | 1 Cup/473ml | 231 | 6.0 | 49 | 2.0 | 7.0 | 1.3 | 0.0 |
| Iced, Caramel Macchiato, Grande, Whole Milk, Starbucks* | 1 Cup/473ml | 257 | 10.0 | 54 | 2.0 | 7.0 | 2.1 | 0.0 |
| Iced, Caramel Macchiato, Tall, Skimmed Milk, Starbucks* | 1 Cup/335ml | 139 | 1.0 | 41 | 2.1 | 7.5 | 0.4 | 0.0 |
| Iced, Caramel Macchiato, Tall, Soy, Starbucks* | 1 Cup/335ml | 152 | 4.0 | 45 | 1.8 | 6.6 | 1.2 | 0.2 |
| Iced, Caramel Macchiato, Tall, SS Milk, Starbucks* | 1 Cup/335ml | 171 | 5.0 | 51 | 2.1 | 7.2 | 1.5 | 0.0 |
| Iced, Caramel Macchiato, Tall, Whole Milk, Starbucks* | 1 Cup/335ml | 191 | 8.0 | 57 | 2.0 | 7.2 | 2.2 | 0.0 |
| Iced, Caramel Macchiato, Venti, Skimmed Milk, Starbucks* | 1 Cup/591ml | 215 | 1.0 | 36 | 1.8 | 6.8 | 0.2 | 0.0 |
| Iced, Caramel Macchiato, Venti, Soy, Starbucks* | 1 Cup/591ml | 234 | 6.0 | 40 | 1.6 | 5.9 | 1.0 | 0.2 |
| Iced, Caramel Macchiato, Venti, SS Milk, Starbucks* | 1 Cup/591ml | 262 | 7.0 | 44 | 1.8 | 6.6 | 1.1 | 0.0 |
| Iced, Caramel Macchiato, Venti, Whole Milk, Starbucks* | 1 Cup/591ml | 291 | 11.0 | 49 | 1.7 | 6.6 | 1.8 | 0.0 |
| Iced, Grande, Starbucks* | 1 Cup/473ml | 4 | 0.0 | 1 | 0.1 | 0.0 | 0.0 | 0.0 |
| Iced, Hazelnut Mocha, with Whip, Grande, Soy, Starbucks* | 1 Cup/473ml | 437 | 19.0 | 92 | 2.2 | 11.8 | 4.1 | 0.1 |
| Iced, Hazelnut Mocha, with Whip, Tall, Soy, Starbucks* | 1 Cup/335ml | 325 | 14.0 | 97 | 2.4 | 12.5 | 4.3 | 0.1 |
| Iced, Hazelnut Mocha, with Whip, Tall, SS Milk, Starbucks* | 1 Cup/335ml | 318 | 14.0 | 95 | 2.4 | 12.1 | 4.2 | 0.0 |
| Iced, Hazelnut Mocha, with Whip, Tall, Wh. Milk, Starbucks* | 1 Cup/335ml | 351 | 17.0 | 105 | 2.5 | 12.8 | 5.0 | 0.0 |
| Iced, Hazelnut Mocha, with Whip, Venti, Soy, Starbucks* | 1 Cup/591ml | 578 | 22.0 | 98 | 2.4 | 13.7 | 3.8 | 0.1 |
| Iced, Hazelnut Mocha, with Whip, Venti, SS Milk, Starbucks* | 1 Cup/591ml | 599 | 23.0 | 101 | 2.6 | 14.2 | 3.9 | 0.0 |
| Iced, Latte, Vanilla, Grande, Skimmed Milk, Starbucks* | 1 Cup/473ml | 155 | 0.0 | 33 | 1.6 | 6.5 | 0.0 | 0.0 |
| Iced, Latte, Vanilla, Grande, Soy, Starbucks* | 1 Cup/473ml | 168 | 3.0 | 36 | 1.3 | 5.7 | 0.7 | 0.2 |
| Iced, Latte, Vanilla, Grande, Whole Milk, Starbucks* | 1 Cup/473ml | 207 | 6.0 | 44 | 1.5 | 6.3 | 1.4 | 0.0 |
| Iced, Latte, Vanilla, Tall, Semi Skimmed Milk, Starbucks* | 1 Cup/335ml | 134 | 3.0 | 40 | 1.6 | 6.5 | 0.9 | 0.0 |
| Iced, Latte, Vanilla, Tall, Soy, Starbucks* | 1 Cup/335ml | 120 | 2.0 | 36 | 1.4 | 5.6 | 0.7 | 0.2 |
| Iced, Latte, Vanilla, Tall, Whole Milk, Starbucks* | 1 Cup/335ml | 149 | 5.0 | 45 | 1.5 | 6.2 | 1.5 | 0.0 |
| Iced, Latte, Vanilla, Venti, Semi Skimmed Milk, Starbucks* | 1 Cup/591ml | 182 | 0.0 | 31 | 1.4 | 6.3 | 0.0 | 0.0 |
| Iced, Latte, Vanilla, Venti, Skimmed Milk, Starbucks* | 1 Cup/591ml | 182 | 0.0 | 31 | 1.4 | 6.3 | 0.0 | 0.0 |
| Iced, Latte, Vanilla, Venti, Soy, Starbucks* | 1 Cup/591ml | 197 | 3.0 | 33 | 1.2 | 5.6 | 0.6 | 0.1 |
| Iced, Latte, Vanilla, Venti, Whole Milk, Starbucks* | 1 Cup/591ml | 240 | 7.0 | 41 | 1.3 | 6.1 | 1.2 | 0.0 |
| Iced, Tall, Starbucks* | 1 Cup/335ml | 3 | 0.0 | 1 | 0.1 | 0.0 | 0.0 | 0.0 |
| Iced, Venti, Starbucks* | 1 Cup/591ml | 5 | 0.0 | 1 | 0.1 | 0.0 | 0.0 | 0.0 |
| Mocha, Peppermint, Skimmed, Grande, Starbucks* | 1 Cup/473ml | 304 | 2.0 | 64 | 2.9 | 13.3 | 0.5 | 0.4 |
| Mocha, Peppermint, Skimmed, Tall, Starbucks* | 1 Cup/354ml | 237 | 1.0 | 67 | 3.1 | 13.6 | 0.4 | 0.4 |
| Mocha, Peppermint, Skimmed, Venti, Starbucks* | 1 Cup/591ml | 385 | 3.0 | 65 | 3.0 | 13.4 | 0.5 | 0.4 |
| Mocha, Peppermint, Skimmed, Whip, Grande, Starbucks* | 1 Cup/473ml | 405 | 21.0 | 86 | 2.9 | 13.7 | 4.4 | 0.4 |
| Mocha, Peppermint, Skimmed, Whip, Tall, Starbucks* | 1 Cup/354ml | 317 | 9.0 | 90 | 3.1 | 13.8 | 2.7 | 0.4 |
| Mocha, Peppermint, Skimmed, Whip, Venti, Starbucks* | 1 Cup/591ml | 486 | 12.0 | 82 | 3.0 | 13.7 | 2.1 | 0.4 |
| Mocha, Peppermint, Whole, Grande, Starbucks* | 1 Cup/473ml | 372 | 11.0 | 79 | 2.7 | 12.9 | 2.4 | 0.4 |
| Mocha, Peppermint, Whole, Tall, Starbucks* | 1 Cup/354ml | 293 | 9.0 | 83 | 2.8 | 13.3 | 2.5 | 0.4 |
| Mocha, Peppermint, Whole, Venti, Starbucks* | 1 Cup/591ml | 475 | 15.0 | 80 | 2.8 | 12.9 | 2.6 | 0.4 |
| Mocha, Peppermint, Whole, Whip, Grande, Starbucks* | 1 Cup/473ml | 473 | 21.0 | 100 | 2.7 | 13.3 | 4.4 | 0.4 |
| Mocha, Peppermint, Whole, Whip, Tall, Starbucks* | 1 Cup/354ml | 373 | 17.0 | 105 | 2.8 | 13.6 | 4.8 | 0.4 |
| Mocha, Peppermint, Whole, Whip, Venti, Starbucks* | 1 Cup/591ml | 576 | 25.0 | 97 | 2.8 | 13.2 | 4.2 | 0.4 |
| Vanilla, with Whip, Grande, Starbucks* | 1 Cup/473ml | 364 | 14.0 | 77 | 1.2 | 11.4 | 3.0 | 0.0 |
| Vanilla, with Whip, Tall, Starbucks* | 1 Cup/335ml | 284 | 10.0 | 85 | 1.3 | 13.1 | 3.1 | 0.0 |
| Vanilla, with Whip, Venti, Starbucks* | 1 Cup/591ml | 412 | 14.0 | 70 | 1.1 | 11.2 | 2.3 | 0.0 |
| Vanilla Latte, Grande, Semi Skimmed Milk, Starbucks* | 1 Cup/473ml | 251 | 6.0 | 53 | 2.4 | 7.6 | 1.3 | 0.0 |

## STARBUCKS

| | Measure INFO/WEIGHT | per Measure | | Nutrition Values per 100g / 100ml | | | | |
|---|---|---|---|---|---|---|---|---|
| | | KCAL | FAT | KCAL | PROT | CARB | FAT | FIBRE |
| **COFFEE** | | | | | | | | |
| Vanilla Latte, Grande, Skimmed Milk, Starbucks* | 1 Cup/473ml | 199 | 0.0 | 42 | 2.5 | 7.8 | 0.1 | 0.0 |
| Vanilla Latte, Grande, Soy, Starbucks* | 1 Cup/473ml | 214 | 5.0 | 45 | 2.0 | 6.5 | 1.0 | 0.2 |
| Vanilla Latte, Grande, Whole Milk, Starbucks* | 1 Cup/473ml | 284 | 11.0 | 60 | 2.4 | 7.6 | 2.2 | 0.0 |
| Vanilla Latte, Short, Semi Skimmed Milk, Starbucks* | 1 Cup/236ml | 127 | 3.0 | 54 | 2.5 | 7.6 | 1.4 | 0.0 |
| Vanilla Latte, Short, Skimmed Milk, Starbucks* | 1 Cup/236ml | 101 | 0.0 | 43 | 2.5 | 8.0 | 0.0 | 0.0 |
| Vanilla Latte, Short, Soy, Starbucks* | 1 Cup/236ml | 108 | 3.0 | 46 | 2.1 | 6.8 | 1.1 | 0.2 |
| Vanilla Latte, Short, Whole Milk, Starbucks* | 1 Cup/236ml | 144 | 5.0 | 61 | 2.4 | 7.6 | 2.3 | 0.0 |
| Vanilla Latte, Tall, Semi Skimmed Milk, Starbucks* | 1 Cup/335ml | 195 | 5.0 | 58 | 2.7 | 8.1 | 1.5 | 0.0 |
| Vanilla Latte, Tall, Skimmed Milk, Starbucks* | 1 Cup/335ml | 152 | 0.0 | 45 | 2.8 | 8.4 | 0.1 | 0.0 |
| Vanilla Latte, Tall, Soy, Starbucks* | 1 Cup/335ml | 165 | 4.0 | 49 | 2.3 | 6.9 | 1.2 | 0.3 |
| Vanilla Latte, Tall, Whole Milk, Starbucks* | 1 Cup/335ml | 221 | 9.0 | 66 | 2.7 | 8.1 | 2.6 | 0.0 |
| Vanilla Latte, Venti, Semi Skimmed Milk, Starbucks* | 1 Cup/591ml | 321 | 9.0 | 54 | 2.5 | 7.8 | 1.4 | 0.0 |
| Vanilla Latte, Venti, Skimmed Milk, Starbucks* | 1 Cup/591ml | 252 | 0.0 | 43 | 2.6 | 7.9 | 0.1 | 0.0 |
| Vanilla Latte, Venti, Soy, Starbucks* | 1 Cup/591ml | 272 | 7.0 | 46 | 2.1 | 6.6 | 1.1 | 0.3 |
| Vanilla Latte, Venti, Whole Milk, Starbucks* | 1 Cup/591ml | 364 | 14.0 | 62 | 2.5 | 7.6 | 2.4 | 0.0 |
| White Mocha, with Whip, Grande, Skim Milk, Starbucks* | 1 Cup/473ml | 425 | 13.0 | 90 | 3.2 | 13.5 | 2.7 | 0.0 |
| White Mocha, with Whip, Grande, Soy, Starbucks* | 1 Cup/473ml | 439 | 17.0 | 93 | 2.8 | 12.3 | 3.6 | 0.2 |
| White Mocha, with Whip, Grande, SS Milk, Starbucks* | 1 Cup/473ml | 471 | 18.0 | 100 | 3.1 | 13.3 | 3.9 | 0.0 |
| White Mocha, with Whip, Grande, Whole Milk, Starbucks* | 1 Cup/473ml | 500 | 22.0 | 106 | 3.1 | 13.1 | 4.7 | 0.0 |
| White Mocha, with Whip, Short, Skimmed, Starbucks* | 1 Cup/236ml | 229 | 8.0 | 97 | 3.3 | 13.6 | 3.4 | 0.0 |
| White Mocha, with Whip, Short, Soy, Starbucks* | 1 Cup/236ml | 236 | 10.0 | 100 | 2.9 | 12.7 | 4.3 | 0.2 |
| White Mocha, with Whip, Short, SS Milk, Starbucks* | 1 Cup/236ml | 252 | 11.0 | 107 | 3.2 | 13.6 | 4.6 | 0.2 |
| White Mocha, with Whip, Short, Whole Milk, Starbucks* | 1 Cup/236ml | 267 | 13.0 | 113 | 3.2 | 13.6 | 5.4 | 0.0 |
| White Mocha, with Whip, Tall, Skimmed Milk, Starbucks* | 1 Cup/335ml | 331 | 10.0 | 99 | 3.5 | 14.3 | 3.1 | 0.0 |
| White Mocha, with Whip, Tall, Soy, Starbucks* | 1 Cup/335ml | 342 | 14.0 | 102 | 3.1 | 13.1 | 4.1 | 0.3 |
| White Mocha, with Whip, Tall, SS Milk, Starbucks* | 1 Cup/335ml | 369 | 15.0 | 110 | 3.5 | 14.3 | 4.5 | 0.0 |
| White Mocha, with Whip, Tall, Whole Milk, Starbucks* | 1 Cup/335ml | 392 | 18.0 | 117 | 3.4 | 14.0 | 5.4 | 0.0 |
| White Mocha, with Whip, Venti, Skimmed Milk, Starbucks* | 1 Cup/591ml | 518 | 14.0 | 88 | 3.3 | 13.5 | 2.4 | 0.0 |
| White Mocha, with Whip, Venti, Soy, Starbucks* | 1 Cup/591ml | 537 | 20.0 | 91 | 2.9 | 12.3 | 3.4 | 0.2 |
| White Mocha, with Whip, Venti, SS Milk, Starbucks* | 1 Cup/591ml | 581 | 22.0 | 98 | 3.2 | 13.4 | 3.7 | 0.0 |
| White Mocha, with Whip, Venti, Whole Milk, Starbucks* | 1 Cup/591ml | 619 | 27.0 | 105 | 3.2 | 13.2 | 4.5 | 0.0 |
| **COOKIES** | | | | | | | | |
| Chocolate, Chunk, Starbucks* | 1 Cookie/90g | 396 | 12.0 | 440 | 6.8 | 69.7 | 13.3 | 0.3 |
| Fruit & Oat, Starbucks* | 1 Cookie/80g | 344 | 14.0 | 430 | 4.2 | 64.0 | 17.5 | 2.2 |
| **CORNFLAKE** | | | | | | | | |
| Chocolate, Square, Starbucks* | 1 Slice/62g | 289 | 14.0 | 466 | 4.0 | 59.7 | 23.0 | 2.2 |
| **CREPE** | | | | | | | | |
| Ham, Mushroom & Tomato, Starbucks* | 1 Pack/153g | 148 | 5.0 | 97 | 4.3 | 14.0 | 3.1 | 1.0 |
| **CRISPS** | | | | | | | | |
| Strong Cheese & Onion, Starbucks* | 1 Bag/50g | 227 | 11.0 | 455 | 7.1 | 56.2 | 22.6 | 4.0 |
| **CROISSANT** | | | | | | | | |
| Almond, Starbucks* | 1 Croissant/92g | 389 | 20.0 | 423 | 7.0 | 48.2 | 21.9 | 2.2 |
| Butter, Starbucks* | 1 Croissant/70g | 279 | 17.0 | 398 | 6.9 | 39.5 | 23.6 | 1.4 |
| Cheese, & Ham, Starbucks* | 1 Pack/114g | 359 | 21.0 | 315 | 13.2 | 24.9 | 18.1 | 0.8 |
| **CUPCAKES** | | | | | | | | |
| Banana & Chocolate Chip, Starbucks* | 1 Cupcake/80g | 342 | 15.0 | 428 | 4.7 | 57.8 | 18.6 | 0.5 |
| Lemon, Sicilian, Starbucks* | 1 Cake/80g | 350 | 18.0 | 437 | 3.3 | 55.3 | 22.5 | 0.5 |
| Strawberry, Starbucks* | 1 Cupcake/83g | 385 | 21.0 | 464 | 4.1 | 55.9 | 25.1 | 0.6 |
| **DOUGHNUT** | | | | | | | | |
| Chocolate & Custard, Mini, Starbucks* | 1 Doughnut/25g | 77 | 3.0 | 307 | 5.8 | 39.8 | 13.8 | 1.6 |
| Jam, Mini, Starbucks* | 1 Donut/24g | 77 | 3.0 | 323 | 6.2 | 49.6 | 11.1 | 1.4 |

| | Measure INFO/WEIGHT | per Measure KCAL | per Measure FAT | Nutrition Values per 100g / 100ml KCAL | PROT | CARB | FAT | FIBRE |
|---|---|---|---|---|---|---|---|---|
| **STARBUCKS** | | | | | | | | |
| **DRIED FRUIT** | | | | | | | | |
| Starbucks* | 1 Av Serving/30g | 88 | 0.0 | 294 | 2.2 | 75.3 | 0.4 | 1.4 |
| **FLAPJACK** | | | | | | | | |
| Banana & Caramel, Starbucks* | 1 Serving/70g | 301 | 15.0 | 430 | 3.3 | 54.4 | 22.0 | 2.5 |
| **FRAPPUCCINO** | | | | | | | | |
| Caramel, Grande, Starbucks* | 1 Cup/473ml | 294 | 4.0 | 62 | 0.0 | 12.5 | 0.8 | 0.0 |
| Caramel, Light, Grande, Starbucks* | 1 Cup/473ml | 158 | 2.0 | 33 | 1.3 | 6.3 | 0.3 | 0.5 |
| Caramel, Light, Tall, Starbucks* | 1 Cup/335ml | 129 | 1.0 | 39 | 1.4 | 7.5 | 0.4 | 0.6 |
| Caramel, Light, Venti, Starbucks* | 1 Cup/591ml | 192 | 2.0 | 32 | 1.2 | 6.4 | 0.3 | 0.5 |
| Caramel, Tall, Starbucks* | 1 Cup/354ml | 228 | 3.0 | 64 | 0.0 | 12.7 | 0.9 | 0.0 |
| Caramel, Venti, Starbucks* | 1 Cup/591ml | 370 | 5.0 | 63 | 0.0 | 12.7 | 0.8 | 0.0 |
| Caramel, with Whip, Grande, Starbucks* | 1 Cup/473ml | 382 | 15.0 | 81 | 1.2 | 12.0 | 3.1 | 0.0 |
| Caramel, with Whip, Tall, Starbucks* | 1 Cup/335ml | 302 | 11.0 | 90 | 1.3 | 13.7 | 3.3 | 0.0 |
| Caramel, with Whip, Venti, Starbucks* | 1 Cup/591ml | 431 | 14.0 | 73 | 1.1 | 11.7 | 2.4 | 0.0 |
| Caramel Cream, Grande, Starbucks* | 1 Cup/473ml | 339 | 5.0 | 72 | 2.8 | 12.7 | 1.1 | 0.0 |
| Caramel Cream, Tall, Starbucks* | 1 Cup/354ml | 261 | 4.0 | 74 | 2.8 | 13.0 | 1.1 | 0.0 |
| Caramel Cream, Venti, Starbucks* | 1 Cup/591ml | 409 | 6.0 | 69 | 2.6 | 12.3 | 1.0 | 0.0 |
| Caramel Cream, with Whip, Grande, Starbucks* | 1 Cup/473ml | 470 | 17.0 | 99 | 2.8 | 13.1 | 3.7 | 0.0 |
| Caramel Cream, with Whip, Tall, Starbucks* | 1 Cup/354ml | 355 | 13.0 | 100 | 2.8 | 13.6 | 3.6 | 0.0 |
| Caramel Cream, with Whip, Venti, Starbucks* | 1 Cup/591ml | 540 | 18.0 | 91 | 2.6 | 12.7 | 3.1 | 0.0 |
| Chocolate, Grande, Starbucks* | 1 Cup/473ml | 338 | 6.0 | 71 | 3.0 | 12.7 | 1.2 | 0.0 |
| Chocolate, Tall, Starbucks* | 1 Cup/354ml | 260 | 4.0 | 73 | 3.0 | 13.0 | 1.3 | 0.0 |
| Chocolate, Venti, Starbucks* | 1 Cup/591ml | 413 | 7.0 | 70 | 2.8 | 12.7 | 1.2 | 0.0 |
| Chocolate, with Whip, Grande, Starbucks* | 1 Cup/473ml | 469 | 18.0 | 99 | 3.0 | 13.1 | 3.8 | 0.1 |
| Chocolate, with Whip, Tall, Starbucks* | 1 Cup/354ml | 354 | 13.0 | 100 | 3.0 | 13.6 | 3.7 | 0.2 |
| Chocolate, with Whip, Venti, Starbucks* | 1 Cup/591ml | 544 | 19.0 | 92 | 2.8 | 13.0 | 3.3 | 0.2 |
| Coffee, Grande, Starbucks* | 1 Cup/473ml | 261 | 9.0 | 55 | 1.2 | 11.0 | 2.0 | 0.0 |
| Coffee, Light, Grande, Starbucks* | 1 Cup/473ml | 128 | 1.0 | 27 | 1.3 | 5.3 | 0.2 | 0.5 |
| Coffee, Light, Tall, Starbucks* | 1 Cup/335ml | 91 | 1.0 | 27 | 1.3 | 5.4 | 0.2 | 0.5 |
| Coffee, Light, Venti, Starbucks* | 1 Cup/591ml | 151 | 1.0 | 26 | 1.2 | 4.9 | 0.2 | 0.5 |
| Coffee, Tall, Starbucks* | 1 Cup/335ml | 184 | 2.0 | 55 | 1.2 | 11.0 | 0.7 | 0.0 |
| Coffee, Venti, Starbucks* | 1 Cup/591ml | 278 | 4.0 | 47 | 1.0 | 9.5 | 0.6 | 0.0 |
| Cream, Caramel, with Whip, Tall, Starbucks* | 1 Cup/335ml | 329 | 10.0 | 98 | 2.7 | 14.9 | 3.1 | 0.0 |
| Cream, Chocolate, with Whip, Grande, Starbucks* | 1 Cup/473ml | 425 | 14.0 | 90 | 2.7 | 13.5 | 3.0 | 0.1 |
| Cream, Chocolate, with Whip, Tall, Starbucks* | 1 Cup/335ml | 322 | 10.0 | 96 | 2.9 | 14.6 | 3.1 | 0.2 |
| Cream, Chocolate, with Whip, Venti, Starbucks* | 1 Cup/591ml | 480 | 14.0 | 81 | 2.5 | 13.0 | 2.4 | 0.2 |
| Cream, Chocolate Chip, with Whip, Grande, Starbucks* | 1 Cup/473ml | 498 | 18.0 | 105 | 2.8 | 15.6 | 3.8 | 0.3 |
| Cream, Chocolate Chip, with Whip, Tall, Starbucks* | 1 Cup/335ml | 368 | 13.0 | 110 | 3.0 | 16.7 | 3.8 | 0.4 |
| Cream, Chocolate Chip, with Whip, Venti, Starbucks* | 1 Cup/591ml | 562 | 19.0 | 95 | 2.6 | 14.9 | 3.2 | 0.4 |
| Cream, Vanilla, with Whip, Grande, Starbucks* | 1 Cup/473ml | 431 | 14.0 | 91 | 2.6 | 13.5 | 3.0 | 0.0 |
| Cream, Vanilla, with Whip, Tall, Starbucks* | 1 Cup/335ml | 310 | 10.0 | 93 | 2.7 | 14.0 | 2.9 | 0.0 |
| Cream, Vanilla, with Whip, Venti, Starbucks* | 1 Cup/591ml | 470 | 13.0 | 80 | 2.3 | 12.7 | 2.2 | 0.0 |
| Espresso, Grande, Starbucks* | 1 Cup/473ml | 209 | 3.0 | 44 | 1.0 | 8.9 | 0.6 | 0.0 |
| Espresso, Tall, Starbucks* | 1 Cup/335ml | 146 | 2.0 | 44 | 1.0 | 8.7 | 0.6 | 0.0 |
| Espresso, Venti, Starbucks* | 1 Cup/591ml | 243 | 3.0 | 41 | 0.9 | 8.1 | 0.5 | 0.0 |
| Grande, Starbucks* | 1 Cup/473ml | 239 | 3.0 | 51 | 1.1 | 10.1 | 0.7 | 0.0 |
| Java Chip, with Whip, Grande, Starbucks* | 1 Cup/473ml | 456 | 19.0 | 96 | 1.5 | 14.6 | 3.9 | 0.3 |
| Java Chip, with Whip, Tall, Starbucks* | 1 Cup/335ml | 345 | 14.0 | 103 | 1.7 | 16.1 | 4.1 | 0.4 |
| Java Chip, with Whip, Venti, Starbucks* | 1 Cup/591ml | 650 | 24.0 | 110 | 1.8 | 17.5 | 4.1 | 0.5 |
| Mango Passion, Grande, Starbucks* | 1 Cup/473ml | 191 | 0.0 | 40 | 0.2 | 9.7 | 0.1 | 0.3 |
| Mango Passion, Tall, Starbucks* | 1 Cup/335ml | 157 | 0.0 | 47 | 0.2 | 11.3 | 0.1 | 0.3 |
| Mango Passion, Venti, Starbucks* | 1 Cup/591ml | 228 | 0.0 | 39 | 0.1 | 9.3 | 0.0 | 0.2 |
| Mocha, Light, Grande, Starbucks* | 1 Cup/473ml | 144 | 1.0 | 30 | 1.3 | 6.1 | 0.3 | 0.6 |

## STARBUCKS

### FRAPPUCCINO

| | Measure INFO/WEIGHT | KCAL | FAT | KCAL | PROT | CARB | FAT | FIBRE |
|---|---|---|---|---|---|---|---|---|
| Mocha, Light, Tall, Starbucks* | 1 Cup/335ml | 113 | 1.0 | 34 | 1.5 | 6.9 | 0.3 | 0.7 |
| Mocha, Light, Venti, Starbucks* | 1 Cup/591ml | 184 | 2.0 | 31 | 1.3 | 6.3 | 0.3 | 0.6 |
| Mocha, White Chocolate, with Whip, Grande, Starbucks* | 1 Cup/473ml | 408 | 16.0 | 86 | 1.4 | 12.9 | 3.3 | 0.0 |
| Mocha, White Chocolate, with Whip, Venti, Starbucks* | 1 Cup/591ml | 481 | 16.0 | 81 | 1.4 | 13.0 | 2.7 | 0.0 |
| Mocha, with Whip, Grande, Starbucks* | 1 Cup/473ml | 378 | 15.0 | 80 | 1.3 | 12.0 | 3.1 | 0.1 |
| Mocha, with Whip, Tall, Starbucks* | 1 Cup/335ml | 283 | 11.0 | 84 | 1.4 | 12.8 | 3.2 | 0.1 |
| Mocha, with Whip, Venti, Starbucks* | 1 Cup/591ml | 428 | 15.0 | 72 | 1.3 | 11.7 | 2.5 | 0.1 |
| Raspberry, Black Currant, with Zen Tea, Grande, Starbucks* | 1 Cup/473ml | 192 | 0.0 | 41 | 0.1 | 9.9 | 0.0 | 0.1 |
| Raspberry, Black Currant, with Zen Tea, Tall, Starbucks* | 1 Cup/335ml | 158 | 0.0 | 47 | 0.1 | 11.6 | 0.0 | 0.2 |
| Raspberry, Black Currant, with Zen Tea, Venti, Starbucks* | 1 Cup/591ml | 229 | 0.0 | 39 | 0.1 | 9.5 | 0.0 | 0.1 |
| Raspberry Tea, Grande, Starbucks* | 1 Cup/473ml | 200 | 0.0 | 42 | 0.1 | 11.0 | 0.0 | 0.2 |
| Raspberry Tea, Tall, Starbucks* | 1 Cup/354ml | 144 | 0.0 | 41 | 0.1 | 10.4 | 0.0 | 0.2 |
| Raspberry Tea, Venti, Starbucks* | 1 Cup/591ml | 261 | 0.0 | 44 | 0.1 | 11.3 | 0.0 | 0.2 |
| Strawberries & Cream, Grande, Starbucks* | 1 Cup/473ml | 424 | 5.0 | 90 | 2.9 | 17.3 | 1.1 | 0.0 |
| Strawberries & Cream, Tall, Starbucks* | 1 Cup/354ml | 299 | 4.0 | 84 | 2.7 | 16.4 | 1.0 | 0.0 |
| Strawberries & Cream, Venti, Starbucks* | 1 Cup/591ml | 543 | 7.0 | 92 | 3.0 | 17.6 | 1.1 | 0.0 |
| Strawberries & Cream, with Whip, Grande, Starbucks* | 1 Cup/473ml | 555 | 17.0 | 117 | 2.9 | 17.8 | 3.7 | 0.1 |
| Strawberries & Cream, with Whip, Tall, Starbucks* | 1 Cup/354ml | 393 | 12.0 | 111 | 2.7 | 16.9 | 3.5 | 0.1 |
| Strawberries & Cream, with Whip, Venti, Starbucks* | 1 Cup/591ml | 674 | 19.0 | 114 | 3.0 | 17.9 | 3.2 | 0.1 |
| Tazo Chai, Grande, Starbucks* | 1 Cup/473ml | 405 | 5.0 | 86 | 2.9 | 16.5 | 1.1 | 0.0 |
| Tazo Chai, Tall, Starbucks* | 1 Cup/354ml | 294 | 4.0 | 83 | 2.9 | 15.8 | 1.1 | 0.0 |
| Tazo Chai, Venti, Starbucks* | 1 Cup/591ml | 487 | 6.0 | 82 | 2.7 | 16.1 | 1.0 | 0.0 |
| Tazo Chai, with Whip, Grande, Starbucks* | 1 Cup/473ml | 536 | 17.0 | 113 | 2.9 | 16.9 | 3.7 | 0.0 |
| Tazo Chai, with Whip, Tall, Starbucks* | 1 Cup/354ml | 388 | 12.0 | 110 | 2.9 | 16.4 | 3.5 | 0.0 |
| Tazo Chai, with Whip, Venti, Starbucks* | 1 Cup/591ml | 618 | 18.0 | 105 | 2.7 | 16.4 | 3.1 | 0.0 |
| Tropical Citrus Tea, Grande, Starbucks* | 1 Cup/473ml | 178 | 0.0 | 38 | 0.3 | 9.3 | 0.1 | 0.3 |
| Tropical Citrus Tea, Tall, Starbucks* | 1 Cup/354ml | 128 | 0.0 | 36 | 0.3 | 9.0 | 0.1 | 0.3 |
| Tropical Citrus Tea, Venti, Starbucks* | 1 Cup/591ml | 232 | 0.0 | 39 | 0.3 | 9.8 | 0.1 | 0.3 |
| Vanilla, with Whip, Grande, Starbucks* | 1 Cup/473ml | 460 | 17.0 | 97 | 2.8 | 12.7 | 3.6 | 0.0 |
| Vanilla, with Whip, Tall, Starbucks* | 1 Cup/354ml | 344 | 12.0 | 97 | 2.8 | 13.0 | 3.5 | 0.0 |
| Vanilla, with Whip, Venti, Starbucks* | 1 Cup/591ml | 530 | 18.0 | 90 | 2.6 | 12.3 | 3.0 | 0.0 |
| White Chocolate Mocha, with Whip, Tall, Starbucks* | 1 Cup/335ml | 319 | 12.0 | 95 | 1.5 | 14.6 | 3.5 | 0.0 |

### FRUIT SALAD

| | Measure INFO/WEIGHT | KCAL | FAT | KCAL | PROT | CARB | FAT | FIBRE |
|---|---|---|---|---|---|---|---|---|
| Starbucks* | 1 Salad/170g | 66 | 0.0 | 39 | 0.6 | 9.5 | 0.2 | 1.2 |

### HOT CHOCOLATE

| | Measure INFO/WEIGHT | KCAL | FAT | KCAL | PROT | CARB | FAT | FIBRE |
|---|---|---|---|---|---|---|---|---|
| Signature, with Whip, Grande, Skimmed Milk, Starbucks* | 1 Cup/473ml | 505 | 27.0 | 107 | 3.3 | 12.5 | 5.7 | 1.4 |
| Signature, with Whip, Grande, Soy, Starbucks* | 1 Cup/473ml | 515 | 30.0 | 109 | 3.0 | 11.8 | 6.3 | 1.6 |
| Signature, with Whip, Grande, SS Milk, Starbucks* | 1 Cup/473ml | 537 | 31.0 | 114 | 3.2 | 12.5 | 6.5 | 6.5 |
| Signature, with Whip, Grande, Whole Milk, Starbucks* | 1 Cup/473ml | 556 | 33.0 | 118 | 3.2 | 12.5 | 7.1 | 1.4 |
| Signature, with Whip, Short, Skimmed Milk, Starbucks* | 1 Cup/236ml | 267 | 15.0 | 113 | 3.3 | 12.7 | 6.4 | 1.4 |
| Signature, with Whip, Short, Soy, Starbucks* | 1 Cup/236ml | 272 | 16.0 | 115 | 3.0 | 11.9 | 6.9 | 1.6 |
| Signature, with Whip, Short, SS Milk, Starbucks* | 1 Cup/236ml | 283 | 17.0 | 120 | 3.3 | 12.7 | 7.2 | 1.4 |
| Signature, with Whip, Short, Whole Milk, Starbucks* | 1 Cup/236ml | 293 | 18.0 | 124 | 3.2 | 12.7 | 7.7 | 1.4 |
| Signature, with Whip, Tall, Semi Skimmed Milk, Starbucks* | 1 Cup/335ml | 418 | 24.0 | 125 | 3.5 | 13.4 | 7.2 | 1.5 |
| Signature, with Whip, Tall, Skimmed Milk, Starbucks* | 1 Cup/335ml | 393 | 21.0 | 117 | 3.5 | 13.7 | 6.4 | 1.5 |
| Signature, with Whip, Tall, Soy, Starbucks* | 1 Cup/335ml | 401 | 23.0 | 120 | 3.2 | 12.8 | 7.0 | 1.7 |
| Signature, with Whip, Tall, Whole Milk, Starbucks* | 1 Cup/335ml | 433 | 26.0 | 129 | 3.5 | 13.4 | 7.8 | 1.5 |
| Signature, with Whip, Venti, Skimmed Milk, Starbucks* | 1 Cup/591ml | 624 | 32.0 | 106 | 3.3 | 12.7 | 5.5 | 1.4 |
| Signature, with Whip, Venti, Soy, Starbucks* | 1 Cup/591ml | 637 | 36.0 | 108 | 3.0 | 12.0 | 6.1 | 1.6 |
| Signature, with Whip, Venti, SS Milk, Starbucks* | 1 Cup/591ml | 665 | 37.0 | 113 | 3.3 | 12.7 | 6.3 | 1.4 |
| Signature, with Whip, Venti, Whole Milk, Starbucks* | 1 Cup/591ml | 690 | 40.0 | 117 | 3.2 | 12.5 | 6.8 | 1.4 |
| Skimmed Milk, Grande, Starbucks* | 1 Cup/473ml | 261 | 2.0 | 55 | 3.3 | 10.6 | 0.5 | 0.4 |

| | Measure INFO/WEIGHT | per Measure | | Nutrition Values per 100g / 100ml | | | | |
|---|---|---|---|---|---|---|---|---|
| | | KCAL | FAT | KCAL | PROT | CARB | FAT | FIBRE |
| **STARBUCKS** | | | | | | | | |
| **HOT CHOCOLATE** | | | | | | | | |
| Skimmed Milk, Tall, Starbucks* | 1 Cup/354ml | 209 | 1.0 | 59 | 3.5 | 11.3 | 0.4 | 0.4 |
| Skimmed Milk, Venti, Starbucks* | 1 Cup/591ml | 340 | 3.0 | 58 | 3.3 | 11.2 | 0.5 | 0.4 |
| White, Skimmed Milk, Grande, Starbucks* | 1 Cup/442ml | 361 | 17.0 | 82 | 3.8 | 13.9 | 3.8 | 0.0 |
| White, Skimmed Milk, Tall, Starbucks* | 1 Cup/354ml | 301 | 4.0 | 85 | 4.1 | 14.4 | 1.1 | 0.0 |
| White, Skimmed Milk, Venti, Starbucks* | 1 Cup/591ml | 493 | 7.0 | 83 | 4.0 | 14.2 | 1.2 | 0.0 |
| White, Skimmed Milk, with Whip, Grande, Starbucks* | 1 Cup/443ml | 456 | 14.0 | 103 | 3.8 | 14.4 | 3.2 | 0.0 |
| White, Skimmed Milk, with Whip, Tall, Starbucks* | 1 Cup/354ml | 381 | 12.0 | 108 | 4.1 | 14.7 | 3.4 | 0.0 |
| White, Skimmed Milk, with Whip, Venti, Starbucks* | 1 Cup/553ml | 556 | 15.0 | 101 | 4.0 | 14.5 | 2.8 | 0.0 |
| White, Whole Milk, Grande, Starbucks* | 1 Cup/443ml | 449 | 17.0 | 101 | 3.5 | 13.3 | 3.8 | 0.0 |
| White, Whole Milk, Tall, Starbucks* | 1 Cup/354ml | 377 | 14.0 | 106 | 3.8 | 13.8 | 4.0 | 0.0 |
| White, Whole Milk, Venti, Starbucks* | 1 Cup/591ml | 618 | 24.0 | 105 | 3.7 | 13.5 | 4.1 | 0.0 |
| White, Whole Milk, with Whip, Grande, Starbucks* | 1 Cup/443ml | 543 | 25.0 | 123 | 3.5 | 13.7 | 5.7 | 0.0 |
| White, Whole Milk, with Whip, Tall, Starbucks* | 1 Cup/354ml | 457 | 22.0 | 129 | 3.8 | 14.1 | 6.3 | 0.0 |
| White, Whole Milk, with Whip, Venti, Starbucks* | 1 Cup/553ml | 673 | 31.0 | 122 | 3.7 | 13.9 | 5.6 | 0.0 |
| Whole Milk, Grande, Starbucks* | 1 Cup/473ml | 347 | 14.0 | 73 | 3.0 | 9.9 | 3.0 | 0.4 |
| Whole Milk, Tall, Starbucks* | 1 Cup/354ml | 277 | 11.0 | 78 | 3.1 | 10.7 | 3.0 | 0.4 |
| Whole Milk, Venti, Starbucks* | 1 Cup/591ml | 448 | 18.0 | 76 | 3.0 | 10.7 | 3.0 | 0.4 |
| Whole Milk, with Whip, Grande, Starbucks* | 1 Cup/443ml | 420 | 22.0 | 95 | 3.0 | 10.4 | 5.0 | 0.4 |
| Whole Milk, with Whip, Tall, Starbucks* | 1 Cup/354ml | 357 | 19.0 | 101 | 3.1 | 11.0 | 5.3 | 0.4 |
| Whole Milk, with Whip, Venti, Starbucks* | 1 Cup/553ml | 514 | 25.0 | 93 | 3.0 | 11.0 | 4.6 | 0.4 |
| **HOUMOUS** | | | | | | | | |
| with Crunchy Vegetables, Starbucks* | 1 Pot/219g | 359 | 10.0 | 164 | 4.7 | 26.4 | 4.4 | 2.9 |
| with Tomato, Vegetables, Red Pepper, Starbucks* | 1 Pack/218g | 405 | 14.0 | 186 | 5.4 | 26.2 | 6.6 | 2.0 |
| **JUICE** | | | | | | | | |
| Orange, Starbucks* | 1 Bottle/250ml | 112 | 0.0 | 45 | 0.8 | 11.4 | 0.1 | 0.3 |
| **MUFFIN** | | | | | | | | |
| Banana & Walnut, Starbucks* | 1 Muffin/125g | 469 | 25.0 | 375 | 5.7 | 42.9 | 20.1 | 4.2 |
| Blueberry, Starbucks* | 1 Muffin/125g | 561 | 23.0 | 449 | 5.8 | 46.5 | 18.4 | 1.1 |
| Chocolate, Belgian Chocolate Sauce Centre, Starbucks* | 1 Muffin/135g | 551 | 29.0 | 408 | 6.2 | 49.5 | 21.3 | 2.5 |
| Raspberry, White Chocolate Icing, Starbucks* | 1 Muffin/121g | 397 | 18.0 | 328 | 4.9 | 43.2 | 15.1 | 1.1 |
| Skinny, Ginger Iced, Starbucks* | 1 Muffin/140g | 405 | 5.0 | 289 | 3.9 | 62.3 | 3.4 | 0.9 |
| Skinny, Lemon, Poppy Seed, Starbucks* | 1 Muffin/130g | 365 | 6.0 | 281 | 4.3 | 56.2 | 4.3 | 4.2 |
| Skinny Blueberry, Starbucks* | 1 Muffin/130g | 323 | 6.0 | 249 | 4.3 | 51.7 | 4.3 | 1.6 |
| Skinny Peach & Raspberry, Starbucks* | 1 Muffin/140g | 321 | 5.0 | 229 | 4.4 | 49.0 | 3.3 | 1.6 |
| Skinny Sunrise, Starbucks* | 1 Muffin/131g | 255 | 4.0 | 194 | 4.6 | 36.7 | 3.0 | 1.3 |
| Sunrise, Starbucks* | 1 Muffin/150g | 592 | 35.0 | 395 | 5.5 | 40.8 | 23.1 | 1.9 |
| **PAIN AU CHOCOLAT** | | | | | | | | |
| Starbucks* | 1 Pastry/70g | 296 | 17.0 | 423 | 6.7 | 43.8 | 24.4 | 2.8 |
| **PAIN AU RAISIN** | | | | | | | | |
| Starbucks* | 1 Pastry/120g | 445 | 22.0 | 371 | 5.3 | 45.6 | 18.5 | 1.8 |
| **PANINI** | | | | | | | | |
| Beef Pastrami, & Roast Chicken, Starbucks* | 1 Panini/220g | 443 | 13.0 | 201 | 12.3 | 25.1 | 5.7 | 1.4 |
| Cheese & Marmite, Breakfast, Starbucks* | 1 Serving/115g | 298 | 10.0 | 259 | 14.5 | 30.3 | 8.8 | 1.7 |
| Chicken, & Green Pesto, Starbucks* | 1 Panini/203g | 351 | 9.0 | 173 | 12.3 | 21.2 | 4.4 | 1.2 |
| Chicken, Mediterranean Style, with Green Pesto, Starbucks* | 1 Panini/224g | 387 | 9.0 | 173 | 11.4 | 22.6 | 4.1 | 1.3 |
| Croque Monsieur, Starbucks* | 1 Av Panini/190g | 441 | 17.0 | 232 | 12.4 | 25.3 | 9.0 | 1.2 |
| Egg & Bacon, Breakfast, Starbucks* | 1 Panini/163g | 302 | 10.0 | 185 | 10.0 | 22.0 | 6.4 | 1.5 |
| Egg Mayo, Breakfast, Starbucks* | 1 Panini/146g | 327 | 12.0 | 224 | 12.3 | 25.4 | 8.1 | 1.7 |
| Falafel, Starbucks* | 1 Pack/213g | 384 | 7.0 | 180 | 6.8 | 30.9 | 3.3 | 2.7 |
| Grilled Chicken Salsa, Lightly Spiced, Starbucks* | 1 Panini/238g | 385 | 8.0 | 162 | 7.9 | 25.0 | 3.4 | 2.0 |
| Grilled Chicken Salsa, with Creme Fraiche, Starbucks* | 1 Panini/180g | 385 | 8.0 | 214 | 10.4 | 32.9 | 4.5 | 0.0 |
| Ham, Cheese & Roasted Vegetable, Starbucks* | 1 Panini/217g | 388 | 8.0 | 179 | 11.0 | 25.4 | 3.7 | 1.4 |

## STARBUCKS

| | Measure INFO/WEIGHT | per Measure KCAL | FAT | Nutrition Values per 100g / 100ml KCAL | PROT | CARB | FAT | FIBRE |
|---|---|---|---|---|---|---|---|---|
| **PANINI** | | | | | | | | |
| Mozzarella, & Slow Roast Tomato, Starbucks* | 1 Panini/180g | 461 | 21.0 | 256 | 11.1 | 27.1 | 11.5 | 2.1 |
| Pesto Chicken, with Sunblush Tomato, Starbucks* | 1 Panini/208g | 399 | 10.0 | 192 | 13.1 | 24.1 | 4.8 | 3.0 |
| Roasted Vegetable & Taw Valley Cheddar, Starbucks* | 1 Panini/226g | 485 | 20.0 | 215 | 9.2 | 25.1 | 8.8 | 1.7 |
| Roasted Vegetables & Cheese, Starbucks* | 1 Panini/215g | 542 | 32.0 | 252 | 8.7 | 20.6 | 15.1 | 0.0 |
| Sausage, Egg & Baked Bean, Starbucks* | 1 Panini/100g | 395 | 10.0 | 395 | 16.9 | 59.8 | 9.8 | 1.5 |
| Steak, & Cheese, Starbucks* | 1 Panini/219g | 451 | 15.0 | 206 | 12.3 | 24.2 | 6.7 | 1.3 |
| Tuna Melt, Starbucks* | 1 Panini/197g | 486 | 21.0 | 247 | 13.5 | 24.1 | 10.8 | 1.6 |
| **PASTA SALAD** | | | | | | | | |
| Salmon & Dill, Starbucks* | 1 Pack/260g | 614 | 35.0 | 236 | 7.8 | 21.0 | 13.4 | 1.0 |
| **SALAD** | | | | | | | | |
| Chicken, Roasted, Starbucks* | 1 Pack/157g | 165 | 10.0 | 105 | 7.1 | 5.1 | 6.5 | 1.2 |
| Chicken Caesar, Starbucks* | 1 Pack/233g | 403 | 18.0 | 173 | 8.7 | 18.0 | 7.9 | 1.2 |
| Mozarella & Cherry Tomato, Starbucks* | 1 Pack/172g | 322 | 29.0 | 187 | 5.5 | 2.9 | 17.0 | 17.0 |
| Pasta, Chicken & Red Pesto, Starbucks* | 1 Av Pack/300g | 390 | 13.0 | 130 | 7.1 | 15.3 | 4.4 | 1.2 |
| Salmon Nicoise, Starbucks* | 1 Pack/260g | 291 | 18.0 | 112 | 6.9 | 7.2 | 7.0 | 1.0 |
| Tuna & Bean Salad, Starbucks* | 1 Pack/326g | 254 | 4.0 | 78 | 7.1 | 9.9 | 1.1 | 2.5 |
| Tuna Nicoise, Starbucks* | 1 Pack/184g | 175 | 10.0 | 95 | 7.8 | 4.6 | 5.3 | 1.2 |
| **SANDWICH** | | | | | | | | |
| Atlantic Prawn, Starbucks* | 1 Pack/185g | 348 | 12.0 | 188 | 10.1 | 22.0 | 6.7 | 2.7 |
| BLT, Starbucks* | 1 Pack/181g | 483 | 27.0 | 267 | 9.6 | 22.9 | 15.2 | 1.9 |
| Cheddar, & Italian Style Roasted Vegetables, Starbucks* | 1 Pack/223g | 553 | 31.0 | 248 | 5.3 | 25.8 | 13.7 | 0.0 |
| Cheddar Cheese & Pickle, Starbucks* | 1 Pack/190g | 504 | 30.0 | 265 | 10.2 | 20.5 | 15.7 | 1.6 |
| Cheese, & Tomato, & Apple Chutney, Half Fat, Starbucks* | 1 Pack/200g | 318 | 8.0 | 159 | 8.8 | 21.3 | 4.2 | 0.0 |
| Chicken, & Bacon, Club, Starbucks* | 1 Pack/252g | 590 | 39.0 | 234 | 11.5 | 12.8 | 15.3 | 0.0 |
| Chicken, Club, Starbucks* | 1 Pack/206g | 422 | 19.0 | 205 | 12.6 | 17.8 | 9.4 | 1.7 |
| Chicken, in Lemon Pepper Dressing, Starbucks* | 1 Pack/198g | 307 | 7.0 | 155 | 11.8 | 19.4 | 3.5 | 1.6 |
| Chicken, Lightly Spiced, Starbucks* | 1 Pack/200g | 286 | 5.0 | 143 | 11.2 | 18.2 | 2.4 | 0.0 |
| Egg Mayonnaise, & Cress, Starbucks* | 1 Pack/200g | 410 | 20.0 | 205 | 10.5 | 17.4 | 10.2 | 1.9 |
| Egg Mayonnaise, on Gluten Free Bread, Starbucks* | 1 Pack/227g | 340 | 12.0 | 150 | 6.2 | 20.3 | 5.1 | 2.9 |
| Falafel & Houmous, in Flatbread, Starbucks* | 1 Pack/250g | 467 | 9.0 | 187 | 7.0 | 34.8 | 3.8 | 3.6 |
| Ham, & Tomato, Smoked, Starbucks* | 1 Pack/206g | 297 | 8.0 | 144 | 5.2 | 22.0 | 3.9 | 0.0 |
| Ham, Yorkshire, Starbucks* | 1 Pack/208g | 374 | 11.0 | 180 | 10.0 | 23.0 | 5.3 | 2.3 |
| Houmous, with Crunchy Vegetables, Starbucks* | 1 Pack/219g | 359 | 10.0 | 164 | 4.7 | 26.4 | 4.4 | 2.9 |
| Prawn, Mayo, Starbucks* | 1 Sandwich/183g | 386 | 20.0 | 211 | 9.8 | 18.3 | 11.0 | 1.6 |
| Salmon, Oak Smoked, & Soft Cheese, Starbucks* | 1 Pack/221g | 523 | 24.0 | 236 | 9.6 | 12.6 | 10.9 | 1.9 |
| Soft Cheese, & Tomato, Extra Light, Starbucks* | 1 Pack/186g | 283 | 5.0 | 152 | 8.0 | 24.0 | 2.7 | 3.1 |
| Tuna, Mayonnaise, Starbucks* | 1 Pack/184g | 333 | 11.0 | 181 | 9.4 | 22.8 | 5.8 | 1.8 |
| Turkey, & Salad, Smoked, Starbucks* | 1 Pack/198g | 303 | 5.0 | 153 | 10.8 | 22.3 | 2.4 | 1.5 |
| Turkey, Pork & Herb, Starbucks* | 1 Pack/198g | 465 | 21.0 | 235 | 11.7 | 22.6 | 10.8 | 2.1 |
| **SCONE** | | | | | | | | |
| Berry, Starbucks* | 1 Scone/90g | 301 | 15.0 | 335 | 5.6 | 40.3 | 16.3 | 2.1 |
| Blueberry, Starbucks* | 1 Scone/128g | 460 | 18.0 | 359 | 3.9 | 53.1 | 14.1 | 2.3 |
| Extremely Fruity, Starbucks* | 1 Scone/100g | 325 | 8.0 | 325 | 5.7 | 57.1 | 8.5 | 2.3 |
| Raisin, Jumbo, Starbucks* | 1 Scone/150g | 564 | 22.0 | 376 | 5.9 | 54.9 | 14.8 | 2.1 |
| **SHORTBREAD** | | | | | | | | |
| Chocolate, Chunk, Fairtrade, Starbucks* | 1 Serving/90g | 484 | 28.0 | 538 | 5.7 | 57.9 | 31.5 | 1.4 |
| Chocolate Caramel, Starbucks* | 1 Bar/62g | 319 | 18.0 | 515 | 3.7 | 59.0 | 29.3 | 0.8 |
| **SLICES** | | | | | | | | |
| Apricot, Pastry, Starbucks* | 1 Pastry/115g | 279 | 15.0 | 243 | 4.7 | 26.1 | 13.3 | 1.1 |
| Belgian Chocolate & Orange, Swirl, Pastry, Starbucks* | 1 Pastry/140g | 525 | 18.0 | 375 | 7.5 | 57.4 | 13.2 | 2.6 |
| Cheese, Savoury, Pastry, Starbucks* | 1 Pastry/120g | 497 | 31.0 | 414 | 11.8 | 32.2 | 26.2 | 1.2 |
| Cinnamon Swirl, Pastry, Starbucks* | 1 Pastry/140g | 434 | 8.0 | 309 | 7.0 | 57.9 | 5.5 | 2.8 |

| | Measure INFO/WEIGHT | per Measure | | Nutrition Values per 100g / 100ml | | | | |
|---|---|---|---|---|---|---|---|---|
| | | KCAL | FAT | KCAL | PROT | CARB | FAT | FIBRE |
| **STARBUCKS** | | | | | | | | |
| **SYRUP** | | | | | | | | |
| Hazelnut Flavoured, Starbucks* | 1 Pump/10g | 20 | 0.0 | 200 | 0.0 | 50.0 | 0.0 | 0.0 |
| Mocha, 1 Pump, Starbucks* | 1 Pump/17g | 26 | 1.0 | 153 | 3.5 | 35.3 | 3.5 | 5.9 |
| **TEA** | | | | | | | | |
| Brewed, Grande, Starbucks* | 1 Cup/473ml | 0 | 0.0 | 0 | 0.0 | 0.0 | 0.0 | 0.0 |
| Brewed, Short, Starbucks* | 1 Cup/236ml | 0 | 0.0 | 0 | 0.0 | 0.0 | 0.0 | 0.0 |
| Brewed, Tall, Starbucks* | 1 Cup/335ml | 0 | 0.0 | 0 | 0.0 | 0.0 | 0.0 | 0.0 |
| Brewed, Venti, Starbucks* | 1 Cup/591ml | 0 | 0.0 | 0 | 0.0 | 0.0 | 0.0 | 0.0 |
| Chai, Latte, Tazo, Grande, Semi Skimmed Milk, Starbucks* | 1 Cup/473ml | 236 | 4.0 | 50 | 1.6 | 9.3 | 0.8 | 0.0 |
| Chai, Latte, Tazo, Grande, Skimmed Milk, Starbucks* | 1 Cup/473ml | 204 | 0.0 | 43 | 1.6 | 9.3 | 0.0 | 0.0 |
| Chai, Latte, Tazo, Grande, Soy, Starbucks* | 1 Cup/473ml | 213 | 3.0 | 45 | 1.3 | 8.7 | 0.7 | 0.2 |
| Chai, Latte, Tazo, Grande, Whole Milk, Starbucks* | 1 Cup/473ml | 255 | 6.0 | 54 | 1.5 | 9.1 | 1.4 | 0.0 |
| Chai, Latte, Tazo, Short, Semi Skimmed Milk, Starbucks* | 1 Cup/236ml | 119 | 2.0 | 50 | 1.6 | 9.3 | 0.8 | 0.0 |
| Chai, Latte, Tazo, Short, Skimmed Milk, Starbucks* | 1 Cup/236ml | 103 | 0.0 | 44 | 1.6 | 9.3 | 0.0 | 0.0 |
| Chai, Latte, Tazo, Short, Soy, Starbucks* | 1 Cup/236ml | 108 | 2.0 | 46 | 1.4 | 8.5 | 0.7 | 0.2 |
| Chai, Latte, Tazo, Short, Whole Milk, Starbucks* | 1 Cup/236ml | 129 | 3.0 | 55 | 1.6 | 9.3 | 1.4 | 0.0 |
| Chai, Latte, Tazo, Tall, Semi Skimmed Milk, Starbucks* | 1 Cup/335ml | 179 | 3.0 | 53 | 1.7 | 9.8 | 0.9 | 0.0 |
| Chai, Latte, Tazo, Tall, Skimmed Milk, Starbucks* | 1 Cup/335ml | 154 | 0.0 | 46 | 1.7 | 9.8 | 0.1 | 0.0 |
| Chai, Latte, Tazo, Tall, Soy, Starbucks* | 1 Cup/335ml | 162 | 2.0 | 48 | 1.4 | 9.2 | 0.7 | 0.2 |
| Chai, Latte, Tazo, Tall, Whole Milk, Starbucks* | 1 Cup/335ml | 194 | 5.0 | 58 | 1.6 | 9.8 | 1.5 | 0.0 |
| Chai, Latte, Tazo, Venti, Semi Skimmed Milk, Starbucks* | 1 Cup/591ml | 297 | 5.0 | 50 | 1.6 | 9.3 | 0.8 | 0.0 |
| Chai, Latte, Tazo, Venti, Skimmed Milk, Starbucks* | 1 Cup/591ml | 256 | 0.0 | 43 | 1.6 | 9.5 | 0.0 | 0.0 |
| Chai, Latte, Tazo, Venti, Soy, Starbucks* | 1 Cup/591ml | 268 | 4.0 | 45 | 1.3 | 8.6 | 0.7 | 0.2 |
| Chai, Latte, Tazo, Venti, Whole Milk, Starbucks* | 1 Cup/591ml | 322 | 8.0 | 54 | 1.5 | 9.3 | 1.4 | 0.0 |
| Iced, Chai, Latte, Tazo, Grande, Skimmed Milk, Starbucks* | 1 Cup/473ml | 205 | 0.0 | 43 | 1.6 | 9.3 | 0.0 | 0.0 |
| Iced, Chai, Latte, Tazo, Grande, Soy, Starbucks* | 1 Cup/473ml | 219 | 3.0 | 46 | 1.4 | 8.7 | 0.7 | 0.2 |
| Iced, Chai, Latte, Tazo, Grande, SS Milk, Starbucks* | 1 Cup/473ml | 238 | 4.0 | 50 | 1.6 | 9.3 | 0.9 | 0.0 |
| Iced, Chai, Latte, Tazo, Grande, Whole Milk, Starbucks* | 1 Cup/473ml | 259 | 7.0 | 55 | 1.5 | 9.3 | 1.5 | 0.0 |
| Iced, Chai, Latte, Tazo, Tall, Semi Skimmed, Starbucks* | 1 Cup/335ml | 176 | 3.0 | 53 | 1.6 | 9.8 | 0.9 | 0.0 |
| Iced, Chai, Latte, Tazo, Tall, Skimmed Milk, Starbucks* | 1 Cup/335ml | 152 | 0.0 | 45 | 1.6 | 9.8 | 0.1 | 0.0 |
| Iced, Chai, Latte, Tazo, Tall, Soy, Starbucks* | 1 Cup/335ml | 153 | 2.0 | 46 | 1.3 | 8.7 | 0.7 | 0.2 |
| Iced, Chai, Latte, Tazo, Tall, Whole Milk, Starbucks* | 1 Cup/335ml | 191 | 5.0 | 57 | 1.6 | 9.5 | 1.5 | 0.0 |
| Iced, Chai, Latte, Tazo, Venti, Skimmed Milk, Starbucks* | 1 Cup/591ml | 242 | 0.0 | 41 | 1.4 | 9.0 | 0.0 | 0.0 |
| Iced, Chai, Latte, Tazo, Venti, Soy, Starbucks* | 1 Cup/591ml | 256 | 3.0 | 43 | 1.2 | 8.5 | 0.6 | 0.2 |
| Iced, Chai, Latte, Tazo, Venti, SS Milk, Starbucks* | 1 Cup/591ml | 277 | 4.0 | 47 | 1.3 | 9.0 | 0.7 | 0.0 |
| Iced, Chai, Latte, Tazo, Venti, Whole Milk, Starbucks* | 1 Cup/591ml | 299 | 7.0 | 51 | 1.3 | 9.0 | 1.2 | 0.0 |
| **TOASTIE** | | | | | | | | |
| Ham & Cheese, Mini, Starbucks* | 1 Av Pack/126g | 328 | 11.0 | 260 | 13.3 | 31.7 | 8.8 | 1.8 |
| **TOPPING** | | | | | | | | |
| Caramel, Starbucks* | 1 Serving/4g | 15 | 1.0 | 375 | 0.0 | 50.0 | 15.0 | 0.0 |
| Chocolate, Starbucks* | 1 Serving/4g | 6 | 0.0 | 150 | 2.5 | 25.0 | 2.5 | 2.5 |
| Sprinkles, Starbucks* | 1 Sprinkle/1g | 4 | 0.0 | 400 | 0.0 | 100.0 | 0.0 | 0.0 |
| Whipped Cream, Cold, Grande Beverage, Starbucks* | 1 Serving/35g | 114 | 11.0 | 326 | 1.7 | 8.6 | 32.0 | 0.0 |
| Whipped Cream, Cold, Tall Beverage, Starbucks* | 1 Serving/25g | 81 | 8.0 | 324 | 1.6 | 8.0 | 32.0 | 0.0 |
| Whipped Cream, Cold, Venti Beverage, Starbucks* | 1 Serving/32g | 104 | 10.0 | 325 | 1.9 | 9.4 | 31.9 | 0.0 |
| Whipped Cream, Hot, Grande/venti, Starbucks* | 1 Serving/22g | 72 | 7.0 | 327 | 1.8 | 9.1 | 31.8 | 0.0 |
| Whipped Cream, Hot, Short Beverage, Starbucks* | 1 Serving/16g | 52 | 5.0 | 325 | 1.9 | 6.2 | 31.9 | 0.0 |
| Whipped Cream, Hot, Tall Beverage, Starbucks* | 1 Serving/19g | 62 | 6.0 | 326 | 1.6 | 10.5 | 32.1 | 0.0 |
| **TUNA** | | | | | | | | |
| Minted Pea, & Potato Salad, Starbucks* | 1 Packet/290g | 276 | 13.0 | 95 | 5.4 | 8.5 | 4.4 | 2.2 |
| **TZATZIKI** | | | | | | | | |
| with Vegetable Sticks, Starbucks* | 1 Tub/140g | 73 | 4.0 | 52 | 2.0 | 4.8 | 2.8 | 1.7 |

| | Measure INFO/WEIGHT | per Measure KCAL | FAT | Nutrition Values per 100g / 100ml KCAL | PROT | CARB | FAT | FIBRE |
|---|---|---|---|---|---|---|---|---|

## STARBUCKS

### WAFFLES

| | | | | | | | | |
|---|---|---|---|---|---|---|---|---|
| Caramel, Starbucks* | 1 Waffle/30g | 140 | 6.0 | 467 | 4.3 | 66.7 | 20.3 | 1.3 |

### WRAP

| | | | | | | | | |
|---|---|---|---|---|---|---|---|---|
| Chicken, Breast, in Honey Mustard, Starbucks* | 1 Pack/200g | 332 | 8.0 | 166 | 7.3 | 25.8 | 3.9 | 1.4 |
| Chicken, Chargrilled, Tomato & Pepper Salsa, Starbucks* | 1 Pack/187g | 320 | 8.0 | 171 | 10.4 | 22.5 | 4.4 | 1.6 |
| Chicken, Roasted, Starbucks* | 1 Pack/197g | 374 | 13.0 | 190 | 11.6 | 21.2 | 6.6 | 2.2 |
| Chicken, with Lightly Spiced Salsa, Starbucks* | 1 Pack/187g | 320 | 8.0 | 171 | 10.4 | 22.5 | 4.4 | 1.6 |
| Chicken with Salad, Starbucks* | 1 Wrap/223g | 362 | 10.0 | 162 | 10.1 | 21.9 | 4.3 | 2.1 |
| Emmental Cheese, & Roasted Aubergines, Starbucks* | 1 Pack/225g | 517 | 26.0 | 230 | 8.9 | 22.3 | 11.4 | 0.0 |
| Greek Salad, Starbucks* | 1 Pack/182g | 265 | 7.0 | 146 | 6.1 | 21.5 | 4.0 | 2.0 |
| Houmous, & Roasted Vegetable, Starbucks* | ½ Pack/102g | 205 | 7.0 | 200 | 6.2 | 29.2 | 6.7 | 3.5 |
| Houmous & Falafel, Starbucks* | 1 Wrap/213g | 383 | 9.0 | 180 | 6.4 | 30.0 | 4.0 | 2.8 |
| Prawn Caesar, Starbucks* | 1 Pack/173g | 464 | 27.0 | 268 | 11.4 | 20.2 | 15.7 | 1.1 |
| Roasted Chicken Salad, with Mange Tout, Starbucks* | 1 Pack/184g | 294 | 4.0 | 160 | 12.2 | 23.5 | 2.0 | 1.7 |

### YOGHURT

| | | | | | | | | |
|---|---|---|---|---|---|---|---|---|
| Blueberry, Starbucks* | 1 Pot/130g | 116 | 0.0 | 89 | 4.4 | 17.8 | 0.0 | 0.0 |
| Blueberry with Mixed Seeds, Organic, Starbucks* | 1 Pot/180g | 194 | 6.0 | 108 | 3.6 | 15.1 | 3.6 | 0.6 |
| Greek, with Crunchy Granola, & Honey, Starbucks* | 1 Pot/150g | 267 | 15.0 | 178 | 1.7 | 20.5 | 10.0 | 1.1 |
| Strawberry, Starbucks* | 1 Pot/180g | 176 | 6.0 | 98 | 3.6 | 12.4 | 3.6 | 1.7 |
| Strawberry with Mixed Seeds, Organic, Starbucks* | 1 Pot/180g | 178 | 6.0 | 99 | 3.6 | 12.6 | 3.6 | 1.1 |

## SUBWAY

### BACON

| | | | | | | | | |
|---|---|---|---|---|---|---|---|---|
| Strips, Subway* | 2 Strips/9g | 40 | 3.0 | 444 | 33.3 | 0.2 | 32.2 | 0.0 |

### BREAD

| | | | | | | | | |
|---|---|---|---|---|---|---|---|---|
| Roll, Hearty Italian, 6", Subway* | 1 Roll/79g | 189 | 2.0 | 239 | 8.9 | 46.8 | 2.9 | 3.2 |
| Roll, Honey Oat, 6", Subway* | 1 Roll/91g | 224 | 3.0 | 246 | 9.9 | 45.0 | 3.3 | 3.6 |
| Roll, Italian, Herbs & Cheese, Subway* | 1 Roll/86g | 220 | 5.0 | 256 | 10.5 | 41.9 | 6.0 | 0.5 |
| Roll, Parmesan & Oregano, 6", Subway* | 1 Roll/79g | 190 | 3.0 | 241 | 8.9 | 45.6 | 3.4 | 3.5 |
| Roll, Wheat, 6", Subway* | 1 Roll/80g | 183 | 2.0 | 229 | 10.0 | 43.7 | 2.9 | 3.5 |
| Roll, Wheat, Mini, Subway* | 1 Roll/53g | 122 | 2.0 | 230 | 8.1 | 49.1 | 3.0 | 3.4 |
| Roll, White, Italian, 6", Subway* | 1 Roll/75g | 178 | 2.0 | 237 | 9.3 | 46.7 | 2.8 | 2.7 |
| Roll, White, Italian, Mini, Subway* | 1 Roll/50g | 117 | 1.0 | 234 | 9.6 | 46.0 | 2.4 | 2.6 |

### CHEESE

| | | | | | | | | |
|---|---|---|---|---|---|---|---|---|
| Cheddar, Sliced, Processed, Subway* | 1 Serving/24g | 88 | 7.0 | 367 | 16.7 | 0.0 | 30.0 | 0.0 |

### COOKIES

| | | | | | | | | |
|---|---|---|---|---|---|---|---|---|
| Chocolate Chip, Subway* | 1 Cookie/45g | 214 | 10.0 | 476 | 4.4 | 68.9 | 22.9 | 2.7 |
| Chocolate Chip & Candy, Subway* | 1 Cookie/45g | 218 | 10.0 | 484 | 4.4 | 68.9 | 21.6 | 2.2 |
| Chocolate Chunk, Subway* | 1 Cookie/45g | 226 | 10.0 | 502 | 4.4 | 68.9 | 22.4 | 2.2 |
| Double Chocolate Chip, Subway* | 1 Cookie/45g | 212 | 9.0 | 471 | 4.4 | 66.7 | 21.1 | 2.2 |
| Oatmeal & Raisin, Subway* | 1 Cookie/45g | 206 | 8.0 | 458 | 6.7 | 68.9 | 18.2 | 3.1 |
| Rainbow, Subway* | 1 Cookie/48g | 209 | 10.0 | 435 | 5.0 | 62.5 | 20.2 | 4.8 |
| Sugar, Subway* | 1 Cookie/45g | 231 | 12.0 | 513 | 4.4 | 64.4 | 26.2 | 1.3 |
| White Chip Macadamia Nut, Subway* | 1 Cookie/45g | 222 | 11.0 | 493 | 4.4 | 64.4 | 24.0 | 1.6 |

### DOUGHNUTS

| | | | | | | | | |
|---|---|---|---|---|---|---|---|---|
| Chocolate, Subway* | 1 Doughnut/55g | 243 | 15.0 | 442 | 7.3 | 38.2 | 28.2 | 2.2 |
| Sugared, Subway* | 1 Doughnut/49g | 207 | 12.0 | 422 | 6.1 | 42.9 | 23.7 | 1.0 |

### DRESSING

| | | | | | | | | |
|---|---|---|---|---|---|---|---|---|
| Ranch, Subway* | 1 Serving/21g | 42 | 4.0 | 200 | 0.0 | 0.0 | 20.5 | 0.0 |

### MAYONNAISE

| | | | | | | | | |
|---|---|---|---|---|---|---|---|---|
| Light, Subway* | 1 Serving/15g | 56 | 6.0 | 373 | 0.0 | 6.7 | 40.0 | 0.0 |
| Subway* | 1 Serving/15g | 108 | 12.0 | 720 | 0.0 | 0.0 | 79.3 | 0.0 |

### MEATBALLS

| | | | | | | | | |
|---|---|---|---|---|---|---|---|---|
| Bowl, Subway* | 1 Bowl/206g | 314 | 20.0 | 153 | 9.4 | 8.9 | 9.5 | 1.4 |

## SUBWAY

| | Measure INFO/WEIGHT | per Measure KCAL | FAT | Nutrition Values per 100g / 100ml KCAL | PROT | CARB | FAT | FIBRE |
|---|---|---|---|---|---|---|---|---|
| **MUFFIN** | | | | | | | | |
| Blueberry, Subway* | 1 Muffin/111g | 352 | 21.0 | 317 | 4.5 | 36.0 | 18.6 | 2.7 |
| Chocolate Chunk, Subway* | 1 Muffin/111g | 394 | 23.0 | 355 | 5.4 | 39.6 | 20.6 | 2.6 |
| Double Chocolate Chip, Subway* | 1 Muffin/111g | 389 | 22.0 | 350 | 5.0 | 40.5 | 19.8 | 2.8 |
| **OIL** | | | | | | | | |
| Olive, Blend, Subway* | 1 Serving/5g | 44 | 5.0 | 880 | 0.0 | 0.0 | 100.0 | 0.0 |
| **SALAD** | | | | | | | | |
| Beef, No Dressing, Subway* | 1 Salad/371g | 127 | 2.0 | 34 | 4.8 | 1.9 | 0.7 | 1.2 |
| Chicken, Breast, No Dressing, Subway* | 1 Salad/385g | 152 | 3.0 | 39 | 5.7 | 2.1 | 0.9 | 1.1 |
| Club, No Dressing, Subway* | 1 Salad/404g | 153 | 3.0 | 38 | 5.7 | 2.0 | 0.8 | 1.1 |
| Ham, No Dressing, Subway* | 1 Salad/371g | 113 | 3.0 | 30 | 3.5 | 2.2 | 0.8 | 1.2 |
| Sweet Onion Chicken Teriyaki, No Dressing, Subway* | 1 Serving/427g | 206 | 4.0 | 48 | 5.4 | 4.7 | 0.9 | 1.1 |
| Turkey, Breast, No Dressing, Subway* | 1 Salad/371g | 111 | 2.0 | 30 | 3.8 | 1.9 | 0.7 | 1.2 |
| Turkey Breast & Ham, No Dressing, Subway* | 1 Serving/380g | 121 | 3.0 | 32 | 3.9 | 2.1 | 0.8 | 1.2 |
| Veggie Delite, No Dressing, Subway* | 1 Salad/314g | 58 | 1.0 | 18 | 1.0 | 2.2 | 0.3 | 1.4 |
| **SANDWICH** | | | | | | | | |
| Italian BMT, & Cheese, White Bread, 6", Subway* | 1 Sub/240g | 424 | 21.0 | 177 | 9.6 | 16.2 | 8.7 | 1.3 |
| Sub, Bacon, & Egg, Breakfast, With Cheese, 6", Subway* | 1 Sub/135g | 331 | 13.0 | 245 | 12.6 | 25.9 | 10.0 | 1.7 |
| Sub, Bacon, Breakfast, Wheat Bread, 6", Subway* | 1 Sub/98g | 268 | 7.0 | 273 | 15.3 | 34.7 | 7.6 | 2.2 |
| Sub, Bacon, Breakfast, White Bread, 6", Subway* | 1 Sub/93g | 259 | 8.0 | 278 | 15.0 | 38.7 | 8.5 | 2.1 |
| Sub, Bacon, Egg & Cheese, Breakfast, White, 6", Subway* | 1 Sub/179g | 432 | 23.0 | 241 | 11.7 | 20.7 | 12.8 | 1.3 |
| Sub, Beef, Wheat Bread, 6", Subway* | 1 Sub/233g | 276 | 3.0 | 118 | 9.4 | 15.9 | 1.5 | 1.4 |
| Sub, Beef, White Bread, Lite, 6, Subway* | 1 Sub/221g | 267 | 4.0 | 121 | 10.4 | 17.6 | 1.8 | 1.4 |
| Sub, Beef, White Bread, Mini, Subway* | 1 Sub/145g | 176 | 2.0 | 121 | 11.4 | 15.9 | 1.6 | 1.4 |
| Sub, BMT, Wheat Bread, 6", Subway* | 1 Sub/252g | 430 | 21.0 | 171 | 9.5 | 15.1 | 8.2 | 1.3 |
| Sub, Chicken & Bacon Ranch, Cheese, Wheat, 6", Subway* | 1 Sub/306g | 496 | 20.0 | 162 | 12.7 | 13.1 | 6.7 | 1.1 |
| Sub, Chicken & Bacon Ranch, Cheese, White, 6", Subway* | 1 Sub/294g | 484 | 21.0 | 165 | 12.9 | 13.9 | 7.0 | 1.1 |
| Sub, Chicken Breast, Wheat Bread, 6", Subway* | 1 Sub/247g | 302 | 4.0 | 122 | 11.3 | 15.4 | 1.7 | 1.3 |
| Sub, Chicken Breast, White Bread, Lite, 6", Subway* | 1 Sub/235g | 293 | 5.0 | 125 | 11.5 | 17.0 | 2.0 | 1.4 |
| Sub, Chicken Teriyaki, Sweet Onion, Wheat, 6", Subway* | 1 Sub/290g | 356 | 5.0 | 123 | 10.0 | 17.2 | 1.6 | 1.2 |
| Sub, Chicken Teriyaki, Sweet Onion, White, 6", Subway* | 1 Sub/278g | 347 | 5.0 | 125 | 10.1 | 18.3 | 1.8 | 1.3 |
| Sub, Chipotle Southwest Cheese Steak, 6", Subway* | 1 Sub/271g | 411 | 17.0 | 152 | 8.5 | 14.8 | 6.3 | 1.5 |
| Sub, Club, Wheat Bread, 6", Subway* | 1 Sub/266g | 303 | 4.0 | 114 | 10.5 | 14.3 | 1.6 | 1.2 |
| Sub, Club, White Bread, Lite, 6", Subway* | 1 Sub/254g | 294 | 5.0 | 116 | 11.0 | 15.3 | 1.9 | 1.3 |
| Sub, Egg & Cheese, Breakfast, Wheat Bread, 6", Subway* | 1 Sub/162g | 352 | 17.0 | 217 | 10.5 | 22.8 | 10.2 | 1.9 |
| Sub, Egg & Cheese, Breakfast, White Bread, 6", Subway* | 1 Sub/157g | 347 | 16.0 | 221 | 10.2 | 23.6 | 10.4 | 1.5 |
| Sub, Ham, Wheat Bread, 6", Subway* | 1 Sub/233g | 263 | 4.0 | 113 | 8.1 | 16.3 | 1.7 | 1.4 |
| Sub, Ham, White Bread, Lite, 6", Subway* | 1 Sub/221g | 254 | 4.0 | 115 | 8.1 | 17.6 | 1.9 | 1.4 |
| Sub, Ham, White Bread, Mini, Subway* | 1 Sub/135g | 157 | 2.0 | 116 | 8.5 | 17.0 | 1.7 | 1.6 |
| Sub, Italian, Bmt, & Cheese, Wheat Bread, 6", Subway* | 1 Sub/245g | 429 | 21.0 | 175 | 9.8 | 15.9 | 8.6 | 1.6 |
| Sub, Meatball Marinara, & Cheese, Wheat, 6", Subway* | 1 Sub/382g | 520 | 22.0 | 136 | 7.3 | 14.9 | 5.9 | 1.8 |
| Sub, Meatball Marinara, & Cheese, White, 6", Subway* | 1 Sub/377g | 515 | 22.0 | 137 | 7.2 | 15.1 | 5.9 | 1.6 |
| Sub, Meatball Marinara, Wheat Bread, 6", Subway* | 1 Sub/331g | 510 | 21.0 | 154 | 8.2 | 16.6 | 6.3 | 1.9 |
| Sub, Mega Breakfast, With Cheese, Wheat, 6", Subway* | 1 Sub/211g | 512 | 26.0 | 243 | 13.3 | 19.9 | 12.3 | 1.8 |
| Sub, Mega Breakfast & Cheese, White Bread, 6, Subway* | 1 Sub/242g | 569 | 32.0 | 235 | 12.4 | 17.8 | 13.1 | 1.6 |
| Sub, Melt, & Cheese, Wheat Bread, 6", Subway* | 1 Sub/263g | 351 | 10.0 | 133 | 10.3 | 14.4 | 4.0 | 1.2 |
| Sub, Melt, & Cheese, White Bread, 6", Subway* | 1 Sub/252g | 346 | 11.0 | 137 | 10.3 | 15.9 | 4.3 | 1.3 |
| Sub, Reggae Reggae, Cheese, Wheat Bread, 6", Subway* | 1 Sub/257g | 361 | 8.0 | 140 | 11.5 | 17.3 | 3.0 | 0.9 |
| Sub, Sausage, Breakfast, Wheat Bread, 6", Subway* | 1 Sub/156g | 368 | 14.0 | 236 | 12.2 | 25.6 | 9.0 | 2.3 |
| Sub, Sausage, Breakfast, White Bread, 6", Subway* | 1 Sub/151g | 359 | 14.0 | 238 | 11.9 | 27.8 | 9.5 | 2.2 |
| Sub, Sausage, Egg & Cheese, White, 6", Subway* | 1 Sub/233g | 528 | 29.0 | 227 | 11.6 | 18.4 | 12.3 | 1.6 |
| Sub, Spicy Italian, & Cheese, Wheat Bread, 6", Subway* | 1 Sub/229g | 461 | 26.0 | 201 | 9.6 | 17.0 | 11.4 | 1.7 |
| Sub, Spicy Italian, & Cheese, White Bread, 6", Subway* | 1 Sub/224g | 456 | 26.0 | 204 | 9.4 | 17.4 | 11.6 | 1.4 |

| | Measure INFO/WEIGHT | per Measure KCAL | FAT | Nutrition Values per 100g / 100ml KCAL | PROT | CARB | FAT | FIBRE |
|---|---|---|---|---|---|---|---|---|
| **SUBWAY** | | | | | | | | |
| **SANDWICH** | | | | | | | | |
| Sub, Spicy Italian, Wheat Bread, 6", Subway* | 1 Sub/247g | 506 | 29.0 | 205 | 9.7 | 15.4 | 11.8 | 1.3 |
| Sub, Steak, & Cheese, Wheat Bread, 6", Subway* | 1 Sub/259g | 337 | 9.0 | 130 | 9.6 | 15.4 | 3.5 | 1.6 |
| Sub, Steak & Cheese, White Bread, 6, Subway* | 1 Sub/248g | 331 | 10.0 | 133 | 9.7 | 16.5 | 3.9 | 1.3 |
| Sub, Tuna, & Cheese, Wheat Bread, 6", Subway* | 1 Sub/253g | 402 | 19.0 | 159 | 8.7 | 16.2 | 7.3 | 1.6 |
| Sub, Tuna, & Cheese, Wheat Bread, Mini, Subway* | 1 Sub/158g | 256 | 12.0 | 162 | 8.2 | 17.1 | 7.3 | 1.6 |
| Sub, Tuna, & Cheese, White Bread, 6", Subway* | 1 Sub/248g | 397 | 18.0 | 160 | 8.5 | 16.5 | 7.4 | 1.3 |
| Sub, Tuna, & Lite Mayonnaise, Wheat Bread, 6", Subway* | 1 Sub/259g | 402 | 18.0 | 155 | 8.1 | 15.1 | 6.9 | 1.3 |
| Sub, Tuna & Cheese, White Bread, Mini, Subway* | 1 Sub/155g | 251 | 11.0 | 162 | 8.7 | 15.5 | 7.2 | 1.3 |
| Sub, Turkey, & Ham, Wheat Bread, 6", Subway* | 1 Sub/244g | 271 | 4.0 | 111 | 7.8 | 16.0 | 1.6 | 1.6 |
| Sub, Turkey Breast, Wheat Bread 6", Subway* | 1 Sub/233g | 260 | 3.0 | 112 | 8.6 | 15.9 | 1.5 | 1.4 |
| Sub, Turkey Breast, White Bread, Lite, 6", Subway* | 1 Sub/221g | 251 | 4.0 | 114 | 8.6 | 17.6 | 1.8 | 1.4 |
| Sub, Turkey Breast & Ham, White Bread, Lite, 6", Subway* | 1 Sub/231g | 262 | 4.0 | 113 | 8.7 | 16.9 | 1.9 | 1.4 |
| Sub, Veggie Delite, Wheat Bread, 6", Subway* | 1 Sub/176g | 207 | 2.0 | 118 | 5.1 | 20.4 | 1.1 | 1.9 |
| Sub, Veggie Delite, White Bread, Lite, 6", Subway* | 1 Sub/164g | 198 | 2.0 | 121 | 4.9 | 23.2 | 1.5 | 1.9 |
| Sub, Veggie Patty, & Cheese, Wheat Bread, 6", Subway* | 1 Sub/273g | 414 | 13.0 | 152 | 8.4 | 16.8 | 4.6 | 1.2 |
| Sub, Veggie Patty, & Cheese, White Bread, 6, Subway* | 1 Sub/262g | 409 | 13.0 | 156 | 8.4 | 17.9 | 5.0 | 1.2 |
| **SAUCE** | | | | | | | | |
| Chipotle Southwest, Subway* | 1 Serving/21g | 88 | 9.0 | 419 | 0.0 | 9.5 | 42.9 | 0.9 |
| Honey & Mustard, Subway^ | 1 Serving/21g | 32 | 0.0 | 152 | 0.0 | 33.3 | 0.9 | 0.5 |
| Sweet Onion, Subway* | 1 Serving/21g | 38 | 0.0 | 181 | 0.0 | 42.9 | 0.9 | 0.5 |
| **TOASTIE** | | | | | | | | |
| Cheese, Subway* | 1 Toastie/66g | 198 | 10.0 | 301 | 15.8 | 27.5 | 15.2 | 1.5 |
| Pepperoni Pizza, Subway* | 1 Toastie/95g | 240 | 12.0 | 251 | 11.8 | 22.1 | 13.1 | 1.3 |
| **WRAP** | | | | | | | | |
| Breakfast, All Day, Mini, Subway* | 1 Wrap/162g | 345 | 15.0 | 214 | 9.0 | 23.8 | 9.2 | 2.1 |
| Chicken, & Bacon Ranch, Subway* | 1 Wrap/256g | 374 | 20.0 | 146 | 13.3 | 3.9 | 7.8 | 5.0 |
| Tuna, & Cheese, Subway* | 1 Wrap/210g | 406 | 31.0 | 193 | 10.0 | 3.8 | 14.8 | 6.1 |
| Tuna, Subway* | 1 Wrap/210g | 310 | 19.0 | 148 | 10.0 | 3.8 | 9.0 | 6.2 |
| Turkey, Subway* | 1 Wrap/184g | 157 | 4.0 | 85 | 10.9 | 4.3 | 2.0 | 7.1 |
| Turkey & Bacon, with Chipotle Sauce, Melt, Subway* | 1 Wrap/242g | 386 | 23.0 | 159 | 12.0 | 5.0 | 9.5 | 5.3 |
| Turkey Breast & Bacon Melt, Subway* | 1 Wrap/242g | 386 | 24.0 | 159 | 12.0 | 5.0 | 9.9 | 5.4 |
| **WIMPY** | | | | | | | | |
| **BAGUETTE** | | | | | | | | |
| Beef, Big, Wimpy* | 1 Serving/240g | 578 | 30.0 | 241 | 13.2 | 19.3 | 12.3 | 1.2 |
| BLT, Best, Wimpy* | 1 Serving/177g | 320 | 7.0 | 181 | 9.9 | 25.1 | 3.9 | 1.6 |
| Cheese, Big, Wimpy* | 1 Serving/185g | 474 | 23.0 | 256 | 11.8 | 24.0 | 12.5 | 1.5 |
| Chicken, Hot 'n' Spicy, Wimpy* | 1 Serving/230g | 522 | 23.0 | 227 | 9.5 | 24.9 | 9.9 | 1.8 |
| Sausage, Sizzler, Wimpy* | 1 Serving/193g | 519 | 24.0 | 269 | 10.8 | 28.6 | 12.4 | 1.7 |
| Spicy Beanburger, Wimpy* | 1 Serving/254g | 597 | 27.0 | 235 | 5.9 | 29.3 | 10.5 | 2.5 |
| **BEANS** | | | | | | | | |
| Baked, Wimpy* | 1 Portion/110g | 82 | 0.0 | 75 | 4.7 | 13.6 | 0.2 | 3.7 |
| **BREAKFAST** | | | | | | | | |
| All Day, Wimpy* | 1 Serving/410g | 730 | 40.0 | 178 | 8.3 | 14.5 | 9.7 | 2.0 |
| Big Breakfast, Wimpy* | 1 Serving/216g | 404 | 26.0 | 187 | 12.7 | 5.6 | 12.2 | 0.5 |
| The Country Breakfast, Wimpy* | 1 Serving/265g | 339 | 17.0 | 128 | 8.5 | 8.8 | 6.4 | 1.8 |
| The Great, Wimpy* | 1 Breakfast/443g | 793 | 41.0 | 179 | 9.7 | 14.2 | 9.3 | 1.3 |
| Wimpy* | 1 Serving/301g | 451 | 25.0 | 150 | 10.6 | 7.7 | 8.3 | 1.6 |
| **BURGERS** | | | | | | | | |
| Cheeseburger, Bacon, Wimpy* | 1 Burger/145g | 345 | 15.0 | 238 | 13.2 | 22.3 | 10.5 | 0.0 |
| Cheeseburger, Wimpy* | 1 Burger/118g | 317 | 15.0 | 269 | 14.7 | 24.7 | 12.5 | 1.3 |
| Chicken, Fillet, Gourmet, Wimpy* | 1 Burger/327g | 513 | 14.0 | 157 | 14.8 | 15.3 | 4.2 | 0.8 |
| Chicken, Hot 'n' Spicy, in a Bun, Wimpy* | 1 Burger/188g | 414 | 20.0 | 220 | 9.7 | 20.7 | 10.9 | 1.6 |

## WIMPY

| INFO/WEIGHT | Measure | | per Measure | | Nutrition Values per 100g / 100ml | | | | |
|---|---|---|---|---|---|---|---|---|---|
| | | | KCAL | FAT | KCAL | PROT | CARB | FAT | FIBRE |
| **BURGERS** | | | | | | | | | |
| Chicken, in a Bun, Wimpy* | 1 Burger/154g | | 411 | 22.0 | 267 | 11.3 | 22.0 | 14.5 | 1.5 |
| Chicken & Bacon, Melt, Wimpy* | 1 Burger/174g | | 447 | 22.0 | 257 | 13.9 | 21.0 | 12.5 | 1.3 |
| Double Decker, Wimpy* | 1 Burger/270g | | 830 | 51.0 | 307 | 19.0 | 15.7 | 19.0 | 2.5 |
| Gourmet, Wimpy* | 1 Burger/291g | | 675 | 33.0 | 232 | 14.4 | 18.8 | 11.2 | 1.0 |
| Half Pounder, Wimpy* | 1 Burger/299g | | 852 | 54.0 | 285 | 18.5 | 12.8 | 17.9 | 1.6 |
| Hamburger, Wimpy* | 1 Burger/104g | | 277 | 12.0 | 266 | 14.2 | 27.3 | 11.1 | 1.4 |
| Leanburger, Wimpy* | 1 Burger/191g | | 315 | 12.0 | 165 | 12.4 | 14.6 | 6.4 | 0.9 |
| Quarter Pounder, Wimpy* | 1 Burger/200g | | 548 | 31.0 | 274 | 15.3 | 18.9 | 15.6 | 2.4 |
| Quarter Pounder, with Cheese, Wimpy* | 1 Burger/214g | | 588 | 34.0 | 275 | 15.4 | 17.9 | 16.0 | 2.2 |
| Spicy Bean, Wimpy* | 1 Burger/221g | | 526 | 24.0 | 238 | 6.3 | 29.1 | 11.0 | 3.8 |
| Spicy Bean, with Cheese, Wimpy* | 1 Burger/205g | | 520 | 22.0 | 254 | 7.8 | 33.5 | 10.7 | 7.8 |
| The Classic, Kingsize, Wimpy* | 1 Burger/229g | | 559 | 32.0 | 244 | 16.4 | 13.1 | 14.0 | 0.8 |
| The Classic, Wimpy* | 1 Burger/159g | | 343 | 16.0 | 216 | 12.8 | 18.4 | 10.1 | 1.1 |
| The Classic, with Cheese, Wimpy* | 1 Burger/173g | | 386 | 19.0 | 223 | 13.2 | 17.3 | 11.2 | 1.0 |
| The Classic, with Cheese & Bacon, Wimpy* | 1 Burger/194g | | 411 | 20.0 | 212 | 14.0 | 15.5 | 10.3 | 0.9 |
| **BURGERS VEGETARIAN** | | | | | | | | | |
| Quorn, in a Bun, Wimpy* | 1 Burger/170g | | 380 | 18.0 | 224 | 9.8 | 22.1 | 10.7 | 0.0 |
| **CHICKEN &** | | | | | | | | | |
| Chips, Chunks, Wimpy* | 1 Serving/317g | | 713 | 42.0 | 225 | 7.9 | 19.5 | 13.2 | 1.9 |
| **CHIPS** | | | | | | | | | |
| Large, Wimpy* | 1 Serving/143g | | 335 | 17.0 | 234 | 3.0 | 30.4 | 12.0 | 3.0 |
| Standard, Wimpy* | 1 Serving/114g | | 267 | 14.0 | 234 | 3.0 | 30.5 | 12.0 | 3.0 |
| **COOKIES** | | | | | | | | | |
| Chocolate, Triple, Wimpy* | 1 Serving/80g | | 377 | 17.0 | 471 | 7.9 | 60.9 | 21.8 | 2.3 |
| Milk Chocolate, Wimpy* | 1 Serving/70g | | 311 | 10.0 | 444 | 6.9 | 69.6 | 15.0 | 1.4 |
| White Chocolate, Wimpy* | 1 Serving/80g | | 383 | 17.0 | 479 | 10.5 | 60.3 | 21.8 | 1.0 |
| **DESSERT** | | | | | | | | | |
| Apple Pie, with Ice Cream, Wimpy* | 1 Serving/194g | | 483 | 25.0 | 249 | 3.2 | 31.7 | 13.0 | 1.4 |
| Apple Pie. with Cream, Wimpy* | 1 Dessert/174g | | 459 | 25.0 | 264 | 3.0 | 32.4 | 14.4 | 1.6 |
| Chocolate Fudge Cake, with Cream, Wimpy* | 1 Dessert/95g | | 315 | 6.0 | 332 | 3.6 | 65.5 | 6.2 | 0.4 |
| Chocolate Fudge Cake, with Ice Cream, Wimpy* | 1 Dessert/115g | | 340 | 6.0 | 296 | 3.7 | 58.6 | 5.2 | 0.3 |
| Spotted Dick, with Cream, Wimpy* | 1 Dessert/140g | | 466 | 19.0 | 333 | 4.1 | 48.9 | 13.7 | 0.6 |
| Spotted Dick, with Custard, Wimpy* | 1 Dessert/280g | | 602 | 21.0 | 215 | 3.6 | 33.6 | 7.5 | 0.3 |
| Spotted Dick, with Ice Cream, Wimpy* | 1 Dessert/160g | | 490 | 19.0 | 306 | 4.2 | 46.1 | 12.1 | 0.6 |
| Treacle Sponge Pudding, with Cream, Wimpy* | 1 Dessert/140g | | 533 | 24.0 | 381 | 3.8 | 52.6 | 17.2 | 0.4 |
| Treacle Sponge Pudding, with Custard, Wimpy* | 1 Dessert/280g | | 669 | 26.0 | 239 | 3.4 | 35.4 | 9.3 | 0.2 |
| Treacle Sponge Pudding, with Ice Cream, Wimpy* | 1 Pudding/160g | | 558 | 24.0 | 349 | 3.9 | 49.3 | 15.2 | 0.3 |
| **FISH** | | | | | | | | | |
| in a Bun, Wimpy* | 1 Serving/245g | | 515 | 13.0 | 210 | 14.0 | 26.1 | 5.5 | 1.5 |
| **FISH & CHIPS** | | | | | | | | | |
| Wimpy* | 1 Serving/266g | | 519 | 28.0 | 195 | 7.6 | 18.2 | 10.6 | 2.4 |
| **GRILL** | | | | | | | | | |
| Bacon, Classic, Wimpy* | 1 Grill/306g | | 719 | 45.0 | 235 | 12.0 | 14.6 | 14.8 | 1.3 |
| Classic, Wimpy* | 1 Grill/314g | | 754 | 51.0 | 240 | 11.1 | 14.1 | 16.2 | 1.2 |
| Double Egg & Chips, Wimpy* | 1 Grill/214g | | 445 | 28.0 | 208 | 7.9 | 16.3 | 12.9 | 1.6 |
| Frankfurter, Wimpy* | 1 Grill/308g | | 684 | 45.0 | 222 | 8.8 | 14.4 | 14.7 | 1.2 |
| Quarterpounder, Wimpy* | 1 Grill/395g | | 955 | 64.0 | 242 | 12.8 | 11.7 | 16.1 | 0.0 |
| The International, Wimpy* | 1 Grill/400g | | 896 | 59.0 | 224 | 12.8 | 11.2 | 14.7 | 1.0 |
| **HASH BROWNS** | | | | | | | | | |
| Wimpy* | 1 Serving/55g | | 93 | 8.0 | 169 | 2.2 | 19.6 | 14.2 | 1.8 |
| **HOT DOG** | | | | | | | | | |
| Frankfurter, in a Bun, with Cheese, Wimpy* | 1 Hotdog/172g | | 432 | 24.0 | 251 | 10.3 | 20.6 | 14.1 | 1.1 |

| | Measure INFO/WEIGHT | per Measure KCAL | per Measure FAT | Nutrition Values per 100g / 100ml KCAL | PROT | CARB | FAT | FIBRE |
|---|---|---|---|---|---|---|---|---|
| **WIMPY** | | | | | | | | |
| **HOT DOG** | | | | | | | | |
| Frankfurter, in a Bun, with Chips, Wimpy* | 1 Meal/158g | 389 | 21.0 | 246 | 9.7 | 22.0 | 13.3 | 1.2 |
| Wimpy* | 1 Hot Dog/146g | 412 | 21.0 | 282 | 11.0 | 27.1 | 14.4 | 1.4 |
| **ICE CREAM** | | | | | | | | |
| Banana Longboat, with Dairy Ice Cream, Wimpy* | 1 Serving/199g | 285 | 9.0 | 143 | 2.4 | 24.0 | 4.6 | 0.7 |
| Banana Longboat, with Soft Ice Cream, Wimpy* | 1 Serving/209g | 259 | 6.0 | 124 | 2.3 | 23.9 | 2.9 | 0.7 |
| Brown Derby, with Dairy Ice Cream, Wimpy* | 1 Serving/125g | 399 | 21.0 | 319 | 5.4 | 36.9 | 16.6 | 1.5 |
| Brown Derby, with Soft Ice Cream, Wimpy* | 1 Serving/138g | 397 | 20.0 | 288 | 5.1 | 35.2 | 14.3 | 1.4 |
| Chocolate, Wimpy* | 1 Serving/67g | 177 | 7.0 | 264 | 7.0 | 32.1 | 10.6 | 0.0 |
| Ice Mountain, Wimpy* | 1 Serving/230g | 531 | 27.0 | 231 | 3.9 | 27.7 | 11.8 | 0.4 |
| Knickerbockerglory, with Dairy Ice Cream, Wimpy* | 1 Serving/194g | 386 | 15.0 | 199 | 2.5 | 30.3 | 7.8 | 0.3 |
| Knickerbockerglory, with Soft Ice Cream, Wimpy* | 1 Serving/136g | 196 | 6.0 | 144 | 2.7 | 25.1 | 4.4 | 4.4 |
| Mint, Choc Chip, Wimpy* | 1 Serving/67g | 187 | 13.0 | 279 | 4.0 | 24.9 | 19.4 | 0.0 |
| Strawberry, Wimpy* | 1 Serving/67g | 148 | 6.0 | 221 | 4.0 | 29.6 | 9.6 | 0.0 |
| Sundae, Mint Chocolate, Wimpy* | 1 Serving/113g | 325 | 16.0 | 288 | 4.1 | 36.6 | 13.8 | 0.4 |
| Sundae, Neopolitan, Wimpy* | 1 Sundae/135g | 329 | 14.0 | 244 | 4.1 | 33.0 | 10.3 | 0.2 |
| Sundae, Strawberry, Triple, with Dairy Ice Cream, Wimpy* | 1 Serving/170g | 394 | 18.0 | 232 | 3.4 | 31.6 | 10.4 | 0.5 |
| Sundea, Strawberry, with Soft Ice Cream, Wimpy* | 1 Serving/78g | 123 | 3.0 | 158 | 2.9 | 28.5 | 4.2 | 0.3 |
| Vanilla, Wimpy* | 1 Serving/67g | 150 | 8.0 | 224 | 4.6 | 25.2 | 11.6 | 0.0 |
| **MUSHROOMS** | | | | | | | | |
| Wimpy* | 1 Serving/114g | 179 | 18.0 | 157 | 2.4 | 0.3 | 16.2 | 1.5 |
| **NUGGETS** | | | | | | | | |
| Veg & Cheese, with Chips, Wimpy* | 1 Meal/234g | 571 | 34.0 | 244 | 3.9 | 25.4 | 14.5 | 2.1 |
| **ONION RINGS** | | | | | | | | |
| 12, Wimpy* | 1 Portion/180g | 401 | 23.0 | 223 | 3.2 | 23.6 | 12.9 | 3.0 |
| 6, Wimpy* | 1 Serving/90g | 201 | 12.0 | 223 | 3.2 | 23.6 | 12.9 | 3.0 |
| **POTATO JACKET** | | | | | | | | |
| Plain, with Butter, Wimpy* | 1 Serving/328g | 453 | 7.0 | 138 | 3.5 | 28.0 | 2.2 | 2.4 |
| with Baked Beans, Wimpy* | 1 Serving/448g | 547 | 7.0 | 122 | 3.8 | 24.3 | 1.6 | 2.8 |
| with Coleslaw, Wimpy* | 1 Serving/456g | 776 | 39.0 | 170 | 2.9 | 21.8 | 8.5 | 2.2 |
| with Tuna Mayo, Wimpy* | 1 Serving/456g | 777 | 36.0 | 170 | 5.9 | 20.5 | 7.9 | 0.0 |
| **RIBS** | | | | | | | | |
| Pork, Wimpy* | 1 Rib/189g | 455 | 22.0 | 241 | 12.9 | 21.1 | 11.6 | 1.4 |
| **ROLL** | | | | | | | | |
| Bacon, Breakfast, Wimpy* | 1 Roll/144g | 278 | 5.0 | 193 | 13.3 | 24.7 | 3.5 | 1.5 |
| Bacon, in a Bun, Wimpy* | 1 Roll/105g | 218 | 5.0 | 208 | 13.1 | 26.9 | 4.4 | 1.5 |
| Bacon & Egg, Breakfast, Wimpy* | 1 Roll/194g | 369 | 12.0 | 190 | 13.4 | 18.3 | 6.2 | 1.1 |
| Bacon & Egg, in a Bun, Wimpy* | 1 Roll/155g | 308 | 11.0 | 199 | 13.3 | 18.2 | 7.4 | 1.0 |
| Quorn, in a Bun, Wimpy* | 1 Roll/165g | 379 | 18.0 | 230 | 10.1 | 22.8 | 11.0 | 3.5 |
| Sausage, Breakfast, Wimpy* | 1 Roll/161g | 436 | 22.0 | 271 | 11.3 | 26.6 | 13.4 | 1.6 |
| Sausage & Egg, Breakfast, Wimpy* | 1 Roll/211g | 527 | 28.0 | 250 | 11.8 | 20.3 | 13.5 | 1.2 |
| **SALAD** | | | | | | | | |
| Chicken, Gourmet, Wimpy* | 1 Serving/383g | 253 | 4.0 | 66 | 11.1 | 2.7 | 1.1 | 0.4 |
| Chicken, Hot 'n' Spicy, Wimpy* | 1 Salad/310g | 267 | 13.0 | 86 | 4.9 | 7.3 | 4.3 | 1.0 |
| Fish, Wimpy* | 1 Serving/320g | 262 | 12.0 | 82 | 5.8 | 6.5 | 3.7 | 1.4 |
| Side, Wimpy* | 1 Salad/155g | 143 | 13.0 | 92 | 0.9 | 2.7 | 8.6 | 0.9 |
| Spicy Beanburger, Wimpy* | 1 Serving/320g | 330 | 19.0 | 103 | 1.8 | 11.3 | 5.8 | 1.7 |
| **TEACAKE** | | | | | | | | |
| with Butter, Wimpy* | 1 Serving/62g | 239 | 9.0 | 385 | 8.1 | 56.7 | 14.6 | 2.6 |
| **TOAST** | | | | | | | | |
| Butter & Jam, Wimpy* | 1 Serving/89g | 278 | 8.0 | 312 | 7.3 | 52.8 | 9.4 | 1.7 |

# Useful Resources

### Beating Bowel Cancer
Beating Bowel Cancer is a leading UK charity for bowel cancer patients, working to raise awareness of symptoms, promote early diagnosis and encourage open access to treatment choice for those affected by bowel cancer.
Tel: 020 8892 5256  Email: info@beatingbowelcancer.org
Website: http://www.beatingbowelcancer.org

### Cancer Research
Cancer Research UK is the leading UK charity dedicated to research, education and fundraising for all forms of cancer.
Tel: 0207 242 0200  Email: via their website
Website: www.cancerresearchuk.org

### Diabetes Advice
Diabetes UK is the leading charity working for people with diabetes. Their mission is to improve the lives of people with diabetes and to work towards a future without diabetes
Tel : 0845 120 2960 Email: info@diabetes.org.uk
Website: www.diabetes.org.uk

### Dietary Advice
The British Dietetic Association has helpful food fact leaflets and information on how to contact a registered dietitian.
Tel:  0121 200 8080 Email: webmaster@bda.uk.com
Website: www.bda.uk.com

### Exercise Equipment for Home
Diet and Fitness Resources has a range of equipment for exercise at home, from pedometers to treadmills and fitballs to weights. As well as diet tools such as food diaries, a weight loss kit and diet plates.
Tel: 01733 345592  Email: helpteam@dietandfitnessresources.co.uk
Website: www.dietandfitnessresources.co.uk

### Healthy Eating
The British Nutrition Foundation has lots of in depth scientifically based nutritional information, knowledge and advice on healthy eating for all ages.
Tel: 0207 404 6504  Email: postbox@nutrition.org.uk
Website: www.nutrition.org.uk

### Healthy Heart

The British Heart Foundation provides advice and information for all on all heart aspects from being healthy, to living with heart conditions, research and fundraising.
Tel: 0845 070 8070  Email: via their website
Website: www.bhf.org.uk

### Safety and Standards

The Food Standards Agency is an independent watchdog, set up to protect the public's health and consumer interests in relation to food.
Tel: 0207 276 8000  Email: helpline@foodstandards.gsi.gov.uk
Website: www.foodstandards.gov.uk

### Weight Loss

Weight Loss Resources is home to the UK's largest calorie and nutrition database along with diaries, tools and expert advice for weight loss and health.
Tel: 01733 345592   Email: helpteam@weightlossresources.co.uk
Website: www.weightlossresources.co.uk

## Feedback

If you have any comments or suggestions about The Calorie, Carb & Fat Bible, or would like further information on Weight Loss Resources, please call, email, or write to us:

Tel:        01733 345592
Email:      helpteam@weightlossresources.co.uk
Address:    Pat Wilson,
            Weight Loss Resources Ltd,
            29 Metro Centre,
            Woodston,
            Peterborough,
            PE2 7UH.

# Reviews for The Calorie Carb & Fat Bible

'What a brilliant book. I know I'll be sinking my teeth into it.'
**GMTV Nutritionist Amanda Ursell, BSc RD**

'To help you make low-cal choices everyday, invest in a copy.'
**ZEST magazine**

'There is no doubt that the food listings are extremely helpful
for anyone wishing to control their calorie intake in order to lose
pounds or maintain a healthy weight.'
**Women's Fitness magazine**

'Useful if you don't want to exclude any overall food groups.'
**Easy Living magazine**

'Quite simply an astonishing achievement by the authors.'
**Evening Post, Nottingham**

'The book gives you all the basic information so you can work out
your daily calorie needs.'
**Woman magazine**

'This is a welcome resource in view of the 'national epidemic of obesity.'

**Bryony Philip, Bowel Cancer UK**

'The authors seem to understand the problems of slimming.'

**Dr John Campion**

'Jam-packed with info on dieting, and full to bursting point with the calorie, carbohydrate and fat values of thousands of different foods, it's the perfect weight loss tool.'

**Evening Express, Aberdeen**

'Excellent resource tool - used by myself in my role as a Practice Nurse.'

**Pam Boal, Sunderland**

'I recently bought your book called the Calorie, Carb & Fat Bible and would love to tell you what a brilliant book it is. I have recently started a weight management programme and I honestly don't know where I'd be without your book. It has helped me a lot and given me some really good advice.'

**Rachel Mitchell**

# About Weight Loss Resources

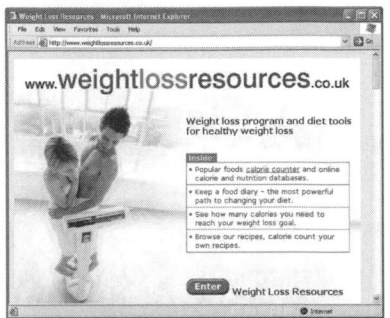

"What this does is put you in control with no guilt, no awful groups and no negativity! Fill in your food diary, get support on the boards and watch it fall off!"

LINDAB, Weight Loss Resources Member

## How Does It Work?

Weight Loss Resources is home to the UK's biggest online calorie and nutrition database. You simply tap in your height, weight, age and basic activity level - set a weight loss goal, and the programme does all the necessary calculations.

## What Does It Do?

The site enables you to keep a food diary which keeps running totals of calories, fat, fibre, carbs, proteins and portions of fruit and veg. You can also keep an exercise diary which adds the calories you use during exercise. At the end of a week, you update your weight and get reports and graphs on your progress.

## How Will It Help?

You'll learn a great deal about how your eating and drinking habits affect your weight and how healthy they are. Using the diaries and other tools you'll be able to make changes that suit your tastes and your lifestyle. The result is weight loss totally tailored to your needs and preferences. A method you can stick with that will help you learn how to eat well for life!

## Try It Free!

Go to **www.weightlossresources.co.uk** and take a completely free, no obligation, 24 hour trial. If you like what you see you can sign up for membership from £7.95 per month.